American
DRUG INDEX

36th Edition

American DRUG INDEX

1992

36th Edition

NORMAN F. BILLUPS, R.Ph., M.S., Ph.D.

Dean and Professor of Pharmacy
College of Pharmacy
The University of Toledo

Associate Editor

SHIRLEY M. BILLUPS, R.N., B.Ed., M.Ed.

Oncology Nurse
The Toledo Hospital

facts and comparisons

A Wolters Kluwer Company

Facts and Comparisons Staff

C. Sue Sewester
publisher

Bernie R. Olin, PharmD
editor-in-chief

Charles E. Dombek, BS, MA
assistant editor

Mary K. Hulbert, BA
coordinating editor

ISBN 0-932686-29-X
ISSN 0065-8111

Library of Congress Catalog Card Number 55-6286

Printed in the United States of America

Published by
Facts and Comparisons
111 West Port Plaza, Suite 423,
St. Louis, Missouri 63146-3098

Preface

The 36th Edition of the *American Drug Index* (ADI) has been prepared for the identification, explanation and correlation of the many pharmaceuticals available to the medical, pharmaceutical and allied health professions. The need for this index has become acute as the variety and number of drugs and drug products have continued to multiply. Hence, the *ADI* should be useful to pharmacists, nurses, physicians, medical transcriptionists, dentists, sales personnel, students and teachers in the fields incorporating pharmaceuticals.

Special note to medical transcriptionists: Although all names in the *ADI* appear in bold capitalized type, trade products are easily identifiable by the manufacturer's name in parentheses immediately following the trade name. The names for official products are preceded by a bullet (•) and should appear in lower case in transcription.

The organization of the *ADI* falls into 13 major sections:

- Monographs of Drug Products
- Common Abbreviations Used in Medical Orders
- Common Systems of Weight and Measure
- Approximate Practical Equivalents
- International System of Units
- Normal Laboratory Values
- Trademark Glossary
- Glossary
- Container Requirements for U.S.P. XXII Drugs
- Container and Storage Requirements for Sterile U.S.P. XXII Drugs
- Oral Dosage Forms That Should Not Be Crushed
- Pharmaceutical Company Labeler Code Index Numbers
- Pharmaceutical Manufacturer and Drug Distributor Addresses

MONOGRAPHS: The organization of the monograph section of the *ADI* is alphabetical with extensive cross-indexing. Names listed are generic (also called nonproprietary, public name or common name); brand (also called trademark, proprietary or specialty); and chemical. Synonyms that are in general use also are included. All names used for a pharmaceutical appear in alphabetical order with the pertinent data given under the brand name by which it is made available.

The monograph for a typical brand name product consists of the manufacturer, generic and/or chemical names, composition and strength, pharmaceutical forms available, package size, and use.

Generic names appear in alphabetical order, followed by the corresponding recognition of the drug to the U.S.P. (United States Pharmacopeia), N.F. (National Formulary) and USAN (United States Adopted Names). Each of these official generic names is preceded by a bullet (•) at the beginning of each entry. The information is in accord with the U.S.P. XXII and N.F. XVII and through Supplement 4, which became official on May 15, 1991; and the USAN-1992.

British Approved Names (B.A.N.) and Veterinary British Approved Names (V.B.A.N.) are also included in this edition.

Because of the multiplicity of brand names used for the same therapeutic agent or the same combination of therapeutic agents, it was apparent that some correlation could be done. As an example of this, please turn to tetracycline HCl. Here under the generic name are listed the various brand names. Following are combinations of tetracycline HCl organized in a manner to point out relationships among the many products. Reference then is made to the brand name or names having the indicated composition. Under the brand name are given manufacturer, composition, available forms, sizes, dosage and use.

The multiplicity of generic names for the same therapeutic agent has complicated the nomenclature of these agents. Examples of multiple generic names for the same chemical substance are (1) parabromdylamine, brompheniramine; (2) acetaminophen, p-hydroxy acetanilid, N-acetyl-p-aminophenol; (3) guaifenesin, glyceryl guaiacolate, glyceryl guaiacol ether, guaianesin, guaifylline, guaiphenesin, guayanesin, methphenoxydiol; (4) pyrilamine, pyranisamine, pyranilamine, pyraminyl, anisopyradamine.

The cross-indexing feature of the *ADI* permits the finding of drugs or drug combinations when only one major ingredient is known. For example, a combination of aluminum hydroxide gel and magnesium trisilicate is available. This combination can be found by looking under the name of either of the two ingredients, and in each case the brand names are given. A second form of cross-indexing lists drugs under various therapeutic and pharmaceutical classes (i.e., antacids, antihistamines, diuretics, laxatives, etc.).

ABBREVIATIONS: The listing of Common Abbreviations used in Medical Orders is included as an aid in interpreting medical orders. The Latin or Greek word and abbreviation are both given with the meaning.

CONVERSION FACTORS: A listing of Approximate Practical Equivalents is added as an aid in calculating and converting dosages among the metric, apothecary and avoirdupois systems.

WEIGHT AND MEASURE: Tables containing the Common Systems of Weight and Measure are included to aid the practitioner in calculating dosages in the metric, apothecary and avoirdupois systems, as well as the International System of Units.

NORMAL LABORATORY VALUES: Tables containing normal reference values for commonly requested laboratory tests are included as a guideline for the health-care practitioner.

TRADEMARK GLOSSARY: An alphabetical listing of trademarked dosage forms and package types is included to aid in the identification of drug products listed in the *ADI*.

GLOSSARY: Commonly used terms are listed and defined as an aid in interpreting the use given for drug monographs included in the *ADI*.

CONTAINER AND STORAGE REQUIREMENTS FOR U.S.P. XXII DRUGS AND STERILE DRUGS: These sections have been added on container and storage requirements specified by the U.S.P. XXII for compendial drugs, to aid the practitioner in storing and dispensing.

ORAL DOSAGE FORMS THAT SHOULD NOT BE CRUSHED: This section has been added to alert the health-care practitioner about oral dosage forms that should not be crushed, and to serve as an aid in consulting with patients. Examples of products falling into the "non-crush" category are extended-release, enteric-coated, encapsulated beads, wax matrix, sublingual and encapsulated liquid formulations.

LABELER CODE INDEX: The Pharmaceutical Labeler Code Index is presented to aid in the identification of drug products. The codes are listed in numerical order followed by the name of the manufacturer.

MANUFACTURER ADDRESSES: The name, address and zip code of virtually every American Pharmaceutical Manufacturer and/or Drug Distributor are listed in alphabetical order in this section. Additionally, a pharmaceutical labeler code number appears before the address of each company as a further aid in the identification of drug products.

Special appreciation and acknowledgment is given to my wife, Shirley, who served again this year as my Associate Editor—and to Dr. Bernie R. Olin, Editor-in-Chief, and Mary K. Hulbert, Coordinating Editor of Facts and Comparisons, for compiling the monograph section of this volume. Special thanks are also extended to the manufacturers who supplied product information, to Dr. Kenneth S. Alexander for organizing the Container and Storage Requirements information, to Dr. John F. Mitchell and Ms. Kathleen S. Pawlicki for the table on Oral Dosage Forms That Should Not Be Crushed, and to Drs. Charles O. Wilson and Tony E. Jones for their earlier contributions to the *ADI*.

Correspondence or communication with reference to a drug or drug products listed in the *American Drug Index* should be directed to Bernie R. Olin, PharmD, Editor-in-Chief, Facts and Comparisons; 111 West Port Plaza; St. Louis, Missouri 63146, or call 1-800-223-0554.

Norman F. Billups, R.Ph., M.S., Ph.D.

Contents

[•] Denotes official name: Generic name or chemical name approved by F.D.A. or recognized by the U.S.P., N.F., or USAN.

Monographs

A

A-200 PYRINATE. (Norcliff Thayer) **Liq.:** Pyrethrins 0.33%, piperonyl butoxide technical 4%, petroleum distillate. Bot. 2 fl oz, 4 fl oz. **Gel:** Pyrethrins 0.33%, piperonyl butoxide technical 4%, petroleum distillate. Tube oz.
Use: Pediculicide.

A.A.A. OINTMENT. (Jenkins) Ammoniated mercury 2%, salicylic acid 1.25%, boric acid 1%, zinc oxide 15%. Jar oz, lb.
Use: Impetigo, nonspecific eczema, minor skin irritations.

A AND D OINTMENT. (Kenyon) Vitamins A & D in lanolin-petrolatum base. Jar lb.
Use: Emollient.

A AND D OINTMENT. (Schering) Fish liver oil, cholecalciferol. Tube 1.5 oz, 4 oz. Jar lb.
Use: Emollient.

A & D TABLETS. (Barth's) Vitamins A 10,000 IU, D 400 IU/Tab. Bot. 100s, 500s.
Use: Vitamin supplement.

A AND D VITAMIN CAPSULES. (Lannett) Vitamins A 5000 IU, D 400 IU/Cap. Bot. 500s, 1000s.
Use: Vitamin supplement.

A AND D VITAMIN OINTMENT. (Lannett) Petrolatum-lanolin base. Jar 1 lb, 5 lb.
Use: Emollient.

AAS INFANTIL W/VITAMIN C. (Winthrop) Acetylsalicylic acid, vitamin C.
Use: Salicylate analgesic, vitamin C supplement.

AAS TABLETS. (Winthrop) Acetylsalicylic acid.
Use: Salicylate analgesic.

•**ABAMECTIN.** USAN.
Use: Antiparasitic.

ABBOKINASE. (Abbott) Urokinase 250,000 IU/5 ml. Lyophilized pow. Vial 5 ml.
Use: Thrombolytic enzyme.

ABBOKINASE OPEN-CATH. (Abbott) Urokinase for catheter clearance 5000 IU/ml. Univial 1 ml.
Use: Thrombolytic enzyme.

ABBOTT AFP-EIA. (Abbott Diagnostics) Enzyme immunoassay for the quantitative measurement of alpha-fetoprotein (AFP) in human serum and amniotic fluid. Test kits 100s.
Use: Diagnostic aid.

ABBOTT AFP-EIA MONOCLONAL. (Abbott Diagnostics) Enzyme immunoassay for the quantitative measurement of alpha-fetoprotein (AFP) in human serum and amniotic fluid.
Use: Diagnostic aid.

ABBOTT ANTI-DELTA. (Abbott Diagnostics) Radioimmunoassay for the detection of antibody to delta antigen (HDAg) in human serum or plasma. For research only. Not for use in diagnostic procedures.
Use: Research.

ABBOTT ANTI-DELTA EIA. (Abbott Diagnostics) Enzyme immunoassay for the detection of antibody to hepatitis delta antigen in human serum or plasma. For research only. Not for use in diagnostic procedures.
Use: Research.

ABBOTT β-HCG 15/15. (Abbott Diagnostics) Enzyme immunoassay for the quantitative determination of human chorionic gonadotropin in human serum.
Use: Diagnostic aid.

ABBOTT CA125-EIA. (Abbott Diagnostics) Enzyme immunoassay for the quantitative measurement of cancer antigen (CA) 125 in human serum. For research only. Not for use in diagnostic procedures.
Use: Research.

ABBOTT CEA-EIA MONOCLONAL. (Abbott Diagnostics) Enzyme immunoassay for the quantitative measurement of carcinoembryonic antigen (CEA) in human serum or plasma to aid in the management of cancer patients and assessing prognosis.
Use: Diagnostic aid.

ABBOTT CEA-RIA. (Abbott Diagnostics) Solid phase radioimmunoassay for the quantitative measurement of carcinoembryonic antigen (CEA) in human serum or plasma to aid in the management of cancer patients and assessing prognosis.
Use: Diagnostic aid.

ABBOTT CMV TOTAL AB EIA. (Abbott Diagnostics) Enzyme immunoassay for the detection of antibody to cytomegalovirus in human serum, plasma, and whole blood. Test kits 100s.
Use: Diagnostic aid.

ABBOTT DIAGNOSTIC REAGENTS. (Abbott Diagnostics) A series of diagnostic tests for cancer, cardiovascular, hepatitis, infectious disease and immunology, metabolic and digestive disease, OB/GYN, rubella, and thyroid.
Use: Diagnostic aid.

ABBOTT ER-EIA MONOCLONAL. (Abbott Diagnostics) Enzyme immunoassay for the quantitative measurement of human estrogen receptor in tissue cytosol. For research only. Not for use in diagnostic procedures.
Use: Research.

ABBOTT ER-ICA MONOCLONAL. (Abbott Diagnostics) Immunoassay for the detection of estrogen receptor. For research only. Not for use in diagnostic procedures.
Use: Research.

ABBOTT-HB EIA. (Abbott Diagnostics) Enzyme immunoassay for the detection of hepatitis Be antigen and/or antibody to hepatitis Be antigen.
Use: Diagnostic aid.

ABBOTT-HBe TEST. (Abbott Diagnostics) Radioimmunoassay or enzyme immunoassay for detection of hepatitis Be antigen and/or antibody to hepatitis Be antigen. Test kits 100s.
Use: Diagnostic aid.

ABBOTT HTLV III ANTIGEN EIA. (Abbott Diagnostics) Enzyme immunoassay for the detection of Human T-Lymphotropic Virus Type III (HIV)

antigens. For research only. Not for use in diagnostic procedures.
Use: Research.

ABBOTT HTLV III EIA. (Abbott Diagnostics) Enzyme immunoassay for the detection of antibody to Human T-Lymphotropic Virus Type III (HIV) in human serum or plasma. Test kits 1s.
Use: Diagnostic aid.

ABBOTT IgE EIA. (Abbott Diagnostics) Enzyme immunoassay for quantitative determination of IgE in human serum and plasma. Test kits 100s.
Use: Diagnostic aid.

ABBOTT PAP-EIA. (Abbott Diagnostics) Enzyme immunoassay for the measurement of prostatic acid phosphatase (PAP) in serum or plasma.
Use: Diagnostic aid.

ABBOTT RSV-EIA. (Abbott Diagnostics) Enzyme immunoassay for the detection of respiratory syncytial virus (RSV) in nasopharyngeal washes and aspirates.
Use: Diagnostic aid.

ABBOTT SCC-RIA. (Abbott Diagnostics) Radioimmunoassay for the quantitative measurement of squamous cell carcinoma associated antigen in human serum. For research only. Not for use in diagnostic procedures.
Use: Research.

ABBOTT TdT EIA. (Abbott Diagnostics) Enzyme immunoassay for the quantitative measurement of terminal deoxynucleotidyl transferase (TdT), in extracts of human whole blood or isolated mononuclear cells.
Use: Diagnostic aid.

ABBOTT TESTPACK HCG-SERUM. (Abbott Diagnostics) Monoclonal antibody, enzyme immunoassay for the qualitative determination of human chorionic gonadotropin (HCG) in serum. No instrumentation required.
Use: Diagnostic aid.

ABBOTT TESTPAK HCG-URINE. (Abbott Diagnostics) Monoclonal antibody, enzyme immunoassay for the qualitative determination of human chorionic gonadotropin (HCG) in urine. No instrumentation required.
Use: Diagnostic aid.

ABBOTT TESTPACK-STREP A. (Abbott Diagnostics) A rapid screening and confirmatory test for the detection of Group A beta-hemolytic streptococci from throat swabs. No instrumentation required.
Use: Diagnostic aid.

ABBOTT TOXO-G EIA. (Abbott Diagnostics) Enzyme immunoassay for the qualitative and quantitative determination of IgG antibody to toxoplasma gondii in human serum and plasma.
Use: Diagnostic aid.

ABBOTT TOXO-M EIA. (Abbott Diagnostics) Enzyme immunoassay for the qualitative determination of IgM antibody to toxoplasma gondii in human serum.
Use: Diagnostic aid.

ABCDG VITAMIN CAPSULES. (Lannett) Vitamins A 5000 IU, D 400 IU, B_1 1 mg, B_2 2 mg, C 30 mg/Cap. Bot. 1000s.
Use: Vitamin supplement.

ABC to Z. (Nature's Bounty) Vitamins A 5000 IU, D 400 IU, E 30 mg, iron 27 mg, B_1 2.25 mg, B_2 2.6 mg, B_3 20 mg, B_5 10 mg, B_6 3 mg, B_{12} 9 mcg, C 90 mg, folic acid 0.4 mg, biotin 45 mcg, vitamin K 25 mcg, zinc 15 mg/Tab. Bot. 100s.
Use: Vitamin/mineral supplement.

ABITREXATE. (International Pharm. Products) Methotrexate sodium 25 mg/ml. Vial 2 ml, 4 ml, 8 ml.
Use: Antineoplastic agent.

•**ABLUKAST.** USAN.
Use: Antiallergic; antiasthmatic.

•**ABLUKAST SODIUM.** USAN.
Use: Antiallergic; antiasthmatic.

ABORTIFACIENTS.
See: Prostin E 2, Supp. (Upjohn).
Prostin F 2 alpha, Inj. (Upjohn).
Prostin/15 M, Inj. (Upjohn).
20% Sodium Cl, Inj. (Abbott).

ABSORBABLE CELLULOSE COTTON OR GAUZE.
See: Oxidized Cellulose (Various Mfr.).

•**ABSORBABLE DUSTING POWDER,** U.S.P. XXII.

•**ABSORBABLE GELATIN FILM,** U.S.P. XXII. Sterile nonantigenic, absorbable, water-insoluble, gelatin film.
Use: Hemostatic, topical.
See: Gelfilm (Upjohn).

•**ABSORBABLE GELATIN SPONGE,** U.S.P. XXII. Gelatin sponge.
Use: Surgical aid.
See: Gelfoam (Upjohn).

•**ABSORBABLE SURGICAL SUTURE,** U.S.P. XXII. (Various Mfr.) Surgical Gut, Surgical Catgut, Catgut suture.
Use: Surgical aid.

•**ABSORBENT GAUZE,** U.S.P. XXII.
Use: Surgical aid.

ABSORBENT RUB RELIEF FORMULA. (DeWitt) Green soap 11.64%, camphor 1.63%, menthol 1.63%, pine tar soap 0.87%, wintergreen oil 0.71%, sassafras oil 0.54%, benzocaine 0.48%, capsicum 0.03%, wormwood oil 0.6%, isopropyl alcohol 75%. Bot. 2 oz.
Use: External analgesic.

ABSORBINE ARTHRITIC PAIN LOTION. (W.F. Young) Bot. 2 oz, 4 oz.

ABSORBINE FOOT POWDER. (W.F. Young) Zinc stearate, parachloroxylenol, aluminum chlorhydroxy, allantonate, benzethonium Cl, menthol. Plastic bot. 3 oz w/shaker top.
Use: Antifungal, external.

ABSORBINE, JR. (W.F. Young) Wormwood, thymol, chloroxylenol, menthol, acetone, zinc stearate, parachloroxylenol, aluminum chlorhydroxy, allantonate, benzethonium Cl, menthol. Liq. Bot. 1 oz, 2 oz, 4 oz, 12 oz w/applicator.

Use: External analgesic, antifungal.

ABUSCREEN. (Roche Diagnostics) An immunological and radiochemical assay for morphine and morphine glucuronide in nanogram levels. Utilizes I-125 labeled morphine requiring gamma scintillation equipment. Tests 100s.
Use: Diagnostic aid.

•**ACACIA,** N.F. XVII. Syr. N.F. XVII: Acacia senegal, arabic gum. (Penick) Pow. 0.25 lb, 1 lb; tears, 0.25-1 lb; whole, 0.25-1 lb.
Use: Demulcent, emulsifier, suspending agent.

A-CAINE. (A.V.P.) Diperodon HCl 0.25%, pyrilamine maleate 0.1%, phenylephrine HCl 0.25%, bismuth subcarbonate 0.2%, zinc oxide 5%, in cod liver oil and petrolatum base. Oint. Tube 1.25 oz.
Use: Local anesthetic.

A-CAPS. (Drug Industries) Vitamin A 50,000 IU/Cap. Bot. 100s, 500s.
Use: Vitamin A supplement.

•**ACARBOSE.** USAN.
Use: Alpha-glucosidase inhibitor.

ACCURBRON. (Merrell Dow) Theophylline, anhydrous 10 mg/ml. Bot. pt.
Use: Bronchodilator.

ACCUSENS T TASTE FUNCTION KIT. (Westport) Test for ability to distinguish among salty, sweet, sour and bitter tastants. Kit contains 15 bottles (60 ml) tastants and 30 taste record forms.
Use: Diagnostic aid.

ACCUTANE. (Roche) Isotretinoin 10 mg, 20 mg, or 40 mg/Cap. Prescription Pak 30s.
Use: Anti-acne, oral.

A-C-D SOLUTION, U.S.P. Sodium citrate, citric acid and dextrose in sterile pyrogen-free solution.
Baxter: 600 ml bot. with 70 ml, 120 ml, 300 ml soln.; 1000 ml bot. with 500 ml soln.
Cutter: 500 ml bot. with 75 ml, 120 ml soln.; 650 ml bot. with 80 ml, 130 ml soln.
Diamond: (Abbo-Vac) 250 ml, 500 ml.
Use: Anticoagulant for preparation of plasma or whole blood.

A-C-D SOLUTION MODIFIED. (Squibb) Acid citrate dextrose anticoagulant solution modified.
Use: Anticoagulant for use in radiolabeling red blood cells.

•**ACEBUTOLOL.** USAN. (±)-1-(2-Acetyl-4-butyramidophenoxy)-3-isopropylaminopropan-2-ol. (Ives) (±)-N-[3-Acetyl-4-[2-hydroxy-3-[(1-methylethyl)amino]propoxy]-phenyl]butamide.
Use: Beta-adrenergic receptor blocking agent.
See: Sectral, Cap. (Ives).

•**ACECAINIDE HYDROCHLORIDE.** USAN.
Use: Cardiac depressant.

•**ACECLIDINE.** USAN. 3-Quinuclidinol acetate (ester). Glaucostat. Under study.
Use: Parasympathomimetic.

•**ACEDAPSONE.** USAN. 4′,4″-Sulfonylbis (acetanilide).
Use: Antimalarial; antibacterial (leprostatic).

ACEDOVAL. (Vale) Dover's powder 15 mg, ipecac 1.5 mg, aspirin 162 mg, caffeine anhydrous 8.1 mg/Tab. Bot. 1000s, 5000s.
Use: Analgesic, antispasmodic, antiperistaltic.

ACEFYLLINE PIPERAZINE. Acepifylline. B.A.N.

•**ACEGLUTAMIDE ALUMINUM.** USAN.
Use: Anti-ulcerative.

•**ACEMANNAN.** USAN.
Use: Antiviral, systemic; immunomodulator; bowel disease, inflammatory, suppressant.

ACEPHEN. (G&W) **Adult:** Acetaminophen 650 mg/Supp. Box 12s, 100s. **Pediatric:** Acetaminophen 120 mg/Supp. Box 12s, 100s.
Use: Analgesic.

ACEPIFYLLINE. B.A.N. Piperazine theophyllin-7-ylacetate. Acefylline Piperazine (I.N.N.). Etophylate.
Use: Spasmolytic.

ACEPROMAZINE. 10(3-Dimethylaminopropyl)-3-acetylphenothiazine maleate. Plegicil. (Wyeth-Ayerst) 1-(10-(3-(Dimethylamino)propyl)-10H-phenothiazin-2-yl)ethanon e(Z)-2-butenedioate.
Use: Tranquilizer.

ACEPROMAZINE. B.A.N. 2-Acetyl-10-(3-di- methylaminopropyl)phenothiazine. Notensil maleate.
Use: Tranquilizer.

•**ACEPROMAZINE MALEATE.** USAN.
Use: Sedative.

ACEROLA-C. (Barth's) Vitamin C 300 mg/Wafer. Bot. 30s, 90s, 180s, 360s.
Use: Vitamin C supplement.

ACEROLA-PLEX. (Barth's) Vitamin C 100 mg, bioflavonoids 50 mg/Tab. Bot. 100s, 500s.
Use: Vitamin supplement.

ACETA. (Century) Acetaminophen 325 mg or 500 mg/Tab. Bot. 100s, 1000s.
Use: Analgesic.

ACETA W/CODEINE. (Century) Acetaminophen 300 mg, codeine phosphate 30 mg/Tab. Bot. 100s, 1000s.
Use: Narcotic analgesic combination.

ACETA-GESIC. (Rugby) Acetaminophen 325 mg, phenyltoloxamine citrate/Tab. Bot. 24s, 100s, 1000s.
Use: Analgesic, antihistamine.

•**ACETAMINOPHEN,** U.S.P. XXII. For Effervescent Oral Soln., Tab., Cap. U.S.P. XXII. Elix. U.S.P. XXI. N-Acetyl-p-amino-phenol. Acetamide, N-(4-hydroxyphenyl)-. 4′-Hydroxyacetanilide. APAP.
Use: Analgesic, antipyretic.
*See:*Acephen, Supp. (G&W).
Aceta, Tab., Elix., Supp. (Century).
Acetaminophen Uniserts, Supp. (Upsher-Smith).
Actamin, Tab. (Buffington).
Actamin Extra, Tab. (Buffington).
Aminodyne, Elix. (Bowman).
Anacin-3, Chew. tab., Tab., Elix., Drops (Whitehall).
Anapap, Tab. (Forest).

Apap, Cap., Tab. (Various Mfr.).
Banesin, Tab. (Forest).
Chlor-A-Tyl (Jenkins).
Dapa, Tab. (Ferndale).
Datril 500, Tab. (Bristol-Myers).
Dolanex, Elix. (Lannett).
Dorcol, Prods. (Sandoz Consumer).
Fendon, Tab. (APC).
G-1 (Hauck).
Genapap, Chew. tab. (Goldline).
Genebs, Tab., Cap. (Goldline).
Halenol, Tab., Elix. (Halsey).
Lestemp, Elix. (Reid-Rowell).
Liquiprin, Soln. (SmithKline Beecham).
Meda Cap, Cap. (Circle).
Meda Tab, Tab. (Circle).
Neopap, Supp. (Webcon).
Nilprin 7.5, Tab. (AVP).
Panadol, Chew. tab., Tab., Drops (Glenbrook).
Panex, Tab. (Mallard).
Parten, Tab. (Parmed).
Phenaphen, Cap., Tab. (Robins).
Proval, Cap., Elix., Drops, Tab. (Reid-Rowell).
Suppap-120, 325, 650, Supp. (Raway).
Tapanol Extra Strength, Tab. (Republic).
Tapar, Tab. (Parke-Davis).
Temetan, Elix., Tab. (Nevin).
Tempra, Drops, Syr., (Mead Johnson).
Ty-Caplets, Tab. (Major).
Ty-Caps, Cap. (Major).
Tylenol, Drops, Elix., Liq., Tab., Chew. tab. (McNeil).
Tylenol Extra-Strength, Tab., Cap. (McNeil).
Ty-Pap, Supp., Elix. (Major).
Ty-Tabs, Tab. (Major).
Valadol, Tab., Liq. (Squibb Mark).
Valorin, Tab. (Otis Clapp).

ACETAMINOPHEN W/COMBINATIONS

Aceta w/Codeine, Tab. (Century).
Akes-N-Pain, Cap. (E. J. Moore).
Al-Ay Modified, Tab. (Bowman).
Allerest Headache Strength, Tab. (Pharmacraft).
Alumadrine, Tab. (Fleming).
Amaphen, Cap. (Trimen).
Aminodyne, Elix. (Bowman).
Anodynos-DHC, Tab. (Berlex).
Anodynos Forte, Tab. (Buffington).
Apap w/Codeine, Tab. (Central).
Arthol, Tab. (Towne).
Arthralgen, Tab. (Robins).
Bancaps (Westerfield).
Banesin-Forte, Tab. (Westerfield).
Blanex, Cap. (Edwards).
Bowman Cold, Tab. (Bowman).
B-Pap, Liq. (Wren).
BQ Cold, Tab. (Bristol-Myers).
Bromo-Seltzer, Gran. (Warner-Lambert).
Capital and Codeine, Susp. (Carnrick).
Chexit, Tab. (Sandoz Consumer).
Codalan, Tab. (Lannett).
Codimal, Tab. (Central).
Colrex Compound, Elix. (Reid-Rowell).
Comtrex, Cap., Liq., Tab. (Bristol-Myers).
Conar-A, Tab., Susp. (Beecham Labs).
Conex, Preps. (Westerfield).
Congesprin, Liq., Tab. (Bristol-Myers).
Contac, Prods. (SmithKline Prods).
Coricidin Sinus Headache, Tab. (Schering).
Corzans, Tab. (Moore Kirk).
Co-Tylenol, Liq., Tab. (McNeil).
Darvocet-N, Tab. (Lilly).
Darvocet-N 100, Tab. (Lilly).
Demerol APAP, Tab. (Winthrop Pharm).
Dengesic, Tab. (Scott-Alison).
Desa-Hist AT, Tab. (Pharmics).
Dilone, Tab. (Vicks).
Dolene AP-65, Tab. (Lederle).
Drinacet, Cap. (Philips Roxane).
Drinophen, Cap. (Lannett).
Duoprin, Tab. (Dunhall).
Empracet with Codeine, Tab. (Burroughs Wellcome).
Esgic, Tab. (Gilbert).
Excedrin, Cap., Tab. (Bristol-Myers).
F.C.A.H., Cap. (Scherer).
Fendol, Tab. (Buffington).
Histogesic, Tab. (Century).
Histosal #2, Tab. (Ferndale).
Hycomine Compound, Tab. (Du Pont).
Hydrocet, Cap. (Carnrick).
Kiddies Sialco, Tab. (Foy).
Kleer, Syr. (Scrip).
Koryza, Tab. (Forest).
Midrin, Cap. (Carnrick).
Myocalm, Tab. (Parmed).
N-D Gesic, Tab. (Hyrex).
Nyquil, Liq. (Vicks).
Ornex, Cap. (SmithKline Prods).
Pamprin, Tab. (Chattem Labs.).
Panitol H.M.B., Tab. (Wesley).
Panritis, Tab. (Pan Amer.).
Parafon Forte, Tab. (McNeil).
Partuss-A, Tab. (Parmed).
Partuss T.D., Tab. (Parmed).
Pedric, Elix., Wafer (Vale).
Percogesic, Tab. (DuPont).
Phenaphen #2, #3, #4 (Robins).
Phenaphen-650, Tab. (Robins).
Phrenilin, Tab. (Carnrick).
Phrenilin Forte, Cap. (Carnrick).
Phrenilin w/Codeine, Cap. (Carnrick).
Presalin, Tab. (Mallard).
Proval No. 3, Tab. (Reid-Rowell).
Renpap, Tab. (Wren).
Rentuss, Cap., Syr. (Wren).
Repan, Tab. (Everett).
Rhinex, D. Lay, Tab. (Lemmon).
Rhinidrin, Tab. (Central).
Rhinogesic, Tab. (Vale).
S.A.C. Sinus, Tab. (Towne).
Saleto, Tab. (Mallard).
Saleto-D, Tab. (Mallard).
Salphenyl, Cap., Liq. (Mallard).

Santussin, Preps. (Sandia).
Sootgesic, Cap., Elix. (Scott/Cord).
Scotuss Pediatric Cough, Syr. (Scott/Cord).
Sedacane, Cap. (E. J. Moore).
Sedalgesic, Tab. (Table Rock).
Sedragesic, Tab. (Lannett).
Sialco, Tab. (Foy).
Sinarest, Tab. (Pharmacraft).
Sine-Aid, Tab. (McNeil).
Sine-Off, Prods (SmithKline Prods).
Sinubid, Tab. (Warner Chilcott).
Sinulin, Tab. (Carnrick).
Sinus Tab. (Zenith).
Sinutab, Prods. (Warner-Lambert).
Spantuss, Liq. (Arco).
Super-Anahist, Tab. (Warner-Lambert).
Talacen, Cap. (Winthrop Pharm).
Tega-Code, Cap. (Ortega).
Tegapap, Liq., Tab. (Ortega).
Triaminicin, Tab. (Sandoz Consumer).
Triaprin, Cap. (Dunhall).
Tussagesic, Tab., Susp. (Sandoz Consumer).
Two-Dyne, Tab. (Hyrex).
Tylenol, Preps. (McNeil).
Tylenol with Codeine, Elix., Tab. (McNeil).
Tylox, Cap. (McNeil).
Valihist, Cap. (Clapp).
Vicks Daycare, Liq. (Vicks).
Wygesic, Tab. (Wyeth-Ayerst).

•**ACETAMINOPHEN AND ASPIRIN TABLETS,** U.S.P. XXII.
Use: Analgesic.

•**ACETAMINOPHEN AND CAFFEINE CAPSULES,** U.S.P. XXII, Cap., Tab.

•**ACETAMINOPHEN, ASPIRIN AND CAFFEINE,** U.S.P. XXII, Cap., Tab., U.S.P. XXII.
Use: Analgesic.

ACETAMINOPHEN BUFFERED.
Use: Analgesic.
See: Bromo-Seltzer (Warner-Lambert).

ACETAMINOPHEN W/CODEINE. (Various Mfr.) **Tab.:** Codeine phosphate 15 mg, acetaminophen 300 mg/Tab. Bot. 100s, 500s, 1000s, UD 100s. Codeine phosphate 30 mg, acetaminophen 300 mg/Tab. **Elix.:** Codeine phosphate 12 mg, acetaminophen 120 mg/5 ml. Bot. 10 ml, 120 ml, 500 ml, pt, gal, UD 5 ml, 12.5 ml, 15 ml (100s).
Use: Narcotic analgesic combination.

•**ACETAMINOPHEN AND CODEINE PHOSPHATE ELIXIR,** U.S.P. XXII.
Use: Analgesic.

•**ACETAMINOPHEN AND DIPHENHYDRAMINE CITRATE TABLETS,** U.S.P. XXII.
Use: Analgesic, antihistamine.

•**ACETAMINOPHEN ORAL SUSPENSION,** U.S.P. XXII.
Use: Analgesic.

•**ACETAMINOPHEN SUPPOSITORIES),** U.S.P. XXII.

•**ACETAMINOPHEN ORAL SOLUTION,** U.S.P. XXII.
Use: Analgesic.

ACETAMINOPHEN UNISERTS. (Upsher-Smith) Acetaminophen **120 mg or 325 mg/Supp.:** Ctn. 12s, 50s; **650 mg/Supp.:** Ctn. 12s, 50s, 500s.
Use: Analgesic.

ACETAMINOPHENOL.
See: Acetaminophen.

ACETANILID. (Various Mfr.) (Acetylaminobenzene, acetylaniline, antifebrin) N-phenylacetamide cry.
Use: Analgesic.

ACETARSOL.
See: Acetarsone.

ACETARSONE. 3-Acetamido-4-hydroxy-phenylarsonic acid. Acetarsol, Acetphenarsine, Amarsan, Dynarsan, Ehrlich 594, Limarsol, Orarsan, Osarsal, Osvarsan, Paroxyl, Stovarsol.

ACETARSONE SALT OF ARECOLINE.
See: Drocarbil.

ACETASOL HC OTIC. (Goldline) Hydrocortisone 1%, acetic acid 2%. Bot. 10 ml.
Use: Otic corticosteroid, anti-infective.

ACETASOL OTIC. (Goldline) Acetic acid (nonaqueous) 2%. Bot. 5 ml.
Use: Anti-infective, otic.

•**ACETAZOLAMIDE,** U.S.P. XXII B.A.N. N-(5-Sulfamoyl-1,3,4-thiadiazol-2-yl)acetamide. Acetamide, N-[5-(aminosulfonyl)-1,3,4-thiadiazol-2-yl].
Use: Carbonic anhydrase inhibitor.
See: Diamox, Tab., Sequels (Lederle).

•**ACETAZOLAMIDE SODIUM, STERILE,** U.S.P. XXII.
Use: Carbonic anhydrase inhibitor.
See: Diamox, Inj. (Lederle).

ACET-DIA-MER-SULFONAMIDE. Sulfacetamide, sulfadiazine and sulfamerazine, Susp.
Use: Antibacterial, sulfonamide.

ACETEST REAGENT TABLETS. (Ames) Sodium nitroprusside, disodium phosphate, aminoacetic acid, lactose. Tab. Bot. 100s, 250s.
Use: Diagnostic aid.

•**ACETIC ACID,** U.S.P. XXII, Glacial, Otic soln., U.S.P. XXII. Diluted, N.F. XVII.
Use: Pharmaceutic aid (acidifying agent).

•**ACETIC ACID IRRIGATION,** U.S.P. XXII. 0.25% soln. (Abbott) 250 ml glass cont.; 250 ml, 1000 ml.
Use: Irrigating solution.

ACETIC ACID, POTASSIUM SALT. Potassium Acetate, U.S.P. XXII.

ACETICYL.
See: Acetylsalicylic Acid.

ACETILUM ACIDULATUM.
See: Acetylsalicylic Acid (Various Mfr.).

•**ACETOHEXAMIDE,** U.S.P. XXII. Tab., U.S.P. XXII. N-(p-acetylphenylsulfonyl)-N′-cyclo-hexylurea. 1-((p-acetylphenyl)sulfonyl)-3-cyclohexylurea. Benzenesulfonamide, 4-acetyl-N-[[cyclohexylamino]carbonyl].
Use: Blood sugar-lowering compound; antidiabetic agent.

See: Dymelor, Tab. (Lilly).
•**ACETOHYDROXAMIC ACID,** U.S.P. XXII. Tab., U.S.P. XXII.
Use: Enzyme inhibitor.
See: Lithostat (Mission).
ACETOL.
See: Acetylsalicylic Acid. (Various Mfr.).
ACETOLAX. (Mills) Acetphenylisatin 5 mg, Vitamins B_1 1 mg, sodium carboxymethyl cellulose 500 mg/Tab. Bulk Pkg. 1000s.
Use: Laxative.
ACETOMEROCTOL. Acetato [2-hydroxy-5-(1,1,-3,3-tetramethylbutyl) phenyl] mercury. Under study.
Use: Antiseptic, topical.
•**ACETONE,** N.F. XVII.
ACETONE or DIACETIC ACID TEST.
See: Acetest, Tab. (Ames).
ACETOPHEN C.T. GREEN. (Jenkins) Aspirin 3.5 gr, phenacetin 2.5 gr, caffeine 0.25 gr/Tab. Bot. 1000s.
•**ACETOPHENAZINE MALEATE,** U.S.P. XXII. Tab., U.S.P. XXII. 2-Acetyl-10- {3-[4-(-β-hydroxyethyl)-piperazinyl] propyl} phenothiazine dimaleate. 10-[3-[4-(2-Hydroxyethyl)-1-piperazinyl]-propyl]-phenothia-zin-2-yl methyl ketone maleate (1:2).
Use: Tranquilizer.
See: Tindal Maleate, Tab. (Schering-Plough).
ACETOPHENETIDIN. Phenacetin, U.S.P. XXII. Ethoxyacetanilide.
Use: Analgesic, antipyretic.
ACETORPHINE. B.A.N. O^3-Acetyl-7,8-dihydro-7α[1(R)-hydroxy-1-methylbutyl]-O^6-methyl-6,-14-endoethenomorphine.
Use: Narcotic analgesic.
ACETOSAL.
See: Acetylsalicylic Acid (Various Mfr.).
ACETOSALIC ACID.
See: Acetylsalicylic Acid (Various Mfr.).
ACETOSALIN.
See: Acetylsalicylic Acid (Various Mfr.).
ACETOSULFONE. 4,4′-Diaminodiphenylsulfone-2-N-acetylsulfonamide sodium. (N^1-acetyl-6-sulfanilylmetanilamido) sodium.
•**ACETOSULFONE SODIUM.** USAN.
Use: Antibacterial.
ACETOXYPHENYLMERCURY.
See: Phenylmercuric acetate.
ACETPHENARSINE.
See: Acetarsone, Tab. (City Chemical).
ACETPHENOLISATIN.
See: Oxyphenisatin Acetate Preps.
ACETRIZOATE SODIUM. 3-Acetamido-2,4,6,-triiodobenzoate sodium.
ACETRIZOIC ACID. 3-Acetylamino-2,4,6,-triiodobenzoic acid.
See: Acetrizoate, Sodium.
ACET-THEOCIN SODIUM.
See: Theophylline Sodium acetate (Various Mfr.).
ACETYL ADALIN.
See: Acetylcarbromal (Various Mfr.).
p-ACETYLAMINOBENZALDEHYDE THIOSEMICARBAZONE. (Amithiozone, Antib, Berculon A, Benzothiozon, Conteben, Myuizone, Neustab, Tebethion, Thiomicid, Thioparamizone, Thiacetazone).
Use: Antituberculous.
ACETYLAMINOBENZENE.
See: Acetanilid (Various Mfr.).
N-ACETYL-p-AMINOPHENOL. Acetaminophen, U.S.P. XXII.
ACETYLANILINE.
See: Acetanilid (Various Mfr.).
ACETYL-BETA-METHYLCHOLINE CHLORIDE.
ACETYL-BROMO-DIETHYLACETYL-CARBAMIDE.
See: Acetylcarbromal (Various Mfr.).
ACETYLCARBROMAL. Acetyladalin, acetylbromodiethylacetylcarbamide. Pow. for manufacturing.
Use: Sedative.
See: Paxarel, Tab. (Circle).
W/Bromisovalum, scopolamine aminoxide HBr.
See: Tranquinal, Tab. (Barnes-Hind).
•**ACETYLCHOLINE CHLORIDE,** U.S.P. XXII. For Ophthalmic Soln., U.S.P. XXII. Ethananinium,2-(acetyloxy)-N, N, N-trimethyl chloride. Choline chloride acetate.
Use: S.C., I.M., I.V. Parasympathomimetic agent, vasodilator. Paroxysmal tachycardia.
See: Miochol Ophthalmic (CooperVision).
ACETYLCHOLINE-LIKE THERAPEUTIC AGENTS.
See: Cholinergic agents.
•**ACETYLCYSTEINE,** U.S.P. XXII. Soln., U.S.P. XXII. B.A.N. N-Acetyl-L-cysteine.
Use: Mucolytic agent.
See: Mucomyst, Soln. (Bristol).
•**ACETYLCYSTEINE AND ISOPROTERENOL HYDROCHLORIDE INHALATION SOLUTION,** U.S.P. XXII.
Use: Mucolytic agent.
ACETYLDIHYDROCODEINONE. Thebacon. B.A.N.
ACETYLIN.
See: Acetylsalicylic Acid (Various Mfr.).
ACETYLMETHADOL, I.N.N. Methadyl acetate. B.A.N.
ACETYLPHENYLISATIN.
See: Oxyphenisatin Acetate.
ACETYLRESORCINOL.
See: Resorcinol Monoacetate (Various Mfr.).
ACETYLSAL.
See: Acetylsalicylic Acid.
ACETYLSALICYLATE ALUMINUM.
See: Aluminum Aspirin.
ACETYLSALICYLIC ACID. Aspirin, U.S.P. XXII. Acidum acetylsalicylicum, 2-acetoxybenzoic acid, Acetilum Acidulatum, Acetophen, Acetol, Acetosal, Acetosalic Acid, Acetosalin, Aceticyl,

Acetylsal, Acylpryin, Aspro, Helicon, Rhodine, Salacetin, Salcetogen, Saletin.
See: Aspirin Preps. (Various Mfr.).

ACETYLSALICYLIC ACID, ACETOPHENETIDIN AND CAFFEINE.
See: A.P.C., Preps. (Various Mfr.).

ACETYL SULFAMETHOXYPYRIDAZINE. 3-(N-Acetylsulfanilamido)-6-methoxypyridazine.

N[1]-ACETYLSULFANILAMIDE. (Albucid; p-Aminobenzenesulfonacetamide; Sulfacet; Sulfacetamide, N-Sulfanilylacetamide).
Use: Sulfonamide therapy.

ACETYL SULFISOXAZOLE. Sulfisoxazole Acetyl, U.S.P. XXII.

ACETYLTANNIC ACID. Tannic acid acetate.
Use: Antiperistaltic.

AC EYE DROPS. (Walgreen) Tetrahydrozoline HCl 0.05%, zinc sulfate 0.25%. Bot. 0.75 oz.
Use: Decongestant combination, ophthalmic.

ACHES-N-PAIN. (Lederle) Ibuprofen 200 mg. Tab. Bot. 50s.
Use: Nonsteroidal anti-inflammatory drug, analgesic.

ACHLORHYDRIA DETERMINATION.
See: Diagnex Blue, Preps. (Squibb).

ACHLORHYDRIA THERAPY.
See: Acidol (Various Mfr.).
Glutamic Acid HCl (Various Mfr.).
Muripsin, Tab. (Norgine).
Normacid, Tab. (Stuart).

ACHOL. (Enzyme Process) Vitamin A 4000 units, ketocholanic acids 62 mg/Tab. Bot. 100s, 250s.
Use: Vitamin A supplement.

ACHROMYCIN. (Lederle) Tetracycline HCl.
Intramuscular: 100 mg or 250 mg, sterile, buffered w/ascorbic acid. Vial Box 1s.
Intravenous: 250 mg or 500 mg, sterile, buffered w/ascorbic acid. Vial.
Ophth. Oint.: 10 mg/Gm 1%. Tube 3.75 Gm.
Ophth. Susp. 1%, Plastic dropper bot. 1 ml, 4 ml.
Use: Antibacterial.

ACHROMYCIN-V. (Lederle) Tetracycline HCl.
Cap: 250 mg: Bot. 100s, 1000s, UD 10 × 10s, Unit-of-use 12 × 20s, 12 × 28s, 12 × 40s, 12 × 100s; **500 mg:** Bot. 100s, 1000s, Unit-of-use 12 × 20s; UD 10 × 10s. **Oral Susp:** 125 mg/5 ml w/methylparaben 0.12%, propylparaben 0.03%. Bot. 2 oz, pt.
Use: Antibacterial, tetracycline.

ACID ACRIFLAVINE.
See: Acriflavine HCl (Various Mfr.).

ACID CITRATE DEXTROSE SOLUTION.
See: A.C.D. Soln. (Various Mfr.).

ACID CITRATE DEXTROSE ANTICOAGULANT SOLUTION MODIFIED.
See: A-C-D Solution Modified (Squibb).

ACID HISTAMINE PHOSPHATE.
See: Histamine Phosphate (Various Mfr.).

ACID MANTLE CREME. (Sandoz Consumer) Aluminum acetate in specially prepared water-soluble hydrophilic cream at pH 4.2. Tube 1 oz, Jar 4 oz, lb.
Use: Prophylactic agent, topical.

ACIDOL.
See: Betaine HCl (Various Mfr.).

ACIDOPHILUS W/PECTIN. (Barth's) *Lactobacillus acidophilus* w/natural citrus pectin 100 mg/Cap. Bot. 100s.
Use: Antidiarrheal.

ACID TRYPAFLAVINE.
See: Acriflavine HCl. (Various Mfr.).

ACIDULATED PHOSPHATE FLUORIDE. (Scherer) Fluoride ion 0.31% in 0.1 molar phosphate. Soln. Bot. 64 oz. (Office Product).
Use: Dental caries preventative.

ACIDULIN. (Lilly) Glutamic acid HCl 340 mg/Pulv. Bot. 100s, 1000s.
Use: Gastric acidifier.

•**ACIFRAN.** USAN.
Use: Antihyperlipoproteinemic.

ACIGLUMIN.
See: Glutamic Acid HCl. (Various Mfr.).

ACI-JEL. (Ortho) Glacial acetic acid 0.92%, ricinoleic acid 0.7%, oxyquinoline sulfate 0.025%, glycerin 5%. Tube 85 Gm w/dose applicator.
Use: Vaginal preparation.

ACINITRAZOLE. B.A.N. 2-Acetamido-5-nitrothiazole, Aminitrozole (I.N.N.).
Use: Treatment of trichomoniasis.
See: Trichorad.
Tritheon.

•**ACITRETIN.** USAN.
Use: Antipsoriatic.

•**ACLARUBICIN.** USAN.
Use: Antineoplastic.

ACLOPHEN. (Nutripharm) Phenylephrine HCl 40 mg, chlorpheniramine maleate 8 mg, acetaminophen 500 mg/S. R. tab. Dye free. Bot. 100s.
Use: Decongestant, antihistamine, analgesic.

ACLOVATE. (Glaxo) Alclometasone dipropionate 0.05%. Cream or Oint. Tube 15 Gm, 45 Gm.
Use: Anti-inflammatory, topical.

A.C.N. (Person & Covey) Vitamin A 25,000 IU, ascorbic acid 250 mg, niacinamide 25 mg/Tab. Bot. 100s.
Use: Vitamin supplement.

ACNAVEEN. (CooperCare)
See: Aveenobar Medicated (CooperCare).

ACNA-VITE. (Cenci) Vitamins A 10,000 IU, C 250 mg, hesperidin 50 mg, niacinamide 25 mg/Cap. Bot. 75s.
Use: Anti-acne, Vitamin supplement.

ACNE-5. (Goldline) Benzoyl peroxide 5%. Bot. oz.
Use: Anti-Acne.

ACNE-10. (Various Mfr.) Benzoyl peroxide 10%. Bot. 30 ml.
Use: Anti-Acne.

ACNE-AID CLEANSING BAR. (Stiefel) Neutral soap of 6.3% surfactant blend. Non-medicated. Bar 112 Gm, 174 Gm.
Use: Skin cleanser.

ACNE-AID CREAM. (Stiefel) Benzoyl peroxide 10%. Tube 54 Gm.
Use: Anti-acne.

ACNEDERM. (Lannett) **Lot.:** Dispersable sulfur 5%, zinc sulfate 1%, zinc oxide 10%, isopropyl alcohol 21%. Bot. 60 ml. **Soap:** Zinc oxide 2%, zinc sulfate 1%, colloidal sulfur 5%. Cake 3.2 oz.
Use: Anti-acne.

ACNE LOTION. (Weeks & Leo) Benzoyl peroxide 10% in odorless, greaseless, vanishing lotion. Bot. 2 oz.
Use: Anti-acne.

ACNO CLEANSER. (Baker/Cummins) Isopropyl alcohol 60%, laureth-23, tetrasodium EDTA. Bot. 240 ml.
Use: Anti-acne.

ACNO LOTION. (Baker/Cummins) Micronized sulfur 3%, salicylic acid 2%. Bot. 120 ml.
Use: Anti-acne.

ACNOMEL. (SmithKline Prods) Resorcinol 2%, sulfur 8%, alcohol 11%.
Cream Tube 28 Gm.
Use: Anti-acne.

ACNOPHILL. (Torch) Sulfur 5%, Potassium and zinc sulfides and polysulfides 5%, zinc oxide 10% in hydrophilic vehicle. Plain or tinted. Jar lb, 60 Gm.
Use: Anti-acne.

ACNOTEX. (C & M Pharmacal) Sulfur 8%, salicylic acid 2.25%, isopropyl alcohol 22%, acetone. In lotion base. Bot. 60 ml.
Use: Anti-acne.

•**ACODAZOLE HYDROCHLORIDE.** USAN.
Use: Antineoplastic.

ACOTUS. (Whorton) Phenylephrine HCl 5 mg, guaiacol glyceryl ether 100 mg, menthol 1 mg, alcohol by volume 10%/5 ml. Bot. 4 oz, 12 oz, gal.
Use: Decongestant, antitussive.

ACR. (Western Research) Ammonium Cl 7.5 gr/Tab. Handicount 28s (36 bags of 28 tab.).
Use: Diuretic.

ACRIFLAVINE. Euflavine, Gonacrine, Neutroflavine Acriflavine neutral; a mixture of 2, 8-diamino-10-methylacridinium Cl and 2,8-diaminoacridine. (Lilly) Tab. 1.5 gr. Bot. 100s.
Use: Antiseptic.

ACRIFLAVINE HYDROCHLORIDE. (Various Mfr.) Hydrochloride form of acriflavine. Acid acriflavine, acid trypaflavine, flavine, trypaflavine.
National Aniline-Pow., Bot. (1 Gm, 5 Gm, 10 Gm, 25 Gm, 50 Gm). Tab. (1.5 gr). Bot. 50s, 100s.
Use: Antibacterial.

•**ACRIVASTINE.** USAN.
Use: Antihistamine.

•**ACRONINE.** USAN. 3, 12-Dihydro-6-methoxy-3,3,12-trimethyl-7H-pyrano[2,3,-c]acridin-7-one. Under study.
Use: Antineoplastic.

ACT. Dactinomycin, U.S.P. XXII.
Use: Antineoplastic.
See: Actinomycin D.

ACT. (J & J) **Rinse:** 0.02% (from 0.05% sodium fluoride). **Mint:** Tartrazine, alcohol 8%. **Cinnamon:** Alcohol 7%. Bot. 360 ml, 480 ml.
Use: Dental Rinse.

A-C TABLET. (Century) Aspirin 6 gr, caffeine 0.5 gr/Tab.
Bot. 100s, 1000s.
Use: Salicylate analgesic.

ACTACIN TABLETS. (Vangard) Triprolidine HCl 2.5 mg, pseudoephedrine HCl 60 mg/Tab. Bot. 100s, 1000s.
Use: Antihistamine, decongestant.

ACTACIN-C SYRUP. (Vangard) Codeine phosphate 10 mg, triprolidine HCl 2 mg, pseudoephedrine HCl 20 mg, guaifenesin 100 mg/5 ml. Bot. pt, gal.
Use: Antitussive, antihistamine, decongestant, expectorant.

ACTAGEN SYRUP. (Goldline) Triprolidine HCl 1.25 mg, pseudoephedrine HCl 30 mg/5 ml. Bot. 120 ml, pt, gal.
Use: Antihistamine, decongestant.

ACTAGEN TABLETS. (Goldline) Triprolidine HCl 2.5 mg, pseudoephedrine HCl 60 mg/Tab. Bot. 100s, 1000s.
Use: Antihistamine, decongestant.

ACTAGEN-C COUGH SYRUP. (Goldline) Triprolidine HCl 1.25 mg, pseudoephedrine HCl 30 mg, codeine phosphate 10 mg/5 ml, alcohol 4.3%. Bot. 120 ml, pt, gal.
Use: Antihistamine, decongestant, antitussive.

ACTAL SUSPENSION. (Winthrop Products) Aluminum hydroxide.
Use: Antacid.

ACTAL PLUS TABLETS. (Winthrop Products) Aluminum hydroxide, magnesium hydroxide.
Use: Antacid.

ACTAL TABLETS. (Winthrop Products) Aluminum hydroxide.
Use: Antacid.

ACTAMIN. (Buffington) Acetaminophen 325 mg/Tab. Dispens-A-Kit 100s, 200s, 500s.
Use: Analgesic.

ACTAMIN EXTRA. (Buffington) Acetaminophen 500 mg/Tab. Bot. 100s, 200s, 500s.
Use: Analgesic.

ACTAMIN SUPER. (Buffington) Acetaminophen 500 mg, caffeine. Sugar, salt, and lactose free. Tab. Dispens-A-Kit 500s, Medipak 200s.
Use: Analgesic.

ACTAMINE. (H. L. Moore) **Tab.:** Pseudoephedrine HCl 60 mg, triprolidine HCl 2.5 mg. Bot. 100s, 1000s. **Syr.:** Pseudoephedrine HCl 30 mg, triprolidine HCl 1.25 mg/5 ml. Bot. 120 ml, pt, gal.
Use: Decongestant, antihistamine.

•**ACTAPLANIN.** USAN.
Use: Growth stimulant.

ACTH-ACTEST GEL. (Forest) Repository corticotropin 40 units or 80 units/ml. Vial 5 ml.

Use: Corticosteroid.

ACTH. (Adrenocorticotropic hormone. Adrenocorticotropin).
Use: Corticosteroid.
See: Corticotropin, U.S.P.
Mallard (40 units/ml, 5 ml).
Forest (40 units or 80 units/ml, 5 ml).
Parke-Davis (25 units/vial; 40 units/vial).
Pharmex (40 units or 80 units/ml, 5 ml).

ACTH GEL, PURIFIED. (Arcum) 40 or 80 units/ml, vial 5 ml. (Conal) 40 or 80 units/ml, vial 5 ml. (Hart Labs.) 40 units/ml, vial 5 ml. (Bowman) Adrenocorticotropic hormone 40 units, aqueous gelatin 16%, phenol 0.5%/ml. Vial 5 ml.
Use: Repository corticotropin.
(Arcum) 40 or 80 units/ml, 5 ml.
(Bell) 40 or 80 units/ml, 5 ml.
(Bowman) 40 units/ml, 5 ml.
(Hyrex) 40 or 80 units/ml, 5 ml.
(Jenkins) 40 or 80 units/ml, 5 ml.
(Rocky Mtn. Pharmacal) 40 or 80 units/ml, vial 5 ml.
(Wesley Pharm.) 40 or 80 units/ml, vial 5 ml.
(Wyeth-Ayerst) 40 or 80 units/ml or Tubex.

ACTHAR. (Armour) Corticotropin for inj. Vial 25 units, 40 units/vial. (Lyophilized w/gelatin).
Use: Corticosteroid.

ACTICORT 100 LOTION. (Baker/Cummins) Hydrocortisone 1%. Bot. 60 ml.
Use: Corticosteroid, topical.

ACTIDIL. (Burroughs Wellcome) Triprolidine HCl. **Tab.:** 2.5 mg. Bot. 100s. **Syr.:** 1.25 mg/5 ml. Bot. pt.
Use: Antihistamine.

ACTIDOSE. (Paddock) Activated charcoal. Soln. 25 Gm/120 ml or 50 Gm/240 ml.
Use: Antidote.

ACTIDOSE-AQUA. (Paddock) Activated charcoal. Aqueous susp. 25 Gm/120 ml or 50 Gm/240 ml.
Use: Antidote.

ACTIDOSE W/SORBITOL. (Paddock) Activated charcoal. Liq: 25 Gm in 120 ml susp. w/sorbitol, 50 Gm in 240 ml susp. w/sorbitol.
Use: Antidote.

ACTIFED. (Burroughs Wellcome) **Tab.:** Triprolidine HCl 2.5 mg, pseudoephedrine HCl 60 mg/Tab. Bot. 100s, 1000s, Box 12s, 24s, UD pack 100s. **Cap.:** Triprolidine HCl 2.5 mg, pseudoephedrine HCl 60 mg/Cap. Box 10s, 20s. **Syr.:** Triprolidine HCl 1.25 mg, pseudoephedrine HCl 30 mg/5 ml. Bot. 120 ml, pt.
Use: Antihistamine, decongestant.

ACTIFED 12-HOUR CAPSULES. (Burroughs Wellcome) Triprolidine HCl 5 mg, pseudoephedrine HCl 120 mg/Cap. Box 10s, 20s.
Use: Antihistamine, decongestant.

ACTIFED PLUS. (Burroughs Wellcome) Pseudoephedrine HCl 30 mg, triprolidine HCl 1.25 mg, acetaminophen 500 mg/Tab. or Cap. Bot. 20s, 40s.
Use: Decongestant, antihistamine, analgesic.

ACTIFED WITH CODEINE COUGH SYRUP. (Burroughs Wellcome) Codeine phosphate 10 mg, triprolidine HCl 1.25 mg, pseudoephedrine HCl 30 mg/5 ml, alcohol 4.3%. Bot. pt, gal.
Use: Antitussive, antihistamine, decongestant.

ACTIGALL. (Ciba) Ursodiol (Ursodeoxycholic acid) 300 mg/Cap. Bot. 100s.
Use: Gallstone solubilizing agent.

ACTIMMUNE. (Genentech) Inteferon gamma-1b 100 mcg (3 million units)/vial.
Use: Biologic response modifier.

ACTINOMYCIN. B.A.N. Antimicrobial substances with antitumor activity produced by *Streptomyces antibioticus* and *Streptomyces chrysomallus*. *Use:* Antineoplastic.

ACTINOMYCIN C. Name previously used for Cactinomycin.

ACTINOMYCIN D. Dactinomycin, U.S.P. XXII.
Use: Antineoplastic.
See: Cosmegen (Merck Sharp & Dohme).

•**ACTINOQUINOL SODIUM.** USAN.
Use: Ultraviolet screen.

ACTINOSPECTOCIN. Name previously used for Spectinomycin.

•**ACTISOMIDE.** USAN.
Use: Cardiac depressant (anti-arrhythmic).

ACTIVASE. (Genentech) Alteplase recombinant. Inj. Vial 20 mg, 50 mg.
Use: Thrombolytic enzyme.

ACTIVATED ATTAPULGITE.
W/Aluminum hydroxide, magnesium carbonate coprecipitate, compressed gel.
See: Hykasil, Cream (Philips Roxane).
W/Polysorbate 80, colloidal sulfur, salicylic acid, propylene glycol.
Use: Anti-Acne.
See: Sebasorb Lotion (Summers Labs.).

ACTIVATED CHARCOAL TABLETS. (Cowley) 5 gr/Tab. Bot. 1000s.
Use: Antidote.

ACTIVATED 7-DEHYDROCHOLESTEROL.
See: Vitamin D-3 (Various Mfr.).

ACTIVATED ERGOSTEROL.
See: Calciferol.

ACTOQUINOL SODIUM. 8-Ethoxy-5-quinolinesulfonic acid sodium salt.
Use: Ultraviolet screen.

ACTRAPID HUMAN INSULIN. (Squibb/Novo) Human insulin 100 units/ml. Vial 10 ml.
Use: Human insulin (rapid action).

ACTYLATE. (Kinney) Ammonium salicylate 80 mg, potassium salicylate 80 mg, strontium salicylate 80 mg, potassium para-aminobenzoate 0.32 Gm, ascorbic acid 20 mg/Tab. Bot. 100s.
Use: Rheumatoid arthritis.

ACUCRON. (Seatrace) Acetaminophen 300 mg, salicylamide 200 mg, phenyltoloxamine 20 mg/Tab. Bot. 100s, 1000s, 5000s.
Use: Analgesic, antihistamine.

ACU-DYNE. (Acme-United) **Douche:** Povidone-

iodine. Pkt. 195 ml. **Oint.:** Povidone-iodine. Jar. lb. Pkt. 1.2, 2.7 (100s). **Perineal wash conc:** Available iodine 1%. Bot. 40 ml. **Prep. Soln.:** Povidone-iodine. Bot. 240 ml, pt, qt, gal. Pkt. 30 ml, 60 ml. **Skin Cleanser:** Povidone-iodine. Bot. 60 ml, 240 ml, pt, qt, gal. **Soln, prep. swabs:** Available iodine 1%. Bot. 100s. **Soln, swabsticks:** Povidone-iodine. Pkt. 1 or 3 in 25s. **Whirlpool conc:** Available iodine 1%. Bot. gal.
Use: Antiseptic, germicide.

ACUTRIM LATE DAY. (Ciba Consumer) Phenylpropanolamine HCl 75 mg. Tab, precision release Bot. 20s.
Use: Diet aid.

ACUTRIM MAXIMUM STRENGTH. (Ciba Consumer) Phenylpropanolamine HCl 75 mg. Tab, precision release Bot. 20s, 40s.
Use: Diet aid.

•**ACYCLOVIR.** USAN. U.S.P. XXII. 9-(2-hydroxyethoxymethyl)-guanine.
Use: Antiviral.
See: Zovirax Cap., Oint. (Burroughs Wellcome).

•**ACYCLOVIR SODIUM.** USAN.
Use: Antiviral.

ACYLPYRIN.
See: Aspirin.

ADAGEN. (Enzon) Pegademase bovine 250 units/ml. Vial 1.5 ml.
Use: Enzyme (ADA) replacement therapy.

ADALAN LANATABS. (Lannett) Amobarbital 50 mg, homatropine methylbromide 7.5 mg, methamphetamine HCl 10 mg/T.D. Tab. Bot. 100s, 1000s.
Use: Sedative/hypnotic, cycloplegic mydriatic, CNS stimulant.

ADALAT. (Miles Pharm) Nifedipine 10 mg or 20 mg/Cap. Bot. 100s, 300s. UD 100s.
Use: Calcium channel blocking agent.

ADAMANTANAMINE HCl. Amantadine HCl. Antiflu capsule. This drug is thought to protect cells against entry of the flu virus without actually destroying the virus. Also used in the treatment of Parkinson's disease.
See: Symmetrel, Cap., Syr. (Du Pont).

ADAPETTES FOR SENSITIVE EYES. (Alcon Surgical) EDTA 0.1%, sorbic acid 0.1%. Pkg. 15 ml.
Use: Contact lens care.

ADAPIN. (Fisons) Doxepin HCl. **10 mg**: Bot. 100s, 1000s, UD 100s. **25 mg**: Bot. 100s, 1000s, 5000s, UD 100s. **50 mg**: Bot. 100s, 1000s, 5000s, UD 100s. **75 mg**: Bot. 100s, 1000s, UD 100s. **100 mg**: Bot. 100s, 1000s, UD 100s. **150 mg**: Bot. 50s, UD 100s.
Use: Antianxiety, antidepressant.

•**ADAPROLOL MALEATE.** USAN.
Use: Antihypertensive (β-blocker, ophthalmic).

ADAPT. (Alcon) Povidone, EDTA 0.1%, thimerosal 0.004%. Bot. 15 ml.
Use: Contact lens care.

ADAVITE. (Nature's Bounty) Vitamins A 5,500 IU, D 400 IU, E 30 mg, B_1 3 mg, B_2 3.4 mg, B_3 30 mg, B_5 10 mg, B_6 3 mg, B_{12} 9 mcg, C 120 mg, folic acid 0.4 mg, biotin 15 mcg. Tab. Bot. 100s.
Use: Vitamin supplement.

ADAVITE-M. (Nature's Bounty) Iron 27 mg, Vitamins A 5,500 IU, D 400 IU, E 30 mg, B_1 3 mg, B_2 3.4 mg, B_3 30 mg, B_5 10 mg, B_6 3 mg, B_{12} 9 mcg, C 120 mg, folic acid 0.4 mg, Cl, Cr, Cu, I, K, Mg, Mn, Mo, Se, Zinc 15 mg, biotin 15 mcg Tab. Bot. 130s.
Use: Vitamin/mineral supplement.

ADEECON. (CMC) Vitamins A 5000 IU, D 1000 IU/Cap. Bot. 1000s.
Use: Vitamin supplement.

ADEFLOR CHEWABLE. (Upjohn) Fluoride 0.5 mg or 1 mg, Vitamins A 4000 IU, D 400 IU, C 75 mg, B_1 2 mg, B_2 2 mg, B_3 18 mg, B_5 5 mg, B_6 1 mg, B_{12} 2 mcg/Chew. tab. 0.5 mg, 1 mg. Bot. 100s.
Use: Vitamin supplement, dental caries preventative.

ADEFLOR DROPS. (Upjohn) Vitamins A 2000 IU, D 400 IU, C 50 mg, B_6 1 mg, fluoride 0.5 mg/0.6 ml. Bot. 50 ml w/dropper.
Use: Vitamin supplement, dental caries preventative.

ADEFLOR M TABLETS. (Upjohn) Vitamins A 6000 IU, D 400 IU, B_1 1.5 mg, B_2 2.5 mg, C 100 mg, B_3 20 mg, B_5 10 mg, B_6 10 mg, B_{12} 2 mcg, folic acid 0.1 mg, fluoride 1 mg, calcium 250 mg, iron 30 mg/Tab. Bot. 100s, 500s.
Use: Vitamin supplement, dental caries preventative.

•**ADENINE,** U.S.P. XXII. 6-Aminopurine.

ADENO TWELVE GEL INJECTION. (Forest Pharm) Adenosine-5-monophosphate 25 mg, methionine 25 mg, niacin 10 mg/ml. Vial 10 ml.
Use: Arthritis, bursitis, tendinitis and other degenerative diseases.

ADENOCARD. (Lyphomed) Adenosine 6 mg/2 ml. Inj. Vial 2 ml.
Use: Antiarrhythmic.

ADENOCREST. (Nutrition) Adenosine-5-monophosphate sodium 25 mg, nicotinic acid as sodium salt 25 mg, gelatin 100 mg, benzyl alcohol 1.5%/ml. Vial 10 ml.
Use: Capillary and arterial vasodilator.

ADENOLIN FORTE. (Lincoln) Adenosine-5-monophosphate 25 mg, methionine 25 mg, niacin 10 mg/ml. Vial 15 ml.
Use: Arthritis, bursitis, tendinitis and other degenerative diseases.

•**ADENOSINE.** USAN. 6-Amino-9-beta-D-Ribofuranosyl-9H-purine.
Use: Antiarrhythmic.
See: Adenocard (Lyphomed).

ADENOSINE IN GELATIN. (Forest Pharm) **Forte:** Adenosine-5-monophosphate 50 mg/ml. **Super:** Adenosine-5-monophosphate 100 mg/ml.
Use: Treatment of varicose vein complications.

ADENOSINE-5-MONOPHOSPHATE AS THE SODIUM SALT.
See: Adenocrest, Amp. (Nutrition).

•**ADENOSINE PHOSPHATE.** USAN. 5-Adenylic acid. B.A.N. Adenosine-5′-(dihydrogen phosphate). Adenosine monophosphate, AMP.
Use: Nutrient.
See: Cobalasine, Inj. (Keene).
My-B-Den (Miles Pharm).

ADEPSINE OIL.
See: Petrolatum Liquid (Various Mfr.).

ADEQUATE IMPROVED. (Ortega) Calcium 125 mg, iron 65 mg, Vitamins A 6,000 IU, D 400 IU, E 25 mg, B_1 1.1 mg, B_2 1.8 mg, B_3 15 mg, B_6 2.5 mg, B_{12} 5 mcg, C 60 mg, folic acid 1 mg/Tab. Bot. 100s.
Use: Vitamin/mineral supplement.

ADICILLIN. B.A.N. 6-[D(+)-5-Amino-5-carboxyvaleramido]penicillanic acid. Penicillin N.
Use: Antibiotic.

•**ADINAZOLAM.** USAN.
Use: Antidepressant, sedative.

•**ADINAZOLAM MESYLATE.** USAN.
Use: Antidepressant, sedative.

ADIPEX-P. (Lemmon) **Cap.:** Phentermine HCl 37.5 mg. Bot. 100s, 400s. **Tab.:** Phentermine HCl 37.5 mg. Bot. 100s, 400s, 1000s.
Use: Anorexiant.

ADIPHENINE HYDROCHLORIDE. USAN. 2-Diethylaminoethyl diphenylacetate hydrochloride.
Use: Antispasmodic.

ADIPOST. (Ascher) Phendimetrazine tartrate 105 mg/S.R. Cap. Bot. 100s.
Use: Anorexiant.

ADISOL TAB. (Major) Disulfiram **250 mg/Tab:** Bot. 100s. **500 mg/Tab:** Bot. 50s.
Use: Antialcoholic agent.

ADLERIKA. (Last) Magnesium sulfate 4 Gm/15 ml. Bot. 12 oz.
Use: Laxative.

ADOLPH'S SALT SUBSTITUTE. (Adolph's) Potassium Cl 2480 mg/5 Gm, silicon dioxide, tartaric acid. Gran. Bot. 99.2 Gm.
Use: Salt substitute.

ADOLPH'S SEASONED SALT SUBSTITUTE. (Adolph's) Potassium Cl 1360 mg/5 Gm, silicon dioxide, tartaric acid. Gran. Bot. 92.1 Gm.
Use: Salt substitute.

ADONIDINE. (City Chem.) Bot. Gm.
Use: Cardiac stimulant.

•**ADOZELESIN.** USAN.
Use: Antineoplastic.

ADR.
Use: Antineoplastic agent.
See: Doxorubicin HCl.

ADRENALIN(E).
See: Epinephrine. (Various Mfr.).

ADRENALIN CHLORIDE SOLUTION. (Parke-Davis) Epinephrine HCl. Principle of the medullary portion of suprarenal glands. **Amp:** 1:1000-1 ml Epinephrine 1 mg/ml with not more than 0.1% sodium bisulfite as antioxidant. Amp. 10s. **Steri-Vial 1:1000:** Epinephrine 100 mg/ml in isotonic sodium Cl solution with 0.5% chlorobutanol as preservative and not more than 0.15% sodium bisulfite as antioxidant. Vial 30 ml. **Soln. 1:1000:** Bot. 30 ml. (Same as Steri-Vial). **Soln. 1:100:** Each 100 ml contains 1 Gm epinephrine HCl dissolved in sodium Cl citrate buffer soln w/ phemerol Cl 0.2 mg/ml as preservative, sodium bisulfite 0.2% as antioxidant. Bot. 0.25 oz.
Use: Sympathomimetic agent.

ADRENALINE HYDROCHLORIDE.
See: Epinephrine Hydrochloride. (Various Mfr.).

•**ADRENALONE.** USAN. 3′,4′-Dihydroxy-2-(methylamino)-acetophenone.
Use: Adrenergic (ophthalmic).

ADRENAMINE.
See: Epinephrine (Various Mfr.).

ADRENERGIC AGENTS.
See: Sympathomimetic agents.

ADRENERGIC-BLOCKING AGENTS.
See: Sympatholytic agents.

ADRENINE.
See: Epinephrine (Various Mfr.).

ADRENOCHROMAZONE.
See: Carbazochrome Salicylate.

ADRENOCHROME.
See: Carbazochrome Salicylate.

ADRENOCHROME MONOSEMICARBAZONE.
See: Carbazochrome Salicylate.

ADRENOCORTICOTROPIC HORMONE. ACTH acts by stimulating the endogenous production of cortisone and the final result is similar whichever substance is administered. The nature of action of each is unknown. Both are necessary in the metabolism of carbohydrates, protein and fat. They exert profound effects on neuromuscular metabolism.
See: ACTH gel, Inj. (Bowman).
Corticotropin, U.S.P.
Cortigel (Savage).

ADRENOMIST INHALANT AND NEBULIZERS. (Nephron) Epinephrine 1%, Bot. 0.5 oz, 1.25 oz.
Use: Bronchodilator.

ADRENUCLEO. (Enzyme Process) Vitamin C 250 mg, d-calcium pantothenate 12.5 mg, bioflavonoids 62.5 mg/Tab. Bot. 100s, 250s.
Use: Vitamin C supplement.

ADRIAMYCIN. (Adria) Doxorubicin HCl 20 mg/vial.
Use: Antineoplastic agent.

ADRIAMYCIN PFS. (Adria) Doxorubicin HCl 2 mg/ml. Inj. Vial: 5 ml, 10 ml, 25 ml.
Use: Antineoplastic agent.

ADRIAMYCIN RDF. (Adria) Doxorubicin HCl. **10 mg:** Methylparaben 1 mg, lactose 50 mg/Vial. Pkg. 10s. **20 mg:** Methylparaben 2 mg, lactose 100 mg/Vial. Pkg. 5s. **50 mg:** Methylparaben 5 mg, lactose 250 mg/Vial. Ctn. 1s. **150 mg:** Methylparaben 15 mg, lactose 750 mg/multi-dose vial. Rapid dissolution formula.
Use: Antineoplastic agent.

ADRIN TABS. (Major) Nylidrin 6 mg or 12 mg/Tab. Bot. 100s, 1000s.
Use: Vasodilator.

ADRUCIL. (Adria) Fluorouracil 50 mg/10 ml. Amp. 10 ml.
Use: Antineoplastic agent.

ADSORBOCARPINE. (Alcon) Pilocarpine HCl 1%, 2% or 4% in adsorbobase, water polymers, polyvinylpyrrolidone. Vial 15 ml.
Use: Miotic.

ADSORBONAC OPHTH. SOLUTION. (Alcon) Sodium Cl 2% or 5% in vehicle of polyvinylpyrrolidone, water-soluble polymers, EDTA 0.1%, thimerosal 0.004%. Dropper Vial 15 ml.
Use: Hyperosmolar preparation.

ADSORBOTEAR. (Alcon) Hydroxyethylcellulose, polyvinylpyrrolidone 1.67%, water-soluble polymers, thimerosal 0.004%, EDTA 0.1%. Soln. Bot. dropper 15 ml.
Use: Artificial tears solution.

ADVANCE. (Ross) **Ready-to-Feed infant formula:** (16 cal/fl oz).
Can 13 fl oz. **Conc. liq:** 32 fl oz.
Use: Enteral nutritional supplement.

ADVANCE PREGNANCY TEST. (Advanced Care) Can be used as early as 3 days after a missed period. Gives results in 30 min. Test kit 1s.
Use: Diagnostic aid.

ADVIL. (Whitehall) Ibuprofen 200 mg/Tab or Capl. In 8s, 24s, 50s, 100s, 165s, 250s (Tab.).
Use: Nonsteroidal anti-inflammatory drug; analgesic.

AER PADS. (Birchwood) Witch hazel-glycerin impregnated rayon pad. Jar pad. 40s.
Use: Astringent.

AERDIL. (Econo Med) Triprolidine HCl 1.25 mg, pseudoephedrine HCl 30 mg/5 ml. Bot. pt, gal.
Use: Antihistamine, decongestant.

AEROAID MERTHIOLATE. (Health & Medical Techniques) Merthiolate (Lilly) 1:1000, alcohol 72%. Spray bot. 3 oz.
Use: Antiseptic.

AEROBID. (Forest) Flunisolide in an inhaler system. Canister 7 Gm, 100 metered inhalations.
Use: Bronchodilator.

AEROCAINE. (Health & Medical Techniques) Benzocaine 13.6%, benzethonium Cl 0.5%. Spray bot. 0.5 oz, 2.5 oz.
Use: Local anesthetic.

AEROCELL. (Health & Medical Techniques) Exfoliative cytology fixative spray. Bot. 3.5 oz.
Use: Exfoliative cytology fixative spray.

AERODINE. (Health & Medical Techniques) Povidone-iodine. Bot. 3 oz.
Use: Antiseptic.

AEROFREEZE. (Health & Medical Techniques) Trichloromonofluoromethane and dichlorodifluoromethane. Aerosol cont. 8 oz. (12s).
Use: Local anesthetic.

AEROLATE. (Fleming) Theophylline 150 mg/15 ml. Soln. Bot. pt.
Use: Bronchodilator.

AEROLATE-III. (Fleming) Theophylline 65 mg/T.D. Cap. Bot. 100s, 1000s.
Use: Bronchodilator.

AEROLATE SR. & JR. (Fleming) **Cap.:** Theophylline 4 gr for Sr., 2 gr for Jr./Cap. Bot. 100s, 1000s. **Syr.:** 160 mg/15 ml. Bot. pt, gal.
Use: Bronchodilator.

AEROPURE. (Health & Medical Techniques) Isopropanol 7.8%, triethylene glycol 3.9%, essential oils 3%, methyldodecyl benzyl trimethyl ammonium Cl 0.12%, methyldodecylxylene bis (trimethyl ammonium Cl) 0.03%, inert ingredients, 85.15%. Bot. 0.8 oz, 4.5 oz.
Use: Air sanitizer, deodorizer.

AEROSAN. (Ulmer) Aerosol 16.6 oz.
Use: Air sanitizer, deodorizer.

AEROSEB-DEX. (Herbert) Dexamethasone 0.01%, alcohol 65.1%. Aerosol 58 Gm.
Use: Corticosteroid, topical.

AEROSEB-HC. (Herbert) Hydrocortisone 0.5%, alcohol 64.6%. Aerosol 58 Gm.
Use: Corticosteroid, topical.

AEROSEPT. (Dalin) Lidocaine, cetyltrimethylammonium bromide, hexachlorophene. Aerosol 6 oz.
Use: Anesthetic, antiseptic.

AEROSIL. (Health & Medical Techniques) Dimethylpolysiloxane. Bot. 4.5 oz.
Use: Silicone lubricant, protectant.

AEROSOL OT.
See: Docusate Sodium, U.S.P.

AEROSOLV. (Health & Medical Techniques) Isopropyl alcohol, methylene Cl, silicone. Aerosol 5.5 oz.
Use: Adhesive tape remover.

AEROSPORIN STERILE POWDER. (Burroughs Wellcome) Polymyxin B sulfate 500,000 units/vial. Multidose vial 20 ml.
Use: Antibacterial.

AEROSPORIN SULFATE. (Burroughs Wellcome) Polymyxin B sulfate 50 mg, 500,000 units. **Pow.:** Vial 20 ml. **Otic Soln.:** Bot. 10 ml.
Use: Antibacterial.
See: Polymyxin B sulfate, U.S.P.

W/Bacitracin.
See: Polysporin, Oint. (Burroughs Wellcome).

W/Bacitracin and neomycin sulfate.
See: Neosporin, Oint. and Ophth. Oint. (Burroughs Wellcome).

W/Bacitracin, neomycin, hydrocortisone.
See: Cortisporin, Prep. (Burroughs Wellcome).

AEROTHERM. (Health & Medical Techniques) Benzethonium Cl 0.5%, benzocaine 13.6%. Spray bot. 5 oz.
Use: Local anesthetic.

AEROZOIN. (Health & Medical Techniques) Comp. tr. of benzoin 30%, isopropyl alcohol 44.8%. Spray bot. 3.5 oz.
Use: Skin protectant.

AETHYLIS CHLORIDIUM.
See: Ethyl Cl (Various Mfr.).

AFAXIN CAPSULES. (Winthrop Products) Vitamin A Palmitate 10,000 IU or 50,000 IU/Cap.
Use: Vitamin A supplement.
A-FIL. (GenDerm) Methyl anthranilate 5%, titanium dioxide 5% in vanishing cream base. Tube 45 Gm. Neutral or dark.
Use: Sunscreen.
AFKO-LUBE. (APC) Docusate sodium 100 mg/Cap. Bot. 100s.
Use: Laxative.
AFKO-LUBE LAX. (APC) Docusate sodium 100 mg, casanthranol 30 mg/Cap. Bot. 100s.
Use: Laxative.
AFRIKOL. (Citroleum) Bot. 4 oz.
Use: Sunscreen.
AFRIN. (Schering) Oxymetazoline HCl 0.05%. **Nose Drops:** Drop. Bot. 20 ml. **Nasal Spray:** Reg.: Bot. 15 ml, 30 ml; Menthol: Bot. 15 ml. **Pediatric Nose Drops:** Oxymetazoline HCl 0.025%. Drop. Bot. 20 ml.
Use: Decongestant.
AFRINOL REPETABS. (Schering) Pseudoephedrine sulfate 120 mg/Repeat Action Tab. Box 12s. Bot. 100s, dispensary pack 48s.
Use: Decongestant.
AFTATE. (Plough) Tolnaftate 1%. **Gel:** Tube 15 Gm **Pump Spray Liq.:** 45 ml (with alcohol 83%). **Pow.:** 67.5 Gm, 45 Gm squeeze bot. **Aerosol pow.:** 105 Gm (with alcohol 14% and talc). **Aerosol liq.:** 120 ml (with alcohol 36%).
Use: Antifungal, external.
AFTER BITE. (Tender) Ammonium hydroxide 3.5% in aqueous solution. Pen-like dispenser.
Use: Antipruritic, external analgesic.
AFTER BURN. (Tender) Lidocaine 0.5% in aloe vera 98% solution.
Use: Local anesthetic, topical.
•**AGAR,** N.F. XVII. (Various Mfr.) Agar-agar, Bengal Gelatin, Ceylon.
Use: Laxative.
W/Mineral oil.
See: Agoral, Emulsion (Parke-Davis Prods).
Petrogalar (Wyeth-Ayerst).
AGENTS FOR MIGRAINE. Agents used to prevent or cure a headache usually of the recurring type over the region of the external carotid artery.
See: Cafergot, Supp., Tab. (Sandoz).
DHE-45, Inj. (Sandoz).
Gynergen, Amp., Tab. (Sandoz).
Sansert, Tab. (Sandoz).
Wigraine, Tab., Supp. (Organon).
AGGREGATED ALBUMIN.
See: Albumotope-LS (Squibb).
AGOFOLLIN.
See: Estradiol (Various Mfr.).
AGORAL. (Parke-Davis) Phenolphthalein 0.2 Gm, mineral oil 4.2 Gm/15 ml in an emulsion containing agar, tragacanth, egg-albumin, acacia, glycerin. Marshmallow and raspberry flavor. Bot. 240 ml, 480 ml.
Use: Laxative.
AGORAL, PLAIN. (Parke-Davis) Emulsion of mineral oil 1.4 Gm/5 ml with agar, tragacanth, egg albumin, acacia, glycerin. Bot. 480 ml.
Use: Laxative.
A/G-PRO. (Miller) Protein hydrolysate 50 gr w/essential and nonessential amino acids 45%, l-lysine 300 mg, methionine 75 mg, Vitamins C, B_6, Fe, Cu, I, Mn, K, Zn, Mg/6 Tab. Bot. 180s.
Use: Nutritional supplement.
AGURIN.
See: Theobromine Sodium Acetate (Various Mfr.).
AHAN. (Eric, Kirk & Gary) Vitamin A acetate 25,000 IU, 50,000 IU, 100,000 IU/Cap. Bot. 100s.
Use: Vitamin A supplement.
AHF.
See: Antihemophilic factor.
A-HYDROCORT. (Abbott Hospital Prods) Hydrocortisone sodium succinate. 100 mg or 250 mg/2 ml Univial, with benzyl alcohol; 500 mg/4 ml Univial with benzyl alcohol; 1000 mg/8 ml Univial with benzyl alcohol.
Use: Corticosteroid.
•**AIR, MEDICAL.** U.S.P. XXII.
AIR & SURFACE DISINFECTANT. (Health & Medical Techniques) Dimethylbenzylammonium Cl 0.33%, o-phenylphenol 0.25%, n-alkyl (50% C-14, 40% C-12, 10% C-16), ethyl alcohol 44.25%. Aerosol 16 oz.
Use: Air sanitizer, deodorizer.
AKARPINE. (Akorn) Pilocarpine HCl 1%, 2% or 4%. Also contains hydroxyethyl cellulose, benzalkonium Cl 0.01%, EDTA 0.01%. Soln. Bot. 15 ml.
Use: Miotic.
AK-CHLOR. (Akorn) Chloramphenicol 10 mg/Gm, mineral oil, parabens in white petrolatum base. Oint. Tube 3.5 Gm.
Use: Antibiotic, ophthalmic.
AK-CIDE. (Akorn) **Drops, susp.:** Prednisolone acetate 0.5%, sodium sulfacetamide 10%, hydroxypropyl methylcellulose, polysorbate 80, sodium thiosulfate, benzalkonium Cl 0.01%. Dropper bot. 5 ml, 15 ml. **Oint.:** Prednisolone acetate 0.5%, sodium sulfacetamide 10%, mineral oil, white petrolatum, lanolin, parabens. Tube 3.5 Gm.
Use: Ophthalmic corticosteroid, anti-infective.
AK-CON. (Akorn) Naphazoline HCl 0.1%, benzalkonium Cl 0.01%, EDTA 0.01%. Soln. Bot. 15 ml.
Use: Vasoconstrictor/mydriatic.
AK-CON-A. (Akorn) Naphazoline HCl 0.025%, pheniramine maleate 0.3%, benzalkonium Cl 0.01%, EDTA. Soln. Bot. 15 ml.
Use: Ophthalmic antihistamine, decongestant.
AK-DEX. (Akorn) Dexamethasone phosphate (as sodium phosphate). **Oint.:** 0.05% in white petrolatum and mineral oil base with lanolin, parabens, PEG-400. Tube 3.5 Gm. **Soln.:** 0.1% with benzalkonium Cl, EDTA. Dropper bot 5 ml.

Use: Corticosteroid, ophthalmic.

AK-DILATE. (Akorn) Phenylephrine HCl 10%. Soln. Bot. 2 ml, 5 ml; 2.5% Bot. 15 ml. Also contains benzalkonium Cl 0.01%, EDTA, sodium bisulfite.
Use: Vasoconstrictor/mydriatic.

AKES-N-PAIN. (E. J. Moore) Acetaminophen 120 mg, salicylamide 210 mg, caffeine 30 mg, calcium gluconate 60 mg/Cap. Bot. 30s.
Use: Analgesic combination.

AKES-N-PAIN RUB. (E. J. Moore) Histamine dihydrochloride, methyl nicotinate, oleoresin capsicum, glycomonosalicylate. Tube 1.25 oz.
Use: Analgesic, external.

AK-FLUOR. (Akorn) Fluorescein sodium. **10%:** Amp. 5 ml; **25%:** Amp. 2 ml, Vial.
Use: Ophthalmic diagnostic.

AK-HOMATROPINE. (Akorn) Homatropine HBr 5%, benzalkonium Cl 0.01%, hydroxyethyl cellulose, EDTA. Soln. Bot. 15 ml.
Use: Cycloplegic mydriatic.

AKINETON. (Knoll) Biperiden HCl 2 mg/Tab. Bot. 100s, 1000s.
Use: Antiparkinson agent.

AKINETON LACTATE. (Knoll) Biperiden lactate 5 mg in aqueous 1.4% sodium lactate soln/ml. Amp 1 ml, Box 10s.
Use: Antiparkinson agent.

•**AKLOMIDE.** USAN.
Use: Coccidiostat.

AK-MYCIN. (Akorn) Erythromycin 5 mg/Gm with white petrolatum, mineral oil. Oint. Tube 3.5 Gm.
Use: Anti-infective, ophthalmic.

AK-NACL. (Akorn) Sodium Cl hypertonic 5%, mineral oil, white petrolatum, anhydrous lanolin. Oint. Tube 3.5 Gm.
Use: Ophthalmic hyperosmolar preparation.

AKNE DRYING LOTION. (Alto) Zinc oxide 12%, urea 10%, sulfur 6%, salicylic acid 2%, benzalkonium Cl 0.2%, isopropyl alcohol 70%, in a base containing menthol, silicon dioxide, iron oxide, perfume. Bot. ¾ oz, 2.25 oz.
Use: Anti-acne.

AK-NEFRIN. (Akorn) Phenylephrine HCl 0.12%, benzalkonium Cl 0.01%, hydroxyethyl cellulose 0.5%, EDTA. Soln. Bot. 15 ml.
Use: Vasoconstrictor/mydriatic.

AKNE-MYCIN. (Hermal) Erythromycin. **Oint.:** 2%. Tube 25 Gm. **Soln.:** 2%. Bot. 60 ml.
Use: Anti-acne.

AK-NEO-CORT. (Akorn) Hydrocortisone acetate 1.5%, neomycin sulfate equivalent to 0.35% neomycin base, polysorbate 80, carboxymethylcellulose, sodium metabisulfite, chlorobutanol 0.5%. Susp. Dropper bot. 5 ml.
Use: Ophthalmic corticosteroid, anti-infective.

AKNE SCRUB. (Alto) Povidone iodine with polyethylene granules. Bot. ¾ oz.
Use: Anti-acne.

AKOLINE C.B. (Akorn) Choline bitartrate 111 mg, inositol 111 mg, methionine 28 mg, Vitamins B_1 0.3 mg, B_2 0.3 mg, B_3 3.3 mg, B_5 0.39 mg, B_6 0.3 mg, B_{12} 1.7 mcg, C 100 mg, lemon bioflavonoids complex 100 mg/Cap. Bot. 100s.
Use: Lipotropics with vitamins.

AK-PENTOLATE. (Akorn) Cyclopentolate HCl. **0.5%:** Soln. Bot. 15 ml; **1%:** Soln. Bot. 2 ml, 15 ml. Also contains benzalkonium Cl 0.01%, EDTA.
Use: Cycloplegic mydriatic.

AK-POLY-BAC. (Akorn) Polymyxin B sulfate 10,000 units, bacitracin zinc 500 units/Gm in a white petrolatum and mineral oil base. Oint. Tube 3.5 Gm.
Use: Anti-infective, ophthalmic.

AK-PRED. (Akorn) Prednisolone sodium phosphate 0.125% or 1%, benzalkonium Cl 0.01%, EDTA, hydroxyethyl cellulose, sodium bisulfite. **0.125%:** Soln. Bot w/dropper 5 ml. **0.1%:** Soln. Bot. w/dropper 5 ml, 15 ml.
Use: Corticosteroid, ophthalmic.

AK-RAMYCIN. (Akorn) Doxycycline hyclate 100 mg/Cap. Bot. 50s, 100s, 200s, 250s, 500s, UD 100s.
Use: Antibacterial, tetracycline.

AK-RATABS. (Akorn) Doxycycline hyclate 100 mg/Tab. Bot. 50s.
Use: Antibacterial, tetracycline.

AK-RINSE. (Akorn) Sodium Cl 0.49%, potassium Cl 0.075%, calcium Cl 0.048%, magnesium Cl 0.03%, sodium acetate 0.39%, sodium citrate 0.17%, benzalkonium Cl 0.013%. Soln. Bot. 30 ml, 118 ml.
Use: Ophthalmic irrigation solution.

AK-SPORE. (Akorn) **Oint.:** Polymyxin B sulfate 10,000 units, neomycin (as sulfate) 3.5 mg, bacitracin zinc 400 units/Gm in a white petrolatum and mineral oil base. Tube 3.75 Gm. **Soln.:** Polymyxin B sulfate 10,000 units, neomycin sulfate 1.75 mg, gramicidin 0.025 mg/ml, thimerosal 0.001%, alcohol 0.5%, propylene glycol, polyoxyethylene, polyoxypropylene. Soln. Dropper bot. 10 ml.
Use: Anti-infective, ophthalmic.

AK-SPORE H.C. OTIC. (Akorn) **Susp.:** Hydrocortisone 1%, neomycin sulfate 5 mg, polymyxin B sulfate 10,000 units/ml. Bot. w/dropper 10 ml. **Soln.:** Hydrocortisone 1%, neomycin sulfate 5 mg, polymyxin B sulfate 10,000 units/ml. Bot. w/dropper 10 ml.
Use: Corticosteroid, anti-infective combination.

AK-SULF. (Akorn) **Soln.:** Sodium sulfacetamide 10% or 15%, hydroxyethyl cellulose, sodium thiosulfate 0.2%, chlorobutanol 0.2%, parabens. 10%: Dropper Bot. 2 ml, 5 ml, 15 ml. 15%: Dropper Bot. 15 ml; **Oint.:** Sodium sulfacetamide 10%, parabens, petrolatum base. Tube 3.5 Gm.
Use: Anti-infective, ophthalmic.

AK-SULF Forte. (Akorn) Sodium sulfacetamide 30%, hydroxyethyl cellulose, sodium thiosulfate 0.2%, chlorobutanol 0.2%, parabens. Soln. Dropper bot. 5 ml.

Use: Anti-infective, ophthalmic.
AK-TAINE. (Akorn) Proparacaine HCl 0.5%, glycerin, chlorobutanol, benzalkonium Cl. Dropper bot. 2 ml, 15 ml.
Use: Local anesthetic, ophthalmic.
AK-TATE. (Akorn) Prednisolone acetate 1%, benzalkonium Cl, EDTA, polysorbate 80, polyvinyl alcohol, hydroxyethyl cellulose. Susp. Dropper bot. 5 ml, 10 ml, 15 ml.
Use: Corticosteroid, ophthalmic.
AK-TRACIN. (Akorn) Bacitracin 500 units/Gm. Oint. Tube 3.5 Gm.
Use: Anti-infective, ophthalmic.
AK-TROL. (Akorn) **Susp.:** Dexamethasone 0.1%, neomycin sulfate equivalent to 0.35% neomycin base, polymyxin B sulfate 10,000 units/ml, hydroxypropyl methylcellulose, polysorbate 20, benzalkonium Cl. Bot. w/dropper 5 ml. **Oint.:** Dexamethasone 0.1%, neomycin sulfate equivalent to 0.35% neomycin base, polymyxin B sulfate 10,000 units/Gm, white petrolatum, liquid lanolin, mineral oil, parabens. Tube 3.5 Gm.
Use: Ophthalmic corticosteroid, anti-infective.
AK-VERNACON. (Akorn) Phenylephrine HCl 0.125%, pheniramine maleate 0.5%, benzalkonium Cl, polyvinyl alcohol, EDTA. Bot. 15 ml.
Use: Decongestant, ophthalmic.
AKWA TEARS. (Akorn) **Soln.:** Polyvinyl alcohol, sodium Cl, benzalkonium Cl 0.01%, EDTA. Bot. 2 ml, 15 ml. **Oint.:** White petrolatum, mineral oil, lanolin.
Use: Artificial tears.
AK-ZOL. (Akorn) Acetazolamide 250 mg/Tab. Bot. 100s, 1000s.
Use: Anticonvulsant, diuretic.
ALA-BATH. (Del-Ray) Bath oil. Bot. 8 oz.
Use: Emollient.
ALA-CORT. (Del-Ray) Hydrocortisone 1%. **Cream:** Tube 1 oz, 3 oz. **Lot.:** Bot. 4 oz.
Use: Corticosteroid.
ALA-DERM. (Del-Ray) Lot. Bot 8 oz, 12 oz.
Use: Emollient.
ALADRINE. (Scherer) Ephedrine sulfate 8.1 mg, secobarbital sodium 16.2 mg/Tab. Bot. 100s.
Use: Decongestant, sedative/hypnotic.
ALAMAG. (Barre) Magnesium-aluminum hydroxide gel. Susp. Bot. pt.
Use: Antacid.
W/Belladonna alkaloid. Susp. Bot. 8 oz.
ALAMAG ANTACID SUSPENSION. (Goldline) Bot. 12 oz.
Use: Antacid.
ALAMAG PLUS ANTACID. (Goldline) Magnesium hydroxide 200 mg, aluminum hydroxide 225 mg, simethicone 25 mg/5 ml. Bot. 12 oz.
Use: Antacid.
ALAMECIN. USAN.
Use: Antibacterial.
ALANINE, U.S.P. XXII. $C_3H_7NO_2$. L-Alanine.
Use: Amino acid.
ALAPROCLATE. USAN.
Use: Antidepressant.
ALA-QUIN 0.5%. (Del-Ray) Hydrocortisone, iodochlorhydroxyquin cream. Tube 1 oz.
Use: Corticosteroid, topical.
ALA-SCALP HP 2%. (Del-Ray) Hydrocortisone lotion. Bot. 1 oz.
Use: Corticosteroid, topical.
ALA-SEB SHAMPOO. (Del-Ray) Bot. 4 oz, 12 oz.
Use: Antiseborrheic.
ALA-SEB T SHAMPOO. (Del-Ray) Bot. 4 oz, 12 oz.
Use: Antiseborrheic.
ALASULF. (Major) Sulfanilamide 15%, aminacrine HCl 0.2%, allantoin 2%. Vaginal Cream Tube w/applicator 120 Gm.
Use: Anti-infective, vaginal.
ALA-TET. (Del-Ray) Tetracycline HCl 250 mg or 500 mg/Cap. Bot. 100s, 1000s.
Use: Antibacterial, tetracycline.
ALATONE. (Major) Spironolactone 25 mg/Tab. Bot. 100s, 250s, 500s, 1000s, UD 100s.
Use: Antihypertensive.
ALAXIN. (Delta) Oxyethlene oxypropylene polymer 240 mg/Cap. Bot. 100s.
Use: Laxative.
AL-AY. (Bowman) **Green Oblong Tube:** Phenylephrine HCl 5 mg, chlorpheniramine maleate 2 mg, aspirin 162 mg, caffeine 15 mg, aminoacetic acid 162 mg/Tab. Bot. 100s, 1000s. **Dark Green S.C:** Phenylephrine HCl 5 mg, chlorpheniramine maleate 2 mg, acetaminophen 160 mg, caffeine 15 mg/Tab. Bot. 100s, 1000s.
Use: Decongestant, antihistamine, analgesic.
ALAZANINE TRICHLORPHATE. 3-Ethyl-2-[3-(3-ethyl-2-benzothiazolinylidene) propenyl]-benzothiazolium 2,4,5-trichlorophenoxide salt with two formula weights of 2,4,5[trichlorophenol].
Use: Anthelmintic.
ALAZIDE TABS. (Major) Spironolactone w/hydrochlorothiazide. Bot. 250s, 1000s.
Use: Antihypertensive.
ALAZINE TABS. (Major) Hydralazine 10 mg, 25 mg or 50 mg/Cap. Bot. 100s, 1000s.
Use: Antihypertensive.
ALBA-DEX. (Pharma-Serv) Dexamethasone phosphate (as sodium phosphate) solution 4 mg/ml, methyl and propyl parabens, sodium bisulfite. Inj. Vial 1 ml, 5 ml, 30 ml.
Use: Corticosteroid.
ALBALON LIQUIFILM. (Allergan) Naphazoline HCl 0.1%, polyvinyl alcohol 1.4%, benzalkonium Cl 0.004%, edetate disodium, citric acid, sodium citrate, sodium Cl, sodium hydroxide, purified water. Bot. 5 ml, 15 ml.
Use: Vasoconstrictor, ophthalmic.
ALBALON-A LIQUIFILM. (Allergan) Naphazoline HCl 0.05%, antazoline phosphate 0.5%, polyvinyl alcohol 1.4%, benzalkonium Cl 0.004%, edetate disodium, povidone, sodium Cl, sodium acetate, acetic acid and/or sodium hydroxide, purified water. Bot. 5 ml, 15 ml.
Use: Decongestant, ophthalmic.

ALBAMYCIN. (Upjohn) Novobiocin sodium 250 mg/Cap. Bot. 100s.
Use: Anti-infective.

ALBAY. (Hollister-Stier) Freeze-dried venom (honeybee) 500 mcg and venom protein (yellow jacket, yellow hornet, white faced hornet, wasp and mixed vespid). Inj. Vial 10 ml.
Use: Allergenic extract.

•**ALBENDAZOLE.** USAN.
Use: Anthelmintic.

ALBOLENE CREAM. (Norcliff Thayer) Unscented or scented. Jar 6 oz, 12 oz.

ALBUCID.
See: Sulfacetamide.

ALBUCONN 25% SOLUTION. (Cryosan) Normal serum albumin (human) 12.5 Gm in 50 ml solution for IV administration. Vial 50 ml.
Use: Treatment of plasma or blood volume deficit, acute hypoproteinemia, oncotic deficit.

•**ALBUMIN, AGGREGATED.** USAN.
Use: Diagnostic aid.

•**ALBUMIN, AGGREGATED IODINATED 1 131 SERUM.** USAN.
Use: Radioactive agent.

•**ALBUMIN, CHROMATED Cr 51 SERUM.** USAN. Radio-Chromated Serum Albumin Human.
Use: Radioactive agent.
See: Chromalbin (Squibb).

•**ALBUMIN HUMAN,** U.S.P. XXII. Normal Human Serum Albumin.
Use: Plasma protein fraction.
See: Proserum 5, Inj. (Merrell Dow).

ALBUMIN HUMAN, 5%. (Immuno-US) Normal serum albumin 5%. Inj. Vial 250 ml.
Use: Plasma protein fraction.

ALBUMIN HUMAN, 25%. (Immuno-US) Normal serum albumin 25%. Inj. Vial 10 ml, 50 ml.
Use: Plasma protein fraction.

•**ALBUMIN, IODINATED I-125 SERUM.** USAN. Radio-iodinated (I-125) Serum Albumin Human.
Use: Diagnostic aid.

•**ALBUMIN, IODINATED I-131 SERUM,** U.S.P. XXII. Radio-iodinated (^{131}I) Serum Albumin Human. Aggregated Radio-Iodinated (I-131) Albumin Human.
Use: Diagnostic aid.
See: Albumotope-LS (Squibb).

•**ALBUMIN, IODINATED I-131 AGGREGATED INJECTION,** U.S.P. XXII.
Use: Diagnostic aid.

ALBUMIN-SALINE DILUENT. (Hollister-Stier) Dilute allergenic extracts and venom products for patient testing and treating. Pre-measured vials 1.8 ml, 4 ml, 4.5 ml, 9 ml, 30 ml. Vial 2 ml, 5 ml, 10 ml, 30 ml.
Use: Diagnostic aid, treatment.

ALBUMINAR-5 AND ALBUMINAR-25. (Armour) Albumin, (human) U.S.P. 5% solution with administration set. Bot. 50 ml, 250 ml, 500 ml, 1000 ml. 25% solution. Vial 20 ml, 50 ml, 100 ml with administration set.
Use: Plasma protein fraction.

ALBUMOTOPE I-131. (Squibb) Albumin, Iodinated I-131 Serum (50 uCi).
Use: Diagnostic aid.

ALBUSTIX REAGENT STRIPS. (Ames) Firm paper reagent strips impregnated with tetrabromphenol blue, citrate buffer and a protein-adsorbing agent. Bot. 50s, 100s.
Use: Diagnostic aid.

ALBUTEIN 5%. (Alpha Therapeutic) Normal serum albumin 5%. Inj. Vial w/IV set: 250 ml, 500 ml.
Use: Plasma protein fraction.

ALBUTEIN 25%. (Alpha Therapeutic) Normal serum albumin 25%. Inj. Vial w/IV set: 50 ml.
Use: Plasma protein fraction.

•**ALBUTEROL.** USAN.
Use: Bronchodilator.
See: Ventolin, Inh (Allen & H).

•**ALBUTEROL SULFATE.** USAN.
Use: Bronchodilator.
See: Proventil, Tab., Soln., Syr. (Schering).
Ventolin, Soln., Syr., Tab. (Allen & H).
Ventolin Rotacaps (Allen & H).

•**ALBUTOIN.** USAN. 3-Allyl-5-isobutyl-2-thiohydantoin.
Use: Anticonvulsant.

ALCAINE. (Alcon) Proparacaine HCl 0.5%, glycerin, sodium Cl, benzalkonium Cl. Bot. 15 ml.
Use: Local anesthetic, ophthalmic.

ALCARE. (Vestal) Ethyl alcohol 62%. Foam Bot. 210 ml, 300 ml, 600 ml.
Use: Antiseptic.

ALCLEAR EYE LOTION. (Walgreen) Sterile isotonic fluid. Bot. 8 oz.
Use: Eye irritation relief.

•**ALCLOFENAC.** USAN. 4-Allyloxy-3-chlorophenylacetic acid.
Use: Analgesic, anti-inflammatory.
See: Prinalgin.

•**ALCLOMETASONE DIPROPIONATE.** USAN.
Use: Anti-inflammatory.
See: Aclovate, Cream, Oint. (Glaxo).

ALCLOXA. USAN. Tetrahydroxychloro-[(2- hydroxy-5-oxo-2-imidazolin-4-yl)ureato]-dialuminum.
Use: Astringent, keratolytic.

•**ALCOHOL,** U.S.P. XXII. Ethanol, ethyl alcohol.
Use: Topical anti-infective; pharmaceutic aid (solvent).

•**ALCOHOL, DEHYDRATED,** U.S.P. XXII.
Use: Solvent, vehicle.

•**ALCOHOL, DEHYDRATED INJECTION,** U.S.P. XXII.

•**ALCOHOL IN DEXTROSE INJECTION,** U.S.P. XXII.

•**ALCOHOL, DILUTED,** N.F. XVII.
Use: Solvent, vehicle.

•**ALCOHOL, RUBBING,** U.S.P. XXII.
Use: Rubefacient.

ALCOHOL 5% AND DEXTROSE 5%. (Abbott Hospital Prods) Alcohol 5 ml, dextrose 5 Gm/100 ml. Bot. 1000 ml.

Use: Parenteral nutritional supplement.
ALCOJET. (Alconox) Biodegradable machine washing detergent and wetting agent. Ctn. 9 × 4 lb, 25 lb, 50 lb, 100 lb, 300 lb.
Use: Detergent, wetting agent.
ALCOLEC. (American Lecithin) Lecithin w/choline base, cephalin, lipositol. Cap. 100s. Gran. 8 oz, lb.
Use: Nutritional supplement.
ALCONEFRIN 12 AND 50. (Webcon) Phenylephrine HCl 0.16% w/benzalkonium Cl. Dropper bot. 30 ml.
Use: Nasal decongestant.
ALCONEFRIN 25. (Webcon) Phenylephrine HCl 0.25% w/benzalkonium Cl. Dropper bot. 30 ml. Spray Pkg. 30 ml.
Use: Nasal decongestant.
ALCON ENZYMATIC CLEANING TABLETS FOR EXTENDED WEAR. (Alcon Lenscare) Pancreatin tablets. Pkg. 12s.
Use: Contact lens care.
ALCON LENS CASE. (Alcon Lenscare) Two lens cases. Ctn. 12s.
Use: Contact lens care.
ALCON OPTI-PURE STERILE SALINE SOLUTION. (Alcon Lenscare) Sterile unpreserved saline solution. Aerosol 8 oz.
Use: Soft contact lens care.
ALCON SALINE SOLUTION FOR SENSITIVE EYES. (Alcon Lenscare) Sodium Cl edetate disodium, sorbic acid 0.1%. Bot. 4 oz, 8 oz, 12 oz.
Use: Soft contact lens care.
ALCONOX. (Alconox) Biodegradable detergent and wetting agent. Box 4 lb, Container 25 lb, 50 lb, 100 lb, 300 lb.
Use: Anionic detergent, wetting agent.
ALCOTABS. (Alconox) Tab. Box 6s, 100s.
Use: Test tube cleaner.
•**ALCURONIUM CHLORIDE.** USAN. Diallyldinortoxiferin dichloride.
Use: Muscle relaxant.
See: Alloferin (Roche).
Toxiferene (Roche).
ALDACTAZIDE TABLETS. (Searle) Spironolactone and hydrochlorothiazide. **25 mg/25 mg:** Bot. 100s, 500s, 1000s, 2500s, UD 100s. **50 mg/50 mg:** Bot. 100s, UD 32s, UD 100s.
Use: Antihypertensive.
ALDACTONE TABLETS. (Searle) Spironolactone. **25 mg/Tab.:** Bot. 100s, 500s, 1000s, UD 100s. **50 mg/Tab.:** Bot. 100s, UD 100s. **100 mg/Tab.:** Bot. 100s, UD 100s.
Use: Antihypertensive.
ALDERLIN HYDROCHLORIDE. Pronethalol, B.A.N.
ALDESLEUKIN. USAN
Use: Biological response modifier; antineoplastic; immunostimulant.
ALDINAMIDE. 2-Carbamoyl pyrazine.
ALDIOXA. USAN. Aluminum dihydroxy allantoinate. Dihydroxy-[(2-hydroxy-5-oxo-2-imidazolin-4-yl)ureato] aluminum.
Use: Astringent, keratolytic.
ALDOCLOR 150. (Merck Sharp & Dohme) Methyldopa 250 mg, chlorothiazide 150 mg/Tab. Bot. 100s.
Use: Antihypertensive.
ALDOCLOR 250. (Merck Sharp & Dohme) Methyldopa 250 mg, chlorothiazide 250 mg/Tab. Bot. 100s.
Use: Antihypertensive.
ALDOMET. (Merck Sharp & Dohme) Methyldopa. **125 mg/Tab.:** Bot. 100s. **250 mg/Tab.:** Bot. 100s, 1000s, UD 100s, Unit-of-use 100s. **500 mg/Tab.:** Bot. 100s, 500s, UD 100s, Unit-of-use 60s, 100s.
Use: Antihypertensive.
W/Chlorothiazide.
See: Aldoclor, Tab. (Merck Sharp & Dohme).
W/Hydrochlorothiazide.
See: Aldoril, Tab. (Merck Sharp & Dohme).
ALDOMET ESTER HCl. (Merck Sharp & Dohme) Methyldopate HCl 250 mg/5 ml, citric acid anhydrous 25 mg, sodium bisulfite 16 mg, disodium edetate 2.5 mg, monothioglycerol 10 mg, sodium hydroxide to adjust pH, methylparaben 0.15%, propylparaben 0.02% w/water for inj. q.s. to 5 ml. Vial 5 ml.
Use: Antihypertensive.
ALDOMET ORAL SUSPENSION. (Merck Sharp & Dohme) Methyldopa 250 mg/5 ml, alcohol 1%, benzoic acid 0.1%, sodium bisulfite 0.2%. Bot. 473 ml.
Use: Antihypertensive.
ALDORIL-15. (Merck Sharp & Dohme) Methyldopa 250 mg, hydrochlorothiazide 15 mg/Tab. Bot. 100s, 1000s, UD 100s.
Use: Antihypertensive.
ALDORIL-25. (Merck Sharp & Dohme) Methyldopa 250 mg, hydrochlorothiazide 25 mg/Tab. Bot. 100s, 1000s, UD 100s.
Use: Antihypertensive.
ALDORIL D30. (Merck Sharp & Dohme) Methyldopa 500 mg, hydrochlorothiazide 30 mg/Tab. Bot. 100s.
Use: Antihypertensive.
ALDOSTERONE B.A.N. 11β,21-Dihydroxy-3,-20-di-oxopregn-4-en-18-al. Aldocorten. Electrocortin.
Use: Corticosteroid.
ALDOSTERONE RIA DIAGNOSTIC KIT. (Abbott Diagnostics) Test kits 50s.
Use: Diagnostic aid.
•**ALENDRONATE SODIUM.** USAN.
Use: Bone resorption inhibitor.
•**ALENTEMOL HYDROBROMIDE.** USAN
Use: Antipsychotic.
ALERSULE CAPSULES. (Misemer) Chlorpheniramine maleate 8 mg, phenylephrine HCl 20 mg/Cap. Bot. 100s.
Use: Antihistamine, decongestant.

ALERT-PEP. (Approved) Caffeine 200 mg/Cap. Bot. 16s.
Use: CNS stimulant.

•**ALETAMINE HYDROCHLORIDE.** USAN.
Use: Antidepressant.

•**ALEXIDINE.** USAN. 1,1′-Hexamethylenebis[5-(2-ethylhexyl) biguanide].
Use: Antibacterial.

•**ALFAPROSTOL.** USAN.
Use: Prostaglandin (veterinary).

ALFENTA. (Janssen) Alfentanil 0.5 mg/ml. Amp. 2 ml, 5 ml, 10 ml, 20 ml.
Use: Narcotic analgesic, anesthetic.

•**ALFENTANIL HYDROCHLORIDE.** USAN.
Use: Analgesic, narcotic; anesthetic.
See: Alfenta, Inj. (Janssen).

ALFERON N. (Purdue Frederick) Interferon alfa-n3 5 mIU/vial. Vial 1 ml.
Use: Antineoplastic agent.

•**ALFUZOSIN HYDROCHLORIDE.** USAN.
Use: Antihypertensive.

ALGEL. (Faraday) Magnesium trisilicate 0.5 Gm, aluminum hydroxide 0.25 Gm/Tab. Bot. 100s. Susp. Bot. gal.
Use: Antacid.

ALGEMIN. (Thurston) Macrocystis pyrifera alga. Pow. Jar 8 oz. Tab. Bot. 300s.
Use: Dietary aid.

ALGENIC ALKA LIQUID. (Rugby) Aluminum hydroxide 31.7 mg/ml, magnesium carbonate 137 mg/ml, sodium alginate, sorbitol. Bot. 355 ml.
Use: Antacid.

ALGENIC ALKA IMPROVED TABLETS. (Rugby) Aluminum hydroxide 240 mg, magnesium hydroxide 100 mg/Chew. Tab. Bot. 100s, 500s.
Use: Antacid.

•**ALGESTONE ACETONIDE.** USAN. 16α,-17α-Isopropylidenedioxypregn-4-ene-3,20-dione.
Use: Progestin.

•**ALGESTONE ACETOPHENIDE.** USAN. (R)-16α, 17-Dihydroxypregn-4-ene-3,20-dione cyclic acetal with acetophenone.
Use: Progestin.

ALGEX LINIMENT. (Approved) Menthol, camphor, methylsalicylate, eucalyptus. Bot. 4 oz.
Use: External analgesic.

ALGICON. (Rorer Consumer) Aluminum hydroxide 360 mg, magnesium carbonate 320 mg, sodium 5.1 mg/Chew. Tab. Box 50s.
Use: Antacid.

ALGIN.
See: Sodium Alginate, N.F. XVII.

ALGIN-ALL. (Barth's) Sodium alginate from kelp. Tab. Bot. 100s, 500s.

•**ALGINIC ACID,** N.F. XVII.
Use: Pharmaceutic aid (tablet binder, thickening agent).

ALGINIC ACID. W/Aluminum hydroxide dried gel, magnesium trisilicate, sodium bicarbonate.
Use: Antacid.
See: Gaviscon Foamtabs (Marion).

•**ALGRELDRATE.** USAN.
Use: Antacid.

ALIDINE DIHYDROCHLORIDE OR PHOSPHATE. Anileridine, N.F.

•**ALIFLURANE.** USAN.
Use: Anesthetic.

ALIKAL POWDER. (Winthrop Products) Sodium bicarbonate, tartaric acid powder.
Use: Antacid.

ALIMENTUM. (Ross) Casein hydrolysate, sucrose, tapioca starch, MCT (fractionated coconut oil), safflower oil, soy oil. Qt ready-to-use.
Use: Enteral nutritional supplement.

•**ALIPAMIDE.** USAN. 4-Chloro-3- sulfamoylbenzoic acid 2,2-dimethylhydrazide.
Use: Diuretic, antihypertensive.

ALIPAMIDE. B.A.N. 4-Chloro-2′,2′-dimethyl-3-sulfamoylbenzohydrazide.
Use: Diuretic.

ALISOBUMAL.
See: Butalbital, U.S.P. XXII.

ALKALOL. (Alkalol Co.) Thymol, eucalyptol, menthol, camphor, benzoin, potassium alum, potassium chlorate, sodium bicarbonate, sodium Cl, sweet birch oil, spearmint oil, pine and cassia oil, alcohol 0.05%. Bot. pt. Nasal douche cup pkg. 1s.
Use: Eyes, nose, throat and all inflamed mucous membranes.

ALKA-MED LIQUID. (Blue Cross) Aluminum hydroxide 200 mg, magnesium hydroxide 200 mg/ 5 ml. Bot. 8 oz.
Use: Antacid.

ALKA-MED TABLETS. (Blue Cross) Magnesium hydroxide, aluminum hydroxide. Bot. 60s.
Use: Antacid.

ALKA-MINTS. (Miles) Calcium carbonate 850 mg/Chew. tab. Carton 30s, 60s.
Use: Antacid.

ALKA-SELTZER. (Miles) Heat treated sodium bicarbonate 1916 mg, citric acid 1000 mg, acetylsalicylic acid 324 mg/Tab. Bot. 8s, 26s; foil pack 12s, 36s, 72s, 100s.
Use: Effervescent antacid, analgesic.

ALKA-SELTZER, ADVANCED FORMULA. (Miles) Heat treated sodium bicarbonate 465 mg, citric acid 900 mg, acetaminophen 325 mg, potassium bicarbonate 300 mg, calcium carbonate 280 mg/Tab. Foil pack 36s.
Use: Effervescent antacid, analgesic.

ALKA-SELTZER, EXTRA STRENGTH. (Miles) Aspirin 500 mg, sodium bicarbonate 1985 mg, citric acid 1000 mg, sodium 588 mg/Tab. Foil pack 12s.
Use: Effervescent antacid, analgesic.

ALKA-SELTZER FLAVORED EFFERVESCENT ANTACID-ANALGESIC. (Miles) Aspirin 324 mg, heat treated sodium bicarbonate 1710 mg, citric acid 1220 mg, sodium 506 mg/Tab. Foil pack 12s, 24s, 36s.
Use: Effervescent antacid, analgesic.

ALKA-SELTZER PLUS. (Miles) Chlorpheniramine maleate 2 mg, phenylpropanolamine bitartrate 24 mg, aspirin 324 mg, sodium 506 mg/Tab. Foil pack 20s, 36s.
Use: Antihistamine, decongestant, analgesic.

ALKA-SELTZER PLUS NIGHT-TIME COLD TABLETS. (Miles) Phenylpropanolamine bitartrate 24 mg, diphenhydramine citrate 38 mg, aspirin 324 mg, sodium 506 mg. Tab. 20s, 36s.
Use: Decongestant, antihistamine, analgesic.

ALKA-SELTZER SPECIAL EFFERVESCENT ANTACID. (Miles) Heat treated sodium bicarbonate 958 mg, citric acid 832 mg, potassium bicarbonate 312 mg, sodium 284 mg/Tab. Foil pack 12s, 20s, 36s.
Use: Effervescent antacid.

ALKERAN. (Burroughs Wellcome) Melphalan 2 mg/Tab. Bot. 50s.
Use: Antineoplastic agent.

ALKETS. (Upjohn) Calcium carbonate 780 mg, magnesium carbonate 130 mg, magnesium oxide 65 mg/Tab. Bot. 100s.
Use: Antacid.

ALKYLBENZYLDIMETHYLAMMONIUM CHLORIDE. Benzalkonium Cl, N.F. XVII.
W/Methylrosaniline Cl, polyoxyethylenenonylphenol, polyethylene glycol tert-dodecylthioether.
See: Hyva, Tab. (Holland-Rantos).

ALLANTOIN. USAN.
Use: Emollient.
See: Cutemol, (Summers).
W/Aminacrine, sulfanilamide.
See: Par Cream (Parmed).
Vagidine, Cream (Elder).
Vagitrol, Cream (Syntex).
W/Balsam, Lano-sil, silicone.
See: Balmex Med. Lot. (Macsil).
W/Camphor, menthol, tincture benzoin.
See: Siltex, Oint. (E. J. Moore).
W/p-Chloro-m-xylenol.
See: Cebum, Shampoo (Dermik).
W/Coal tar extract, hexachlorophene, glycerin, lanolin.
See: Pso-Rite, Cream (DePree).
W/Coal tar in cream base.
See: Tegrin Cream (Block Drug).
W/Coal tar solution, isopropyl myristate, psorilan.
See: Psorelief, Soln. (Quality Generics).
W/Dienestrol, sulfanilamide, aminacrine HCl.
See: AVC/Dienestrol Cream, Supp. (Merrell Dow).
W/Hydrocortisone.
See: Tarcortin, Cream (Reed & Carnrick).
W/Nitrofurazone.
See: Eldezol, Oint. (Elder).
W/Pramoxine HCl, benzalkonium Cl.
See: Perifoam, Aerosol (Rowell Labs.).
W/Resorcinol, hexachlorophene, menthol.
See: Tackle, Gel. (Colgate-Palmolive).
W/Salicylic acid, sulfur.
See: Neutrogena Disposables (Neutrogena).
W/Sulfanilamide, 9-aminoacridine HCl.
Nil Vaginal Cream (Century).
Vagisan, Creme (Sandia).
Vagisul, Creme (Sheryl).
W/Sulfisoxazole, Aminoacridine.
Use: Topically, aid in the promotion of granulation.
See: Vagilia, Cream, Supp. (Lemmon).
W/Tarbonis.
See: Sebical, Shampoo (Carnrick & Reed).
W/Vitamins A, D.
See: A-D Dressing (LaCrosse).

ALLAY. (LuChem) Acetaminophen 650 mg, hydrocodone bitartrate 7.5 mg/Cap. Bot. 100s.
Use: Narcotic analgesic combination.

ALLBEE C-800. (Robins) Vitamins E 45 IU, C 800 mg, B_1 15 mg, B_2 17 mg, niacin 100 mg, B_6 25 mg, B_{12} 12 mcg, pantothenic acid 25 mg/Tab. Bot. 60s.
Use: Vitamin supplement.

ALLBEE C-800 PLUS IRON. (Robins) Vitamins E 45 IU, C 800 mg, B_1 15 mg, B_2 17 mg, niacin 100 mg, B_6 25 mg, B_{12} 12 mcg, pantothenic acid 25 mg, iron 27 mg, folic acid 0.4 mg/Tab. Bot. 60s.
Use: Vitamin/mineral supplement.

ALLBEE W/VITAMIN C. (Robins) Vitamins B_1 15 mg, B_6 5 mg, B_2 10.2 mg, niacin 50 mg, pantothenic acid 10 mg, C 300 mg/Cap. Bot. 30s, 100s, 1000s. Dis-co pack 10x100s.
Use: Vitamin supplement.

ALLBEE-T. (Robins) Vitamins B_1 15.5 mg, B_2 10 mg, B_6 8.2 mg, pantothenic acid 23 mg, niacin 100 mg, C 500 mg, B_{12} 5 mcg/Tab. Bot. 100s, 500s.
Use: Vitamin supplement.

ALLBEX. (Approved) Vitamins B_1 5 mg, B_2 2 mg, B_6 0.25 mg, calcium pantothenate 3 mg, niacinamide 20 mg, ferrous sulfate 194.4 mg, inositol 10 mg, choline 10 mg, B_{12} (concentrate) 3 mcg/Cap. Bot. 100s, 1000s.
Use: Vitamin/mineral supplement.

ALL-DAY B-COMPLEX. (Barth's) Vitamins B_{12} 25 mcg, B_1 7 mg, B_2 14 mg, niacin 4.67 mg, B_6, pantothenic acid, folic acid, choline, aminobenzoic acid, inositol, biotin, Mg, Mn, Cu/Cap. Bot. 30s, 90s, 180s, 360s.
Use: Vitamin/mineral supplement.

ALL-DAY-C. (Barth's) Vitamin C 200 mg/Cap. or 500 mg/Tab. with rose hip extract. Bot. 30s, 90s, 180s, 360s.
Use: Vitamin supplement.

ALL-DAY IRON YEAST. (Barth's) Iron 20 mg, Vitamins B_1 2 mg, B_2 4 mg, niacin 0.57 mg/Cap. Bot. 30s, 90s, 180s.
Use: Vitamin/mineral supplement.

ALL-DAY-VITES. (Barth's) Vitamins A 10,000 IU, D 400 IU, B_1 3 mg, B_2 6 mg, niacin 1 mg, C 120 mg, B_{12} 10 mcg, E 30 IU/Cap. Bot. 30s, 90s, 180s, 360s.
Use: Vitamin supplement.

ALLEGRON. Nortriptyline.
Use: Antidepressant.

ALLENT. (Ascher) Pseudoephedrine HCl 120 mg, brompheniramine maleate 12 mg. Slow-release cap. Bot. 100s.
Use: Decongestant, antihistamine.

ALLERBEN INJECTION. (Forest) Diphenhydramine 10 mg/ml. Vial 30 ml.
Use: Antihistamine.

ALLERCHLOR INJECTION. (Forest) Chlorpheniramine maleate 10 mg/ml. Vial 30 ml.
Use: Antihistamine.

ALLER-CHLOR. (Rugby) Chlorpheniramine maleate. **Tab.:** 4 mg. Bot. 24s, 100s, 1000s. **Syr.:** 2 mg/5 ml. Bot. 4 oz, pt, gal.
Use: Antihistamine.

ALLERCREME SKIN. (Owen/Galderma) Mineral oil, petrolatum, lanolin, lanolin oil, lanolin alcohols, glycerin, triethanolamine, cetyl alcohol, stearic acid, parabens. Lot. Bot. 240 ml.
Use: Emollient.

ALLERCREME ULTRA EMOLLIENT. (Owen/Galderma) Mineral oil, petrolatum, lanolin, lanolin alcohol, lanolin oil, glycerin, glyceryl stearate, PEG-100 stearate, squalane, cetyl alcohol, sorbitan laurate, quaternium-15, parabens. Cream Bot. 60 Gm.
Use: Emollient.

ALLERDEC CAPSULES. (Towne) Phenylpropanolamine HCl 25 mg, chlorpheniramine maleate 1 mg, pyrilamine maleate 5 mg/Cap. Bot. 25s, 50s.
Use: Decongestant, antihistamine.

ALLEREST. (Pharmacraft) **Tab.:** Phenylpropanolamine HCl 18.7 mg, chlorpheniramine maleate 2 mg/Tab. Sleeve Pack 24s, 48s. Bot. 72s. **Chew. Tab. for Children:** Phenylpropanolamine HCl 9.4 mg, chlorpheniramine maleate 1 mg/Tab. Sleeve Pack 24s. **Eye Drops:** Naphazoline HCl 0.012%, benzalkonium Cl 0.01%, disodium edetate 0.1% w/boric acid, sodium borate. Bot. 0.5 oz. **Headache Strength Tab.:** Acetaminophen 325 mg, phenylpropanolamine HCl 18.7 mg, chlorpheniramine maleate 2 mg/Tab. Sleeve Pack 24s. **Nasal Spray:** Oxymetazoline HCl 0.05%. Bot. 0.5 oz.
Use: Decongestant, antihistamine; analgesic (Headache strength Tab only).

ALLEREST 12-HOUR CAPLETS. (Pharmacraft) Phenylpropanolamine HCl 75 mg, chlorpheniramine maleate 12 mg/Capl. Pkg. 10s.
Use: Decongestant, antihistamine.

ALLEREST 12-HOUR CAPSULES. (Pharmacraft) Phenylpropanolamine HCl 75 mg, chlorpheniramine maleate 8 mg/Cap. Sleeve pak 10s.
Use: Decongestant, antihistamine.

ALLEREST NO DROWSINESS. (Pharmacraft) Pseudoephedrine 30 mg, acetaminophen 325 mg/Tab. Bot. 20s.
Use: Decongestant, analgesic.

ALLEREST SINUS PAIN FORMULA. (Pharmacraft) Acetaminophen 500 mg, phenylpropanolamine HCl 18.7 mg, chlorpheniramine maleate 2 mg/Tab. Sleeve pack 20s.
Use: Analgesic, decongestant, antihistamine.

ALLERFRIN. (Rugby) **Tab.:** Pseudoephedrine HCl 60 mg, triprolidine HCl 2.5 mg. Bot. 24s, 100s, 1000s. **Syr.:** Pseudoephedrine HCl 30 mg, triprolidine HCl 1.25 mg. Bot. 120 ml, pt.
Use: Decongestant, antihistamine.

ALLERFRIN W/CODEINE. (Rugby) Pseudoephedrine HCl 30 mg, triprolidine HCl 1.25 mg, codeine phosphate 10 mg, alcohol 4.3%. Syr. Bot. 120 ml, pt, gal.
Use: Decongestant, antihistamine, antitussive.

ALLERGAN ENZYMATIC. (Allergan) Papain, sodium Cl, sodium carbonate, sodium borate, edetate disodium. Kits 12s, 48s.
Use: Soft contact lens care.

ALLERGAN HYDROCARE CLEANING & DISINFECTING SOLUTION. (Allergan) tris(2-hydroxyethyl)tallow ammonium Cl 0.013%, thimerosal 0.002%, bis(2-hydroxyethyl)tallow ammonium Cl, sodium bicarbonate, dibasic, monobasic and anhydrous sodium phosphate, hydrochloric acid, propylene glycol, polysorbate 80, special soluble polyhema. Bot. 4 oz, 8 oz, 12 oz.
Use: Soft contact lens care.

ALLERGAN HYDROCARE PRESERVED SALINE SOLUTION. (Allergan) Sodium Cl, sodium hexametaphosphate, sodium hydroxide, boric acid, sodium borate, EDTA 0.01%, thimerosal 0.001%. Bot. 8 oz, 12 oz.
Use: Soft contact lens care.

ALLERGAN SORBI-CARE SALINE SOLUTION. (Allergan) Saline solution. Bot. 8 oz.
Use: Soft contact lens care.

ALLERGEN EAR DROPS. (Goldline) Benzocaine 1.4%, antipyrine 5.4%, glycerin, oxyquinoline sulfate. Bot. 0.5 oz.
Use: Otic preparation.

ALLERGENIC EXTRACTS}. (Center) Allergenic extracts of pollen, mold, house dust, inhalants, epidermals, insects in saline 0.9% and phenol 0.4% up to 1:10 w/v or 40,000 PNU/ml in sets or vials up to 30 ml.
Use: Diagnosis of specific allergies, relief of allergic symptoms.

ALLERGENIC EXTRACTS. (Hollister-Stier) Allergenic extracts of pollens, foods, inhalants, epidermals, fungi, insects, miscellaneous antigens.
Use: Diagnosis of specific allergies, relief of allergic symptoms.

ALLERGEX. (Hollister-Stier) Silicones, polyethylene and triethylene glycol, antioxidants, mineral oil concentrate. Bot. pt. Aerosol pt.
Use: Control of house dust allergens.

ALLERGY DROPS. (Bausch & Lomb) Naphazoline HCl 0.012%, PEG 300 0.2%. Bot. 0.5 oz.
Use: Mydriatic/vasoconstrictor, ophthalmic.

ALLERGY PREPARATIONS.
See: Antihistamine Preparations.

ALLERGY RELIEF MEDICINE.
Use: Decongestant, antihistamine.

See: A.R.M. Caplets (SmithKline Prods).

ALLERGY TABLETS. (Weeks & Leo) Phenylpropanolamine HCl 37.5 mg, chlorpheniramine 4 mg/Tab. Bot. 30s.
Use: Decongestant, antihistamine.

ALLERID. (Murdock) Pseudoephedrine HCl 60 mg/Cap. Bot. 30s.
Use: Decongestant.

ALLERMAX. (Pfeiffer) Diphenhydramine HCl 50 mg/Cap. 20s.
Use: Antihistamine.

ALLERSONE. (Mallard) Hydrocortisone 0.5%, diperodon HCl 0.5%, zinc oxide 5%, sodium lauryl sulfate, propylene glycol, cetyl alcohol, petrolatum, methyl and propyl parabens. Oint. Tube 15 Gm.
Use: Corticosteroid, topical.

ALLERSULE FORTE. (Misemer) Phenylephrine HCl 20 mg, chlorpheniramine maleate 8 mg, methscopolamine nitrate 2.5 mg/Cap. Bot. 100s.
Use: Decongestant, antihistamine, anticholinergic.

ALLETORPHINE. B.A.N. N-Allyl-7,8-dihydro-7α-(1(R)-hydroxy-1-methylbutyl)-0^6-methyl-6,14-endoethenonormorphine. N-Allylnoretorphine.
Use: Analgesic.

ALL-NITE COLD FORMULA. (Major) Pseudoephedrine HCl 10 mg, doxylamine succinate 1.25 mg, dextromethorphan HBr 5 mg, acetaminophen 167 mg/5 ml. Liq. Bot. 177 ml.
Use: Decongestant, antihistamine, antitussive, analgesic.

•**ALLOBARBITAL.** USAN. 5,5-Diallylbarbituric acid.
Use: Hypnotic.
W/Acetaminophen, salicylamide, caffeine.
See: Allylvon, Cap. (Elder).
W/Aspirin, acetaminophen, aluminum aspirin.
See: Allylgesic, Tab. (Elder).
W/Ergotamine tartrate.
See: Allylgesic w/Ergotamine, Cap. (Elder).

ALLOBARBITONE.
See: Diallylbarbituric Acid (Various Mfr.).

ALLOMETHADIONE. (I.N.N.) Aloxidone. B.A.N.

•**ALLOPURINOL,** U.S.P. XXII. Tablets, U.S.P. XXII. 1 H-Pyrazolo-[3, 4-d] pyrimidin-4-ol.
Use: Antigout, xanthine oxidase inhibitor.
See: Lopurin, Tab. (Boots Pharm).
Zyloprim, Tab. (Burroughs Wellcome).

ALLPYRAL. (Miles Pharm) Allergenic extracts, alum-precipitated. For subcutaneous inj. pollens, molds, epithelia, house dust, other inhalants, stinging insects.
Use: Diagnosis of specific allergies, relief of allergic symptoms.

ALLYLBARBITURIC ACID. Allylisobutyl-barbituric acid, butalbital. Tab. (Various Mfr.).
Use: Sedative.
W/A.P.C.
See: Anti-Ten, Tab. (Century).
Fiorinal, Cap., Tab. (Sandoz).
Salipral, Tab. (Kenyon).
Tenstan (Standex).
W/Acetaminophen, homatropine methylbromide.
See: Panitol H.M.B., Tab. (Wesley).
W/Acetaminophen, salicylamide, caffeine.
See: Renpap, Tab. (Wren).

ALLYLESTRENOL. 17a-Allyl-17b-hydroxy-4-estrene.

ALLYL-ISOBUTYLBARBITURIC ACID.
See: Allyl Barbituric Acid.

ALLYLISOPROPYLMALONYLUREA.
See: Aprobarbital.

ALLYL ISOTHIOCYANATE, Oil of mustard. (Various Mfr.).
Use: Counterirritant in neuralgia.

4-ALLYL-2-METHOXYPHENOL. Eugenol, U.S.P. XXII.

N-ALLYLNOROXYMORPHONE HCl. Naloxone Hydrochloride, U.S.P. XXII.

ALLYLOESTRENOL. B.A.N. 17α-Allyloestr-4-en-17β-ol. Gestanin.
Use: Progestational steroid.

ALLYLPRODINE. B.A.N. 3-Allyl-1-methyl-4-phenyl-4-propionyloxypiperidine.
Use: Analgesic.

5-ALLYL-SEC-BUTYLBARBITURIC ACID.
See: Talbutal.

ALMACONE. (Rugby) **Chew tab.:** Aluminum hydroxide 200 mg, magnesium hydroxide 200 mg, simethicone 20 mg/Bot. 100s, 1000s. **Liq.:** Aluminum hydroxide 200 mg, magnesium hydroxide 200 mg, simethicone 20 mg, sodium 0.75 mg/5 ml. Bot. 360 ml, gal.
Use: Antacid.

ALMACONE 2. (Rugby) Aluminum hydroxide 400 mg, magnesium hydroxide 400 mg, simethicone 30 mg, sodium 1.5 mg/5 ml. Bot. 360 ml, gal.
Use: Antacid.

•**ALMADRATE SULFATE.** USAN. Aluminum magnesium hydroxide-oxide-sulfate-hydrate.
Use: Antacid.

•**ALMAGATE.** USAN.
Use: Antacid.

ALMAGUCIN. Gastric mucin, dried aluminum hydroxide gel, magnesium trisilicate.
Use: Antacid.

ALMA-MAG #4 IMPROVED. (Rugby) Aluminum hydroxide 200 mg, magnesium hydroxide 200 mg, simethicone 25 mg/Chew. tab. Bot. 100s, 1000s.
Use: Antacid.

ALMA-MAG LIQUID IMPROVED. (Rugby) Aluminum hydroxide 200 mg, magnesium hydroxide 200 mg, simethicone 25 mg/5 ml. Bot. 360 ml.
Use: Antacid.

ALMATRI. (Robinson) Aluminum hydroxide gel 4 gr, magnesium trisilicate 7.5 gr/Tab. Bot. 100s, 1000s, Bulk pack 5000s.
Use: Antacid.

ALMEBEX PLUS B12. (Dayton) Vitamins B_1 1 mg, B_2 2 mg, B_3 5 mg, B_6 0.4 mg, B_{12} 5 mcg,

choline 33 mg/5 ml, alcohol 5%. Pt. (with B_{12} in separate container).
Use: Vitamin supplement.

•**ALMOND OIL,** N.F. XVII.
Use: Pharmaceutical aid (emollient and perfume).

ALMORA. (Forest) Magnesium gluconate 0.5 Gm/Tab. Pkg. 100s.
Use: Mineral supplement.

ALNYTE. (Mayer) Scopolamine aminoxide HBr 0.2 mg, salicylamide 250 mg/Tab. Pkg. 16s.
Use: Anticholinergic, analgesic.

ALOCASS LAXATIVE. (Western Research) Aloin 0.25 gr, cascara sagrada 0.5 gr, rhubarb 0.5 gr, ginger 1/32 gr, powdered extract of belladonna 1/20 gr/Tab. Bot. 1000s. Pak 28s.
Use: Laxative.

ALODOPA-15 TABLETS. (Major) Hydrochlorothiazide 15 mg, methyldopa 250 mg. Bot. 100s.
Use: Antihypertensive.

ALODOPA-25 TABLETS. (Major) Hydrochlorothiazide 25 mg, methyldopa 250 mg. Bot. 100s.
Use: Antihypertensive.

•**ALOE,** U.S.P. XXII.
Use: See Compound Benzoin Tincture.

ALOE GRANDE CREME. (Gordon) Aloe, vitamins E 1500 IU, A 100,000 units/oz in cream base. Jar 2.5 oz.
Use: Emollient.

ALOE VERA ACTIVE PRINCIPLE.
See: Alvagel, Oint. (Kenyon).

ALOE VESTA. (Vestal Labs) Solution of sodium C14-16 olefin sulfonate, amphoteric 2, propylene glycol, aloe vera gel, TEA-COCO hydrolyzed protein with sorbitol, DMDM hydantoin, cetethyl morpholinium ethosulfate, citric acid. Bot. 120 ml, 240 ml, gal.
Use: Perianal hygiene.

•**ALOFILCON A.** USAN.
Use: Contact lens material.

ALOIN. (Baker, J.T.) A mixture of crystalline pentosides from various aloes. Bot. oz.
Use: Laxative.

W/Ox bile (desiccated), phenolphthalein, cascara sagrada extract, podophyllin.
See: Bilgon (Reid-Rowell).

•**ALONIMID.** USAN.
Use: Sedative.

ALOPHEN PILLS. (Warner-Lambert Consumer) Phenolphthalein 60 mg/Tab. Bot. 100s.
Use: Laxative.

ALOTONE. (Major) Triamcinolone 4 mg/Tab. Bot. 100s.
Use: Corticosteroid.

ALOXIDONE. B.A.N. 3-Allyl-5-methyloxazolidine-2,4-dione. Allomethadione (I.N.N.) Malidone.
Use: Anticonvulsant.

ALOXIPRIN. B.A.N. Polymeric condensation product of aluminum oxide and O-acetylsalicylic acid. Palaprin.
Use: Antirheumatic.

•**ALPERTINE.** USAN.
Use: Antipsychotic.

•**ALPHA AMYLASE.** USAN. A concentrated form of alpha amylase produced by a strain of nonpathogenic bacteria.
Use: Digestive aid.
See: Kutrase, Cap. (Kremers-Urban).
Ku-Zyme, Cap. (Kremers-Urban).

ALPHA-AMYLASE W-100. W/Proteinase W-300, cellase W-100, lipase, estrone, testosterone, vitamins, minerals.
Use: Digestive aid.
See: Geramine, Tab. (Brown).

ALPHA-BEL. (Moore Kirk) Phenobarbital 50 mg, hyoscyamine sulfate 0.3 mg, hyoscine HBr 0.02 mg, atropine sulfate 0.06 mg/T.D. Cap. Bot. 100s, 1000s.
Use: Sedative/hypnotic, anticholinergic/antispasmodic.

$ALPHA_{1}$-ADRENERGIC BLOCKERS.
Use: Antihypertensive.
See: Cardura (Roerig).

ALPHACETYLMETHADOL. B.A.N. α-4-Dimethylamino-1-ethyl-2,2-diphenylpentyl acetate.
Use: Analgesic.

ALPHA-CHYMOTRYPSIN.
See: Alpha Chymar, Vial (Armour).
Zolyse, Vial (Alcon).

ALPHADERM. (Lemmon) Hydrocortisone 1%. Cream 30 Gm, 100 Gm.
Use: Corticosteroid, topical.

ALPHADOLONE. B.A.N. 3α,21-Dihydroxy-5α-pregnane-11,20-dione.
Use: Anesthetic component.

ALPHA-E. (Barth's) d-Alpha tocopherol. **50 IU or 100 IU:** Cap. Bot. 100s, 500s, 1000s. **200 IU:** Cap. Bot. 100s, 250s. **400 IU:** Cap. Bot. 100s, 250s, 500s.
Use: Vitamin E Supplement.

ALPHA-ESTRADIOL. Known to be beta-estradiol.
See: Estradiol (Various Mfr.).

ALPHA-ESTRADIOL BENZOATE.
See: Estradiol benzoate (Various Mfr.).

ALPHA FAST. (Eastwood) Bath oil. Bot. 16 oz.
Use: Emollient.

ALPHA-HYPOPHAMINE.
See: Oxytocin Inj.

ALPHA INTERFERON-2A.
See: Roferon-A (Roche).

ALPHA INTERFERON-2B.
See: Intron A (Schering).

ALPHA-KERI. (Westwood) **Therapeutic Bath:** Mineral oil, lanolin oil, PEG-4-dilaurate, benzophenone-3, D & C green #6, fragrance. Bot. 4 oz, 8 oz, 16 oz. **Spray:** 5 oz. **Cleansing Bar:** Bar containing sodium tallowate, sodium cocoate, water, mineral oil, fragrance, PEG-75, glycerin, titanium dioxide, lanolin oil, sodium Cl, BHT, EDTA, D & C green #5, D & C yellow # 10.
Use: Emollient.

ALPHAMEPRODINE. B.A.N. α-3-Ethyl-1-methyl-4-propionyloxypiperidine.
Use: Analgesic.

ALPHAMETHADOL. B.A.N. α-6-Dimethyl-amino-4,4-diphenylheptan-3-ol.
Use: Analgesic.

ALPHA-METHYLDOPA. Name previously used for Methyldopa.

ALPHAMUL. (Lannett) Castor oil 60% w/v, emulsifying agent. Bot. 3 fl oz, gal.
Use: Laxative.

ALPHA-PHENOXYETHYL PENICILLIN, POTASSIUM.
See: Phenethicillin Potassium.

ALPHAPRODINE. B.A.N. U.S.P. XXI. α-1,3-Dimethyl-4-phenyl-4-propionyloxypiperidine.
Use: Analgesic.

ALPHA-1-PROTEINASE INHIBITOR.
Use: Treatment of Alpha-1-antitrypsin deficiency.
See: Prolastin (Cutter).

ALPHASONE ACETOPHENIDE. Name previously used for Algestone acetonide.

ALPHA-TOCOPHEROL.
See: Dalfatol, Cap. (Reid-Rowell).
Tocopherol, Alpha (Various Mfr.).

dl-ALPHA-TOCOPHEROL SUCCINATE.
See: D'Alpha-E, Cap. (Alto).

ALPHATREX. (Savage) **Cream and Oint.:** Betamethasone dipropionate 0.05%. Tube 15 Gm, 45 Gm. **Lot.:** Betamethasone dipropionate 0.05%. Bot. 60 ml.
Use: Corticosteroid, topical.

ALPHA VEE-12. (Schlicksup) Hydroxocobalamin 1000 mcg/ml. Vial 10 ml.
Use: Vitamin B_{12} supplement.

ALPHAXALONE. B.A.N. 3α-Hydroxy-5α-pregnane-11,20-dione.
Use: Anesthetic component.

ALPHOSYL. (Reed & Carnrick) Allantoin 1.7%, special crude coal tar extracts 5%. **Lot.:** Bot. 8 fl oz. **Cream:** 2 oz.
Use: Antipruritic.

ALPIDEM. USAN.
Use: Antianxiety agent (anxiolytic).

ALPRAZOLAM, U.S.P. XXII. Tab., U.S.P. XXII. 8-Chloro-1-methyl-6-phenyl-4H-s- triazolo (4,3-a)(1,4)benzodiazepine.
Use: Management of anxiety disorders.
See: Xanax, Tab. (Upjohn).

ALPRENOLOL. B.A.N. 1-(2-Allylphenoxy)-3-isopropylaminopropan-2 ol. Betaptin hydrochloride.
Use: Beta-adrenergic receptor blocking agent.

ALPRENOLOL HYDROCHLORIDE. USAN.
Use: Anti-adrenergic.

ALPRENOXIME HYDROCHLORIDE. USAN.
Use: Antiglaucoma agent.

ALPROSTADIL, U.S.P. XXII. Inj., U.S.P. XXII. (11α, 13E,15S)-11,15 dihydroxy-9-oxoprost-13-en-1-oic acid.
Use: Palliative therapy to maintain patency of the ductus arteriosus in neonates with congenital heart defects.
See: Prostin VR, Inj. (Upjohn).

AL-R. (Saron) Chlorpheniramine maleate 6 mg or 12 mg/S.R. Cap. Bot. 100s.
Use: Antihistamine.

ALRAMUCIL. (Alra) Psyllium.
Use: Laxative.

•**ALRESTATIN SODIUM.** USAN.
Use: Enzyme inhibitor.

ALSEROXYLON-ALKAVERVIR. A mixture of partially purified extracts of Rauwolfia serpentina and Veratrum viride.

ALSORB GEL. (Standex) Magnesium and aluminum hydroxide. Colloidal Susp.
Use: Antacid.

ALSORB GEL, C.T. (Standex) Calcium carbonate 2 gr, glycine 3 gr, magnesium trisilicate 3 gr/Tab.
Use: Antacid.

ALTACE. (Hoechst-Roussel) Ramipril.
Use: Antihypertensive.

•**ALTANSERIN TARTRATE.** USAN.
Use: Serotonin antagonist.

ALTEPLASE, RECOMBINANT. Tissue plasminogen activator; tPA.
Use: Thrombolytic.
See: Activase.

ALTERNAGEL. (Stuart) Aluminum hydroxide 600 mg, sodium $>$ 2.5 mg/5 ml. Bot. 1 oz, 5 oz, 12 oz.
Use: Antacid.

ALTEX. (Cenci) Spironolactone 25 mg/Tab. Bot. 100s, 1000s.
Use: Diuretic, antihypertensive.

ALTEXIDE. (Cenci) Spironolactone 25 mg, hydrochlorothiazide 25 mg/Tab. Bot. 100s, 1000s.
Use: Diuretic, antihypertensive.

ALTHIAZIDE. USAN. 3-Allylthiomethyl-3-4-dihydro-6-chloro-7-sulfamoyl-1,2,4-benzothiadiazine-1-dioxide.
Use: Hypotensive, diuretic.

•**ALTRENOGEST.** USAN.
Use: Progestin (veterinary).

•**ALTRETAMINE.** USAN.
Use: Antineoplastic.
See: Hexalen (US Bioscience).

ALU-CAP. (Riker) Aluminum hydroxide dried gel 475 mg, silicon dioxide, talc/Cap. Bot. 100s.
Use: Antacid.

AL-U-CREME. (MacAllister) Aluminum hydroxide equivalent to 4% aluminum oxide. Susp. Bot. pt, gal.
Use: Antacid.

ALUDROX. (Wyeth-Ayerst) Aluminum hydroxide gel 307 mg, magnesium hydroxide 103 mg/5 ml. Susp. Bot. 12 fl oz, Box 12s.
Use: Antacid.

ALUKALIN. Activated kaolin.
Use: Antidiarrheal.
See: Lusyn, Tab. (Pennwalt).

ALULEX. (Lexington) Magnesium trisilicate 3.25 gr, aluminum hydroxide gel 3.5 gr, phenobarbital 1/8 gr, homatropine methylbromide 1/60 gr/Tab. Bot. 100s.
Use: Agent for peptic ulcer.

•**ALUM,** U.S.P. XXII. Sulfuric acid, aluminum ammonium salt (2:1:1), dodecahydrate. Sulfuric acid, aluminum potassium salt (2:1:1), dodecahydrate.
Use: Astringent.

•**ALUM, AMMONIUM,** U.S.P. XXII.
Use: Astringent.

•**ALUM, POTASSIUM,** U.S.P. XXII.
Use: Astringent.

ALUMADRINE. (Fleming) Acetaminophen 500 mg, phenylpropanolamine HCl 25 mg, chlorpheniramine maleate 4 mg/Tab. Bot. 100s, 1000s.
Use: Analgesic, decongestant, antihistamine.

ALUMATE-HC. (Dermco) Hydrocortisone 1/8%, 0.25%, 0.5% or 1%. Cream 1/8% Pkg. 4 oz. 0.25% Pkg. 1 oz. 0.5% Pkg. 0.5 oz, 1 oz. 1% Pkg. 0.5 oz.
Use: Corticosteroid, topical.

ALUMATE MIXTURE. (Schlicksup) Aluminum hydroxide gel, milk of magnesia/5 ml. Bot. 12 oz, gal.
Use: Antacid.

ALUMID PLUS LIQUID. (Vangard) Aluminum hydroxide 200 mg, magnesium hydroxide 200 mg, simethicone 20 mg, sodium 0.75 mg/5 ml. Bot. 12 oz, gal.
Use: Antacid, antiflatulent.

ALUMINA HYDRATED POWDER.
W/Activated attapulgite, pectin.
Use: Antidiarrheal.
See: Polymagma, Plain, Tab. (Wyeth-Ayerst).

•**ALUMINA, MAGNESIA, AND CALCIUM CARBONATE TABLETS,** U.S.P. XXII.
Use: Antacid.

•**ALUMINA, MAGNESIA, CALCIUM CARBONATE, AND SIMETHICONE TABLETS,** U.S.P. XXII.

•**ALUMINA, MAGNESIA, AND CALCIUM CHLORIDE ORAL SUSPENSION,** U.S.P. XXII.
Use: Antacid.

•**ALUMINA AND MAGNESIA ORAL SUSPENSION,** U.S.P. XXII.
Use: Antacid.

•**ALUMINA AND MAGNESIA TABLETS,** U.S.P. XXII.
Use: Antacid.

•**ALUMINA, MAGNESIA AND SIMETHICONE,** U.S.P. XXII, Susp., Tab., U.S.P. XXII.
Use: Antacid, antiflatulent.

•**ALUMINA AND MAGNESIUM CARBONATE ORAL SUSPENSION,** U.S.P. XXII.
Use: Antacid.

•**ALUMINA, MAGNESIUM CARBONATE, AND MAGNESIUM OXIDE TABLETS,** U.S.P. XXII.
Use: Antacid.

•**ALUMINA AND MAGNESIUM TRISILICATE ORAL SUSPENSION,** U.S.P. XXII.
Use: Antacid.

•**ALUMINA AND MAGNESIUM TRISILICATE TABLETS,** U.S.P. XXII.
Use: Antacid.

ALUMINETT. (Lannett) Aluminum hydroxide 10 gr/Tab. Bot. 1000s.
Use: Antacid.

ALUMINOSTOMY. (Richards Pharm.) Aluminum pow. 18%, zinc oxide, zinc stearate in a bland water repellent ointment. Jar 2 oz, 6 oz, lb.
Use: Skin protectant.

ALUMINUM.
See: Aluminostomy (Richards Pharm.).

ALUMINUM ACETATE.
Use: Astringent.
See: Acid Mantle Creme (Sandoz Consumer).
Buro-Sol pow. (Doak).
W/Phenol, zinc oxide, boric acid, eucalyptol, ichthammol.
See: Lanaburn, Oint. (Lannett).
W/Salicylic acid, boric acid.

•**ALUMINUM ACETATE TOPICAL SOLUTION,** U.S.P. XXII. (Various Mfr.). Burow's Solution.
Use: Astringent.
See: Bluboro Powder (Herbert).
Buro-Sol Powder Conc. (Doak).
Burotor, Emul. (Torch).
Domeboro, Pow. (Miles Pharm).

ALUMINUM AMINOACETATE, DIHYDROXY.
See: Dihydroxy aluminum aminoacetate (Various Mfr.).

ALUMINUM CARBONATE BASIC.
Use: Antacid.
See: Basaljel, Susp. (Wyeth-Ayerst).

•**ALUMINUM CARBONATE, DRIED BASIC, GEL,** U.S.P. XXII, Cap., Tab., U.S.P. XXII.
Use: Antacid.

•**ALUMINUM CARBONATE GEL, BASIC,** U.S.P. XXII.
Use: Antacid.
See: Basaljel, Susp. (Wyeth-Ayerst).

ALUMINUM CHLORHYDROXY ALLANTOINATE.
See: Alcloxa (Schuylkill).

•**ALUMINUM CHLORIDE,** U.S.P. XXII. Aluminum Cl hexahydrate.
Use: Astringent.
W/Oxyquinoline sulfate, benzalkonium Cl.
See: Alochor Stypic (Gordon Labs.).

ALUMINUM CHLORIDE HEXAHYDRATE.
Use: Astringent.
See: Drysol (Person & Covey).

•**ALUMINUM CHLOROHYDRATE.** USAN.
Use: Anhidrotic.

•**ALUMINUM CHLOROHYDREX.** USAN.
Use: Astringent.

ALUMINUM CLOFIBRATE. B.A.N. Di-[2-(4-chlorophenoxy)-2-methylpropionato] hydroxyaluminum.
Use: Treatment of arteriosclerosis.

ALUMINUM DIHYDROXYAMINOACETATE.

See: Dihydroxy Aluminum Aminoacetate, U.S.P. XXII. (Various Mfr.).

ALUMINUM GLYCINATE, BASIC.
See: Dihydroxy Aluminum Aminoacetate, U.S.P. XXII.
W/Aspirin, Magnesium carbonate.
See: Bufferin, Tab. (Bristol-Myers).

ALUMINUM HYDROXIDE GEL, U.S.P. XXII.
Aqueous susp. of aluminum hydroxide equivalent to 4% aluminum oxide.
Use: Antacid.
See: ALterna GEL, Gel (Stuart).
Al-U-Creme, Susp. (MacAllister).
Aluminett, Tab. (Lannett).
Alu-Cap, Cap. (Riker).
Alu-Tab, Tab. (Riker).
Amphojel, Susp., Tab. (Wyeth-Ayerst).
Dialume, Cap. (Armour).
Nutrajel (Cenci).
W/Aminoacetic acid, magnesium trisilicate.
See: Maracid-2, Tab. (Marin).
W/Aminophylline.
See: Asmadrin, Tab. (Jenkins).
W/Belladonna extract, magnesium hydroxide.
See: Trialka, Liq., Tab. (Commerce).
W/Calcium carbonate.
See: Alkalade, Susp., Tab. (DePree).
W/Calcium carbonate, magnesium carbonate, magnesium trisilicate.
See: Marblen, Susp., Tab. (Fleming).
W/Clioquinol, methylcellulose, atropine sulfate, hyoscine HBr, hyoscyamine sulfate.
See: Enterex, Tab. (Person & Covey).
W/Dicyclomine HCl, magnesium hydroxide, methylcellulose.
See: Triactin Liq., Tab. (Norwich).
W/Gastric mucin, magnesium glycinate.
See: Mucogel, Liq., Tab. (Inwood).
W/Kaolin, pectin.
See: Metropectin, Liq. (Pennwalt).
W/Magnesium carbonate.
See: Algicon, Tab. (Rorer Consumer).
Estomul-M Liq., Tab. (Riker).
W/Magnesium carbonate, calcium carbonate, amino-acetic acid.
See: Glycogel Tab., Susp. (Central).
W/Magnesium hydroxide.
See: Alsorb Gel (Standex).
Aludrox, Susp., Tab. (Wyeth-Ayerst).
Delcid, Liq. (Merrell Dow).
Kolantyl, Gel, Wafer (Merrell Dow).
Maalox, Susp. (Rhone-Poulenc Rorer).
Mylanta, Tab. (Stuart).
Mylanta II, Tab. (Stuart).
Neutralox, Susp. (Lemmon).
Nutramag, Liq. (Cenci).
WinGel, Liq., Tab. (Winthrop Consumer Products).
W/Magnesium hydroxide, aspirin.
See: Ascriptin, Tab. (Rhone-Poulenc Rorer).
Ascriptin Extra Strength, Tab. (Rorer Consumer).
Calciphen, Tab. (Westerfield).
Cama, Tab. (Dorsey).
Cama Inlay-Tab. (Sandoz Consumer).
W/Magnesium hydroxide, belladonna extract
W/Magnesium hydroxide, calcium carbonate.
See: Camalox, Susp. (Rhone-Poulenc Rorer).
W/Magnesium hydroxide, glycine, magnesium trisilicate, belladonna extract.
W/Magnesium hydroxide and simethicone.
See: DI-GEL, Liq. (Plough).
Maalox Plus, Susp. (Rhone-Poulenc Rorer).
Mylanta, Liq. (Stuart).
Mylanta-II, Liq. (Stuart).
Silain-Gel, Liq., Tab. (Robins).
Simeco, Liq. (Wyeth-Ayerst).
W/Magnesium trisilicate.
See: Antacid G, Tab. (Walgreen).
Antacid Tablets, Tab. (Panray).
Arcodex Antiacid, Tab. (Arcum).
Gacid, Tab. (Arcum).
Malcogel, Susp. (Upjohn).
Malcotabs (Upjohn).
Manalum, Tab. (Paddock).
Trisogel, Pulv., Susp. (Lilly).
W/Paregoric, kaolin (colloidal), bismuth subcarbonate, pectin, aromatics.
See: Kapinal, Tab. (Jenkins).
W/Phenindamine tartrate, phenylephrine HCl, aspirin, caffeine, magnesium carbonate.
See: Dristan, Tab. (Whitehall).
W/Phenol, zinc oxide, camphor, eucalyptol, ichthammol.
See: Almophen, Oint. (Bowman).
W/Prednisolone.
See: Fernisolone-B (Ferndale).
Predoxine, Tab. (Mallard).
W/Sodium salicylate, acetaminophen, vitamin C.
See: Gaysal-S., Tab. (Geriatric).

•**ALUMINUM HYDROXIDE GEL, DRIED,** U.S.P. XXII. Tab. U.S.P. XXII.
Use: Antacid.
See: Amphojel, Tab. (Wyeth-Ayerst).

•**ALUMINUM HYDROXIDE GEL, DRIED, CAPSULES,** U.S.P. XXII.
Use: Antacid.

ALUMINUM HYDROXIDE GEL, DRIED W/COMBINATIONS.
Use: Antacid.
See: Aludrox, Susp., Tab. (Wyeth-Ayerst).
Alurex, Tab. (Rexall).
Banacid, Tab. (Buffington).
Camalox, Tab. (Rhone-Poulenc Rorer).
Delcid, Liq. (Merrell Dow).
Eulcin, Tab. (Leeds).
Fermalox, Tab. (Rhone-Poulenc Rorer).
Gas-Eze, Tab. (E. J. Moore).
Gaviscon, Foamtab (Marion).
Gelusil, Preps. (Parke-Davis).
Kolantyl, Wafers (Merrell Dow).
Maalox, Tab. (Rhone-Poulenc Rorer).
Maalox Plus, Tab. (Rhone-Poulenc Rorer).
Magnatril, Tab., Susp. (Lannett).

Malcotabs, Tab. (Upjohn).
Mylanta, Tab., Liq. (Stuart).
Mylanta II, Tab., Liq. (Stuart).
Phencaset Improved, Tab. (Elder).
Presalin, Tab. (Mallard).
Silmagel, Tab. (Lannett).
Spasmasorb, Tab. (Hauck).

ALUMINUM HYDROXIDE GLYCINE.
See: Dihydroxy aluminum aminoacetate.

ALUMINUM HYDROXIDE MAGNESIUM CARBONATE.
Use: Antacid.
See: Aloxine (Forest).
DI-GEL, Tab. (Plough).
Magnagel, Susp., Tab. (Mallard).
W/Aminoacetic acid, calcium carbonate.
See: Eugel, Tab., Liq. (Reid-Rowell).
W/Dicyclomine HCl, magnesium trisilicate, methylcellulose.
See: Triactin, Liq., Tab. (Norwich).
W/Magnesium trisilicate.
See: Escot, Cap. (Reid-Rowell).
W/Magnesium trisilicate, bismuth aluminate.
See: Escot, Cap. (Reid-Rowell).

•**ALUMINUM MONOSTEARATE,** N.F. XVII. Aluminum, dihydroxy(octadecanoato-O-)-,Dihydroxy (stearato)aluminum.

ALUMINUM OXIDE.
See: Epi-Clear Scrub Cleanser (Squibb).

ALUMINUM PASTE. (Torch) Zinc oxide 85%, aluminum 10%, mineral oil 5%. Jar 60 Gm, lb.
Use: Skin protectant.

ALUMINUM PHENOSULFONATE
See: AR-EX Cream Deodorant (Ar-Ex).

•**ALUMINUM PHOSPHATE GEL,** U.S.P. XXII. Aluminum phosphate 4.15%.
Use: Antacid.
See: Phosphaljel, Susp. (Wyeth-Ayerst).

•**ALUMINUM SESQUICHLOROHYDRATE.** USAN.
Use: Anhidrotic.

ALUMINUM SODIUM CARBONATE HYDROXIDE.
See: Dihydroxyaluminum Sodium Carbonate.

•**ALUMINUM SUBACETATE TOPICAL SOLUTION,** U.S.P. XXII. (Various Mfr.) Aluminum acetate basic solution, aluminum subacetate solution.
Use: Astringent wash.

•**ALUMINUM SULFATE,** U.S.P. XXII.
Use: Pharmaceutic necessity for preparation of aluminum subacetate solution.

•**ALUMINUM ZIRCONIUM TETRACHLOROHYDREX GLY.** USAN.
Use: Anhidrotic.

•**ALUMINUM ZIRCONIUM TRICHLOROHYDREX GLY.** USAN.
Use: Anhidrotic.

ALUPENT. (Boehringer Ingelheim) Metaproterenol sulfate. **Metered dose inhaler:** 225 mg in 15 ml. **Tab.:** 10 mg or 20 mg. Bot. 100s. **Syr.:** 10 mg/5 ml. Bot. pt. **Inhalant Soln.: 0.4%**: 2.5 ml UD vial. **0.6%:** 2.5 ml UD vial. **5%**: Bot. 10 ml, 30 ml UD.
Use: Bronchodilator.

ALURATE. (Roche) Aprobarbital 40 mg/5 ml. Alcohol 20%. Elix. Bot. pt.
Use: Sedative/hypnotic.

ALUREX. (Rexall) Magnesium-aluminum hydroxide. **Susp.:** (200 mg-150 mg/5 ml) Bot. 12 oz. **Tab:** (400 mg-300 mg) Box 50s.
Use: Antacid.

ALU-TAB. (Riker) Aluminum hydroxide gel 600 mg/Tab. Bot. 250s.
Use: Antacid.

ALVAGEL. (Kenyon) Aloe vera active principle 55% in ointment base. Tube 2 oz, 4 oz.
Use: Skin protectant.

ALVEDIL CAPS. (Luly-Thomas) Theophylline 4 gr, pseudoephedrine HCl 50 mg, butabarbital 15 mg/Cap. Bot. 100s.
Use: Bronchodilator, decongestant, sedative/hypnotic.

•**ALVERINE CITRATE.** USAN. N-ethyl-3,3′-diphenyl dipropylamine citrate.
Use: Anticholinergic.
See: Spacolin, Tab. (Philips Roxane).

AL-VITE. (Drug Industries) Vitamins A 10,000 IU, D_3 400 IU, E 25 IU, C 200 mg, B_1 20 mg, B_2 10 mg, B_6 6 mg, calcium pantothenate 20 mg, niacinamide 100 mg, B_{12} w/intrinsic factor concentrate 0.5 units/Tab. Bot. 100s, 500s.
Use: Vitamin/mineral supplement.

ALZAPAM. (Major) Lorazepam 0.5 mg, 1 mg or 2 mg/Tab. Bot. 100s, 500s.
Use: Antianxiety agent.

AMA. (Wampole-Zeus) Antimitochondrial antibodies test by IFA. Test 48s.
Use: Diagnostic aid.

•**AMACETAM SULFATE.** USAN.
Use: Cognition adjuvant.

AMACID. (Kenyon) An acid protein hydrolysate prepared from casein and lactalbumin by special process which retains l-tryptophan and other essential amino acids. Bot. 4 oz, pt, gal.

AMACODONE. (Trimen) Hydrocodone bitartrate 5 mg, acetaminophen 500 mg/Tab. Bot. 100s.
Use: Narcotic analgesic combination.

•**AMADIMONE ACETATE.** USAN.
Use: Progestin.

AMANOZINE HCl. 2-Amino-4-anilino-s-triazine HCl.

AMANTADINE. B.A.N. 1-Adamantanamine.
Use: Antiviral agent, treatment of Parkinson's disease.
See: Symadine (Reid-Rowell).
Symmetrel, Cap. (Du Pont).

•**AMANTADINE HYDROCHLORIDE,** U.S.P. XXII. Caps., Syr., U.S.P. XXII. 1-Adamantanamine HCl. Tricylo [3.3.1.1^{3,7}] decan-1-amine, HCl.
Use: Antiviral agent, treatment of Parkinson's disease.
See: Symmetrel, Cap., Syr. (DuPont).

AMAPHEN. (Trimen) Butalbital 50 mg, caffeine 40 mg, acetaminophen 325 mg/Cap. Bot. 100s.
Use: Sedative/hypnotic, analgesic.

AMAPHEN W/CODEINE #3. (Trimen) Codeine phosphate 30 mg, acetaminophen 325 mg, caffeine 40 mg, butalbital 50 mg Cap. Bot. 100s.
Use: Narcotic analgesic combination, sedative/hypnotic.

AMARANTH. 3-Hydroxy-4-[(4-sulfo-1-naphthyl)azo]-2,7-naphthalene-disulfonic acid trisodium salt. F.D. and C. Red No. 2.
Use: Color (Not for internal use).

AMARSAN.
See: Acetarsone.

AMAZONE. 1:4-Benzoquinone amidinohydrazine thiosemicarbazone hydrate. Iversal.

AMBAZONE. B.A.N. 1,4-Benzoquinone amidinohydrazone thiosemicarbazone.
Use: Antiseptic.

AMBENONIUM CHLORIDE. N,N′-bis-(2-Diethyl aminoethyl) oxamide bis-2-chlorobenzyl Cl. [Oxalylbis (iminoethylene)] bis [(o-chlorobenzyl)-diethylammonium] dichloride. B.A.N. NN′-Di-[2-(N-2-chlorobenzyldiethylammonio) ethyl] oxamide dichloride.
Use: Cholinergic for treatment of myasthenia gravis.
See: Mytelase, Cap. (Winthrop Pharm).

AMBENOXAN. B.A.N. 2-(2-Methoxyethoxyethylaminomethyl)-1,4-benzodioxan.
Use: Muscle relaxant.

AMBENYL COUGH SYRUP. (Forest) Codeine phosphate 10 mg, bromodiphenhydramine HCl 12.5 mg/5 ml, alcohol 5%. Bot. 4 oz, pt, gal.
Use: Antitussive, antihistamine.

AMBENYL-D. (Forest) Guaifenesin 200 mg, pseudoephedrine HCl 60 mg, dextromethorphan HBr 30 mg/10 ml, alcohol 9.5%. Bot. 4 oz.
Use: Expectorant, decongestant, antitussive.

AMBERLITE, I.R.P.-64. (Rohm and Haas). Polacrilin.

AMBERLITE, I.R.P.-88. (Rohm and Haas). Polacrilin potassium.

AMBOMYCIN. USAN. Isolated from filtrates of *Streptomyces ambofaciens.*
Use: Antineoplastic.

AMBROSIACEAE POLLENS. (Parke-Davis) Ragweed and related pollens.
See: Allergenic extracts.

AMBRUTICIN. USAN.
Use: Antifungal.

AMBUCAINE. Ambutoxate HCl.

AMBUCETAMIDE. 2-(di-n-Butylamino)-2-(p-methoxyphenyl)acetamide.

AMBUCETAMIDE. B.A.N. α-Dibutylamino-4-methoxyphenylacetamide.
Use: Antispasmodic.

AMBUPHYLLINE. USAN. Theophylline compound with 2-amino-2-methyl-1-propanol. Bufylline.
Use: Diuretic, smooth muscle relaxant.

AMBUSIDE. USAN. 5-Allylsulfamoyl-2-chloro-4-(3-hydroxybut-2-enylideneamino)benzenesulfonamide.
Use: Diuretic.
See: Novohydrin.

AMBUTONIUM BROMIDE. Ethyl-dimethylammonium(3-carbamyl-3,3-diphenyl propyl)-ethyl dimethylammonium bromide.
Use: Antispasmodic.

AMBUTONIUM BROMIDE. B.A.N. (3-Carbamoyl-3,3-diphenylpropyl)ethyldimethylammonium bromide.
Use: Antispasmodic.

AMBUTOXATE HYDROCHLORIDE. 2-Diethylaminoethyl-4-amino-2-butoxybenzoate HCl. Ambucaine.

AMC. (Schlicksup) Ammonium Cl 7.5 gr/Tab. Bot. 1000s.
Use: Diuretic, expectorant.

AMCILL. (Parke-Davis) **Cap.:** Ampicillin trihydrate 250 mg or 500 mg/Cap. Bot. 100s, 500s, UD pkg 100s. **Oral Susp.:** 125 mg or 250 mg/5 ml. Bot. 100 ml, 200 ml.
Use: Antibacterial, penicillin.

•**AMCINAFAL.** USAN. 9-Fluoro-11β, 16α,17,21-tetrahydroxypregna-1,4-diene-3, 20-dione cyclic 16, 17-acetal with 3-pentanone.
Use: Anti-inflammatory agent.

•**AMCINAFIDE.** USAN. (R)-9-Fluoro-11β, 16α,17,21-tetrahydroxypregna-1, 4-diene-3,20-dione cyclic 16,17-acetal with acetophenone.
Use: Anti-inflammatory agent.

•**AMCINONIDE,** U.S.P. XXII. Cream, Oint., U.S.P. XXII.
Use: Glucocorticoid.
See: Cyclocort, Cream, Oint. (Lederle).

AMCORT. (Keene) Triamcinolone diacetate 40 mg/ml. Vial 5 ml.
Use: Corticosteroid.

•**AMDINOCILLIN.** USAN. 6-β-amidinopenicillanic acid.
Use: Antibacterial.
See: Coactin, Inj. (Roche).

AMEBAN.
See: Carbarsone.

AMEBICIDES.
See: Acetarsone (Various Mfr.).
Aralen HCl, Inj. (Winthrop Pharm).
Aralen Phosphate, Tab. (Winthrop Pharm).
Carbarsone, Pulv., Tab. (Lilly).
Chiniofon, Tab. (Various Mfr.).
Diiodohydroxyquin (Various Mfr.).
Diodoquin, Tab. (Searle).
Emetine HCl (Various Mfr.).
Flagyl, Tab. (Searle).
Humatin, Kapseal, Syr. (Parke-Davis).
Yodoxin, Tab. (Glenwood).

AMECHOL.
Use: Diagnostic aid.
See: Methacholine Cl.

•**AMEDALIN HCl.** USAN. 3-Methyl-3-[3-(methylamino)propyl]-1-phenyl-2-indolinone monohydrochloride.
Use: Antidepressant.

•**AMELTOLIDE.** USAN.
Use: Anticonvulsant.

AMEN. (Carnrick) Medroxyprogesterone acetate 10 mg/Tab. Bot. 50s, 100s, 1000s.
Use: Progestin.

AMERICAINE AEROSOL. (DuPont Critical Care) Benzocaine 20% in a water-soluble vehicle. Bot. 0.67 oz, 2 oz, 4 oz.
Use: Local anesthetic.

AMERICAINE ANESTHETIC LUBRICANT. (DuPont Critical Care) Benzocaine 20%, benzethonium Cl 0.1% in a water-soluble polyethylene glycol base. Foil pack 2.5 Gm, Pkg. 144s. Tube oz.
Use: Local anesthetic.

AMERICAINE FIRST AID BURN OINTMENT. (DuPont Critical Care) Benzocaine 20%, benzethonium Cl 0.1% in a water-soluble polyethylene glycol base. Tube 0.75 oz.
Use: Local anesthetic.

AMERICAINE HEMORRHOIDAL OINTMENT. (DuPont Critical Care) Benzocaine 20%, benzethonium Cl 0.1% in a water-soluble polyethylene glycol base. Tube oz w/rectal applicator.
Use: Local anesthetic.

AMERICAINE OTIC. (DuPont Critical Care) Benzethonium Cl 0.1%, benzocaine 20% in a water-soluble base of 1% (w/w) glycerin, polyethylene glycol 300. Bot. 0.5 oz.
Use: Otic preparation.

AMER-TET. (Robinson) Tetracycline HCl 250 mg or 500 mg/Cap. Bot. 100s, 1000s.
Use: Anti-infective.

AMER-TET SUSPENSION. (Robinson) Tetracycline HCl Susp. 125 mg/5 ml. Bot. pt.
Use: Anti-infective.

AMES DEXTRO SYSTEM LANCETS. (Ames) Sterile disposable lancet. Box 100s.
Use: Diagnostic aid.

•**AMETANTRONE ACETATE.** USAN.
Use: Antineoplastic.

AMETAZOLE. B.A.N. 3-(2-Aminoethyl)pyrazole. Betazole (I.N.N.). Histalog, hydrochloride.
Use: To stimulate gastric secretion in diagnostic tests.

A-METHAPRED UNIVIAL. (Abbott Hospital Prods) Methylprednisolone sodium succinate. **40 mg/ml:** Pkg. 1s, 25s, 50s, 100s; 125 mg/2 ml Pkg. 1s, 5s, 25s, 50s, 100s; **500 mg/4 ml:** Pkg. 1s, 5s, 25s, 100s; **1000 mg/8 ml:** Pkg. 1s, 5s, 25s 100s.
Use: Corticosteroid.

AMETHOCAINE HYDROCHLORIDE.
Use: Local anesthetic.
See: Tetracaine HCl.

AMETHOPTERIN.
Use: Antineoplastic.
See: Methotrexate (Lederle).

AMFECLORAL. B.A.N. α-Methyl-N(2,2,2-trichloroethylidene)-phenethylamine.
Use: Appetite suppressant.

•**AMFENAC SODIUM.** USAN.
Use: Anti-inflammatory.

•**AMFILCON A.** USAN.
Use: Contact lens material (hydrophilic).

•**AMFLUTIZOLE.** USAN.
Use: Treatment of gout.

AMFODYNE.
See: Imidecyl iodine.

•**AMFONELIC ACID.** USAN. 7-Benzyl-1-ethyl-4-oxo-1,8-naphthyridine-3-carboxylic acid.
Use: Central nervous system stimulant.

AMGENAL COUGH SYRUP. (Goldline) Bromodiphenhydramine HCl 12.5 mg, codeine phosphate 10 mg/5 ml, alcohol 5%. Bot. 120 ml, pt, gal.
Use: Antihistamine, antitussive.

AMIBIARSON.
See: Carbarsone (Various Mfr.).

AMICAR. (Lederle) Aminocaproic acid. **Syr.:** 25%. Bot. pt. **Inj.:** 250 mg/ml. Vial 20 ml, 96 m **Tab.:** 500 mg. Bot. 100s.
Use: Antifibrinolytic agent.

AMICARBALIDE. B.A.N. 3,3′-Diamidino-carbanilide. Diampron, isethionate.
Use: Antiprotozoan (veterinary).

•**AMICLORAL.** USAN. 6-0-(2,2,2-Trichloro-1-hydroxyethyl)-α-D-glucopyranosel-4 polymer with a-D-glucopyranose.
Use: Food additive (veterinary).

•**AMICYCLINE.** USAN.
Use: Antibacterial.

•**AMIDAPSONE.** USAN. p-Sulfanilylphenyl urea.
Use: Antiviral (for poultry).

AMIDATE. (Abbott Hospital Prods) Etomidate 2 mg/ml, propylene glycol 35%. Single dose Amp 20 mg/10 ml or 40 mg/20 ml;Abboject syringe 40 mg/20 ml .
Use: General anesthetic.

AMIDEPHRINE. B.A.N. 3-(1-Hydroxy-2-methylaminoethyl)methanesulfonanilide. Dricol.
Use: Vasoconstrictor, nasal decongestant.

•**AMIDEPHRINE MESYLATE.** USAN.
Use: Adrenergic.

AMIDOFEBRIN.
See: Aminopyrine (Various Mfr.).

AMIDONE HYDROCHLORIDE.
Use: Narcotic agonist analgesic.
See: Methadone HCl (Various Mfr.).

AMIDOPYRAZOLINE.
See: Aminopyrine (Various Mfr.).

AMIDOTRIZOATE, SODIUM.
See: Diatrizoate sodium.

AMIDOTRIZOIC ACID. Diatrizoic Acid. B.A.N.

•**AMIFLOXACIN.** USAN.
Use: Antibacterial.

AMIFLOXACIN MESYLATE. USAN.
Use: Antibacterial.
AMIGEN. (Baxter) Protein hydrolysate. **5%:** Bot. 500 ml, 1000 ml; **10%:** Bot. 500 ml, 1000 ml. **5% w/dextrose 5%:** Bot. 500 ml, 1000 ml. **5% w/dextrose 5%, alcohol 5%:** Bot. 1000 ml. **5% w/fructose 10%:** Bot. 1000 ml. **5% w/fructose 12.5%, alcohol 2.4%:** Bot. 1000 ml.
Use: Nutritional supplement.
AMIGESIC. (Amide) Salsalate 500 mg/Cap or Tab. Salsalate 75 mg/capl. Bot. 100s, 500s.
Use: Salicylate analgesic.
AMIKACIN, U.S.P. XXII.
Use: Antibacterial.
AMIKACIN SULFATE INJECTION, U.S.P. XXII. 0-3-Amino-3-deoxy-α-D-glucopyranosyl(1-6)-0-[6-amino-6-deoxy-α-D-glucopyranosyl(1-4)]-N-[(S)-4-amino- 2-hydroxyl-1-oxobutyl]-2-deoxy-D-streptamine sulfate.
Use: Antibacterial.
See: Amikin, Inj. (Bristol).
AMIKIN. (Bristol) Amikacin sulfate inj. Vial 100 mg, 500 mg, 1 Gm, disposable syringes 500 mg.
Use: Anti-infective.
AMILORIDE. B.A.N. N-Amidino-3,5-diamino-6-chloropyrazine-2-carboxamide.
Use: Diuretic.
See: Midamor, Tab. (Merck Sharp & Dohme).
W/Hydrochlorthiazide.
See: Moduretic, Tab. (Merck Sharp & Dohme).
AMILORIDE HYDROCHLORIDE, U.S.P. XXII. Tab., U.S.P. XXII. Pyrazinecarboxamide,3,5-diamino-N-(ami-noiminomethyl)-6-chloro-, monochloride.
Use: Antikaliuretic diuretic, antihypertensive.
See: Midamor, Tab. (Merck Sharp & Dohme).
AMILORIDE HYDROCHLORIDE AND HYDROCHLORTHIAZIDE TABLETS, U.S.P. XXII.
Use: Antikaliuretic diuretic, antihypertensive.
See: Moduretic, Tab. (Merck Sharp & Dohme).
AMIN-AID INSTANT DRINK POWDER. (Kendall McGaw) Essential amino acids, maltodextrin, sucrose, partially hydrogenated soybean oil, lecithin, mono and diglycerides. Packet 162 Gm.
Use: Enteral nutritional supplement.
AMINA-21. (Miller) L-form amino acids 600 mg/Cap. Bot. 100s, 300s.
Use: Tissue repair.
AMINACRINE. F.D.A. 9-Aminoacridine.
Use: Anti-infective, topical.
AMINACRINE HYDROCHLORIDE. USAN. 9-Aminoacridine hydrochloride.
Use: Anti-infective, topical.
W/Dienestrol, sulfanilamide, allantoin.
See: AVC/Dienestrol Cream, Supp. (Merrell Dow).
Use: Bacteriostatic agent.
W/Oxyquinoline benzoate.
See: Triva, Vaginal Jelly (Boyle).
W/Sulfanilamide, allantoin.
See: AVC, Cream, Supp. (Merrell Dow).
Femguard Vaginal Cream (Reid Rowell).
Sulfem Vaginal Cream (Federal Pharm.).
Vagidine, Cream (Elder).
Vagitrol, Cream, Supp. (Lemmon).
AMIN-AID. (American McGaw) Instant drinks, puddings.
Use: Enteral nutritional supplement.
AMINARSONE.
See: Carbarsone (Various Mfr.).
AMINE RESIN.
See: Polyamine Methylene Resin.
AMINESS. (Clintec) Essential amino acids. 10 Tab. = adult amino acid MDR. Jar 300s.
Use: Parenteral nutitional supplement.
AMINESS 5.2%. (Clintec) Amino acids and electrolytes, Inj.
Use: Parenteral nutritional supplement.
AMINICOTIN.
Use: Vitamin supplement.
See: Nicotinamide (Various Mfr.).
AMINOACETIC ACID. Glycerine, U.S.P. XXII. (Various Mfr.). (Glycine, glycocoll) available as elix., pow., tab.
Use: Myasthenia gravis, irrigating solution.
W/Aluminum hydroxide, magnesium hydroxide, calcium carbonate.
See: Eugel, Tab., Liq. (Reid-Rowell).
W/Calcium carbonate.
See: Antacid pH, Tab. (Towne).
Eldamint, Tab. (Elder).
W/Calcium carbonate, aluminum hydroxide, magnesium carbonate.
See: Glytabs, Tab. (Pharmics).
W/Calcium carbonate, magnesium carbonate, bismuth subcarbonate, dried aluminum hydroxide gel.
See: Buffer-Tabs (Forest).
W/Magnesium trisilicate, aluminum hydroxide.
See: Maracid-2, Tab. (Marin).
W/Phenylephrine HCl, pyrilamine maleate, acetylsalicylic acid, caffeine.
See: Al-Ay, Tab. (Bowman).
W/Phenylephrine HCl, chlorpheniramine maleate, acetaminophen, caffeine.
See: Codimal, Tab. (Central).
AMINOACETIC ACID & CALCIUM CARBONATE.
W/Lysine.
See: Lycolan, Elix. (Lannett).
AMINO ACID & PROTEIN PREP.
See: Aminoacetic Acid, U.S.P. XXII.
Glutamic Acid.
Histidine HCl.
Lysine.
Phenylalanine.
Thyroxine.
AMINO ACIDS.
Use: Amino acid supplement.
See: Aminosol, Soln. (Abbott).
Aminosyn, Soln. (Abbott).
W/Estrone, testosterone, vitamins, minerals.
See: Geramine, Tab., Inj. (Brown).

W/Vitamin B_{12}.
See: Stuart Amino Acids and B_{12}, Tab. (Stuart).
AMINOACRIDINE.
Use: Bacteriostatic agent.
See: 9-aminoacridine.
9-AMINOACRIDINE HCl. (Various Mfr.).
Aminacrine HCl.
Use: Anti-infective, vaginal.
See: Vagisec Plus (J. Schmid).
W/Hydrocortisone acetate, tyrothricin, phenylmercuric acetate, polysorbate-80, urea, lactose.
See: Aquacort, Vaginal Supp. (Webcon).
W/Iodoquinol.
See: Vagitric, Oint. (Elder).
W/Phenylmercuric acetate, tyrothricin, urea, lactose.
See: Trinalis, Vaginal Supp. (Webcon).
W/Polyoxyethylene nonyl phenol, sodium edetate, docusate sodium.
See: Vagisec Plus, Supp. (Schmid).
W/Pramoxine HCl, acetic acid, parachlorometaxylenol, methyl-dodecylbenzyltrimethyl ammonium Cl.
See: Drotic No. 2, Drops (Ascher).
W/Sulfanilamide, allantoin.
See: AVC Cream, Supp. (Merrell Dow).
Nil Vaginal Cream (Century).
Par Cream (Parmed).
Vagisan, Creme (Sandia).
Vagisul, Creme (Sheryl).
W/Sulfisoxazole, allantoin.
See: Vagilia, Cream (Lemmon).
p-AMINOBENZENE-SULFONYLACETYLIMIDE.
See: Sulfacetamide.
•**AMINOBENZOATE POTASSIUM,** U.S.P. XXII. Cap., for Oral Soln., Tab., U.S.P. XXII.
Use: Analgesic.
See: Potaba, Pow., Tab. (Glenwood).
W/Hydrocortisone, ammonium salicylate, ascorbic acid.
See: Neocylate sodium free, Tab. (Central).
W/Potassium salicylate.
See: Pabalate-SF, Tab. (Robins).
W/Potassium salicylate, ascorbic acid.
See: Pabalan, Tab. (Lannett).
•**AMINOBENZOATE SODIUM,** U.S.P. XXII.
Use: Analgesic.
See: PABA sodium, Tab. (Various Mfr.).
W/Phenobarbital, colchicine salicylate, Vitamin B_1, aspirin.
See: Doloral, Tab. (Alamed).
W/Salicylamide, ascorbic acid.
See: Sylapar, Tab. (Forest).
W/Salicylamide, sodium salicylate, ascorbic acid, butabarbital sodium.
See: Bisalate, Tab. (Allison Lab).
W/Sodium salicylate.
See: Pabalate, Tab. (Robins).
Salpara, Tab. (Reid-Rowell).
•**AMINOBENZOIC ACID,** U.S.P. XXII. Gel, Topical Soln., U.S.P. XXII. Benzoic acid, 4-amino. PABA. Available as Cap., Bot., Pow., Soln., Tab. Massengill Soln. (10%) Bot. pt.
Use: Topical protectant (sunscreening agent).
See: Pabafilm (Owen/Galderma).
Pabanol, Lot. (Elder).
W/Mephenesin, salicylamide.
See: Sal-Phenesin, Tab. (Marion).
W/Sodium salicylate, ascorbic acid.
See: Nucorsal, Tab. (Westerfield).
p-AMINOBENZOIC ACID, SALTS.
See: p-Aminobenzoate potassium and p-Aminobenzoate sodium.
•**AMINOCAPROIC ACID,** U.S.P. XXII. Syr., Inj., Tab., U.S.P. XXII. 6-Aminohexanoic acid.
Use: Antifibrinolytic, hemostatic.
See: Amicar, Syr., Tab., Vial (Lederle).
•**AMINOCAPROIC ACID.** USAN. 6-Aminohexanoic acid. Amicar. Epsikapron.
Use: Inhibitor of fibrinolytic activity.
AMINOCARDOL.
Use: Bronchodilator.
See: Aminophylline. (Various Mfr.).
AMINO CERV. (Milex) Urea 8.34%, sodium propionate 0.5%, methionine 0.83%, cystine 0.35%, inositol 0.83%, benzalkonium Cl 0.000004%, buffered to pH 5.5. Tube with applicator 2.75 oz.
Use: Vaginal preparation.
AMINODYNE COMPOUND. (Bowman) Acetaminophen 2.5 gr, aspirin 3.5 gr, caffeine 0.5 gr/Tab. Bot. 100s, 1000s.
Use: Analgesic combination.
AMINO-ETHYL-PROPANOL.
See: Aminoisobutanol.
W/Bromotheophyllin.
See: Pamabrom (Various Mfr.).
AMINOFEN. (Dover) Acetaminophen 325 mg/Tab. Sugar, lactose and salt free. UD Box 500s.
Use: Analgesic.
AMINOFEN MAX. (Dover) Acetaminophen 500 mg/Tab. Sugar, lactose and salt free. UD Box 500s.
Use: Analgesic.
AMINOFORM.
Use: Anti-infective, urinary.
See: Methenamine (Various Mfr.).
AMINOGEN. (Christina) Vitamin B complex, folic acid. Amp. 2 ml Box 12s, 24s, 100s. Vial 10 ml.
Use: Vitamin B supplement.
•**AMINOGLUTETHIMIDE,** U.S.P. XXII. Tab., U.S.P. XXII. 2-(p-Aminophenyl)-2-ethylglutarimide.
Use: Treatment of Cushing's syndrome.
See: Cytadren, Prods. (Ciba).
•**AMINOHIPPURATE SODIUM,** U.S.P. XXII. Inj., U.S.P. XXII. Glycine, N-(4-aminobenzoyl), monosodium salt. Monosodium p-aminohippurate. (Merck Sharp & Dohme) 2 Gm/10 ml. Amp. 10 ml, 50 ml.
Use: I.V., diagnostic aid for renal plasma flow.
•**AMINOHIPPURIC ACID,** U.S.P. XXII. Glycine, N-(4-aminobenzoyl)-.

Use: Diagnostic aid (renal function determination).

AMINOISOBUTANOL. 2-Amino-2-methylpronanol-1.
See: Butaphyllamine.
Pamabrom for combinations.

AMINOISOMETRADINE. DL-2-Amino-4-(methylthio) butyric acid.
See: Methionine.

AMINOMETRADINE. B.A.N. 1-Allyl-6-amino-3-ethyl-pyrimidine-2,4-dione. Mictine.
Use: Diuretic.

AMINONAT. Protein hydrolysates (oral).

AMINONITROZOLE. N-(5-Nitro-2-thiazolyl) acetamide.
Use: Antitrichomonal.

AMINOPENTAMIDE SULFATE. 4-(Dimethylamino)-2,2-diphenylvaleramide sulfate.
Use: Anticholinergic.

AMINOPHYLLIN. (Searle) Trademark for Aminophylline. **100 mg/Tab.** Bot. 100s, 1000s, UD 100s. **200 mg**/Tab. Bot. 100s, 1000s, UD 100s.
Use: Bronchodilator.

AMINOPHYLLIN INJECTION. (Searle) Trademark for Aminophylline. Amp. **250 mg:** 10 ml; 25s, 100s; **500 mg:** 20 ml; 25s, 100s.
Use: Bronchodilator.

•**AMINOPHYLLINE,** U.S.P. XXII. Enema, Inj., Supp., Tab., U.S.P. XXII. Theophylline compound w/ethylenediamine (2:1). (Aminocardol, Ammophyllin, Cardophyllin, Carena, Diophyllin, Genophyllin, Ionphylline, Metaphyllin, Phyllindon, Teholamine, Theophyldine.).
Use: Smooth muscle relaxant (bronchodilator).
See: Aminodur, Dura-Tab. (Berlex).
Lixaminol, Elix. (Ferndale).
Phyllocontin, Tab. (Purdue Frederick).
Rectalad-Aminophylline (Wallace).
Somophyllin Oral Liq. (Fisons).
Somophyllin Rectal Soln. (Fisons).

AMINOPHYLLINE COMBINATIONS.
Amphedrine Compound, Cap. (Lannett).
Asmadrin (Jenkins).
Asminorel, Tab. (Reid-Rowell).
B.M.E., Elix. (Brothers).
Bronchovent, Tab. (Mills).
Lixaminol AT/5 ml (Ferndale).
Mudrane GG-2, Tab. (Poythress).
Orthoxine and Aminophylline, Cap. (Upjohn).
Quinamm, Tab. (Merrell Dow).
Quinite, Tab. (Reid-Rowell).
Romaphed, Tab. (Robinson).
Strema, Cap. (Foy).
Theo-Kaps (Scrip).

AMINOPHYLLINE INJECTION, U.S.P. XXII. (Abbott) Amp. 250 mg/10 ml, 500 mg/20 ml; Fliptop vial 10 mg/20 ml, 20 mg/50 ml.
Use: Bronchodilator.

AMINOPHYLLINE INJECTION, U.S.P. XXII. Theophylline ethylenediamine. Amp. 3¾ gr, 7.5 gr (Various Mfr.).
Use: Smooth muscle relaxant.

•**AMINOPHYLLINE SUPPOSITORIES,** U.S.P. XXII. 3⅜ gr, 7.5 gr (Various Mfr.).
Use: Smooth muscle relaxant.

•**AMINOPHYLLINE TABLETS,** U.S.P. XXII. Plain or enteric coated 1.5 gr, 3 gr (Various Mfr.).
Use: Smooth muscle relaxant.

AMINOPHYLLINE-PHENOBARBITAL. (Robinson) Aminophylline 1.5 gr, phenobarbital 0.25 gr or 0.5 gr/Tab. Bot. 100s, 1000s, Bulk Pack 5000s. Aminophylline 3 gr, phenobarbital 0.25 gr or 0.5 gr/Tab. Bot. 100s, 1000s, Bulk Pack 5000s.
Use: Bronchodilator, sedative/hypnotic.

AMINOPHYLLINE WITH PHENOBARBITAL COMBINATIONS.
Amodrine, Tab. (Searle).
Mudrane, Tab. (Poythress).
Mudrane GG, Tab. (Poythress).

AMINOPREL. (Pasadena) L-lysine 60 mg, dl-methionine 15 mg, hydrolyzed protein 750 mg, iron 2 mg, Cu, I, K, Mg, Mn, Zn. Cap. Bot. 180s.
Use: Nutritional supplement.

AMINOPROMAZINE (I.N.N.). Proquamezine. B.A.N.

AMINOPTERIN SODIUM. B.A.N. Sodium N-[4-(2,4-diaminopteridin-6-ylmethyl)aminobenzoyl]-L-glutamate. Sodium N-[p-[[2,4,-(diamino-6-pteridinyl)methyl]amino]benzoyl]-L-glutamate.
Use: Antineoplastic agent.

AMINOPYRINE. Amidofebrin, Amidopyrazoline, Anafebrina, Novamidon, Pyradone. Dimethylamino-phenyl-dimethylpyrazolone.
Use: Antipyretic, analgesic.
See: Dipyrone, Vial (Maurry).

AMINOQUIN NAPHTHOATE.
See: Pamaquine Naphthoate.

4-AMINOQUINOLINE DERIVATIVES.
Use: Antimalarial.
See: Aralen HCl (Winthrop Pharm).
Chloroquine Phosphate (Various Mfr.).
Plaquenil Sulfate (Winthrop Pharm).

8-AMINOQUINOLINE DERIVATIVES.
Use: Antimalarial.
See: Primaquine Phosphate, U.S.P.
Primaquine Phosphate (Winthrop Pharm).

•**AMINOREX.** USAN. 2-Amino-5-phenyl-2-oxazoline.
Use: Appetite suppressant.
See: Apiquel fumarate.

AMINOSALICYLATE CALCIUM, U.S.P. XXI. Cap., Tab., U.S.P. XXI. Calcium 4-Aminosalicylate (1:2) trihydrate. (Dumas-Wilson) 7.5 gr, Bot. 1000s.
Use: Tuberculosis therapy.
W/Isoniazid, pyridoxine HCl.
See: Calpas-Inah-6, Tab. (Amer. Chem. & Drug).

AMINOSALICYLATE POTASSIUM. Monopotassium 4-aminosalicylate.
Use: Antibacterial (tuberculostatic).
See: Paskalium, Tab., Pow. (Glenwood).

•**AMINOSALICYLATE SODIUM,** U.S.P. XXII. Tab., U.S.P. XXII. Aminosalicylate sodium Benzoic acid, 4-amino-2-hydroxy-, monosodium salt, dihydrate. Monosodium 4-amino-salicylate dihydrate.
Use: Tuberculostatic.
See: Neopasalate, Tab. (Mallinckrodt).
P.A.S., Pow. (Century).
Pasara Sodium, Pow., Tab. (Dorsey).
Pasdium, Tab. (Kasar).

p-AMINOSALICYLIC ACID SALTS.
See: Aminosalicylate Calcium.
Aminosalicylate Potassium.
Aminosalicylate Sodium.

AMINOSYN. (Abbott Hospital Prods) Crystalline amino acid solution. **3.5%:** 1000 ml; **5%:** Container 250 ml, 500 ml, 1000 ml; **7%:** 500 ml; 7% kit (cs/3); **8.5%:** Single dose container 500 ml, 1000 ml. **10%:** 500 ml, 1000 ml.
W/Dextrose.
W/Electrolytes.
7%: 500 ml; **8.5%:** 500 ml.
Use: Parenteral nutritional supplement.

AMINOSYN (pH6). (Abbott) Crystalline amino acid infusion. **8.5%:** 500 ml, 1000 ml; **10%:** 500 ml, 1000 ml.
Use: Parenteral nutritional supplement.

AMINOSYN-HBC 7%. (Abbott) Crystalline amino acid infusion for high metabolic stress. 500 ml, 1000 ml.
Use: Parenteral nutritional supplement.

AMINOSYN M 3.5%. (Abbott) Crystalline amino acid infusion with electrolytes. 1000 ml.
Use: Parenteral nutritional supplement.

AMINOSYN-PF. (Abbott) Crystalline amino acid infusions for pediatric use. **7%:** 250 ml, 500 ml; **10%:** 1000 ml.
Use: Parenteral nutritional supplement.

AMINOSYN-RF. (Abbott) Crystalline amino acid infusion for renal failure patients. **5.2%:** 300 ml.
Use: Parenteral nutritional supplement.

AMINOSYN II, (Abbott) Crystalline amino acid infusion. **3.5%:** 1000 ml; **5%:** 1000 ml; **7%:** 500 ml; **8.5%:** 500 ml, 1000 ml; **10%:** 500 ml, 1000 ml.
W/Dextrose:
3.5% in 5% dextrose: 1000 ml; **3.5% in 25% dextrose:** 1000 ml; **5% in 25% dextrose:** 1000 ml.
W/Dextrose and electrolytes.
3.5% in 5% dextrose: 1000 ml; **3.5% in 25% dextrose:** 1000 ml; **4.25% in 10% dextrose:** 1000 ml; **4.25% in 25% dextrose:** 1000 ml.
W/Electrolytes.
7%: 1000 ml; **8.5%:** 1000 ml; **10%:** 1000 ml.
Use: Parenteral nutritional supplement.

AMINOSYN II M. (Abbott) Crystalline amino acid infusion with maintenance electrolytes, 10% dextrose. Soln. 1000 ml.
Use: Parenteral nutritional supplement.

AMINO-THIOL. (Marcen) Sulfur 10 mg, casein 50 mg, sodium citrate 5 mg, phenol 5 mg, benzyl alcohol 5 mg/ml. Vial 10 ml, 30 ml.
Use: Treatment of arthritis, neuritis.

AMINOTRATE PHOSPHATE. Trolnitrate phosphate.
See: Triethanolamine, Preps.

AMINOXYTROPINE TROPATE HCl. Atropine-N-oxide HCl.

•**AMIODARONE.** USAN.
Use: Antiarrhythmic agent.

AMIODARONE HYDROCHLORIDE.
Use: Antiarrhythmic agent.
See: Cordarone, Tab. (Wyeth-Ayerst).

AMIPAQUE. (Winthrop Pharm) Metrizamide 18.75%/20 ml Vial.
Use: Radiopaque agent.

AMIPHENAZOLE. B.A.N. 2,4-Diamino-5-phenylthiazole.
Use: Respiratory stimulant.

AMIPHENAZOLE HCl. 2,4-Diamino-5-phenylthiazole HCl. Daptazole.

•**AMIPRILOSE HYDROCHLORIDE.** USAN.
Use: Antibacterial, antifungal, anti-inflammatory, antineoplastic, antiviral, immunomodulator.

•**AMIQUINSIN HYDROCHLORIDE.** USAN. 4-Amino-6,7-dimethoxyquinoline hydrochloride monohydrate. Under study.
Use: Antihypertensive.

AMISOMETRADINE. B.A.N. 6-Amino-1,2-methylallyl-3-methylpyrimidine-2,4-dione. Rolicton.
Use: Diuretic.

AMI-TEX LA. (Amide) Phenylpropanolamine HCl 75 mg, guaifenesin 400 mg/tab. Bot. 100s, 500s, 1000s.
Use: Decongestant, expectorant.

AMITIN. (Thurston) Vitamin C 200 mg, lemon bioflavonoid 100 mg, niacinamide 60 mg, methionine 100 mg/Tab. Bot. 100s, 500s.
Use: Vitamin supplement.

AMITONE. (Norcliff Thayer) Calcium carbonate 350 mg/Tab. Bot. 100s.
Use: Antacid.

•**AMITRAZ.** USAN.
Use: Scabicide.

AMITRIPTYLINE. B.A.N. 3-(3-Dimethylamino-propylidene)dibenzo[a,d]cyclohepta-1,4-diene. Amitriptyline hydrochloride. Laroxyl, Lenitzol, Saroten, Tryptizol.
Use: Antidepressant.
See: Elegen-G, Tab. (Grafton).

•**AMITRIPTYLINE HCl.** U.S.P. XXII. Inj., Tab. U.S.P. XXII. 10,11-dihydro-N, N-dimethyl-5H-dibenzo[a,d]cycloheptene-Δ^5,-propylamine hydrochloride.
Use: Antidepressant.
See: Amitril, Tab. (Parke-Davis).
Elavil HCl, Tab., Inj. (Merck Sharp & Dohme).
Emitrip, Tab. (Major).
Endep, Tab. (Roche).
W/Chlordiazepoxide.
See: Limbitrol, Tab. (Roche).

W/Perphenazine.
See: Etrafon, Prods. (Schering).
Triavil, Tab. (Merck Sharp & Dohme).
•**AMLODIPINE MALEATE.** USAN.
Use: Antianginal, antihypertensive.
AMMENS MEDICATED POWDER. (Bristol-Myers) Boric acid 4.55%, zinc oxide 9.10%, talc, starch. Can 6.25 oz, 11 oz.
Use: Skin protectant.
AMMOIDIN. Methoxsalen.
Use: Psoralen.
AMMONIA. Aromatic Ammonia Spirit, U.S.P. XXII. Strong soln., N.F. XVII. (Lilly) 0.4 ml; pt; Aspirols 0.4 ml Pkg. 12s. (Burroughs-Wellcome). Vaporoles 5.41 min in crushable glass capsule. Box 12s, 100s (Glenwood) Amp 0.33 ml. Box 10s.
Use: Source of ammonia for fainting spells.
•**AMMONIA N 13.** USAN.
Use: Diagnostic radiopharmaceutical.
•**AMMONIA SOLUTION, STRONG,** N.F. XVII.
Use: Pharmaceutic aid (source of ammonia).
•**AMMONIATED MERCURY,** U.S.P. XXII. Oint., Ophth. Oint., U.S.P. XXII. (Various Mfr.).
Use: Anti-infective, topical.
See: Mercuronate 5% Oint. (Bowman).
W/Salicylic acid.
See: Emersal, Liq. (Medco).
AMMONIUM BENZOATE.
Use: Urinary antiseptic.
•**AMMONIUM CARBONATE,** N.F. XVII.
Use: Source of ammonia.
•**AMMONIUM CHLORIDE,** U.S.P. XXII. Inj., Delayed Release Tab., U.S.P. XXII. **Delayed Release Tab.:** (Various Mfr.) Plain or E.C. (5 gr or 7.5 gr). **Inj.:** (Cutter) 120 mEq/30 ml Vial.
Use: Diuretic, expectorant, alkalosis.
See: Nodema, Tab. (Towne).
AMMONIUM CHLORIDE, ENSEALS. (Lilly) Ammonium Cl. Tab. Enseal 7.5 gr. Bot. 100s.
Use: Urinary acidifier.
AMMONIUM MANDELATE. Ammonium salt of mandelic acid. Syr. 8 Gm/fl oz. Bot. pt, gal.
Use: Urinary antiseptic, oral.
AMMONIUM MOLYBDATE, U.S.P. XXII. Inj., U.S.P. XXII.
AMMONIUM NITRATE.
See: Reditemp-C, Cold Pack (Wyeth-Ayerst).
AMMONIUM PHOSPHATE, N.F. XVII. Phosphoric acid diammonium salt. Diammonium phosphate.
AMMONIUM VALERATE.
Use: Sedative.
AMMOPHYLLIN.
Use: Bronchodilator.
See: Aminophylline, U.S.P. XXII. (Various Mfr.).
AMMORID. (Kinney) Benzethonium Cl, zinc oxide in a lanolin absorption base. Oint. Tube 2 oz.
Use: Dermatologic agent.
AMMORID DIAPER RINSE. (Kinney) Methylbenzethonium Cl 5%, deionizing and buffering agents in dry powder form, readily soluble in water. Bot. 240 Gm.
Use: Skin protectant.
•**AMOBARBITAL,** U.S.P. XXII. Tab., U.S.P. XXII. Elix., U.S.P. XXI. (Various Mfr.). 5-Ethyl-5-isoamylbarbituric acid.
Use: Hypnotic of intermediate duration.
See: Amytal, Elix., Pulv. (Lilly).
AMOBARBITAL W/COMBINATIONS.
Amodex, Cap. (Forest).
Amoseco, Cap. (Robinson).
Bronchovent, Tab. (Mills).
Dextrobar, Tab. (Lannett).
Ectasule, Cap. (Fleming).
Obalan Lanatabs, Tab. (Lannett).
Obe-Slim, Tab. (Jenkins).
Penta-E W/Amobarb, Cap. (Recsei).
Trimex, Cap. (Mills).
•**AMOBARBITAL SODIUM,** U.S.P. XXII. Cap., Sterile, XXII. (Various Mfr.) 2,4,6(1H,3H,5H)-Pyrimidinetrione, 5-ethyl-5-(3-me-thylbutyl)-, monosodium salt. Sodium 5-ethyl-5-isopentylbarbiturate.
Cap. **1 gr:** Bot. 100s, 500s; **3 gr:** Bot. 100s, 500s, 1000s. (Various Mfr.).
Pow. Bot. 15 Gm, 30 Gm. (Lannett).
Tab. **30 mg:** Bot. 100s; **50 mg:** Bot. 100s; **100 mg:** Bot. 100s. (Lilly).
Vial 250 mg, 500 mg. (Lilly).
Use: Hypnotic of intermediate duration, sedative.
See: Amytal sodium (Lilly).
W/Ephedrine HCl, theophylline, chlorpheniramine maleate.
See: Theo-Span, Cap. (Scrip).
W/Secobarbital sodium.
See: Amsee, Tab. (Kenyon).
Compobarb, Cap. (Vitarine).
Dusotal, Cap. (Harvey).
Lanabarb, Cap. (Lannett).
AMOBARBITAL-EPHEDRINE CAPSULES. (Lannett) Amobarbital 50 mg, ephedrine sulfate 25 mg/Cap. Bot. 500s, 1000s.
Use: Sedative/hypnotic combination.
AMOCAL JR. (Jenkins) Pyrilamine maleate 3 mg, phenylephrine HCl 1 mg, tartar emetic 1/136 gr, benzoic acid 1/68 gr, ipecac pow. 1/16 gr, ammonium Cl 0.5 gr, iodized calcium 1/16 gr, licorice extract 1 gr/Tab. Bot. 1000s.
Use: Antihistamine, decongestant.
AMO-DERM. (High) Mineral abrasive, lecithin soap base, 3,4,4′-trichlorocarbanilide 1%, allantoin 2%. Pkg. Bar 3.5 oz.
Use: Skin cleanser.
AMODEX. (Fellows) Dextroamphetamine HCl 5 mg, amobarbital 20 mg/Tab. Bot. 100s, 1000s.
Use: CNS stimulant, sedative/hypnotic.
•**AMODIAQUINE,** U.S.P. XXII. 7-Chloro-4-(3-diethyl-aminomethyl-4-hydroxyanilino)quinoline.
Use: Antimalarial.
•**AMODIAQUINE HYDROCHLORIDE,** U.S.P. XXII.

Tab., U.S.P. XXII. 4-(7-Chloro-4-quinolylamino)-a-(Diethylamino)-o-cresol-di-HCl.
Use: Antimalarial.

AMODOPA. (Major) Methyldopa 125 mg, 250 mg or 500 mg. **125 mg:** 100s, UD 100s. **250 mg:** 100s, 1000s, UD 100s. **500 mg:** 100s, 500s, UD 100s.
Use: Antihypertensive.

AMOL. Mono-n-amyl-hydroquinone ether.
See: B-F-I, Pow. (Calgon).

AMOLINE. (Major) Aminophylline 100 mg or 200 mg/Tab. Bot. 100s, 1000s, UD 100s.
Use: Bronchodilator.

AMONIDRIN. (Forest) Ammonium Cl 200 mg, guaifenesin 100 mg/Tab. Bot. 1000s.
Use: Expectorant.

AMOPYROQUIN HCl. 4-(7-Chloro-4-quinolylamino)-a-1-pyrrolidyl-o-cresoldihydrochloride.
See: Propoquin.

•**AMOROLFINE.** USAN.
Use: Antimycotic.

AMOSAN. (Oral-B) Sodium perborate. Single-dose packet box 20s, 40s.
Use: Mouth and gum product.

AMOSECO. (Robinson) Secobarbital, amobarbital. Bot. 100s, 1000s.
Use: Sedative/hypnotic.

AMOTRIPHENE. 2,3,3-Tris(p-methoxy-phenyl)-N,N-
dimethylallylamine, 3-Dimethylamino-1, 1.2-tris(4-methoxyphenyl)-1-propene HCl.
Use: Coronary vasodilator.

•**AMOXAPINE.** USAN. 2-Chloro-II-(l-piperazinyl)dibenz[b,f][1,4]oxazepine.
Use: Antidepressant.
See: Asendin, Tab. (Lederle).

•**AMOXICILLIN.** U.S.P. XXII. Cap., Oral Susp., For Susp., Tab., U.S.P. XXII. 6-[D-(-)2-Amino-2-(p-hydroxyphenyl)acetamido]-3,3-dimethyl-7-oxo-4-thia-1-azabicy-clo[3.2.0]heptane-2-carboxylic acid.
Use: Antibiotic.
See: Amoxil, Preps. (Beecham Labs).
Polymox, Preps. (Bristol).
Sumox, Preps. (Reid-Rowell).

•**AMOXICILLIN AND CLAVULANATE POTASSIUM FOR ORAL SUSPENSION,** U.S.P. XXII.
Use: Antibiotic, inhibitor (β-*lactamase*).
See: Augmentin (Beecham Labs).

•**AMOXICILLIN AND CLAVULANATE POTASSIUM TABLETS,** U.S.P. XXII.
Use: Antibiotic, inhibitor (β-*lactamase*).
See: Augmentin (Beecham Labs).

•**AMOXICILLIN INTRAMAMMARY INFUSION,** U.S.P. XXII.
Use: Antibiotic.

AMOXICILLIN TRIHYDRATE.
Use: Antibiotic.
See: Amoxil Chew. Tab. (Beecham Labs).
Polymox, Cap., Susp. (Bristol).
Trimox, Preps. (Squibb Mark).
Utimox, Cap, Susp. (Parke-Davis).
Wymox, Cap, Liq. (Wyeth-Ayerst).
W/Clavulanate Potassium.
See: Augmentin, Tab., Chew. tab., Pow. for susp. (Beecham Labs).

AMOXIL. (Beecham Labs) Amoxicillin. **Cap.:** 250 mg. Bot. 100s, 500s, UD 10 × 10; 500 mg Bot. 50s, 500s. UD 10 × 10; **Pow. for Oral Susp.:** 125 mg or 250 mg/5 ml. Bot. 80 ml, 100 ml, 150 ml, UD 5 ml.
Use: Antibacterial, penicillin.

AMOXIL CHEWABLE TABLETS. (Beecham Labs) Amoxicillin trihydrate. 125 mg or 250 mg/Tab. Bot. 60s.
Use: Antibacterial, penicillin.

AMOXIL PEDIATRIC DROPS. (Beecham Labs) Amoxicillin 50 mg/ml. Bot. 15 ml, 30 ml.
Use: Antibacterial, penicillin.

AMP. Adenosine Phosphate. USAN.
Use: Nutrient.

AMPERIL. (Geneva) Ampicillin trihydrate 250 mg or 500 mg/Cap. Bot. 100s, 500s.
Use: Antibacterial, penicillin.

•**AMPHECLORAL.** USAN. α-Methyl-N-(2,2,2- trichloroethylidene) phenethylamine.
Use: Sympathomimetic.

AMPHEDRINE COMPOUND CAPSULES. (Lannett) Aminophylline-ephedrine compound. Bot. 1000s.
Use: Agent for varicose veins.
See: Cobalasine (Keene).

AMPHENIDONE. l-(m-Aminophenyl)-2-(lH)-pyridone.
Use: CNS stimulant.

AMPHETAMINE HYDROCHLORIDE. Racemic amphetamine HCl, methylphenethylamine HCl, dl-1-phenyl-2-aminopropane HCl, dl-methylphen-ethylamine HCl, racemic desoxynorephedrine HCl. **Amp:** 20 mg/ml, 1 ml (Various Mfr.). **Cap:** (Various Mfr.).
Use: Vasoconstrictor, CNS stimulant.

AMPHETAMINE, LEVO.
Use: CNS stimulant.
See: Levamphetamine.

AMPHETAMINE PHOSPHATE. Monobasic dl-a-methyl-phenethylamine phosphate. Monobasic racemic amphetamine phosphate.
Use: CNS stimulant.

•**AMPHETAMINE PHOSPHATE, DEXTRO,** U.S.P. XXII. Tab., U.S.P. XXII. Dextroamphetamine phosphate. (Various Mfr.).
Use: CNS stimulant.

AMPHETAMINE PHOSPHATE, DIBASIC, Racemic amphetamine phosphate. **Cap:** 5 mg or 10 mg. **Tab:** 5 mg or 10 mg. (Various Mfr.).
Use: CNS stimulant.

AMPHETAMINES.
See: Amphetamine Sulfate, Tab. (Lannett).
Biphetamine, Cap. (Pennwalt).
Desoxyn, Tab. (Abbott).
Desoxyn Gradumets, Long-acting tab. (Abbott).
Dexampex, Cap., Tab. (Lemmon).

Dexedrine, Elix., Tab., S.R. Cap. (SKF).
Dextroamphetamine Sulfate, Tab., S.R. Cap. (Various Mfr.).
Ferndex, Tab. (Ferndale).
Methampex, Tab. (Lemmon).
Obetrol, Tab. (Obetrol).

•**AMPHETAMINE SULFATE,** U.S.P. XXII. Tab., U.S.P. XXII. dl-a-Methyl-phenethylamine sulfate. (Racemic or dl form). **Cap:** 5 mg or 10 mg (Various Mfr.). **Tab:** 5 mg or 10 mg (Various Mfr.). **Vial:** 20 mg/ml (Various Mfr.).
Use: CNS stimulant.

AMPHETAMINE SULFATE, DEXTRO.
Use: CNS stimulant.
See: Dextroamphetamine Sulfate, U.S.P. XXII.

AMPHETAMINE WITH DEXTROAMPHETAMINE AS RESIN COMPLEXES.
Use: Appetite depressant.
See: Biphetamine, Cap. (Pennwalt).

AMPHOCAPS. (Blue Cross) Ampicillin 250 mg or 500 mg/Cap. Bot. 100s.
Use: Antibacterial, penicillin.

AMPHODEX. (Jamieson-McKames) d-Amphetamine sulfate 15 mg, amobarbital 45 mg, Vitamins A 6600 IU, D 400 IU, B_1 1.6 mg, B_2 2.5 mg, niacinamide 15.5 mg, C 30 mg, iron sulfate 20 mg, copper sulfate 2.8 mg, sodium molybdate 0.45 mg, zinc sulfate 2.8 mg, potassium iodide 0.13 mg/T.R. Cap. Bot. 100s.
Use: CNS stimulant, sedative/hypnotic, vitamin/mineral supplement.

AMPHOJEL. (Wyeth-Ayerst) Aluminum hydroxide (320 mg/5 ml), equivalent to aluminum oxide 4%. **Aqueous Susp.:** Bot. 12 fl oz. **Tab.:** 5 gr Bot. 100s, 10 gr Ctn. 100s. **Susp.:** Without flavor. Bot. 12 fl oz.
Use: Antacid.

•**AMPHOMYCIN.** USAN. An antibiotic produced by *Streptomyces canus.* Amphocortrin.
Use: Anti-infective.
See: Ecomytrin.

AMPHOTERICIN.
Use: Antifungal.
See: Fungizone, Preps. (Squibb).

•**AMPHOTERICIN B,** U.S.P. XXII. Cream, Inj., Lot., Oint., U.S.P. XXII. B.A.N. A polyene antibiotic substance obtained from cultures of *Streptomyces nodosus.*
Use: Antifungal.
See: Amphotericin B (Lyphomed).
Fungizone, Preps. (Squibb).
W/Tetracycline and K metaphosphate.
See: Mysteclin-F, Preps. (Squibb).

AMPHOTERICIN B. (Lyphomed) Polyene antibiotic obtained from cultures of *Streptomyces nodosus.* Inj. 50 mg/15 ml.
Use: Antifungal.

•**AMPICILLIN,** U.S.P. XXII. Cap., Pow. for Oral Susp., Soln. Pow., Pow. for Sterile Susp., Tab., U.S.P. XXII. 6[(D)-α-aminophenyl-acetamido] penicillanic acid. 6-(D-2-amino-2-phenylacetamido)-3, 3-dimethyl 7-oxo-4-thia-1-azabicyclo [3.2.0] heptane-2-carboxylic acid.
Use: Antibiotic.
See: Omnipen, Preps. (Wyeth-Ayerst).
Polycillin, Preps. (Bristol).
Principen, Preps. (Squibb Mark).
Roampicillin, Tab. (Robinson).
Roampicillin Pow., Inj. (Robinson).
Totacillin, Preps. (Beecham Labs).
W/Probenecid.
See: Polycillin-PRB, UD (Bristol).
Principen W/Probenecid Cap. (Squibb).
Probampacin (Robinson).

•**AMPICILLIN AND PROBENECID.** Cap., Oral Susp., U.S.P. XXII.
Use: Antibiotic.
See: Principen w/Probenecid (Squibb).
Polycillin PRB (Bristol).
Probanpacin (Various Mfr.).

•**AMPICILLIN SODIUM STERILE,** U.S.P. XXII.
Use: Antibiotic.
See: Omnipen-N, Inj. (Wyeth-Ayerst).
Polycillin-N (Bristol Labs).
Totacillin-N, Vial (Beecham Labs).

AMPICILLIN SODIUM/SULBACTAM SODIUM.
Use: Antibacterial, penicillin.
See: Unasyn (Roerig).

AMPICILLIN TRIHYDRATE. Cap., Oral Susp. Marketed by various manufacturers.
Use: Antibacterial, penicillin.
See: Amcil, Cap., Susp. (Parke-Davis).
D-Amp, Cap., Susp. (Dunhall).
Omnipen, Cap., Susp. (Wyeth-Ayerst).
Polycillin Preps. (Bristol).
Principen, Cap., Susp. (Squibb).
Totacillin, Cap., Susp. (Beecham Labs).

•**AMPROLIUM,** U.S.P. XXII. Oral pow., Soluble pow., U.S.P. XXII. 1-(4-amino-2-propyl-5-pyrimidinylmethyl)-2-picolinium Cl.
Use: Coccidiostat, (veterinary).

AMPROTROPINE PHOSPHATE. 2-Diethylamino-2,2-dimethylpropyl tropate.

•**AMQUINATE.** USAN.
Use: Antimalarial.

•**AMRINONE.** USAN.
Use: Cardiotonic.
See: Inocor Lactate Inj. (Winthrop Products).

•**AMSA.** Amsacrine (Orphan Drug).
Use: Antineoplastic agent.

•**AMSACRINE.** USAN.
Use: Antineoplastic agent.

AMSEE. (Kenyon) Amobarbital sodium ¾ gr, secobarbital sodium ¾ gr/Cap. Bot. 100s, 1000s.
Use: Sedative/hypnotic.

AMSEE #2. (Kenyon) Amobarbital sodium 1.5 gr, secobarbital sodium 1.5 gr/Cap. Bot. 100s, 1000s.
Use: Sedative/hypnotic.

AMSIDYL. Amsacrine (Orphan Drug).
Use: Antineoplastic agent.
Sponsor: Warner-Lambert.

AM-TUSS ELIXIR. (T.E. Williams) Codeine phosphate 10 mg, phenylephrine HCl 10 mg, phenylpropanolamine HCl 5 mg, prophenpyridamine maleate 12.5 mg, guaifenesin 44 mg, fluid extract of ipecac 0.17 min., citric acid 60 mg, sodium citrate 197 mg/5 ml, alcohol 5%. Bot. pt, gal.
Use: Antitussive, decongestant, antihistamine, expectorant.

AMVISC. (Precision-Cosmet) **Inj.:** Sodium hyaluronate 10 mg/ml. Disp. syringe: 0.25 ml, 0.5 ml, 0.8 ml, 4 ml.
Use: Viscoelastic agent.

AMVISC PLUS. (Precision-Cosmet) **Inj.:** Sodium hyaluronate 16 mg/ml. Disp. syringe: 0.25 ml, 0.5 ml, 0.8 ml.
Use: Viscoelastic agent.

AM-WAX. (Amlab) Urea, benzocaine, propylene glycol, glycerin. Bot. 10 ml.
Use: Otic preparation.

AMYL. Phenyl phenol, phenyl mercuric nitrate.
See: Lubraseptic Jelly (Guardian).

αAMYLASE.
W/Calcium carbonate, glycine, belladonna extract.
See: Trialka, Tab. (Commerce).
W/Pancreatin, protease, lipase.
See: Dizymes, Cap. (Recsei).
W/Pepsin, homatropine methyl bromide, lipase, protease, bile salts.
See: Digesplen, Tab., Elix. (Med. Prod. Panamericana).
W/Pepsin, pancreatin, ox bile extract.
See: Gourmase, Cap. (Reid-Rowell).
W/Phenobarbital, belladonna, pepsin, amylase, pancreatin, ox bile extract.
See: Gourmase-PB, Cap. (Reid-Rowell).

•**AMYLENE HYDRATE,** N.F. XVII. Tertiary amyl alcohol. Tert-pentyl alcohol. 2-Methyl-2-butanol. (Various Mfr.).
Use: Pharmaceutic aid (solvent).

•**AMYL NITRITE,** U.S.P. XXII. Inhalant, U.S.P. XXII. Isoamyl nitrite. Isopentyl nitrite. Burroughs Wellcome Vaporole 0.18 ml or 0.3 ml. Box 12s. Lilly Aspirols 0.3 ml. Box 12s.
Use: Inhalation, coronary vasodilator in angina pectoris.
W/Sodium nitrite, sodium thiosulfate.
See: Cyanide Antidote Pkg. (Lilly).

AMYLOLYTIC ENZYME.
W/Butabarbital sodium, belladonna extract, cellulolytic enzyme, proteolytic enzyme, lipolytic enzyme, iron ox bile.
See: Butibel-Zyme, Tab. (McNeil).
W/Calcium carbonate, glycine, proteolytic and cellulolytic enzymes.
See: Co-Gel, Tab. (Arco).
W/Cellulolytic, proteolytic and lipolytic enzymes, hyoscyamine sulfate.
See: Converspaz, Tab. (Ascher).
W/Lipase, proteolytic, cellulolytic enzymes, phenobarbital, hyoscyamine sulfate, atropine sulfate.
See: Arco-Lipase Plus, Tab. (Arco).
W/Proteolytic, cellulolytic enzymes.
See: Trienzyme, Tab. (Fellows-Testagar).
W/Proteolytic, cellulolytic, lipolytic enzymes, iron, ox bile.
See: Spaszyme, Tab. (Dooner).
W/Proteolytic enzyme, d-sorbitol.
See: Kuzyme, Cap. (Kremers-Urban).
W/Proteolytic, cellulolytic, lipolytic enzymes.
See: Arco-Lase, Tab. (Arco).
Zymme, Tab. (Scrip).
W/Proteolytic enzyme (Papain), homatropine methylbromide, d-sorbitol.
See: Converzyme, Liq. (Ascher).
W/Proteolytic enzyme, lipolytic enzyme, cellulolytic enzyme, belladonna extract.
See: Mallenzyme Improved, Tab. (Mallard).

AMYTAL. (Lilly) Amobarbital. 4 gr/fl oz., alcohol 34%. Elix. Bot. 16 fl oz.
Use: Sedative/hypnotic.

AMYTAL SODIUM. (Lilly) Amobarbital sodium. **Pow.:** 15 Gm, 30 Gm. **Vial:** 250 mg/vial or 500 mg/vial. Traypak 10s, 25s.
Use: Sedative/hypnotic.

ANA. (Wampole-Zeus) Antinuclear antibodies test by IFA. Test 54s.
Use: Diagnostic aid.

ANA HEp-2. (Wampole-Zeus) Antinuclear antibodies test by IFA. Tests 60s.
Use: Diagnostic aid.

ANABOLIC AGENTS. These agents stimulate constructive processes leading to retention of nitrogen and increasing the body protein.
See: Adroyd, Tab. (Parke-Davis).
Anabolin-IM, Vial (Alto).
Anadrol, Tab. (Syntex).
Anavar, Tab. (Searle).
Android, Tab. (Brown).
Androlone, Vial (Keene).
Crestabolic, Vial (Nutrition).
Deca-Durabolin, Amp., Vial (Organon).
Dianabol, Tab. (Ciba).
Di Genik, Vial (Savage).
Drolban, Vial (Lilly).
Durabolin, Amp., Vial (Organon).
Halotestin, Tab. (Upjohn).
Hybolin, Vial (Hyrex).
Maxibolin, Elix., Tab. (Organon).
Nandrobolic, Vial (Forest Pharm).
Ora-Testryl, Tab. (Squibb).
Os-Cal-Mone, Tab. (Marion).
Winstrol, Tab. (Winthrop Pharm).
W/Vitamins and minerals.
See: Dumogran, Tab. (Squibb).

ANABOLIN. (Alto) Nandrolone phenpropionate 50 mg, benzyl alcohol 2%, sesame oil q.s./ml. Vial 2 ml.
Use: Anabolic steroid.

ANABOLIN-IM. (Alto) Nandrolone phenpropionate 50 mg, benzyl alcohol 2%, sesame oil q.s./ml. Vial 2 ml.
Use: Anabolic steroid.

ANABOLIN LA-100. (Alto) Nandrolone decanoate 100 mg/ml. Vial 2 ml.
Use: Anabolic, steroid.

ANACAINE. (Gordon) Benzocaine 10%. Jar oz, lb.
Use: Local anesthetic.

ANACIN TABLETS. (Whitehall) Aspirin 400 mg, caffeine 32 mg. **Tab.:** Tin 12s, bot. 30s, 50s, 100s, 200s. **Cap.:** Bot. 30s, 50s, 100s.
Use: Analgesic.

ANACIN MAXIMUM STRENGTH. (Whitehall) Aspirin 500 mg, caffeine 32 mg/Tab. Bot. 12s, 20s, 24s, 40s, 72s, 150s.
Use: Analgesic.

ANACIN-3 CHILDREN'S. (Whitehall) Acetaminophen. **Elix.:** 160 mg/5 ml Bot. 2 oz, 4 oz. **Chew. tab:** 80 mg/Tab. Bot. 30s.
Use: Analgesic.

ANACIN-3 INFANTS. (Whitehall) Acetaminophen 100 mg/ml. Soln. Bot. 0.5 oz.
Use: Analgesic.

ANACIN-3 MAXIMUM STRENGTH. (Whitehall) Acetaminophen 500 mg. **Tab or Cap.:** Tin 12s, bot. 24s, 30s, 60s, 100s.
Use: Analgesic.

ANACIN-3 REGULAR STRENGTH. (Whitehall) Acetaminophen 325 mg/Tab. Bot. 24s, 50s, 100s.
Use: Analgesic.

ANADROL-50. (Syntex) Oxymetholone 50 mg/Tab. Bot. 100s.
Use: Anabolic steroid.

ANAFEBRINA.
See: Aminopyrine (Various Mfr.).

ANAFER. (British Drug House) Ferrous sulfate 200 mg, vitamin C 10 mg, menadione as diacetyl derivative 1.5 mg/Tab. Bot. 100s, 1000s.
Use: Vitamin/mineral supplement.

ANAFRANIL. (Ciba) Clomipramine HCl 25 mg, 50 mg or 75 mg/Cap. Bot. 100s, UD 100s.
Use: Antidepressant.

ANAGESTONE ACETATE. USAN. 17-Hydroxy-6α-methylpregn-4-en-20-one acetate.
Use: Progestin.
See: Anatropin (Ortho).

ANAGRELIDE HYDROCHLORIDE. USAN.
Use: Antithrombotic.

ANAIDS. (Forest) Calcium carbonate 300 mg, sodium phenobarbital 9 mg/Tab. Bot. 1000s.
Use: Antacid combination.

ANA-KIT. (Hollister-Stier) Syringe which allows administration of epinephrine 1:1000 in 1 ml; four Chlo-amine tablets, each 2 mg chlorpheniramine maleate; two sterilized swabs, tourniquet, instructions/kit.
Use: Emergency kit.

ANALBALM IMPROVED FORMULA. (Central) Methyl salicylate 10%, menthol 1.25%, camphor 3%. Liq. Bot. **Green**: 4 oz, gal. **Pink:** 4 oz, pt, gal.
Use: Counter-irritant.

ANALEPTICS. Usually a term applied to agents with stimulant action, particularly on the central nervous system. See also central nervous system stimulants.
See: Amphetamine salts (Various Mfr.).
Caffeine (Various Mfr.).
Cylert, Tab. (Abbott).
Dextroamphetamine salts (Various Mfr.).
Dopram, Vial (Robins).
Ephedrine Salts (Various Mfr.).
Methamphetamine salts (Various Mfr.).
Ritalin HCl, Tab. (Ciba).
Sodium Succinate (Various Mfr.).

ANALGESIC BALM. (Various Mfr.) Menthol w/ methyl salicylate in a suitable base.
Use: Counter-irritant.
A.P.C., 1.5 oz, lb.
Fougera, oz.
Horton & Converse, oz, lb.
Lilly, oz.
Musterole (Plough).
Stanlabs, oz, pt.
Wisconsin, 1 lb, 5 lb.

ANALGESIC LIQUID. (Weeks & Leo) Triethanolamine salicylate 20% in an alcohol base. Bot. 4 oz.
Use: External analgesic.

ANALGESIC LOTION. (Weeks & Leo) Methyl nicotinate 1%, methyl salicylate 10%, camphor 0.1%, menthol 0.1%. Bot. 4 oz.
Use: External analgesic.

ANALGESIC OINTMENT "LANNETT". (Lannett) Camphor, menthol syn., methyl salicylate in lanolin petrolatum base. Tube oz, Jar 1 lb, 5 lb.
Use: External analgesic.

ANALGESICS.
See preparations of: Acetanilid-type, Antipyrine-type, Aspirin, Salicylamide.

ANALGIC-C. (Kenyon) Salicylamide 250 mg, acetaminophen 250 mg, ascorbic acid 25 mg/Tab. Bot. 100s, 1000s.
Use: Analgesic combination.

ANALPRAM-HC. (Ferndale Labs) Hydrocortisone acetate 1%, pramoxine HCl 1%. Cream Tube 30 Gm.
Use: Topical corticosteroid, local anesthetic.

ANALUCIN. (Lincoln) Pentetrazol 100 mg/ml. Vial 10 ml.
Use: Senile confusion.

ANALVAL TABLETS. (Vale) Aspirin 227 mg, acetaminophen 162 mg, caffeine 32 mg/Tab. Bot. 1000s.
Use: Analgesic combination.

ANAMINE. (Mayrand) Pseudoephedrine HCl 30 mg, chlorpheniramine maleate 2 mg/5 ml. Syr. Bot. 473 ml.
Use: Decongestant, antihistamine.

ANAMINE HD SYRUP. (Mayrand) Phenylephrine HCl 5 mg, chlorpheniramine maleate 2 mg, hydrocodone bitartrate 1.67 mg. 10 ml tid or qid.
Use: Decongestant, antihistamine, antitussive.

ANAMINE T.D. CAPSULES. (Mayrand) Chlorpheniramine maleate 8 mg, pseudoephedrine HCl 120 mg/T.D. Cap. Bot. 100s.
Use: Antihistamine, decongestant.

ANAPROX. (Syntex) Naproxen sodium 275 mg (naproxen base 250 mg with sodium 25 mg)/Tab. Bot. 100s, 500s, Blister pkg. 100s.
Use: Nonsteroidal anti-inflammatory agent.

ANAPROX DS. (Syntex) Naproxen sodium 550 mg (naproxen base 500 mg with sodium 50 mg)/Tab. Bot. 100s.
Use: Nonsteroidal anti-inflammatory agent.

ANAREL. Guanadrel sulfate.

•**ANARITIDE ACETATE.** USAN.
Use: Antihypertensive, diuretic.

ANAROL. (Kenyon) Acetaminophen 120 mg/5 ml. Bot. 4 oz.
Use: Analgesic.

ANASPAZ. (Ascher) l-Hyoscyamine sulfate 0.125 mg/Tab. Bot. 100s, 500s.
Use: Anticholinergic, antispasmodic.

ANATUSS SYRUP. (Mayrand) Dextromethorphan HBr 15 mg, phenylpropanolamine HCl 25 mg, guaifenesin 100 mg/10 ml. Bot. 120 ml, 480 ml.
Use: Antitussive, decongestant, expectorant.

ANATUSS TABS. (Mayrand) Guaifenesin 100 mg, acetaminophen 325 mg, dextromethorphan HBr 15 mg, phenylpropanolamine HCl 25 mg/Tab. Bot. 100s, 500s.
Use: Expectorant, analgesic, antitussive, decongestant.

ANATUSS W/CODEINE. (Mayrand) **Syr.:** Phenylpropanolamine HCl 25 mg, codeine phosphate 10 mg, guaifenesin 100 mg/5 ml. Bot. 120 ml, 480 ml. **Tab.:** Phenylpropanolamine HCl 25 mg, codeine phosphate 10 mg, guaifenesin 100 mg, acetaminophen 300 mg. Bot. 100s.
Use: Decongestant, antitussive, expectorant, analgesic (Tab.).

ANAVAR. (Searle) Oxandrolone 2.5 mg/Tab. Bot. 100s.
Use: Anabolic steroid.

ANAYODIN.
See: Chiniofon.

•**ANAZOLENE SODIUM.** USAN. 4-[(4-Anilino-5-sulfo-1-naphthyl)azo]-5-hydroxy-2,7-naphthalenedisulfonic acid trisodium salt. (2) C.I. acid blue 92 trisodium salt. Sodium Anoxynaphthonate. B.A.N.
Use: Diagnostic aid.
See: Coomassie Blue (Wyeth-Ayerst).

ANBESOL BABY GEL. (Whitehall) Benzocaine 7.5%. Tube 0.25 oz.
Use: Local anesthetic.

ANBESOL GEL. (Whitehall) Benzocaine 6.3%, phenol 0.5%, alcohol 70%. Tube 7.2 Gm.
Use: Local anesthetic, topical combination.

ANBESOL LIQUID. (Whitehall) Benzocaine 6.3%, phenol 0.5%, povidone-iodine 0.04%, alcohol 70%. Bot. 9 ml, 22 ml.
Use: Local anesthetic topical combination.

ANCEF. (SmithKline) Cefazolin sodium. **Vial:** Equivalent to 250 mg, 500 mg or 1 Gm of cefazolin. **Multi Pack:** 500 mg or 1 Gm/Pack. 25s. **Bulk Vial:** 5 Gm, 10 Gm. **Piggyback Vial:** 500 mg or 1 Gm/100 ml. **Minibag:** 1 Gm/50 ml w/ 5% dextrose inj. (D5W). 500 mg/50 ml D5W.
Use: Antibacterial, cephalosporin.

ANCID TABLET AND SUSPENSION. (Sheryl) Calcium aluminum carbonate, di-amino acetate complex. Tab. 100s. Susp. pt.
Use: Antacid.

ANCOBON. (Roche) Flucytosine 250 mg or 500 mg/Cap. Bot. 100s.
Use: Anti-infective.

•**ANCROD.** USAN. An active principle obtained from the venom of the Malayan pit viper *Agkistrodon rhodostoma*.
Use: Anticoagulant.
See: Arvin.

ANDESTERONE SUSPENSION. (Lincoln) Estrone 2 mg, testosterone 6 mg/ml. Vial 15 ml. **Forte:** Estrone 1 mg, testosterone 20 mg/ml. Inj. Vial 15 ml.
Use: Estrogen, androgen combination.

ANDREST 90-4. (Seatrace) Testosterone enanthate 90 mg, estradiol valerate 4 mg/ml. Vial 10 ml.
Use: Androgen, estrogen combination.

ANDRO 100. (Forest) Testosterone 100 mg/ml. Vial 10 ml.
Use: Androgen.

ANDROCUR. Cyproterone acetate (Orphan Drug).
Use: Hirsutism, severe.
Sponsor: Berlex.

ANDRO-CYP 100. (Keene) Testosterone cypionate 100 mg/ml. Vial 10 ml.
Use: Androgen.

ANDRO-CYP 200. (Keene) Testosterone cypionate 200 mg/ml. Vial 10 ml.
Use: Androgen.

ANDRO-ESTRO 90-4. (Rugby) Estradiol valerate 4 mg, testosterone enanthate 90 mg/ml with chlorobutanol in sesame oil. Inj. Vial. 10 ml.
Use: Estrogen, androgen combination.

ANDRO FEM. (Pasadena Research) Testosterone cypionate 50 mg, estradiol cypionate 2 mg, chlorobutanol 0.5%, cottonseed oil/ml. Vial 10 ml.
Use: Androgen, estrogen combination.

ANDROGENS. Substances which possess masculinizing activities.
See: Methyltestosterone.
Testosterone.
Testosterone cyclopentylpropionate.
Testosterone enanthate.
Testosterone heptanoate.
Testosterone phenylacetate.
Testosterone propionate.

ANDROGEN-ESTROGEN THERAPY.
See: Dienestrol with Methyltestosterone.
Estradiol Esters with Methyltestosterone.

Estradiol Esters with Testosterone.
Estrogenic Substance, Conjugated with Methyltestosterone.
Estrogenic Substance Mixed with Methyltestosterone.
Estrogenic Substance Mixed with Testosterone.
Estrone with Testosterone.
Gynetone, Tab. (Schering).

ANDROGYN L.A. (Forest) Testosterone enanthate 90 mg, estradiol valerate 4 mg/ml in sesame oil. Vial 10 ml.
Use: Androgen, estrogen combination.

ANDROID-5, 10 and 25. (Brown) Methyltestosterone 5 mg/Buccal Tab., 10 mg/Tab. or 25 mg/Tab. Bot. 60s.
Use: Androgen.

ANDROID-F. (Brown) Fluoxymesterone 10 mg/Tab. Bot. 60s.
Use: Androgen.

ANDRO L.A. 200. (Forest) Testosterone enanthate 200 mg/ml. Vial 10 ml.
Use: Androgen.

ANDROLAN AQUEOUS. (Lannett) Testosterone 25 mg, 50 mg or 100 mg/ml. Susp. Vial 10 ml.
Use: Androgen.

ANDROLAN IN OIL. (Lannett) Testosterone propionate 25 mg, 50 mg or 100 mg/ml in oil. Vial 10 ml.
Use: Androgen.

ANDROLIN. (Lincoln) Testosterone 100 mg/ml. Vial 10 ml.
Use: Androgen.

ANDROLONE. (Keene) Nandrolone phenpropionate 25 mg/ml in sesame oil. Vial 5 ml.
Use: Anabolic steroid.

ANDRONAQ-50. (Central) Testosterone 50 mg/ml, sodium carboxymethylcellulose, methylcellulose, povidone, DSS, thimerosal. Inj. Vial. 10 ml.
Use: Androgen.

ANDRONAQ LA. (Central) Testosterone cypionate 100 mg, benzyl alcohol 0.9% in cottonseed oil. Vial 10 ml. Bot. 12s.
Use: Androgen.

ANDRONATE 100. (Pasadena Research) Testosterone cypionate 100 mg/ml with benzyl alcohol in cottonseed oil. Vial 10 ml.
Use: Androgen.

ANDRONATE 200. (Pasadena Research) Testosterone cypionate 200 mg/ml with benzyl alcohol, benzyl benzoate in cottonseed oil. Vial 10 ml.
Use: Androgen.

ANDRONE. (Rocky Mtn.) Testosterone 25 mg, estrone 2 mg/ml. Vial 10 ml.
Use: Androgen, estrogen combination.

ANDROPOSITORY 100. (Rugby) Testosterone enanthate 100 mg/ml in sesame oil with chlorobutanol. Inj. Vial 10 ml.
Use: Androgen.

ANDROSTANAZOLE.
See: Stanozolol.

ANDROSTANE-17-(beta)-ol-3-one.
See: Stanolone.

ANDROSTANOLONE. (I.N.N.) Stanolone.

ANDROSTENOPYRAZOLE. Anabolic steroid; pending release.

ANDROTEST P.
See: Testosterone propionate.

ANDRYL 200. (Keene) Testosterone enanthate 200 mg/ml. Vial 10 ml.
Use: Androgen.

ANDYLATE FORTE. (Vita Elixir) Acetaminophen 3 gr, salicylamide 3 gr, caffeine 0.25 gr/Tab.
Use: Analgesic combination.

ANDYLATE RUB. (Vita Elixir) Methylnicotinate, methylsalicylate, camphor, dipropyleneglycol salicylate, oil of cassia, oleoresin of capsicum, oleoresin of ginger.
Use: External analgesic.

ANDYLATE TABLETS. (Vita Elixir) Sodium salicylate 10 gr/Tab.
Use: Salicylate analgesic.

ANECAL CREAM. (Lannett) Benzocaine 3%, calamine 5%, zinc oxide 5%. Jar lb.
Use: Local anesthetic, antiseptic, skin protectant.

ANECTINE. (Burroughs Wellcome) Succinylcholine Cl. Soln. 20 mg/ml. Multidose Vial 10 ml. Sterile Pow. Flo-Pak 500 mg or 1000 mg. Box 12s.
Use: Muscle relaxant.

ANEFRIN NASAL SPRAY, LONG ACTING. (Walgreen) Oxymetazoline HCl 0.05%. Bot. 0.5 oz.
Use: Nasal decongestant.

ANELEP-O.D. (Trimen) Phenytoin 250 mg/Cap. Bot. 100s.
Use: Anticonvulsant.

ANERGAN 25. (Forest) Promethazine HCl 25 mg/ml. Vial 10 ml.
Use: Antihistamine.

ANERGAN 50. (Forest) Promethazine HCl 50 mg/ml. Vial 10 ml.
Use: Antihistamine.

ANERTAN.
See: Testosterone propionate.

ANESTACON. (Webcon) Lidocaine HCl 20 mg/ml. Bot. 15 ml, 240 ml.
Use: Local anesthetic.

ANESTHESIN. Ethyl-p-aminobenzoate.
Use: Local anesthetic.
See: Benzocaine, U.S.P. XXII.

ANETHAINE.
See: Tetracaine HCl.

•**ANETHOLE,** N.F. XVII. p-Propenylanisole. Benzene, 1-methoxy-4-(1-propenyl).
Use: Flavor.

ANEURINE HYDROCHLORIDE.
See: Thiamine HCl, Preps. (Various Mfr.).

ANEXSIA. (Beecham Labs) Hydrocodone bitartrate 5 mg, acetaminophen 500 mg/Tab. Bot. 100s, 1000s.

Use: Narcotic analgesic combination.
ANEXSIA 7.5. (Beecham Labs). Hydrocodone bitartrate 7.5 mg, acetaminophen 650 mg/Tab. Bot. 100s, 1000s.
Use: Narcotic analgesic combination.
ANGEL SWEET. (Garrett) Vitamins A and D_2. Cream 90 Gm.
Use: Skin protectant.
ANGEN. (Davis & Sly) Estrone 2 mg, testosterone 25 mg/ml Aqueous susp. Vial 10 ml.
Use: Estrogen, androgen combination.
ANGERIN. (Kingsbay) Nitroglycerin 1 mg/Cap. Bot. 60s.
Use: Coronary vasodilator.
ANGEX. (Janssen) Lidoflazine.
Use: Coronary vasodilator.
ANGIJEN GREEN. (Jenkins) Pentaerythritol tetranitrate 10 mg or 20 mg/Tab. Bot. 1000s.
Use: Antianginal.
ANGIJEN S.C. SALMON. (Jenkins) Pentaerythritol tetranitrate 10 mg, phenobarbital 8 mg/Tab. Bot. 1000s.
Use: Antianginal, sedative/hypnotic.
ANGIJEN NO. 1. (Jenkins) Pentaerythritol tetranitrate 20 mg, phenobarbital 15 mg/Tab. Bot. 1000s.
Use: Antianginal, sedative/hypnotic.
ANGIL. (Kenyon) Pentaerythritol tetranitrate 10 mg, mephobarbital 0.25 gr, phenobarbital 1/8 gr/Tab. Bot. 100s, 1000s.
Use: Antianginal, sedative/hypnotic.
ANGIO-CONRAY. (Mallinckrodt) Iothalamate sodium 80% (48% iodine), EDTA. Inj. Vial 50 ml.
Use: Radiopaque agent.
•**ANGIOTENSIN AMIDE.** USAN. 1-L-asparaginyl-5-L-valyl angiotensin octapeptide. 1L-asparagine-5-L-Valine angiotensin.
Use: Vasoconstrictor.
See: Hypertensin (Ciba).
ANGIOTENSIN CONVERTING ENZYME INHIBITORS.
Use: Antihypertensive.
See: Altace (Hoechst-Roussel)
Capoten, Tab. (Squibb).
Prinivil, Tab. (MSD).
Vasotec, Tab. (MSD).
Vasotec I.V., Inj. (MSD).
Zestril, Tab. (Stuart).
ANGIOVIST 282. (Berlex) Diatrizoate meglumine 60% (iodine 28%).
Vial 50 ml, 100 ml or 150 ml. Box 10s.
Use: Radiopaque agent.
ANGIOVIST 292. (Berlex) Diatrizoate meglumine 52%, diatrizoate sodium 8% (iodine 29.2%).
Vial 30 ml, 50 ml or 100 ml. Box 10s.
Use: Radiopaque agent.
ANGIOVIST 370. (Berlex) Diatrizoate meglumine 66%, diatrizoate sodium 10%, (iodine 37%).
Vial 50 ml, 100 ml, 150 ml or 200 ml. Box 10s.
Use: Radiopaque agent.
ANHYDROHYDROXYPROGESTERONE. Ethisterone.
•**ANIDOXIME.** USAN. 3-Diethylaminopropiophenone-O-(p-methoxyphenylcarbamoyl)oxime.
Use: Analgesic.
See: Bamoxine (U.S.V. Pharm.).
A-NIL. (Vangard) Codeine phosphate 10 mg, bromodiphenhydramine HCl 3.75 mg, diphenhydramine HCl 8.75 mg, ammonium Cl 80 mg, potassium guaiacolsulfonate 80 mg, menthol 0.5 mg/5 ml, alcohol 5%. Bot. pt. gal.
Use: Antitussive, expectorant.
•**ANILERIDINE HCl,** U.S.P. XXII. Tab., U.S.P. XXII. 1-(4-aminophenethyl)-4-phenylisonipecotic acid ethyl ester.
Use: Analgesic.
See: Leritine HCl, Tab. (Merck Sharp & Dohme).
•**ANILOPAM HYDROCHLORIDE.** USAN.
Use: Analgesic.
ANION EXCHANGE RESINS.
See: Polyamine-Methylene Resin.
•**ANIRACETAM.** USAN.
Use: Mental performance enhancer.
•**ANIROLAC.** USAN.
Use: Anti-inflammatory, analgesic.
•**ANISE OIL,** N.F. XVII.
Use: Flavor.
ANISINDIONE.
See: Miradon (Schering).
ANISOPYRADAMINE.
See: Pyrilamine Maleate.
•**ANISOTROPINE.** F.D.A. Tropine 2-propylvalerate.
•**ANISOTROPINE METHYLBROMIDE.** USAN. Octatropine Methylbromide, B.A.N. 2-Propylpentanoyl tropinium methylbromide. 8-Methyltropinium bromide 2 Propylvalerate.
Use: Anticholinergic.
See: Valpin 50, Tab. (Du Pont).
•**ANISTREPLASE.** USAN.
Use: Fibrinolytic, thrombolytic.
See: Eminase (Beecham).
•**ANITRAZAFEN.** USAN.
Use: Anti-inflammatory.
ANOCAINE. (Mallard) Benzocaine, zinc oxide, bismuth subgallate, balsam Peru in a vegetable oil base. Supp. Box 12s.
Use: Local anesthetic.
ANODYNINE. Antipyrine (Orphan Drug).
ANODYNON.
See: Ethyl Cl.
ANODYNOS. (Buffington) Aspirin 420.6 mg, salicylamide 34.4 mg caffeine 34.4 mg/Tab. Sugar, lactose and salt free. Dispens-A-Kit 500s, Bot. 100s, 500s, Medipak 200s.
Use: Analgesic combination.
ANODYNOS-DHC TABLETS. (Forest) Hydrocodone bitartrate 5 mg, acetaminophen 500 mg/Tab. Bot. 100s.
Use: Narcotic analgesic combination.
ANODYNOS FORTE. (Buffington) Chlorpheniramine maleate, phenylephrine HCl, salicylamide, acetaminophen, caffeine/Tab. Sugar, lac-

tose and salt free. Dispens-A-Kit 500s, Bot. 100s.
Use: Antihistamine, decongestant, analgesic.

ANOQUAN. (Mallard) Butalbital 50 mg, caffeine 40 mg, acetaminophen 325 mg/Cap. Bot. 100s, 1000s.
Use: Sedative/hypnotic, analgesic.

ANOREX. (Dunhall) Phendimetrazine 35 mg/Tab. Bot. 100s.
Use: Anorexiant.

ANOREXIGENIC AGENTS. Appetite depressants.
See: Amphetamine Preps.
Didrex, Tab. (Upjohn).
Plegine, Tab. (Wyeth-Ayerst).
Preludin HCl (Boehringer Ingelheim).
Sanorex, Tab. (Sandoz).
Tenuate (Merrell Dow).
Tepanil, Tab. (Riker).
Wilpo, Tab. (Dorsey).

ANOVLAR. Norethindrone plus ethinyl estradiol.
Use: Oral contraceptive.

•**ANOXOMER.** USAN.
Use: Pharmaceutic aid.

ANOXYNAPHTHONATE SODIUM. Anazolene Sodium.

ANSAID. (Upjohn) Flurbiprofen 50 mg or 100 mg. Tab. 100s, 500s, UD 100s.
Use: Nonsteroidal anti-inflammatory agent.

ANSPOR. (SmithKline) Cephradine (a semisynthetic cephalosporin) **Cap.:** 250 mg. Bot. 100s, UD 100s; 500 mg. Bot. 20s, 100s, UD 100s. **Oral Susp.:** 125 mg or 250 mg/5 ml. Bot. 100 ml.
Use: Antibacterial, cephalosporin.

ANSWER. (Carter Products) Reagent in-home pregnancy test kit for urine testing. Test kit box 1s.
Use: Diagnostic aid.

ANSWER 2. (Carter Products) Reagent in-home pregnancy test kit for urine testing. Test kit box 2s.
Use: Diagnostic aid.

ANSWER PLUS. (Carter Products) Reagent in-home pregnancy test kit for urine testing. Test kit box 1s.
Use: Diagnostic aid.

ANSWER PLUS 2. (Carter Products) Reagent in-home pregnancy test kit for urine testing. Test kit box 2s.
Use: Diagnostic aid.

ANTABUSE. (Wyeth-Ayerst) Disulfiram. **250 mg/Tab.** Bot. 100s; **500 mg/Tab.** Bot. 50s, 1000s.
Use: Antialcoholic agent.

ANTACID. (Walgreen) Calcium carbonate 500 mg/Tab. Bot. 75s.
Use: Antacid.

ANTACID #2. (Richlyn) Calcium carbonate 5.5 gr, magnesium carbonate 2.5 gr/Tab. Bot. 100s.
Use: Antacid.

ANTACID M LIQUID. (Walgreen) Aluminum oxide 225 mg, magnesium hydroxide 200 mg/5 ml. Bot. 12 oz, 26 oz.
Use: Antacid.

ANTACID NO. 6. (Bowman) Calcium carbonate 0.42 Gm, glycine 0.18 Gm/Tab. Bot. 100s.
Use: Antacid.

ANTACID RELIEF TABLETS. (Walgreen) Dihydroxyaluminum sodium carbonate 334 mg/Tab. Bot. 75s.
Use: Antacid.

ANTACIDS. Drugs that neutralize excess gastric acid.
See: Alka-Seltzer, Tab. (Miles).
Alka-Seltzer Plus, Tab. (Miles).
Alka-Seltzer Special Effervescent Antacid, Tab.(Miles).
Alka-2 Chewable Antacid, Tab. (Miles).
Aluminum Hydroxide Gel (Various Mfr.).
Aluminum Hydroxide Gel w/Combinations (Various Mfr.).
Aluminum Hydroxide Gel Dried (Various Mfr.).
Aluminum Hydroxide Gel Dried w/Combinations (Various Mfr.).
Aluminum Hydroxide Magnesium Carbonate, Tab. (Various Mfr.).
Aluminum Phosphate Gel (Wyeth-Ayerst).
Aluminum Proteinate, Tab. (Reid-Rowell).
Amitone, Tab. (Smith-Kline Beecham).
Calcium Carbonate, Precipitated (Various Mfr.).
Calcium Carbonate Tab. (Various Mfr.).
Carbamine (Key Pharm.).
Ceo-Two, Supp. (Beutlich).
Chooz, Gum Tab. (Schering-Plough).
Citrocarbonate, Liq. (Upjohn).
Dicarbosil, Tab. (Arch).
Di-Gel, Liq., Tab. (Schering-Plough).
Dihydroxyaluminum Aminoacetate (Various Mfr.).
Dihydroxyaluminum Sodium Carbonate Tab. (Warner-Lambert).
Magaldrate, Tab., Susp. (Wyeth-Ayerst).
Magnesium Carbonate (Various Mfr.).
Magnesium Glycinate, Tab. (Various Mfr.).
Magnesium Hydroxide (Various Mfr.).
Magnesium Oxide, Tab., Cap. (Various Mfr.).
Magnesium Trisilicate (Various Mfr.).
Neutralox, Susp. (Lemmon).
Oxaine, Susp. (Wyeth-Ayerst).
Ratio, Tab. (Adria).
Rolaids, Tab. (Warner-Lambert).
Romach, Tab. (ROR Pharmacal).
Sodium Bicarbonate, Inj., Tab. (Various Mfr.).
Tums, Tab. (Smith-Kline Beeecham).

ANTACID SPECIAL NO. 1. (Jenkins) Magnesium carbonate 3 gr, calcium carbonate 2 gr, bismuth subcarbonate 1 gr, cerium oxalate 0.5 gr/Tab. Bot. 1000s.
Use: Antacid.

ANTACID W/PHENOBARBITAL. (Archer-Taylor) Magnesium hydroxide 0.3 Gm, calcium carbon-

ate 9.3 Gm, atropine 0.2 mg, phenobarbital 8 mg/Tab. Bot. 1000s.
Use: Antacid, sedative/hypnotic.

ANTA-GEL. (Halsey) Aluminum hydroxide 200 mg, magnesium hydroxide 200 mg, simethicone 20 mg/5 ml. Bot. 12 oz.
Use: Antacid, antiflatulent.

ANTA-GEL II. (Halsey) Aluminum hydroxide 400 mg, magnesium hydroxide 400 mg, simethicone 30 mg/5 ml. Bot. 12 oz.
Use: Antacid, antiflatulent.

ANTAGONISTS OF CURARIFORM DRUGS.
See: Neostigmine Methylsulfate.
Tensilon Cl (Roche).

ANTASTAN.
See: Antazoline Hydrochloride, U.S.P. XXII.

ANTAZOLINE. B.A.N. N-Phenylbenzylamino-methyl-2-imidazoline.
Use: Antihistamine.

ANTAZOLINE HYDROCHLORIDE. Antastan. 2(N-Benzylanilinomethyl)-2-imidazoline HCl.
See: Arithmin, Tab. (Lannett).

•**ANTAZOLINE PHOSPHATE,** U.S.P. XXII. 2-[(N-Benzylanilino)methyl]-2-imidazoline dihydrogen phosphate.
Use: Antihistamine.
See: Arithmin, Inj. (Lannett).
W/Naphazoline, boric acid, phenylmercuric acetate, sodium Cl, sodium carbonate anhydrous.
See: Vasocon-A Ophthalmic, Soln. (Smith, Miller & Patch).
W/Naphazoline HCl, polyvinyl alcohol.
See: Albalon-A Liquifilm, Ophth. Soln. (Allergan).

ANTERIOR PITUITARY.
See: Pituitary, Anterior.

ANTHELMINTIC. A remedy for worms.
See: Antiminth, Susp. (Roerig).
Atabrine, Tab. (Winthrop Pharm).
Betanaphthol Benzoate (Various Mfr.).
Biltricide, Tab. (Miles Pharm).
Carbon Tetrachloride (Various Mfr.).
Gentian Violet (Various Mfr.).
Jayne's PW Vermifuge (Glenbrook).
Jayne's RW, Tab. (Glenbrook).
Mintezol, Tab., Susp. (Merck Sharp & Dohme).
Niclocide, Chew. tab. (Miles Pharm.).
Piperazine Preps. (Various Mfr.).
Povan, Tab., Susp. (Parke-Davis).
Terramycin (Various Mfr.).
Tetrachloroethylene.
Vansil, Cap. (Pfipharmecs).
Vermox, Chew tab., Oral Susp. (MSD).

•**ANTHELMYCIN.** USAN.
Use: Anthelmintic.

ANTHELVET. Tetramisole HCl.

ANTHRA-DERM. (Dermik) Anthralin 0.1%, 0.25%, 0.5% or 1% in petrolatum ointment base. Tube 1.5 oz.
Use: Antipsoriatic.

•**ANTHRALIN,** U.S.P. XXII. Cream, Oint., U.S.P. XXII. 1,8,9-Anthracenetriol. Cignolin, Dithranol, Dihydroxy-Anthranol.
Use: Treatment of psoriasis.
See: Anthra-Derm Oint. (Dermik)
Lasan, Cream (Stiefel)
W/Mineral oil.
See: Lasan Pomade (Stiefel).

ANTHRALIN PASTE 0.2%. (Durel) Anthralin 0.2%, salicylic acid 0.2%, paraffin 5%, Lassar's paste q.s. Jar oz, lb.
Use: Enzyme metabolism inhibitor.

ANTHRALIN POMADE 0.4%. (Durel) Anthralin 0.4%, salicylic acid 0.4%, sodium lauryl sulfate 2.1%, cetyl alcohol 21.9%, mineral oil q.s. Bot. 1 oz, 4 oz.
Use: Enzyme metabolism inhibitor.

•**ANTHRAMYCIN.** USAN.
Use: Antineoplastic agent.

ANTHRAQUINONE OF CASCARA.
See: Cascara Sagrada, Prods.

ANTIACID. (Hillcrest North) Aluminum hydroxide, magnesium trisilicate, calcium carbonate/Tab. Bot. 100s.
Use: Antacid.

ANTI-ALLERGY CAPSULES. (Robinson) Phenylephrine HCl 2.5 mg, phenylpropanolamine HCl 25 mg, pyrilamine maleate 10 mg, chlorpheniramine maleate 2 mg, phenylpyridine HCl 10 mg/Cap. Bot. 100s, 1000s.
Use: Decongestant, antihistamine.

ANTI-ALLERGY TABLET. (Walgreen) Phenylpropanolamine HCl 18.7 mg, chlorpheniramine maleate 2 mg/Tab. Bot. 24s.
Use: Decongestant, antihistamine.

ANTIASTHMATIC COMBINATIONS.
See: Cromolyn Sodium, Cap. (Various Mfr.).
Decadron Respihaler, Aerosol. (Merck Sharp & Dohme).
Ephedrine HCl (Various Mfr.).
Ephedrine Sulfate (Various Mfr.).
Isoephedrine HCl (Various Mfr.).
Isoetharine (Winthrop Pharm).
Isoetharine HCl (Winthrop Pharm).
Isoetharine Mesylate (Winthrop Pharm).
Isoproterenol HCl (Various Mfr.).
Isoproterenol Sulfate (Various Mfr.).
Methoxyphenamine HCl (Various Mfr.).
Phenylephrine HCl (Various Mfr.).
Phenylpropanolamine HCl (Various Mfr.).
Pseudoephedrine HCl (Various Mfr.).
Racephedrine HCl (Various Mfr.).

ANTIASTHMATIC INHALANT.
See: AsthmaHaler (Smith-Kline Beecham).
AsthmaNefrin, Soln. (Smith-Kline Beecham).

ANTIBACTERIAL SERUMS.
See: Hypertussis Serum.
Influenzae Antihaemophilus Type B Serum.

ANTIBASON.
See: Methylthiouracil (Various Mfr.).

ANTIBIOTICS.
See: Amoxicillin (Various Mfr.).

Amphotericin B (Squibb).
Ampicillin (Various Mfr.).
Ampicillin Sodium (Various Mfr.).
Ampicillin Trihydrate (Various Mfr.).
Anspor, Cap., Susp. (SmithKline).
Bacitracin (Various Mfr.).
Benzathine Penicillin G (Various Mfr.).
Carbenicillin Indanyl Sodium, Tab. (Roerig).
Cefadroxil (Bristol, Mead Johnson).
Cefazolin Sodium, Vial (Various Mfr.).
Ceftin, Tabs. (Glaxo).
Cephalexin (Lilly).
Cephalexin Monohydrate, Pulv., Susp. (Lilly).
Cephalothin, Sodium, Vial (Lilly).
Ceptaz, Inj. (Glaxo).
Chloramphenicol (Various Mfr.).
Chloramphenicol Sodium Succinate, Inj. (Various Mfr.).
Clindamycin (Upjohn).
Cloxapen, Cap. (Beecham Labs).
Colistimethate Sodium, Inj. (Parke-Davis).
Colistin Sulfate, Ophth., Susp. (Various Mfr.).
Demeclocycline (Lederle).
Demethylchlortetracycline HCl (Lederle).
Dicloxacillin, Cap., Susp. (Various Mfr.).
Doxycycline (Various Mfr.).
Duricef, Cap. (Mead Johnson).
Erythromycin (Various Mfr.).
Erythromycin Ethylsuccinate (Abbott, Ross).
Erythromycin Lactobionate for Inj. (Abbott).
Erythromycin Stearate, Tab. (Various Mfr.).
Flucytosine, Cap. (Roche).
Fortaz, Inj. (Glaxo).
Gentamicin Sulfate (Schering-Plough).
Griseofulvin, Tab., Susp. (Various Mfr.).
Griseofulvin Microcrystalline, Tab., Cap. (Various Mfr.).
Kanamycin Sulfate, Cap., Inj. (Bristol-Myers).
Ledercillin VK, Prods. (Lederle).
Lincomycin (Upjohn).
Mefoxin, Inj. (Merck Sharp & Dohme).
Methacycline HCl, Cap., Syr. (Wallace).
Methicillin Sodium, Vial, Pow. (Various Mfr.).
Minocycline, Cap. (Lederle).
Nafcillin Sodium, Vial, Cap., Pow. (Wyeth-Ayerst).
Nalidixic Acid, N.F.
NegGram, Prods. (Winthrop Pharm).
Neomycin Sulfate, Tab., Soln. (Various Mfr.).
Novobiocin (Various Mfr.).
Novobiocin Calcium (Upjohn).
Novobiocin Sodium, Cap. (Upjohn).
Nystatin (Various Mfr.).
Oxacillin, Sodium (Various Mfr.).
Oxytetracycline (Pfizer).
Paromomycin, Cap., Syr. (Parke-Davis).
Penicillin G, Potassium (Various Mfr.).
Penicillin G, Potassium w/Comb. (Various Mfr.).
Penicillin G, Procaine (Various Mfr.).
Penicillin G, Procaine w/Comb. (Various Mfr.).
Penicillin G, Sodium (Various Mfr.).
Penicillin V Potassium (Various Mfr.).
Phenethicillin Potassium, Tab., Pow., Soln. (Various Mfr.).
Phenoxymethyl Penicillin (Various Mfr.).
Polymyxin B Sulfate (Various Mfr.).
Primaxin, Inj. (Merck Sharp & Dohme).
Rifampin, Cap. (Various Mfr.).
Seromycin, Pulv. (Lilly).
Sodium Cloxacillin, Cap., Soln. (Bristol-Myers)
Streptomycin Sulfate (Various Mfr.).
Tetracycline (Various Mfr.).
Tetracycline HCl (Various Mfr.).
Tetracycline Phosphate Complex (Various Mfr.).
Troleandomycin, Cap., Susp. (Various Mfr.).
Vancomycin HCl (Lilly).
Zinacef, Inj. (Glaxo).

ANTIBIOTICS, VETERINARY USE.
See: Oxytetracycline (Merck Animal Health).
Penstrep (Merck Animal Health).
Pro-Penstrep (Merck Animal Health).
Sulfastrep w/sulfonamides (Merck Animal Health).
Tresaderm w/thiabendazole, dexamethasone and neomycin (Merck Animal Health).
Vetstrep (Merck Animal Health).

ANTICHOLINERGIC AGENTS. Parasympatholytic agents.
See: Akineton (Knoll).
Antrenyl Bromide (Ciba).
Artane HCl (Lederle).
Atropine Preps.
Banthine Bromide (Searle).
Belladonna Preps.
Cantil Preps. (Merrell Dow).
Cogentin (Merck Sharp & Dohme).
Daricon, Tab. (Beecham Labs).
Dicyclomine HCl (Various Mfr.).
Disipal (Riker).
Donabarb Sr., Cap. (Elder).
Homatropine methylbromide.
Hybephen, Prods. (Beecham Labs).
Kemadrin, Tab. (Burroughs Wellcome).
Kinesed, Tab. (Stuart).
L-Hyoscyamine, Tab. (Kremers-Urban).
Murel, Amp. (Wyeth-Ayerst).
Norflex, Inj., Tab. (Riker).
Oxyphencyclimine HCl (Various Mfr.).
Pagitane HCl, Tab. (Lilly).
Pamine Bromide, Tab., Soln. (Upjohn).
Panparnit HCl.
Parsidol HCl, Tab. (Parke-Davis).
Pathilon (Lederle).
Phenoxene HCl (Marion Merrell Dow).
Prantal Methylsulfate, Tab. (Schering-Plough).
Pro-Banthine Bromide, Preps. (Searle).
Robinul, Tab., Inj. (Robins).
Scopolamine methylbromide.
Scopolamine methylbromide HBr.
Tral, Preps. (Abbott).
Trihexyphenidyl HCl (Various Mfr.).
Trocinate, Tab. (Poythress).
Valpin 50, Tab. (DuPont).

Valpin 50-PB, Tab. (DuPont).

•**ANTICOAGULANT CITRATE DEXTROSE SOLUTION,** U.S.P. XXII.
Use: Anticoagulant for storage of whole blood.
See: A.C.D. Solution. (Various Mfr.).

•**ANTICOAGULANT CITRATE PHOSPHATE DEXTROSE ADENINE SOLUTION,** U.S.P. XXII.
Use: Anticoagulant for storage of whole blood.

•**ANTICOAGULANT CITRATE PHOSPHATE DEXTROSE SOLUTION,** U.S.P. XXII.
Use: Anticoagulant for storage of whole blood.

•**ANTICOAGULANT HEPARIN SOLUTION,** U.S.P. XXII.
Use: Anticoagulant for storage of whole blood.

ANTICOAGULANTS.
See: Acenocoumarin.
Anisindione.
Bishydroxycoumarin (Various Mfr.).
Calciparine, Inj. (American Critical Care).
Coumadin, Amp., Tab. (DuPont).
Depo-Heparin, Sodium (Upjohn).
Dicumarol (Various Mfr.).
Dipaxin, Tab. (Upjohn).
Diphenadione.
Eridione, Tab. (Eric, Kirk & Gary).
Ethyl Biscoumacetate, Tab.
Hedulin, Tab. (Merrell Dow).
Heparin, Sodium (Various Mfr.).
Liquaemin Sodium, Vial (Organon).
Liquamar, Tab. (Organon).
Miradon, Tab. (Schering-Plough).
Panheprin, Amp., Vial (Abbott).
Panwarfin, Tab. (Abbott).
Phenindione, Tab. (Various Mfr.).
Warfarin (Various Mfr.).

•**ANTICOAGULANT SODIUM CITRATE SOLUTION,** U.S.P. XXII. Anticoagulant (plasma and blood, fractionation).

ANTICONVULSANTS. Agents that inhibit muscular spasms originating in the central nervous system.
See: Amytal Sodium, Amp. (Lilly).
Celontin, Cap. (Parke-Davis).
Depakene, Liq., Tab. (Abbott).
Dilantin, Preps. (Parke-Davis).
Gemonil, Tab. (Abbott).
Glutamic Acid (Various Mfr.).
Magnesium sulfate.
Mephobarbital.
Mesantoin, Tab. (Sandoz).
Milontin, Cap. (Parke-Davis).
Paradione, Cap., Soln. (Abbott).
Peganone, Tab. (Abbott).
Phenobarbital (Various Mfr.).
Phenurone, Tab. (Abbott).
Phenytoin, Susp., Tab. (Various Mfr.).
Phenytoin Sodium, Cap. (Various Mfr.).
Tegretol, Tab. (Geigy).
Tridione, Cap., Dulcet, Soln., Tab. (Abbott).
Valium, Tab. (Roche).
Zarontin, Cap., Syr. (Parke-Davis).

ANTIDEPRESSANTS.
See: Amitid, Tab. (Squibb).
Amitriptyline HCl (Various Mfr.).
Aventyl HCl, Pulv., Liq. (Lilly).
Deaner, Tab. (Riker).
Deprol, Tab. (Wallace).
Desipramine HCl, Cap., Tab. (Various Mfr.).
Elavil Tab., Inj. (Merck Sharp & Dohme).
Imipramine HCl, Amp., Tab. (Various Mfr.).
Imipramine Pamoate, Cap. (Geigy).
Marplan, Tab. (Roche).
Monoamine oxidase inhibitors.
Nardil, Tab. (Parke-Davis).
Niamid, Tab. (Pfizer).
Norpramin, Preps. (Merrell Dow).
Pamelor, Cap., Liq. (Sandoz).
Parnate Sulfate, Tab. (SmithKline).
Pertofrane, Cap. (USV).
Presamine, Tab. (USV).
Protriptyline HCl (Merck Sharp & Dohme).
Ritalin, Tab., Vial (Ciba).
Sinequan, Cap. (Pfizer).
Tofranil, Amp., Tab. (Geigy).
Tofranil-PM, Cap. (Geigy).
Triavil, Tab. (Merck Sharp & Dohme).
Vivactil, Tab. (Merck Sharp & Dohme).

ANTIDIARRHEALS.
See: Attapulgite, Activated (Various Mfr.).
Cantil, Liq., Tab. (Merrell Dow).
Coly-Mycin S, Oral Susp., (Parke-Davis).
Corrective Mixture, Liq. (Beecham Labs).
Corrective Mixture with Paregoric, Liq. (Beecham Labs).
DIA-Quel Liq. (Inter. Pharm. Corp.).
Diastay, Tab. (Elder).
Diastop, Liq. (Elder).
Diatrol, Tab. (Otis Clapp).
Donnagel, Susp. (Robins).
Donnagel-PG (Robins).
Furoxone Liq., Tab. (Eaton).
Homapin, Preps. (Mission).
Infatol Pink, Liq. (Scherer).
Kaolin (Various Mfr.).
Kaolin Colloidal (Various Mfr.).
Kaomin, Pow. (Lilly).
Kaopectate, Susp. (Upjohn).
Lactinex, Tab., Gran. (Hynson, Westcott & Dunning).
Lactobacillus acidophilus & *bulgaricus* mixed culture, Tab. (Hynson, Westcott & Dunning).
Lactobacillus acidophilus, viable culture (Various Mfr.).
Lomotil, Liq., Tab., (Searle & Co.).
Milk of Bismuth (Various Mfr.).
Mycifradin Sulfate, Soln., Tab. (Upjohn).
Palsorb Improved, Liq. (Hauck).
Paocin, Susp. (Massengill).
Paregel, Liq. (Ferndale).
Parelixer, Liq. (Purdue-Frederick).
Parepectolin, Susp. (Rhone-Poulenc Rorer).
Pectocel, Susp. (Lilly).
Pektamalt, Susp. (Warren-Teed).

Pepto-Bismol, Liq., Tab. (Norwich).
Sorboquel, Tab. (Schering-Plough).

ANTIDIURETICS.
See: Pitressin, Amp. (Parke-Davis).
Pitressin Tannate In Oil, Amp. (Parke-Davis).
Pituitary Post. Inj. (Various Mfr.).

ANTIEMETIC/ANTIVERTIGO AGENTS.
See: Antinauseants Supprettes "WANS" (Webcon).
Atarax, Tab., Syr. (Roerig).
Bendectin, Tab. (Merrell Dow).
Bucladin-S, Softab Tab. (Stuart).
Cesamet, Cap. (Lilly).
Compazine, Preps. (SmithKline).
Dramamine, and Dramamine-D, Preps. (Searle).
Emesert, Rectal Insert (American Critical Care).
Emetrol, Liq. (Rhone-Poulenc Rorer).
Marezine, Preps. (Burroughs Wellcome).
Marinol, Cap. (Roxane).
Meclizine HCl, Tab. (Various Mfr.).
Mepergan, Inj. (Wyeth-Ayerst).
Naus-A-Tories, Supp. (Table Rock).
Nausetrol, Syr. (Medical Chemicals).
Phenergan, Preps. (Wyeth-Ayerst).
Pyridoxine HCl, Preps. (Various Mfr.).
Thorazine, Preps. (SmithKline).
Tigan, Preps. (Beecham Labs).
Torecan Amp., Supp., Tab. (Sandoz).
Trilafon, Preps. (Schering-Plough).
Vistaril, Cap., Susp., Soln. (Pfizer).
Zofran, Inj. (Glaxo).

ANTIEPILEPTIC AGENTS.
See: Anticonvulsants.

ANTIESTROGEN. Tamoxifen citrate.
Use: Hormone for cancer therapy.
See: Nolvadex (ICI Pharma).

ANTIFEBRIN.
See: Acetanilid (Various Mfr.).

ANTIFLATULENTS.
See: Di-Gel, Prods. (Schering-Plough).
Silain, Tab., Gel (Robins).
Simethicone Prods.

ANTIFOAM A COMPOUND. (Merrell Dow).
Use: Antiflatulent.
See: Simethicone, U.S.P. XXII.

ANTIFOLIC ACID.
See: Methotrexate, Tab. (Lederle).

ANTIFORMIN. Sodium hypochlorite in sodium hydroxide 7.5%, available chlorine 5.2%; may be colored with meta cresol purple.
Use: Antiseptic, germicide.

ANTIFUNGAL AGENTS.
See: Fungicides.

•**ANTIHEMOPHILIC FACTOR,** U.S.P. XXII. Human antihemophilic factor. (Hyland & Alpha Therapeutics) Antihemophilic Factor, human. Method for Syringe Administration 10 ml 450 A.H.F. or 300 A.H.F. units/Pkg. W/Syringe 30 ml or 900 A.H.F. units/Pkg.
Use: Antihemophilic.
See: Hemofil, Vial (Hyland).
Koate-HS, Vial (Cutter).
Koate-HT, Vial (Cutter).

ANTIHEPARIN. Protamine Sulfate.

ANTIHISTAMINE CREAM. (Towne) Methapyrilene HCl 10 mg, pyrilamine maleate 5 mg, allantoin 2 mg, diperodon HCl 2.5 mg, benzocaine 10 mg, menthol 2 mg/Gm. Cream Jar 2 oz.
Use: Antihistamine, topical.

ANTIHISTAMINES.
See: Actidil, Tab., Syr. (Burroughs Wellcome).
Ambodryl, Kapseal (Parke-Davis).
Benadryl HCl, Preps. (Parke-Davis).
Chlorpheniramine Maleate (Various Mfr.).
Chlorpheniramine Maleate w/Comb. (Various Mfr.).
Clistin, Elix., Tab. (McNeil).
Co-Pyronil, Pulv., Susp. (Lilly).
Diafen, Tab. (Riker).
Dimetane, Preps. (Robins).
Diphenhydramine HCl (Various Mfr.).
Diphenylpyraline HCl (Various Mfr.).
Disophrol, Prods. (Schering-Plough).
Doxylamine Succinate (Merrell Dow).
Drixoral, Prods. (Schering-Plough).
Forhistal Maleate, Syr., Tab. (Ciba).
Inhiston, Tab. (Plough).
Novahistine LP, Tab. (Merrell Dow).
Optimine, Prods. (Schering-Plough).
PBZ, Tab. (Geigy).
PBZ-SR, Tab. (Geigy).
Periactin, Syr., Tab. (Merck Sharp & Dohme).
Promethazine HCl (Various Mfr.).
Prophenpyridamine Maleate (Various Mfr.).
Pyrilamine Maleate (Various Mfr.).
Tripelennamine HCl (Various Mfr.).
Triprolidine HCl (Various Mfr.).

ANTIHYPERLIPIDEMICS.
See: Atromid-S, Cap. (Wyeth-Ayerst).
Choloxin, Tab. (Flint).
Clofibrate, Cap. (Various Mfr.).
Colestid, Gran (Upjohn).
Lopid, Cap. (Parke-Davis).
Lorelco, Tab. (Merrell Dow).
Lovastatin.
Mevacor, Tab. (MSD).
Questran, Pow. (Bristol-Myers U.S. Pharm.).

ANTIHYPERTENSIVES.
See: Hypertension Therapy.

ANTI-INHIBITOR COAGULANT COMPLEX.
Use: Antihemophilic agent.
See: Autoplex T. (Hyland Therapeutic).
Feiba VH. (Immuno-U.S.).

ANTI-ITCH CREAM. (Spencer-Mead) Burow's solution 5%, phenol 0.5%, menthol 0.5%, camphor 1% in washable base. Tube oz.
Use: Antipruritic, counter-irritant.

ANTILEPROTICS.
Use: Local anesthetic, antipruritic.
See: Hansen's disease.

ANTILERGE. (Metz) Chlorpheniramine maleate 8 mg, phenylephrine HCl 12 mg/Tab. Bot. 30s.
Use: Antihistamine, decongestant.
ANTILEUKEMIA.
See: Antineoplastic agents.
ANTILIRIUM. (Forest) Physostigmine salicylate 2 mg/2 ml. Amp. Box. 12s.
Use: Antidote.
ANTIMALARIAL AGENTS.
See: Amodiaquin HCl.
Aralen HCl, Inj. (Winthrop Pharm).
Aralen Phosphate (Winthrop Pharm).
Aralen Phosphate w/Primaquine (Winthrop Pharm).
Atabrine HCl, Tab. (Winthrop Pharm).
Chloroguanide HCl.
Daraprim Tab. (Burroughs Wellcome).
Hydroxychloroquine Sulfate.
Paludrine HCl, Tab. (Wyeth-Ayerst).
Pamaquine Naphthoate.
Plaquenil Sulfate, Tab. (Winthrop Pharm).
Plasmochin Naphthoate.
Primaquine Phosphate, Tab. (Winthrop Pharm).
Pyrimethamine.
Quinacrine HCl, Tab.
Quinine Salts (Various Mfr.).
Quinine Sulfate (Various Mfr.).
Totaquine, Pow.
ANTIME. (Rand) Pentaerythritol tetranitrate 30 mg or 80 mg/Cap. Bot. 60s, 500s.
Use: Smooth muscle relaxant.
ANTIME FORTE. (Rand) Pentaerythritol tetranitrate 30 mg, secobarbital 50 mg/Cap. Bot. 60s, 500s.
Use: Smooth muscle relaxant, sedative/hypnotic.
ANTIMINTH. (Pfizer Laboratories) Pyrantel pamoate 250 mg/5 ml. Bot. 60 ml.
Use: Anthelmintic.
•**ANTIMONY POTASSIUM TARTRATE,** U.S.P. XXII. Antimonate (2-),bis[u-[2,3-dihydroxybutanedioato(4-)-0,0:0,0]] dipotassium, trihydrate, stereoisomer. Dipotassium bis[u-tar-trato(4-)] diantimonate (2-) trihydrate. Tartar emetic. (Various Mfr.).
Use: Schistosomiasis, leishmaniasis, expectorant, emetic.
W/Cocillana, euphorbia pilulifera, squill, senega.
See: Cylana, Syr. (Bowman).
W/Guaifenesin, codeine phosphate.
See: Cheracol, Syr. (Upjohn).
W/Guaifenesin, dextromethorphan HBr.
See: Cheracol-D, Syr. (Upjohn).
W/Paregoric, glycyrrhiza fluid extract.
See: Brown Mixture (Lilly).
W/Thenylpyramine HCl, ammonium Cl, sodium citrate, menthol, aromatics.
See: Histacomp, Syr., Tab. (Approved Pharm.).
ANTIMONY PREPARATIONS.
See: Antimony Potassium Tartrate (Various Mfr.).
Antimony Sodium Thioglycollate (Various Mfr.).
Tartar Emetic (Various Mfr.).
•**ANTIMONY SODIUM TARTRATE,** U.S.P. XXII.
ANTIMONY SODIUM THIOGLYCOLLATE. (Various Mfr.).
Use: Schistosomiasis, leishmaniasis, filariasis.
•**ANTIMONY TRISULFIDE COLLOID.** USAN.
Use: Pharmaceutic aid.
ANTIMONYL POTASSIUM TARTRATE.
See: Antimony Potassium Tartrate, U.S.P. XXII.
ANTINAUSEANTS.
See: Antiemetic/antivertigo agents.
ANTINEA. (American Dermal) Benzoic acid 6%, salicylic acid 3% in water-washable cream base. Tube oz.
Use: Antifungal, topical.
ANTINEOPLASTIC AGENTS.
See: Adriamycin, Vial (Adria).
Alkeran, Tab. (Burroughs Wellcome).
Blenoxane, Amp. (Bristol).
Cosmegen, Inj. (Merck Sharp & Dohme).
Cytosar, sterile (Upjohn).
Cytoxan, Tab., Vial (Mead Johnson).
Dicorvin, Tab. (Amfre-Grant).
Drolban, Inj. (Lilly).
Elspar, Inj. (Merck Sharp & Dohme).
Estinyl, Tab. (Schering-Plough).
Estradurin, Inj. (Wyeth-Ayerst).
5-Fluorouracil, Amp. (Roche).
FUDR, Vial (Roche).
Hexalen (US Bioscience).
Hydrea, Cap. (Squibb).
Idamycin (Adria).
Leukeran, Tab. (Burroughs Wellcome).
Lysodren, Tab. (Calbio).
Matulane, Cap. (Roche).
Medroxyprogesterone Acetate Tab., Vial (Various Mfr.).
Megace, Tab. (Mead Johnson).
Mercaptopurine, Tab. (Burroughs Wellcome).
Methosarb, Tab. (Upjohn).
Methotrexate, Tab. (Lederle).
Methotrexate Sodium, Vial (Lederle).
Meticorten, Tab. (Schering-Plough).
Mithracin, Vial (Pfizer).
Mustargen, Inj. (Merck Sharp & Dohme).
Myleran, Tab. (Burroughs Wellcome).
Oncovin, Amp. (Lilly).
Progynon, Pellets, Susp. (Schering-Plough).
Purinethol, Tab. (Burroughs Wellcome).
TACE, Cap. (Merrell Dow).
Teslac, Tab., Vial (Squibb).
Thioguanine, Tab. (Burroughs Wellcome).
Thio-Tepa, Vial (Lederle).
Triethylene Melamine, Tab. (Lederle).
Uracil Mustard, Cap. (Upjohn).
Velban, Amp. (Lilly).
Vercyte, Tab. (Abbott).
ANTI-OBESITY AGENTS.
See: Thyroid.
Amphetamine Preps. (Various Mfr.).

Dextroamphetamine Preps. (Various Mfr.).
Diethylpropion HCl.
Fastin, Cap. (Beecham Labs).
Ionamin, Cap. (Pennwalt).
Levo-Amphetamine.
Methamphetamine Preps. (Various Mfr.).
Plegine, Tab. (Wyeth-Ayerst).
Preludin, Tab. (Boehringer Ingelheim).
Sanorex, Tab. (Sandoz).
Statobex, Tab. (Lemmon).
Tenuate, Tab. (Merrell Dow).
Tepanil, Tab. (Riker).

ANTI-OXIDANT. (Murdock) Vitamins A 5000 IU, E 134 mg, C 90 mg, zinc 15 mg, selenium 100 mg, glutathione 30 mg. Cap. Bot. 90s.
Use: Vitamin/mineral supplement.

ANTIOXIDANT FORMULA. (Life's Finest) Vitamins E 134 mg, C 250 mg, selenium 100 mcg. Cap. Bot. 100s, 200s, 250s.
Use: Vitamin supplement.

ANTI-PAK COMPOUND. (Lowitt) Phenylephrine HCl 5 mg, salicylamide 0.23 Gm, acetophenetidin 0.15 gr, caffeine 0.03 Gm, ascorbic acid 50 mg, hesperidin complex 50 mg, chlorprophenpyridamine maleate 2 mg/Tab. Bot. 30s, 100s.
Use: Decongestant, analgesic, antihistamine combination.

ANTIPARASYMPATHOMIMETICS.
See: Parasympatholytic agents.

ANTI-PELLAGRA VITAMIN.
See: Nicotinic acid.

ANTI-PERNICIOUS ANEMIA PRINCIPLE.
See: Vitamin B_{12}.

ANTIPHLOGISTINE. (Denver) Medicated poultice. Jar 5 oz, lb. Tube 8 oz. Can 5 lb.

ANTIPROTOZOAN AGENTS.
See: Antimony Preps.
Arsenic Preps.
Bismuth Preps.
Chiniofon (Various Mfr.).
Diiodohydroxyquinoline.
Emetine HCl (Various Mfr.).
Furazolidone.
Iodocholohydroxyquinoline.
Iodohydroxyquinoline Sulfonate Sodium.
Levofuraltadone.
Ornidyl (Marion Merrell Dow).
Quinoxyl.
Suramin Sodium.

ANTIPYRINE, U.S.P. XXII. 2,3-Dimethyl-1-phenyl-3-pyrazolin-5-one. (Various Mfr.) Analgesine, anodynine, dimethyloxyquinazine, oxydimethylquinizine, parodyne, phenazone, phenylone, pyrazoline, sedatine.
Use: Analgesic, antipyretic.
W/Benzocaine, chlorobutanol.
See: G.B.A., Drops (Scrip).
W/Carbamide, benzocaine, cetyldimethylbenzylammonium HCl.
See: Auralgesic, Liq. (Elder).
W/Phenylephrine HCl, benzocaine.
See: Tympagesic, Liq. (Adria).
W/Pyrilamine maleate, phenylephrine, benzalkonium.
See: Prefrin-A Ophthalmic (Allergan).

•**ANTIPYRINE AND BENZOCAINE OTIC SOLUTION,** U.S.P. XXII.
Use: Local anesthetic.
See: Auro Ear Drops (Commerce).
Lanaurine, Drops (Lannett).
Pyrocaine Eardrop, Liq. (Med. Chem.).

•**ANTIPYRINE, BENZOCAINE AND PHENYLEPHRINE HYDROCHLORIDE OTIC SOLUTION,** U.S.P. XXII.
Use: Local anesthetic, decongestant eardrop.

ANTIRABIES SERUM. (Sclavo) Antirabies serum, equine origin (ARS) 125 IU/ml with m-Cresol 0.3%. Inj. Vial 1000 units.
Use: Rabies prophylaxis.

ANTIRHEUMATIC PREPARATIONS.
See: p-Aminobenzoic Acid and salts (calcium, potassium, sodium).
Ammonium Salicylate.
Colchicine, Preps.
Gentisate Sodium.
Gold Sodium Thiosulfate, Preps. (Various Mfr.).
Myochrysine, Inj. (Merck Sharp & Dohme).
Salicylamide, Preps.
Sodium Salicylate.
Solganal, Vial (Schering-Plough).

ANTIRICKETTSIAL AGENTS.
See: p-Aminobenzoic Acid (Various Mfr.).
p-Aminobenzoate Sodium (Various Mfr.).
Aureomycin, Preps. (Lederle).
Chloromycetin, Preps. (Parke-Davis).
Rocky Mountain Spotted Fever Serum (Rabbit), Vial (Lederle).
Terramycin, Preps. (Pfizer).

ANTI-RUST TABLETS. (Lannett) Not for medicinal use. For use with benzalkonium aqueous sterilizing solution. Sodium carbonate monohydrate 1.15 Gm, sodium nitrate 0.5 Gm for a total of 1.66 Gm/Tab. Bot. 500s.
Use: Rust preventative.

ANTI-RUST TABLETS. (Winthrop Pharm) Sodium nitrite 0.5 Gm, sodium bicarbonate 1.16 Gm for a total of 1.66 Gm/Tab. Bot. 50s, 500s.
Use: Rust preventative.

ANTISCORBUTIC VITAMIN.
See: Ascorbic Acid.

ANTISEPTIC, CHLORINE, ACTIVE.
See: Antiseptic, N-Chloro Compounds, Hypochlorite Preps.

ANTISEPTIC, DYES.
See: Acriflavine (Various Mfr.).
Aminoacridine HCl.
Bismuth Violet, Preps. (Table Rock).
Brilliant Green.
Crystal Violet.
Fuchsin.
Gentian Violet (Various Mfr.).
Methylrosaniline Cl (Various Mfr.).
Methyl Violet.

Pyridium, Tab. (Parke-Davis).
Serenium, Tab. (Squibb).

ANTISEPTIC, MERCURIALS.
See: Mercresin (Upjohn).
Merthiolate, Preps. (Lilly).
Phenylmercuric Acetate (Various Mfr.).
Phenylmercuric Borate (Various Mfr.).
Phenylmercuric Nitrate (Various Mfr.).
Phenylmercuric Picrate (Various Mfr.).
Thimerosal.

ANTISEPTIC, N-CHLORO COMPOUNDS.
See: Chloramine-T (Various Mfr.).
Chlorazene, Pow., Tab. (Badger).
Dichloramine-T (Various Mfr.).
Halazone, Tab. (Abbott).

ANTISEPTIC, PHENOLS.
See: Anthralin (Various Mfr.).
Bithionol.
Coal Tar Products (Various Mfr.).
Creosote (Various Mfr.).
Cresols (Various Mfr.).
Guaiacol (Various Mfr.).
Hexachlorophene (Various Mfr.).
Hexylresorcinol (Various Mfr.).
Methylparaben (Various Mfr.).
o-Phenylphenol (Various Mfr.).
Oxyquinoline Salts (Various Mfr.).
Parachlorometaxylenol (Various Mfr.).
Phenol (Various Mfr.).
Picric Acid (Various Mfr.).
Propylparaben (Various Mfr.).
Pyrogallol (Various Mfr.).
Resorcinol (Various Mfr.).
Resorcinol Monoacetate (Various Mfr.).
Thymol (Various Mfr.).
Trinitrophenol (Various Mfr.).

ANTISEPTICS.
See: Furacin, Preps. (Eaton).
Iodine Products.
Mercurials.
N-Chloro Compounds.
Phenols.
Surface-Active Agents.

ANTISEPTIC, SURFACE-ACTIVE AGENTS.
See: Bactine, Preps. (Miles).
Benzalkonium Cl (Various Mfr.).
Benzethonium Cl (Various Mfr.).
Ceepryn (Merrell Dow).
Cēpacol Preps. (Merrell Dow).
Cetylpyridinium Cl (Various Mfr.).
Diaparene Cl, Preps. (Glenbrook).
Methylbenzethonium Cl (Various Mfr.).
Zephiran Cl, Preps. (Winthrop Pharm).

ANTISPAS. (Keene) Dicyclomine HCl 10 mg/ml. Vial 10 ml.
Use: Antispasmodic.

ANTISPASMODICS. Usually refers to agents that combat the muscarinic effect of liberated acetylcholine. Relief of smooth muscle spasms. Parasympatholytic agents.
See: Anticholinergic Agents.
Spasmolytic Agents.

ANTISPASMODIC CAPSULES. (Lemmon) Phenobarbital 16.2 mg, hyoscyamine sulfate 0.1037 mg, atropine sulfate 0.0194 mg, scopolamine HBr 0.0065 mg/Cap. Bot. 1000s.
Use: Sedative/hypnotic, anticholinergic/antispasmodic.

ANTISTEREPTOLYSIN-O. Titration procedure.
See: Also (Wampole Labs).

ANTISTERILITY VITAMIN.
See: Vitamin E.

ANTI-TEN. (Century) Allylisobutylbarbituric acid ¾ gr, aspirin 3 gr, phenacetin 2 gr, caffeine ⅔ gr/Tab. Bot. 100s, 1000s.
Use: Sedative, analgesic, CNS stimulant.

ANTITHROMBIN III. (Human).
Use: Thromboembolic agent
See: ATnativ (Hyland).

ANTITHYROID AGENTS.
See: Iothiouracil Sodium.
Methimazole.
Methylthiouracil (Various Mfr.).
Propylthiouracil (Various Mfr.).
Tapazole, Tab. (Lilly).

ANTITOXINS.
See: Botulism Antitoxin.
Diphtheria Antitoxin.
Gas Gangrene Antitoxin.
Tetanus Antitoxin.

ANTITRYPSIN, ALPHA 1.
See: Prolastin (Cutter).

ANTITUBERCULOSIS AGENTS.
See: Aminosalicylates (Na, Ca, K) (Various Mfr.).
Benzapas, Pow., Tab. (Dorsey).
Calcium Benzoylpas (Various Mfr.).
Capastat Sulfate, Amp. (Lilly).
Cycloserine, Pulv. (Lilly).
Diasone Sodium, Tab. (Abbott).
Dihydrosteptomycin (Various Mfr.).
Isoniazid (Various Mfr.).
Myambutol, Tab. (Lederle).
Natri-Pas, Pow., Tab. (Glenwood).
Niadox, Tab. (Barnes-Hind).
Niconyl, Tab. (Parke-Davis).
P.A.S. Acid, Tab. (Kasar).
Pasara Sodium, Pow., Tab. (Dorsey).
Pasdium, Tab. (Kasar).
Pyrazinamide, Tab. (Lederle).
Rifadin, Cap. (Merrell Dow).
Rimactane, Cap. (Ciba).
Seromycin, Pulv. (Lilly).
Streptomycin (Various Mfr.).
Trecator-SC, Tab. (Wyeth-Ayerst).
Triniad, Tab. (Kasar).
Uniad, Tab. (Kasar).
Uniad-Plus 5,10, Tab. (Kasar).

ANTI-TUSS. (Century) Guaifenesin 100 mg/5 ml. Bot. 4 oz, gal.
Use: Expectorant.

ANTI-TUSS D.M. (Century) Guaifenesin 100 mg, dextromethorphan HBr 15 mg/5 ml. Bot. 4 oz, pt, gal.

Use: Expectorant, antitussive.

ANTI-TUSSIVE. (Canright) Dextromethorphan HBr 10 mg, potassium guaiacol sulfonate 125 mg, terpin hydrate 100 mg, phenylpropanolamine HCl 12.5 mg, pyrilamine maleate 12.5 mg/ Tab. Bot. 60s.
Use: Antitussive, expectorant, decongestant, antihistamine.

ANTITUSSIVE COUGH SYRUP. (Weeks & Leo) Chlorpheniramine 2 mg, phenylephrine HCl 5 mg, dextromethorphan 15 mg, ammonium Cl 50 mg/5 ml.
Use: Antihistamine, decongestant, antitussive, expectorant.

ANTITUSSIVE COUGH SYRUP WITH CODEINE. (Weeks & Leo) Chlorpheniramine maleate 2 mg, phenylephrine HCl 5 mg, codeine phosphate 10 mg, ammonium Cl 50 mg/5 ml. Bot. 4 oz.
Use: Antihistamine, decongestant, antitussive, expectorant.

ANTITUSSIVE-DECONGESTANT.
See: St. Joseph Cough Syrup for Children (Schering-Plough).
Tussend, Tab., Liq. (Merrell Dow).

•**ANTIVENIN (CROTALIDAE) POLYVALENT,** U.S.P. XXII. Polyvalent crotaline antivenin. Rattlesnake antivenin for four species of pit vipers.
Use: Passive immunizing agent for treatment of rattlesnake bite.

•**ANTIVENIN (LATRODECTUS MACTANS),** U.S.P. XXII. (Merck Sharp & Dohme) Black widow spider antivenin. Each vial contains not less than 6000 antivenin units. Thimerosal (mercury derivative) 1:10,000 added as preservative. Vial 2.5 ml.
Use: Treatment of black widow spider bites.

•**ANTIVENIN (MICRURUS FULVIUS),** U.S.P. XXII. (Wyeth-Ayerst) Lyophilized antivenin of animal origin (*Micrurus fulvius*) with phenol 0.25% and thimerosal 0.005% as preservatives. Bacteriostatic water w/phenylmercuric nitrate 1:100,000 as preservative. Combination package. Vial 10 ml.
Use: Bites of North American coral snake and Texas coral snake.

ANTIVENIN, CROTALIDAE, POLYVALENT. (Wyeth-Ayerst) Antivenin Crotalidae, Polyvalent, U.S.P. XXII. (*Crotalidae*) Rattlesnake, copperhead and moccasin antitoxic serum. Pkg. Comb w/Phenol 0.25%, thimerosal 0.005% as preservatives. One disposable syringe, 10 ml of bacteriostatic water for inj. w/preservative phenyl mercuric nitrate 0.001%; one applicator vial iodine tincture. Normal horse serum 1:10, as sensitivity testing material w/preservatives thimerosal 0.005% and phenol 0.35%.
Use: Bites of crotalid snakes of the United States.

ANTIVERT. (Roerig) Meclizine HCl 12.5 mg, 25 mg or 50 mg/Tab., 25 mg/Chew. Tab. **12.5 mg:** Bot. 100s, 1000s, UD 100s; **25 mg:** Bot. 100s, 1000s, UD 100s. **50 mg:** Bot. 100s. **Chew. tab.:** Bot. 100s, 500s.
Use: Antiemetic/antivertigo.

ANTIVIRAL AGENTS.
See: Cytovene, Inj. (Syntex).
Retrovir, Cap. (Burroughs Wellcome).
Symmetrel, Cap., Syr. (DuPont).
Vira-A, Inj. (Parke-Davis).
Virazole, Pow. for Reconstitution for aerosol (ICN).
Zovirax, Cap, Inj. (Burroughs Wellcome).

ANTIXEROPHTHALMIC VITAMIN.
See: Vitamin A.

ANTRIZINE TABS. (Major) Meclizine 12.5 mg, 25 mg or 50 mg/Tab. **12.5 mg:** 100s, 500s, 1000s. **25 mg:** 100s, 500s, 1000s, UD 100s. **50 mg:** 100s.
Use: Antiemetic/antivertigo.

ANTROCOL. (Poythress) Atropine sulfate 0.195 mg, phenobarbital 16 mg/Tab. or Cap. Tab. Bot, 100s. Cap. Bot. 100s, 500s.
Use: Anticholinergic/antispasmodic, sedative/ hypnotic.

ANTROCOL ELIXIR. (Poythress) Atropine sulfate 0.039 mg, phenobarbital 3 mg, alcohol 20%/5 ml. Bot. oz. w/dropper. Bot. pt.
Use: Anticholinergic/antispasmodic, sedative/ hypnotic.

ANTURANE. (Ciba) Sulfinpyrazone, U.S.P. **100 mg/Tab.:** Bot 100s. **200 mg/Cap.:** Bot. 100s.
Use: Agent for gout.

ANUCAINE. (Calvin) Procaine 50 mg, butyl-p-aminobenzoate 200 mg, benzyl alcohol 265 mg in sweet almond oil/5 ml. Amp. 5 ml. Box 6s, 24s, 100s.
Use: Anorectal preparation.

ANUJECT. (Hauck) Procaine. Soln. Vial 5 ml or 10 ml.
Use: Anorectal preparation.

ANULAN SUPPOSITORIES. (Lannett) Bismuth resorcin compound, bismuth subgallate, zinc oxide, boric acid, balsam Peru. Supp. Box 12s.
Use: Anorectal preparation.

ANUMED. (Major) Bismuth subgallate 2.25%, bismuth resorcin compound 1.75%, benzyl benzoate 1.2%, zinc oxide 11%, balsam Peru 1.8% in a hydrogenated vegetable oil base. Supp. Box 12s.
Use: Anorectal preparation.

ANUMED HC. (Major) Bismuth subgallate 2.25%, bismuth resorcin compound 1.75%, benzyl benzoate 1.2%, balsam Peru 1.8%, zinc oxide 11%. Supp. Box 12s.
Use: Anorectal preparation.

ANUSOL. (Parke-Davis Prods) Bismuth subgallate 2.25%, bismuth resorcin compound 1.75%, balsam Peru 1.8%, zinc oxide 11%, benzyl benzoate 1.2%, in hydrogenated vegetable oil/ Supp. Box 12s, 24s, 48s.
Use: Anorectal preparation.

ANUSOL OINTMENT. (Parke-Davis Prods) Balsam Peru 18 mg, zinc oxide 110 mg/Gm, ben-

zyl benzoate 1.2%, pramoxine HCl 1% in a mineral oil glyceryl stearate and water base. Tube 1 oz, 2 oz.
Use: Anorectal preparation.

ANUSOL-HC. (Parke-Davis Prods) Hydrocortisone acetate 25 mg/Supp. Box 12s, 24s.
Use: Anorectal preparation.

ANXANIL. (Econo Med) Hydroxyzine HCl 25 mg/Tab. Bot. 100s.
Use: Antianxiety agent.

AORACILLIN-B. (Vita Elixir) Penicillin G 200,000 units or 500,000 units/Tab. Bot. 50s.
Use: Antibacterial, penicillin.

AOSEPT. (Ciba Vision) Hydrogen peroxide 3%, sodium Cl 0.85%, sodium stannate, sodium nitrate, phosphate buffer. Soln. Bot. 120 ml.
Use: Contact lens care.

APACET. (Parmed) Acetaminophen 80 mg/Chew. tab. Bot. 100s.
Use: Analgesic.

•**APALCILLIN SODIUM.** USAN.
Use: Antibacterial.

APATATE LIQUID. (Kenwood) Vitamins B_1 15 mg, B_{12} 25 mcg, B_6 0.5 mg/5 ml. Liq. Bot. 4 oz, 8 oz.
Use: Vitamin supplement.

APATATE TABLETS. (Kenwood) Vitamins B_1 15 mg, B_{12} 25 mcg, B_6 0.5 mg/Tab. Bot. 50s.
Use: Vitamin supplement.

•**APAZONE.** USAN. 5-(Dimethylamino)-9-methyl-2-propyl-lH-pyrazolo[1,2,-a][1,2,4] benzotriazine-1,-3(2H)-dione.
Use: Anti-inflammatory agent.

A.P.C. (Various Mfr.) Aspirin, phenacetin, caffeine. Cap., Tab.
Use: Analgesic combination.
See: A.S.A. Compound, Preps. (Lilly).
P.A.C. Compound, Cap., Tab. (Upjohn).
Pan-APC, Tab. (Panray).
Phensal, Tab. (Merrell Dow).
W/Codeine phosphate. (Various Mfr.).
See: Anexsia w/Codeine, Tab. (Beecham Labs).
Anexsia D, Tab. (Beecham Labs).

A.P.C. W/GELSEMIUM COMBINATIONS
See: Aidant, Tab. (Noyes).
Ansemco, No. 2, Tab. (Elder).
Asphac-G, Tab. (Central).
Valacet, Tab. (Vale).

APCOGESIC. (Apco) Sodium salicylate 5 gr, colchicine 1/320 gr, calcium carbonate 65 mg, dried aluminum hydroxide gel 130 mg, phenobarbital ⅛ gr/Tab. Bot. 100s.
Use: Agent for gout, sedative/hypnotic.

APCOHIST. (APC) Phenylpropanolamine HCl 25 mg, chlorpheniramine maleate 1 mg/Tab. Bot. 100s.
Use: Decongestant, antihistamine.

APCORETIC. (APC) Caffeine anhydrous 100 mg, ammonium Cl 325 mg/Tab. Bot. 90s.
Use: Diuretic.

AP CREME. (T.E. Williams) Hydrocortisone 0.5%, iodochlorhydroxyquin 3%. Tube oz.
Use: Corticosteroid, antifungal (topical).

APF. (Whitehall).
Use: Salicylate analgesic.
See: Arthritis Pain Formula. (Whitehall).

APHCO HEMORRHOIDAL COMBINATION. (APC) Combination package of Aphco Hemorrhoidal Ointment 1.5 oz tube, Aphco Hemorrhoidal Supp. Box 12s, 1000s.
Use: Anorectal preparation.

APHEN TABS. (Major) Trihexyphenidyl 2 mg or 5 mg/Tab. Bot. 250s, 1000s.
Use: Antiparkinson agent.

APHRODYNE. (Star) Yohimbine HCl 5.4 mg/Tab. Bot. 100s, 1000s.
Use: Alpha-adrenergic blocking agent.

APICILLIN. D-(-)-α-Aminobenzyl penicillin.
See: Ampicillin.

APIQUEL FUMARATE. Aminorex. B.A.N.

A.P.L. (Wyeth-Ayerst) Chorionic Gonadotropin for Injection. Dry form, package vial 1s containing 5000 U.S.P. units, 10,000 U.S.P. units or 20,000 U.S.P. units, sterile diluent, w/benzyl alcohol, phenol, lactose.
Use: Chorionic gonadotropin therapy.

APLISOL. (Parke-Davis) Tuberculin purified protein derivative diluted 5 units/0.1 ml, polysorbate 80, potassium and sodium phosphates, phenol. Vial 1 ml (10 tests), 5 ml (50 tests).
Use: Diagnostic aid.

APLITEST. (Parke-Davis) Purified tuberculin protein derivative buffered with potassium and sodium phosphates, phenol 0.5%/single-use, multipuncture unit. 25s.
Use: Diagnostic aid.

•**APOMORPHINE HYDROCHLORIDE,** U.S.P. XXII. Tab. U.S.P. XXII. 4H-Dibenzo[de,g] quinoline-10,11-diol, 5,6,6a,7-tetrahydro-6-methyl HCl hemihydrate. 6α,β-Aporphine-10,11-diol HCl, hemihydrate. (Lilly) Soln. Tab. 6 mg Bot. 100s.
Use: Emetic.

APORPHINE-10, 11-DIOL HYDROCHLORIDE.
See: Apomorphine HCl.

APPEDRINE. (Thompson Medical) Phenylpropanolamine HCl 25 mg, multivitamins, caffeine 100 mg/Tab.
Use: Diet aid.

APPETITE-DEPRESSANTS.
See: Anorexiants.

APPG.
See: Penicillin G, Procaine, Aqueous.

APRACLONIDINE HCl.
Use: Agent for glaucoma.
See: Iopidine (Alcon).

•**APRACLONIDINE OPHTHALMIC SOLUTION,** U.S.P. XXII.

•**APRAMYCIN.** USAN. B.A.N. An antibiotic produced by *Streptomyces tenebrarius*.
Use: Antibacterial (veterinary).

APRAZONE. (Major) Sulfinpyrazone. **Cap.:** 200 mg. Bot. 100s, 500s, 1000s. **Tab.:** 100 mg. Bot. 100s.
Use: Agent for gout.

APRESAZIDE. (Ciba) **25/25:** Hydralazine HCl 25 mg, hydrochlorothiazide 25 mg/Cap. **50/50:** Hydralazine HCl 50 mg, hydrochlorothiazide 50 mg/Cap. **100/50:** Hydralazine 100 mg, hydrochlorothiazide 50 mg/Cap. Bot. 100s.
Use: Antihypertensive.
APRESODEX. (Rugby) Hydrochlorothiazide 15 mg, hydralazine HCl 25 mg. Tab. Bot. 100s, 1000s.
Use: Antihypertensive.
APRESOLINE. (Ciba) Hydralazine HCl. **Amp.:** 20 mg w/propylene glycol, methyl and propyl parabens/ml. Pkg. 5s. **Tab.:** 10 mg Bot. 100s, 1000s; 25 mg or 50 mg Bot. 100s, 500s, 1000s; 100 mg Bot. 100s. Consumer pack 100s.
Use: Antihypertensive.
W/Serpasil.
See: Serpasil Prods., Preps. (Ciba).
APRESOLINE-ESIDRIX. (Ciba) Hydralazine HCl 25 mg, hydrochlorothiazide 15 mg/Tab. Bot. 100s.
Use: Antihypertensive.
APRINDINE. USAN. 3-[N-(Indan-2-yl)-N-phenylamino]propyldiethylamine. (Lilly) N-(2,3-Dihydro-1H-inden-2-yl)-N′,N′-diethyl-N-phenyl-1,3-propanediamine.
Use: Antiarrhythmic.
APROBARBITAL. 5-Allyl-5-isopropylbarbituric acid, Allylisopropylmalonylurea. Pow.
Use: Sedative/hypnotic.
See: Alurate, Elix. (Roche).
APROBEE W/C. (Approved) Vitamins B_1 15 mg, B_2 10 mg, B_6 5 mg, niacinamide 50 mg, calcium pantothenate 10 mg, C 250 mg/Cap. or Tab. **Cap.:** Bot. 100s, 1000s. **Tab.:** Bot. 50s, 100s, 1000s.
Use: Vitamin supplement.
APRODINE. (Major) **Tab.:** Pseudoephedrine HCl 60 mg, triprolidine HCl 2.5 mg. Bot. 24s, 100s, 1000s, UD 100s. **Syr.:** Pseudoephedrine HCl 30 mg, triprolidine HCl 1.25 mg/15 ml. Bot. 120 ml, pt.
Use: Decongestant, antihistamine.
APROTININ. USAN. A polypeptide proteinase inhibitor.
Use: Enzyme inhibitor (proteinase).
See: Trasylol.
APROZIDE 25/25 CAPSULES. (Major) Hydralazine 25 mg, hydrochlorothiazide 25 mg/Cap. Bot. 100s, 250s.
Use: Antihypertensive.
APROZIDE 50/50 CAPSULES. (Major) Hydrochlorothiazide 50 mg, hydralazine 50 mg/Cap. Bot. 100s, 250s.
Use: Antihypertensive.
A.P.S. Aspirin, phenacetin and salicylamide.
APTAZAPINE MALEATE. USAN.
Use: Antidepressant.
APTOCAINE. B.A.N. 2-Pyrrolidin-1-ylpropiono-o-toluidide.
Use: Local anesthetic.
See: Pirothesin HCl.
APYRON.
See: Magnesium acetylsalicylate.
AQ-4B. (Western Research) Trichlormethiazide 4 mg/Tab. Bot. 1000s.
Use: Diuretic.
AQUA-BAN. (Thompson Medical) Caffeine 100 mg, ammonium Cl 325 mg/Tab. Bot. 60s.
Use: Diuretic.
AQUA-BAN PLUS. (Thompson Medical) Ammonium Cl 650 mg, caffeine 200 mg, iron 6 mg/Tab. Bot. 30s.
Use: Diuretic, CNS stimulant, mineral supplement.
AQUABASE. (Vale) Cetyl alcohol, propylene glycol, sodium lauryl sulfate, white wax, purified water. Jar lb.
Use: Hydrophilic ointment base.
AQUACARE CREAM. (Herbert) Urea 2%, benzyl alcohol, carbomer 934, cetyl esters wax, fragrance, glycerin, oleth-3 phosphate, petrolatum, phenyl dimethicone, water, sodium hydroxide. Tube 2.5 oz.
Use: Emollient.
AQUACARE/HP. (Herbert) Urea 10%, benzyl alcohol. **Cream:** Tube 2.5 oz. **Lot.:** Bot. 8 oz, 16 oz.
Use: Emollient.
AQUACARE LOTION. (Herbert) Benzyl alcohol, oleth-3 phosphate, phenyl dimethicone, fragrance. Bot. 8 oz.
Use: Emollient.
AQUACHLOR. (Geneva) Chlortetracycline.
Use: Antibacterial, tetracycline.
AQUACHLORAL. (Webcon) Chloral hydrate, polyethylene glycol, spreading agent. Supp. 5 gr, 10 gr. Strip 12s.
Use: Sedative/hypnotic, rectal.
AQUA-CILLIN 250. (Kenyon) Crystalline penicillin G potassium 3 million units buffered w/sodium citrate/60 ml vial.
Use: Antibacterial, penicillin.
AQUACILLIN G. (Geneva) Penicillin G.
Use: Antibacterial, penicillin.
AQUACYCLINE. (Geneva) Tetracycline HCl.
Use: Antibacterial, tetracycline.
AQUADERM. (C & M Pharmacal) Purified water, glycerin 25%, salicylic acid 0.1%, octoxynol-9 0.03%, FD&C Red #40 0.0001%. Bot. 2 oz.
Use: Emollient.
AQUAFLEX ULTRASOUND GEL PAD. (Parker) Clear, solid, flexible, moist, standoff gel pad for use where transducer movement is impeded by bony or irregular body surfaces. 2 cm × 9 cm.
Use: Ultrasound agent.
AQUAFUREN. (Geneva) Nitrofurantoin.
Use: Anti-infective, urinary.
AQUAKAY.
See: Menadione (Various Mfr.).
AQUA LACTEN LOTION. (Herald Pharmacal) Demineralized water, urea, petrolatum, propylene glycol monostearate, sorbitan monostearate, lactic acid. Bot. 8 oz.

Use: Emollient.
AQUAMEPHYTON INJECTION. (Merck Sharp & Dohme) Phytonadione 2 mg/ml or 10 mg/ml, vitamin K-1, w/polyoxyethylated fatty acid derivative 70 mg, dextrose 37.5 mg, benzyl alcohol 0.9%, water for injection q.s. to 1 ml. Inj. Amp. 1 mg/0.5 ml Box 25s; 10 mg/1 ml Box 6s, 25s. Vial 10 mg/ml 2.5 ml, 5 ml.
Use: Anticoagulant.
AQUA MIST. (Faraday) Nasal spray. Squeeze Bot. 20 ml.
AQUAMUCIL. (Cenci) Psyllium hydrophilic mucilloid. Bot. 7 oz, 14 oz.
Use: Laxative.
AQUAMYCIN. (Geneva) Erythromycin.
Use: Antibacterial.
AQUANIL. (Sig) Mersalyl 100 mg, theophylline (hydrate) 50 mg, methylparaben 0.18%, propylparaben 0.02%. Vial 10 ml.
Use: Diuretic, bronchodilator.
AQUANINE. (Geneva) Quinine HCl.
Use: Antimalarial.
AQUAOXY. (Geneva) Oxytetracycline HCl.
Use: Antibacterial, tetracycline.
AQUAPHENICOL. (Geneva) Chloramphenicol.
Use: Anti-infective.
AQUAPHILIC OINTMENT. (Medco Lab) Hydrated hydrophilic oint. Jar 16 oz.
Use: Emollient, ointment base.
AQUAPHILIC OINTMENT WITH CARBAMIDE 10% and 20%. (Medco Lab) Stearyl alcohol, white petrolatum, sorbitol, propylene glycol, sodium lauryl sulfate, lactic acid, methylparaben, propylparaben.
Use: Prescription compounding, emollient.
AQUAPHOR. (Beiersdorf) Cholesterolized anhydrous petrolatum ointment base. Tube 1.75 oz, 3.25 oz, 16 oz, Jar 5 lb, Bar 3 oz.
Use: Water-miscible ointment base.
See: Eucerin, Emulsion (Duke).
AQUAPHYLLIN SYRUP. (Ferndale) Theophylline anhydrous 80 mg/15 ml UD pk. 15 ml, 30 ml. Bot. 16 oz, gal.
Use: Bronchodilator.
AQUAPOOL CONCENTRATE. (Parker) Color additive for hydrotherapy to control foaming. Bot. pt, gal.
AQUASOL A. (Armour) Water-miscible Vitamin A. **Inj.:** 50,000 U.S.P. units/ml. Vial 2 ml Box 10s. **Cap.:** 25,000 U.S.P. units/Cap. Bot. 100s. 50,000 U.S.P. units/Cap. Bot. 100s, 500s. **Drops:** 5000 U.S.P. units/0.1 ml. Bot. 30 ml w/ dropper.
Use: Vitamin A supplement.
AQUASOL E. (Armour) Vitamin E. **Cap.:** 73.5 mg Bot. 100s; 400 IU Bot. 30s. **Drops:** 50 mg/ml Bot. 12 ml, 30 ml w/dropper.
Use: Vitamin E supplement.
AQUASONIC 100. (Parker) Water-soluble, viscous, contact medium gel for ultrasonic transmission. Bot. 250 ml, 1 L, 5 L.
Use: Ultrasound agent.
AQUASONIC 100 STERILE. (Parker) Water-soluble, sterile gel for ultrasonic transmission. Overwrapped Foil Pouches 15 Gm, 50 Gm.
Use: Ultrasound agent.
AQUASULF. (Geneva) Triple sulfa tablet.
Use: Anti-infective.
AQUATAR THERAPEUTIC TAR GEL. (Herbert) Coal tar extract (BioTar) 2.5% w/DEA oleth-3 phosphate, glycerin, imidurea, methylparaben, mineral oil, oleth-3, oleth-10, oleth-20, poloxamer 407, polysorbate 80, propylparaben, purified water. Tube 3 oz.
Use: Antipruritic, keratoplastic, antipsoriatic.
AQUATENSEN. (Wallace) Methyclothiazide 5 mg/Tab. Bot. 100s, 500s.
Use: Diuretic, antihypertensive.
AQUAVITE. (Geneva) Soluble multivitamin.
Use: Vitamin supplement.
AQUAZIDE. (Western Research) Trichlormethiazide 4 mg/Tab. Bot. 100s.
Use: Antihypertensive, diuretic.
AQUAZIDE H. (Western Research) Hydrochlorothiazide 50 mg/Tab. Bot. 1000s.
Use: Diuretic.
AQUAZOL. (Geneva) Sulfisoxazole.
Use: Anti-infective.
AQUEOUS ALLERGENS. (Miles Pharm).
Use: Hyposensitizing agents.
AQUEST. (Dunhall) Estrone 20,000 IU. 2 mg/ml. Vial 30 ml.
Use: Estrogen.
AQUEX TABLETS. (Lannett) Trichlormethiazide 4 mg/Tab. Bot. 100s. 1000s.
Use: Diuretic.
AQUINONE.
See: Menadione, U.S.P. XXII.
AQUOL BATH OIL. (Lamond) Vegetable oil, olive oil. Bot. 4 oz, 6 oz, 16 oz, qt, gal.
Use: Emollient, antipruritic.
ARA-A.
See: Vidarabine.
ARA-C.
See: Cytarabine.
ARALEN HYDROCHLORIDE (Winthrop Pharm) Chloroquine HCl 50 mg/ml. Amp 5 ml. Box 5s.
Use: Antimalarial, amebicide.
ARALEN PHOSPHATE. (Winthrop Pharm) Chloroquine phosphate 500 mg/Tab. Bot. 25s.
Use: Antimalarial, amebicide.
ARALEN PHOSPHATE W/PRIMAQUINE PHOSPHATE. (Winthrop Pharm) Aralen phosphate 500 mg, primaquine phosphate 79 mg/Tab. Bot. 100s.
Use: Antimalarial.
ARALIS TABLETS. (Winthrop Products) Glycobiarsol, chloroquine phosphate.
Use: Amebicide.
ARAMINE (Merck Sharp & Dohme) Metaraminol bitartrate (equivalent to metaraminol) 10 mg/ml sodium Cl 4.4 mg, water for injection q.s. ad. 1 ml, methylparaben 0.15%, propylparaben 0.02%, sodium bisulfite 0.2%. Vial 10 ml.

Use: Sympathomimetic.

ARANOTIN. USAN.
Use: Antiviral.

ARBAPROSTIL. USAN.
Use: Antisecretory.

ARBOLIC. (Burgin-Arden) Methandriol dipropionate 50 mg/ml. Vial 10 ml.
Use: Anabolic steroid.

ARBON. (Forest) Iron 18 mg, Vitamins A 5000 IU, D 400 IU, E 30 IU, B_1 1.5 mg, B_2 1.7 mg, B_3 20 mg, B_5 10 mg, B_6 2 mg, B_{12} 6 mcg, C 60 mg, folic acid 0.4 mg, Ca, Cu, I, Mg, P, Zn. Bot. 100s, 1000s.
Use: Vitamin/mineral supplement.

ARBON PLUS. (Forest) Iron 27 mg, Vitamins A 5000 IU, D 400 IU, E 30 IU, C 90 mg, folic acid 400 mcg, B_1 2.25 mg, B_2 2.6 mg, niacinamide 20 mg, B_6 3 mg, B_{12} 9 mcg, pantothenic acid 10 mg, biotin 150 mcg, calcium 162 mg, phosphorus 125 mg, iodine 150 mcg, magnesium 100 mg, copper 3 mg, manganese 7.5 mg, potassium 7.5 mg, zinc 22.5 mg/Tab. Bot. 100s.
Use: Vitamin/mineral supplement.

ARBUTAL. (Arcum) Butalbital ¾ gr, phenacetin 2 gr, aspirin 3 gr, caffeine ⅔ gr/Tab. Bot. 100s, 1000s.
Use: Sedative/hypnotic, analgesic.

ARCLOFENIN. USAN.
Use: Diagnostic aid for hepatic function determination.

ARCOBAN TABLETS. (Arcum) Meprobamate 400 mg/Tab. Bot. 50s, 1000s.
Use: Antianxiety agent.

ARCOBEE W/C. (Nature's Bounty) Vitamins B_1 15 mg, B_2 10.2 mg, B_3 50 mg, B_5 10 mg, B_6 5 mg, C 300 mg, tartrazine. Cap. Box UD 100s.
Use: Vitamin supplement.

ARCOBEX EXTRA STRENGTH CAPS. (Arcum) Vitamins B_1 100 mg, B_2 2 mg, B_6 5 mg, niacinamide 125 mg, panthenol 10 mg, B_{12} 30 mcg, benzyl alcohol 1%, genistic acid ethanolamide 2.5%/ml. Vial 30 ml.
Use: Vitamin B supplement.

ARCOCILLIN. (Arcum) Crystalline penicillin G potassium 400,000 units/Tab. Bot. 100s, 1000s. Pow. 400,000 units/5 ml. Bot. 80 ml.
Use: Antibacterial, penicillin.

ARCODEX ANTACID TABLETS. (Arcum) Magnesium trisilicate 500 mg, aluminum hydroxide 250 mg/Tab. Bot. 100s, 1000s.
Use: Antacid.

ARCO-LASE. (Arco) Trizyme 38 mg (amylase 30 mg, protease 6 mg, cellulase 2 mg), lipase 25 mg/Tab. Bot. 50s.
Use: Digestive aid.

ARCO-LASE PLUS. (Arco) Phenobarbital 8 mg, hyoscyamine sulfate 0.1 mg, atropine sulfate 0.02 mg, trizyme 38 mg, lipase 25 mg/Tab. Bot. 50s.
Use: Sedative/hypnotic, digestive aid.

ARCOSTERONE. (Arcum) Methyltestosterone.
Oral: 10 mg or 25 mg/Tab. Bot. 100s, 1000s.
Sublingual: 10 mg/Tab. Bot. 100s, 1000s.
Use: Androgen.

ARCO-THYROID. (Arco) Thyroid 1.5 gr/Tab. Bot. 1000s.
Use: Thyroid hormone.

ARCOTINIC. (Arco) Iron 106 mg, liver fraction 200 mg, Vitamin C 250 mg Tab. Bot. 100s.
Use: Vitamin/mineral supplement.

ARCOTRATE. (Arcum) Pentaerythritol tetranitrate 10 mg/Tab. **No. 2:** Pentaerythritol tetranitrate 20 mg/Tab. **No. 3:** Pentaerythritol tetranitrate 20 mg, phenobarbital ⅛ gr/Tab. Bot. 100s, 1000s.
Use: Antianginal.

ARCOVAL IMPROVED. (Arcum) Vitamin A palmitate 10,000 IU, D 400 IU, thiamine mononitrate 15 mg, B_2 10 mg, nicotinamide 150 mg, B_6 5 mg, calcium pantothenate 10 mg, B_{12} 5 mcg, C 150 mg, E 5 IU/Cap. Bot. 100s, 1000s.
Use: Vitamin supplement.

ARCUM R-S. (Arcum) Reserpine 0.25 mg/Tab. Bot. 100s, 1000s.
Use: Antihypertensive.

ARCUM V-M. (Arcum) Vitamin A palmitate 5000 IU, D 400 IU, B_1 2.5 mg, B_2 2.5 mg, B_6 0.5 mg, B_{12} 2 mcg, C 50 mg, niacinamide 20 mg, calcium pantothenate 5 mg, iron 18 mg/Cap. Bot. 100s, 1000s.
Use: Vitamin/mineral supplement.

A-R-D. (Birchwood) Anatomically shaped dressing. Dispenser 24s.
Use: Rectal counter-irritant, antipruritic.

ARDEBEN. (Burgin-Arden) Diphenhydramine HCl 10 mg, chlorobutanol 0.5%. Inj. Vial 30 ml.
Use: Antihistamine.

ARDECAINE 1%. (Burgin-Arden) Lidocaine HCl 1%. Inj. Vial 30 ml.
Use: Local anesthetic.

ARDECAINE 2%. (Burgin-Arden) Lidocaine HCl 2%. Inj. Vial 30 ml.
Use: Local anesthetic.

ARDECAINE 1% W/EPINEPHRINE. (Burgin-Arden) Lidocaine HCl 1%, epinephrine. Inj. Vial 30 ml.
Use: Local anesthetic.

ARDECAINE 2% W/EPINEPHRINE. (Burgin-Arden) Lidocaine HCl 2%, epinephrine. Inj. Vial 30 ml.
Use: Local anesthetic.

ARDEFEM 10. (Burgin-Arden) Estradiol valerate 10 mg/ml. Vial 10 ml.
Use: Estrogen.

ARDEFEM 20. (Burgin-Arden) Estradiol valerate 20 mg/ml. Vial 10 ml.
Use: Estrogen.

ARDEFEM 40. (Burgin-Arden) Estradiol valerate 40 mg/ml. Vial 10 ml.
Use: Estrogen.

ARDEPRED SOLUBLE. (Burgin-Arden) Prednisolone 20 mg, niacinamide 25 mg, disodium ed-

etate 0.5 mg, sodium bisulfite 1 mg, phenol 5 mg/ml. Vial 10 ml.
Use: Corticosteroid combination.

ARDERONE 100. (Burgin-Arden) Testosterone enanthate 100 mg/ml. Vial 10 ml.
Use: Androgen.

ARDERONE 200. (Burgin-Arden) Testosterone enanthate 200 mg/ml. Vial 10 ml.
Use: Androgen.

ARDEVILA TABLETS. (Winthrop Products) Inositol hexanicotinate.
Use: Vasodilator.

ARDIOL 90/4. (Burgin-Arden) Testosterone enanthate 90 mg, estradiol valerate 4 mg/ml. Vial 10 ml.
Use: Androgen/estrogen combination.

ARDUAN. (Organon) Pipecuronium Br 10 mg/10 ml. Vial.
Use: Neuromuscular blocking agent.

ARECA. Ether-soluble alkaloids 0.35%, as arecoline.
Use: Anthelmintic (veterinary).

ARECOLINE ACETARSONE SALT.
See: Drocarbil.

AR-EX Products. (Ar-Ex) A series of hypo-allergenic products for sensitive skin including:

Skin Care Products:
- Body Lotion.
- Chap Cream.
- Cleansing Cream.
- Cold Cream.
- Cream For Dry Skin.
- Enriched Night Cream.
- Eye Cream.
- Moisture Cream.
- Moisture Lotion.

Personal Care Products:
- Bath Oil.
- Bath Soap.
- Cream Deodorant.
- Roll-On Deodorant.
- Safe Suds (liquid detergent).
- Shampoo.
- Soap.

Cosmetics and Eye Make-up:
- Brush-On.
- Disappear (blemish stick).
- Eye Make-Up Remover Pads.
- Eye Pencil.
- Face and Compact Powder.
- Foundation Lotion.
- Lip Gloss.
- Lipstick.
- Mascara.

ARFONAD. (Roche) Trimethaphan camsylate 50 mg/ml, sodium acetate 0.013%. Amp. 10 ml. Box 10s.
Use: Vasodilator.
Note: Refrigerate between 2° and 8° C.

•**ARGININE,** U.S.P. XXII. $C_6H_{14}N_4O_2$. L-Arginine.
Use: Ammonia detoxicant, diagnostic aid (pituitary function determination).

•**ARGININE GLUTAMATE.** USAN. L(+)-arginine salt of L(+)-glutamic acid.
Use: Aid in ammonia intoxication due to hepatic failure.
See: Modumate (Abbott).

•**ARGININE HYDROCHLORIDE,** U.S.P. XXII. Inj., U.S.P. XXII.
Use: Ammonia detoxicant.

ARGIPRESSIN. B.A.N. 8-Argininevasopressin.
Use: Antidiuretic hormone.

•**ARGIPRESSIN TANNATE.** USAN.
Use: Antidiuretic.

ARGYN.
See: Mild Silver Protein (Various Mfr.).

ARGYROL S.S. 20%. (CooperVision) Mild silver protein 20%. Dropperette 1 ml. Box 12s.
Use: Anti-infective, ophthalmic.

ARIDOL. (MPL) Pamabrom 52 mg, pyrilamine maleate 30 mg, homatropine methylbromide 1.2 mg, hyoscyamine sulfate 0.10 mg, scopolamine HBr 0.02 mg, methamphetamine HCl 1.5 mg/Tab. Bot. 100s.
Use: Diuretic, anticholinergic/antispasmodic, CNS stimulant.

•**ARILDONE.** USAN.
Use: Antiviral.

ARIS PHENOBARBITAL REAGENT STRIPS. (Ames) Box 25s.
Use: Diagnostic aid.

ARIS PHENYTOIN REAGENT STRIPS. (Ames) Box 25s.
Use: Diagnostic aid.

ARISTOCORT. (Lederle) Triamcinolone. **Tab.:** 1 mg Bot. 50s; 2 mg Bot. 100s; 4 mg Bot. 30s, 100s; 8 mg Bot. 50s. **Syr.:** Diacetate w/methylparaben 0.08%, propylparaben 0.02%) 2 mg/5 ml. Bot. 4 oz.
Use: Corticosteroid.

ARISTOCORT A CREAM. (Lederle) Triamcinolone acetonide w/emulsifying wax, isopropyl palmitate, glycerin, sorbitol, lactic acid, benzyl alcohol. **0.025% w/Aquatain:** Tube 15 Gm, 60 Gm. **0.1%:** Tube 15 Gm, 60 Gm, Jar 240 Gm. **0.5%:** Tube 15 Gm, Jar 240 Gm.
Use: Corticosteroid.

ARISTOCORT ACETONIDE, SODIUM PHOSPHATE SALT. (Lederle)
Use: Corticosteroid.
See: Aristocort Preps.
Sodium Phosphate Triamcinolone Acetonide.

ARISTOCORT CREAM. (Lederle) Triamcinolone acetonide w/emulsifying wax, polysorbate 60, mono and diglycerides, squalane, sorbitol soln., sorbic acid, potassium sorbate. **LP: 0.025%:** Tube 15 Gm, 60 Gm, Jar 240 Gm, 480 Gm; **R: 0.1%:** Tube 15 Gm, 60 Gm, Jar 240 Gm, 480 Gm; **HP: 0.5%:** Tube 15 Gm, Jar 240 Gm.
Use: Corticosteroid.

ARISTOCORT FORTE. (Lederle) Triamcinolone diacetate 40 mg/ml. Vial 1 ml, 5 ml.
Use: Corticosteroid.

ARISTOCORT INTRALESIONAL. (Lederle) Triamcinolone diacetate 25 mg/ml. Vial 5 ml.
Use: Corticosteroid.

ARISTOCORT A OINTMENT. (Lederle) Triamcinolone acetonide 0.1%. Tube 15 Gm, 60 Gm.
Use: Corticosteroid.

ARISTOCORT OINTMENT. (Lederle) Triamcinolone acetonide. **R: 0.1%:** Tube 15 Gm, 60 Gm, Jar 240 Gm. **HP: 0.5%:** Tube 15 Gm, Jar 240 Gm.
Use: Corticosteroid.

ARISTO-PAK. (Lederle) Triamcinolone 4 mg/Tab. 16s.
Use: Corticosteroid.

ARISTOSPAN INTRALESIONAL. (Lederle) Triamcinolone hexacetonide 5 mg/ml, polysorbate 80 0.2% w/v, sorbitol soln. 64% w/v, water q.s., benzyl alcohol 0.9% w/v. Vial 5 ml.
Use: Corticosteroid.

ARISTOSPAN INTRA-ARTICULAR. (Lederle) Triamcinolone hexacetonide 20 mg/ml micronized susp., polysorbate 80 0.4% w/v, sorbitol soln. 64% w/v, water q.s., benzyl alcohol 0.9% w/v. Vial 1 ml, 5 ml.
Use: Corticosteroid.

ARITHMIN INJECTABLE. (Lannett) Antazoline phosphate 100 mg/2 ml. Amp. 12s, 100s.
Use: Antihistamine.

ARITHMIN TABLETS. (Lannett) Antazoline HCl 100 mg or 200 mg/Tab. Bot. 100s.
Use: Antihistamine.

ARLACEL 83. (ICI Americas) Sorbitan Sesquioleate.
Use: Surface-active agent.

ARLACEL 165. (ICI Americas) Glyceryl monostearate, PEG-100 stearate nonionic self-emulsifying.
Use: Surface-active agent.

ARLACEL C. (ICI Americas) Sorbitan Sesquioleate. Mixture of oleate esters of sorbitol and its anhydrides.
Use: Surface-active agent.

ARLAMOL E. (ICI Americas) Polyoxypropylene (15), stearyl ether, BHT 0.1%.
Use: Emollient.

ARLATONE 507. (ICI Americas) Padimate O.
Use: Sunscreen.

ARLIDIN. (Rhone-Poulenc Rorer) Nylidrin HCl 6 mg or 12 mg/Tab. Bot. 100s, 1000s, UD 100s.
Use: Vasodilator.

ARLIX. (Hoechst) Piretanide HCl.
Use: Diuretic, antihypertensive.

ARM-A-MED. (Armour) Isoproterenol HCl inhalation 0.031%, 0.062% Soln. Plastic vial 4 ml. Box 100s.
Use: Bronchodilator.

ARM-A-MED ISOETHARINE HCl. (Armour) Soln. for nebulization: Isoetharine 0.125%, sodium metabisulfite, glycerin. Bot. UD 4 ml.
Use: Bronchodilator.

ARM-A-MED METAPROTERENOL SULFATE. (Armour) Soln. for nebulization: Metaproterenol sulfate 0.4% or 0.6% with sodium Cl, EDTA. Vial UD 2.5 ml for use with IPPB device.
Use: Bronchodilator.

ARM-A-VIAL. (Armour) Sterile water, sodium Cl 0.45% or 0.9%. Box 100s. Plastic vial 3 ml, 5 ml.
Use: Electrolyte.

A.R.M. TABLETS. (SmithKline Prods) Chlorpheniramine maleate 4 mg, phenylpropanolamine HCl 25 mg/Tab. Pkg. 20s, 40s.
Use: Antihistamine, decongestant.

ARMOUR THYROID. (Rorer) Desiccated animal thyroid glands (active thyroid hormones: T-4 thyroxine, T-3 thyronine 0.25 gr, 0.5 gr, 1 gr, 1.5 gr, 2 gr, 3 gr, 4 gr or 5 gr/Tab. Bot. 100s, 1000s, Handy Hundreds, Carton Strip 100s.
Use: Thyroid hormone.

ARNICA TINCTURE. (Lilly) Arnica 20% in alcohol 66%. Bot. 120 ml, 480 ml.
Use: External analgesic.

•**AROMATIC AMMONIA SPIRIT,** U.S.P. XXII (Lilly) Bot. 16 oz. Aspirols 0.4 ml. Box 12s.
Use: Source of ammonia for fainting spells.
See: Ammonia.

AROMATIC AMMONIA VAPOROLE. (Burroughs Wellcome) Inhalant. Vial 5 min. Box 10s, 12s, 100s.
Use: Respiratory/CNS stimulant.

•**AROMATIC ELIXIR,** N.F XVII. (Lilly) Alcohol 22%. Bot. 16 fl. oz.
Use: Flavored vehicle.

•**ARPRINOCID.** USAN.
Use: Coccidiostat.

ARSAMBIDE.
See: Carbarsone (Various Mfr.).

ARSANILIC ACID. B.A.N. p-Aminophenylarsonic acid.
Use: Treatment of enteritis, growth promotion (veterinary medicine).
See: Maize Pro-Gen.

ARSECLOR.
See: Dichlorophenarsine HCl (Various Mfr.).

ARSENIC COMPOUNDS.
Use: Rarely employed in modern medicine; there are no longer any official compounds.
See: Acetarson.
Arsphenamine.
Carbarsone (Various Mfr.).
Dichlorophenarsine HCl.
Ferric Cacodylate.
Glycobiarsol.
Neoarsphenamine.
Oxophenarsine HCl.
Sodium Cacodylate (Various Mfr.).
Tryparsamide.

ARSENOBENZENE.
See: Arsphenamine.

ARSENPHENOLAMINE.
See: Arsphenamine.

ARSPHENAMINE. 3, 3′-diamino-4, 4′ dihydroxy-

arsenobenzene dihydrochloride. Arsenobenzene, arsenobenzol, arsenphenolamine, Ehrlich 606, salvarsan.
Use: Formerly used as antisyphilitic.

ARSTHINOL. Cyclic (hydroxymethyl)ethylene-3-acetamido-4-hydroxydithiobenzenearsonite.
Use: Antiprotozoal.

ARTANE. (Lederle) Trihexyphenidyl HCl. **Elix.:** 2 mg/5 ml w/methylparaben 0.08%, propylparaben 0.02%, Bot. pt. **Tab.:** 2 mg or 5 mg, Bot. 100s, 1000s, UD 10×10 in 10s. **Sequel:** 5 mg Bot. 60s, 500s.
Use: Anti-parkinson agent.

ARTARAU. (Archer-Taylor) Rauwolfia serpentina 50 mg or 100 mg/Tab. Bot. 100s, 1000s.
Use: Antihypertensive.

ARTA-VI-C. (Archer-Taylor) Multivitamins with Vitamin C 100 mg/Tab. Bot. 100s.
Use: Vitamin supplement.

ARTAZYME. (Archer-Taylor) Bot. 13 ml.
Use: Autolyzed proteolytic enzyme.

•**ARTEGRAFT.** USAN. Arterial graft composed of a section of bovine carotid artery that has been subjected to enzymatic digestion with ficin and tanned with dialdehyde starch.
Use: Prosthetic aid (arterial).

ARTERENOL.
See: Norepinephrine bitartrate.

ARTERIAL GRAFT. (Johnson & Johnson) Bovine origin.
Use: Arterial grafting.

ARTHA-G. (T.E. Williams) Salsalate 750 mg/Tab. Bot. 120s.
Use: Salicylate analgesic.

ARTHRALGEN. (Robins) Salicylamide 250 mg, acetaminophen 250 mg/Tab. Bot. 30s, 100s, 500s.
Use: Analgesic.

ARTHRITIC PAIN LOTION. (Walgreen) Triethanolamine salicylate 10%. Bot. 6 oz.
Use: External analgesic.

ARTHRITIS BAYER TIMED RELEASE ASPIRIN. (Glenbrook) Aspirin 650 mg/TR Tab. Bot. 30s, 72s, 125s.
Use: Salicylate analgesic.

ARTHRITIS PAIN FORMULA. (Whitehall) Aspirin 486 mg, aluminum hydroxide gel 20 mg, magnesium hydroxide 60 mg/Tab. Bot. 40s, 100s, 175s.
Use: Analgesic combination.

ARTHRITIS PAIN FORMULA, ASPIRIN FREE. (Whitehall) Acetaminophen 500 mg/Tab. Bot. 30s, 75s.
Use: Analgesic.

ARTHRITIS VACCINES.
See: Streptococcus Vaccine (Lilly).

ARTHROPAN LIQUID. (Purdue Frederick) Choline salicylate 870 mg/5 ml. Bot. 8 oz, 16 oz.
Use: Analgesic.

ARTHROTRIN TABLETS. (Whiteworth) Enteric coated aspirin 325 mg/Tab. Bot. 100s.
Use: Salicylate analgesic.

ARTICULOSE-50. (Seatrace) Prednisolone acetate 50 mg/ml. Vial 10 ml, 30 ml.
Use: Corticosteroid.

ARTICULOSE L. A. (Seatrace) Triamcinolone diacetate 40 mg/ml. Vial 5 ml.
Use: Corticosteroid.

ARTIFICIAL TANNING AGENT.
See: QT, Prods. (Schering-Plough).
Sudden Tan, Prods. (Schering-Plough).

ARTIFICIAL TEAR INSERT.
See: Lacrisert (Merck Sharp & Dohme).

ARTIFICIAL TEARS. (Various Mfr.).
Use: Lubricant, ophthalmic.

ARTIFICIAL TEARS. (Rugby) **Soln.:** Polyvinyl alcohol 1.4%, EDTA, chlorobutanol. Bot. 15 ml. **Oint.:** White petrolatum, mineral oil, lanolin. Tube 3.75 Gm.
Use: Lubricant, ophthalmic.

ARTRA BEAUTY BAR. (Schering-Plough) Triclocarban 1% in soap base. Cake 3.6 oz.
Use: Skin cleanser.

ARTRA SKIN TONE CREAM. (Schering-Plough) Hydroquinone 2%. Oint. Tube 1 oz. (normal only), 2 oz, 4 oz.
Use: Skin bleaching agent.

ASA. (Wampole-Zeus) Anti-skin antibodies test by IFA. Test 48s.
Use: Diagnostic aid.

A.S.A. (Lilly) Aspirin. Acetylsalicylic acid. **Enseal:** 5 gr or 10 gr. Bot. 100s, 1000s. **Supp.:** 5 gr or 10 gr. Pkg. 6s, 144s.
Use: Salicylate analgesic.

ASAFETIDA, EMULSION OF. Milk of Asafetida.

ASALCO NO. 1. (Jenkins) Acetylsalicylic acid 3.5 gr, acetophenetidin 2.5 gr, caffeine 0.5 gr/Tab. or Cap. Bot. 1000s.
Use: Analgesic.

ASAPED TABLETS. (Winthrop Products) Acetylsalicylic acid.
Use: Analgesic.

ASAWIN TABLETS. (Winthrop Products) Acetylsalicylic acid.
Use: Analgesic.

A.S.B. (Femco) Calcium carbonate, magnesium carbonate, bismuth subcarbonate, sodium bicarbonate, kaolin. Pow., Can 3 oz. Tabs. 50s.
Use: Antacid.

ASBRON G. (Sandoz) **Tab.:** Theophylline sodium glycinate 300 mg, guaifenesin 100 mg. Bot. 100s. **Elix.:** Theophylline sodium glycinate 300 mg, guaifenesin 100 mg, alcohol 15%/15 ml. Bot. pt.
Use: Bronchodilator, expectorant.

ASCLEROL. (Spanner) Liver injection crude (2 mcg/ml) 50%, Vitamins B_1 20 mg, B_2 3 mg, B_6 1 mg, B_{12} 30 mcg, niacinamide 100 mg, panthenol 2.8 mg, choline Cl 20 mg, inositol 10 mg/ml. Multiple dose vial 10 ml.
Use: Vitamin supplement.

ASCORBATE SODIUM. Antiscorbutic vitamin.

•**ASCORBIC ACID,** U.S.P. XXII. Inj., Oral Soln., U.S.P. XXII. Tab., U.S.P. XXII. 3-Oxo-L-gulofu-

ranolactone (enol form). Antiscorbic vitamin; Vitamin C.
Cap.: (Various Mfr.) 25 mg, 100 mg, 250 mg, 500 mg. **Inj.:** (Various Mfr.) Amp. (100 mg/ml) 1 ml, 2 ml, 5 ml; (200 mg/ml) 5 ml, (500 mg) 2 ml, 5 ml, 10 ml, 30 ml, (250 mg/ml) 10 ml; (1000 mg/ml) 10 ml. **Tab.:** (Various Mfr.) 50 mg, 100 mg, 250 mg, 500 mg. **Chew. Tab.:** (Various Mfr.) 100 mg, 250 mg, 500 mg. **SR Tab.:** (Various Mfr.) 500 mg, 1500 mg. **SR Cap.:** 500 mg. **Pow.:** (Various Mfr.) 4 Gm/5 ml. **Soln.:** (Various Mfr.) 35 mg/0.6 ml or 100 mg/ml.
Use: Vitamin C supplement.
See: Ascorbajen, Tab. (Jenkins).
Ascorbicap, Cap. (ICN).
Ascorbineed, Cap. (Hanlon).
C-Caps 500 (Drug Industries).
Cecon, Soln. (Abbott).
Cenolate, Amp. (Abbott).
Cetane, Cap., Vial (Forest).
Cevalin, Tab., Amp. (Lilly).
Cevi-Bid, Cap. (Geriatric).
Ce-Vi-Sol, Drops (Mead Johnson).
C-Syrup-500 (Ortega).
Neo-Vadrin, Preps. (Scherer).
Solucap C, Cap. (Jamieson-McKames).
Tega-C Tab. (Ortega).

•**ASCORBIC ACID INJECTION,** U.S.P. XXII.
Use: Vitamin C supplement.
See: Cevalin, Amp. (Lilly).

ASCORBIC ACID SALTS.
See: Bismuth Ascorbate.
Calcium Ascorbate.
Sodium Ascorbate.

ASCORBICAP. (ICN) Ascorbic acid 500 mg/S.R. Cap. Bot. 50s.
Use: Vitamin C supplement.

ASCORBIN/11. (Pasadena Research) Lemon bioflavonoids 110 mg, Vitamin C 1 Gm, rose hips powder 50 mg, rutin 25 mg/S.R. Tab. Bot. 100s.
Use: Vitamin supplement.

ASCORBINEED. (Hanlon) Vitamin C 500 mg/T-Cap. Bot. 100s.
Use: Vitamin C supplement.

ASCORBOCIN POWDER. (Paddock) Vitamin C 500 mg, niacin 500 mg, B_1 50 mg, B_6 50 mg, d-a-tocopheryl, polyethylene glycol 1000 succinate 50 IU, lactose/3 Gm. Bot. lb.
Use: Vitamin supplement.

ASCORBYL PALMITATE, N.F. XVII. L-Ascorbic acid 6-palmitate.
Use: Preservative, antioxidant.

ASCORVITE S.R. (Vitarine) Vitamin C 500 mg/S.R. Cap.
Use: Vitamin C supplement.

ASCRIPTIN. (Rorer Consumer) Aspirin 325 mg, magnesium hydroxide 50 mg, aluminum hydroxide 50 mg/Tab. Bot. 50s, 100s, 225s, 500s.
Use: Analgesic, antacid.

ASENDIN. (Lederle) Amoxapine. **25 mg/Tab.:** Bot. 100s; **50 mg/Tab.:** Bot. 100s, 500s, UD 100s; **100 mg/Tab.:** Bot. 100s, UD 100s; **150 mg/Tab.:** Bot. 30s.
Use: Antidepressant.

ASEPTICHROME.
See: Merbromin (Various Mfr.).

ASLUM. (Drug Products) Carbolic acid 1%, aluminum acetate, ichthammol, zinc oxide, aromatic oils in a petrolatum-stearin base. Tube oz. Jar lb.
Use: Astringent, dressing.

ASMA. (Wampole-Zeus) Anti-smooth muscle antibody test by IFA. Test 48.
Use: Diagnostic aid.

ASMADRIN. (Jenkins) Aminophylline 4 gr, aluminum hydroxide gel, dried, 4 gr, ephedrine HCl 3/8 gr, "trio-bar" 0.25 gr (representing 33⅓% each of pentobarbital sodium, butabarbital sodium, phenobarbital sodium)/Tab. Bot. 100s.

ASMALIX. (Century) Theophylline 80 mg, alcohol 20%/15 ml. Bot. qt, gal.
Use: Bronchodilator.

ASMATEX. (Kenyon) Chlorpheniramine 1.25 mg, phenylephrine HCl 2.5 mg, acetylsalicylic acid 150 mg buffered w/aluminum and magnesium hydroxide/Tab. Bot. 100s.
Use: Antihistamine, decongestant.

ASMA-TUSS. (Blue Cross) Phenobarbital 4 mg, theophylline 15 mg, ephedrine sulfate 12 mg, guaifenesin 50 mg/5 ml. Bot. 4 oz.
Use: Bronchodilator.

ASOLECTIN. (Associated Conc.) Chemical lecithin 25%, chemical cephalin 22%, inositol phosphatides 16%, soybean oil 2.5%, other miscellaneous sterols and lipids 34.5%.
Use: Diet supplement.

•**ASPARAGINASE.** USAN. L-asparagine amidohydrolase.
Use: Antineoplastic agent.
See: Elspar, Inj. (Merck Sharp & Dohme).

•**ASPARTAME,** N.F. XVII. 3-Amino-N-(α-methoxycarbonyl-phenethyl)succinamic acid. L-Aspartyl-L-phenyl-alanine methyl ester.
Use: Sweetening agent.

•**ASPARTIC ACID.** USAN. Aspartic acid; aminosuccinic acid.
Use: Management of fatigue.

•**ASPARTOCIN.** USAN.
Use: Antibacterial.

A-SPAS. (Hyrex) Dicyclomine HCl 10 mg/ml. Vial 10 ml.
Use: Antispasmodic.

ASPERCIN. (Otis Clapp) Aspirin 325 mg/Tab. Sugar, caffeine, lactose, and salt free. Safety pack 500s.
Use: Salycylate analgesic.

ASPERCIN EXTRA. (Otis Clapp) Aspirin 500 mg/Tab. Sugar, caffeine, lactose, and salt free. Safety pack 500s.
Use: Salicylate analgesic.

ASPERCREME. (Thompson Medical) Triethanolamine salicylate 10% in cream base.
Use: External analgesic

ASPERGILLUS ORYZAE ENZYME. Diastase.
See: Taka-Diastase, Preps. (Parke-Davis).

ASPERGUM. (Schering-Plough) Aspirin 227.5 mg/1 Gum. Tab. Orange or Cherry flavor. Box 16s, 40s.
Use: Salicylate analgesic.

ASPERKINASE. Proteolytic enzyme mixture derived from *aspergillus oryzae.*

•**ASPERLIN.** USAN.
Use: Antibacterial, antineoplastic agent.

ASPERMIN. (Buffington) Aspirin 325 mg/Tab. Sugar, caffeine, lactose, and salt free. Dispens-A-Kit 500s.
Use: Salicylate analgesic.

ASPERMIN EXTRA. (Buffington) Aspirin 500 mg/Tab. Sugar, caffeine, lactose, and salt free. Dispens-A-Kit 500s.
Use: Salicylate analgesic.

ASPIRBAR. (Lannett) Phenobarbital 0.25 gr, aspirin 10 gr/Tab. Bot. 1000s.
Use: Sedative/hypnotic, salicylate analgesic.

ASPIR-CODE. (Robinson) Salicylamide 3.5 gr, phenacetin 2.5 gr, caffeine 0.5 gr, codeine phosphate 2 mg/Tab. Bot. 36s, 100s.
Use: Analgesic combination.

ASPIR-D COMPOUND CAPSULES. (Lannett) Cap. Bot. 100s.

•**ASPIRIN,** U.S.P. XXII. Cap., Supp., Tab., U.S.P. XXII. A.S.A., Acetophen, Acetol, Acetosal, Acetosalin, Aceticyl, Acetylin, Acetylsal, Empirin, Saletin. Acetylsalicylic acid, Benzoic acid, 2-(acetyloxy)-., Salicyclic acid acetate.
Use: Analgesic, antipyretic, antirheumatic. Prophylactic to reduce risk of death or non-fatal MI in patients with a previous infarction or unstable angina pectoris (*FDA Drug Bull*, Dec. 1985).
See: A.S.A., Preps. (Lilly).
Aspergum, Gum, Tab. (Schering-Plough).
Aspirjen Jr., Tab. (Jenkins).
BC Tablets (Block Drug).
Buffinol, Tab. (Otis Clapp).
Ecotrin, Tab. (SmithKline Prods).
Empirin, Tab. (Burroughs Wellcome).
Measurin, Tab. (Winthrop Pharm).
Norwich Aspirin, Tab. (Norwich Eaton).
St. Joseph, Prods. (Schering-Plough).

•**ASPIRIN, ALUMINA, AND MAGNESIA TABLETS,** U.S.P. XXII.
Use: Analgesic, antacid.

•**ASPIRIN, ALUMINA, AND MAGNESIUM OXIDE TABLETS,** U.S.P. XXII.
Use: Analgesic, antacid.

ASPIRIN-BARBITURATE COMBINATIONS.
Use: Analgesic, sedative/hypnotic.
See: Amytal w/Acetylsalicylic acid, Cap. (Lilly).
Aspirbar, Tab. (Lannett).
Axotal, Tab. (Warren-Teed).
Brogesic, Tab. (Brothers).
Buff-A Comp., Cap., Tab. (Mayrand).
Cefinal, Tab. (Alto).
Doloral, Tab. (Alamed).
Fiorinal, Cap., Tab. (Sandoz).
Palgesic, Tab., Cap. (Pan Amer.).
Rotense, Tab. (Robinson).
Salibar Jr., Tab. (Jenkins).
Sedalgesic, Tab. (Table Rock).

•**ASPIRIN, CAFFEINE AND DIHYDROCODEINE CAPSULES,** U.S.P. XXII.
Use: Analgesic.

ASPIRIN W/CODEINE No. 2. (Halsey) Codeine phosphate 15 mg, aspirin 325 mg Tab. Bot. 100s, 1000s.
Use: Narcotic analgesic.

ASPIRIN W/CODEINE No. 3. (Halsey) Codeine phosphate 30 mg, aspirin 325 mg Tab. Bot. 100s, 1000s.
Use: Narcotic analgesic.

ASPIRIN W/CODEINE No. 4. (Halsey) Codeine phosphate 60 mg, aspirin 325 mg Tab. Bot. 100s, 1000s.
Use: Narcotic analgesic.

•**ASPIRIN, CODEINE, PHOSPHATE ALUMINA, AND MAGNESIA TABLETS,** U.S.P. XXII.
Use: Analgesic.

•**ASPIRIN AND CODEINE PHOSPHATE TABLETS,** U.S.P. XXII.
Use: Analgesic.

•**ASPIRIN DELAYED-RELEASE CAPSULES,** U.S.P. XXII.
Use: Analgesic.

•**ASPIRIN DELAYED-RELEASE TABLETS,** U.S.P. XXII.
Use: Analgesic.

ASPIRIN, ENTERIC COATED.
Use: Analgesic.
See: A.S.A., Preps. (Lilly).
Ecotrin, Tab. (SmithKline Prods).

ASPIRIN-FREE ST. JOSEPH COMPLETE NIGHTTIME COLD RELIEF. (Schering-Plough) Pseudoephedrine 15 mg, Chlorpheniramine maleate 1 mg, dextromethorphan HBr 5 mg, acetaminophen 160 mg. Bot. 120 ml.
Use: Decongestant, antihistamine, antitussive, analgesic.

ASPIRIN W/O.T.C. COMBINATIONS.
See: Alka Seltzer, Tab. (Miles).
Alka Seltzer Plus, Tab. (Miles).
A.P.C., Tab., Cap. (Various Mfr.).
A.S.A. Comp., Cap., Tab. (Lilly).
Ascriptin, Tab. (Rhone-Puolenc Rorer Consumer).
Ascriptin A/D, Tab. (Rhone-Puolenc Rorer Consumer).
Ascriptin, Extra Strength, Tab. (Rhone-Puolenc Rorer Consumer).
Ascriptin Codeine, Tab. (Rhone-Puolenc Rorer).
Bayer Aspirin Preps. (Glenbrook).
Bayer Prods. (Glenbrook).
BC Powder (Block Drug).
Buffaprin, Tab. (Buffington).

Bufferin, Tab. (Bristol-Myers).
Buffinol, Tab. (Otis Clapp).
Cama, Tab. (Sandoz Consumer).
Capathyn, Cap. (Scrip).
Damason, Preps. (Mason).
Emagrin, Tab. (Otis Clapp).
Excedrin, Cap., Tab. (Bristol-Myers).
4-Way, Tab., Spray (Bristol-Myers).
Liquiprin, Tab. (Mitchum-Thayer).
Midol, Cap., Spray (Glenbrook).
PAC, Cap., Tab. (Upjohn).
Pap, Cap. (Zenith).
Presalin, Tab. (Mallard).
Saleto, Preps. (Mallard).
Salocol, Tab. (Mallard).
Sine-Off Tablets (Menley & James).
Stanback, Pow., Tab. (Stanback).
St. Joseph Cold Tablets For Children (Schering-Plough).
Trigesic, Tab. (Squibb).
Vanquish, Cap. (Glenbrook).

ASPIRIN PLUS. (Walgreen) Aspirin 400 mg, caffeine 32 mg/Tab. Bot. 100s.
Use: Nonnarcotic analgesic combination.

ASPIRIN SALTS.
See: Calcium Acetylsalicylate.

•**ASPIRIN TABLETS, BUFFERED,** U.S.P. XXII.
Use: Salicylate Analgesic.

ASPIRIN UNISERTS. (Upsher-Smith) Aspirin 125 mg, 300 mg or 600 mg/supp. Ctn. 12s, 50s.
Use: Salicylate Analgesic.

ASPIRJEN Jr. (Jenkins) Aspirin 2.5 gr/Tab. Bot. 1000s.
Use: Salicylate Analgesic.

ASPIR-PHEN. (Robinson) Aspirin 5 gr, phenobarbital 0.5 gr/Tab. Bot. 100s, 1000s, Bulk Pack 5000s.
Use: Analgesic, sedative/hypnotic.

ASPIRTAB. (Dover) Aspirin 325 mg/Tab. Sugar, lactose, and salt free. UD Box 500s.
Use: Salicylate Analgesic.

ASPIRTAB MAX. (Dover) Aspirin 500 mg/Tab. Sugar, lactose, and salt free. UD Box 500s.
Use: Salicylate analgesic.

ASPOGEN. Dihydroxyaluminum aminoacetate.

ASPRO.
See: Acetylsalicylic acid.

ASPROJECT. (Mayrand) Sodium thiosalicylate 50 mg/ml. Inj. Vial. 30 ml.
Use: Analgesic.

ASTARIL TABLETS. (Winthrop Products) Theophylline anhydrous, ephedrine sulphate.
Use: Bronchodilator.

•**ASTEMIZOLE.** USAN.
Use: Antihistamine.

ASTEROL. 6-(2-Diethylaminoethoxy)-2-dimethylaminobenzothiazole dihydrochloride. Diamthazole Dihydrochloride, B.A.N.
Use: Antifungal.

ASTHMAHALER. (Norcliff Thayer) Epinephrine bitartrate 0.3 mg/ml in an inert propellant. Oral inhaler, 15 ml with mouthpiece; 15 ml refills.
Use: Bronchodilator.

ASTHMALIXIR. (Reese) Theophylline 45 mg, ephedrine sulfate 36 mg, guaifenesin 150 mg, phenobarbital 12 mg/15 ml. Alcohol 19%. Bot.
Use: Bronchodilator, expectorant, sedative/hypnotic.

ASTHMANEFRIN SOLUTION & NEBULIZER. (Norcliff Thayer) Racepin (racemic epinephrine) as HCl equivalent to epinephrine base 2.25%, chlorobutanol 0.5%. Bot. 0.5 fl oz. With sodium bisulfite. Bot. 1 fl oz.
Use: Bronchodilator.

•**ASTIFICON A.** USAN.
Use: Contact lens material (hydrophilic).

ASTRAMORPH PF. (Astra) Morphine sulfate 0.5 mg/ml or 1 mg/ml preservative free. Amp. 10 ml, Vial 10 ml.
Use: Narcotic analgesic.

•**ASTROMICIN SULFATE.** USAN.
Use: Antibacterial.

ASTRO-VITES. (Faraday) Vitamins A 3500 IU, D 400 IU, C 60 mg, B_1 0.8 mg, B_2 1.3 mg, niacinamide 14 mg, B_6 1 mg, B_{12} 2.5 mcg, folic acid 0.05 mg, pantothenic acid 5 mg, iron 12 mg/Tab. Bot. 100s, 250s.
Use: Vitamin/mineral supplement.

AST/SGOT REAGENT STRIPS. (Ames) Seralyzer reagent strip. A quantitative strip test for asparate transaminase/serum glutamic oxaloacetic transaminase in serum or plasma. Bot. Strip 25s.
Use: Diagnostic aid.

ASUPIRIN. (Suppositoria) Aspirin 60 mg, 120 mg, 200 mg, 300 mg, 600 mg or 1.2 Gm/Supp. Box 12s, 100s, 1000s.
Use: Salicylate analgesic.

A.T. 10.
See: Dihydrotachysterol.

ATABEE TD. (Defco) Vitamins C 500 mg, B_1 15 mg, B_2 10 mg, B_6 2 mg, nicotinamide 50 mg, calcium pantothenate 10 mg/Cap. Bot. 30s, 1000s.
Use: Vitamin supplement.

ATABRINE HYDROCHLORIDE. (Winthrop Pharm) Quinacrine HCl 100 mg Tab. Bot. 100s.
Use: Antimalarial, anthelmintic.

ATARAX. (Roerig) Hydroxyzine HCl. **Tab.:** 10 mg or 25 mg Bot. 100s, 500s, UD 10 × 10s, Unit-of-use 40s; 50 mg Bot. 100s, 500s, UD 10 × 10s; 100 mg Bot. 100s, UD 10 × 10s. **Syr.:** 10 mg/5 ml, alcohol 0.5%. Bot. pt.
Use: Antianxiety agent.
W/Ephedrine sulfate, theophylline.
See: Marax, Tab., Syr. (Roerig).
W/Penta-erythrityltetranitrate.
See: Cartrax, Tab. (Roerig).

ATARAXIC AGENTS.
See: Tranquilizers.

ATARVET. Acepromazine.

ATENOLOL. USAN. 4-(2-Hydroxy-3-isopropylaminopropoxy) phenylacetamide.
Use: Beta-adrenergic blocking agent.

See: Tenormin, Tab. (Stuart).

ATGAM. (Upjohn) Lymphocyte immune globulin, antithymocyte globulin 250 mg protein (50 mg/ml). Amp. 5 ml.
Use: Management of allograft rejection in renal transplant patients.

ATHLETE'S FOOT OINTMENT. (Walgreen) Zinc undecylenate 20%, undecylenic acid 5%. Tube 1.5 oz.
Use: Antifungal, external.

•**ATIPAMEZOLE.** USAN.
Use: Antiadrenergic.

•**ATIPROSIN MALEATE.** USAN.
Use: Antihypertensive.

ATIVAN INJECTION. (Wyeth-Ayerst) Lorazepam 2 mg/ml or 4 mg/ml. Vial 1 ml, 10 ml/2 ml Tubex (w/1 ml fill). Pkg. 10s.
Use: Antianxiety agent.

ATIVAN TABLETS. (Wyeth-Ayerst) Lorazepam 0.5 mg, 1 mg or 2 mg/Tab. **0.5 mg:** Bot. 100s, 500s, 1000s, Redipak 25s. **1 mg:** Bot. 100s, 500s, 1000s, Redipak 25s. **2 mg:** Bot. 100s, 500s, 1000s, Redipak 25s.
Use: Antianxiety agent.

•**ATOLIDE.** USAN. 2-Amino-4′-(diethylamino)-o-benzotoluidide. Under study.
Use: Anticonvulsant.

ATOLONE. (Major) Triamcinolone 4 mg/Tab. Bot. 100s, Uni-Pak 16s.
Use: Corticosteroid.

•**ATOSIBAN.** USAN.
Use: Antagonist, oxytocin.

ATOZINE TABS. (Major) Hydroxyzine HCl 10 mg, 25 mg or 50 mg/Tab; **10 and 25 mg:** Bot. 100s, 250s, 1000s, UD 100s; **50 mg:** Bot. 100s, 250s, 500s, UD 100s.
Use: Antianxiety agent.

ATPEG. (ICI Americas) Polyethylene glycol available as 300, 400, 600 or 4000.
Use: Surfactant, humectant.

•**ATRACURIUM BESYLATE.** USAN.
Use: Skeletal muscle relaxant.
See: Tracrium (Burroughs Wellcome).

ATRIDINE. (Interstate) Triprolidine 2.5 mg, pseudoephedrine HCl 60 mg/Tab. Bot. 100s, 1000s.
Use: Antihistamine, decongestant.

ATROCAP. (Freeport) Atropine sulfate 0.06 mg, hyoscyamine sulfate 0.3 mg, hyoscine hydrobromide 0.02 mg, phenobarbital 50 mg/T.R. Cap. Bot. 1000s.
Use: Sedative/hypnotic, anticholinergic/antispasmodic.

ATROCHOLIN TABLETS. (Glaxo) Dehydrocholic acid 130 mg/Tab. Bot. 100s.
Use: Laxative.

ATROHIST LA. (Adams) Pseudoephedrine HCl 120 mg, brompheniramine maleate 4 mg, phenyltoloxamine citrate 50 mg/SR Tab with atropine sulfate 0.0242 mg available for immediate release. Bot. 100s.
Use: Decongestant, antihistamine.

ATROHIST SPRINKLE. (Adams) Pseudoephedrine HCl 120 mg, brompheniramine maleate 2 mg, phenytoloxamine citrate 25 mg/SR Cap. Bot. 100s.
Use: Decongestant, antihistamine.

ATROMID-S. (Wyeth-Ayerst) Clofibrate 500 mg/Cap. Bot. 100s.
Use: Antihyperlipidemic.

ATROPEN AUTO-INJECTER. (Survival Technology) Atropine sulfate, phenol 2 mg. In prefilled automatic injection device.
Use: For toxic exposure to organophosphorus or carbamate insecticides.

ATROPHYSINE. (Lannett) Physostigmine salicylate 0.6 mg, atropine sulfate 0.6 mg/ml. Vial 30 ml.
Use: Antispasmodic.

•**ATROPINE,** U.S.P. XXII. 1αH, 5αH-Tropan-3α-ol dl-Tropate (Ester) (dl-Hyoscyamine)dl-Tropyltropate.
Use: Anticholinergic.
See: Atropine Combinations.

ATROPINE AND DEMEROL INJECTION. (Winthrop Pharm) Atropine sulfate 0.4 mg, meperidine HCl 50 mg or 75 mg/Carpuject.
Use: Preoperative sedative.

ATROPINE-CARE. (Akorn) Atropine sulfate 1%, benzalkonium Cl 0.01%, hydroxypropyl methylcellulose. Soln. Bot. 2 ml, 5 ml, 15 ml.
Use: Cycloplegic mydriatic.

ATROPINE-HYOSCINE-HYOSCYAMINE COMBINATIONS. (See also Belladonna Products)
See: Barbella, Tab., Elix. (Forest).
Barbeloid, Tab. (Vale).
Bar-Don, Tab., Elix. (Warren-Teed).
Belakoids TT, Tab. (Philips Roxane).
Belbutal No. 2 Kaptabs. (Churchill).
Brobella-P.B., Tab. (Brothers).
Buren, Tab. (Ascher).
Donnacin, Elix., Tab. (Pharmex).
Donnagel, Susp. (Robins).
Donnamine, Elix., Tab. (Tennessee Pharm.).
Donnatal, Cap., Elix., Tab. (Robins).
Donnatal #2, Tab. (Robins).
Donnatal Extentabs, Tab. (Robins).
Donnazyme, Tab. (Robins).
Eldonal, Preps. (Canright).
Haponal, Cap. (Jenkins).
Hyatal, Elix. (Winsale).
Hybephen, Preps. (Beecham Labs).
Hyonal, Preps. (Paddock).
Hyonatol B, Preps. (Bowman).
Hytrona, Tab. (Webcon).
Kinesed, Tab. (Stuart).
Koryza, Tab. (Forest).
Maso-Donna, Elix., Tab. (Mason).
Nilspasm, Tab. (Parmed).
Sedamine, Tab. (Dunhall).
Sedapar, Tab. (Parmed).
Seds, Tab. (Pasadena Research).
Spabelin, Elix. (Arcum).

Spasdel, Cap. (Marlop).
Spasloids, Tab. (G.F. Harvey).
Spasmolin, Tab. (Bell).
Spasquid, Elix. (Geneva).
Uriseptin, Tab. (Blaine).
Urogesic, Tab. (Edwards).

ATROPINE METHYLNITRATE. (Various Mfr.) dl-Hyoscyamine methylnitrate.
See: Harvatrate, Tab. (Forest Pharm.).
Thitrate W.P., Tab. (Blaine).
W/Hyoscine HBr, hyoscyamine sulfate, amobarbital sodium.
See: Amocine, Tab. (Mallard).
W/Methenamine mandelate and phenylazodiaminopyridine HCl.
See: Uritral, Cap. (Central).
W/Phenobarbital and dihydroxyaluminum aminoacetate.
See: Atromal, Tab. (Blaine).
Harvatrate A, Tab. (Forest Pharm.).

ATROPINE-N-OXIDE HCl.
See: Atropine Oxide HCl.

•**ATROPINE OXIDE HYDROCHLORIDE.** USAN. Atropine N-oxide HCl.
Use: Anticholinergic.
See: X-Tro (Xttrium).

•**ATROPINE SULFATE,** U.S.P. XXII. Inj., Ophth., Oint., Ophth. Soln., Tab, U.S.P. XXII. (Various Mfr.) Benzeneacetic acid, α-(hydroxymethyl)-8-methyl-8-azabicyclo-[3.2.1.]oct-3-yl ester, endo-(±)-, sulfate (2:1) (salt), monohydrate. l-αH, 5-α-H-Tropan-3-α-ol (±)-tropate (ester), sulfate (2:1) (salt) monohydrate. **Pediatric Inj.:** 0.05 mg/ml 5 ml Abboject. **Tab, Hypodermic:** 0.3 mg, 0.4 mg and 0.6 mg/Tab. Bot. 100s. **Tab, Oral:** 0.4 mg/Tab. Bot. 100s. **Inj.:** 0.1 mg/ml 5 ml and 10 ml Abboject 0.3 mg/ml. Vial 1 ml; 0.4 mg/ml. Amp. 1 ml, vial 20 ml; 0.8 mg/ml. Amp. 1 ml, dosette 0.5 ml; 1 mg/ml. Amp., vial 1 ml, syringe 10 ml; 1.2 mg/ml. Vial 1 ml syringe. **Lyophilized:** Lyopine (Hyrex). **Ophth. Oint:** 0.5% Tube 3.5 Gm.; 1% Tube 3.5 Gm., 3.75 Gm. **Ophth. Soln:** 0.5% Bot. 1 ml, 5 ml; 1% Bot. 1 ml, 2 ml, 5 ml, 15 ml; 2% Bot. 1 ml, 2 ml; 3% Bot. 5 ml.
Use: Anticholinergic, antidote to cholinesterase inhibitors.
See: Isopto-Atropine (Alcon).
Lyopine, Inj. (Hyrex).
Parasympatholytic and antispasmodic.
W/Ephedrine sulfate.
See: Enuretrol, Tab. (Berlex).

ATROPINE SULFATE AND MEPERIDINE HCl.
See: Atropine and Demerol. (Winthrop Pharm.).

ATROPINE SULFATE AND MORPHINE SULFATE.
See: Morphine and Atropine Sulfates. (Beecham Labs).

ATROPINE SULFATE W/PHENOBARBITAL.
See: Antrocol, Tab., Cap. (Poythress).
Arco-Lase Plus, Tab. (Arco).
Barbeloid, Tab. (Vale).
Briabell, Tab. (Briar).
Brobella-P.B., Tab. (Brothers).
Donnatal, Cap., Extentab, Tab., Elix. (Robins).
Donnatal #2, Tab. (Robins).
Haponal, Cap. (Jenkins).
Hyatal Elix. (Winsale).
Palbar No. 2, Tab. (Hauck).
Ro Trim, Cap. (Rocky Mtn.).
Seds, Tab. (Pasadena Research).
Spabelin, Elix. (Arcum).
Spasdel, Cap. (Marlop).
Spasmolin, Tab. (Kenyon).
Stannitol (Standex).

ATROPISOL. (CooperVision) Atropine sulfate soln. **Dropperette:** 0.5%, 1% or 2%. 1 ml Box 12s. **Dropper Bot.:** 1%. 5 ml. **Bot.:** 1%. 15 ml.
Use: Cycloplegic mydriatic.

ATROSED. (Freeport) Atropine sulfate 0.0195 mg, hyoscine HBr 0.0065 mg, hyoscyamine sulfate 0.104 mg, phenobarbital 0.25 gr/Tab. Bot. 1000s, 5000s.
Use: Anticholinergic/antispasmodic, sedative/hypnotic,.

ATROSEPT. (Geneva Generics) Methenamine 40.8 mg, phenyl salicylate 18.1 mg, atropine sulfate 0.03 mg, hyoscyamine 0.03 mg, benzoic acid 4.5 mg, methylene blue 5.4 mg/Tab. Bot. 100s, 1000s.
Use: Urinary anti-infective.

ATROVENT. (Boehringer Ingelheim) Ipratropium bromide 18 mcg/dose. Inhalation aerosol 15 ml.
Use: Bronchodilator.

AT-SOLUTION. (Winthrop Products) Dihydrotachysterol solution.
Use: Hypocalcemic tetany.

A/T/S TOPICAL SOLUTION. (Hoechst) Erythromycin 2% topical soln. Bot. 60 ml w/applicator.
Use: Anti-acne.

ATTAIN LIQUID. (Sherwood). Sodium caseinate, calcium caseinate, maltodextrin, corn oil, soy lecithin. Can 250 ml and 1000 ml closed system.
Use: Enteral nutritional supplement.

ATTAPULGITE, ACTIVATED.
Use: Antidiarrheal.
See: Quintess, Susp. (Lilly).
W/Pectin, hydrated alumina powder.
See: Polymagma Plain Tab. (Wyeth-Ayerst).
W/Polysorbate 80, salicylic acid, propylene glycol.
See: Sebasorb Lot. (Summer).

ATTENUVAX. (Merck Sharp & Dohme) Measles virus vaccine, live, attenuated w/neomycin 25 mcg/Vial. Single-dose vial w/diluent. Pkg. 1s, 10s.
Use: Agent for immunization.
W/Meruvax.
See: M-R-Vax-II, Vial (Merck Sharp & Dohme).
W/Mumpsvax, Meruvax.
See: M-M-R II, Vial (Merck Sharp & Dohme).

ATUSSIN-D.M. EXPECTORANT. (Amfre-Grant) Chlorpheniramine maleate 2 mg, phenylephrine HCl 5 mg, phenylpropanolamine HCl 5 mg,

guaifenesin 100 mg, dextromethorphan HBr 15 mg/5 ml Syr. Bot. 4 oz, pt, gal.
Use: Antihistamine, decongestant, expectorant, antitussive.

W/Pentobarbital sodium, 2-diethylaminoethyl diphenyl-acetate HCl, aluminum hydroxide.
See: Spasmasorb, Tab. (Hauck).

AUGMENTIN CHEWABLE TABLETS. (Beecham Labs) **125:** Amoxicillin 125 mg, clavulanic acid 31.25 mg/Tab. Ctn. 30s. **250:** Amoxicillin 250 mg, clavulanic acid 62.5 mg/Tab. Ctn. 30s.
Use: Antibacterial, penicillin.

AUGMENTIN ORAL SUSPENSION. (Beecham Labs) **125:** Amoxicillin 125 mg, clavulanic acid (as potassium salt) 31.25 mg/5 ml. Bot. 75 ml, 150 ml. **250**: Amoxicillin 250 mg, clavulanic acid (as potassium salt) 62.5 mg/5 ml. Bot. 75 ml, 150 ml.
Use: Antibacterial, penicillin.

AUGMENTIN TABLETS. (Beecham Labs) Amoxicillin trihydrate 250 mg or 500 mg, clavulanic acid (as potassium salt) 125 mg/Tab. **250:** Bot. 30s, UD 100s. **500:** Bot. 30s, 100s.
Use: Antibacterial, penicillin.

AURAL ACUTE. (Saron) Polymyxin B sulfate 10,000 units, neomycin sulfate 5 mg, hydrocortisone 10 mg/10 ml, alcohol 0.1%.
Use: Corticosteroid combination.

AURALGAN OTIC SOLUTION. (Wyeth-Ayerst) Antipyrine 54 mg, benzocaine 14 mg/ml w/oxyquinoline sulfate in dehydrated glycerin (contains not more than 0.6% moisture). Bot. w/ dropper 15 ml.
Use: Otic preparation.

AURALGESIC. (Wesley) Carbamide 10%, antipyrine 5%, benzocaine 2.5%, cetyldimethylbenzylammonium HCl 0.2%. Bot. 0.5 oz.
Use: Otic preparation.

•**AURANOFIN.** USAN.
Use: Antirheumatic.

AUREOMYCIN PREPARATIONS. (Lederle) Chlortetracycline HCl.
Ophth. Oint.: 1% (10 mg/Gm) Tube 0.125 oz.
Topical Oint.: 3% (30 mg/Gm) in white petrolatum, anhydrous lanolin base. Tube 0.5 oz, 1 oz.
Use: Anti-infective.

AUREOQUIN DIAMATE. Name previously used for Quinetolate.

AUROCAINE. (Republic) Carbamide, glycerin, propylene glycol with chlorobutanol 0.5%. Bot. 15 ml.
Use: Otic preparation.

AUROCAINE 2. (Republic) Boric acid in isopropyl alcohol 2.75%. Soln. Bot. 30 ml.
Use: Otic preparation.

AUROCEIN. (Christina) Gold naphthyl sulfhydryl derivative. 5% or 12.5% Amp. 10 ml.
Use: Antirheumatic agent.

AURO-DRI. (Commerce) Boric acid 2.75% in isopropyl alcohol. Bot. oz.
Use: Otic preparation.

AURO EAR DROPS. (Commerce) Carbamide peroxide 6.5% in a specially prepared base. Bot. 15 ml.
Use: Otic preparation.

AUROLIN.
See: Gold sodium thiosulfate.

AUROPIN.
See: Gold sodium thiosulfate.

AUROSAN.
See: Gold sodium thiosulfate.

AUROTHIOBLYCANIDE. 2-Mercaptoacetanilide S-gold (1+) salt.
Use: Antirheumatic agent.

AUROTHIOGLUCOSE INJECTION.
See: Sterile aurothioglucose suspension.

AUROTHIOMALATE, SODIUM.
See: Gold Sodium Thiomalate, U.S.P. XXII.

AUSAB. (Abbott Diagnostics) Radioimmunoassay or enzyme immunoassay for detection of antibody to hepatitis B surface antigen. Test kit 100s.
Use: Diagnostic aid.

AUSAB EIA. (Abbott Diagnostics) Enzyme immunoassay for the detection of antibody to hepatitis B surface antigen.
Use: Diagnostic aid.

AUSCELL. (Abbott Diagnostics) Reverse passive hemagglutination test for hepatitis B surface antigen. Test kit 110s, 450s, 1800s.
Use: Diagnostic aid.

AUSRIA II-125. (Abbott Diagnostics) Radioimmunoassay for detection of hepatitis B surface antigen. Test kit 100s, 500s, 600s, 700s, 800s, 900s, 1000s.
Use: Diagnostic aid.

AUSZYME II. (Abbott Diagnostics) Enzyme immunoassay for detection of hepatitis B surface antigen (HBsAg) in human serum or plasma. Test kit 100s, 500s.
Use: Diagnostic aid.

AUSZYME MONOCLONAL. (Abbott Diagnostics) Qualitative third generation enzyme immunoassay for the detection of hepatitis B surface antigen (HBsAg) in human serum or plasma.
Use: Diagnostic aid.

AUTOANTIBODY SCREEN. (Wampole-Zeus) Autoantibody screening system. To screen serum for the presence of a variety of autoantibodies. Test 48s.
Use: Diagnostic aid.

AUTOLET KIT. (Ames) Automatic blood letting spring-loaded device to obtain capillary blood samples from fingertips, earlobes or heels.
Use: Diagnostic aid.

AUTOPLEX. (Hyland) Anti-inhibitor coagulant complex prepared from pooled human plasma. Vial 30 ml.
Use: Diagnostic aid.

AUTOPLEX T. (Hyland) Dried anti-inhibitor coagulant complex. With a maximum of heparin 2 units and polyethylene glycol 2 mg per ml re-

constituted material. Inj. Vial with diluent and needles.
Use: Diagnostic aid.

AUTRINIC. Intrinsic factor concentrate.
Use: To increase absorption of Vitamin B_{12}.

AUXOTAB ENTERIC 1 & 2. (Colab) Rapid identification of enteric bacteria and *pseudomonas.* Test contains capillary units with selective biochemical reagents.
Use: Diagnostic aid.

AVAIL. (SmithKline Beecham) Elemental iron 18 mg, vitamin A 5000 IU, D 400 IU, E 30 mg, B_1 2.25 mg, B_2 2.55 mg, B_3 20 mg, B_6 3 mg, B_{12} 9 mcg, C 90 mg, folic acid 0.4 mg, Ca, Cr, I, Mg, Se and zinc 22.5 mg/Tab. Bot. 60s, 100s.
Use: Vitamin/mineral supplement.

AVALGESIC LOTION. (Various Mfr.) Methyl salicylate, menthol, camphor, methyl nicotinate, dipropylene glycol salicylate, oil of cassia, oleoresins capsicum and ginger. Bot. 120 ml, pt, gal.
Use: External analgesic.

A-VAN. (Stewart-Jackson) Dimenhydrinate 50 mg/Cap. Bot. 100s.
Use: Antivertigo agent.

AVC CREAM. (Merrell Dow) Sulfanilamide 15% in a water-miscible base of propylene glycol, stearic acid, diglycol stearate to acid pH. Tube 4 oz. w/applicator.
Use: Anti-infective, vaginal.

AVC SUPPOSITORIES. (Merrell Dow) Sulfanilamide 1.05 Gm in a base made from polyethylene glycol 400, polysorbate 80, polyethylene glycol 3350, glycerin, inert glycerin-gelatin covering. Box 16s w/inserter.
Use: Anti-infective, vaginal.

AVEENOBAR MEDICATED. (Rydell) Aveeno colloidal oatmeal 50%, sulfur 2%, salicylic acid 2%, in soap-free cleansing bar. Formerly Acnaveen. Bar 3.5 oz.
Use: Antipruritic.

AVEENOBAR OILATED. (Rydell) Vegetable oils, lanolin derivative, glycerine 29%, aveeno colloidal oatmeal 30% in soap-free base. Formerly Emulave. Bar. 3 oz.
Use: Emollient.

AVEENOBAR REGULAR. (Rydell) Colloidal oatmeal 50%, anionic sulfonate, hypo-allergenic lanolin. Formerly Aveeno Bar. Bar 3.2 oz, 4.4 oz.
Use: Skin cleanser.

AVEENO BATH. (Rydell) Colloidal oatmeal. Box 1 lb, 4 lb.
Use: Emollient.

AVEENO COLLOIDAL OATMEAL. (Rydell) Colloidal oatmeal. Box 1 lb, 4 lb.
Use: Emollient.

AVEENO LOTION. (Rydell) Colloidal oatmeal in aqueous lotion base. Bot. 6 oz.
Use: Emollient.

AVEENO OILATED. (Rydell) Aveeno colloidal oatmeal impregnated with 35% liquid petrolatum, refined olive oil. Box 8 oz, 2 lb.
Use: Emollient.

AVENTYL HCl. (Lilly) Nortriptyline HCl. **Liq.:** Equivalent to 10 mg base/5 ml in alcohol 4%. Bot. 16 fl. oz. **Pulv.:** Equivalent to 10 mg base or 25 mg base/Cap. Bot. 100s, 500s, Blisterpak 10 × 10s.
Use: Antidepressant.

AVERTIN. Tribromoethanol (Various Mfr.).

•**AVILAMYCIN.** USAN.
Use: Antibacterial.

AVINAR. Uredepa.
Use: Antineoplastic agent.

AVITENE. (Alcon Surgical) Hydrochloric acid salt of purified bovine corium collagen. **Fibrous Form:** Jar 1 Gm, 5 Gm. **Web Form:** Blister Pak. Sheets of 70 mm × 70 mm, 70 mm × 35 mm.
Use: Topical hemostat.

•**AVOBENZONE.** USAN.
Use: Sunscreen.

AVONIQUE. (Geneva) Vitamins A 4000 IU, D 400 IU, B_1 1 mg, B_2 1.2 mg, B_6 2 mg, B_{12} 2 mcg, calcium pantothenate 5 mg, B_3 10 mg, C 30 mg, calcium 100 mg, phosphorous 76 mg, iron 10 mg, manganese 1 mg, magnesium 1 mg, zinc 1 mg.
Use: Vitamin/mineral supplement.

•**AVOPARCIN.** USAN.
Use: Antibacterial.

A.V.P. CILLIN TABS AND POWDER FOR SYRUP. (A.V.P.) Potassium penicillin G. **Syr.:** (400,000 units) 250 mg/5 ml. Bot. 80 ml. **Tab.:** 250 mg. Bot. 100s.
Use: Antibacterial, penicillin.

A.V.P. NATAL-FA. (A.V.P.) Vitamins A 5000 IU, elemental iron 200 mg, ferrous fumarate 65 mg, calcium 165 mg, phosphorus 75 mg, C 100 mg, B_6 10 mg, folic acid 1 mg/Tab. Bot. 100s.
Use: Vitamin/mineral supplement.

•**AVRIDINE.** USAN.
Use: Antiviral.

AWAKE. (Walgreen) Caffeine 100 mg/Tab. Bot. 36s.
Use: CNS stimulant.

AXEROPHTHOL.
See: Vitamin A.

AXID. (Lilly) Nizatidine 150 mg or 300 mg/Cap. Bot. 60s, UD 30s.
Use: H_2 antagonist.

AXON THROAT SPRAY. (McKesson) Bot. 5 Gm.
Use: Throat preparation.

AXOTAL. (Adria) Butalbital 50 mg, aspirin 650 mg/Tab. Bot. 100s, 500s.
Use: Sedative/hypnotic, salicylate analgesic.

AXSAIN. (Galen Pharma) Capsaicin 0.075%. 60 Gm.
Use: Pain reliever.

AXSINATE. (Lannett) Styramate 200 mg, salicylamide 210 mg, acetophenetidin 150 mg, caffeine 30 mg/Tab. Bot. 50s.
Use: Analgesic.

AYDS APPETITE SUPPRESSANT CANDY. (Jeffrey Martin) Benzocaine 5 mg in chewy candy base w/25 cal./Cube. Ctn. 12s, 48s, 96s.
Use: Diet aid.

AYGESTIN. (Wyeth-Ayerst) Norethindrone acetate 5 mg/Tab. Bot. 50s, Cycle pack 10s.
Use: Progestin.

AYR SALINE NASAL DROPS. (Ascher) Sodium Cl 0.65% adjusted with phosphate buffers to proper tonicity and pH to prevent nasal irritation. **Drops:** Bot. 20 ml. **Mist:** Bot. 50 ml.
Use: Moisture replenisher.

•**AZABON.** USAN.
Use: Stimulant.

•**AZACHLORZINE HYDROCHLORIDE.** USAN.
Use: Vasodilator.

•**AZACITIDINE.** USAN.
Use: Antineoplastic agent.

AZACTAM FOR INJECTION. (Squibb) L-arginine 780 mg/Gm aztreonam. **Single dose 15 ml vial:** 500 mg/Vial Pkg. 10s, 25s. 1 Gm/Vial Pkg. 10s, 25s. 2 Gm/vial Pkg. 10s, 25s. **Single dose 100 ml IV infusion bottle w/ball bands:** 500 mg/Bot. Pkg. 10s. 1 Gm/vial Pkg. 10s. 12 Gm/vial Pkg. 10s.
Use: Antibacterial.

AZACYCLONOL. B.A.N. α-4-Piperidylbenzhydrol. Frenquel HCl.
Use: Tranquilizer.

AZACYCLONOL HCl. Alpha, alpha-diphenyl-4-piperidine-methanol HCl.

AZALINE TABS. (Major) Sulfasalazine 500 mg/Tab. Bot. 100s, 500s, 1000s.
Use: Agent for ulcerative colitis.

AZALOMYCIN. B.A.N. A mixture of related antibiotics produced by *Streptomyces hygroscopicus var. azalomyceticus*.
Use: Antibacterial.

•**AZALOXAN FUMARATE.** USAN.
Use: Antidepressant.

AZAMETHONIUM BROMIDE. B.A.N. 3-Methyl-3-azapentamethylenedi(ethyldimethylammonium bromide). Pendiomide.
Use: Ganglionic blocking agent.

AZAMETHONIUM BROMIDE. (Ciba) 3-Methyl-3-azapentamethylenebis (ethyldimethyl-ammonium) dibromide. Pendiomide, Pentamin.
Use: Ganglionic blocking agent.

•**AZANATOR MALEATE.** USAN.
Use: Bronchodilator.

•**AZANIDAZOLE.** USAN.
Use: Antiprotozoal.

•**AZAPERONE.** USAN. 4′-Fluoro-4-[4-(2-pyridyl)-piperazin-l-yl]butyrophenone. Stresnil. Suicalm.
Use: Tranquilizer, (veterinary).

AZAPETINE. B.A.N. 6-Allyl-5,7-dihydrodibenz-[c,e]azepine. Ilidar phosphate.
Use: Vasodilator.

AZAPETINE PHOSPHATE. 6-Allyl-6,7-dihydro-5H-dibenz(c,e)azepine, azephine.

AZAPROPAZONE. B.A.N. 5-Dimethylamino-9-methyl-2-propyl-1H-pyrazolo[1,2-α][1,2,4]-benzotriazine-1,3(2H)-dione.
Use: Analgesic, anti-inflammatory.

•**AZARIBINE.** USAN. 2-β-D-Ribofuranosyl-1,2,4-triazine-3,5-(2H,4H)dione2,3′,5′-triacetate. 6-Azauridine 2′,3′,5′-triacetate. Triazure.
Use: Treatment of psoriasis.

•**AZAROLE.** USAN.
Use: Immunoregulator.

•**AZASERINE.** USAN.
Use: Antifungal.

•**AZATADINE MALEATE,** U.S.P. XXII. 5-H-Benzo (5-6) cyclohepta (1,2-b) pyridine, 6,11-dihydro-11-(1-methyl-4-piperidylidene)-5H-benzo(5,6)-cyclohepta (1,2-b) pyridine maleate (1:2).
Use: Antihistamine.
See: Optimine, Tab. (Schering-Plough).
Trinalin, Tab. (Schering-Plough).

•**AZATHIOPRINE,** U.S.P. XXII. Tab., U.S.P. XXII. (Burroughs Wellcome) 6-(1-Methyl-4-nitroimidazol-5-ylthio) purine. lH-Purine, 6-[(l-methyl-4-nitro-lH-imidazol-5-yl)thio]-.6-[(l-Methyl-4-nitroimidazolyl-5-)thio]purine.
Use: Anti-leukemic compound.
See: Imuran, Inj., Tab. (Burroughs Wellcome).

AZATHIOPRINE. B.A.N. 6-(1-Methyl-4-nitroimidazol-5-ylthio)purine.
Use: Antimetabolite.

AZATHIOPRINE SODIUM, U.S.P. XXII.
Use: Anti-leukemic compound.

5-AZC.
See: Azacitidine.

AZDONE. (Central) Hydrocodone bitartrate 5 mg, aspirin 500 mg/Tab. Bot. 100s, 1000s.
Use: Narcotic analgesic combination.

•**AZELASTINE HYDROCHLORIDE.** USAN.
Use: Antiallergic, antiasthmatic.

•**AZEPINDOLE.** USAN.
Use: Antidepressant.

•**AZETEPA.** USAN. PP-Diaziridin-1-yl-N-ethyl-1,3,4-thiadiazol-2-ylphosphinamide.
Use: Antimetabolite.

AZIDOCILLIN. B.A.N. 6-[D()-α-Azidophenyl-acetamido]penicillanic acid.
Use: Antibiotic.

AZIDOTHYMIDINE
See: Zidovudine.

•**AZIPRAMINE HYDROCHLORIDE.** USAN.
Use: Antidepressant.

•**AZITHROMYCIN.** USAN.
Use: Antibacterial.

AZLIN. (Miles Pharm) Azlocillin sodium. Vial 2 Gm, 3 Gm, 4 Gm.
Use: Antibacterial; penicillin.

•**AZLOCILLIN.** USAN.
Use: Antibacterial.
See: Azlin, Inj. (Miles).

•**AZLOCILLIN SODIUM, STERILE,** U.S.P. XXII.
Use: Antibacterial.

AZMA-AID. (Purepac) Theophylline 118 mg, ephedrine 24 mg, phenobarbital 8 mg/Tab. Bot. 100s, 250s, 1000s.
Use: Bronchodilator.
AZMACORT INHALER. (Rhone-Puolenc Rorer) Triamcinolone acetonide ≈ 100 mcg delivered from the collapsible expansion chamber activator. Canister 20 Gm, contains triamcinolone acetonide 60 mg w/oral adapter.
Use: Bronchodilator.
AZO-100. (Scruggs) Phenylazodiaminopyridine HCl 100 mg/Tab. Bot. 100s, 1000s.
Use: Urinary tract analgesic.
•**AZOCONAZOLE.** USAN.
Use: Antifungal.
AZO-CYST. (Moore Kirk) Phenylazodiaminopyridine HCl 50 mg, calcium mandelate 120 mg, acid sodium phosphate 120 mg, methenamine 120 mg, hyoscyamine HBr 0.1037 mg, hyoscine HBr 0.0065 mg, atropine sulfate 0.0194 mg/Tab. Bot. 100s, 1000s.
Use: Urinary tract sterilization.
AZODYNE.
Sulfadiazine, sulfamethizole.
See: Suladyne, Tab. (Stuart).
AZODYNE HCl
See: Pyridium, Tab. (Parke-Davis).
AZO-GAMAZOLE TABS. (Major) Bot. 100s, 1000s.
Use: Urinary anti-infective.
AZO GANTANOL. (Roche) Sulfamethoxazole 500 mg, phenazopyridine HCl 100 mg/Tab. Bot. 100s, 500s.
Use: Urinary anti-infective.
AZO GANTRISIN. (Roche) Sulfisoxazole 500 mg, phenazopyridine HCl 50 mg/Tab. Bot. 100s, 500s.
Use: Urinary anti-infective.
•**AZOLIMINE.** USAN.
Use: Diuretic.
AZO NEGACIDE TABLETS. (Winthrop Products) Nalidixic acid, phenazopyridine HCl.
Use: Urinary anti-infective.
•**AZOSEMIDE.** USAN.
Use: Diuretic.
AZO-STANDARD. (Webcon) Phenazopyridine HCl 100 mg/Tab. Bot. 360s.
Use: Urinary anti-infective.
AZOSTIX REAGENT STRIPS. (Ames) Bromthymol blue, urease, buffers. Colorimetric test for blood urea nitrogen level. Bot 25 strips.
Use: Diagnostic aid.
AZO-SULFISOXAZOLE. (Forest Pharm.) Sulfisoxazole 500 mg, phenazopyridine HCl 50 mg/Tab. Bot. 100s, 1000s.
Use: Urinary anti-infective.
AZO-SULFISOXAZOLE. (Richlyn) Sulfisoxazole 500 mg, phenazopyridine HCl 50 mg/Tab. Bot. 1000s.
Use: Urinary anti-infective.
•**AZOTOMYCIN.** USAN. Antibiotic isolated from broth filtrates of *Streptomyces ambofaciens.*
Use: Antineoplastic agent.
AZO-URIZOLE. (Jenkins) Sulfisoxazole 0.5 Gm, phenazopyridine HCl 50 mg/Tab. Bot. 1000s.
Use: Urinary anti-infective.
AZOVAN BLUE. Tetrasodium salt of 4:4′-di-[7-(1-amino-8-hydroxy-2:4-disulpho)-naphthylazo]-3:3′-bitolyl.
See: Evans Blue Dye, Amp. (City Chemical; Harvey).
AZOVAN BLUE. B.A.N. Tetrasodium salt of 4,4′-di-(8-amino-1-hydroxy-5,7-disulfo-2-naphthylazo)-3,3′-bitolyl.
Use: Diagnostic aid.
See: Evans Blue.
AZO WINTOMYLON. (Winthrop Products) Nalidixic acid, phenazopyridine HCl.
Use: Urinary anti-infective.
AZT.
See: Zidovudine.
•**AZTREONAM,** U.S.P. XXII. Inj.
Use: Antimicrobial.
See: Azactam, Vial (Squibb).
AZULFIDINE ORAL SUSPENSION. (Pharmacia) Sulfasalazine 250 mg/5 ml. Bot. pt.
Use: Agent for ulcerative colitis.
AZULFIDINE TABLETS and EN-TABS. (Pharmacia) Sulfasalazine (salicylazosulfapyridine) 500 mg/Tab or En-tab. Bot. 100s, 500s, UD 100s, 1000s.
Use: Agent for ulcerative colitis.
•**AZUMOLENE SODIUM.** USAN.
Use: Relaxant.
AZURESIN. B.A.N. Prepared from carbacrylic cation exchange resin and azure A dye (3-amino-7-dimethylaminophenazathionium Cl). Diagnex Blue. (Squibb UK).
Use: Diagnostic aid.

B

B_1. Thiamine HCl.
B_2. Riboflavin.
B_3. Niacinamide.
B_6. Pyridoxine HCl.
B_6 50. (Western Research) Vitamin B_6 50 mg/Tab. Bot. 1000s.
Vitamin B_6 supplement.
B_{12}. Cyanocobalamin.
B50. (Nature's Bounty) Vitamins B_1 50 mg, B_2 50 mg, B_3 50 mg, B_5 50 mg, B_6 50 mg, B_{12} 50 mcg, folic acid 0.1 mg, d-biotin 50 mcg, PABA 50 mg, choline bitartrate 50 mg, inositol 50 mg, lecithin/Tab. Bot. 100s.
Use: Vitamin/mineral supplement.
B50 TIME RELEASE. (Nature's Bounty) Vitamins B_1 50 mg, B_2 50 mg, B_3 50 mg, B_5 50 mg, B_6 50 mg, B_{12} 50 mcg, folic acid 0.1 mg, d-biotin 50 mcg, PABA 50 mg, choline bitartrate 50 mg, inositol 50 mg, lecithin/Tab. Bot. 100s.
Use: Vitamin/mineral supplement.
B100. (Nature's Bounty) Vitamins B_1 100 mg, B_2

100 mg, B_3 100 mg, B_5 100 mg, B_6 100 mg, B_{12} 100 mcg, folic acid 0.1 mg, d-biotin 100 mcg, PABA 100 mg, choline bitartrate 100 mg, inositol 100 mg, lecithin. Tab. Bot. 100s.
Use: Vitamin/mineral supplement.

B125. (Nature's Bounty) Vitamins B_1 125 mg, B_2 125 mg, B_3 125 mg, B_5 125 mg, B_6 125 mg, B_{12} 125 mcg, folic acid 0.1 mg, d-biotin 125 mcg, PABA 125 mg, choline bitartrate 125 mg, inositol 125 mg, lecithin. Tab. Bot. 100s.
Use: Vitamin/mineral supplement.

B150. (Nature's Bounty) Vitamins B_1 150 mg, B_2 150 mg, B_3 150 mg, B_5 150 mg, B_6 150 mg, B_{12} 150 mcg, folic acid 0.1 mg, d-biotin 150 mcg, PABA 150 mg, choline bitartrate 150 mg, inositol 150 mg, lecithin. Tab. Bot. 100s.
Use: Vitamin/mineral supplement.

B & A. (Eastern Research) Sodium bicarbonate, potassium, aluminum, borax. Hygenic pow. Jar. 8 oz, 5 lb.
Use: Vaginal preparation.

B.A. GRADUAL. (Federal) Theophylline 260 mg, pseudoephedrine HCl 50 mg, butabarbital 15 mg/Gradual. Bot. 50s, 1000s.
Use: Bronchodilator, decongestant, sedative/hypnotic.

BABEE TEETHING. (Pfeiffer) Benzocaine 2.5%, cetalkonium Cl 0.02%, alcohol 20%, hamamelis water, propylene glycol, sodium benzoate, urea, menthol, camphor. Soln. Bot. 15 ml.
Use: Local anesthetic.

BABY COUGH SYRUP. (Towne) Ammonium Cl 300 mg, sodium citrate 600 mg/oz w/citric acid. Bot. 4 oz.
Use: Antitussive.

BAC.
See: Benzalkonium Cl.

B-A-C. (Mayrand) Aspirin 650 mg, caffeine 40 mg, butalbital 50 mg/Tab. Bot. 100s.
See: Analgesic combination.

B-A-C #3. (Mayrand) Codeine phosphate 30 mg, aspirin 325 mg, caffeine 40 mg, butalbital 50 mg/Tab. Bot. 100s.
Use: Analgesic combination.

•**BACAMPICILLIN HYDROCHLORIDE,** U.S.P. XXII. for Oral Soln., Tab., U.S.P. XXII.
Use: Antibiotic.
See: Spectrobid (Roerig).

BACARATE. (Solvay) Phendimetrazine tartrate 35 mg/Tab. Bot. 100s, 1000s.
Use: Anorexiant.

BACCO-RESIST. (Vita Elixir) Lobeline sulfate 1/64 gr.
Use: Antismoking lozenge.

BACID. (Fisons) A specially cultured strain of human *Lactobacillus acidophilus,* sodium carboxymethylcellulose 100 mg, sodium 0.5 mEq/Cap. Bot. 50s, 100s.
Use: Antidiarrheal.

BACIGUENT ANTIBIOTIC OINTMENT. (Upjohn) Bacitracin 500 units/Gm. Oint. Tube 0.5 oz, 1 oz, 4 oz.
Use: Anti-infective, external.

•**BACITRACIN,** U.S.P. XXII. Oint., Ophth., Oint., Sterile, U.S.P. XXII. B.A.N. An antibiotic produced by a strain of *Bacillus subtilis.*}
Available forms (Various Mfr.).
Diagnostic Tabs.
Oint.
Ophthalmic Oint.
Soluble Tab.
Systemic Use, Vial.
Topical Use, Vial.
Troche.
Vaginal Tab.
Use: Antibacterial.
See: Baciquent, Oint. (Upjohn).
W/Neomycin sulfate.
See: Bacimycin, Oint. (Merrell Dow).
Bacitracin-Neomycin, Oint., Ophth. Oint. (Various Mfr.).
W/Neomycin, polymyxin B sulfate.
See: Baximin, Oint. (Quality Generics).
BPN Ointment (Norwich Eaton).
Mycitracin, Oint., Ophth. Oint. (Upjohn).
Neosporin, Oint., Ophth. Oint., Aerosol, Pow. (Burroughs Wellcome).
Neo-Thrycex, Oint. (Commerce).
P.B.N., Oint. (Jenkins).
Tigo, Oint. (Burlington).
Tri-Biotic Oint. (Burgin-Arden).
Tri-Biotic, Oint. (Standex).
Tri-Bow Oint. (Bowman).
Triple Antibiotic Oint. (Kenyon, Towne).
W/Neomycin sulfate, polymyxin B sulfate, diperodon HCl.
See: Epimycin A, Oint. (Delta).
Mity-Mycin, Oint. (Solvay).
W/Neomycin sulfate, polymyxin B sulfate, hydrocortisone acetate.
See: Neopolycin-HC, Oint., Ophth. Oint. (Merrell Dow).
W/Polymyxin B sulfate.
See: Polysporin, Oint., Ophth. Oint. (Burroughs Wellcome).
W/Polymyxin B sulfate and neomycin sulfate.
See: Trimixin, Oint. (Hance).
W/Polymyxin B sulfate, neomycin sulfate and hydrocortisoce-free alcohol.
See: Biotic-Ophth. W/HC, Oint. (Scrip).
Cortisporin, Preps. (Burroughs Wellcome).

•**BACITRACIN METHYLENE DISALICYLATE,** U.S.P. XXII. Soluble, Soluble Pow., U.S.P. XXII.
Use: Antibiotic.

BACITRACIN-NEOMYCIN OINTMENT. (Various Mfr.) Neoycin sulfate equivalent to 3.5 mg base, bacitracin 500 units/Gm. Topical Oint. Tube 0.5 oz, 1 oz, Ophth. Oint. 1/8 oz.
Use: Anti-infective, external.

•**BACITRACIN AND POLYMYXIN B SULFATE,** U.S.P. XXII. Topical Aerosol.
Use: Antibiotic.

See: Polysporin Spray (Burroughs Wellcome).

•**BACITRACIN ZINC,** U.S.P. XXII. Sterile, Soluble Pow., U.S.P. XXII. (Upjohn) Sterile pow. 10,000 units, 50,000 units/Vial.
Use: Antibiotic.
W/Neomycin sulfate, polymyxin B sulfate.
See: Neomixin, Oint. (Hauck).
Neosporin, Prods. (Burroughs Wellcome).
Neotal, Oint. (Hauck).
W/Neomycin sulfate, polymyxin B, benzalkonium Cl.
See: Biotres, Oint. (Central Pharmacal).
W/Neomycin sulfate, polymyxin B sulfate, hydrocortisone acetate.
See: Biotres HC, Cream (Central).
Coracin, Oint. (Hauck).
W/Polymyxin B sulfate, neomycin sulfate.
See: Ophthel, Ophth. Oint. (Elder).

•**BACITRACIN ZINC OINTMENT,** U.S.P. XXII. Bacitracin zinc in an anhydrous ointment base.
Use: Antibiotic.

•**BACITRACIN ZINC AND POLYMYXIN B SULFATE OINTMENT,** U.S.P. XXII. Ophth. Oint., U.S.P. XXII.
Use: Antibiotic.

BACIT-WHITE. (Whiteworth) Bacitracin. Oint. Tube 0.5 oz, 1 oz.
Use: Anti-infective, external.

•**BACLOFEN.** USAN. 4-Amino-3-(4-chlorophenyl) butyric acid. β-Aminomethyl-p-chlorohydrocinnamic acid. 10 mg or 20 mg/Tab. Bot. 100s, UD 100s.
Use: Muscle relaxant.
See: Lioresal, Tab. (Geigy).
Baclofen, Tab. (Vitarine).

BAC-NEO-POLY OINTMENT. (Burgin-Arden) Bacitracin 400 units, neomycin sulfate 5 mg, polymyxin B sulfate 5000 units/Gm. Tube 0.5 oz.
Use: Anti-infective, external.

BACTERIOSTATIC SODIUM CHLORIDE. (Various Mfr.) Sodium Cl 0.9%. Also contains benzyl alcohol or parabens. Inj. Bot. 10 ml, 20 ml, 30 ml.
Use: Parenteral diluent.

•**BACTERIOSTATIC WATER FOR INJECTION.** U.S.P. XXII. (Abbott) 30 ml. Multiple-dose Fliptop Vial (plastic).
Use: Pharmaceutic acid for diluting and dissolving drugs for injection.

BACTICORT. (Rugby) Hydrocortisone 1%, neomycin sulfate equivalent to 0.35% neomycin base, polymyxin B sulfate 10,000 units/ml, benzalkonium Cl, cetyl alcohol, glyceryl monostearate, mineral oil, polyoxyl 40 stearate, propylene glycol. Ophth. Soln. Bot. 7.5 ml.
Use: Ophth. corticosteroid, anti-infective.

BACTIGEN GROUP A STREPTOCOCCUS. (Wampole) Latex agglutination slide test for the qualitative detection of group A streptococcal antigen directly from throat swabs. Test kit 60s.
Use: Diagnostic aid.

BACTIGEN GROUP A STREPTOCOCCUS WITH FAST TRAK SLIDES. (Wampole) Latex agglutination slide test for qualitative detection of group A streptococcal antigen directly from throat swabs. Test 24s. Test kit 48s.
Use: Diagnostic aid.

BACTIGEN GROUP B STREPTOCOCCUS. (Wampole) Latex agglutination slide test for the qualitative detection of group B streptococcus antigen in urine, cerebrospinal fluid and serum. Test kit 15s.
Use: Diagnostic aid.

BACTIGEN H. INFLUENZAE. (Wampole) Rapid latex agglutination slide test for the qualitative detection of *Hemophilus influenzae,* type b antigen in cerebrospinal fluid, serum and urine. Test kit 15s, 30s.
Use: Diagnostic aid.

BACTIGEN MENINGITIS PANEL. (Wampole) Rapid latex agglutination slide test for the qualitative detection of *Hemophilus influenzae* type b, *Neisseria meningitidis* A/B/C/Y/W135 and Streptococcus pneumoniae antigens in cerebrospinal fluid, serum and urine. Test kit 18.
Use: Diagnostic aid.

BACTIGEN N. MENINGITIDIS. (Wampole) Rapid latex agglutination slide test for the qualitative detection of *Neisseria meningitidis,* serogroups A/B/C/Y/W135 antigens in cerebrospinal fluid, serum and urine. Test kit 15s, 30s.
Use: Diagnostic aid.

BACTIGEN S. PNEUMONIAE. (Wampole) Rapid latex agglutination slide test for the qualitative detection of *Streptococcus pneumoniae* antigens in cerebrospinal fluid, serum and urine. Test kit 15s, 30s.
Use: Diagnostic aid.

BACTINE ANTISEPTIC/ANESTHETIC FIRST AID SPRAY. (Miles) Benzalkonium Cl 0.13%, lidocaine 2.5%. **Squeeze Bot.:** 2 oz, 4 oz. **Liq.:** 16 oz. **Aerosol:** 3 oz.
Use: Antiseptic, anesthetic.

BACTINE FIRST AID ANTIBIOTIC. (Miles) Polymyxin B sulfate 5,000 units, bacitracin 500 units, neomycin sulfate 5 mg/Gm in mineral oil, white petrolatum. Oint. Tube 15 Gm.
Use: Anti-infective, external.

BACTINE HYDROCORTISONE SKIN CREAM. (Miles) Hydrocortisone 0.5%. Tube 0.5 oz.
Use: Corticosteroid.

BACTOCILL. (Beecham Labs) Oxacillin sodium. **Cap.:** 250 mg or 500 mg Bot. 100s. **Vial:** (w/dibasic sodium phosphate 40 mg, methylparaben 3.6 mg, propylparaben 0.4 mg, sodium 3.1 mEq/Gm) 500 mg, 1 Gm, 2 Gm or 4 Gm/Vial; 10s. Piggyback vial 1 Gm, 2 Gm; 25s. Bulk pharm pkg 10 Gm; Box 25s.
Use: Antibacterial; penicillin.

BACTRIM. (Roche) Sulfamethoxazole 400 mg, trimethoprim 80 mg/Tab. Bot. 100s, 500s, Teledose 100s, Prescription Pak 40s.
Use: Anti-infective combination.

BACTRIM DS. (Roche) Trimethoprim 160 mg, sulfamethoxazole 800 mg/Tab. Bot. 100s, 500s, Tel-E-Dose 100s, Prescription Pak 20s.
Use: Anti-infective combination.

BACTRIM IV INFUSION. (Roche) Sulfamethoxazole 400 mg, trimethoprim 80 mg/5 ml. Amp. Box 10 × 5 ml. Vials Box 10 × 5 ml, 10 × 10 ml. Multidose vials. Box 1 × 30 ml.
Use: Anti-infective.

BACTRIM PEDIATRIC SUSPENSION. (Roche) Trimethoprim 40 mg, sulfamethoxazole 200 mg/ 5 ml. Bot. 100 ml, 480 ml.
Use: Anti-infective combination.

BACTRIM SUSPENSION. (Roche) Sulfamethoxazole 200 mg, trimethoprim 40 mg/5 ml. Bot. 16 oz.
Use: Anti-infective.

BACTROBAN. (Beecham) Mupirocin 2% in a polyethylene glycol base. Oint. Tube 15 Gm.
Use: Anti-infective, external.

BACTURCULT. (Wampole) A urinary bacteria culture medium diagnostic urine culture system for urine collection, bacteriuria screening and presumptive bacterial identification. Test kit 10s, 100s.
Use: Diagnostic aid.

BAFIL CREAM. (Scruggs) Hydrocortisone 0.5%, clioquinol 3%, lidocaine 3%, pH adjusted to 6. Tube oz.
Use: Corticosteroid, antifungal, local anesthetic.

BAKERS BEST. (Scherer) Water, alcohol 38%, propylene glycol, extract of capsicum, glycerin, boric acid, Tween 80, diethylphthalate, rose oil, pyrilamine maleate, glacial acetic acid, Uvinul MS 40, hexetidine, benzalkonium Cl 50%, sodium hydroxide 76%. Bot. 8 oz.
Use: Antipruritic, antiseborrheic.

BAL IN OIL. (Hynson, Westcott & Dunning) 2,3-dimercaptopropanol 100 mg, benzyl benzoate 210 mg, peanut oil 680 mg/ml. Amp. 3 ml Box 10s.
Use: Antidote.

BALANCED B_{100}. (Fibertone) Vitamins B_1 100 mg, B_2 100 mg, B_3 100 mg, B_5 100 mg, B_6 100 mg, B_{12} 100 mcg, folic acid 0.1 mg, PABA 100 mg, inositol 100 mg, d-biotin 100 mcg/SR Tab. Bot. 50s, 90s.
Use: Vitamin/mineral supplement.

BALANCED SALT SOLUTION. (Various Mfr.) Sodium Cl 0.64%, potassium Cl, 0.075%, calcium Cl 0.036%, magnesium Cl 0.03% in sodium acetate-sodium citrate buffer system. Soln. Drop-tainer 15 ml, 30 ml, 250 ml, 300 ml, 500 ml.
Use: Intraocular irrigant.

BALDEX OPHTHALMIC OINTMENT. (Bausch & Lomb) Dexamethasone phosphate 0.05%. 3.75 Gm.
Use: Corticosteroid, ophthalmic.

BALDEX OPHTHALMIC SOLUTION. (Bausch & Lomb) Dexamethasone phosphate 0.01%. Dropper bot 5 ml.
Use: Corticosteroid, ophthalmic.

BALMEX BABY POWDER. (Macsil) Specially purified balsam Peru, zinc oxide, starch, calcium carbonate. Shaker top can. 4 oz.
Use: Adsorbent, emollient.

BALMEX EMOLLIENT LOTION. (Macsil) Fraction of lanolin, allantoin, specially purified balsam Peru, silicone in a non-mineral oil base. Bot. 6 fl. oz.
Use: Emollient.

BALMEX OINTMENT. (Macsil) Specially purified balsam Peru, Vitamins A and D, zinc oxide, bismuth subnitrate in a base w/silicone. Tube 1 oz, 2 oz, 4 oz. Jar lb.
Use: Emollient.

BALNEOL. (Solvay) Water, mineral oil, propylene glycol, glyceryl stearate, PEG-100 stearate, PEG-40 stearate, laureth-4, PEG-4-dilaurate, lanolin oil, sodium acetate, carbomer-934, triethanolamine, methylparaben, docusate sodium, acetic acid, fragrance. Bot. 120 ml.
Use: Anorectal preparation.

BALNETAR. (Westwood) Tar equivalent to 2.5% coal tar, U.S.P. Bot. 8 oz.
Use: Bath dermatological.

BALSAN. Specially purified balsam Peru.
See: Balmex Prods. (Macsil).

•**BAMBERMYCINS.** USAN.
Use: Antibacterial.

BAMETHAN. B.A.N. 2-Butylamino-1-(4-hydroxyphenyl)ethanol.
Use: Vasodilator.

•**BAMETHAN SULFATE.** USAN. α-[(Butylamino) methyl]-p-hydroxybenzyl alcohol sulfate.
Use: Vasodilator.

BAMIFYLLINE. B.A.N. 8-Benzyl-7-[2-(N-ethyl-2-hy- droxy-ethylamino)ethyl]theophylline. Trentadil HCl.
Use: Bronchodilator.

BAMIFYLLINE HYDROCHLORIDE. USAN. 8-Benzyl-7-[2-[ethyl (2-hydroxyethyl) amino]ethyl]-theophylline HCl.
Use: Bronchodilator.

BAMIPINE. B.A.N. 4-(N-Benzylanilino)-1-methylpiperidine.
Use: Antihistamine.

•**BAMNIDAZOLE.** USAN.
Use: Antiprotozoal.

BANACID TABLETS. (Buffington) Magnesium trisilicate 220 mg. Bot. 100s, 200s, 500s.
Use: Antacid.

BANALG. (Forest) Menthol, camphor, methyl salicylate, eucalyptus oil in a greaseless base. Regular liniment and hospital strength. Bot. 2 oz, pt, gal.
Use: External analgesic.

BANALG HOSPITAL STRENGTH LINIMENT. (Forest) Methyl salicylate 14%, menthol 3%. Bot. 60 ml.
Use: External analgesic.

BANATIL. (Trimen) Butabarbital 32.4 mg, hyoscyamine sulfate 0.25 mg, scopolamine methyl-

nitrate 0.05 mg, atropine sulfate 0.006 mg/D.R. Tab. Bot. 100s. Elix. pt.
Use: Sedative/hypnotic, anticholinergic/antispasmodic.

BANCAP. (Forest) Acetaminophen 325 mg, butalbital 50 mg/Cap. Bot. 100s, 500s.
Use: Analgesic, sedative/hypnotic.

BANCAP HC. (Forest) Acetaminophen 500 mg, hydrocodone bitartrate 5 mg/Cap. Bot. 100s, 500s, UD 100s.
Use: Narcotic analgesic combination.

•**BANDAGE, ADHESIVE,** U.S.P. XXII.
Use: Surgical aid.

•**BANDAGE, GAUZE,** U.S.P. XXII.
Use: Surgical aid.

BANESIN. (Forest) Acetaminophen 500 mg/Tab. Bot. 1000s.
Use: Analgesic.

BANEX CAPSULES. (LuChem) Phenylpropanolamine HCl 45 mg, phenylephrine HCl 5 mg, guaifenesin 200 mg. Bot. 100s, 500s.
Use: Decongestant, expectorant.

BANEX-LA TABLETS. (LuChem) Phenylpropanolamine HCl 75 mg, guaifenesin 400 mg. Bot. 100s, 500s.
Use: Decongestant, expectorant.

BANFLEX. (Forest) Orphenadrine citrate 30 mg/ml. Inj. Vial 10 ml.
Use: Skeletal muscle relaxant.

BANGESIC. (H.L. Moore) Menthol, camphor, methyl salicylate, eucalyptus oil in non-greasy base. Bot. 2 oz, gal.
Use: External analgesic.

BANOCIDE.
See: Diethylcarbamazine Citrate, U.S.P.

BANOPHEN. Diphenhydramine 25 or 50 mg/Cap. **25 mg:** In 100s, 1000s, UD 100s. **50 mg:** In 100s, 250s, 1000s, UD 100s.
Use: Antihistamine.

BANTHINE. (Searle) Methantheline bromide 50 mg/Tab. Bot. 100s.
Use: Anticholinergic.

BANTRON BRAND SMOKING DETERRENT TABLETS. (Jeffrey Martin) Magnesium carbonate 129.6 mg, lobeline sulfate 2 mg, tribasic calcium phosphate 129.6 mg/Tab. Carton 18s, 36s.
Use: Smoking deterrent.

BARBASED. (Major) **Tab.:** Butabarbital 0.25 gr or 0.5 gr/Tab. Bot. 1000s. **Elix.:** Butabarbital 30 mg/5 ml, alcohol 7%. Bot. 480 ml.
Use: Sedative/hypnotic.

BARBATOSE NO. 2 TABLETS. (Vale) Barbital 64.8 mg/Tab. w/hyoscyamus sulfate, passiflora, valarian. Bot. 1000s.
Use: Sedative.

BARBELLA ELIXIR. (Forest) Phenobarbital 0.25 gr, hyoscyamine sulfate 0.1037 mg, atropine sulfate 0.0194 mg, scopolamine HBr 0.0065 mg, alcohol 23%/5 ml. Bot. 4 oz, gal.
Use: Sedative/hypnotic, anticholinergic/antispasmodic.

BARBELLA TABLETS. (Forest) Phenobarbital 16.2 mg, atropine sulfate 0.0194 mg, hyoscyamine sulfate 0.1037 mg, hyoscine HBr 0.0065 mg/Tab. Bot. 100s, 1000s, 5000s.
Use: Sedative/hypnotic, anticholinergic/antispasmodic.

BARBELOID. (Vale) Phenobarbital 16.2 mg, hyoscyamine sulfate 0.1037 mg, atropine sulfate 0.0194 mg, scopolamine HBr 0.0065 mg/Tab. Bot. 100s, 1000s.
Use: Sedative/hypnotic, anticholinergic/antispasmodic.

BARBENYL.
See: Phenobarbital.

BARBIDONNA. (Wallace) **Elix.:** Phenobarbital 21.6 mg, hyoscyamine sulfate 0.174 mg, atropine sulfate 0.034 mg, scopolamine HBr 0.01 mg, alcohol 15%/5 ml. Bot. pt. **Tab.:** Phenobarbital 16 mg, hyoscyamine sulfate 0.1286 mg, atropine sulfate 0.025 mg, scopolamine HBr 0.0074 mg/Tab. Bot. 100s, 500s.
Use: Sedative/hypnotic, anticholinergic/antispasmodic.

BARBIDONNA NO. 2. (Wallace) Phenobarbital 32 mg, hyoscyamine sulfate 0.1286 mg, atropine sulfate 0.025 mg, scopolamine HBr 0.0074 mg/Tab. Bot. 100s.
Use: Sedative/hypnotic, anticholinergic/antispamodic.

BARBINAL CAPSULES. (Forest) Phenobarbital 0.5 gr, acetophenetidin 2 gr, aspirin 3 gr, hyoscyamus 0.25 gr/Cap. Bot. 100s, 500s.
Use: Sedative/hypnotic, analgesic combination, anticholinergic/antispasmodic.

BARBINAL NO. 3. (Forest) Phenobarbital 0.25 gr, codeine phosphate 0.5 gr, acetophenetidin 2 mg, aspirin 3 gr, hyoscyamine sulfate 0.031 mg/Cap. Bot. 100s, 500s.
Use: Sedative/hypnotic, analgesic combination, anticholinergic/antispasmodic.

BARBIPHENYL.
See: Phenobarbital.

BARBITAL. Barbitone, Deba, Dormonal, Hypnogene, Malonal, Sedeval, Uronal, Veronal, Vesperal, diethylbarbituric acid, diethylmalonylurea.
Use: Sedative/hypnotic.
W/Aspirin, caffeine, niacinamide.
See: Mentran, Tab.(Pasadena Research).

BARBITAL SODIUM. Barbitone Sodium, diethylbarbiturate monosodium, diethylmalonylurea sodium, Embinal, Medinal, Veronal Sodium.
Use: Sedative/hypnotic.

BARBITONE.
See: Barbital.

BARBITONE SODIUM.
See: Barbital Sodium.

BARBITURATE-ASPIRIN COMBINATIONS.
See: Aspirin-Barbiturate Combination.

BARBITURATES, INTERMEDIATE DURATION.
See: Butabarbital (Various Mfr.).
Butethal (Various Mfr.).
Diallylbarbituric Acid (Various Mfr.).

Lotusate, Cap. (Winthrop Pharm).
Vinbarbital. (Various Mfr.).

BARBITURATES, LONG DURATION.
See: Barbital (Various Mfr.).
Mebaral, Tab. (Winthrop Pharm).
Mephobarbital (Various Mfr.).
Phenobarbital (Various Mfr.).
Phenobarbital Sodium (Various Mfr.).

BARBITURATES, SHORT DURATION.
See: Amobarbital (Various Mfr.).
Amobarbital Sodium (Various Mfr.).
Butalbital (Various Mfr.).
Butallylonal (Various Mfr.).
Cyclobarbital (Various Mfr.).
Cyclopal.
Pentobarbital Salts (Various Mfr.).
Sandoptal.
Secobarbital (Various Mfr.).

BARBITURATES, TRIPLE.
See: Butseco, S.C.T., Tab. (Bowman).
Ethobral, Cap. (Wyeth-Ayerst).

BARBITURATES, ULTRASHORT DURATION.
See: Hexobarbital.
Neraval.
Pentothal Sodium, Amp. (Abbott).
Surital Sodium, Amp., Vial (Parke-Davis).
Thiopental Sodium (Various Mfr.).

BARC GEL. (Commerce) Pyrethrins 0.18%, piperonyl butoxide technical 2.2%, petroleum distillate 4.8% in gel base. Tube oz.
Use: Pediculicide.

BARC LIQUID. (Commerce) Pyrethrins 0.18%, piperonyl butoxide technical 2.2%, petroleum distillate 5.52%. Bot. 2 oz.
Use: Pediculicide.

BARC NON-BODY LICE CONTROL SPRAY. (Commerce) Resmethrin-5-(phenylmethyl)-3-furanyl] methyl-2, 2-dimethyl-3-(2-methyl-1-propanyl) cyclopropanecarboxylate. Spray can 5 oz.
Use: Pediculicide.

BARICON. (Lafayette) Barium sulfate 95% pow. for susp. In UD 340 Gm.
Use: Gastrointestinal contrast agent.

BARIDIUM. (Pfeiffer) Phenazopyridine HCl 100 mg/Tab. Bot. 32s.
Use: Urinary analgesic.

BARI-STRESS M. (Barre) Vitamins B_1 10 mg, B_2 10 mg, niacinamide 100 mg, C 300 mg, B_6 2 mg, B_{12} 4 mcg, folic acid 1.5 mg, calcium pantothenate 20 mg/Cap or Tab. **Cap.:** Bot. 30s, 100s, 1000s. **Tab.:** Bot. 100s, 1000s.
Use: Vitamin/mineral supplement.

•**BARIUM HYDROXIDE LIME,** U.S.P. XXII.
Use: Carbon dioxide absorbant.

BARIUM SULFATE PREPARATION.
See: Baroflave, Pow. (Lannett).
Barotrast, Pow., Cream (Barnes-Hind).
Fleet Barobag, Liq. (Fleet).
Raybar, Susp. (Fleet).
Redi-Flow, Susp. (Berlex).
Rugar, Susp. (McKesson).

BARLEVITE. (Barth's) Vitamins B_6 0.6 mg, B_{12} 3 mcg, pantothenic acid 0.6 mg, D 3 IU, l-lysine 20 mg/0.6 ml. 100-Day Supply.
Use: Vitamin/mineral supplement.

BARNES-HIND CLEANING AND SOAKING SOLUTION. (Barnes-Hind) Cleaning and buffering agents, benzalkonium Cl 0.01%, disodium edetate 0.2%. Bot. 1.2 oz, 4 oz.
Use: Hard contact lens care.

BARNES-HIND WETTING & SOAKING SOLUTION. (Barnes-Hind) Polyvinyl alchohol, povidone, hydroxyethyl cellulose, octylphenoxy (oxyethylene) ethanol, benzalkonium Cl, edetate disodium. Bot. 4 oz.
Use: Hard contact lens care.

BARNES-HIND WETTING SOLUTION. (Barnes-Hind) Polyvinyl alcohol, edetate disodium 0.02%, benzalkonium Cl 0.004%. Bot. 35 ml, 60 ml.
Use: Hard contact lens care.

BAROBAG. (Lafayette) Disposable prefilled barium enema bag. 12 oz, 16 oz with or without retention catheter.
Use: Barium enema.

BAROBAG, EMPTY. (Lafayette) Disposable enema kit.
Use: Barium enema.

BARO-CAT. (Lafayette) Barium sulfate 1.5% susp. 300 ml, 900 ml.
Use: Gastrointestinal contrast agent.

BAROFLAVE POWDER. (Lannett) Barium sulfate for diagnostic X-ray use. Bot. 5 lb, Fibre drum 25 lb.
Use: Gastrointestinal contrast agent.

BAROPHEN. (Various Mfr.) **Elix.:** Atropine sulfate 0.0194 mg, scopolamine HBr 0.0065 mg, hyoscyamine HBr or SO_4 0.1037 mg, phenobarbital 16.2 mg/5 ml w/alcohol 23%. Elix. Bot. 120 ml, pt, gal.
Use: Anticholinergic/antispasmodic, sedative/hypnotic.

BAROSET. (Lafayette) Air contrast stomach. Unit-of-use kit. Case 12s.
Use: Radiopaque agent.

BAROSMIN.
See: Diosmin.

BAROSPERSE. (Lafayette) Barium sulfate 95%, suspending agent. Susp. 25 lb.
Use: Radiopaque agent.

BAROSPERSE 110. (Lafayette) Barium sulfate 95%. Susp. 900 Gm.
Use: Radiopaque agent.

Iron. Ferric pyrophosphate 250 mg/5 ml plus Barovite liquid formula.

BARTONE. (Rand) Phenobarbital 16.2 mg, scopolamine HBr 0.0065 mg, atropine sulfate 0.0194 mg, hyoscyamine sulfate 0.1037 mg/Tab. or 5 ml. **Tab.:** Bot. 100s, 1000s. **Elix.:** Pt, gal.
Use: Sedative/hypnotic, anticholinergic/antispasmodic.

BASA. (Freeport) Acetylsalicylic acid 324 mg/Tab. Bot. 1000s.
Use: Salicylate analgesic.

BASALJEL. (Wyeth-Ayerst) Aluminum carbonate gel. **Susp.:** Equivalent to aluminum hydroxide 400 mg/5 ml. Extra strength: Equivalent to 1000 mg aluminum hydroxide gel. Bot. 12 fl oz. **Cap.:** Equivalent to 608 mg dried aluminum hydroxide gel or 500 mg aluminum hydroxide. Bot. 100s, 500s. **Tab.:** Equivalent to 608 mg dried aluminum hydroxide gel or 500 mg aluminum hydroxide. Bot. 100s.
Use: Antacid.

BASIC ALUMINUM AMINOACETATE.
See: Dihydroxyaluminum Aminoacetate.

BASIC ALUMINUM CARBONATE.
See: Basaljel, Susp. (Wyeth-Ayerst).

BASIC ALUMINUM GLYCINATE.
See: Dihydroxyaluminum aminoacetate.

BASIC BISMUTH CARBONATE.
See: Bismuth Subcarbonate.

BASIC BISMUTH GALLATE.
See: Bismuth Subgallate (Various Mfr.).

BASIC BISMUTH NITRATE.
See: Bismuth Subnitrate (Various Mfr.).

BASIC BISMUTH SALICYLATE.
See: Bismuth Subsalicylate.

BASIC FUCHSIN.
See: Carbol-Fuchsin Topical Soln., U.S.P. XXII.

BASIS, GLYCERIN SOAP. (Beiersdorf) **Bar:** Tallow, coconut oil, glycerin. **Sensitive:** Bar 90 Gm, 150 Gm. **Normal to dry:** Bar 90 Gm, 150 Gm.
Use: Therapeutic skin cleanser.

BASIS, SUPERFATTED SOAP. (Beiersdorf) **Bar:** Sodium tallowate, sodium cocoate, petrolatum, glycerin, zinc oxide, sodium Cl, titanium dioxide, lanolin, alcohol, beeswax, BHT, EDTA. Bar 99 Gm, 225 Gm.
Use: Therapeutic skin cleanser.

BATANOPRIDE HYDROCHLORIDE. USAN.
Use: Antiemetic.

BATELAPINE MALEATE. USAN.
Use: Antipsychotic.

BAYER ASPIRIN, GENUINE. (Glenbrook) Aspirin 325 mg/Tab. Bot. 50s, 100s, 200s, 300s. Pkg. 12s, 24s.
Use: Salicylate analgesic.

BAYER ASPIRIN, MAXIMUM. (Glenbrook) Aspirin 500 mg/Tab. Bot. 30s, 60s, 100s.
Use: Salicylate analgesic.

BAYER CHILDREN'S CHEWABLE ASPIRIN. (Glenbrook) Aspirin 1.25 gr (81 mg)/Tab. Bot. 30s.
Use: Salicylate analgesic.

BAYER CHILDREN'S COLD TABLETS. (Glenbrook) Phenylpropanolamine HCl 3.125 mg, aspirin 1.25 gr (81 mg)/Tab. Bot. 30s.
Use: Decongestant, salicylate analgesic.

BAYER COUGH SYRUP FOR CHILDREN. (Glenbrook) Phenylpropanolamine HCl 9 mg, dextromethorphan HBr 7.5 mg/5 ml w/alcohol 5%. Bot. 3 oz.
Use: Decongestant, antitussive.

BAYER 8-HOUR TIMED-RELEASE ASPIRIN. (Glenbrook) Aspirin 10 gr (650 mg)/T.R. Tab. Bot. 30s, 72s, 125s.
Use: Salicylate analgesic.

BAYER 205.
See: Suramin Sodium. (No Mfr. currently listed.).

BAYER 2502.
See: Nifurtimox. (No Mfr. currently listed.).

BAYLOCAINE 4%. (Bay Labs) Lidocaine 4% w/methylparaben. Soln. Bot. 50 ml, 100 ml.
Use: Local anesthetic.

BAYLOCAINE 2% Viscous. (Bay Labs) Lidocaine 2% w/sodium carboxymethylcellulose. Soln. Bot. 100 ml.
Use: Local anesthetic.

BC-1000. (Solvay) Vitamins B_1 50 mg, B_2 5 mg, B_{12} 1000 mcg, B_6 5 mg, d-panthenol 6 mg, niacinamide 125 mg, ascorbic acid 50 mg, benzyl alcohol 1%/ml. Vial 10 ml.
Use: Vitamin supplement.

B-C-BID CAPSULES. (Geriatric) Vitamins B_1 15 mg, B_2 10 mg, B_6 5 mg, niacinamide 50 mg, calcium pantothenate 10 mg, C 300 mg, B_{12} 5 mcg/Cap. Bot. 30s, 100s, 500s.
Use: Vitamin/mineral supplement.

B•C•E & ZINC. (Schein) Vitamins E 45 mg, B_1 15 mg, B_2 10.2 mg, B_3 100 mg, B_5 25 mg, B_6 10 mg, B_{12} 6 mcg, C 600 mg, zinc 22.5 mg, tartrazine/Tab. Bot. 60s, 250s.
Use: Vitamin/mineral supplement.

•**BCG VACCINE,** U.S.P. XXII. (Various Mfr.) Prepared from a Glaxo culture of a Danish strain of BCG bacillus. Amp. ml.
Use: Immunization against tuberculosis.
See: Theracys (Connaught).

BCNU. 1,3-bis(2-Chloroethyl)-1-nitrosourea.
Use: Antineoplastic agent.
See: BiCNU, Inj. (Bristol).

BCO. (Western Research) Vitamins B_1 10 mg, B_2 2 mg, B_6 1.5 mg, B_{12} 25 mcg, niacinamide 50 mg/Tab. Bot. 1000s.
Use: Vitamin supplement.

B-COM. (Century) Vitamins B_1 3 mg, B_2 3 mg, B_6 0.5 mg, niacinamide 20 mg, calcium pantothenate 5 mg, B_{12} 1 mcg, desiccated liver (undefatted) 60 mg, debittered brewer's dried yeast 60 mg/Cap. Bot. 100s, 1000s.
Use: Vitamin/mineral supplement.

B-COMPLEX 2. (Kenyon) Vitamins B_1 3 mg, B_2 3 mg, B_6 0.5 mg, calcium pantothenate 5 mg, niacinamide 20 mg, dried yeast N.F. 60 mg/Cap. Bot. 100s.
Use: Vitamin supplement.

B-COMPLEX NO. 5. (Pharmex) Vitamins B_1 100 mg, B_2 2 mg, B_6 4 mg, panthenol 10 mg, niacinamide 100 mg, benzyl alcohol 1%, propylparaben 0.02%, methylparaben 0.18%/ml. Vial 30 ml.
Use: Vitamin supplement.

B-COMPLEX 25-25 INJ. (Forest) Niacinamide 100 mg, Vitamins B_1 25 mg, B_2 1 mg, B_6 2 mg, pantothenic acid 2 mg/ml. Vial 30 ml.
Use: Vitamin supplement.

B-COMPLEX 100. (Kenyon) Vitamins B_1 100 mg, B_2 2 mg, B_6 4 mg, d-panthenol 4 mg, niacinamide 100 mg/ml. Vial 30 ml.
Use: Vitamin supplement.

B COMPLEX #100 (Medical Chem) Vitamins B_1 100 mg, B_2 2 mg, B_6 4 mg, d-panthenol 4 mg, niacinamide 100 mg/ml. Vial 30 ml.
Use: Vitamin supplement.

B COMPLEX 100. (Rabin-Winters) Vitamins B_1 100 mg, B_2 2 mg, B_6 2 mg, niacinamide 125 mg, panthenol 10 mg/ml. Vial 30 ml.
Use: Vitamin supplement.

B-COMPLEX 100/100. (Sandia) Vitamins B_1 100 mg, B_2 2 mg, B_6 2 mg, niacinamide 100 mg/ml. Inj. Vial 30 ml.
Use: Vitamin supplement.

B COMPLEX CAPSULES. (Arcum) Vitamins B_1 1.5 mg, B_2 2 mg, niacinamide 10 mg, B_6 0.1 mg, calcium pantothenate 1 mg, desiccated liver 70 mg, dried yeast 100 mg/Cap. Bot. 100s, 1000s.
Use: Vitamin/mineral supplement.

B COMPLEX CAPSULES J.F. (Bryant) Vitamins B_1 1 mg, B_2 0.3 mg, nicotinic acid 0.3 mg, B_6 0.25 mg, desiccated liver 0.15 Gm, yeast powder, dried 0.15 Gm/Cap. Bot. 100s, 1000s.
Use: Vitamin/mineral supplement.

B COMPLEX INJECTION WITH VITAMIN C.
Use: Vitamin supplement.
See: Cplex Cap. (Arcum).

B COMPLEX AND B_{12}. (Nature's Bounty) Vitamins B_1 7 mg, B_2 14 mg, B_3 4.5 mg, B_{12} 25 mcg, protease 10 mg/Tab. Bot. 90s.
Use: Vitamin supplement.

B COMPLEX WITH B_{12} CAPSULES. (Bryant) Vitamins B_1 2 mg, B_2 2 mg, B_6 0.5 mg, niacinamide 10 mg, B_{12} 2 mcg, biotin 10 mcg, calcium pantothenate 1.5 mg, choline dihydrogen citrate 40 mg, inositol 30 mg, desiccated liver 1 gr, brewer's yeast 3 gr/Cap. Bot. 100s, 1000s.
Use: Vitamin/mineral supplement.

B-COMPLEX + C. (Nature's Bounty) Vitamins C 200 mg, B_1 10 mg, B_2 10 mg, B_3 50 mg, B_5 10 mg, B_6 5 mg/Tab. Bot. 100s.
Use: Vitamin supplement.

BC POWDER. (Block) Aspirin 650 mg, salicylamide 195 mg, caffeine 32 mg/Pow. Pkg. 2s, 6s, 24s, 50s.
Use: Salicylate analgesic.

BC POWDER, ARTHRITIS STRENGTH. (Block) Aspirin 742 mg, salicylamide 222 mg, caffeine 36 mg/Powder. Pkg. 6s, 24s, 50s.
Use: Salicylate analgesic.

BC TABLETS. (Block) Aspirin 325 mg, salicylamide 95 mg, caffeine 16 mg/Tab. Bot. 12s, 50s, 100s.
Use: Salicylate analgesic.

BC-VITE. (Drug Industries) Vitamins B_1 25 mg, B_2 5 mg, B_3 50 mg, B_5 10 mg, B_6 1 mg, B_{12} 2 mcg, C 150 mg/Tab. Bot. 100s, 500s.
Use: Vitamin supplement.

B-C WITH FOLIC ACID. (Geneva Marsam) Vitamins B_1 15 mg, B_2 15 mg, B_3 100 mg, B_5 18 mg, B_6 4 mg, B_{12} 5 mcg, C 500 mg, folic acid 0.5 mg/Tab. Bot. 100s.
Use: Vitamin/mineral supplement.

B-DAY TABLETS. (Barth's) Vitamins B_1 7 mg, B_2 14 mg, niacin 4.67 mg, B_{12} 5 mcg/Tab. Bot. 100s, 500s.
Use: Vitamin B supplement.

BDEP.
See: Benzathine Penicillin G.

B-DOX. (Lannett) Vitamins B_1 100 mg, B_6 100 mg/ml. Vial 10 ml.
Use: Vitamin B supplement.

B DOZEN. (Standex) Vitamin B_{12} 25 mcg/Tab. Bot. 1000s.
Use: Vitamin B supplement.

B-DRAM w/C COMPUTABS. (Dram) Vitamins B_2 10 mg, B_6 5 mg, nicotinamide 50 mg, calcium pantothenate 20 mg, B_1 5 mg/Tab. Bot. 100s.
Use: Vitamin supplement.

BEBATAB NO. 2. (Freeport) Belladonna ⅙ gr, phenobarbital 0.25 gr/Tab. Bot. 1000s.
Use: Anticholinergic/antispasmodic, sedative/hypnotic.

•**BECANTHONE HYDROCHLORIDE.** USAN.
Use: Antischistosomal.

BECAUSE. (Schering) Nonoxynol 98%. Vaginal foam. Bot. 10 Gm (6 dose contraceptor unit).
Use: Spermicide.

BECEEVITE CAPSULES. (Blue Cross) Vitamins C 300 mg, B_1 15 mg, B_2 10 mg, niacin 50 mg, B_6 5 mg, pantothenic acid 10 mg/Tab. Bot. 100s.
Use: Vitamin supplement.

BE-CE FORTE. (Kenyon) Vitamins B_1 15 mg, B_2 10 mg, niacinamide 80 mg, B_6 20 mg, d-panthenol 23 mg, C 100 mg/2 ml. Vial 20 ml.
Use: Vitamin supplement.

BECLAMIDE. B.A.N. N-Benzyl-3-chloropropionamide.
Use: Anticonvulsant.

BECLOMETHASONE. B.A.N. 9α-Chloro-11β, 17α, 21-trihydroxy-16β-methylpregna-1, 4-diene-3,20-dione. 9α-Chloro-16β-methylprednisolone.
Use: Corticosteroid.

•**BECLOMETHASONE DIPROPIONATE.** USAN.
Use: Corticosteroid.
See: Beclovent Aerosol (Allen & H).
Beconase Aerosol (Allen & H).
Beconase AQ Nasal Spray (Allen & H).
Vancenase Nasal Inhaler (Schering).
Vanceril Inhaler (Schering).

•**BECLOMYCIN DIPROPIONATE,** U.S.P. XXII.
Use: Corticosteroid.

BECLOVENT AEROSOL. (Allen & H). Beclomethasone dipropionate 42 mcg/actuation. Aerosol canister (16.8 Gm) containing 200 metered inhalations. Canister 16.8 Gm w/oral adapter. Refill canister 16.8 Gm.

Use: Corticosteroid.

BECOMP-C. (Cenci) Vitamins C 250 mg, B_1 25 mg, B_2 10 mg, nicotinamide 50 mg, B_6 2 mg, calcium pantothenate 10 mg, hesperidin complex 50 mg/Cap. Bot. 100s, 500s.
Use: Vitamin supplement.

BECONASE AQ NASAL SPRAY. (Allen & H). Beclomethasone dipropionate 42 mcg/metered spray. Pump aerosol bot. 25 Gm (200 metered inhalations) w/nasal adapter.
Use: Corticosteroid.

BECONASE INHALATION AEROSOL. (Allen & H). Beclomethasone dipropionate 42 mcg/actuation. Aerosol canister (16.8 Gm) containing 200 meterd inhalations. Canister 16.8 Gm w/compact actuator. Refill 16.8 Gm.
Use: Corticosteroid.

BECOTIN. (Dista) Vitamins B_1 10 mg, B_2 10 mg, B_6 4.1 mg, niacinamide 50 mg, pantothenic acid 25 mg, B_{12} 1 mcg/Pulv. Bot. 100s.
Use: Vitamin supplement.

BECOTIN-T. (Dista) Vitamins B_1 15 mg, B_2 10 mg, B_6 5 mg, niacinamide 100 mg, pantothenic acid 20 mg, B_{12} 4 mcg, C 300 mg/Tab. Bot. 100s, 1000s, Blister pkg. 10 × 10s.
Use: Vitamin supplement.

BECOTIN W/VITAMIN C. (Dista) Vitamins B_1 10 mg, B_2 10 mg, B_6 4 mg, niacinamide 50 mg, pantothenic acid 25 mg, B_{12} 1 mcg, C 150 mg/Pulv. Bot. 100s, 500s, Blister pkg. 10 × 10s.
Use: Vitamin supplement.

BEDOCE. (Lincoln) Crystalline anhydrous vitamin B_{12} 1000 mcg/ml. Vial 10 ml.
Use: Vitamin B_{12} supplement.

BEDOCE-GEL. (Lincoln) Vitamin B_{12} 1000 mcg/ml in 17% gelatin soln. Vial 10 ml.
Use: Vitamin B_{12} supplement.

BEDSIDE CARE. (Sween) Bot. 8 oz, gal.
Use: Non-rinsing shampoo, body wash.

BEECEEVITES CAPSULES. (Halsey)
Use: Vitamin supplement.

BEECHWOOD CREOSOTE.
See: Creosote, N.F.

BEE-FORTE W/C. (Rugby) Vitamins B_1 25 mg, B_2 12.5 mg, B_3 50 mg, B_5 10 mg, B_6 3 mg, B_{12} 2.5 mcg, C 250 mg/Cap. Bot. 100s.
Use: Vitamin supplement.

BEEF PEPTONES. (Sandia) Water soluble peptones derived from beef 20 mg/2 ml. Inj. Vial 30 ml.
Use: Nutritional supplement.

BEELITH. (Beach) Pyridoxine HCl 20 mg, magnesium oxide 600 mg/Tab. Bot. 100s.
Use: Vitamin/mineral supplement.

BEEPEN-VK. (Beecham Labs) Penicillin VK. **Tab.:** 250 mg. Bot. 1000s; 500 mg. Bot. 500s. **Oral Susp.:** 125 mg/5 ml Bot. 100 ml, 200 ml; 250 mg/5 ml Bot. 100 ml, 200 ml.
Use: Antibacterial; penicillin.

BEESIX INJECTION. (Forest) Pyridoxine HCl 100 mg/ml. Vial 10 ml.
Use: Vitamin B supplement.

BEE-THI. (Burgin-Arden) Cyanocobalamin 1000 mcg, thiamine HCl 100 mg in isotonic soln. of sodium Cl/ml. Vial 10 ml, 20 ml.
Use: Vitamin B supplement.

BEE-T-VITES. (Rugby) Vitamins B_1 15 mg, B_2 10 mg, B_3 100 mg, B_5 20 mg, B_6 5 mg, B_{12} 4 mcg, C 300 mg/Tab. Bot. 100s.
Use: Vitamin supplement.

BEE-TWELVE 1000. (Burgin-Arden) Cyanocobalamin 1000 mcg/ml. Vial 10 ml, 30 ml.
Use: Vitamin B supplement.

BEE-ZEE. (Rugby) Vitamins E 45 mg, B_1 15 mg, B_2 10.2 mg, B_3 100 mg, B_5 25 mg, B_6 10 mg, B_{12} 6 mcg, C 600 mg, zinc 22.5 mg/Tab. Bot. 60s.
Use: Vitamin/mineral supplement.

BEFERRIC. (Kenyon) Ferric ammonium citrate 500 mg, vitamins B_1 12 mg, B_2 6 mg, B_6 0.6 mg, folic acid 0.5 mg, calcium pantothenate 6 mg, niacinamide 15 mg, magnesium 1 mg, cobalt 0.1 mg, zinc 2 mg/fl oz. Bot. 4 oz.
Use: Vitamin/mineral supplement.

BEHEPAN.
See: Vitamin B_{12}.

BELATOL NO. 1; NO. 2. (Cenci) **No. 1:** Belladonna leaf extract ⅛ gr, phenobarbital 0.25 gr/Tab. 100s, 1000s. **No. 2:** Belladonna leaf extract ⅛ gr, phenobarbital 0.5 gr/Tab. Bot. 100s, 1000s.
Use: Anticholinergic/antispasmodic, sedative/hypnotic.

BELATOL ELIXIR. (Cenci) Phenobarbital 20 mg, belladonna 6.75 min./5 ml w/alcohol 45%. Elix. Bot. pt, gal.
Use: Sedative/hypnotic, anticholinergic/antispasmodic.

BELBUTAL NO. 2 KAPTABS. (Churchill) Phenobarbital 32.4 mg, hyoscyamine sulfate 0.1092 mg, atropine sulfate 0.0215 mg, hyoscine HBr 0.0065 mg/Tab. Bot. 100s.
Use: Sedative/hypnotic, anticholinergic/antispasmodic.

BELDIN. (Blue Cross) Diphenhydramine HCl 12.5 mg/5 ml w/alcohol 5%. Bot. gal.
Use: Antitussive.

BELEXAL. (Vale) Vitamins B_1 1.5 mg, B_2 2 mg, B_6 0.167 mg, calcium pantothenate 1 mg, niacinamide 10 mg/Tab. w/brewer's yeast. Bot. 1000s, 5000s.
Use: Vitamin supplement.

BELEXON FORTIFIED IMPROVED. (APC) Liver fraction No. 2 3 gr, yeast extract 3 gr, vitamins B_1 5 mg, B_2 6 mg, niacinamide 10 mg, calcium pantothenate 2 mg, cyanocobalamin 1 mcg, iron 10 mg/Cap. Bot. 100s.
Use: Vitamin/mineral supplement.

BELFER. (Forest) Vitamins B_1 2 mg, B_2 2 mg, B_{12} 10 mcg, B_6 2 mg, C 50 mg, iron 17 mg/Tab. Bot. 100s.

Use: Vitamin/mineral supplement.

•**BELFOSDIL.** USAN.
Use: Antihypertensive (calcium channel blocker).

BELIX ELIXIR. (Blue Cross) Diphenhydramine HCl 12.5 mg/5 ml. Bot. 118 ml.
Use: Antihistamine.

BELLADENAL. (Sandoz) Bellafoline 0.25 mg, phenobarbital 50 mg/Tab. Bot. 100s.
Use: Anticholinergic/antispasmodic, sedative/hypnotic.

BELLADENAL S. (Sandoz) Bellafoline 0.25 mg, phenobarbital 50 mg w/tartrazine/Tab. Bot. 100s.
Use: Anticholinergic/antispasmodic, sedative/hypnotic.

BELLADONNA ALKALOIDS.
Use: Anticholinergic/antispasmodic.
W/Combinations.
See: Accelerase-PB, Cap. (Organon).
Belladenal, Preps. (Sandoz).
Belphen, Tab. (Robinson).
Belphen Elix. (Robinson).
Belphen Timed Cap. (Robinson).
Coryztime, Cap. (Elder).
Decobel, Lanacap (Lannett).
Fitacol Stankap (Standex).
Nilspasm, Tab. (Parmed).
Ultabs, Tab. (Burlington).
Urised, Tab. (Webcon).
U-Tract, Tab. (Bowman).
Wigraine, Tab., Supp. (Organon).
Wyanoids, Supp. (Wyeth-Ayerst).

BELLADONNA ALKALOIDS W/PHENOBARBITAL. (Various Mfr.) Atropine sulfate 0.0194 mg, scopolamine HBr 0.0065 mg, hyoscyamine HBr or SO_4 0.1037 mg, phenobarbital 16.2 mg/Tab. Bot. 20s, 1000s, UD 100s.
Use: Anticholinergic/antispasmodic, sedative/hypnotic.

•**BELLADONNA EXTRACT,** U.S.P. XXII. (Lilly) 15 mg (0.187 mg belladonna)/Tab.
Use: Intestinal antispasmodic.

BELLADONNA EXTRACT COMBINATIONS.
Use: Anticholinergic/antispasmodic.
See: Amobell, Cap. (Bock).
Amsodyne, Tab. (Elder).
B & O Supprettes (Webcon).
Belap, Tab. (Lemmon).
Bellafedrol A-H, Tab. (Lannett).
Bellkatal, Tab. (Ferndale).
Butibel, Tab., Elix. (McNeil).
Gelcomul, Liq. (Commerce).
Hycoff Cold, Cap. (Saron).
Lanothal, Pills (Lannett).
Phebe (Western Research).
Rectacort, Supp. (Century).

•**BELLADONNA LEAF,** U.S.P. XXII.
Use: Intestinal antispasmodic.
W/Phenobarbital and benzocaine.
Use: Anticholinergic.
See: Gastrolic, Tab. (Hauck).

BELLADONNA PRODUCTS AND PHENOBARBITAL COMBINATIONS.
Use: Anticholinergic/antispasmodic, sedative/hypnotic.
See: Accelerase-PB, Cap. (Organon).
Alised, Tab. (Elder).
Atrocap, Cap. (Freeport).
Atrosed, Tab. (Freeport).
Bebatab, Tab. (Freeport).
Belap, Tab., Elix. (Lemmon).
Belatol, Tab., Elix. (Cenci).
Belladenal, Tab., Spacetab, Elix. (Sandoz).
Bellergal, Tab., Spacetab. (Dorsey).
Bellkatal, Tab. (Ferndale).
Bellophen, Tab. (Richlyn).
B-Sed, Tab. (Scrip).
Chardonna, Tab. (Rorer).
Donabarb, Tab., Elix. (Elder).
Donnafed Jr., Tab. (Jenkins).
Donnatal, Tab., Extentab, Cap., Elix. (Robins).
Donnatal #2, Tab. (Robins).
Donnazyme, Tab. (Robins).
Gastrolic, Tab. (Hauck).
Hypnaldyne, Tab. (North American Pharm).
Kinesed, Tab. (Stuart).
Mallenzyme, Tab. (Hauck).
Medi-Spas, Elix. (Medical Chemicals).
Phenobarbital and Belladonna, Tab. (Lilly).
Sedapar, Tab. (Parmed).
Spabelin, Tab. (Arcum).
Spabelin No. 2, Tab. (Arcum).
Spasnil, Tab. (Rhode).

•**BELLADONNA TINCTURE,** U.S.P. XXII. (Lilly) Bot. 4 oz, 16 oz.
Use: Intestinal antispasmodic.

BELLAFEDROL A-H TABLETS. (Lannett) Pyrilamine maleate 12.5 mg, chlorpheniramine maleate 1 mg, phenylephrine HCl 2.5 mg, belladonna extract 6 mg/Tab. Bot. 100s, 500s, 1000s.
Use: Antihistamine, decongestant, anticholinergic/antispasmodic.

BELLAFOLINE. (Sandoz) Levorotatory alkaloids of belladonna. **0.25 mg/Tab.:** Bot. 100s. **0.5 mg/ml.:** Amp 1 ml.
Use: Anticholinergic/antispasmodic.

BELLANEED. (Hanlon) Belladonna, phenobarbital 16 mg/Cap. Bot. 100s.
Use: Anticholinergic/antispasmodic, sedative/hypnotic.

BELL/ANS. (C.S. Dent) Sodium bicarbonate 520 mg, sodium content 144 mg/Tab. Bot. 30s, 60s.
Use: Antacid.

BELLASTAL. (Wharton) Atropine sulfate 0.0194 mg, scopolamine HBr 0.0065 mg, hyoscyamine HBr or SO_4 0.1037 mg, phenobarbital 16.2 mg Cap. Bot. 1000s.
Use: Anticholinergic/antispasmodic.

BELLERGAL-S. (Sandoz) Ergotamine tartrate 0.6 mg, bellafoline 0.2 mg, phenobarbital 40 mg, tartrazine/SR Tab. Bot. 100s.

Use: Anticholingergic/antispasmodic, sedative/hypnotic.

•**BELOXAMIDE.** USAN.
Use: Antihyperlipoproteinemic.

BELPHEN. (Robinson) Belladonna alkaloids, phenobarbital. Tab. Bot. 100s, 1000s.
Use: Anticholinergic/antispasmodic, sedative/hypnotic.

BELPHEN ELIXIR. (Robinson) Belladonna alkaloids, phenobarbital. Elix. Bot. pt, gal.
Use: Anticholinergic/antispasmodic, sedative/hypnotic.

BELPHEN TIMED CAPS. (Robinson) Belladonna alkaloids, phenobarbital. T.D. Cap. Bot. 100s, 500s, 1000s.
Use: Anticholinergic/antispasmodic, sedative/hypnotic.

•**BEMARINONE HYDROCHLORIDE.** USAN.
Use: Cardiotonic (positive inotropic, vasodilator).

BEMEGRIDE. B.A.N. 3-Ethyl-3-methylglutarimide.
Use: Medullary respiratory stimulant.

BEMINAL 500. (Wyeth-Ayerst) Vitamins B_1 25 mg, B_2 12.5 mg, niacinamide 100 mg, B_6 10 mg, calcium pantothenate 20 mg, C 500 mg, cyanocobalamin 5 mcg/Tab. Bot. 100s.
Use: Vitamin supplement.

BEMINAL FORTE W/VIT. C. (Wyeth-Ayerst) Vitamins B_1 25 mg, B_2 12.5 mg, niacinamide 50 mg, B_6 3 mg, calcium pantothenate 10 mg, C 250 mg, B_{12} 2.5 mcg/Cap. Bot. 100s.
Use: Vitamin supplement.

BEMINAL STRESS PLUS IRON. (Wyeth-Ayerst) Vitamins B_1 25 mg, B_2 12.5 mg, B_3 100 mg, B_5 20 mg, B_6 10 mg, B_{12} 25 mcg, folic acid 400 mcg, C 700 mg, E 45 IU, iron 27 mg. Dye-free. Tab. Bot. 60s.
Use: Vitamin/mineral supplement.

BEMINAL STRESS PLUS ZINC. (Wyeth-Ayerst) Vitamins B_1 25 mg, B_2 12.5 mg, B_3 100 mg, B_5 20 mg, B_6 10 mg, B_{12} 25 mcg, C 700 mg, E 45 IU, zinc 45 mg/Tab. Bot. 60s, 250s.
Use: Vitamin/mineral supplement.

•**BEMITRADINE.** USAN.
Use: Antihypertensive, diuretic.

•**BEMORADAN.** USAN.
Use: Cardiotonic.

BEMOTE. (Everett) Dicyclomine. **Cap.:** 10 mg. **Tab.:** 20 mg. In 100s.
Use: Anticholinergic/antispasmodic.

BENACEN. (Cenci) Probenecid 0.5 Gm/Tab. Bot. 100s, 1000s.
Use: Agent for gout.

BENACOL. (Cenci) Dicyclomine HCl 20 mg/Tab. Bot. 100s, 1000s.
Use: Anticholinergic/antispasmodic.

BENACTYZINE. B.A.N. 2-Diethylaminoethyl benzilate.
Use: Tranquilizer.

BENACTYZINE HYDROCHLORIDE. 2-Diethylaminoethyl benzilate HCl.
Use: Tranquilizer.
W/Meprobamate.
See: Deprol, Tab. (Wallace).

BENA-D-10. (Seatrace) Diphenhydramine HCl 10 mg/ml. Vial 30 ml.
Use: Antihistamine.

BENA-D-50. (Seatrace) Diphenhydramine HCl 50 mg/ml. Vial 10 ml.
Use: Antihistamine.

BENADRYL. (Parke-Davis) Diphenhydramine HCl.
Cap.: 25 mg. Bot. 100s, 1000s, UD 100s.
Cream: 1%. Tube 1 oz.
Elix. (w/alcohol 14%): 12.5 mg/5 ml. Bot. 4 oz, pt, gal, UD 5 ml × 100s.
Kapseal: 50 mg. Bot. 100s, 1000s, UD 100s.
Spray: 1%. Bot. 2 oz.
Tab.: 25 mg. Bot. 100s.
Use: Antihistamine.

BENADRYL-25 CAPSULES. (Parke-Davis) Diphenhydramine HCl 25 mg/Cap. Box 24s.
Use: Antihistamine.

BENADRYL COUGH PREPARATION.
See: Benylin Cough Syrup (Parke-Davis).

BENADRYL DECONGESTANT CAPSULES. (Parke-Davis) Diphenhydramine HCl 25 mg, pseudoephedrine HCl 60 mg/Cap. Box 24s.
Use: Antihistamine, decongestant.

BENADRYL DECONGESTANT ELIXIR. (Parke-Davis) Diphenhydramine HCl 5 ml, pseudoephedrine HCl 30 mg/5 ml, alcohol 5%. Bot. 4 oz.
Use: Antihistamine, decongestant.

BENADRYL ELIXIR. (Parke-Davis) Diphenhydramine HCl 12.5 mg/5 ml, alcohol 14%. Bot. 4 oz, pt, gal, UD (5 ml) 100s.
Use: Antihistamine.

BENADRYL INJECTION. (Parke-Davis) Diphenhydramine HCl.
Amp: 50 mg/ml. Amp. 1 ml. Box 10s.
Steri-Dose: 50 mg/ml, pH adjusted w/HCl or sodium hydroxide. Amp. 1 ml. Box 10s. Disposable syringe 1 ml.
Steri-Vial: . Phemerol benzethonium Cl as germicidal agent. pH adjusted w/sodium hydroxide or HCl. **10 mg/ml:** 10 ml, 30 ml. **50 mg/ml:** 10 ml.
Use: Antihistamine.

BENADRYL PLUS. (Parke-Davis) Pseudoephedrine 30 mg, diphenhydramine 12.5 mg, acetaminophen 500 mg/Tab. 24s.
Use: Decongestant, antihistamine, analgesic.

BENADRYL PLUS NIGHTTIME. (Parke-Davis). Pseudoephedrine 30 mg, diphenhydramine 25 mg, acetaminophen 500 mg/5 ml. 180 ml, 300 ml.
Use: Decongestant, antihistamine, analgesic.

BENAHIST 10. (Keene) Diphenhydramine 10 mg/ml. Vial 30 ml.
Use: Antihistamine.

BENAHIST 50. (Keene) Diphenhydramine 50 mg/ml. Vial 10 ml.
Use: Antihistamine.

BEN-ALLERGIN-50. (Mayrand) Diphenhydramine HCl 50 mg/ml w/chlorobutanol. Inj. Vial 10 ml.
Use: Antihistamine.

BENANEERIN HCl. 3-(2-Aminoethyl)-1-benzyl-5-methoxy-2-methylindole HCl.

BENANSERIN HYDROCHLORIDE. 3-(2-Aminoethyl)-1-benzyl-5-methoxy-2-methylindole monohydrochloride.
Use: Serotonin antagonist.

BENAPEN.
See: Benethamine.

BENAPHEN CAPS. (Major) Diphenhydramine 25 mg or 50 mg/Cap. Bot. 100s, 1000s.
Use: Antihistamine.

BENAPRYZINE. B.A.N. 2-(N-Ethylpropylamino)-ethyl benzilate.
Use: Treatment of Parkinsonism.

•**BENAPRYZINE HYDROCHLORIDE.** USAN.
Use: Anticholinergic.

BEN-AQUA. (Syosset) **Gel:** Benzoyl peroxide 5% or 10% w/polyoxyethylene laurylether. Tube 45 Gm, 120 Gm. **Lot.:** Benzoyl peroxide 5% or 10%: Bot. 60 ml.
Use: Anti-acne.

BENASE. (Ferndale) Proteolytic enzymes extracted from Carica papaya 20,000 units enzyme activity. Tab. Bot. 1000s.
Use: Reduction of edema, relief of episiotomy.

BENAT-12. (Hauck) Cyanocobalamin 30 mcg, liver injection 0.5 ml, vitamins B_1 10 mg, B_2 2 mg, niacinamide 50 mg, d-panthenol 1 mg, B_6 1 mg/ml, benzyl alcohol 4%, phenol 0.5%. Vial 10 ml.
Use: Vitamin/mineral supplement.

•**BENAZEPRIL HYDROCHLORIDE.** USAN.
Use: ACE inhibitor.

•**BENAZEPRILAT.** USAN.
Use: ACE inhibitor.

•**BENDACALOL MESYLATE.** USAN.
Use: Antihypertensive.

•**BENDAZAC.** USAN. [l-Benzyl-(H-indazol-3yl)oxy] acetic acid.
Use: Anti-inflammatory.

BENDROFLUAZIDE. B.A.N. 3-Benzyl-3,4-dihydro-6-trifluoromethylbenzo-1,2,4-thiadiazine-7-sulfonamide 1,1-dioxide. Bendroflumethiazide (I.N.N.).
Use: Diuretic.

•**BENDROFLUMETHIAZIDE,** U.S.P. XXII. Tab., U.S.P. XXII. 3-Benzyl-3:4-dihydro-7-sulphamoly-6-tri-fluoromethylbenzo-1:2:4-thiadiazine 1:1-dioxide. 6-(Trifluoromethyl)-2H-1,2,4-benzothiadiazine-7-sulfonamide 1, 1-dioxide.
Use: Diuretic, antihypertensive.
See: Naturetin, Tab. (Squibb).
W/Potassium Cl.
See: Naturetin W-K, Tab. (Squibb).
W/Rauwolfia serpentina.
See: Rauzide, Tab.
W/Rauwolfia serpentina, potassium Cl.
See: Rautrax-N, Tab. (Squibb).
Rautrax-N Modified, Tab. (Squibb).

BENEMID. (Merck Sharp & Dohme) Probenecid 0.5 Gm/Tab. Bot. 100s, 1000s, UD 100s.
Use: Agent for gout.
W/Colchicine.
See: Colbenemid, Tab. (Merck Sharp & Dohme).

BENEPHEN ANTISEPTIC MEDICATED POWDER. (Halsted) Methylbenzethonium Cl 1:1800, magnesium carbonate in cornstarch base. Shaker can 3.56 oz.
Use: Deodorant, antiseptic.

BENEPHEN ANTISEPTIC OINTMENT W/COD LIVER OIL. (Halsted) Methylbenzethonium Cl 1:1000, water-repellent base of zinc oxide, cornstarch. Tube 1.5 oz, jar lb.
Use: Antiseptic.

BENEPHEN ANTISEPTIC VITAMIN A & D CREAM. (Halsted) Methylbenzethonium Cl 1:1000, cod liver oil w/vitamins A and D in petrolatum and glycerin base. Tube 2 oz, jar lb.
Use: Antiseptic.

BENEPRO TABS. (Major) Probenecid 500 mg/Tab. Bot. 100s, 1000s.
Use: Agent for gout.

BENETHAMINE PENICILLIN. B.A.N. N-Benzylphenethylammonium 6-phenylacetamidopenicillanate. N-Benzylphenethylamine salt of benzylpenicillin.
Use: Antibiotic.

BENGAL GELATIN.
See: Agar.

BEN-GAY CHILDREN'S VAPORIZING RUB. (Leeming) Camphor, menthol, w/oils of turpentine, eucalyptus, cedar leaf, nutmeg, thyme in stainless white base. Jar 1.125 oz.
Use: External analgesic.

BEN-GAY EXTRA STRENGTH BALM. (Leeming) Methylsalicylate 30%, menthol 8%. Jar 3.75 oz.
Use: External analgesic.

BEN-GAY EXTRA STRENGTH SPORTS BALM. (Leeming) Methylsalicylate 28%, menthol 10%. Tube 1.25 oz, 3 oz.
Use: External analgesic.

BEN-GAY GEL. (Leeming) Methylsalicylate 15%, menthol 7%, alcohol 40%. Tube 1.25 oz, 3 oz.
Use: External analgesic.

BEN-GAY GREASELESS OINTMENT. (Leeming) Methylsalicylate 18.3%, menthol 16%. Tube 1.25 oz, 3 oz, 5 oz.
Use: External analgesic.

BEN-GAY LOTION. (Leeming) Methylsalicylate 15%, menthol 7% in lotion base. Bot. 2 oz, 4 oz.
Use: External analgesic.

BEN-GAY OINTMENT. (Leeming) Methylsalicylate 15%, menthol 10% in ointment base. Tube 1.25 oz, 3 oz, 5 oz.
Use: External analgesic.

BEN-GAY SPORTSGEL. (Leeming) Methylsalicylate, menthol, alcohol 40%. Tube 1.25 oz, 3 oz.
Use: External analgesic.

BENOJECT. (Mayrand) Diphenhydramine HCl 50 mg/ml. Vial 10 ml.
Use: Antihistamine, anticholinergic.

BENOQUIN. (Elder) Monobenzone 20% in cream base. Tube 35 Gm, 453.6 Gm.
Use: Treatment of vitiligo.

BENORAL CAPSULES. (Winthrop) Benorylate.
Use: Analgesic, antipyretic.

BENORAL SUSPENSION. (Winthrop) Benorylate.
Use: Analgesic, antipyretic.

BENORAL TABLETS. (Winthrop) Benorylate.
Use: Analgesic, antipyretic.

•**BENORTERONE.** USAN. 17 β-Hydroxy-17-methyl-β-norandrost-4-en-3-one.
Use: Antiandrogen.

BENORYLATE. B.A.N. 4-Acetamidophenyl O-acetylsalicylate.
Use: Analgesic.

•**BENOXAPROFEN.** USAN. 2-(2-p-Chlorophenyl-benzoxazol-5-yl)propionic acid.
Use: Anti-inflammatory, analgesic.

•**BENOXINATE HYDROCHLORIDE,** U.S.P. XXII. Ophth. Soln., U.S.P. XXII. 2-(Diethylaminoethyl)4-amino-3-butoxybenzoate HCl.
Use: Ophth. anesthesia.
See: Fluress (Barnes-Hind).

•**BENOXYL LOTION.** (Stiefel) Benzoyl peroxide 5% or 10% in mild lotion base. Bot. 1 oz, 2 oz.
Use: Anti-acne.

•**BENPERIDOL.** USAN. 1-{1-[3-(4-Fluorobenzoyl)-propyl]-4-piperidyl}benzimidazolin-2-one.
Use: Tranquilizer.
See: Anquil.

•**BENSALAN.** USAN. 3,5-Dibromo-N-p-bromo-benzyl)salicylamide. Under study.
Use: Germicide.

•**BENSERAZIDE.** USAN. DL-2-Amino-3-hydroxy-2′-(2,3,4-trihydroxybenzyl)propionohydrazide.
Use: Treatment of Parkinson's disease.

•**BENSULDAZIC ACID.** V.B.A.N. (5-Benzyl-6-thioxo-1,3,5-thiadiazin-3-yl)acetic acid. Defungit sodium salt.
Use: Fungicide, veterinary medicine.

•**BENSULFOID.** (Poythress) Colloidal sulfur 33%. **Tab.:** Elemental sulfur 130 mg by weight, fused on colloidal bentonite. 2 gr. Bot. 100s. **Pow.:** 1 oz.
Use: Prescription compounding.
W/Phenobarbital.
See: Solfoton, Tab. or Cap. (Poythress).

•**BENSULFOID CREAM.** (Poythress) Sulfur 8%, resorcinol 2%, alcohol 10%. 15 Gm.
Use: Anti-acne.

•**BENSULFOID LOTION.** (Poythress) Bensulfoid 6% (33% colloidal sulfur), thymol 0.5%, methyl salicylate 5%, zinc oxide 6%, alcohol (by vol.) 12%, perfume, cosmetic colors, emulsifiers. Bot. 2 oz.
Use: Anti-acne.

•**BENTAZEPAM.** USAN.
Use: Sedative.

BENTICAL. (Lamond) Bentonite, zinc oxide, zinc carbonate, titanium dioxide. Bot. 4 oz, 6 oz, 8 oz, 16 oz, 32 oz, 0.5 gal, gal.
Use: Bland lotion.

•**BENTIROMIDE.** USAN.
Use: Diagnostic aid.
See: Chymex, Soln. (Adria).

•**BENTONITE,** N.F. XVII.
Use: Pharmaceutical aid (suspending agent).

•**BENTONITE, PURIFIED,** N.F. XVII.
Use: Pharmaceutical aid.

•**BENTONITE MAGMA,** N.F. XVII.
Use: Pharmaceutical aid (suspending agent).

BENTRAC 25, 50. (Kenyon) Diphenhydramine HCl 25 mg or 50 mg/Cap. Bot. 100s.
Use: Antihistamine.

BENTRAC-ELIXIR. (Kenyon) Diphenhydramine HCl 10 mg/4 ml. Alcohol 14%. Bot. 4 oz.
Use: Antihistamine.

BENTRAC EXPECTORANT. (Kenyon) Diphenhydramine HCl 80 mg, ammonium Cl 12 gr, sodium citrate 5 gr, chloroform 2 gr, menthol 1/10 gr, alcohol 5%/fl oz. Bot. 4 oz.
Use: Antitussive, expectorant.

BENTYL. (Lakeside) Dicyclomine HCl. **Cap.:** 10 mg. Bot. 100s, 500s, UD 100s. **Tab.:** 20 mg. Bot. 100s, 500s, 1000s, UD 100s. **Syr.:** 10 mg/5 ml. Bot. pt. **Inj.:** 10 mg/ml. Amp. 2 ml, syringe 2 ml. Vial 10 ml (also contains chlorobutanol).
Use: Anticholinergic/antispasmodic.

•**BENURESTAT.** USAN.
Use: Enzyme inhibitor.

BENYLIN COUGH SYRUP. (Parke-Davis) Diphenhydramine HCl 12.5 mg, alcohol 5%. Bot. 4 oz, 8 oz, UD 5 ml, 10 ml. Box 100s.
Use: Antitussive.

BENYLIN DECONGESTANT LIQUID. (Parke-Davis) Pseudoephedrine HCl 30 mg, diphenhydramine HCl 12.5 mg, alcohol 5%, saccharin. Bot. 120 ml.
Use: Decongestant, antihistamine.

BENYLIN DM COUGH SYRUP. (Parke-Davis) Dextromethorphan HBr 10 mg/5 ml, alcohol 5%. Bot. 4 oz, 8 oz.
Use: Antitussive.

BENYLIN DME. (Parke-Davis) **Liq.:** Dextromethorphan HBr 5 mg, guaifenesin 100 mg, alcohol 5%, saccharin, menthol. Bot. 240 ml.
Use: Antitussive, expectorant.

BENZA. (Century) Benzalkonium Cl 1:5000 and 1:750. Bot. 2 oz, 4 oz.
Use: Antiseptic, germicide.

BENZAC 5 & 10. (Owen/Galderma) Benzoyl peroxide 5% or 10% w/polyoxyethylene lauryl ether 6%, alcohol 12%. Tube 60 Gm, 90 Gm.
Use: Anti-acne.

BENZAC w 2.5, 5 & 10. (Owen/Galderma) Benzoyl peroxide 2.5%, 5% or 10% gel in water base w/carbomer 940.
Use: Anti-acne.

BENZAC w WASH. (Owen/Galderma) Benzoyl peroxide 5% or 10% in vehicle of sodium C14-

16 olefin sulfonate, carbomer 940, purified water. **5%**: Bot. 4 oz, 8 oz. **10%**: Bot. 8 oz.
Use: Anti-acne.

BENZAGEL. (Dermik) Benzoyl peroxide 5% or 10% in gel base of water, carbomer 940, alcohol 14%, sodium hydroxide, docusate sodium, fragrance. Tube 1.5 oz, 3 oz.
Use: Anti-acne.

•**BENZALDEHYDE,** N.F. XVII. Cpd. Elix., N.F. XVII.
Use: Pharmaceutic aid (flavor).

•**BENZALKONIUM CHLORIDE,** N.F. XVII. Soln., N.F. XVII. Alkyldimethylbenzylammonium Cl. Zephirol. Soln. 1:5000. ammonium, alkyldimethyl(phenylmethyl)-, Cl.
Use: Surface antiseptic, antimicrobial preservative.
See: Benz-All, Liq. (Xytrium).
Econopred, Susp. (Alcon).
Eye-Stream (Alcon).
Germicin, Soln. (Consolidated Mid.).
Hyamine 3500 (Rohm & Haas).
Otrivin Spray (Geigy).
Ultra Tears (Alcon).
Zalkon Conc., Liq. (Gordon).
Zephiran Chloride Preps. (Winthrop Pharm).
W/Aluminum Cl, oxyquinoline sulfate.
See: Alochor Styptic, Liq. (Gordon).
W/Bacitracin zinc, polymyxin B, neomycin sulfate.
See: Biotres, Oint. (Central).
W/Benzocaine, benzyl alcohol.
See: Aerocain, Oint. (Aeroceuticals).
W/Benzocaine, orthohydroxyphenyl-mercuric Cl, parachlorometaxylenol.
See: Unguentine, Aerosol (Norwich).
W/Berberine HCl, sodium borate, phenylephrine HCl, sodium Cl, boric acid.
See: Ocusol, Eye Lotion, Drops (Norwich).
W/Boric acid, potassium Cl, sodium carbonate anhydrous, disodium edetate.
See: Swim-Eye, Drops (Savage).
W/Chlorophyll.
See: Mycomist, Spray Liq. (Gordon).
W/Hydrocortisone.
See: Barseb Thera-Spray, Soln. (Barnes-Hind).
W/Diperodon HCl, carbolic acid, ichthammol, thymol, camphor, juniper tar.
See: Boro Oint. (Scrip).
W/Disodium edetate, potassium Cl, isotonic boric acid.
See: Dacriose (Smith, Miller & Patch).
W/Epinephrine.
See: Epinal, Soln. (Alcon).
W/Epinephrine bitartrate, pilocarpine HCl, mannitol.
See: E-Pilo Ophth., Preps. (Smith, Miller & Patch).
W/Ethoxylated lanolin, methylparaben, hamamelis water, glycerin.
See: Mediconet, clothwipes. (Medicone).
W/Gentamicin sulfate, disodium phosphate, monosodium, phosphate, sodium Cl.
See: Garamycin Ophth. Soln., Preps. (Schering).
W/Hydroxypropyl methylcellulose.
See: Isopto Plain & Tears (Alcon).
W/Hydroxypropyl methylcellulose, disodium edetate.
See: Goniosol (Smith, Miller & Patch).
W/Isopropyl alcohol, methyl salicylate.
See: Cydonol Massage Lotion (Gordon).
W/Lidocaine, phenol.
See: Unguentine, spray (Norwich).
W/Methylcellulose.
See: Tearisol (Smith, Miller & Patch).
W/Methylcellulose, phenylephrine HCl.
See: Efricel ⅛% (Professional Pharmacal).
W/Oxyquinolin sulfate, distilled water.
See: Oxyzal Wet Dressing, Soln. (Gordon).
W/Phenylephrine, pyrilamine maleate, antipyrine.
See: Prefrin-A, Ophth. (Allergan).
W/Pilocarpine HCl, epinephrine bitartrate, mannitol.
See: E-Pilo Ophth., Preps. (Smith, Miller & Patch).
W/Polymyxin B, neomycin sulfate, zinc bacitracin.
See: Biotres, Oint. (Central).
W/Polyoxyethylene ethers.
See: Ionax, Aerosol Can (Owen/Galderma).
W/Polyvinyl alcohol.
See: Contique Artificial Tears (Alcon).
W/Pramoxine HCl, allantoin.
See: Perifoam, Aerosol (Solvay).
W/Pramoxine HCl, hydrocortisone, parachlorometaxylenol, acetic acid.
See: My Cort Otic #2, Ear Drops (Scrip).
Steramine Otic, Drops. (Mayrand).
W/Pramoxine HCl, hydrocortisone, parachlorometaxylenol, acetic acid, propylene glycol.
See: Otostan H.C. (Standex).
W/Pyrilamine maleate, pheniramine maleate, chlorpheniramine maleate, menthol.
See: Trigelamine, Oint. (E.J. Moore).
W/Sodium borate, sodium bicarbonate, sodium Cl.
See: Zalkon Wet Dressing, Liq. (Gordon).
W/Tripelennamine HCl, methapyrilene.
See: Didelamine, Cream (Commerce).
W/Zinc oxide, urea, sulfur, salicylic acid, isopropyl alcohol in a base containing menthol, silicon dioxide, iron oxide and perfume.
See: Akne Drying Lotion, Bot. (Alto).

BENZ-ALL. (Xttrium) Benzalkonium Cl 12.9%. Bot. 10 ml, 40 ml. 15s.
Use: Germicidal concentrate with anti-rust factor.

BENZALOIDS. (Jenkins) Benzocaine 5 mg, cal. iodized 12 mg, eucalyptol 0.35 mg, methenamine 6.5 mg, menthol 0.2 mg/Loz. Bot. 1000s.

BENZAMYCIN TOPICAL GEL. (Dermik) Erythromycin 3%, benzoyl peroxide 5%. Jar 23.3 Gm.
Use: Anti-acne.

BENZATHINE PENICILLIN. B.A.N. NN′-Dibenzylethylenedi(ammonium 6-phenylacetamido-penicillanate). NN′-Dibenzylethylenediamine di-(benzylpenicillin).
Use: Antibiotic.

•**BENZATHINE PENICILLIN G,** U.S.P. XXII. Oral Susp. Sterile, Tab., U.S.P. XXII. N,N′-Dibenzylethylenediamine di(benzylpenicillin) Benzethacil. 3,3-Dimethyl-7-oxo-6-(2-phenylacetamido)-4-thia-1-azabicyclo [3.2.0] heptaine-2-carboxylic acid compound with N,N-Dibenzylethylene-diamine (2:1). Dibencil, Penidural.
Use: Antibiotic.
See: Permapen, Disp. Syringe (Roerig).
Isoject Permapen, Aq. Susp. (Pfizer).
W/Procaine penicillin G.
See: Bicillin P.A.B., Disp. Syr. (Wyeth-Ayerst).

BENZAZOLINE HYDROCHLORIDE.
See: Tolazoline HCl.

BENZBROMARONE. USAN.
Use: Uricosuric.

BENZCHLORPROPAMID.
Used in Europe under:
Nydrane.
Posedrine.

BENZ-EASE. (Novocol) Benzocaine, oil of clove, oxyquinoline benzoate. Oint. Tube 0.25 oz, 6s, 36s.
Use: Anesthetic, antiseptic, adhesive.

BENZEDREX INHALER. (SmithKline Products) Propylhexedrine 250 mg, menthol and lavender oil. Single plastic tube 12s.
Use: Nasal decongestant.

BENZEHIST. (Pharmex) Diphenhydramine HCl 10 mg/ml. Vial 30 ml.
Use: Antihistamine.

BENZENE HEXACHLORIDE, GAMMA.
See: Lindane U.S.P. XXII.

BENZESTROL. 4,4′-(1,2-Diethyl-3-methyltrimethylene) diphenol.

BENZETHACIL. Dibenzylethylenediamine dipenicillin G DBED.
See: Penicillin G Benzathine, U.S.P. XXII.

BENZETHIDINE. B.A.N. Ethyl 1-(2-benzyloxyethyl)-4-phenylpiperidine-1-carboxylate.
Use: Narcotic analgesic.

BENZETHONIUM CHLORIDE, U.S.P. XXII. Tincture, Topical Soln., U.S.P. XXII. Benzyldimethyl [2-[2-[p-(1,1,3,3-tetramethylbutyl)phenoxy]ethoxy]ethyl]ammonium Cl.
Use: Surface antiseptic, antimicrobial preservative.
See: Ammorid Diaper Rinse, Oint. (Kinney).
Hyacide, Soln. (Niltig).
Hyamine 1622 (Rohm & Haas).
Phemerol Chloride, Soln., Tr. (Parke-Davis).
Phemithyn, Liq. (Davis & Sly).
W/Benzocaine.
See: Americaine, Oint., Aerosol (Arnar-Stone).
Dermoplast, Spray (Wyeth-Ayerst).
W/Nonyl phenoxypolyoxyethylene ethanol.
See: Dalkon Foam (Robins).
Emko Pre-Fil, Foam (Emko).
W/Zinc oxide.
See: Ammorid, Oint. (Kinney).

BENZETHONIUM CHLORIDE. B.A.N. Benzyldimethyl-2-{2-[4-(1,1,3,3-tetramethylbutyl)-phenoxy]ethoxy}ethylammonium Cl.
Use: Antibacterial.

•**BENZETIMIDE HCl.** USAN. (1)2-(l-Benzyl-4-piperidyl)-2-phenylglutarimide monohydrochloride.
Use: Anticholinergic.

BENZHEXOL. B.A.N. 1-Cyclohexyl-1-phenyl-3-piperidinopropan-1-ol. Trihexyphenidyl (I.N.N.).
Use: Treatment of Parkinson's disease.

alpha-BENZHYDROL HCl. Diphenylhydroxy-carbinol.

BENZIDE. (Canright) Benzthiazide 50 mg/Tab. Bot. 100s, 1000s.
Use: Diuretic, antihypertensive.

•**BENZILONIUM BROMIDE.** USAN. 1-Ethyl-3-pyrrolidinyl benzilate ethylbromide.
Use: Anticholinergic.

BENZILONIUM BROMIDE. B.A.N. 3-Benziloyloxy-1, 1-diethylpyrrolidinium bromide.
Use: Inhibition of gastric secretion.

BENZINDAMINE HCl. Benzydamine HCl.

•**BENZINDOPYRINE HYDROCHLORIDE.** USAN. 1-Benzyl-3-[2-(4-pyridyl)-ethyl] indole HCl. Pyrbenzindole.
Use: Tranquilizer.

BENZIODARONE. B.A.N. 2-Ethyl-3-(4-hydroxy-3,5-di-iodobenzoyl-benzofuran.
Use: Coronary vasodilator.

BENZO-C. (Freeport) Benzocaine 5 mg, cetalkonium Cl 5 mg, ascorbic acid 50 mg/Troche. Bot. 1000s, cello-packed boxes 1000s.
Use: Local anesthetic.

•**BENZOCAINE,** U.S.P. XXII. Cream, Oint., Otic Soln., Topical Aerosol, Topical Soln., U.S.P. XXII. Ethyl-p-aminobenzoate. Anesthesin, orthesin, parathesin.
Use: Local anesthetic.
W/Combinations.
See: Aerotherm, Oint. (Aeroceuticals).
Aerocaine, Oint. (Aeroceuticals).
Americaine, Oint., Aerosol (American Critical Care).
Anacaine, Oint. (Gordon).
Anecal, Cream (Lannett).
Aura-Aid, Liq. (E.J. Moore).
Auralgan, Otic Drops (Wyeth-Ayerst).
Auralgesic, Liq. (Elder).
Benadex, Oint. (Fuller).
Benzo-C, Troche (Freeport).
Benzocol, Oint. (Hauck).
Benzodent, Oint. (Vicks).
Biscolan, Supp. (Lannett).
Boilaid, Oint. (E.J. Moore).
Bonal Itch Cream, Cream (E.J. Moore).

Bowman Drawing Paste, Oint. (Bowman).
Boil-Ease Anesthetic Drawing Salve (Commerce).
Burn Gon, Oint. (E.J. Moore).
20-Cain Burn Relief, (Alto).
Calamatum, Preps. (Blair).
Cēpacol, Troches (Merrell Dow).
Cetacaine, Preps. (Cetylite).
Chiggerex, Oint. (Scherer).
Chiggertox, Liq. (Scherer).
Chloraseptic Children's Lozenges (Norwich Eaton).
CPI Hemorrhoidal, Supp. (Century).
Culminal, Cream (Culminal).
D.D.D. Cream (Campana).
Dent's Dental Poultice (C.S. Dent).
Dent's Lotion, Jel (C.S. Dent).
Dent's Toothache Gum (C.S. Dent).
Derma Medicone (Medicone).
Derma Medicone-HC (Medicone).
Dermoplast, Spray (Wyeth-Ayerst).
Diplan, Cap. (Solvay).
Dulzit, Cream (Commerce).
Epinephricaine, Oint. (Upjohn).
Erase, Supp. (LaCrosse).
E.R.O. Forte, Liq. (Scherer).
Extend, Tab. (E.J. Moore).
Foille, Preps. (Carbisulphoil).
Formula 44 Cough Control Discs, Loz. (Vicks).
Fung-O-Spray (Scrip).
G.B.A. Drops (Scrip).
Hemocaine, Oint. (Hauck).
Hurricaine, Liq. or Gel (Beutlich).
Isodettes Loz. (Norcliff-Thayer).
Jiffy, Drops (Block Drug).
Kanalka, Tab. (Lannett).
Kankex, Liq. (E.J. Moore).
Lanaurine, Drop. (Lannett).
Lanazets, Loz. (Lannett).
Listerine Cough Control Lozenges (Warner-Lambert).
Medicone Dressing (Medicone).
Meditrating Throat Lozenge, Loz. (Vicks).
My-Cort Drops (Scrip).
Myringacaine, Liq. (Upjohn).
Nilatus, Loz. (Bowman).
Off-Ezy Corn Remover, Liq. (Commerce).
Oracin, Loz. (Vicks).
Oradex-C, Troche (Commerce).
Ora-Jel, Gel. (Commerce).
Pain-Eze, Oint. (E.J. Moore).
Pazo, Oint., Supp. (Bristol-Myers).
Pyrogallic Acid Oint. (Gordon).
Rectal Medicone (Medicone).
Rectal Medicone-HC, Supp. (Medicone).
Rectal Medicone Unguent (Medicone).
Ridupois Capsule (Elder).
Rite-Diet, Cap. (E.J. Moore).
Robitussets, Troche (Robins).
Salicide, Oint. (Gordon).
Scrip, Preps. (Scrip).
Sepo, Loz. (Otis Clapp).
Solarcaine, Lot. (Schering).
Soretts, Loz. (Lannett).
Spec-T Sore Throat-Cough Suppressant Loz. (Squibb).
Spec-T Sore Throat-Decongestant Loz. (Squibb).
Sucrets Cold Decongestant Lozenge (Calgon).
Sucrets Cough Control Lozenge (Calgon).
Tanac, Liq. (Commerce).
Tympagesic, Liq. (Adria).
Tyro-Loz, Loz. (Kenyon).
Unguentine Aerosol (Norwich).
Vicks Cough Silencers, Loz. (Vicks).
Vicks Formula 44 Cough Control Discs, Loz. (Vicks).
Vicks Medi-Trating Throat Lozenges, Loz. (Vicks).
Vicks Oracin, Loz. (Vicks).

BENZOCHLOROPHENE SODIUM. The sodium salt of ortho-benzyl-para-chlorophenol.

BENZOCOL. (Hauck) Benzocaine 5%. Tube oz.
Use: Local anesthetic.

BENZOCTAMINE. B.A.N. N-Methyl-9,10-ethanoanthracene-9(10H)-methylamine.
Use: Tranquilizer.

•**BENZOCTAMINE HYDROCHLORIDE.** USAN. N-Methyl-9,10-ethanoanthracene-9(10H)-methylamine HCl.
Use: Muscle relaxant, sedative.

BENZODENT. (Vicks Products) Benzocaine 20%, eugenol 0.4%, hydroxyquinoline sulfate 0.1% in an adhesive ointment base. Tube 0.25 oz, 1 oz.
Use: Local anesthetic.

BENZODEPA. USAN. Benzyl[bis(aziridinyl)-phosphinyl] carbamate.
Use: Antineoplastic.

BENZOIC ACID. (Various Mfr.) Pkg. 0.25 lb, 1 lb.
Use: Fungistatic, fungicidal.
W/Boric acid, zinc oxide, zinc stearate.
See: Ting, Cream, Pow. (Pharmacraft).
W/Salicylic acid.
See: Whitfield's Oint. (Various Mfr.).

BENZOIC ACID, 2-HYDROXY. Salicylic Acid, U.S.P. XXII.

•**BENZOIC AND SALICYLIC ACIDS OINTMENT,** U.S.P. XXII.
Use: Antifungal (topical).
See: Whitfield's Oint. (Various Mfr.).

•**BENZOIN,** U.S.P. XXII. Tincture, Compound, U.S.P. XXII.
Use: Topical protectant, expectorant.
See: Arcum—Bot. 2 oz, 4 oz, pt, gal.
Lilly—Bot. 4 fl oz, pt.
Rals—Aerosol 12 oz.
Stanlabs—Bot. 2 oz, 4 oz, pt, Compound. Bot. 1 oz, 4 oz, pt.
W/Methyl salicylate, guaiacol.
See: Methagul, Oint. (Gordon).
W/Podophyllum resin.

See: Podoben, Liq. (Maurry).
W/Polyoxyethylene dodecanol, aromatics.
See: Vicks Vaposteam, Liq. (Vicks).
BENZOIN SPRAY. (Morton) Benzoin, tolu balsam, styrax, alcohol w/propellant. Aerosol can 7 oz.
Use: Skin protectant.
BENZOL. Usually refers to benzene.
BENZO-MENTH TABLETS. (Vale) Benzocaine 2.2 mg/Tab. Bot. 1000s.
Use: Topical anesthetic.
•**BENZONATATE,** U.S.P. XXII. Cap., U.S.P. XXII. o-Meth-oxypoly-(ethyleneoxy)ethyl-p-butylaminobenzoate. 2,5,8,11,14,17,20,23,26-Nonaoxaoctacosan-28-yl p-(butylamino)benzoate. B.A.N.: 3,6,9,12,15,18,21,24,27-non-aoxaoctacosyl 4-N-butylaminobenzoate.
Use: Cough suppressant.
See: Tessalon, Perles (DuPont).
BENZOPHENONE.
See: Pan Ultra, Lot., Lipstick (Cummins).
Oxybenzone, dioxybenzone.
See: Solbar Lotion (Person & Covey).
BENZOPYRROLATE.
See: Benzopyrronium.
BENZOQUINOLIMINE.
See: Emete-Con (Pfizer).
BENZOQUINONIUM CHLORIDE.
Use: Skeletal muscle relaxant (No mfr. listed).
BENZOSULFIMIDE.
See: Saccharin, U.S.P. XXII.
BENZOSULPHINIDE SODIUM. Name previously used for Saccharin Sodium.
BENZOXIQUINE. USAN.
Use: Disinfectant.
BENZOYL p-AMINOSALICYLIC
See: Benzapas, Pow., Tab. (Dorsey).
BENZOYLPAS CALCIUM Benzoic acid, 4-(benzoylamino)-2-hydroxy-calcium salt (2:1), pentahydrate. Calcium 4-benzamidosalicylate (1:2) pentahydrate.
Use: Antitubercular.
See: Benzapas, Tab., Pow. (Dorsey).
•**BENZOYL PEROXIDE, HYDROUS,** U.S.P. XXII. Gel., Lot., U.S.P. XXII. Peroxide, dibenzoyl.
Use: Keratolytic.
See: Benzagel-5 & 10, Oint. (Dermik).
Benoxyl, Lot. (Stiefel).
Clearasil Acne Treatment, Cream (Vicks).
Clearasil Antibacterial Acne Lotion (Vicks).
Epi-Clear Antiseptic Lotion, Scrub (Squibb).
Oxy-5 Acne Pimple Medication (Norcliff Thayer).
Oxy-10 Maximum Strength Acne-Pimple Medication (Norcliff Thayer).
Oxy Wash Antibacterial Skin Wash (Norcliff Thayer).
Panoxyl, Bar (Stiefel).
Persadox, Cream, Lot. (Ortho).
Persadox HP, Cream, Lot. (Owen/Galderma).
Persa-Gel, Gel (Ortho).
Topex, Lot. (Vicks).
W/Chlorhydroxyquinoline, hydrocortisone.
See: Loroxide-HC, Lot. (Dermik).
Vanoxide-HC, Lot. (Dermik).
W/Polyoxyethylene lauryl ether.
See: Benzac 5 & 10, Gel (Owen/Galderma).
Desquam-X, Gel (Westwood).
W/Sulfur.
See: Sulfoxyl Lotion (Stiefel).
N'-BENZOYLSULFANILAMIDE.
See: Sulfabenzamide.
W/Sulfacetamide, sulfathiazole, urea.
See: Sultrin, Tab, Cream (Ortho).
BENZPHETAMINE HCl. N-Benzyl-N-α-dimethylphenethylamine HCl, dextro.
Use: Anorexiant.
See: Didrex, Tab. (Upjohn).
BENZPYRINIUM BROMIDE. 1-Benzyl-3-hydroxypyridinium bromide dimethylcarbamate.
•**BENZQUINAMIDE.** USAN. B.A.N. N,N-diethyl-1,3,4,6,7,11b-hexahydro-2-hydroxy-9,10-dimethoxy-2H-benzo[a]quinolizine-3-carboxamide acetate.
Use: Antiemetic agent.
See: Emete-Con, Vial (Roerig).
Quantril (Roerig).
BENZQUINAMIDE HCl.
See: Emete-Con. (Roerig).
BENZTHIANIDE. 3-Benzylthiomethyl-6-chloro-7-sulfamyl-2H-1,2,4-benzothiadiazine-1,1-di-oxide. Urease.
•**BENZTHIAZIDE,** U.S.P. XXII. Tabs., U.S.P. XXII. B.A.N. 3-Benzylthiomethyl-6-chloro-7-sulfamyl-1,2,4-benzothiadiazine 1,1-dioxide. 3-((benzylthio)-methyl)-6-chloro-2H-1,2,4,benzothiadiazine-7-sulfonamide 1,1-dioxide. 6-chloro-3[(phenylmethyl) thio] methyl -2H-1,2,4, benzothiadiazine-7-sulfonamide 1,1-dioxide.
Use: Diuretic, antihypertensive.
See: Aquatag, Tab. (Solvay).
Exna, Tab. (Robins).
Hydrex, Tab. (Trimen).
Proaqua, Tab. (Solvay).
Urazide, Tab. (Hauck).
W/Reserpine.
*See:*Exna-R, Tab. (Robins).
BENZTROPINE. B.A.N. 3-Benzhydryloxytropane.
Use: Treatment of Parkinson's disease.
•**BENZTROPINE MESYLATE,** U.S.P. XXII., Inj., Tab., U.S.P. XXII., Methanesulfonate, 3α-(Diphenylmethoxy)-1αH,5αH-tropane methanesulfonate.
Use: Parasympatholytic, antiparkinsonism.
W/sodium Cl.
See: Cogentin, Tab., Amp. (MSD).
BENZTROPINE METHANESULFONATE.
See: Benztropine Mesylate.
BENZYDAMINE. B.A.N. 1-Benzyl-3-(3-dimethylaminopropoxy)indazole.
Use: Anti-inflammatory, analgesic.

BENZYDAMINE HCl. USAN. 1-Benzyl-3- [3-(dimethylamino)-propoxyl]-1H-indazole HCl. Tantum.
Use: Analgesic, anti-inflammatory, antipyretic.
BENZYDROFLUMETHIAZIDE. 3-Benzyl-3,4-dihydro-6-(trifluoromethyl)-1,2,4-benzthiadiazine-7-sulfonamide, 1,1-dioxide.
See: Bendroflumethiazide.
•**BENZYL ALCOHOL,** N.F. XVII. Phenylcarbinol.
Use: Antiseptic, local anesthetic.
See: Topic, Gel (Ingram).
Vicks Blue Mint, Regular & Wild Cherry Medicated Cough Drops (Vicks).
N-BENZYHYDRYL-N-METHYLPIPERAZINE HCl. Cyclizine HCl, U.S.P. XXII.
•**BENZYL BENZOATE,** U.S.P. XXII. Lot., U.S.P. XXII. Benzoic acid, phenylmethyl ester.
Use: 10% to 30% emulsion in scabies; pharmaceutical necessity.
BENZYL BENZOATE SAPONATED. Triethanolamine 20 Gm, oleic acid 80 Gm, benzyl benzoate q.s. 1000 ml.
BENZYL CARBINOL.
See: Phenylethyl Alcohol, U.S.P. XXII.
BENZYLPENICILLIN-C-14. (Nuclear-Chicago) Carbon-14 labelled penicillin; prepared from phenyl-(acetic acid-1-C-14), 6-aminopenicillanic acid as the potassium salt. 23.4 mc/mM (62.9 mc/mg); radiochemical purity is 100%. Vacuum-sealed glass vial 50 microcuries, 0.5 millicuries.
Use: Radioisotope.
BENZYL PENICILLIN G, POTASSIUM.
See: Penicillin G Potassium.
•**BENZYLPENICILLOYL POLYLYSINE CONCENTRATE,** U.S.P. XXII. Inj., U.S.P. XXII.
Use: Skin test antigen.
See: Pre-Pen (Kremers-Urban).
BENZYL PENICILLIN G, SODIUM.
See: Penicillin G Sodium.
BEPANTHEN.
See: Panthenol.
BEPHEDIN. Benzyl ephedrine.
BEPHENIUM BROMIDE. N-Benzyl-N, N-dimethyl-N-(2-phenoxyethyl)ammonium bromide.
BEPHENIUM HYDROXYNAPHTHOATE, U.S.P. XXI. For Oral Susp., U.S.P. XXI. Benzyldimethyl (2-phenoxy-ethyl)ammonium-3-hydroxy-2-naphthoate. Benzenemethanaminium,N,N-dimethyl-N-(2-phenoxy-ethyl)-, salt with 3-hydroxy-2-naphthalenecarboxylic acid (1:1).
Use: Anthelmintic (hookworms).
BEPHENIUM HYDROXYNAPHTHOATE. B.A.N. Benzyldimethyl-2-phenoxyethylammonium 3-hydroxy-2-naphthoate.
Use: Treatment of ancylostomiasis and ascariasis.
•**BEPRIDIL HYDROCHLORIDE.** USAN.
Use: Vasodilator.
See: Vascor (McNeil).
BERACTANT.
Use: Lung surfactant.
See: Survanta (Ross).
BERBERINE.
W/Hydrastine, glycerin.
See: Murine, Ophth. Soln.
BERBERINE HYDROCHLORIDE.
W/Borax, sodium Cl, boric acid, camphor water, cherry laurel water, rose water, thimerosol.
See: Lauro, eye irrigator and drops (Otis Clapp).
BER-EX. (Dolcin) Calcium succinate 2.8 gr, acetylsalicylic acid 3.7 gr/Tab. Bot. 100s, 500s.
Use: Anti-arthritic, antirheumatic.
BEROCCA PARENTERAL NUTRITION. (Roche) Vitamins B_1 3 mg, biotin 60 mcg, B_2 3.6 mg, niacinamide 40 mg, B_6 4 mg, d-panthenol 15 mg, C 100 mg, folic acid 0.4 mg/ml. Inj. **Amp.:** Duplex pkg. containing 1 ml Soln. 1 and 1 ml Soln. 2. Box 25s.; **Vial:** Duplex pkg. containing 20 ml vial (10 ml fill) of Soln 1 plus a 10 ml vial of Soln 2. Box 1s.
Use: Vitamin/mineral supplement.
BEROCCA PLUS TABLETS. (Roche) Vitamins A 5000 IU, E 30 IU, C 500 mg, B_1 20 mg, B_2 20 mg, niacinamide 100 mg, B_6 25 mg, biotin 0.15 mg, pantothenic acid 25 mg, folic acid 0.8 mg, B_{12} 50 mcg, iron 27 mg, cromium 0.1 mg, magnesium 50 mg, manganese 5 mg, copper 3 mg, zinc 22.5 mg/Tab. Bot. 100s.
Use: Vitamin/mineral supplement.
BEROCCA TABLETS. (Roche) Vitamins B_1 15 mg, B_2 15 mg, B_6 4 mg, niacinamide 100 mg, calcium pantothenate 18 mg, B_{12} 5 mcg, folic acid 0.5 mg, C 500 mg/Tab. Bot. 100s, 500s.
Use: Vitamin/mineral supplement.
BERPLEX-C. (Alton) Vitamins B and C. Bot. 100s, 1000s.
Use: Vitamin supplement.
BERSOTRIN. (Kenyon) Vitamins B_1 15 mg, B_2 10 mg, C 300 mg, calcium pantothenate 10 mg, niacinamide 50 mg, B_6 5 mg/Cap. Bot. 100s.
Use: Vitamin supplement.
BERVITE. (Alton) Multiple vitamin. Bot. 100s, 1000s.
Use: Vitamin supplement.
•**BERYTHROMYCIN.** USAN. (1) 12-Deoxyery-thromycin; (2) Erythromycin B.
Use: Antiamebic, antibacterial.
BESAPRIN TABLETS. (Winthrop) Aspirin, chlormezanone.
Use: Salicylate, analgesic, tranquilizer, muscle relaxant.
BESEROL TABLETS. (Winthrop) Acetaminophen, chlormezanone.
Use: Analgesic, tranquilizer, muscle relaxant.
BESITEX B1. (Mills) Ephedrine ethylenediamine HCl 6 mg/Tab. Bot. 100s.
Use: Diet aid.
BESITEX B3. (Mills) Ephedrine ethylenediamine HCl 6 mg/Tab. Bot. 100s.
Use: Diet aid.
BESTA CAPSULES. (Hauck) Vitamins B_1 20 mg, B_2 15 mg, niacinamide 100 mg, calcium panto-

thenate 20 mg, E 50 IU, magnesium sulfate 70 mg, zinc 18.4 mg, B_{12} 4 mcg, B_6 25 mg, C 300 mg/Cap. Bot. 100s.
Use: Vitamin/mineral supplement.

BEST C CAPS. (Hauck) Ascorbic acid 500 mg/TR Cap. Bot. 100s.
Use: Vitamin C supplement.

BESTRONE INJECTION. (Bluco) Estrone in aqueous susp. 2 mg or 5 mg/ml. Vial 10 ml.
Use: Estrogen.

BETA-2. (Nephron) Isoetharine HCl 1% with glycerin, sodium bisulfite, parabens. Bot. 10 ml, 30 ml.
Use: Respiratory therapy, oral inhalant.

BETA-ADRENERGIC BLOCKERS.
See: Brevibloc, Inj. (DuPont).
Blocadren, Tab. (MSD).
Cartrol, Tab. (Abbott).
Corgard, Tab. (Princeton).
Inderal, Tab., Inj. (Wyeth-Ayerst).
Inderal LA, Sustained Release Cap. (Wyeth-Ayerst).
Levatol, Tab. (Reed-Carnrick).
Lopressor, Tab., Inj. (Geigy).
Propranolol HCl, Tab. (Various Mfr.).
Propranolol HCl, Inj. (SoloPak).
Sectral, Cap. (Wyeth-Ayerst).
Tenormin, Tab. (ICI Pharm.).
Visken, Tab. (Sandoz).

BETA-ADRENERGIC BLOCKERS, OPHTHALMIC.
See: Betagan Liquifilm, Soln. (Allergan).
Betoptic, Soln. (Alcon).
Timoptic in Ocudose, Soln. (MSD).
Timoptic, Soln. (MSD).

BETA CAROTENE, U.S.P. XXII. Cap., U.S.P. XXII. β,β-Carotene. All-trans-B-Carotene. (All-E)-1,1-(3,7,12,16-Tetramethyl-1,3,5,7,9,11,13,15,17-octadecanonaene-1,18-diyl) bis (2,6,6-trimethylcyclohexene).
Use: Ultraviolet screen.
See: Max-Caro (Marlyn).
Provatene (Solgar).
Solatene (Roche).

BETACETYLMETHADOL. B.A.N. β-4-Dimethylamino-1-ethyl-2,2-diphenylpentyl acetate.
Use: Narcotic analgesic.

BETACREST. (Nutrition) **Kapule:** Vitamins B_1 15 mg, B_2 10 mg, B_6 5 mg, B_{12} 4 mcg, calcium pantothenate 20 mg, niacinamide 100 mg, C 600 mg, liver 125 mg. Bot. 60s. **Inj.:** Vitamins B_1 100 mg, B_2 2 mg, B_6 5 mg, B_{12} 30 mcg, niacinamide 125 mg, panthenol 10 mg, benzyl alcohol 1.5%/ml. Vial 30 ml.
Use: Vitamin supplement.

BETACREST KAPULE. (Nutrition) Vitamins B_1 30 mg, B_2 20 mg, B_6 10 mg, B_{12} 8 mcg, calcium pantothenate 40 mg, niacinamide 200 mg, C 600 mg, liver 250 mg/2 Cap. Bot. 60s.
Use: Vitamin/mineral supplement.

BETADINE. (Purdue Frederick) Povidone-iodine.
Aerosol Spray, Bot. 3 oz.
Antiseptic Gauze Pads 3″ × 9″. Box 12s.
Antiseptic Lubricating Gel, Tube 5 Gm.
Disposable Medicated Douche, concentrated packette w/cannula and 6 oz water.
Douche, Bot. 1 oz, 4 oz, 8 oz.
Douche Packette, 0.5 oz (6 per carton).
Helafoam Solution Canister 250 Gm.
Mouthwash/Gargle, Bot. 6 oz.
Oint., Tube 1 oz, Jar 1 lb, 5 lb.
Oint., packette 1/32 oz, 1/8 oz.
Perineal Wash Conc. Kit, Bot. 8 oz w/dispenser.
Skin Cleanser, Bot. 1 oz, 4 oz.
Skin Cleanser Foam, Canister 6 oz.
Solution, 0.5 oz, 8 oz, 16 oz, 32 oz, gal.
Solution Packette, oz.
Solution Swab Aid, 100s.
Solution Swabsticks, 1s Box 200s; 3s Box 50s.
Surgical Scrub, Bot. pt, pt w/dispenser, qt, gal, packette 0.5 oz.
Surgi-prep Sponge-Brush 36s.
Vaginal Suppositories, Box 7s w/vaginal applicator.
Viscous Formula Antiseptic Gauze Pads: 3″ × 9″, 5″ × 9″. Box 12s.
Whirlpool Concentrate, Bot. gal.
Use: Antiseptic for uses indicated in product labeling.

BETA-ESTRADIOL.
See: Estradiol, U.S.P. XXII.

BETAEUCAINE HCl. Name previously used for Eucaine HCl.

BETAGAN. (Allergan) Levobunolol HCl 0.5% w/ polyvinyl alcohol, benzalkonium Cl, sodium metabisulfite, EDTA. Bot. 5 ml, 10 ml, 15 ml.
Use: Beta-adrenergic blocking agent, ophthalmic.

BETAGEN. (Enzyme Process) Vitamins B_1 1 mg, B_2 1.2 mg, niacin 15 mg, B_6 18 mg, pantothenic acid 18 mg, choline 1.8 Gm, betaine 96 mg/6 Tab. Bot. 100s, 250s.
Use: Vitamin supplement.

BETAGEN OINTMENT. (Goldline) Povidone iodine. Oint. Tube oz. Jar lb.
Use: Antiseptic.

BETAGEN SOLUTION. (Goldline) Povidone iodine. Bot. pt, gal.
Use: Antiseptic.

BETAGEN SURGICAL SCRUB. (Goldline) Povidone iodine. Bot. pt, gal.
Use: Antiseptic.

•**BETAHISTINE HYDROCHLORIDE.** USAN. 2-(2-Methylaminoethyl) pyridine dihydrochloride.
Use: Meniere's disease. A diamine oxidase inhibitor. Increase microcirculation.

BETA-HYPOPHAMINE.
See: Vasopressin.

•**BETAINE HYDROCHLORIDE,** U.S.P. XXII. Acidol HCl, lycine HCl.
Use: Replenisher adjunct (electrolyte).
W/Ferrous fumarate, docusate sodium, desiccated liver, vitamins, minerals.

See: Hemaferrin, Tab. (Western Research).
W/Pancreatin, pepsin, ammonium Cl.
See: Zypan, Tab. (Standard Process).
W/Pepsin.
See: Normacid, Tab. (Stuart).

BETALIN S. (Lilly) Thiamine HCl.
50 mg or 100 mg. Tab. Bot. 100s.
Use: Vitamin B_1 supplement.

BETALIN 12 CRYSTALLINE. (Lilly) Vitamin B_{12} 1000 mcg/ml, sodium Cl 0.25%, benzyl alcohol 2%. Vial 10 ml.
Use: Vitamin B_{12} supplement.

BETAMEPRODINE. B.A.N. β-3-Ethyl-1-methyl-4-phenyl-4-propionyloxypiperidine.
Use: Narcotic analgesic.

BETAMETHADOL. B.A.N. β-6-Dimethylamino-4,4-diphenylheptan-3-ol.
Use: Narcotic analgesic.

•**BETAMETHASONE,** U.S.P. XXII. Cream, Syr., Tab., U.S.P. XXII. 9-α-Fluoro-11β, 17,21-trihydroxy16β-methylpregna-1,4-diene-3,20-dione. 9α-Fluoro16β-methylprednisolone. Acetate and sodium phosphate.
Use: Glucocorticoid.
See: Celestone, Inj., Syr., Tab. (Schering).

•**BETAMETHASONE ACETATE,** U.S.P. XXII. Pregna-1,4-diene-3,20-dione, 9-fluoro-11, 17-dihydroxy-16-methyl-21-(acetyloxy)-, (11β, 16β)-. 9-Fluoro-11β,17,21-trihydroxy-16β-methylpregna-1,4-diene-3,20-dione 21-acetate.
Use: Glucocorticoid.

BETAMETHASONE ACIBUTATE. B.A.N. 21-Acetoxy-9α-fluoro-11β-hydroxy-16β-methyl-17-(2-methylpropionyloxy)pregna-1,4-diene-3,20-dione.
Use: Corticosteroid.

•**BETAMETHASONE BENZOATE,** U.S.P. XXII. Gel, U.S.P. XXII. 9-Fluoro-11β 17,21-trihydroxy-16β-methylpregna-1,4-diene-3,20-dione 17 benzoate.
Use: Glucocorticoid.
See: Benisone. (Warner-Chilcott).
Flurobate (Texas Pharmacal).
Uticort, Prods. (Parke-Davis).

•**BETAMETHASONE DIPROPIONATE,** U.S.P. XXII. Topical Aerosol, Cream, Lot., Oint., U.S.P. XXII.
Use: Glucocorticoid.
See: Alphatrex Prods. (Savage).
Diprolene Prods. (Schering).
Diprosone Prods. (Schering).

•**BETAMETHASONE SODIUM PHOSPHATE,** U.S.P. XXII. Inj., U.S.P. XXII. Pregna-1,4-diene-3,20-dione, 9-fluoro-11,17-dihydroxy-16-methyl-21-(phosphonoxy)-, disodium salt, (11β, 16β). 9-Fluoro-11β,17,21-trihydroxy-16β-methylpregna-1,4-diene-3,20-dione 21-(disodium phosphate).
See: Celestone Phosphate Inj. (Schering).

•**BETAMETHASONE SODIUM PHOSPHATE AND BETAMETHASONE ACETATE SUSPENSION, STERILE,** U.S.P. XXII.
See: Celestone Soluspan (Schering).

•**BETAMETHASONE VALERATE,** U.S.P. XXII. Cream, Lot., Oint., U.S.P. XXII. Topical Aerosol U.S.P. XXI. Pregna-1,4-diene-3,20-dione,9-fluoro-11,21-dihydroxy-16-methyl-17-[(1-oxopentyl)oxy]-,(11β,16β)-. 9-Fluoro-11β,17,21-trihydroxy-16β-methylpregna-1,4-diene-3,20-dione 17-valerate.
See: Betatrex Prods. (Savage).
Beta-Val Prods. (Lemmon).
Valisone Prods. (Schering).
Valnac Prods. (Schering).

•**BETAMICIN SULFATE.** USAN.
Use: Antibacterial.

BETANAPHTHOL. 2-Naphthol.
Use: Parasiticide.

BETAPEN-VK. (Bristol) Penicillin V potassium.
Oral Soln.: 125 mg/ml Bot. 100 ml. 250 mg/5 ml Bot. 100 ml, 200 ml. **Tab.:** 250 mg/Tab. Bot. 100s, 1000s; 500 mg/Tab. Bot. 100s.
Use: Antibacterial; penicillin.

BETAPRODINE. B.A.N. β-1,3-Dimethyl-4-phenyl-4-propionyloxypiperidine.
Use: Narcotic analgesic.

BETA-ADRENERGIC BLOCKERS, OPTHALMIC.
See: OptiPranolol, Soln. (Bausch & Lomb).

BETA-PROPIOLACTONE.
See: Betaprone, Vial (Forest).

BETA-PYRIDYL-CARBINOL. Nicotinyl alcohol. Alcohol corresponding to nicotinic acid.
See: Roniacol, Elix., Tab. (Roche Lab.).

BETATREX. (Savage) Betamethasone valerate 0.1%. Cream, Oint. Tube 15 Gm, 45 Gm; Lot. Bot. 60 ml.
Use: Corticosteroid.

BETA-VAL CREAM. (Lemmon) Betamethasone valerate equivalent to 0.1% betamethasone base in cream base. Tube 15 Gm, 45 Gm.
Use: Corticosteroid.

BETA-VAL LOTION. (Lemmon) Betamethasone valerate equivalent to 0.1% betamethasone in lotion base. Bot. 60 ml.
Use: Corticosteroid.

BETA-VAL OINTMENT. (Lemmon) Betamethasone valerate equivalent to 0.1% betamethasone base in ointment base. Tube 15 Gm, 45 Gm.
Use: Corticosteroid.

•**BETAXOLOL HYDROCHLORIDE.** USAN.
Use: Antianginal, antihypertensive.
See: Betoptic, Ophth. (Alcon).
Kerlone (Searle).

•**BETAXOLOL OPHTHALMIC SOLUTION,** U.S.P XXII.

•**BETHANECHOL CHLORIDE,** U.S.P. XXII. Inj., Tab., U.S.P. XXII. (2-Hydroxypropyl) trimethylammonium Cl Carbamate. Carbamylmethylcholine Cl.
Use: Parasympathomimetic.
See: Duvoid, Tab. (Norwich Eaton).
Myotonachol, Tab., Amp. (Glenwood).

Urabeth, Tab. (Major).
Urecholine, Tab., Amp. (MSD).
Vesicholine, Tab. (Star).

•**BETHANIDINE.** USAN. 2-Benzyl-1,3-dimethylguanidine.
Use: Hypotensive.

BETHAPRIM. (Major) Trimethoprim 40 mg, sulfamethoxazole 200 mg/5 ml, alcohol 0.26%, saccharin and sorbitol. Susp.
Use: Anti-infective.

BETHAPRIM DS TABS. (Major) Trimethoprim 160 mg, sulfamethoxazole 800 mg/Tab. Bot. 100s, 500s, UD 100s.
Use: Anti-infective.

BETHAPRIM SS TABS. (Major) Trimethoprim 80 mg, sulfamethoxazole 400 mg/Tab. Bot. 100s, 500s.
Use: Anti-infective.

•**BETIATIDE.** USAN.
Use: Pharmaceutic aid.

BETOPTIC. (Alcon) Betaxolol HCl 0.5%. Bot. 2.5 ml, 5 ml, 10 ml, 15 ml.
Use: Beta-adrenergic blocking agent, ophthalmic.

BETULINE. (Ferndale) Methyl salicylate, camphor, menthol, peppermint oil in a water soluble base. Lot. Bot. 60 ml, pt.
Use: External analgesic.

BEVANTOLOL HYDROCHLORIDE. USAN.
Use: Antianginal, antihypertensive, cardiac depressant.

BEVONIUM METHYLSULFATE. B.A.N. 2-Benziloyloxy-methyl-1,1-dimethylpiperidinium methylsulfate.
Use: Antispasmodic.

BEXOMAL-C. (Hauck) Vitamins B_1 6 mg, B_2 7 mg, B_3 80 mg, B_5 10 mg, B_6 5 mg, B_{12} 6 mcg, C 250 mg/Tab. Bot. 50s.
Use: Vitamin supplement.

BEXOPHENE. (Hauck) Propoxyphene HCl 65 mg, aspirin 389 mg, caffeine 32.4 mg. Cap. Bot. 500s.
Use: Analgesic combination.

•**BEZAFIBRATE.** USAN.
Use: Antihyperlipoproteinemic.
See: Bezalip (Norwich Eaton).

BEZITRAMIDE. B.A.N. 4-[4-(2-Oxo-3-propionylbenzimidazolin-1-yl)piperidino]-2,2-diphenylbutyronitrile.
Use: Narcotic analgesic.

BEZON. (Whittier) Vitamins B_1 5 mg, B_2 3 mg, niacinamide 20 mg, pantothenic acid 3 mg, B_6 0.5 mg, C 50 mg, B_{12} 1 mcg/Cap. Bot. 30s, 100s.
Use: Vitamin supplement.

BEZON FORTE. (Whittier) Vitamins B_1 25 mg, B_2 12.5 mg, niacinamide 50 mg, pantothenic acid 10 mg, B_6 5 mg, C 250 mg/Cap. Bot. 30s, 100s.
Use: Vitamin supplement.

B-F-I POWDER. (Beecham Products) Bismuth-formic-iodide, zinc phenolsulfonate, bismuth subgallate, amol, potassium alum, boric acid, menthol, eucalyptol, thymol and inert diluents. Can 0.25 oz, 1.25 oz, 8 oz.
Use: Antiseptic.

B.G.O. (Calotabs) Iodoform, salicylic acid, sulfur, zinc oxide, phenol (liquefied) 1%, calamine, menthol, petrolatum, lanolin, mineral oil, undecylenic acid 1%. Jar ⅞ oz, Tube 1⅛ oz.
Use: Antiseptic, antifungal.

BIALAMICOL. B.A.N. 3,3′-Diallyl-5,5′-bisdiethylaminomethyl-4,4′-dihydroxybiphenyl. Biallylamicol.
Use: Treatment of amebiasis.

•**BIALAMICOL HCl.** USAN. 5,5′-Diallyl-α,α′-bis-(diethylamino)-m,m′-bitolyl-4,4′-diol HCl.
Use: Antiamebic.

BIAPHASIC INSULIN INJECTION. A suspension of insulin crystals in a solution of insulin buffered at pH 7. Insulin Novo Rapitard.

BIAVAX-II. (MSD) Rubella and mumps virus vaccine, live. See details under Meruvax-II and Mumpsvax. Single-dose vial w/diluent. Pkg. 1s, 10s.
Use: Agent for immunization.

BIBENZONIUM BROMIDE. B.A.N. 2-(1,2-Diphenylethoxy) ethyltrimethylammonium bromide.
Use: Cough suppressant.

BICALMA TABLETS. (Ferndale) Calcium Carbonate 250 mg, magnesium trisilicate 300 mg. Chewable. In 100s, 1000s.
Use: Antacid.

BICILLIN. (Wyeth-Ayerst) Penicillin G benzathine 200,000 units/Tab. Bot. 36s.
Use: Antibacterial; penicillin.

BICILLIN C-R. (Wyeth-Ayerst) Penicillin G benzathine 150,000 units, penicillin G procaine 150,000 units/ml w/lecithin, povidone, methyl and propylparabens. Vial 10 ml. Bicillin 300,000 units, penicillin G procaine 300,000 units/1 ml w/lecithin, povidone, methyl and propylparaben. Tubex cartridge 1 ml. Pkg. 10s. Bicillin 600,000 units, penicillin G procaine 600,000 units with parabens, lecithin and povidone/2 ml Tubex cartridge. Pkg. 10s. Bicillin 1,200,000 units, penicillin G procaine 1,200,000 units with parabens, lecithin and povidone/4 single-dose disposable syringe, 10s, 4 ml.
Use: Antibacterial; penicillin.

BICILLIN C-R 900/300 INJECTION. (Wyeth-Ayerst) Penicillin G benzathine 900,000 units, penicillin G procaine 300,000 units with parabens, lecithin and povidone/2 ml. Tubex. Pkg. 10s.
Use: Antibacterial; penicillin.

BICILLIN LONG-ACTING. (Wyeth-Ayerst) Penicillin G benzathine 300,000 units/ml w/lecithin, povidone, methyl and propylparabens. 300,000 units/ml. Vial 10 ml 600,000 units/Tubex. 1,200,000 units/2 ml Tubex 10s. 2,400,000 units/4 ml single dose disposable syringe, 10s.
Use: Antibacterial; penicillin.

BICITRA. (Willen) Sodium citrate dihydrate 500 mg, citric acid monohydrate 334 mg, 5 mEq sodium ion/5 ml. Shohl's Solution. Bot. 4 oz, pt, gal, Unit-dose 15 ml, 30 ml.
Use: Systemic alkalinizer.

•**BICLODIL HYDROCHLORIDE.** USAN.
Use: Antihypertensive (vasodilator).

BiCNU. (Bristol-Myers/Bristol Oncology) Carmustine (BCNU) 100 mg, sterile diluent (dehydrated alcohol USP inj.) 3 ml/Vial.
Use: Antineoplastic agent.

BICOZENE CREAM. (Sandoz) Benzocaine 6%, resorcinol 1.66% in cream base. Tube oz.
Use: Local anesthetic.

BICYCLINE. (Knight) Tetracycline HCl 250 mg/Cap. Bot. 100s.
Use: Antibacterial; tetracycline.

BIDIMAZIUM IODIDE. B.A.N. 4-(Biphenyl-4-yl)- 2-(4-dimethylaminostyryl)-3-methylthiazolium iodide.
Use: Anthelmintic.

BIDISOMIDE. USAN.
Use: Antiarrhythmic.

BIFE. (Jenkins) Thiamine HCl 1 mg, ferrous sulfate 3 gr/Tab. Bot. 1000s.
Use: Vitamin/iron supplement.

BIFLURANOL. B.A.N. erythro-4,4′-(1-Ethyl-2-methylethylene)di-(2-fluorophenol).
Use: Benign hypertrophy of the prostate.

•**BIFONAZOLE.** USAN.
Use: Antifungal.

BILAX. (Drug Industries) Dehydrocholic acid 50 mg, docusate sodium 100 mg/Cap. Bot. 100s, 500s.
Use: Laxative.

BILE ACIDS, OXIDIZED. Note also dehydrocholic acid.

W/Atropine methyl nitrate, ox and hog bile extract, phenobarbital.
See: G.B.S., Tab.(Forest).

W/Bile whole (desiccated), dessicated whole pancreas, homatropine methylbromide.
See: Pancobile, Tab. (Solvay).

W/Ox bile, steapsin, phenobarbital, homatropine methylbromide.
See: Oxacholin, Tab. (Roxane).

BILE EXTRACT. (Various Mfr.) Pow. 0.25 lb, 1 lb.

W/Cascara sagrada, dandelion root, podophyllin, nux vomica.
See: Oxachol, Liq. (Roxane).

W/Dehydrocholic acid, homatropine methylbromide, phenobarbital.
See: Neocholan, Tab. (Merrell Dow).

W/Pancreatic substance, dl-methionine, choline bitartrate.
See: Licoplex, Tab. (Mills).

BILE EXTRACT, OX. Purified ox gall.
Lilly—Enseal 5 gr, Bot. 100s, 500s, 1000s.
C. D. Smith—Tab. 5 gr, Bot. 1000s.
Stoddard—Tab. 3 gr, Bot. 100s, 500s, 1000s.

W/Cellulase, pepsin, glutamic acid HCl, pancreatin.
See: Kanulase, Tab. (Dorsey).

W/Cellulase, pepsin, glutamic acid HCl, pancreatin, methscopolamine nitrate, pentobarbital.
See: Kanumodic, Tab. (Dorsey).

W/Colcynth compound extract, cascara sagrada extract, podophyllin, hyoscyamus extract.
See: Bileo-Secrin Compound Tablets (First Texas).

W/Dehydrocholic acid, homatropine methylbromide, phenobarbital.
See: Bilamide, Tab. (Norgine).

W/Dehydrocholic acid, pepsin, homatropine methylbromide.
See: Biloric, Cap. (Arcum).

W/Desoxycholic acid, oxidized bile acids, pancreatin.
See: Bilogen, Tab. (Organon).

W/Enzyme concentrate, pepsin, dehydrocholic acid, belladonna extract.
See: Ro-Bile, Tab. (Solvay).

W/Oxidized bile acids, steapsin, phenobarbital, homatropine methylbromide.
See: Oxacholin, Tab. (Philips).

W/Pepsin, pancreatic enzyme concentrate.
See: Konzyme, Tab. (Brunswick).
Nu'Leven, Tab. (Lemmon).
Nu'Leven Plus, Tab. (Lemmon).

W/Sodium salicylate, phenolphthalein, chionanthus extract, cascara sagrada extract, sodium glycocholate, sodium taurocholate.
See: Glycols, Tab. (Bowman).

BILEIN. Bile salts obtained from ox bile.

BILE-LIKE PRODUCTS.
See: Zanchol, Tab. (Searle).

BILE PRODUCTS.
See: Bile Salts.
Dehydrocholic Acid.
Desoxycholic Acid.
Ketocholanic Acid.

BILE SALTS. Sodium glycocholate and taurocholate. Note also Bile Extract, Ox and oxidized bile acids.
Lilly—Enseal 5 gr, Bot. 100s.
See: Bilein.
Bisol, Tab. (Paddock).
Ox Bile Extract.
Oxidized Bile Acids.

W/Belladonna, nux vomica compound Bile salts 60 mg, belladonna leaf extract 5 mg, nux vomica extract 2 mg, phenolphthalein 30 mg, sodium salicylate 15 mg, aloin 15 mg/Tab. Bot. 1000s.
Use: Laxative, antispasmodic.

W/Cascara extract, phenolphthalein, capsicum oleoresin.

See: Bilocomp, Tab. (Lannett).
W/Cascara sagrada, phenolphthalein, capsicum oleoresin, peppermint oil.
See: Torocol, Tab. (Plessner).
W/Cellulase, calcium carbonate, pancrelipase.
See: Accelerase, Cap. (Organon).
W/Cellulase, pancrelipase, calcium carbonate, belladonna alkaloids, phenobarbital.
See: Accelerase-PB, Cap. (Organon).
W/Dehydrocholic acid, pancreatic substance.
See: Depancol, Tab. (Parke-Davis).
W/Dehydrocholic acid, pepsin, pancreatin.
See: Progestive, Tab. (NCP).
W/Iron.
See: Bilron, Pulv. (Lilly).
W/Pancreatin, pepsin, dehydrocholic acid, desoxycholic acid.
See: Pepsatal, Tab. (Kenyon).
W/Pancrelipase, cellulase.
See: Cotazym-B, Tab. (Organon).
W/Papain, cascara sagrada extract, phenolphthalein, capsicum oleoresin.
See: Torocol Compound, Tab. (Plessner).
W/Pepsin, homatropine, methylbromide, amylase, lipase, protease.
See: Digesplen, Tab., Elix., Drops (Med. Prod.).
W/Phenolphthalein, chionanthus extract.
See: Bile Anthus Compound, Cap. (Scrip).
W/Sodium salicylate, phenolphthalein, chionanthus extract, bile extract, cascara sagrada extract.
See: Glycols, Tab. (Bowman).

BILE, WHOLE DESICCATED.
W/Pancreatin, mycozyme diastase, pepsin, nux vomica extract.
See: Enzobile, Tab. (Hauck).

BILEZYME. (Geriatric) Amylolytic enzyme 30 mg, proteolytic enzyme 6 mg, dehydrocholic acid 200 mg, desoxycholic acid 50 mg/Tab. Bot. 42s, 100s, 500s.
Use: Digestive aid.

BILI-LABSTIX REAGENT STRIPS. (Ames) Reagent strips. Bot. 100s.
Test for pH, protein, glucose, ketones, bilirubin and blood in urine.
Use: Diagnostic aid.

BILI-LABSTIX SG REAGENT STRIPS. (Ames) Bot. 100s.
Urinalysis reagent strip test for specific gravity, pH, protein, glucose, ketone, bilirubin, and blood.
Use: Diagnostic aid.

BILIRUBIN REAGENT STRIPS. (Ames) Seralyzer reagent strip. Bot. 25s.
Quantitative strip test for total bilirubin in serum or plasma.
Use: Diagnostic aid.

BILIRUBIN TEST.
See: Ictotest.(Ames).

BILIVIST. (Berlex) Ipodate sodium 500 mg/Cap. Bot. 120s.
Use: Radiopaque agent.

BILOCOMP TABLETS. (Lannett) Bile salts 1.5 gr, cascara extract 0.5 gr, phenolphthalein 0.5 gr, oleoresin capsicum 1/20 min/Tab. Bot. 1000s.
Use: Laxative.

BILOGEST. (Mills) Mixed oxidized bile acids 65 mg, desoxycholic acid 60 mg, extract ox bile 40 mg, pepsin 100 mg, pancreatin 100 mg, inositol 40 mg, dimethionine 120 mg, betaine HCl 75 mg, choline bitartrate 100 mg, diazyme 10 mg/Tab. Bot. 100s.
Use: Gallbladder disorders, indigestion, cirrhosis, obesity.

BILOPAQUE. (Winthrop) Tyropanoate sodium 750 mg/Cap. Catchcovers of 4 cap. Box 20s, Bot. 100s, 500s.
Use: Radiopaque agent.

BILORIC. (Arcum) Pepsin 9 mg, ox bile 160 mg/Cap. Bot. 100s, 1000s.
Use: Antispasmodic.

BILRON. (Lilly) Iron bile salts. Pulv. **150 mg/Cap.:** Bot. 100s. **300 mg/Cap.:** Bot. 100s, 500s.
Use: Laxative.

BILSTAN. (Standex) Bile salts 0.5 gr, cascara sagrada powder extract 0.5 gr, phenolphthalein 0.5 gr, aloin 1/8 gr, podophyllin 1/20 gr/Tab. Bot. 100s.
Use: Laxative.

BILTRICIDE. (Miles) Praziquantel 600 mg/Tab. Bot. 6s.
Use: Anthelmintic.

BIMETHOXYCAINE LACTATE. Bis-[b-(o-methoxy-phenyl) isopropyl] amine lactate. Isocaine Lactate.

BINDAZAC. B.A.N. 1-Benzylindazol-3-yloxyacetic acid. Bendazac (I.N.N.).
Use: Anti-inflammatory.

BINEX-C. (Scruggs) B complex formula with C vitamins. Tab. Bot. 100s, 1000s.
Use: Vitamin supplement.

•**BINIRAMYCIN.** USAN.
Use: Antibiotic.

BINTRON TABLETS. (Madland) Liver fraction 4.6 gr, ferrous sulfate 5 gr, vitamins B_1 3 mg, B_2 0.5 mg, B_6 0.15 mg, C 20 mg, calcium pantothenate 0.3 mg, niacinamide 10 mg/Tab. Bot. 100s, 1000s.
Use: Vitamin/mineral supplement.

BIOBRANE. (Winthrop) A temporary skin substitute available in various sizes.
Use: Temporary skin substitute.

BIOCAL 250. (Miles) Calcium 250 mg/Chew. Tab. Bot. 75s.
Use: Calcium supplement.

BIOCAL 500. (Miles) Calcium 500 mg/Tab. Bot. 75s.
Use: Calcium supplement.

BIO-CREST. (Nutrition) Citrus bioflavonoid complex 200 mg, vitamin C 250 mg, rutin 50 mg/Tabseal. Bot. 100s.
Use: Vitamin supplement.

BIOCULT-GC. (Medical Technology Corp.) Swab Test for gonorrhea. For endocervical, urethral, rectal and pharyngeal cultures. Box 1 test per kit.
Use: Diagnostic aid.

BIODINE. (Major) Iodine 1%. Soln. Bot. pt, gal.
Use: Antiseptic, germicide.

BIO-FLAVONOID COMPOUNDS. Vitamins P.}
BIO-FLAVONOID COMPOUND, CITRUS.
W/Vitamins C.
See: C.V.P. Syr., Cap. (USV Pharm).
Mevanin-C, Cap. (Beutlich).
Mevatinic-C, Tab. (Beutlich).
Peridin-C, Tab. (Beutlich).
Pregent, Tab. (Beutlich).

BIOGASTRONE.
See: Carbenoxolone.

•**BIOLOGICAL INDICATOR FOR DRY-HEAT STERILIZATION, PAPER STRIP,** U.S.P. XXII.
Use: Indicator.

•**BIOLOGICAL INDICATOR FOR ETHYLENE OXIDE STERILIZATION, PAPER STRIP,** U.S.P.XXII.
Use: Indicator.

•**BIOLOGICAL INDICATOR FOR STEAM STERILIZATION,** U.S.P. XXII.
Use: Indicator.

BIO-MEDI-PEC. (Medi-Rx) Neomycin sulfate 300 mg, kaolin 6 Gm, pectin 0.13 Gm/fl oz. Bot. pt, gal.
Use: Antidiarrheal.

BIONATE 50-2. (Seatrace) Testosterone cypionate 50 mg, estradiol cypionate 2 mg/ml. Vial 10 ml.
Use: Androgen, estrogen combination.

BIOPAR, FORTE. (Rhone-Poulenc Rorer) Vitamin B_{12} w/intrinsic factor concentrate 0.5 units, cobalamin 25 mcg/Tab. Bot. 30s.
Use: Vitamin B_{12} supplement.

BIORAL.
See: Carbenoxolone.

BIOS I.
See: Inositol.

BIOTEXIN.
See: Novobiocin.

BIOTHESIN. (Pal-Pak). Phosphorated carbohydrate solution cerium oxalate 120 mg, bismuth subnitrate 120 mg, benzocaine 15 mg, aromatics/Tab. 1000s.
Use: Antiemetic/antivertigo combination.

•**BIOTIN,** U.S.P. XXII.
Use: Vitamin.

BIO-TYTRA. (Approved) Neomycin sulfate 2.5 mg, gramicidin 0.25 mg, benzocaine 10 mg/Troche. Box 10s.
Use: Anti-infective.

BIPECTOL TABLETS. (Vale) Opium 1.2 mg, bismuth hydroxide 32.4 mg, kaolin colloidal 162 mg, pectin 32.4 mg/Tab. Bot. 1000s.
Use: Antidiarrheal.

•**BIPENAMOL HYDROCHLORIDE.** USAN.
Use: Antidepressant.

•**BIPERIDEN,** U.S.P. XXII. 1-Piperidinepropanol,α-bicyclo[2.2.1]hept-5-en-2-yl-α-phenyl-α-5-Norbornen-2-yl-α-phenyl-1-piperidinepropanol.
Use: Anticholinergic.

•**BIPERIDEN HYDROCHLORIDE,** U.S.P. XXII. Tab., U.S.P. XXII. 1-Piperidinepropanol, -α-bicyclo[2.2.1]-hept-5-en-2-yl-α-phenyl-, hydrochloride. α-5-Norbornen-2-yl-α-phenyl-1-piperidinepropanol HCl.
Use: Anticholinergic, antiparkinson agent.

•**BIPERIDEN LACTATE INJECTION,** U.S.P. XXII. 1- Piperidinepropanol, α-bicyclo[2.2.1]hept-5-en-2-yl-α-phenol, compound with 2-hydroxypropanoic acid (1:1). α-5-Norbornen-2-yl-α-phenyl-1-piperidine- propanol lactate (salt).
Use: Anticholinergic, antiparkinson agent.

BIPERIDEN HCl and LACTATE. (Alpha-(Bicyclo[2,2,1] hept-5-en-2-yl)-alpha-phenyl-1-piperidine propanol.
Use: Anticholinergic, antiparkinson agent.
See: Akineton, Amp., Tab. (Knoll).

BIPHASIC INSULIN INJECTION. B.A.N. A suspension of bovine and porcine insulin crystals in a solution of insulin buffered at pH 7.
Use: Hypoglycemic agent.

•**BIPHENAMINE HYDROCHLORIDE.** USAN. 2-Diethylaminoethyl-3-phenylsalicylate HCl.
Use: Topical anesthetic, antibacterial, antifungal.

BIPHETAMINE 12.5. (Pennwalt) Dextroamphetamine (as resin complex) 6.25 mg, amphetamine (as resin complex) 6.25 mg/Cap. Bot. 100s.
Use: Diet aid.

BIPHETAMINE 20. (Pennwalt) Dextroamphetamine (as resin complex) 10 mg, amphetamine (as resin complex) 10 mg/Cap. Bot. 100s.
Use: Diet aid.

BIPOLE-S. (Spanner) Testosterone 25 mg, estrone 2 mg/ml. Vial 10 ml.
Use: Androgen, estrogen combination.

BIRTH CONTROL.
See: Oral Contraceptive.

BIS (ACETOXYPHENYL) OXINDOL.
See: Oxyphenisatin.

•**BISACODYL,** U.S.P. XXII. Supp., Tab., U.S.P. XXII. Phenol, 4,4′-(2-pyridinylmethylene) bis-,diacetate (ester). Di-(p-acetoxyphenyl)-2-pyridylmethane. 4-4′-(2-pyridylmethylene) diphenol diacetate (ester).
Use: Cathartic.
See: Bisacodyl Uniserts, Supp. (Upsher-Smith).
Bisco-Lax, Supp. (Raway).
Dacodyl, Tab., Supp. (Major).
Deficol, Tab., Supp. (Vangard).
Delco-Lax, Tab. (Delco).
Dulcolax, Tab., Supp. (Boehringer Ingelheim).

Fleet Bisacodyl, Tab., Supp. (Fleet).
Theralax, Tab., Supp. (Beecham Labs).

BISACODYL TANNEX. USAN. Water-soluble complex of bisacodyl and tannic acid.
Use: Contact laxative.
See: Clysodrast, packet (Barnes-Hind).

BISACODYL UNISERTS. (Upsher-Smith) Bisacodyl. Supp. **5 mg**: 12s. **10 mg**: 12s, 50s, 500s.
Use: Laxative.

BISALATE. (Allison) Sodium salicylate 5 gr, salicylamide 2.5 gr, sodium paraminobenzoate 5 gr, ascorbic acid 50 mg, butabarbital sodium 1/8 gr/Tab. Bot. 100s, 1000s.
Use: Antirheumatic.

BISANTRENE HYDROCHLORIDE. USAN.
Use: Antineoplastic.

BISATIN.
See: Oxyphenisatin.

BISCOLAN SUPPOSITORIES. (Lannett) Bismuth subgallate, benzocaine, resorcin, cod liver oil, lanolin, zinc oxide/Supp. Box 12s.

BISCOLAN HC SUPPOSITORIES. (Lannett) Same as Biscolan Supp. w/hydrocortisone acetate 10 mg/Supp. Box 12s.

BISCO-LAX. (Raway) Bisacodyl 10 mg/Supp. Box of foil UD 4s, 12s, 50s, 100s, 500s, 1000s.
Use: Laxative.

BISHYDROXYCOUMARIN.
See: Dicumarol, U.S.P. XXII.

BISMAPEC TABLETS. (Vale) Bismuth hydroxide 137.7 mg, colloidal kaolin 648 mg, citrus pectin 129.6 mg/Tab. Bot. 1000s.
Use: Antidiarrheal.

BISMU-KINO. (Denver) Bismuth oxycarbonate 10 gr, eucalyptus gum 6 gr, phenyl salicylate, camphor, menthol, carminative oils of nutmeg and clove in soothing, demulcent base w/alcohol 2%/fl oz. Bot. 4 oz, pt.
Use: Stomach and intestinal upset.

BISMUTH ALUMINATE Magnesium trisilicate, aluminum hydroxide, magnesium carbonate coprecipitate.
See: Escot, Cap. (Solvay).

BISMUTH GLYCOLLYLARSANILATE. B.A.N. Bismuthyl N-glycoloylarsanilate. Glycobiarsol(I.N.N.).
Use: Treatment of amebiasis.

BISMUTH GLYCOLYLARSANILATE. Bismuthyl N-glycollylarsanilate.
Use: Antiamebic.
See: Glycobiarsol, N.F. XVII.

BISMUTH HYDROXIDE.
See: Milk of Bismuth, U.S.P. XXII.

BISMUTH, INSOLUBLE PRODUCTS.
See: Bismuth Subgallate (Various Mfr.).
Bismuth Subsalicylate (Various Mfr.).
Bismuth Tribromophenate (N.Y. Quinine).

BISMUTH, MAGMA. Name previously used for Milk of Bismuth.

BISMUTH, MILK OF, N.F. XVII.
Use: Astringent, antacid.

BISMUTH OXYCARBONATE.
See: Bismuth Subcarbonate.

BISMUTH POTASSIUM TARTRATE. Basic bismuth potassium bismuthotartrate.
Brewer—25 mg/ml Amp. 2 ml.
Miller—0.016 Gm/ml Amp. 2 ml, Box 12s, 100s; Bot. 30 ml, 60 ml.
Raymer—2.5% Amp. 2 ml, Box 12s, 100s.
Use: Agent for syphilis.

BISMUTH RESORCIN COMPOUND.
W/Bismuth subgallate, balsam Peru, benzocaine, zinc oxide, boric acid.
See: Bonate, Supp. (Suppositoria).
W/Bismuth subgallate, balsam Peru, zinc oxide, boric acid.
See: Versal, Supp. (Suppositoria).
W/Bismuth subgallate, zinc oxide, boric acid, balsam Peru.
See: Anulan, Supp. (Lannett).

BISMUTH SODIUM TARTRATE.
Use: I.M., syphilis.

BISMUTH SUBBENZOATE.
Use: Dusting powder for wounds.

BISMUTH SUBCARBONATE.
Use: Gastroenteritis, diarrhea.
W/Benzocaine, zinc oxide, boric acid.
See: Aracain Rectal Supp. (Commerce).
W/Calcium carbonate, magnesium carbonate.
See: Dimacid, Tab. (Otis Clapp).
W/Calcium carbonate, magnesium carbonate, aminoacetic acid, dried aluminum hydroxide gel.
See: Buffertabs, Tab. (Forest).
W/Charcoal and ginger.
See: Harv-a-carbs, Tab. (Forest).
W/Hydrocortisone acetate, belladonna extract, ephedrine sulfate, zinc oxide, boric acid, balsam Peru, cocoa butter.
See: Rectacort, Supp. (Century).
W/Kaolin, pectin.
See: K-C, Liq. (Century).
Paregoric, kaolin (colloidal), aluminum hydroxide, pectin.
See: Kapinal, Tab. (Jenkins).
W/Paregoric, phenyl salicylate, zinc phenolsulfonate, pepsin.
See: Bismuth, salol, zincand paregoric. (Bowman).
W/Pectin, kaolin, opium powder.
See: KBP/O, Cap. (Cole).
W/Phenyl salicylate, zinc phenolsulfonate, pepsin.
See: Bismuth, salol, zinc compound (Bowman).
W/Phenyl salicylate, chloroform, eucalyptus gum, camphor.
See: Bismu-Kino, Liq. (Denver Chem.).
W/Ephedrine sulfate, belladonna extract, zinc oxide, boric acid, bismuth oxyiodide, balsam Peru.
See: Wyanoids, Preps. (Wyeth-Ayerst).

BISMUTH SUBGALLATE, U.S.P. XXII, (Various Mfr.) Dermatol.

Use: Topically for skin conditions; orally as an antidiarrheal.
W/Balsam Peru, zinc oxide, cod liver oil.
See: Pile-Gon, Oint. (E.J. Moore).
W/Benzocaine, resorcin, cod liver oil, lanolin, zinc oxide.
See: Biscolan, Supp. (Lannett).
W/Benzocaine, zinc oxide, boric acid, balsam Peru.
See: Anocaine, Supp. (Hauck).
W/Bismuth oxyiodide, bismuth resorcin compound, benzocaine, boric acid.
See: Bonate, Supp. (Suppository).
W/Bismuth resorcin compound, balsam Peru, benzocaine, zinc oxide, boric acid.
See: Bonate, Supp. (Suppository).
W/Bismuth resorcin compound, zinc oxide, boric acid, balsam Peru.
See: Anulan, Supp. (Lannett).
Versal, Supp. (Suppository).
W/Cod liver oil, benzocaine, lanolin, zinc oxide, resorcin, balsam Peru, hydrocortisone.
See: Doctient HC, Supp. (Suppository).
W/Hydrocortisone acetate, bismuth resorcin compound, zinc oxide, balsam Peru, benzyl benzoate.
See: Anusol-HC, Supp. (Parke-Davis).
W/Diethylaminoacet-2,6-xylidide, zinc oxide, aluminum subacetate, balsam Peru.
See: Xylocaine Suppositories (Astra).
W/Kaolin, colloidal.
See: Diastop, Liq. (Elder).
W/Kaolin colloidal, calcium carbonate, magnesium trisilicate, papain, atropine sulphate.
See: Kaocasil, Tab. (Jenkins).
W/Kaolin, opium, zinc phenolsulfonate, pectin.
See: Cholactabs, Tab. (Roxane).
W/Kaolin, pectin, zinc phenolsulfonate, opium powder.
See: Diastay, Tab. (Elder).
W/Opium powder, pectin, kaolin, zinc phenolsulfonate.
See: Bismuth, Pectin, Paregoric (Lemmon).
W/Zinc oxide, bismuth resorcin compound, balsam Peru, benzyl benzoate.
See: Anugesic, Supp., Oint. (Parke-Davis).
Anusol, Supp., Oint. (Parke-Davis).
BISMUTH SUBIODIDE.
See: Bismuth oxyiodide.
•**BISMUTH SUBNITRATE,** U.S.P. XXII.
Use: Gastroenteritis, amebic dysentery, locally for wounds.
W/Calcium carbonate, magnesium carbonate.
See: Antacid No. 2, Tab. (Bowman).
Maygel, Tab. (Century).
W/Sodium bicarbonate, magnesium carbonate, diastase, papain.
Panacarb, Tab. (Lannett).

BISMUTH SUBSALICYLATE. Basic bismuth salicylate.
Use: Agent for syphilis.
W/Calcium carbonate, glycocoll.
See: Pepto-Bismol, Tab. (Norwich).
W/Pectin, salol, kaolin, zinc sulfocarbolate, aluminum hydroxide.
See: Wescola Antidiarrheal-Stomach Upset (Western Research).
W/Phenylsalicylate, zinc phenolsulfonate, methylcellulose, magnesium aluminum silicate.
See: Pepto-Bismol, Liq. (Norwich).
BISMUTH TANNATE. (Various Mfr.) Tanbismuth.
Use: Astringent and protective in G.I. disorders.
BISMUTH TRIBROMOPHENATE.
Use: Intestinal antiseptic.
BISMUTH VIOLET. (Table Rock) Bismuth Violet. **Oint.** 1%. Jar oz, lb. **Soln.** 0.5%. Bot. 0.5 oz, 6 oz, pt, gal. **Tr.** 0.5%. Bot. 6 oz, pt, also 1% w/ benzoic and salicylic acid. Bot. 0.5 oz, 6 oz, pt.
Use: Antibacterial, antifungal.
BISMUTH, WATER-SOLUBLE PRODUCTS.
See: Bismuth Potassium Tartrate (Various Mfr.).
•**BISOBRIN LACTATE.** USAN. Meso-1,1′-tetramethlenebis[1,2,3,4-tetrahydro-6,7-dimethoxyisoquinoline]dilactate.
Use: Fibrinolytic.
BISODOL POWDER. (Whitehall) Sodium bicarbonate 644 mg, magnesium carbonate 475 mg/5 ml. Bot. 3 oz, 5 oz.
Use: Antacid.
BISODOL TABLETS. (Whitehall) Calcium carbonate 194 mg, magnesium hydroxide 178 mg/Chew. tab. Bot. 30s, 100s.
Use: Antacid.
•**BISOPROLOL.** USAN.
Use: Antihypertensive.
•**BISOPROLOL FUMARATE.** USAN.
Use: Antihypertensive.
BISOXATIN. B.A.N. 2,3-Dihydro-2,2-di(4-hydroxyphenyl)-1,4-benzoxazin-3-one.
Use: Laxative.
•**BISOXATIN ACETATE.** USAN.
Use: Cathartic.
•**BISPYRITHIONE MAGSULFEX.** USAN.
Use: Antibacterial, antidandruff.
BISQUADINE. (Sterwin) Alexidine.
BIS-TROPAMIDE. Tropicamide.
See: Mydriacyl, Soln. (Alcon).
BITE & ITCH LOTION. (Weeks & Leo) Pramoxine HCl 1%, pyrilamine maleate 2%, pheniramine maleate 0.2%, chlorpheniramine maleate 0.2%. Bot. 4 oz.
Use: Minor skin irritations.
BITHIONOL. 2,2′-Thiobis(4,6-dichlorophenol) B.A.N.
Use: Local anti-infective.
See: Actamer (Monsanto Chem.).
W/Allantoin, salicylic acid.
See: Domerine, Shampoo (Miles).
Bitin (No Mfr. currently listed).

Lorothidol (No Mfr. currently listed).
W/Resorcinol monoacetate, sulfur.
See: Acne-Dome, Preps. (Miles).

•**BITHIONOLATE SODIUM.** USAN. Disodium 2,2′-thiobis-(4,6-dichlorophenoxide).
Use: Topical anti-infective.

•**BITOLTEROL MESYLATE.** USAN.
Use: Bronchodilator.

BITRATE. (Arco) Phenobarbital 15 mg, pentaerythritol tetranitrate 20 mg/Tab. Bot. 100s.
Use: Sedative/hypnotic, antianginal.

B-JECT-100.(Hyrex) Vitamins B_1, 100 mg B_2, 2 mg, B_3 100 mg, B_5 2 mg, B_6 2 mg/ml. Inj. Vial 10 ml, 30 ml.
Use: Vitamin B supplement.

BLACK AND WHITE BLEACHING CREAM. (Schering-Plough) Hydroquinone 2%. 0.75 oz, Tube 1.5 oz.
Use: Skin bleaching agent.

BLACK AND WHITE OINTMENT. (Schering-Plough) Resorcinol 3%. Tube 0.62 oz, 2.25 oz.
Use: Antiseptic, antipruritic.

BLACK DRAUGHT. (Chattem) Powdered senna extract. **Tab.:** 600 mg. Bot. 30s. **Gran.:** 1.65 Gm/½ tsp. Jar 22.5 Gm.
Use: Laxative.

BLACK DRAUGHT SYRUP. (Chattem) Casanthranol 90 mg w/senna, rhubarb, anise, methyl salicylate, ginger, peppermint oil, spearmint oil, menthol, alcohol 5%, tartrazine/Tbsp. Bot. 2 oz, 5 oz.
Use: Laxative.

BLACK WIDOW SPIDER, ANTIVENIN.
See: Antivenin (Lactrodectus mactens), Inj. (MSD).

BLAIREX STERILE SALINE SOLUTION. (Blairex) Normal saline 0.9%. Aerosol can 90 ml, 240 ml, 360 ml.
Use: Soft contact lens care.

BLAIREX SYSTEM. (Blairex Labs) Sodium Cl 135 mg/Tab. 200s, 365s w/15 ml bot.
Use: Soft contact lens care.

BLAIREX SYSTEM II. (Blairex Labs) Sodium Cl 250 mg/Tab. 90s, 180s w/27.7 ml bot.
Use: Soft contact lens care.

BLAUD STRUBEL. (Strubel) Ferrous sulfate 5 gr/Cap. Bot. 100s.
Use: Iron supplement.

BLEFCON. (Madland) Sodium sulfacetamide 30%. Oint. Tube ⅛ oz.
Use: Ophthalmic preparation.

BLENOXANE. (Bristol-Myers/Mead Johnson Oncology) Bleomycin sulfate 15 units/Vial. 1s, 10s.
Use: Antineoplastic agent.

BLEOMYCIN SULFATE, STERILE, U.S.P. XXII. Antibiotic obtained from cultures of *Streptomyces verticillus.*}
Use: Antineoplastic.
See: Blenoxane, Inj. (Bristol).

BLEPH-10 LIQUIFILM. (Allergan) Sulfacetamide sodium 10%, polyvinyl alcohol 1.4%, thimerosal 0.005%, polysorbate 80, sodium thiosulfate, EDTA, purified water. Plastic dropper bot. 2.5 ml, 5 ml, 15 ml.
Use: Anti-infective, ophthalmic.

BLEPH-10 S.O.P. STERILE OPHTHALMIC OINTMENT. (Allergan) Sulfacetamide sodium 10%, phenylmercuric acetate 0.0008%, white petrolatum, mineral oil, nonionic lanolin derivatives. Tube 3.5 Gm.
Use: Anti-infective, ophthalmic.

BLEPHAMIDE LIQUIFILM. (Allergan) Sulfacetamide sodium 10%, prednisolone acetate 0.2%, polyvinyl alcohol 1.4%, EDTA, polysorbate 80, sodium thiosulfate, benzalkonium Cl. Dropper bot. 2.5 ml, 5 ml, 10 ml.
Use: Anti-inflammatory, anti-infective, ophthalmic.

BLEPHAMIDE S.O.P. STERILE OPHTHALMIC OINTMENT. (Allergan) Prednisolone acetate 0.2%, sulfacetamide sodium 10%, phenylmercuric acetate 0.0008%, mineral oil, white petrolatum, nonionic lanolin derivatives. Tube 3.5 Gm.
Use: Anti-inflammatory, anti-infective, ophthalmic.

BLINK-N-CLEAN. (Allergan) Polyoxyl 40 stearate, polyethylene glycol 300, chlorobutanol 0.5%. Bot. 7.5 ml, 15 ml, UD 1 ml.
Use: Hard contact lens care.

BLINX. (Barnes-Hind) Sterile, isotonic, alkaline borate buffer, boric acid, sodium borate, phenylmercuric acetate 0.004%. Bot. 1 oz, 4 oz.
Use: Ophthalmic preparation.

BLIS. (Commerce) Boric acid 47.5%, salicylic acid 17%. Bot. 7 oz.
Use: Foot preparation.

BLISTEX. (Blistex) Camphor 0.5%, phenol 0.5%, allantoin 1% in a lanolin and mineral oil base. Oint. Tube 4.2 Gm, 10.5 Gm.
Use: Lip balm.

BLISTIK. (Blistex) Padimate O 6.6%, oxybenzone 2.5%, dimethicone 2%. Lip balm stick 4.5 Gm.
Use: Lip protectant.

BLIS-TO-SOL. (Chattem) **Liq.:** Salicylic acid, undecylenic acid. Bot. 1 oz, 2 oz. **Pow.:** Benzoic acid, salicylic acid. Bot. 2 oz.
Use: Antifungal, external.

BLM.
See: Bleomycin sulfate.

BLOCADREN. (MSD) Timolol maleate 5 mg, 10 mg or 20 mg/Tab. **5 mg:** Bot. 100s; **10 mg:** Bot. 100s, UD 100s; **20 mg:** Bot. 100s.
Use: Beta-adrenergic blocking agent.

BLOCK OUT BY SEA & SKI. (Carter) Padimate O, octyl methoxycinnamate, oxybenzone. Cream. Tube 120 Gm.
Use: Sunscreen.

BLOCK OUT CLEAR BY SEA & SKI. (Carter) Padimate O, octyl methoxycinnamate, octyl salicylate, SD alcohol 40. Lot. Bot. 120 ml.
Use: Sunscreen.

BLOOD, ANTICOAGULANTS.
See: Anticoagulants.

•**BLOOD CELLS, RED.** U.S.P. XXII.
Use: Blood replenisher.
BLOOD COAGULATION.
See: Hemostatics.
BLOOD FRACTIONS.
See: Albumin (Human) Salt-Poor (Armour; Hyland).
BLOOD GLUCOSE CONCENTRATOR.
See: Glucagon (Lilly).
BLOOD GLUCOSE TEST.
See: Chemstrip bG Strips. (Boehringer Mannheim).
Dextrostix Reagent Strips. (Ames).
Glucostix Strips. (Ames).
Visidex II Reagent Strips. (Ames).
•**BLOOD GROUPING SERUMS.** U.S.P. XXII. Anti-Rh. (Anti-D) 85%-Tubes, 10 tests; Vial, with pipette, 5 ml Anti-Rh. (Anti C plus D) 17%-Tube, 10 tests; Vial, with pipette, 5 ml.
Use: Diagnostic aid in the determination of Rh. (D) and Rh. (C plus D) factors in red blood cells.
•**BLOOD GROUPING SERUM, ANTI-A.** U.S.P. XXII.
Use: Diagnostic aid (in vitro, blood).
•**BLOOD GROUPING SERUM, ANTI-B,** U.S.P. XXII.
Use: Diagnostic aid (in vitro, blood).
•**BLOOD GROUP SPECIFIC SUBSTANCES A, B AND AB,** U.S.P. XXII.
Use: Blood neutralizer (isoagglutinins, group O blood).
BLOOD PLASMA.
See: Normal Human Plasma.
BLOOD PLASMA SUBSTITUTES.
See: Dextran (Cutter; Pharmachem).
BLOOD UREA NITROGEN TEST.
See: Azostix Strips. (Ames).
BLOOD VOLUME DETERMINATION.
See: Evans Blue, dye (City Chem).
•**BLOOD, WHOLE HUMAN,** U.S.P. XXII.
Use: Blood replenisher.
BLU-6. (Bluco) Pyridoxine HCl 100 mg/ml. Vial 30 ml.
Use: Vitamin B supplement.
BLU-12 100. (Bluco) Cyanocobalamin 100 mcg/ml. Vial 30 ml.
Use: Vitamin B supplement.
BLU-12 1000. (Bluco) Cyanocobalamin 1000 mcg/ml. Vial 30 ml.
Use: Vitamin B supplement.
BLUBORO POWDER. (Herbert) Aluminum sulfate 53.9%, calcium acetate 43% w/boric acid, FD&C Blue 1. Packet 1.9 Gm. Box 12s.
Use: Astringent.
BLUDEX. (Burlington) Methenamine 40.8 mg, methylene blue 5.4 mg, phenyl salicylate 18.1 mg, atropine sulfate 0.03 mg, hyoscyamine 0.03 mg, benzoic acid 4.5 mg/Tab. Bot. 100s, 1000s.
Use: Urinary antiseptic, antispasmodic.
BLUE. (Various Mfr.) Pyrethrins 0.3%, piperonyl butoxide 3%, petroleum distillate 1.2%. Gel Bot. 30 Gm, 480 Gm.
Use: Pediculicide.
BLUE STAR OINTMENT. (McCue Labs.) Salicylic acid, benzoic acid, methyl salicylate, camphor, lanolin, petrolatum. Jar 2 oz.
Use: Minor skin irritations, ringworm, corn or callus removal.
BLUTENE CHLORIDE. Tolonium chloride, Toluidine blue O chloride, 3-amino-7-dimethylamino-2-methyl-phenazathonium salt.
B-MAJOR. (Barth's) Vitamins B_1 7 mg, B_2 14 mg, niacin 2.35 mg, B_{12} 7.5 mcg, B_6 0.15 mg, pantothenic acid 0.37 mg, choline 85 mg, inositol 6 mg, biotin, folic acid, aminobenzoic acid/Cap. Bot. 1s, 3s, 6s, 12s.
Use: Vitamin/mineral supplement.
B.M.E. (Brothers) Aminophylline 32 mg, ephedrine sulfate 8 mg, phenobarbital 8 mg, chlorpheniramine maleate 2 mg, alcohol 15%/5 ml. Bot. pt.
Use: Bronchodilator, decongestant, sedative/hypnotic, antihistamine.
B-N. (Eric, Kirk & Gary). Bacitracin 500 units, neomycin sulfate 5 mg. Oint. Tube 0.5 oz.
Use: Anti-infective, external.
B-NUTRON TABLETS. (Nion) Vitamins B_1 2 mg, niacinamide 18 mg, B_2 3 mg, B_6 2.2 mg, cyanocobalamin 3 mcg, folic acid 0.4 mg, iron 6 mg, pantothenic acid 3.3 mg, B complex as provided by 150 mg Brewer's yeast/Tab. Bot. 100s, 500s.
Use: Vitamin/mineral supplement.
B and O SUPPRETTES NO. 15A & NO. 16A. (Webcon) Opium 30 mg or 60 mg, belladonna extract 15 mg/Supp. Jar 12s.
Use: Narcotic analgesic, antispasmodic.
BOBID. (Boyd) Phenylpropanolamine HCl 50 mg, chlorpheniramine maleate 8 mg, methscopolamine bromide 2.5 mg/Cap. Bot. 100s.
Use: Decongestant, antihistamine, anticholinergic.
BO-CAL. (Fibertone) Calcium^{++} 250 mg, magnesium^{++} 125 mg, vitamin D_3 100 IU, boron 0.75 mg/tab. Bot. 120s.
Use: Vitamin/mineral supplement.
BOILAID. (E.J. Moore) Benzocaine, tetracaine, ichthammol, resin cerate, thymol iodide. Jar oz.
Use: Anesthetic drawing salve.
BOIL-EASE ANESTHETIC DRAWING SALVE. (Commerce) Benzocaine 0.5%, ichthammol 1.86%, sulfur 0.44%, camphor 1.6%, juniper tar 0.11%, phenol 0.42%. Tube oz.
Use: Anesthetic drawing salve.
BOILnSOAK. (Alcon) Sodium Cl 0.7%, boric acid, sodium borate, thimerosal 0.001%, disodium edetate 0.1%. Bot. 8 oz, 12 oz.
Use: Soft contact lens care.
•**BOLANDIOL DIPROPIONATE.** USAN.
Use: Anabolic.
•**BOLASTERONE.** USAN.

Use: Anabolic.

BOLAX. (Boyd) Docusate sodium 240 mg, phenolphthalein 30 mg, dihydrocholic acid ¾ gr/Cap. Bot. 100s.
Use: Laxative.

BOLDENONE. B.A.N. 17β-Hydroxyandrosta-1,4-dien-3-one.
Use: Anabolic steroid.

•**BOLDENONE UNDECYLENATE.** USAN. 17β Hydroxyandrosta-1,4-dien-3-one 10 undecenoate. Parenabol. Under study.
Use: Anabolic.

•**BOLENOL.** USAN. 19-Nor-17-α-pregn-5-en-17-ol. 17α-ethyl-5-estren-17-ol. Under study.
Use: Anabolic.

•**BOLMANTALATE.** USAN. 17β-Hydroxyestr-4-en-3-one adamantane-1-carboxylate.
Use: Anabolic steroid.

BONACAL PLUS TABLETS. (Kenwood) Vitamins A 5000 IU, D 400 IU, C 100 mg, B_1 3 mg, B_2 3 mg, B_6 10 mg, B_{12} 4 mcg, niacinamide 20 mg, d-calcium pantothenate 3.3 mg, iron 42 mg, calcium 350 mg, manganese 0.33 mg, zinc 0.1 mg, magnesium 1.67 mg, potassium 1.67 mg/Tab. Bot. 100s.
Use: Vitamin/mineral supplement.

BONAL ITCH CREAM. (E.J. Moore) Benzocaine, dibucaine, tetracaine in water-washable base. Tube oz.
Use: Local anesthetic.

BONATE. (Suppositoria) Bismuth subgallate, balsam Peru, benzocaine, zinc oxide/Supp. Box 12s, 100s, 1000s.
Use: Anorectal preparation.

BONINE. (Pfipharmecs) Meclizine HCl 25 mg/Chew. tab. Pkg. 8s, 48s.
Use: Antiemetic/antivertigo.

BONTRIL PDM. (Carnrick) Phendimetrazine tartrate 35 mg/3 layer Tab. Bot. 100s, 1000s.
Use: Anorexiant.

BONTRIL SLOW RELEASE CAPSULES. (Carnrick) Phendimetrazine tartrate 105 mg/Cap. Bot. 100s.
Use: Anorexiant.

BOPEN-VK. (Boyd) Potassium phenoxymethyl penicillin 400,000 units/Tab. Bot. 100s.
Use: Antibacterial; penicillin.

BORAX. Sodium Borate, N.F. XVII.

•**BORIC ACID,** N.F. XVII. Cryst. or Pow.
Use: Mild antiseptic.
See: Borofax, Oint. (Burroughs Wellcome).
W/Combinations.
See: Saratoga Ointment (Blair).

BORIC ACID OINTMENT. (Various Mfr.) Topical ointment 5% or 10%. Tube, Jar 30 Gm, 52.5 Gm, 60 Gm, 120 Gm, 454 Gm. Ophth. oint. 0.5% or 10%. Tube, Jar. 3.5 Gm, 3.75 Gm, 30 Gm, 60 Gm, 480 Gm.
Use: Minor skin irritations.

2-BORNANONE. Camphor, U.S.P. XXII.

BORNAPRINE. B.A.N. 3-Diethylaminopropyl 2-phenylbicyclo[2.2.1]-heptane-2-carboxylate.
Use: Spasmolytic.
See: Sormodren.

•**BORNELONE.** USAN.
Use: Ultraviolet screen.

•**BOROCAPTATE SODIUM B10.** USAN.
Use: Antineoplastic.

BOROFAIR. (Pharmafair) Acetic acid 2% in aluminum acetate soln. Bot. 60 ml.
Use: Otic preparation.

BOROFAX OINTMENT. (Burroughs Wellcome) Boric acid 5%. Tube 1.75 oz.
Use: Minor skin irritations.

BOROGLYCERIN. Glycerol borate. (Emerson) Bot. pt.

BOROGLYCERIN GLYCERITE. Boric acid 31 parts, glycerin 96 parts.
Use: Agent for dermatitis.

BOROTANNIC COMPLEX. Boric acid 31 mg, tannic acid 50 mg.
W/salicylic acid, ethyl alcohol.
See: Onycho-Phytex, Liq. (Unimed).

BOSTON CLEANER. (Polymer Tech) Anionic sulfate surfactant with friction-enhancing agents, sodium Cl. Soln. Bot. 30 ml.
Use: Hard contact lens care.

BOSTON RECONDITIONING DROPS. (Polymer Tech) Hydrophilic polyelectrolyte, polyvinyl alcohol, hydroxyethylcellulose, chlorhexidine gluconate, EDTA. Soln. Bot. 120 ml.
Use: Contact lens care.

BOTULINUM TOXIN TYPE A.
Use: Treatment of strabismus and blepharospasm.
See: Occulinum (Allergan).

•**BOTULISM ANTITOXIN,** U.S.P. XXII.
Use: Prophylaxis and treatment of the toxins of C. botulinum, Types A or B; passive immunizing agent.

BOUNTY BEARS. (Nature's Bounty) Vitamins A 2500 IU, D 400 IU, E 15 IU, C 60 mg, B_1 1.05 mg, B_2 1.2 mg, B_3 13.5 mg, B_6 1.05 mg, B_{12} 4.5 mcg, folic acid 0.3 mg/Tab. Bot. 100s.
Use: Vitamin/mineral supplement.

BOUNTY BEARS PLUS IRON. (Nature's Bounty) Vitamins A 2500 IU, D 400 IU, E 15 IU, C 60 mg, B_1 1.05 mg, B_2 1.2 mg, B_3 13.5 mg, B_6 1.05 mg, B_{12} 4.5 mcg, folic acid 0.3 mg, iron 15 mg/Tab. Bot. 100s.
Use: Vitamin/mineral supplement.

BOURBONAL.
See: Ethyl Vanillin, N.F. XVII.

BOWMAN COLD TABS. (Bowman) Acetaminophen 324 mg, phenylpropanolamine HCl 24.3 mg, caffeine 16.2 mg/Tab. Bot. 1000s, 5000s.
Use: Analgesic, decongestant.

BOWMAN'S POISON ANTIDOTE KIT. (Bowman) Syrup of ipecac 1 oz, 1 bottle; activated charcoal liquid 2 oz, 3 bottles.
Use: Antidote.

BOWSTERAL. (Bowman) Isopropanol 60%. Bot. pt, gal.

Use: Anti-rust disinfectant for surgical instruments.

•**BOXIDINE.** USAN. 1-[2-[[4′-(Trifluoromethyl)-4-biphenylyl]-oxy]ethyl]pyrrolidine.
Use: Adrenal steroid blocker.

BOYLEX. (Approved) Diperodon, hexachlorophene, rosin cerate, ichthammol, carbolic acid, thymol, camphor, juniper tar. Tube oz.
Use: Drawing salve.

BOYOL. (Pfeiffer) Ichthammol 10%, benzocaine, lanolin and petrolatum base. Salve Tube 30 Gm.
Use: Antiseptic, local anesthetic.

B-PAP. (Wren) Acetaminophen 120 mg, sodium butabarbital 15 mg/5 ml. Bot. pt, gal.
Use: Analgesic, sedative.

B-PAS.
See: Calcium Benzoylpas.

B-PLEX. (Goldline) Vitamins B_1 15 mg, B_2 15 mg, B_3 100 mg, B_5 18 mg, B_6 4 mg, B_{12} 5 mcg, C 500 mg, folic acid 0.5 mg/Tab. Bot. 100s.
Use: Vitamin/mineral supplement.

B-PLEX 100, INJECTABLE. (Jenkins) Vitamins B_1 100 mg, B_2 2 mg, B_6 2 mg, panthenol 10 mg, niacinamide 125 mg, ethanolamide of gentisic acid 2.5%/ml. Vial 30 ml.
Use: Vitamin/mineral supplement.

B-PLEX 100 W/B_{12}. (Jenkins) Vitamins B_1 100 mg, B_2 2 mg, B_6 5 mg, niacinamide 125 mg, panthenol 10 mg, B_{12} 30 mcg, ethanolamide of gentisic acid 2.5%/ml. Vial 30 ml, 12s.
Use: Vitamin/mineral supplement.

B-P-M CREAM. (Durel) Burow's solution 5%, phenol 0.5%, menthol 0.5%, camphor 1% in Duromantel cream. Jar oz, 1 lb, 6 lb.
Use: Agent for eczema.

BP-PAPAVERINE. (Burlington) Papaverine HCl 150 mg/S.R. Cap. Bot. 50s.
Use: Vasodilator.

BQ COLD TABLETS. (Bristol-Myers) Acetaminophen 325 mg, phenylpropanolamine HCl 12.5 mg, chlorpheniramine maleate 2 mg/Tab. Card 16s, Bot. 16s, 30s, 50s.
Use: Analgesic, decongestant, antihistamine.

B.Q.R. (Calotabs) Fluid extract Cascara sagrada aromatic, sodium salicylate, syrup of ipecac, menthol, balsam Peru in elixir, lactated pepsin base, alcohol 8.5%. Bot. 2 fl oz.
Use: Cold discomforts.

BRACE. (Norcliff Thayer) Denture adhesive. Tube 1.4 oz, 2.4 oz.

BRADOSOL BROMIDE. (Ciba) Domiphen bromide.

BRANCHAMIN 4%. (Travenol) Isoleucine 1.38 Gm, leucine 1.38 Gm, valine 1.25 Gm, phosphate 31.6 mOsm/100 ml. Bot. 500 ml.
Use: Adjunct to regular TPN therapy for highly stressed or traumatized patients.

BRASIVOL FINE, MEDIUM AND ROUGH. (Stiefel) Aluminum oxide scrub particles in a surfactant cleansing base. **Fine:** Jar 5.1 oz. **Medium:** Jar 6 oz. **Rough:** Jar 6.5 oz.
Use: Scrub cleanser.

BRASIVOL BASE. (Stiefel) Cleansing paste containing polyoxyethylene lauryl ether and a surfactant cleanser. Jar 4.1 oz.
Use: Degreasing skin cleanser.

BREACOL DECONGESTANT COUGH MEDICATION. (Glenbrook) Dextromethorphan HBr 10 mg, phenylpropanolamine HCl 37.5 mg, alcohol 10%, chlorpheniramine maleate 4 mg/5 ml. Bot. 3 oz, 6 oz.
Use: Antitussive, decongestant, antihistamine.

BREATHEASY. (Pascal) Racemic epinephrine HCl soln. 2.2% inhaled by use of nebulizer. Bot. 0.25 oz, 0.5 oz, 1 oz.
Use: Bronchodilator.

BREEZEE MIST. (Pedinol) Aluminum chlorhydrate, undecylenic acid, menthol. Aerosol Bot. 4 oz.
Use: Antifungal, deodorant, antiperspirant, foot powder.

BREONESIN. (Winthrop-Breon) Guaifenesin 200 mg/Cap. Bot. 100s.
Use: Expectorant.

•**BREQUINAR SODIUM.** USAN.
Use: Antineoplastic.

•**BRETAZENIL.** USAN
Use: Antianxiety agent.

BRETHAIRE. (Geigy) Terbutaline sulfate inhaler 7.5 ml. (10.5 Gm) w/mouthpiece.
Use: Bronchodilator.

BRETHANCER. (Geigy) Inhaler (complete unit to be used with Brethaire).

BRETHINE. (Geigy) Terbutaline sulfate. **Tab.:** 2.5 mg. Bot. 100s, 1000s, UD 100s, Gy-Pak 90s, 100s. 5 mg. Bot. 100s, 1000s, UD 100s, Gy-Pak 90s, 100s. **Amp.:** 1 mg/ml. Box 10s, 100s.
Use: Bronchodilator.

•**BRETYLIUM TOSYLATE.** USAN. 2-Bromobenzyl-ethyldimethylammonium toluene-p-sulfonate.
Use: Hypotensive.
See: Bretylol, Inj. (American Critical Care).

BRETYLOL. (American Critical Care) Bretylium tosylate 50 mg/ml. Amp. 10 ml.
Use: Antiarrhythmic agent.

BREVIBLOC. (DuPont) Esmolol HCl 10 mg/ml or 250 mg/ml, propylene glycol 25%. **10 mg/ml:** Vial 10 ml. **250 mg/ml:** Amp 10 ml.
Use: Beta-adrenergic blocking agent.

BREVICON. (Syntex) Norethindrone 0.5 mg, ethinyl estradiol 0.035 mg/Tab. 21 and 28 day (7 inert tabs) Wallette.
Use: Oral contraceptive.

BREVITAL SODIUM. (Lilly) Methohexital sodium. **Vial:** 500 mg/50 ml, 500 mg/50 ml w/diluent, 2.5 Gm/250 ml, 5 Gm/500 ml. **Amp.:** 2.5 Gm, 5 Gm.
Use: General anesthetic.

BREWER'S YEAST. (Various Mfr.) Pow., Tab. 6 gr, 7.5 gr, 1 lb.
W/Docusate sodium.
See: Doss or Super Doss, Tab., Cap. (Ferndale).

W/Psyllium seed, plantago ovata, karaya gum.
See: Plantamucin Granulo, (Elder).

BREXIN EX LIQUID. (Savage) Pseudoephedrine HCl 30 mg, guaifenesin 200 mg/5 ml.
Use: Decongestant, expectorant.

BREXIN EX TABLET. (Savage) Pseudoephedrine HCl 60 mg, guaifenesin 400 mg/Tab. Bot. 100s.
Use: Decongestant, expectorant.

BREXIN L.A. (Savage) Chlorpheniramine maleate 8 mg, pseudoephedrine HCl 120 mg/L.A. Tab. Bot. 100s.
Use: Antihistamine, decongestant.

BRICANYL INJECTION. (Lakeside) Terbutaline sulfate 1 mg/Amp. 1 ml. 10s.
Use: Bronchodilator.

BRICANYL TABLETS. (Lakeside) Terbutaline sulfate 2.5 mg or 5 mg/Tab. Bot. 100s, 1000s, UD 100s.
Use: Bronchodilator.

•**BRIFENTANIL HYDROCHLORIDE.** USAN.
Use: Analgesic.

BRIGEN-G. (Grafton) Chlordiazepoxide 5 mg, 10 mg or 25 mg/Tab. Bot. 500s.
Use: Antianxiety agent.

BRIJ 96 and 97. (ICI Americas) Polyoxyl 10 oleyl ether available as 96 and 97.
Use: Surface-active agent.

BRIJ-721. (ICI Americas) Polyoxyethylene 21 stearyl ether (100% active).
Use: Surface-active agent.

BRINOLASE. USAN. Fibrinolytic enzyme produced by *Aspergillus oryzae.*}
Use: Fibrinolytic.

BRIREL W/SUPERINONE. (Winthrop) Hexahydropyrazine, hexahydrate.
Use: Anthelmintic.

BRISTOJECT. (Bristol) Prefilled disposable syringes w/needle.
- Aminophylline:250 mg/10 ml.
- Atropine Sulfate:5 mg/5 ml or 1 mg/ml. 10s.
- Calcium Cl:10%. 10 ml. 10s.
- Dexamethasone:20 mg/5 ml.
- Dextrose:50%. 50 ml. 10s.
- Diphenhydramine:50 mg/5 ml.
- Dopamine HCl:200 mg/5 ml, 400 mg/10 ml.
- Ephedrine:50 mg/10 ml.
- Epinephrine:1:10,000. 10 ml. 10s.
- Lidocaine HCl.:1%: 5 ml, 10 ml; 2%: 5 ml; 4%: 25 ml, 50 ml; 20%: 5 ml, 10 ml.
- Magnesium Sulfate:5 Gm/10 ml. 10s.
- Metaraminol:1%. 10 ml.
- Sodium Bicarbonate:7.5%: 50 ml; 8.4%: 50 ml. 10s.

BRITISH ANTI-LEWISITE. Dimercaprol.
See: BAL.

BROBELLA-P.B. (Brothers) Atropine sulfate 0.0195 mg, hyoscine HBr 0.0065 mg, hyoscyamine sulfate 0.1040 mg, phenobarbital 0.25 gr/Tab. Bot. 100s, 1000s.
Use: Anticholinergic/antispasmodic, sedative/hypnotic.

BROCILLIN. (Brothers) Potassium penicillin G 400,000 units/Tab. or 5 ml. Bot. 100s. Bot. 80 ml.
Use: Antibacterial; penicillin.

•**BROCRESINE.** USAN. 0-(4-Bromo-3-hydroxybenzyl)hydroxylamine. Alpha(amino-oxy)-6-bromo-m-cresol.
Use: Histidine decarboxylase inhibitor.
See: Contramine phosphate.

•**BROCRINAT.** USAN.
Use: Diuretic.

BROCYCLINE. (Brothers) Tetracycline HCl 250 mg/Cap. Bot. 100s, 1000s.
Use: Antibacterial; tetracycline.

BROFEZIL. B.A.N. 2-(4-p-Bromophenylthiazol-2-yl)propionic acid.
Use: Anti-inflammatory.

•**BROFOXINE.** USAN.
Use: Antipsychotic.

BROLADE. (Brothers) Chlorpheniramine maleate 8 mg, phenylephrine HCl 20 mg, methscopolamine nitrate 2.5 mg/Cap. Bot. 50s, 500s.
Use: Antihistamine, decongestant, anticholinergic.

BROMACRYLIDE. N-(acrylamidomethyl)-3-bromopropionamide.

•**BROMADOLINE MALEATE.** USAN.
Use: Analgesic.

BROMALEATE. A mixture of 2-amino-2-methyl-1-propanol and 8-bromotheophylline.
See: Pamabrom.

BROMALIX. (Century) Bromphenramine maleate 4 mg, phenylephrine HCl 5 mg, phenylpropanolamine HCl 5 mg, alcohol 2.3%/5 ml. Bot. 4 oz, pt, gal.
Use: Antihistamine, decongestant.

BROMANATE DC COUGH SYRUP. (Various Mfr.) Phenylpropanolamine HCl 12.5 mg, brompheniramine maleate 2 mg, codeine phosphate 10 mg, alcohol 0.95%. Syr. Bot. 120 ml, pt, gal.
Use: Decongestant, antihistamine, antitussive.

BROMANYL. (Various Mfr.) Bromodiphenhydramine HCl 12.5 mg, codeine phosphate 10 mg, alcohol 5%. Syr. Bot. pt, gal.
Use: Antihistamine, antitussive.

BROMATANE D.C. COUGH SYRUP. (Goldline) Brompheniramine maleate, phenylpropanolamine HCl, codeine phosphate. Bot. gal.
Use: Antihistamine, decongestant, antitussive.

BROMATAPP ELIXIR. (Goldline) Brompheniramine maleate 2 mg, phenylephrine HCl 12.5 mg, alcohol 2.3%/5 ml. Bot. 4 oz, 8 oz, pt, gal.
Use: Antihistamine, decongestant.

BROMATAPP TABLETS. (Goldline) Brompheniramine maleate 12 mg, phenylpropanolamine HCl 75 mg/Tab. Bot. 100s, 1000s.
Use: Antihistamine, decongestant.

BROMAURIC ACID. Hydrogen tetrabromoaurate.

•**BROMAZEPAM.** USAN. 7-Bromo-1,3-dihydro-5-(2-Pyridyl)-2H-1,4-benzodiazepin-2-one.
Use: Antianxiety agent.

BROMAZINE.
See: Ambodryl HCl, Elix., Kapseal (Parke-Davis).

BROMBAY ELIXIR. (PBI) Brompheniramine maleate 2 mg/5 ml, alcohol 3%. Bot. 4 oz, pt, gal.
Use: Antihistamine.

•**BROMCHLORENONE.** USAN. 6-Bromo-5-chloro-2-benzoxazolinone. (Maumee) Vinyzene.
Use: Local anti-infective.

BROMEBRIC ACID. B.A.N. cis-3-Bromo-3-p-anisoylacrylic acid.
Use: Cytotoxic agent.

BROMENZYME. (Barth's) Bromelain 40 mg/Tab. Bot. 100s, 250s, 500s.
Use: Digestive aid.

BROMETHOL.
See: Avertin.

BROMEZYME. (Barth's) Bromelain 40 mg, papaya fruit, papain enzyme/Tab. Bot. 100s, 250s, 500s.
Use: Digestive aid.

BROMFED CAPSULES. (Muro) Brompheniramine maleate 12 mg, pseudoephedrine HCl 120 mg/TR Cap. Bot. 100s, 500s.
Use: Antihistamine, decongestant.

BROMFED-DM SYRUP. (Muro) Brompheniramine maleate 2 mg, pseudoephedrine HCl 30 mg, dextromethorphan HBr 10 mg/5 ml. Bot. 120 ml, 240 ml, 480 ml.
Use: Antihistamine, decongestant, antitussive.

BROMFED-PD CAPSULES. (Muro) Brompheniramine maleate 6 mg, pseudoephedrine HCl 60 mg/TR Cap. Bot. 100s, 500s.
Use: Antihistamine, decongestant.

BROMFED SYRUP. (Muro) Brompheniramine maleate 2 mg, pseudoephedrine HCl 30 mg/5 ml. Bot. 480 ml.
Use: Antihistamine, decongestant.

BROMFED TABLETS. (Muro) Brompheniramine maleate 4 mg, pseudoephedrine HCl 60 mg/Tab. Bot. 100s.
Use: Antihistamine, decongestant.

•**BROMFENAC SODIUM.** USAN.
Use: Analgesic.

BROMHEXINE. B.A.N. N-(2-Amino-3,5-dibromobenzyl)-N-cyclohexylmethylamine.
Use: Bronchial mucolytic.

•**BROMHEXINE HCl.** USAN. (1) 3,5-Dibromo-Nα-cyclohexyl-Nα-methyltoluene-α, 2-diamine monohydrochloride. (2) N-cyclohexyl-N-methyl-(2-amino-3,-5-dibromobenzyl) ammonium Cl.
Use: Expectorant, mucolytic.
See: Bisolvon (Boehringer Ingelheim).

BROMIDES.
See: Lanabrom, Elix. (Lannett).
Peacocks Bromides, Liq. (Natcon).

BROMIDE SALTS.
See: Calcium Bromide.
Ferrous Bromide.
Potassium Bromide.
Sodium Bromide.
Strontium Bromide.

BROMI-LOTION. (Gordon) Aluminum hydroxychloride 20%, emollient base. Bot. 1.5 oz, 4 oz.
Use: Antiperspirant.

•**BROMINDIONE.** USAN. 2-(4-Bromophenyl)(2)2-(p-Bromophenyl)-1,3-indandione.
Use: Anticoagulant.
See: Circladin.

BROMI-TALC. (Gordon) Potassium alum, bentonite, talc. Shaker can 3.5 oz, 1 lb, 5 lb.
Use: Bromidrosis, hyperhidrosis.

•**BROMOCRIPTINE.** USAN. 2-Bromo-α-ergocryptine.
Use: Prolactin inhibitor.

•**BROMOCRIPTINE MESYLATE.** USAN 2-Bromo-a-ergocryptine mesylate.
Use: Prolactin inhibitor.
See: Parlodel, Tab. (Sandoz).

•**BROMOCRIPTINE MESYLATE,** U.S.P. XXII. Tab., U.S.P. XXII.
Use: Prolactin inhibitor.

BROMOCYCLEN. V.B.A.N. 5-Bromomethyl-1,2,3,4,7,7-hexachloronorborn-2-ene.
Use: Insecticide, acaricide, veterinary medicine.

BROMODIETHYLACETYLUREA.
See: Carbromal.

BROMODIPHENHYDRAMINE. B.A.N. USAN N-2-(4-Bromobenzhydryloxy)ethyldimethylamine. Bromazine (I.N.N.).
Use: Antihistamine.

BROMOFROM. Tribromomethane.

BROMOISOVALERYL UREA. Alpha, bromoisovaleryl urea.
See: Bromisovalum.

BROMOPHEN T.D. (Rugby) Phenylpropanolamine HCl 15 mg, phenylephrine HCl 15 mg, brompheniramine maleate 12 mg/Tab. Bot. 100s, 1000s.
Use: Decongestant, antihistamine.

BROMOPHIN.
See: Apomorphine HCl (Various Mfr.).

BROMO QUININE COLD TABLETS.
See: BQ Cold Tablets (Bristol-Myers).

BROMO-SELTZER. (Warner-Lambert) Acetaminophen 325 mg, sodium bicarbonate 2.78 Gm, citric acid 2.22 Gm (when dissolved, forms sodium citrate 2.85 Gm)/Dose. Large (2⅝ oz), King (4.25 oz), Giant (9 oz), Foil pack, single dose 48s.
Use: Antacid, analgesic.

8-BROMOTHEOPHYLLINE W/2-amino-2-methyl-1-propanol.
See: Pamabrom.

BROMOTHEOPHYLLINATE AMINOISOBUTANOL.
See: Pamabrom.

BROMOTHEOPHYLLINATE PYRILAMINE.
See: Pyrabrom.

BROMOTHEOPHYLLINATE PYRANISAMINE.
See: Pyrabrom.

BROMOTUSS W/CODEINE. (Rugby) Bromodiphenhydramine HCl 12.5 mg, codeine phosphate 10 mg, alcohol 5 %. Syr. Bot. 120 ml, pt, gal.
Use: Antihistamine, antitussive.

•**BROMOXANIDE.** USAN.
Use: Anthelmintic.

•**BROMPERIDOL.** USAN.
Use: Antipsychotic.

BROMPHEN DC W/CODEINE COUGH SYRUP. (Various Mfr.) Phenylpropanolamine HCl 12.5 mg, brompheniramine maleate 2 mg, codeine phosphate 10 mg, alcohol 0.95%. Syr. Bot. 120 ml, pt, gal.
Use: Decongestant, antihistamine, antitussive.

BROMPHEN EXPECTORANT. (Various Mfr.) Phenylpropanolamine HCl 5 mg, phenylephrine HCl 5 mg, brompheniramine maleate 2 mg, guaifenesin 100 mg, alcohol 3.5%. Liq. Bot. 120 ml, pt, gal.
Use: Decongestant, antihistamine, expectorant.

BROMPHENIRAMINE. B.A.N. 3-(4-Bromophenyl)-3-(2-pyridyl) propyldimethylamine.
Use: Antihistamine.

•**BROMPHENIRAMINE MALEATE,** U.S.P. XXII. Elix., Inj., Tab., U.S.P. XXII. 2-{p-Bromo-α-[2-dimethylamino)ethyl]-benzyl]}-pyridine maleate.
Use: Antihistamine.
See: Dimetane, Tab., Elix., Inj. (Robins).
Rolabromophen, Tab. (Robinson).
Rolabromophen Decongestant Elixir (Robinson).
Rolabromophen Elixir (Robinson).
Rolabromophen Expectorant (Robinson).
Rolabromophen Forte, Tab. (Robinson).
Rolabromophen Injection (Robinson).
Rolabromophen Timed, Tab. (Robinson).
Symptom 3, Liq. (Parke-Davis).
Veltane (Lannett).

BROMPHENIRAMINE MALEATE W/COMBINATIONS.
See: Bro-Expectorant W/Codeine, Liq. (Solvay).
Bromepaph, Preps. (Quality Generics).
Cortane, Preps. (Standex).
Cortapp, Elix. (Standex).
Dimetane Decongestant, Tab., Elix. (Robins).
Dimetane Expectorant, Liq. (Robins).
Dimetane Expectorant-DC, Liq. (Robins).
Dimetapp Extentabs, Elix. (Robins).
Eldatapp, Tab., Liq. (Elder).

BROMTAPP. (Blue Cross) Brompheniramine maleate 4 mg, phenylephrine HCl 5 mg, phenylpropanolamine HCl 5 mg/5 ml. Bot. 16 oz, gal.
Use: Antihistamine, decongestant.

BRONCAJEN. (Jenkins) Pyrilamine maleate 10 mg, phenylephrine HCl 2 mg, potassium guaiacol sulfonate 2 gr, ammonium Cl 2 gr, ipecac 1/8 gr/Tab. Bot. 1000s.
Use: Antihistamine, decongestant, expectorant.

BRONCHOLATE CAPSULES. (Bock) Ephedrine HCl 12.5 mg, guaifenesin 200 mg/Cap. Bot. 100s, 1000s.
Use: Bronchodilator, expectorant.

BRONCHOLATE CS. (Bock) Codeine phosphate 10 mg, ephedrine HCl 6.25 mg, guaifenesin 100 mg/5 ml. Bot. pt.
Use: Antitussive, bronchodilator, expectorant.

BRONCHOLATE SYRUP. (Bock) Ephedrine HCl 6.25 mg, guaifenesin 100 mg/5 ml. Bot. pt.
Use: Bronchodilator, expectorant.

BRONCHO SALINE. (Blairex) 0.9% sodium Cl for diluting bronchodilator solutions for inhalation. Soln. 90 ml, 240 ml w/metered dispensing valve.
Use: Inhalation diluent.

BRONCHOVENT. (Mills) Aminophylline 90 mg, guaifenesin 50 mg, amobarbital 16 mg/coated Tab. Bot. 100s.
Use: Bronchodilator, expectorant, sedative.

BRONDECON. (Parke-Davis) **Tab.:** Oxtriphylline 200 mg, guaifenesin 100 mg/Tab. Bot. 100s. **Elix.:** Oxtriphylline 100 mg, guaifenesin 50 mg/5 ml w/alcohol 20%. Bot. 8 oz, 16 oz.
Use: Bronchodilator, expectorant.

BRONDELATE. (Various Mfr.) Oxtriphylline 300 mg, guaifenesin 150 mg, alcohol 20%/5 ml. Elix. Bot. pt, gal.
Use: Bronchodilator, expectorant.

BRONICOF. (Jenkins) Ethylmorphine HCl 2.5 mg, syrup hydriodic acid 50%, potassium citrate 438 mg, sodium benzoate 10 mg, aromatics/5 ml. Bot. 3 oz, 4 oz, gal.
Use: Cough sedative, expectorant.

BRONITIN. (Whitehall) Theophylline hydrous 120 mg, guaifenesin 100 mg, ephedrine HCl 24.3 mg, pyrilamine maleate 16.6 mg/Tab. Bot. 24s, 60s.
Use: Bronchodilator.

BRONKAID MIST. (Winthrop Consumer) Epinephrine 0.5% in inhalation aerosol. Each spray releases 0.25 mg epinephrine. Aerosol 10 Gm or 16.7 Gm w/adapter; 15 Gm, 25 Gm refills.
Use: Bronchodilator.

BRONKAID MIST SUSPENSION. (Winthrop Consumer) Epinephrine bitartrate 0.7%. Each spray releases 0.3 mg epinephrine bitartrate equivalent to 0.16 mg epinephrine base. Bot. 10 ml, 15 ml with and without adapter.
Use: Bronchodilator.

BRONKAID TABLETS. (Winthrop Consumer) Ephedrine sulfate 24 mg, guaifenesin 100 mg, theophylline 100 mg/Tab. Box 24s, 60s.
Use: Bronchodilator, expectorant.

BRONKASMA TABLETS. (Winthrop) Theophylline anhydrous, ephedrine sulphate, thenyldiamine.
Use: Bronchodilator.

BRONKEPHRINE. (Winthrop) Ethylnorepinephrine HCl 2 mg/ml in a sterile isotonic solution of sodium chloride 0.7% w/sodium acetone bisulfite 0.2%, sodium hydroxide or HCl to adjust pH to 2.9-4.5. Amp. 1 ml. Box 25s.
Use: Bronchodilator.

BRONKODYL. (Winthrop) Theophylline 100 mg or 200 mg/Cap. Bot. 100s. Theophylline 300 mg/SR Cap. Bot. 100s.
Use: Bronchodilator.

BRONKOLATE "G". (Parmed) Dyphylline 200 mg, guaifenesin 200 mg/Tab. Bot. 100s, 1000s.
Use: Bronchodilator, expectorant.

BRONKOLIXIR. (Winthrop) Guaifenesin 50 mg, ephedrine sulfate 12 mg, theophylline 15 mg, phenobarbital 4 mg/5 ml. Bot. pt.
Use: Expectorant, bronchodilator, sedative/hypnotic.

BRONKOMETER. (Winthrop) Isoetharine mesylate 0.61%, saccharin, menthol, alcohol 30%. Metered dose of 340 mcg isoetharine in fluoro hydrocarbon propellant. Bot. w/nebulizer 10 ml, 15 ml. Refill 10 ml, 15 ml.
Use: Bronchodilator.

BRONKOSOL. (Winthrop) Isoetharine HCl 1% w/ glycerin, sodium bisulfite, parabens for oral inhalation. Bot. 10 ml, 30 ml.
Use: Bronchodilator.

BRONKOTABS. (Winthrop) Ephedrine sulfate 24 mg, theophylline 100 mg, guaifenesin 100 mg, phenobarbital 8 mg/Tab. Bot. 100s, 1000s.
Use: Bronchodilator, expectorant, sedative/hypnotic.

BRONKOTUSS. (Hyrex) Chlorpheniramine maleate 4 mg, guaifenesin 100 mg, ephedrine sulfate 8.216 mg, hydriodic acid syrup 1.67 mg/ 5 ml w/alcohol 5%. Bot. pt, gal.
Use: Antihistamine, expectorant, decongestant.

BRONOPOL. B.A.N. 2-Bromo-2-nitropropane-1,3-diol.
Use: Antiseptic, preservative.

•**BROPERAMOLE.** USAN.
Use: Anti-inflammatory.

•**BROPIRIMINE.** USAN.
Use: Antineoplastic, antiviral.

BROSERPINE. (Brothers) Reserpine 0.25 mg/ Tab. Bot. 250s, 1000s.
Use: Antihypertensive.

BRO-T'S. (Brothers) Bromisovalum 0.12 Gm, carbromal 0.2 Gm/Tab. Bot. 100s, 1000s.
Use: Sedative, tranquilizer.

BROTANE ELIXIR. (Halsey) Bot. 16 oz, gal.
Use: Decongestant.

BROTANE EXPECTORANT. (Blue Cross) Guaifenesin 100 mg, brompheniramine maleate 2 mg, phenylephrine HCl 5 mg, phenylpropanolamine HCl 5 mg/5 ml, alcohol 3.5%. Bot. 16 oz.
Use: Expectorant, antihistamine, decongestant.

BROTIANIDE. V.B.A.N. 2-Bromo-4-chloro-6-(4-bromophenylthiocarbamoyl)phenyl acetate.
Use: Anthelmintic, veterinary medicine.

•**BROTIZOLAM.** USAN.
Use: Hypnotic.

BRO-TUSS. (Brothers) Dextromethorphan HBr 15 mg, chlorpheniramine maleate 2 mg, phenylephrine HCl 5 mg, ammonium Cl 100 mg, sodium citrate 150 mg, vitamin C 30 mg/10 ml. Bot. 4 oz, pt, gal.
Use: Antitussive, antihistamine, decongestant, expectorant.

BRO-TUSS A.C. (Brothers) Acetaminophen 120 mg, codeine phosphate 10 mg, phenylephrine HCl 5 mg, chlorpheniramine maleate 2 mg, menthol 1 mg, alcohol 10%/5 ml. Bot. pt, gal.
Use: Analgesic, antitussive, decongestant, antihistamine.

BROWN MIXTURE. (Various Mfr.) Paregoric 12%, glycyrrhiza fluid extract, antimony potassium tartrate, alcohol. Liq. Bot. 120 ml, pt, gal.
Use: Antidiarrheal.

BRUCELLA VACCINE. Undulant fever vaccine.
Use: I.M., S.C., undulant fever.

BRYREL SYRUP. (Winthrop) Piperazine citrate anhydrous 110 mg/ml. Bot. oz.
Use: Anthelmintic.

B-SCORBIC. (Pharmics) Vitamins C 300 mg, B_1 25 mg, B_2 10 mg, calcium pantothenate 10 mg, niacinamide 50 mg, lemon flavored complex 200 mg/Tab. Bot. 100s, 1000s.
Use: Vitamin supplement.

BSS.
See: Balanced Salt Solution.

BSS PLUS. (Alcon Surgical) Balanced salt solution with bicarbonate dextrose and glutathione. Two part solution reconstituted within 6 hrs. of surgery. Bot. 500 ml.
Use: Intraocular irrigating solution.

•**BUCAINIDE MALEATE.** USAN.
Use: Cardiac depressant.

BUCETIN. B.A.N. N-3-Hydroxybutyryl-p-phenetidine.
Use: Analgesic.

BUCHU.
See: Barosmin.

•**BUCINDOLOL HYDROCHLORIDE.** USAN. A Mead Johnson investigational drug.
Use: Investigative, antihypertensive.

BUCLADIN-S. (Stuart) Buclizine HCl 50 mg. Softab. Tab. Bot. 100s.
Use: Antiemetic/antivertigo.

BUCLIZINE. B.A.N. 1-(4-t-Butylbenzyl)-4-(4-chlorobenzhydryl) piperazine.
Use: Antiemetic.

•**BUCLIZINE HYDROCHLORIDE.** USAN. 1-(p-tert Butylbenzyl)-4-(p-chloro-alpha-phenylbenzyl) piperazine dihydrochloride.
Use: Antiemetic, antinauseant.
See: Bucladin-S, Tab. (Stuart).

BUCLOSAMIDE. B.A.N. N-Butyl-4-chlorosalicylamide.
Use: Antimycotic.

•**BUCROMARONE.** USAN.
Use: Cardiac depressant (antiarrhythmic).

•**BUCRYLATE.** USAN.
Use: Surgical aid.

•**BUDESONIDE.** USAN.
Use: Anti-inflammatory.

BUFACET. (Jenkins) Acetylsalicylic acid 3.5 gr, acetophenetidin 2.5 gr, caffeine alkaloid 0.5 gr, aromatics, buffered w/aluminum hydroxide gel/ Tab. Bot. 1000s.
Use: Analgesic.

BUF ACNE CLEANSING BAR. (3M Products) Salicylic acid 1%, sulfur 1% in detergent cleansing bar. 3.5 oz.
Use: Anti-acne.

BUF BODY SCRUB. (3M Products) Round cleansing sponge on plastic handles.
Use: Cleansing sponge.

BUFEXAMAC. B.A.N. 4-Butoxyphenylacetohydroxamic acid.
Use: Anti-inflammatory.

BUFF-A. (Mayrand) Aspirin acid 5 gr. buffered w/ magnesium hydroxide, aluminum hydroxide dried gel. Tab. Bot. 100s, 1000s.
Use: Analgesic.

BUFF-A-COMP. (Mayrand) Aspirin 648 mg, caffeine 40 mg, butalbital 50 mg/Tab. Bot. 100s.
Use: Analgesic combination.

BUFF-A-COMP NO. 3. (Mayrand) Butalbital 50 mg, aspirin 325 mg, caffeine 40 mg, codeine phosphate 30 mg/Tab. Bot. 100s.
Use: Analgesic combination.

BUFFAPRIN. (Buffington) Aspirin 325 mg. buffered with magnesium oxide. Sugar, caffeine, lactose, salt free. Tab. Dispens-A-Kit 500s.
Use: Salicylate analgesic.

BUFFASAL. (Dover) Aspirin 325 mg/Tab. w/magnesium oxide. Sugar, lactose, salt free. UD Box 500s.
Use: Salicylate analgesic.

BUFFASAL MAX. (Dover) Aspirin 500 mg/Tab w/ magnesium oxide. Sugar, lactose, salt free.
Use: Salicylate analgesic.

BUFFERIN ANALGESIC TABLETS. (Bristol-Myers) Aspirin 324 mg buffered with aluminum glycinate, magnesium carbonate. Tab. Blister pkg. 12s. Bot. 12s, 36s, 60s, 100s, 165s, 225s, 375s, 1000s, UD 12s, 400s.
Use: Salicylate analgesic.

BUFFERIN ARTHRITIS STRENGTH TABLETS. (Bristol-Myers) Aspirin 486 mg buffered w/aluminum glycinate and magnesium carbonate. Tab. Bot. 40s, 100s.
Use: Salicylate analgesic.

BUFFERIN, ARTHRITIS STRENGTH TRI-BUFFERED. (Bristol-Myers) Aspirin 500 mg w/calcium carbonate, magnesium oxide, magnesium carbonate. Capl. Bot. 40s.
Use: Salicylate analgesic.

BUFFERIN EXTRA STRENGTH COATED TABLETS. (Bristol-Myers) Aspirin 500 mg buffered w/magnesium carbonate, aluminum glycinate. Tab. Bot. 30s, 60s, 100s.
Use: Salicylate analgesic.

BUFFERIN, EXTRA STRENGTH TRI-BUFFERED. (Bristol-Myers) Aspirin 500 mg, calcium carbonate, magnesium oxide, magnesium carbonate. Tab. Bot. 30s.
Use: Salicylate analgesic.

BUFFERIN, TRI-BUFFERED. (Bristol-Myers) Aspirin 325 mg, calcium carbonate, magnesium oxide, magnesium carbonate. Capl. Bot. 60s.
Use: Salicylate analgesic.

BUFFETS II. (JMI) Aspirin 226 mg, acetaminophen 162 mg, caffeine 32.4 mg, aluminum hydroxide 50 mg/Tab. Bot. 1000s.
Use: Analgesic combination.

BUFFEX. (Hauck) Aspirin 325 mg w/dihydroxyaluminum aminoacetate. Tab. Bot. 1000s, Sanipack 1000s.
Use: Salicylate analgesic.

BUFFINOL. (Otis Clapp) Aspirin 324 mg buffered w/magnesium oxide. Sugar, caffeine, lactose, salt free. Tab. Bot. 100s, 200s, 500s.
Use: Salicylate analgesic.

BUFFINOL EXTRA. (Otis Clapp) Aspirin 500 mg/ Tab. Sugar, caffeine, lactose, salt free. Safety pack 500s.
Use: Salicylate analgesic.

BUF FOOT CARE KIT. (3M Products) Cleansing system for the feet.
Use: Foot preparation.

BUF FOOT CARE LOTION. (3M Products) Moisturizing lotion for feet.
Use: Foot preparation.

BUF FOOT CARE SOAP. (3M Products) Bar 3.5 oz.
Use: Foot preparation.

BUFILCON A. USAN.
Use: Contact lens material.

BUF KIT FOR ACNE. (3M Products) Cleansing sponge, cleansing bar. 3.5 oz w/booklet, holding tray.
Use: Anti-acne.

BUF LOTION. (3M Products) Moisturizing lotion.
Use: Emollient.

•**BUFORMIN.** USAN. 1-Butylbiguanide. Silubin.
Use: Oral hypoglycemic agent.

BUFOSAL. (Table Rock) Sodium salicylate 15 gr/ dram w/calcium carbonate, sodium bicarbonate as granulated effervescent powder. Bot. 4 oz.
Use: Salicylate analgesic.

BUF-PED NON MEDICATED CLEANSING SPONGE. (3M Products) Abrasive cleansing sponge.
Use: Cleansing skin on feet.

BUF PUF BODYMATE. (3M Products) Oval two-sided cleansing sponge. Abrasive/gentle.
Use: Cleansing all areas of the body.

BUF-PUF NON-MEDICATED CLEANSING SPONGE. (3M Products) Abrasive cleansing sponge.
Use: Skin cleansing.

BUFROLIN. B.A.N. 6-Butyl-1,4,7,10-tetrahydro-4,10-dioxo-1,7-phenanthroline-2,8-dicarboxylic acid.
Use: Mast-cell stabilizer.

BUF-SUL TABLETS AND SUSPENSION. (Sheryl) Sulfacetamide 167 mg, sulfadiazine 167

mg, sulfamerazine 167 mg. Tab. 100s. Susp. pt.
Use: Antibacterial, sulfonamide.

BUF-TABS. (Blue Cross) Aspirin 5 gr/Tab. w/aluminum hydroxide, glycine magnesium carbonate. Bot. 100s.
Use: Salicylate analgesic.

BUFURALOL. B.A.N. 2-tert-Butylamino-1-(7-ethylbenzofuran-2-yl)ethanol.
Use: Beta adrenergic blocking agent.

BUFYLLINE. B.A.N. Theophylline compound with 2-amino-2-methylpropan-1-ol (1:1).
Use: Bronchodilator.

BUG-PRUF. (Scherer) n, n diethyl-m-toluamide (DEET) 94.525%, other isomers 4.975%, fragrance 0.5%. Bot. 2 oz.
Use: Insect repellent.

BUGS BUNNY. (Miles) Vitamins A 2500 IU, E 15 IU, C 60 mg, folic acid 0.3 mg, B_1 1.05 mg, B_2 1.2 mg, niacin 13.5 mg, B_6 1.05 mg, B_{12} 4.5 mcg, D 400 IU/Tab. Bot. 60s.
Use: Vitamin/mineral supplement.

BUGS BUNNY CHEWABLE VITAMINS AND MINERALS. (Miles) Vitamins A 5000 IU, D 400 IU, E 30 IU, C 60 mg, folic acid 0.4 mg, B_1 1.5 mg, B_2 1.7 mg, niacin 20 mg, B_6 2 mg, B_{12} 6 mcg, biotin 40 mcg, pantothenic acid 10 mg, iron 18 mg, calcium 100 mg, phosphorus 100 mg, iodine 150 mcg, magnesium 20 mg, copper 2 mg, zinc 15 mg/Tab. Bot 60s.
Use: Vitamin/mineral supplement.

BUGS BUNNY PLUS IRON. (Miles) Vitamins A 2500 IU, E 15 IU, C 60 mg, folic acid 0.3 mg, B_1 1.05 mg, B_2 1.2 mg, niacin 13.5 mg, B_6 1.05 mg, B_{12} 4.5 mcg, D 400 IU, iron 15 mg/Chew. tab. Bot. 60s.
Use: Vitamin/mineral supplement.

BUGS BUNNY WITH EXTRA C. (Miles) Vitamins A 2500 IU, D 400 IU, E 15 IU, C 250 mg, folic acid 0.3 mg, B_1 1.05 mg, B_2 1.2 mg, niacin 13.5 mg, B_6 1.05 mg, B_{12} 4.5 mcg/Tab. Bot. 60s.
Use: Vitamin/mineral supplement.

BULKOGEN. A mucin extracted from the seeds of *Cyanopsis tetragonaloba.*}

BULLFROG SUNBLOCK. (Chattem) Octocrylene 10%, ethyl dihydroxypropyl PABA 5%. Bot. 1 oz.
Use: Sunscreen.

•**BUMETANIDE.** U.S.P. XXII, Tab., Inj., 3-Butylamino-4-phenoxy-5-sulfamoylbenzoic acid.
Use: Diuretic.
See: Bumex, Tab. (Roche).

•**BUMETRIZOLE.** USAN.
Use: Ultraviolet screen.

BUMEX. (Roche) Bumetanide 0.5 mg, 1 mg or 2 mg/Tab. 0.5 mg and 1 mg Bot. 30s, 100s, 500s, UD 100s. 2 mg Bot. 100s, UD 100s. Amp 2 ml, 0.25 mg/ml. Box 10s. Vial 2 ml, 4 ml or 10 ml, 0.25 mg/ml. Box 10s.
Use: Loop diuretic.

BUMINATE. (Hyland) Normal serum albumin (human) **25%** soln. in 20 ml w/o administration set; 50 ml and 100 ml w/administration set. **5%** soln. in 250 ml and 500 ml w/administration set.
Use: Albumin replacement.

BUN REAGENT STRIPS. (Ames) Seralyzer reagent strips. A quantitative strip test for BUN in serum or plasma. Bot 25s.
Use: Diagnostic aid.

BUNAMIDINE. V.B.A.N. NN-Dibutyl-4-hexyloxy-1-naphthamidine.
Use: Anthelmintic, veterinary medicine.

•**BUNAMIDE HYDROCHLORIDE.** USAN.
Use: Anthelmintic.

BUNAMIODYL SODIUM. Sodium 3-butyramido-a-ethyl-2,4,6-triiodocinnamate.
Use: Diagnostic aid (radiopaque medium).

BUNIODYL. B.A.N. 3-(3-Butyramido-2,4,6-triiodophenyl)-2-ethylacrylic acid. Bunamiodyl (I.N.N.).
Use: Radio-opaque substance.

•**BUNOLOL HCl.** USAN. (±)-5-[3-(tert)- butylamino)-2-hydroxypropoxy]-3,4-dihydro-1-(2H)-naphthalenone HCl.
Use: Antiadrenergic (β-receptors).

BUPHENINE. B.A.N. 1-(4-Hydroxyphenyl)-2-(1-methyl-3-phenylpropylamino)propan-1-ol.
Use: Peripheral vasodilator.
See: Perdilatal HCl.

•**BUPICOMIDE.** USAN.
Use: Antihypertensive.

BUPIVACAINE. B.A.N. USAN 1-Butyl-2-(2,6-xylylcarbamoyl)piperidide. 1-Butyl-2′,6′-pipecoloxylidide. (Abbott) **0.25%**: Amp. 20 ml, syr. 50 ml. **0.5%**: Amp. 20 ml, syr. 30 ml. **0.75%**: Amp. 20 ml, syr. 20 ml.
Use: Local anesthetic.

•**BUPIVACAINE IN DEXTROSE INJECTION,** U.S.P. XXII.
Use: Local anesthetic.

•**BUPIVACAINE AND EPINEPHRINE INJECTION,** U.S.P. XXII.
Use: Local anesthetic.
See: Marcaine w/Epinephrine, Inj. (Winthrop).

•**BUPIVACAINE HYDROCHLORIDE,** U.S.P. XXII. Inj. U.S.P. XXII. 2-piperidinecarboxamide, 1-butyl-N-(2, 6-dimethylphenyl)-, monohydrochloride, monohydrate.
Use: Local anesthetic.
See: Marcaine, Injectable (Winthrop).
Sensorcaine, Inj. (Astra).

BUPRENEX INJECTION. (Norwich Eaton) Buprenorphine HCl 0.3 mg/ml w/50 mg anhydrous dextrose. Amp. 1 ml.
Use: Narcotic analgesic.

BUPRENORPHINE. B.A.N. N-Cyclopropylmethyl-7,8-dihydro-7α-(1-(S)-hydroxy-1,2,2-trimethylpropyl)-O^6-methyl-6,14-endoethanonormorphine.
Use: Analgesic.
See: Buprenex, Inj. (Norwich Eaton).

•**BUPRENORPHINE HYDROCHLORIDE.** USAN.
Use: Analgesic.

•**BUPROPION HYDROCHLORIDE.** USAN.
Use: Antidepressant.
See: Wellbutrin (Burroughs Wellcome).

•**BUQUINOLATE.** USAN. Ethyl 4-hydroxy-6,7-diisobutoxy-3-quinolinecarboxylate.
Use: Coccidiostat for poultry.

•**BURAMATE.** USAN. 2-Hydroxyethyl benzylcarbamate. Hyamate.
Use: Anticonvulsant, tranquilizer.
See: Hyamate (Xttrium).

BURDEO. (Hill) Aluminum subacetate 100 mg, boric acid 300 mg/oz. Bot. 3 oz. Roll-on 8 oz.
Use: Deodorant.

BURN GON. (E.J. Moore) Benzocaine, cod liver oil, boric acid, lanolin. Tube 1.25 oz.
Use: Burn remedy.

BURN THERAPY.
See: Americaine, Preps. (American Critical Care).
Amertan, Jelly (Lilly).
Burn-A-Lay, Cream (Ken-Gate).
Burnicin, Oint. (Quality Generics).
Burn-Quel, Aerosol (Halperin).
Butesin Picrate Oint. (Abbott).
Foille, Preps. (Carbisulphoil).
Kip, Preps. (Youngs Drug Prod.).
Nupercainal, Oint. (Ciba).
Silvadene, Cream (Marion).
Solarcaine, Preps. (Schering-Plough).
Sulfamylon, Cream (Winthrop).
Unguentine, Preps. (Norwich).

BURN-A-LAY. (Ken-Gate) Chlorobutanol 0.75% oxyquinoline benzoate 0.025%, zinc oxide 2%, thymol 0.5%. Cream Tube oz.
Use: Burn remedy.

BURNATE. (Burlington) Vitamins A 4000 IU, D-2 400 IU, thiamine HCl 3 mg, riboflavin 2 mg, niacinamide 10 mg, pyridine HCl 2 mg, cyanocobalamin 5 mcg, calcium pantothenate 0.5 mg, folic acid 0.4 mg, ascorbic acid 50 mg, ferrous fumarate 300 mg, calcium 200 mg, iodine 0.15 mg, copper 1 mg, magnesium 5 mg, zinc 1.5 mg/Tab. Bot. 100s.
Use: Vitamin/mineral supplement.

BURN-QUEL. Halperin aerosol dispenser. 1 oz, 2 oz.
Use: Burn remedy.

BURNTAME SPRAY. (Otis Clapp) Benzocaine, in spray. Aerosol can 2.5 oz.
Use: Anesthetic/antiseptic burn remedy.

BUR-OIL-ZINC. (Durel) Zinc oxide, talcum, lanolin, olive oil, Burow's solution. Bot. 4 oz, pt, gal.
Use: Generalized and widespread eczematous eruptions, acute and subacute inflammatory processes, exfoliative dermatitis.

BUR-OIL-ZINC LOTION PLUS. (Durel) Menthol 0.25%, phenol 0.5% added to Bur-oil-zinc compound. Bot. 4 oz, pt, gal.
Use: Antipruritic.

BURO-SOL ANTISEPTIC POWDER. (Doak) Contents make a diluted Burow's Solution. aluminum acetate topical soln. plus benzethonium Cl. Pkg. (2.36 Gm) 12s, 100s. Bot. Pow. 4 oz, 1 lb, 5 lb.
Use: Astringent wet dressing.

BUROTIC. (Parnell) Acetic acid 2% in aluminum acetate solution. Soln. Bot. 60 ml.
Use: Otic preparation.

BUROW'S SOLUTION. Aluminum Acetate Topical Solution, U.S.P. XXII.
See: Buro-Sol Pow. (Doak).
Domeboro, Pow., Tab. (Miles).
Boric acid, acetic acid.
See: Star-Otic, Drops (Star).

BURSUL. (Burlington) Sulfamethiazole 500 mg/Tab. Bot. 100s.
Use: Antibacterial; sulfonamide.

BUR-TUSS. (Burlington) Chlorpheniramine maleate 2 mg, phenylephrine HCl 5 mg, phenylpropanolamine HCl 5 mg, guaifenesin 100 mg, alcohol 2.5%/5 ml. Bot. pt, gal.
Use: Antihistamine, decongestant, expectorant.

BUR-ZIN. (Lamond) Aluminum acetate solution 2%, zinc oxide 10%. Bot. 4 oz, 8 oz, pt, qt, gal. Also w/o lanolin.
Use: Antipruritic, counter-irritant.

•**BUSERELIN ACETATE.** USAN.
Use: Gonad-stimulating principle.

BUSPAR TABLETS. (Mead Johnson) Buspirone HCl 5 mg or 10 mg/Tab.
Use: Antianxiety agent.

•**BUSPIRONE HYDROCHLORIDE.** USAN.
Use: Antianxiety agent.
See: BuSpar, Tab. (Mead Johnson).

•**BUSULFAN,** U.S.P. XXII. Tabs, U.S.P. XXII. Tetramethylene dimethanesulfonate. 1-4-Dimethanesulphonyloxybutane. 1,4-Butanediol dimethanesulfonate.
Use: Chronic myeloid leukemia.
See: Myleran, Tab. (Burroughs Wellcome).

BUSULPHAN. B.A.N. Tetramethylene di(methanesulphonate).
Use: Antineoplastic agent.

•**BUTABARBITAL,** U.S.P. XXII 5-sec-Butyl-5-ethylbarbituric acid.
Use: Sedative/hypnotic.
See: BBS, Tab. (Solvay).
Butisol, Prods. (Wallace).
Da-Sed, Tab. (Sheryl).
Expansatol, Cap. (Merit).
Medarsed, Elix., Tab. (Medar).
W/Acetaminophen.
See: G-3, Tab. (Hauck).
Sedapap, Elix. (Mayrand).
Sedapap-10, Tab. (Mayrand).
W/Acetaminophen, codeine phosphate.
See: G-3, Cap. (Hauck).
W/Acetaminophen, mephenesin.
See: T-Caps, Cap. (Burlington).
W/Acetaminophen, phenacetin, caffeine.
See: Windolor, Tab. (Winston).
W/Acetaminophen, salicylamide, phenyltoloxamine citrate.
See: Dengesic, Tab. (Scott-Alison).
Scotgesic, Cap., Elix. (Scott/Cord).

W/Ambutonium bromide, aluminum hydroxide, magnesium hydroxide.
See: Aludrox, Susp., Tab. (Wyeth-Ayerst).
W/Aminophylline, phenylpropanolamine HCl, chlorpheniramine maleate, aluminum hydroxide, magnesium trisilicate.
See: Asmacol, Tab. (Vale).
W/Carboxyphen.
See: Bontril Timed No. 2, Tab. (G. W. Carnrick).
W/Chlorpheniramine maleate, hyoscine HBr.
See: Pedo-Sol, Tab., Elix. (Warren Pharmacal).
W/Dihydroxypropyl theophylline, ephedrine HCl.
See: Airet R, Tab. (Baylor).
W/Ephedrine sulfate, theophylline.
See: Airet Y, Tab., Elix. (Baylor).
W/Ephedrine HCl, theophylline, guaifenesin.
See: Quibron Plus, Cap., Elix. (Bristol).
W/Ephedrine HCl, theophylline, isoproterenol.
W/Ephedrine sulfate, theophylline, guaifenesin.
See: Broncholate, Cap., Elix. (Bock).
W/l-Hyoscyamine.
See: Cystospaz-SR, Cap. (Webcon).
W/Hyoscyamine sulfate, atropine sulfate, hyoscine HBr, homatropine methylbromide.
See: Butabell HMB, Tab., Elix. (Saron).
W/Hyoscyamine sulfate, scopolamine methylnitrate, atropine sulfate.
See: Banatil, Cap., Elix. (Trimen).
W/Nitroglycerin.
See: Nitrodyl-B, Cap. (Bock).
W/Pentaerythritol tetranitrate.
See: Petn Plus (Saron).
W/Pentobarbital, phenobarbital.
See: Quiess, Tab. (Forest).
W/Phenazopyridine, hyoscyamine HBr.
See: Pyridium Plus, Tab. (Parke-Davis).
W/Phenazopyridine, scopolamine HBr, atropine sulfate, hyoscyamine sulfate.
See: Buren, Tab. (Ascher).
W/Phenobarbital, pentobarbital, hyoscyamine sulfate, hyoscine HBr, atropine sulfate.
See: Neoquess, Tab. (Forest).
W/Salicylamide.
See: Dapco, Tab. (Mericon).
W/Secobarbital.
See: Monosyl, Tab. (Arcum).
W/Secobarbital, pentobarbital, phenobarbital.
See: Quad-Set, Tab. (Kenyon).
W/Theophylline.
See: Theobid, Cap. (Meyer).
W/Theophylline, pseudoephedrine HCl.
See: Asmadil, Cap. (Solvay).
Ayr, Liq. (Ascher).
Ayrcap, Cap. (Ascher).
Az-Kap, Cap. (Keene).
B. A., Prods. (Federal).
Bronchobid, Duracap (Meyer).

•**BUTABARBITAL SODIUM.** U.S.P. XXII. Cap., Elix., Tab., U.S.P. XXII. Sodium 5-sec-butyl-5-ethylbarbiturate.
Use: Sedative/hypnotic.
See: BBS, Tab. (Solvay).
Butalan, Elix. (Lannett).
Buticaps, Cap. (Wallace).
Butisol Sodium, Elix., Tab. (Wallace).
Expansatol, Cap. (Merit).
Quiebar, Spantab, Tab (Nevin).
Renbu, Tab. (Wren).
Soduben Tab., Elix. (Arcum).
W/Acetaminophen.
See: Amino-Bar, Tab. (Bowman).
Minotal, Tab. (Carnrick).
W/Acetaminophen, aspirin, caffeine.
See: Dolor Plus, Tab. (Geriatric).
W/Acetaminophen, caffeine.
See: Dularin-TH, Tab. (Donner).
Phrenilin, Tab. (Carnrick).
W/Acetaminophen, mephenesin, codeine phosphate.
See: Bancaps-C, Cap. (Westerfield).
W/Acetaminophen, salicylamide.
See: Banesin Forte, Tab. (Westerfield).
Indogesic, Tab. (Century).
W/Acetaminophen, salicylamide, d-amphetamine sulfate, hexobarbital, secobarbital sodium, phenobarbital.
See: Sedragesic, Tab. (Lannett).
W/d-Amphetamine sulfate.
See: Bontril, Tab. (Carnrick).
W/Ascorbic acid, sodium p-aminobenzoate, salicylamide, sodium salicylate.
See: Bisalate, Tab. (Allison).
W/Atropine sulfate, hyoscyamine HBr, alcohol, hyoscine HBr.
See: Hyonatol Tab., Hyonatol B Elix., Hexett, Tab. (Bowman).
W/Belladonna extract
See: Butibel, Tab., Elix. (McNeil).
Quiebel, Elix., Cap. (Nevin).
W/Dehydrocholic acid, belladonna extract.
See: Decholin-BB, Tab. (Miles).
W/Methscopolamine bromide, aluminum hydroxide gel, dried, magnesium trisilicate.
See: Eulcin, Tab. (Leeds).
W/Pentobarbital sodium, phenobarbital sodium.
See: Trio-Bar, Tab. (Jenkins).
W/Salicylamide, mephenesin.
See: Metrogesic, Tab. (Metric).
W/Secobarbital sodium.
See: Monosyl, Tab. (Arcum).
W/Secobarbital sodium, pentobarbital sodium, phenobarbital.
See: Nidar, Tab. (Armour).
W/Secobarbital sodium, phenobarbital.

See: S.B.P., Tab. (Lemmon).
W/Simethicone, hyoscyamine sulfate, atropine sulfate, hyoscine HBr.
See: Sidonna, Tab. (Reed & Carnrick).
W/Theophylline, pseudoephedrine HCl.
See: Dilorbron, Cap. (Hauck).
BUTABELL HMB. (Saron) Butabarbital 15 mg, hyoscyamine sulfate 0.1037 mg, atropine sulfate 0.0194 mg, hyoscine HBr 0.0065 mg/Tab. Bot. 100s, 1000s.
Use: Sedative/hypnotic, anticholinergic/antispasmodic.
BUTACAINE.
Use: Local anesthetic.
See: Butyn Dental Oint. (Abbott).
BUTACE. (American Urologicals) Acetaminophen 325 mg, caffeine 40 mg, butalbital 50 mg. Cap. Bot. 100s.
Use: Analgesic, sedative/hypnotic.
•**BUTACETIN.** USAN. 4′-Tert-butoxyacetanilide.
Use: Analgesic.
•**BUTACLAMOL HYDROCHLORIDE.** USAN.
Use: Antipsychotic.
BUTAGEN CAPS. (Goldline) Phenylbutazone 100 mg/Cap. Bot. 100s, 500s.
Use: Antirheumatic.
BUTALAMINE. B.A.N. 5-(2-Dibutylaminoethyl)-amino-3-phenyl-1,2,4-oxadiazole.
Use: Vasodilator.
BUTALAN. (Lannett) Butabarbital sodium 33.3 mg/5 ml, alcohol 7%. Elix. Bot. pt, gal.
Use: Sedative/hypnotic.
•**BUTALBITAL,** U.S.P. XXII. 5-Allyl-5-isobutyl-barbituric acid. Allylbarbituric Acid.
Use: Nonnarcotic analgesic.
See: Buff-A-Comp #3 (Mayrand).
Lotusate, Cap. (Winthrop).
Sandoptal, Preps. (Sandoz).
W/Acetaminophen.
See: Phrenilin, Tab. (Carnrick).
Phrenilin Forte, Cap. (Carnrick).
W/Acetaminophen, codeine.
See: Phrenilin w/Codeine, Cap. (Carnrick).
W/Acetaminophen, caffeine.
See: Arbutal, Tab. (Arcum).
Buff-A-Comp, Tab., Cap. (Mayrand).
Esgic, Tab. (Gilbert).
Cefinal, Tab. (Alto).
Protension, Tab. (Blaine).
Repan, Tab. (Everett).
W/Aspirin, caffeine.
See: Duogesic, Cap. (Western Research).
Fiorinal, Cap., Tab. (Sandoz).
W/Aspirin, caffeine, codeine phosphate.
See: Buff-A-Comp, Tab w/Codeine. (Mayrand).
Fiorinal With Codeine, Cap. (Sandoz).
W/Caffeine, aspirin, acetaminophen.
See: Anaphen, Cap. (Hauck).
•**BUTALBITAL, ACETAMINOPHEN AND CAFFEINE TABLETS,** U.S.P. XXII.
Use: Analgesic.
•**BUTALBITAL AND ASPIRIN TABLETS,** U.S.P. XXII.
Use: Analgesic, sedative.
BUTALBITAL COMPOUND. (Various Mfr.) Tab., Cap. Bot. 100s, 500s, 1000s.
Use: Nonnarcotic analgesic.
W/Acetaminophen, butalbital.
See: Phrenilin (Carnrick).
Bancap (Forest).
Triaprin (Dunhall).
Sedapap-10 (Mayrand).
W/Acetaminophen, caffeine, butalbital.
See: Esgic (Forest).
Fioricat (Sandoz).
Repan (Everett).
Amaphen (Trimen).
Butace (American Pharm.).
Endolor (Keene).
G-1 (Hauck).
Medigesic Plus (U.S. Pharm. Corp.).
Phrenilin Forte (Carnrick).
Sedapap-10 (Mayrand).
W/Aspirin, butalbital.
See: Axotal (Adria).
W/Aspirin, caffeine, butalbital.
See: Fiorgen PF (Goldline).
Fiorinal (Sandoz).
Isollyl Improved (Rugby).
Lanorinal (Lannett).
Lorprn (Russ Pharm.).
B-A-C (Mayrand).
BUTALGIN.
See: Methadone HCl (Various Mfr.).
BUTALAN ELIXIR. (Lannett) Sodium butabarbital 0.2 Gm/30 ml. Bot. pt, gal.
Use: Sedative/hypnotic.
BUTALLYLONAL. 5-(2-Bromoallyl)-5-sec-butyl-barbituric acid. (Pernocton).
Use: Hypnotic.
•**BUTAMBEN,** U.S.P. XXII. Benzoic acid, 4-amino-,butyl ester. Butyl p-aminobenzoate.
Use: Local anesthetic.
•**BUTAMBEN PICRATE.** USAN.
Use: Topical anesthetic.
See: Butesin Picrate, Oint. (Abbott).
•**BUTAMIRATE CITRATE.** USAN.
Use: Antitussive.
•**BUTAMISOLE HYDROCHLORIDE.** USAN.
Use: Anthelmintic.
BUTAMYRATE. B.A.N. 2-(2-Diethylaminoethoxy)-ethyl 2-phenylbutyrate.
Use: Cough suppressant.
•**BUTANE,** N.F. XVII.
Use: Aerosol propellant.
BUTANILICAINE. B.A.N. 2-Butylamino-6′-chloroacet-o-toluidide.
Use: Local anesthetic.
BUTANISAMIDE. 1-Butyl-1-(o-methoxyphenyl) urea.
•**BUTAPERAZINE MALEATE.** USAN.
Use: Antipsychotic.

BUTAPHYLLAMINE. Ambuphylline. Theophylline aminoisobutanol. Theophylline with 2-amino-2-methyl-1-propanol.

BUTAPRO ELIXIR. (Approved) Butabarbital sodium 0.2 Gm/30 ml. Bot. pt, gal.
Use: Sedative/hypnotic.

•**BUTAPROST.** USAN.
Use: Bronchodilator.

BUTAZOLIDIN CAPSULES. (Geigy) Phenylbutazone 100 mg/Cap. Bot. 100s, 1000s, UD 100s, Gy-Pak 100s.
Use: Antirheumatic.

BUTAZOLIDIN TABLETS. (Geigy) Phenylbutazone 100 mg/Tab. Bot. 100s, 1000s, UD 100s.
Use: Antirheumatic.

BUTAZONE. (Major) Phenylbutazone. **Cap.:** 100 mg. Bot. 100s, 500s. **Tab.:** 100 mg. Bot. 500s.
Use: Antirheumatic.

•**BUTEDRONATE TETRASODIUM.** USAN.
Use: Diagnostic aid (bone imaging).

BUTELLINE.
See: Butacaine Sulfate (Various Mfr.).

•**BUTERIZINE.** USAN.
Use: Vasodilator.

BUTESIN PICRATE. n-Butyl-p-aminobenzoate. Butamben picrate.

BUTESIN PICRATE OINTMENT. (Abbott) Butamben picrate 1%. Tube oz.
Use: Local anesthetic.

BUTETHAL. (Various Mfr.) 5-Ethyl-5-butylbarbituric acid.
Use: Sedative/hypnotic.

BUTETHAMATE. B.A.N. 2-Diethylaminoethyl 2-phenylbutyrate.
Use: Antispasmodic.

BUTETHAMINE FORMATE. 2-Isobutyl aminoethyl-p-aminobenzoate formate.

BUTETHAMINE HYDROCHLORIDE. 2-(Isobutylamino) ethyl-p-amino benzoate HCl.
See: Dentocaine (Amer. Chem. & Drug).

BUTETHANOL.
See: Tetracaine.

BUTHALITONE SODIUM. B.A.N. A mixture of 100 parts by weight of the monosodium derivative of 5-allyl-5-isobutyl-2-thiobarbituric acid and 6 parts by weight of dried sodium carbonate.
Use: Sedative/hypnotic.

•**BUTHIAZIDE.** USAN. 6-Chloro-3, 4-dihydro-3-isobutyl-2H-1,2,4-benzothiadiazine-7-sulfonamide 1,1-dioxide.
Use: Diuretic, antihypertensive.

BUTIBEL. (Wallace) Butabarbital sodium 15 mg, belladonna extract 15 mg/Tab or 5 ml. **Tab.** Bot. 100s. **Elix.:** (w/alcohol 7%) Bot. pt.
Use: Sedative/hypnotic, anticholinergic/antispasmodic.

BUTICAPS. (Wallace) Butabarbital sodium 15 mg, 30 mg, 50 mg or 100 mg/Cap. Bot. 100s.
Use: Sedative/hypnotic.

•**BUTIKACIN.** USAN.
Use: Antibacterial.

•**BUTIFENIN.** USAN.
Use: Diagnostic aid.

•**BUTIROSIN SULFATE.** USAN. A mixture of the sulfates of the A and B forms of an antibiotic produced by *Bacillus circularis.*}
Use: Antibacterial.

BUTISOL SODIUM. (Wallace) Butabarbital sodium. **Elix.:** 30 mg/5 ml. Bot pt, gal. **Tab.:** 15 mg, 30 mg, 50 mg or 100 mg. Bot. 100s, 1000s.
Use: Sedative/hypnotic.
See: Buticaps, Cap. (Wallace).
W/Belladonna extract.
See: Butibel, (Wallace).

•**BUTIXIRATE.** USAN.
Use: Analgesic, antirheumatic.

•**BUTOCONAZOLE NITRATE.** USAN.
Use: Antifungal.
See: Femstat, Cream (Syntex).

BUTOLAN. Benzylphenyl carbamate.

•**BUTONATE.** USAN.
Use: Anthelmintic.

•**BUTOPAMINE.** USAN.
Use: Cardiotonic.

BUTOPYRONOXYL. (Indalone) Butylmesityl oxide.
Use: Insect repellant.

•**BUTORPHANOL.** USAN.
Use: Analgesic, antitussive.

•**BUTORPHANOL TARTRATE,** U.S.P. XXII. Inj., U.S.P. XXII.
Use: Analgesic.
See: Stadol, Inj. (Bristol).

BUTOXAMINE. B.A.N. (±)-erythro-1-(2,5-Dimethoxyphenyl)-2-t-butylaminopropan-1-ol.
Use: Inhibitor of fatty acid mobilization.

•**BUTOXAMINE HCl.** USAN.α-[1-(Tertbutylamino)ethyl]-2,5-dimethoxybenzyl alcohol HCl.
Use: Oral hypoglycemic, antilipemic.

BUTRIPTYLINE. B.A.N. DL-3-(10,11-Dihydro-5H-diben- zo[a,d]cycloheptene-5-yl)-2-methyl-propyldimethylamine.
Use: Antidepressant.

•**BUTRIPTYLINE HYDROCHLORIDE.** USAN. dl-10, 11-Dihydro-N, N, β-trimethyl-5H-dibenzo (a,d)cycloheptene-5-propylamine HCl.
Use: Antidepressant.

•**BUTYL ALCOHOL,** N.F. XVII. Butyl alcohol is *n*-butyl alcohol.
Use: Pharmaceutic aid (solvent).

BUTYL AMINOBENZOATE. n-Butyl p-Aminobenzoate. Scuroforme.
Use: Local anesthetic.
W/Benzocaine, tetracaine HCl.
See: Cetacaine, Preps. (Cetylite).
W/Benzyl alcohol, phenylmercuric borate, benzocaine.
See: Dermathyn, Oint. (Davis & Sly).
W/Procaine, benzyl alcohol, in sweet almond oil.
See: Anucaine, Amp. (Calvin).
W/Tetracaine.
See: Pontocaine, Oint. (Winthrop Pharm).
m).

•**BUTYLATED HYDROXYANISOLE,** N.F. XVII. tert-Butyl-4-methoxyphenol.
Use: Pharmaceutic aid (antioxidant).

•**BUTYLATED HYDROXYTOLUENE,** N.F. XVII. B.A.N. 2,6-Di-tert-butyl-P-cresolution
Use: Pharmaceutic aid (antioxidant).

•**BUTYLPARABEN,** N.F. XVII. Butyl p-Hydroxybenzoate.
Use: Pharmaceutical aid (antifungal preservative).

BUTYLPHENAMIDE. N-n-butyl-3-phenyl-salicylamide.

BUTYLPHENYLSALICYLAMIDE.
See: Butylphenamide.

BUTYN DENTAL OINTMENT. (Abbott) Butacaine 4%, benzyl alcohol 1%, eugenol. Tube 7.5 Gm.
Use: Local anesthetic.

B-VITE INJECTION. (Bluco) Vitamins B_1 50 mg, B_2 5 mg, B_6 5 mg, niacinamide 125 mg, B_{12} 1000 mcg, dexpanthenol 6 mg, C 50 mg/10 ml. Mono vial w/benzyl alcohol 1% in water for injection.
Use: Vitamin supplement.

BVU.
See: Bromisovalum.

BYCLOMINE. (Major) Dicyclomine. **Cap.:** 10 mg. Bot. 100s, 250s, 1000s. **Tab.:** 20 mg. Bot. 100s, 250s, 1000s.
Use: Antispasmodic.

BYCLOMINE W/PHENOBARBITAL. (Major) **Cap.:** Dicyclomine HCl 10 mg, phenobarbital 15 mg. Bot. 250s, 1000s. **Tab.:** Dicyclomine HCl 20 mg, phenobarbital 15 mg. Bot. 100s, 250s, 1000s.
Use: Antispasmodic, sedative/hypnotic.

BYDRAMINE. (Major) Diphenhydramine HCl 12.5 mg/5 ml, alcohol 5%. Syr. Bot. 118 ml, pt, gal.
Use: Antihistamine.

BYDRAMINE COUGH. (Major) Diphenhydramine HCl 12.5 mg/5 ml, alcohol 5%. Syr. Bot. 118 ml, pt, gal.
Use: Antitussive.

C

C VITAMIN.
See: Ascorbic Acid, Prep.

•**CABUFOCON B.** USAN.
Use: Contact lens material.

CACODYLIC ACID SALTS.
Ferric Salt.
Iron Salt.
Sodium Salt.

•**CACTINOMYCIN.** USAN. Dactinomycin 10%, actinomycin C_2 45%, actinomycin C_3 45%. Actinomycin C.
Use: Antineoplastic agent.
See: Sanamycin (FBA Pharm).

CADE OIL.
See: Juniper Tar.

CADE OIL CREAM NO. 26. (Durel) Cade oil 3%, ammoniated mercury 2%, in Duromantel cream. Jar 1 oz, 1 lb, 6 lb.
Use: Antipsoriatic.

CADE OIL CREAM NO. 27. (Durel) Cade oil 5%, sulfur 5%, salicylic acid 3% in Duromantel cream. Jar 1 oz, 1 lb, 6 lb.
Use: Antipsoriatic, keratolytic.

•**CADEXOMER IODINE.** USAN.
Use: Antiseptic, antiulcerative.

CAD-O-BATH. (Durel) Oil of cade 35%, polysorbate "20" 35%. Bot. 8 oz, pt, gal.
Use: Antipruritic, antipsoriatic.

CAFATINE PB. (Major) Ergotamine tartrate 2 mg, caffeine 100 mg, belladonna alkaloids 0.25 mg, pentobarbital 60 mg/Supp. Box foil 10s.
Use: Agent for migraine.

CAFEDRINE. B.A.N. L-7-[2-(β-Hydroxy-α-methylphenethylamino)ethyl]-theophylline.
Use: Analeptic.

CAFENOL. (Winthrop Products) Aspirin, caffeine.
Use: Salicylate analgesic.

CAFERGOT P-B SUPPOSITORIES. (Sandoz) Ergotamine tartrate 2 mg, caffeine 100 mg, bellafoline 0.25 mg, pentobarbital 60 mg/Supp. Box 12s.
Use: Agent for migraine.

CAFERGOT P-B TABLETS. (Sandoz) Ergotamine tartrate 1 mg, caffeine 100 mg, bellafoline 0.125 mg, pentobarbital sodium 30 mg/Tab. SigPak dispensing pkg. of 90s, 250s.
Use: Agent for migraine.

CAFERGOT SUPPOSITORIES. (Sandoz) Ergotamine tartrate 2 mg, caffeine 100 mg in cocoa butter base. Box 12s.
Use: Agent for migraine.

CAFERGOT TABLETS. (Sandoz) Ergotamine tartrate 1 mg, caffeine 100 mg/S.C. Tab. Bot. 250s. SigPak dispensing pkg. of 90s.
Use: Agent for migraine.

CAFFEDRINE. (Thompson) Caffeine 200 mg/T.R. Cap. Bot. 20s.
Use: CNS stimulant.

•**CAFFEINE,** U.S.P. XXII. 1H-purine-2,6-dione,3,-7-dihydro-1,3,7-trimethyl-xanthine. Guaranine; Methyltheobromine; Thein.
Use: CNS stimulant.
See: Enerjets, Loz. (Chilton).
Femicin, Tab. (Norcliff Thayer).
Nodoz, Tab. (Bristol-Myers).
Stim 250, Cap. (Scrip).
Tirend (Norcliff-Thayer).
Vivarin, Tab. (J.B. Williams).

CAFFEINE CITRATED.
Use: CNS stimulant.

CAFFEINE SODIO-BENZOATE.
See: Caffeine sodium benzoate.

•**CAFFEINE SODIUM BENZOATE INJECTION,** U.S.P. XXII. Approximately equal parts of caffeine and sodium benzoate. (Various Mfr.) Amp. (3¾ gr and 7.5 gr) 2 ml, Box 12s, 100s. Hypo Tab. (1 gr) Tube 20s, 100s and Pow.

Use: Orally, I.M. central nervous system stimulant.

CAFFEINE SODIUM SALICYLATE. (Various Mfr.) Bot. 1 oz; Pkg. 0.25 lb, 1 lb.
Use: See caffeine.

CAFFEINE-THEOPHYLLINE COMPOUND. w/ Nux Vomica Ext.
See: Xanthinux, Tab. (Cole).

CAFFIN-T.D. (Kenyon) Caffeine 250 mg/Cap. Bot. 100s.
Use: CNS stimulant.

CAGOL. (Harvey) Guaiacol 0.1 Gm, eucalyptol 0.08 Gm, iodoform 0.2 Gm, camphor 0.05 Gm/2 ml in olive oil. Vial 30 ml.
Use: Expectorant.

CALADRYL. (Parke-Davis) Benadryl HCl 1% in specially prepared calamine base. **Cream:** Tube 1.5 oz, **Lot.:** Bot. 6 oz Plastic Squeeze Bot. 2.5 oz
Use: Minor skin irritations.

CALAFORMULA. (Eric, Kirk & Gary) Ferrous gluconate 130 mg, calcium lactate 130 mg, vitamins A 1000 IU, D 400 IU, B_1 2 mg, B_2 2 mg, niacinamide 5 mg, ascorbic acid 20 mg, folic acid 0.13 mg, magnesium 0.25 mg, copper 0.25 mg, zinc 0.25 mg, manganese 0.25 mg, potassium 0.075 mg/Cap. Bot. 50s, 100s, 500s, 1000s, 5000s.
Use: Vitamin/mineral supplement.

CALAFORMULA WITH AMPHETAMINE. (Eric, Kirk & Gary) Calaformula with amphetamine sulfate 5 mg/Cap. Bot. 100s.
Use: Vitamin/mineral supplement, CNS stimulant.

CALAFORMULA F. (Eric, Kirk & Gary) Calaformula plus fluorine 0.333 mg/Tab. Bot. 100s.
Use: Vitamin/mineral supplement, dental caries preventative.

CALAHIST LOTION. (Walgreen) Diphenhydramine HCl 1%, calamine 8.1%, camphor 0.1%. Bot. 6 oz.
Use: Minor skin irritations.

CALAMATUM. (Blair) **Lot.:** Calamine, zinc oxide, phenol, camphor, benzocaine 3%, nongreasy base. Bot. 1125 ml. **Oint:** Calamine, zinc oxide, phenol, camphor, benzocaine. Tube 45 Gm.
Use: Minor skin irritations.

CALAMATUM AEROSOL SPRAY. (Blair) Benzocaine 3%, zinc oxide, calamine, phenol, camphor. Spray can 3 oz.
Use: Minor skin irritations.

•**CALAMINE,** U.S.P. XXII. (Various Mfr.) : Calamine 8%, zinc oxide 8%, glycerin 2%, bentonite magma, calcium hydroxide soln. Lot. Bot. 120 ml, 240 ml, pt, gal.
Use: Astringent, mild antiseptic.

CALAMOX. (Hauck) Prepared calamine 0.17 Gm. Oint. Tube 60 Gm.
Use: Astringent, mild antiseptic.

CALAMYCIN. (Pfeiffer) Pyrilamine maleate, zinc oxide 10%, calamine 10%, benzocaine, chloroxylenol, zirconium oxide, isopropyl alcohol 10%. Lot. Bot. 120 ml.
Use: Minor skin irritations.

CALAN. (Searle) Verapamil HCl 40 mg, 80 mg or 120 mg/Tab. Bot. 100s, 500s, 1000s, UD 100s.
Use: Calcium channel blocking agent.

CALAN SR. (Searle) Verapamil HCl 180 mg or 240 mg/SR Capl. Bot. 60s, 100s, UD 100s.
Use: Calcium channel blocking agent.

CAL-BID. (Geriatric) Elemental calcium 250 mg, ascorbic acid 100 mg, vitamin D 125 IU/Tab. Bot. 100s.
Use: Vitamin/mineral supplement.

CALCET. (Mission) Elemental calcium 153 mg, vitamin D 100 units/Tab. Bot. 100s.
Use: Vitamin/mineral supplement.

CALCET PLUS. (Mission) Elemental calcium 152.8 mg, elemental iron 18 mg, vitamins A 5000 IU, D 400 IU, E 24.8 mg, B_1 2.25 mg, B_2 2.55 mg, B_3 30 mg, B_5 15 mg, B_6 3 mg, B_{12} 9 mcg, C 500 mg, folic acid 0.8 mg, zinc 15 mg/Tab. Bot 100s.
Use: Vitamin/mineral supplement.

CALCIBIND. (Mission) Inorganic phosphate content ≈ 34%, sodium content ≈ 11%. Packets: Cellulose sodium phosphate 25 Gm. Single dose 90 packets, 300 Gm bulk pack.
Use: Urinary tract product.

CALCICAPS. (Nion) Calcium (dibasic calcium phosphate, calcium gluconate, calcium carbonate) 125 mg, vitamin D 67 IU, phosphorus 60 mg/Tab. Bot. 100s, 500s.
Use: Vitamin/mineral supplement.

CALCICAPS WITH IRON. (Nion) Calcium 125 mg, phosphorus 60 mg, vitamin D 67 IU, ferrous gluconate 7 mg, tartrazine/Tab. Bot. 100s, 500s.
Use: Vitamin/mineral supplement.

CALCICAPS, SUPER. (Nion) Calcium 400 mg, phosphorus 41.7 mg, vitamin D 100 IU/Tab. Bot. 90s.
Use: Vitamin/mineral supplement.

CALCI-CHEW. (R & D) Calcium carbonate 1.25 Gm (500 mg calcium)/Chew. Tab. Bot. 100s.
Use: Antacid.

CALCIDAY-667. (Nature's Bounty) Calcium carbonate 667 mg (266.8 mg calcium)/Tab. Bot. 60s.
Use: Antacid.

CALCIDRINE SYRUP. (Abbott) Codeine 8.4 mg, calcium iodide anhydrous 152 mg, alcohol 6%/5 ml. Bot. 120 ml, 480 ml.
Use: Antitussive, expectorant.

•**CALCIFEDIOL,** U.S.P. XXII. Cap., U.S.P. XXII. 25-hydroxycholecalciferol; 25[OH]$-D_3$.
Use: Calcium regulator.
See: Calderol (Organon).

CALCIFEROL, U.S.P. XXII. Ergosterol. (D_2) **Liq:** 8000 IU/ml. Bot. 60 ml. **Tab:** 50,000 IU. Bot. 100s. **Inj:** 500,000 IU/ml. Amp. 1 ml.
Use: Vitamin D (antirachitic).

CALCIJEX. (Abbott) Calcitriol injection 1 mcg or 2 mcg/ml. Amp. 1 ml.
Use: Vitamin supplement.

CALCILAC. (Schein) Calcium carbonate 420 mg, glycine 180 mg/Tab. Bot. 1000s.
Use: Antacid.

CALCIMAR INJECTION, SYNTHETIC. (Rorer) Calcitonin solution (Salmon origin) containing 200 IU/ml. Vial 2 ml.
Use: Treatment of Paget's disease.

CALCIPARINE. (DuPont Critical Care) Heparin calcium in water for injection. **5000** units/0.2 ml prefilled syringe. **12,500** units/0.5 ml Amp. **20,000** units/0.8 ml Amp.
Use: Anticoagulant.

CALCITONIN.
Use: Treatment of Paget's disease.
See: Calcimar (USV).
Cibacalcin (Ciba).
Miacalcin (Sandoz).

•**CALCITONIN HUMAN.** USAN. Hormone from thyroid gland.
Use: Plasma hypocalcemic hormone.
See: Cibacalcin (Ciba).

CALCITONIN SALMON.
See: Calcimar (USV).
Miacalcin (Sandoz).

•**CALCITRIOL.** USAN. 9,10-seco(5Z,7E)-5,7,10(19)-cholestatriene-1a, 3b, 25-triol.
Use: Management of hypocalcemia in chronic renal dialysis patients.
See: Calcijex, Inj. (Abbott).
Rocaltrol, Cap. (Roche).

CALCIUM ACETYLSALICYLATE. Kalmopyrin, kalsetal, soluble aspirin, tylcalsin.
Use: Salicylate analgesic.

CALCIUM ALUMINUM CARBONATE. W/DI-Amino acetate complex.
See: Ancid Tab., Susp. (Sheryl).

CALCIUM AMINOSALICYLATE. Aminosalicylate calcium, N.F. XVII.

CALCIUM AMPHOMYCIN.
See: Amphomycin.

•**CALCIUM AND MAGNESIUM CARBONATES TABLETS,** U.S.P. XXII.
Use: Antacid.

CALCIUM ASCORBATE. (Freeda) **Tab.:** Calcium ascorbate 610 mg (equivalent to 500 mg ascorbic acid). Bot. 100s, 250s, 500s. **Pow.:** Calcium ascorbate 1 Gm (equivalent to 826 mg ascorbic acid) per ¼ tsp. Bot. 120 Gm, 448 Gm.
Use: Calcium supplement.

CALCIUM 4-BENZAMIDOSALICYLATE. Calcium Aminacyl B-PAS. Benzoylpas Calcium.
See: Benzapas, Pow., Tab. (Dorsey).

CALCIUM BENZAMIDOSALICYLATE. B.A.N. Calcium 4-benzamido-2-hydroxybenzoate.
Use: Treatment of tuberculosis.

CALCIUM BENZOYL-p-AMINOSALICYLATE.
See: Benzoylpas calcium.

CALCIUM BENZOYLPAS.
See: Benzoylpas calcium.

CALCIUM BIS-DIOCTYL SULFOSUCCINATE.
See: Dioctyl Calcium Sulfosuccinate.

•**CALCIUM CARBONATE AND MAGNESIA TABLETS,** U.S.P. XXII.
Use: Antacid.

•**CALCIUM CARBONATE, MAGNESIA, AND SIMETHICONE,** U.S.P. XXII. Tab

CALCIUM CARBONATE, AROMATIC. (Lilly) Calcium carbonate 10 gr/Tab. Bot. 100s, 1000s.
Use: Antacid.

•**CALCIUM CARBONATE, PRECIPITATED,** U.S.P. XXII. (Various Mfr.) Precipitated chalk; carbonic acid, calcium salt (1:1).
Use: Antacid.
See: Amitone, Tab. (Norcliff Thayer).
Biocal Prods. (Miles).
Cal-Sup, Tab. (Riker).
Dicarbosil, Tab. (Arch).
Mallamint, Tab. (Mallard).
Tums, Tab. (Norcliff Thayer).

CALCIUM CARBONATE W/COMBINATIONS
See: Accelerase, Cap. (Organon).
Alkets, Tab. (Upjohn).
Anti-Acid No. 1, Tab. (Vortech).
Camalox, Tab., Susp. (Rorer Consumer).
Ca-Plus, Tab. (Miller).
Co-Gel, Tab. (Arco).
Diatrol, Tab. (Otis Clapp).
Dimacid, Tab. (Otis Clapp).
Gas-Eze, Tab. (E.J. Moore).
Kanalka, Tab. (Lannett).
Kaocasil, Tab. (Jenkins).
Lactocal, Tab. (Laser).
Natabec, Prep. (Parke-Davis).
Titralac, Liq., Tab. (Riker).

•**CALCIUM CARBONATE ORAL SUSPENSION,** U.S.P. XXII.
Use: Antacid.

CALCIUM CARBIMIDE. Calcium cyanamide.

CALCIUM CASEINATE.
See: Casec, Pow. (Mead Johnson).

CALCIUM CHANNEL BLOCKERS.
Use: Angina pectoris, vasospastic and unstable angina.
See: Adalat, Cap. (Miles).
Calan, Inj., Tab, (Searle).
Calan SR, SR Cap. (Searle).
Cardizem, Tab. (Marion).
DynaCirc (Sandoz).
Isoptin, Inj., Tab. (Knoll).
Isoptin SR, SR Cap. (Knoll).
Procardia, Cap. (Pfizer).
Vasor (McNeil).
Verapamil HCl, Inj., Tab. (Various Mfr.).

CALCIUM CHEL 330. (Geigy).
Use: Heavy metal antagonist.
See: Calcium Trisodium Pentetate.

•**CALCIUM CHLORIDE,** U.S.P. XXII. Inj., U.S.P. XXII. 1 Gm (10 ml) contains 272 mg (13.6 mEq) calcium. Inj: 10% soln. Amp., vial, syringe 10 ml.
Use: Electrolyte.

•**CALCIUM CHLORIDE CA 45.** USAN.
Use: Radioactive agent.
•**CALCIUM CHLORIDE CA 47.** USAN.
Use: Radioactive agent.
•**CALCIUM CHLORIDE INJECTION,** U.S.P. XXII. (Upjohn) 1 Gm Amp. 10 ml, 25s. (Torigian) 1 Gm Amp. 10 ml 12s, 25s, 100s. (Trent) 10% Amp. 10 ml (Cutter) 13.6 mEq./10 ml Vial.
Use: IV, hypocalcemic tetany.
•**CALCIUM CITRATE,** U.S.P. XXII.
Use: Calcium supplement.
CALCIUM CYCLAMATE. Calcium cyclohexanesulfamate.
CALCIUM CYCLOBARBITAL. Calcium 5-(l-cyclohexen-l-yl)-5-ethylbarbiturate.
Use: Central depressant.
CALCIUM CYCLOHEXANESULFAMATE.
See: Calcium Cyclamate.
CALCIUM DL-PANTOTHENATE. Calcium Pantothenate, Racemic, U.S.P. XXII.
CALCIUM DIOCTYL SULFOSUCCINATE. Docusate Calcium, U.S.P. XXII.
See: Surfak (Hoechst).
CALCIUM DISODIUM EDATHAMIL.
See: Edetate Calcium Disodium, U.S.P. XXII.
CALCIUM DISODIUM EDETATE. Edetate Calcium Disodium, U.S.P. XXII.
Use: Antidote for acute and chronic lead poisoning, lead encephalopathy.
See: Calcium Disodium Versenate (Riker).
CALCIUM DISODIUM VERSENATE. (Riker) Calcium Disodium Edetate U.S.P. Inj.: 200 mg/ml. Amp 5 ml.
Use: IV or IM for lead poisoning and/or lead encephalopathy.
CALCIUM EDETATE SODIUM. Edetate Calcium Disodium, U.S.P. XXII.
Use: Antidote for acute and chronic lead poisoning or lead encephalopathy.
CALCIUM EDTA.
See: Calcium Disodium Versenate, Amp. (Riker).
CALCIUM FOLINATE. B.A.N. Calcium N-[4-(2-amino-5-formyl-5,6,7,8-tetrahydro-4-hydroxypteridinyl-6-methyl-aminobenzoyl]-L-glutamate.
Use: Antidote to folic acid antagonists.
See: Leucovorin Calcium.
•**CALCIUM GLUBIONATE.** USAN. 6.5% Calcium.
Use: Calcium replenisher.
See: Neo-Calglucon (Sandoz).
•**CALCIUM GLUCEPTATE,** U.S.P. XXII. (Various Mfr.) 1.1 Gm (5 ml) contains 90 mg (4.5 mEq) calcium. Inj.: 1.1 Gm/5 ml. Amp. 5 ml. Vial 50 ml.
Use: Calcium electrolyte replacement.
See: Calcium Gluceptate (Abbott).
Calcium Gluceptate (I.M.S).
Calcium Gluceptate (Lilly).
CALCIUM GLUCOHEPTONATE. (Various Mfr.) Cal. D-glucoheptonate O.
Use: Calcium supplement.
•**CALCIUM GLUCONATE,** U.S.P. XXII. 9% Calcium. Tab.: 500 mg (calcium 45 mg), 650 mg (calcium 58.5 mg), 975 mg (calcium 87.75 mg) or 1 Gm (calcium 90 mg). Bot. 100s, 200s, 500s, 1000s, UD 100s.
Use: Calcium replacement.
CALCIUM GLYCEROPHOSPHATE. Neurosin. (Various Mfr.).
•**CALCIUM HYDROXIDE,** U.S.P. XXII. Topical Soln. U.S.P. XXII.
Use: Astringent; pharmaceutic necessity for calamine lotion.
CALCIUM HYDROXIDE POWDER. (Lilly) Powder 4 oz/Bot.
Use: Preparation of lime water solution.
CALCIUM HYPOPHOSPHITE. (N.Y. Quinine & Chem. Works).
CALCIUM IODIDE.
W/Codeine phosphate.
See: Calcidrine Syr. (Abbott).
W/Chloral hydrate, ephedrine HCl.
See: Iophed, Syr. (Marsh Labs).
CALCIUM IODIZED.
See: Cal-Lime-1, Tab. (Scrip).
W/Calcium creosotate.
See: Niocrese, Tab. (Noyes).
W/Ipecac, hyoscyamus extract, licorice extract.
See: Kaldifane, Tab. (Noyes).
CALCIUM IODOBEHENATE. Calioben. (Various Mfr.).
CALCIUM IPODATE. Ipodate Calcium, U.S.P. XXII.
See: Oragrafin Calcium, Granules (Squibb).
CALCIUM KINATE GLUCONATE. Kinate is hexahydrotetrahydroxybenzoate. Calcium Quinate.
•**CALCIUM LACTATE,** U.S.P. XXII. 13% Calcium. Tab.: 325 mg (42.25 mg Calcium) or 650 mg (84.5 mg Calcium). Bot. 100s, 1000s, UD 100s.
Use: Calcium deficiency and prophylaxis.
W/Calcium glycerophosphate.
See: Calphosan, Amp., Vial (Carlton).
W/Calcium glycerophosphate, phenol, sodium Cl solution.
See: Calpholac, Vial (Century).
Calphosan, Inj. (Brown).
W/Niacinamide, folic acid, ferrous gluconate, vitamins.
See: Pergrava No. 2, Cap. (Arcum).
W/Phenobarbital, extract hyoscyamus, terpin hydrate, guaifenesin.
See: Gylanphen, Tab. (Lannett).
W/Theobromine sodium salicylate, phenobarbital.
See: Theolaphen, Tab. (Elder).
W/Thiamine HCl.
See: Nycralan, Tab. (Lannett).
W/Zinc sulfate.
See: Zinc-220, Cap. (Alto).
•**CALCIUM LACTOBIONATE,** U.S.P. XXII.
Use: Calcium supplement.
CALCIUM LACTOPHOSPHATE. Lactic acid hydrogen phosphate calcium salt.

CALCIUM LEUCOVORIN. Leucovorin Calcium, U.S.P. XXII. Inj., tab., powder for oral, powder for inj.
Use: Overdosage folic acid antagonists, megalobastic anemias.
See: Leucovorin Calcium (Lederle).
Wellcovorin (Burroughs Wellcome).
CALCIUM MANDELATE. Urisept (Grail).
Use: Urinary antiseptic, acidifier.
CALCIUM NOVOBIOCIN. Calcium salt of an antibacterial substance produced by *Streptomyces niveus.*
Use: Anti-infective.
CALCIUM OROTATE.
See: Calora, Tab. (Miller).
CALCIUM OXYTETRACYCLINE. Oxytetracycline Calcium, N.F. XIV.
CALCIUM OYSTER SHELL. (Schein) $Calcium^{++}$ 250 mg, vitamin D 125 IU/Tab. Bot. 250s, 1000s.
Use: Calcium supplement.
•**CALCIUM PANTOTHENATE,** U.S.P. XXII. Tab., U.S.P. XXII. β-Alanine, N-(2,4-dihydroxy-3,3-dimethyl-1-oxobutyl)-,calcium salt (2:1). vitamin B_5. D(+)-N-(alpha, gamma dihydroxy-beta,beta-dimethyl-butyryl)-beta aminopropionic acid, calcium salt, dextro form. Pantothenic Acid. Tab.
Use: Pantothenic acid (B_5) deficiency, coenzyme A precursor.
See: Calcium Pantothenate (Freeda).
Calcium Pantothenate (Fibertone).
W/Ascorbic acid, niacinamide, vitamins B_1, B_2, B_6, B_{12}, A, D, E.
See: Tota-Vi-Caps Gelatin Capsule, Cap. (Elder).
W/Calcium carbonate.
See: Ilomel, Pow. (Warren-Teed).
W/Calcium carbonate, ferrous fumarate, niacinamide.
See: Prenatag, Tab. (Reid-Rowell).
W/Danthron.
See: Modane, Tab., Liq. (Warren-Teed).
Parlax, Tab. (Parmed).
W/Docusate sodium.
See: Pantyl, Tab. (McGregor).
W/Docusate sodium, acetphenolisatin.
See: Android-Plus, Tab. (Brown).
Peri-Pantyl, Tab. (McGregor).
W/Methoscopolamine nitrate, mephobarbital.
See: Ilocalm, Tabs. (Warren-Teed).
W/Niacinamide and vitamins.
See: Allbee C-800, Prods. (Robins).
Allbee T, Cap. (Robins).
Allbee with C, Cap. (Robins).
Ferrovite, Tab. (Laser).
Fumatinic, Tab. (Laser).
Maintenance Vitamin Formula, Tab. (Burgin-Arden).
Mulvidren, Tab. (Stuart).
OB-Tabs, Tab. (Laser).
Probec, Tab. (Stuart).
Probec-T, Tab. (Stuart).
Stuart Hematinic, Tab. (Stuart).
Stuart Therapeutic Multivitamin, Tab. (Stuart).
Vita Cebus, Tab. (Cenci).
W/Niacinamide, vitamins B_1, B_2, B_6.
See: Noviplex Capsules, Cap. (Elder).
W/Vitamins B_1, B_2, B_6, B_{12}, niacinamide, choline Cl, inositol, dl-methionine, testosterone, estrone, procaine.
See: Gerihorm, Inj. (Burgin-Arden).
W/Vitamin complex, ferrous fumarate, folic acid, calcium lactate, niacinamide.
See: Vitanate, Tab. (Century).
W/Vitamins A, D, B_1, B_2, C, niacinamide, calcium phosphorus, iron, B_6, B_{12}, E, magnesium, manganese, potassium, zinc, choline bitartrate, inositol.
See: Geriatric Vitamin Formula, Tab. (Burgin-Arden).
W/Vitamins A, E, C, zinc sulfate, magnesium sulfate, niacinamide, B_1, B_2, manganese Cl, B_6, folic acid, B_{12}.
See: Vicon Forte, Cap. (Glaxo).
W/Vitamin C, niacin, zinc sulfate, vitamins E, B_1, B_2, B_6, B_{12}.
See: Z-Bec, Tab. (Robins).
W/Vitamin complex, iron.
See: Vita-iron, Tab. (Century).
W/Vitamins,minerals, niacinamide.
See: Arcum-VM, Cap. (Arcum).
Capre, Tab. (Marion).
Orovimin, Tab. (Reid-Rowell).
Os-Cal Forte, Tab. (Marion).
Os-Vim, Tab. (Marion).
Stuartinic, Tab. (Stuart).
Theramin, Tab. (Arcum).
Theron, Tab. (Stuart).
Uplex, Cap. (Arcum).
W/Vitamins, minerals, methyl testosterone, ethinyl estradiol, niacinamide.
See: Geritag, Cap. (Reid-Rowell).
W/Vitamin C, niacinamide, zinc sulfate, magnesium sulfate, vitamins B_1, B_2, B_6.
See: Vicon-C, Cap. (Glaxo).
W/Zinc sulfate, niacinamide, magnesium sulfate, manganese sulfate, vitamin complex.
See: Vicon Plus, Cap. (Glaxo).
•**CALCIUM PANTOTHENATE, RACEMIC,** U.S.P. XXII. β-Alanine, N-(2,4-dihydroxy-3,3-dimethyl-1-oxo- butylO-, calcium salt (2:1), (±-Calcium DL-pan- tothenate (1:2).
Use: Vitamin B (enzyme cofactor).
See: Pantholin (Lilly).
•**CALCIUM PHOSPHATE, DIBASIC,** U.S.P. XXII. Tab., U.S.P. XXII.
Use: Calcium replenisher.
See: Dicalcium Phosphate.
Diostate D, Tab. (Upjohn).
CALCIUM PHOSPHATE, MONOCALCIUM.
See: Dicalcium Phosphate.
•**CALCIUM PHOSPHATE, TRIBASIC.** Tricalcium Phosphate, N.F. XVII. 39% Calcium. Tab.
Use: Calcium replacement.

See: Posture (Wyeth-Ayerst).
CALCIUM-PHOSPHORUS-FREE.
See: Fosfree, Tab. (Mission).
•**CALCIUM POLYCARBOPHIL,** U.S.P. XXII. Tab.
Use: Cathartic.
See: Fibercon, Tab. (Lederle).
Mitrolan (Robins).
CALCIUM POLYSULFIDE.
Use: Wet dressing, soak.
See: Vlemasque, Cream. (Permik).
Vleminckx', Soln. (Ulmer).
CALCIUM PROPIONATE.
See: Propionate-caprylate mixtures.
CALCIUM QUINATE.
See: Calcium Kinate Gluconate.
•**CALCIUM SACCHARATE,** U.S.P. XXII.
Use: Sweetening agent.
CALCIUM SACCHARIN. Saccharin Calcium, U.S.P. XXII.
Use: Sweetening agent.
CALCIUM SALICYLATE, THEOBROMINE.
See: Theocalcin, Tab., Pow. (Knoll).
CALCIUM SALTS OF SENNOSIDES A & B.
Use: Laxative.
See: Gentle Nature, Tab. (Sandoz).
Nytilax, Tab. (Mentholatum).
•**CALCIUM SILICATE,** N.F. XVII. A compound of calcium oxide and silicon dioxide.
Use: Pharmaceutic aid (tablet excipient).
•**CALCIUM STEARATE,** N.F. XVII.
Use: Pharmaceutic aid (tablet lubricant).
CALCIUM SUCCINATE.
W/Aspirin.
See: Ber-Ex, Tab. (Dolcin).
Dolcin, Tab. (Dolcin).
W/Phenobarbital, salicylamide, vitamin C.
See: Calsuxaphen, Cap., Tab. (Lannett).
•**CALCIUM SULFATE,** N.F. XVII.
Use: Pharmaceutic aid (tablet diluent).
CALCIUM THIOSULFATE.
Use: Wet dressing, soak.
See: Vlemasque Cream (Dermik).
Vleminckx', Soln. (Ulmer).
CALCIUM TRISODIUM PENTETATE. Calcium trisodium (carboxymethylimino)-bis(ethyl-enenitrilo) tetra-acetic acid.
Use: Heavy metal antagonist.
See: Calcium Chel 330 (Geigy).
CALCIUM TRISODIUM PENTETATE. B.A.N. Calcium chelate of the trisodium salt of diethylenetriamine-NNN'N"N"-penta-acetic acid.
Use: Chelating agent.
CALCIUM UNDECYLENATE. 10% calcium undecylenate Pow.
Use: Antifungal.
See: Caldesene, Pow. (Pharmacraft).
Cruex Squeeze Pow. (Pharmacraft).
CALCIUM WITH VITAMIN D. (Schein) Calcium^{++} 600 mg, vitamin D 125 IU Bot. 60s.
Use: Calcium supplement.
CALDECORT CREAM. (Pharmacraft) Hydrocortisone acetate equivalent to hydrocortisone 0.5% in lanolin, white petroleum, mineral oil base. Tube 15 Gm, 30 Gm.
Use: Corticosteroid, topical.
CALDECORT LIGHT CREAM. (Pharmacraft) Hydrocortisone acetate equivalent to hydrocortisone 0.5% w/aloe cream. Tube 15 Gm.
Use: Corticosteroid, topical.
CALDECORT SPRAY. (Pharmacraft) Hydrocortisone 0.5%. Aerosol can 1.5 oz
Use: Corticosteroid, topical.
CALDEE. (Jenkins) Ascorbic acid (sodium ascorbate equivalent to 10 mg vitamin C) 10 mg, vitamin D 200 IU, dicalcium phosphate 7.5 gr, irradiated yeast/Tab. Bot. 1000s.
Use: Vitamin/mineral supplement.
CALDEROL. (Organon) Calcifediol 20 mcg or 50 mcg/Tab. Bot. 60s.
Use: Calcium supplement.
CALDESENE. (Pharmacraft) **Oint.:** Cod liver oil (vitamins A, D) zinc oxide 15%, lanolin, petroleum 54%, talc. Tube 37.5 Gm. **Pow.:** Calcium undecylenate 10%. Bot. 60 Gm, 120 Gm.
Use: Antifungal.
•**CALDIAMIDE SODIUM.** USAN.
Use: Pharmaceutic aid.
CAL-D-MINT. (Enzyme Process) Calcium 800 mg, magnesium 150 mg, iron 18 mg, iodine 0.1 mg, copper 2 mg, vitamin D 200 IU/2 Tab. Bot. 100s, 250s.
Use: Vitamin/mineral supplement.
CAL-D-PHOS. (Archer-Taylor) Dicalcium phosphate 4.5 gr, calcium gluconate 3 gr, vitamin D/ Tab. Bot. 1000s.
Use: Vitamin/mineral supplement.
CALEL-D TABLETS. (Rorer) Calcium 500 mg, vitamin D 200 IU/Tab. Bot. 60s, 75s.
Use: Vitamin/mineral supplement.
CALFER-VITE. (Drug Industries) Iron (ferrous fumarate) 30 mg, vitamins A 5000 IU, D 400 IU, B_1 3 mg, B_2 3 mg, B_3 20 mg, B_5 5 mg, B_6 2 mg, B_{12} 2 mcg, C 75 mg, Cu, I, Mg, Zn, lemon bioflavonoid complex/Tab. Bot. 100s, 500s.
Use: Vitamin/mineral supplement.
CALFOS D TABLETS. (Pal-Pak) Dibasic calcium phosphate 486 mg, vitamin D 100 IU/Tab. Bot. 1000s.
Use: Vitamin/mineral supplement.
CALGLYCINE TABLETS. (Rugby) Calcium carbonate 420 mg, glycine 180 mg, saccharin/ Chew. Tab. Bot. 250s, 1000s.
Use: Antacid.
CALICARB. (Jenkins) Calcium carbonate 0.25 Gm, magnesium carbonate 0.15 Gm, bismuth subnitrate 60 mg, powdered ipecac 0.25 mg, aromatics/Tab. Bot. 1000s.
Use: Antacid.
CALICYLIC CREME. (Gordon) Salicylic acid 10%, mineral oil, cetyl alcohol, propylene glycol white wax, sodium lauryl sulfate, oleic acid, methyl and propyl parabens, triethanolamine. 6 Gm.
Use: Keratolytic.

CAL-IM. (Standex; Kenyon) Calcium glycerophosphate 1%, calcium levulinate 1.5%. Vial 30 ml.
Use: Calcium supplement.

CALINATE-FA. (Reid-Rowell) Calcium 250 mg, vitamins A 4000 IU, D 400 IU, B_1 3 mg, B_2 3 mg, B_6 5 mg, B_{12} 1 mcg, folic acid 1 mg, C 50 mg, B_3 (niacinamide) 20 mg, B_5 (d-panthenol 1 mg), iron 60 mg, iodine 0.02 mg, manganese 0.2 mg, magnesium 0.2 mg, zinc 0.1 mg, copper 0.15 mg/Tab. Bot. 100s.
Use: Vitamin/mineral supplement.

CALIOBEN.
See: Calcium Iodobehenate.

CALIVITE. (Apco) Calcium carbonate 885 mg, ferrous sulfate 199 mg, vitamins A 3600 IU, D 400 IU, C 75 mg, B_1 1.5 mg, B_2 1.95 mg, B_6 0.75 mg, nicotinic acid 15 mg, B_{12} activity 0.025 mcg, choline 1500 mcg, inositol 2500 mcg, pantothenic acid 75 mcg, folic acid 25 mcg, p-aminobenzoic acid 12 mcg, potassium 10 mg, magnesium 1 mg, zinc 0.075 mg, manganese 0.02 mg, copper 0.01 mg, cobalt 0.02 mcg/Tab. Bot. 100s.
Use: Vitamin/mineral supplement.

CAL-LIME-1. (Scrip) Calcium iodized 1 gr/Tab. Bot. 1000s.

CALMOL 4. (Mentholatum) **Supp.:** Cocoa butter 80%, zinc oxide 10%, bismuth subgallate. Box 12s, 24s. **Cream:** Zinc oxide 5%. In 28 Gm.
Use: Anorectal preparation.

CALMOSIN. (Spanner) Calcium gluconate, strontium bromide. Amp. 10 ml. 100s.

CALOCARB TABLETS. (Vale) Calcium carbonate 648 mg/Tab. w/cinnamon flavor. Bot. 1000s.
Use: Antacid.

CALOMEL. MercurousCl.
Use: Cathartic.

CALOTABS. Reformulated. (Calotabs) Docusate sodium 100 mg, casanthranol 30 mg/Tab. Box 10s.
Use: Laxative.

CALOXIDINE (IODIZED CALCIUM).
See: Calcium Iodized.

CALPHOSAN. (Glenwood) Calcium glycerophosphate 50 mg, calcium lactate 50 mg/10 ml sodium Cl solution. Contains calcium 0.08 mEq/ml. Inj. Amp. 10 ml, Vial 60 ml.
Use: Calcium supplement.

CAL-PLUS. (Geriatric) Calcium carbonate 1500 mg/Tab. Bot. 100s.
Use: Calcium supplement.

CALSAN. (Burgin-Arden) Calcium glycerophosphate 10 mg, calcium levulinate 15 mg, chlorobutanol 0.5%/ml. Inj. Vial 100 ml.
Use: Calcium supplement.

CAL SUP INSTANT 1000. (3M Personal Care Products) Elemental calcium 1000 mg, vitamins D 400 IU, C 60 mg. Pow. Packet 12s.
Use: Vitamin/mineral supplement.

CAL SUP 600 PLUS. (3M Personal Care Products) Elemental calcium 600 mg, vitamins D 200 IU, C 30 mg/Tab. Bot. 60s.
Use: Vitamin/mineral supplement.

CALSUXAPHEN. (Lannett) Calcium succinate 2.5 gr, salicylamide 4 gr, phenobarbital ⅛ gr, vitamin C 30 mg/Cap., Tab. Bot. 250s, 500s, 1000s.
Use: Analgesic, sedative/hypnotic.

•**CALTERIDOL CALCIUM.** USAN.
Use: Pharmaceutic aid.

CALTRATE 600. (Lederle) Calcium carbonate 1.5 Gm (calcium 600 mg). Bot. 60s, 120s.
Use: Calcium supplement.

CALTRATE 600 + D. (Lederle) Calcium carbonate 1.5 Gm (elemental calcium 600 mg), vitamin D 125 IU/Tab. Bot. 60s.
Use: Vitamin/mineral supplement.

CALTRATE 600 + IRON. (Lederle) Calcium carbonate 600 mg, iron 18 mg, vitamin D 125 IU/Tab. Bot. 60s.
Use: Vitamin/mineral supplement.

CALTRATE JR. (Lederle) Calcium carbonate 750 mg (300 mg calcium)/Chew. Tab. Bot. 60s.
Use: Calcium supplement.

CALTRO. (Geneva Generics) Elemental calcium 250 mg, vitamin D 125 IU/Tab. Bot. 100s, 1000s.
Use: Vitamin/mineral supplement.

CAMA ARTHRITIS STRENGTH. (Sandoz Consumer) Aspirin 500 mg, magnesium oxide 150 mg, aluminum hydroxide gel 150 mg/Tab. Bot. 100s, 250s.
Use: Salicylate analgesic.

CAMALOX. (Rorer Consumer) **Liq.:** Aluminum hydroxide 225 mg, magnesium hydroxide 200 mg, calcium carbonate 250 mg/5 ml. Sodium content 1.2 mg/5 ml (0.05 mEq), vanilla-mint flavor. Bot. 360 ml. **Tab.:** Aluminum hydroxide 225 mg, magnesium hydroxide 200 mg, calcium carbonate 250 mg, sodium 1 mg, saccharin, sorbitol, vanilla-mint flavor. Bot. 50s.
Use: Antacid.

CAM-AP-ES. (Camall) Hydrochlorothiazide 15 mg, reserpine 0.1 mg, hydralazine HCl 25 mg/Tab. Bot. 100s.
Use: Antihypertensive.

•**CAMBENDAZOLE.** USAN. Isopropyl 2-(4-thiazolyl)-5-benzi-midazolecarbamate.
Use: Anthelmintic, veterinary medicine.

CAMELLIA LOTION. (O'Leary) Moisturizer lotion for face, hands and body. For normal to oily skin. Bot. 4 oz
Use: Emollient.

CAMEO OIL. (Medco Lab) Mineral oil, isopropyl myristate, lanolin oil, PEG-8-Dioleate. Plastic Bot. 8 oz, 16 oz, 32 oz.
Use: Emollient.

CAMOUFLAGE CRAYON. (O'Leary) Coverup for minor skin discolorations, under eye concealer, lipstick fixer. Available 6 shades. Crayon 0.05 oz.
Use: Skin coverup.

CAMPHO-PHENIQUE. (Winthrop Consumer) Camphor 10.8%, phenol 4.7%. **Liq.:** 22.5 ml, 45 ml, 120 ml. **Gel:** 6.9 Gm, 15 Gm.
Use: External analgesic, antiseptic.

•**CAMPHOR,** U.S.P. XXII. Spirit U.S.P. XXII. Bicyclo- [2.2.1.]heptane-2-one, 1,7,7-trimethyl. 2-Bornanone.
Use: Topical antipruritic; anti-infective; pharmaceutic necessity for camphorated phenol, paregoric and flexible collodion, antitussive, expectorant, local counterirritant, nasal decongestant.
See: Vicks Inhaler (Vicks).
Vicks Regular and Wild Cherry Medicated Cough Drops (Vicks).
Vicks Medi-Trating Throat Lozenges (Vicks).
Vicks Sinex, Nasal Spray (Vicks).
Vicks Vaporub, Oint. (Vicks).
Vicks Vaposteam, Liq. (Vicks).
Vicks Va-Tro-Nol, Nose Drops (Vicks).

CAMPHOR, MONOBROMATED. 3-Bromo-2-bornanone.

•**CAMPHORATED, PARACHLOROPHENOL.** U.S.P. XXII.
Use: Anti-infective (dental).

CAMPHORIC ACID. 1,2,2-Trimethyl-1,3-cyclopentanedicarboxylic acid.

CAMPHORIC ACID ESTER. Ester of p-Tolylmethylcarbinal as Diethanolamine Salt.

CAMPTROPIN. (Jenkins) Caffeine alkaloid 5 mg, camphor 12 mg, atropine sulfate 0.1 mg/Tab. Bot. 1000s.
Use: Expectorant, anticholinergic/antispasmodic.

•**CANDICIDIN,** U.S.P. XXII. Oint., Vag. Tab., U.S.P. XXII. An antifungal antibiotic derived from *Strep. griseus.*
Use: Local antifungal.
See: Candeptin, Vaginal Tab., Oint. (Julius Schmid).
Vanobid, Oint., Vaginal Tab. (Merrell Dow).

CANDYCON. (Allison) Chlorprophenpyridamine maleate 2 mg, phenylephrine HCl 5 mg/Tab. Bot. 50s.
Use: Antihistamine, decongestant.

CANKAID. (Becton Dickinson) Carbamide peroxide 10% in anhydrous glycerol. Soln. Bot. 22.5 ml.
Use: Oral mucosal analgesic and anti-inflammatory.

CANNABINOL. B.A.N. 6,6,9-Trimethyl-3-pentyl-ben-zo[c]chromen-l-ol.

CANOPAR. (Burroughs Wellcome).
See: Thenium closylate.

•**CANRENOATE POTASSIUM.** USAN.
Use: Aldosterone antagonist.

•**CANRENONE.** USAN.
Use: Aldosterone antagonist.

CANTHARIDIN.
Use: Keratolytic.

CANTHARONE. (Seres) Cantharidin 0.7% in a film-forming vehicle containing acetone, pyroxylin, castor oil, camphor. Liq. Bot. 7.5 ml.
Use: Keratolytic.

CANTHARONE PLUS. (Seres) Salicylic acid 30%, podophyllin 5%, cantharidin 1% in a film-forming vehicle containing octylphenyl polyethylene glycol 0.5%, cellosolve, ethocel, collodion, castor oil and acetone. Liq. Bot. 7.5 ml.
Use: Keratolytic.

CANTIL. (Merrell Dow) Mepenzolate bromide 25 mg/Tab. Bot. 100s.
Use: Anticholinergic/antispasmodic.

CANTRI. (Hauck) Sulfisoxazole 10%, aminacrine HCl 0.2%, allantoin 2%. Cream. Tube with applicator 90 Gm.
Use: Antibacterial, sulfonamide.

CA-OROTATE. (Miller) Calcium (as calcium orotate) 50 mg/Tab. Bot. 100s.
Use: Calcium supplement.

C-A-P. (Eastman) Cellulose acetate phthalate.

CAPAHIST-DMH. (Freeport) Chlorpheniramine maleate 8 mg, phenylpropanolamine HCl 50 mg, atropine sulfate 1/180 gr, dextromethorphan HBr 20 mg/T.R. Cap.
Use: Antihistamine, decongestant, anticholinergic/antispasmodic, antitussive.

CAPASTAT SULFATE. (Lilly) Capreomycin sulfate 1 Gm/5 ml. Vial 5 ml.
Use: Antituberculous agent.

CAPITAL WITH CODEINE. (Carnrick) **Liq.:** Acetaminophen 120 mg, codeine phosphate 12 mg/5 ml. Bot. pt. **Tab.:** Codeine phosphate 30 mg, acetaminophen 325 mg/Tab. scored. Bot. 100s.
Use: Narcotic analgesic combination.

CAPITROL CREAM SHAMPOO. (Westwood) 5,7-dichloro-8-hydroxyquinoline. Chloroxine 2% in a shampoo base, sodium octoxynol-3 sulfonate, PEG-6 lauramide, dextrin, stearyl alcohol/ceteareth-20, sodium lauryl sulfoacetate, docusate sodium, magnesium aluminum silicate, PEG-14M, EDTA, benzyl alcohol 1%, citric acid, water, color, fragrance. Tube 85 Gm.
Use: Antiseborrheic.

Ca-PLUS-PROTEIN. (Miller) Calcium (as contained in a calcium-protein complex made with specially isolated soy protein) 280 mg/Tab. Bot. 100s.
Use: Calcium supplement.

CAPNITRO. (Freeport) Nitroglycerin 6.5 mg/TR Cap. Bot. 100s.
Use: Antianginal agent.

•**CAPOBENATE SODIUM.** USAN. Sodium 6-(3,4,5-trimethoxybenzamido) Hexanoate.
Use: Cardiac depressant (antiarrhythmic).

•**CAPOBENIC ACID.** USAN. 6-(3,4,5-Trimethoxybenzamido)-hexanoic acid.
Use: Cardiac depressant (antiarrhythmic).

CAPOTEN. (Squibb) Captopril 12.5 mg, 25 mg, 37.5 mg, 50 mg or 100 mg/Tab. Bot 100s, UD 100s.
Use: Antihypertensive.

CAPOZIDE. (Squibb) Captopril/hydrochlorothiazide 25/15 mg, 25/25 mg, 50/15 mg or 50/25 mg/Tab. Bot. 100s.
Use: Antihypertensive.

CAPREOMYCIN. B.A.N.
Use: Antituberculosis agent.
See: Capastat sulfate (Lilly).
•**CAPREOMYCIN SULFATE STERILE,** U.S.P. XXII. An antibiotic derived from *Streptomyces capreolus.* Caprocin.
Use: Antibiotic (tuberculostatic).
See: Capastat Sulfate, Amp. (Lilly).
CAPROCHLORONE. Levo-gamma-(o-chlorobenzyl)-delta-oxo-gamma-phenylcaproic acid.
CAPROXAMINE. B.A.N. (E)-3′-Amino-4′-methylhexanophenone O-(2-aminoethyl)oxime.
Use: Antidepressant.
CAPRYLATE-PROPIONATE MIXTURES.
See: Sopronol, Preps. (Wyeth-Ayerst).
CAPRYLATE, SALTS.
See: Sodium Caprylate.
Zinc Caprylate.
CAPRYLATE SODIUM, INJECTION. Ingram—Amp. 33%, 1 ml Pkg. 12s, 25s, 100s.
Use: Antifungal.
See: Sodium Caprylate Preps.
CAPSAICIN.
Use: External analgesic.
See: Axsain (Galen Pharma).
Zostrix Cream (GenDerm).
CAPSICUM OLEORESIN.
W/Alcohol, benzocaine, oxyquinoline, thymol, capsicum oleoresin.
See: Dent's Dental Poultice (C. S. Dent).
W/Alcohol, chlorobutanol hydrous (chloroform derivative), phenol, eugenol, cresol.
See: Dent's Toothache Drops Treatment (C. S. Dent).
W/Benzocaine, phenol.
See: Dent's Toothache Gum (C. S. Dent).
W/Methyl salicylate, oil of camphor, oil of pine, turpentine oil.
See: Sloan's Liniment, Liq. (Warner-Lambert).
CAPSULES, EMPTY GELATIN. (Lilly) Lilly markets clear empty gelatin capsules in sizes 000,00,0,1,2,3,4,5.
CAPTAMINE HYDROCHLORIDE. USAN. N-(2-mercaptoethyl)dimethylamine hydrochloride.
Use: Cutaneous depigmenting activity.
CAPTODIAME. B.A.N. 4-Butylthiobenzhydryl 2-dimethylaminoethyl sulfide.
Use: Tranquilizer.
See: Covatin hydrochloride.
CAPTODIAME HCl. 4-Butylthio-a-phenylbenzyl 2-dimethylaminoethyl sulfide. Covatin hydrochloride.
CAPTOPRIL, U.S.P. XXII. Tab., U.S.P. XXII. Angiotensin I converting enzyme inhibitor.
Use: Antihypertensive agent.
See: Capoten, Tab. (Squibb).
CAPURIDE. USAN.
Use: Hypnotic.
CAQUIN. (Forest) Hydrocortisone 1%, iodochlorhydroxyquin 3%, hydrophilic base. Cream. Tube 20 Gm.
Use: Corticosteroid, topical.

•**CARACEMIDE.** USAN.
Use: Antineoplastic.
CARAFATE. (Marion) Sucralfate 1 Gm/Tab. Bot. 100s. UD, Ctn. 100s.
Use: Anti-ulcer agent.
•**CARAMEL,** N.F. XVII.
Use: Pharmaceutic aid (Color).
CARAMIPHEN. B.A.N. 2-Diethylaminoethyl 1-phenylcyclopentane-1-carboxylate.
Use: Treatment of the parkinsonian syndrome.
See: Parpanit hydrochloride.
Taoryi edisylate.
CARAMIPHEN EDISYLATE.
W/Phenylpropanolamine.
See: Tuss-Ornade, Prods. (SmithKline).
CARAMIPHEN ETHANEDISULFONATE.
W/Phenylephrine HCl, phenindamine tartrate.
See: Dondril, Tab. (Whitehall).
CARAMIPHEN HYDROCHLORIDE. 1-Phenylcyclo- pentanecarboxylic acid 2-diethyl-aminoethyl ester hydrochloride.
Use: Proposed antiparkinson agent.
•**CARAWAY,** N.F. XVII. Oil, N.F. XVII.
Use: Flavor.
CARBACHOL, U.S.P. XXI. Intraocular Soln., Ophth. Soln., U.S.P. XXI. Ethanaminium, 2-(aminocarbonyl)oxy-N,N,N-trimethyl-,Cl. CarbamycholineCl. CholineCl carbamate, Lentin, Carbolin.
Use: Parasympathomimetic agent; cholinergic.
See: Miostat Intraocular, Soln. (Alcon).
Murocarb, Soln. (Muro).
W/Methylcellulose.
See: Isopto Carbachol, Soln. (Alcon).
CARBACRYLAMINE RESINS.
Use: Cation-exchange resin.
•**CARBADOX.** USAN. Methyl 3-quinoxalin-2-yl-methylenecarbazate N^1N^4-dioxide.
Use: Antibacterial, veterinary medicine.
CARBAMATE.
See: Valmid, Tab. (Lilly).
•**CARBAMAZEPINE,** U.S.P. XXII. Tab., U.S.P. XXII. 5H-dibenz[b,f]azepine-5-carboxamide.
Use: Treatment of epilepsy and trigeminal neuralgia.
See: Carbamazepine (Rugby).
Tegretol, Tab. (Geigy).
CARBAMIDE. (Various Mfr.) Urea. Cream, Lot.
Use: Emollient.
See: Aquacare (Herbert).
Carmol 20 (Syntex).
Elaqua XX (Elder).
Nutraplus (Owen/Allercreme).
Rea-Lo (Whorton).
Ultra Mide Moisturizer (Baker/Cummins).
Ureacin-20 (Pedinol).
Ureacin-40 (Pedinol).
CARBAMIDE COMPOUNDS.
See: Acetylcarbromal (Various Mfr.).
Bromisovalum (Various Mfr.).
Bromural, Tab. (Knoll).
Carbrital, Elix., Kap. (Parke-Davis).

Carbromal (Various Mfr.).
Sedamyl, Tab. (Riker).

•**CARBAMIDE PEROXIDE TOPICAL SOLUTION,** U.S.P. XXII. Urea compound w/hydrogen peroxide (1:1).
Use: Local anti-infective, anti-inflammatory, analgesic, dental discomfort.
See: Cankaid (Becton Dickinson).
Gly-Oxide (Marion).
Orajel Brace-aid Rinse (Commerce).
Proxigel (Reed & Carnick).

CARBAMIDE PEROXIDE. 6.5% IN GLYCERIN.
Use: Otic preparation.
See: Murine Ear Drops (Abbott).
Murine Ear Wax Removal System (Abbott).

CARBAMYLCHOLINE CHLORIDE.
See: Carbachol.

CARBAMYLMETHYLCHOLINE CHLORIDE.
See: Urecholine, Tab., Inj. (Merck Sharp & Dohme).

•**CARBANTEL LAURYL SULFATE.** USAN.
Use: Anthelmintic.

CARBARSONE, U.S.P. XXI. Caps., U.S.P. XXI. (Various Mfr.) N-carbamoylarsanilic acid. Amabevan, ameban, amibiarson, arsambide, fenarsone, leucarsone, aminarsone, amebarsone. p-Ureidobenzenearsonic acid.
Use: Acute and chronic amebiasis and trichomoniasis.

•**CARBASPIRIN CALCIUM.** USAN.
Use: Analgesic.

•**CARBAZERAN.** USAN.
Use: Cardiotonic.

•**CARBENICILLIN DISODIUM, STERILE,** U.S.P. XXII. Sterile, U.S.P. XXII. 4-Thia-1-azabicyclo[3.2.0]-heptane-2-carboxylic acid, 6-[(carboxyphenylacetyl)-amino]-3,3-dimethyl-7-oxo-, disodium salt. N-(2-Carboxy-3,3-dimethyl-7-oxo-4-thia-1-azabicyclo-[3.2.0]-hept-6-yl)-2-phenylmalonamic acid disodium salt.
Use: Antibacterial.
See: Geopen, Vial (Roerig).
Pyopen, Inj. (Beecham Labs).

•**CARBENICILLIN INDANYL SODIUM,** U.S.P. XXII. Tabs., U.S.P. XXII.
Use: Antibacterial.
See: Geocillin, Tab. (Roerig).

•**CARBENICILLIN PHENYL SODIUM.** USAN.
Use: Antibacterial.

•**CARBENICILLIN POTASSIUM.** USAN.
Use: Antibacterial.

•**CARBENOXOLONE SODIUM.** USAN.
Use: Glucocorticoid.

CARBETAPENTANE CITRATE. 2-[2-(Diethylamino)ethoxy] ethyl 1-phenyl-cyclopentyl-1-carboxylate dihydrogen citrate.
Use: Antitussive.
W/Codeine phosphate, chlorpheniramine maleate, guaifenesin.
See: Tussar-2, Syr. (Rorer).
Tussar SF, Liq. (Rorer).
W/Terpin hydrate, menthol, alcohol, sodium citrate, citric acid, glycerin.
See: Toclonol Expectorant, Liq. (Cenci).
W/Terpin hydrate, sodium citrate, citric acid, menthol glycerin, alcohol, codeine.
See: Toclonol W/Codeine, Liq. (Cenci).

CARBETHOXYSYRINGOYL METHYLRESERPATE.
See: Singoserp, Tab. (Ciba).

CARBETHYL SALICYLATE.
See: Sal-Ethyl Carbonate, Tab. (Parke-Davis).

•**CARBETIMER.** USAN.
Use: Antineoplastic.

•**CARBIDOPA,** U.S.P. XXII. 2-(3,4-Dihydroxybenzyl)-2-hydrazinopropionic acid; (-)-Lα-hydrazino-a-methyl-β-(3,4-dihydroxybenzene) propanoic acid monohydrate.
Use: Decarboxylase inhibitor.
See: Lodosyn, Tab. (Merck Sharp & Dohme).
W/Levodopa.
See: Sinemet, Tab. (Merck Sharp & Dohme).

•**CARBIDOPA AND LEVODOPA TABLETS,** U.S.P. XXII.
Use: Treatment of parkinson's disease.
See: Sinemet, Tab. (Merck Sharp & Dohme).

CARBIMAZOLE. B.A.N. Ethyl 3-methyl-2-thioimidazoline-1-carboxylate.
Use: Antithyroid substance.
See: Bimazol.
Neo-Mercazole.

CARBIMAZOLE. 1-Ethoxycarbonyl-2:3-di-hydro-3- methyl-2-thioimidazole. Neo-Mercazole.

•**CARBINOXAMINE MALEATE,** U.S.P. XXII. Tabs., U.S.P. XXII. 2-[p-Chloro-alpha-[(2-(dimethyl-amino-ethoxy[benzyl]pyridine bimaleate.
Use: Antihistamine.
See: Clistin Elix., Tab. (McNeil).
W/Ammonium Cl, potassium guaiacol sulfonate, sodium citrate.
See: Clistin Expectorant (McNeil).
W/Pseudoephedrine HCl.
See: Rondec Prods. (Ross).
W/Pseudoephedrine HCl, dextromethorphan HBr.
See: Rondec DM, Drops, Syr. (Ross).

CARBIPHENE. B.A.N. α-Ethoxy-N-methyl-N [2-(N-methylphenethylamino)ethyl]diphenyl- acetamide.
Use: Analgesic.

•**CARBIPHENE HCl.** USAN. 2-Ethoxy-N-methyl-n-[2-(methylphenethylamino)ethyl]-2, 2-diphenylacetamide HCl.
Use: Analgesic.

CARBISET TABLETS. (Nutripharm) Pseudoephedrine 60 mg, carbinoxamine maleate 4 mg/Tab. Bot. 100s.
Use: Decongestant, antihistamine.

CARBOCAINE. (Cook-Waite) Mepivacaine HCl 3%. Inj. Dental cartridge 1.8 ml.
Use: Local anesthetic.

CARBOCAINE. (Winthrop Pharm) Mepivacaine HCl. **1%:** Vial 30 ml, 50 ml. **1.5%:** Vial 30 ml. **2%:** Vial 20 ml, 50 ml.

Use: Local anesthetic.
CARBOCAINE WITH NEO-COBEFRIN. (Cook-Waite) Mepivacaine HCl 2% with levonorefrin 1:20,000. Inj. Dental cartridge 1.8 ml.
Use: Local anesthetic.
•**CARBOCLORAL.** USAN. Ethyl (2,2,2,-trichloro-1-hydroxyethyl)carbamate.
Use: Hypnotic.
See: Chloralurethane.
Prodorm (Parke-Davis).
•**CARBOCYSTEINE.** USAN.
Use: Mucolytic.
CARBODEC. (Rugby) Pseudoephedrine HCl 60 mg, carbinoxamine maleate 4 mg/5 ml. Syr. Bot. pt, gal.
Use: Decongestant, antihistamine.
CARBODEC DM PRODUCTS. (Rugby) **Syr.:** Pseudoephedrine HCl 60 mg, carbinoxamine maleate 4 mg, dextromethorphan HBr 15 mg, alcohol >0.6%/5 ml. Bot. 30 ml, 120 ml, pt, gal. **Drops (Pediatric):** Pseudoephedrine HCl 25 mg, carbinoxamine maleate 2 mg, dextromethorphan HBr 4 mg, alcohol >0.6%/ml. Bot. 30 ml.
Use: Decongestant, antihistamine, antitussive.
CARBOL-FUCHSIN PAINT. Original fuchsin formula known as Castellani's Paint. Basic Fuchsin 0.3%, phenol 4.5%, resorcinol 10%, acetone 5%, alcohol 10%. Bot. 30 ml, 120 ml, 480 ml.
Use: Local antifungal.
See: Carfusin, Soln. (Rorer).
Castaderm, Lot. (Lannett).
Castellani's Paint (Various Mfr.).
CARBOLONIUM BROMIDE. B.A.N. Hexamethylenedi(carbamoylcholine bromide). Hexcarbacholine Bromide (I.N.N.).
Use: Muscle relaxant.
CARBOMER, N.F. XVII. A polymer of acrylic acid, crosslinked with a polyfunctional agent.
Use: Pharmaceutic aid (suspending agent); emulsifying agent.
See: Carbopol 934 P (Goodrich).
CARBOMER. B.A.N. A polymer of acrylic acid crosslinked with allyl sucrose.
Use: Pharmaceutic aid.
See: Carbopol 934.
CARBOMER 910, N.F. XVII, USAN.
Use: Pharmaceutic aid.
CARBOMER 934. N.F. XVII, USAN.
Use: Pharmaceutic aid.
CARBOMER 934P. USAN.
Use: Pharmaceutic aid.
CARBOMER 940, N.F. XVII, USAN.
Use: Pharmaceutic aid.
CARBOMER 941, N.F. XVII, USAN.
Use: Pharmaceutic aid.
CARBOMER 1342, N.F. XVII.
Use: Pharmaceutic aid.
CARBOMYCIN. An antibiotic from *Streptomyces halstedii.*
Use: Anti-infective.
CARBON DIOXIDE, U.S.P. XXII.
Use: Inhalation, respiratory stimulant.
See: Ceo-Two, Supp. (Beutlich).
•**CARBON TETRACHLORIDE,** N.F. XVII. Benzinoform. (Various Mfr.).
Use: Pharmaceutic aid (solvent).
CARBONIC ACID, DILITHIUM SALT. Lithium Carbonate, U.S.P. XXII.
CARBONIC ACID, DISODIUM SALT. Sodium Carbonate, N.F. XVII.
CARBONIC ACID, MONOSODIUM SALT. Sodium Bicarbonate, U.S.P. XXII.
CARBONIC ANHYDRASE INHIBITORS.
See: Acetazolamide, Tab. (Various Mfr.).
AK-ZOL, Tab. (Akorn).
Daranide, Tab. (Merck Sharp & Dohme).
Dazamide, Tab. (Major).
Diamox, Tab., Sequel, Vial (Lederle).
Neptazane, Tab. (Lederle).
CARBONIS DETERGENS, LIQUOR.
See: Coal Tar Solution.
CARBONYL DIAMIDE.
See: Chap Cream (Ar-Ex).
CARBOPHENOTHION. V.B.A.N. S-(4)Chlorophenylthiomethyl)00)diethyl phosphorodithioate.
Use: Insecticide, veterinary medicine.
•**CARBOPLATIN.** USAN.
Use: Antineoplastic.
•**CARBOPROST.** USAN.
Use: Oxytocic.
•**CARBOPROST TROMETHAMINE,** U.S.P. XXII. Inj., U.S.P. XXII.
Use: Oxytocic.
See: Prostin, Amp. (Upjohn).
CARBOSE D.
See: Carboxymethylcellulose sodium, Prep.
CARBOTABS. (Jenkins) Sodium bicarbonate 3⅓ gr, magnesium carbonate 1 gr, calcium carbonate ¾ gr, papain 1/32 gr, pancreatin 1/32 gr/Tab. Bot. 1000s.
Use: Antacid.
CARBOWAX. 300, 400, 1540, 4000. Polyethylene glycol 300, 400, 1540, 4000.
CARBOXYMETHYLCELLULOSE SALT OF DEXTROAMPHETAMINE. Carboxyphen.
See: Bontril Timed Tab. (Carnrick).
•**CARBOXYMETHYLCELLULOSE SODIUM,** U.S.P. XXII. Paste, Tab., U.S.P. XXII. Cellulose, carboxymethyl ester, sodium salt. Carbose D, C.M.C. (Hercules Pow. Co.).
Use: Pharmaceutic aid (suspending agent, tablet excipient, viscosity-increasing agent); cathartic.
W/Acetphenolisatin, docusate sodium.
See: Scrip-Lax, Tab. (Scrip).
W/Alginic acid, sodium bicarbonate.
See: Pretts, Tabs. (Marion).
W/Belladonna extract, kaolin, pectin, zinc phenosulfonate.
See: Gelcomul, Liq. (Commerce).
W/Digitoxin.
See: Foxalin, Cap. (Standex).
Thegitoxin (Standex).

W/Docusate sodium.
See: Dialose, Cap. (Stuart).
W/Docusate sodium, casanthranol.
See: Dialose Plus, Cap. (Stuart).
Disolan Forte, Cap. (Lannett).
Tri-Vac, Cap. (Rhode).
W/Docusate sodium, oxyphenisatin acetate.
See: Dialose Plus, Cap. (Stuart).
W/Methylcellulose.
See: Ex-Caloric, Wafer (Eastern Research).
W/Testosterone, estrone, sodium Cl.
See: Tostestro, Inj. (Bowman).

•**CARBOXYCELLULOSE SODIUM 12,** N.F. XVII.
Use: Pharmaceutic aid (suspending agent, viscosity increasing agent).

CARBOXYMETHYLCYSTEINE. B.A.N. S-Carboxymethylcysteine.
Use: Mucolytic agent.

CARBOXYPHEN.
W/Butabarbital.
See: Bontril, Timed Tab. (Carnrick).

CARBROMAL. (Various Mfr.) Bromodiethylacetylurea, bromadel, nyctal, planadalin, uradal.
Use: Sedative/hypnotic.
W/Bromisovalum (Bromural).
See: Bro-T's, Tab. (Brothers).

CARBUTAMIDE. B.A.N. 1-Butyl-3-sulphanilylurea.
Use: Hypoglycemic agent.

CARBUTAMIDE. N-Butyl-N′-sulfanilyl-urea. BZ. 55; Invenol; Nadisan.
Use: Hypoglycemic agent.

•**CARBUTEROL HYDROCHLORIDE.** USAN.
Use: Bronchodilator.

CARDABID. (Saron) Nitroglycerine 2.5 mg/SR Tab. Bot. 60s, 100s.
Use: Antianginal agent.

•**CARDAMON,** N.F. XVII. Oil, seed, Cpd. Tincture; N.F. XVII.
Use: Flavor.

CARDEC DM SYRUP. (Various Mfr.) Carbinoxamine maleate 4 mg, pseudoephedrine HCl 60 mg, dextromethorphan HBr 15 mg, alcohol $>$0.6%/5 ml. Bot. 30 ml, 120 ml, pt, gal.
Use: Antihistamine, decongestant, antitussive.

CARDEC DM DROPS. (Various Mfr.) Carbinoxamine maleate 2 mg, pseudoephedrine HCl 25 mg, dextromethorphan HBr 4 mg, alcohol $>$0.6%/ml. Drop. Bot. 30 ml.
Use: Antihistamine, decongestant, antitussive.

CARDEC-S. (Various Mfr.) Pseudoephedrine HCl 60 mg, carbinoxamine maleate 4 mg/5 ml. Syr. Bot. pt, gal.
Use: Decongestant, antihistamine.

CARDENE. (Syntex) Nicardipine 20 mg or 30 mg/Cap. Bot. 100s, 500s, UD 100s.
Use: Calcium channel blocking agent.

CARDENZ. (Miller) Vitamins C 25 mg, E 5 mg, inositol 30 mg, p-aminobenzoic acid 9 mg, A 2000 IU, B_6 1.5 mg, B_{12} 1 mcg, D 100 IU, niacinamide 20 mg, magnesium 23 mg, iodine 0.05 mg, potassium 8 mg/Tab. Bot. 100s.
Use: Vitamin/mineral supplement.

CARDIAMID.
See: Nikethamide. (Various Mfr.).

CARDIAZOL.
See: Metrazol, Preps. (Knoll).

CARDILATE. (Burroughs Wellcome) Erythrityl tetranitrate 10 mg/Tab. Bot. 100s.
Use: Antianginal agent.

CARDIO-GREEN. (Hynson, Westcott & Dunning) Indocyanine Green. Vial 25 mg, 50 mg, with diluent. CG disposable units/10 mg, 40 mg.
Use: Diagnostic aid.

CARDIO-GREEN DISPOSABLE UNIT. (Hynson, Westcott & Dunning) Vial Cardio-Green, ampule aqueous solvent and calibrated syringe. 10 mg.
Use: Diagnostic aid.

CARDI-OMEGA 3. (Thompson Medical) EPA 180 mg, DHA 120 mg, cholesterol 5 mg, less than 2% RDA of vitamins A, B_1, B_2, B_3, C, D, Fe, Ca/Cap. Bot. 60s.
Use: Vitamin/mineral supplement.

CARDIOPLEGIC SOLUTION.
Use: During open heart surgery.
See: Plegisol, Soln. (Abbott).

CARDIOQUIN TABLETS. (Purdue Frederick) Quinidine polygalacturonate 275 mg equivalent to quinidine sulfate 200 mg/Tab. Bot. 100s, 500s.
Use: Antiarrhythmic agent.

CARDIOTROL-CK. (Roche Diagnostics) Lyophilized human serum containing three CK isoenzymes from human tissue source. 10x2 ml.
Use: Suitable for use as a quality control for immunochemical or electrophoretic assays.

CARDIOTROL-LD. (Roche Diagnostics) Lyophilized human serum containing all LD isoenzymes from human tissue source. 10x1 ml.
Use: Suitable for use as a quality control for immunochemical or electrophoretic assays.

CARDIZEM. (Marion) Diltiazem HCl 30 mg, 60 mg, 90 mg or 120 mg/Tab. Bot. 100s, UD 100s.
Use: Calcium channel blocking agent.

CARDIZEM SR. (Marion) Diltiazem 60 mg, 90 mg or 120 mg/S.R. Cap. Bot. 100s, UD 100s.
Use: Calcium channel blocking agent.

CARDOPHYLLIN.
See: Aminophylline. (Various Mfr.).

CARDOXIN. (Vita Elixir) Digoxin 0.25 mg/Tab.
Use: Cardiotonic.

CARENA.
See: Aminophylline (Various Mfr.).

CARFECILLIN. B.A.N. 6-(α-Phenoxycarbonylphenylacetamido) penicillanic acid.
Use: Antibiotic.

•**CARFENTANIL CITRATE.** USAN.
Use: Narcotic analgesic.

CARFIN TABS. (Major) Warfarin sodium 2 mg, 2.5 mg, 5 mg, 7.5 mg or 10 mg/Tab. Bot. 100s, 200s (5 mg only).
Use: Anticoagulant.

CARGENTOS.
See: Silver Protein, Mild.

CARGESIC. (Rand) Bot. 2 oz
Use: Analgesic, counterirritant.

CARINDACILLIN. B.A.N. 6-(α-Indan-5-yloxycarbonylphenylacetamido)penicillanic acid.
Use: Antibiotic.

CARISOPRODOL, U.S.P. XXII. Tab., U.S.P. XXII. N-isopropyl meprobamate. Isomeprobamate, N-isopropyl-2-methyl-2-propyl-1, 3 propanediol dicarbamate. B.A.N. 2-Carbamoyloxymethyl-2-N-isopropylcarbamoyloxymethylpentane.
Use: Skeletal muscle relaxant.
See: Rela, Tab. (Schering).
Soma, Tab. (Wallace).

•**CARISOPRODOL AND ASPIRIN TABLETS,** U.S.P. XXII.
Use: Analgesic, muscle relaxant.
See: Soma Compound Tab. (Wallace).

•**CARISOPRODOL, ASPIRIN, AND CODEINE PHOSPHATE TABLETS,** U.S.P. XXII.
Use: Analgesic, muscle relaxant.
See: Soma Compound w/Codeine Tab. (Wallace).

CARISOPRODOL COMPOUND. (Various Mfr.) Carisoprodol 200 mg, aspirin 325 mg/Tab. Bot. 15s, 30s, 40s, 100s, 500s, 1000s.
Use: Skeletal muscle relaxant, salicylate analgesic.

CARI-TAB. (Jones Medical) Fluoride 0.5 mg, vitamins A 2000 IU, D 200 IU, C 75 mg/Softab. Bot. 100s.
Use: Vitamin supplement, dental caries preventative.

•**CARMANTADINE.** USAN.
Use: Treatment of parkinson's disease.

CARMOL 10. (Syntex) Urea (carbamide) 10% in hypoallergenic water-washable lotion base. Bot. 6 fl oz.
Use: Emollient.

CARMOL 20. (Syntex) Urea (carbamide) 20% in hypoallergenic vanishing cream base. Tube 3 oz, Jar lb.
Use: Emollient.

CARMOL-HC CREAM 1%. (Syntex) Micronized hydrocortisone acetate 1%, urea 10% in water-washable base. Tube 1 oz, Jar 4 oz.
Use: Corticosteroid.

•**CARMUSTINE.** USAN. 1,3bis-(2-chloroethyl)-1-nitrosourea.
Use: Antineoplastic.
See: Bicnu, Inj. (Bristol).

CARNATION INSTANT BREAKFAST. (Carnation) Non-fat instant breakfast containing 280 K calories w/15 Gm protein and 8 oz whole milk. Pkt. 35 Gm, Ctn. 6s. Six flavors.
Use: Enteral nutritional supplement.

•**CARNIDAZOLE.** USAN. Methyl-nitro-imidazole.
Use: Antiparasitic, antiprotozoal.

L-CARNITINE. (R & D Labs) Levocarnitine 250 mg/Cap. Bot. 60s.
Use: Vitamin supplement.

CARNITOR. (Sigma-Tau) Levocarnitine. **Liq.:** 100 mg/ml. Bot. 10 ml. **Tab.:** 330 mg. Bot. 90s.
Use: Vitamin supplement.

•**CAROXAZONE.** USAN.
Use: Antidepressant.

CARPERIDINE. B.A.N. Ethyl 1-(2-carbamoylethyl)-4-phenylpiperidine-4-carboxylate.

CARPHENAZINE. B.A.N. 10-{3-[4-(2-Hydroxyethyl)piperazin-1-yl]propyl}-2-propionylphenothiazine.
Use: Tranquilizer.

CARPROFEN.
Use: Nonsteroidal anti-inflammatory drug; analgesic.
See: Rimadyl. (Roche).

•**CARRAGEENAN,** N.F. XVII.
Use: Pharmaceutic aid (suspending agent, viscosity increasing agent).

CARSALAM. B.A.N. 1,3-Benzoxazine-2,4-dione. O-Carbamoylsalicylic acid lactam.
Use: Analgesic.

•**CARTAZOLATE.** USAN.
Use: Antidepressant.

•**CARTEOLOL HYDROCHLORIDE.** USAN.
Use: Anti-adrenergic.

CARTER'S LITTLE PILLS. (Carter Products) Bisacodyl 5 mg/Pill. Vial 30s, 85s.
Use: Laxative.

CARTICAINE. B.A.N. Methyl 4-methyl-3-(2- propylaminopropionamido)thiophene-2-carboxylate.
Use: Local anesthetic.

CARTROL. (Abbott) Carteolol 2.5 mg or 5 mg/Tab. Bot. 100s.
Use: Beta-adrenergic blocking agent.

CARTUCHO COOK WITH RAVOCAINE. (Winthrop Products) Ravocaine, novocaine, levophed or neo-cobefrin.
Use: Dental anesthetic.

•**CARUBICIN.** USAN.
Use: Antineoplastic.

•**CARUMONAM SODIUM.** USAN.
Use: Antibacterial.

•**CARVEDILOL.** USAN.
Use: Antianginal, antihypertensive.

CAR-VIT. (Mericon) Ascorbic acid 60 mg, vitamins A acetate 4000 IU, D-2 400 IU, ferrous fumarate 90 mg (elemental iron 30 mg), oyster shell 600 mg (calcium 230 mg)/Cap. Bot. 90s, 1000s.
Use: Vitamin/mineral supplement.

CARZENIDE. p-Sulfoamoylbenozoic acid.
Use: Carbonic anhydrase inhibitor.

CASA-DICOLE. (Blue Cross) Docusate sodium 100 mg, casanthrol 30 mg/Cap. Bot. 100s.
Use: Laxative.

•**CASANTHRANOL.** USAN. U.S.P. XXII. A purified mixture of the anthranol glycosides derived from Cascara sagrada.
Use: Cathartic.
See: Black Draught, Prods. (Chattem Labs.).
W/Docusate sodium.
See: Bu-Lax-Plus, Cap. (Ulmer).
Calotabs, Tab. (Calotabs).
Comfolax-Plus, Cap. (Rorer).

Comfolax-Plus, Cap. (Searle).
Comfula-Plus (Searle).
Constiban, Cap. (Quality Generics).
Diolax, Cap. (Century).
Dio-Soft (Standex).
Disanthrol, Cap. (Lannett).
Disulans, Cap. (Noyes).
Easy-Lax Plus, Cap. (Walgreen).
Genericace, Cap. (Forest Pharm.).
Neo-Vardin D-S-S-C, Cap. (Scherer).
Nuvac, Cap. (LaCrosse).
Peri-Colace, Cap., Syr. (Mead Johnson).
Sodex, Cap. (Mallard).
Stimulax, Cap. (Geriatric).
Tonelax Plus, Cap. (A.V.P.).

W/Docusate sodium, sodium carboxymethylcellulose.
See: Dialose Plus, Cap. (Stuart).
Disolan Forte, Cap. (Lannett).
Tri-Vac, Cap. (Rhode).

W/Mineral oil, irish moss.
See: Neo-Kondremul, Liq. (Fisons).

CASCARA. (Lilly) Cascara 150 mg/Tab. Bot. 100s.
Use: Cathartic.

•**CASCARA FLUIDEXTRACT, AROMATIC,** U.S.P. XXII.
Use: Cathartic.

W/Psyllium husk powder, prune powder.
See: Casyllium, Pow. (Upjohn).

CASCARA GLYCOSIDES.
Use: Cathartic.

•**CASCARA SAGRADA,** U.S.P. XXII. Extract, Fluidextract, U.S.P. XXII. (Various Mfr.) 325 mg/Tab. Bot. 100s, 1000s.
Use: Cathartic.

•**CASCARA SAGRADA EXTRACT,** U.S.P. XXII.
Use: Cathartic.

W/Bile salts, papain, phenolphthalein, capsicum oleoresin.
See: Torocol Compound, Tab. (Plessner).

W/Bile salts, phenolphthalein, capsicum oleoresin, peppermint oil.
See: Torocol, Tab. (Plessner).

W/Ox bile (desiccated), phenolphthalein, aloin, podophyllin.
See: Bilgon, Tab. (Reid-Rowell).

W/Oxgall, dandelion root, podophyllin, tincture nux vomica.
See: Oxachol, Liq. (Philips Roxane).

W/Pancreatin, pepsin, sodium salicylate.
See: Bocresin, Liq. (Scrip).

W/Phenolphthalein, sodium glycocholate, sodium taurocholate, aloin.
See: Bicholax, Tab. (Elder).
Oxiphen, Tab. (Webcon).

W/Sodium salicylate, phenolphthalein, chionanthus extract, bile extract, sodium glycocholate, sodium taurocholate.
See: Glycols, Tab. (Bowman).

•**CASCARA SAGRADA FLUIDEXTRACT,** U.S.P. XXII. (Parke-Davis) Alcohol 18%. Bot. pt, gal, UD 5 ml.
Use: Cathartic.
See: Cas-Evac, Liq. (Parke-Davis).
Bilstan (Standex).

CASCARA SAGRADA FLUIDEXTRACT AROMATIC. Aromatic Cascara Fluid extract, U.S.P. XXII. Liq. Alcohol ≈ 18%/5 ml. Bot. 60 ml, 120 ml, pt, gal, UD 5 ml.
Use: Cathartic.

W/Psyllium husk powder, prune powder.
See: Casyllium, Granules (Upjohn).

CASCARIN.
See: Casanthranol (Various Mfr.).

CASEC. (Mead Johnson Nutrition) Calcium caseinate (derived from skim milk curd and calcium carbonate). Pow. Can 2.5 oz.
Use: Enteral nutritional supplement.

CASOATE-A. (Marcen) Hydrolyzed casein 100 mg, histidine monohydrochloride 4 mg, benzyl alcohol 5 mg, phenol 5 mg/ml. Vial 10 ml.
Use: Anti-ulcer agent.

CAST. (NMS) Color Allergy Screening Test: A visual ELISA test for quantitative determination of Human Immunoglobulin E in serum.
Use: Diagnostic aid.

CASTADERM. (Lannett) Resorcin, boric acid, acetone, fuchsin basic, phenol, alcohol 9%. Liq. Bot. 30 ml, 120 ml, 480 ml.
Use: Antifungal, external.

CASTEL MINUS. (Syosset) Resorcinol 10%, acetone, basic fuchsin, hydroxyethyl cellulose, alcohol 10%. Non-staining. Liq. Bot. 30 ml.
Use: Antifungal, external.

CASTEL PLUS. (Syosset) Resorcinol 10%, acetone, basic fuchsin, hydroxyethyl cellulose, alcohol 10%. Liq. Bot. 30 ml.
Use: Antifungal, external.

CASTELLANI PAINT. (Pedinol) Basic fuchsin, phenol resorcinol, acetone, alcohol. Bot. 30 ml, 120 ml, 480 ml. Also available as colorless solution without basic fuchsin. Bot. 30 ml, 120 ml, 480 ml.
Use: Antifungal, external.

CASTELLANI'S PAINT. (Archer-Taylor) Bot. 4 oz, 16 oz.
Use: Antifungal, external.

CASTELLANI'S PAINT. (Penta) Carbol-fuchsin solution. Fuchsin 0.3%, phenol 4.5%, resorcinol 10%, acetone 1.5%, alcohol 13%. Bot. 1 oz, 4 oz, pt.
Use: Antifungal, external.

•**CASTOR OIL,** U.S.P. XXII. Aromatic, Caps., U.S.P. XXII. (Various Mfr.) Liq., emulsion.
Use: Cathartic; pharmaceutic aid (plasticizer).
See: Neoloid (Lederle).

•**CASTOR OIL EMULSION,** U.S.P. XXII.
Use: Cathartic.

•**CASTOR OIL, HYDROGENATED,** N.F. XVII.
Use: Cathartic.

CATAPRES. (Boehringer Ingelheim) Clonidine HCl 0.1 mg, 0.2 mg or 0.3 mg/Tab. Bot. 100s. 0.1 mg, 0.2 mg: Bot. 1000s, UD 100s.
Use: Antihypertensive.

CATAPRES-TTS. (Boehringer Ingelheim) Clonidine 2.5 mg, 5 mg or 7.5 mg/Transdermal patch. Pkg. 4s, 12s.
Use: Antihypertensive.

CATARASE. (Iolab) Chymotrypsin 1:5,000 (300 units) in a 2 chamber vial with 2 ml sodium Cl; Chymotrypsin 1:10,000 (150 units) in a 2 chamber vial with 2 ml sodium Cl.
Use: Ophthalmic enzyme.

CATARRHALIS, KILLED NEISSERIA.
W/*Klebsiella pneumoniae, Diplococcus pneumoniae,* Streptococci, staphylococci.
See: Combined Vaccine No. 4 W/Catarrhalis, Inj. (Lilly).

CATHOMYCIN CALCIUM. Calcium novobiocin.
Use: Anti-infective.

CATHOMYCIN SODIUM. Novobiocin sodium.
Use: Anti-infective.

CATIONIC RESINS.
See: Resins, Sodium Removing.

CAV-X FLUORIDE TREATMENT. (Palisades) Stannous fluoride 0.4% gel. Bot. 121.9 Gm.
Use: Dental caries preventative.

C-BIO. (Barth's) Vitamin C 150 mg, citrus bioflavonoid complex 100 mg, rutin 50 mg/Tab. Bot. 100s, 500s, 1000s.
Use: Vitamin supplement.

C-B TIME. (Arco) Ascorbic acid 200 mg, vitamins B_1 10 mg, B_2 10 mg, B_6 5 mg, B_{12} 10 mcg, niacinamide 50 mg, calcium pantothenate 10 mg/Tab. Bot. 40s, 120s, 500s.
Use: Vitamin supplement.

C-B TIME 500. (Arco) Vitamins C 500 mg, B_1 10 mg, B_2 10 mg, B_6 5 mg, cyanocobalamin 10 mg, niacinamide 50 mg, calcium pantothenate 10 mg/Tab. Bot. 30s, 100s, 500s.
Use: Vitamin supplement.

C-CAPS 500. (Drug Industries) Vitamin C 500 mg/Cap. Bot. 100s.
Use: Vitamin C supplement.

CCNU. Lomustine.
Use: Antineoplastic agent.
See: CeeNu, Tab. (Bristol).

CDDP.
Use: Antineoplastic agent.
See: Cisplatin.

C.D.M. EXPECTORANT. (Lannett) Dextromethorphan HBr 10 mg, chlorpheniramine maleate 1 mg, phenylephrine HCl 5 mg, sodium citrate 15 mg, guaifenesin 25 mg/5 ml. Bot. pt, gal.
Use: Antitussive, antihistamine, decongestant, expectorant.

C.D.P. CAPS. (Goldline) Chlordiazepoxide HCl 5 mg, 10 mg or 25 mg/Cap. Bot. 100s, 500s, 1000s.
Use: Antianxiety agent.

CEA. (Abbott Diagnostics) Radioimmunoassay or enzyme immunoassay for quantitative measurement of carcinoembryonic antigen in human serum or plasma. Test kit 100s.
Use: Diagnostic aid.

CEA-ROCHE. (Roche Diagnostics) Radioimmunoassay capable of detecting and measuring plasma levels of CEA in the nanogram range. Sensitivity-0.5 ng./ml of CEA.
Use: Diagnostic aid.

CEA-ROCHE TEST KIT. (Roche Diagnostics) Carcinoembryonic antigen, a glycoprotein which is a constituent of the glycocalyx of embryonic entodermal epithelium. Test kit.
Use: Diagnostic aid.

CEBID TIME CELLES. (Hauck) Ascorbic acid 500 mg/Cap. Bot. 100s.
Use: Vitamin C supplement.

CEB NUGGETS. (Scott/Cord) Vitamins B_1 15 mg, B_2 15 mg, B_6 5 mg, B_{12} 5 mcg, C 600 mg, niacinamide 100 mg, E 40 IU, calcium pantothenate 20 mg, folic acid 0.1 mg/Nugget. Bot. 60s.
Use: Vitamin supplement.

CEBO-CAPS. (Forest) Placebo capsules.

CEBRALAN-M TABLETS. (Lannett) Vitamin B_1 10 mg, niacinamide 30 mg, B_{12} 3 mcg, C 100 mg, E 5 IU, A 10,000 IU, D 1000 IU, iron 15 mg, copper 1 mg, iodine 0.15 mg, manganese 1 mg, magnesium 5 mg, zinc 1.5 mg/Tab. Bot. 100s, 1000s.
Use: Vitamin/mineral supplement.

CEBRALAN M.T. TABLETS. (Lannett) Vitamins B_1 15 mg, B_2 10 mg, B_6 2 mg, pantothenic acid 10 mg, niacinamide 100 mg, B_{12} 7.5 mcg, C 150 mg, E 5 IU, A 25,000 IU, copper 1 mg, iron 15 mg, iodine 0.15 mg, manganese 1 mg, magnesium 5 mg, zinc 1.5 mg/Tab. Bot. 100s, 1000s.
Use: Vitamin/mineral supplement.

CECLOR. (Lilly) **Pulv.**: Cefaclor 250 mg or 500 mg. Bot. 15s, Rx Pak 100s, Blister pkg. 10 × 10s. **Oral Susp.:** Cefaclor 125 mg, 187 mg, 250 mg or 375 mg/5 ml. Bot. 75 ml, 150 ml.
Use: Antibacterial, cephalosporin.

CECON SOLUTION. (Abbott) Ascorbic acid 10% in propylene glycol. Each drop from enclosed dropper supplies 2.5 mg ascorbic acid; each ml contains 100 mg Bot. w/dropper 50 ml.
Use: Vitamin C supplement.

CEDILANID-D. (Sandoz) Deslanoside (desacetyl lanatoside C.) 0.4 mg/2 ml w/citric acid, sodium phosphate, alcohol 9.8%, glycerin 15%, Water for injection qs 2 ml/Amp.
Use: Cardiac glycoside.

CEEBEVIM. (Nature's Bounty) Vitamins B_1 15 mg, B_2 10.2 mg, B_3 50 mg, B_5 10 mg, B_6 5 mg, C 300 mg/Cap. Bot. 100s, 300s.
Use: Vitamin supplement.

CeeNU. (Bristol-Myers/Bristol Oncology) Lomustine (CCNU) 10 mg, 40 mg or 100 mg/Cap. Dose pk. of two cap. each of all three strengths.
Use: Antineoplastic agent.

CEEPA. (Geneva) Theophylline 130 mg, ephedrine HCl 24 mg, phenobarbital 8 mg/Tab. Bot. 100s, 1000s.
Use: Bronchodilator, decongestant, sedative/hypnotic.

CEEPRYN. Cetylpyridinium Cl.
Use: Antiseptic.
See: Cēpacol Lozenges, Soln., Troches (Merrell Dow).

CEETOLAN CONCENTRATE. (Lannett) Cetyldimethylbenzyl ammonium Cl 1:5500/2 oz. Bot. diluted w/1 gal water. Bot. 2 oz.
Use: Mouthwash.

CEE WITH BEE. (Wesley) Vitamins B_1 15 mg, B_2 10.2 mg, B_3 50 mg, B_5 10 mg, B_6 5 mg, C 300 mg, tartrazine. Bot. 100s, 1000s.
Use: Vitamin supplement.

•**CEFACLOR,** U.S.P. XXII. Capsules, For Oral Susp., For Oral Susp., U.S.P. XXII.
Use: Antibacterial.
See: Ceclor, Cap. (Lilly).

•**CEFACTOR.** USAN.
Use: Anti-infective.

•**CEFADROXIL,** U.S.P. XXII. Caps., Tabs., Oral Susp., U.S.P. XXII. 7-[[D-2-amino-2-(4 hydroxyphenyl) acetyl] amino]-3-methyl-8-oxo-5-thia-1-azabicyclo [4.2.0] Oct-2-ene-2-carboxylic acid monohydrate.
Use: Antibiotic.
See: Duricef, Cap., Tab., Susp. (Mead Johnson).

CEFADYL. (Bristol) Cephapirin sodium 500 mg, 1 Gm or 2 Gm/Vial.; Piggyback vial 1 Gm, 2 Gm or 4 Gm; Bulk vial 20 Gm.
Use: Antibacterial, cephalosporin.

•**CEFAMANDOLE.** USAN.
Use: Antibacterial.

•**CEFAMANDOLE NAFATE, STERILE,** U.S.P. XXII. For Inj. U.S.P. XXII. 5-Thia-1-azabicyco(4.2.0)oct-2-ene-2-carboxylic acid,7-(((formyloxy,)phenylacetyl)amino)-3-(((1-methyl-1H-tetrazol-5-yl)thio)methyl)-8-oxo-monosodium salt,(6R-(6a, 7 b (R))).
Use: Antibiotic.
See: Mandol, Amp. (Lilly).

•**CEFAMANDOLE SODIUM,** U.S.P. XXII. For Inj., U.S.P., Sterile, U.S.P. XXII.
Use: Antibiotic.

CEFANEX. (Bristol) Cephalexin monohydrate 250 mg or 500 mg/Cap. Bot. 100s.
Use: Antibacterial, cephalosporin.

•**CEFAPAROLE.** USAN.
Use: Antibacterial.

CEFAPIRIN. B.A.N. 7-[α-(4-Pyridylthioacetamido)]- cephalosporanic acid.
Use: Antibiotic.

•**CEFATRIZINE.** USAN.
Use: Antibacterial.

•**CEFAZAFLUR SODIUM.** USAN.
Use: Antibacterial.

•**CEFAZOLIN,** U.S.P. XXII.
Use: Antibiotic.

•**CEFAZOLIN SODIUM, STERILE,** U.S.P. XXII. Inj., U.S.P. XXII. Sodium salt of 3-[(5-methyl-1, 3, 4-thiadiazol-2-yl) thio]-methyl -8-oxo 7-[2-(1H-tetrazol-1-yl) acetanido]-5-thia-1-azabicyclo[4-2.0]oct-2-ene-2-carboxylic acid.
Use: Antibiotic.
See: Ancef, Vial (SmithKline).
Kefzol, Amp. (Lilly).

•**CEFBUPERAZONE.** USAN.
Use: Antibacterial.

•**CEFEPIME.** USAN.
Use: Antibacterial.

•**CEFETAMET.** USAN.
Use: Antibacterial.

•**CEFETECOL.** USAN.
Use: Antibacterial.

CEFINAL II. (Alto) Salicymide 150 mg, acetaminophen 250 mg, doxylamine succinate 25 mg/Tab. Bot. 100s.
Use: Analgesic combination.

•**CEFIXIME.** USAN. U.S.P. XXII. Tab., Oral Susp., U.S.P. XXII.
Use: Antibacterial, cephalosporin.
See: Suprax (Lederle).

CEFIZOX. (SmithKline) Semisynthetic cephalosporin equivalent to: **Vials:** 1 Gm, 2 Gm, 10 Gm of ceftizoxime/Vial. **Piggyback Vials:** 1 Gm, 2 Gm/100 ml. **Minibags:** 1 Gm, 2 Gm/50 ml w/dextrose injection (D5W).
Use: Antibacterial, cephalosporin.

•**CEFMENOXINE HYDROCHLORIDE.** USAN. U.S.P. XXII. Sterile, Inj. U.S.P. XXII.
Use: Antibacterial.
See: Takeda (Abbott).

•**CEFMETAZOLE SODIUM.** USAN.
Use: Antibacterial.
See: Zefazone (Upjohn).

•**CEFMETAZOLE SODIUM STERILE),** U.S.P. XXII.

CEFOBID. (Roerig) Cefoperazone sodium 1 Gm or 2 Gm/Vial. 1 Gm, 2 Gm PBU 10 pack.
Use: Antibacterial, cephalosporin.

CEFOL FILMTAB. (Abbott) Vitamins B_1 15 mg, B_2 10 mg, B_6 5 mg, B_{12} 6 mcg, C 750 mg, E 30 mg, calcium pantothenate 20 mg, niacinamide 100 mg, folic acid 500 mcg/Tab. Bot. 100s.
Use: Vitamin/mineral supplement.

•**CEFONICID MONOSODIUM.** USAN.
Use: Antibacterial.

•**CEFONICID SODIUM.** USAN.
Use: Antibacterial.

•**CEFONICID SODIUM, STERILE,** U.S.P. XXII.
Use: Antibacterial.

•**CEFOPERAZONE SODIUM, STERILE,** U.S.P. XXII.
Use: Antibacterial.
See: Cefobid, Inj. (Roerig).

•**CEFORANIDE.** USAN.
Use: Antibacterial.
See: Precef, Inj. (Bristol).

•**CEFORANIDE FOR INJECTION,** U.S.P. XXII.
Use: Antibacterial.

EFORANIDE, STERILE, U.S.P. XXII.
Use: Antibacterial.
EFOTAN. (Stuart) Cefotetan disodium 1 Gm/10 ml, 1 Gm/100 ml or 2 Gm/100 ml. Vial.
Use: Antibacterial, cephalosporin.
EFOTAXIME SODIUM, U.S.P XXII. Inj., U.S.P. XXII.
Use: Antibacterial.
See: Claforan, Inj. (Hoechst).
EFOTETAN STERILE, U.S.P. XXII, USAN.
Use: Antibacterial.
EFOTETAN DISODIUM STERILE, U.S.P. XXII, USAN.
Use: Antibacterial.
See: Cefotan, Inj. (Stuart).
EFOTIAM HYDROCHLORIDE. USAN.
Use: Antibacterial.
EFOXITIN. USAN.
Use: Antibacterial.
EFOXITIN SODIUM, U.S.P. XXII.
Use: Antibacterial.
EFOXITIN SODIUM INJECTION, U.S.P. XXII.
Use: Antibacterial.
EFOXITIN SODIUM, STERILE, U.S.P. XXII. 5-Thia-1-azabicyclo (4.2.0) oct-2-ene-2-carboxylic acid, 3-((aminocarbonyl) oxy) methyl)-7-methoxy-8-oxo-7-((2-thienylacetyl)-amino)-, sodium salt (6R-cis)-.
Use: Antibacterial.
See: Mefoxin, Inj. (Merck Sharp & Dohme).
EFPIMIZOLE. USAN.
Use: Antibacterial.
EFPIMIZOLE SODIUM. USAN.
Use: Antibacterial.
EFPIRAMIDE, U.S.P. XXII, Inj., USAN.
Use: Antibacterial.
EFPIRAMIDE SODIUM. USAN.
Use: Antibacterial.
EFPIROME SULFATE. USAN.
Use: Antibacterial.
EFPROZIL. USAN.
Use: Antibacterial.
EFROXADINE. USAN.
Use: Antibacterial.
EFSULODIN SODIUM, STERILE, U.S.P. XX1.
Use: Antibacterial.
EFTAZIDIME, U.S.P. XXII, Inj., USAN.
Use: Antibacterial.
See: Ceptaz, Inj. (Glaxo).
Fortaz, Inj. (Glaxo).
Tazicef, Inj. (SmithKline Beecham).
Tazidime, Inj. (Lilly).
EFTIOFUR HYDROCHLORIDE. USAN.
Use: Antibacterial (veterinary).
EFTIOFUR SODIUM. USAN.
Use: Antibacterial (veterinary).
EFTIN. (A & H). Cefuroxime axetil 125 mg, 250 mg or 500 mg/Tab. Bot. 20s, 60s, UD 100s.
Use: Antibacterial, cephalosporin.
EFTIZOXIME SODIUM, U.S.P. XXII.
Use: Antibacterial.

•**CEFTRIAXONE SODIUM, STERILE,** U.S.P. XXII.
Use: Antibacterial.
See: Rocephin, Inj. (Roche).
•**CEFUROXIME.** USAN. U.S.P. XXII (6R, 7R)-3-Carbamoyloxymethyl-7-[(2Z)-2-(2-furyl)-2-methoxyiminoacetamido]-ceph-3-em-1-carboxylic acid.
Use: Antibiotic.
•**CEFUROXIME AXETIL.** USAN. U.S.P. XXII. Tab.
Use: Antibiotic.
See: Ceftin, Tab. (Allen & Hanburys).
•**CEFUROXIME PIVOXETIL.** USAN
Use: Antibacterial.
•**CEFUROXIME SODIUM,** U.S.P. XXII. Inj., U.S.P. XXII.
•**CEFUROXIME SODIUM, STERILE,** U.S.P. XXII.
Use: Antibiotic.
See: Kefurox, Inj. (Lilly).
Zinacef, Inj. (Glaxo).
CELESTONE. (Schering) **Tab.:** Betamethasone 0.6 mg. Bot. 100s, 500s, UD 21s. **Syr.:** Betamethasone 0.6 mg/5 ml, alcohol $<$ 1%. Bot. 120 ml.
Use: Corticosteroid.
CELESTONE PHOSPHATE INJECTION. (Schering) Betamethasone sodium phosphate 4 mg/ml equivalent to betamethasone alcohol 3 mg/ml. Vial 5 ml.
Use: Corticosteroid.
CELESTONE SOLUSPAN. (Schering) Betamethasone sodium phosphate 3 mg, betamethasone acetate 3 mg, dibasic sodium phosphate 7.1 mg, monobasic sodium phosphate 3.4 mg, edetate disodium 0.1 mg, benzalkonium Cl 0.2 mg/ml. Vial 5 ml.
Use: Corticosteroid.
CELLABURATE. (Eastman) Cellulose acetate butyrate.
Use: Pharmaceutic aid (plastic filming agent).
•**CELIPROLOL HYDROCHLORIDE.** USAN.
Use: Anti-adrenergic.
CELLACEPHATE. B.A.N. A partial mixed acetate and hydrogen phthalate ester of cellulose.
Use: Enteric coating.
CELLASE W-100. W/Alpha-amylase W-100, proteinase W-300, lipase, estrone, testosterone, vitamins, minerals.
See: Geramine, Tab. (Brown).
CELLEPACBIN. (Arthrins) Vitamins A 1200 IU, B_1 1.5 mg, B_2 1.5 mg, B_6 0.75 mg, niacinamide 7.5 mg, panthenol 3 mg, C 20 mg, B_{12} 2 mcg, E 1 IU/Cap. Bot. 180s.
Use: Vitamin supplement.
CELLOTHYL. (Numark) Methylcellulose 0.5 Gm/Tab. Bot. 100s, 1000s.
Use: Laxative.
•**CELLULASE.** USAN. A concentrate of cellulose-splitting enzymes derived from *Aspergillus niger* and other sources.
Use: Digestive aid.
W/Bile salts, mixed conjugated, pancrelipase.

See: Cotazym-B, Tab. (Organon).
W/Mylase, prolase, calcium carbonate, magnesium glycinate.
See: Zylase, Tab. (Vitarine).
W/Mylase, prolase, lipase.
See: Ku-Zyme, Cap. (Kremers-Urban).
W/Pepsin, glutamic acid, pancreatin, ox bile extract.
See: Kanulase, Tab. (Sandoz Consumer).
W/Pepsin, pancreatin, dehydrocholic acid.
See: Gastroenterase, Tab. (Wallace).

CELLULOSE.
W/Hexachlorophene.
See: ZeaSorb, Pow. (Stiefel).

•**CELLULOSE ACETATE,** N.F. XVII.
Use: Polymer membrane, insoluble.

•**CELLULOSE ACETATE PHTHALATE,** N.F. XVII. Cellulose, acetate, 1,2-benzenedicarboxylate.
Use: Pharmaceutic aid (tablet-coating agent).

CELLULOSE, CARBOXYMETHYL, SODIUM SALT. Carboxymethylcellulose Sodium, U.S.P. XXII.

CELLULOSE, HYDROXYPROPYL METHYL ETHER. Hydroxypropyl Methylcellulose, U.S.P. XXII.

CELLULOSE METHYL ETHER.
See: Methylcellulose, Prep. (Various Mfr.).

•**CELLULOSE MICROCRYSTALLINE,** N.F. XVII.
Use: Tablet diluent.

CELLULOSE, NITRATE. Pyroxylin, U.S.P. XXII.

CELLULOSE, OXIDIZED. Oxidized Cellulose, U.S.P. XXII.
Use: Local hemostatic.

CELLULOSE, OXIDIZED REGENERATED, U.S.P. XXII.

•**CELLULOSE, POWDERED,** N.F. XVII.
Use: Tablet and capsule diluent.

•**CELLULOSE SODIUM PHOSPHATE,** U.S.P. XXII.
Use: Antiurolithic.
See: Calcibind (Mission).

CELLULOSIC ACID.
See: Oxidized Cellulose. (Various Mfr.).

CELLULOLYTIC.
W/Amylolytic, proteolytic.
See: Trienzyme, Tab. (Forest Pharm.).

CELLULOLYTIC ENZYME.
See: Cellulase (Various Mfr.).
W/Amylolytic, proteolytic enzymes, lipase, phenobarbital, hyoscyamine sulfate, atropine sulfate.
See: Arco-Lipase Plus, Tab. (Arco).
W/Amylolytic enzyme, proteolytic enzyme, lipolytic enzyme, butisol sodium, belladonna.
See: Butibel-zyme, Tab. (McNeil).
W/Calcium carbonate, glycine, amylolytic and proteolytic enzymes.
See: Co-Gel, Tab. (Arco).
W/Proteolytic enzyme, amylolytic enzyme, lipolytic enzyme.
See: Ku-Zyme, Cap. (Kremers-Urban).
Zymme, Cap. (Scrip).
W/Proteolytic, amylolytic, lipolytic enzymes, iron, ox bile.
See: Spaszyme, Tab. (Dooner).

CELLUVISC. (Allergan) Carboxymethylcellulose 1% ophthalmic soln. Single use containers 0.01 fl oz
Use: Artificial tear solution.

CELONTIN. (Parke-Davis) Methsuximide 150 mg or 300 mg/Kapseal. Bot. 100s.
Use: Anticonvulsant.

CEL-U-JEC. (Mallard) Betamethasone sodium phosphate 4 mg (equivalent to betamethasone alcohol 3 mg)/ml. Soln. Inj. Vial 5 ml.
Use: Corticosteroid.

CENAFED. (Century) **Tab.:** Pseudoephedrine HCl 30 mg or 60 mg. Bot. 100s, 1000s. **Syr.:** Pseudoephedrine HCl 30 mg/5 ml. Bot. 120 ml, pt, gal.
Use: Decongestant.

CENAFED PLUS. (Century Pharm.) Pseudoephedrine HCl 60 mg, triprolidine HCl 25 mg/Tab. Bot. 100s, 1000s.
Use: Decongestant, antihistamine.

CENA-K. (Century) Potassium and Cl 20 mEq/15 ml (10% KCl), saccharin. Bot. pt, gal.
Use: Potassium supplement.

CENALAX. (Century) Bisacodyl. **Tab.:** 5 mg. Bot. 100s, 1000s. **Supp.:** 10 mg. Pkg. 12s, 1000s.
Use: Laxative.

CENOCORT A-40. (Central) Triamcinolone acetonide 40 mg/ml. Inj. Vial 1 ml, 5 ml.
Use: Corticosteroid.

CENOCORT FORTE. (Central) Triamcinolone diacetate 40 mg/ml. Inj. Vial 5 ml. Box 12s.
Use: Corticosteroid.

CENOLATE. (Abbott Hospital Prods) Sodium ascorbate 562.5 mg/ml (equivalent to 500 mg/ml ascorbic acid), sodium hydrosulfate 0.5%. Inj. Amp. 1 ml, 2 ml.
Use: Vitamin C supplement.

CENTER-AL. (Center) Allergenic extracts, alum precipitated 10,000 PNU/ml or 20,000 PNU/ml. Vial 10 ml, 30 ml.
Use: Treatment of allergy due to pollens or house dust.

CENTRAFREE. (Nature's Bounty) Iron 27 mg, vitamins A 5000 IU, D 400 IU, E 30 IU, B_1 2.25 mg, B_2 2.6 mg, B_3 20 mg, B_5 10 mg, B_6 3 mg, B_{12} 9 mcg, C 90 mg, folic acid 0.4 mg, biotin 45 mcg, Ca, Cl, Cr, Cu, I, K, Mg, Mn, Mo, P, Se, Zn/Tab. Bot. 100s.
Use: Vitamin/minera supplement.

CENTRAL NERVOUS SYSTEM DEPRESSANTS.
See: Sedatives.

CENTRAL NERVOUS SYSTEM STIMULANTS.
See: Amphetamine (Various Mfr.).
D-Amphetamine (Various Mfr.).
Anorexigenic agents.
Caffeine (Various Mfr.).
Coramine, Liq., Inj. (Ciba).
Desoxyephedrine HCl, Tab. (Various Mfr.).

Desoxyn HCl, Tab. Gradumet. (Abbott).
Dexedrine, Preps. (SmithKline).
Methamphetamine HCl (Various Mfr.).
Ritalin HCl, Tab., Inj. (Ciba).

CENTRAX. (Parke-Davis) Prazepam. **Cap.**: 5 mg or 10 mg. Bot. 100s, 500s. 20 mg. Bot. 100s. **Tab.:** 10 mg. Bot. 100s, UD 100s.
Use: Antianxiety agent.

CENTROVITE JR. (Rugby) Iron 18 mg, vitamins A 5000 IU, D 400 IU, E 15 IU, B_1 1.5 mg, B_2 1.7 mg, B_3 20 mg, B_5 10 mg, B_6 2 mg, B_{12} 6 mcg, C 60 mg, folic acid 0.4 mg, biotin 45 mcg, Cr, Cu, I, Mg, Mn, Mo, Zn/Chew. Tab. Bot. 60s.
Use: Vitamin/mineral supplement.

CENTRUM. (Lederle) Vitamins A 5000 IU, E 30 IU, C 90 mg, folic acid 400 mcg, B_1 2.25 mg, B_2 2.6 mg, B_6 3 mg, niacinamide 20 mg, B_{12} 9 mcg, D 400 IU, biotin 45 mcg, pantothenic acid 10 mg, calcium 162 mg, phosphorus 125 mg, iodine 150 mcg, iron 27 mg, magnesium 100 mg, potassium 30 mg, manganese 5 mg, chromium 25 mcg, selenium 25 mcg, molybdenum 25 mcg, zinc 15 mg, copper 2 mg, K 25 mcg, Cl 27.2 mg/Tab.
Use: Vitamin/mineral supplement.

CENTRUM JR. (Lederle) Vitamins A 5000 IU, D 400 IU, E 30 IU, C 60 mg, folic acid 400 mcg, B_1 1.5 mg, B_6 2 mg, B_{12} 6 mcg, riboflavin 1.7 mg, niacinamide 20 mg, iron 18 mg, magnesium 25 mg, copper 2 mg, zinc 10 mg, biotin 45 mcg, panthothenic acid 10 mg, molybdenum 20 mcg, chromium 20 mcg, iodine 150 mcg, manganese 1 mg/Chew. Tab. Bot. 60s.
Use: Vitamin/mineral supplement.

CENTRUM JR. + EXTRA C. (Lederle) Vitamins A 5000 IU D 400 IU, E 30 IU, C 300 mg, folic acid 400 mcg, biotin 45 mcg, B_1 1.5 mg, pantothenic acid 10 mg, B_2 1.7 mg, nicacinamide 20 mg, B_6 2 mg, B_{12} 6 mcg, K-1 10 mcg, iron 18 mg, magnesium 40 mg, iodine 150 mcg, copper 2 mg, phosphorous 50 mg, calcium 108 mg, zinc 15 mg, manganese 1 mg, molybdenum 20 mcg, chromium 20 mcg/Chew. Tab. Cherry, orange, grape, lemon lime flavors. Bot. 15s.
Use: Vitamin/mineral supplement.

CENTRUM, JR. + EXTRA CALCIUM. (Lederle) Calcium 160 mg, iron 18 mg, vitamins A 5000 IU, D 400 IU, E 30 IU, B_1 1.5 mg, B_2 20 mg, B_3 20 mg, B_5 10 mg, B_6 2 mg, B_{12} 6 mcg, C 60 mg, folic acid 400 mcg, Cr, Cu, I, Mn, Mg, Mo, P, Zn, K 10 mcg, biotin 45 mcg/Chew. Tab. Bot. 15s.
Use: Vitamin/mineral supplement.

CENTRUM, JR. + IRON. (Lederle) Iron 18 mg, vitamins A 5000 IU, D 400 IU, E 30 IU, B_1 1.5 mg, B_2 20 mg, B_3 1.7 mg, B_5 10 mg, B_6 2 mg, B_{12} 6 mcg, C 60 mg, folic acid 0.4 mg, Ca, Cr, Cu, I, Mg, Mn, Mo, P, zinc 15 mg, biotin 45 mcg, K 10 mcg/Chew. Tab. Bot. 75s.
Use: Vitamin/mineral supplement.

CENTUSS. (Century) Dextromethorphan HBr 10 mg, salicylamide 227 mg, phenacetin 100 mg, caffeine 10 mg, ascorbic acid 20 mg, phenylephrine HCl 5 mg, chlorpheniramine maleate 2 mg/MLT Tab. Bot. 100s, 1000s.
Use: Antitussive, analgesic, decongestant, antihistamine.

CEO-TWO. (Beutlich) Potassium bitartrate, sodium bicarbonate in polyethylene glycol base/ Supp. 10s.
Use: Laxative.

CEPACOL. (Lakeside) Cetylpyridinium Cl 0.05%, alcohol 14%, tartrazine, saccharin. Liq. Bot. 360 ml, 540 ml, 720 ml, 960 ml.
Use: Antiseptic.

CEPACOL ANESTHETIC LOZENGES. (Lakeside) Benzocaine 10 mg, cetylpyridinium Cl 0.07%, tartrazine, aromatics in citrus flavored hard candy base. Pkg. 18s, 324s.
Use: Anesthetic, antiseptic.

CEPACOL THROAT LOZENGES. (Lakeside) Cetylpyridinium Cl 0.07%, benzyl alcohol 0.3%, tartrazine, aromatics in mint flavored hard candy base. Pkg. 27s, 400s.
Use: Antiseptic.

CEPASTAT LOZENGES. (Lakeside) Phenol 1.45%, menthol 0.12%/Lozenge w/sorbitol, saccharin, eucalyptus oil. Pkg. 18s.
Use: Anesthetic.

CEPASTAT CHERRY FLAVOR LOZENGES. (Lakeside) Phenol 0.72%, menthol 0.12%, sorbitol saccharin. Box 18s.
Use: Anesthetic.

CEPHACETRILE SODIUM. Sodium 7-(2-cyanoacetamido)-3-(hydroxy-methyl)-8-oxo-5-thia-1-aza-bicyclo [4.3.0]oct-2-ene-2-carboxylate acetate (ester).
Use: Antibacterial.

•**CEPHADRINE TABLETS,** U.S.P. XXII.

•**CEPHALEXIN,** U.S.P. XXII. Caps., Oral Susp., Tabs., U.S.P. XXII. 7-(D-2-Amino-2-phenyl-acetamido)-3-methyl-8-oxo-5-thia-1-azabicyclo-[4.2.0]oct-2-3n3-2-carboxylic acid. 5-Thia-1-azabicyclo[4.2.0.]oct-2-ene-2-carboxylic acid,7-[(aminophenylacetyl)amino]-3-methyl-8oxo-, monohydrate.
Use: Antibiotic.
See: Ceporex.
Keflex (Lilly).
Keforal (Lilly).

•**CEPHALEXIN HYDROCHLORIDE.** USAN.
Use: Antibacterial.
See: Keftab (Lilly).

CEPHALEXIN MONOHYDRATE.
See: Keflex, Pulvule, Susp. (Lilly).

CEPHALIN.
W/Lecithin with choline base, lipositol.
See: Alcolec, Cap., Granules (American Lecithin).

CEPHALONIUM. V.B.A.N. 3-(4-Carbamoyl-1-pyridinio-methyl)-7-(2-thienylacetamido)-3-cephem-4-carboxylate.
Use: Veterinary antibiotic.

CEPHALORAM. B.A.N. 7-Phenylacetamidocephalosporanic acid.
Use: Antibiotic.

CEPHALORIDINE, STERILE. USAN 1-[[2-Carboxy-8-oxo-7-[2-(2-thienyl)acetamido]-5-thia-1-azabicyclo[4.2.0]oct-2-en-3-yl]methyl]pyridinium hydroxide inner salt.
Use: Antibacterial.

CEPHALOSPORIN C. B.A.N. 7-(5-Amino-5-carboxy- valeramido)cephalosporanic acid.
Use: Antibiotic.

•**CEPHALOTHIN SODIUM,** U.S.P. XXII. Inj., Sterile, For Inj., U.S.P. XXII. 7-(2-Thienyl acetamido) cephalosporanic acid sodium salt. 5-Thia-1-azabicyclo[4.2.0]oct-2-ene-2-carboxylic acid,3-[(acetyloxy)methyl]-8-oxo-7-[(2-thienylacetyl)-amino]-,monosodium salt.
Use: Antibacterial, antibiotic.
See: Keflin, Vial (Lilly).
Cephapirin Sodium (Lyphomed).

•**CEPHAPIRIN SODIUM, STERILE,** U.S.P. XXII. Sodium 3-(hydroxymethyl)-8-oxo-7-[2-(4-pyridylthio) acetamido]-5-thia-1-azabicyclo[4.2.0]oct-2-ene-2-carboxylate acetate (ester).
Use: Antibiotic.
See: Cefadyl, Vial (Bristol).

CEPHAZOLIN SODIUM.
See: Ancef (SmithKline).
Kefzol (Lilly).

CEPHOXAZOLE. V.B.A.N. 7-(3-o-Chlorophenyl-5-methylisoxazole-4-carboxamido)-cephalosporanic acid.
Use: Veterinary antibiotic.

•**CEPHRADINE,** U.S.P. XXII. Cap., Inj., Oral Susp., Sterile U.S.P. XXII. 7-[D-2-Amino-2-(1,4-cyclohexadien-1-yl-acetamido]-3-methyl-8-oxo-5-thia-1-azabicyclo[4.2.0]oct-2-ene-2-carboxylic acid monohydrate.
Use: Antibiotic.
See: Anspor, Cap., Susp. (SmithKline).
Eskacef.
Velosef, Cap., Inj., Susp. (Squibb).

CEPHULAC. (Merrell Dow) Lactulose syrup 10 Gm/15 ml (less than galactose 2.2 Gm, lactose 1.2 Gm, other sugars 1.2 Gm). Bot. 473 ml, 1890 ml, UD 15 ml, 30 ml. Box 100s.
Use: Laxative.

CERAPON. Triethanolamine Polypeptide Oleate-Condensate. (Purdue-Frederick).
See: Cerumenex, Drops (Purdue-Frederick).

CEREBID-150. (Saron) Papaverine HCl 150 mg/SR Cap. Bot. 100s, 1000s.
Use: Peripheral vasodilator.

CEREBID-200. (Saron) Papaverine HCl 200 mg/SR Tab. Bot. 100s, 1000s.
Use: Peripheral vasodilator.

CERELOSE.
See: Glucose (Various Mfr.).

CERESPAN. (Rorer) Papaverine HCl 150 mg/SR Cap. Bot. 100s, 1000s.
Use: Peripheral vasodilator.

CERETEX. (Enzyme Process) Iron 15 mg, vitamins B_{12} 10 mcg, B_1 2 mg, B_6 1 mg, niacinamide 1 mg, pantothenic acid 0.15 mg, B_2 2 mg, iodine 15 mg/2 ml. Bot. 60 ml, 8 oz.
Use: Vitamin/mineral supplement.

•**CERONAPRIL.** USAN.
Use: Antihypertensive.

CEROSE-DM. (Wyeth-Ayerst) Dextromethorphan HBr 15 mg, chlorpheniramine maleate 4 mg, phenylephrine HCl 10 mg/5 ml, alcohol 2.4%, saccharin. Sugar free. Liq. Bot. 120 ml, 480 ml.
Use: Antitussive, antihistamine, decongestant.

CERTAGEN. (Goldline) Iron 27 mg, vitamins A 5000 IU, D 400 IU, E 30 IU, B_1 2.25 mg, B_2 2.6 mg, B_3 20 mg, B_5 10 mg, B_6 3 mg, B_{12} 9 mcg, C 90 mg, folic acid 0.4 mg, biotin 45 mcg, Ca, Cl, Cr, Cu, I, K, Mg, Mn, Mo, P, Se, Zn, vitamin K. Bot. 30s, 100s, 130s, 1000s.
Use: Vitamin/mineral supplement.

CERUBIDINE. (Wyeth-Ayerst) Daunorubicin HCl 5 mg/ml once reconstituted w/4 ml water for injection. Vial 20 mg.
Use: Antineoplastic agent.

•**CERULETIDE.** USAN.
Use: Stimulant.

CERUMENEX DROPS. (Purdue Frederick) Triethanolamine polypeptide oleate-condensate 10%, chlorobutanol in propylene glycol 0.5%. Liq. Dropper bot. 6 ml, 12 ml.
Use: Otic preparation.

CES. (I.C.N.) Conjugated estrogens 0.625 mg, 1.25 mg or 2.5 mg/Tab.
Use: Estrogen.

CESAMET. (Lilly) Nabilone 1 mg/Cap. UD 20s.
Use: Antiemetic/antivertigo.

•**CESIUM CHLORIDE.** USAN.
Use: Myocardial scanning.

•**CETABEN SODIUM.** USAN.
Use: Antihyperlipoproteinemic.

CETACAINE. (Cetylite) Benzocaine 14%, butyl aminobenzoate 2%, tetracaine HCl 2%, benzalkonium Cl 0.5%, cetyl dimethyl ethyl ammonium bromide 0.005%. **Aerosol Spray:** 56 Gm. **Liq.:** 56 Gm. **Oint.:** Jar 37 Gm, flavored. **Hosp. Gel:** 29 Gm.
Use: Local anesthetic.

CETACIN. (Jenkins) Cetylpyridinium Cl 4 mg, sodium propionate 10 mg, benzocaine 6 mg/Tab. Bot. 1000s.
Use: Anesthetic, antiseptic.

CETACORT LOTION. (Owen) Hydrocortisone in concentrations of 0.25%, 0.5%, 1% w/cetyl alcohol, propylene glycol, stearyl alcohol, sodium lauryl sulfate, butylparaben, methylparaben, propylparaben, purified water. Bot. 120 ml (0.25% only), 60 ml (0.5%, 1%).
Use: Corticosteroid.

•**CETALKONIUM.** F.D.A. Benzylhexadecyldimethylammonium ion.

•**CETALKONIUM CHLORIDE.** USAN. Cetyldimethylbenzyl ammoniumCl.
Use: Antibacterial agent.

W/Phenylephrine, pyrilamine maleate, thimerosal.
See: Anti-B Mist (DePree).
CETAMIDE. (Alcon) Sulfacetamide sodium 10%, with parabens in white petrolatum, mineral oil, liquid lanolin. Sterile ophthalmic oint. Tube 3.5 Gm.
Use: Anti-infective, ophthalmic.
•**CETAMOLOL HYDROCHLORIDE.** USAN.
Use: Anti-adrenergic.
CETANE. (Forest) Ascorbic acid 500 mg/T.R. Cap. Bot. 100s.
Use: Vitamin C supplement.
CETAPHIL. (Owen) Cetyl alcohol, stearyl alcohol, propylene glycol, sodium lauryl sulfate, methylparaben, propylparaben, butylparaben, purified water. Cream, Lot. Bot. 480 Gm (cream), 240 ml, 480 ml (lotion).
Use: Skin cleanser.
CETAPRED. (Alcon) Sulfacetamide sodium 10%, prednisolone acetate, mineral oil, white petrolatum, liquid lanolin, parabens. 0.25% Soln., Ophth. Oint. Tube 3.5 Gm.
Use: Anti-infective, ophthalmic.
CETAZOL. (Professional Pharmacal) Acetazolamide 250 mg/Tab. Bot. 100s.
Use: Anticonvulsant, diuretic.
•**CETIEDIL CITRATE.** USAN.
Use: Vasodilator.
•**CETIRIZINE HYDROCHLORIDE.** USAN.
Use: Antihistamine.
•**CETOCYCLINE HYDROCHLORIDE.** USAN.
Use: Antibacterial.
CETOMACROGOL 1000. B.A.N. Polyethylene glycol 1000 monocetyl ether. Polyoxyethylene glycol 1000 monocetyl ether.
Use: Pharmaceutical aid.
•**CETOPHENICOL.** USAN. D-threo-N-p-[acetyl-β-hydroxy-α-(hydroxymethyl)-phenethyl]}- 2,2-dichloroacetamide.
Use: Antibacterial agent.
•**CETOSTEARYL ALCOHOL,** N.F. XVII.
Use: Pharmaceutic aid (emulsifying agent).
CETOXIME. B.A.N. N-Benzylanilinoacetamidoxime.
Use: Antihistamine.
•**CETRAXATE HYDROCHLORIDE.** USAN.
Use: Anti-ulcerative.
CETRIMONIUM CHLORIDE. B.A.N. HexadecyltrimethylammoniumCl.
Use: Antiseptic detergent.
•**CETYL ALCOHOL,** N.F. XVII. 1-Hexadecanol. *Use:* Emulsifying and stiffening agent.
•**CETYL ESTERS WAX,** N.F. XVII.
Use: Pharmaceutic aid (stiffening agent).
CETYLCIDE SOLUTION. (Cetylite) Cetyldimethylethyl ammonium bromide 6.5%, benzalkonium Cl 6.5%, isopropyl alcohol 13%. Inert ingredients 74%, including sodium nitrite. Bot. 16 oz, 32 oz.
Use: Disinfectant.
CETYLDIMETHYL BENZYL AMMONIUM CHLORIDE.
See: Ceetolan Concentrate, Liq. (Lannett).
W/Benzocaine, ascorbic acid.
See: Locane, Troches (Reid-Rowell).
W/Phenylephrine HCl, pyrilamine maleate.
See: Dalihist, Nasal Spray (Dalin).
•**CETYLPYRIDINIUM CHLORIDE,** U.S.P. XXII. Topical Soln., Loz, U.S.P. XXII. 1-HexadecylpyridiniumCl.
Use: Local anti-infective.
See: Bactalin (LaCrosse).
W/Benzocaine.
See: Axon Throat Loz. (McKesson).
Cēpacol, Throat Loz., (Merrell Dow).
Coirex, Preps. (Reid-Rowell).
Lanazets, Loz. (Lannett).
Oradex-C, Troches (Commerce).
Semets, Troches (Beecham Labs).
Spec-T Sore Throat Loz. (Squibb).
Tyro-Loz (Kenyon).
Vicks Medi-Trating Throat Lozenges (Vicks).
W/Benzocaine.
See: Cepacol Antiseptic Lozenges (Merrell Dow).
W/Benzocaine, menthol, camphor, eucalyptus oil.
See: Vicks Medi-Trating Throat Lozenges (Vicks).
W/Dextromethorphan HBr, benzocaine.
See: Thorzettes (Towne).
W/d-Methorphan HBr, phenyltoloxamine dihydrogen citrate, sodium citrate.
See: Exo-Kol, Cough Syrup, Spray, Tab. (Inwood).
W/Phenylephrine HCl, methapyrilene HCl, menthol, eucalyptol, camphor, methyl salicylate.
See: Vicks Sinex Nasal Spray (Vicks).
W/Phenylpropanolamide HCl, benzocaine, terpin hydrate.
See: S.A.C. Throat Lozenges (Towne).
CETYLTRIMETHYL AMMONIUM BROMIDE. (Bio Labs.) Cetrimide B.P., Cetavlon, CTAB.
Use: Antiseptic.
W/Hydrocortisone, phenylephrine, methapyrilene, chlorobutanol.
See: T-Spray (Saron).
W/Lidocaine, hexachlorophene.
See: Aerosept, Aerosol (Dalin).
CEVALIN. (Lilly) Ascorbic acid 100 mg or 500 mg/ml. Inj. Amp. 10 ml (100 mg), 1 ml (500 mg).
Use: Vitamin C supplement.
CEVI-BID. (Geriatric) Ascorbic acid 500 mg/TR Caps. Bot. 30s, 100s, 500s.
Use: Vitamin C supplement.
CEVI-FER. (Geriatric) Ascorbic acid 300 mg, ferrous fumarate 20 mg, folic acid 1 mg/Cap. Bot. 30s, 100s.
Use: Vitamin/mineral supplement.
CE-VI-SOL. (Mead Johnson Nutrition) Ascorbic acid 35 mg/0.6 ml, alcohol 5%. Bot. w/dropper 50 ml.
Use: Vitamin C supplement.
CEVITAMIC ACID.

See: Ascorbic acid.
CEVITAN.
See: Ascorbic acid.
CEWIN TABLETS. (Winthrop Products) Ascorbic acid.
Use: Vitamin C supplement.
CEYLON GELATIN.
See: Agar.
C.G. (Sig) Chorionic gonadotropin (lyophilized) 10,000 units, mannitol 100 mg, supplied with diluent. Univial 10 ml.
Use: Chorionic gonadotropin.
CG DISPOSABLE UNIT.
See: Cardio Green, Vial (Hynson, Westcott & Dunning).
CG RIA. (Abbott Diagnostics) Radioimmunoassay for the quantitative measurement of total circulating serum cholylglycine.
Use: Diagnostic aid.
CHAP CREAM. (Ar-Ex) Carbonyl diamide. Tube 1.5 oz, 3.25 oz. Jar 4 oz, 9 oz, 18 oz.
Use: Emollient.
CHAPOLINE CREAM LOTION. (Wade) Glycerine, boric acid, chlorobutanol 0.5%, alcohol 10%. Bot. 4 oz, pt, gal.
Use: Emollient.
CHAPSTICK SUNBLOCK 15. (Robins Consumer) Padimate O 0.7%, oxybenzone 3%. Stick 4.25 Gm.
Use: Lip protectant, sunscreen.
CHARCOAID. (Requa) Activated charcoal 30 Gm/150 ml in sorbitol. Bot. 150 ml.
Use: Antidote.
CHARCOAL. (Various Mfr.) Cap., Tab.
Use: Antiflatulent.
See: Charcoal (Paddock).
Charcoal (Rugby).
•**CHARCOAL, ACTIVATED,** U.S.P. XXII.
Use: Antidote: Drug, chemical poisoning.
See: Actidose-Aqua (Paddock).
Charcoaid (Requa).
Liqui-Char (Jones Medical).
Superchar (Gulf-Bio-Systems).
W/Nux vomica, bismuth subgallate, pepsin, berberis, diastase, pancreatin, hydrastis, papain.
See: Charcocaps, Cap. (Requa).
Charcotabs, Tab. (Requa).
Digestalin, Tab. (Vortech).
CHARCOCAPS. (Requa) Activated charcoal 260 mg/Cap. Bot. 36s.
Use: Antiflatulent.
CHARDONNA-2. (Kremers-Urban) Belladonna extract 15 mg, phenobarbital 15 mg/Tab. Bot. 100s.
Use: Anticholinergic/antispasmodic, sedative/hypnotic.
CHARO SCATTER-PAKS. (Requa) Activated charcoal 5 Gm/Packet.
Use: Odor absorber.
CHAZ SCALP TREATMENT DANDRUFF SHAMPOO. (Revlon) Zinc pyrithione 1% in liquid shampoo.
Use: Antiseborrheic.
CHECKMATE. (Oral-B) Acidulated phosphate fluoride 1.23%. Bot. 2 oz, 16 oz.
Use: Dental caries preventative.
CHEK-STIX URINALYSIS CONTROL STRIPS. (Ames) Bot. 25s.
Use: Diagnostic aid.
CHEALAMIDE INJECTION. (Vortech) Disodium edetate 150 mg/ml. Vial 20 ml.
Use: Chelating agent.
CHELAFRIN.
See: Epinephrine.
CHELATED CALCIUM MAGNESIUM. (Nature's Bounty) Calcium^{++} 500 mg, magnesium 250 mg/Tab. Protein coated. Bot. 50s.
Use: Mineral supplement.
CHELATED CALCIUM MAGNESIUM ZINC. (Nature's Bounty) Calcium^{++} 333 mg, magnesium 133 mg, zinc 8.3 mg/Tab. Bot. 100s.
Use: Mineral supplement.
CHELATED MAGNESIUM. (Freeda) Magnesium amino acids chelate 500 mg (magnesium 100 mg)/Tab. Bot. 100s, 250s, 500s.
Use: Magnesium supplement.
CHELATED MANGANESE. (Freeda) Manganese 20 mg or 50 mg/Tab. Bot. 100s, 250s, 500s.
Use: Manganese supplement.
CHELATING AGENT.
See: BAL, Amp. (Hynson, Westcott & Dunning).
Calcium Disodium Versenate, Amp., Tab. (Riker).
Desferal, Amp. (Ciba).
Endrate Disodium, Amp. (Abbott).
Magora, Tab. (Miller).
CHELEN.
See: Ethyl Chloride.
CHEL-IRON. (Kinney) Iron choline citrate complex (ferrocholinate) 0.33 Gm equivalent to 40 mg of elemental iron/Tab. Bot. 100s.
Use: Iron supplement.
CHEL-IRON LIQUID. (Kinney) Ferrocholinate 0.417 Gm equivalent to 50 mg of elemental iron. Bot. 8 fl oz.
Use: Iron supplement.
CHEL-IRON PEDIATRIC DROPS. (Kinney) Ferrocholinate 0.208 Gm equivalent to 25 mg of elemental iron/ml. Bot. 60 ml with calibrated dropper.
Use: Iron supplement.
CHEL-IRON PLUS. (Kinney) Ferrocholinate 200 mg (equivalent to 24 mg elemental iron), vitamin B_{12} with intrinsic factor concentrate ⅓ units, vitamins C 50 mg, B_1 2 mg, B_2 2 mg, B_6 HCl 2 mg, niacin 25 mg/Tab. Bot. 100s.
Use: Vitamin/mineral supplement.
CHEMIPEN. Potassium phenethicillin.
Use: Antibacterial, penicillin.
CHEMOVAG SUPPS. (Forest Pharm.) Sulfisoxazole 0.5 Gm/Supp. Bot. 12s w/applicators.
Use: Antibacterial, sulfonamide.
CHEMOZINE. (Tennessee Pharm.) Sulfadiazine, 0.167 Gm, sulfamerazine 0.167 Gm, sulfame-

thazine 0.167 Gm/Tab. Bot. 100s, 1000s. Susp. Bot. pt, gal.
Use: Antibacterial, sulfonamide.

CHEMSTRIP 9. (Boehringer Mannheim) Broad range test for glucose, protein, pH, blood, ketones, bilirubin, urobilinogen, nitrite and leukocytes in urine. Bot. strip 100s.
Use: Diagnostic aid.

CHEMSTRIP bG. (Boehringer Mannheim) For measuring glucose in blood. Bot. strip 25s, 50s.
Use: Diagnostic aid.

CHEMSTRIP GP. (Boehringer Mannheim) Broad range test for glucose and protein. Bot. strip 100s.
Use: Diagnostic aid.

CHEMSTRIP-K. (Boehringer Mannheim) Reagent papers for ketones in urine. Bot. paper 25s, 100s.
Use: Diagnostic aid.

CHEMSTRIP 5L. (Boehringer Mannheim) Broad range test for glucose, protein, pH, blood, ketones and leukocytes. Bot. strip 100s.
Use: Diagnostic aid.

CHEMSTRIP 6L. (Boehringer Mannheim) Broad range test for glucose, protein, pH, blood, ketones, bilirubin and leukocytes. Bot. strip 100s.
Use: Diagnostic aid.

CHEMSTRIP 7L. (Boehringer Mannheim) Broad range test for glucose, protein, pH, blood, ketones, bilirubin, urobilinogen and leukocytes. Bot. strip 100s.
Use: Diagnostic aid.

CHEMSTRIP LN. (Boehringer Mannheim) Broad range test for nitrite and leukocytes. Bot. strip 100s.
Use: Diagnostic aid.

CHEMSTRIP uG. (Boehringer Mannheim) Use to test for glucose in urine using the glucose oxidase method. Bot. strip 100s.
Use: Diagnostic aid.

CHEMSTRIP uGK. (Boehringer Mannheim) Broad range test for glucose and ketones. Bot. strip 50s, 100s.
Use: Diagnostic aid.

CHENATAL. (Miller) Calcium 580 mg, magnesium 200 mg, vitamins C 100 mg, folic acid 0.4 mg, A 5000 IU, D 400 IU, B_1 3 mg, B_2 3 mg, B_6 5 mg, B_{12} 9 mcg, niacinamide 30 mg, pantothenic acid 5 mg, tocopherols (mixed) 10 mg, iron 20 mg, copper 1 mg, manganese 2 mg, potassium 10 mg, zinc 25 mg, iodine 0.1 mg/2 Tabs. Bot. 100s.
Use: Vitamin/mineral supplement.

CHENIX. (Reid-Rowell) Chenodiol 250 mg/Tab. Bot. 100s.
Use: Gallstone solubilizing agent.

CHENODEOXYCHOLIC ACID.
Use: Gallstone solubilizing agent.
See: Chenodiol.

•**CHENODIOL.** USAN.
Use: Anticholelithogenic.
See: Chenix, Tab. (Reid-Rowell).

CHERACOL. (Upjohn) Codeine phosphate 10 mg, guaifenesin 100 mg/5 ml, alcohol 4.75%. Bot. 2 oz, 4 oz, pt.
Use: Antitussive, expectorant.

CHERACOL D. (Upjohn) Dextromethorphan HBr 10 mg, guaifenesin 100 mg/5 ml, alcohol 4.75%. Bot. 2 oz, 4 oz, 6 oz.
Use: Antitussive, expectorant.

CHERACOL PLUS. (Upjohn) Phenylpropanolamine HCl 8.3 mg, dextromethorphan HBr 6.7 mg, chlorpheniramine maleate 1.3 mg/5 ml. Bot. 4 oz, 6 oz.
Use: Decongestant, antitussive, antihistamine.

CHERALIN EXPECTORANT LIQUID. (Lannett) Potassium guaiacolsulfonate 88 mg, ammonium Cl 88 mg, antimony potassium tartrate 1 mg, alcohol 3%. Bot. pt, gal.
Use: Expectorant.

CHERALIN SYRUP. (Lannett) Potassium guaiacolsulfonate 88 mg, ammonium Cl 88 mg, antimony potassium tartrate 1 mg, codeine phosphate 10 mg/5 ml. Bot. pt, gal.
Use: Antitussive, expectorant.

CHERALIN W/CODEINE SYRUP. (Lannett) Codeine phosphate 10 mg, potassium guaiacolsulfonate 80 mg, ammonium Cl 80 mg, antimony potassium tartrate 0.8 mg, alcohol 3%. Bot. pt, gal.
Use: Antitussive, expectorant.

CHERASULFA PEDIATRIC. (Cenci) Triple sulfa (5 gr): Sulfadiazine 1.67 gr, sulfamethazine 1.67 gr, sulfamerazine 1.67 gr, sodium citrate 6 gr/5 ml. Bot. 16 oz. **F.S. Liq.**: 7.5 gr. Bot. 16 oz. **Tab.**: 7.5 gr. Bot. 100s, 1000s, 5000s.
Use: Antibacterial, sulfonamide.

CHERATUSSIN COUGH SYRUP. (Towne) Dextromethorphan HBr 45 mg, ammonium Cl 575 mg, citrate sodium 280 mg/Fl oz. Bot. 4 oz.
Use: Antitussive, expectorant.

CHERI-APRO. (Approved) Codeine phosphate 1 gr, potassium guaiacolsulfonate 8 gr, tartar emetic 1/12 gr/Fl oz. Bot. 4 oz, gal.
Use: Antitussive, expectorant.

CHERIJEN MORPHINE SULFATE. (Jenkins) Alcohol 7%, morphine sulfate 2.5 mg, ammonium Cl 88 mg, potassium guaiacolsulfonate 88 mg, tartar emetic 0.9 mg/5 cc. Syr. 4 oz, gal.
Use: Narcotic analgesic, expectorant.

CHERO-TRISULFA-V. (Vita Elixir) Sulfadiazine 0.166 Gm, sulfacetamide 0.166 Gm, sulfamerazine 0.166 Gm, sodium citrate 0.5 Gm/5 ml. Susp. Bot. pt.
Use: Antibacterial, sulfonamide.

•**CHERRY JUICE,** N.F. XVII.
Use: Flavor.

•**CHERRY SYRUP,** N.F. XVII.
Use: Pharmaceutic aid (Vehicle).

CHEST THROAT LOZENGES. (Lane) Eucalyptol, anise, horehound, tolu balsam, benzoin tincture, sugar, corn syrup. Pkg. 30s.
Use: Antiseptic.

CHESTAMINE. (Leeds) Chlorpheniramine maleate 8 mg or 12 mg/Cap. Bot. 50s.
Use: Antihistamine.

CHEW HIST. (Kenyon) Phenylephrine HCl 7.5 mg, chlorpheniramine maleate 2 mg, vitamin C 50 mg/Wafer. Bot. 100s.
Use: Decongestant, antihistamine.

CHEW-VIMS. (Barth's) Vitamins A 5000 IU, D 400 IU, B_1 3 mg, B_2 6 mg, niacin 1.71 mg, C 100 mg, B_{12} 5 mcg, E 5 IU/Tab. Bot. 30s, 90s, 180s, 360s.
Use: Vitamin supplement.

CHEW-VI-TAB. (Blue Cross) Vitamins A 2500 IU, D 400 IU, E 15 IU, C 60 mg, folic acid 0.3 mg, B_1 1.05 mg, B_2 1.2 mg, niacin 13.5 mg, B_6 1.05 mg, B_{12} 4.5 mcg/Tab. Bot. 100s.
Use: Vitamin supplement.

CHEW-VI-TAB WITH IRON. (Blue Cross) Vitamins A 5000 IU, C 60 mg, E 15 IU, folic acid 0.4 mg, B_1 1.5 mg, B_2 1.7 mg, niacin 20 mg, B_6 2 mg, B_{12} 6 mcg, D 400 IU, iron 18 mg/Tab. Bot. 100s.
Use: Vitamin/mineral supplement.

CHEW VITES. (Kenyon) Vitamins A 5000 IU, D 500 IU, B_1 2 mg, B_2 2 mg, B_6 1 mg, B_{12} 2 mcg, calcium pantothenate 2 mg, C 50 mg, niacinamide 10 mg, fluoride 0.05 mg/Tab. Bot. 100s.
Use: Vitamin/mineral supplement.

CHIGGEREX. (Scherer) Benzocaine 0.02%, camphor, menthol, peppermint oil, olive oil, clove oils, pegosperse, methylparaben, distilled water. Oint. Jar 50 Gm.
Use: Local anesthetic, counterirritant.

CHIGGERTOX. (Scherer) Benzocaine 2.1%, benzyl benzoate 21.4%, soft soap, isopropyl alcohol. Liq. Bot. oz.
Use: Local anesthetic.

CHILDREN'S ADVIL. (Whitehall) Ibuprofen 100 mg/5 ml. Bot. 119 ml, 473 ml.
Use: Nonsteroidal anti-inflammatory drug; analgesic.

CHILDREN'S FEVERNOL. (Upsher-Smith) Acetaminophen 120 mg or 325 mg/Supp. Pkg. 6s.
Use: Analgesic.

CHILDREN'S HOLD 4-HOUR COUGH SUPPRESSANT & DECONGESTANT. (Beecham Products) Dextromethorphan HBr 3.75 mg, phenylpropanolamine HCl 6.25 mg/Loz. Pkg. 10s.
Use: Antitussive, decongestant.

CHILDREN'S NO ASPIRIN ELIXIR. (Walgreen) Acetaminophen 80 mg/2.5 ml. Non-alcoholic. Bot. 4 oz.
Use: Analgesic.

CHILDREN'S NO-ASPIRIN TABLETS. (Walgreen) Acetaminophen 80 mg/Tab. Bot. 30s.
Use: Analgesic.

CHILDREN'S NYQUIL. (Vicks) Pseudoephedrine HCl 10 mg, chlorpheniramine maleate 0.6 mg, dextromethorphan HBr 5 mg/5 ml. Bot. 120 ml, 240 ml.
Use: Decongestant, antihistamine, antitussive.

CHINESE GELATIN.
See: Agar.

CHINESE ISINGLASS. 7-Iodo-8-hydroxyquinoline-5-sulfonic acid sodium salt. Yatren.
Use: Amebicide.

CHINIOFON. 7-Iodo-8-hydroxyquinoline-5-sulfonic acid, anayodin, yatren, quinoxyl.
Use: Amebicide.

CHINOSOL. (Vernon) 8-Hydroxyquinoline sulfate 7.5 gr/Tab. Vial 6s. Trit. Tab. (3/5 gr) Bot. 50s. Vial 110s. Pow. 1 oz.
Use: Antiseptic.

CHLAMYDIA TRACHOMATIS TEST.
Use: Diagnostic aid.
See: MicroTrak (Syva).

CHLAMYDIAZYME. (Abbott Diagnostics) Enzyme immunoassay for detection of *Chlamydia trachomatis* from urethral or urogenital swabs. Test kit 100s.
Use: Diagnostic aid.

CHLO-AMINE. (Hollister-Stier) Chlorpheniramine maleate 2 mg/Chew. Tab. Box 24x4 mg Tab. Packages.
Use: Antihistamine.

•**CHLOPHEDIANOL.** F.D.A. 2-Chloro-alpha-[2-(dimethylamino)ethyl] benzhydrol.

•**CHLOPHEDIANOL HCl.** USAN. a-(2-Dimethylaminoethyl)-o-chlorobenzyhydrol HCl.
Use: Antitussive.

CHLOR-4. (Mills) Chlorpheniramine maleate 4 mg/Tab. Bot. 100s.
Use: Antihistamine.

CHLORACOL 0.5%. (Horizon) Chloramphenicol 5 mg/ml with chlorobutanol, hydroxypropyl methylcellulose. Dropper bot. 7.5 ml.
Use: Anti-infective, ophthalmic.

CHLORAFED. (Hauck) Chlorpheniramine maleate 2 mg, pseudoephedrine HCl 30 mg/5 ml, alcohol, dye, sugar and corn free. Bot. 120 ml, 480 ml.
Use: Antihistamine, decongestant.

CHLORAFED H.S. TIMECELLES. (Hauck) Chlorpheniramine maleate 4 mg, pseudoephedrine HCl 60 mg/SR Cap. Bot. 100s, 500s, UD 50s.
Use: Antihistamine, decongestant.

CHLORAFED TIMECELLES. (Hauck) Chlorpheniramine maleate 8 mg, pseudoephedrine HCl 120 mg/SA timecelles. Bot. 100s, 500s. UD 50s.
Use: Antihistamine, decongestant.

CHLORAHIST. (Evron) Chlorpheniramine maleate **4 mg/Tab.:** Bot. 100s, 1000s. **8 mg or 12 mg/Cap.:** Bot. 250s, 1000s. **Syr. 2 mg/4 ml.:** Bot. qt.
Use: Antihistamine.

CHLORALFORMAMIDE. N-(2,2,2-trichloro-l-hydrox-yethyl) formamide.

•**CHLORAL HYDRATE,** U.S.P. XXII. Caps., Syr. U.S.P. XXII. 1,1-Ethanediol, 2,2,2-trichloro-ethanol. Chloral.
Use: Hypnotic and sedative.
See: Aquachloral Supprettes, Supp. (Webcon). Felsules, Cap. (Forest Pharm.).

Maso-Chloral, Cap. (Mason).
Noctec, Cap., Syr. (Squibb).
Oradrate, Cap. (Coast Labs.).
Rectules, Supp. (Forest Pharm.).
SK-Chloral Hydrate, Cap. (SmithKline).
Somnos, Elixir. (Merck Sharp & Dohme).
Generic Products:
Quality Generics (7.5 gr) Bot. 100s.
G.F. Harvey-Cap. (3¾ gr) Bot. 100s; (7.5 gr) Bot. 100s.
Lederle-Cap. (500 mg) 100s.
Pacific Pharm. Corp.-Cap. (7.5 gr) Bot. 100s, 1000s.
Parke, Davis-Cap. (500 mg) Bot. 100s, UD 100s.
Stayner-Cap. (250 mg or 500 mg) Bot. 100s, (500 mg) Bot. 1000s, Crystals Bot. 1 lb. and 5 lbs.
West-Ward-Cap. (3¾ gr, 7.5 gr) Bot. 100s.

CHLORAL HYDRATE BETAINE (1:1) COMPOUND. Chloral Betaine.

CHLORAL-METHYLOL OINTMENT. (Ulmer) Methyl salicylate, methol. Jar 2 oz, lb.
Use: External analgesic.

CHLORALPYRINE DICHLORALPYRINE.
See: Dichloralantipyrine.

CHLORALURETHANE. Name used for Carbochloral.

CHLORAMAN. (Rasman) Chlorpheniramine maleate 12 mg/Tab. Bot. 100s, 500s, 1000s.
Use: Antihistamine.

•**CHLORAMBUCIL,** U.S.P. XXII. Tab. U.S.P. XXII. 4-{p-[Bis(2-chlorethyl)-amino]-phenylbutyric acid. Benzenebutanoic acid. 4-[bis(2-chloroethyl)-amino]-.
Use: Antineoplastic.
See: Leukeran, Tab. (Burroughs Wellcome).

CHLORAMINE-T. Sodium paratoluenesulfan chloramide, chloramine, chlorozone.
Lilly-Tab. (0.3 Gm), Bot. 100s, 1000s.
Robinson, Pow., 1 oz.
Use: Antiseptic, deodorant.
See: Chlorazene (Badger).

•**CHLORAMPHENICOL,** U.S.P. XXII. Caps., Cream, Oral Soln., Tab., Otic Soln., Sterile, Ophth. Soln., Ophth. Oint., for Ophth. Soln. Inj., U.S.P. XXII. D(-)-threo-2, 2-Dichloro-N[Beta-hydroxy-alpha-(hy-droxymethyl)-p-nitrophenethyl]acetamide.
Use: Antibacterial, antirickettsial.
See: Chlorcetin.
Chloromycetin, Preps. (Parke-Davis).
Chloroptic Ophth. Oint. (Allergan).
Chloroptic S.O.P. Ophth. Oint. (Allergan).
Econochlor, Soln., Oint. (Alcon).
Kemicetine.
Mychel, Cap. (Rachelle).
Ophthochlor, Soln. (Parke-Davis).
Paraxin.
W/Polymixin B.
Use: Treatment of superficial ocular infections involving the conjunctiva and/or cornea caused by susceptible organisms.
See: Chloromyxin Ophthalmic Oint. (Parke-Davis).
W/Polymyxin B, Hydrocortisone.
See: Ophthocort, Oint. (Parke-Davis).

•**CHLORAMPHENICOL AND HYDROCORTISONE ACETATE FOR OPHTHALMIC SUSPENSION,** U.S.P. XXII.
Use: Antibiotic, anti-inflammatory.
See: Chloromycetin, Prods. (Parke-Davis).

•**CHLORAMPHENICOL AND POLYMYXIN B SULFATE OPHTHALMIC OINTMENT,** U.S.P. XXII.
Use: Antibiotic.

•**CHLORAMPHENICOL, POLYMIXIN B SULFATE, AND HYDROCORTISONE ACETATE OPHTHALMIC OINTMENT,** U.S.P. XXII.
Use: Antibiotic, anti-inflammatory.
See: Chloromycetin, Prods. (Parke-Davis).

•**CHLORAMPHENICOL AND PREDNISOLONE OPHTHALMIC OINTMENT,** U.S.P. XXII.
Use: Antibiotic, steroid combination.
See: Chloromycetin, Prods. (Parke-Davis).

•**CHLORAMPHENICOL PALMITATE,** U.S.P. XXII. Oral Susp. U.S.P. XXII.
Use: Antibacterial, antirickettsial.
See: Chloromycetin Palmitate, Oral Susp. (Parke-Davis).

•**CHLORAMPHENICOL PANTOTHENATE COMPLEX.** USAN. A complex consisting of 4 parts of chloramphenicol to one part of calcium pantothenate. Pantofenicol.
Use: Antibiotic.

•**CHLORAMPHENICOL SODIUM SUCCINATE, STERILE,** U.S.P. XXII.
Use: Antibacterial, antirickettsial.
See: Chloromycetin Succinate, Inj., (Parke-Davis).
Mychel-S, IV. (Rachelle).

CHLORANIL. 2,3,5,6-Tetrachloro-1,4-benzoquinone.

CHLORASEPTIC CHILDREN'S LOZENGES. (Vicks) Benzocaine 5 mg/Loz. Pkg. 18s.
Use: Local anesthetic.

CHLORASEPTIC LIQUID. (Vicks) Total phenol 1.4% as phenol and sodium phenolate, saccharin. Menthol and cherry flavors. Bot. 180 ml, 360 ml (mouthwash/gargle); 45 ml, 240 ml, 360 ml (throat spray).
Use: Antiseptic, anesthetic.

CHLORASEPTIC LOZENGE. (Vicks) Total phenol 32.5 mg/lozenge as phenol and sodium phenolate. Menthol and cherry flavors. Pkg. 18s, 36s.
Use: Anesthetic, antiseptic.

CHLORATE. (Major) Chlorpheniramine maleate 4 mg/Tab. Bot. 24s, 100s, 1000s.
Use: Antihistamine.

CHLORAZANIL HCl. 2-Amino-4-(p-chloroanilino)-s-triazine HCl. Daquim.

CHLORAZENE. (Badger) Chloramine-T, sodium p-toluene-sulfonchloramide. **Pow.:** UD Pkg. 20 Gm, 38 Gm, 50 Gm, 88 Gm, 200 Gm, 240 Gm, 320 Gm, Bot. 1 lb, 5 lb. **Aromatic Pow. (5%):** Bot. 1 lb, 5 lb. **Tab. (0.3 Gm):** Bot. 20s, 100s, 1000s, 5000s.
Use: Antiseptic, deodorant.

CHLORAZEPATE DIPOTASSIUM.
Use: Antianxiety agent, anticonvulsant.
See: Tranxene Prods. (Abbott).

CHLORAZEPATE MONOPOTASSIUM.
Use: Antianxiety agent, anticonvulsant.

CHLORAZINE TABS. (Major) Prochlorperazine 5 mg or 10 mg/Tab. Bot. 100s.
Use: Antiemetic/antivertigo, antipsychotic.

CHLORAZONE.
See: Chloramine-T.

CHLOR BENZO MOR, A AND D OINTMENT. (Wade) Vitamins A and D fortified, chlorobutanol 3%, benzocaine 2%, benzyl alcohol 3%, actamer 1%, in lanolin and petrolatum base. Tube 1 oz, Jar 1 oz, lb.
Use: Antiseptic, local anesthetic.

CHLOR BENZO MOR SPRAY. (Wade) Vitamin A and D fortified, chlorobutanol 3%, benzocaine 2%, benzyl alcohol 3%, and actamer 1%, in lanolin and mineral oil base. Bot. 2 oz, 11 oz.
Use: Antiseptic, anesthetic.

CHLORBETAMIDE. B.A.N. Dichloro-N-(2,4-dichlorobenzyl)-N-(2-hydroxyethyl)acetamide.
Use: Treatment of amebiasis.

CHLORBUTANOL.
See: Chlorobutanol, N.F. XVII.

CHLORBUTOL.
See: Chlorobutanol, N.F. XVII.

CHLORCYCLIZINE. B.A.N. 1-(4-Chlorobenzhydryl)-4-methylpiperazine.
Use: Antihistamine.

CHLORCYCLIZINE HYDROCHLORIDE, N.F. XVI. 1-(p-Chloro-α-phenylbenzyl)-4-methylpiperazine HCl. 1-(p-Chlorobenzhydryl)-4-methylpiperazine HCl. Histantin.
Use: Antihistamine.
W/Hydrocortisone acetate.
See: Mantadil, Cream (Burroughs Wellcome).
W/Pseudoephedrine HCl.
See: Fedrazil, Tab. (Burroughs Wellcome).

•**CHLORDANTOIN.** F.D.A. 5-(1-Ethylpentyl)-3-[(trichloromethyl) thio] hydantoin.

•**CHLORDANTOIN.** USAN. 5-(1-Ethylamyl)-3-trichloro- methyl thiohydantoin.
Use: Antifungal.
See: Sporostacin Cream (Ortho).

•**CHLORDIAZEPOXIDE,** U.S.P. XXII. Tab., U.S.P. XXII. 3H-1, 4-Benzodiazepin-2-amine, 7-chloro-N-methyl-5-phenyl-, 4-oxide; 7-chloro-2-(methylamino)-5-phenyl-3H-1, 4-benzodiazepine 4-oxide.
Use: Antianxiety agent.
See: A-poxide, Cap. (Abbott).
Brigen-G, Tab. (Grafton).
Libritabs, Tab. (Roche).
Menrium, Tab. (Roche).
W/Amitriptyline.
See: Limbitrol, Tab. (Roche).

•**CHLORDIAZEPOXIDE HCl,** U.S.P. XXII., Caps, Sterile U.S.P. XXII. 7-Chloro-2-methylamino-5-phenyl-3H-1, 4-benzodiazepine-4-oxide HCl. Metha- minodiazepine HCl.
Use: Tranquilizer, sedative.
See: A-poxide, Cap. (Abbott).
Chlordiazachel, Cap. (Rachelle).
Librium, Cap., Inj. (Roche).
Screen, Cap. (Foy).
Zetran, Cap. (Hauck).
W/Clidinium bromide.
See: Librax, Cap. (Roche).

•**CHLORDIAZEPOXIDE AND AMITRIPTYLINE HCL TABLETS,** U.S.P. XXII.
Use: Antianxiety agent.
See: Limbitrol, Tab. (Roche).

CHLOREN 4. (Wren) Chlorpheniramine maleate 4 mg/Tab. Bot. 100s, 1000s.
Use: Antihistamine.

CHLOREN 8 T.D. (Wren) Chlorpheniramine maleate 8 mg/Tab. Bot. 100s, 1000s.
Use: Antihistamine.

CHLOREN 12 T.D. (Wren) Chlorpheniramine maleate 12 mg/Tab. Bot. 100s, 1000s.
Use: Antihistamine.

CHLORESIUM. (Rystan) **Oint.:** Chlorophyllin copper complex 0.5% in hydrophilic base. Tube 1 oz, 4 oz, Jar lb. **Soln.:** Chlorophyllin copper complex 0.2% in isotonic saline soln. Bot. 60 ml, 240 ml, qt.
Use: Healing agent, deodorizer.

CHLORESIUM TABLETS. (Rystan) Chlorophyllin copper complex 14 mg/Tab. Bot. 100s, 1000s.
Use: Oral deodorant.

CHLORESIUM TOOTH PASTE. (Rystan) Chlorophyllin copper complex. Tube 3.25 oz.
Use: Oral deodorant.

CHLORETHYL.
See: Ethyl Chloride.

CHLORGUANIDE HYDROCHLORIDE.
See: Chloroguanide HCl (Various Mfr.).

CHLORHEXADOL. 2-Methyl-4-(2′,2′,2′,-trichlor-1′-hydroxyethoxy)-2-pentanol. Lora.

CHLORHEXADOL. B.A.N. 2-Methyl-4-(2,2,2-trichloro-1-hydroxyethoxy)pentan-2-ol.
Use: Hypnotic, sedative.

•**CHLORHEXIDINE.** F.D.A. 1,1′-Hexamethylenebis-[5-(ρ-chlorophenyl) biguanide]
Use: Antiseptic.
See: Hibiclens.
Hibiscrub.
Hibitane.
Lisium.
Rotersept.

•**CHLORHEXIDINE GLUCONATE.** USAN. 1,1′-Hex-amethylenebis [5-(ρ-chlorophenyl)biguanide] dihydro-Cl. Oral rinse or topical skin cleanser.
Use: Antimicrobial.

See: Hibiclens, Liq. (Stuart).
Hibistat, Liq. (Stuart).
Peridex (Procter & Gamble).

•**CHLORHEXIDINE HYDROCHLORIDE.** USAN.
Use: Anti-infective, topical.

CHLORHYDROXYQUINOLIN.
See: Quinolor Compound, Oint. (Squibb).

CHLORINATED AND IODIZED PEANUT OIL. Chloriodized Oil.

•**CHLORINDANOL.** USAN. 7-Chloro-4-indanol.
Use: Antiseptic, spermaticide.

CHLORINE COMPOUND, ANTISEPTIC. Antiseptics, Chlorine.

CHLORIODIZED OIL. Chlorinated and iodized peanut oil.

CHLORISONDAMINE CHLORIDE. 4,5,6,7-Tetrachloro-2-(2-dimethylaminoethyl)-isoindoline dimethoCl.

CHLORISONDAMINE CHLORIDE. B.A.N. 4,5,6,7-Tetrachloro-2-(2-trimethylammonioethyl)-isoindolinium diCl.
Use: Hypotensive.

•**CHLORMADINONE ACETATE.** USAN. 6-Chloro-6-dehydro-17α-acetoxyprogesterone. 6-Chloro-17-hydroxypregna-4,6-diene-3,20 dione acetate.
Use: Progestin.

CHLOR MAL w/SAL + APAP S.C. (Richlyn) Chlorpheniramine maleate 2 mg, acetaminophen 150 mg, salicylamide 175 mg/Tab. Bot. 1000s.
Use: Antihistamine, analgesic.

CHLORMENE. (Robinson) Chlorpheniramine maleate 4 mg/Tab. Bot. 100s, 1000s.
Use: Antihistamine.

CHLORMENE INJECTION. (Robinson) Chlorpheniramine maleate injection. 10 mg/30 ml Vial; 100 mg/10 ml Vial.
Use: Antihistamine.

CHLORMENE REPEAT ACTION. (Robinson) Chlorpheniramine 8 mg or 12 mg/Tab. Bot. 100s, 1000s.
Use: Antihistamine.

CHLORMENE TIMECAPS. (Robinson) Chlorpheniramine maleate time disintegration 8 mg or 12 mg/Tab. Bot. 100s, 500s, 1000s.
Use: Antihistamine.

CHLORMERODRIN. 3-Chloro-mercuri-2-methoxypropylurea. Chloro (2-methoxy-3-ureidopropyl) mercury. Mercloran.
Use: Diuretic.

CHLORMERODRIN Hg 197 INJECTION. Mercury-^{197}HG, [3-[(aminocarbonyl)amino]-2- methoxypropyl]-chloro-. Chloro(2-methoxy-3-ureidopropyl)mercury-^{197}Hg.
Use: Diagnostic aid (renal scanning).

CHLORMERODRIN Hg 203 INJECTION. Mercury-^{203}Hg,[3-[(aminocarbonyl)amino]-ureidopropyl)mercury-^{203}Hg.
Use: Diagnostic aid (tumor localization).

CHLORMETHIAZOLE. B.A.N. 5-(2-Chloroethyl)-4-methylthiazole.
Use: Hypnotic, sedative.

CHLORMEZANONE. Chlormethazanone. 2-(4-Chlorophenyl)-3-methyl-4-methathiazanone-1-2-dioxide.
Use: Antianxiety agent.
See: Trancopal, Cap. (Winthrop Pharm).

CHLORMIDAZOLE. B.A.N. 1-(4-Chlorobenzyl)-2-methylbenzimidazole.
Use: Antifungal agent.

CHLOR-NIRAMINE ALLERGY TABS. (Whiteworth) Chlorpheniramine maleate 4 mg/Tab. Bot. 24s, 100s.
Use: Antihistamine.

CHLOROAZODIN. Alpha, alpha, Azobis-(chloroformamidine).

•**CHLOROBUTANOL,** N.F. XVII. 1,1,1-Trichloro-2-methyl-2-propanol. Sedaform. (Various Mfr.).
Use: Anesthetic, antiseptic, hypnotic; pharmaceutic aid (antimicrobial preservative).
See: Cerumenex, Drops (Purdue-Frederick).
Pre-Sert (Allergan).
W/Atropine sulfate, chlorpheniramine maleate, phenylpropanolamine HCl.
See: Decongestant, Inj. (Century).
W/Benzocaine, camphor.
See: Eardro, Liq. (Jenkins).
W/Calcium glycerophosphate, calcium levulinate.
See: Cal San, Inj. (Burgin-Arden).
W/Cetyltrimethylammonium Br, methapyrilene HCl, phenylephrine HCl, hydrocortisone.
See: T-Spray, Liq. (Saron).
W/Diphenhydramine HCl.
See: Ardeben, Inj. (Burgin-Arden).
W/Ephedrine HCl, sodium Cl.
See: Efedron HCl Nasal Jelly (Hart).
W/Estradiol cypionate, testosterone cypionate.
See: Depo-Testadiol, Vial (Upjohn).
Depotestogen, Vial (Hyrex).
W/Glycerin, anhydrous.
See: Ophthalgan, Liq. (Wyeth-Ayerst).
W/Liquifilm.
See: Liquifilm Tears (Allergan).
W/Methylcellulose.
See: Lacril (Allergan).
W/Myristyl-gamma-picolinium Cl.
See: Wet Tone, Soln. (Riker).
W/Nonionic lanolin derivative.
See: Lacri-Lube, Ophthalmic Ointment (Allergan).
W/Polyethylene glycol, polyoxyl 40 stearate.
See: Blink-N-Clean (Allergan).
W/Sodium Cl.
See: Ocean, Liq. (Fleming).
W/Tannic acid, isopropyl alcohol.
See: Outgro, Soln. (Whitehall).
W/Vitamins B_1, B_2, B_6, niacinamide, calcium pantothenate, benzyl alcohol.
See: Lanoplex, Inj. (Lannett).

•**CHLOROCRESOL,** U.S.P. XXII.
Use: Antiseptic, disinfectant.

CHLOROETHANE.
See: Ethyl Chloride.

CHLORODRI. (Kenyon) Chlorpheniramine maleate 5 mg, phenylpropanolamine HCl 12.5 mg, atropine sulfate 0.2 mg/ml. Vial 10 ml.
Use: Antihistamine, decongestant, anticholinergic/antispasmodic.

CHLOROFAIR. (Pharmafair) **Soln.:** Chloramphenicol 5 mg/ml. Bot. 7.5 ml **Oint.:** Chloramphenicol 10 mg/Gm in white petrolatum base with mineral oil, polysorbate 60. Tube 3.5 Gm.
Use: Anti-infective, ophthalmic.

CHLOROFON-F. (Rugby) Chlorzoxazone 250 mg, acetaminophen 300 mg/Tab. Bot. 100s, 1000s.
Use: Skeletal muscle relaxant, analgesic.

•**CHLOROFORM,** N.F. XVII. Bot. 1 lb, 5 lb.
Use: Inhalation anesthetic; solvent.

CHLOROGUANIDE HYDROCHLORIDE. (Various Mfr.) (Proguanil HCl) 1-(p-Chlorophenyl)-5-isopropylbiguanidine HCl. Guanatol HCl.
Use: Antimalarial.

CHLOROHIST-LA. (Hauck) Xylometazoline HCl 0.1%. Soln. Spray 15 ml.
Use: Nasal decongestant.

CHLORO-IODOHYDROXYQUINOLINE.
See: Clioquinol, U.S.P. XXII.

p-CHLOROMETAXYLENOL.
W/Benzocaine, benzyl alcohol, propylene glycol.
See: 20-Cain Burn Relief (Alto).
W/Hydrocortisone, pramoxine HCl.
See: Orlex HC, Otic (Baylor).

CHLOROMETHAPYRILENE CITRATE.
See: Chlorothen Citrate.

CHLOROMYCETIN. (Parke-Davis) Chloramphenicol.
Cream: (1%) w/cetyl alcohol, sodium lauryl sulfate, liquid petrolatum, buffered with sodium phosphate, propylparaben. Tube 30 Gm.
Ophth. Oint.: (1%) in base of petrolatum, polyethylene. Tube 3.5 Gm.
Ophth. Soln.: (25 mg) Bot. w/dropper 15 ml (dry). Soln. 5 mg/ml Plastic dropper Bot. 5 ml.
Otic Drops: (0.5%) 5 mg/ml w/propylene glycol. Bot. 15 ml.
Use: Anti-infective.

CHLOROMYCETIN-HYDROCORTISONE. (Parke-Davis) Hydrocortisone acetate 0.5% (2.5% as powder), chloramphenicol 0.25% (1.25% as powder), cholesterol, methylcellulose, benzethonium Cl 0.01%. Pow. Bot. with dropper 5 ml. Reconstitute with water.
Use: Anti-infective, ophthalmic.

CHLOROMYCETIN SODIUM SUCCINATE I.V. (Parke-Davis) Chloramphenicol sodium succinate dried powder which when reconstituted contains chloromycetin 100 mg/ml. Steri-vial 1 Gm, 10s.
Use: Anti-infective.

CHORON 10. (Forest) Chorionic gonadotropin 1000 units. Vial 10 ml.
Use: Chorionic gonadotropin.

p-CHLOROPHENOL.
See: Parachlorophenol.

CHLOROPHENOTHANE. 1,1,1-Trichloro-2,2-bis(p-chlorophenyl) ethane. Gesarol, Neocid, Dicophane.
Use: Pediculicide.

CHLOROPHYLL. (Freeda Vitamins) Chlorophyll 20 mg/Tab. Bot. 100s, 250s, 500s.
Use: Deodorizer.

CHLOROPHYLL "A" OINTMENT.
See: Chloresium Oint. (Rystan).

CHLOROPHYLL "A" SOLUTION (Chlorophyllin).
See: Chloresium Soln. (Rystan).

CHLOROPHYLL COMPLEX PERLES. (Standard Process) Natural chlorophyll extracted from alfalfa and tillandsia. Vitamin K 3.3 mg/6 Perles. Bot. 60s, 350s. Oint. Tube 1.5 oz, Jar 3 oz.
Use: Healing agent, deodorizer.

CHLOROPHYLL TABLETS.
See: Derifil, Tab. (Rystan).
Nullo, Tab. (Depree).

CHLOROPHYLL, WATER-SOLUBLE. (Various Mfr.) Chlorophyllin.
See: Chloresium Prep. (Rystan).
Derifil, Pow. (Rystan).

CHLOROPHYLLIN.
Use: Healing agent, deodorizer.

•**CHLOROPHYLLIN COPPER COMPLEX.** USAN.
Use: Deodorant.

•**CHLOROPROCAINE HCl,** U.S.P. XXII. Inj., U.S.P. XXII. beta, Diethylamino-ethyl 2-chloro-4-amino-benzoate HCl. 4-amino-2-chloro-, 2-(diethylamino) ethyl ester, HCl. 2-(Diethylamino) ethyl 4-amino-2-chlorobenzoate HCl. (Abbott) 2% or 3%. Concentration in Abboject Syringe, Ampule or Vial.
Use: Anesthetic (local).
See: Nesacaine, Vial (Pennwalt).
Nescaine-CE, Vial (Pennwalt).

CHLOROPTIC STERILE OPHTHALMIC SOLUTION. (Allergan) Chloramphenicol 0.5%, chlorobutanol 0.5%. Dropper bot. 2.5 ml, 7.5 ml.
Use: Anti-infective, ophthalmic.

•**CHLOROQUINE,** U.S.P. XXII. 7-Chloro-4-[[4-(diethylamino)-1-methyl butyl]amino]quinoline.
Use: Pharmaceutic necessity for chloroquine HCl.
See: Aralen HCl Prods. (Winthrop Pharm).
Roquine, Tab. (Robinson).

•**CHLOROQUINE HYDROCHLORIDE INJ.,** U.S.P. XXII.
Use: Antiamebic, antimalarial.
See: Aralen HCl (Winthrop).

•**CHLOROQUINE PHOSPHATE,** U.S.P. XXII. Tab. U.S.P. XXII. Nivaquine.
Use: Febrile attacks of malaria; antiamebic; lupus erythematosus suppressant.
See: Aralen Phosphate, Tab. (Winthrop Pharm).

CHLOROQUINE PHOSPHATE W/PRIMAQUIN PHOSPHATE.
See: Aralen Phosphate W/Primaquine Phosphate (Winthrop Pharm.).

5-CHLORO-SALICYLANILIDE.

CHLOROSERPIN. (Various Mfr.) Chlorothiazide 250 mg or 500 mg, reserpine 0.125 mg/Tab. Bot. 100s, 1000s.
Use: Antihypertensive.

CHLOROTHEN. 2-[(5-Chloro-2-thenyl)(2-di- methylaminoethyl)amino]pyridine hydrochloride, citrate salts (Chlorothenylpyramine, chloromethapyrilene, pyrithen).
Use: Antihistamine.

CHLOROTHEN CITRATE. (Whittier) 2-[-(5-Chloro-2-thenyl)]2-dimethylamino)-ethyl]amino]pyridine dihydrogen citrate. Chloromethapyrilene, chlorothenylpyramine, pyrithen. Tab., Bot. 100s.
Use: Antihistamine.
W/Pyrilamine, thenylpyramine.
See: Derma-Pax, Liq. (Recsei).

CHLOROTHENYLPYRAMINE. Chlorothen, Prep.

CHLOROTHEOPHYLLINATE W/BENADRYL.
See: Dramamine, Prep. (Searle).

•**CHLOROTHIAZIDE,** U.S.P. XXII. Oral Susp., Tabs., U.S.P. XXII. 6-Chloro-2H-1,2,4-benzothiadiazine-7-sulfonamide 1,1-dioxide.
Use: Diuretic.
See: Diuril, Tab., Susp. (Merck Sharp & Dohme).
W/Methyldopa.
See: Aldoclor, Tab. (Merck Sharp & Dohme).
W/Reserpine. Tab.: Chlorothiazide 250 mg or 500 mg, reserpine 0.125 mg. Bot. 100s, 1000s.
See: Diupres, Tab. (Merck Sharp & Dohme).
Use: Diuretic.

•**CHLOROTHIAZIDE SODIUM FOR INJECTION,** U.S.P. XXII.
Use: Diuretic.
See: Sodium Diuril, Vial (Merck Sharp & Dohme).

CHLOROTHYMOL. 6-Chlorothymol.
Use: Antibacterial.

•**CHLOROTRIANISENE,** U.S.P. XXII. Cap., U.S.P. XXII. Chlorotris (p-methoxyphenyl)ethylene. Chlorotri-(4-methoxyphenyl)ethylene.
Use: Estrogen.
See: TACE, Cap. (Merrell Dow).

β-CHLOROVINYL ETHYNYL CARBINOL.
See: Placidyl, Cap. (Abbott).

•**CHLOROXINE,** USAN.
Use: Antiseborrheic.

•**CHLOROXYLENOL,** U.S.P. XXII. 4-Chloro-3,5-xylenol. p-Chloro-m-xylenol; parachloro-metaxylenol; benzytol.
Use: Antiseptic.
W/Benzocaine, menthol, lanolin.
See: Unburn, Spray, Cream, Lot. (Leeming-Pacquin).
W/Hexachlorophene.
See: Desitin, Preps. (Leeming-Pacquin).
W/Methyl salicylate, menthol, camphor, thymol, eucalyptus oil, isopropyl alcohol.
See: Gordobalm, Balm (Gordon).

CHLORPAZINE. (Major) Prochlorperazine maleate 5 mg, 10 mg or 25 mg/Tab. Bot. 100s, UD 100s (5 mg, 10 mg only).
Use: Antipsychotic.

CHLORPHED INJECTION. (Hauck) Brompheniramine maleate 10 mg/ml. Vial 10 ml.
Use: Antihistamine.

CHLORPHED-LA. (Hauck) Oxymetazoline 0.05%. Soln. Spray 15 ml.
Use: Decongestant.

•**CHLORPHENESIN.** F.D.A. 3-(p-Chlorophenoxy)-1,2-propanediol.

CHLORPHENESIN. B.A.N. 3-(4-Chlorophenoxyl)-propane-1,2-diol.
Use: Antifungal agent.

•**CHLORPHENESIN CARBAMATE.** USAN. 3-(p-Chlorophenoxy)-2-hydroxypropyl carbamate.
Use: Muscle relaxant.
See: Maolate, Tab. (Upjohn).

•**CHLORPHENIRAMINE MALEATE,** U.S.P. XXII. Inj., Syr., Tab., U.S.P. XXII. 2-[p-Chloro-alpha(2-dime-thylaminoethyl)benzyl]pyridine maleate, chlorprophenpyridamine maleate. 2-Pyridinepropanamine, gamma-(4-chlorophenyl)-N,N-dimethyl-,(Z)-2-butenedioate(1:1).
Use: Antihistamine.
See: Alermine, Tab. (Reid-Rowell).
Chestamine, Cap. (Leeds).
Chlo-Amine, Tab. (Hollister-Stier).
Chloraman, Tab. (Rasman).
Chloren, Preps. (Wren).
Chlor-4, Tab. (Mills).
Chlormene, Tab. (Robinson).
Chlormene Inj. (Robinson).
Chlormene Repeat Action, Tab. (Robinson).
Chlormene Timecaps, Tab. (Robinson).
Chlor-Niramine, Tab. (Whiteworth).
Chlorophen, Vial (Medical Chem.).
Chlor-pen, Tab., Vial (American Chemical & Drug).
Chlor-Span, Cap. (Burlington).
Chlortab, Tab., Cap., Inj. (North American Pharmacal).
Chlor-Trimeton Maleate, Preps. (Schering).
Cosea, Preps. (Center).
Histacon, Tab., Syr. (Marsh Labs).
Histaspan, Cap. (Rorer).
Histex, Cap. (Hauck).
Nasahist (Keene).
Phenetron, Preps. (Lannett).
Polaramine, Tab., Syr. (Schering).
Pyranistan Tab. (Standex).
Rhinihist, Elix. (Central).
Teldrin, Spansule (SmithKline Prods).
Trymegen (Medco).

CHLORPHENIRAMINE MALEATE W/COMBINATIONS.
See: Al-Ay, Preps. (Bowman).
Alka-Seltzer Plus, Tab. (Miles).
Allerdec, Cap. (Towne).
Allerest, Prods. (Pharmacraft).
Alumadrine, Tab. (Fleming).

A.R.M., Tab. (SmithKline Prods).
Atussin-D.M. Expectorant, Liq. (Federal).
Bellafedrol A-H, Tab. (Lannett).
B.M.E., Liq. (Brothers).
Bobid, Cap. (Boyd).
Breacol Cough Medication, Liq. (Glenbrook).
Brolade, Cap. (Brothers).
Bur-Tuss Expectorant (Burlington).
CDM Expectorant (Lannett).
Cenahist, Cap. (Century).
Cenaid, Tab. (Century).
Centuss, Tab. (Century).
Chew-Hist, Wafer (Kenyon).
Chlorodri, Vial (Kenyon).
Chlorpel, Cap. (Santa).
Chlor-Trimeton, Preps. (Schering).
Codimal, Tab. (Central).
Col-Decon, Tab. (Quality Generics).
Colrex Compound, Preps. (Reid-Rowell).
Comtrex, Tab., Cap., Liq. (Bristol-Myers).
Conalsyn Croncap, Cap. (Cenci).
Contac, Cap. (SmithKline Prods).
Cophene No. 2, Cap. (Dunhall).
Cophene-S, Syr. (Dunhall).
Coricidin, Preps. (Schering).
Corilin, Liq. (Schering).
Corizahist, Preps. (Mason).
Coryban-D, Cap. (Leeming).
Co-Tylenol, Preps. (McNeil).
Dallergy, Tab., Cap., Syr. (Laser).
Decobel, Cap. (Lannett).
Decojen, Tab., Vial (Jenkins).
Deconamine, Tab., Cap., Syr. (Berlex).
Dehist, Cap. (Forest).
Demazin, Tab., Syr. (Schering).
Derma-Pax, Lot. (Recsei).
Dezest, Cap. (Geneva Drugs).
Donatussin, Liq., Syr. (Laser).
Dristan, Preps. (Whitehall).
Drucon, Elix. (Standard Drug).
Efricon Expectorant (Lannett).
Extendryl, Tab., Cap., Syr. (Fleming).
F.C.A.H., Cap. (Scherer).
Fedahist, Prods. (Donner).
Fitacol (Standex).
Formadrin, Liq. (Kenyon).
Histabid, Cap. (Glaxo).
Hista-Compound #5, Tab. (Vortech).
Histacon, Tab., Syr. (Marsh Labs).
Histapco, Tab. (Apco).
Histaspan-D, Cap. (Rorer).
Histaspan Plus, Cap. (Rorer).
Hista-Vadrin, Tab., Cap., Syr. (Scherer).
Histine Prods. (Freeport).
Histogesic, Tab. (Century).
Hycomine Compound, Tab. (Du Pont).
Infantuss, Liq. (Scott/Cord).
Koryza, Tab. (Forest Pharm.).
Kronofed-A, Cap. (Ferndale).
Lanatuss Expectorant (Lannett).
Marhist (Marlop).
Neo-Pyranistan, Tab. (Standex).
Nilcol, Tab., Elix. (Parke-Davis).
Nolamine, Tab. (Carnrick).
Novafed A, Cap., Liq. (Merrell Dow).
Novahistine, Preps. (Merrell Dow).
Oraminic, Preps. (Vortech).
Partuss, Liq. (Parmed).
Partuss T.D., Tab. (Parmed).
Phenahist, Preps. (Amid).
Phenchlor, Prods. (Freeport).
Phenetron Compound, Tab. (Lannett).
Polytuss-DM, Liq. (Rhode).
Pyma, Cap., Vial (Forest Pharm.).
Pyristan, Cap., Elix. (Arcum).
Pyranistan (Standex).
Quelidrine, Syr. (Abbott).
Rentuss, Cap., Syr. (Wren).
Rhinex D M, Tab., Syr. (Lemmon).
Rhinogesic, Tab. (Vale).
Rinocidin, Cap., Liq. (Cenci).
Rohist-D, Cap. (Rocky Mtn.).
Rolanade, Cap. (Robinson).
Ryna, Liq. (Wallace).
Ryna-tussadine, Tab., Liq. (Wallace).
Salphenyl, Cap. (Hauck).
Scotcof, Liq. (Scott/Cord).
Scotnord (Scott/Cord).
Scotuss Liq. (Scott/Cord).
Shertus, Liq. (Sheryl).
Sialco, Tab. (Foy).
Sinarest, Tab. (Pharmacraft).
Sine-Off, Prods. (SmithKline Prods).
Sino-Compound, Tab. (Bio-Factor).
Sinovan Timed, Cap. (Drug Ind.).
Sinucol, Cap., Vial (Tennessee).
Sinulin, Tab. (Carnrick).
Sinutab Extra Strength, Cap. (Warner-Lambert).
Spantuss, Tab., Liq. (Arco).
Statomin Maleate CC, Tab. (Bowman).
Sudafed Plus, Tab., Syr. (Burroughs Wellcome).
Symptrol, Cap. (Saron).
T.A.C., Cap. (Towne).
Tonecol, Tab., Syr. (A.V.P.).
Triamininc, Prods. (Sandoz Consumer).
Triamincin Chewables (Sandoz Consumer).
Trigelamine, Oint. (E.J. Moore).
Turbilixir, Liq. (Burlington).
Turbispan Leisurecaps, Cap. (Burlington).
Tusquelin, Syr. (Circle).
Tussar, Prods. (Rorer).
Valihist, Cap. (Otis Clapp).

d-CHLORPHENIRAMINE MALEATE.
See: Polarmine Expectorant, Tab., Syr. (Schering).

•**CHLORPHENIRAMINE POLISTIREX.** USAN.
Use: Antihistamine.

CHLORPHENIRAMINE RESIN W/COMBINATIONS.
See: Omni-Tuss, Liq. (Pennwalt).

CHLORPHENIRAMINE TANNATE.

W/Carbetapentane tannate, ephedrine tannate, phenylephrine tannate.
See: Rynatuss Tab., Susp. (Wallace).
W/Phenylephrine tannate, pyrilamine tannate.
See: Rynatan, Tab., Susp. (Wallace).

CHLORPHENOCTIUM AMSONATE. B.A.N. 2,4-Di- chlorophenoxymethyldimethyloctylammonium 4,4′-diaminostilbene-2,2′-disulfonate.
Use: Antifungal agent.

CHLORPHENOXAMINE. B.A.N. N-2-(4-Chloro-α-methylbenzhydryloxy)ethyldimethylamine.
Use: Antiparkinson agent.

CHLORPHTHALIDONE. 1-Oxo-3-(3′-sulfanyl-4′-chlorphenyl)-3-hydroxy-isoindoline.
See: Chlorthalidone.

CHLOR-PRO 10. (Schein) Chlorpheniramine maleate 10 mg/ml, benzyl alcohol. Inj. Vial 30 ml.
Use: Antihistamine.

CHLORPROGUANIL. B.A.N. 1-(3,4-Dichlorophenyl)-5-isopropylbiguanide.
Use: Antimalarial.

•**CHLORPROMAZINE,** U.S.P. XXII. Supp. U.S.P. XXII. 2-Chloro-10-[3-(dimethylamino)propyl]-phenothiazine. 10H-Phenothiazine-10-propanamine,2-chloro-N,N-dimethyl
Use: Antiemetic, tranquilizer.
See: Chloractil.
Largactil.

•**CHLORPROMAZINE HCl,** U.S.P. XXII. Inj., Syr., Tab., Cap., Supp. U.S.P. XXII.
Use: Antiemetic, tranquilizer.
See: Chlorzine, Inj. (Hauck).
Promachlor, Tab. (Geneva).
Promapar, Tab. (Parke-Davis).
Promaz, Inj. (Keene).
Sonazine, Tab. (Reid-Rowell).
Terpium, Tab. (Scrip).
Thorazine, Tab., Cap., Liq., Syr., Supp., Amp. (SmithKline).

CHLORPROMAZINE HCL INTENSOL ORAL SOLUTION. (Roxane) Chlorpromazine HCl concentrated oral soln. **30 mg/ml:** Bot. 120 ml. **100 mg/ml:** Bot. 240 ml.
Use: Antiemetic, antipsychotic.

•**CHLORPROPAMIDE,** U.S.P. XXII. Tabs. U.S.P. XXII. 1-[(p-Chlorophenyl)-sulfonyl]-3-propylurea. Benzene-sulfonamide, 4-chloro-N-[(propylamino)carbonyl]-.
Use: Hypoglycemic agent.
See: Diabinese, Tab. (Pfizer Laboratories).

CHLORPROPHENPYRIDAMINE MALEATE.
See: Chlorpheniramine Maleate, U.S.P. XXII.

•**CHLORPROTHIXENE,** U.S.P. XXII. Inj., Oral Susp., Tab., U.S.P. XXII. 1-Propanamine, 3-(2-chloro-9H-thioxanthene-9-ylidene)-N,N-dimethyl-,(Z)-; (Z)-2-Chloro-N,N-dimethylthioxanthene-Δ^9-propylamine.
Use: Tranquilizer; antiemetic.
See: Taractan, Tab., Conc., Inj. (Roche).

CHLORQUINALDOL. 5,7-Dichloro-8-hydroxyquinal-dine.

CHLORQUINALDOL. B.A.N. 5,7-Dichloro-8-hydroxy-2-methylquinoline.
Use: Antiseptic, fungicide.

CHLORQUINOL. A mixture of the chlorinated products of 8-hydroxyquinoline containing about 65% of 5,7-dichloro-8-hydroxyquinoline. Quixalin.

CHLOR-REST. (Rugby) Phenylpropanolamine HCl 18.7 mg, chlorpheniramine maleate 2 mg/Tab. Bot. 24s, 100s, 1000s.
Use: Decongestant, antihistamine.

CHLOR-SPAN. (Burlington) Chlorpheniramine maleate 8 mg/S.R. Cap. Bot. 60s.
Use: Antihistamine.

CHLORSPAN-12. (Vortech) Chlorpheniramine maleate 12 mg/Cap. Bot. 1000s.
Use: Antihistamine.

CHLORTAB. (Vortech) Chlorpheniramine maleate **4 mg or 8 mg/Tab.:** Bot. 1000s. **Vial 100 mg/ml:** 10 ml. **Spancap:** 12 mg/Cap.
Use: Antihistamine.

•**CHLORTETRACYCLINE AND SULFAMETHAZINE BISULFATES SOLUBLE POWDER,** U.S.P XXII.
Use: Antibiotic.

•**CHLORTETRACYCLINE BISULFATE,** U.S.P. XXII.
Use: Antibiotic.

•**CHLORTETRACYCLINE HYDROCHLORIDE,** U.S.P. XXII. Caps., Oint., Ophth. Oint., Soluble Powder, Sterile, Tab., U.S.P. XXII. 7-Chlorotetracycline hydrochloride.
Use: Antibiotic.
See: Aureomycin, Prep. (Lederle).

•**CHLORTHALIDONE,** U.S.P. XXII. Tabs. U.S.P. XXII. 2-Chloro-5-(1-hydroxy-3-oxo-1-isoindolinyl)benzenesulfonamide. Benzenesulfonamide, 2-chloro-5-(2,3-dihydro-1-hydroxy-3-oxo-1H-isoindol-1-yl)-.
Use: Diuretic, antihypertensive.
See: Combipres, Tab. (Boehringer-Ingelheim).
Hygroton, Tab. (Rorer).
W/Reserpine.
See: Demi-Regroton, Tab. (Rorer).
Regroton, Tab. (Rorer).

CHLORTHENOXAZIN. B.A.N. 2-(2-Chloroethyl)-2,3-dihydro-1,3-benzoxazin-4-one.
Use: Anti-inflammatory, analgesic.

CHLORTRIANISENE, U.S.P. XXI.

CHLOR-TRIMETON. (Schering) Chlorpheniramine maleate. **Inj.:** 10 mg/ml. Amp. 1 ml 100s. **Tab.:** 4 mg. Box 24s. Bot. 100s, 1000s. **Repetabs:** 8 mg. Box 24s, 48s. Bot. 100s, 1000s. 12 mg. Bot. 100s, 1000s. Blister packs 12s, 24s. **Syr.:** 2 mg/5 ml. Bot. 4 oz, pt, gal.
Use: Antihistamine.

CHLOR-TRIMETON W/COMBINATIONS. (Schering) Chlorpheniramine maleate.
W/Acetaminophen.
See: Coricidin, Tab. (Schering).
W/Acetaminophen, phenylpropanolamine.
See: Coricidin "D", Prods. (Schering).

W/Phenylephrine HCl.
See: Demazin, Prods. (Schering).
W/Pseudoephedrine sulfate.
See: Chlor-Trimeton Decongestant Tab. (Schering).
Chlor-Trimeton Decongestant Repetabs (Schering).
W/Salicylamide, phenacetin, caffeine, vitamin C.
See: Coriforte, Cap. (Schering).
W/Sodium salicylate, amino acetic acid.
See: Corilin, Liq. (Schering).

CHLOR-TRIMETON DECONGESTANT REPETABS. (Schering) Chlorpheniramine maleate 8 mg, pseudoephedrine sulfate 120 mg/SR Tab. Box 24s, 48s. UD 96s.
Use: Antihistamine, decongestant.

CHLOR-TRIMETON DECONGESTANT TABLETS. (Schering) Chlorpheniramine maleate 4 mg, pseudoephedrine sulfate 60 mg/Tab. Box 24s, 48s.
Use: Antihistamine, decongestant.

CHLOR-TRIMETON SINUS. (Schering) Phenylpropanolamine HCl 12.5 mg, chlorpheniramine maleate 2 mg, acetaminophen 500 mg/Capl. Box 12s, 24s.
Use: Decongestant, antihistamine, analgesic.

CHLORTRON. (Pharmex) Chlorpheniramine maleate 10 mg/Vial. Vial 30 ml.
Use: Antihistamine.

CHLORZIDE. (Foy) Hydrochlorothiazide 50 mg/Tab. Bot. 1000s.
Use: Diuretic.

CHLORZONE FORTE. (Schein) Chlorzoxazone 250 mg, acetaminophen 300 mg/Tab. Bot. 100s, 1000s.
Use: Skeletal muscle relaxant, analgesic.

•**CHLORZOXAZONE,** U.S.P. XXII. Tab., U.S.P. XXII. 5-Chlorobenzoxazolin-2-one. 5-Chlorobenzoxazolinone.
Use: Muscle relaxant.
See: Paraflex, Tab. (McNeil).
W/Acetaminophen.
See: Blanex, Cap. (Edwards).
Parafon Forte, Tab. (McNeil).

•**CHLORZOXAZONE AND ACETAMINOPHEN CAPSULES,** U.S.P. XXII.
Use: Muscle relaxant, analgesic.

CHLORZOXAZONE AND ACETAMINOPHEN TABLETS, U.S.P. XXI.
Use: Muscle relaxant, analgesic.

CHOICE 10. (Whiteworth) Potassium Cl 10% soln., unflavored. Bot. gal.
Use: Potassium supplement.

CHOICE 20. (Whiteworth) Potassium Cl 20% soln., unflavored. Bot. gal.
Use: Potassium supplement.

CHOLAC. (Alra) Lactulose 10 Gm/15 ml. Bot. 240 ml, pt, UD 30 ml.
Use: Laxative.

CHOLACRYLAMINE RESIN. An anion exchange resin consisting of a water soluble polymer having a molecular weight equivalent between 350 and 360 in which aliphatic quaternary amine groups are attached to an acrylic backbone by ester linkages.

CHOLAJEN. (Jenkins) Ox bile extract 3.5 gr, desoxycholic acid ⅛ gr, dehydrocholic acid ⅛ gr, pancreatin 1 gr, betaine HCl 1 gr. Bot. 1000s.
Use: Laxative.

CHOLALIC ACID.
See: Cholic Acid.

CHOLAN-DH. (Pennwalt) Dehydrocholic acid 250 mg/Tab. Bot. 100s.
Use: Laxative.

CHOLAN-HMB. (Pennwalt) Dehydrocholic acid 250 mg/Tab. Bot. 100s.
Use: Laxative.

CHOLANIC ACID. Dehydrodesoxycholic acid.

CHOLEBRINE. (Mallinckrodt) Iocetamic acid (62% iodine) 750 mg/Tab. Bot. 100s, 150s.
Use: Radiopaque agent.

•**CHOLECALCIFEROL,** U.S.P. XXII. Vitamin D-3, activated 5,7-Cholestadien-3β-ol. 9,10-Secocholesta-5,7,- 10(19)-trien-3-ol.
Use: Vitamin D deficiency.
See: Decavitamin Cap., Tab.

CHOLECYSTOGRAPHY AGENTS.
See: Bilopaque, Cap. (Winthrop Pharm).
Iodized Oil (Various Mfr.).
Iophendylate Inj.
Pantopaque, Amp. (LaFayette).
Telepaque, Tab. (Winthrop Pharm).

CHOLEDYL. (Parke-Davis) Oxtriphylline. **Tab.:** 100 mg. Bot. 100s; 200 mg. Bot. 100s, 1000s, UD 100s. **Elix.:** 100 mg/5 ml, alcohol 20%. Bot. pt. **Pediatric Syr.:** 50 mg/5 ml. Bot. pt.
Use: Bronchodilator.

CHOLEDYL SA. (Parke-Davis) Oxtriphylline 400 mg or 600 mg/Tab. Bot. 100s, UD 100s.
Use: Bronchodilator.

•**CHOLERA VACCINE,** U.S.P. XXII. (Lederle) India Strains, Vial 1.5 ml (Lilly) Vial 1.5 ml (Wyeth-Ayerst) Vial 1.5 ml, 20 ml.
Use: Active immunizing agent.

CHOLERETIC. Bile salts.
See: Bile Preps. and Forms.
Dehydrocholic Acid.
Desoxycholic Acid.
Tocamphyl, Tab. (Various Mfr.).

CHOLESTERIN.
See: Cholesterol.

•**CHOLESTEROL.** N.F. XVII. Cholest-5-en-3β-ol. 5,6-Cholesten-3-Ol(Cholesterin). (Various Mfr.).
Use: Pharmaceutic aid (emulsifying agent).

CHOLESTEROL REAGENT STRIPS. (Ames) A quantitative strip test for cholesterol in serum. Seralyzer reagent strips. Bot. 25s.
Use: Diagnostic aid.

•**CHOLESTYRAMINE RESIN,** U.S.P. XXII. A styryl-divinyl-benzene copolymer (about 2% divinylbenzene) containing quaternary ammonium groups.

Use: Resin producing insoluble bile acid complexes.
See: Questran, Pow. (Bristol).

•**CHOLESTYRAMINE FOR ORAL SUSPENSION,** U.S.P. XXII.
Use: Ion-exchange resin (bile salts), antihyperlipoproteinemic.

CHOLIC ACID. 3,7,12-Trihydroxycholanic acid. Cholalic acid. Dehydrocholic Acid.

CHOLIDASE. (Freeda) Choline 185 mg, inositol 150 mg, vitamins B_6 2.5 mg, B_{12} 5 mcg, E 7.5 mg/Tab. Bot. 100s, 250s, 500s.
Use: Lipotropic/vitamin supplement.

CHOLINATE. (Cenci) Choline dihydrogen citrate 1 Gm/4 ml. Bot. 16 oz, gal.
Use: Lipotropic.

CHOLINE. (Various Mfr.) Choline. Tab.: **250 mg:** Bot. 100s, 250s, 500s, 1000s. **500 mg:** Bot. 100s. **650 mg:** Bot. 90s, 100s, 250s, 500s.
Use: Lipotropic.

CHOLINE BITARTRATE.
W/Bile extract, pancreatic substance, dl-methionine.
See: Licoplex, Tab. (Mills).
W/Inositol, B-vitamins.
See: Lipotriad Cap. (Smith, Miller & Patch).
W/Lemon bioflavonoid complex, inositol, vitamin C, B-vitamins.
See: Lipoflavonoid, Cap. (Smith, Miller & Patch).
W/Methionine, inositol, desiccated liver, vitamin B_{12}.
See: Limvic, Tab. (Briar).
W/Mucopolysaccharide, epinephrine neutralizing factor, pancreatic lipotropic fraction, dl-methionine, inositol, bile extract.
See: Lipo-K, Cap. (Marcen).
W/d-Pantothenyl alcohol.
See: Ilopan-Choline, Tab. (Adria).
W/Pentylenetetrazol, nicotinic acid, methyl-testosterone, ethinyl estradiol, vitamins B_1, B_2, B_6, B_{12}, C, panthenol, inositol.
See: Benizol Plus, Elix., Tab. (ICN).
W/Safflower oil, whole liver, soybean, lecithin, inositol, methionine, natural tocopherols, vitamins B_6, B_{12}, panthenol.
See: Nutricol, Cap., Vial (Nutrition Control).

CHOLINE CHLORIDE. (Various Mfr.).
Use: Liver supplement.
W/Inositol, methionine, vitamin B_{12}.
See: Cho-Meth, Vial (Kenyon).
Lychol-B, Inj. (Burgin-Arden).
W/Methionine, vitamins, niacinamide, panthenol.
See: Minoplex, Vial (Savage).
W/Panthenol, inositol, vitamins, minerals, estrone, testosterone.
See: Geramine, Inj. (Brown).
W/Panthenol, inositol, vitamins, minerals, estrone, testosterone, polydigestase.
See: Geramine, Tab. (Brown).
W/Vitamin B_1, niacinamide, B_2, B_6, calcium pantothenate, cyanocobalamin, B_{12}, inositol, dl-methionine, testosterone, estrone, procaine.
See: Gerihorm, Inj. (Burgin-Arden).

CHOLINE CHLORIDE, CARBAMATE. Carbachol, U.S.P. XXII.

CHOLINE CHLORIDE SUCCINATE.
See: Succinylcholine Chloride, U.S.P. XXII.

CHOLINE CITRATE, TRICHOLINE CITRATE.
W/Inositol, methionine, vitamin B_{12}.
See: Cholimeth Tab. (Central).

CHOLINE DIHYDROGEN CITRATE. 2-Hydroxyethyl trimethylammonium citrate-U.S. vitamin 0.5 Gm. Bot. 100s, 500s.
Use: Lipotropic.
See: Cholinate, Liq. (Cenci).

CHOLINE MAGNESIUM TRISALICYLATE.
Use: Salicylate analgesic.
See: Trilisate, Tab. (Purdue Frederick).

CHOLINE SALICYLATE. B.A.N. Choline salt of salicylic acid.
Use: Analgesic, antipyretic.

CHOLINE THEOPHYLLINATE.
See: Oxtriphylline.

CHOLINE THEOPHYLLINATE. B.A.N. Choline salt of theophylline.
Use: Bronchodilator.

CHOLINERGIC AGENTS.
(Parasympathomimetic Agents).
See: Mecholyl Cl, Inj. (Baker).
Mestinon, Tab., Syr., Amp. (Roche).
Mytelase, Cap. (Winthrop Pharm).
Pilocarpine Nitrate (Various Mfr.).
Prostigmin Bromide, Tab. (Roche).
Prostigmin Methylsulfate, Inj. (Roche).
Tensilon, Inj. (Roche).
Urecholine, Inj., Tab. (Merck Sharp & Dohme).

CHOLINERGIC BLOCKING AGENTS.
See: Parasympatholytic agents.

CHOLINOID. (Goldline) Choline 111 mg, inositol 111 mg, vitamins B_1 0.3 mg, B_2 0.3 mg, B_3 3.3 mg, B_5 1.7 mg, B_6 0.3 mg, B_{12} 1.7 mcg, C 100 mg, lemon bioflavonoid complex 100 mg/Cap. Bot. 100s.
Use: Lipotropic/vitamin supplement.

CHO-LIV-12. (Jenkins) Choline 100 mg, cyanocobalamin 200 mcg, liver equal to vitamin B_{12} 10 mcg/ml. Vial 10 ml, 12s.
Use: Lipotropic/vitamin supplement.

CHOL METH IN B. (Esco) Choline bitartrate 235 mg, inositol 112 mg, methionine 70 mg, betaine anhydrous 50 mg, vitamins B_{12} 6 mcg, B_1 6 mg, B_6 3 mg, niacin 10 mg/Cap. Bot. 500s, 1000s.
Use: Vitamin supplement.

CHOLOGRAFIN MEGLUMINE. (Squibb) Iodipamide meglumine **10.3%** (iodine 5.1%)/100 ml, Vial 100 ml. **52%** (26% iodine)/20 ml, Vial 20 ml.
Use: Cholangiography, cholecystography.

CHOLOGRAFIN SODIUM. Disodium salt of N,N′-adipyl bis-(3-amino-2:4:6 triodobenzoic acid).

CHOLOXIN. (Flint) Sodium dextrothyroxine 1 mg, 2 mg, 4 mg or 6 mg/Tab. Tartrazine (2 mg, 4 mg only). Bot. 100s, Bot. 250s (2 mg, 4 mg only).
Use: Antihyperlipidemic.
CHOLYBAR. (Parke-Davis) Anhydrous cholestyramine resin 4 Gm/bar. 25s.
Use: Antihyperlipidemic.
CHOLYGLYCINE.
See: CG RIA, Kit (Abbott).
CHO-METH. (Kenyon) Methionine 30 mg, choline Cl 200 mg, inositol 100 mg, vitamin B_{12} 12 mcg/2 ml. Vial 30 ml.
Use: Nutritional supplement.
CHONDODENDRON TOMENTOSUM.
See: Curare.
CHONDRUS. Irish Moss.
W/Petrolatum, Liq.
See: Kondremul, Liq. (Fisons).
CHOO E PLUS C. (Stayner) Vitamin E 100 IU, C 250 mg/Tab. Bot. 100s.
Use: Vitamin supplement.
CHOOZ ANTACID GUM. (Plough) Calcium carbonate 500 mg/Gum tab. Pkg. 16s.
Use: Antacid.
CHOREX 5. (Hyrex) Chorionic gonadotropin 5000 units, urea 100 mg, thimerosal 1 mg, sodium phosphate buffer/Vial 10 ml.
Use: Chorionic gonadotropin.
CHOREX 10. (Hyrex) Chorionic gonadotropin 10,000 units, urea 100 mg, thimerosal 1 mg, sodium phosphate buffer/Vial 10 ml.
Use: Chorionic gonadotropin.
CHORIGON. (Dunhall) Chorionic gonadotropin (dried) 1000 units/ml. Vial 10 ml.
Use: Chorionic gonadotropin.
CHORION-PLUS. (Pharmex) Chorionic gonadotropin 10,000 units/Vial. Diluent: Glutamic acid 52 mcg, vitamin B_1 25 mg, procaine 1%/ml. Vial 10 ml.
Use: Chorionic gonadotropin.
•**CHORIONIC GONADOTROPIN,** U.S.P. XXII. Inj., U.S.P. XXII. 5000 IU/Vial w/diluent 10 ml, 10,000 IU/Vial w/diluent 10 ml (Serono) hCG 10,000 IU, mannitol 100 mg, benzyl alcohol 0.9%/10 ml Vial.
Use: Prepubertal cryptorchidism or induction of ovulation and pregnancy in anovulatory women.
See: Antuitrin-S (Parke-Davis).
A.P.L., Inj. (Wyeth-Ayerst).
C-G-10, Vial (Scrip).
Chorigon, Amp. (Dunhall).
Chorex 5, Vial (Hyrex).
Chorex 10, Vial (Hyrex).
Chorion-Plus, Vial (Pharmex).
Follutein, Vial (Squibb).
Gonadex (Continental Dist.).
Khorion (Hickam).
Neovital-Diluent, Inj. (Pasadena Research).
Rochoric, Inj. (Rocky Mtn.).
CHORON 10. (Forest Pharm.) Chorionic gonadotropin 10,000 units/vial with diluent 10 ml. Also contains mannitol. Inj. Vial 10 ml.
Use: Chorionic gonadotropin.
CHROMAGEN. (Savage) **Cap.:** Ferrous fumarate 66 mg, vitamins C 250 mg, B_{12} activity 10 mcg, desiccated stomach substances 100 mg/soft gelatin cap. Bot. 100s, 500s. **Inj.:** Iron peptonized 100 mg, vitamin B_{12} 5 mcg, cyanocobalamin 25 mcg, lidocaine HCl 1%/2 ml. Vial 10 ml, 30 ml.
Use: Vitamin/mineral supplement.
CHROMAGEN OB CAPSULES. (Savage) Calcium 125 mg, iron 33 mg, vitamins A 4000 IU, D 200 IU, E 15 mg, B_1 1.5 mg, B_2 1.7 mg, B_3 10 mg, B_6 5 mg, B_{12} 6 mcg, C 75 mg, folic acid 0.4 mg, Cu, docusate sodium, Fe, Mg, zinc 12.5 mg/Cap. Bot. 100s.
Use: Vitamin/mineral supplement.
CHROMALBIN. (Squibb) 100 uCi containing chromium CR 51 and human albumin.
CHROMA-PAK. (SoloPak) Chromium **4 mcg/ml:** Vial 10 ml, 30 ml. **20 mcg/ml:** Vial 5 ml.
Use: Parenteral nutritional supplement.
CHROMARGYRE.
See: Merbromin (Various Mfr.).
•**CHROMATE Cr-51, SODIUM FOR INJECTION,** U.S.P. XXII.
CHROMATED SOLUTION (^{51}Cr).
See: Chromitope sodium (Squibb).
CHROMELIN COMPLEXION BLENDER. (Summers) Dihydroxyacetone 5%, alcohol 50%. Bot. oz.
Use: Agent for vitiligo.
CHROMIC ACID, DISODIUM SALT. Sodium Chromate Cr^{51} Inj., U.S.P. XXII.
•**CHROMIC CHLORIDE,** U.S.P. XXII. Inj., U.S.P. XXII. Chromium Cl (CrCl3) hexahydrate. Chromium (3+) Cl hexahydrate.
Use: Chromium deficiency treatment.
See: Chrometrace, Inj. (Armour).
•**CHROMIC CHLORIDE Cr^{51}.** USAN.
Use: Radioactive agent.
See: Chromitope Cl (Squibb).
•**CHROMIC PHOSPHATE Cr^{51}.** USAN.
Use: Radioactive agent.
•**CHROMIC PHOSPHATE P^{32} SUSPENSION,** U.S.P. XXII.
Use: Radioactive agent.
CHROMITOPE SODIUM. (Squibb) Chromate Cr^{51}, Sodium for Inj. 0.25 mCi.
Use: Radioactive agent.
CHROMIUM TRACE METAL ADDITIVE. (IMS) Chromium 10 mcg/ml. Inj. Vial 10 ml.
Use: Parenteral nutritional supplement.
•**CHROMONAR HCl.** USAN. Ethyl[[3-[-2-(di- ethylamino)-ethyl]-4-methyl-2-oxo-2H-1-benzopyran-7-yl]oxy]acetate HCl. Intensain.
Use: Recommended as coronary vasodilator, upon release.
CHRONULAC. (Merrell Dow) Lactulose 10 Gm/15 ml (> 2.2 Gm galactose, > 1.2 Gm lactose,

> 1.2 Gm other sugars). Bot. 473 ml, 1890 ml, UD 15 ml, 30 ml. Box 100s.
Use: Laxative.

CHRYSAZIN.
See: Danthron, N.F. XVII.

CHUR-HIST. (Churchill) Chlorpheniramine 4 mg/ Kaptab. Bot. 100s.
Use: Antihistamine.

CHYMEX. (Adria) Bentiromide 500 mg/7.5 ml w/ propylene glycol 40%. Screening test for pancreatic exocrine insufficiency.
Use: Diagnostic aid.

CHYMODIACTIN. (Smith) 4 nKat units, 1.4 mg sodium L-cysteinate HCl with diluent. Pow. for Inj. Vial 2 ml.
Use: Proteolytic enzyme.

•**CHYMOPAPAIN.** USAN. Proteolytic enzyme isolated from papaya latex, differing from papain in electrophoretic mobility, solubility and substrate specificity.
Use: Proteolytic enzyme.

•**CHYMOTRYPSIN,** U.S.P. XXII. Ophth. Soln. U.S.P. XXII. An enzyme, α-Chymotrypsin obtained in crystalline form from mammalian pancreas by aqueous acid extraction of its proenzyme, chymotrypsinogen, and subsequent conversion with trypsin to chymotrypsin.
Use: Proteolytic enzyme.
See: Catarase, Soln. (CooperVision).
W/Trypsin.
Orenzyme, Tab. (Merrell Dow).
W/Trypsin, neomycin palmitate.
See: Biozyme, Oint. (Armour).

C.I. BASIC VIOLET 3. Gentian Violet, U.S.P. XXII.

CIBA VISION CLEANER. (Ciba Vision) Cocoamphocarboxyglycinate, sodium lauryl sulfate, sorbic acid 0.1%, hexylene glycol, EDTA 0.2%. Soln. 15 ml.
Use: Soft contact lens care.

CIBACALCIN. (Ciba) Calcitonin-human for inj. Double-chambered syringe: 0.5 mg/vial with mannitol. UD (blister-pack) Ctn. 5s.
Use: Treatment of Paget's disease.

CIBALITH-S. (Ciba) Lithium 8 mEq (as citrate equivalent to lithium carbonate 300 mg)/5 ml, alcohol 0.3%, saccharin, sorbitol. Syr. Bot. 480 ml.
Use: Antipsychotic.

CIBENZOLINE.
See: Cifenline Succinate. USAN.

•**CICLAFRINE HYDROCHLORIDE.** USAN.
Use: Antihypotensive.

•**CICLAZINDOL.** USAN. 10-m-Chlorophenyl-2,3,4,-10-tetrahydropyrimido[1,2-α]-indol-10-ol.
Use: Antidepressant.

•**CICLETANINE.** USAN.
Use: Antihypertensive.

•**CICLOPIROX OLAMINE,** U.S.P. XXII. Cream, U.S.P. XXII.
Use: Antifungal.
See: Loprox, Cream (Hoechst).

•**CICLOPROFEN.** USAN. 2-(2-Fluorenyl)propionic acid.
Use: Anti-inflammatory.

•**CICLOPROLOL HYDROCHLORIDE.** USAN.
Use: Anti-adrenergic (beta receptor).

CICLOXOLONE. B.A.N. 3β-(cis-2-Carboxycyclohexylcarbonyloxy)-11-oxo-olean-12-en-30-oic acid.
Use: Treatment of gastric ulcers.

CIDEX. (Surgikos) Activated dialdehyde soln. Bot. qt, gal, 2½ gal.
Use: Sterilizing, disinfecting agent.

CIDEX-7. (Surgikos) Glutaraldehyde 2% and vial of activator with aqueous potassium salt as buffer and sodium nitrite as a corrosive inhibitor. Soln. Bot. qt, 1 gal, 5 gal.
Use: Sterilizing, disinfecting agent.

CIDEXPLUS. (Surgikos) 3.2% glutaraldehyde. Soln. Gal.
Use: Sterilizing, disinfecting agent.

C.I. DIRECT BLUE 53 TETRASODIUM SALT. Evans Blue, U.S.P. XXII.

•**CIDOXIEPIN HCl.** USAN.
Use: Psychotherapeutic.

•**CIFENLINE SUCCINATE.** USAN. Formerly Cibenzoline.
Use: Cardiac depressant (antiarrhythmic).

•**CIGLITAZONE.** USAN.
Use: Antidiabetic.

CIGNOLIN.
See: Anthralin (Various Mfr.).

•**CILADOPA HYDROCHLORIDE.** USAN.
Use: Treatment of Parkinson's disease.

•**CILASTATIN SODIUM.** USAN.
Use: Enzyme inhibitor.
W/Imipenem.
See: Primaxin, Inj. (Merck Sharp & Dohme).

•**CILAZAPRIL.** USAN.
Use: Antihypertensive.

CILFOMIDE TABLETS. (Winthrop Products) Inositol hexanicotinate.
Use: Hypolipidimic, peripheral vasodilator.

CILLIUM. (Whiteworth) Psyllium seed husk pow. 4.94 Gm, 14 calories/rounded tsp. Bot. 420 Gm, 630 Gm.
Use: Laxative.

•**CIMATEROL.** USAN.
Use: Repartitioning agent.

•**CIMETIDINE,** U.S.P. XXII. Tab., U.S.P. XXII. 1-Methyl-3-[2-(5-methylimidazol-4-ylmethylthio)ethyl]guanidine-2-carbonitrile.
Use: H_2 receptor histamine antagonist.
See: Tagamet, Tab., Inj. (SmithKline).

•**CIMETIDINE HYDROCHLORIDE.** USAN.
Use: H_2 receptor histamine antagonist.

CINACORT SPAN. (Foy) Triamcinolone acetonide 40 mg/ml. Vial 5 ml.
Use: Corticosteroid.

•**CINANSERIN HYDROCHLORIDE.** USAN. 2′-[[3-(Dimethylamino)-propyl]thio]cinnamanilide HCl.
Use: Serotonin antagonist.

CINCHONA BARK. (Various Mfr.).

Use: Antimalarial, tonic.
W/Anhydrous quinine, cinchonidine, cinchonine, quinidine, quinine.
See: Totaquine, Pow. (Various Mfr.).
W/Iron oxide, nux vomica, vitamin B_1, alcohol.
See: Briatonic, Liq. (Briar).
CINCHONIDINE SULFATE.
CINCHONINE SALTS. (Various Mfr.).
Use: Quinine dihydrochloride.
CINCHOPHEN. 2-Phenylcinchoninic acid.
Use: Analgesic.
CINEPAZATE. B.A.N. Ethyl 4-(3,4,5-trimethoxy-cinnamoyl)piperazin-1-ylacetate.
Use: Treatment of angina.
•**CINEPAZET MALEATE.** USAN.
Use: Antianginal.
CINEPAZIDE. B.A.N. 1-Pyrrolidin-1-ylcarbonyl-methyl-4-(3,4,5-trimethoxycinnamoyl)-piperazine.
Use: Peripheral vasodilator.
•**CINFLUMIDE.** USAN.
Use: Muscle relaxant.
•**CINGESTOL.** USAN. 19-Nor-17α-pregn-5-en-20-yn-17-ol.
Use: Progestogen.
CINNAMALDEHYDE.
•**CINNAMEDRINE.** USAN. a-[1-(Cinnamyl-methyl-amine)-ethyl] benzyl alcohol.
Use: Uterine antispasmodic.
See: Midol, Tab. (Glenbrook).
CINNAMIC ALDEHYDE. Name previously used for Cinnamaldehyde.
•**CINNAMON,** N.F. XVII.
Use: Flavoring agent.
•**CINNAMON OIL,** N.F. XVII. (Various Mfr.).
Use: Pharmaceutic aid.
CINNAMYL EPHEDRINE HCl.
W/Acetaminophen, homatropine methylbromide.
See: Periodic, Cap. (Towne).
•**CINNARIZINE.** USAN. 1-Diphenylmethyl-4-trans-cinnamylpiperazine; 1-Benzhydryl-4-cinnamylpiperazine; F.D.A. 1-Cinnamyl-4-diphenyl-methyl-piperazine.
Use: Antihistamine.
CINNOPENTAZONE. INN for Cintazone.
CINOBAC. (Dista) Cinoxacin **250 mg/Pulv.:** Bot. 40s. **500 mg/Pulv.:** Bot. 50s.
Use: Urinary anti-infective.
•**CINODINE HYDROCHLORIDE.** USAN.
Use: Antibacterial.
•**CINOXACIN,** U.S.P. XXII. Cap., U.S.P. XXII. 1-Ethyl-4-oxo[1,3]dioxolo-[4,5-g]cinnoline-3-carboxylic acid.
Use: Antibacterial.
See: Cinobac, Cap. (Dista).
•**CINOXATE,** U.S.P. XXII. Lot., U.S.P. XXII. 2-Ethoxyethyl p-methoxycinnamate.
Use: Ultraviolet screen.
See: Sundare Prods. (Cooper).
W/Methyl anthranilate.
See: Maxafil Cream (Cooper).
CINOXOLONE. B.A.N. Cinnamyl 3β-acetoxy-11-oxo-olean-12-en-30-oate.
Use: Treatment of gastric ulcer.
•**CINPERENE.** USAN. 1-Cinnamyl-4-(2,6-dioxo-3-phenyl-3-piperidyl)piperidine.
Use: Tranquilizer.
CIN-QUIN. (Reid-Rowell) Quinidine sulfate. (Contains 83% anhydrous quinidine alkaloid.) **Tab.:** 100 mg, 200 mg or 300 mg. Bot. 100s, 1000s, UD 100s. **Cap.:** 200 mg. Bot. 100s. 300 mg. Bot. 100s, 1000s, UD 100s.
Use: Antiarrhythmic.
•**CINROMIDE.** USAN.
Use: Anticonvulsant.
•**CINTAZONE.** USAN. 2-Pentyl-6-phenyl-1H-pyrazolo [1,2-a] cinnoline-1,3(2H)-dione.
Use: Anti-inflammatory.
•**CINTRIAMIDE.** USAN.
Use: Antipsychotic.
•**CIPREFADOL SUCCINATE.** USAN.
Use: Analgesic.
CIPRO. (Miles Pharm.) Ciprofloxacin HCl 250 mg, 500 mg or 750 mg/Tab. Bot. 50s, UD 100s.
Use: Antibacterial, fluoroquinolone.
•**CIPROCINONIDE.** USAN.
Use: Adrenocortical steroid.
•**CIPROFIBRATE.** USAN.
Use: Antihyperlipoproteinemic.
•**CIPROFLOXACIN.** USAN. U.S.P. XXII
Use: Antibacterial.
•**CIPROFLOXACIN HYDROCHLORIDE.** USAN. U.S.P. XXII
Use: Antibacterial.
See: Cipro (Miles).
•**CIPROSTENE CALCIUM.** USAN.
Use: Platelet anti-aggregatory agent.
•**CIRAMADOL.** USAN.
Use: Analgesic.
•**CIRAMADOL HYDROCHLORIDE.** USAN.
Use: Analgesic.
CIRBED. (Boyd) Papaverine HCl 150 mg/Cap. Bot. 100s.
Use: Antispasmodic.
CIRCAVITE-T. (Circle) Iron 12 mg, vitamins A 10,000 IU, D 400 IU, E 15 mg, B_1 10.3 mg, B_2 10 mg, B_3 100 mg, B_5 18.4 mg, B_6 4.1 mg, B_{12} 5 mcg, C 200 mg, Cu, Mg, Mn, zinc 1.5 mg. Bot. 100s.
Use: Vitamin/mineral supplement.
•**CIROLEMYCIN.** USAN.
Use: Antibacterial, antineoplastic.
•**CISAPRIDE.** USAN.
Use: Peristaltic stimulant.
•**CISPLATIN,** U.S.P. XXII.
Use: Antineoplastic agent.
See: Platinol, Inj. (Bristol).
CIS-RETINOIC ACID. (13-cis-Retinoic Acid).
Use: Anti-acne.
See: Isotretinoin.
Accutane (Roche).
CITANEST HCl. (Astra) **Plain:** Prilocaine HCl 4%/1.8 ml dental cartridge.
Use: Local anesthetic.

CITANEST HCl FORTE. (Astra) Prilocaine HCl 4% with epinephrine 1: 200,000. Contains sodium metabisulfite. Dental cartridge 1.8 ml. Inj.
Use: Local anesthetic.

•**CITENAMIDE.** USAN.
Use: Anticonvulsant.

CITHAL CAPSULES. (Table Rock) Watermelon seed extract 2 gr, theobromine 4 gr, phenobarbital 0.25 gr/Cap. Bot. 100s, 500s.
Use: Antihypertensive.

CITRACAL. (Mission) Calcium citrate 950 mg/Tab. Bot. 100s.
Use: Calcium supplement.

CITRACAL 1500 + D. (Mission) Calcium citrate 1500 mg, vitamin D 200 IU/Tab. Bot. 60s.
Use: Vitamin/calcium supplement.

CITRACAL LIQUITAB. (Mission) Calcium citrate 2376 mg/Effervescent tab. Box. 30s.
Use: Calcium supplement.

CITRA FORTE. (Boyle) Hydrocodone bitartrate 5 mg, ascorbic acid 30 mg, pheniramine maleate 2.5 mg, pyrilamine maleate 3.33 mg, potassium citrate 150 mg/5 ml. Bot. pt, gal.
Use: Antitussive, vitamin C supplement, antihistamine.

CITRAMIN-500. (Thurston) Vitamin C 500 mg, rose hips, acerola with mixed bioflavonoids/Loz. Bot. 100s, 250s, 1000s.
Use: Vitamin/mineral supplement.

CITRANOX. (Alconox)
Use: Liquid acid detergent for manual and ultrasonic washers.

CITRASAN B. (Sandia) Lemon bioflavonoid complex 300 mg, vitamins C 300 mg, B_1 30 mg, B_2 10 mg, B_6 5 mg, B_{12} 4 mcg, calcium pantothenate 10 mg, niacinamide 50 mg/Tab. Bot. 100s, 1000s.
Use: Vitamin supplement.

CITRASAN K LIQUID. (Sandia) Vitamins C 125 mg, K 0.66 mg, lemon bioflavonoid complex 125 mg/5 ml. Bot. pt, gal.
Use: Vitamin supplement.

CITRASAN K-250. (Sandia) Vitamins C 250 mg, K 1 mg, lemon bioflavonoid 250 mg/Tab. Bot. 100s, 1000s.
Use: Vitamin supplement.

CITRATE ACID.
See: Bicitra Soln. (Willen).

CITRATE AND CITRIC ACID SOLUTION.
Use: Alkalinizer.
See: Polycitra (Willen).
Polycitra-LC (Willen).
Polycitra-K (Willen).
Oracit (Carolina Medical Products.).
Bicitra (Willen).

CITRATE OF MAGNESIA. (Various Mfr.) Magnesium citrate. Soln. Bot. 300 ml.
Use: Laxative.

CITRATED CAFFEINE.
See: Caffeine Citrate.

CITRATED NORMAL HUMAN PLASMA.
See: Plasma, Normal Human.

CITRESCO-K. (Esco) Vitamins C 100 mg, K 0.7 mg, citrus bioflavonoid complex 100 mg/Cap. Bot. 100s, 500s, 1000s.
Use: Vitamin supplement.

•**CITRIC ACID,** U.S.P. XXII. 1,2,3-Propanetricarboxylic acid, 2-hydroxy-.
Use: Component of anticoagulant solutions and drug products.

CITRIC ACID AND D-GLUCONIC ACID IRRIGANT.
Use: Genitourinary irrigant.
See: Renacidin (Guardian).

•**CITRIC ACID, MAGNESIUM OXIDE, AND SODIUM CARBONATE IRRIGATION,** U.S.P. XXII.
Use: Irrigating solution.

CITRIN.
See: Vitamin P.

CITRIN CAPSULES. (Table Rock) Watermelon seed extract 4 gr/Cap. Bot. 100s, 500s.
Use: Antihypertensive.

CITROCARBONATE. (Upjohn) Sodium bicarbonate 0.78 Gm, sodium citrate anhydrous 1.82 Gm/3.9 Gm. Bot. 4 oz, 8 oz.
Use: Antacid.

CITRO CEE, SUPER. (Marlyn) Bioflavonoids 500 mg, rutin 50 mg, vitamin C 500 mg, rose hips powder 500 mg/Tab. Bot. 50s, 100s.
Use: Vitamin supplement.

CITRO-FLAV 200. (Goldline) Citrus bioflavonoid compound 200 mg/Cap. Bot. 100s, 1000s.
Use: Vitamin supplement.

CITROHIST. (Robinson) Prophenpyridamine 6.75 mg, pyrilamine maleate 8.33 mg, hesperidin 50 mg, C 50 mg, ephedrine sulfate 16.2 mg, salicylamide 3.5 gr, phenacetin 2 gr, caffeine alkaloid 0.5 gr, atropine sulfate 1/600 gr/Cap. Bot. 100s, 1000s, Bulk Pack 5000s. Vial 20s.
Use: Antihistamine, decongestant, analgesic, anticholinergic.

CITROLEUM SUNBURN CREME. (Citroleum) Bot. 4 oz.

CITROLITH. (Beach) Potassium citrate 50 mg, sodium citrate 950 mg/Tab. Bot. 100s, 500s.
Use: Urinary alkalinizer.

CITROMA. (Century) Magnesium citrate. Oral soln. Bot. 10 oz.
Use: Laxative.

CITROMA LOW SODIUM. (National Magnesia) Magnesium citrate. Oral soln w/lemon or cherry flavor in sugar-free vehicle. Bot. l0 oz.
Use: Laxative.

CITRO-NESIA. (Century) Magnesium citrate. Soln. Bot. 296 ml.
Use: Laxative.

CITROPAM. (Jenkins) No. 1 Ammonium Cl 0.5 Gm, citric acid 0.5 Gm, potassium guaiacolsulfonate 0.5 Gm/fl oz. Bot. 3 oz, 4 oz, gal. Also Citropam No. 2 w/codeine phosphate 30 mg/fl oz. Bot. 3 oz, 4 oz, gal.
Use: Expectorant.

CITROTEIN. (Sandoz Nutrition) Sucrose, pasteurized egg white solids, amino acids, maltodex-

trin, citric acid, natural and artificial flavors, mono and diglycerides, partially hydrogenated soybean oil, 0.66 cal/ml, protein 40.7 Gm, carbohydrate 120.7 Gm, fat 1.55 Gm, sodium 698 mg, potassium 698 mg/L. Tartrazine (orange flavor only). Pow. 1.57 oz/packet, Can 14.16 oz. Orange, grape and punch flavors.
Use: Enteral nutritional supplement.

CITROVORUM FACTOR. Leucovorin Calcium, U.S.P. XXII.
See: Leucovorin Calcium (Lederle) Folinic Acid.

CITRUCEL. (Lakeside) Methylcellulose 2 Gm/heaping tbsp. dose w/citric acid. Bot. 16 oz, 30 oz.
Use: Laxative.

CITRUS BIOFLAVONOID COMPOUND.
See: Bioflavonoid Compounds (Various Mfr.).
C.V.P., Syr. (USV Pharm.).
Vitamin P.
W/Ascorbic acid, phenyltoloxamine dihydrogen citrate, salicylamide, acetyl p-aminophenol, caffeine, racemic amphetamine sulfate.
See: Euphenex, Tab. (Westerfield).

C-JECT. (Lincoln) Ascorbic acid 2000 mg, sodium bisulfite 0.1%, disodium sequestrene 0.01%/10 ml. Amp. 10 ml, "Score-Break" Box 25s.

C-JECT WITH B. (Lincoln) When mixed with 10 ml of diluent, each vial contains: Vitamins C 2000 mg, B_1 50 mg, B_2 5 mg, B_6 10 mg, nicotinamide 100 mg, methylparaben 0.89 mg, propylparaben 0.22 mg, sodium bisulfite 10 mg, disodium sequestrene 1 mg. Box of 6 lyophilized plugs and 6 10 ml vials of Sterile Diluent.

CKA CANKER AID. (Pannett Prod.) Benzocaine, aluminum hydrate, magnesium trisilicate, sodium acid carbonate. Pow.
Use: Cold-canker sore.

CK(CPK) REAGENT STRIPS. (Ames) Seralyzer reagent strips for creatnine phosphokinase in serum or plasma. Bot. 25s.
Use: Diagnostic aid.

CLAFORAN. (Hoechst) Cefotaxime sodium 1 Gm, 2 Gm or 10 Gm/Vial. Infusion Bot.: 1 Gm, 2 Gm. Viaflex (pre-mixed frozen) Bag: 1 Gm, 2 Gm. Add-Vantage System: Vial 1 Gm, 2 Gm.
Use: Antibacterial, cephalosporin.

CLAMIDOXIC ACID. B.A.N. [2-(3,4-Dichlorobenzamido)phenoxy]acetic acid.
Use: Antirheumatic.

•**CLAMOXYQUIN HYDROCHLORIDE.** USAN. 5-Chloro-7-(((3-(diethylamino)propyl)-amino)methyl)-8-quinolinol dihydrochloride.
Use: Amebicide.

CLARETIN-12.
See: Vitamin B_{12}.

CLAVULANIC ACID/AMOXICILLIN.
Use: Antibacterial, penicillin.
See: Augmentin Tab. (Beecham Labs).

CLAVULANIC ACID/TICARCILLIN.
Use: Antibacterial, penicillin.
See: Timentin Pow. for Inj. (Beecham Labs).

•**CLAVULANATE POTASSIUM,** U.S.P. XXII.
Use: Inhibitor (β-*lactamase*).

•**CLAVULANATE POTASSIUM, STERILE,** U.S.P. XXII.
Use: Inhibitor (β-*lactamase*).

•**CLAZOLAM.** USAN.
Use: Tranquilizer.

•**CLAZOLIMINE.** USAN.
Use: Diuretic.

•**CLAZURIL.** USAN.
Use: Coccidiostat.

CLEAN-N-SOAK. (Allergan) Cleaning agent with phenylmercuric nitrate 0.004%. Bot. 4 oz.
Use: Hard contact lens care.

CLEARASIL DOUBLE CLEAR. (Richardson-Vicks) **Regular strength:** Salicylic acid 1.25%, alcohol 40% in pads. Bot. 32s. **Maximum strength:** Salicylic acid 2.5%, alcohol 40% in pads. Bot. 32s.
Use: Anti-acne.

CLEARASIL MAXIMUM STRENGTH ACNE TREATMENT CREAM. (Vicks Prods) Benzoyl peroxide 10% in tinted or vanishing base. Tube 19.5 Gm, 30 Gm.
Use: Anti-acne.

CLEARASIL 10%. (Vicks Prods) Benzoyl peroxide 10%. Bot. oz.
Use: Anti-acne.

CLEARASIL ANTIBACTERIAL SOAP. (Vicks Prods) Triclosan 0.75%, glycerin, bentonite, titanium dioxide. 3.25 oz.
Use: Skin cleanser.

CLEARASIL MEDICATED ASTRINGENT. (Vicks Prods) Salicylic acid 0.5%, alcohol 43%. Bot. 4 oz.
Use: Anti-acne.

CLEARASIL ADULT CARE MEDICATED BLEMISH STICK. (Vicks Prods) Sulfur 8%, resorcinol 1%, bentonite 4%, laureth-4, titanium dioxide. Stick ⅛ oz.
Use: Anti-acne.

CLEARBLUE PREGNANCY TEST. (VLI) Dip stick for pregnancy test. Kit 2s.
Use: Diagnostic aid.

CLEAR BY DESIGN. (Herbert) Benzoyl peroxide 2.5% in an invisible, greaseless gel base. Tube 1.5 oz, 3 oz.
Use: Anti-acne.

CLEAREX ACNE CREAM. (Approved) Allantoin, sulfur, resorcinol, d-panthenol, isopropanol. Tube 1.5 oz.
Use: Anti-acne.

CLEAR EYES EYE DROPS. (Ross) Naphazoline HCl 0.012%, benzalkonium Cl 0.01%, disodium edetate 0.1%, glycerin 0.2%, boric acid, sodium borate. Bot. 0.5 oz, 1 oz.
Use: Ophthalmic vasoconstrictor, lubricant.

CLEARPLAN. (VLI) Ovulation prediction test. Bot. 10s.
Use: Diagnostic aid.

•**CLEBOPRIDE.** USAN.
Use: Antiemetic.

CLEFAMIDE. B.A.N. αα-Dichloro-N-(2-hydroxyethyl)-N-[4-(4-nitrophenoxy)benzyl]acetamide.
Use: Treatment of amebiasis.

•**CLEMASTINE.** USAN. (+)-2-[2-(4-Chloro-α-methyl- benzhydryloxy)ethyl]-1-methylpyrrolidine. Tavegil hydrogen fumarate.
Use: Antihistamine.
See: Tavist, Tab., Syr. (Sandoz).

•**CLEMASTINE FUMARATE.** USAN.
Use: Antihistamine.

•**CLEMASTINE FUMARATE TABLETS,** U.S.P. XXII.
Use: Antihistamine.

CLEMIZOLE. B.A.N. 1-(4-chlorobenzyl)-2-pyrrolidin-1-ylmethylbenzimidazole.
Use: Antipruritic.

CLEMIZOLE HCl. 1-p-Chlorobenzyl-2-pyrrolidylmethyl benzimidazole. Reactrol.

CLEMIZOLE PENICILLIN. B.A.N. Benzylpenicillin combined with 1-(4-chlorobenzyl)-2-pyrrolidin-1-ylmethylbenzimidazole. Neopenyl.
Use: Antibiotic.

CLENPYRIN. V.B.A.N. 1-Butyl-2-(3,4-dichlorophenylimino)pyrrolidine.
Use: Insecticide (veterinary).

CLENS. (Alcon) Cleansing agent with benzalkonium Cl 0.02%, EDTA 0.1%. Soln. Bot. 60 ml.
Use: Hard contact lens care.

CLENTIAZEM MALEATE. USAN.
Use: Antianginal, antihypertensive.

CLEOCIN HCl. (Upjohn) Clindamycin HCl 75 mg, 150 mg or 300 mg/Cap. Tartrazine. Bot. 100s. (75 mg); 16s, 100s, UD 100s (150 mg, 300 mg).
Use: Anti-infective.

CLEOCIN PEDIATRIC. (Upjohn) Clindamycin palmitate HCl equivalent to clindamycin 75 mg/5 ml when reconstituted as directed. Bot. 100 ml.
Use: Anti-infective.

CLEOCIN PHOSPHATE. (Upjohn) Clindamycin phosphate equivalent to clindamycin 150 mg/ml. **300 mg**: Vial 2 ml w/disodium edetate 1 mg, benzyl alcohol 18.9 mg. Pack 25s, 100s. **600 mg:** Vial 4 ml w/disodium edetate 2 mg, benzyl alcohol 37.8 mg. Pack 25s, 100s. **900 mg:** Vial 6 ml. Pack 25s, 100s. **9000 mg:** Bulk Vial 60 ml. Pack 5s.
Use: Anti-infective.

CLEOCIN T. (Upjohn) Clindamycin phosphate 10 mg/ml. Topical soln., gel. Bot. 30 ml, 60 ml, pt. (topical soln.). Bot. 7.5 Gm, 30 Gm (gel).
Use: Anti-infective.

CLERZ DROPS FOR HARD LENSES. (Ciba Vision) Hypertonic solution with hydroxyethyl cellulose, sorbic acid, poloxamer 407, EDTA 0.1%, thimerosal 0.001%. Soln. Bot. 25 ml.
Use: Hard contact lens care.

CLERZ DROPS FOR SOFT LENSES. (Ciba Vision) Hypertonic solution with hydroxyethyl cellulose, sodium borate, poloxamer 407, sorbic acid, thimerosal 0.001%, EDTA 0.1%. Soln. Bot. 25 ml.
Use: Soft contact lens care.

CLERZ 2 FOR HARD LENSES. (Ciba Vision) Isotonic solution with hydroxyethyl cellulose, poloxamer 407, sodium Cl, potassium Cl, sodium borate, boric acid, sorbic acid, EDTA. Soln. Bot. 5 ml, 15 ml.
Use: Hard contact lens care.

CLERZ 2 FOR SOFT LENSES. (Ciba Vision) Isotonic solution with sodium Cl, potassium Cl, hydroxyethyl cellulose, poloxamer 407, sodium borate, boric acid, sorbic acid, EDTA. Soln. Bot. 5 ml, 15 ml.
Use: Soft contact lens care.

CLETOQUINE. B.A.N. 7-Chloro-4-[4-(2-hydroxyethylamino)-1-methylbutyl]aminoquinoline.
Use: Anti-inflammatory.

•**CLIDINIUM BROMIDE,** U.S.P. XXII. Cap., U.S.P. XXII. 1-Methyl-3-benzil-oyloxy-quinuclidinium bromide. 3-Hydroxy-1-methyl-quinuclidinium bromide benzilate.
Use: Anticholinergic.
See: Quarzan, Cap. (Roche).
W/Chlordiazepoxide.
See: Librax, Cap. (Roche).

•**CLINDAMYCIN.** USAN. Methyl 7-chloro-6,7,8-trideoxy-6-(trans-1-methyl-4-propyl-L-2-pyrrolidinecarboxamido)-1-thio-L-threo-α-D-galactooctopyranoside.
Use: Topical antibiotic for acne. Oral as antibiotic.
See: Cleocin T (Upjohn).
Cleocin (Upjohn).

•**CLINDAMYCIN HYDROCHLORIDE,** U.S.P. XXII. Cap. U.S.P. XXII.
Use: Antibacterial.
See: Cleocin HCl A.D.T., Cap. (Upjohn).

•**CLINDAMYCIN PALMITATE HYDROCHLORIDE,** U.S.P. XXII. Oral Soln., U.S.P. XXII.
Use: Antibacterial.
See: Cleocin Pediatric (Upjohn).
Cleocin T, Liq. (Upjohn).

•**CLINDAMYCIN PHOSPHATE,** U.S.P. XXII. Inj., Topical Soln., Sterile, Topical Susp., Gel, U.S.P. XXII.
Use: Antibacterial.
See: Cleocin phosphate, Inj. (Upjohn).

CLINDEX. (Rugby) Clidinium bromide 2.5 mg, chlordiazepoxide HCl 5 mg/Cap. Bot. 100s, 500s, 1000s.
Use: Anticholinergic/antispasmodic.

CLINISTIX REAGENT STRIPS. (Ames) Glucose oxidase, peroxidase and orthotolidine. Diagnostic test for glucose in urine. Bot. 50s.
Use: Diagnostic aid.

CLINITEST. (Ames) 2-drop and 5-drop combination packages w/color charts for both 2-drop and 5-drop use. Reagent tablets containing copper sulfate, sodium hydroxide, heat-producing agents. Patient's plastic set; Tab. refills. **Box:** 100s, 500s, sealed in foil. **Child-resistant bot.:** 36s, 100s.
Use: Diagnostic aid.

CLINOCAINE HCl.
See: Procaine HCl.
CLINORIL. (Merck Sharp & Dohme) Sulindac 150 mg or 200 mg/Tab. Bot. 100s, UD 100s. Unit-of-use 60s, 100s.
Use: Nonsteroidal anti-inflammatory drug; analgesic.
•**CLIOQUINOL,** U.S.P. XXII. Comp. Pow., Cream, Oint., U.S.P. XXII. 5-Chloro-7-iodo-8-quinolinol. Quinambicide, Rometin. Iodohydroxyquin.
Use: Topical antifungal.
See: HCV Creame (Saron).
Quin III, Cream (Lemmon).
Quinoform, Oint., Cream, Lot. (C & M Pharmacal).
Torofor, Cream, Oint. (Torch).
Vioform, Prep. (Ciba).
W/Aluminum acetate solution, hydrocortisone.
See: Hydrelt, Cream, Oint. (Elder).
W/Hydrocortisone acetate.
See: Viotag Cream (Reid-Rowell).
W/Hydrocortisone acetate, lidocaine.
See: Lidaform-HC, Creme, Lot. (Miles Pharm).
W/Hydrocortisone, coal tar solution.
See: Tar-Quin-HC, Oint. (Jenkins).
W/Hydrocortisone, lidocaine.
See: Bafil Lotion (Scruggs).
HIL-20 Lotion (Reid-Rowell).
W/Hydrocortisone, chlorobutanol.
See: Hc-Form, Jelly (Recsei).
W/Hydrocortisone, coal tar extract.
See: Racet LCD, Cream (Lemmon).
W/Hydrocortisone and pramoxine HCl.
See: Dermarex Cream (Hyrex).
Sherform-HC, Oint. (Sheryl).
Stera-Form Creme (Mayrand).
V-Cort, Cream (Scrip).
W/Methylcellulose, aluminum hydroxide, atropine sulfate, hyoscine HBr, hyoscyamine sulfate.
See: Enterex, Tab. (Person & Covey).
W/Nystatin.
See: Nystaform, Oint. (Miles Pharm).
•**CLIOQUINOL AND HYDROCORTISONE CREAM,** U.S.P. XXII.
Use: Topical antifungal.
See: Bafil, Cream (Skruggs).
Caquin Cream (Forest).
Coidocort Cream (Coast).
Corticoid, Cream (Jenkins).
Cort Nib V, Cream (Cenci).
Domeform-HC, Cream (Miles Pharm).
Hi-Form Cream (Blaine).
Hydrelt, Cream (Elder).
Hysone, Cream (Hauck).
Ido-Cortistan Oint. (Standex).
Iodocort, Cream (Ulmer).
Iohydro, Cream (Freeport).
Kencort, Cream (Kenyon).
Lanvisone, Cream (Lannett).
Maso-Form, Cream (Mason).
Mity-Quin Cream (Reid-Rowell).
Racet, Cream (Lemmon).
Racet Forte, Cream (Lemmon).
Vioform-Hydrocortisone, Cream, Oint., Lot. (Ciba).
Vio-Hydrocort, Cream, Oint. (Quality Generics).
•**CLIOQUINOL AND HYDROCORTISONE OINTMENT,** U.S.P. XXII.
Use: Topical antifungal.
See: Hysone, Cream (Hauck).
Vioform-Hydrocortisone, Cream, Oint., Lot. (Ciba).
Vio-Hydrocort, Cream, Oint. (Quality Generics).
CLINOXIDE. (Geneva G) Clidinium bromide 2.5 mg, chlordiazepoxide HCl 5 mg/Cap. Bot. 100s, 500s.
Use: Anticholinergic/antispasmodic.
•**CLIOXANIDE.** USAN. 2-(4-Chlorophenylcarbamoyl)-4,6-di-iodophenylacetate.
Use: Anthelmintic (veterinary).
See: Tremerad.
CLIPOXIDE. (Schein) Clidinium bromide 2.5 mg, chlordiazepoxide HCl 5 mg/Cap. Bot. 100s, 500s.
Use: Anticholinergic/antispasmodic.
•**CLIPROFEN.** USAN.
Use: Anti-inflammatory.
CLISTIN. (McNeil Pharm) Carbinoxamine maleate 4 mg/Tab. Bot. 100s.
Use: Antihistamine.
•**CLOBAMINE MESYLATE.** USAN.
Use: Antidepressant.
•**CLOBAZAM.** USAN. 7-Chloro-1-methyl-5-phenyl-1,5-benzodiazepine-2,4-dione.
Use: Tranquilizer.
CLOBENZTROPINE. 3-(p-Chloro-a-phenylbenzyloxy)tropane.
•**CLOBETASOL PROPIONATE.** USAN.
Use: Corticosteroid.
See: Temovate, Cream, Oint. (Glaxo).
CLOBETASONE. B.A.N. 21-Chloro-9α-fluoro-17α-hydroxy-16β-methylpregna-1,4-diene-3,11,20-trione.
Use: Corticosteroid.
•**CLOBETASONE BUTYRATE.** USAN.
Use: Corticosteroid.
CLOCIGUANIL. B.A.N. 4,6-Diamino-1-(3,4-dichlorobenzyloxy)-1,2-dihydro-2,2-dimethyl-1,3,5-triazine.
Use: Antimalarial.
•**CLOCORTOLONE ACETATE.** USAN.
Use: Glucocorticoid.
•**CLOCORTOLONE PIVALATE,** U.S.P. XXII. Cream, U.S.P. XXII.
Use: Glucocorticoid.
CLOCREAM. (Upjohn) Vitamins A and D in vanishing base. Tube oz.
Use: Emollient.
•**CLODANOLENE.** USAN.
Use: Relaxant (skeletal muscle).
•**CLODAZON HYDROCHLORIDE.** USAN.
Use: Antidepressant.

CLODERM. (Hermal) Clocortolone pivalate cream 0.1%. Tube 15 Gm, 45 Gm.
Use: Corticosteroid.
CLODRONIC ACID. USAN.
Use: Regulator.
CLOFAZIMINE. USAN. 3-(p-Chloroanilino) 10-(p-chlorophenyl)-2,10-dihydro-2-(isopropylimino)-phena-zine.
Use: Tuberculostatic, leprostatic.
See: Lamprene, Cap. (Geigy).
CLOFIBRATE, U.S.P. XXII. Cap., U.S.P. XXII. Ethyl 2-(p-chlorophenoxy-2-methyl-propionate. Propanoic acid, 2-(4-chlorophenoxy)-2-methyl-, methyl ester.
Use: Antihyperlipidemic.
See: Atromid S, Cap. (Wyeth-Ayerst).
CLOFILIUM PHOSPHATE. USAN.
Use: Cardiac depressant.
CLOFLUCARBAN. USAN. 4,4′-Dichloro-3-(trifluoro-methyl)-carbanilide. Irgasan, CF3.
Use: Recommended as antiseptic on release.
CLOFLUPEROL. B.A.N. 4-(4-Chloro-3-trifluoromethylphenyl)-1-[3-(4-fluorobenzoyl)propyl]piperidin-4-ol.
Use: Neuroleptic.
CLOGESTONE ACETATE. USAN. 6-Chloro-3β, 17-dihydroxypregna-4,6-dien-20-one diacetate. Under study.
Use: Progesterone.
CLOGUANAMILE. B.A.N. 1-Amidino-3-(3-chloro-4- cyanophenyl)urea.
Use: Antimalarial.
CLOMACRAN. B.A.N. NN-Dimethyl-3-(2-chloro-9, 10-dihydroacridin-9-yl)propylamine.
Use: Tranquilizer.
CLOMACRAN PHOSPHATE. USAN. 2-Chloro-9-[3-dimethyl-amino)propyl] acridan phosphate (1:1). Under study.
Use: Tranquilizer.
CLOMEGESTONE ACETATE. USAN. 6-Chloro-17-acetoxy-1,6α-methyl-4,6-pregnadiene-3,20-dione. Under study.
Use: Progestin.
CLOMETHERONE. USAN. 6α-Chloro-16α-methyl-pregn-4-ene-3,20-dione.
Use: Anti-estrogen.
CLOMID. (Merrell Dow) Clomiphene citrate 50 mg/Tab. Carton 30s.
Use: Ovulation stimulant.
CLOMINOREX. USAN.
Use: Anorexic.
CLOMIPHENE CITRATE, U.S.P. XXII. Tab., U.S.P. XXII. 2-[p-(2-Chloro-1,2-diphenyl-vinyl)phenoxy]triethylamine dihydrogen citrate. Ethanamine, 2-[4-(2-chloro-1,2-diphenylethenyl)-phenoxy]-N,N-diethyl-,2-hydroxy-1,2,3-propanetricarboxylate(1:1).
Use: Ovulation stimulant.
See: Clomid, Tab. (Merrell Dow).
Serophene, Tab. (Serono).
CLOMIPRAMINE HCl. USAN. 3-Chloro-5-[3-(dimethyl-amino)propyl]-10, 11-dihydro-5H-dibenz-[b,f] azepine monohydrochloride.
Use: Antidepressant.
See: Anafranil (Ciba).
CLOMOCYCLINE. B.A.N. N^2-(Hydroxymethyl)-chlortetracycline.
Use: Antibiotic.
•**CLONAZEPAM,** U.S.P. XXII. Tab., U.S.P. XXII. 5-(o-Chlorophenyl)-1,3-dihydro-7-nitro-2H-1,4-benzodiazepin-2-one. B.A.N. 5-(2-Chlorophenyl)-1,3-dihydro-7-nitro-2H-1,4-benzodiazepin-2-one. Rivotril.
Use: Anticonvulsant.
See: Klonopin, Tab. (Roche).
•**CLONIDINE.** USAN. 2-(2,6-Dichloroanilino)-2-imida-zoline.
Use: Antihypertensive.
See: Catapres (Boehringer Ingelheim).
•**CLONIDINE HYDROCHLORIDE,** U.S.P. XXII. Tabs., U.S.P. XXII. Benzamine, 2,6-dichloro-N-2-imidazolidinyl-idene-, monoCl. (1)2-(2,6-Dichloranilino)-2-imidazoline monohydrochloride. (2)2-(2,6-Dichloro-phenylamino)-2-imidazoline HCl.
Use: Hypotensive.
See: Catapres, Tab. (Boehringer Ingelheim).
•**CLONIDINE HYDROCHLORIDE AND CHLORTHALIDONE TABLETS,** U.S.P. XXII.
Use: Antihypertensive, diuretic.
See: Combipres, Tab. (Boehringer Ingelheim).
CLONITAZENE. B.A.N. 2-(4-Chlorobenzyl)-1-(2-diethylaminoethyl)-5-nitrobenzimidazole.
Use: Narcotic analgesic.
•**CLONITRATE.** USAN. 3-Chloro-1,2-propanediol dinitrate. Dylate.
Use: Coronary vasodilator.
•**CLONIXERIL.** USAN.
Use: Analgesic.
•**CLONIXIN.** USAN.
Use: Analgesic.
•**CLOPAMIDE.** USAN. **(1)** 4-Chloro-N-(2,6-dimethylpiperidino)-3-sulfamoylbenzamide; **(2)** 4-chloro-3-sulfamoylbenzoic acid 1,5-dimethylpentamethylenehydrazide.
Use: Antihypertensive, diuretic.
See: Aquex, Tab. (Lannett).
•**CLOPENTHIXOL.** USAN. BAN. 4-[3-(2-Chlorothioxanthen-9-ylidene)propyl]-1-piperazine-ethanol.
Use: Antipsychotic.
See: Sordinol (Wyeth-Ayerst).
•**CLOPERIDONE HYDROCHLORIDE.** USAN. 3-[3-[4-(m-Chlorophenyl)-1-piperazinyl] propyl]-2,-4-(IH, 3H)-quinazolinedione HCl.
Use: Sedative, tranquilizer.
CLOPHEDIANOL HCl.
See: Acutuss, Tab., Expect. (Philips Roxane).
CLOPHENOXATE HCl. 2-Dimethylamino-ethyl p-chlorphenoxyacetate HCl.
Use: Cerebral stimulant.
•**CLOPIDOL.** USAN. 3,5-Dichloro-4-hydroxy-2,6-dimethylpyridine.

Use: Antiprotozoan (veterinary).
See: Coyden 25.
•**CLOPIMOZIDE.** USAN.
Use: Antipsychotic.
•**CLOPIPAZAN MESYLATE.** USAN.
Use: Antipsychotic.
CLOPRA. (Quantum) Metoclopramide 10 mg (as monohydrochloride monohydrate)/Tab. Bot. 100s, 500s, 1000s.
Use: Antiemetic, gastrointestinal stimulant.
CLOPIRAC. USAN. 1-p-Chlorophenyl-2,5-dimethylpyrrol-3-ylacetic acid.
Use: Anti-inflammatory.
CLOPONONE. B.A.N. β,4-Dichloro-α-dichloroacetamidopropiophenone.
Use: Antiseptic.
•**CLOPREDNOL.** USAN.
Use: Glucocorticoid.
CLOPROSTENOL. V.B.A.N. (±)-7-(1R,2R,3R,5S)-2- [(3R)-4-(3-Chlorophenoxy)-3-hydroxybut-1-(E)-enyl]-3,5-dihydroxycyclopent-1-yl hept-5-(Z) enoic acid.
Use: Synchronization of estrus; infertility, veterinary medicine.
•**CLOPROSTENOL SODIUM.** USAN.
Use: Prostaglandin.
CLOQUINATE. B.A.N. Chloroquine di-(8-hydroxy-7-iodoquinoline-5-sulfonate).
Use: Treatment of amebiasis.
•**CLORAZEPATE DIPOTASSIUM.** USAN. 7-Chloro-2,3-dihydro-2,2-dihydroxy-5-phenyl-IH-1,4-benzodiazepine-3-carboxylic acid dipotassium salt.
Use: Antianxiety, minor tranquilizer, anticonvulsant.
See: Tranxene, Cap. (Abbott).
•**CLORAZEPATE MONOPOTASSIUM.** USAN.
Use: Minor tranquilizer.
CLORAZEPIC ACID. B.A.N. 7-Chloro-2,3-dihydro-2,2-dihydroxy-5-phenyl-1H-1,4-benzodiazepine-3-carboxylic acid.
Use: Sedative.
•**CLORETHATE.** USAN.
Use: Sedative/hypnotic.
•**CLOREXOLONE.** USAN. 5-Chloro-2-cyclohexyl-6-sulfamoylisoindolin-1-one.
Use: Diuretic.
See: Nefrolan.
CLORFED II. (Stewart-Jackson) Chlorpheniramine 4 mg, pseudoephedrine 60 mg/Tab. Bot. 100s.
Use: Antihistamine, decongestant.
CLORFED CAPSULES. (Stewart-Jackson) Chlorpheniramine 8 mg, pseudoephedrine 120 mg/Cap. Bot. 100s.
Use: Antihistamine, decongestant.
CLORFED EXPECTORANT. (Stewart-Jackson) Pseudoephedrine 30 mg, guaifensen 100 mg, codeine 10 mg. Bot. pt.
Use: Decongestant, expectorant, antitussive.
CLORGYLINE. B.A.N. N-3-(2,4-Dichlorophenoxy) propyl-N-methylprop-2-ynylamine.
Use: Monoamine oxidase inhibitor, antidepressant.
CLORINDIONE. B.A.N. 2-(4-Chlorophenyl)indane-1,3-dione.
Use: Anticoagulant.
•**CLOROPERONE HYDROCHLORIDE.** USAN.
Use: Antipsychotic.
CLORPACTIN WCS-90. (Guardian) Sodium oxychlorosene. Bot. 2 Gm, 5s.
Use: Antiseptic.
CLORPACTIN XCB. (Guardian) Oxychlorosene 5 Gm. Pow. for soln. Box of bot. 4s.
Use: Antiseptic, germicide.
•**CLOROPHENE.** USAN. 4-Chloro-alpha-phenyl-o-cresol.
Use: Disinfectant.
See: Santophen 1 (Monsanto).
•**CLORPRENALINE HYDROCHLORIDE.** USAN. (formerly Isoprophenamine HCl) 1-(α-Chlorophenyl)-2-isopropyl-aminoethanol hydrochloride hydrate. Vortel.
Use: Bronchodilator.
•**CLORSULON.** USAN.
Use: Antiparasitic, fasciolicide.
•**CLORTERMINE HCl.** USAN. o-Chloro-α,α-dimethylphenethylamine HCl.
Use: Anorexic.
•**CLOSANTEL.** USAN.
Use: Anthelmintic.
•**CLOSIRAMINE ACETURATE.** USAN.
Use: Antihistamine.
CLOSTEBOL ACETATE. B.A.N. 17β-Acetoxy-4-chloroandrost-4-en-3-one.
Use: Anabolic steroid.
•**CLOTHIAPINE.** USAN. 2-Chloro-11-(4-methyl-piperazin-1-yl)dibenzo[b,f][1,4]thiazepine.
Use: Tranquilizer.
•**CLOTHIXAMIDE MALEATE.** USAN. 4-[3-(2-Chlorothioxanthen-9-ylidene)propyl]-N-methyl-1-piperazinepropionamide dimaleate.
Use: Tranquilizer.
•**CLOTICASONE PROPIONATE.** USAN.
Use: Anti-inflammatory.
•**CLOTRIMAZOLE,** U.S.P. XXII. Cream, Lot., Topical Soln., Vaginal Tab., U.S.P. XXII. I-(o-Chloro-α,α-diphenylbenzyl)-imidazole.
Use: Antifungal, candida infections.
See: Gyne-Lotrimin, Cream, Vaginal Tab. (Schering).
Lotrimin, Cream, Soln. (Schering).
Myclex, Cream, Soln. (Miles Pharm).
Myclex-G, Vaginal Supp. (Miles Pharm).
•**CLOTRIMAZOLE AND BETAMETHASONE DIPROPIONATE CREAM,** U.S.P. XXII.
Use: Antifungal, anti-inflammatory.
•**CLOVE OIL,** N.F. XVII.
Use: Pharmaceutic aid (flavor).
CLOVERINE. (Medtech) White salve. Tin oz.
Use: Minor skin irritations.
CLOVOCAIN. (Vita Elixir) Benzocaine, oil of cloves.
Use: Local anesthetic.

•**CLOXACILLIN BENZATHINE,** U.S.P. XXII. Intramammary Soln., Sterile, U.S.P. XXII.
Use: Antibiotic.

•**CLOXACILLIN SODIUM,** U.S.P. XXII., Cap., Intramammary Soln., Sterile, For Oral Soln., U.S.P. XXII. 4-Thia-1-azabicyclo[3.2.0]heptane-2-carboxylic acid,6-[[[3-(2-chlorophenyl)-5-methyl-4-isoxazoly]carbonyl]amino]-3,3-dimethyl-7-oxo-,monosodium salt, monohydrate. Monosodium 6-[3-(o-chlorophenyl)-5-methyl-4-isoxazolecarboxamido]-3,3-dimethyl-7-oxo-4-thia-1-azabicyclo[3.2.0]heptane-2-carboxylate monohydrate.
Use: Antibiotic for resistant staph infections.
See: Cloxapen, Cap. (Beecham Labs).
Tegopen, Cap., Granules (Bristol).

CLOXAPEN. (Beecham Labs) Cloxacillin sodium 250 mg or 500 mg/Cap. Bot. 100s.
Use: Antibacterial, penicillin.

CLOXYQUIN. USAN.
Use: Antibacterial.

CLOZAPINE. USAN. 8-Chloro-11-(4-methylpiperazin-1-yl)-5H-dibenzo[b,e][1,4]-diazepine.
Use: Antipsychotic.
See: Clozaril (Sandoz).

CLOZARIL. (Sandoz) Clozapine 25 mg or 100 mg/Tab. UD 100s, total daily dose packages of 150 mg, 200 mg, 250 mg, 300 mg, 400 mg, 500 mg, 600 mg/day.
Use: Antipsychotic.

CLUSIVOL SYRUP. (Whitehall) Vitamins A 2500 U.S.P. units, D-2 400 U.S.P. units, C 15 mg, B_{12} 2 mcg, B_1 1 mg, B_2 1 mg, niacinamide 5 mg, d-panthenol 3 mg, B_6 0.6 mg, manganese, 0.5 mg, zinc 0.5 mg, magnesium 3 mg/5 ml. Bot. 8 fl oz, 16 fl oz.
Use: Vitamin/mineral supplement.

C.M.C. CELLULOSE GUM.
See: Carboxymethylcellulose Sodium, Preps.

CMV. (Wampole-Zeus) Cytomegalovirus antibody test system for the qualitative and semi-quantitative detection of CMV antibody in human serum. Test 100s.
Use: Diagnostic aid.

COACTIN. (Roche) Amdinocillin 500 mg or 1 Gm. Inj. Vial. Box 10s.
Use: Antibacterial, penicillin.

COADVIL. (Whitehall) Ibuprofen 200 mg, pseudoephedrine HCl 30 mg/Tab. Bot. 100s.
Use: Analgesic, decongestant.

OAGULANTS.
See: Hemostatics.

COAL TAR. U.S.P. XXII. Oint., Soln., U.S.P. XXII.
Use: Topical antieczematic; antipsoriatic.
See: Balnetar, Liq. (Westwood).
Estar, Gel (Westwood).
L.C.D. Compound, Oint., Soln. (Almay).
Polytar Bath, Liq. (Stiefel).
Tarbonis, Cream (Reed & Carnrick).
Zetar, Preps. (Dermik).
W/Allantoin, hydrocortisone.
See: Alphosyl-HC, Lot., Cream (Reed & Carnrick).
W/Hydrocortisone.
See: Doak Oil Forte, Liq. (Doak).
Tarcortin, Cream (Reed & Carnrick).
W/Iodoquinol, hydrocortisone.
See: ZeTar-Quin, Cream (Dermik).
W/Mercury oleate, salicylic acid, phenol, p-nitrophenol.
See: Prosol, Emulsion (Torch).
W/Zinc oxide.
See: Tarpaste, Paste (Doak).

COAL TAR BATH. (Durel) Coal tar solution 20%, polysorbate "20" 5%, isopropanol 75%. Bot. 8 oz, pt, gal.
Use: Tar-containing preparation, topical.

COAL TAR CREAM COTASOL. (Durel) Coal tar solution 5% in Duromantel cream. Jar 1 oz, 1 lb, 6 lb.
Use: Tar-containing preparation, topical.

COAL TAR, DISTILLATE.
Use: Tar-containing preparation, topical.
See: Lavatar, Liq. (Doak).
Syntar, Cream (Elder).
W/Sulfur, salicylic acid.
See: Pragmatar, Oint. (Menley & James).

COAL TAR EXTRACT.
Use: Tar-containing preparation, topical.
W/Allantoin, hexachlorophene.
See: Sebical Cream (Reed & Carnrick).
W/Allantoin, hexachlorophene, glycerin, lanolin.
See: Pso-Rite, Cream (DePree).
W/Allantoin, salicylic acid, perhydrosqualine.
See: Skaylos Cream (Ambix).
Skaylos Lotion (Ambix).
W/Salicylic acid, resorcinol, benzoic acid.
See: Mazon Cream (Norcliff-Thayer).

COAL TAR PASTE.
Use: Tar-containing preparation, topical.
W/Zinc paste.
See: Tarpaste, Paste (Doak).

•**COAL TAR TOPICAL SOLUTION,** U.S.P. XXII. Liquor Carbonis Detergens. L.C.D.
Use: Anti-eczematic, topical.
See: Balnetar, Liq. (Westwood).
Estar, Gel (Westwood).
L.C.D. Compound Oint., Soln. (Almay).
Psorigel, Gel (Owen).
Wright's Soln. (Fougera).
Zetar, Emulsion, Shampoo (Dermik).
W/Allantoin, psorilan, myristate.
See: Iocon, Shampoo (Owen).
Psorelief, Cream (Quality Generics).
W/Hydrocortisone, iodoquinol.
See: Cor-Tar-Quin, Cream, Lot. (Miles Pharm).
W/Hydrocortisone alcohol, clioquinololine, diperodon HCl, vitamins A, D.
See: Pentarcort, Cream (Dalin).
W/Robane (perhydrosqualene).
See: Skaylos Shampoo (Ambix).
W/Salicylic acid.
See: Epidol, Soln. (Spirt).

Ionil T, Shampoo (Owen).
W/Salicylic acid, sulfur, protein.
See: Vanseb-T Tar Shampoo (Herbert).
CO-APAP. (Various Mfr.) Pseudoephedrine HCl 30 mg, chlorpheniramine maleate 2 mg, dextromethorphan HBr 15 mg, acetaminophen 325 mg/Tab. Bot. 24s, 50s, 100s, 1000s.
Use: Decongestant, antihistamine, antitussive, analgesic.
COBALAMINE CONCENTRATE, U.S.P. XXI.
Use: Hematopoietic vitamin.
See: Vitamin B_{12} (Various Mfr.).
COBALT CHLORIDE.
W/Ferrous gluconate, vitamin B_{12}, duodenum whole desiccated.
See: Bitrinsic-E, Cap. (Elder).
COBALT GLUCONATE.
W/Ferrous gluconate, vitamin B_{12} activity, desiccated stomach substance, folic acid.
See: Chromagen, Cap., Inj. (Savage).
COBALT STANDARDS FOR VITAMIN B_{12}.
See: Cobatope-57, and Cobatope-60 (Squibb).
COBALT-LABELED VITAMIN B_{12}.
See: Rubratope-57 (Squibb).
•**COBALTOUS CHLORIDE Co 57.** USAN.
Use: Radioactive agent.
•**COBALTOUS CHLORIDE Co 60.** USAN.
Use: Radioactive agent.
COBATOPE-57. (Squibb) Cobaltous Cl Co 57.
COBEX 1000. (Standex) Vitamin B_{12} 1000 mcg/10 ml. Vial 30 ml.
Use: Vitamin B_{12} supplement.
CO-BILE. (Western Research) Hog bile 64.8 mg, pancreas substance 64.8 mg, papain-pepsin complex 97.2 mg, diatase malt 16.2 mg, papain 48.6 mg, pepsin 48.6 mg/Tab. Bot. 1000s.
Use: Digestive enzyme.
COBIRON. (Pharmex) Cyanocobalamin 100 mcg, hydroxycobalamine 50 mcg, ferrous gluconate 60 mg, liver inj. 5 mcg/2 ml, procaine HCl 2%, phenol 0.5%. Vial 30 ml.
Use: Vitamin/mineral supplement.
•**COCAINE,** U.S.P. XXII. Methyl 3β-Hydroxy-1αH,-5αH-tropane-2β-carboxylate Benzoate (Ester) Alkaloid.
Use: Anesthetic (topical).
•**COCAINE HYDROCHLORIDE,** U.S.P. XXII. Tab., for Topical Soln., U.S.P. XXII. 8-Azabicyclo[3.2.1]octane-2-carboxylic acid, 3-(benzoyloxy)-8-methyl-, methyl ester, hydrochloride. Methyl 3β-hydroxy-1αH,5αH-tropan-2β-carboxylate, benzoate (ester) HCl.
Use: Mucosal anesthetic (topical).
CO-CARBOXYLASE. B.A.N. Pyrophosphoric ester of aneurine.
Use: Co-enzyme.
COCCIDIOIDIN.
See: Spherulin (Berkeley Biologicals).
COCCULIN.
See: Picrotoxin, Inj. (Various Mfr.).
COCILAN SYRUP. (Approved) Euphorbia, wild lettuce, cocillana, squill, senega, cascarin (bitterless). Bot. gal. Available w/codeine. Bot. gal.
COCILLANA.
W/Euphorbia pilulifera, squill, antimony potassium tartrate, senega.
See: Cylana Syr. (Bowman).
•**COCOA,** N.F. XVII. Syr., N.F. XVII.
Use: Pharmaceutic aid (flavor; flavored vehicle).
•**COCOA BUTTER,** N.F. XVII.
Use: Pharmaceutic aid (suppository base).
CODACTIDE. B.A.N. D-Ser^{1}-Lys^{17,18}-β$^{1-18}$-corticotrophin amide.
Use: Corticotrophic peptide.
CODALAN NO. 1. (Lannett) Codeine phosphate 8 mg, acetaminophen 500 mg, caffeine 30 mg/Tab. Bot. 100s, 500s, 1000s.
Use: Narcotic analgesic combination.
CODALAN NO. 2 (Lannett) Codeine phosphate 15 mg/Tab. Bot. 100s, 500s, 1000s.
Use: Narcotic analgesic combination.
CODALAN NO. 3 (Lannett) Codeine phosphate 30 mg/Tab. Bot. 100s, 500s, 1000s.
Use: Narcotic analgesic combination.
CODAMINE PEDIATRIC SYRUP. (Goldline) Hydrocodone bitartrate. Bot. pt.
Use: Antitussive.
CODAMINE SYRUP. (Goldline) Hydrocodone bitartrate 5 mg, phenylpropanolamine HCl 25 mg/5 ml. Bot. pt, gal.
Use: Antitussive, decongestant.
CODANOL OINTMENT. (A.P.C.) Vitamins A, D, hexachlorophene, zinc oxide. Tube 1.5 oz, 4 oz Jar lb.
Use: Minor skin irritations.
CODAP. (Reid-Rowell) Codeine phosphate 32 mg, acetaminophen 325 mg/Tab. Bot. 250s.
Use: Narcotic analgesic combination.
CODAPRIN. (Cenci) APC w/codeine. **No. 2:** 0.25 gr. **No. 3:** 0.5 gr. **No. 4:** 1 gr. Bot. 100s, 1000s
Use: Narcotic analgesic.
CODASA I. (Stayner) Codeine phosphate 0.25 gr, aspirin 5 gr/Cap. Bot. 100s, 500s.
Use: Narcotic analgesic combination.
CODASA II. (Stayner) Codeine phosphate 0.5 gr aspirin 5 gr/Cap. Bot. 100s, 500s.
Use: Narcotic analgesic combination.
CODASA FORTE. (Stayner) Codeine phosphate 0.5 gr, aspirin 10 gr/Cap. Bot. 100s, 500s.
Use: Narcotic analgesic combination.
CODASA TABS. (Stayner) Codeine phosphate 0.25 gr or 0.5 gr, aspirin 5 gr/Tab. Bot. 100s, 1000s.
Use: Narcotic analgesic combination.
CODEHIST DH ELIXIR. (Geneva Generics) Pseudoephedrine 30 mg, chlorpheniramine maleate 2 mg, codeine phosphate 10 mg, alcohol 5%. Bot. 120 ml, 480 ml.
Use: Decongestant, antihistamine, antitussive.
•**CODEINE,** U.S.P. XXII. 7,8-Didehydro-4,5α-epoxy-3-methoxy-17-methylmorphinan-6α-ol monohydrate. Crystal or Pow. Bot. ⅛ oz, 1 oz.

Use: Analgesic (narcotic); antitussive.

CODEINE COMBINATIONS.

See: Actifed-C, Expectorant, Syr. (Burroughs-Wellcome).
- Anexsia w/Codeine, Tab. (Beecham Labs).
- APAP w/Codeine, Tab. (Central).
- A.P.C. w/Codeine, Tab. (Various Mfr.).
- Ascriptin W/Codeine No. 2, Tab. (Rorer).
- Ascriptin W/Codeine No. 3, Tab. (Rorer).
- Buff-A-Compound, Tab. (Mayrand).
- Calcidrine Syr. (Abbott).
- Capital w/Codeine, Susp. (Carnrick).
- Cheracol, Syr. (Upjohn).
- Chlor-Trimeton Expectorant (Schering).
- Codalan, Tab. (Lannett).
- Codasa I and II, Cap. (Stayner).
- Colrex Compound, Cap., Elix. (Reid-Rowell).
- Cosanyl Cough Syrup (Health Care Ind.).
- Drucon w/Codeine, Liq. (Standard Drug).
- Empirin No. 1, No. 2, No. 3, No. 4, Tab. (Burroughs-Wellcome).
- Fiorinal w/Codeine, Cap. (Sandoz).
- G-3, Cap. (Hauck).
- Golacol, Syr. (Arcum).
- Isoclor, Expectorant (Arnar-Stone).
- Novahistine, Expectorant (Merrell Dow).
- Nucofed, Liq. (Beecham).
- Partuss AC (Parmed).
- Pediacof, Syr. (Winthrop Pharm).
- Phenaphen #2, #3, #4, Cap. (Robins).
- Phenaphen-650, Cap. (Robins).
- Phenatuss, Liq. (Dalin).
- Phenergan Expectorant w/Codeine, Troches (Wyeth-Ayerst).
- Proval No. 3, Tab. (Reid-Rowell).
- Prunicodeine, Syr. (Lilly).
- Robitussin A-C, DAC (Robins).
- Tega-Code, Cap. (Ortega).
- Tolu-Sed, Elix. (Scherer).
- Tussar-2, Syr. (Rorer).
- Tussar SF, Liq. (Rorer).
- Tussi-Organidin, Liq. (Wallace).
- Tylenol w/Codeine No. 1, No. 2, No. 3, No. 4 Tab. (McNeil).
- Tylenol w/Codeine, Elix. (McNeil).
- Vasotus, Liq. (Sheryl).

CODEINE METHYLBROMIDE. Eucodin.
Use: Antitussive.

•**CODEINE PHOSPHATE,** U.S.P. XXII. Inj., Tab., U.S.P. XXII. (Various Mfr.) Pow. Bot. 1/8 oz, 0.25 oz, 0.5 oz, 1 oz.
Use: Narcotic analgesic, antitussive.

•**CODEINE POLISTIREX.** USAN.
Use: Antitussive.

CODEINE RESIN COMPLEX COMBINATIONS.
See: Omni-Tuss, Liq. (Pennwalt).

•**CODEINE SULFATE,** U.S.P. XXII. Tab., U.S.P. XXII. 7,8-Didehydro-4,5α-epoxy-3-methoxy-17-methyl-morphinan-6α-ol sulfate.
Use: Narcotic analgesic, antitussive.

CODELCORTONE.
See: Prednisolone.

CODICLEAR DH SYRUP. (Central) Hydrocodone bitartrate 5 mg, potassium guaiacolsulfonate 300 mg/5 ml. Bot. 4 oz, pt.
Use: Antitussive, expectorant.

CODIMAL. (Central) Chlorpheniramine maleate 2 mg, pseudoephedrine HCl 30 mg, acetaminophen 325 mg/Cap. Bot. 24s, 100s, 1000s.
Use: Antihistamine, decongestant, analgesic.

CODIMAL DH SYRUP. (Central) Hydrocodone bitartrate 1.66 mg, phenylephrine HCl 5 mg, pyrilamine maleate 8.33 mg/5 ml. Bot. 4 oz, pt, gal.
Use: Antitussive, decongestant, antihistamine.

CODIMAL DM. (Central) Dextromethorphan HBr 10 mg, phenylephrine HCl 5 mg, pyrilamine maleate 8.33 mg/5 ml, alcohol 4%, saccharin, sorbitol. Sugar free. Bot. 4 oz, pt, gal.
Use: Antitussive, decongestant, antihistamine.

CODIMAL EXPECTORANT. (Central) Phenylpropanolamine HCl 25 mg, guaifenesin 100 mg/5 ml. Menthol. Bot. 4 oz, pt.
Use: Decongestant, expectorant.

CODIMAL PH SYRUP. (Central) Codeine phosphate 10 mg, phenylephrine HCl 5 mg, pyrilamine maleate 8.33 mg/5 ml. Bot. 4 oz, pt, gal.
Use: Antitussive, decongestant, antihistamine.

CODIMAL TABLETS. (Central) Chlorpheniramine maleate 2 mg, pseudoephedrine HCl 30 mg, acetaminophen 325 mg/Tab. Bot. 24s, 100s, 1000s.
Use: Antihistamine, decongestant, analgesic.

CODIMAL-A. (Central) Brompheniramine maleate 10 mg/ml, methylparaben 0.18%, propylparaben 0.02%. Inj. Vial 10 ml.
Use: Antihistamine.

CODIMAL-L.A. (Central) Chlorpheniramine maleate 8 mg, pseudoephedrine HCl 120 mg/SR Cap. Bot. 100s, 1000s.
Use: Antihistamine, decongestant.

•**COD LIVER OIL,** U.S.P. XXII. Emulsion.
Use: Vitamin A and D therapy.
See: Cod Liver Oil Concentrate Cap. (Schering).

W/Anesthesin, zinc oxide, hydroxyquinoline.
See: Medicone Dressing. (Medicone).

W/Benzocaine.
See: Morusan, Oint. (Beecham Labs).

W/Creosote. (Bryant) Cod liver oil 9 min, creosote 1 min/Cap. Bot. 100s.

W/Malt extract (Burroughs Wellcome) Vitamins A 6450 IU, D 645 IU. Bot. 10 fl oz, 20 fl oz.

W/Methylbenzethonium Cl.
See: Benephen, Prods. (Halsted).

W/Viosterol.
(Abbott) Vitamins A 2800 IU, D 255 IU/Gm. Bot. 12 fl oz.
(Squibb) Vitamins A 2000 IU, D 440 IU/Gm. Bot. 4 fl oz, 12 fl oz.

W/Zinc oxide.
See: Desitin, Preps. (Leeming).

COD LIVER OIL CONCENTRATE. (Schering) Concentrate of cod liver oil with vitamins A and

D added. **Cap.:** Bot. 40s, 100s. **Tab.:** Bot. 100s, 240s. Also W/Vitamin C. Bot. 100s.
Use: Vitamin supplement.

COD LIVER OIL OINTMENT.
See: Moruguent, Oint. (Beecham Labs).

•**CODORPHONE HYDROCHLORIDE.** USAN.
Use: Analgesic.

•**CODOXIME.** USAN.
Use: Antitussive.

•**CODOXY.** (Halsey) Oxycodone HCl 4.5 mg, oxycodone terephthalate 0.38 mg, aspirin 325 mg/Tab. Bot. 100s.
Use: Narcotic analgesic combination.

CODROXOMIN INJECTION. (Forest Pharm.) Crystalline hydroxocobalamin 1000 mcg/ml. Vial 10 ml.
Use: Vitamin B_{12} supplement.

CO-ESTRO. (Robinson) Conjugated estrogen 0.625 mg, 1.25 mg or 2.5 mg/Tab. Bot. 100s, 500s, 1000s.
Use: Estrogen.

COFFEE BREAK. (O'Connor) Anhydrous caffeine 200 mg/Cap. and Capl. Bot. 20s.
Use: Analeptic.

COGENTIN. (Merck Sharp & Dohme) Benztropine Mesylate **Tab.:** 0.5 mg Bot. 100s; 1 mg Bot. 100s, UD 100s; 2 mg Bot. 100s, 1000s, UD 100s. **Inj.:** Benztropine mesylate 1 mg/ml w/ sodium Cl 9 mg and water for injection q.s. to 1 ml Amp. 2 ml, Box 6s.
Use: Antiparkinson agent.

CO-GESIC. (Central) Hydrocodone bitartrate 5 mg, acetaminophen 500 mg/Tab. Bot. 100s, 500s.
Use: Narcotic analgesic combination.

COGNEX. (Parke-Davis) Tacrine HCl. Investigational cholinergic agent.
Use: Alzheimer's disease.

CO-HEP-TRAL. (Davis & Sly) Folic acid 10 mg, vitamin B_{12} 100 mcg, liver injection q.s./ml. Vial 10 ml.
Use: Vitamin/mineral supplement.

COLABID TABS. (Major) Probenecid 500 mg, colchicine 0.5 mg/Tab. Bot. 100s, 1000s.
Use: Agent for gout.

COLACE. (Bristol-Myers) Docusate sodium. **Cap.:** 50 mg or 100 mg. Bot. 30s, 60s, 250s, 1000s, UD 100s. **Syr.:** 60 mg/15 ml with alcohol > 1%. Bot. 240 ml, 480 ml. **Liq.:** 150 mg/15 ml. Bot. 30 ml, 480 ml with calibrated droppers.
Use: Laxative.

COLAGYN. (Smith) Zinc sulfocarbolate, potassium, oxyquinoline sulfate, lactic acid, boric acid. Jelly. Tube w/applicator and refill 6 oz. Douche Pow. 3 oz, 7 oz, 14 oz.

COLANA SYRUP. (Hance) Euphorbia pilulifera tincture 8 ml, wild lettuce syrup 8 ml, cocillana tincture 2.5 ml, squill compound syrup 1.5 ml, cascara 0.25 Gm, menthol 4.8 mg/fl oz. Bot. 4 fl oz, gal. Also w/Dionin 15 mg/fl oz. Bot. gal.

COLASPASE. B.A.N. L-Asparagine amidohydrolase obtained from cultures of *Escherichia coli.*
See: Crasnitin.

COLAX. (Rugby) Docusate sodium 100 mg, phenolphthalein 65 mg/Tab. Bot. 30s.
Use: Laxative.

COLBENEMID. (Merck Sharp & Dohme) Probenecid 0.5 Gm, colchicine 0.5 mg/Tab. Bot. 100s.
Use: Agent for gout.

COLBENI-MOR. (H.L. Moore) Probenecid 0.5 mg/Tab. Bot. 100s, 1000s.
Use: Agent for gout.

•**COLCHICINE,** U.S.P. XXII. Tab., Inj. U.S.P. XXII. Acetamide, N-(5,6,7,9-tetrahydro-1,2,3,10-tetrame-thoxy-9-oxobenzo[a]heptalen-7-yl)-.(Various Mfr.).
Use: Gout suppressant.

W/Benemid.
See: Colbenemid, Tab. (Merck Sharp & Dohme).

W/Methyl salicylate. (Parke-Davis) Colchicine 1/250 gr, methyl salicylate 3 min/Cap. Bot. 100s, 500s, 1000s.
Use: Orally, gout therapy.

W/Probenecid.
See: Benn-C, Tab. (Scrip).
Colbenemid, Tab. (Merck Sharp & Dohme).
Robenecid with colchicine, Tab. (Robinson).

W/Sodium salicylate.
See: Salcoce, Tab. (Cole).

W/Sodium salicylate, calcium carbonate, dried aluminum hydroxide gel, phenobarbital.
See: Apcogesic, Tabs. (Apco).

W/Sodium salicylate, potassium iodide.
See: Bricolide, Tab. (Briar).
Colsalide, Tab. (Vortech).

COLCHICINE SALICYLATE.
W/Phenobarbital, sodium p-aminobenzoate, vitamin B_1, aspirin.
See: Doloral, Tab. (Alamed).

COLD CREAM, U.S.P. XXI.
Use: Emollient; water in oil emulsion ointment base.

COLDONYL. (Dover) Acetaminophen, phenylephrine HCl/Tab. Sugar, lactose and salt free. UD Box 500s.
Use: Analgesic, decongestant.

COLDRAN. (Blue Cross) Phenylephrine HCl 5 mg, chlorpheniramine maleate 2 mg, salicylamide 1.5 gr, acetaminophen 0.5 gr, caffeine/Tab. Bot. 30s.
Use: Decongestant, antihistamine, analgesic.

COLDRINE. (Hauck) Acetaminophen 200 mg, pseudoephedrine HCl 30 mg/Tab. Bot. 1000s.
Use: Analgesic, decongestant.

COLD SORE LOTION. (McKesson) Bot. 0.25 oz.
Use: Cold sores.

COLD SORE LOTION. (Purepac) Camphor, benzoin, aluminum Cl. Bot. 0.5 oz.
Use: Cold sores.

COLD TABLETS. (Walgreen) Phenylephrine HCl 5 mg, chlorpheniramine maleate 2 mg, acetaminophen 325 mg/Tab. Bot. 50s.
Use: Decongestant, antihistamine, analgesic.

COLD TABLETS MULTIPLE SYMPTOM. (Walgreen) Acetaminophen 500 mg, pseudoephedrine HCl 30 mg, chlorpheniramine maleate 2 mg, dextromethorphan HBr 10 mg/Tab. Bot. 50s.
Use: Analgesic, decongestant, antihistamine, antitussive.

COLD VACCINES, ORAL. (Sherman) Oral Tabs.
See: Entoral, Pulvule (Lilly).

COLESTID. (Upjohn) Colestipol HCl 5 Gm/pkt. Box 30s, Bot. 500 Gm.
Use: Antihyperlipidemic.

COLESTIPOL HYDROCHLORIDE, U.S.P. XXII. For Oral Susp., U.S.P. XXII.
Use: Antihyperlipoproteinemic.
See: Colestid (Upjohn).

COL-EVAC. (Forest) Potassium bitartrate, bicarbonate of soda and a blended base of polyethylene glycols. Supp. 2s, 12s.

COLEXUSS. (Jenkins) White pine 56.7 mg, wild cherry 56.7 mg, American spikenard 6 mg, poplar bud 6 mg, sanguinaria 5 mg, menthol 0.5 mg/fldr. Bot. 3 oz, 4 oz, gal.
Use: Cough syrup.

COLFANT. (Jenkins) Paregoric 2 min (pow. opium 1/125 gr), sodium bicarbonate 1 gr, magnesium trisilicate 5/8 gr, catnip extract 1/50 gr, chamomile extract 1/100 gr (Matricaria), oil fennel q.s./Tab. Bot. 1000s.
Use: Narcotic analgesic, antacid.

COLFORSIN. USAN.
Use: Antiglaucoma agent.

COLIMYCIN SODIUM METHANESULFONATE. (Parke-Davis).
See: Colistimethate Sodium.

COLIMYCIN SULFATE. (Parke-Davis).
See: Coly-Mycin, Preps. (Parke-Davis).

COLISTIMETHATE SODIUM, STERILE, U.S.P. XXII. Sodium Colistin Methanesulfonate. Colistin methane sulfonic acid, pentasodium salt. Pentasodium colistin methanesulfonate.
Use: Antibiotic.
See: Coly-Mycin-M, Injectable (Parke-Davis).

COLISTIN. B.A.N. A mixture of polypeptides produced by strains of *Bacillus polymyxa var. colistinus*.
Use: Antibiotic.

COLISTIN BASE.
W/Neomycin base, hydrocortisone acetate, thonzonium bromide, polysorbate 80, acetic acid, sodium acetate.
See: Coly-Mycin Otic W/Neomycin and Hydrocortisone, Liq. (Parke-Davis).

COLISTIN AND NEOMYCIN SULFATES AND HYDROCORTISONE ACETATE OTIC SUSPENSION, U.S.P. XXII.
Use: Antibiotic, anti-inflammatory.

COLISTIN METHANESULFONATE.
See: Colistimethate Sodium.

COLISTIN SULFATE, U.S.P. XXII. Oral Susp., U.S.P. XXII. The sulfate salt of an antibiotic substance elaborated by Aerobacillus colistinus.
Use: Antibacterial.
See: Colymycin-S Ophthalmic (Parke-Davis).
Coly-Mycin S Susp. (Parke-Davis).

COLISTIN SULFOMETHATE. B.A.N. An antibiotic obtained from colistin sulfate by sulfomethylation with formaldehyde and sodium bisulfite.
Use: Anti-infective.

CO-LIVER. (Standex) Folic acid 1 mg, vitamin B_{12} 100 mcg, liver 10 mcg/ml. Vial 10 ml.
Use: Vitamin/mineral supplement.

COLLADERM. (C & M Pharmacal) Purified water, glycerin, soluble collagen, hydrolysed elastin, allantoin, ethylhydroxycellulose, sorbic, octoxynol-9. Bot. 2.3 oz.
Use: Emollient.

COLLAGENASE.
See: Santyl (Knoll).

COLLAGENASE ABC OINTMENT. (Advance Biofactures) Collagenase 250 units/Gm in white petrolatum. 25 Gm, 50 Gm.
Use: Topical enzyme preparation.

COLLAGEN IMPLANT.
See: Zyderm I. (Collagen Corp.).
Zyderm II. (Collagen Corp.).

•**COLLODION,** U.S.P. XXII. Flexible, U.S.P. XXII.
Use: Topical protectant.

COLLOIDAL ALUMINUM HYDROXIDE.
See: Aluminum Hydroxide Gel, U.S.P. XXII.

COLLOIDAL GOLD.
See: Aureotope (Squibb).

COLLOIDAL SILVER IODIDE.
See: Neo-Silvol, Soln. (Parke-Davis).

COLOCTYL. (Vitarine) Docusate sodium 100 mg/Cap. Bot. 100s, 1000s, UD 1000s.
Use: Laxative.

COLOGEL. (Lilly) Methylcellulose 450 mg/5 ml, alcohol 5%, saccharin. Bot. 16 fl oz.
Use: Laxative.

COLONY STIMULATING FACTOR.
Use: Adjunct during antineoplastic therapy.
See: Leukine (Immunex).
Neupogen (Amgen).
Prokine (Hoechst-Roussel).

COLOSCREEN. (Helena Labs) Occult blood screening test. Kit 12s, 25s, 50s. 3 tests per kit.
Use: Diagnostic aid.

COLOSCREEN/VPI. (Helena Labs) Occult blood screening test. Box 100s, 1000s.
Use: Diagnostic aid.

COLOVAGE. (Dyna Pharm) Formerly Colonlite. Powder for reconstitution to produce 1 gal soln. Containing sodium Cl 5.53 Gm, potassium Cl 2.82 Gm, sodium bicarbonate 6.36 Gm, sodium sulfate anhydrous 21.5 Gm, polyethylene glycol 3350. Pkg. 1s.
Use: Laxative.

COL-PROBENECID. (Various Mfr.) Probenecid 500 mg, colchicine 0.5 mg/Tab. Bot. 100s, 1000s, UD 100s.
Use: Agent for gout.

COLREX. (Reid-Rowell) Chlorpheniramine maleate 2 mg, phenylephrine HCl 5 mg, acetaminophen 325 mg/Cap. Bot. 24s, 100s.
Use: Antihistamine, decongestant, analgesic.

COLREX COMPOUND. (Reid-Rowell) Codeine phosphate 16 mg, acetaminophen 325 mg, phenylephrine HCl 10 mg, chlorpheniramine maleate 2 mg/Cap. Bot. 100s, 500s.
Use: Antitussive, analgesic, decongestant, antihistamine.

COLREX COMPOUND ELIXIR. (Reid-Rowell) Codeine phosphate 8 mg, acetaminophen 120 mg, chlorpheniramine maleate 1 mg, phenylephrine HCl 5 mg/5 ml, alcohol 9.5%. Sugar free elixir. Bot. pt, gal.
Use: Antitussive, analgesic, antihistamine, decongestant.

COLREX EXPECTORANT. (Reid-Rowell) Guaifenesin 100 mg/5 ml, alcohol 4.7%. Bot. 120 ml, 480 ml. Sugar free base.
Use: Expectorant.

COLREX SYRUP. (Reid-Rowell) Dextromethorphan HBr 10 mg, phenylephrine HCl 5 mg, chlorpheniramine maleate 2 mg/5 ml, alcohol 4.5%. Sugar free base. Bot. 120 ml.
Use: Antitussive, decongestant, antihistamine.

COLREX TROCHES. (Reid-Rowell) Benzocaine 10 mg, cetylpyridinium Cl 2.5 mg/Troche. 20s.
Use: Anesthetic, antiseptic.

COLSALIDE. (Vortech) Colchicine 0.65 mg/Tab. Bot. 1000s.
Use: Agent for gout.

COLTAB CHILDREN'S. (Hauck) Phenylephrine HCl 2.5 mg, chlorpheniramine maleate 1 mg/Chew. tab. Bot. 30s.
Use: Decongestant, antihistamine.

•**COLTEROL MESYLATE.** USAN.
Use: Bronchodilator.

COLY-MYCIN M PARENTERAL. (Parke-Davis) Colistimethate sodium equivalent 150 mg colistin base per vial.
Use: Anti-infective.

COLY-MYCIN S ORAL SUSPENSION. (Parke-Davis) Colistin sulfate 300 mg/60 ml. For oral susp. Bot. 300 mg.
Use: Anti-infective.

COLY-MYCIN S OTIC DROPS W/NEOMYCIN AND HYDROCORTISONE. (Parke-Davis) Colistin base as the sulfate 3 mg, neomycin base as the sulfate 3.3 mg, hydrocortisone acetate 10 mg, thonzonium bromide 0.5 mg/ml, polysorbate 80, acetic acid, sodium acetate, thimerosal. Dropper bot. 5 ml, 10 ml.
Use: Anti-infective.

COLYTE. (Reed & Carnrick)
2L: PEG (Polyethylene glycol-electrolyte solution) 3350 120 Gm, sodium sulfate 11.36 Gm, sodium bicarbonate 3.36 Gm, sodium Cl 2.92 Gm, potassium Cl 1.49 Gm.
1 gal: PEG 3350 227.1 Gm, sodium sulfate 21.5 Gm, sodium bicarbonate 6.36 Gm, sodium Cl 5.53 Gm, potassium Cl 2.82 Gm.
6 L: PEG 3350 360 Gm, sodium sulfate 34.08 Gm, sodium bicarbonate 10.08 Gm, sodium Cl 8.76 Gm, potassium Cl 4.47 Gm. Pack 5. Bot. 2 L, gal, 4L, 6L.
Use: Cathartic, GI exams.

COMBICAL D. (Mills) Calcium 375 mg, vitamin D 400 IU, phosphorus 180 mg, magnesium 144 mg/3 Tab. Bot. 1000s.
Use: Vitamin/mineral supplement.

COMBICHOLE. (Trout) Dehydrocholic acid 2 gr, desoxycholic acid 1 gr/Tab. Bot. 100s, 1000s.
Use: Hydrocholeretic.

COMBIPRES TABLETS. (Boehringer Ingelheim) **0.1 mg:** Clonidine HCl 0.1 mg, chlorthalidone 15 mg/Tab. Bot. 100s, 1000s. **0.2 mg:** Clonidine HCl 0.2 mg, chlorthalidone 15 mg/Tab. Bot. 100s, 1000s. **0.3 mg:** Clonidine HCl 0.3 mg, chlorthalidone 15 mg/Tab. Bot. 100s.
Use: Antihypertensive.

COMBISTIX REAGENT STRIPS. (Ames) Protein test-tetrabromphenol blue, citrate buffer, protein-absorbing agent; glucose test area-glucose oxidase, orthotolidin and a catalyst; pH test area methyl red and bromthymol blue. Box, strips, 100s.
Use: Diagnostic aid.

COMFORT DROPS. (Barnes-Hind) Isotonic solution containing naphazoline 0.03%, benzalkonium Cl 0.005%, edetate disodium 0.02%. Bot. 15 ml.
Use: Hard contact lens care.

COMFORT EYE DROPS. (Barnes-Hind) Naphazoline HCl 0.03%, disodium edetate 0.02%, benzalkonium Cl 0.005%. Plastic dropper bot. 15 ml.
Use: Ophthalmic decongestant.

COMFORT GEL LIQUID. (Walgreen) Aluminum hydroxide compressed gel 200 mg, magnesium hydroxide 200 mg, simethicone 20 mg/5 ml. Bot. 12 oz.
Use: Antacid, antiflatulent.

COMFORT GEL TABLETS. (Walgreen) Magnesium hydroxide 85 mg, simethicone 25 mg, aluminum hydroxide-magnesium carbonate codried gel 282 mg/Tab. Bot. 100s.
Use: Antacid, antiflatulent.

COMFORTINE. (Dermik) Zinc oxide 12%, vitamins A and D, lanolin in protective base. Oint. Tube 1.5 oz, 4 oz.
Use: Emollient.

COMFORT TEARS. (Barnes-Hind) Hydroxyethyl cellulose, benzalkonium Cl 0.005%, edetate disodium 0.02%. Bot. 15 ml.
Use: Soft contact lens care.

COMHIST L.A. CAPSULES. (Norwich Eaton) Phenylephrine HCl 20 mg, chlorpheniramine maleate 4 mg, phenyltoloxamine citrate 50 mg/Cap. Bot. 100s.
Use: Decongestant, antihistamine.

COMHIST TABLETS. (Norwich Eaton) Phenylephrine HCl 10 mg, chlorpheniramine maleate 2

mg, phenyltoloxamine citrate 25 mg/Tab. Bot. 100s.
Use: Decongestant, antihistamine.

COMPAL. (Reid-Rowell) Dihydrocodeine 16 mg, acetaminophen 356.4 mg, caffeine 30 mg/Cap. Bot. 100s.
Use: Analgesic combination.

COMPAT NUTRITION ENTERAL DELIVERY SYSTEM. (Sandoz Nutrition) Top fill feeding containers 600 ml, 1400 ml. Gravity delivery set. Pump delivery set. Compat enteral feeding pump.
Use: Enteral nutritional supplement.

COMPAZINE. (SmithKline) Prochlorperazine as the maleate. **Tab.:** 5 mg, 10 mg or 25 mg. Bot. 100s, 1000s, UD 100s (except for 25 mg). **Inj.:** Edisylate salt 5 mg/ml. Amp. 2 ml, vial 10 ml, disposable syringe 2 ml. **SR Spansule:** Maleate salt 10 mg, 15 mg or 30 mg. Bot. 50s, 500s, UD 100s. **Supp.:** 2.5 mg, 5 mg or 25 mg. Box 12s. **Syr.:** Edisylate salt 5 mg/5 ml. Bot. 4 fl oz.
Use: Antiemetic, antipsychotic.

COMPETE. (Mission) Iron 27 mg, vitamins A 5000 IU, D 400 IU, E 45 IU, B_1 2.25 mg, B_2 2.6 mg, B_3 30 mg, B_6 25 mg, B_{12} 9 mcg, C 90 mg, folic acid 0.4 mg, Zn/Tab. Bot. 100s.
Use: Vitamin/mineral supplement.

COMPLEAT-B MEAT BASE FORMULA. (Sandoz Nutrition) Beef, nonfat milk, hydrolyzed cereal solids, maltodextrin, pureed fruits and vegetables, corn oil, mono and diglycerides. Bot. 250 ml, Can 250 ml.
Use: Enteral nutritional supplement.

COMPLEAT-MODIFIED FORMULA MEAT BASE. (Sandoz Nutrition) Hydrolyzed cereal solids, calcium caseinate, pureed fruits and vegetables, corn oil, beef puree, mono and diglycerides. Can 250 ml.
Use: Enteral nutritional supplement.

COMPLEAT-REGULAR FORMULA. (Sandoz Nutrition) Deionized water, beef puree, hydrolyzed cereal solids, green bean puree, pea puree, nonfat milk, corn oil, maltodextrin, peach puree, orange juice, mono and diglycerides, carrageenan, vitamins, minerals. Bot. 250 ml, Can 250 ml.
Use: Enteral nutritional supplement.

COMPLETE. (Mission) Vitamins A 5000 IU, D 400 IU, E 45 IU, C 90 mg, B_1 2.25 mg, folic acid 0.4 mg, B_2 2.6 mg, B_3 30 mg, B_6 25 mg, B_{12} 9 mcg, ferrous gluconate 233 mg, zinc 22.5 mg/Tab. Bot. 100s, 1000s.
Use: Vitamin/mineral supplement.

COMPLETONE ELIXIR FORT. (Winthrop Products) Ferrous gluconate.
Use: Iron supplement.

COMPLEX 15 CREAM. (Baker/Cummins) Jar 4 oz.
Use: Emollient.

COMPLEX 15 LOTION. (Baker/Cummins) Bot. 8 oz.
Use: Emollient.

COMPLY LIQUID. (Sherwood) Sodium caseinate, calcium caseinate, hydrolyzed cornstarch, sucrose, corn oil, soy lecithin, vitamins A, B_1, B_2, B_3, B_5, B_6, B_{12}, C, D, E, K, folic acid, biotin, choline, Ca, Cl, Cu, Fe, I, Mg, Mn, P, Zn. Can 250 ml, Bot. 200 ml.
Use: Enteral nutritional supplement.

COMPOUND 42.
See: Warfarin (Various Mfr.).

COMPOUND B.
See: Corticosterone (Various Mfr.).

COMPOUND CB3025.
See: Alkeran, Tab. (Burroughs Wellcome).

COMPOUND E. (Kendall).
See: Cortisone Acetate. (Various Mfr.).

COMPOUND F.
See: Hydrocortisone (Various Mfr.).

COMPOUND S.
Use: Antiviral.
See: Retrovir (Burroughs).
Zidovudine.

COMPOUND W. (Whitehall) Salicylic acid 17% w/w in flexible collodion vehicle w/ether 63.5%. Bot. 0.31 oz.
Use: Keratolytic.

COMPOZ. (Medtech) Diphenhydramine HCl 50 mg/Tab. Ctn. 24s.
Use: OTC sleep aid.

COMTREX A/S. (Bristol-Myers) **Tab.:** Pseudoephedrine HCl 30 mg, chlorpheniramine maleate 2 mg, acetaminophen 500 mg. Bot. 24s, 50s. **Capl.:** Pseudoephedrine HCl 30 mg, chlorpheniramine maleate 2 mg, acetaminophen 500 mg. Bot. 16s, 36s.
Use: Decongestant, antihistamine, analgesic.

COMTREX CAPLETS. (Bristol-Myers) Acetaminophen 325 mg, pseudoephedrine HCl 30 mg, chlorpheniramine maleate 2 mg, dextromethorphan HBr 10 mg/Capl. Bot. 24s, 50s.
Use: Analgesic, decongestant, antihistamine, antitussive.

COMTREX COUGH FORMULA. (Bristol-Myers) Pseudoephedrine HCl 15 mg, dextromethorphan 7.5 mg, guaifenesin 67 mg, acetaminophen 125 mg/5 ml, alcohol 20%. Bot. 120 ml, 240 ml.
Use: Decongestant, antitussive, expectorant, analgesic.

COMTREX LIQUID MULTI-SYMPTOM COLD RELIEVER. (Bristol-Myers) Acetaminophen 650 mg, phenylpropanolamine HCl 25 mg, chlorpheniramine maleate 4 mg, dextromethorphan HBr 20 mg/30 ml, alcohol 20%. Bot. 6 oz, 10 oz.
Use: Analgesic, decongestant, antihistamine, antitussive.

COMTREX LIQUI-GELS. (Bristol-Myers) Acetaminophen 325 mg, phenylpropanolamine HCl 12.5 mg, chlorpheniramine maleate 2 mg, dextromethorphan HBr 10 mg/Tab. Blister pkg. 24s, 50s.
Use: Analgesic, decongestant, antihistamine, antitussive.

COMTREX. (Bristol-Myers) Acetaminophen 325 mg, pseudoephedrine HCl 30 mg, chlorpheniramine maleate 2 mg, dextromethorphan HBr 10 mg/Tab. Bot. 24s, 50s.
Use: Analgesic, decongestant, antihistamine, antitussive.

CONALSYN. (Cenci) Chlorpheniramine maleate 8 mg, phenylephrine HCl 20 mg, methscopolamine nitrate 2.5 mg/TR Cap. Bot. 30s, 250s, 500s.
Use: Antihistamine, decongestant, anticholinergic/antispasmodic.

CONAR-A TAB. (Beecham Labs) Dextromethorphan HBr 15 mg, phenylephrine HCl 10 mg, acetaminophen 300 mg, guaifenesin 100 mg/Tab. Bot. 100s. UD 20s.
Use: Antitussive, decongestant, analgesic, expectorant.

CONAR. (Beecham Labs) Dextromethorphan HBr 15 mg, phenylephrine HCl 10 mg/5 ml. Bot. pt.
Use: Antitussive, decongestant.

CONAR EXPECTORANT. (Beecham Labs) Dextromethorphan HBr 15 mg, phenylephrine HCl 10 mg, guaifenesin 100 mg/5 ml. Bot. 4 oz, pt.
Use: Antitussive, decongestant, expectorant.

CONCENTRATED OLEOVITAMIN A & D.
See: Oleovitamin A & D, Concentrated, Cap. (Various Mfr.).

CONCENTRATED TUBERCULIN.

CONCENTRIN CAPS. (Parke-Davis) Dextromethorphan HBr 15 mg, pseudoephedrine HCl 30 mg, guaifenesin 100 mg/Cap. Bot. 12s.
Use: Antitussive, decongestant, expectorant.

CONCEPTROL CREAM. (Ortho) Nonoxynol-9 5%, in an oil-in-water emulsion at pH 4.5. Tube 70 Gm with applicator.
Use: Contraceptive.

CONCEPTROL DISPOSABLE CONTRACEPTIVE GEL. (Ortho) Nonoxynol-9 100 mg. Each applicator contains 2.5 Gm Conceptrol. Pkg. 6, 10 disposable applicators.
Use: Contraceptive.

CONDOL SUSPENSION. (Winthrop Products) Dipyrone, chlormezanone.
Use: Analgesic, muscle relaxant.

CONDOL TABLETS. (Winthrop Products) Dipyrone, chlormezanone.
Use: Analgesic, muscle relaxant.

CONDOMMATE. (Upsher-Smith) Blend of polyethylene glycols, a surfactant and a glyceride. Box 12s.
Use: Vaginal lubricant.

CONDRIN-LA. (Hauck) Phenylpropanolamine HCl 75 mg, chlorpheniramine maleate 12 mg. Bot. 1000s.
Use: Decongestant, antihistamine.

CONDYLOX. (Oclassen) Podofilox.
Use: Keratolytic.

CONEST. (Grafton) Conjugated estrogens 0.625 mg, 1.25 mg or 2.5 mg/Tab. Bot. 100s, 1000s.
Use: Estrogen.

CONEX-DA. (Forest) Phenylpropanolamine HCl 37.5 mg, chlorpheniramine maleate 4 mg/Tab. Bot. 100s, 1000s.
Use: Decongestant, antihistamine.

CONEX LOZENGE CT. (Forest) Benzocaine 5 mg, methylparaben 2 mg, propylparaben 0.5 mg, cetylpyridinium Cl 0.5 mg/Loz. Bot. 1000s.
Use: Anesthetic, antiseptic.

CONEX PLUS. (Forest) Phenylpropanolamine HCl 25 mg, chlorpheniramine maleate 4 mg, acetaminophen 325 mg/Tab. Bot. 1000s.
Use: Decongestant, antihistamine, analgesic.

CONEX SYRUP. (Forest) Phenylpropanolamine HCl 12.5 mg, guaifenesin 100 mg/5 ml. Bot. 4 oz.
Use: Decongestant, expectorant.

CONEX WITH CODEINE. (Forest) Codeine phosphate 10 mg, guaifenesin 100 mg, phenylpropanolamine HCl 12.5 mg/5 ml. Bot. 4 oz.
Use: Antitussive, expectorant, decongestant.

CONFIDENT. (Block) Carboxymethylcellulose gum, ethylene oxide polymer, petrolatum/mineral oil base. Tube 0.7 oz, 1.4 oz, 2.4 oz.
Use: Denture adhesive.

CONGESPIRIN FOR CHILDREN. ASPIRIN-FREE CHEWABLE COLD TABLETS. (Bristol-Myers) Acetaminophen 81 mg, phenylephrine HCl 1.25 mg, saccharin/Chew. Tab. Bot. 24s.
Use: Analgesic, decongestant, antipyretic.

CONGESPIRIN FOR CHILDREN, ASPIRIN-FREE LIQUID COLD MEDICINE. (Bristol-Myers) Acetaminophen 130 mg, phenylpropanolamine HCl 6.25 mg/15 ml, alcohol 10%. Bot. 3 oz.
Use: Analgesic, decongestant.

CONGESPIRIN FOR CHILDREN, COUGH SYRUP. (Bristol-Myers) Dextromethorphan hydrobromide 5 mg/5 ml. Bot. 3 oz.
Use: Antitussive.

CONGESTAC. (SmithKline Prods) Pseudoephedrine HCl 60 mg, guaifenesin 400 mg/Tab. Bot. 12s, 24s.
Use: Decongestant, expectorant.

CONGESTERONE. (Kenyon) Conjugated estrogens 0.625 mg, 1.25 mg or 2.5 mg/Tab. Bot. 100s.
Use: Estrogen.

CONGO RED. Injection.
Use: Hemostatic in hemorrhagic disorders.

CONGESS. (Fleming) **Sr.:** Guaifenesin 250 mg, pseudoephedrine HCl 120 mg/SR Cap. **Jr.:** Guaifenesin 125 mg, pseudoephedrine HCl 60 mg/TR Cap. Bot. 100s, 1000s.
Use: Expectorant, decongestant.

CONJUGATED ESTROGENS.
See: Estrogens, Conjugated (Various Mfr.).
Use: Estrogen.

CONJUNCTAMIDE. (Horizon) Prednisolone acetate 0.5%, sodium sulfacetamide 10%, hydroxypropyl methylcellulose, polysorbate 80, sodium thiosulfate, benzalkonium Cl 0.01%. Susp. Dropper bot. 5 ml, 15 ml.

Use: Corticosteroid, anti-infective, ophthalmic.

CONJUTABS. (Rand) **Conjutabs 62:** Estrogens 0.625 mg/Tab. **Conjutabs 125:** Estrogens 1.25 mg/Tab. **Conjutabs 250:** Estrogens 2.5 mg/Tab. (Enteric coated) Bot. 100s, 500s.
Use: Estrogen.

CONRAY. (Mallinckrodt) Iothalamate meglumine 60% (28.2% iodine), EDTA. Inj. Vial 20 ml, 30 ml, 50 ml, 100 ml, 150 ml.
Use: Radiopaque agent.

CONRAY-30. (Mallinckrodt) Iothalamate meglumine 30% (14.1% iodine), EDTA. Inj. Vial 300 ml.
Use: Radiopaque agent.

CONRAY-43. (Mallinckrodt) Iothalamate meglumine 43% (20.2% iodine), EDTA. Inj. Vial 50 ml, 100 ml, 250 ml.
Use: Radiopaque agent.

CONRAY-325. (Mallinckrodt) Iothalamate sodium 54.3% (32.5% iodine), EDTA. Inj. Vial 30 ml, 50 ml.
Use: Radiopaque agent.

CONRAY-400. (Mallinckrodt) Iothalamate sodium 66.8% (40% iodine), EDTA. Inj. Vial 25 ml, 50 ml.
Use: Radiopaque agent.

CONSIN COUMOUND SALVE. (Wisconsin) Carbolic acid ointment. Jar 2 oz, lb.
Use: Minor skin irritations.

CONSTAB 100. (Kenyon) Docusate sodium 100 mg/Tab. Bot. 100s, 1000s.
Use: Laxative.

CONSTANT-T. (Geigy) Theophylline (anhydrous) 200 mg, 300 mg/SR Tab. Bot. 100s, UD 100s, Gy-Pak 60s.
Use: Bronchodilator.

CONSTILAC. (Alra) Lactulose syrup 10 Gm/15 ml. Bot. 8 oz, 16 oz, UD 30 ml.
Use: Laxative.

CONSTONATE 60. Docusate sodium 100 mg, 250 mg/Cap. Bot. 100s, 1000s.
Use: Laxative.

CONSTULOSE. (Barre-National) Lactulose 10 Gm, galactose > 2.2 Gm, lactose > 1.2 Gm, other sugars ≤ 1.2 Gm/15 ml. Syr. Bot. 237 ml, 946 ml.
Use: Laxative.

CONTAC COUGH FORMULA. (SmithKline Prods.) Dextromethorphan HBr 10 mg, guaifenesin 67 mg/5 ml. Bot. 120 ml.
Use: Expectorant, antitussive.

CONTAC COUGH AND SORE THROAT FORMULA. (SmithKline Prods.) Dextromethorphan HBr 10 mg, guaifenesin 67 mg, acetaminophen 217 mg/5 ml. Bot. 120 ml.
Use: Expectorant, antitussive, analgesic.

CONTAC JR. (SmithKline Prods.) Pseudoephedrine HCl 15 mg, acetaminophen 160 mg, dextromethorphan HBr 5 mg, saccharin, sorbitol/5 ml. Bot. 4 oz.
Use: Decongestant, analgesic, antitussive.

CONTAC NIGHTTIME COLD. (SmithKline Prods.) Acetaminophen 167 mg, dextromethorphan HBr 5 mg, pseudoephedrine HCl 10 mg, doxylamine succinate 1.25 mg/5 ml, alcohol 25%. Bot. 177 ml.
Use: Analgesic, antitussive, decongestant, antihistamine.

CONTAC SEVERE COLD FORMULA. (SmithKline Prods.) Phenylpropanolamine HCl 12.5 mg, acetaminophen 500 mg, chlorpheniramine maleate 2 mg, dextromethorphan HBr 15 mg/Capl. Pkg. 10s, 20s.
Use: Decongestant, analgesic, antihistamine, antitussive.

CONTAC-12 HOUR CAPLETS. (SmithKline Prods.) Phenylpropanolamine HCl 75 mg, chlorpheniramine maleate 12 mg/Capl. Bot. 10s, 20s.
Use: Decongestant, antihistamine.

CONTAC-12 HOUR CAPSULES. (SmithKline Prods.) Phenylpropanolamine HCl 75 mg, chlorpheniramine maleate 8 mg/CA Cap. Pkg. 10s, 20s.
Use: Decongestant, antihistamine.

CONTE-PAK-4. (SoloPak) Zinc 5 mg, copper 1 mg, manganese 0.5 mg, chromium 10 mcg. Vial 1 ml, 10 ml, 30 ml.
Use: Parenteral nutritional supplement.

CONTRACEPTIVES.
See: Oral Contraceptives (Various Mfr.).
Foams, Vaginal.
See: Delfen, Vaginal Foam (Ortho Pharm.).
Emko, Vaginal Foam (Emko).
Jellies & Creams, Vaginal.
See: Colagyn, Jel (Smith).
Colagyn, Jel (Smith).
Conceptrol, Cream, Gel (Ortho).
Gynol II, Gel (Ortho).
Immolin, Cream-Jel (Schmid).
Koromex-A, Jelly (Holland-Rantos).
Koromex, Cream or Jelly (Holland-Rantos).
Ortho-Creme (Ortho).
Ortho-Gynol, Jelly (Ortho).
Miscellaneous.
See: Norplant (Wyeth-Ayerst).
Suppositories, Vaginal.
See: Intercept, Inserts (Ortho).
Lorophyn, Supp., Jelly (Eaton).

CONTROL. (Thompson) Phenylpropanolamine HCl 75 mg/TR Cap. Bot. 14s, 28s, 56s.
Use: OTC diet aid.

CONVATEC PRODUCTS. (Conva-Tec) A series of health care products for the convalescent patient including:
Accuseal Bedside Drainage Bag w/Washport or Filter;
Accuseal Leg Bag;
Active Life Ostomy Pouch, Closed Open;
Duoderm Hydroactive Dressing w/Adhesive Border, Burnpak, Granules or Ulcerpak;
Durahesive Wafer w/low profile flange;

Stomahesive, Paste, Powder, Wafers, Wafer w/Sure Fit Accordian Flange;
Sur-Fit, Closed Pouch, Disposable Convex Inserts, Drainable Pouch, Flexible, Irrigation Sleeve, O.R. Set, System, Pouch Covers, Urostomy Pouch w/Covers;
Urihesive, System, System w/Accuseal Connection;
Wound Manager Drainage Pouch;
Visi-Flow Irrigation Starter Set.

CONVERSPAZ. (Ascher) Cellulase 5 mg, protease 10 mg, amylase 30 mg, lipase 13 mg, l-hyoscyamine sulfate 0.0625 mg/Cap. Bot. 100s.
Use: Digestive enzymes.

CONVERZYME CAPS. (Ascher) Cellulase 5 mg, protease 10 mg, amylase 30 mg, lipase 13 mg/Cap. Bot. 100s.
Use: Digestive enzymes.

COOPERVISION BALANCED SALT SOLUTION. (CooperVision) Sterile intraocular irrigation soln. Bot. 15 ml, 500 ml.
Use: Intraocular irrigating solution.

COPAVIN PULVULES. (Lilly) Codeine sulfate 15 mg, papaverine HCl 15 mg/Cap. Bot. 100s.
Use: Antitussive.

COPE. (Mentholatum) Aspirin 421.2 mg, magnesium hydroxide 50 mg, aluminum hydroxide 25 mg, caffeine 32 mg/Tab. Bot. 36s, 60s.
Use: Salicylate analgesic, antacid.

COPHENE #2. (Dunhall) Chlorpheniramine maleate 12 mg, pseudoephedrine HCl 120 mg/Time Cap. Bot. 100s, 500s.
Use: Antihistamine, decongestant.

COPHENE INJECTABLE. (Dunhall) Atropine sulfate 0.2 mg, phenylpropanolamine HCl 12.5 mg, chlorpheniramine maleate 5 mg/ml. Pkg. 10 ml.
Use: Anticholinergic/antispasmodic, decongestant, antihistamine.

COPHENE-PL. (Dunhall) Phenylephrine HCl 20 mg, phenylpropanolamine HCl 20 mg, chlorpheniramine maleate 5 mg/5 ml. Bot. 16 oz.
Use: Decongestant, antihistamine.

COPHENE-S. (Dunhall) Dihydrocodone bitartrate 3 mg, phenylephrine HCl 20 mg, phenylpropanolamine HCl 20 mg, chlorpheniramine maleate 5 mg/5 ml. Bot. pt.
Use: Antitussive, decongestant, antihistamine.

COPHENE-X. (Dunhall) Carbetapentane citrate 20 mg, phenylephrine HCl 10 mg, phenylpropanolamine HCl 10 mg, chlorpheniramine maleate 2.5 mg, potassium guaiacolsulfonate 45 mg/Cap. Bot. 100s.
Use: Antitussive, decongestant, antihistamine, expectorant.

COPHENE-XP SYRUP. (Dunhall) Carbetapentane citrate 20 mg, phenylephrine HCl 10 mg, phenylpropanolamine HCl 20 mg, chlorpheniramine maleate 2.5 mg, potassium guaiacolsulfonate 45 mg/5 ml. Bot. pt.
Use: Antitussive, decongestant, antihistamine, expectorant.

COPPER. (Abbott) Copper 0.4 mg/ml (as 0.85 mg cupric Cl.) Inj. Vial 10 ml, 30 ml.
Use: Parenteral nutritional supplement.

•**COPPER GLUCONATE,** U.S.P. XXII.
Use: Copper supplement.

COPPERHEAD BITE THERAPY.
See: Antivenin, Snake Polyvalent Inj. (Wyeth-Ayerst).

COPPERIN. (Vernon) Iron ammonium citrate, copper (6 gr). "A" adult dose, "B" children dose. Bot. 30s, 100s, 500s.
Use: Mineral supplement.

COPPERTONE. (Plough) A series of sun-care products marketed under the Coppertone name including Waterproof Lotions SPF 4, 6, 8, 15 and 25. Bot. 4 fl oz, 8 fl oz. Oil SPF 2: Bot. 4 fl oz, 8 fl oz; Lite Formula Oil SPF 2: Bot. 4 fl oz; Lite Lotion SPF 4: Bot. 4 fl oz; Dark Tanning Body Mousse SPF 4: Tube 4 oz; Suntanning Gel SPF 4: Tube 3 oz; Noskote SPF 8: Tube 0.44 oz, Jar 1 oz; Noskote SPF-15: Jar 1 oz. Contain one or more of the following ingredients: Padimate O, oxybenzone, homosalate, ethylhexyl p-methocinnamate.
Use: Sunscreen.

COPPERTONE FACE. (Plough) A series of sunscreen lotions with SPF 2, 4, 6 and 15 in a non-greasy base with Padimate O, oxybenzone (SPF 15 only).
Use: Sunscreen.

COPPERTONE NOSKOTE. (Plough) Homosalate 8%, oxybenzone 3%. (SPF 8) Oint. Jar 13.2 Gm, 30 Gm.
Use: Sunscreen.

COPPERTONE SPF-25 SUNBLOCK LOTION. (Plough) Ethylhexyl p-methoxycinnamate, oxybenzone, padimate 0 in lotion base (SPF-25). Bot. 4 fl oz.
Use: Sunscreen.

COPPERTONE DARK TANNING SPRAY. (Plough) Padimate 0 in spray base (SPF 2). Bot. 8 fl oz.
Use: Sunscreen.

COPPER TRACE METAL ADDITIVE. (IMS) Copper 1 mg. Inj. Vial 10 ml.

COPPER UNDECYLENATE.
W/Sodium propionate, sodium caprylate, propionic acid, undecylenic acid, salicylic acid.

CO-PYRONIL 2. (Dista) Chlorpheniramine maleate 4 mg, pseudoephedrine HCl 60 mg/Pulvule. Bot. 100s, 1000s.
Use: Antihistamine, decongestant.

CORAB. (Abbott Diagnostics) Radioimmunoassay for detection of antibody to hepatitis B core antigen. Test kit 100s.
Use: Diagnostic aid.

CORAB-M. (Abbott Diagnostics) Radioimmunoassay for the qualitative determination of specific IgM antibody to hepatitis B virus core antigen (Anti-HBc IgM) in human serum or plasma and may be used as an aid in the diagnosis of acute or recent hepatitis B infection.

Use: Diagnostic aid.

CORACE INJECTION. (Forest Pharm.) Cortisone acetate 50 mg/ml. Vial 10 ml.
Use: Glucocorticoid.

CORACIN. (Hauck) Hydrocortisone acetate 1%, neomycin sulfate 0.5%, bacitracin zinc 400 units, polymyxin B sulfate 10,000 units/Gm in white petrolatum and mineral oil base. Oint. Tube 3.75 Gm.
Use: Corticosteroid, anti-infective, ophthalmic.

CORAL. (Lorvic) Fluoride ion 1.23%, 0.1 molar phosphate. Jar 250 Gm, Coral II: 180 disposable cup units//carton.
Use: Phosphate/fluoride prophylaxis paste.

CORAL/PLUS. (Lorvic) Free fluoride ion 2.2%, recrystallized kaolinite. Tube 250 Gm.

CORAL SNAKE (NORTH AMERICAN) ANTIVENIN.
See: Antivenin (Micrurus fulvius). (Wyeth-Ayerst).

CORANE CAPSULES. (Forest Pharm.) Pyrilamine maleate 25 mg, pheniramine maleate 10 mg, phenylpropanolamine HCl 25 mg, phenylephrine HCl 10 mg/Cap. Bot. 100s, 500s, 1000s.
Use: Antihistamine, decongestant.

CORBICIN-125. (Arthrins) Vitamin C 125 mg/Cap. Bot. 100s.
Use: Vitamin C supplement.

CORDARONE. (Wyeth-Ayerst) Amiodarone HCl 200 mg/Tab. Bot. 60s.
Use: Antiarrhythmic.

CORDRAN. (Dista) Flurandrenolide 0.025%, 0.05% in emulsified petrolatum base/Gm. **0.025%:** Tube 30 Gm, 60 Gm, Jar 225 Gm. **0.05%:** Tube 15 Gm, 30 Gm, 60 Gm, Jar 225 Gm.
Use: Corticosteroid.

CORDRAN LOTION. (Dista) Flurandrenolide 0.05%, cetyl alcohol, benzyl alcohol, stearic acid, glyceryl monostearate, polyoxyl 40 stearate, glycerin, mineral oil, menthol, purified water. Squeeze bot. 15 ml, 60 ml.
Use: Corticosteroid.

CORDRAN-N CREAM & OINTMENT. (Dista) Flurandrenolide 0.5 mg, neomycin sulfate 5 mg/Gm. Tube 15 Gm, 30 Gm, 60 Gm.
Use: Corticosteroid.

CORDRAN SP. (Dista) Flurandrenolide 0.025%, 0.05% in emulsified base w/cetyl alcohol, stearic acid, polyoxyl 40 stearate, mineral oil, propylene glycol, sodium citrate, citric acid, purified water. **0.025%:** Tube 30 Gm, 60 Gm, Jar 225 Gm. **0.05%:** Tube 15 Gm, 30 Gm, 60 Gm, Jar 225 Gm.
Use: Corticosteroid.

CORDRAN TAPE. (Dista) Flurandrenolide 4 mcg/sq. cm. Roll 7.5 cm × 60 cm, 7.5 cm × 200 cm.
Use: Corticosteroid.

CORDROL. (Vita Elixir) Prednisolone 5 mg, 10 mg or 20 mg/Tab. Bot. 100s.
Use: Corticosteroid.

COREGA POWDER. (Block) Denture adhesive containing polyethyleneoxide polymer w/peppermint oil, karaya gum. Pkg.: pocket 0.7 oz; medium 1.15 oz; economy 3.55 oz.
Use: Denture adhesive.

CORGARD. (Princeton) Nadolol 20 mg, 40 mg, 80 mg, 120 mg or 160 mg/Tab. Bot 100s, 1000s, UD 100s.
Use: Beta-adrenergic blocker.

CORGONJECT-5. (Mayrand) Human chorionic gonadotropin 500 units/ml with mannitol, benzyl alcohol. Vial 10 ml.
Use: Chorionic gonadotropin.

•**CORIANDER OIL,** N.F. XVII.
Use: Pharmaceutic aid (flavor).

CORICIDIN. (Schering) Chlorpheniramine maleate 2 mg, acetaminophen 325 mg/Tab. Bot. 12s, 24s, 48s, 100s, 1000s.
Use: Antihistamine, analgesic.

CORICIDIN "D" DECONGESTANT TABLETS. (Schering) Chlorpheniramine maleate 2 mg, acetaminophen 325 mg, phenylpropanolamine HCl 12.5 mg/Tab. Bot. 12s, 24s, 48s, 100s. Dispensary pack 200s.
Use: Antihistamine, analgesic, decongestant,

CORICIDIN EXTRA STRENGTH SINUS HEADACHE TABLETS. (Schering) Acetaminophen 500 mg, phenylpropanolamine HCl 12.5 mg, chlorpheniramine maleate 2 mg/Tab. Box 24s.
Use: Analgesic, decongestant, antihistamine.

CORICIDIN NASAL MIST. (Schering) Oxymetazoline HCl 0.05%. Soln. Bot. 20 ml.
Use: Decongestant.

CORILIN INFANT LIQUID. (Schering) Chlorpheniramine maleate 0.75 mg, sodium salicylate 80 mg/ml, alcohol >1%. Bot. 30 ml.
Use: Antihistamine, salicylate analgesic.

CORMED.
See: Nikethamide (Various Mfr.).

•**CORMETHASONE ACETATE.** USAN.
Use: Anti-infammatory.

CORN FIX. (Last) Turpentine oil 2.4%, liquefied phenol 2.25%. Bot. 0.3 oz.
Use: Cauterizing agent.

CORN HUSKERS LOTION. (Warner-Lambert Prods.) Glycerin 6.7%, SD alcohol, algin, TEA-oleoyl sarcosinate, guar gum, methylparaben, calcium sulfate, calcium Cl, TEA-fumarate, TEA-borate. Bot. 4 oz, 7 oz.
Use: Emollient.

•**CORN OIL,** N.F. XVII.
Use: Pharmaceutic aid (solvent, oleaginous vehicle).
See: G. B. Prep Emulsion (Gray).
Lipomul-Oral, Liq. (Upjohn).

CORNS-O-POPPIN. (Ries-Hamly) Salicylic acid 6.5%, benzoic acid 12%.
Use: Cauterizing agent.

COR-OTICIN. (Americal) Hydrocortisone acetate 1.5%, neomycin sulfate equivalent to 0.35% neomycin base, polysorbate 80, carboxymethyl-

cellulose, sodium metabisulfite, sodium Cl, chlorobutanol 0.5%. Dropper bot. 5 ml.
Use: Corticosteroid, anti-infective, ophthalmic.

COROTROPE. (Winthop Pharm.) Milrinone for IV use.
Use: Cardiotonic agent.

CORPUS LUTEUM, EXTRACT (WATER SOLUBLE).
See: Progesterone, Preps. (Various Mfr.).

CORQUE. (Geneva Generics) Hydrocortisone 1%, iodochlorhydroxyquin 3%. Cream. Tube 20 Gm.
Use: Corticosteroid.

CORRECTIVE MIXTURE W/PAREGORIC. (Beecham Labs) Zinc sulfocarbolate 10 mg, phenyl salicylate 22 mg, bismuth subsalicylate 85 mg, pepsin 45 mg, paregoric 0.6 ml/5 ml, alcohol 2%. Bot. Gal.
Use: Antidiarrheal.

CORRECTOL TABLETS. (Plough) Docusate sodium 100 mg, yellow phenolphthalein 65 mg/Tab. Box 15s, 30s, 60s, 90s.
Use: Laxative.

CORTAID. (Upjohn) Hydrocortisone acetate 0.5%. **Cream:** Tube 0.5 oz, 1 oz. **Lot.:** Bot. 1 oz, 2 oz. **Oint. W/Aloe:** Tube 0.5 oz. **Spray:** 1.5 fl oz, alcohol 46%. Bot. 45 ml.
Use: Corticosteroid.

CORTAN. (Blue Cross) Prednisone 5 mg/Tab. Bot. 1000s.
Use: Corticosteroid.

CORTANE D.C. EXPECTORANT. (Standex) Brompheniramine maleate 2 mg, guaifenesin 100 mg, phenylephrine HCl 5 mg, phenylpropanolamine HCl 5 mg, codeine phosphate 10 mg, alcohol 3.5%/5 ml. Bot. pt.
Use: Antihistamine, expectorant, decongestant, antitussive.

CORTANE EXPECTORANT. (Standex) Brompheniramine maleate 2 mg, guaifenesin 100 mg, phenylephrine 5 mg, phenylpropanolamine HCl 5 mg, alcohol 3.5%/5 ml. Bot. pt.
Use: Antihistamine, expectorant, decongestant.

CORTAPP ELIXIR. (Standex) Brompheniramine maleate 5 mg, phenylephrine HCl 5 mg, phenylpropanolamine HCl 5 mg, alcohol 2.3%/5 ml. Bot. pt.
Use: Antihistamine, decongestant.

CORTATRIGEN EAR SUSPENSION. (Goldline) Hydrocortisone 1%, neomycin sulfate 5 mg, polymyxin B sulfate 10,000 units/ml. Bot. 10 ml.
Use: Corticosteroid, anti-infective, otic.

CORTATRIGEN MODIFIED EAR DROPS. (Goldline) Bot. 10 ml.
Use: Corticosteroid, anti-infective, otic.

CORT-DOME. (Miles Pharm) Hydrocortisone alcohol. **Cream:** 0.25%: 1 oz, 4 oz; 0.5%: 1 oz; 1%: 1 oz. **Lot.:** 0.25%: 4 oz; 0.5%: 4 oz; 1%: 1 oz.
Use: Corticosteroid.

CORT-DOME HIGH POTENCY. (Miles Pharm.) Hydrocortisone acetate 25 mg in a monoglyceride base. Supp. Box foil 12s.
Use: Corticosteroid.

CORTEF ACETATE OINTMENT. (Upjohn) Hydrocortisone acetate 10 mg/Gm, lanolin (anhydrous), white petrolatum, mineral oil. Tube 20 Gm (10 mg/Gm).
Use: Corticosteroid.

CORTEF FEMININE ITCH CREAM. (Upjohn) Hydrocortisone acetate equivalent to hydrocortisone 5 mg/Gm. Tube 0.5 oz.
Use: Corticosteroid.

CORTEF ORAL SUSPENSION. (Upjohn) Hydrocortisone 10 mg/5 ml (as 13.4 mg hydrocortisone cypionate). Oral susp. Bot. 4 oz.
Use: Corticosteroid.

CORTEF TABLETS. (Upjohn) Hydrocortisone. **5 mg/Tab.:** Bot. 50s; **10 mg or 20 mg/Tab.:** Bot. 100s.
Use: Corticosteroid.

CORTENEMA. (Reid-Rowell) Hydrocortisone 100 mg in aqueous solution w/carboxypolymethylene, polysorbate 80, methylparaben 0.18%/60 ml. Bot. w/applicator. UD 1s.
Use: Corticosteroid.

CORTENIL.
See: Desoxycorticosterone Acetate, Preps. (Various Mfr.).

CORTICAINE CREAM. (Whitby) Hydrocortisone acetate 0.5%, dibucaine 0.5%. Tube 1 oz w/rectal applicator.
Use: Corticosteroid, anesthetic.

CORTICAL HORMONE PRODUCTS.
See: Adrenal Cortex Extract (Various Mfr.).
Aristocort, Preps. (Lederle).
Corticotropin, Preps. (Various Mfr.).
Hydrocortisone, Preps. (Various Mfr.).
Cortisone Acetate, Preps. (Various Mfr.).
Decadron LA, Inj. (Merck Sharp & Dohme).
Decadron, Tab., Elix., Inj. (Merck Sharp & Dohme).
Desoxycorticosterone Acetate, Preps. (Various Mfr.).
Dexamethasone, Tab. (Various Mfr.).
Fludrocortisone (Various Mfr.).
Hydeltrasol, Inj. (Merck Sharp & Dohme).
Hydrocortone Acetate, Inj. (Merck Sharp & Dohme).
Hydrocortone Phosphate, Inj. (Merck Sharp & Dohme).
Kenacort, Prep. (Squibb).
Lipo-Adrenal Cortex, Inj. (Upjohn).
Medrol, Preps. (Upjohn).
Methylprednisolone, Tab. (Various Mfr.).
Prednisolone, Tab. (Various Mfr.).
Prednisone, Tab. (Various Mfr.).
Triamcinolone, Tab. (Various Mfr.).

CORTICOID. (Jenkins) Hydrocortisone alcohol 10 mg, clioquinol 30 mg, methylparaben 0.5 mg, propylparaben 0.5 mg/Gm. Tube 20 Gm.
Use: Corticosteroid, antifungal, anti-infective.

CORTICORELIN OVINE TRIFLUTATE. USAN.
Use: Diagnostic aid for adrenal cortical function and Cushings syndrome.

CORTICOTROPIN HIGHLY PURIFIED.
See: H. P. Acthar Gel. Vial. (Armour).

CORTICOTROPIN INJECTION, U.S.P. XXII. ACTH, Adrenocorticotropic hormone or adrenocorticotrop(h)in or corticotropin.
Use: Adrenal corticotropic hormone; adrenocortical steroid (anti-inflammatory); diagnostic aid (adrenocortical insufficiency).
See: Cortrophin Gel, Vial, Amp. (Organon).

CORTICOTROPIN FOR INJECTION, U.S.P. XXII.
Use: Adrenal corticotropic hormone; adrenocortical steroid (anti-inflammatory); diagnostic aid (adrenocortical insufficiency).
See: ACTH.
Acthar (Armour).

CORTICOTROPIN INJECTION, REPOSITORY, U.S.P. XXII. (Various Mfr.).
Use: IM anterior pituitary hormone therapy; adrenocortical steroid (anti-inflammatory); diagnostic aid (adrenocortical insufficiency).
See: Acthar Gel Vial (Armour).
ACTH Gel Purified (Various Mfr.).
Cortrophin Gel Amp., Vial (Organon).
H.P. Acthar Gel, Vial (Armour).

CORTICOTROPIN ZINC HYDROXIDE.
See: Cortrophin-Zinc, Vial (Organon).

CORTICOTROPIN-ZINC HYDROXIDE SUSPENSION, STERILE, U.S.P. XXII. Absorbed on zinc hydroxide.
Use: Adrenal corticotropic hormone; adrenocortical steroid (anti-inflammatory); diagnostic aid (adrenocortical insufficiency).

CORTIFOAM. (Reed & Carnrick) Hydrocortisone acetate 10% in an aerosol foam w/propylene glycol, emulsifying wax, steareth 10, cetyl alcohol, methylparaben, propylparaben, trolamine, water, inert propellants. Container 20 Gm w/rectal applicator for 14 applicatorfuls.
Use: Corticosteroid.

CORTIN 1% CREAM. (C & M Pharmacal) Hydrocortisone 1%, clioquinol 3%. Tube 20 Gm.
Use: Corticosteroid, antifungal, anti-infective.

CORTINAL. (Kenyon) Micronized hydrocortisone alcohol in a nonallergenic water washable base 5 mg/Gm. Tube 1 oz.
Use: Corticosteroid.

CORTISOL.
See: Hydrocortisone, U.S.P. XXII.
Note: Cortisol was the official published name for hydrocortisone in U.S.P. XXII. The name was changed back to Hydrocortisone, U.S.P. in Supplement 1 to the U.S.P. XXII.

CORTISOL CYCLOPENTYLPROPIONATE.
See: Cortef Fluid, Susp., Tab. (Upjohn).

CORTISONE ACETATE, U.S.P. XXII. Sterile Susp., Tab., U.S.P. XXII. 17,21-Dihydroxypregn-4-ene 3,11,20-trione 21 acetate. (Kendall's Compound E) (Upjohn) 5 mg, 10 mg, 25 mg/Tab. Bot. 50s, 100s, 500s.
Use: Adrenocortical steroid (anti-inflammatory).
See: Cortistan (Standex).
Cortone Acetate, Tab. (Merck Sharp & Dohme).
Pantisone, Tab. (Panray).

CORTISPORIN CREAM. (Burroughs Wellcome) Polymyxin B sulfate 10,000 units, neomycin sulfate 5 mg, hydrocortisone acetate 5 mg/Gm, methylparaben 0.25%. Tube 7.5 Gm.
Use: Anti-infective, corticosteroid.

CORTISPORIN OINTMENT. (Burroughs Wellcome) Polymyxin B sulfate 5000 units, bacitracin zinc 400 units, neomycin sulfate 5 mg, hydrocortisone (1%) 10 mg/Gm in petrolatum base. Tube 30 Gm.
Use: Anti-infective, corticosteroid.

CORTISPORIN OPHTHALMIC OINTMENT. (Burroughs Wellcome) Polymyxin B sulfate 10,000 units, bacitracin 400 units, neomycin sulfate 5 mg, hydrocortisone (1%) 10 mg/Gm in petrolatum base. Tube 3.75 Gm.
Use: Anti-infective, corticosteroid, ophthalmic.

CORTISPORIN OPHTHALMIC SUSPENSION. (Burroughs Wellcome) Polymyxin B sulfate 10,000 units, neomycin sulfate 5 mg, hydrocortisone (1%) 10 mg, in sterile, isotonic saline, thimerosal, cetyl alcohol, glyceryl monostearate, liquid petrolatum, polyoxyl 40 stearate, propylene glycol/ml. Dropper bot. 7.5 ml Sterile.
Use: Anti-infective, corticosteroid, ophthalmic.

CORTISPORIN OTIC SOLUTION STERILE. (Burroughs Wellcome) Polymyxin B sulfate 10,000 units, neomycin sulfate 5 mg, hydrocortisone 10 mg/ml, glycerin, propylene glycol, vitamin K metabisulfite 0.1%. Dropper bot. 10 ml Sterile.
Use: Anti-infective, corticosteroid, otic.

CORTISPORIN OTIC SUSPENSION. (Burroughs Wellcome) Polymyxin B sulfate 10,000 units, neomycin sulfate 5 mg, hydrocortisone free alcohol 10 mg/ml, cetyl alcohol, propylene glycol, polysorbate 80, thimerosal. Dropper bot. 10 ml Sterile.
Use: Anti-infective, corticosteroid, otic.

CORTISTAN. (Standex) Cortisone 25 mg/10 ml.
Use: Corticosteroid.

•**CORTIVAZOL.** USAN. 11B,17,21-trihydroxy-6,16α-dimethyl-2′-phenyl-2′H-pregna-2,4,6-trieno[3,2-c]-pyrazol-20-one 21-acetate.
Use: Anti-inflammatory.

CORTIZONE-5. (Thompson Med.) Hydrocortisone 0.5%, glycerin, mineral oil, white petrolatum. Tube 30 Gm.
Use: Corticosteroid.

CORTIZONE-S, MAXIMUM STRENGTH. (Thompson Medical) Hydrocortisone 0.5%. Tube.
Use: Corticosteroid.

CORT-NIB CREAM. (Cenci) Hydrocortisone alcohol 0.25%, 0.5% or 1%. Cream. Tube oz, Jar lb.
Use: Corticosteroid.

CORT-NIB V CREAM. (Cenci) Hydrocortisone alcohol 0.5%, clioquinol 3%. Tube 1 oz.
Use: Corticosteroid, antifungal, anti-infective.

•**CORTODOXONE.** USAN. 17,21-Dihydroxy-pregn-4-ene-3,20-dione. Cortexolone.
Use: Anti-inflammatory.

CORTOGEN ACETATE. Cortisone acetate.

CORTONE ACETATE. (Merck Sharp & Dohme) Cortisone acetate. **5 mg/Tab.:** Bot. 50s. **10 mg/Tab.:** Bot. 100s. **25 mg/Tab.:** Bot. 100s, 500s, 1000s, UD 100s.
Use: Corticosteroid.

CORTOXIDE GEL. (Syosset) Hydrocortisone 0.5% or 1% in gel base. Bot. 1.5 oz.
Use: Corticosteroid.

CORTRIL TOPICAL OINTMENT 1%. (Pfizer Laboratories) Hydrocortisone 1%, cetyl and stearyl alcohol, propylene glycol, sodium lauryl sulfate, petrolatum, cholesterol, mineral oil, methyl and propyl parabens in ointment base. Tube 0.5 oz.
Use: Corticosteroid.

CORTROPHIN-ZINC. (Organon) Corticotropin zinc 40 units/ml. Vial 5 ml.
Use: Corticosteroid.

CORTROSYN INJECTION. (Organon) Cosyntropin 0.25 mg, mannitol 10 mg, lyophilized powder/ml. Vial. Pkg. w/1 ml amp. diluent. Box 10s. Vial.
Use: Corticosteroid.

CORT-TOP OINTMENT. (Standex) Topical hydrocortisone 1%. Tube 20 Gm.
Use: Corticosteroid.

CORUBEEN. (Spanner) Vitamin B_{12} crystalline 1000 mcg/ml. Vial 10 ml.
Use: Vitamin B_{12} supplement.

CORYZA BRENGLE. (Hauck) Pseudoephedrine HCl 30 mg, acetaminophen 200 mg/Cap. Bot. 1000s.
Use: Decongestant, analgesic.

CORZIDE. (Princeton) Nadolol 40 mg, bendroflumethiazide 5 mg/Tab or Nadolol 80 mg, bendroflumethiazide 5 mg/Tab. Bot. 100s.
Use: Antihypertensive.

CORZYME. (Abbott Diagnostics) Enzyme immunoassay for detection of antibody to hepatitis B core antigen in serum or plasma. Test kit 100s.
Use: Diagnostic aid.

CORZYME-M. (Abbott Diagnostics) Enzyme immunoassay for the detection of IgM antibody to hepatitis B core antigen. (Anti-HBc IgM) in human serum or plasma. Test kit 100s.
Use: Diagnostic aid.

COSANYL. (Health Care Industries) Codeine sulfate 10 mg, d-pseudoephedrine HCl 30 mg/5 ml, alcohol 6% in peach flavored base. Bot. 4 oz, pt, gal.
Use: Antitussive, decongestant.

COSANYL-DM. (Health Care Industries) Dextromethorphan HBr 15 mg, d-pseudoephedrine HCl 30 mg/5 ml, alcohol 6% in a peach flavor. Bot. 4 oz, gal.
Use: Antitussive, decongestant.

COSMEGEN. (Merck Sharp & Dohme) Actinomycin D (dactinomycin) 0.5 mg (lyophilized powder)/3 ml.
Use: Antineoplastic agent.

COSMOLINE.
See: Petrolatum.

COSULID. (Ciba) Sulfachloropyridazine.

•**COSYNTROPIN.** USAN.
Use: Adrenal corticotropic hormone.
See: Cortrosyn, Vial (Organon).

COTAPHYLLINE TABS. (Major) Oxtriphylline 100 mg or 200 mg/Tab. Bot. 100s, 500s.
Use: Bronchodilator.

COTARNINE CHLORIDE. Cotarnine hydrochloride.

COTARNINE HYDROCHLORIDE.
See: Cotarnine Chloride.

COTAZYM. (Organon) Pancrelipase, lipase 8000 units, protease 30,000 units, amylase 30,000 units, calcium carbonate 25 mg/Cap. Bot. 100s, 500s.
Use: Digestive enzymes.

COTAZYM-S. (Organon) Pancrelipase spheres, lipase 5,000 units, protease 20,000 units, amylase 20,000 units/Cap. Bot. 100s, 500s.
Use: Digestive enzymes.

COTININE FUMARATE. (-)-1-Methyl-5-(3-pyridyl)-2 pyrrolidinone compound (2:1) with fumaric acid.
Use: Psychomotor stimulant.

COTOLATE TABS. (Major) Benztropine 1 mg or 2 mg/Tab. Bot. 100s, 1000s.
Use: Antiparkinson agent.

COTRIM. (Lemmon) Sulfamethoxazole 400 mg, trimethoprim 80 mg/Tab. Bot. 100s, 500s.
Use: Anti-infective.

COTRIM D.S. (Lemmon) Sulfamethoxazole 800 mg, trimethoprim 160 mg/Tab. Bot. 100s, 500s, UD 100s.
Use: Anti-infective.

COTRIM PEDIATRIC. (Lemmon) Sulfamethoxazole 200 mg, trimethoprim 40 mg/5 ml. Bot. 480 ml.
Use: Anti-infective.

COTRIM S.S. (Lemmon) Sulfamethoxazole 400 mg, trimethoprim 800 mg/Tab. Bot. 100s.
Use: Anti-infective.

CO-TRIMOXAZOLE. B.A.N. Compounded preparations of trimethoprim and sulfamethoxazole in the proportions of 1 part to 5 parts.
Use: Antibacterial.

•**COTTON, PURIFIED,** U.S.P. XXII.
Use: Surgical aid.

•**COTTONSEED OIL,** N.F. XVII.
Use: Pharmaceutic aid, solvent, oleaginous vehicle.

COTYLENOL CHEWABLE COLD TABLET. (McNeil Prods.) Acetaminophen 80 mg, phenylpropanolamine HCl 3.125 mg, chlorpheniramine maleate 0.5 mg/Tab. Bot. 24s.
Use: Analgesic, decongestant, antihistamine.

COTYLENOL CHILDREN'S CHEWABLE COLD TABLET. (McNeil Prods.) Acetaminophen 80 mg, chlorpheniramine maleate 0.5 mg, pseudoephedrine HCl 7.5 mg/Tab. Bot. 24s.
Use: Analgesic, antihistamine, decongestant.

COTYLENOL CHILDREN'S LIQUID COLD FORMULA. (McNeil Prods.) Acetaminophen 160 mg, chlorpheniramine maleate 1 mg, pseudoephedrine HCl 15 mg, sorbitol/5 ml. Bot. 4 oz.
Use: Analgesic, antihistamine, decongestant.

COTYLENOL COLD FORMULA. (McNeil Prods.) Chlorpheniramine maleate 2 mg, dextromethorphan HBr 15 mg, pseudoephedrine HCl 30 mg, acetaminophen 325 mg/Tab. or Capl. **Tab.:** Box 24s, Bot. 50s, 100s. **Capl.:** Bot. 24s, 50s.
Use: Antihistamine, antitussive, decongestant, analgesic.

COTYLENOL LIQUID COLD FORMULA. (McNeil Prods.) Acetaminophen 650 mg, chlorpheniramine maleate 4 mg, pseudoephedrine HCl 60 mg, dextromethorphan HCl 30 mg/30 ml, alcohol 7.5%, sorbitol. Bot. 5 oz.
Use: Analgesic, antihistamine, decongestant, antitussive.

COUMADIN. (Du Pont) Warfarin sodium crystalline. **Tab.:** 2 mg, 2.5 mg, 5 mg, 7.5 mg or 10 mg/Tab. Bot. 100s, 1000s, UD 100s. **Inj.:** 50 mg/Vial w/diluent sodium Cl, thimerosal, sodium hydroxide to adjust pH. Vial 50 mg with 2 ml amp. diluent. Box 6s.
Use: Antibiotic.

COUMARIN.
Use: Antibiotic.

•**COUMERMYCIN.** USAN. Antibiotic derived from *Streptomyces rishiriensis.*
Use: Antibiotic.

•**COUMERMYCIN SODIUM.** USAN.
Use: Antibiotic.

COUNTERPAIN RUB. (Squibb Mark) Methyl salicylate, eugenol, menthol. Oint. Tube 1 oz.
Use: External analgesic.

COVANGESIC. (Wallace) Phenylpropanolamine HCl 12.5 mg, phenylephrine HCl 7.5 mg, chlorpheniramine maleate 2 mg, pyrilamine maleate 12.5 mg, acetaminophen 275 mg, tartrazine/Tab. Bot. 24s.
Use: Decongestant, antihistamine, analgesic.

COVERMARK. (O'Leary) Neutral cream, hypoallergenic, opaque, greaseless. Jars 1 oz, 3 oz, available in eleven shades.
Use: Conceals birthmarks and skin discolorations.

COVERMARK STICK. (O'Leary) For normal to oily skin, available in 7 shades.
Use: Conceals birthmarks and skin discolorations.

COVICONE CREAM. (Abbott) Silicone (dimethicone), nitrocellulose, castor oil suspended in vanishing cream base. Tube 1 oz.
Use: Skin protectant.

CO-XAN SYRUP. (Central) Theophylline anhydrous 150 mg, ephedrine HCl 25 mg, guaifenesin 100 mg, codeine phosphate 15 mg, alcohol 10%/15 ml. Bot. 1 pt.
Use: Bronchodilator, decongestant, expectorant, antitussive.

CPI HEMORRHOIDAL SUPPS. (Century) Bismuth subgallate 2.25%, benzyl benzoate 1.2%, bismuth resorcin compound 1.2%, balsam Peru 1.8%, zinc oxide 11%, hydrogenated vegetable oil base. Pkg. 12s.
Use: Antihemorrhoidal.

CPLEX. (Arcum) Vitamins B_1 10 mg, B_2 10 mg, B_6 5 mg, B_{12} 10 mcg, niacinamide 100 mg, calcium pantothenate 25 mg, C 150 mg, liver 50 mg, dried yeast 50 mg/Cap. Bot. 100s, 1000s.
Use: Vitamin/mineral supplement.

C.P.M. TABLETS. (Goldline) Chlorpheniramine 4 mg/Tab. Bot. 1000s.
Use: Antihistamine.

C-REACTIVE PROTEIN TEST.
See: LA test-CRP kit. (Fisher).

CREAM CAMELLIA. (O'Leary) Jar 2 oz.
Use: Emollient.

CREATININE REAGENT STRIPS. (Ames) Seralyzer reagent strips. A quantitative strip test for creatinine in serum or plasma. Bot. 25s.
Use: Diagnostic aid.

CREMAGOL. (Cremagol) Emulsion of liquid petrolatum, agar agar, acacia, glycerin. Bot. 14 oz. W/cascara 11 gr/oz, Bot. 14 oz. W/phenolphthalein 2 gr/oz, Bot. 14 oz.
Use: Laxative.

CREMESONE. (Dalin) Hydrocortisone alcohol 5 mg/Gm. Tube 1 oz.
Use: Corticosteroid.

CREOMULSION COUGH MEDICINE. (Creomulsion) Beechwood creosote, cascara, ipecac, menthol, white pine, wild cherry w/alcohol. For Adults. Bot. 4 fl oz, 8 fl oz.
Use: Coughs and bronchial irritations due to colds.

CREOMULSION FOR CHILDREN. (Creomulsion) Beechwood creosote, cascara, ipecac, menthol, white pine, wild cherry w/alcohol. For Children. Bot. 4 fl oz, 8 fl oz.
Use: Coughs and bronchial irritations due to colds.

CREON. (Reid-Rowell) Porcine pancreatic enzymes: Lipase 8000 units, amylase 30,000 units, protease 13,000 units/Cap. Bot. 100s, 250s.
Use: Digestive enzymes.

CREOSOTE. Wood creosote, creosote, beechwood creosote.
W/Ipecac, menthol, licorice, white pine, wild cherry, cascara, vitamin C.
See: Creozets, Loz. (Creomulsion).

CREOTERP. (Jenkins) Terpin hydrate 2 gr, potassium iodide 1/8 gr, creosote 1/10 min, eucalyptol 1/10 min/Tab. Bot. 1000s.
Use: Antitussive.

CREO-TERPIN. (Denver) Creosote 0.12 ml, sodium glycerophosphate 259 mg, terpin hydrate 130 mg, chloroform 0.06 ml, alcohol 25%/30 ml. Bot. 3 oz, 6 oz.
Use: Antitussive.

CRESCORMON. (KabiVitrum) Somatotropin 4 IU/Vial. IM administration.
Use: Growth hormone.
Note: Crescormon will be available only for patients who qualify for treatment; full documentation for prospective patients to be submitted to Kabi Group Inc. for approval.

•**CRESOL,** N.F. XVII. Mixture of 3 isomeric cresols. Phenol, methyl cresol.
Use: Antiseptic, disinfectant.

CRESOL PREPARATIONS.
Use: Antiseptic, disinfectant.
See: Cresol, Soln. (Various Mfr.).
Cresylone, Liq. (Parke-Davis).
Saponated Cresol Soln.

CRESTABOLIC. (Nutrition) Protein anabolic steroid, methandriol dipropionate 50 mg/ml, benzyl alcohol 5% in sesame oil. Vial 10 ml.
Use: Anabolic steroid.

m-CRESYL-ACETATE.
See: Cresylate, Liq. (Recsei).

CRESYLATE. (Recsei) M-cresyl-acetate 25%, isopropanol 25%, chlorobutanol 1%, benzyl alcohol 1%, castor oil 5%, propylene glycol/15 ml. Bot. 15 ml, pt.
Use: Otic preparation.

CRESYLIC ACID. Same as Cresol.

•**CRISNATOL MESYLATE.** USAN.
Use: Antineoplastic.

CRITICARE HN. (Mead Johnson Nutrition) High nitrogen elemental diet. Protein 14%, fat 4.3%, carbohydrate 81.5%. Bot. 8 oz.
Use: Enteral nutritional supplement.

CROFERRIN. (Forest Pharm.) Iron peptonate 50 mg, liver injection 2.5 mcg, vitamin B_{12} 12.5 mcg, lidocaine HCl 1%, phenol 0.5%, sodium citrate 0.125%, sodium bisulfite 0.009%/ml. Vial 10 ml, 30 ml.
Use: Vitamin/mineral supplement.

•**CROFILCON A.** USAN.
Use: Contact lens material.

•**CROMITRILE SODIUM.** USAN.
Use: Antihistamine.

CROMOGLYCIC ACID. B.A.N. 1,3-Di-(2-carboxy-4-oxochromen-5-yloxy)propan-2-ol.
Use: Treatment of allergic airway obstruction.

•**CROMOLYN SODIUM,** U.S.P. XXII. For Inhalation, Inhalation Nasal Soln., Ophth. Soln., U.S.P. XXII. Disodium 5,5′-[(2-hydroxytrimethylene)dioxy]bis[4-oxo-4H-1-benzopyran-2-carboxylate].
Use: Treatment of allergic airway obstruction.
Gastrocrom, Cap. (Fisons).
See: Intal, Cap. (Fisons).
Opticrom, Soln. (Fisons).

CROMORAL. Cromolyn sodium (Orphan Drug).
Use: Mastocytosis, vernal keratoconjunctivitis.
Sponsor: Fisons.

CRONETAL.
See: Disulfiram.

CROPROPAMIDE. B.A.N. NN-Dimethyl-2-(N-propyl- crotonamido)butyramide.
Use: Respiratory stimulant.

C ROSE HIPS. (Robinson) 100 mg, 250 mg or 500 mg/Tab. Bot. 100s, 250s, 1000s.

•**CROSCARMELLOSE SODIUM,** N.F. XVII.
Use: Tablet disintegrant.

•**CROSPOVIDONE,** N.F. XVII.
Use: Pharmaceutic aid (tablet excipient).

CROSS ASPIRIN. (Cross) Aspirin 325 mg/Tab. Sugar, salt and lactose free. Bot. 100s, 1000s.
Use: Salicylate analgesic.

CROTALINE ANTIVENIN, POLYVALENT. Antivenin Crotalidae Polyvalent, U.S.P. XXII. North and South American Antisnakebite serum.
Use: Passive immunizing agent.

•**CROTAMITON,** U.S.P. XXII. Cream, U.S.P. XXII. N-Crotonyl-N-ethyl-o-toluidine.
Use: Antipruritic.
See: Eurax, Cream, Lot. (Geigy).

CROTETHAMIDE. B.A.N. 2-(N-Ethylcrotonamido)-NN-dimethylbutyramide.
Use: Respiratory stimulant.

CRPA, CRPA LATEX TEST. (Laboratory Diagnostics) Rapid latex agglutination test for the qualitative determination of C reactive protein. CRPA, 1 ml—CRP Positest Control, 0.5 ml CRPA Latex Test Kit.
Use: Diagnostic aid.

CRUDE TUBERCULIN.
See: Tuberculin, Old, Vial (Parke-Davis).

CRUEX CREAM. (Pharmacraft) Total undecylenate 20% as undecylenic acid and zinc undecylenate. Tube 0.5 oz.
Use: Antifungal, external.

CRUEX SPRAY POWDER. (Pharmacraft) Undecylenic acid 2% and zinc undecylenate 20%. Aerosol can 1.8 oz, 3.5 oz, 5.5 oz.
Use: Antifungal, external.

CRUEX SQUEEZE POWDER. (Pharmacraft) Calcium undecylenate 10%. Plastic squeeze bot. 1.5 oz.
Use: Antifungal, external.

•**CRUFOMATE.** USAN. 4-tert-Butyl-2-chlorophenyl methyl methylphosphoramidate.
Use: Insecticide; anthelmintic, veterinary medicine.
See: Ruelene.

CRYPTOLIN. (Hoechst) Gonadorelin in nasal spray.
Use: Cryptorchism treatment.

CRYSPEN-400. (Knight) Buffered penicillin G potassium 400,000 units/Tab. Bot. 100s.
Use: Antibacterial, penicillin.

CRYSTALLINE TRYPSIN. Highly purified preparation of enzyme as derived from mammalian pancreas glands.
See: Tryptar, Inj. (Armour).

CRYSTAL VIOLET.
See: Methylrosaniline Chloride, U.S.P.

CRYSTAMINE. (Dunhall) Cyanocobalamin 100 mcg or 1000 mcg/ml, benzyl alcohol. Vial 10 ml, 30 ml.
Use: Vitamin B_{12} supplement.

CRYSTICILLIN 300 A.S. (Squibb Marsam) Sterile procaine penicillin G suspension U.S.P. 300,000 units/ml, lecithin, povidone, sodium citrate, sodium formaldehyde sulfoxylate, sodium carboxymethylcellulose, methylparaben, propylparaben. Vial 10 ml.
Use: Antibacterial, penicillin.

CRYSTICILLIN 600 A.S. (Squibb Marsam) Sterile procaine penicillin G suspension 600,000 units/1.2 ml, lecithin, phenol, povidone, sodium citrate, sodium carboxymethylcellulose, sodium formaldehyde sulfoxylate, methylparaben, propylparaben. Vial 12 ml.
Use: Antibacterial, penicillin.

CRYSTI-LIVER. (Hauck) Liver injection (equivalent to B_{12} 10 mcg), crystalline B_{12} 100 mcg, folic acid 0.4 mg, phenol. Vial 10 ml.
Use: Vitamin/mineral supplement.

CRYSTOGRAFIN. Meglumine diatrizoate.
Use: Contrast medium.

C-SOLVE. (Syosset) Alcohol 36%, glycerin, polysorbate 20, laureth-4, water soluble cellulose gum, PVA, collagen, gelatin hydrolysate, midazolidinyl urea, sorbic acid. Lot. Bot. 50 ml.
Use: Lotion base.

C-SOLVE 2. (Syosset) Erythromycin 2%, alcohol 81%, propylene glycol, lauramide DEA, zinc acetate, hydroxypropyl cellulose. Soln. Bot. 60 ml.
Use: Anti-acne.

C SPERIDIN. (Marlyn) Hesperidin 100 mg, lemon bioflavonoids 100 mg, vitamin C 500 mg/SR Tab. Bot. 100s.
Use: Vitamin supplement.

C.S.R. UNIT. Unit represents the amount of veratrum viride extract per kg of body weight which will just abolish the pressor response to the carotid sinus reflex resulting from occlusion of the carotid arteries in dogs.
See: Cryptenamine.

CS-T. (Helena Labs.) Occult blood screening test. Test kit 3s.
Use: Diagnostic aid.

C-SYRUP-500. (Ortega) Ascorbic acid 500 mg/5 ml. Bot. pt, gal.
Use: Vitamin C supplement.

CTAB.
See: Cetyl Trimethyl Ammonium Bromide.

C-TUSSIN. (Century) Codeine phosphate 10 mg, pseudoephedrine HCl 30 mg, guaifenesin 100 mg/5 ml, alcohol 7.5%. Bot. 120 ml, gal.
Use: Antitussive, decongestant, expectorant.

CULMINAL. (Culminal) Benzocaine 3% in water miscible cream base. Tube oz.
Use: Local anesthetic.

CULTURETTE 10 MINUTE GROUP A STEP ID. (Marion) Latex slide agglutination test for group A streptococcal antigen on throat swabs. Kit 55 determinations.
Use: Diagnostic aid.

CUMETHAROL. B.A.N. 4,4′-Dihydroxy-3,3′-(2-methoxy-ethylidene)dicoumarin.
Use: Anticoagulant.

•**CUPRIC ACETATE Cu 64.** USAN.
Use: Radioactive agent.

•**CUPRIC CHLORIDE,** U.S.P. XXII., Inj., U.S.P. XXII.
Use: Copper deficiency treatment.
See: Coppertrace, Inj. (Armour).

•**CUPRIC SULFATE,** U.S.P. XXII. Inj., U.S.P. XXII.
Use: Antidote to phosphorus.
W/Zinc sulfate, camphor.
See: Dalibour, Pow. (Doak).

CUPRID. (Merck Sharp & Dohme) Trientine HCl 250 mg/Cap. Bot. 100s.
Use: Chelating agent.

CUPRIMINE. (Merck Sharp & Dohme) Penicillamine 125 mg or 250 mg/Cap. Bot. 100s.
Use: Penicillamine.

•**CUPRIMYXIN.** USAN.
Use: Antibacterial.

CUPRI-PAK. (SoloPak) Copper **0.4 mg/ml:** Vial 10 ml, 30 ml. **2 mg/ml:** Vial 5 ml.
Use: Parenteral nutritional supplement.

CURARE.
Use: Muscle relaxant.
See: d-Tubocurarine Salts (Various Mfr.).

CURARE ANTAGONIST.
See: Neostigmine Methylsulfate Inj. (Various Mfr.).
Tensilon, Amp. (Roche).

CUREL MOISTURIZING. (Rydelle) **Lot.:** Glycerin, quaternium-5, petrolatum, isopropyl palmitate, 1-hexadecanol, dimethicone, parabens. Bot. 180 ml, 300 ml. **Cream:** Glycerin, quaternium-5, petrolatum, isopropyl palmitate, 1-hexadecanol, dimethicone, parabens. Bot. 90 Gm.
Use: Emollient.

CURITY INCONTINENT CARE PRODUCTS. (Kendall).
Use: Management of adult bladder control problems.

CURRAL.
See: Diallyl Barbituric Acid, Tab. (Various Mfr.).

CURRETAB. (Reid-Rowell) Medroxyprogesterone acetate 10 mg/Tab. Bot. 50s.
Use: Progestin.

CUTAR BATH OIL. (Summers) Liquor carbonis detergens 7.5% in liquid petrolatum, isopropyl myristate, acetylated lanolin, lanolin alcohols extract. Bot. 180 ml.
Use: Emollient.

CUTEMOL EMOLLIENT CREAM. (Summers) Allantoin 0.2%, liquid petrolatum, acetylated lano-

lin, lanolin alcohols extract, isopropyl myristate, water. Jar 2 oz.
Use: Emollient.

CUTICURA ACNE CREAM. (DEP Corp.) Benzoyl peroxide 5%. Bot. 30 Gm.
Use: Anti-acne.

CUTICURA MEDICATED SHAMPOO. (Jeffrey Martin) Sodium lauryl sulfate, sodium stearate, salicylic acid, protein, sulfur. Tube 3 oz.
Use: Antidandruff shampoo.

CUTICURA MEDICATED SOAP. (DEP Corp.) Triclocarban 1%, petrolatum, sodium tallowate, sodium cocoate, glycerin, mineral oil, sodium Cl, tetrasodium EDTA, sodium bicarbonate, magnesium silicate, iron oxides. Bar 3.5 oz, 5.5 oz.
Use: Antibacterial skin care.

CUTICURA OINTMENT. (DEP Corp.) Precipitated sulfur 0.5%, phenol 0.1%, oxyquinoline 0.05%. Tube 52.5 Gm.
Use: Anti-acne.

CUTIVATE. (Glaxo) Fluticasone propionate.
Use: Corticosteroid, topical.

CUTTER INSECT REPELLENT. (Miles) N,N-Diethyl-meta-toluamide 28.5%, other isomers 1.5%. Vial 1 oz; Foam, Can 2 oz; Spray 7 oz, 14 oz aerosol can; Assortment Pack; First Aid Kits, Trial Pack, 6s; Marine Pack 3s; Camp Pack 4s; Pocket Pack, Travel Pack.
Use: Insect repellent.

CYACETAZIDE. V.B.A.N. Cyanoacetohydrazide.
Use: Anthelmintic, veterinary medicine.

CYADE-GEL. (Kenyon) Adenosine-5-monophosphate 100 mg, vitamin B_{12} 100 mcg/ml. Vial 10 ml.
Use: Adenosine phosphate.

CYANIDE ANTIDOTE PACKAGE. (Lilly) 2 Amp. (300 mg/10 ml) sodium nitrite; 2 Amp. (12.5 Gm/50 ml) w/sodium thiosulfate; 12 aspirols amyl nitrite 5 min/Pkg. Check exact dosage before administration.
Use: Antidote.

CYANOCOB. (Paddock) Vitamin B_{12} 1000 mcg/ml. Bot. 1000 ml, Vial 10 ml.
Use: Vitamin B_{12} supplement.

•**CYANOCOBALAMIN,** U.S.P. XXII. Inj. U.S.P. XXII.α-(5,6-Dimethyl-benzimidazol-1-yl)cobamide cyanide. Vitamin B_{12}.
Use: Vitamin B_{12} supplement.
See: Redisol, Inj., Tab. (Merck Sharp & Dohme).

•**CYANOCOBALAMIN CO 57,** USP XXII. Cap., Oral Soln., U.S.P. XXII.
Use: Diagnostic aid (pernicious anemia).

•**CYANOCOBALAMIN CO 60,** U.S.P. XXII. Cap., Oral Soln., U.S.P. XXII.
Use: Diagnostic aid (pernicious anemia).

CYANOJECT. (Mayrand) Vitamin B_{12} 1000 mcg/ml, benzyl alcohol. Vial 10 ml, 30 ml.
Use: Vitamin B_{12} supplement.

CYANOVER. (Research Supplies) Cyanocobalamin 100 mcg, liver injection 10 mcg, folic acid 10 mg/ml. Lyo-layer vial 10 ml with vial of diluent 10 ml.
Use: Vitamin/mineral supplement.

CYCLAMATE SODIUM. Cyclohexanesulfamate dihydrate salt.

•**CYCLAMIC ACID.** USAN. N-Cyclohexylsulfamic acid. Hexamic Acid. Cyclohexanesulfamic acid. Currently banned in U.S.
Use: Sweetening agent.

CYCLAN CAPS. (Major) Cyclandelate 200 mg or 400 mg/Tab. Bot. 100s, 1000s, UD 100s. 400 mg: Bot. 250s also.
Use: Vasodilator.

CYCLANDELATE. 3,3,5-Trimethylcyclohexyl mandelate.
Use: Vasodilator.
See: Cyclan, Cap. (Major).
Cyclospasmol, Tab., Cap. (Wyeth-Ayerst).

CYCLARBAMATE. B.A.N. 1,1-Di(phenylcarbamoyl-oxymethyl)cyclopentane.
Use: Muscle relaxant; tranquilizer.

•**CYCLAZOCINE.** USAN. 3-(Cyclopropylmethyl)-1,2,3,4,5,6-hexahydro-6, 11-dimethyl-2,6-methano-3-benzazocin-8-ol. This product is under study.
Use: Analgesic.

•**CYCLINDOLE.** USAN.
Use: Antidepressant.

•**CYCLIRAMINE MALEATE.** USAN.
Use: Antihistamine.

•**CYCLIZINE.** U.S.P. XXII. Piperazine, 1-(diphenylmethyl)-4-methyl-1-(Diphenylmethyl)-4-methyl piperazine.
Use: Anticholinergic.
See: Marzine (hydrochloride).
Valoid (hydrochloride or lactate).

•**CYCLIZINE HYDROCHLORIDE,** U.S.P. XXII. Tab. U.S.P. XXII. 1-Diphenylmethyl-4-methylpiperazine. N-Benzhydryl-N-methyl piperazine. Piperazine, 1-(diphenylmethyl)-4-methyl-,monohydrochloride.
Use: Antiemetic.
See: Marezine HydroCl and lactate, Preps. (Burroughs Wellcome).
W/Ergotamine tartrate, caffeine.
See: Migral, Tab. (Burroughs Wellcome).

•**CYCLIZINE LACTATE INJECTION,** U.S.P. XXII. A sterile soln. of cyclizine lactate in water for injection.
Use: Antihistamine, antiemetic.

CYCLOBARBITAL. 5-(1-Cyclohexen-1-yl)-5-ethylbarbituric acid.
Use: Central depressant.

CYCLOBARBITAL CALCIUM. Cyclobarbitone, namuron, palinum, cyclobarbital Cal. 5-(1-Cyclohexenyl)-5-Ethylbarbituric Acid.
Use: Sedative/hypnotic.

CYCLOBARBITONE. B.A.N. 5-(Cyclohex-1-enyl)-5-ethylbarbituric acid.
Use: Hypnotic; sedative.

•**CYCLOBENDAZOLE.** USAN.
Use: Anthelmintic.

CYCLOBENZAPRINE HCl, U.S.P. XXII. Tab., U.S.P. XXII. 5-(3-Dimethylamino-propylidene)-dibenzo(a.e.)cycloheptatriene HCl.
Use: Musculoskeletal relaxant.
See: Flexeril, Tab. (Merck Sharp & Dohme).

CYCLOCORT CREAM. (Lederle) Amcinonide 0.1% in Aquatain hydrophilic base. Tubes 15 Gm, 30 Gm, 60 Gm.
Use: Corticosteroid.

CYCLOCORT OINTMENT. (Lederle) Amcinonide 0.1% in ointment base. Tube 15 Gm, 30 Gm, 60 Gm.
Use: Corticosteroid.

CYCLOCUMAROL. 3,4-Dihydro-2-methoxy-2-methyl-4-phenyl-2H,5H-pyrano[3,2c][1]benzopyran-5-one.
Use: Anticoagulant.

CYCLOFENIL. B.A.N. 4,4′-Diacetoxybenz-hydrylidenecyclohexane.
Use: Treatment of infertility.

•**CYCLOFILCON A.** USAN.
Use: Contact lens material.

CYCLOGEN. (Central) Dicyclomine HCl 10 mg, sodium Cl 0.9%, chlorobutanol hydrate 0.5%. Vial 10 ml, Box 12s.
Use: Antispasmodic.

CYCLOGUANIL EMBONATE. B.A.N. 4,6-Diamino-1-(4-chlorophenyl)-1,2-dihydro-2,2-dimethyl-1,3,5-triazine compound with 4,4′-methylenedi-(3-hydroxy-2-naphthoic acid) (2:1).
Use: Antimalarial.

•**CYCLOGUANIL PAMOATE.** USAN. 4,6-Diamino-1-(p-chlorophenyl)-1,2-dihydro-2,2-dimethyl-s-triazine compound (2:1) with 4,4′-methylenebis-[3-hydroxy-2-naphthoic acid].
Use: Antimalarial.

CYCLOGYL. (Alcon) Cyclopentolate HCl Soln. 0.5%, 1% or 2%. Droptainer 2 ml, 5 ml, 15 ml.
Use: Cycloplegic, mydriatic.

•**CYCLOHEXIMIDE.** USAN.
Use: Antipsoriatic.

•**CYCLOMETHICONE,** N.F. XVII.
Use: Pharmaceutic aid (wetting agent).

CYCLOMETHYCAINE. B.A.N. 3-(2-Methylpiperidino)propyl 4-cyclohexyloxybenzoate.
Use: Local anesthetic.

CYCLOMETHYCAINE AND METHAPYRILENE.
Use: Topical anesthetic.
See: Surfadil Cream, Lot. (Lilly).

CYCLOMETHYCAINE SULFATE, U.S.P. XXI. Creme, Jelly, Oint., Supp., U.S.P. XXI. 3-(2-Methylpiperidino) propyl p-(cyclohexyloxy) benzoate sulfate.
Use: Topical anesthetic.
See: Surfacaine, Prep. (Lilly).
W/Methapyrilene.
See: Surfadil, Cream, Lot. (Lilly).

CYCLOMETHYCAINE AND THENYLPYRAMINE.
See: Surfadil Cream, Lot. (Lilly).

CYCLOMYDRIL. (Alcon) Phenylephrine HCl 1%, cyclopentolate HCl 0.2%, benzalkonium Cl 0.01%, EDTA. Droptainer 2 ml, 5 ml.
Use: Mydriatic.

CYCLONIL. (Seatrace) Dicyclomine HCl 10 mg/ml. Vial 10 ml.
Use: Anticholinergic/antispasmodic.

CYCLOPAL. 5-Allyl-5(2-cyclopenten-1-yl)-barbituric acid. Cyclopentenyl allylbarbituric acid.

CYCLOPAR. (Parke-Davis) Tetracycline HCl 250 mg or 500 mg/Cap. **250 mg:** Bot. 100s, 1000s. **500 mg:** Bot. 100s, UD 100s.
Use: Antibacterial, tetracycline.

CYCLOPENTAMINE HYDROCHLORIDE, U.S.P. XXI. Nasal Soln., U.S.P. XXI. N-a-Dimethylcyclopentaneethylamine HCl.
Use: Adrenergic (vasoconstrictor).
See: Clopane Hydrochloride, Nasal Soln. (Dista).
W/Aludrine.
See: Aerolone Compound, Soln. (Lilly).
W/Chlorpheniramine.
See: Hista-Clopane, Pulvule (Lilly).

CYCLOPENTENYL - ALLYL - BARBITURIC ACID.
See: Cyclopal.

•**CYCLOPENTHIAZIDE.** USAN. 6-Chloro-3-(cyclopentylmethyl)-3,4-dihydro-2H-1,2,4-benzothiadiazine-7-sulfonamide 1,1-dioxide.
Use: Diuretic, anti-hypertensive.
See: Navidrex.

•**CYCLOPENTOLATE HYDROCHLORIDE,** U.S.P. XXII. Ophth. Soln., U.S.P. XXII. β-Di-methylaminoethyl (1-hydroxycyclopentyl) phenylacetate HCl. 2-(Dimethylamino)ethyl 1-Hydroxy-α-phenylcyclopentane- acetate HCl. Benzeneacetic acid, α-(1-hydroxy- cyclopentyl)-,2-(dimethylamino)ethyl ester, hydrochloride.
Use: Anticholinergic (ophthalmic).
See: Cyclogyl, Soln. (Alcon).
W/Phenylephrine HCl.
See: Cyclomydril, Soln. (Alcon).

CYCLOPENTYLPROPIONATE.
See: Depo-Testosterone, Vial (Upjohn).

•**CYCLOPHENAZINE HYDROCHLORIDE.** USAN.
Use: Antipsychotic.

•**CYCLOPHOSPHAMIDE,** U.S.P. XXII. Inj., Tabs., U.S.P. XXII. N,N-bis(2-Chloroethyl)-tetrahydro-,2- oxide, monodydrate. 2 H-1,3,2-Oxazaphosphorin-2-amine. phordiamidic acid cyclic ester monohydrate. 2-[bis(2-Chloroethyl) amino] tetrahydro-2H-1,3,2-oxazaphosphorine-2-Oxide.
Use: Antineoplastic, immunosuppressive.
See: Cytoxan, Tab., Vial (Bristol Oncology).

•**CYCLOPROPANE,** U.S.P. XXII. Trimethylene.
Use: Inhalation anesthetic.

CYCLO-PROSTIN. (Orphan drug).
Use: Hypertension, replacement of heparin in some hemodialysis patients.
Sponsors: Burroughs Wellcome, Upjohn.

•**CYCLOSERINE,** U.S.P. XXII. Caps., U.S.P. XXII. D-(+)-4-Amino-3-isoxazolidinone. 3-Isoxazolidi-

none, 4-amino-, (R)-. An antibiotic produced by *Streptomycin orchidaceus.* Oxamycin.
Use: Antibacterial (tuberculostatic).
See: Seromycin, Cap. (Lilly).

CYCLOSPASMOL CAPSULES. (Wyeth-Ayerst) Cyclandelate 200 mg or 400 mg/Cap. Bot. 100s.
Use: Vasodilator.

CYCLOSPASMOL TABLETS. (Wyeth-Ayerst) Cyclandelate 100 mg/Tab. Bot. 100s, 500s.
Use: Vasodilator.

CYCLOSPORIN A.
Use: Immunosuppressant.
See: Cyclosporine, U.S.P. XXII.

•**CYCLOSPORINE,** U.S.P. XXII.
Use: Immunosuppressive.
See: Sandimmune, Inj., Oral Soln. (Sandoz).

CYCLO-TAB. (Jenkins) Butabarbital sodium 5.4 mg, pentobarbital sodium 5.4 mg, phenobarbital sodium 5.4 mg, hyoscyamine HBr 0.1037 mg, scopolamine HBr 0.0065 mg, atropine sulfate 0.0194 mg/Tab. Bot. 1000s.
Use: Sedative/hypnotic, anticholinergic/antispasmodic.

CYCLOTHIAZIDE, U.S.P. XXI. Tab., U.S.P. XXI. 6-Chloro-3-(2-norbornenyl-5)-7-sulfamyl-3,4-dihydro-1,2,4-benzothiadiazine-1, 1-dioxide,-6-Chloro-3,4-dihydro-3-(5-norbornen-2-yl)-2H-1,2,4-benzothiadiazine-7-sulfonamide-1,-1-Dioxide. Bot. 100s, 1000s.
Use: Diuretic.
See: Anhydron, Tab. (Lilly).

CYCRIMINE. B.A.N. 1-Cyclopentyl-1-phenyl-3- piperidinopropan-1-ol.
Use: Treatment of the parkinsonian syndrome.

CYCRIN. (Wyeth-Ayerst) Medroxyprogesterone acetate 10 mg/Tab. Bot. 100s.
Use: Progestin.

CYDONOL MASSAGE LOTION. (Gordon) Isopropyl alcohol 14%, methyl salicylate, benzalkonium Cl. Bot. 4 oz, gal.
Use: Counterirritant.

•**CYHEPTAMIDE.** USAN.
Use: Anticonvulsant.

CYKLOKAPRON. (KabiVitrum) **Tab.:** Tranexamic acid 500 mg. Bot. 100s. **Inj.:** 100 mg/ml. Amp. 10 ml.
Use: Hemostatic.

CYLERT CHEWABLE TABLETS. (Abbott) Pemoline 37.5 mg/Tab. Bot. 100s.
Use: Psychotherapeutic agent.

CYLERT TABLETS. (Abbott) Pemoline 18.75, 37.5 or 75 mg/Tab. Bot. 100s.
Use: Psychotherapeutic agent.

CYNOBAL. (Arcum) Cyanocobalamin 100 mcg or 1000 mcg/ml. Inj. **100 mcg:** Vial 30 ml. **1000/ mcg/ml.:** Inj. Vial 10 ml, 30 ml.
Use: Vitamin B_{12} supplement.

CYOMIN. (Forest) Cyanocobalamin 1000 mcg/ml. Vial 10 ml, 30 ml.
Use: Vitamin B_{12} supplement.

•**CYPENAMINE HCl.** USAN. 2-Phenylcyclopentylamine HydroCl.
Use: Antidepressant.

•**CYPOTHRIN.** USAN.
Use: Insecticide.

•**CYPRAZEPAM.** USAN.
Use: Sedative.

CYPRENORPHINE. B.A.N. N-Cyclopropylmethyl-7,8-dihydro-7α-(1-hydroxy-1-methylethyl)-O^6-methyl-6, 14-endoethenonormorphine.
Use: Narcotic antagonist.

•**CYPROHEPTADINE HYDROCHLORIDE,** U.S.P. XXII. Syrup, Tabs., U.S.P. XXII. 4-(5H-Dibenzo-[a,d]cyclohepten-5-ylidene)-1-methylpiperidene HydroCl. 1-Methyl-4-(5-dibenzo-[a,e]cycloheptatrienylidene) piperidine HCl monohydrate.
Use: Antihistamine, antipruritic.
See: Periactin, Tab., Syr. (Merck Sharp & Dohme).

•**CYPROLIDOL HYDROCHLORIDE.** USAN. Diphenyl (2-(4-pyridyl)cyclo-propyl)-methanol hydrochloride.
Use: Psychotherapeutic agent.

•**CYPROQUINATE.** USAN.
Use: Coccidiostat (for poultry).

CYPROTERON. Cyproterone acetate (Orphan Drug).
Use: Severe hirsutism.
Sponsor: Berlex.

•**CYPROTERONE ACETATE.** USAN. 6-Chloro-17-hydroxy-1α-2α-methylenepregna-4,6-diene-3, 20-dione acetate.
Use: Anti-androgen.

•**CYPROXIMIDE.** USAN.
Use: Antidepressant.

CYREN A.
See: Diethylstilbestrol Prep. (Various Mfr.).

CYRIMINE HCl. 1-Phenyl-1-cyclopentyl-3-piperidino-1-propanol HCl.
Use: Antispasmodic.
See: Pagitane HCl, Tab. (Lilly).

CYRONINE. (Major) Liothyronine sodium 25 mcg/ Tab. Bot. 100s.
Use: Thyroid hormone.

CYSTAMIN.
See: Methenamine, Tab. (Various Mfr.).

CYSTAMINE. (Tennessee) Methenamine 2 gr, phenyl salicylate 0.5 gr, phenazopyridine HCl 10 mg, benzoic acid 1/8 gr, hyoscyamine sulfate 1/2000 gr, atropine sulfate 1/2000 gr/SC Tab. Bot. 100s, 1000s.
Use: Urinary anti-infective.

•**CYSTEAMINE.** USAN.
Use: Antiurolithic, cysteine calculi.

•**CYSTEINE HCl,** U.S.P. XXII. Lotion, U.S.P. XXII. L-Cysteine hydrochloride monohydrate.
Use: Amino acid for replacement therapy.
See: Cysteine HCl (Abbott).

CYSTEX. (Numark) Methenamine 162 mg, salicylamide 65 mg, sodium salicylate 97 mg, benzoic acid 32 mg/Tab. Bot. 40s, 100s.
Use: Urinary anti-infective.

•**CYSTINE.** USAN. An essential amino acid. Delta—Bot. 100 Gm; Mann—Bot. 25 Gm; Abbott—50 mg/ml HCl salt solution.
Use: Amino acid replacement therapy, an additive for infants on TPN.

CYSTITOL. (Vortech) Atropine sulfate 0.03 mg, hyoscyamine 0.03 mg, gelsemium 6.1 mg, methenamine 40.8 mg, salol 18.1 mg, benzoic acid 4.5 mg/Tab. Bot. 1000s.
Use: Urinary anti-infective.

CYSTO. (Freeport) Methenamine 40.8 mg, methylene blue 5.4 mg, phenyl salicylate 18.1 mg, atropine sulfate 0.03 mg, hyoscyamine 0.03 mg, benzoic acid 4.5 mg/Tab. Bot. 1000s.
Use: Urinary anti-infective.

CYSTO-CONRAY. (Mallinckrodt) Iothalamate meglumine 43% (iodine 20.2%) with EDTA. Soln. Vial 50 ml, 100 ml. Bot. 250 ml.
Use: Radiopaque agent.

CYSTO-CONRAY II. (Mallinckrodt) Iothalamate meglumine 17.2% (iodine 8.1%) with EDTA. Soln. Bot. 250 ml, 500 ml.
Use: Radiopaque agent.

CYSTOGRAFIN. (Squibb) Meglumine diatrizoate 30% (bound iodine 14%), EDTA 0.04%. Bot. 100 ml, 300 ml.
Use: Radiopaque agent.

CYSTOGRAFIN-DILUTE. (Squibb) Diatrizoate meglumine 18% (organically-bound iodine 85 mg)/ml. Vial 300 ml, 500 ml.
Use: Radiopaque agent.

CYSTO-SPAZ. (Webcon) l-Hyoscyamine 0.15 mg/Tab. Bot. 100s.
Use: Anticholinergic/antispasmodic.

CYSTO-SPAZ-M. (Webcon) Hyoscyamine sulfate 375 mcg/Cap. Bot. 100s.
Use: Anticholinergic/antispasmodic.

CYSTREA. (Moore Kirk) Methenamine 2 gr, phenyl salicylate 0.5 gr, methylene blue 1/5 gr, benzoic acid 1/10 gr, hyoscyamine alkaloid 1/2000 gr, atropine sulfate 1/2000 gr/Tab. Bot. 100s, 1000s.
Use: Urinary anti-infective.

CYTADREN. (Ciba) Aminoglutethimide 250 mg/Tab. Bot. 100s.
Use: Adrenal steroid inhibitor.

•**CYTARABINE,** U.S.P. XXII. Sterile, U.S.P. XXII. 2(1H)-Pyrimidihone, 4-amino-1-β- -arabinofuranosyl-. 1-β- -Arabinofuranosylcytosine.
Use: Antineoplastic agent.
See: Cytosar, Inj. (Upjohn).

•**CYTARABINE HYDROCHLORIDE.** USAN. 1-Arabinoluranosylcytosine hydrochloride.
Use: Management of acute leukemias.
See: Cytosar-U, Vial (Upjohn).

CYRONINE TABS. (Major) Liothyronine sodium 25 mcg or 50 mcg/Tab. Bot. 100s.
Use: Thyroid hormone.

CYTOMEL. (SmithKline) Liothyronine sodium 5 mcg, 25 mcg or 50 mcg/Tab. Bot. 100s. 25 mcg: Bot. 1000s.
Use: Thyroid hormone.

CYTOSAR-U. (Upjohn) Cytarabine 20 mg/ml in powder, 50 mg/ml reconstituted. Vial 100 mg, 500 mg.
Use: Antineoplastic agent.

CYTOSINE ARABINOSIDE HCl. Cytarabine HCl.
See: Cytosar-U (Upjohn).

CYTOTEC. (Searle) Misoprostol 200 mcg/Tab. Bot. 100s, UD 100s.
Use: Prostaglandins.

CYTOX. (MPL) Cyanocobalamin 500 mcg, vitamins B_6 20 mg, B_1 100 mg, benzyl alcohol 2% in isotonic solution of sodium Cl/ml. Inj. Vial 10 ml.
Use: Vitamin supplement.

CYTOXAN LYOPHILIZED. (Bristol-Myers/Mead Johnson Oncology) Cyclophosphamide. Vial 500 mg.
Use: Antineoplastic agent.

CYTOXAN POWDER. (Bristol-Myers/Mead Johnson Oncology) Cyclophosphamide powder 100 mg, 200 mg, 500 mg, 1 Gm or 2 Gm/Vial.
Use: Antineoplastic agent.

CYTOXAN TABLETS. (Bristol-Myers/Mead Johnson Oncology) Cyclophosphamide 25 mg or 50 mg/Tab. **25 mg/Tab.:** Bot. 100s; **50 mg/Tab.:** Bot. 100s, 1000s, UD 100s.
Use: Antineoplastic agent.

D

D_2. One of the D vitamins.
See: Ergocalciferol.

D_3. One of the D vitamins.
See: Cholecalciferol.

DAA.
See: Dihydroxy Aluminum Aminoacetate.

•**DACARBAZINE,** U.S.P. XXII. Inj., U.S.P. XXII. 5-(3,3-Dimethyltriazeno) imidazole-4-carboxamide.
Use: Antineoplastic.
See: Dtic-Dome, Inj. (Miles Pharm).

DACODYL. (Major) **Tab.:** Bisacodyl 5 mg/Tab. Bot. 100s, 250s, 1000s. UD 100s. **Supp.:** Bisacodyl 10 mg. Box 12s, 100s.
Use: Laxative.

DACRIOSE. (Iolab) Isotonic, buffered solution of purified water, sodium Cl, potassium Cl, sodium hydroxide, sodium phosphate, benzalkonium CL 0.01%, edetate disodium 0.03%. Bot. 0.5 oz, 1 oz, 4 oz.
Use: Irrigating solution, ophthalmic.

•**DACTINOMYCIN,** U.S.P. XXII. Inj., U.S.P. XXII. Actinomycin D.
Use: Antineoplastic.
See: Cosmegen, Vial (Merck Sharp & Dohme).

DACURONIUM BROMIDE. B.A.N. 3α-Acetoxy-17β-hydroxy-5α-androstan-2β,16β-di-(1-methyl-1-piperidinium) dibromide.
Use: Neuromuscular blocking agent.

DAILY CLEANER. (Bausch & Lomb) Isotonic solution with sodium Cl, sodium phosphate, tylox-

apol, hydroxyethyl cellulose, polyvinyl alcohol with thimerosal 0.004%, EDTA 0.2%. Soln. Bot. 45 ml.
Use: Soft contact lens care.

DAILY CONDITIONING TREATMENT. (Blistex) Padimate O 7.5%, oxybenzone 3.5%, petrolatum. Stick 11.4 Gm. SPF 15.
Use: Lip protectant, sunscreen.

DAILY/JET. (Kirkman) Bot. 100s.
Use: Vitamin supplement.

DAILY VITAMIN LIQUID. (PBI) Vitamins A 2500 IU, D 400 IU, E 15 IU, C 60 mg, B_1 1.2 mg, B_2 1.2 mg, B_6 1.05 mg, B_{12} 4.5 mcg, niacinamide 13.5 mg/5 ml. Bot. 8 oz, pt, gal.
Use: Vitamin supplement.

DAILY VITAMINS. (Kirkman) Vitamins A 5000 IU, D 400 IU, C 50 mg, B_1 3 mg, B_2 2.5 mg, B_6 1 mg, B_{12} 1 mcg, niacinamide 20 mg, d-calcium pantothenate 1 mg/Tab. Bot. 100s.
Use: Vitamin supplement.

DAILY VITAMINS W/IRON. (Kirkman) Vitamins A 5000 IU, D 400 IU, B_1 2 mg, B_2 2.5 mg, B_6 1 mg, B_{12} 1 mcg, niacinamide 20 mg, d-calcium pantothenate 1 mg, iron 18 mg/Tab. Bot. 100s.
Use: Vitamin/mineral supplement.

DAILY-VITE W/IRON & MINERALS. (Rugby) Elemental iron 18 mg, vitamins A 5000 IU, D 400 IU, E 30 mg, B_1 1.5 mg, B_2 1.7 mg, B_3 20 mg, B_5 10 mg, B_6 2 mg, B_{12} 6 mcg, C 60 mg, folic acid 0.4 mg, Ca, Cl, Cr, Cu, I, K, Mg, Mn, Mo, P, Se, zinc 15 mg, biotin 30 mcg, vitamin K 50 mcg/Tab. Bot. 100s, 365s, 1000s.
Use: Vitamin/mineral supplement.

DAISY 2 PREGNANCY TEST. (Advanced Care) Home pregnancy test. Test kit 2s.
Use: Diagnostic aid.

DAKIN'S SOLUTION.
See: Sodium Hypochlorite Solution Diluted.

DAKIN'S SOLUTION-FULL STRENGTH. (Century) Sodium hypochlorite 0.5%. Soln. Bot. pt, gal.
Use: Anti-infective, external.

DAKIN'S SOLUTION-HALF STRENGTH. (Century) Sodium hypochlorite 0.25%. Soln. Bot. pt.
Use: Anti-infective, external.

DALALONE. (Forest) Dexamethasone sodium phosphate 4 mg/ml, methyl and propyl parabens, sodium bisulfite. Vial 5 ml.
Use: Corticosteroid.

DALALONE D.P. (Forest) Dexamethasone acetate 16 mg/ml, polysorbate 80, carboxymethylcellulose, sodium bisulfite, EDTA, benzyl alcohol. Vial 1 ml, 5 ml.
Use: Corticosteroid.

DALALONE L.A. (Forest) Dexamethasone 8 mg/ml, polysorbate 80, carboxymethylcellulose, sodium bisulfite, EDTA, benzyl alcohol. Vial 5 ml.
Use: Corticosteroid.

DALCAINE. (Forest) Lidocaine HCl 2%. Inj. Vial 5 ml.
Use: Local anesthetic.

DALEDALIN TOSYLATE. USAN. 3-Methyl-3-[3-(methylamino) ropyl]-1-phenylindoline mono-p-toluene sulfonate.
Use: Antidepressant.

DALEX. (Dalin) Dextromethorphan HBr 45 mg, phenylephrine HCl 15 mg, chlorpheniramine maleate 6 mg, guaifenesin 180 mg, ammonium Cl 600 mg/fl oz. **Syr.:** Bot. 4 oz, pt. **Loz.:** 10s, 18s. **Cap.:** 20s. **Pediatric:** Bot. 4 oz. **TR:** 15s.
Use: Antitussive, decongestant, antihistamine, expectorant.

DALGAN. (Wyeth-Ayerst) Dezocine 5 mg, 10 mg or 15 mg/ml. **5 mg/ml:** Vial (SD) 1 ml. **10 mg/ml:** Vial (SD) 1 ml, Vial (MD) 10 ml, syringes (prefilled) 1 ml. **15 mg/ml:** Vial (SD) 1 ml, syringes (prefilled) 1 ml.
Use: Narcotic analgesic.

DALICOTE. (Dalin) Hexachlorophene, pyrilamine maleate, diperodon HCl 0.25%, dimethyl polysiloxane, silicone, zinc oxide, camphor. Lot. Bot. 4 fl oz.
Use: Antihistamine, antipruritic, anesthetic.

DALICREME. (Dalin) Vitamins A 750 IU, D 75 IU, diperodon HCl 0.25%, quaternary ammonium compound. Tube 1.5 oz, 4 oz. Jar 16 oz.
Use: Vitamin supplement.

DALIDERM LIQUID. (Dalin) Ethyl alcohol 66%, quaternium ammonium compound, carbolic acid, benzoic acid, salicylic acid, resorcin, camphor, tannic acid, coal tar solution, chlorothymol. Bot. 0.5 oz, 1 oz.
Use: Antipruritic, antifungal, keratolytic.

DALIDERM POWDER. (Dalin) Zinc undecylenate, sodium propionate, quaternium ammonium compound, salicylic acid, boric acid, aluminum acetate, alum. Can 2 oz, 3.5 oz.
Use: Antipruritic, antifungal, keratolytic.

DALIDYNE. (Dalin) Methylbenzethonium Cl, tannic acid, benzocaine, ethyl alcohol, benzyl alcohol, camphor, menthol, chlorothymol. Lot. Bot. 0.25 oz, 0.5 oz, 1 oz.
Use: Counterirritant for mouth.

DALIDYNE JEL. (Dalin) Benzocaine, cherry-flavored base. Tube 10 Gm.
Use: Local anesthetic, topical.

DALIDYNE THROAT SPRAY. (Dalin) Lidocaine, cetyldimethylbenzyl ammonium Cl, ethyl alcohol. Aerosol ⅓ oz.
Use: Anesthetic, antiseptic.

DALIFORT. (Dalin) Vitamins A 25,000 IU, D 400 IU, C 500 mg, B_1 10 mg, B_2 5 mg, B_6 5 mg, B_{12} 5 mcg, niacinamide 100 mg, d-calcium pantothenate 20 mg, iron 10 mg, magnesium oxide 5 mg, zinc sulfate 1.5 mg, copper sulfate 1 mg/Tab. Bot. 30s, 100s.
Use: Vitamin/mineral supplement.

DALIHIST. (Dalin) Phenylephrine HCl 0.5%, pyrilamine maleate 0.15%, cetyl benzyldimethyl ammonium Cl 0.04% in aqueous isotonic solution. Spray 20 ml.
Use: Decongestant, antihistamine.

DALIMYCIN. (Dalin) Oxytetracycline HCl 250 mg/Cap. Bot. 24s, 100s.
Use: Antibacterial, tetracycline.

DALISEPT. (Dalin) Vitamins A 750 IU, D 75 IU, diperodon HCl 1%, methylbenzethonium Cl 0.1%. Tube 2 oz, 4 oz. Jar 16 oz.
Use: Anesthetic, topical w/vitamins.

DALIVIM FORTE. (Dalin) Iron ammonium citrate 18 gr, liver fraction 3 gr, vitamins B_{12} 60 mcg, A palmitate 10,000 IU, D 1000 IU, B_1 12 mg, B_2 4 mg, niacinamide 20 mg, B_6 2 mg, calcium pantothenate 12 mg, mixed tocopherols 30 mg, calcium glycerophosphate 65 mg, manganese glycerophosphate 17.5 mg/oz. Bot. 4 oz, 8 oz, 16 oz.
Use: Vitamin/mineral supplement.

DALIVIM FORTE TABLETS. (Dalin) Iron 100 mg, desiccated liver 150 mg, vitamins B_{12} 10 mcg, A palmitate 1667 IU, D 167 IU, C 50 mg, B_1 3 mg, B_2 3 mg, niacinamide 10 mg, B_6 0.5 mg, calcium pantothenate 2 mg, calcium glycerophosphate 11 mg, manganese glycerophosphate 3 mg/Tab. Bot. 50s, 100s.
Use: Vitamin/mineral supplement.

DALLERGY CAPSULES. (Laser) Chlorpheniramine maleate 8 mg, phenylephrine HCl 20 mg, methscopolamine nitrate 2.5 mg/Cap. Bot. 100s, 1000s.
Use: Antihistamine, decongestant, antisecretory.

DALLERGY-D CAPSULES. (Laser) Chlorpheniramine maleate 12 mg, pseudoephedrine HCl 120 mg/Cap. Bot. 12s, 100s.
Use: Antihistamine, decongestant.

DALLERGY-D SYRUP. (Laser) Chlorpheniramine maleate 2 mg, phenylephrine HCl 5 mg/5 ml. Bot. 4 oz.
Use: Antihistamine, decongestant.

DALLERGY-JR CAPSULES. (Laser) Brompheniramine maleate 6 mg, pseudoephedrine HCl 60 mg/Cap. Bot. 100s, 1000s.
Use: Antihistamine, decongestant.

DALLERGY SYRUP. (Laser) Chlorpheniramine maleate 2 mg, phenylephrine HCl 10 mg, methscopolamine nitrate 0.625 mg/5 ml. Bot. pt, gal.
Use: Antihistamine, decongestant, anticholinergic/antispasmodic.

DALLERGY TABLETS. (Laser) Chlorpheniramine maleate 4 mg, phenylephrine HCl 10 mg, methscopolamine nitrate 1.25 mg/Tab. Bot. 100s, 1000s.
Use: Antihistamine, decongestant, anticholinergic/antispasmodic.

DALMANE. (Roche) Flurazepam HCl 15 mg or 30 mg/Cap. Bot. 100s, 500s, Prescription Pak 300s. RNP (Reverse Numbered Packages) 4 rolls × 25 cap. or 4 cards × 25 cap. UD 100s.
Use: Sedative/hypnotic.

•**DALTROBAN.** USAN.
Use: Platelet aggregation inhibitor.

DAMACET-P. (Mason) Hydrocodone bitartrate 5 mg, acetaminophen 500 mg/Tab. Bot. 100s, 500s.
Use: Narcotic analgesic combination.

DAMASON-P. (Mason) Hydrocodone bitartrate 5 mg, aspirin 224 mg, caffeine 32 mg/Tab. Bot. 100s, 500s.
Use: Narcotic analgesic combination.

DAMBOSE.
See: Inositol, Tabs.

D-AMP. (Dunhall) Ampicillin trihydrate 500 mg/Cap. Bot. 100s.
Use: Antibacterial, penicillin.

DANATROL CAPSULES. (Winthrop Products) Danazol.
Use: Gonadotropin inhibitor.

•**DANAZOL,** U.S.P. XXII. Cap., U.S.P. XXII. 17α-Pregna-2,4-dien-20-yno-[2,3-d]isoxazol-17-ol.
Use: Pituitary gonadotropin suppressant.
See: Danocrine, Cap. (Winthrop Pharm).

DANDRUFF SHAMPOO. (Walgreen) Zinc pyrithione 2 Gm/100 ml. Bot. 11 oz. Tube 7 oz.
Use: Antiseborrheic..

DANEX PROTEIN ENRICHED DANDRUFF SHAMPOO. (Herbert) Pyrithione zinc 1%. Bot. 4 oz.
Use: Antiseborrheic.

DANOCRINE. (Winthrop Pharm) Danazol 50 mg, 100 mg or 200 mg/Cap. Bot. 100s.
Use: Gonadotropin inhibitor.

•**DANOFLOXACIN MESYLATE.** USAN.
Use: Antibacterial (veterinary).

DANOGAR TABLETS. (Winthrop Products) Danazol.
Use: Gonadotropin inhibitor.

DANOL CAPSULES. (Winthrop Products) Danazol.
Use: Gonadotropin inhibitor.

DANTRIUM. (Norwich Eaton) Dantrolene sodium. **25 mg/Cap.:** Bot. 100s, 500s, UD 100s; **50 mg/Cap.:** Bot. 100s; **100 mg/Cap.:** Bot. 100s, UD 100s.
Use: Skeletal muscle relaxant.

DANTRIUM I.V. (Norwich Eaton) Dantrolene sodium 20 mg/Vial. Vial 70 ml.
Use: Skeletal muscle relaxant.

•**DANTROLENE.** USAN. 1(((5-(4-nitrophenyl)-2-furanyl) methylene) amino) 2,4-nidazolidinedione.
Use: Skeletal muscle relaxant.

•**DANTROLENE SODIUM.** USAN.
Use: Skeletal muscle relaxant.
See: Dantrium, Cap. (Norwich Eaton).

DAPA TABLETS. (Ferndale) Acetaminophen 324 mg/Tab. Bot. 100s, 1000s, UD 100s.
Use: Analgesic.

DAPA EXTRA STRENGTH TABLETS. (Ferndale) Acetaminophen 500 mg/Tab. Bot. 100s, 1000s, UD 100s.
Use: Analgesic.

DAPACIN COLD CAPSULES. (Ferndale) Phenylpropanolamine 12.5 mg, chlorpheniramine maleate 2 mg, acetaminophen 325 mg. Bot. 100s.
Use: Decongestant, antihistamine, analgesic.

DAPCO. (Schlicksup) Salicylamide 300 mg, butabarbital 15 mg/Tab. Bot. 100s, 1000s.
Use: Salicylate analgesic, sedative/hypnotic.

DAPEX. (Ferndale) Phentermine HCl 37.5 mg/Cap. Bot. 100s.
Use: Anorexiant.

•**DAPSONE,** U.S.P. XXII. Tab., U.S.P. XXII. Benzenamine, 4,4′-sulfonyl-bis-. Diaminodiphenylsulfone. 4,4′-Sulfonyldianiline.
Use: Treatment of leprosy; dermitis herpetiformis suppressant.

DARAGEN. (Owen/Galderma) Collagen polypeptide, benzalkonium Cl in a mild amphoteric base. Shampoo. Bot. 8 oz.
Use: Hair repair.

DARA SOAPLESS SHAMPOO. (Owen/Galderma) Purified water, potassium coco hydrolyzed protein, sulfated castor oil, pentasodium triphosphate, sodium benzoate, sodium lauryl sulfate, fragrance. Shampoo. Bot. 8 oz, 16 oz.
Use: Scalp protectant.

DARANIDE. (Merck Sharp & Dohme) Dichlorphenamide 50 mg/Tab. Bot. 100s.
Use: Agent for glaucoma.

DARAPRIM. (Burroughs Wellcome) Pyrimethamine 25 mg/Tab. Bot. 100s.
Use: Antimalarial.

DARBID. (SmithKline) Isopropamide iodide 5 mg/Tab. Bot. 50s.
Use: Anticholinergic/antispasmodic.

DARCO G-60. (ICI Americas) Activated carbon from lignite.
Use: Purifier.

DARICON. (Beecham Labs) Oxyphencyclimine HCl 10 mg/Tab. Bot. 60s, 500s.
Use: Antispasmodic.

•**DARODIPINE.** USAN.
Use: Antihypertensive, bronchodilator, vasodilator.

DARVOCET-N 50. (Lilly) Propoxyphene napsylate 50 mg, acetaminophen 325 mg/Tab. Bot. 100s (Rx Pak) 500s; Blister pkg. 10 × 10s.
Use: Narcotic analgesic combination.

DARVOCET-N 100. (Lilly) Propoxyphene napsylate 100 mg, acetaminophen 650 mg/Tab. Bot. 100s (Rx Pak) 500s; Blister pkg. 10 × 10s; 500 single cut blisters; UD rolls 20 × 25s.
Use: Narcotic analgesic combination.

DARVON. (Lilly) Propoxyphene HCl 65 mg/Pulv. Bot. 100s. Rx Pak 500s; Blister pkg. 10 × 10s; UD 20 rolls × 25s.
Use: Narcotic analgesic.

DARVON COMPOUND-65. (Lilly) Propoxyphene HCl 65 mg, aspirin 389 mg, caffeine 32.4 mg/Pulv. Bot. 100s (Rx Pak) 500s; Blister pkg. 10 × 10s.
Use: Narcotic analgesic combination.

DARVON-N. (Lilly) Propoxyphene napsylate. **Tab.:** 100 mg. Bot. 100s (Rx Pak), 500s; Blister pkg. 10 × 10s; Rx Pak 20 × 50s. **Susp.:** 50 mg/5 ml. Bot. 16 fl oz.
Use: Narcotic analgesic.

DA-SED TABLET. (Sheryl) Butabarbital 0.5 gr/Tab. Bot. 100s.
Use: Sedative/hypnotic.

DASIN. (SmithKline/Beecham) Ipecac 3 mg, acetylsalicylic acid 130 mg, camphor 15 mg, caffeine 8 mg, atropine sulfate 0.13 mg/Cap. Bot. 100s, 500s.
Use: Analgesic, anticholinergic/antispasmodic.

DATRIL EXTRA STRENGTH TABLETS. (Bristol-Myers) Acetaminophen 500 mg/Tab. Bot. 30s, 60s, 100s.
Use: Analgesic.

DATURINE HBr.
See: Hyoscyamine Salts (Various Mfr.).

•**DAUNORUBICIN HCL,** U.S.P. XXII. For Inj., U.S.P. XXII. An antibiotic produced by *Streptomyces ceruleorubidus.* 3-Acetyl-1,2,3,-4,6,11-hexahydro-3,5, 12-trihydroxy-10-methoxy-6,11-dioxonaphthacen-1-yl-3-amino-2,3,6-trideoxy-β-D-galactopyranoside.
Use: Antineoplastic.
See: Cerubidine, Inj. (Wyeth-Ayerst).

•**DAUNORUBICIN HYDROCHLORIDE.** USAN.
Use: Antineoplastic.

DAVITAMON K.
See: Menadione Inj., Tab. (Various Mfr.).

DAVOSIL. (Hoyt) Silicon carbide in glycerin base. Jar 8 oz, 10 oz.
Use: Agent for oral hygiene.

DAYALETS. (Abbott) Vitamins B_1 1.5 mg, B_2 1.7 mg, A 5000 IU, C 60 mg, D 400 IU, niacinamide 20 mg, B_6 2 mg, B_{12} 6 mcg, E 30 IU, folic acid 0.4 mg/Filmtab. Bot. 100s.
Use: Vitamin supplement.

DAYALETS PLUS IRON. (Abbott) Vitamins B_1 1.5 mg, B_2 1.7 mg, niacinamide 20 mg, B_6 2 mg, C 60 mg, A 5000 IU, D 400 IU, E 30 IU, B_{12} 6 mcg, iron 18 mg, folic acid 0.4 mg/Filmtab. Bot. 100s.
Use: Vitamin/mineral supplement.

DAY CAPS. (Towne) Vitamins A 5500 IU, D 400 IU, B_1 3 mg, B_2 3 mg, B_6 0.5 mg, B_{12} 4 mcg, C 50 mg, calcium pantothenate 5 mg, niacinamide 20 mg/Cap. Bot. 120s, 300s.
Use: Vitamin supplement.

DAY CAP TABS-M. (Towne) Vitamins A 5500 IU, D 400 IU, B_1 3 mg, B_2 3 mg, B_6 0.5 mg, B_{12} 4 mcg, C 50 mg, niacinamide 20 mg, calcium pantothenate 5 mg, l-Lysine HCl 15 mg, iron 10 mg, zinc 1.5 mg, manganese 1 mg, iodine 0.1 mg, copper 1 mg, potassium 5 mg, magnesium 6 mg/Cap. or tab. Bot. 100s, 250s.
Use: Vitamin/mineral supplement.

DAYCARE. (Vicks Health Care) **Capl.:** Pseudoephedrine HCl 30 mg, dextromethorphan HBr 10 mg, guaifenesin 100 mg, acetaminophen 325 mg. Bot. 20s, 36s. **Expectorant Liq.:** Pseudoephedrine HCl 10 mg, dextromethorphan HBr 3.3 mg, guaifenesin 33.3 mg, acetaminophen 108 mg, alcohol 10% and saccharin. Bot. 180 ml, 300 ml.

Use: Decongestant, antitussive, expectorant, analgesic.

DAY TAB. (Towne) Vitamins A 5000 IU, D 400 IU, B_1 15 mg, B_2 10 mg, C 600 mg, niacinamide 20 mg, B_6 5 mg, folic acid 400 mcg, pantothenic acid 10 mg, zinc 15 mg, copper 2 mg, B_{12} 5 mcg/Tab. Bot. 100s, 200s.
Use: Vitamin/mineral supplement.

DAY TAB ESSENTIAL. (Towne) Vitamins A 5000 IU, D 400 IU, E 15 IU, C 60 mg, folic acid 0.4 mg, B_1 1.5 mg, B_2 1.7 mg, niacin 20 mg, B_6 2 mg, B_{12} 6 mcg/Tab. Bot. 200s.
Use: Vitamin supplement.

DAY TABS, NEW. (Towne) Vitamins A 5000 IU, E 15 IU, D 400 IU, C 60 mg, folic acid 0.4 mg, B_1 1.5 mg, B_2 1.7 mg, niacin 20 mg, B_6 20 mg, B_{12} 6 mcg/Tab. Bot 100s, 250s.
Use: Vitamin supplement.

DAY TAB PLUS IRON. (Towne) Iron 18 mg, vitamins A 5000 IU, D 400 IU, B_1 1.5 mg, B_2 1.7 mg, niacinamide 20 mg, C 60 mg, B_6 2 mg, pantothenic acid 10 mg, B_{12} 6 mcg, folic acid 0.1 mg/Tab. Bot. 100s.
Use: Vitamin/mineral supplement.

DAY TAB STRESS COMPLEX. (Towne) Vitamins A 5000 IU, C 600 mg, B_1 15 mg, B_2 10 mg, niacin 100 mg, D 400 IU, E 30 IU, B_6 5 mg, folic acid 400 mcg, B_{12} 6 mcg, pantothenic acid 20 mg, iron 18 mg, zinc 15 mg, copper 2 mg/Tab. Bot. 60s.
Use: Vitamin/mineral supplement.

DAY TABS PLUS IRON, NEW. (Towne) Vitamins A 5000 IU, E 15 IU, D 400 IU, C 60 mg, folic acid 0.4 mg, B_1 1.5 mg, B_2 1.7 mg, niacin 20 mg, B_6 20 mg, B_{12} 6 mcg, iron 18 mcg/Tab. Bot. 250s.
Use: Vitamin/mineral supplement.

DAY TAB WITH IRON. (Towne) Vitamins A 5000 IU, D 400 IU, E 15 IU, C 60 mg, folic acid 1.5 mg, B_1 15 mg, B_2 1.7 mg, niacin 20 mg, B_6 2 mg, B_{12} 6 mcg, iron 18 mg/Tab. Bot. 200s.
Use: Vitamin/mineral supplement.

DAYTO-ANASE. (Dayton) Bromelains 50,000 IU (protease activity). Tab. Bot. 60s.
Use: Enzyme.

DAYTO HIMBIN. (Dayton) Yohimbine 5.4 mg/Tab. Bot. 60s.
Use: Alpha adrenergic blocker.

DAYTO SULF. (Dayton) Sulfathiazole 3.42%, sulfacetamide 2.86%, sulfabenzamide 3.7%, urea 0.64%. Cream. Tube 78 Gm with 8 disposable applicators.
Use: Anti-infective, vaginal.

DAY-VITE. (Drug Industries) Vitamins A 10,000 IU, D-3 1000 IU, E 6.7 mg, C 100 mg, B_1 5 mg, B_2 5 mg, B_6 2 mg, B_{12} 2 mcg, niacinamide 25 mg, calcium pantothenate 10 mg/Tab. Bot. 100s, 500s.
Use: Vitamin supplement.

DAZAMIDE TABS. (Major) Acetazolamide 250 mg/Tab. Bot. 100s, 250s, 1000s, UD 100s.
Use: Diuretic.

•**DAZANDROL MALEATE.** USAN.
Use: Antidepressant.

•**DAZEPINIL HYDROCHLORIDE.** USAN.
Use: Antidepressant.

•**DAZMEGREL.** USAN.
Use: Inhibitor (thromboxane synthetase).

•**DAZOPRIDE FUMARATE.** USAN.
Use: Peristaltic stimulant.

•**DAZOXIBEN HYDROCHLORIDE.** USAN.
Use: Antithrombotic.

DB ELECTRODE PASTE. (Day-Baldwin) Tube 5%.

DBED. Dibenzylethylenediamine dipenicillin G.
Use: Antibacterial, penicillin.
See: Benzathine penicillin G Susp.

DCA
See: Desoxycorticosterone acetate preps. (Various Mfr.).

DCP. (Towne) Calcium 180 mg, phosphorus 105 mg, vitamins D 66.7 IU/Tab. Bot. 100s.
Use: Vitamin/mineral supplement.

DC 240. (Goldline) Docusate calcium 240 mg/Cap. Bot. 100s, 500s.
Use: Laxative.

DDAVP. (Rhone-Poulenc Rorer) Desmopressin acetate 0.1 mg, chlorobutanol 5 mg, sodium Cl 9 mg/ml. Vial 2.5 ml w/applicator tubes for nasal administration.
Use: Antidiuretic.

DDAVP INJECTION. (Rhone-Poulenc Rorer). Desmopressin acetate 4 mcg, chlorobutanol 5 mg, sodium Cl 9 mg/ml. Amp. 1 ml.
Use: Antidiuretic.

D-DIOL. (Burgin-Arden) Testosterone cypionate 50 mg, estradiol cypionate 2 mg/ml. Vial 10 ml.
Use: Androgen, estrogen.

DDS.
See: Dapsone Tab., U.S.P. XXII.

DDT.
See: Chlorophenothane.

DEACETYLLANATOSIDE C.
See: Deslanoside, U.S.P. XXII.

DEADLY NIGHTSHADE LEAF, U.S.P.
See: Belladonna Leaf, U.S.P. XXII.

DEBA.
See: Barbital (Various Mfr.).

DEBRISAN. (Johnson & Johnson) Dextranomer. **Beads:** Spherical hydrophilic 0.1-0.3 mm diameter. Bot. 25 Gm, 60 Gm, 120 Gm. Pk. 7 × 4 Gm, 14 × 14 Gm. U.S. distributor Johnson & Johnson Products. **Paste:** 10 Gm. Foil packets 6s.
Use: Wound and ulcer cleansing.

•**DEBRISOQUIN SULFATE.** USAN. 3,4-Dihydro-2(IH) isoquinolinecarboxamidine sulfate. Formerly Isocaramidine Sulfate.
Use: Hypotensive agent.

DEBROX. (Marion) Carbamide peroxide 6.5% in anhydrous glycerol. Plastic squeeze bot. 0.5 oz, 1 oz.
Use: Otic preparation.

DECABID. (Lilly) Indecainide HCl 50 mg, 75 mg or 100 mg/SR tab. Bot. 100s, UD 100s. [Approved but not marketed].
Use: Antiarrhythmic.

DECA-BON. (Barrows) Vitamins A 3000 IU, D 400 IU, C 60 mg, B_1 1 mg, B_2 1.2 mg, niacinamide 8 mg, B_6 1 mg, panthenol 3 mg, B_{12} 1 mcg, biotin 30 mcg/0.6 ml. Drops Bot. 50 ml.
Use: Vitamin supplement.

DECADERM. (Merck Sharp & Dohme) Dexamethasone 0.1% w/isopropyl myristate gel, wood alcohols, refined lanolin alcohol, microcrystalline wax, anhydrous citric acid, anhydrous sodium phosphate dibasic. Tube 30 Gm.
Use: Corticosteroid.

DECADROL. (Paddock) Dexamethasone sodium phosphate 4 mg/ml. Vial 5 ml.
Use: Corticosteroid.

DECADRON. (Merck Sharp & Dohme) Dexamethasone. **Tab.:** 0.25 mg: Bot. 100s; 0.5 mg: Bot. 100s, UD 100s; 0.75 mg: 100s, UD 100s; 1.5 mg: Bot. 50s, UD 100s; 4 mg: Bot. 50s, UD 100s; 6 mg: Bot. 50s, UD 100s. **Elix.:** 0.5 mg/5 ml, benzoic acid 0.1%, alcohol 5% Bot. w/dropper 100 ml, Bot. w/out dropper 237 ml.
Use: Corticosteroid.
W/Neomycin sulfate.
See: NeoDecadron, Ophth. Soln., Ophth. Oint., Topical, Cream (Merck Sharp & Dohme).

DECADRON-LA SUSPENSION. (Merck Sharp & Dohme) Dexamethasone acetate equivalent to 8 mg dexamethasone/ml w/sodium Cl 6.67 mg, creatinine 5 mg, disodium edetate 0.5 mg, sodium carboxymethylcellulose 5 mg, polysorbate 80 0.75 mg, sodium hydroxide to adjust pH, benzyl alcohol 9 mg, sodium bisulfite 1 mg, water for injection q.s. 1 ml. Vial 1 ml, 5 ml.
Use: Corticosteroid.

DECADRON PHOSPHATE. (Merck Sharp & Dohme) Dexamethasone sodium phosphate equivalent in various forms:
Ophth. Soln.: 0.1% w/creatinine, sodium citrate, sodium borate, polysorbate 80, hydrochloric acid to adjust pH, disodium edetate, sodium bisulfite 0.1%, water for injection, phenylethanol 0.25%, benzalkonium Cl 0.02%. Ocumeter dispenser 5 ml.
Use: Ophthalmic and otic anti-inflammatory agent.
Ophth. Oint.: 0.05% w/white petrolatum and mineral oil. Tube 3.5 Gm.
Use: Ophthalmic and otic corticosteroid.
Cream: 0.1% w/stearyl alcohol, cetyl alcohol, mineral oil, polyoxyl 40 stearate, sorbitol solution, methyl polysilicone emulsion, creatinine, purified water, sodium citrate, disodium edetate, sodium hydroxide to adjust pH, methylparaben 0.15%, sorbic acid 0.1%. Tube 15 Gm, 30 Gm.
Use: Topical corticosteroid.
Turbinaire: Dexamethasone sodium phosphate 0.1 mg equivalent to dexamethasone 0.084 mg w/fluorochlorohydrocarbons as propellants and alcohol 2%. Aerosol w/nasal applicator. Container 170 sprays; refill package without nasal applicator.
Use: Nasal corticosteroid.
W/Neomycin.
Use: Corticosteroid, anti-infective.
See: NeoDecadron, Ophth. Soln., Ophth. Oint., Topical Cream (Merck Sharp & Dohme)
W/Xylocaine **Inj.:** Dexamethasone sodium phosphate equivalent to dexamethasone phosphate 4 mg, lidocaine HCl 10 mg, citric acid 10 mg, creatinine 8 mg, sodium bisulfite 0.5 mg, disodium edetate 0.5 mg, sodium hydroxide to adjust pH, water for injection, methylparaben 1.5 mg, propylparaben 0.2 mg/ml. Vial 5 ml.
Use: Corticosteroid.

DECADRON PHOSPHATE INJECTION. (Merck Sharp & Dohme) Dexamethasone sodium phosphate 4 mg or 24 mg/ml, creatinine 8 mg, sodium citrate 10 mg, disodium edetate 0.5 mg (24 mg/ml only), sodium hydroxide to adjust pH, sodium bisulfite 1 mg, methylparaben 1.5 mg, propylparaben 0.2 mg/ml. **4 mg/ml:** Vial 1 ml, 5 ml, 25 ml. **24 mg/ml** (for I.V. use only): Vial 5 ml, 10 ml.
Use: Corticosteroid.

DECADRON PHOSPHATE RESPIHALER. (Merck Sharp & Dohme) Dexamethasone sodium phosphate equivalent to 0.1 mg dexamethasone phosphate (approximately 0.084 mg dexamethasone) w/fluorochlorohydrocarbons as propellants, alcohol 2%. Aerosol for oral inhalation, 170 sprays in 12.6 Gm pressurized container.
Use: Bronchodilator.

DECA-DURABOLIN. (Organon) Nandrolone decanoate injection w/benzyl alcohol 10%. **50 mg/ml:** Multidose vial 2 ml. **100 mg/ml:** Multidose vial 2 ml, syringe 1 ml. **200 mg/ml:** Multidose vial 1 ml, syringe 1 ml.
Use: Anabolic steroid.

DECA-DURABOLIN REDIJECT SYRINGES. (Organon) Nandrolone decanoate 50 mg, 100 mg or 200 mg/ml. Syringe 1 ml Box 25s.
Use: Anabolic steroid.

DECAGEN. (Goldline) Elemental iron 30 mg, vitamins A 9000 IU, D 400 IU, E 30 mg, B_1 10 mg, B_2 10 mg, B_3 20 mg, B_5 20 mg, B_6 5 mg, B_{12} 10 mcg, C 90 mg, folic acid 0.4 mg, Ca, Cr, Cu, I, K, Mg, Mn, Mo, P, Se, zinc 15 mg, vitamin K 25 mcg, biotin 45 mcg/Tab. Bot. 130s, 1000s.
Use: Vitamin/mineral supplement.

DECAJECT. (Mayrand) Dexamethasone sodium phosphate 4 mg/ml. Vial 5 ml, 10 ml.
Use: Corticosteroid.

DECAJECT-L.A. (Mayrand) Dexamethasone acetate 8 mg/ml suspension, polysorbate 80, carboxymethylcellulose, sodium bisulfite, EDTA, benzyl alcohol. Inj. vial 5 ml.
Use: Corticosteroid.

DECAJEST LA. (Mayrand) Dexamethasone acetate 8 mg/ml. Vial 5 ml.

Use: Corticosteroid.
DECALIX. (Pharmed) Dexamethasone 0.5 mg/5 ml Bot. 100 ml.
Use: Corticosteroid.
DECAMETH. (Foy) Dexamethasone sodium phosphate injection 4 mg/5 cc vial.
Use: Corticosteroid.
DECAMETH L.A. (Foy) Dexamethasone sodium phosphate injection. 8 mg/ml. Vial/5 ml.
Use: Corticosteroid.
DECAMETH TABLETS. (Foy) Dexamethasone 0.75 mg/Tab. Bot. 1000s.
Use: Corticosteroid.
DECAMETHONIUM IODIDE. B.A.N. Decamethylenedi(trimethylammonium iodide)
Use: Muscle relaxant.
DECAPRYN. (Merrell Dow) Doxylamine succinate 12.5 mg/Tab. Bot. 100s.
Use: Antihistamine.
W/Pyridoxine HCl.
See: Bendectin, Tab. (Merrell Dow).
DECASONE INJECTION. (Forest Pharm.) Dexamethasone sodium phosphate equivalent to dexamethasone phosphate 4 mg/ml. Vial 5 ml.
Use: Corticosteroid.
DECASPRAY. (Merck Sharp & Dohme) Topical dexamethasone aerosol. Every second of spray dispenses approximately 0.075 mg of dexamethasone. Dexamethasone 10 mg, isopropyl myristate, isobutane in pressurized container 25 Gm.
Use: Corticosteroid, topical.
DECAVITAMIN CAPSULES AND TABLETS, U.S.P. XXI. Vitamins A 4000 IU, D 400 IU, C 70 mg, calcium pantothenate 10 mg, B_{12} 5 mcg, folic acid 100 mcg, nicotinamide 20 mg, B_6 2 mg, B_2 2 mg, B_1 2 mg/Cap. or Tab.
Use: Vitamin therapy.
DECCASOL-T. (Kenyon) Vitamins B_1 10 mg, B_2 5 mg, B_6 2 mg, pantothenic acid 10 mg, niacinamide 30 mg, B_{12} 3 mcg, C 100 mg, E 5 IU, A 10,000 IU, D 1000 IU, iron 15 mg, copper 1 mg, manganese 1 mg, magnesium 5 mg, zinc 1.5 mg/Tab. Bot. 100s.
Use: Vitamin/mineral supplement.
DECHOLIN. (Miles Pharm) Dehydrocholic acid 250 mg/Tab. Bot. 100s, 500s.
Use: Hydrocholeric.
DECHLORISON ACETATE. 9-alpha, 11-beta, dichloro-1,4-pregnadiene-17-alpha, 21-diol-3,20-dione-21 acetate. Diloderm.
DECICAIN. Tetracaine HCl.
DECITABINE. USAN.
Use: Antineoplastic.
DECLABEN. USAN.
Use: Antiarthritic, emphysema therapy adjunct.
DECLENPERONE. USAN.
Use: Sedative.
DECLOMYCIN HCl. (Lederle) Demeclocycline HCl. **Cap.:** 150 mg Bot. 100s. **Tab.:** 150 mg Bot. 100s; 300 mg Bot. 48s.
Use: Antibacterial, tetracycline.
DECOBEL LANACAPS. (Lannett) Belladonna alkaloids 0.128 mg, phenylpropanolamine HCl 50 mg, chlorpheniramine maleate 1 mg, pheniramine maleate 12.5 mg/Cap. Bot. 100s, 1000s.
Use: Decongestant, antihistamine.
DECOFED. (Various Mfr.) Pseudoephedrine HCl 30 mg/5 ml. Syr. Bot. 120 ml, 240 ml, pt, gal.
Use: Decongestant.
DECOHIST CAPSULES. (Towne) Chlorpheniramine maleate 1 mg, phenylpropanolamine HCl 12.5 mg, salicylamide 180 mg, caffeine 15 mg/Cap. Bot. 18s.
Use: Antihistamine, decongestant, analgesic.
DECOJEN INJECTION. (Jenkins) Atropine sulfate 0.2 mg, phenylpropanolamine HCl 12.5 mg, chlorpheniramine maleate 5 mg, water for injection q.s./ml. Vial 10 ml, 12s.
Use: Anticholinergic/antispasmodic, decongestant, antihistamine.
DE-COMBEROL. (Schein) Estradiol cypionate 2 mg and testosterone cypionate 50 mg/ml in oil. Inj. Vial 10 ml.
Use: Estrogen, androgen combination.
DECONADE. (H.L. Moore) Phenylpropanolamine HCl 75 mg, chlorpheniramine maleate 12 mg/Cap. Bot. 100s, 1000s.
Use: Decongestant, antihistamine.
DECONAMINE SR CAPSULES. (Berlex) Chlorpheniramine maleate 8 mg, d-pseudoephedrine HCl 120 mg/Cap. Bot. 100s, 500s.
Use: Antihistamine, decongestant.
DECONAMINE SYRUP, DYE FREE. (Berlex) Chlorpheniramine maleate 2 mg, d-pseudoephedrine HCl 30 mg/5 ml, sorbitol. Bot. 473 ml.
Use: Antihistamine, decongestant.
DECONAMINE TABLETS, DYE-FREE. (Berlex) Chlorpheniramine maleate 4 mg, d-pseudoephedrine HCl 60 mg/Tab. Bot. 100s.
Use: Antihistamine, decongestant.
DECONGESTANT FORMULA MEDIQUELL. (Parke-Davis Prods) Dextromethorphan HBr 30 mg, pseudoephedrine HCl 60 mg/Square.
Use: Antitussive, decongestant.
DECONSAL II CAPSULES. (Adams) Pseudoephedrine 60 mg, guaifenesin 600 mg/Cap. Bot. 100s.
Use: Decongestant, expectorant.
DECONSAL SPRINKLE CAPSULE. (Adams) Phenylephrine 10 mg, guaifenesin 200 mg/S.R. Cap. Bot. 100s.
Use: Decongestant, expectorant.
•**DECOQUINATE.** USAN. Ethyl 6-decyloxy-7-ethoxy-4-hydroxyquinoline-3-carboxylate.
Use: Antiprotozoan, veterinary medicine.
See: Deccox.
•**DECTAFLUR.** USAN.
Use: Dental caries prophylactic.
DECUBITEX. (I.C.P) **Oint.:** Biebrich scarlet red sulfonated 0.1%, balsam Peru, castor oil, zinc oxide, starch, sodium propionate, parabens. Jar 15 Gm, 60 Gm, 120 Gm, lb. **Pow.:** Biebrich scarlet red sulfonated 0.1%, starch, zinc oxide,

sodium propionate, parabens. Bot. 30 Gm, UD 1 Gm.
Use: Wound-healing agent, emollient, antipruritic.

DECYLENES. (Rugby) Undecylenic acid, zinc undecylenate. Oint. Tube 30 Gm, lb.
Use: Antifungal, external.

DEEP DOWN PAIN RELIEF RUB. (Beecham Products) Methyl salicylate 15%, menthol 5%, camphor 0.5%. Tube 1.25 oz, 3 oz.
Use: External analgesic.

DEEP STRENGTH MUSTEROLE. (Schering-Plough) Methyl salicylate 30%, menthol 3%, methyl nicotinate 0.5% Tube 1.25 oz, 3 oz.
Use: External analgesic.

DEFED-60. (Ferndale) Pseudoephedrine 60 mg/Tab. Bot 1000s.
Use: Decongestant.

•**DEFEROXAMINE.** USAN.
Use: Chelating agent for iron.

•**DEFEROXAMINE HYDROCHLORIDE.** USAN.
Use: Chelating agent for iron.

•**DEFEROXAMINE MESYLATE,** U.S.P. XXII. Sterile, U.S.P. XXII. *N*-[5-[3-[(5-aminopentyl) hydroxycar- bamoyl]propionamido]-pentyl]-3-[[5-(*N*-hydroxyacetamido) entyl]-carbamoyl]-propionohydroxamic acid.
Use: Iron depleter.
See: Desferal, Amp. (Ciba).

DEFICOL. (Vangard) Bisacodyl 5 mg/Tab. Bot. 100s, 1000s.
Use: Laxative.

•**DEFLAZACORT.** USAN.
Use: Anti-inflammatory.

DEGEST-2. (Barnes-Hind) Naphazoline HCl 0.012%, benzalkonium Cl 0.0067%, disodium edetate 0.02%. Bot. 15 ml.
Use: Ophthalmic decongestant.

DEHIST. (Forest) **S.R. Cap:** Phenylpropanolamine HCl 75 mg, chlorpheniramine maleate 8 mg Bot. 100s, 1000s. **Inj:** Brompheniramine maleate 10 mg/ml, methyl and propyl parabens. Vial 10 ml.
Use: Decongestant, antihistamine.

•**DEHYDROACETIC ACID,** N.F. XVII.
Use: Pharmaceutic aid (preservative).

DEHYDROCHOLATE SODIUM INJ., U.S.P. XXI. Sodium 3,7,12-trioxo-5B-Cholan-24-oate.
Use: Relief of liver congestion; diagnosis of cardiac failure.
See: Decholine Sodium, Inj. (Miles Pharm).

7-DEHYDROCHOLESTEROL, ACTIVATED. (Various Mfr.) Vitamin D-3.

•**DEHYDROCHOLIC ACID,** U.S.P. XXII. Tab., U.S.P. XXII. 3,7,12-Trioxo-5β-cholan-24-oic acid.
Ketocholanic acid, oxidized cholic acid, bile acids oxidized.
Use: Orally, hydrocholeretic and choleretic.
See: Atrocholin,Tab. (Glaxo).
Cholan-DH, Tab. (Pennwalt).
Ketocholanic acid.
Neocholan, Tab. (Merrell Dow).
W/Amyloytic and proteolytic enzymes, desoxycholic acid.
See: Bilezyme, Tab. (Geriatric).
W/Bile, homatropine methylbromide, pepsin.
See: Biloric, Caps. (Arcum).
W/Bile, homatropine methylbromide, phenobarbital.
See: Bilamide, Tab. (Norgine).
W/Bile extract, pepsin, pancreatin.
See: Progestive, Tab. (NCP).
W/Desoxycholic acid.
See: Combichole, Tab. (F. Trout).
Ketosox, Tab. (Ascher).
W/Docusate sodium.
See: Dubbalax-B, Cap. (Redford).
Dubbalax-N, Cap. (Redford).
Neolax, Tab. (Central).
W/Docusate sodium, phenolphthalein.
See: Bolax, Cap. (Boyd).
Sarolax (Saron).
Tripalax, Cap. (Redford).
W/Homatropine methylbromide.
See: Cholan V, Tab. (Pennwalt).
Dranochol, Tab. (Marin).
W/Homatropine methylbromide, sodium pentobarbital.
See: Homachol, Tab. (Lemmon).
W/Methscopolamine, ox bile, amobarbital.
See: Hydrochol Plus, Tab. (Elder).
W/Ox bile, homatropine methylbromide, phenobarbital.
See: Bilamide, Tab. (Norgine).
W/Pancreatin, pepsin, bile salts, desoxycholic acid.
See: Pepsatal, Tab. (Kenyon).
W/Pancreatin, pepsin, ox bile, belladonna extract.
See: Ro-Bile, Tab. (Solvay).
W/Pepsin, pancreatin, ox bile extract, papain.
See: Canz, Tab. (Cole).
W/Pepsin, pancreatin enzyme concentrate, cellulase.
See: Gastroenterase, Tab (Wallace).
W/Phenobarbital, homatropine methylbromide.
See: Cholan-HMB, Tab. (Pennwalt).
W/Phenobarbital, homatropine methylbromide, gerilase, geriprotase, desoxycholic acid.
See: Bilezyme Plus, Tabs. (Geriatric).
W/Phenolphthalein, docusate sodium.
See: Sarolax, Cap. (Saron).

DEHYDROCHOLIN.
Use: Hydrocholeretic.
See: Dehydrocholic acid.

DEHYDRODESOXYCHOLIC ACID.
See: Cholanic acid.

DEHYDROEMETINE. B.A.N. 3-Ethyl-1,6,7,11b-tetrahydro-9,10-dimethoxy-2-(1,2,3,4-tetrahydro-6,7-dimethoxy-1-isoquinolylmethyl)-4H-benzo[a]-quinolizine. 2,3-Dehydroemetine.
Use: Treatment of amebiasis.

DEKASOL. (Seatrace) Dexamethasone phosphate 4 mg/ml. Vial 5 ml, 10 ml.

Use: Corticosteroid.
DEKASOL L.A. (Seatrace) Dexamethasone acetate 8 mg/ml. Vial 5 ml.
Use: Corticosteroid.
DE-KOFF. (Whiteworth) Terpin hydrate w/dextromethorphan. Elix. Bot. 4 oz.
Use: Antitussive, expectorant.
DELACORT LOTION. (Mericon) Hydrocortisone 0.5%. Bot. 4 oz.
Use: Corticosteroid, topical.
DELADIOL-40. (Dunhall) Estradiol valerate 40 mg/ml, castor oil, benzyl benzoate, benzyl alcohol. Vial 10 ml.
Use: Estrogen.
DELADUMONE. (Squibb Mark) Testosterone enanthate 90 mg, estradiol valerate 4 mg in sesame oil/ml, chlorobutanol 0.5%. Vial 5 ml, 1 dose (1 ml).
Use: Androgen, estrogen combination.
•**DELAPRIL HYDROCHLORIDE.** USAN.
Use: Antihypertensive, enzyme inhibitor.
DEL-AQUA-5. (Del-Ray) Benzoyl peroxide 5%. Tube 1.5 oz.
Use: Anti-acne.
DEL-AQUA-10. (Del-Ray) Benzoyl peroxide 10%. Tube 1.5 oz.
Use: Anti-acne.
DELAQUIN LOTION. (Schlicksup) Hydrocortisone 0.5%, iodoquin 3%. Bot. 3 oz.
Use: Corticosteroid, anti-fungal.
DELATEST. (Dunhall) Testosterone enanthate 100 mg/ml, chlorobutanol in sesame oil. Amp. 10 ml.
Use: Androgen.
DELATESTADIOL. (Dunhall) Testosterone enanthate 90 mg, estradiol valerate 4 mg/ml, chlorobutanol in sesame oil. Amp. 10 ml.
Use: Androgen, estrogen combination.
DELATESTRYL. (Squibb Mark) Testosterone enanthate 200 mg/ml in sesame oil, chlorobutanol 0.5%. Vial 5 ml.
Use: Androgen.
DELCID. (Lakeside) Aluminum hydroxide 600 mg, magnesium hydroxide 665 mg/5 ml, alcohol 0.3%, saccharin. Bot. 8 oz.
Use: Antacid.
DEL-CLENS. (Del-Ray) Soapless cleanser. Bot. 8 oz.
Use: Skin cleanser.
DELCO-LAX. (Delco) Bisacodyl 5 mg/Tab. Bot. 1000s.
Use: Laxative.
DELCOZINE. (Delco) Phendimentrazine tartrate 70 mg/Tab. Bot. 1000s, 5000s.
Use: Anorexiant.
DELESTREC. Estradiol 17-undecanoate.
Use: Estrogen.
DELESTROGEN. (Squibb Mark) Estradiol valerate **10 mg/ml:** In sesame oil, chlorobutanol 0.5%. Vial 5 ml. **20 mg/ml:** In castor oil, benzyl benzoate 20%, benzyl alcohol 2%. Vial 5 ml. **40 mg/ml:** In castor oil, benzyl benzoate 40%, benzyl alcohol 2%. Vial 5 ml.
Use: Estrogen.
DELFEN CONTRACEPTIVE FOAM. (Ortho) Nonoxynol-9 12.5% in an oil-in-water emulsion at pH 4.5 to 5.0. Starter can with applicator 20 Gm. Refill 20 Gm, 50 Gm.
Use: Spermicide.
DELINAL. Propenzolate HydroCl.
•**DELMADINONE ACETATE.** USAN. 6-Chloro-17-hydroxypregna-1, 4, 6-triene-3, 20-dione acetate.
Use: Progestin.
See: Delmate (Syntex).
DELSYM COUGH SUPPRESSANT LIQUID. (McNeil Prods) Dextromethorphan HBr 30 mg/5 ml. Bot. 3 oz.
Use: Antitussive.
DELTA-CORTEF. (Upjohn) Prednisolone 5 mg/Tab. Bot. 100s, 500s.
Use: Corticosteroid.
DELTACORTONE. Prednisone.
Use: Corticosteroid.
DELTA-CORTRIL. Prednisolone.
Use: Corticosteroid.
DELTA-D. (Freeda) Vitamin D_3 400 IU/Tab. Bot. 250s, 500s.
Use: Vitamin D supplement.
•**DELTAFILCON A.** USAN.
Use: Contact lens material.
•**DELTAFILCON B.** USAN.
Use: Contact lens material.
DELTA-1-CORTISONE.
Use: Corticosteroid.
See: Deltasone, Tab. (Upjohn).
DELTA-1-HYDROCORTISONE.
Use: Corticosteroid.
See: Prednisolone (Various Mfr.).
DELTAPEN. (Trimen) Potassium penicillin G (U.S.P.) 400,000 units/5 ml. Oral Susp. Bot. "16 dose." Tab. Bot. 100s.
Use: Antibacterial, penicillin.
DELTASONE. (Upjohn) Prednisone. **2.5 mg:** Tab. Bot. 100s. **5 mg:** Tab. Bot. 100s, 500s, UD 100s, Dosepak 21s. **10 mg, 20 mg:** Tab. Bot. 100s, 500s, UD 100s. **50 mg:** Tab. Bot. 100s, UD 100s.
Use: Corticosteroid.
DELTAVAC. (Trimen) Sulfanilamide 15%, aminacrine HCl 0.2%, allantoin 2%. Vaginal cream: Tube with applicator 113.4 Gm.
Use: Vaginal anti-infective, antiseptic.
DEL-TRAC. (Del-Ray) Acne lotion. Bot. 2 oz.
Use: Anti-acne.
DELTRA-STAB.
Use: Corticosteroid.
See: Prednisolone (Various Mfr.).
DEL-STAT. (Del-Ray) Abradent cleaner. Jar 2 oz.
Use: Anti-acne.
DEL-VI-A. (Del-Ray) Vitamin A 50,000 IU/Cap. Bot. 100s.
Use: Vitamin A supplement.

DELYSID. Lysergic acid diethylamide.
Use: Potent psychotogenic.

DEMAZIN. (Schering-Plough) **Syr.:** Chlorpheniramine maleate 2 mg, phenylpropanolamine HCl 12.5 mg/5 ml, alcohol 7.5%, menthol. Bot. 4 oz. **Tab.:** Chlorpheniramine maleate 4 mg, phenylpropanolamine HCl 25 mg. Box 24s. Bot. 100s, 1000s.
Use: Antihistamine, decongestant.

•**DEMECARIUM BROMIDE,** U.S.P. XXII. Ophth. Soln. U.S.P. XXII.
Use: Cholinergic, (ophthalmic).
See: Humorsol, Soln. (Merck Sharp & Dohme).

•**DEMECLOCYCLINE,** U.S.P. XXII. Oral susp., U.S.P. XXII. 7-Chloro-4-(dimethylamino)-1,4,4α,5,5α,6,11,12α-octahydro-3,6,10,-12,12α-pentahydroxy-1,11-dioxo-2-naphthacene-carboxamide.
Use: Antibacterial.
See: Declomycin Prods. (Lederle).
Ledermycin Prods. (Lederle).

•**DEMECLOCYCLINE HYDROCHLORIDE,** U.S.P. XXII. Cap., Tab., U.S.P. XXII.
Use: Antibacterial.
See: Declomycin HCl, Preps. (Lederle).

•**DEMECLOCYCLINE HYDROCHLORIDE AND NYSTATIN CAPSULES,** U.S.P. XXII.
Use: Antibacterial.
See: Declostatin, Cap. (Lederle).

•**DEMECLOCYCLINE HYDROCHLORIDE AND NYSTATIN TABLETS,** U.S.P. XXII.
Use: Antibacterial.
See: Declostatin, Tab. (Lederle).

DEMECOLCINE. B.A.N. N-Methyl-N-deacetyl-colchicine.
Use: Antimitotic, leukemia therapy.

•**DEMECYCLINE.** USAN.
Use: Antibacterial.

DEMEROL APAP. (Winthrop Pharm) Meperidine HCl 50 mg, acetaminophen 300 mg/Tab. Bot. 100s.
Use: Narcotic analgesic combination.

DEMEROL HYDROCHLORIDE. (Winthrop Pharm) Meperidine HCl. **Syr.:** 50 mg/5 ml, saccharin. Bot. 16 fl oz. **Inj.:** Detecto-Seal, Carpuject, Sterile Cartridge-Needle Unit. **2.5%** (25 mg/ml), **5%** (50 mg/ml), **7.5%** (75 mg/ml), **10%** (100 mg/ml), Box 10s. **Uni-Amp 5%:** 0.5 ml (25 mg)/Amp., 1 ml (50 mg)/Amp., 1.5 ml (75 mg)/Amp., 2 ml (100 mg)/Amp. Box 25s; **10%:** 1 ml (100 mg)/Amp. Box 25s. **Uni-Nest 5%:** 0.5 ml (25 mg)/Amp., 1 ml (50 mg)/Amp., 1.5 ml (75 mg)/Amp., 2 ml (100 mg)/Amp. Box 25s; **10%:** 1 ml/Amp. Box 25s. **Vial: 5%** multiple-dose vial/30 ml Box 1s. **Tab.:** 50 mg or 100 mg. Bot. 100s, 500s.
Use: Narcotic analgesic.

DEMETHYLCHLORTETRACYCLINE HCl.
Use: Antibacterial, tetracycline.
See: Demeclocycline HCl, U.S.P. XXII.

DEMI-REGROTON. (Rhone-Poulenc Rorer) Chlorthalidone 25 mg, reserpine 0.125 mg/Tab. Bot. 100s, 1000s.
Use: Antihypertensive, diuretic.

•**DEMOXEPAM.** USAN. 7-Chloro-1, 3-dihydro-5-phenyl-2H-1, 4-benzodiazepin-2-one-4-oxide.
Use: Minor tranquilizer.

DEMSER. (Merck Sharp & Dohme) Metyrosine 250 mg/Cap. Bot. 100s.
Use: Antihypertensive.

DEMULEN 1/35-21. (Searle) Ethynodiol diacetate 1 mg, ethinyl estradiol 35 mcg/Tab. Compack disp. 21s, 6×21, 24×21. Refill 21s, 12×21.
Use: Oral contraceptive.

DEMULEN 1/35-28. (Searle) Ethynodiol diacetate 1 mg, ethinyl estradiol 35 mcg/Tab.Compack 28s: 21 active tabs, 7 placebo tabs. Compack 6×28, 24×28. Refill 28s, 12×28.
Use: Oral contraceptive.

DEMULEN 1/50-21. (Searle) Ethynodiol diacetate 1 mg, ethinyl estradiol 50 mcg/Tab. Compack Disp. 21s, 6×21, 24×21. Refill 21s, 12×21.
Use: Oral contraceptive.

DEMULEN 1/50-28. (Searle) Ethynodiol diacetate 1 mg, ethinyl estradiol 50 mcg/Tab. Compack 28s: 21 active tabs, 7 placebo tabs. Compack Disp. of 28, 6×28, 24×28. Refill 28s, 12×28.
Use: Oral contraceptive.

DENALAN DENTURE CLEANSER. (Whitehall) Sodium percarbonate 30%. Bot. 7 oz., 13 oz.
Use: Agent for oral hygiene.

•**DENATONIUM BENZOATE,** N.F. XVII. Bitrex (MacFarlan Smith, Ltd. Scotland) Benzyldiethyl [(2, 6-xylylcarbamoyl) methyl] ammonium benzoate.
Use: Denaturant for ethyl alcohol.
See: Bitrex.

DENCORUB. (Last) Methyl salicylate 20%, menthol 0.75%, camphor 1%, eucalyptus oil 0.5%. Tube 1.25 oz, 2.75 oz.
Use: External analgesic.

DENCORUB ANALGESIC LIQUID. (Last) Oleoresin capsicum suspension in aqueous vehicle. Bot. 6 oz.
Use: External analgesic.

DENGESIC. (Scott-Alison) Salicylamide 100 mg, acetaminophen 240 mg, phenyltoloxamine dihydrogen citrate 30 mg, butabarbital ⅛ gr/Tab. Bot. 60s, 500s.
Use: Analgesic, sedative/hypnotic.

•**DENOFUNGIN.** USAN.
Use: Antifungal, antibacterial.

DENOREX. (Whitehall) Coal tar solution 9%, menthol 1.5%. Shampoo Bot. 4 oz, 8 oz.
Use: Antiseborrheic.

DENOREX MOUNTAIN FRESH. (Whitehall) Coal tar solution 9%, menthol 1.5%. Bot. 4 oz, 8 oz.
Use: Antiseborrheic.

DENOREX WITH CONDITIONERS. (Whitehall) Coal tar solution 9%, menthol 1.5%. Bot 4 oz, 8 oz.
Use: Antiseborrheic.

DENQUEL. (Procter & Gamble) Potassium nitrate 5%, calcium carbonate, glycerin, flavors. Tube 1.6 oz, 3 oz, 4.5 oz.
Use: Agent for oral hygiene, preparation for sensitive teeth.

DENTAL CARIES PREVENTIVE. (Hoyt) Fluoride ion 1.2%, alumina abrasive. 2 Gm Box 200s, Jar 9 oz.
Use: Dental caries preventative.

DENTAL TYPE SILICA, U.S.P. XXII.

DENTROL. (Block) Carboxymethylcellulose, polyethelyne oxide homopolymer, peppermint and spearmint in mineral oil base. Bot. 0.9 oz, 1.8 oz.
Use: Denture adhesive.

DENT'S DENTAL POULTICE. (C.S. Dent) Glycerin mineral oil, polyoxyethylene sorbitan monooleate. Bot. 0.125 oz, 0.25 oz.
Use: Dental poultice.

DENT'S EAR WAX DROPS. (C.S. Dent) Glycerin, mineral oil, polyoxyethylene sorbitan monooleate. Bot. 0.125 oz, 0.25 oz.
Use: Otic preparation.

DENT'S LOTION-JEL. (C.S. Dent) Benzocaine in special base. Tube 0-2 oz.
Use: Local anesthetic, oral.

DENT'S TOOTHACHE DROPS TREATMENT. (C.S. Dent) Alcohol 60%, chlorobutanol anhydrous (chloroform derivative) 0.09%, propylene glycol, eugenol. Bot. 0.125 oz.
Use: Local anesthetic, oral.

DENT'S TOOTHACHE GUM. (C.S. Dent) Benzocaine, eugenol, petrolatum in base of cotton and wax. Box 0.035 oz.
Use: Local anesthetic, oral.

DENT-ZEL-ITE. (Last) **Oral Mucosal Analgesic:** Benzocaine 5%, alcohol, glycerin. Bot. 1/16 oz,. **Temporary Dental Filling:** Sandarac gum, alcohol. Bot. 1/16 oz,. **Toothache Drops:** Eugenol 85% in alcohol. Bot. 1/16 oz.
Use: Local anesthetic, oral.

DENYL SODIUM.
Use: Anticonvulsant.
See: Diphenylhydantoin Sodium, Cap. (Various Mfr.).

DEOXYCHOLIC ACID.
See: Desoxycholic Acid, Tab. (Various Mfr.).

DEPAKENE. (Abbott) Valproic acid. **Cap.:** 250 mg. Bot. 100s, UD 100s. **Syr.:** 250 mg/5 ml, sorbitol. Bot. 480 ml.
Use: Anticonvulsant.

DEPAKOTE. (Abbott) Divalproex sodium 125 mg, 250 mg or 500 mg/enteric coated tab and 125 mg/sprinkle cap. **125 mg:** Bot. 100s. **250 mg:** Bot. 100s, UD 100s. **500 mg:** Bot. 100s, UD 100s. **125 mg sprinkle:** Bot. 100s, UD 100s.
Use: Anticonvulsant.

dep ANDRO 100. (Forest) Testosterone cypionate in cottonseed oil 100 mg/ml, benzyl alcohol. Vial 10 ml.
Use: Androgen.

dep ANDRO 200. (Forest) Testosterone cypionate in cottonseed oil 200 mg/ml, benzyl benzoate, benzyl alcohol. Vial 10 ml.
Use: Androgen.

dep ANDROGYN. (Forest) Testosterone cypionate 50 mg, estradiol cypionate 2 mg/ml, chlorobutanol, cottonseed oil. Vial 10 ml.
Use: Androgen, estrogen combination.

DEPA-SYRUP. (Alra) Valproic acid syrup 250 mg/5 ml. Bot. 4 oz, 16 oz.
Use: Anticonvulsant.

DEPEN TITRATABLE TABLETS. (Wallace) Penicillamine 250 mg/Tab. Bot. 100s.
Use: Penicillamine.

DEPEPSEN. Amylosulfate sodium.
Use: Digestive aid.

DEP-ESTRADIOL. (Rocky Mtn.) Estradiol cypionate 5 mg/ml. Vial 10 ml.
Use: Estrogen.

dep GYNOGEN. (Forest) Estradiol cypionate in cottonseed oil 5 mg/ml, cottonseed oil, chlorobutanol. Vial 10 ml.
Use: Estrogen.

dep MEDALONE 40. (Forest) Methylprednisolone acetate in aqueous suspension 40 mg/ml, polyethylene glycol, myristyl-gamma-picolinium Cl. Vial 5 ml.
Use: Corticosteroid.

dep MEDALONE 80. (Forest) Methylprednisolone acetate 80 mg/ml, polyethylene glycol, myristyl-gamma-picolinium Cl. Vial 5 ml.
Use: Corticosteroid.

DEPOESTRA. (Tennessee Pharm.) Estradiol cypionate 5 mg/ml. Vial 10 ml.
Use: Estrogen.

DEPO-ESTRADIOL. (Upjohn) Estradiol cypionate 1 mg or 5 mg/ml, chlorobutanol anhydrous 5.4 mg/ml, cottonseed oil. **1 mg/ml:** Vial 10 ml. **5 mg/ml:** Vial 5 ml.
Use: Estrogen.

DEPOGEN. (Sig) Estradiol valerate 10 mg or 20 mg/ml in oil. Vial 10 ml.
Use: Estrogen.

DEPOGEN. (Hyrex) Estradiol cypionate 5 mg/ml, cottonseed oil, chlorobutanol. Vial 10 ml.
Use: Estrogen.

DEPOJECT. (Mayrand) Methylprednisolone acetate 40 mg or 80 mg/ml suspension with polyethylene glycol and myristyl-gamma-picolinium Cl. Inj. Vial 5 ml.
Use: Corticosteroid.

DEPONIT. (Wyeth-Ayerst) Nitroglycerin transdermal delivery system containing 5 mg or 10 mg/24 Hrs. Box 30s.
Use: Vasodilator, antianginal.

DEPO-PRED 40. (Hyrex) Methylprednisolone acetate suspension 40 mg/ml, polyethylene glycol, myristyl-gamma-picolinum Cl. Vial 5 ml, 10 ml.
Use: Corticosteroid.

DEPO-PROVERA. (Upjohn) Medroxyprogesterone acetate 100 mg or 400 mg/ml. **100 mg/ml:** Suspended in polyethylene glycol 3350 27.6

mg, polysorbate 80 1.84 mg, sodium Cl 8.3 mg, methylparaben 1.75 mg, propylparaben 0.194 mg/ml. Vial 5 ml. **400 mg/ml:** Suspended in polyethylene glycol 3350 20.3 mg, sodium sulfate (anhydrous) 11 mg, myristyl-gamma-picolinium Cl 1.69 mg/ml. Vial 2.5 ml, 10 ml, 1 ml U-Ject.
Use: Progestin.

DEPOTEST. (Hyrex) Testosterone cypionate. **100 mg:** With cottonseed oil, benzyl alcohol. **200 mg:** With cottonseed oil, benzyl benzoate, benzyl alcohol. Vial 10 ml.
Use: Androgen.

DEPO-TESTADIOL. (Upjohn) Testosterone cypionate 50 mg, estradiol cypionate 2 mg, chlorobutanol 5.4 mg, cottonseed oil 874 mg/ml. Vial 1 ml, 10 ml.
Use: Androgen estrogen combination.

DEPOTESTOGEN. (Hyrex) Testosterone cypionate 50 mg, estradiol cypionate 2 mg, chlorobutanol 5 mg/ml in cottonseed oil. Vial 10 ml.
Use: Androgen, estrogen combination.

DEPO-TESTOSTERONE. (Upjohn) Testosterone cypionate. **100 mg/ml:** In benzyl alcohol 9.45 mg, cottonseed oil 736 mg/ml. Vial 1 ml, 10 ml. **200 mg/ml:** In benzyl benzoate 0.2 ml, benzyl alcohol 9.45 mg, cottonseed oil 560 mg/ml. Vial 1 ml, 10 ml.
Use: Androgen.

DEPRENYL. Selegiline HCl (Orphan Drug).
Use: Adjuvant in parkinsonism.
See: Eldepryl (Somerset).
Sponsor: Farmacon.

DEPRODONE. B.A.N. 11 β 17α-Dihydroxypregna-1, 4-diene-3,20-dione.
Use: Corticosteroid.

DEPROIST EXPECTORANT WITH CODEINE. (Geneva Marsam) Pseudoephedrine HCl 30 mg, codeine phosphate 10 mg, guaifenesin 100 mg/5 ml. Bot. 120 ml, 480 ml.
Use: Decongestant, antitussive, expectorant.

DEPROL TABLETS. (Wallace) Meprobamate 400 mg, benactyzine HCl 1 mg/Tab. Bot. 100s, 500s.
Use: Antidepressant.

•**DEPROSTIL.** USAN.
Use: Antisecretory.

DEP-TEST. (Sig) Testosterone cypionate 100 mg/ml. Vial 10 ml.
Use: Androgen.

DEP-TESTOSTERONE. (Rocky Mtn.) Testosterone cypionate. **100 mg/ml:** Vial 1 ml. **200 mg/ml:** Vial 10 ml.
Use: Androgen.

DEP-TESTRADIOL. (Rocky Mtn.) Estradiol cypionate 2 mg, testosterone cypionate 50 mg/ml. Vial 10 ml.
Use: Estrogen, androgen combination.

DEPTROPINE. B.A.N. 3-(10, 11-Dihydrodibenzo-[a, d]cycloheptadien-5-yloxy)tropane.
Use: Bronchodilator.

DEQUALINIUM CHLORIDE. B.A.N. Decamethylenedi-(4-aminoquinaldinium Cl).
Use: Antiseptic.

DEQUASINE. (Miller) L-lysine 20 mg, l-cysteine 100 mg, dl-methionine 50 mg, vitamin C 200 mg, iron 5 mg, Cu, I, Mg, Mn, Zn. Tab. Bot. 100s.
Use: Vitamin/mineral supplement.

DERIFIL. (Rystan) Chlorophyllin copper complex 100 mg/Tab. Bot. 30s, 100s, 1000s.
Use: Internal deodorant.

DERMACARE. (Jenkins) Hexachlorophene, camphor, menthol, lanolin. Lot. Bot. 2 oz, 6 oz, pt, gal.
Use: Antiseptic.

DERMACOAT AEROSOL SPRAY. (Century) Benzocaine 4.5%. Bot. 7 oz.
Use: Local anesthetic, topical.

DERMACORT CREAM. (Solvay) Hydrocortisone 0.5% or 1% in a water soluble cream of stearyl alcohol, cetyl alcohol, isopropyl palmitate, citric acid, polyoxyethylene 40 stearate, sodium phosphate, propylene glycol, water, benzyl alcohol, buffered to pH 5.0. 0.5% in 30 Gm, 1% in 1 lb.
Use: Corticosteroid, topical.

DERMACORT LOTION. (Solvay) Hydrocortisone 1% in lotion base, buffered to pH 5.0. Paraben free. Bot. 120 ml.
Use: Corticosteroid, topical.

DERMA-COVER. (Scrip) Sulfur, salicylic acid, hyamine 10x, isopropyl alcohol 22%, in powder film forming base. Bot. 2 oz.
Use: Keratolytic.

DERMA-GUARD. (Greer) Protective adhesive pow. Can w/sifter top, 4 oz. Spray top Bot. 4 oz, pkg. 1 lb. Rings. Pkg. 5s, 10s.
Use: Skin protectant.

DERMAL-RUB BALM. (Hauck) Menthol racemic 7%, camphor 1%, methyl salicylate 1%, cajuput oil 1%. Cream. Jar 1 oz, 1 lb.
Use: External analgesic.

DERMA-MEDICONE. (Medicone) Benzocaine 20 mg, oxyquinoline sulfate 10.5 mg, menthol 4.8 mg, ichthammol 10 mg, zinc oxide 137 mg/Gm w/petrolatum, lanolin, perfume, certified color. Oint. Tube 1 oz, Jar lb.
Use: Local anesthetic, antipruritic, vasoconstrictor.

DERMA MEDICONE-HC. (Medicone) Hydrocortisone acetate 10 mg, benzocaine 20 mg, oxyquinoline sulfate 10.5 mg, ephedrine HCl 1.1 mg, menthol 4.8 mg, ichthammol 10 mg, zinc oxide 137 mg/Gm, petrolatum, lanolin, perfume Oint. Tube 7 Gm, 20 Gm.
Use: Corticosteroid, local anesthetic, antipruritic

DERMANEED. (Hanlon) Zirconium oxide 4.5%, calamine 6%, zinc oxide 4%, actamer 0.1% in bland lotionized base. Bot. 4 oz.
Use: Antipruritic.

DERMA-PAX. (Recsei) Methapyrilene HCl 0.22% chlorothenylpyramine maleate 0.06%, pyrilamine maleate 0.22%, benzyl alcohol 1%, chloro-

butanol 1%, isopropyl alcohol 40%. Liq. 4 oz, pt.
Use: Topical antipruritic, antihistamine.

DERMA-PAX HC. (Recsei) Hydrocortisone 0.5%, pyrilamine maleate 0.2%, pheniramine maleate 0.2%, chlorpheniramine 0.06%, benzyl alcohol 1%. Liq. Bot. 60 ml, 120 ml, 480 ml.
Use: Topical corticosteroid, antihistamine.

DERMAPHILL. (Torch) Aluminum acetate 1%, phenol 1%, menthol 0.5%, camphor 3%, in hydrophilic vehicle. Jar 1 lb, 2 oz.
Use: Skin protectant.

)ERMA-pH SKIN LOTION. (Day-Baldwin) pH 4.6 to 4.9. Mentholated or plain. Plastic squeeze bot. 4 oz, 8 oz. Plastic bot. gal.

)ERMAREX. (Hyrex) Hydrocortisone 1%, clioquinol 3%, pramoxine HCl 0.5%. Cream. Tube 0.5 oz.
Use: Corticosteroid, antifungal, antibacterial agent.

ERMA-SMOOTHE/FS OIL. (Hill) Fluocinolone acetonide 0.01%. Oil. Bot. 4 oz.
Use: Antipsoriatic, antiseborrheic.

ERMA-SMOOTHE OIL. (Hill) Refined peanut oil, mineral oil in lipophilic base.
Use: Antipruritic, skin protectant.

ERMA SOAP. (Ferndale) Dowicil 0.1%. 4 oz w/ dispenser.
Use: Antiseptic.

ERMA-SOFT. (Vogarell) Medicated cream. Salicylic acid, castor oil, triethanolamine. Tube ¾ oz.
Use: Keratolytic.

ERMA-SONE 1%. (Hill) Hydrocortisone 1%, pramoxine HCl 1%, cetyl alcohol, glyceryl monosterate, isopropyl myristate, potassium sorbate, furcelleran.
Use: Corticosteroid, topical.

ERMASORCIN. (Lamond) Resorcin 2%, sulfur 5%. Bot. 1 oz, 2 oz, 4 oz, 8 oz, pt, 32 oz, 0.5 gal.
Use: Anti-acne, antiseborrheic.

ERMASSAGE. (Kendall) Mineral oil, lanolin, menthol 0.11%, TEA-stearate, propylene glycol, stearic acid, diammonium phosphate, triclosan, urea, parabens. Lot. Bot. 180 ml, 300 ml, 450 ml.
Use: Emollient.

ERMASTRINGE. (Lamond) Bot. 4 oz, 6 oz, 8 oz, pt, 32 oz, gal.
Use: Skin cleanser.

ERMASUL. (Lamond) Sulfur 5%. Bot. 1 oz, 2 oz, 4 oz, 8 oz, pt, 32 oz, 0.5 gal, gal.
Use: Anti-acne, antiseborrheic.

ERMATHYN. (Davis & Sly) Benzyl alcohol 3%, benzocaine 3.5%, butyl-p-aminobenzoate 1%, phenylmercuric borate. Tube 1 oz.
Use: Local anesthetic.

ERMATIC BASE. (Whorton) Compounding cream base. Bot. 16 oz.
Use: Cream and lotion base.

ERMATOL.
See: Bismuth subgallate, Preps. (Various Mfr.).

DERMAX. (Dermco) Methphenoxydiol 100 mg, (3-(2-methosyphenoxy)-1, 2-propanediol). Bot. 100s, 1000s.
Use: Tension states.

DERMED. (Holloway) Vitamins A and D with hydrogenated vegetable oil. Cream. Tube 60 Gm, 120 Gm.
Use: Emollient.

DERMEZE. (Premo) Thenylpyramine HCl 2%, benzocaine 2%, tyrothricin 0.25 mg/Gm. Massage Lot. Bot. 5¾ oz.
Use: Topical antihistamine, antibiotic, anesthetic.

DERMOLIN. (Hauck) Menthol racemic, methyl salicylate, camphor, mustard oil, isopropyl alcohol 8%. Bot. 3 oz, pt, gal.
Use: Liniment, topical.

DERMOPLAST AEROSOL SPRAY. (Wyeth-Ayerst) Benzocaine 20%, menthol 0.5%, in water-dispersible base of Tween 85, PEG 400 monolaurate, methylparaben as preservative, propellants. Spray 2.75 oz, 6 oz.
Use: Topical anesthetic, antipruritic.

DERMOVAN. (Owen/Galderma) Glyceryl stearate, spermaceti, mineral oil, glycerin, cetyl alcohol, butylparaben, methylparaben, propylparaben, purified water. Vanishing-type base, Jar 1 lb.
Use: Skin protectant.

DERMTEX HC. (Pfeiffer) Hydrocortisone 0.5% in a glycerin base. Tube 15 Gm.
Use: Corticosteroid, topical.

D.E.S.
See: Diethylstilbestrol.

DESACCHROMIN. A nonprotein bacterial colloidal dispersion of polysaccharide.

•**DESCICLOVIR.** USAN.
Use: Antiviral.

•**DESCINOLONE ACETONIDE.** USAN.
Use: Glucocorticoid.

DESENEX. (Pharmacraft) **Cream:** Undecylenic acid, zinc undecylenate. Tube 0.5 oz, 1 oz. **Oint.:** Undecylenic acid 5%, zinc undecylenate 20%. Tube 0.9 oz, 1.8 oz, Can 1 lb. **Pow.:** Undecylenic acid 2%, zinc undecylenate 20%. Can 1.5 oz, 3 oz, Carton 1 lb. **Liq.:** Undecylenic acid 10%, isopropyl alcohol 47.1%. Pump spray bot. 1.5 oz. **Spray Pow.:** Undecylenic acid 2%, zinc undecylenate 20%. Aerosol can 2.7 oz, 5.5 oz. **Penetrating Foam:** Undecylenic acid 10%, isopropyl alcohol 35.2%. Can 1.5 oz.
Use: Antifungal, external.

DESENEX FOOT & SNEAKER SPRAY. (Pharmacraft) Aluminum chlorhydrex w/alcohol 89.3%. Aerosol can 2.7 oz.
Use: Foot deodorant, antiperspirant.

DE SERPA. (de Leon) Reserpine 0.25 mg or 0.5 mg/Tab. Bot. 100s, 500s, 1000s (0.25 mg only).
Use: Antihypertensive.

DESERPIDINE. B.A.N. 11-Demethoxyreserpine.
Use: Tranquilizer.

DESERPIDINE. An alkaloid derived from *Rauwolfia canescens.* 11-Desmethoxyreserpine (Raunormine).
Use: Antihypertensive.
See: Harmonyl, Tab. (Abbott).
W/Hydrochlorothiazide.
See: Oreticyl, Tab. (Abbott).
W/Methyclothiazide.
See: Enduronyl and Enduronyl Forte, Tab. (Abbott).

DESFERAL. (Ciba) Deferoxamine mesylate 500 mg/5 ml. Amp. 4s.
Use: Antidote.

DESFERRIOXAMINE. B.A.N. 30-Amino-3,14,25-tri- hydroxy-3,9,14,20,25-penta-azatriacontane-2,10,- 13,21,24-pentaone. Deferoxamine (I.N.N.).
Use: Chelating agent.

•**DESFLURANE.** USAN.

•**DESIPRAMINE HYDROCHLORIDE,** U.S.P. XXII. Cap., Tab., U.S.P. XXII. 10, 11-Dihydro-5-[3-(me- thylamiLL) Lropyl]-5H-dibenz[b,f]azepine hydroCl.
Use: Antidepressant.
See: Norpramin, Tab. (Merrell Dow).
Pertofrane, Cap. (USV).

DESITIN. (Leeming) **Pow.:** Talc. Can 3 oz, 7 oz, 10 oz. **Oint.:** Cod liver oil, zinc oxide 40%, talc, petrolatum, lanolin. Tube 1 oz, 2 oz, 4 oz, 8 oz, Jar 1 lb.
Use: Topical astringent, skin protectant.

DESLANOSIDE, U.S.P. XXI. Inj., U.S.P. XXI. Deacetyllanatoside C.
Use: Cardiotonic.
See: Cedilanid-D, Amp. (Sandoz).

•**DESLORELIN.** USAN
Use: Gonadotropin inhibitor.

DESMA. (Tablicaps) Diethylstilbesterol 25 mg/Tab. Patient dispenser 10s.
Use: Estrogen.

•**DESMOPRESSIN ACETATE.** USAN.
Use: Treatment of diabetes insipidus.
See: Stimate (Armour).
DDAVP, Liq. (Rorer).

•**DESOGESTREL.** USAN.
Use: Progestin.

DESOMORPHINE. B.A.N. 7,8-Dihydro-6-deoxymorphine.
Use: Narcotic analgesic.

•**DESONIDE.** USAN. 16-alpha-Hydroxyprednisolone-16, 17 acetonide. B.A.N. 11 β,21-Dihydroxy-16α, 17 α-isopropylidenedioxypregna-1,4-diene-3,20-dione.
Use: Anti-inflammatory, corticosteroid.
See: Tridesilon, Cream (Miles Pharm).

DESONIDE CREAM. (Owen/Galderma) Desonide 0.05% in cream base. Tube 15 Gm, 60 Gm.
Use: Corticosteroid, topical.

DESOWEN. (Owen/Galderma) Desonide 0.05%. Cream. Tube 15 Gm, 60 Gm.
Use: Corticosteroid, topical.

•**DESOXIMETASONE,** U.S.P. XXII. Cream, Gel, Oint., U.S.P. XXII.
Use: Adrenocortical steroid.

•**DESOXYCORTICOSTERONE TRIMETHYLACETATE.** 11-Deoxycorticosterone pivalate.
Use: Adrenocortical steroid (salt-regulating).

DESOXYEPHEDRINE HYDROCHLORIDE. (Various Mfr.) Dextro-l-phenyl-2-methylaminopropane, d-phenylisopropylmethylamine, d-N-methylamphetamine.
Use: CNS stimulant.
See: Methamphetamine HCl, Prep.

dl-DESOXYEPHEDRINE HYDROCHLORIDE.
See: dl-Methamphetamine HCl.

DESOXYMETHASONE. B.A.N. 9α-Fluoro-11β,-21-dihydroxy-16α-methylpregna-1,4-diene-3,20-dione.
Use: Topical corticosteroid.

DESOXYN. (Abbott) Methamphetamine HCl. **Tab.:** 5 mg. Bot. 100s. **Gradumets:** 5 mg. Bot. 100s; 10 mg. Bot. 100s; 15 mg. Bot. 100s, 500s.
Use: CNS stimulant.

DESOXY NOREPHEDRINE.
Use: CNS stimulant.
See: Amphetamine HCl, Preps. (Various Mfr.).

DESOXYRIBONUCLEASE.
W/Fibrinolysin.
Use: Topical enzyme preparation.
See: Elase, prep. (Parke-Davis).

DESQUAM-E. (Westwood) Benzoyl peroxide 2.5%, 5% or 10%. Gel. Tube 42.5 Gm.
Use: Anti-acne.

DESQUAM-X 2.5%, 5% or 10% GEL. (Westwood) Benzoyl peroxide 2.5%, 5% or 10%, water base with laureth-4 6%. Tube 1.5 oz.
Use: Anti-acne.

DESQUAM-X 5% or 10% WASH. (Westwood) Benzoyl peroxide 5% or 10% in a lathering base of sodium oxtoxynol-3 sulfonate, docusate sodium, magnesium aluminum silicate, methylcellulose, EDTA. Bot. 5 oz.
Use: Anti-acne.

D-EST. (Burgin-Arden) Estradiol cypionate 5 mg/ml. Vial 10 ml.
Use: Estrogen.

DE-STAT. (Sherman) Surfactant cleaner, benzalkonium Cl 0.01%, EDTA 0.25%. Soln. Bot. 118 ml.
Use: Hard contact lens care.

DESYREL. (Mead-Johnson) Trazodone HCl 50 mg or 100 mg. **50 mg:** Bot. 100s, 1000s, UD 100s. **100 mg:** Bot. 500s.
Use: Antidepressant.

DESYREL DIVIDOSE. (Mead Johnson) Trazodone HCl 150 mg or 300 mg/Dividose tab. Dividose design breakable into fragments for dosing convenience. Bot. 100s, 500s (150 mg).
Use: Antidepressant.

DETACHOL. (Ferndale) Bland, nonirritating liquid for removing adhesive tape. Pkg. 4 oz.
Use: Adhesive remover.

DE TAL. (de Leon) Phenobarbital 0.25 gr, hyoscyamine sulfate 0.1037 mg, atropine sulfate 0.0194 mg, hyoscine HBr 0.0065 mg/Tab. or 5 ml. **Tab.:** Bot. 100s. **Elix.:** With alcohol 20%. Bot. pt.
Use: Sedative/hypnotic, anticholinergic/antispasmodic.

DETANE. (Commerce) Benzocaine 7.5%. Tube 0.5 oz.
Use: Local anesthetic.

DETERENOL HYDROCHLORIDE. USAN.
Use: Adrenergic.

DETERGENTS, Surface-Active.
See: pHisoDerm, Liq. (Winthrop Pharm).
pHisoHex, Liq. (Winthrop Pharm).
Zephiran, Prods. (Winthrop Pharm).

DETIGON HYDROCHLORIDE.
See: Chlophedianol HCl (Various Mfr.).

DETIRELIX ACETATE. USAN.
Use: Antagonist.

DET-O-JET. (Alconox).
Use: Liquid detergent for mechanical, instrument and cage washers.

DETOMIDINE HYDROCHLORIDE. USAN.
Use: Analgesic (veterinary) sedative.

DETUSS. (Various Mfr.) Phenylpropanolamine HCl 75 mg and caramiphen edisylate 40 mg/TR Cap. Bot. 100s, 500s, 1000s.
Use: Decongestant, antitussive.

DEUTIERIUM OXIDE. USAN.
Use: Radioactive agent.

DEVAZEPIDE. USAN.
Use: Antispasmodic, gastrointestinal.

DEVROM. (Parthenon) Bismuth subgallate 200 mg/Chew. tab. Bot. 100s.
Use: Antidiarrheal.

DEWITT'S PILLS. (DeWitt) Blister Pack 20s, 40s, 80s.
Use: Analgesic, diuretic.

DEXACEN-4. (Central) Dexamethasone phosphate (as dexamethasone sodium phosphate) 4 mg/ml, sodium citrate 10 mg, sodium bisulfite 1 mg, methylparaben 1.5 mg, propylparaben 0.2 mg, creatinine 8 mg/ml, sodium hydroxide to adjust pH. Vial 10 ml.
Use: Corticosteroid.

DEXACEN-LA-8. (Central) Dexamethasone acetate equivalant to dexamethasone 8 mg/ml, sodium Cl 6.67 mg, creatinine 5 mg, disodium edetate 0.5 mg, sodium carboxymethylcellulose 5 mg, polysorbate-80 0.75 mg, benzyl alcohol 9 mg, sodium bisulfite 1 mg/ml. Vial 5 ml. Box 12s.
Use: Corticosteroid.

DEXACIDIN OINTMENT. (Iolab) Neomycin sulfate 3.5 mg, dexamethasone 1 mg, polymyxin B sulfate 10,000 units/Gm. Tube 3.5 Gm.
Use: Anti-infective, corticosteroid, ophthalmic.

DEXACIDIN OPHTHALMIC SUSPENSION. (Iolab) Neomycin 3.5 mg, polymyxin B sulfate 10,000 units, dexamethasone 1 mg/ml. Bot. 5 ml.
Use: Anti-infective, corticosteroid, ophthalmic.

DEX-A-DIET CAFFEINE FREE. (O'Connor) Phenylpropanolamine HCl 75 mg/Cap. or Capl. Pkg. 3s, 6s, 20s, 40s.
Use: Diet aid.

DEX-A-DIET ORIGINAL FORMULA. (O'Connor) Phenylpropanolamine HCl 75 mg, ascorbic acid 200 mg/Cap. Pkg. 3s, 6s, 10s, 24s, 48s.
Use: Diet aid.

DEX-A-DIET PLUS VITAMIN C. (O'Connor) Phenylpropanolamine HCl 75 mg, vitamin C 200 mg/TR Cap. Bot. 16s.
Use: Diet aid.

DEXAFED. (Hauck) Phenylephrine HCl 5 mg, dextromethorphan HBr 10 mg, guaifenesin 100 mg/5 ml. Syr. Bot. 120 ml.
Use: Decongestant, antitussive, expectorant.

DEXAMETH. (Major) **Tab.:** Dexamethasone 0.25 mg, 0.5 mg, 0.75 mg, 1.5 mg or 4 mg. Bot. 100s (0.25 mg, 0.5 mg, 1.5 mg); Bot. 100s, 1000s, Unipak 12s (0.75 mg); Bot. 50s, 100s (4 mg). **Elix.:** 0.5 mg/5 ml, alcohol 5%. Bot. 100 ml, 240 ml.
Use: Corticosteroid.

•**DEXAMETHASONE,** U.S.P. XXII. Tab., Elix., Gel, Ophth. Susp., Topical Aerosol, U.S.P. XXII. Pregna-1,4-diene-3,20-dione,9-fluoro-11,17,21-trihydroxy-16-methyl-, (11β,16α). 9-fluoro-11β, 17,21-trihydroxy-16α-methyl-, pregna-1,4-diene-3,20-dione.
Use: Adrenal corticosteroid (anti-inflammatory). Dose: Individualized according to disease, 0.75 mg is equivalent to 4 mg triamcinolone, 5 mg prednisone/prednisolone, 20 mg hydrocortisone or 25 mg cortisone.
See: Aeroseb-Dex, Aerosol (Herbert).
Decaderm in Estergel (Merck Sharp & Dohme).
Decadron, Tab., Elix. (Merck Sharp & Dohme).
Decameth, Inj. (Foy).
Decameth L.A., Inj. (Foy).
Decaspray, Aerosol (Merck Sharp & Dohme).
Dexaport, Tab. (Freeport).
Dexone TM, Tab. (Solvay).
Dezone, Tab. (Solvay).
Hexadrol, Tab., Elix., Cream (Organon).
Maxidex Ophth. Liq. (Alcon).
W/Neomycin sulfate.
See: NeoDecadron, Prep. (Merck Sharp & Dohme).
NeoDecaspray, Aerosol (Merck Sharp & Dohme).
W/Neomycin sulfate, polymyxin B sulfate.
See: Maxitrol Ophth. Susp., Oint. (Alcon).

•**DEXAMETHASONE ACEFURATE.** USAN.
Use: Anti-inflammatory, topical steroid.

•**DEXAMETHASONE ACETATE,** U.S.P. XXII. Sterile Susp., U.S.P. XXII.
Use: Adrenocortical steroid (anti-inflammatory).
See: Dexone LA, Ind. (Kay).

•**DEXAMETHASONE DIPROPIONATE.** USAN.

Use: Anti-inflammatory.

DEXAMETHASONE INTENSOL ORAL SOLUTION. (Roxane) Dexamethasone 1 mg/ml concentrated oral soln. Bot. 30 ml w/calibrated dropper.
Use: Corticosteroid.

•**DEXAMETHASONE SODIUM PHOSPHATE,** U.S.P. XXII. Inhalation Aerosol, Cream, Ophth. Oint., Ophth. Soln., Inj., U.S.P. XXII. Pregn-4-ene-3,20-dione, 9-fluoro-11, 17-dihydroxy-16-methyl-21-(phosphonooxy)-disodium salt, (11β, 16α)-9-Fluoro-11β, 17,21-trihydroxy-16α-methylpregna-1,4-diene-3,20-dione-21-(dihydrogen phosphate) disodium salt.
Use: Adrenocortical steroid (anti-inflammatory).
See: Decadron Phosphate, Preps. (Merck Sharp & Dohme).
Decadron Phosphate Respihaler (Merck Sharp & Dohme).
Decaject, Vial (Mayrand).
Decameth, Inj. (Foy).
Dexone, Inj. (Keene, Hauck).
Dezone, Inj. (Solvay).
Hexadrol Phosphate, Inj. (Organon).
Savacort D, Inj. (Savage).
Solurex, Inj. (Hyrex).
W/Lidocaine (Xylocaine).
See: Decadron Phosphate w/Xylocaine, Inj. (Merck Sharp & Dohme).
W/Neomycin sulfate.
See: NeoDecadron, Prods. (Merck Sharp & Dohme).
W/Neomycin and polymixin B sulfates.
See: Dexacidin, Prods. (CooperVision).

•**DEXAMISOLE.** USAN.
Use: Antidepressant.

DEXAMPHETAMINE.
See: Dextroamphetamine (Various Mfr.).

DEXAPHEN SA TABLETS. (Major) Pseudoephedrine sulfate 120 mg, dexbrompheniramine maleate 6 mg. In 10s, 20s, 40s, 100s, 500s.
Use: Decongestant, antihistamine.

DEXAPORT. (Freeport) Dexamethasone 0.75 mg/Tab. Bot. 1000s.
Use: Corticosteroid.

DEXASONE. (Various Mfr.) Dexamethasone sodium phosphate 4 mg/ml, methyl and propyl parabens, sodium bisulfite. Vial 5 ml, 10 ml, 30 ml.
Use: Corticosteroid.

DEXASONE INJECTION. (Hauck) Dexamethasone sodium phosphate 4 mg/ml. Vial 5 ml, 30 ml.
Use: Corticosteroid.

DEXASONE-L.A. INJECTION. (Hauck) Dexamethasone acetate 8 mg/ml. Vial 5 ml.
Use: Corticosteroid.

DEXATRIM-15. (Thompson) Phenylpropanolamine HCl 75 mg/TR Cap. Bot. 20s, 40s.
Use: Diet aid.

DEXATRIM-15 W/VITAMIN C. (O'Connor) Phenylpropanolamine HCl 75 mg, vitamin C 180 mg/TR Cap. Bot. 20s.
Use: Diet aid.

DEXATRIM PLUS VITAMINS. (O'Connor) Phenylpropanolamine HCl 75 mg, vitamins B_1 1.5 mg, B_2 1.7 mg, B_3 20 mg, B_5 10 mg, B_6 2 mg, B_{12} 6 mcg, C 60 mg, biotin 30 mcg, folic acid 0.4 mg, cromium 50 mcg, copper 2 mg, iron 7.5 mg, iodine 150 mg, manganese 3 mg, zinc 15 mg/TR Cap. Bot. 16s.
Use: Appetite suppressant, vitamin/mineral supplement.

•**DEXBROMPHENIRAMINE MALEATE,** U.S.P. XXII. (+)-2-[p-Bromo-α-[2-(dimethylamino) ethyl]-[benzyl]pyridine maleate. Dextro form of brompheniramine. Dextroparabromdylamine 1-(p-bromophenyl-1-(2- pyridyl)-3-dimethylamino propane maleate. (+)-2-(p-Bromo-α-(2-(dimethylamithenzyl)-pyridine-Maleate (1:1).
Use: Antihistamine.
W/Pseudoephedrine sulfate.
See: Disophrol Chronotab, Tab. (Schering-Plough).
Drixoral S.A., Tab. (Schering-Plough).

DEXCHLOR. (Schein) Dexchlorpheniramine maleate 4 mg/RA Tab. Bot. 100s.
Use: Antihistamine.

•**DEXCHLORPHENIRAMINE MALEATE,** U.S.P. XXII. Syr., Tab., U.S.P. XXII. d-2-[p-Chloroalpha(2-di- methyl-amino-ethLL) Lenzyl] pyridine bimaleate. (+)-2-(p-Chloro-α-(2-dimethylamino)-ethenzyridine-Maleate (1:1) Dextro-Chlorpheniramine Maleate.
Use: Antihistamine.
See: Polaramine, Repetabs Tab., Tab., Syr. (Schering-Plough).
W/Pseudoephedrine sulfate, guaifenesin, alcohol.
See: Polaramine Expectorant (Schering-Plough).

•**DEXCLAMOL HYDROCHLORIDE.** USAN.
Use: Sedative.

DEXEDRINE. (SmithKline Beecham) Dextroamphetamine sulfate. **Tab.:** 5 mg Bot. 100s, 1000s. **Spansule:** 5 mg Bot. 50s; 10 mg, 15 mg Bot. 50s, 500s.
Use: CNS stimulant.

•**DEXETIMIDE.** USAN. (+)-3-(1-Benzyl-4-piperidyl)-3-phenylpiperidine-2,6-dione.
Use: Treatment of Parkinson's disease.

•**DEXIBUPROFEN LYSINE.** USAN.
Use: Nonsteroidal anti-inflammatory; analgesic.

•**DEXIMAFEN.** USAN.
Use: Antidepressant.

•**DEXIVACAINE.** USAN.
Use: Anesthetic.

•**DEXMEDETOMIDINE.** USAN.
Use: Sedative/hypnotic.

DEXONE. (Solvay) Dexamethasone 0.5 mg, 0.75 mg, 1.5 mg or 4 mg/Tab. Bot. 100s, UD 100s. Box 1s, 10s, 150s.
Use: Corticosteroid.

DEXONE. (Hauck) Dexamethasone sodium phosphate 4 mg/ml. Amp. 5 ml.
Use: Corticosteroid.

DEXONE. (Keene) Dexamethasone sodium phosphate 4 mg/ml, methyl and propyl parabens, sodium bisulfite. Vial 5 ml, 10 ml.
Use: Corticosteroid.

DEXONE L.A. (Keene) Dexamethasone acetate suspension equivalent to dexamethasone 8 mg, polysorbate 80, carboxymethylcellulose, sodium bisulfite, EDTA, benzyl alcohol. Vial 5 ml.
Use: Corticosteroid.

DEXORMAPLATIN. USAN.
Use: Antineoplastic.

DEXOTIC. (Parnell) Dexamethasone phosphate 0.1% (as sodium phosphate), benzalkonium Cl, EDTA. Soln. Bottle w/dropper 5 ml.
Use: Corticosteroid, ophthalmic.

DEXOXADROL HYDROCHLORIDE. USAN. d-2-(2,2-Diphenyl-1,3-dioxolan-4-yl) piperidine hydroCl. Dextro form of dioxadrol HCl.
Use: Antidepressant.

DEXPANTENOL WITH CHOLINE BITARTRATE.
See: Ilopan-choline (Adria).

DEXPANTHENOL, U.S.P. XXII. Preparation, U.S.P. XXII. (+)-2,4-Dihydroxy-N-(3-hydroxypropyl)-3,3-di-methylbutyramide.
Use: Treatment of paralytic ileus and postoperative distention.
See: Ilopan, Inj. (Adria).
Panthoderm (USV).

DEXPROPANOLOL HCl. USAN. (±)-l-(Iso- propylamino)-3-(l-naphthyloxy)-2-propanol HCl.
Use: Cardiac depressant (Antiarrhythmic).

DEXRAZOXANE. USAN.
Use: Cardioprotectant.

DEXTRAN. B.A.N. Polyanhydroglucose.
Use: Blood volume expander.
See: LMWD-Dextran 40 (Pharmchem).
Macrodex, Soln. (Pharmacia).

DEXTRAN ADJUNCT.
Use: Plasma expander.
See: Promit (Pharmacia) Inj.

DEXTRAN 6%. (Abbott).
See: Dextran 75, I.V. (Abbott).

DEXTRAN 40. USAN. Polysaccharide (m.w. 40,000) produced by the action of Leuconostoc mesenteroides on saccharose.
Use: Blood suspension stabilizer.

DEXTRAN 45, 75. Polysaccharide (m.w. 45,000, 75,000) produced by the action of Leuconostoc mesenteroides on saccharose. Rheotran (45).
Use: Blood volume expander, antithrombogenic agent.

DEXTRAN 70. USAN. A polysaccharide.
Macrodex, Soln. (Pharmacia).
Use: Blood volume expander.

DEXTRAN 75. USAN. Dextran 75 6% in 0.9% saline. Flask 500 ml; Dextran 75 6% in 5% dextrose. Flask 500 ml.
Use: Blood plasma expander.

DEXTRANOMER. B.A.N. Dextran cross-linked with epichlorohydrin.
Use: Promoter of wound healing.

•**DEXTRATES,** N.F. XVII. Mixture of sugars (approximately 92% dextrose monohydrate and 8% higher saccharides; dextrose equivalent is 95 to 97%) resulting from the controlled enzymatic hydrolysis of starch.
Use: Pharmaceutic aid (tablet binder and diluent).

DEXTRIFERRON. B.A.N. A colloidal solution of ferric hydroxide in complex with partially hydrolyzed dextrin.
Use: Treatment of iron-deficiency anemias.
See: Imferon, Amp. (Merrell Dow).

•**DEXTRIN,** N.F. XVII.
Use: Pharmaceutic aid (tablet and capsule diluent).

•**DEXTROAMPHETAMINE.** USAN.
Use: Stimulant (central).

DEXTROAMPHETAMINE WITH AMPHETAMINE AS RESIN COMPLEX.
See: Biphetamine 12.5, 20, Cap. (Pennwalt).

DEXTROAMPHETAMINE PHOSPHATE. Monobasic d-a-methylphenethlyamine phosphate. (+)-α-Methylphenethylamine phosphate.
Use: CNS stimulant.
See: d-Amphetamine Phosphate combinations.

•**DEXTROAMPHETAMINE SULFATE,** U.S.P. XXII. Cap., Elix., Tab., U.S.P. XXII. Benzeneethanamine, α-methyl-, sulfate (2:1). (+)-α-Methylphenethylamine sulfate (2:1). d-Amphetamine sulfate, d-Methyl-phenylamine sulfate.
Use: Central stimulant.
See: Dexampex, Cap., Tab. (Lemmon).
Dexedrine, Preps. (SmithKline Beecham).
Diphylets, Granucaps (Solvay).
Robese P., Tab., Vial (Rocky Mtn.).
Tidex Tab. (Allison).

DEXTROAMPHETAMINE SULFATE W/COMBINATIONS.
Use: CNS stimulant.
See: Amphodex, Cap. (Jamieson-McKames).
Delcobese (Delco).
Dextrobar, Tab. (Lannett).
Min-Gera, Tab. (Scrip).
Ro Trim, Cap. (Rocky Mtn.).
Trimex, Trimex #2, Cap. (Mills).

DEXTROBAR. (Lannett) Dextroamphetamine sulfate 5 mg, amobarbital 32 mg/Tab. Bot. 500s, 1000s.
Use: CNS stimulant, sedative/hypnotic.

DEXTRO-CHEK CALIBRATORS. (Ames) Clear liquid soln. containing measured amounts of glucose. Low calibrator contains 0.05% w/v glucose. High calibrator contains 0.30% w/v glucose.
Use: Dextrostix to perform calibration procedure for Glucometer reflectance photometer.

DEXTRO-CHECK NORMAL CONTROL. (Ames) Clear liquid containing measured amount of glucose 0.10% w/v.

Use: Perform check of Glucometer refluctance photometer or Dextrometer refluctance photometer using Dextrostix and Glucometer II Blood Glucose Meter using Glucostix.

DEXTRO-CHLORPHENIRAMINE MALEATE.
Use: Antihistamine.
See: Polaramine, Repetab, Tab., Expect., Syr. (Schering-Plough).

•**DEXTROMETHORPHAN,** U.S.P. XXII. (+)-3-Methoxy-N-methylmorphinan.
Use: Cough suppressant.
See: Benylin DM Cough Syrup(Parke-Davis).
Delsym, Liq. (Pennwalt).
W/Benzocain, menthol, peppermint oil.
See: Vicks Formula 44 Cough Control Discs, Loz. (Vicks).

•**DEXTROMETHORPHAN HYDROBROMIDE,** U.S.P. XXII. Syr., U.S.P. XXII. d-3-Methoxy-N-methylmorphinan. (+)-3-Methoxy-17-methyl-9α, 13α,-14α-morphinan HBr. Dormethan. d-Methorphan.
Use: Antitussive.
See: Benylin DM Cough Syr. (Parke-Davis).
Dicodethal, Elix. (Lannett).
Mediquell, Tab. (Warner-Lambert).
St. Joseph Cough Syr. (Schering-Plough).
Symptom 1, Liq. (Parke-Davis).
Tus-F, Liq. (Orbit).
Tussade Tab. (Westerfield).

DEXTROMETHORPHAN HBr W/COMBINATIONS
See: Ambenyl-D, Liq. (Marion).
Anti-Tuss D.M., Liq. (Century).
Anti-Tussive, Tab. (Canright).
Bayer Prods. (Glenbrook).
Breacol Cough Medication, Liq. (Glenbrook).
Capahist-DMH, Cap. (Freeport).
C.D.M., Expectorant (Lannett).
Centuss, MLT, Tab. (Century).
Cerose-DM, Liq. (Wyeth-Ayerst).
Cheracol-D, Cough Syr. (Upjohn).
Cheratussin, Cough Syr. (Towne).
Chexit, Tab. (Sandoz Consumer).
Children's Hold 4-Hour Cough Suppressant & Decongestant, Loz. (Calgon).
Codimal DM, Liq. (Central).
Colrex, Syr. (Solvay).
Comtrex, Cap., Liq. Tab. (Bristol-Myers).
Congespirin Cough Syrup (Bristol-Myers).
Contac Jr., Liq. (SmithKline Beecham).
Coricidin Children's Cough Syrup (Schering-Plough).
Dimacol, Cap. (Robins).
Donatussin, Syr. (Laser).
Dorcol Ped. Cough Syr. (Sandoz Consumer).
Dristan Cough Formula, Syr. (Whitehall).
End-A-Koff, Jr. Syr. (Quality Generics).
Formula 44 Prods. (Vicks).
Halls Mentho-Lyptus Decongestant Cough Formula, Liq. (Warner-Lambert).
Histalets, DM, Syr. (Reid Provident).
Infantuss, Liq. (Scott/Cord).
Niltuss, Syr. (Minn. Pharm.).
Nyquil, Liq. (Vicks).
Orthoxicol, Syr. (Upjohn).
Partuss, Liq. (Parmed).
Phenergan, Pediatric, Liq. (Wyeth-Ayerst).
Polytuss-DM, Liq. (Rhode).
Rentuss, Tab., Syr. (Wren).
Rentuss, Tab. (Wren).
Robitussin-DM, Syr., Loz. (Robins).
Robitussin-CF (Robins).
Rondec DM, Drops, Syr. (Ross).
Scotcof Liq. (Scott/Cord).
Scotuss, Pediatric Cough Syr. (Scott/Cord).
Shertus, Liq. (Sheryl).
Silexin, Syr. (Clapp).
Sorbase Cough Syr. (Fort David).
Spec-T Sore Throat-Cough Suppressant Loz. (Squibb).
Sudafed Cough Syr. (Burroughs Wellcome).
Synatuss-One, Liq. (Freeport).
Thor, Cough Syr. (Towne).
Tolu-Sed DM, Liq. (Scherer).
Tonecol, Syr., Tab. (A.V.P.).
Triaminic-DM Cough Formula (Sandoz, Consumer).
Triaminicol, Syr. (Sandoz, Consumer).
Trind-DM, Syr. (Mead Johnson).
Tusquelin, Syr. (Circle).
Tussagesic, Tab., Susp. (Sandoz, Consumer).
Tusscidin Expectorant D, Liq. (Cenci).
Unproco, Cap. (Solvay).
Vicks Cough Prods. (Vicks).
Vicks Daycare, Liq. (Vicks).
Vicks Formula 44 Prods. (Vicks).
Vicks Nyquil, Liq. (Vicks).
Wal-Tussin DM, Syr. (Walgreen).

•**DEXTROMETHORPHAN POLISTIREX.** USAN.
Use: Antitussive.

DEXTROMORAMIDE. B.A.N. (+)-1-(3-Methyl-4-morpholino-2, 2-diphenylbutyryl) pyrrolidine.
Use: Narcotic analgesic.

DEXTROMORAMIDE TARTRATE. dl-(3- Methyl-4-morpholino-2, 2-d-phenyl-butyryl) pyrrolidine.
Use: Narcotic analgesic.

DEXTRO-PANTOTHENYL ALCOHOL.
See: Panthenol (Various Mfr.).
Ilopan (Adria).

DEXTROPROPOXYPHENE. B.A.N. α-(+)-4-Dimethylamino-3-methyl-1,2-diphenyl-2-propionyloxy-butane. α-(+)-1-Benzyl-3-dimethylamino-2-methyl-1-phenylpropyl propionate.

DEXTROPROPOXYPHENE HCl.
Use: Analgesic.
See: Propoxyphene HCl, Cap. (Various Mfr.).
W/Acetylsalicylic acid, phenaglycodol.
See: Darvo-Tran, Pulv. (Lilly).

DEXTRORPHAN. B.A.N. (+)-3-Hydroxy-N-methylmorphinan.
Use: Narcotic analgesic.

•**DEXTROSE,** U.S.P. XXII. Inj., U.S.P. XXII. d-Glucose. -Glucose, monohydrate.
Use: Fluid and nutrient replenisher.

W/Calcium ascorbate and benzyl alcohol injection
See: Calscorbate, Amp. (Cole).

W/Psyllium mucilloid.
See: V-lax, Pow. (Century).

DEXTROSE EXCIPIENT, N.F. XVII.
Use: Pharmaceutic aid (tablet excipient).

DEXTROSE 5% AND ELECTROLYTE #48. (Travenol) Dextrose 50 Gm, calories 180/L with Na^+ 25, K^+ 20, Mg^{++} 3, Cl^- 24, phosphate 3, acetate 23 with osmolarity 348 mOsm/L. Soln. Bot. 250 ml, 500 ml, 1000 ml.
Use: Parenteral nutritional supplement.

DEXTROSE 5% AND ELECTROLYTE #75. (Travenol) Dextrose 50 Gm, calories 180/L with Na^+ 40, K^+ 35, Cl^- 48, phosphate 15 and lactate 20 with osmolarity 402 mOsm/L. Soln. Bot. 250 ml, 500 ml, 1000 ml.
Use: Parenteral nutritional supplement.

DEXTROSE LARGE VOLUME PARENTERALS. (Abbott Hospital Prods).
Dextrose 2 0.5% in Water-1000 ml.
Dextrose 2 0.5% in 0.5 Sterile Lactose Ringer's or in 0.5 Sterile Saline-1000 ml.
Dextrose 5% in Water-150 ml, 250 ml, 500 ml, 1000 ml in Abbo-Vac glass or LifeCare flexible plastic container; partial-fill glass: 50 in 200 ml, 50 in 300 ml, 100 in 300 ml, 400 in 500 ml; partial-fill plastic: 50 in 150 ml, 100 in 150 ml.
Dextrose 5% in Lactose Ringer's-250 ml, 500 ml, 1000 ml glass; 500 ml, 1000 ml plastic container.
Dextrose 5% in Ringer's-500 ml, 1000 ml.
Dextrose 5% in Saline 0.9% or in 0.25, 0.33 or 0.5 Sterile Saline-250, 500, 1000 ml glass or plastic container.
Dextrose 10% in Water-250 ml, 500 ml, 1000 ml containers.
Dextrose 20% in Water-500 ml.
Dextrose 50% in Water-500 ml.
Dextrose 20%, 30%, 40%, 50%, 60%, 70% Injections, U.S.P. in partial-fill container, 500 ml in 1000 ml.
Dextrose Injection 50%. Bot. 1000 ml.
Dextrose 50% and Injection w/Electrolytes in partial-fill container, 500 ml in 1000 ml.
Dextrose Injection 70%. Bot. 1000 ml.
Use: Parenteral nutritional supplement.

DEXTROSE SMALL VOLUME PARENTERALS. (Abbott Hospital Prods) **Dextrose 5%:** 50 ml, 100 ml pressurized pintop vial. **Dextrose 10%:** 5 ml amp.; **Dextrose 25%:** 10 ml syringe. **Dextrose 50%:** 50 ml Abboject syringe (18 G X 1.5"), 50 ml Fliptop vial. **Dextrose 70%:** 70 ml pressurized pintop vial.
Use: Parenteral nutritional supplement.

DEXTROSE & SODIUM CHLORIDE INJECTION, U.S.P. XXII. (Abbott) 10% Dextrose and 0.225% Sodium Cl. Inj. Single dose container 500 ml.
Use: Parenteral nutritional supplement.

DEXTROSTIX. (Ames) A cellulose strip containing glucose oxidase and indicator system. Bot. 25s, 100s. Box 10s.
Use: Blood-glucose test.

DEXTROTHYROXINE SODIUM, U.S.P. XXI. Tab., U.S.P. XXI. D-Tyrosine, 0-(4-hydroxy-3, 5-diiodophenyl)- 3, 5-diiod-, monosodium salt hydrate.
Use: Anticholesteremic.
See: Choloxin, Tab. (Flint).

DEXULE. (Approved) Vitamins A 1333 IU, D 133 IU, B_1 0.33 mg, B_2 0.4 mg, C 10 mg, niacinamide 3.3 mg, iron 3.3 mg, calcium 29 mg, phosphorous 15 mg, methylcellulose 100 mg, benzocaine 3 mg/Cap. Bot. 21s, 90s.
Use: Vitamin/mineral supplement.

DEXYL. (Pinex) Dextromethorphan HBr 15 mg, vitamin C 20 mg/Tab. Box 20s.
Use: Antitussive, vitamin C supplement.

DEY-DOSE EPINEPHRINE. (Dey Labs) Racemic epinephrine (as HCl) equal to 2.25% epinephrine base, chlorobutanol, sodium metabisulfite. Soln. for nebulization. Vial 0.25 ml.
Use: Bronchodilator.

DEY-DOSE ISOETHARINE HCl. (Dey Labs) Isoetharine HCl 1% with glycerin, sodium metabisulfite and parabens. Soln. for nebulization. Vial 0.25 ml, 0.5 ml.
Use: Brochodilator.

DEY-DOSE ISOPROTERENOL HCl. (Dey Labs) Isoproterenol HCl 0.5% (1:200). Soln. for nebulization. Vial 0.5 ml.
Use: Bronchodilator.

DEY-DOSE METAPROTERENOL SULFATE. (Dey Labs) Metaproterenol sulfate 0.5%. Inhaler 0.3 ml.
Use: Bronchodilator.

DEY-LUTE. (Dey Labs) Isoetharine HCl with sodium metabisulfite, glycerin. Soln. **0.08%:** UD 3 ml; **0.1%:** UD 5 ml; **0.17%:** UD 3 ml; **0.25%:** UD 2 ml.
Use: Bronchodilator.

DEY-LUTE METAPROTERENOL SULFATE. (Dey Labs) Metaproterenol sulfate 0.6%. Soln. for inhalation 2.5 ml.
Use: Bronchodilator.

•**DEZAQUANINE.** USAN.
Use: Antineoplastic.

•**DEZAQUANINE MESYLATE.** USAN.
Use: Antineoplastic.

DEZEST. (Geneva Marsam) Atropine sulfate, phenylpropanolamine HCl, chlorpheniramine maleate. Bot. 100s.
Use: Anticholinergic/antispasmodic, decongestant, antihistamine.

•**DEZOCINE.** USAN.
Use: Analgesic.
See: Dalgan (Wyeth-Ayerst).

D-FILM. (Ciba Vision) Poloxamer 407, EDTA 0.25%, benzalkonium Cl 0.025%. Gel Tube 25 Gm.
Use: Hard contact lens care.

DFP. Diisopropyl fluorophosphate (Various Mfr.).
DHS CONDITIONING RINSE. (Person & Covey) Conditioning ingredients. Bot. 8 oz.
Use: Dermatological hair conditioner.
DHS SHAMPOO. (Person & Covey) Blend of cleansing surfactants and emulsifiers. Plastic bot. w/dispenser 8 oz, 16 oz.
Use: Dermatological hair and scalp shampoo.
DHS TAR GEL SHAMPOO. (Person & Covey) Coal Tar, U.S.P. 0.5% Bot. 8 oz.
Use: Antiseborrheic, antipsoriatic.
DHS TAR SHAMPOO. (Person & Covey) Coal tar 0.5% in DHS shampoo. Bot. 4 oz, 8 oz, 16 oz.
Use: Antiseborrheic, antipsoriatic.
DHS ZINC SHAMPOO. (Person & Covey) Zinc pyrithione 2% in DHS shampoo. Bot. 6 oz, 12 oz.
Use: Antiseborrheic.
DHT. (Roxane) Dihydrotachysterol. **Tab.:** 0.125 mg, 0.2 mg or 0.4 mg/Tab. Bot. 50s, UD 100s (0.125 mg). 100s, UD 100s (0.2 mg). 50s (0.4 mg). **Intensol:** Dihydrotachysterol 0.2 mg/ml, alcohol 20%. Bot. 30 ml w/dropper.
Use: Calcium regulator.
DIABETA TABLETS. (Hoechst) Glyburide. **1.25 mg:** Bot. 50s. **2.5 mg:** Bot. 100s, UD 100s. **5 mg:** Bot. 100s.
Use: Antidiabetic agent.
DIABINESE. (Pfizer Laboratories) Chlorpropamide. **100 mg/Tab.:** Bot. 100s, UD 100s; **250 mg/Tab.** Bot. 100s, 1000s.
Use: Antidiabetic agent.
DIABISMUL LIQUID. (Forest) Opium 7 mg, pectin 80 mg, kaolin 2500 mg/15 ml. Bot. 8 oz.
Use: Antidiarrheal.
DIABISMUL TABLETS. (Forest) Bismuth subcarbonate 125 mg, powdered opium 1.23 mg, calcium carbonate 125 mg/Tab. Bot. 1000s.
Use: Antidiarrheal.
DIACETAMATE. B.A.N. 4-Acetamidophenyl acetate.
Use: Analgesic.
DIACETIC ACID TEST.
See: Acetest, Tab. (Ames).
DIACETO. (Archer-Taylor) Aspirin 3.5 gr, acetophenetidin 2.5 gr, caffeine 0.5 gr/Tab. Bot. 100s, 1000s.
Use: Analgesic.
DIACETO W/CODEINE. (Archer-Taylor) Codeine 0.25 gr, 0.5 gr/Tab. or Cap. Bot. 500s, 1000s.
Use: Narcotic analgesic.
DIACETO W/GELSEMIUM. (Archer-Taylor) Phenobarbital 0.5 gr, gelsemium 3 min./Tab. Bot. 1000s.
Use: Sedative/hypnotic.
•**DIACETOLOL HYDROCHLORIDE.** USAN.
Use: Anti-adrenergic.
DIACETRIZOATE, SODIUM.
See: Diatrizoate (Various Mfr.).
•**DIACETYLATED MONOGLYCERIDES,** N.F. XVII. Glycerin esterfied with edible fatty acids and acetic acid.
Use: Plasticizer.
DIACETYLCHOLINE CHLORIDE. Succinylcholine Cl.
See: Anectine Chloride, Inj., Pow. (Burroughs-Wellcome).
DIACETYL-DIHYDROXYDIPHENYLISATIN.
See: Oxyphenisatin acetate (Various Mfr.).
DIACETYLDIOXYPHENYLISATIN.
See: Oxyphenisatin acetate (Various Mfr.).
DIACETYLMORPHINE SALTS. Heroin. Illegal in U.S.A. by Federal statute because of its addiction-causing nature.
DIACETYLNALORPHINE. B.A.N. O^3O^6-Diacetyl-N-allylnormorphine.
Use: Narcotic analgesic.
DIACHLOR TABS. (Major) Chlorothiazide 250 mg, 500 mg/Tab. Bot. 100s, 250s, 1000s.
Use: Diuretic.
DI-ADEMIL.
See: Hydroflumethiazide, Tab. (Various Mfr.).
DIAGNIOL.
See: Sodium Acetrizoate.
DIAGNOSTIC AGENTS.
See: Acholest, Kit (Fougera).
Baroflave, Pow. (Lannett).
Cardio-Green, Vial (Hynson Westcott & Dunning).
Cardiografin, Vial (Squibb).
Cea-Roche, Kit (Roche).
Cholografin, Prep. (Squibb).
Coccidioidin, Vial (Cutter).
Dextrostix, Strip (Ames).
Diptheria Toxin for Schick Test (Various Mfr.).
Evans Blue, Amp. (Harvey).
Fertility Tape (Weston Labs.).
Fluorescein Sodium Ophth. Soln. (Various Mfr.).
Fluor-I-Strip (Wyeth-Ayerst).
Fluor-I-Strip A.T. (Wyeth-Ayerst).
Fluress, Ophth. Soln. (Barnes-Hind).
Glucola, Soln. (Ames).
Hema-Combistix Strips (Ames).
Hemastix Strips (Ames).
Histalog, Amp. (Lilly).
Histoplasmin, Vial (Parke-Davis).
Indigo Carmine (Various Mfr.).
Mannitol Soln., Inj. (Merck Sharp & Dohme).
Phenolsulfonphthalein (Various Mfr.).
Phentolamine Methanesulfonate, Inj. (Various Mfr.).
Regitine, Amp., Tab. (Ciba).
Rheumanosticon Slide Test (Organon).
Rocky Mountain Spotted Fever Antigen, Vial (Lederle).
Sodium Dehydrocholate, Inj. (Various Mfr.).
Tes-Tape (Lilly).
See also: Cholecystography Agents.
Kidney Function Agents.
Liver Function Agents.

Urography Agents.
DIAGNOSTIC AGENTS FOR URINE.
See: Acetest, Tab. (Ames).
Albustix, Strip (Ames).
Bumintest, Tab. (Ames).
Clinistix, Strip (Ames).
Clinitest, Tab. (Ames).
Hema-Combistix, Strip (Ames).
Hemastix, Strip (Ames).
Hematest, Tab. (Ames).
Icotest, Tab. (Ames).
Ketostix, Strip (Ames).
Pheniplate, Preps.(Ames).
Phenistix, Strip (Ames).
Uristix, Strip (Ames).
DIAGNOSTIC AGENTS.
See: Persantine IV (DuPont-Merck).
DIALLYLAMICOL. Diallyl-diethylaminoethyl phenol di HCl.
DIALLYBARBITURIC ACID. Allobarbital, Allobarbitone, Curral.
W/Acetaminophen, aluminum aspirin, aspirin.
See: Allylgesic, Tab. (Elder).
DIALLYLNORTOXIFERINE.
See: Alloferin (Roche).
DIALMINATE. Mixture of magnesium carbonate and (alminate) dihydroxyaluminum glycinate.
W/Aspirin.
See: Bufferin, Preps. (Bristol-Myers).
DIALONE TABS. (Major) Methandrostenolone 5 mg/Tab. Bot. 100s.
Use: Anabolic steroid.
DIALOSE. (Stuart) Docusate potassium 100 mg/Cap. Bot. 36s, 100s, UD 100s.
Use: Laxative.
DIALOSE PLUS. (Stuart) Docusate potassium 100 mg, casanthranol 30 mg/Cap. Bot. 36s, 100s, 500s, UD 100s.
Use: Laxative.
DIALUME. (Armour) Aluminum hydroxide gel 500 mg/Cap. Bot. 100s, 500s.
Use: Antacid.
DIALYTE PATTERN LM W/1.5% DEXTROSE. (Gambro) Dextrose 15 g/L, Na^+ 131, Ca^{++} 3.5, Mg^{++} 0.5, Cl^- 94 and lactate 40 with osmolarity 345 mOsm/L. Soln. Bot. 1000 ml, 2000 ml.
Use: Peritoneal dialysis solution.
DIALYTE PATTERN LM W/2.5% DEXTROSE. (Gambro) Dextrose 25 g/L, Na^+ 131.5, Ca^{++} 3.5, Mg^{++} 0.5, Cl^- 94 and lactate 40 with osmolarity 395 mOsm/L. Soln. Bot. 2000 ml.
Use: Peritoneal dialysis solution.
DIALYTE PATTERN LM W/4.25% DEXTROSE. (Gambro) Dextrose 42.5 g/L, Na^+ 131.5, Ca^{++} 3.5, Mg^{++} 0.5, Cl^- 94 and lactate 40 with osmolarity 485 mOsm/L. Soln. Bot. 2000 ml.
Use: Peritoneal dialysis solution.
DIAMETHINE.
See: Dimethyl tubocurarine (Various Mfr.).
DIAMINEDIPENICILLIN G.
See: Benzethacil (Various Mfr.).
DIAMINE T.D. (Major) Brompheniramine maleate 8 mg or 12 mg/TR tab. Bot. 100s, 250s, 1000s.
Use: Antihistamine.
DI-AMINO ACETATE COMPLEX W/CALCIUM ALUMINUM CARBONATE}. Cap. IU.
See: Ancid Tab., Susp. (Sheryl).
DIAMINODIPHENYLSULFONE. Dapsone, U.S.P. XXII.
Use: Treatment of malaria.
See: Avlosulfon, Tab. (Wyeth-Ayerst).
Diasone Sodium, Tab. (Abbott).
Glucosulfone Sodium, Inj. (Various Mfr.).
DIAMINOPROPYL TETRAMETHYLENE.
See: Spermine.
•**DIAMOCAINE CYCLAMATE.** USAN. (1) 1-(2-Anilinoethyl)-4-[2-(diethylamino)-ethoxy]-4-phenylpiperidine bis(cyclohexanesulfamate); (2) Cyclohexanesulfamic acid compound with 1-(2-anilinoethyl)-4-[2-(diethylamino)ethoxy]-4-phenylpiperidine (2:1).
Use: Local anesthetic.
DIAMOX. (Lederle) Acetazolamide. **Tab.:** 125 mg Bot. 100s. 250 mg Bot. 100s, 1000s, UD 10 × 10s. **Inj. Vial:** Sterile sodium salt 500 mg (sodium hydroxide to adjust pH).
Use: Diuretic, anticonvulsant.
DIAMOX SEQUELS. (Lederle) Acetazolamide 500 mg/Cap. Bot. 30s, 100s.
Use: Diuretic, anticonvulsant.
DIAMPHENETHIDE. V.B.A.N. ββ′-Oxydi(aceto-p-phenetidide).
Use: Anthelmintic (veterinary).
DIAMPROMIDE. B.A.N. N-[2-(N-Methylphen-ethylamino)propyl]propionanilide.
Use: Analgesic.
DIAMTHAZOLE. B.A.N. 6-(2-Diethylaminoethoxy)-2-dimethylaminobenzothiazole.
Dimazole (I.N.N.).
Use: Antifungal.
DIAMTHAZOLE DIHYDROCHLORIDE. Asterol.
DIANEAL W/1.5% DEXTROSE. (Travenol) Dextrose 15 Gm/L, Na^+ 141, Ca^{++} 3.5, Mg^{++} 1.5, Cl^- 101, lactate 45 with osmolarity 364 mOsm/L. Soln. Bot. 1000 ml, 2000 ml.
Use: Peritoneal dialysis solution.
DIANEAL 137 W/1.5% DEXTROSE. (Travenol) Dextrose 15 Gm/L, Na^+ 132, Ca^{++} 3.5, Mg^{++} 1.5, Cl^- 102, lactate 35 with osmolarity 347 mOsm/L. Soln. Bot. 2000 ml.
Use: Peritoneal dialysis solution.
DIANEAL W/4.25% DEXTROSE. (Travenol) Dextrose 42.5 Gm/L, Na^+ 141, Ca^{++} 3.5, Mg^{++} 1.5, Cl^- 101, lactate 45 with osmolarity 503 mOsm/L. Soln. Bot. 2000 ml.
Use: Peritoneal dialysis solution.
DIANEAL 137 W/4.25% DEXTROSE. (Travenol) Dextrose 42.5 Gm/L, Na^+ 132, Ca^{++} 3.5, Mg^{++} 1.5, Cl^- 102, lactate 35 with osmolarity 486 mOsm/L. Soln. Bot. 2000 ml.
Use: Peritoneal dialysis solution.
•**DIAPAMIDE.** USAN.
Use: Diuretic, antihypertensive.

DIAPANTIN. (Janssen) Isoprofamide bromide.
Use: Anticholinergic.

DIAPARENE. (Glenbrook) Methylbenzethonium Cl. Pow. Bot. 4 oz, 9 oz, 12.5 oz, 14 oz.
Use: Surface-active disinfectant.

DIAPARENE CRADOL EMULS. (Glenbrook) Methylbenzethonium Cl in petrolatum and lanolin Base. Plastic Bot. 3 oz.
Use: Antimicrobial.

DIAPARENE OINTMENT. (Glenbrook) Methylbenzethonium Cl 0.1% w/petrolatum, glycerin. Tube 1 oz, 2 oz, 4 oz.
Use: Antimicrobial.

DIAPARENE PERI-ANAL CREAM. (Glenbrook) Methylbenzethonium Cl 1:1000, zinc oxide, starch, cod liver oil, white petrolatum, lanolin, calcium caseinate. Cream Tube 1 oz, 2 oz, 4 oz.
Use: Antimicrobial, astringent.

DIAPARESS. (Jenkins) Cod liver oil, diperodon HCl 0.25%, zinc oxide, starch, aluminum acetate, balsam Peru. Tube 1.5 oz.
Use: Skin protectant.

DIAPHENYLSULFONE. Dapsone, U.S.P. XXII.
Use: Leprostatic.

DIAPID. (Sandoz,) Lypressin synthetic lysine-8-vasopressin. Equiv. to 50 U.S.P. units posterior pituitary/ml (0.185 mg/ml). Nasal spray. Bot. 8 ml.
Use: Pituitary hormone.

DI-AP-TROL. (Foy) Phendimetrazine tartrate 35 mg/Tab. Bot. 100s, 1000s.
Use: Anorexiant.

DIAQUA. (Hauck) Hydrochlorothiazide 50 mg/ Tab. Bot. 100s, 1000s.
Use: Diuretic.

DIA-QUEL. (MiLance) Opium 18 mg (equivalent to 4.5 ml paregoric), homatropine MBr 0.9 mg, pectin 144 mg/ml with alcohol 10%. Liq. Bot. 120 ml.
Use: Antidiarrheal.

DIAR AID. (Thompson Medical) Activated attapulgite 750 mg, pectin 150 mg Tab. Bot. 12s, 24s.
Use: Antidiarrheal.

DIARREST. (Dover) Calcium carbonate, pectin/ Tab. Sugar, lactose and salt free. UD box 500s.
Use: Antidiarrheal.

DIARRHEA RELIEF WITH PAREGORIC. (Weeks & Leo) Bismuth subsalicylate 63 mg, kaolin 675 mg, pectin 27 mg, paregoric 0.6 mg/ 5 ml Bot. 4 oz.
Use: Antidiarrheal.

DIARRHEA THERAPY.
See: Antidiarrheals.

DIASERP TABS. (Major) Chlorothiazide 250 mg or 500 mg/Tab. w/reserpine. Bot. 100s.
Use: Antihypertensive.

DIASORB. (Schering) Activated nonfibrous attapulgite. **Liq.:** 750 mg per 5 ml. In 120 ml. **Tab.:** 750 mg. In 24s.
Use: Antidiarrheal.

DIASPORAL CREAM. (Doak) Formerly Sulfur Salicyl Diasporal. Sulfur 3%, salicylic acid 2%, isopropyl alcohol in diasporal base. Cream Jar 3¾ oz.
Use: Antiseptic, topical.

DIASTASE.
See: Aspergillus oryzae enzyme.
W/Bismuth subnitrate, sodium bicarbonate, magnesium carbonate, papain.
See: Panacarb, Tab. (Lannett).
W/Carica papaya enzyme.
See: Caripeptic, Liq. (Upjohn).
W/Sodium bicarbonate, magnesium carbonate, bismuth subnitrate, papain.

DIASTIX REAGENT STRIPS. (Ames) Broad range test for glucose in urine. Containing glucose oxidase, peroxidase, potassium iodide/w blue background dye. Tab. Pkg. 50s, 100s.
Use: Diagnostic aid.

DIATRIZOATE. 3,5-diacetamido-2,4,6-triiodobenzoic acid.

•**DIATRIZOATE MEGLUMINE,** U.S.P. XXII. Inj., U.S.P. XXII. Benzoic acid, 3,5-bis(acetylamino)-2,4,6-triiodo compound with 1-deoxy-1-(methylamino)-glucitol (1:1).
Use: Diagnostic aid (radiopaque medium).
See: Angiovist 282, Inj. (Berlex).
Cardiografin, Vial (Squibb).
Cystographin, Inj. (Squibb).
Gastrografin, Liq. (Squibb).
Hypaque-Cysto, Liq. (Winthrop Pharm).
Hypaque Meglumine (Winthrop Pharm).
Renografin, Inj. (Squibb).
Reno-M-DIP, Inj. (Squibb).
Reno-M-30, Inj. (Squibb).
Reno-M-60, Inj. (Squibb).
Urovist, Prods. (Berlex).
W/Iodipamide methylglucamine.
See: Sinografin, Vial (Squibb).
W/Sodium Diatrizoate.
See: Renovist, Inj. (Squibb).

•**DIATRIZOATE MEGLUMINE AND DIATRIZOATE SODIUM INJECTION,** U.S.P. XXII.
Use: Diagnostic aid (radiopaque medium).
See: Angiorist 292, Inj. (Berlex).
Angiovist 370, Inj. (Berlex).
Gastrovist, Soln. (Berlex).
Hypaque-M Prods. (Winthrop Pharm).

•**DIATRIZOATE MEGLUMINE AND DIATRIZOATE SODIUM SOLUTION,** U.S.P. XXII.
Use: Diagnostic aid (radiopaque medium).
See: Gastrografini Soln. (Squibb).
Renografin-60, Soln. (Squibb).
Renografin-76, Soln. (Squibb).
Renovist, Soln. (Squibb).

DIATRIZOATE METHYLGLUCAMINE.
Use: Diagnostic aid (radiopaque medium).
See: Diatrizoate Meglumine, U.S.P. XXII.

DIATRIZOATE METHYLGLUCAMINE SODIUM. Sodium salt of N-methylglucamine salt of 3,5-diacetamido-2,4,6-triiodobenzoate.
Use: Diagnostic aid (radiopaque medium).

•**DIATRIZOATE SODIUM,** U.S.P. XXII. Inj., Soln., U.S.P. XXII. Benzoic acid, 3,5-bis(acetylamino)-2,4,6-triiodo-, monosodium salt.
Use: Diagnostic aid (radiopaque medium).
See: Hypaque Prods. (Winthrop Pharm).
Urovist Sodium, Inj. (Berlex).
W/Meglumine diatrizoate.
See: Gastrografin, Liq.(Squibb).
Renografin-60, -76, Vial (Squibb).
Renovist II, Vial (Squibb).
W/Methylglucamine diatrizoate, sodium citrate, disodium ethylenediamine tetra-acetate dihydrate, methylparaben, propylparaben.
See: Renovist, Vial (Squibb).

•**DIATRIZOATE SODIUM I-125.** USAN.
Use: Radioactive agent.

•**DIATRIZOATE SODIUM I-131.** USAN.
Use: Radioactive agent.

•**DIATRIZOIC ACID.** USAN. 3,5-Diacetamido-2,4,6-tri-iodobenzoic acid.
Use: Radiopaque substance.
See: Amidotrizoic Acid.
Hypaque sodium salt.

•**DIATRIZOIC ACID,** U.S.P. XXII. Benzoic acid, 3,5-bis(acetylamino)-2,4,6-triiodo-. 3,5-Diacetamido-2,4,6-triiodobenzoic acid.
Use: Radiopaque medium (urographic).

DIATROL. (Otis Clapp) Calcium carbonate 261 mg, pectin 65 mg. In 100s, 200s, 500s.
Use: Antacid.

•**DIAVERIDINE.** USAN. 2,4-Diamino-5-(3,4-dimethoxybenzyl)pyrimidine. Present in Darvisul.
Use: Antiprotozoan, (veterinary).

•**DIAZEPAM,** U.S.P. XXII. Cap., Extended-Release Cap., Inj., Tab: U.S.P. XXII. 2H-1,4-Benzodiazepin-2-one, 7-chloro-1,3-dihydro-1-methyl-5-phenyl-. 7-Chloro-1,3-dihydro-1-methyl-5-phenyl-2H-1,4-benzodiazepin-2-one. B.A.N. 7-Chloro-1,3-dihydro-1-methyl-5-phenyl-2H-1,4-benzodiazepin-2-one.
Use: Agent for control of emotional disturbances; sedative; tranquilizer.
Oral Soln. (Roxane): 5 mg/5 ml. In 500 ml and UD 5 mg, 10 mg patient cups.
Concentrated Oral Soln. (Roxane): 5 mg/ml In 30 ml w/dropper.
See: Valium, Tab. (Roche).
Valrelease, S.R. Cap. (Roche).

•**DIAZIQUONE.** USAN.
Use: Antineoplastic.

DIAZMA. (Pharmex) Diphylline 250 mg/ml. Vial 10 ml.
Use: Antiasthmatic.

DIAZOMYCINS A, B, & C. Antibiotic obtained from *Streptomyces ambofaciens*. Under study.

•**DIAZOXIDE,** U.S.P. XXII. Cap., Oral Susp., Inj., U.S.P. XXII. 7-Chloro-3-methyl-2H-1,-2, 4-benzothiadiazine-1, 1-dioxide.
Use: Glucose elevating agent.
See: Proglycem Capsules (Medical Market Specialists).
Proglycem Suspension (Medical Market Specialists).

•**DIBASIC CALCIUM PHOSPHATE DIHYDRATE,** U.S.P. XXII.
Use: Replenisher (calcium); pharmaceutic aid (tablet base).
See: D.C.P. 340, Tab. (Parke-Davis).
Diostate D, Tab. (Upjohn).

DIBASIC CALCIUM PHOSPHATE w/VITAMIN D. (Lilly) Dibasic calcium phosphate, anhydrous, equiv. to 500 mg of dibasic calcium phosphate dihydrate, Vitamin D synthetic 33 IU (0.825 mcg)/Pulv. Bot. 100s.
Use: Calcium, phosphorus and Vitamin D supplement.

DIBATROL. (Metro Med) Chlorpropamide 100 mg or 250 mg/Tab. Bot. 100s, 1000s.
Use: Antidiabetic agent.

DIBENCIL.
See: Benzathine Penicillin G. (Various Mfr.).

DIBENT. (Hauck) Dicyclomine 10 mg/ml with chlorobutanol. Inj. Vial 10 ml.
Use: GI anticholinergic/antispasmodic.

DIBENZEPIN. B.A.N. 10-(2-Dimethylaminoethyl)-5-methyldibenzo[b,e][1,4]diazepin-11-one.
Use: Antidepressant.

•**DIBENZEPIN HCl.** USAN. 10-[2-Dimethylamino)ethyl]-5,10-dihydro-5-methyl-llH-dibenzo-[b,e][1,4]diazepin-11-one monohydroCl.
Use: Antidepressant.

•**DIBENZOTHIOPHENE.** USAN.
Use: Keratolytic.

DIBENZYLETHYLENEDIAMINE DIPENICILLIN G, U.S.P.
See: Benzethacil.

DIBENZYLINE. (SmithKline Beecham) Phenoxybenzamine HCl 10 mg/Cap. Bot. 100s.
Use: Antihypertensive.

•**DIBROMSALAN.** USAN. 4′, 5-Dibromosalicylanilide. Diaphene.
Use: Germicide.

•**DIBUCAINE,** U.S.P. XXII. Cream, Oint., U.S.P. XXII. 2-Butoxy-N-[2-(diethylamino)ethyl]-cinchoninamide.
Use: Local anesthetic.
See: D-caine, Oint. (Century).
Dulzit, Cream (Commerce).
Nupercainal, Oint. (Ciba).
W/Benzocaine.
See: Extend, Tab. (E.J. Moore).
W/Benzocaine, tetracaine.
See: Bonal Itch Cream, (E.J. Moore).
W/Hydrocortisone.
See: Corticaine Cream (Whitby).
W/Dextrose.
See: Nupercaine Heavy Soln. (Ciba).
W/Sodium bisulfite.
See: Nupercainal, Cream, Oint. (Ciba).
W/Zinc oxide, bismuth subgallate, acetone sodium bisulfite.
See: Nupercainal, Oint., Supp. (Ciba).

•**DIBUCAINE HYDROCHLORIDE,** U.S.P. XXII. Inj., U.S.P. XXII. 2-Butoxy-N-(2-diethylaminoethyl) cinchoninamide HCl. (Cinchocaine, Percaine).
Use: Surface and spinal anesthesia.
See: Nupercaine HCl, soln., (Ciba).
W/Antipyrine, hydrocortisone, polymyxin B sulfate, neomycin sulfate.
See: Otocort, Liq. (Lemmon).
W/Colistin sodium methanesulfonate, citric acid, sodium citrate.
See: Coly-Mycin M, Injectable (Warner-Chilcott).

DIBUPYRONE. B.A.N. Sodium N-(2,3-dimethyl-1-phenyl-5-oxopyrazolin-4-yl)-N-isobutylaminomethanesulphonate.
Use: Analgesic.

DIBUTOLINE SULFATE. Ethyl(2-hydroxy-ethyl)-dimethylammonium sulfate (2:1) bis(dibutyl-carbamate).
Use: Anticholinergic/antispasmodic.

DI-CAL CAPTABS. (Rugby) Calcium 116 mg, vitamin D 133 IU, phosphorus 90 mg. Bot. 1000s.
Use: Calcium, vitamin D supplement.

DI-CAL D. (Abbott) Calcium 117 mg, vitamin D 133 IU, phosphorus 90 mg/Tab. Bot. 100s, 500s.
Use: Calcium, vitamin D supplement.

DICALCIUM PHOSPHATE. Dibasic Calcium Phosphate, U.S.P., Monocalcium Phosphate. (Various Mfr.) **Cap.:** 7.5 gr or 10 gr. **Tab.:** 7.5 gr, 10 gr or 15 gr. **Wafer:** 15 gr.
Use: Calcium supplement.
See: Irophos-D, Cap. (Lannett).
W/Calcium gluconate and Vitamin D. (Various Mfr.) Cap., Tab., Wafer.
See: Calcicaps, Tab. (Nion).
Di-Cal, Cap. (Kenyon).
W/Iron and Vitamin D. (Various Mfr.).
Lilly—Pulv., Bot. 100s.
W/Vitamin D. (Squibb) Calcium 85 mg, phosphorous 60 mg, vitamin D 41 IU.

DICAL-D. (Abbott) Dibasic calcium phosphate containing calcium 116.7 mg, phosphorous 90 mg, vitamin D 133 IU/Cap. Bot. 100s, 500s.
Use: Calcium and phosphorus supplement.

DICAL-D WITH VITAMIN C. (Abbott) Dibasic calcium phosphate containing calcium 116.7 mg, phosphorus 90 mg, vitamin D 133 IU, ascorbic acid 15 mg/Cap. Bot. 100s.
Use: Calcium, phosphorus and Vitamin C supplement.

DICAL-D WAFERS. (Abbott) Dibasic calcium phosphate containing calcium 232 mg, phosphorus 180 mg, vitamin D 200 IU/Wafer. Box 51s.
Use: Calcium, phosphorus supplement.

DICAL-DEE. (Barre) Vitamins D 350 IU, dibasic calcium phosphate 4.5 gr, calcium gluconate 3 gr/Cap. Bot. 100s, 1000s.
Use: Calcium supplement.

DICALDEL. (Faraday) Dibasic calcium phosphate 300 mg, calcium gluconate 200 mg, vitamin D 33 IU/Cap. Bot. 100s, 250s, 500s, 1000s.
Use: Calcium supplement.

DICALTABS. (Faraday) Dibasic calcium phosphate 108 mg, calcium gluconate 140 mg, vitamin D 35 IU/Tab. Bot. 100s, 250s, 1000s.

DICARBOSIL. (Norcliff-Thayer) Calcium carbonate 500 mg/Tab. Roll 12s.
Use: Antacid.

DI-CET. (Sanford & Son) Methylbenzethonium Cl 24.4 Gm, sodium carbonate monohydrate 48.8 Gm, sodium nitrite 24.4 Gm, trisodium ethylenediamine tetra-acetate monohydrate 2.4 Gm. Pow. Pkg. 2.4 Gm, Box 24s.
Use: Dental instrument disinfectant.

DICHLORALANTIPYRINE. Dichloralphenazone. Chloralpyrine. A complex of 2 mol. chloral hydrate with 1 mol. antipyrine. Sominat.
W/Isometheptene mucate, N-acetyl-p-amino-phenol.
See: Midrin, Cap. (Carnrick).

DICHLORALPHENAZONE. B.A.N. A complex of chloral hydrate and phenazone. Dichloralantipyrine (Various Mfr.).
Use: Hypnotic.

DICHLORAMINE T. (Various Mfr.) (1% to 5% in chlorinated paraffin). P-Toluenesulfone-dichloramine.
Use: Antiseptic

DICHLOREN.
See: Mechlorethamine HCl, Sterile Inj. (Various Mfr.).

DICHLORISONE ACETATE. 9a, 11b-dichloro-dl,-4-pregnadiene-17a,21-diol-3,20-dione-21-acetate.

DICHLORMETHAZANONE. 2-(3,4-dichlorophenyl)-3-methyl-4-metathiazanone-1-dioxide.

•**DICHLORODIFLUOROMETHANE,** N.F. XVII.
Use: Aerosol propellant.

DICHLORODIPHENYL TRICHLOROETHANE.
See: Chlorophenothane (Various Mfr.).

DICHLOROPHEN. B.A.N. Di(5-chloro-2-hydroxyphenyl) methane.
Use: Anthelmintic.

DICHLOROPHENARSINE. B.A.N. 3-Amino-4-hydroxyphenyldichloroarsine.
Use: Antifungal.

DICHLOROPHENARSINE HYDROCHLORIDE. (Chlorarsen, Clorarsen, Fontarsol, Halarsol).

DICHLOROPHENE. Didroxane. G-4, bis(5-Chloro-2-hydroxyphenyl) methane. Related to hexachlorophene.
W/Parachlorometaxylenol, propylparaaminobenzoate, hexachlorophene, benzocaine.
See: Triguent, Oint. (Commerce).
W/Undecylenic acid.
See: Fungicidal Talc. (Gordon).
Onychomycetin, Liq. (Gordon).
W/Undecylenic acid, salicylicacid, hexachlorophene.
See: Podiaspray, aerosol pow. (Dalin).

•**DICHLOROTETRAFLUOROETHANE,** N.F. XVII. 1, 2-Dichlorotetrafluoroethane.
Use: Aerosol propellant.

DICHLOROXYLENOL. B.A.N. 2,4-Dichloro-3,5-xylenol.
Use: Bactericide.

DICHLORPHENAMIDE, U.S.P. XXI. Tab. U.S.P. XXI. 1,3-Benzenedisulfonamide, 4,5-di- chloro-. 1,3-Disulfamyl-4-5-dichloro-benzene. B.A.N. 4,5-Dichlorobenzene-1,3-disulfonamide.
Use: Agent for glaucoma.

•**DICHLORVOS.** USAN. 2, 2-Dichlorovinyl dimethyl phosphate.
Use: Anthelmintic, insecticide (veterinary).
See: Atgard.
Canogard.
Equigard.
Vapona.

DICHOLIN. (Kenyon) Ox bile extract ⅜ gr, iron lactate ¾ gr, calumba ¾ gr, chamomile flowers 1⅝ gr, rhubarb 1⅝ gr/Cap. Bot. 100s, 1000s.

DICHROMIUM TRIOXIDE. B.A.N. Chromium sesquioxide.
Use: Diagnostic aid.

•**DICIRENONE.** USAN.
Use: Hypotensive.

DICKEY'S OLD RELIABLE EYE WASH. (Dickey Drug) Berberine sulfate, boric acid, propyl parasept, methyl parasept. Plastic dropper bot. 8 ml, 12 ml, 1 oz.
Use: Counter-irritant, ophthalmic.

•**DICLOFENAC SODIUM.** USAN.
Use: Anti-inflammatory.
See: Voltaren (Geigy).

•**DICLORALUREA.** USAN.
Use: Food additive.

DICLOXACIL. (Goldline) Dicloxacillin sodium 250 mg or 500 mg/Cap. Bot. 100s.
Use: Antibacterial, penicillin.

•**DICLOXACILLIN.** USAN.6-[3-(2,6-Dichlorophenyl)-5-methyl-4-isoxazolecarboxamido]-3,3-dimethyl-7-oxo-4-thia-1-azabicyclo[3.2.0]-heptane-2-carboxylic acid.
Use: Antibiotic.
See: Dynapen, Cap., Susp. (Bristol).
Pathocil, Cap., Susp. (Wyeth-Ayerst).
Veracillin, Cap., Inj. (Wyeth-Ayerst).

•**DICLOXACILLIN SODIUM,** U.S.P. XXII. Cap., Sterile, For Oral Susp. U.S.P. XXII.
Use: Penicillinase-resistant penicillin.
See: Dycill, Cap. (Beecham).
Dynapen, Cap., Soln. (Bristol).

DICODETHAL ELIXIR. (Lannett) Dextromethorphan HBr 10 mg/5 ml in el. terpin hydrate. Bot. pt, gal.
Use: Antitussive, expectorant.

DICOLE. (Blue Cross) Docusate sodium 100 mg/Cap. Bot. 100s.
Use: Laxative.

DICOPHANE.
See: Chlorophenothane (Various Mfr.), DDT.

DICOUMARIN.
See: Dicumarol, Preps. (Various Mfr.).

DICOUMAROL.
See: Dicumarol, U.S.P. XXII.

•**DICUMAROL,** U.S.P. XXII. Tab., U.S.P. XXII. Cap., U.S.P. XXI. 2H-1-Benzopyran-2-one 3,3′-methylenebis 4-hy-droxy-3,3′-methylenebis(4-hydroxycoumarin). Dicoumarol. Dicoumarin. Bishydroxycoumarin. Melitoxin. (Abbott) Tab. 25 mg or 50 mg Bot. 100s, 1000s; 100 mg Bot. 1000s.
Use: Blood anticoagulant.

•**DICYCLOMINE HYDROCHLORIDE,** U.S.P. XXII. Cap., Inj., Syr., Tab., U.S.P. XXII. Bicyclohexyl-1-carboxylic acid, 2-(diethylamino) ethyl 3w534 HCl. 2-(Diethylamino)ethyl (Bicyclohexyl)-1-carboxylate hydroCl.
Use: Antispasmodic.
See: Antispas, Inj. (Keene).
Benacol, Tab. (Cenci).
Bentyl, Amp. Syringe, Cap., Tab., Syr. (Merrell Dow).
Dysaps, Tab., Liq., Inj. (Savage).
Nospaz, Vial (Solvay).
Rocyclo Preps. (Robinson).
Rotyl HCl, Vial (Rocky Mtn.).
Stannitol (Standex).
W/Aluminum hydroxide, magnesium hydroxide, methylcellulose.
See: Triactin Liq., Tab. (Norwich Eaton).
W/Phenobarbital.
See: Bentyl with Phenobarbital, Prods. (Merrell Dow).

DICYCLON-M. (Kenyon) Dicyclomine HCl 10 mg, pyrilamine maleate 10 mg, pyridoxine HCl 10 mg/Tab. Bot. 100s, 1000s.
Use: Anticholinergic/antispasmodic.

DICYCLON NO.1. (Kenyon) Dicyclomine HCl 10 mg/Tab. Bot. 100s, 1000s.
Use: Anticholinergic/antispasmodic.

DICYCLON NO. 2. (Kenyon) Dicyclomine HCl 10 mg, phenobarbital 15 mg/Tab. Bot. 100s, 1000s.
Use: Anticholinergic/antispasmodic, sedative/hypnotic.

DICYCLON NO. 3. (Kenyon) Dicyclomine HCl 20 mg, phenobarbital 15 mg/Tab. Bot. 100s, 1000s.
Use: Anticholinergic/antispasmodic, sedative/hypnotic.

DICYNENE. (Baxter)
Use: Hemostatic agent.
See: Ethamsylate.

DICYSTEINE.
See: Cystine, Pow. (Various Mfr.)

•**DIDANOSINE.** USAN.
Use: Antiviral, systemic.

DI-DELAMINE GEL. (Commerce) Tripelennamine HCl 0.5%, diphenhydramine HCl 1%, benzalkonium Cl 0.12% in clear gel. Tube 1.25 oz.
Use: Antipruritic.

DI-DELAMINE SPRAY. (Commerce) Tripelennamine HCl 0.5%, diphenhydramine HCl 1%, benzalkonium Cl 0.12%. Spray pump 4 oz.
Use: Antipruritic.

DIDREX. (Upjohn) Benzphetamine HCl. **25 mg/Tab.:** Bot. 100s; **50 mg/Tab.:** Bot. 100s, 500s.
Use: Anorexiant.

DIDRONEL. (Norwich Eaton) Etidronate disodium 200 mg or 400 mg/Tab. Bot. 60s. **IV Infusion:** Etidronate disodium 300 mg/6 ml amp.
Use: Hypercalcemia of malignancy.

•**DIENESTROL,** U.S.P. XXII. Cream, U.S.P. XXII. Non-steroid, synthetic estrogen. Dienoestrol. 4,4′-(Diethylideneethylene)diphenol. (Ortho) Dienestrol 0.01%. Tube 78 Gm w/applicator.
Use: Estrogen therapy, atrophic vaginitis.
See: D V, Cream (Merrell Dow).
D V, Supp. (Merrell Dow).
Ortho Dienestrol Cream (Ortho).
W/Sulfanilamide, aminacrine HCl, allantoin.
See: AVC/Dienestrol Cream, Supp. (Merrell Dow).

DIET AYDS. (DEP) Benzocaine 6 mg/square. Bot. 48s.
Use: Diet aid.

DIETHADIONE. B.A.N. 5,5-Diethyloxazine-2,4-dione.
Use: Analeptic agent.

•**DIETHANOLAMINE,** N.F. XVII.
Use: Pharmaceutic acid (alkalizing agent).

DIETHAZINE. B.A.N. 10-(2-Diethylaminoethyl)-Phenothiazine.
Use: Treatment of Parkinsonian syndrome.

DIETHAZINE HCl. 10-(β-Diethylaminoethyl)-pheno-thiazine HCl. Diparcol.

DIETHANOLAMINE.
See: Diolamine.

DIETHOXIN. Intracaine HCl.

•**DIETHYLCARBAMAZINE CITRATE,** U.S.P. XXII. Tab., U.S.P. XXII. Diethylcarbamazine Dihydrogen Citrate. N, N-Diethyl-4-methyl-1-piperazinecarboxamide dihydrogen citrate. 1-Piperazinecarboxamide, N,N-diethyl-4-methyl-, 2-hydroxy-1,2,3-propanetricarboxylate. Banocide, Ethodryl.
Use: Antifilarial.

DIETHYLDITHIOCARBAMATE.
Use: Trial drug for AIDS.
See: Imuthiol.

DIETHYLENEDIAMINE CITRATE. Piperazine Citrate, Piperazine Hexahydrate.
See: Antepar, Syr., Tab., Wafer (Burroughs Wellcome).

DIETHYLMALONYLUREA.
See: Barbital, Tab. (Various Mfr.).

•**DIETHYL PHTHALATE,** N.F. XVII.
Use: Plasticizer.

•**DIETHYLPROPION HCl,** U.S.P. XXII. Tab., U.S.P. XXII. 1-Phenyl-2-diethylaminopropanone-1 HCl. 2-(Di- ethylamino)propiophenone HCl.
Use: Anorexiant.
See: D.E.P.-75
Ro-Diet, Tab. (Robinson).
Ro-Diet Timed (Robinson).
Tenuate, Tab. (Merrell Dow).
Tepanil, Tab. (Riker).
Tepanil Ten-Tab, Tab. (Riker).

•**DIETHYLSTILBESTROL,** U.S.P. XXII. Inj., Tab., U.S.P. XXII. Supp. U.S.P. XXI. Phenol 4,4′-(1,2-diethyl-1,2-ethenediyl)bis-. (Cyren A, Domestrol, Estrobene, Fonatol, New-Oestranol 1, Oestrogenine, Oestromie-nin, Palestrol, Synthoestrin, Stiboestroform, Stilbestrol, Synestrin) alpha, alpha′-Diethyl-4,4′-stilbenediol.
Use: Estrogen.
See: Acnestrol, Lot. (Dermik).
Mase-Bestrol, Tab. (Mason).
W/Clioquinol, sulfanilamide.
See: D.I.T.I. Creme (Dunhall).
W/Nitrofurazone, diperodon HCl.
See: Furacin-E Urethral Inserts (Eaton).

•**DIETHYLSTILBESTROL DIPHOSPHATE,** U.S.P. XXII. Inj., U.S.P. XXII.
Use: Estrogen.
See: Stilphostrol, Inj., Tab. (Miles Pharm).

DIETHYLSTILBESTROL DIPROPIONATE, a,a′-Diethyl-4, 4′ stilbenediol dipropionate. Cyren B, Estilben, Estroben DP, New-Oestranol 11, Orestol, Pabestrol D, Stilbestronate, Stilboestrol DP, Stilronate, Synestrin Amp. (Various Mfr.) Amp. in oil, 0.5 mg, 1 mg or 5 mg/ml. Tab. 0.5 mg, 1 mg or 5 mg.
Use: Estrogen.

DIETHYLTHIAMBUTENE. B.A.N. 3-Diethylamino-1, 1-di(2-thienyl)but-1-ene.
Use: Narcotic analgesic.

•**DIETHYLTOLUAMIDE,** U.S.P. XXII. Topical Soln., U.S.P. XXII. Benzamide, N, N-diethyl-3-methyl-N, N-Diethyl-m-toluamide.
Use: Repellent (arthropod).
See: RV Pellent, Oint. (Elder).

N, N-DIETHYLVANILLAMIDE.
See: Ethamivan, Inj. (Various Mfr.).

DIET-TRIM. (Pharmex) Phenylpropanolamine, carboxymethylcellulose, benzocaine/Tab. Bot. 21s, 90s.
Use: Diet aid.

DIET-TUSS. (Approved) Dextromethorphan 30 mg, thenylpyramine HCl, pyrilamine maleate 80 mg, sodium salicylate 200 mg, sodium citrate 600 mg, ammonium Cl 100 mg/fl oz. Sugar free. Bot. 4 oz.
Use: Antitussive, antihistamine, analgesic, expectorant.

DIEUTRIM T.D. (Legere) Phenylpropanolamine 75 mg, benzocaine 9 mg, sodium carboxymethylcellulose 75 mg/SR Cap. Bot. 100s, 1000s.
Use: Diet aid.

•**DIFENOXIMIDE HYDROCHLORIDE.** USAN.
Use: Antiperistaltic.

•**DIFENOXIN.** USAN. 1-(3-Cyano-3, 3-diphenylpropyl)-4-phenylpiperidine-4-carboxylic acid.
Use: Antidiarrheal.
W/Atropine sulfate.
See: Motofen (Carnrick).

DIFETARSONE. B.A.N. NN′-Ethylene-1, 2-diarsanilic acid.
Use: Arsenicalcium.

•**DIFLORASONE DIACETATE,** U.S.P. XXII. Cream, Oint., U.S.P. XXII. 6α, 9α-difluoro 11β, 17, 21trihydroxy-16β methyl-pregna-1, 4-diene-3, 20-dione 17, 21 diacetate.
Use: Anti-inflammatory, antipruritic.
See: Florone, Cream, Oint. (Upjohn).
Maxiflor, Cream, Oint. (Herbert).

•**DIFLOXACIN HYDROCHLORIDE.** USAN.
Use: Anti-infective (DNA gyrase inhibitor).

•**DIFLUANINE HCl.** USAN. (McNeil) 1-(2-Anilinoethyl)-4-[4, 4-bis(p-fluorophenyl)butyl]-piperazine trihydroCl.
Use: CNS stimulant.

DIFLUCAN. (Roerig) Fluconazole. **Tab.:** 50 mg, 100 mg or 200 mg. Bot. 30s, UD 100s. **Inj.:** 2 mg/ml. Vial 100 ml, 200 ml.
Use: Antifungal.

•**DIFLUCORTOLONE.** USAN. 6α,9-Difluoro-11β, 21-dihydroxy-16α-methylpregna-1, 4-diene-3, 20-dione.
Use: Glucocorticoid.

•**DIFLUCORTOLONE PIVALATE.** USAN.
Use: Glucocorticoid.

•**DIFLUMIDONE SODIUM.** USAN.
Use: Anti-inflammatory agent.

•**DIFLUNISAL,** U.S.P. XXII. Tab., U.S.P. XXII.
Use: Analgesic, anti-inflammatory agent.
See: Dolobid, Tab. (Merck Sharp & Dohme).

•**DIFTALONE.** USAN.
Use: Anti-inflammatory agent.

•**DIFLUPREDNATE.** USAN. 6α, 9-difluoro-11β, 17, 21-trihydroxypregna-1, 4-diene-3, 20-dione 21-acetate-17-butyrate.
Use: Anti-inflammatory agent.

DI-GEL ADVANCED FORMULA. (Schering-Plough) Magnesium hydroxide 128 mg, calcium carbonate 280 mg, simethicone 20 mg/Tab. Bot. 30s, 60s, 90s.
Use: Antacid, antiflatulent.

DI-GEL LIQUID. (Schering-Plough) Aluminum hydroxide (equivalent to dried gel) 200 mg, magnesium hydroxide 200 mg, simethicone 20 mg/5 ml, saccharin, sorbitol. Bot. 6 oz, 12 oz. Mint or lemon-orange.
Use: Antacid, antiflatulent.

DIGESTAMIC. (Metro Med) Pancrealipase 300 mg, pepsin 100 mg/Tab. Bot. 50s.
Use: Digestive aid.

DIGESTAMIC LIQUID. (Metro Med) Belladonna leaf fluid extract 0.64 min./5 ml. Bot. 8 oz.
Use: Anticholinergic/antispasmodic.

DIGESTANT. (Canright) Pancreatin 5.25 gr, ox bile extract 2 gr, pepsin 5 gr, betaine HCl 1 gr/Tab. Bot. 100s, 1000s.
Use: Digestive aid.

DIGESTIVE COMPOUND. (Thurston) Betaine HCl 3.25 gr, pepsin 1 gr, papain 2 gr, mycozyme 2 gr, ox bile 2 gr/2 Tab. Bot. 100s, 500s.
Use: Digestive aid.

DIGESTOZYME TABS. (Goldline) Pancreatin, pepsin, bile salts. Bot. 1000s.
Use: Digestive aid.

DIGIBIND. (Burroughs Wellcome) Digoxin Immune Fab (ovine) fragments 40 mg, sorbitol 75 mg/Vial. Box 1s.
Use: Antidote.

DIGIDOTE. (Orphan Drug)
Use: Antidote.
Sponsor: Boehringer Mannheim.

DIGITALIS GLYCOSIDES.
Use: Cardiotonic.
See: Acylanid, Tab. (Sandoz).
Cedilanid, Tab. (Sandoz).
Cedilanid-D, Amp. (Sandoz).
Crystodigin, Tab. Amp., Vial (Lilly).
Deslanoside, Inj. (Various Mfr.).
Digiglusin, Tab. (Lilly).
Digitaline Nativelle, Soln., Tab., Elix. (Savage).
Digitoxin, Preps. (Various Mfr.).
Digoxin, Preps. (Various Mfr.).
Gitaligin, Tab. (Schering).
Gitalin, Tab. (Various Mfr.).
Lanatoside C, Inj., Tab. (Various Mfr.).
Lanoxin, Tab., Inj., Elix. (Burroughs Wellcome).
Purodigin, Tab. (Wyeth-Ayerst).

DIGITALIS LEAF, POWDERED.
Use: Cardiotonic.
See: Pil-Digis, Pill (Key).

DIGITALIS TINCTURE.
Use: Cardiotonic.

•**DIGITOXIN,** U.S.P. XXII. Inj., Tab., U.S.P. XXII. (Various Mfr.) Amp. (0.2 mg/ml) 1 ml, Cap. in oil, 0.1 mg or 0.2 mg. Tab. 0.1 mg, 0.2 mg.
Use: Digitalis therapy, cardiotonic.
See: Crystodigin, Tab. (Lilly).
De-Tone 0.1, 0.2, Tab. (Scrip).
Digitaline Nativelle, Preps. (Savage).
Maso-Toxin, Tab. (Mason).
W/Carboxymethylcellulose and sodium.
See: Foxalin, Cap. (Standex).

DIGITOXIN, ACETYL.
Use: Cardiotonic.
See: Acylanid, Tab. (Sandoz).

α-DIGITOXIN MONOACETATE.
Use: Cardiotonic.
See: Acetyldigitoxin, Tab. (Various Mfr.).

•**DIGOXIN,** U.S.P. XXII. Elix., Inj., Tab. U.S.P. XXII. Crystalline glycoside isolated from lvs. of digitalis lanata. 0.25 mg/Tab. Bot. 1000s, UD 100s.
Use: Cardiotonic.
See: Lanoxin, Preps. (Burroughs Wellcome).
Masoxin, Tab. (Mason).

DIGOXIN ANTIBODY.
See: Digidote.

DIGOXIN I-125 IMUSAY. (Abbott Diagnostics) Digoxin diagnostic kit for the quantitative determination of serum digoxin. 100s, 300s.
Use: Diagnostic aid.

DIGOXIN IMMUNE FAB (OVINE) FRAGMENTS.
Use: Antidote.
See: Digibind, Inj. (Burroughs Wellcome).
DIGOXIN RIABEAD. (Abbott Diagnostics) Solid-phase radioimmunoassay for quantitative measurement of serum digoxin. Test kit 100s, 300s.
Use: Diagnostic aid.
•**DIHEXYVERINE HYDROCHLORIDE.** USAN.
Use: Anticholinergic.
DIHISTINE D.H. (Goldline) Pseudoephedrine HCl 30 mg, chlorpheniramine maleate 2 mg, codeine phosphate 10 mg. Elix. Bot. 4 oz, pt, gal.
Use: Decongestant, antihistamine, antitussive.
DIHISTINE ELIXIR. (Various Mfr.) Phenylephrine HCl 5 mg, chlorpheniramine maleate 2 mg/5 ml. Bot. pt, gal.
Use: Decongestant, antihistamine.
DIHISTINE EXPECTORANT. (Goldline) Pseudoephedrine HCl 30 mg, codeine phosphate 10 mg, guaifenesin 100 mg, alcohol 7.5%. Bot. 4 oz, pt, gal.
Use: Decongestant, antitussive, expectorant.
DIHYDAN SOLUBLE.
See: Phenytoin Sodium (Various Mfr.).
DIHYDRALLAZINE. B.A.N. 1,4-Dihydrazinophthalazine.
Use: Hypotensive.
DIHYDROCODEINE. Paracodin. Drocode.
Use: Antitussive, analgesic.
DIHYDROCODEINE COMPOUND. (Various Mfr.) Dihydrocodeine bitartrate 16 mg, aspirin 356.4 mg, caffeine 30 mg. Cap. Bot. 100s, 500s.
Use: Narcotic analgesic.
•**DIHYDROCODEINONE BITARTRATE.** U.S.P. XXII.
Use: Narcotic.
See: Hydrocodone Bitartrate, U.S.P. XXII.
W/Caffeine, phenacetin, aspirin.
See: Drocogesic #3, Tab. (Rand).
Duradyne DHC, Liq. (Forest).
W/Caffeine, aspirin.
See: Synalgos-DC, Cap. (Wyeth-Ayerst).
DIHYDROCODEINONE RESIN COMPLEX.
W/Phenyltoloxamine resin complex.
See: Tussionex, Preps. (Pennwalt).
DIHYDRO-DIETHYLSTILBESTROL.
See: Hexestrol, Tab., Vial (Various Mfr.).
DIHYDROERGOCORNINE. Ergot alkaline component of hydergine.
See: Circanol, Tab. (Riker).
Deapril-ST, Tab. (Mead Johnson).
DIHYDROERGOCRISTINE. Ergot alkaloid component of hydergine.
See: Circanol, Tab. (Riker).
Deapril-ST, Tab. (Mead Johnson).
DIHYDROERGOCRYPTINE. Ergot alkaloid component of hydergine.
See: Circanol, Tab. (Riker).
Deapril-ST, Tab. (Mead Johnson).
DIHYDROERGOTAMINE. (D.H.E. 45) (Sandoz) Dihydroergotamine mesylate. Amp.
•**DIHYDROERGOTAMINE MESYLATE,** U.S.P. XXII. Inj., U.S.P. XXII. Dihydroergotamine methanesulfonate.
Use: Agent for migraine, antiadrenergic.
See: DHE 45, Amp. (Sandoz).
W/Scopolamine HBr, phenobarbital sodium, barbital sodium, Sandoptal.
See: Plexonal, Tab. (Sandoz).
•**DIHYDROERGOTAMINE MESYLATE, HEPARIN SODIUM, and LIDOCAINE HYDROCHLORIDE INJECTION,** U.S.P. XXII. Inj.
DIHYDROFOLLICULAR HORMONE.
See: Estradiol (Various Mfr.).
DIHYDROFOLLICULINE.
See: Estradiol (Various Mfr.).
DIHYDROHYDROXYCODEINONE. Oxycodone. (Ducodal, Eukodal, Eucodal).
Use: Narcotic analgesic.
DIHYDROHYDROXYCODEINONE HCl or BITARTRATE. Oxycodone HCl or Bitartrate.
W/Combinations.
See: Cophene-S, Syr. (Dunhall).
Corizahist-D, Syr. (Mason).
Damason-P, Tab. (Mason).
Percobarb, Cap. (Du Pont).
Percodan, Tab. (Du Pont).
Triaprin-DC, Cap. (Dunhall).
DIHYDROMORPHINONE HCl.
See: Dilaudid, Preps. (Knoll).
•**DIHYDROSTREPTOMYCIN SULFATE,** U.S.P. XXII. Boluses, Inj., Sterile, U.S.P. XXII.
Use: Antibiotic.
•**DIHYDROTACHYSTEROL,** U.S.P. XXII. Cap., Oral Soln., Tab., U.S.P. XXII. 9,10-Seco-5,7,22-ergostartien-3-β-ol. (Roxane) 0.2 mg/Tab. Bot. 100s, UD 100s.
Use: Treatment of hypocalcemia.
See: Hytakerol, Cap., Soln. (Winthrop Pharm).
DIHYDROTESTOSTERONE. Androstane-17-beta-ol-3-one.
See: Stanolone.
DIHYDROTHEELIN.
See: Estradiol (Various Mfr.).
DIHYDROXYACETONE.
See: Chromelin, Liq. (Summers).
QT, Liq. (Schering-Plough).
Sudden Tan, Liq. (Schering-Plough).
•**DIHYDROXYALUMINUM AMINOACETATE,** U.S.P. XXII. Cap., Magma, Tab., U.S.P. XXII. Aluminum, (glycinato-N,O) dihydroxy-hydrate. (Glycinato)-dihydroxyaluminum hydrate. Aluminum dihydroxyaminoacetate; basic aluminum aminoacetate. (Glycinato) dihydroxyaluminum.
Use: Antacid.
W/Methscopolamine bromide, sodium lauryl sulfate, magnesium hydroxide.
See: Alu-Scop, Cap., Susp. (Westerfield).
W/Phenobarbital and atropine methyl nitrate.
See: Harvatrate A, Tab. (O'Neal).
W/Salicylsalicylic acid, aspirin.
See: Salsprin, Tab. (Seatrace).

•**DIHYDROXYALUMINUM SODIUM CARBONATE,** U.S.P. XXII. Tab., U.S.P. XXII. Aluminum sodium carbonate hydroxide. Sodium (carbonato)-dihydroxyaluminate(1-)hydrate.
Use: Antacid.
See: Rolaids, Tab. (Warner-Lambert).
DIHYDROXYCHOLECALCIFEROL.
See: Rocaltrol. (Roche).
DIHYDROXYESTRIN.
See: Estradiol (Various Mfr.).
DIHYDROXYFLUORANE. Fluorescein.
DIHYDROXYPHENYLISATIN.
See: Oxyphenisatin (Various Mfr.).
DIHYDROXYPHENYLOXINDOL.
See: Oxyphenisatin (Various Mfr.).
DIHYDROXYPROPYLTHEOPHYLLINE. Dyphylline.
See: Airet, Preps. (Norwich Eaton).
Neothylline, Tab., Elix., Inj. (Lemmon).
W/Ephedrine HCl, butabarbital.
See: Airet R, Tab. (Baylor Labs.).
W/Guaifenesin.
See: Airet G. G., Cap., Elix. (Baylor Labs.).
DIHYDROXY(STEARATO)ALUMINUM. Aluminum Monostearate, N.F. XVII.
DIIODOHYDROXYQUIN.
Use: Amebicide.
See: Iodoquinol, U.S.P. XXII.
DI-IODOHYDROXYQUINOLINE. B.A.N. 8-Hydroxy-5,7-di-iodoquinoline.
Use: Treatment of amebiasis.
DIIODOHYDROXYQUINOLINE.
See: Iodoquinol, U.S.P. XXII.
DIISOPROMINE HCl. N,N-diisopropyl-3,3-diphenylpropylamine HCl. (Lab. for Pharmaceutical Development, Inc.).
See: Desquam-X (Westwood).
•**DIISOPROPANOLAMINE,** N.F. XVII.
Use: Pharmaceutic aid (alkalinizing agent).
DIISOPROPYL PHOSPHOROFLUORIDATE.
See: Isofluorophate, U.S.P. XXII.
Floropryl, Oint. (Merck Sharp & Dohme).
DIISOPROPYL SEBACATE.
See: Delavan, Cream (Miles Pharm).
DILAMINATE. Mixture of magnesium carbide and dihydroxy aluminum glycinate.
Use: Antacid.
DILANTIN. (Parke-Davis) Phenytoin. **30′ Susp.:** 30 mg/5 ml. Bot. 8 oz, UD 5 ml. **125′ Susp.:** 125 mg/5 ml. Bot. 8 oz, UD 5 ml. **Infatab:** 50 mg/Tab. Bot. 100s, UD 100s.
Use: Anticonvulsant.
DILANTIN SODIUM. (Parke-Davis) Extended phenytoin sodium. **Kapseal:** 30 mg, 100 mg. Bot. 100s, 1000s, UD 100s. **Amp.:** (w/propylene glycol 40%, alcohol 10%, sodium hydroxide) 100 mg/2 ml. UD 10s; 250 mg/5 ml. Amp. 10s, UD 10s.
Use: Anticonvulsant.
DILANTIN SODIUM W/PHENOBARBITAL KAPSEAL. (Parke-Davis) Phenytoin sodium 100 mg, phenobarbital 16 mg or 32 mg/Cap. Bot. 100s, 1000s, UD 100s (32 mg only).
Use: Anticonvulsant, sedative/hypnotic.
DILATRATE SR. (Reed & Carnrick) Isosorbide dinitrate 40 mg/SR Cap. Bot. 100s.
Use: Antianginal.
DILAUDID COUGH SYRUP. (Knoll) Hydromorphone HCl 1 mg, guaifenesin 100 mg/5ml. Alcohol 5%. Bot. pt.
Use: Narcotic analgesic, expectorant.
DILAUDID HP AMPULE. (Knoll) Hydromorphone 10 mg/ml. Box 10s; 50 mg/5 ml. Box 1s.
Use: Narcotic analgesic.
DILAUDID HYDROCHLORIDE. (Knoll) Hydromorphone HCl. **Amp.** (w/sodium citrate 0.2%, citric acid soln. 0.2%): 1 mg, 2 mg or 4 mg/ml. Box 10s. 2 mg. Box 25s. **Multiple Dose Vial:** 2 mg/ml. Bot. 20 ml. **Tab.:** 1 mg. Bot. 100s. 2 mg Bot. 100s, 500s. Strip pack 4 × 25s. 3 mg Bot. 100s. 4 mg 100s, 500s. Strip pack 4 × 25s. **Pow:** Vial, 15 gr Multiple dose vial 10 ml, 20 ml. 2 mg/ml. **Rectal Supp.:** (in cocoa butter base, w/colloidal silica 1%): 3 mg/Supp. Box 6s.
Use: Narcotic analgesic.
W/Guaifenesin.
See: Dilaudid Cough Syrup. (Knoll).
•**DILEVALOL HYDROCHLORIDE.** USAN.
Use: Antihypertensive, anti-adrenergic.
DILITHIUM CARBONATE. Lithium Carbonate, U.S.P. XXII.
Use: Antipsychotic.
DILOCAINE. (Hauck) Lidocaine HCl 1% or 2%. Bot. 50 ml.
Use: Local anesthetic.
DILOR. (Savage) Dyphylline. **Tab.:** 200 mg. Bot. 100s, 1000s, UD 100s. **Elix.:** 160 mg/15 ml. Bot. pt.
Use: Bronchodilator.
DILOR 400. (Savage) Dyphylline 400 mg. Bot. 100s, 1000s, UD 100s.
Use: Bronchodilator.
DILOR G LIQUID. (Savage) Dyphylline 300 mg, guaifenesin 300 mg/15 ml. Bot. pt, gal.
Use: Bronchodilator, expectorant.
DILOR G TABLETS. (Savage) Dyphylline 200 mg, guaifenesin 200 mg/Tab. Bot. 100s, 1000s, UD 100s.
Use: Bronchodilator, expectorant.
DILOXANIDE. B.A.N. 4-(N-Methyldichloroacetamido) phenol.
Use: Treatment of amebiasis.
•**DILTIAZEM HYDROCHLORIDE.** USAN.
Use: Vasodilator.
DIMACID. (Otis Clapp) Calcium carbonate 270 mg, magnesium carbonate 97 mg. In 100s, 500s.
Use: Antacid.
DIMACOL. (Robins) Pseudoephedrine HCl 30 mg, dextromethorphan HBr 15 mg, guaifenesin 100 mg/Cap. or 5 ml. **Cap.** Bot. 100s, 500s, Pre-Pack 12s, 24s. **Liq.** (w/alcohol 4.75%) Bot. pt.

Use: Decongestant, nonnarcotic antitussive, expectorant.

DIMAPHEN S.A. (Major) Phenylpropanolamine HCl 15 mg, phenylephrine HCl 15 mg, brompheniramine maleate 12 mg. Tab. Bot. 100s, 1000s.
Use: Decongestant, antihistamine.

DIMAPHEN TIME-TABS. (Major) Phenylpropanolamine HCl 75 mg, brompheniramine maleate 12 mg/Tab. Bot. 12s, 24s.
Use: Decongestant, antihistamine.

DIMAZOLE (I.N.N.). Diamthazole, B.A.N.

•**DIMEFADANE.** USAN. N, N-Dimethyl-3-phenyl-1-indanamine.
Use: Nonnarcotic analgesic.

•**DIMEFLINE HYDROCHLORIDE.** USAN.
Use: Respiratory stimulant.

•**DIMEFOLCON A.** USAN.
Use: Contact lens material.

DIMENEST. (Forest Pharm.) Dimenhydrinate 50 mg/ml. Vial 10 ml.
Use: Antiemetic/antivertigo.

•**DIMENHYDRINATE,** U.S.P. XXII. Syr., Tab., Inj., U.S.P. XXII. Beta-dimethylaminoethyl benzohydryl ether-8-chlorotheophyllinate. 8-Chlorotheophylline 2-(Diphenylmethoxy)-N, N-dimethylethylamine compound (1:1). IH-Purine-2,6-dione,8-chloro-3,7-dihydro-1,3-dimethyl-, compound with 2-(diphenylmethoxy)-N,N-dimethylethanamine (1:1). Gravol.
Use: Antiemetic, antihistamine.
See: Dimenest, Inj. (Forest Pharm.).
Dimentabs, Tab. (Bowman).
Dipendrate, Tab. (Kenyon).
Dramamine, Preps. (Searle).
Dramocen, Inj. (Central).
Dymenate, Inj. (Keene).
Eldadryl, Preps. (Elder).
Eldodram, Tab. (Elder).
Hydrate, Vial (Hyrex).
Reidamine, Inj. (Solvay).
Signate, Inj. (Sig).
Trav-Arex, Cap. (Quality Generics).
Traveltabs, Tab. (Geneva Marsam).

DIMENOXADOLE. B.A.N. 2-Dimethylaminoethyl2-ethoxy-2, 2-diphenylacetate.
Use: Narcotic analgesic.

DIMENTABS. (Bowman) Dimenhydrinate 50 mg/Tab. Bot. 100s.
Use: Antiemetic/antivertigo.

DIMEPHEPTANOL. B.A.N. 6-Dimethylamino-4, 4-diphenylheptan-3-ol.
Use: Narcotic analgesic.

•**DIMEPRANOL ACEDOBEN.** USAN.
Use: Immunomodulator.

DIMEPREGNEN. B.A.N. 3β-Hydroxy-6α, 16α-dimethylpregn-4-en-20-one.
Use: Anti-estrogen.

DIMEPROPION. B.A.N. α-Dimethylaminopropiophenone. Metamfepramone (I.N.N.).
Use: Anorexigenic.

•**DIMERCAPROL,** U.S.P. XXII. Inj. U.S.P. XXII. 2, 3-Dimercaptol-1-propanol.
Use: Antidote to gold, arsenic and mercury poisoning; metal complexing agent.
See: BAL Amp. (Hynson, Wescott & Dunning).

DIMESONE. B.A.N. 9α-Fluoro- 11β, 21-dihydroxy-16α, 17-dimethylpregna-1, 4-diene-3, 20-dione.
Use: Anti-inflammatory steroid.

DIMETANE. (Robins) Brompheniramine maleate. **Tab.:** 4 mg Bot. 100s, 500s, Pre-Pack 24s. **Extentab:** 8 mg or 12 mg Bot. 100s, 500s. **Elix.:** 2 mg/5 ml Bot. 4 oz, pt, gal. **Amp.:** 10 mg/ml, pH adjusted with sodium hydroxide. 1 ml Box 25s.
Use: Antihistamine.
W/Phenylephrine HCl, phenylpropanolamine HCl.
See: Dimetapp Elix., Extentab (Robins).

DIMETANE DECONGESTANT ELIXIR. (Robins) Brompheniramine maleate 2 mg, phenylephrine HCl 5 mg/5 ml, alcohol 2.3%, saccharin. Bot. 4 oz.
Use: Antihistamine, decongestant.

DIMETANE DECONGESTANT TABLETS. (Robins) Brompheniramine maleate 4 mg, phenylephrine HCl 10 mg/Tab. Ctn. 24s, 48s.
Use: Antihistamine, decongestant.

DIMETANE-DC COUGH SYRUP. (Robins) Brompheniramine maleate 2 mg, phenylpropanolamine HCl 12.5 mg, codeine phosphate 10 mg/5 ml w/alcohol 0.95%. Bot. pt, gal.
Use: Antihistamine, decongestant, antitussive.

DIMETANE-DX COUGH SYRUP. (Robins) Pseudoephedrine HCl 30 mg, brompheniramine maleate 2 mg, dextromethorphan HBr 10 mg, alcohol 0.95%, saccharin, sorbitol. Bot. pt.
Use: Decongestant, antihistamine, antitussive.

DIMETAPP ELIXIR. (Robins) Brompheniramine maleate 2 mg, phenylpropanolamine HCl 12.5 mg/5 ml alcohol 2.3%, saccharin, sorbitol. Bot, 4 oz, 8 oz, pt, gal, Dis-Co Pack 5 ml 10 × 10s.
Use: Antihistamine, decongestant.

DIMETAPP EXTENTABS. (Robins) Brompheniramine maleate 12 mg, phenylpropanolamine HCl 75 mg/Tab. Bot. 100s, 500s, Dis-Co Pack 100s. Blister pack 12s, 24s.
Use: Antihistamine, decongestant.

DIMETAPP TABLETS. (Robins) Brompheniramine maleate 4 mg, phenylpropanolamine HCl 12.5 mg/Tab. Blisterpak 24s.
Use: Antihistamine, decongestant.

•**DIMETHADIONE.** USAN. 5, 5-Dimethyl-2, 4-oxazolidine-dione. Eupractone (Travenol).
Use: Anticonvulsant.

DIMETHAZAN. 1, 3-Dimethyl-7-(2-dimethylaminoethyl) xanthine.

•**DIMETHICONE,** N.F. XVII. Dimethylsiloxane polymers. dimethyl polysiloxane.
Use: Prosthetic aid, component of barrier creams.
See: Covicone, Cream (Abbott).
Silicone, Oint. (Various Mfr.).

Silicote, Preps. (Arnar-Stone).

•**DIMETHICONE 350.** USAN.
Use: Prosthetic aid for soft tissue.

DIMETHINDENE. B.A.N. 2- 1-[2-(2-Dimethylaminoethyl) inden-3-yl]ethyl pyridine.
Use: Antihistamine.

DIMETHISOQUIN. B.A.N. 3-Butyl-1-(2-dimethylaminoethoxy)isoquinoline. Quinisocaine (I.N.N.).
Use: Antipruritic.

•**DIMETHISTERONE.** USAN.
Use: Progesterone.

DIMETHOLIZINE PHOSPHATE. 1-(2-Methoxyphenyl)-4-(3-methoxypropyl)piperazine phosphate. Ansiv.

DIMETHOTHIAZINE. B.A.N. 10-(2-Dimethylamino- propyl)-2-dimethysulfamoylphenothiazine.
Use: Agent for migraine.

DIMETHOXANATE. B.A.N. 2-(2-Dimethylaminoethoxy) ethyl phenothiazine-10-carboxylate.
Use: Cough suppressant.

DIMETHOXYPHENYL PENICILLIN SODIUM.
See: Methicillin sodium (Various Mfr.).

DIMETHPYRIDENE MALEATE. Dimethindene Maleate, U.S.P. XXII.
See: Dimethindene Maleate, U.S.P. XXII.

DIMETHYLAMINOPHENAZONE.
See: Aminopyrine (Various Mfr.).

DIMETHYLAMINO PYRAZINE SULFATE.
See: Ampyzine Sulfate.

DIMETHYLCARBAMATE of 3-Hydroxy-1-Methylpyridinium Bromide.
See: Mestinon, Tab. (Roche).

DIMETHYLHEXESTROL DIPROPIONATE. Promethestrol Dipropionate.
See: Meprane Dipropionate, Tab. (Reed & Carnrick).

DIMETHYL POLYSILOXANE.
See: Dimethicone (Various Mfr.).
W/Benzocaine, bismuth subcarbonate, carbamide, hexachlorophene, phenylephrine HCl, pyrilamine maleate, zinc oxide.
W/Hexachlorophene, zinc oxide, pyrilamine maleate, tetracaine HCl, methyl salicylate, zirconium oxide.

•**DIMETHYL SULFOXIDE,** U.S.P. XXII. Irrigation, U.S.P. XXII. Methyl sulfoxide. DMSO.
Use: Anti-inflammatory agent, topical.
See: Demasorb (Squibb).
Demeso (Merck Sharp & Dohme).
Domoso (Syntex).
Dromisol (Merck Sharp & Dohme).
Rimso-50 (Research Ind.).

DIMETHYLTHIAMBUTENE. B.A.N. 3-Dimethylamino-1, 1-di-(2-thienyl)but-1-ene.
Use: Narcotic analgesic.

DIMETHYLTUBOCURARINE. B.A.N. Dimethyl ether of (+)-tubocurarine.
Use: Neuromuscular blocking agent.

DIMETHYL-TUBOCURARINE IODIDE.
Use: Skeletal muscle relaxant.
See: Metocurine Iodide, U.S.P. XXII.

DIMETHYLURETHIMINE.
See: Meturedepa (Armour).

DIMETRIDAZOLE. V.B.A.N. 1, 2-Dimethyl-5- nitroimidazole. Emtryl.
Use: Antiprotoz,oan, (veterinary).

DIMINAZENE. V.B.A.N. pp′-Diamidinodiazoamino-benzene.
Use: Antiprotozoan, antibacterial, (veterinary).

•**DIMOXAMINE HYDROCHLORIDE.** USAN.
Use: Memory adjuvant.

DIMPYLATE. V.B.A.N. 00-Diethyl 0-(2-isopropyl-6-methylpyrimidin-4-yl) phosphorothioate.
Use: Insecticide, (veterinary).

DIMYCOR. (Standard Drug) Pentaerythritol tetranitrate 10 mg, phenobarbital 15 mg/Tab. Bot. 1000s.
Use: Antianginal, sedative/hypnotic.

DINACRIN. (Winthrop Products) Isonicotinic acid, hydrazide.
Use: Antituberculous agent.

DINATE. (Blaine) Dimenhydrinate 50 mg/ml. Vial 10 ml.
Use: Antiemetic/antivertigo.

DINDEVAN.
See: Phenindione (Various Mfr.).

DINITOLMIDE. V.B.A.N. 3, 5-Dinitro-o-toluamide.
Use: Antiprotozoan, (veterinary).

•**DINOPROST.** USAN. 7-[3α,5α-Dihydroxy-2β-[3S-)hydroxy-trans-oct-1-enyl]cyclopent-1-yl]cis-hept-5-enoic acid.
Use: Smooth muscle activator.
See: Prostaglandin F_2.

•**DINOPROSTONE.** USAN. 7-[3α-Hydroxy-2β-[(3S)-hydroxy-trans-oct-1-enyl]-5-oxocyclopent-1-yl]-cis-hept-5-enoic acid.
Use: Smooth muscle activator.
See: Prostaglandin E-2.

•**DINSED.** USAN. N,N′-Ethylenebis (3-nitrobenzenesulfonamide).
Use: Coccidiostat.

DIOCTIN. (Janssen) Difenoxin HCl.
Use: Antidiarrheal.

DIOCTO. (Purepac) Docusate sodium 100 mg or 200 mg/Cap. Bot. 100s.
Use: Laxative.

DIOCTO-C. (Various Mfr.) Docusate sodium 60 mg, casanthranol 30 mg/15 ml. Syr. Bot. 240 ml, pt, gal.
Use: Laxative.

DIOCTO-K. (Rugby) Docusate potassium 100 mg/Cap. Bot. 100s, 1000s.
Use: Laxative.

DIOCTO-K PLUS. (Rugby) Docusate sodium 100 mg, casanthranol 30 mg. Cap. Bot. 100s, 1000s.
Use: Laxative.

DIOCTOLOSE. (Goldline) Docusate potassium 100 mg/Cap. Bot. 100s, 1000s.
Use: Laxative.

DIOCTYL CALCIUM SULFOSUCCINATE. Docusate Calcium, U.S.P. XXII.
Use: Laxative.

DIOCTYL POTASSIUM SULFOSUCCINATE.

W/Glycerin, potassium oleate and stearate.
See: Rectalad, Liq. (Wallace).
DIOCTYL SODIUM SULFOSUCCINATE. B.A.N. Docusate Sodium, U.S.P. XXII.
Use: Non-laxative fecal softener.
DIODONE INJECTION.
See: Iodopyracet injection.
DIOEZE.(Century) Dioctyl sodium sulfosuccinate 250 mg/Cap. Bot. 100s, 1000s.
Use: Laxative.
•**DIOHIPPURIC ACID I-125.** USAN.
Use: Radioactive agent.
•**DIOHIPPURIC ACID I-131.** USAN.
Use: Radioactive agent.
DIO-HIST. (Approved) Dextromethorphan 30 mg, thenylpyramine HCl 80 mg, phenylephrine HCl 20 mg, potassium tartrate 1/24 gr/oz. Bot. 4 oz.
Use: Antihistamine.
DIOLAMINE. Diethanolamine.
DIOLOSTENE.
See: Methandriol.
DIONEX. (Interstate) Docusate sodium 100 mg or 250 mg/Cap. Bot. 100s, 250s, 1000s.
Use: Laxative.
DIONIN. Ethylmorphine HCl.
Use: Orally; cough depressant, ocular lymphagogue.
DIONOSIL OILY. (Glaxo) Propyliodone 60% in peanut oil. Inj. Vial 20 ml.
Use: Bronchographic contrast medium.
DIOPHYLLIN.
See: Aminophylline, Preps. (Various Mfr.).
DIOPTERIN. Pteroyldiglutamic acid, PDGA, Pteroyl-alpha-glutamylglutamic acid.
Use: Antineoplastic agent.
DIORAPIN. (Standex) Estrogenic conjugate 0.625 mg, methyltestosterone 5 mg/Tab. Bot. 100s. Estrone 2 mg, testosterone 25 mg/ml. Inj. Vial 10 ml.
Use: Estrogen, androgen combination.
DIOSATE. (Towne) Docusate sodium. Cap. 100 mg or 250 mg/Tab. Bot. 100s.
Use: Laxative.
DIOSMIN. Buchu resin obtained from lvs. of barosma serratifolia and alliedrutaceae.
DIO-SOFT. (Standex) Docusate sodium 100 mg, casanthranol 30 mg/Cap. Bot. 100s.
Use: Laxative.
DIOSTATE D. (Upjohn) Vitamin D 400 IU, calcium 343 mg, phosphorus 265 mg/3 Tab. Bot. 100s.
Use: Vitamin/mineral supplement.
•**DIOTYROSINE I-125.** USAN.
Use: Radioactive agent.
DIOVAL. (Keene) Estradiol valerate 10 mg/ml. Vial 10 ml.
Use: Estrogen.
DIOVAL XX. (Keene) Estradiol valerate 20 mg/ml. Vial 10 ml.
Use: Estrogen.
DIOVAL 40. (Keene) Estradiol valerate 40 mg/ml. Vial 10 ml.
Use: Estrogen.
DIOVOCYLIN. (Ciba)
See: Estradiol, Preps. (Various Mfr.).
•**DIOXADROL HYDROCHLORIDE.** USAN.
Use: Antidepressant.
DIOXAMATE. B.A.N. 4-Carbamoyloxymethyl-2-methyl-2-nonyl-1,3-dioxolan.
Use: Treatment of Parkinsonian syndrome.
DIOXAPHETYL BUTYRATE. B.A.N. Ethyl 4-morpholino-2,2-diphenylbutyrate.
Use: Narcotic analgesic.
DIOXATHION. B.A.N. A mixture consisting essentially of cis- and trans-SS′-1,4-dioxan-2,3-diyl bis (00-diethyl phosphorodithioate).
Use: Insecticide, acaricide, (veterinary).
See: Delnav.
DIOXINDOL. Diacetylhydroxyphenylisatin.
DIOXYANTHRANOL.
See: Anthralin, N.F. (Various Mfr.).
DIOXYANTHRAQUINONE. 1,8-Dihydroxy-anthraquinone.
See: Danthron, U.S.P. XXII.
•**DIOXYBENZONE,** U.S.P. XXII. Dioxybenzone and Oxybenzone Cream, U.S.P. XXII. Methanone, (2-hydroxy-4-methoxyphenyl)(2-hydroxyphenyl)1.
Use: Sunscreen agent.
W/Oxybenzone, benzophene.
See: Solbar, Lot. (Person & Covey).
DIPARCOL HYDROCHLORIDE. Diethazine.
DIPEGYL.
See: Nicotinamide, Preps. (Various Mfr.).
DIPENICILLIN G.
See: Benzethacil.
DIPENINE BROMIDE. B.A.N. 2-Dicyclopentylacetoxy-ethyltriethylammonium bromide.
Use: Antispasmodic.
See: Diponium Bromide (I.N.N.).
DIPENTUM. (Pharmacia) Osalazine sodium 250 mg/Cap. Bot. 100s, 500s.
Use: Ulcerative colitis.
DIPERODON. B.A.N. 3-Piperidinopropane-1,2-diol di(phenylcarbamate).
Use. Local anesthetic.
DIPERODON, U.S.P. XXII. Oint., U.S.P. XXII. 3-Piperidino-1,2-propanediol dicarbanilate (ester) monohydrate.
Use: Local anesthetic.
DIPERODON HYDROCHLORIDE.
Use: Anesthetic.
See: Diothane Oint. (Merrell Dow).
Proctodon, Cream (Solvay).
W/Bacitracin, neomycin sulfate, polymyxin.
See: Epimycin A, Oint. (Delta).
W/Benzalkonium Cl, ichthammol, thymol, camphor, juniper tar.
See: Boro Oint. (Scrip).
W/Furacin (nitrofurazone).
See: Furacin E Urethral Inserts (Eaton).
Furacin H.C. Urethral Inserts (Eaton).
W/Furacin (nitorfurazone) and Microfur (nituroxime).

See: Furacin Otic, Drops. (Eaton).
W/Hydrocortisone, polymyxin B sulfate, neomycin.
See: My Cort Otic #1, Ear Drops (Scrip).
W/Hydroxyquinoline Benzoate.
See: Diothane, Oint. (Merrell Dow).
W/Methapyrilene HCl, pyrilamine maleate, allantoin, benzocaine, menthol.
See: Antihistamine Cream (Towne).
W/Neomycin sulfate, polymyxin B sulfate.
See: Aural Acute (Saron).
W/Thimerosal, isopropyl alcohol.
See: Earobex, Ear Drops (Hauck).

DIPHEMANIL METHYLSULFATE. B.A.N. 4-Benzhydrylidene-1, 1-dimethylpiperidinium methyl-sulfate.
Use: Parasympatholytic.

DIPHENACEN-50. (Central) Diphenhydramine HCl 50 mg/ml w/chlorobutanol 0.5%. Inj. Vial 10 ml.
Use: Antihistamine.

DIPHENADIONE. 2-(Diphenylacetyl)-1-3, indandione.
Use: Anticoagulant.
See: Dipaxin, Tab. (Upjohn).

DIPHENATIL.
See: Diphemanil methylsulfate.

DIPHENATOL. (Rugby) Diphenoxylate HCl 2.5 mg, atropine sulfate 0.025 mg. Tab. Bot. 100s, 500s, 1000s.
Use: Antidiarrheal.

DIPHEN COUGH. (PBI) Diphenhydramine HCl 12.5 mg/5 ml. Syr. Bot. 118 ml, pt, gal.
Use: Antitussive.

DIPHENHIST. (Rugby) Diphenhydramine. **Captabs:** 25 mg Bot. 100s, UD 24s. **Elix.:** 12.5 mg/5 ml. Bot. 120 ml, pt, gal.
Use: Antihistamine.

•**DIPHENHYDRAMINE AND PSEUDOEPHEDRINE CAPSULES.** U.S.P. XXII.
Use: Antihistamine, decongestant.

•**DIPHENHYDRAMINE CITRATE,** U.S.P. XXII.
Use: Antihistamine.

•**DIPHENHYDRAMINE HYDROCHLORIDE.** U.S.P. XXII. Cap., Elix., Inj., U.S.P. XXII. Ethanamine, 2-(diphenylmethoxy)-N,N-dimethyl-,HCl. 2-Diphenyl- methoxy)-N,N-dimethylethylamine HCl.
Use: Antihistamine.
See: Bax, Cap., Elix., Expectorant (McKesson).
Benachior, Syr. (Jenkins).
Benadryl Hydrochloride, Preps. (Parke-Davis).
Benahist, Preps. (Keene).
Bentrac, Cap. (Kenyon).
Benylin Cough Syrup (Warner-Lambert).
Diphen-Ex, Syr. (Quality Generics).
Diphenhydramine HCl (Weeks & Leo).
Fenylhist, Cap. (Hauck).
Histine Prods. (Freeport).
Hyrexin, Inj. (Hyrex).
Nordryl, Prep. (North. Amer. Pharm.).
Rodryl, Inj. (Rocky Mtn.).
Rodryl-50, Inj. (Rocky Mtn.).
Rohydra, Elix. (Robinson).
Span-Lanin, Cap. (Scrip).
Tusstat, Expectorant (Century).
W/Ammonium Cl, menthol.
See: Bentrac Expectorant, Liq. (Kenyon).
Eldadryl Expectorant, Liq. (Elder).
Fenylex, Expectorant (Hauck).
Tusstat Expectorant (Century).
W/Antihistamines.
See: Symptrol, Syr., Cap., Inj. (Saron).
W/Benzethonium Cl.
See: Bendylate, Inj. (Solvay).
W/Chlorobutanol.
See: Ardeben, Inj. (Burgin-Arden).
W/Pheniramine maleate pyrilamine maleate, phenylephrine HCl, phenylpropanolamine HCl.
See: Symptrol, Syr. (Saron).
W/Zinc oxide.
See: Ziradryl, Lot. (Parke-Davis).

•**DIPHENIDOL.** USAN. α,α-Diphenyl-1-piperidinebutanol.
Use: Antiemetic.
See: Vontrol, Preps. (SmithKline Beecham).

•**DIPHENIDOL HCl.** USAN. αα-Diphenyl-1- piperidinebutanol HCl.
Use: Antiemetic.

•**DIPHENIDOL PAMOATE.** USAN. α,α-Diphenyl-1-piperidinebutanol compound with 4,4′-methylenebis [3-hydroxy-2-naphthoic acid](2:1).
Use: Antiemetic.

DIPHENMETHANIL METHYLSULFATE. 4-Diphenylmethylene-1,1-dimethylpiperidinium methylsulfate.
See: Diphemanil Methylsulfate (Various Mfr.).

•**DIPHENOXYLATE HCl,** U.S.P. XXII. 4-Piperidinecarboxylic acid, 1-(3-cyano-3,3-diphenylpropyl-4-phenyl-, ethyl ester, HCl, 2,2-Diphenyl-4-(4-carbethoxy-4-phenyl-1-pyeridino)butyronitrite ethyl ester HCl. Ethyl 1-(3-Cyano-3,3 diphenylpropyl)-4-phenylisonipecotate Hydrochloride.
Use: Antiperistaltic to treat diarrhea.
W/Atropine.
See: Diaction, Tab. (Boots Pharm.).
Lomotil, Tab., Liq. (Searle).

•**DIPHENOXYLATE HYDROCHLORIDE AND ATROPINE SULFATE,** U.S.P. XXII. Oral Soln., Tab., U.S.P. XXII.
Use: Antiperistaltic.

DIPHENYLAN SODIUM. (Lannett) Phenytoin sodium, prompt 30 mg (27.6 mg phenytoin) or 100 mg (92 mg phenytoin)/Cap. Bot. 500s, 1000s.
Use: Anticonvulsant.

DIPHENYLHYDROXYCARBINOL. Benzhydrol HCl.

DIPHENYLHYDANTOIN. Phenytoin, U.S.P. XXII.
Use: Anticonvulsant.

DIPHENYLHYDANTOIN SODIUM. Phenytoin Sodium, U.S.P. XXII.
Use: Anticonvulsant.

DIPHENYLISATIN.
See: Oxyphenisatin (Various Mfr.).

DIPHOSPHONIC ACID.
See: Etidronic acid.
DIPHOSPHOPYRIDINE (DPN). Antialcoholic. Under study.
DIPHOSPHOTHIAMIN. Cocarboxylase.
See: Coenzyme-B, Cap., and Inj. (Inwood).
DIPHOXAZIDE. N^1-(b-hydroxy-b,b-diphenylpropionyl)-N^2-acetylhdrazine. Inductin.
•**DIPHTHERIA ANTITOXIN,** U.S.P. XXII. (Squibb/Connaught) 20,000 units/Vial. (not > 500 units/ml).
Use: I.M., slow I.V. infusion; protection, treatment of diphtheria.
See: Diphtheria Toxoid, U.S.P. XXII.
•**DIPHTHERIA & TETANUS TOXOIDS,** U.S.P. XXII.
Use: Agent for immunization.
•**DIPHTHERIA & TETANUS TOXOIDS ABSORBED,** U.S.P. XXII. (Dow, Lilly, Squibb/Connaught) Vial 5 ml.
Use: Agent for immunization.
DIPHTHERIA & TETANUS TOXOIDS ADSORBED, ALUMINUM PHOSPHATE ADSORBED. (Wyeth-Ayerst) Tubex 0.5 ml. Vial 5 ml. Pkg. 10s. Available in pediatric and adult strengths. 10 Lf units diphtheria and 5 Lf units tetanus per 0.5 ml dose. 1.5 Lf units diphtheria, 5 Lf units tetanus per 0.5 ml dose.
Use: Agent for immunization.
DIPHTHERIA/TETANUS TOXOIDS, ADSORBED. (Lederle).
Pediatric: 12.5 Lf units diphtheria, 5 Lf units tetanus per 0.5 ml dose. Vial 5 ml.
Adult: 2 Lf units diphtheria, and 5 Lf units tetanus per 0.5 ml dose. Vial 5 ml Disp. syringe 0.5 ml.
Use: Agent for immunization.
•**DIPHTHERIA & TETANUS TOXOIDS & PERTUSSIS VACCINE,** U.S.P. XXII.
Use: Prevention against diphtheria, tetanus and pertussis.
See: Tri-immunol, Vial (Lederle).
Tri-Solgen Vial, Hyporet (Lilly).
DIPHTHERIA & TETANUS TOXOIDS & PERTUSSIS VACCINE ADSORBED. (Lederle) Vaccine Vial 7.5 ml.
Use: Agent for immunization.
DIPHTHERIA & TETANUS TOXOIDS & PERTUSSIS VACCINE COMBINED, ALUMINUM HYDROXIDE ADSORBED.
See: Triogen, Vial (Parke-Davis).
DIPHTHERIA & TETANUS TOXOIDS & PERTUSSIS VACCINE COMBINED, ALUMINUM PHOSPHATE-ADSORBED.
See: Tri-Immunol, Vial (Lederle)-Ramon, Diphtheria Anatoxin).
Use: Agent for immunization.
DIPHTHERIA TOXIN, DIAGNOSTIC. Schick Test.
•**DIPHTHERIA TOXIN FOR SCHICK TEST,** U.S.P. XXII.
Use: Diagnostic aid (dermal reactivity indicator).
See: Diphtheria Toxin, Diagnostic.
DIPHTHERIA TOXIN, INACTIVATED DIAGNOSTIC. Schick test control.
•**DIPHTHERIA TOXOID,** U.S.P. XXII.
Use: Agent for immunization.
•**DIPHTHERIA TOXOID ADSORBED,** U.S.P. XXII. Alum. Precipitated antoxin.
Use: Agent for immunization.
DIPHTHERIA TOXOID & PERTUSSIS VACCINE. (Lilly) Vial test 10s.
Use: Agent for immunization.
DIPHYLLINE.
See: Diazma, Vial (Pharmex).
DIPIMOL. (Everett) Dipyridamole 25 mg, 50 mg or 75 mg/Tab. Bot. 100s, 500s, 1000s.
Use: Antianginal.
DIPIPANONE. B.A.N. 4,4-Diphenyl-6-piperidinoheptan-3-one.
Use: Narcotic analgesic.
DIPIVALYL EPINEPHRINE.
See: Propine (Allergan).
•**DIPIVEFRIN.** USAN.
Use: Adrenergic.
•**DIPIVEFRIN HYDROCHLORIDE,** U.S.P. XXII. Ophth. Soln., U.S.P. XXII.(+)-3,4-dihydroxy-a-(methylamino) methyl benzyl alcohol 3,4-dipivalate HCl.
Use: Treatment of chronic open-angle glaucoma.
See: Propine, Soln. (Allergan).
DIPONIUM BROMIDE (I.N.N.). Dipenine Bromide, B.A.N.
DIPRENORPHINE. B.A.N. N-Cyclopropylmethyl-7,8-dihydro-7 α-(1-hydroxy-1-methylethyl)-0^6-methyl-6,14 endoethanonormorphine.
Use: Narcotic antagonist.
DIPRIDAMOLE. (Foy) Dipyridamole 25 mg/Tab. Bot. 1000s.
Use: Antianginal.
DIPRIVAN. (Stuart) Propofol 10 mg/ml. Inj. Amp. 20 ml.
Use: General anesthetic.
DIPROLENE AF CREAM. (Schering) Betamethasone dipropionate cream equivalent to 0.05% betamethasone. 15 Gm, 45 Gm.
DIPROLENE CREAM 0.05%. (Schering) Betamethasone dipropionate 0.05% in cream base. Tube 15 Gm.
Use: Anti-inflammatory, antipruritic (topical).
DIPROLENE OINTMENT 0.05%. (Schering) Betamethasone dipropionate 0.05%, in ointment base. Tube 15 Gm, 45 Gm.
Use: Anti-inflammatory, antipruritic (topical).
DIPROPHYLLINE. B.A.N. 7-(2,3-Dihydroxypropyl)- theophylline.
Use: Bronchodilator.
DIPROPYLACETIC ACID.
See: Valproic Acid.
DIPROSONE AEROSOL 0.1%. (Schering) Betamethasone dipropionate 6.4 mg (equiv. to 5 mg bethamethasone) in vehicle of mineral oil, caprylic-capric triglyceride w/isopropyl alcohol

10%, inert hydrocarbon propellants. (propane and isobutane). Can 85 Gm.
Use: Anti-inflammatory agent, topical.

DIPROSONE CREAM 0.05%. (Schering) Betamethasone dipropionate 0.64 mg (equiv. to 0.5 mg betamethasone) w/mineral oil, white petrolatum, polyethylene glycol 1000 monocetyl ether, cetostearyl alcohol, phosphoric acid, monobasic sodium phosphate with 4-chloro-m-cresol as preservative. Tube 15 Gm, 45 Gm.
Use: Anti-inflammatory agent, topical.

DIPROSONE LOTION 0.05%. (Schering) Betamethasone dipropionate 0.64 mg (equivalent to 0.5 mg betamethasone) w/isopropyl alcohol (46.8%), purified water. Bot. 20 ml, 60 ml.
Use: Anti-inflammatory agent, topical.

DIPROSONE OINTMENT 0.05%. (Schering) Betamethasone dipropionate 0.64 mg (equivalent to 0.5 mg betamethasone) in white petrolatum and mineral oil base. Tube 15 Gm, 45 Gm.
Use: Anti-inflammatory agent, topical.

•**DIPYRIDAMOLE,** U.S.P. XXII. Tab., U.S.P. XXII. 2,6-Di[di(2-hydroxy-ethyl)-amino]-4,8-dipiperidinopyrimido-[5,4-d]-pyrimidine.
Use: Coronary vasodilator.
See: Persantine.

•**DIPYRIDAMOLE.** USAN. 2,2′,2″-2‴,-[4,8- Dipiperidinopyrimido[5,4-d]pyrimidine-2,6-diyl)-dinitrilo]tetraethanol.
Use: Coronary vasodilator.
See: Dipimol, Tab. (Everett).
Dipridamole, Tab. (Foy).
Persantine, Tab. (Boehringer-Ingelheim).
Persantine IV (DuPont-Merck).

•**DIPYRITHIONE.** USAN.
Use: Antibacterial, antifungal.

•**DIPYRONE.** USAN, FDA. Sodium N-(2,3-dimethyl-1-phenyl-5-oxopyrazolin-4-yl)-N-methylamino-methanesulfonate. Sodium noramidopyrine methanesulfonate. Sodium phenyldimethylpyrazolon-me-thylamino-methane sulfonate, sodium (anti-pyrinylmethylamino)-methane sulfonate hydrate; methylmelubrin, methampyrone,4-Sod. methanesulfonate methylamine-antipyrine.
Use: Analgesic, antipyretic.

DIRIDONE. (Premo) Phenylazo-diamino-pyridine HCl 100 mg/Tab. Bot. 100s, 1000s.
Use: Urinary anesthetic, antiseptic.

DIROX TABLETS. (Winthrop Products) Paracetamol.
Use: Analgesic, antipyretic.

DISALCID. (Riker) Salsalate. **Tab.:** 500 mg or 750 mg. Bot. 100s, 500s, UD 100s. **Cap.:** 500 mg. Bot. 100s.
Use: Salicylate analgesic.

DISANTHROL CAPSULES. (Lannett) Docusate sodium 100 mg, casanthranol 30 mg/Cap. Bot. 100s, 1000s.
Use: Laxative.

DISCASE. (Omnis Surgical) Chymopapain 5 units/2 ml. Vial 5 ml.
Use: Intradiscal injection for herniated lumbar intervertebral discs.

DISINFECTING SOLUTION. (Bausch & Lomb) Sodium Cl, sodium borate, boric acid, chlorhexidine gluconate 0.005%, EDTA 0.1%, thimerosal 0.001%.
Use: Soft contact lens care.

•**DISIQUONIUM CHLORIDE.** USAN.
Use: Antiseptic.

DISMISS DOUCHE. (Schering) Sodium Cl, sodium citrate, citric acid, cetaryl octoate, ceteareth-27, fragrance. Pow. for dilution. Pkg. 2s.
Use: Vaginal preparation.

DISOBROM. (Various Mfr.) Pseudoephedrine sulfate 120 mg, dexbrompheniramine maleate 6 mg Tab. Bot. 30s, 100s, 1000s.
Use: Decongestant, antihistamine.

•**DISOBUTAMIDE.** USAN.
Use: Cardiac depressant.

DISODIUM CARBONATE. Sodium Carbonate, N.F. XVII.

DISODIUM CHROMATE. Sodium Chromate Cr 51 Injection, U.S.P. XXII.

DISODIUM CHROMOGLYCATE.
See: Intal (Fisons).
Nasalcrom (Fisons).

DISODIUM EDATHAMIL.
See: Edathamil Disodium (Various Mfr.).

DISODIUM EDETATE. Disodium ethylenediaminetetra acetate.
See: Edetate Disodium, U.S.P. XXII.

DISODIUM PHOSPHATE.
See: Sodium Phosphate, U.S.P. XXII.

DISODIUM PHOSPHATE HEPTAHYDRATE. Sodium Phosphate, U.S.P. XXII.

DISODIUM THIOSULFATE PENTAHYDRATE. Sodium Thiosulfate, U.S.P. XXII.

DI-SODIUM VERSENATE.
See: Edathamil Disodium (Various Mfr.).

•**DISOFENIN.** USAN.
Use: Diagnostic aid.

DISOLAN. (Lannett) Docusate sodium 100 mg, phenolphthalein 65 mg/Cap. Bot. 100s, 500s, 1000s.
Use: Laxative.

DISOLAN FORTE CAPSULES. (Lannett) Casanthranol 30 mg, sodium carboxymethylcellulose 400 mg, docusate sodium 100 mg/Cap. Bot. 100s, 500s, 1000s.
Use: Laxative.

DISONATE. (Lannett) Docusate sodium. **Cap.:** 60 mg, 100 mg or 240 mg. Bot. 100s, 500s, 1000s. **Liq.:** 10 mg/ml Bot. pt. **Syr.:** 20 mg/5 ml Bot. pt, gal.
Use: Laxative.

DISOPHROL. (Schering) Pseudoephedrine sulfate 60 mg, dexbrompheniramine maleate 2 mg. Tab. Bot. 100s.
Use: Decongestant, antihistamine.

DISOPHROL CHRONOTABS. (Schering) Dexbrompheniramine maleate 6 mg, pseudoephedrine sulfate 120 mg/SA Tab. Bot. 100s.

Use: Antihistamine, decongestant.

DISOPLEX. (Lannett) Docusate sodium 100 mg, sodium carboxymethylcellulose 400 mg. Cap. Bot. 100s, 500s, 1000s.
Use: Laxative.

•**DISOPYRAMIDE.** USAN. 4-Di-isopropylamino-2-phenyl-2-(2-pyridyl)butyramide.
Use: Antiarrhythmic.
See: Rythmodan.

•**DISOPYRAMIDE PHOSPHATE,** U.S.P. XXII. Cap., U.S.P. XXII.
Use: Antiarrhythmic.

•**DISOPYRAMIDE PHOSPHATE EXTENDED-RELEASE CAPSULES,** U.S.P. XXII.
Use: Antiarrhythmic.

DI-SOSUL. (Drug Industries) Docusate sodium 50 mg/Tab. Bot. 100s, 500s.
Use: Laxative.

DI-SOSUL FORTE. (Drug Industries) Docusate sodium 100 mg, casanthranol 30 mg/Tab. Bot. 100s, 500s.
Use: Laxative.

DISOTATE. (Forest) Disodium edetate 150 mg/ml. Vial 20 ml.
Use: Treatment of hypercalcemia.

•**DISOXARIL.** USAN.
Use: Antiviral.

DISPOS-A-MED. (Parke-Davis) Isoetharine HCl 0.5% or 1%, isoproterenol HCl 0.25% or 0.5%. Can of prefilled sterile tubes 0.5 ml, 50s.
Use: Bronchodilator.

DISPOS-A-VIAL. (Parke-Davis) Sodium Cl 0.45% or 0.9%. Container 3 ml, 5 ml. Box 100s.
Use: Oral inhalation.

DISTAQUAINE.
See: Penicillin V.

DISTIGMINE BROMIDE. B.A.N. NN′-Hexamethyl- enedi-[1-methyl-3-(methylcarbamoyloxy)-pyridinium bromide].
Use: Anticholinesterase.

DISTIGMINE BROMIDE. Hexamarium bromide.

DISULFAMIDE. B.A.N. 5-Chlorotoluene-2,4-disulfonamide.
Use: Diuretic.

•**DISULFIRAM,** U.S.P. XXII. Tab., U.S.P. XXII. Bis-(diethylthiocarbamoyl)disulfide. Tetraethylthiuram Disulfide.
Use: Treatment of alcoholism.
See: Antabuse, Tab. (Wyeth-Ayerst).

DISULFONAMIDE.
See: Dia-Mer-Sulfonamides (Various Mfr.).

DITATE D.S. (Savage) Testosterone enanthate 360 mg, estradiol valerate 16 mg, benzyl alcohol 2% in sesame oil. Syringe 2 ml Box 10s. Vial 2 ml.
Use: Androgen, estrogen combination.

•**DITEKIREN.** USAN.
Use: Antihypertensive (renin inhibitor).

DITHIAZANINE. B.A.N. 3-Ethyl-2-[5-(3-ethyl-benzothiazolin-2-ylidene)penta-1,3-dienyl]benzothiazolium.
Use: Anthelmintic.

DITHRANOL.
See: Anthralin, U.S.P. XXII. (Various Mfr.).

D.I.T.I. CREME. (Dunhall) Iodoquinol 100 mg, sulfanilamide 500 mg, diethylstilbestrol 0.1 mg/Gm Jar. 4 oz.
Use: Anti-infective, vaginal.

D.I.T.I.-2 CREME. (Dunhall) Sulfanilamide 15%, aminacrine HCl 0.2%, allantoin 2%. Tube 142 Gm.
Use: Anti-infective, vaginal.

DITOPHAL. B.A.N. SS′-Diethyl dithioisophthalate.
Use: Antileprotic.

DITROPAN. (Marion) Oxybutynin Cl 5 mg/Tab. Bot. 100s, 1000s, UD identification pak 100s.
Use: Urinary tract agent.

DITROPAN SYRUP. (Marion) Oxybutynin Cl. 5 mg/5 ml Bot. 473 ml.
Use: Urinary tract agent.

DIUCARDIN. (Wyeth-Ayerst) Hydroflumethiazide 50 mg/Tab. Bot. 100s.
Use: Diuretic, antihypertensive.

DIULO. (Searle) Metolazone. 2.5 mg, 5 mg or 10 mg/Tab. Bot. 100s.
Use: Diuretic, antihypertensive.

DIUPRES. (Merck Sharp & Dohme) Chlorothiazide 250 mg or 500 mg, reserpine 0.125 mg/Tab. Bot. 100s, 1000s.
Use: Antihypertensive.

DIURESE. (American Urologicals) Trichlormethiazide 4 mg/Tab. Bot. 100s, 1000s.
Use: Diuretic.

DIURETICS, LOOP.
See: Bumex, Inj., Tab. (Roche).
Edecrin, Tab. (MSD).
Edecrin Sodium, Inj. (MSD).
Fumide, Tab. (Everett).
Furomide M.D., Inj. (Hyrex).
Furosemide, Inj., Tab. (Various Mfr.).
Furosemide, Oral Soln. (Roxane).
Lasix, Inj., Oral Soln., Tab. (Hoechst-Roussel).
Luramide, Tab. (Major).

DIURETICS, OSMOTIC.
See: Glyrol, Soln. (Iolab).
Ismotic, Soln. (Alcon).
Mannitol, Inj. (Various Mfr.).
Osmitrol, Inj. (Baxter).
Osmoglyn, Soln. (Alcon).
Ureaphil, Inj. (Abbott).

DIURETICS, POTASSIUM-SPARING.
See: Alatone, Tab. (Major).
Aldactone, Tab. (Searle).
Amiloride HCl, Tab. (Various Mfr.).
Dyrenium, Cap. (SmithKline Beecham).
Midamor, Tab. (MSD).
Spironolactone, Tab. (Various Mfr.).

DIURETICS, THIAZIDES.
See: Anhydron, Tab. (Lilly).
Aquatag, Tab. (Solvay).
Aquatensen, Tab. (Wallace).
Chlorothiazide, Tab. (Various Mfr.).
Chlorthalidone, Tab. (Various Mfr.).
Diachlor, Tab. (Major).

Diaqua, Tab. (Hauck).
Diucardin, Tab. (Wyeth-Ayerst).
Diulo, Tab. (Searle).
Diurese, Tab. (American Urologicals).
Diurigen, Tab. (Goldline).
Diuril, Oral Susp., Tab. (MSD).
Diuril Sodium, Inj. (MSD).
Enduron, Tab. (Abbott).
Esidrix, Tab. (Ciba).
Ethon, Tab. (Major).
Exna, Tab. (Robins).
Hydrex, Tab. (Trimen).
Hydrochlorothiazide, Tab. (Various Mfr.).
Hydrochlorothiazide, Oral Soln. (Roxane).
Hydro DIURIL, Tab. (MSD).
Hydroflumethiazide, Tab. (Various Mfr.).
Hydromal, Tab. (Hauck).
Hydromox, Tab. (Lederle).
Hydro-T, Tab. (Major).
Hydro-Z-50, Tab. (Mayrand).
Hydroz,ide-50, Tab. (T.E. Williams).
Hygroton, Tab. (Rhone-Poulenc Rorer).
Hylidone, Tab. (Major).
Loz,ol, Tab. (Rhone-Poulenc Rorer).
Metahydrin, Tab. (Merrell Dow).
Methyclothiazide, Tab. (Various Mfr.).
Microx, Tab. (Pennwalt).
Mictrin, Tab. (Econo Med).
Naqua, Tab. (Schering).
Naturetin, Tab. (Princeton).
Niazide, Tab. (Major).
Oretic, Tab. (Abbott).
Proaqua, Tab. (Solvay).
Renese, Tab. (Pfizer).
Saluron, Tab. (Bristol Labs.).
Thalitone, Tab. (Boehringer-I).
Thiuretic, Tab. (Warner-Chilcott).
Trichlorex, Tab. (Lannett).
Trichlormethiazide, Tab. (Various Mfr.).
Zaroxolyn, Tab. (Pennwalt).

DIURETIC TABLETS. (Faraday) Buchu leaves 150 mg, uva ursi leaves 150 mg, juniper berries 120 mg, bone meal, parsley, asparagus/Tab. Bot. 100s.
Use: Diuretic.

DIURETTS. (Faraday) Tab. Bot. 84s.
Use: Diuretic.

DIURGEN TABLETS. (Goldline) Chlorothiazide 250 mg or 500 mg/Tab Bot. 100s, 1000s.
Use: Diuretic.

DIURIGEN W/RESERPINE 250 TABLETS. (Goldline). Chlorothiazide 250 mg, reserpine 0.125 mg. Tab. Bot. 100s, 1000s.
Use: Antihypertensive combination.

DIURIGEN W/RESERPINE 500 TABLETS. (Goldline). Chlorothiazide 500 mg, reserpine 0.125 mg. Tab. Bot. 100s, 1000s.
Use: Antihypertensive combination.

DIURIL. (Merck Sharp & Dohme) Chlorothiazide, U.S.P. **Tab.:** 250 mg Bot. 100s, 1000s; 500 mg Bot. 100s, 1000s, UD 100s. **Oral Susp.:** 250 mg/5 ml w/methylparaben 0.12%, propylparaben 0.02%, benzoic acid 0.1%, alcohol 0.5%. Bot. 237 ml.
Use: Diuretic, antihypertensive.
W/Methyldopa.
See Aldoclor, Tab. (Merck Sharp & Dohme).
W/Reserpine.
See: Diupres, Tab. (Merck Sharp & Dohme).

DIURIL SODIUM INTRAVENOUS. (Merck Sharp & Dohme) Chlorothiazide sodium equivalent to 0.5 Gm chlorothiazide w/mannitol 0.25 Gm sodium hydroxide, thimerosal 0.4 mg. Vial 20 ml.
Use: Diuretic, antihypertensive.

DIURSAL. (Harvey) Mersalyl 100 mg, theophylline 50 mg/ml. Amp. 2 ml, Box 25s, 100s.
Use: Diuretic.

DIUTENSEN-R. (Wallace) Methyclothiazide 2.5 mg, reserpine 0.1 mg/Tab. Bot. 100s, 500s.
Use: Antihypertensive combination.

•**DIVALPROEX SODIUM.** USAN.
Use: Anticonvulsant.

DIVINYL OXIDE. Vinyl ether, divinyl ether.
Use: Inhalation anesthetic.

DIZMISS. (Bowman) Meclizine HCl 25 mg/Tab. Bot. 100s, 1000s.
Use: Antiemetic/antivertigo.

DIZYMES. (Recsei) Pancreatin 250 mg, lipase 6,750 units, protease 41,250 units, amylase 43,750 units. E.C. Tab. Bot. 100s, 500s, 1000s.
Use: Digestive aid.

DM COUGH. (PBI) Dextromethorphan HBr 10 mg/5 ml, alcohol 5%. Syr. Bot. 120 ml, pt, gal.
Use: Antitussive.

DMCT. (Lederle) Demethylchlortetracycline.
Use: Anti-infective, tetracycline.
See: Declomycin HCl, Preps. (Lederle).

DML DERMATOLOGICAL MOISTURIZING LOTION. (Person & Covey) Purified water, petrolatum, glycerin, methyl glucose sesquisterate, dimethicone, methyl gluceth-20 sesquisterate, benzyl alcohol, volatile silicone, glyceryl stearate, stearic acid, palmitic acid, cetyl alcohol, xanthan gum, magnesium aluminum silicate carbomer 941, sodium hydroxide. Bot. 8 oz.
Use: Emollient.

DML FORTE. (Person & Covey) Petrolatum, PPG-2 myristyl ether propionate, glyceryl stearate, glycerin, stearic acid, d-panthenol, DEA-cetyl phosphate, simethicone, PVP eicosene copolymer, benzyl alcohol, cetyl alcohol, silica, disodium EDTA, BHA, magnesium aluminum silicate, sodium carbomer 1342. Tube 113 Gm.
Use: Emollient.

DMSA. 2, 3-dimercaptosuccinic acid (Orphan Drug).
Use: Lead poisoning in children.
Sponsor: Johnson & Johnson Baby Products Co.

DMSO.
See: Dimethyl sulfoxide.

DNR.
See: Cerubidine (Wyeth-Ayerst).

DOAK-OIL. (Doak) Tar distillate 2%, in a lanolin, mineral oil suspension. Pl. Bot. 8 oz.
Use: Antiseborrheic.
DOAK OIL FORTE. (Doak) Tar distillate 5%. Bot. 4 oz.
Use: Antiseborrheic.
DOAK TAR LOTION. (Doak) Tar distillate 5%. Bot. 4 oz.
Use: Antiseborrheic.
DOAK TAR SHAMPOO. (Doak) Tar distillate 3% in shampoo base. Bot. 4 oz.
Use: Antiseborrheic.
DOAK TERSASEPTIC. (Doak) Liquid cleanser, pH 6.8. Bot. 4 oz, pt, gal.
Use: Liquid detergent.
DOAN'S BACKACHE SPRAY. (Jeffrey Martin) Methyl salicylate 15%, menthol 8.4%, methyl nicotinate 0.6%. Aerosol can 4 oz.
Use: External analgesic.
DOAN'S PILLS. (DEP Corp.) Magnesium salicylate 325 mg/Tab. Ctn. 24s, 48s.
Use: Analgesic.
•**DOBUTAMINE.** USAN.
Use: Cardiac stimulant.
•**DOBUTAMINE HYDROCHLORIDE.** U.S.P. XXII. For Inj., U.S.P. XXII.
Use: Cardiac stimulant.
See: Dobutrex, Inj. (Lilly).
•**DOBUTAMINE LACTOBIONATE.** USAN.
Use: Cardiac stimulant.
•**DOBUTAMINE TARTRATE.** USAN.
Use: Cardiac stimulant.
DOBUTREX SOLUTION. (Lilly) Dobutamine HCl 250 mg. Inj. Vial 20 ml.
Use: Inotropic agent.
•**DOCEBENONE.** USAN.
Use: Inhibitor (5-lipoxygenase).
See: Antiallergic; antiasthmatic.
•**DOCONAZOLE.** USAN.
Use: Antifungal.
DOCTASE. (Purepac) Docusate sodium 100 mg, casanthranol 30 mg/Cap. Bot. 100s.
Use: Laxative.
DOCTYL. (Approved) Docusate sodium 100 mg/ Tab. Bot. 40s, 100s, 1000s.
Use: Laxative.
DOCTYLAX. (Approved) Docusate sodium 100 mg, acetophenolisatin 2 mg, prune conc. ¾ mg/ Tab. Bot. 40s, 100s, 1000s.
Use: Laxative.
•**DOCUSATE CALCIUM,** U.S.P. XXII. Cap., U.S.P. XXII. 1, 4-Bis(2-ethylhexyl)sulfosuccinate, calcium salt. Calcium bis-dioctyl-sulfosuccinate.
Use: Fecal softener.
See: Surfak, Cap. (Hoechst).
Doxidan, Cap. (Hoechst).
Danthron, Tab. (Goldline).
•**DOCUSATE POTASSIUM,** U.S.P. XXII. Cap., U.S.P. XXII.
Use: Stool softener.
See: Dialose, Cap. (Stuart).
Dialose Plus, Cap. (Stuart).
Kasof, Cap. (Stuart).
•**DOCUSATE SODIUM,** U.S.P. XXII. Cap., Soln., Syr., Tab., U.S.P. XXII. Aerosol OT. (Am. Cyanamid). Bis-(2-ethoxy)-S-sodium sulfosuccinate. Sodium 1, 4-Bis (2-ethylhexyl) Sulfosuccinate.
Use: Pharmaceutical aid (surfactant), stool softener.
See: Colace, Cap., Liq., Syr. (Mead Johnson).
Coloctyl, Cap. (Vitarine).
Comfolax, Cap. (Searle).
Consta B100, Tab. (Kenyon).
Diomedicone, Tab (Medicone).
Diosate Caps. (Towne).
Diosux, Cap. (Jenkins).
Disonate, Cap., Tab. Syr., Liq. (Lannett).
Doss, Super Doss, Tab. (Ferndale).
Doxinate, Cap., Liq. (Hoechst).
DSS (Parke-Davis).
Duosol, Cap. (Kirkman Sales).
Dynoctol, Cap. (Solvay).
Easy-Lax, Cap. (Walgreen).
Konsto, Cap. (Freeport).
Laxatab, Tab. (Freeport).
Liqui-Doss, Liq. (Ferndale).
Modane Soft, Cap. (Adria).
Peri-Doss, Cap. (Ferndale).
Regul-Aid, Syr. (Quality Generics).
Regutol, Tab. (Schering-Plough).
Revac Supprettes, Supp. (Webcon).
Rodox, Caps. (Rocky Mtn.).
Stulex, Tab. (Bowman).
Surfak, Cap. (Hoechst).
W/Ascorbic acid, ferrous fumarate.
See: Hemaspan Cap. (Bock).
W/Betaine HCl, zinc, manganese, molybdenum.
See: Hemaferrin (Western Research).
W/Bisacodyl.
See: Laxadan, Supp. (Lemmon).
W/Brewer's yeast.
See: Doss or Super Doss, Tab. (Ferndale).
W/Casanthranol.
See: Calotabs, Tab. (Calotabs).
Constiban (Quality Generics).
Diolax, Cap. (Century).
Dio-Soft (Standex).
Disanthrol, Cap. (Lannett).
Di-Sosul Forte, Tab. (Drug).
Easy-Lax Plus, Cap. (Walgreen).
Genericace, Cap. (Forest Pharm.).
Neo-Vadrin D-D-S, Cap. (Scherer).
Nuvac, Cap. (LaCrosse).
Peri-Colace, Cap., Syr. (Mead Johnson).
Rodox, Cap. (Rocky Mtn.).
W/Casanthranol, sodium carboxymethylcellulose.
See: Dialose Plus, Cap. (Stuart).
Disolan Forte, Cap. (Lannett).
Tri-Vac, Cap. (Rhode).
W/Dehydrocholic acid.
See: Dubbalax-B, Cap. (Redford).
Dubbalax-N, Cap. (Redford).
Neolax, Tab. (Central).

W/D-calcium pantothenate and acetphenolisatin.
See: Peri-Pantyl, Tab. (McGregor).
W/Ferrous fumarate, Vitamin C.
See: Hemaspan, Cap. (Bock).
Recoup, Tab. (Lederle).
W/Ferrous fumarate, vitamins.
See: Bevitone, Tab. (Lemmon).
W/Ferrous fumarate, betaine HCl, desiccated liver, vitamins, minerals.
See: Hemaferrin, Tab. (Western Research).
W/Glycerin.
See: Rectalad Enema, Liq. (Wampole).
W/Isobornyl thiocyanoacetate.
See: Barc, Cream, Liq. (Commerce).
W/Petrolatum.
See: Milkinol, Liq., Emulsion (Kremers-Urban).
W/Phenolphthalein.
See: Correctol, Tab. (Schering-Plough).
Disolan, Cap. (Lannett).
Ex-Lax Prods. (Sandoz Consumer).
Feen-A-Mint, Pills (Schering-Plough).
W/Phenolphthalein, dehydrocholic acid.
See: Bolax, Cap. (Boyd).
Sarolax, Cap. (Saron).
Tripalax, Cap. (Redford).
W/Polyoxyethylene nonyl phenol, sodium edetate, and 9-aminoacridine HCl.
See: Vagisec Plus Supp. (Schmid).
W/Senna concentrate.
See: Gentlax S, Tab. (Blair).
Sarolax (Saron).
Senokap-DDS, Cap. (Purdue Frederick).
Senokot S, Tab. (Purdue Frederick).
W/sodium propionate, propionic acid, salicylic acid.
See: Prosal, Liq. (Gordon).
W/Vitamin-mineral combination.
See: Geriplex-FS, Kapseal (Parke-Davis).
Materna 1.60, Tab. (Lederle).

DODERLEIN BACILLI.
See: Redoderlein, Vial (Forest Pharm.).

DODICIN. B.A.N. 3,6,9-Triazaheneicosanoic acid. Dodecyldi(aminoethyl)glycine.
Use: Surface active agent.

DOFAMIUM CHLORIDE. B.A.N. 2-(N-Dodecanoyl-N-methylamino)ethyldimethyl-(phenylcarbamoyl- methyl)ammonium Cl.
Use: Antiseptic.

DOFUS. (Miller) Freeze dried *Lactobacillus acidophilus* minimum of 100,000,000 organisms/ Cap. w/*Lactobacillus bifidus* organisms added. Bot. 60s.
Use: To restore intestinal flora.

DOK. (Major) Docusate sodium 100 mg. Cap. Bot. 100s, 1000s, UD 100s.
Use: Laxative.

DOK-250. (Major) Docusate sodium 250 mg. Cap. Bot. 100s.
Use: Laxative.

DOLACET C-3. (Hauck) Hydrocodone bitartrate 5 mg, acetaminophen 500 mg/Cap. Bot. 50s, 100s, 500s.
Use: Narcotic analgesic.

DOLAMIDE TABS. (Major) Chlorpropamide 100 mg or 250 mg/Tab. Bot. 100s, 500s, 1000s.
Use: Antidiabetic agent.

DOLAMIN. (Harvey) Ammonium sulfate 0.75% with sodium Cl, benzyl alcohol. Amp. 10 ml. In 12s, 25s, 100s.
Use: Antineuralgic.

DOLANEX ELIXIR. (Lannett) Acetaminophen 325 mg/5 ml, alcohol 23%. Bot. pt, gal.
Use: Analgesic.

DOLANTIN.
See: Meperidine HCl, U.S.P. XXII.

DOLCIN. (Dolcin) Aspirin 3.7 gr, calcium succinate 2.8 gr/Tab. Bot. 100s, 200s.
Use: Analgesic.

DOLDRAM. (Dram) Salicylamide 7.5 gr/Tab. Bot. 100s.
Use: Salicylate analgesic.

DOLEAR. (Eastwood) Bot. 0.5 oz.
Use: Otic preparation.

DOLENE AP-65. (Lederle) Propoxyphene HCl 65 mg, acetaminophen 650 mg/Tab. Bot. 100s, 500s.
Use: Narcotic analgesic.

DOLENE COMPOUND-65. (Lederle) Propoxyphene HCl 65 mg, aspirin 389 mg, caffeine 32.4 mg/Cap. Bot. 100s, 500s.
Use: Narcotic analgesic.

DOLENE PLAIN. (Lederle) Propoxyphene HCl 65 mg/Cap. Bot. 100s, 500s.
Use: Narcotic analgesic.

DOLOBID. (Merck Sharp & Dohme) Diflunisal 250 mg or 500 mg/Tab. Unit-of-use 60s, UD 100s.
Use: Salicylate analgesic.

DOLOMITE. (Nature's Bounty) Magnesium 78 mg, calcium 130 mg/Tab. Bot. 100s, 250s.
Use: Mineral supplement.

DOLOMITE. (Blue Cross) Calcium 426 mg, magnesium 246 mg/3 Tab. w/guar and acacia gum. Bot. 250s.
Use: Mineral supplement.

DOLOMITE PLUS CAPSULES. (Barth's) Magnesium 37 mg, calcium 187 mg, phosphorous 50 mg, iodine 0.25 mg/Cap. Bot. 100s, 500s, 1000s.
Use: Mineral supplement.

DOLOMITE TABLETS. (Faraday) Calcium 150 mg, magnesium 90 mg/Tab. Bot. 250s.
Use: Mineral supplement.

DOLONIL. (Parke-Davis)
See: Pyridium Plus, Tab. (Parke-Davis).

DOLOPHINE HYDROCHLORIDE. (Lilly) Methadone HCl. **Amp.:** (10 mg/ml; sodium Cl 0.9%) 1 ml 12s, 100s. **Vial:** (10 mg/ml) 20 ml (sodium Cl 0.9%, chlorobutanol 0.5%). 1s, 25s. **Tab.:** 5 mg, Bot. 100s. 10 mg, Bot. 100s.
Use: Narcotic analgesic.

DOLOPIRONA TABLETS. (Winthrop Products) Dipyrone with chlormezanone.

Use: Analgesic, muscle relaxant, antianxiety agent.

DOLORAL. (Progressive Enterprises) Colchicine salicylate 0.1 mg, phenobarbital 8 mg, sodium p-amino-benzoate 15 mg, vitamins B_1 25 mg, aspirin 325 mg/Tab. Bot. 100s, 1000s.
Use: Agent for gout, antiarthritic.

DOLORGON. (Kenyon) Mephenesin 200 mg, salicylamide 75 mg, acetyl-p-aminophenol 75 mg, ascorbic acid 50 mg/Tab. Bot. 100s, 1000s.
Use: Analgesic.

DOLOSAL.
See: Meperidine HCl.

DOLSED. (American Urologicals) Methenamine 40.8 mg, phenylsalicylate 18.1 mg, atropine sulfate 0.03 mg, hyoscyamine 0.03 mg, benzoic acid 4.5 mg, methylene blue 5.4 mg. Tab. Bot. 100s, 1000s.
Use: Urinary anti-infective.

DOLVANOL.
Use: Narcotic analgesic.
See: Meperidine HCl.

•**DOMAZOLINE FUMARATE.** USAN.
Use: Anticholinergic.

DOMEBORO. (Miles Pharm) Aluminum sulfate and calcium acetate when added to water gives therapeutic effect of Burow's. One pkg. or Tab./pt. water approximately equivalent to 1:40 dilution. **Pkg.:** 2.2 Gm, 12s, 100s. **Effervescent Tab.:** Box 12s, 100s, 1000s.
Use: Anti-inflammatory agent, topical.

DOME-PASTE BANDAGE. (Miles Pharm) Zinc oxide, calamine and gelatin bandage. Pkg. 4″ × 10 yd. and 3″ × 10 yd. impregnated gauze bandage.
Use: Treatment of conditions of the extremities.

DOMESTROL.
See: Diethylstilbestrol, Preps. (Various Mfr.).

D.O.M.F.
Use: Germicide.
See: Merbromin (Mercurochrome) (City Chem.).

•**DOMIODOL.** USAN.
Use: Mucolytic.

•**DOMIPHEN BROMIDE.** USAN. Dodecyldimethyl-2-phenoxyethylammonium bromide. Phenododecinium Bromide (I.N.N.).
Use: Antiseptic.
See: Bradosol.
Domibrom.

DOMMANATE. (Forest) Dimenhydrinate 50 mg/ml. Vial 10 ml.
Use: Antiemetic/antivertigo.

DOMOL BATH AND SHOWER OIL. (Miles Pharm.) D_1-isopropyl sebacate, isopropyl myristate with mineral oil. Bot. 240 ml.
Use: Emollient.

•**DOMPERIDONE.** USAN.
Use: Antiemetic.

DONATUSSIN DC SYRUP. (Laser) Hydrocodone bitartrate 2.5 mg, phenylephrine HCl 7.5 mg, guaifenesin 50 mg/5 ml. Bot. 120 ml, 480 ml.
Use: Antitussive, decongestant, expectorant.

DONATUSSIN PEDIATRIC DROPS. (Laser) Guaifenesin 20 mg, chlorpheniramine maleate 1 mg, phenylephrine HCl 2 mg/ml. Drop. bot. 30 ml.
Use: Expectorant, antihistamine, decongestant.

DONATUSSIN SYRUP. (Laser) Phenylephrine 10 mg, chlorpheniramine maleate 2 mg, dextromethorphan HBr 7.5 mg, guaifenesin 100 mg. Bot. pt, gal.
Use: Decongestant, antihistamine, antitussive, expectorant.

DONDRIL. (Whitehall) Dextromethorphan HBr 10 mg, phenylephrine HCl 5 mg, chlorpheniramine maleate 1 mg/Tab. Bot. 24s.
Use: Antitussive, decongestant, antihistamine.

•**DONETIDINE.** USAN.
Use: Antagonist (to Histamine H_2 receptors).

DONNA. (Arcum) Menthol, thymol, eucalyptol, exsiccated alum, boric acid. 4 oz, 14 oz.
Use: Vaginal preparation.

DONNACIN. (Pharmex) Phenobarbital 16.2 mg, hyoscyamine sulfate 0.1037 mg, atropine sulfate 0.194 mg, hyoscine HBr 0.0065 mg/5 ml or Tab. **Elix.:** Bot. pt, gal. **Tab.:** Bot. 1000s.
Use: Anticholinergic/antispasmodic.

DONNAFED Jr. (Jenkins) Ephedrine HCl 1/16 gr, belladonna extract 1/20 gr (total alkaloids, 0.0006 gr), salicylamide 1.25 gr/Tab. Bot. 1000s.
Use: Coryza, rhinitis, asthmatic conditions.

DONNAGEL. (Robins) Hyoscyamine sulfate 0.1037 mg, atropine sulfate 0.0194 mg, scopolamine HBr 0.0065 mg, sodium benzoate (preservative) 60 mg, kaolin 6 Gm, pectin 142.8 mg/30 ml, alcohol 3.8%. Susp. Bot. 120 ml, 240 ml, 480 ml.
Use: Antidiarrheal.

DONNAGEL-PG. (Robins) Powdered opium 24 mg, kaolin 6 Gm, pectin 142.8 mg, hyoscyamine sulfate 0.1037 mg, atropine sulfate 0.0194 mg, scopolamine HBr 0.0065 mg, sodium benzoate 60 mg/30 ml, alcohol 5%. Bot. 180 ml, 480 ml.
Use: Antidiarrheal.

DONNAMOR. (H.L. Moore) Atropine sulfate 0.0194 mg, scopolamine HBr 0.0065 mg, hyoscyamine HBr or SO_4 0.1037 mg, phenobarbital 16.2 mg/5 ml, alcohol 23%. Elix. Bot. 120 ml, pt, gal.
Use: Anticholinergic/antispasmodic.

DONNAPECTOLIN-PG. (Major) Powdered opium 24 mg, kaolin 6 Gm, pectin 142.8 mg, hyoscyamine sulfate 0.1037 mg, atropine sulfate 0.0194 mg, scopolamine HBr 0.0065 mg/30 ml, alcohol 5%. Susp. Bot. 180 ml, pt, gal.
Use: Antidiarrheal.

DONNAPHEN ELIXIR. (Approved) Phenobarbital 16.2 mg, hyoscyamine sulfate 0.1037 mg, atropine sulfate 0.0194 mg, hyoscine HBr 0.0065 mg/5 ml. Bot. pt, gal.
Use: Anticholinergic/antispasmodic.

DONNAPINE TABS. (Major) Belladonna alkaloids, phenobarbital. Bot. 100s, 1000s, UD 100s.
Use: Sedative, anticholinergic/antispasmodic.

DONNATAL. (Robins) Hyoscyamine sulfate 0.1037 mg, atropine sulfate 0.0194 mg, scopolamine HBr 0.0065 mg, phenobarbital 16.2 mg. **Cap. & Tab.:** Bot. 100s, 1000s. **Elix.:** w/alcohol 23%. Bot. 4 oz, pt, gal, Dis-Co pack 5 ml, 100s.
Use: Sedative, anticholinergic/antispasmodic.

DONNATAL DIS-CO UD PACK. (Robins) Hyoscyamine sulfate 0.1037 mg, atropine sulfate 0.0194 mg, hyoscine HBr 0.0065 mg, phenobarbital 16.2 mg (0.25 gr)/Tab. or 5 ml. **Tab.:** UD 100s. **Elix.:** UD (5 ml) 25s.
Use: Sedative, anticholinergic/antispasmodic.

DONNATAL EXTENTABS. (Robins) Hyoscyamine sulfate 0.3111 mg, atropine sulfate 0.0582 mg, scopolamine HBr 0.0195 mg, phenobarbital 48.6 mg (¾ gr)/Tab. Bot. 100s, 500s, Dis-Co pack 100s.
Use: Sedative, anticholinergic/antispasmodic.

DONNATAL #2. (Robins) Phenobarbital 32.4 mg (0.5 gr), hyoscyamine sulfate 0.1037 mg, atropine sulfate 0.0194 mg, scopolamine HBr 0.0065 mg/Tab. Bot. 100s, 1000s.
Use: Sedative, anticholinergic/antispasmodic.

DONNAZYME. (Robins) Hyoscyamine sulfate 0.0518 mg, atropine sulfate 0.0097 mg, scopolamine HBr 0.0033 mg, phenobarbital 8.1 mg (⅛ gr), pepsin 150 mg/Tab. in outer layer, pancreatin 300 mg, bile salts 150 mg/Tab. in core. Bot. 100s, 500s.
Use: Anticholinergic/antispasmodic, digestive aid.

DONPHEN. (Lemmon) Phenobarbital 15 mg, hyoscyamine sulfate 0.1 mg, atropine sulfate 0.02 mg, scopolamine HBr 6 mcg/Tab. Bot. 100s, 1000s.
Use: Sedative, anticholinergic/antispasmodic.

DON'T. (Commerce) Sucrose octa acetate 5%, isopropyl alcohol 54%. Bot. 0.45 oz.
Use: Discourage nail biting and thumb sucking.

•**DOPAMANTINE.** USAN.
Use: Antiparkinsonian.

DOPAMINE. (Astra) Dopamine. **Amp.:** 200 mg/5 ml Amp. Box 10s; 400 mg/10 ml Amp. Box 5s. **Additive Syringe:** 200 mg/5 ml Syr. Box 1s; 400 mg/10 ml Syr. Box 1s.
Use: Inotropic agent.

•**DOPAMINE HYDROCHLORIDE,** U.S.P. XXII. Inj., U.S.P. XXII. 4-(2-Aminoethyl)pyrocatechol HCl.
Use: Adrenergic
Intropin, Amp. (American Critical Care).

•**DOPAMINE HYDROCHLORIDE AND DEXTROSE INJECTION,** U.S.P. XXII.
Use: Adrenergic, emergency treatment of low blood pressure.

DOPAR. (Norwich Eaton) Levodopa 100 mg or 250 mg/Cap. Bot. 100s. 500 mg/Cap. Bot. 100s, 1000s.
Use: Anti-parkinson agent.

DOPASTAT. (Warner Chilcott) Dopamine HCl 40 mg/ml. Vial 5 ml.
Use: Inotropic agent.

•**DOPEXAMINE.** USAN.
Use: Cardiovascular agent.

•**DOPEXAMINE HYDROCHLORIDE.** USAN.
Use: Cardiovascular agent.

DOPRAM. (Robins) Doxapram HCl 20 mg/ml, 0.9% benzyl alcohol. Vial 20 ml.
Use: Respiratory stimulant.

DORAL. (Baker Cummins) Quazepam 7.5 mg or 15 mg/Tab. Bot. 100s, UD 100s.
Use: Sedative/hypnotic.

•**DORAMECTIN.** USAN.
Use: Antiparasitic (veterinary).

DORAPHEN COMPOUND 65. (Cenci) Propoxyphene HCl 65 mg, aspirin 227 mg, phenacetin 162 mg, caffeine 32.4 mg/Cap. Bot. 100s, 500s, 1000s.
Use: Narcotic analgesic.

DORAPHEN HCL. (Cenci) Propoxyphene HCl 65 mg/Cap. Bot. 100s, 1000s.
Use: Narcotic analgesic.

DORCOL CHILDREN'S COUGH SYRUP. (Sandoz Consumer) Dextromethorphan HBr 5 mg, pseudoephedrine HCl 15 mg, guaifenesin 50 mg/5 ml. Bot. 120 ml, 240 ml.
Use: Antitussive, decongestant, expectorant.

DORCOL CHILDREN'S DECONGESTANT LIQUID. (Sandoz Consumer) Pseudoephedrine HCl 15 mg/5 ml. Bot. 4 oz.
Use: Decongestant.

DORCOL CHILDREN'S LIQUID COLD FORMULA. (Sandoz Consumer) Pseudoephedrine HCl 15 mg, chlorpheniramine maleate 1 mg/5 ml. Bot. 4 oz.
Use: Decongestant, antihistamine.

DORCOL FEVER AND PAIN REDUCER. (Dorsey) Acetaminophen 160 mg/5 ml. Bot. 4 oz.
Use: Analgesic.

DORICO DROPS. (Winthrop Products) Paracetamol.
Use: Analgesic, antipyretic.

DORICO TABLETS. (Winthrop Products) Paracetamol.
Use: Analgesic, antipyretic.

DORIGLUTE TABS DEA. (Major) Glutethimide 0.5 Gm/Tab. Bot. 100s, 250s, 1000s.
Use: Nonbarbiturate hypnotic.

DORIMIDE. (Cenci) Glutethimide 0.5 Gm/Tab. Bot. 100s, 1000s.
Use: Sedative/hypnotic.

DORME. (A.V.P.) Promethazine HCl 12.5 mg, 25 mg or 50 mg/Cap. Bot. 100s.
Use: Antihistamine.

DORMEER. (Pasadena Research) Scopolamine aminoxide HBr 0.2 mg/Cap. Bot. 100s, 1000s.
Use: Sedative/hypnotic.

DORMETHAN.
See: Dextromethorphan HBr. (Various Mfr.).

DORMIN SLEEPING CAPSULES. (Randob) 25 mg/Cap. Bot. 32s, 72s.
Use: Sleep aid.

DORMIRAL.
See: Phenobarbital, Preps. (Various Mfr.).

DORMONAL.
See: Barbital, Preps. (Various Mfr.).

DORMUTOL. (Approved) Scopolamine aminoxide HBr 0.2 mg/Cap. Bot. 24s, 60s.
Use: Sedative/hypnotic.

•**DORSATINE HYDROCHLORIDE.** USAN.
Use: Antihistamine.

DORYX PELLETS. (Parke-Davis) Doxycycline hyclate 100 mg/Cap. Bot. 50s.
Use: Anti-infective, tetracycline.

D.O.S. CAPS. (Goldline) Dioctyl sodium sulfosuccinate SG 100 mg or 250 mg/Cap. Bot. 100s, 1000s.
Use: Laxative.

DOSS SYRUP. (PBI) Docusate sodium 20 mg/5 ml. Bot. pt, gal.
Use: Laxative.

•**DOTHIEPIN HCL.** USAN. 11-(3-Dimethylaminopropylidene)-6H-dibenzo[b,e]thiepin hydrochloride. Dosulepin (I.N.N.).
Use: Antidepressant.
See: Prothiaden (hydrochloride).

DOTIROL. (Winthrop Products) Ampicillin trihydrate available in Cap, Susp., Inj. (IV, IM.).
Use: Antibacterial, penicillin.

DOUBLE ACTION TOOTHACHE RELIEF KIT. (C.S. Dent) Toothache drops, acetaminophen 325 mg/Tab. Box 8s.
Use: Treatment of toothache.

DOUBLE SAL TABLETS. (Vale) Sodium salicylate 648 mg/EC Tab. Bot. 1000s.
Use: Salicylate analgesic.

DOUCHE. (Jenkins) Boric acid, borax, tannic acid, sodium salicylate, zinc sulfate, alum, hydrastine HCl, thymol, sodium bicarbonate and tartaric acid/Tab. Bot. 1000s.
Use: Vaginal preparation.

DOVACET CAPSULES. (Vale) Dover's powder 24.3 mg, aspirin 324 mg, caffeine 32.4 mg/Tab. Bot. 1000s.
Use: Analgesic.

DOVAPHEN CAP. (Jenkins) Dover's powder 16.2 mg (opium 1.62 mg), ipecac 1.62 mg, aspirin 2.5 gr, phenacetin 1.5 gr, caffeine ⅛ gr, camphor 0.25 gr, atropine sulfate 1/1000 gr/Cap. Bot. 1000s.
Use: Analgesic.

DOVAPHEN JR. (Jenkins) Dover's powder 8.1 mg, acetophenetidin 0.5 gr, atropine sulfate 1/4000 gr, salicylamide 0.5 gr, caffeine 1/10 gr/Tab. Bot. 1000s.
Use: Analgesic.

DOVER'S POWDER. Ipecac 1 part, opium 1 part, lactose 8 parts.
Use: Analgesic, sedative, diaphoretic.
W/Acetophenetidin, atropine sulfate, aspirin, camphor, caffeine, sodium sulfate, dried.
See: Dovium, Cap. (Hance).
W/Acetophenetidin, atropine sulfate, salicylamide, caffeine.
See: Dovaphen Jr., Tab. (Jenkins).
W/Acetophenetidin, camphor, aspirin, caffeine, atropine sulfate.
See: Analgestine, Cap. (Hauck).
W/Acetophenetidin, sodium citrate, potassium guaiacolsulfonate.
See: Doverlyn, Cap., Tab. (Davis & Sly).
W/A.P.C. camphor monobromated.
See: Coldate, Tab. (Elder).
W/Aspirin, phenacetin, camphor monobromated, caffeine.
See: Coldate, Tab. (Elder).
W/Atropine sulfate, A.P.C., camphor.
See: Dasin, Cap. (Beecham-Massengill).
W/Phenacetin, aspirin, camphor, caffeine alkaloid, atropine sulfate.
See: Analgestine Forte, Cap. (Hauck).
Dovernon, Cap. (Solvay).
Phenacaps, Cap. (Scrip).
W/Phenacetin, camphor, caffeine.
See: Doverlyn Adult, Tab. (Scrip).
W/Pyrilamine maleate, racephedrine HCl, salicylamide, phenacetin.
See: Asphamal-D, Tab. (Central).

DOVIUM. (Hance) Dover's powder 0.5 gr, acetophenetidin 1.5 gr, atropine sulfate 1/500 gr, aspirin 2 gr, camphor 0.25 gr, caffeine ⅛ gr, sodium sulfate, dried, 7.5 gr/Cap. Bot. 100s, 1000s.
Use: Analgesic, antipyretic.

DOWICIL 200.
See: Derma Soap (Ferndale).

DOW-ISONIAZID. (Merrell Dow) Isoniazid 300 mg/Tab. Bot. 30s.
Use: Antituberculous agent.

•**DOXACURIUM CHLORIDE.** USAN.
Use: Neuromuscular blocking agent.
See: Nuromax (Burroughs Wellcome).

DOXAMIN. (Forest) Thiamine HCl 100 mg, vitamin B_6 100 mg/ml. Vial 10 ml.
Use: Vitamin supplement.

DOXAPAP-N TABS. (Major) Propoxyphene napsylate 100 mg, acetaminophen 650 mg Bot. 100s, 500s.
Use: Narcotic analgesic.

DOXAPHENE CAPSULES. (Major) Propoxyphene HCl 65 mg/Cap. Bot. 1000s.
Use: Narcotic analgesic.

DOXAPHENE COMPOUND 65 CAPS. (Major) Propoxyphene HCl, acetaminophen. Bot. 1000s.
Use: Narcotic analgesic.

•**DOXAPRAM HYDROCHLORIDE,** U.S.P. XXII. Inj., U.S.P. XXII. 1-Ethyl-4-(2-morpholinoethyl)-3,3- diphenyl-2-pyrrolidinone HCl.
Use: Respiratory and CNS stimulant.
See: Dopram, Vial (Robins).

•**DOXAPROST.** USAN.
Use: Bronchodilator.

DOXATE. Docusate sodium.

Use: Laxative.

DOXAZOSIN MESYLATE. USAN.
Use: Antihypertensive.

DOXEPIN HYDROCHLORIDE, U.S.P. XXII. Cap., Oral Soln., U.S.P. XXII.
Use: Psychotherapeutic drug.
See: Adapin, Cap. (Pennwalt).
Sinequan, Cap. (Roerig).

DOXIDAN. (Hoechst) Yellow phenolphthalein 65 mg, docusate calcium 60 mg/Cap. Bot. 30s, 100s, 1000s, UD 100s, Display Pack 10s.
Use: Laxative.

DOXINATE. (Hoechst) Docusate sodium. **Cap.:** 240 mg/Cap. Bot. 100s. **Soln:** 50 mg/ml 5% alcohol. Bot. 60 ml, gal.
Use: Laxative.

DOXOFYLLINE. USAN.
Use: Bronchodilator.

DOXORUBICIN. USAN.
Use: Antineoplastic agent.

DOXORUBICIN HYDROCHLORIDE, U.S.P. XXII. Inj., U.S.P. XXII. 14-Hydroxydaunorubicin. An antibiotic produced by *Streptomyces peuceticus* var. caesius.
Use: Antineoplastic agent.
See: Adriamycin (Adria).

DOXPICOMINE HYDROCHLORIDE. USAN.
Use: Analgesic.

DOXY 100. (Lyphomed) Doxycycline hyclate for injection. Pow. 100 mg/Vial.
Use: Anti-infective, tetracycline.

DOXY 200. (Lyphomed) Doxycycline hyclate. Pow. 200 mg/Vial.
Use: Anti-infective, tetracycline.

DOXYBETASOL. B.A.N. 9α-Fluoro-11β, 17α-dihydroxy-16β-methylpregna-1,4-diene-3,20-dione.
Use: Corticosteroid.

DOXY-CAPS. (Edwards) Doxycycline hyclate 100 mg/Cap. Bot. 50s.
Use: Anti-infective, tetracycline.

DOXYCHEL CAPSULES. (Rachelle) Doxycycline hyclate 50 mg or 100 mg/Cap. Bot. 50s, 500s, UD 100s.
Use: Anti-infective, tetracycline.

DOXYCHEL INJECTABLE. (Rachelle) Doxycycline hyclate 100 mg or 200 mg/Vial.
Use: Anti-infective, tetracycline.

DOXYCHEL TABLETS. (Rachelle) Doxycycline hyclate 50 mg or 100 mg/Tab. Bot. 50s, 500s.
Use: Anti-infective, tetracycline.

DOXYCYCLINE, U.S.P. XXII. For Oral Susp. U.S.P. XXII. 4-(Dimethylamino)-1,4,4a,5,5a,6,11,12a-octahydro-3,5,10,12,12a-pentahydroxy-6-methyl-1,11-dioxo-2-naphthacenecarboxamide.
Use: Antibiotic.
See: Vibramycin for Oral Susp. (Pfizer Laboratories).
Vibramycin IV. (Roerig).

•**DOXYCYCLINE CALCIUM ORAL SUSPENSION,** U.S.P. XXII.
Use: Antibiotic.

•**DOXYCYCLINE FOSFATEX.** USAN.
Use: Antibacterial.

•**DOXYCYCLINE HYCLATE,** U.S.P. XXII. Cap., Inj., Sterile, Tab., Delayed Release Tab., U.S.P. XXII. 2-Naphthacenecarboxamide, 4-(dimethylamino)-1,4,4a,5,5a,6,11,12a-octahydro-3,5,10,12-12a-pentahydroxy-6-methyl-1,11-dioxo-, HCl compound with ethanol monohydrate.
Use: Antibacterial.
See: Doxy-Caps, Cap. (Edwards).
Vibra-Tabs, Tab. (Pfizer Laboratories).
Vibramycin, Cap., Tab., Vial (Pfizer Laboratories).
Vivox, Cap., Tab. (Squibb Mark).

•**DOXYLAMINE SUCCINATE,** U.S.P. XXII. Syr., Tab., U.S.P. XXII. 2-[α(2-Dimethylamino-ethoxy)-α-methyl- benzyl]pyridine bisuccinate.
Use: Antihistamine.
See: Decapryn, Prep. (Merrell Dow).
Unisom, Tab. (Leeming-Pacquin).
W/Acetaminophen, ephedrine sulfate, dextromethorphan HBr, alcohol.
See: Nyquil, Liq. (Vick).
W/Dextromethorphan HBr, alcohol.
See: Consotuss Antitussive, Syr. (Merrell Dow).
W/Dextromethorphan HBr, sodium citrate, alcohol.
See: Vicks Formula 44 Cough Mixture, Syr. (Vicks).
W/Mercodol.
See: Mercodol w/Decapryn, Syr. (Merrell Dow).

DOXY-LEMMON CAPSULES. (Lemmon) Doxycycline hyclate equivalent to 100 mg of doxycycline base/Cap. Bot. 50s, 500s, UD 100s.
Use: Anti-infective, tetracycline.

DOXY-LEMMON TABLETS. (Lemmon) Doxycycline hyclate equivalent to 100 mg of doxycycline base/Tab. Bot. 50s, 500s, UD 100s.
Use: Anti-infective, tetracycline.

DOXY-TABS. (Rachelle) Doxycycline hyclate 100 mg/FC Tab. Bot. 50s, 500s.
Use: Anti-infective, tetracycline.

DOXY-TABS-50. (Rachelle) 50 mg/Tab. Bot. 50s.
Use: Anti-infective, tetracycline.

DRAMAJECT. (Mayrand) Dimenhydrinate 50 mg/ml. Vial 10 ml.
Use: Antiemetic/antivertigo.

DRAMAMINE INJECTION. (Searle) Dimenhydrinate. **Amp.:** 50 mg/ml Ctn. 5s, 25s, 100s. **Vial:** 250 mg/5 ml Ctn. 5s, 25s.
Use: Antiemetic/antivertigo.

DRAMAMINE LIQUID. (Searle) Dimenhydrinate 12.5 mg/4 ml Bot. 90 ml, pt.
Use: Antiemetic/antivertigo.

DRAMAMINE TABLETS. (Searle) Dimenhydrinate 50 mg/Tab. Bot. 36s, 100s, 1000s, Blister pkg. 12s, UD 100s.
Use: Antiemetic/antivertigo.

DRAMANATE. (Pasadena) Dimenhydrinate 50 mg/ml. Inj. Vial 10 ml.
Use: Antiemetic/antivertigo.

DRAMARIN.
See: Dramamine, Preps. (Searle).

DRAMOCEN. (Central) Dimenhydrinate 50 mg/ml. Inj. Vial 10 ml Box 12s.
Use: Antiemetic, antivertigo.

DRAMOJECT. (Mayrand) Dimenhydrinate 50 mg/ml, benzyl alcohol, propylene glycol. Inj. Vial 10 ml.
Use: Antiemetic/antivertigo.

DRAMYL.
See: Dramamine, Preps. (Searle).

DRANOCHOL. (Marin) Dehydrocholic acid 200 mg, homatropine methylbromide 5 mg/Tab. Bot. 60s, 500s, 1000s.
Use: Hydrocholeretic, antispasmodic.

DRAWING SALVE. (Whiteworth) Tube oz.
Use: Healing agent, topical.

DRAWING SALVE with TRIQUINODIN. (Towne) Tube 2 oz.
Use: Healing agent, topical.

DR. BERRY'S SKIN TONER. (Last) Hydroquinone 2%. Jar oz.
Use: Skin bleaching agent.

DR. CALDWELL SENNA LAXATIVE. (Mentholatum) Senna 7%, alcohol 4.5%. Bot. 130 ml, 360 ml.
Use: Laxative.

DRC PERI-ANAL CREAM. (Xttrium) Lassar's paste 37.5%, anhydrous lanolin, U.S.P. 37.5%, cold cream 25%. Tube 5 oz.
Use: Skin protectant, perianal.

DR. DRAKE'S COUGH MEDICINE. (Last) Dextromethorphan HBr 10 mg/5 ml Bot. 2 oz.
Use: Antitussive.

•**DRIBENDAZOLE.** USAN.
Use: Anthelmintic.

DRI-A CAPS. (Barth's) Vitamin A 10,000 IU/Cap. Bot. 100s, 500s.
Use: Vitamin A supplement.

DRI A&D CAPS. (Barth's) Vitamins A 10,000 IU, D 400 IU/Cap. Bot. 100s, 500s.
Use: Vitamin A and D supplement.

DRI-E. (Barth's) Vitamin E. **100 IU/Cap.:** Bot. 100s, 500s, 1000s. **200 IU/Cap.:** Bot. 100s, 250s, 500s. **400 IU/Cap.:** Bot. 100s, 250s.
Use: Vitamin E supplement.

DRI/EAR. (Pfeiffer) Boric acid 2.75% in isopropyl alcohol. Soln. Dropper bot. 30 ml.
Use: Otic preparation.

•**DRIED ALUMINUM HYDROXIDE GEL,** U.S.P. XXII.
Use: Antacid.
See: Aluminum Hydroxide Gel, dried.

DRIED YEAST.
See: Yeast, dried.

DRIMINATE TABS. (Major) Dimenhydrinate 50 mg/Tab. Bot. 100s, 1000s.
Use: Antiemetic/antivertigo.

DRINOPHEN CAPSULES. (Lannett) Phenylpropanolamine HCl 15 mg, acetylsalicylic acid 230 mg, acetaminophen 200 mg, caffeine 15 mg/Cap. Bot. 1000s.
Use: Decongestant, analgesic.

DRISDOL. (Winthrop Pharm) Ergocalciferol (Vitamin D) 8000 IU/ml in propylene glycol solvent. Bot. 60 ml.
Use: Treatment of refractory rickets.

DRISDOL 50,000 UNIT CAPSULES. (Winthrop Pharm) Vitamin D-2, 50,000 IU/Cap. Bot. 50s.
Use: Vitamin D supplement.

DRISTAN 12 HOUR. (Whitehall) Chlorpheniramine maleate 4 mg, phenylephrine HCl 20 mg/Cap. Bot. 6s, 10s, 15s.
Use: Antihistamine, decongestant.

DRISTAN-AF. (Whitehall) Phenylephrine HCl 5 mg, chlorpheniramine maleate 2 mg, acetaminophen 325 mg, caffeine 16.2 mg/Tab. Bot. 24s, 50s.
Use: Decongestant, antihistamine, analgesic.

DRISTAN CAPSULES. (Whitehall) Phenylephrine HCl 5 mg, chlorpheniramine maleate 2 mg, acetaminophen 325 mg/Cap. Bot. 16s, 36s, 75s.
Use: Decongestant, antihistamine, analgesic.

DRISTAN LONG LASTING NASAL MIST. (Whitehall) Oxymetazoline HCl 0.05%. Bot. 15 ml, 30 ml. Spray (menthol): 15 ml.
Use: Nasal decongestant.

DRISTAN MAXIMUM STRENGTH CAPLETS. (Whitehall) Pseudoephedrine HCl 30 mg, acetaminophen 500 mg/Capl. Bot. 24s.
Use: Decongestant, analgesic.

DRISTAN MENTHOL NASAL MIST. (Whitehall) Phenylephrine HCl 0.5%, pheniramine maleate 0.2%. Bot. 0.5 oz, 1 oz.
Use: Decongestant, antihistamine.

DRISTAN NASAL MIST. (Whitehall) Phenylephrine HCl 0.5%, pheniramine maleate 0.2%. Regular: 15 ml, 30 ml. Menthol: 15 ml.
Use: Decongestant, antihistamine.

DRISTAN TABLETS. (Whitehall) Phenylephrine HCl 5 mg, chlorpheniramine maleate 2 mg, acetaminophen 325 mg/Tab. Bot. 24s, 50s, 100s.
Use: Decongestant, antihistamine, analgesic.

DRITHO-CREME. (American Dermal) Anthralin 0.1%, 0.25% or 0.5%. Tube 50 Gm.
Use: Antipsoriatic.

DRITHO-CREME HP 1.0%. (American Dermal) Anthralin 1%. Tube 50 Gm.
Use: Antipsoriatic.

DRITHO-SCALP. (American Dermal) Anthralin 0.25% or 0.5%. Tube 50 Gm.
Use: Antipsoriatic.

DRIXORAL. (Schering) Dexbrompheniramine maleate 6 mg, pseudoephedrine sulfate 120 mg/SA Tab. Box 10s, 20s, 40s. Bot. 48s, 100s.
Use: Antihistamine, decongestant.

DRIXORAL PLUS. (Schering) Pseudoephedrine sulfate 60 mg, dexbrompheniramine maleate 3 mg, acetaminophen 500 mg/TR Tab. Bot. 24s.
Use: Decongestant, antihistamine, analgesic.

DRIZE. (Ascher) Phenylpropanolamine HCl 75 mg, chlorpheniramine maleate 12 mg/SR Cap. Bot. 100s.
Use: Decongestant, antihistamine.
DROBULINE. USAN.
Use: Cardiac depressant.
DROCARBIL. Acetarsone salt of arecoline. Arecoline n-acetyl-4-hydroxy-m-arsanilate.
Use: Anthelmintic (veterinary).
DROCINONIDE. USAN.
Use: Anti-inflammatory.
DROCODE.
See: Dihydrocodeine.
DROMORAN, LEVO. Levorphanol, Levorphan.
See: Levo-Dromoran, Vial, Amp., Tab. (Roche).
DRONABINOL. USAN.
Use: Antiemetic.
DROP CHALK. (Various Mfr.) Calcium carbonate, prepared. Prepared Chalk.
DROPERIDOL, U.S.P. XXII. Inj., U.S.P. XXII. 1-{1-[3-(p-Fluorobenzoyl)propyl-1,2,3,6-tetrahydro-4-pyridyl]}-2-benzimidazolinone.
Use: Tranquilizer.
See: Inapsine, Inj. (Janssen).
W/Fentanyl citrate.
Use: Tranquilizer.
See: Innovar, Inj. (Janssen).
DROPRENILAMINE. USAN.
Use: Vasodilator.
DROPROPIZINE. B.A.N. 1-(2,3-Dihydroxypropyl)-4-phenylpiperazine.
Use: Antitussive.
DROSTANOLONE. B.A.N. 17β-Hydroxy-2α-methyl-5α-androstan-3-one.
Use: Anabolic steroid.
DROTEBANOL. B.A.N. 3,4-Dimethoxy-17-methylmorphinan-6β, 14-diol.
Use: Analgesic, antitussive.
DROTIC STERILE OTIC SOLUTION. (Ascher) Hydrocortisone 10 mg (1%), polymyxin B sulfate 10,000 units, neomycin 5 mg/ml, preservatives. Dropper bot. 10 ml.
Use: Otic preparation.
DROXACIN SODIUM. USAN.
Use: Antibacterial.
DROXIFILCON A. USAN.
Use: Contact lens material.
DROXYPROPINE. B.A.N. 1-[2-(2-Hydroxyethoxy)-ethyl]-4-phenyl-4-propionylpiperidine.
Use: Cough suppressant.
DR. SCHOLL'S ATHLETE'S FOOT CREAM. (Scholl) Tolnaftate 1%. Tube 0.5 oz.
Use: Antifungal, external.
DR. SCHOLL'S ATHLETE'S FOOT POWDER. (Scholl) Tolnaftate 1%. Shaker: Plastic bot. 2.5 oz. Spray: Aerosol can 3.5 oz.
Use: Antifungal, external.
DR. SCHOLL'S ATHLETE'S FOOT SPRAY. (Scholl) Tolnaftate 1%. Aerosol can 4 oz.
Use: Antifungal, external.
DR. SCHOLL'S CORN/CALLOUS REMOVER. (Scholl) Salicylic acid 12.6%. Bot. 0.33 oz.
Use: Keratolytic.
DR. SCHOLL'S CORN/CALLOUS SALVE. (Scholl) Salicylic acid 15%. Tube 0.4 oz.
Use: Keratolytic.
DR. SCHOLL'S CORN SALVE. (Scholl) Salicylic acid 15%. Jar 0.4 oz.
Use: Keratolytic.
DR. SCHOLL'S INGROWN TOENAIL RELIEVER. (Scholl) Sodium sulfide 1%. Bot. 0.33 oz.
Use: Foot preparation.
DR. SCHOLL'S PRO COMFORT JOCK ITCH SPRAY. (Scholl) Tolnaftate 1%. Aerosol can 3.5 oz.
Use: Antifungal, external.
DR. SCHOLL'S WART REMOVER KIT. (Scholl) Salicylic acid 17%. Bot. 3.25 oz.
Use: Keratolytic.
DR. SCHOLL'S ZINO PADS/WITH MEDICATED DISKS. (Scholl) Salicylic acid 20% or 40%. Protective pads designed for use with and without salicylic acid-impregnated disks.
Use: Keratolytic.
DRUCON. (Standard Drug) Phenylephrine HCl 5 mg, chlorpheniramine maleate 2 mg, menthol 1 mg, alcohol 5%/5 ml Elix. Bot. pt, gal.
Use: Decongestant, antihistamine.
DRUCON C R. (Standard Drug) Phenylephrine HCl 25 mg, chlorpheniramine maleate 4 mg/Tab. Bot. 100s.
Use: Decongestant, antihistamine.
DRUCON WITH CODEINE. (Standard Drug) Codeine phosphate 10 mg, phenylephrine HCl 10 mg, chlorpheniramine maleate 2 mg, menthol 1 mg, alcohol 5%/5 ml. Bot. pt.
Use: Antitussive, decongestant, antihistamine.
DRY & CLEAR ACNE MEDICATION. (Whitehall) Benzoyl peroxide 5%. Lot. Bot. 30 ml, 60 ml.
Use: Anti-acne.
DRY & CLEAR DOUBLE STRENGTH CREAM. (Whitehall) Benzoyl peroxide 10%. Tube 30 Gm.
Use: Anti-acne.
DRY SKIN CREME. (Gordon) Cetyl alcohol, lubricating oils in a water soluble base. Jar 2 oz, 1 lb, 5 lb.
Use: Emollient.
DRYSOL. (Person & Covey) Aluminum Cl hexahydrate 20% in 93% SD alcohol 40. Bot. 37.5 ml.
Use: Astringent.
DRYSUM SHAMPOO. (Summers) Alcohol 15%, acetone 6%. Plastic bot. 4 oz.
Use: Drying agent for oily hair.
DRYTERGENT. (C & M Pharmacal) TEA-dodecylbenzenesulfonate, boric acid, lauramide DEA, propylene glycol, purified water, color, fragrance. Bot. 8 oz, 16 oz, 1 gal.
Use: Anti-acne.
DRYTEX. (C & M Pharmacal) Salicylic acid 2%, benzalkonium Cl 0.1%, non-ionic wetting agent,

acetone 10%, isopropyl alcohol 40%, purified water, color, perfume. Lot. Bot. 240 ml.
Use: Anti-acne, antiseborrheic.

DSMC PLUS. (Geneva Marsam) Docusate potassium 100 mg. Cap. Bot. 100s.
Use: Laxative.

D-S-S PLUS CAPSULES. (Warner-Chilcott) Docusate sodium 100 mg, casanthranol 30 mg/ Cap. Bot. 100s, 1000s, UD 100s.
Use: Laxative.

DST. Dihydrostreptomycin.
See: Dihydrostreptomycin, Preps. (Various Mfr.).

D-TEST 100. (Burgin-Arden) Testosterone cypionate 100 mg/ml. Vial 10 ml.
Use: Androgen.

D-TEST 200. (Burgin-Arden) Testosterone cypionate 200 mg/ml. Vial 10 ml.
Use: Androgen.

DTIC-DOME. (Miles Pharm) Dacarbazine 100 mg or 200 mg. Vial 10 ml, 20 ml.
Use: Antineoplastic agent.

DUADACIN. (Hoechst) Phenylpropanolamine HCl 12.5 mg, chlorpheniramine maleate 2 mg, acetaminophen 325 mg/Cap. Bot. 100s, 1000s.
Use: Decongestant, antihistamine, analgesic.

DUAL-WET. (Alcon Lenscare) Polyvinyl alcohol, duasorb water soluble polymetric system, benzalkonium Cl 0.01%, disodium edetate 0.05%. Bot. 2 oz.
Use: Hard contact lens care.

•**DUAZOMYCIN.** USAN. Antibiotic isolated from broth filtrates of *Streptomyces ambofaciens.*
Use: Antineoplastic agent.

DUAZOMYCIN A. Name used for Duazomycin.

DUAZOMYCIN B. Name used for Azotomycin.

DUAZOMYCIN C. Name used for Ambomycin.

DUBILE. (Kenyon) Ox bile extract 1.5 gr, mixed oxidized bile acids 1.5 gr, homatropine MBr 1/120 gr/Tab. Bot. 100s, 1000s.

DULCAGEN SUPPOSITORIES. (Goldline) Bisacodyl 10 mg/Supp. Box 12s, 100s.
Use: Laxative.

DULCAGEN TABLETS. (Goldline) Bisacodyl 5 mg/Tab. Bot. 100s, 1000s.
Use: Laxative.

DULCOLAX. (Boehringer Ingelheim) Bisacodyl. **EC Tab.:** 5 mg. Box 10s, 25s, 50s, 100s. Bot. 1000s, UD 100s. **Supp.:** 10 mg. Box 2s, 4s, 8s, 50s, 500s. **Bowel Prep Kit:** 4 tab., 1 supp./Kit. 5s/box.
Use: Laxative.

DULL-C. (Freeda) Ascorbic acid 4 Gm/tsp. Pow. Bot. 100 Gm, 500 Gm, 1000 Gm.
Use: Vitamin supplement.

DUO. (Norcliff Thayer) Surgical adhesive. Tube 0.5 oz.

DUO-CYP. (Keene) Testosterone cypionate 50 mg, estradiol cypionate 2 mg/ml. Vial 10 ml.
Use: Androgen, estrogen combination.

DUODENAL SUBSTANCE.
W/Ox bile extract, pancreatin, papain.
See: Digenzyme, Tab. (Burgin-Arden).

DUODENUM WHOLE, DESICCATED & DEFATTED.
W/Ferrous gluconate, Vitamin B_{12}, cobalt Cl.
See: Bitrinsic-E, Cap. (Elder).

DUODERM. (Conva Tec) **Sterile dressing:** 10 cm × 10 cm. Pack 5s. 20 cm × 20 cm. Pack 3s. **Sterile gran:** Packet 4 Gm. Pack 5s.
Use: Wound-healing agent.

DUOFILM. (Stiefel) Salicylic acid 16.7%, lactic acid 16.7% in flexible collodion. Bot. 15 ml w/ applicator.
Use: Keratolytic.

DUO-FLOW. (CooperVision) Poloxamer 188, benzalkonium Cl 0.013%, EDTA 0.25%. Soln. Bot. 120 ml.
Use: Hard contact lens care.

DUO-K. (Various Mfr.) Potassium 20 mEq, chloride 3.4 mEq/15 ml (from potassium gluconate and potassium Cl). Bot. pt, gal.
Use: Mineral supplement.

DUOLUBE. (Bausch & Lomb) White petrolatum, mineral oil. Sterile, preservative and lanolin free. Oint. Tube 3.5 Gm.
Use: Lubricant, ophthalmic.

DUO-MEDIHALER. (Riker) Isoproterenol HCl 0.16 mg, phenylephrine bitartrate 0.24 mg. In 15 ml (300 metered doses) or 22.5 ml (450 metered doses) medihaler. Refill vial 15 ml, 22.5 ml.
Use: Bronchodilator.

DUOMINE. (Kenyon) Dextromethorphan HBr 7.5 mg, chlorpheniramine maleate 10 mg, ammonium Cl 80 mg, potassium guaiacolate 80 mg, tartar emetic 0.8 mg/5 ml. Bot. 4 oz, pt, gal.
Use: Antitussive, antihistamine, expectorant.

DUOMYCIN.
See: Aureomycin, Preps. (Lederle).

•**DUOPERONE FUMARATE.** USAN.
Use: Neuroleptic.

DUOSOL. (Kirkman Sales) Docusate sodium 100 mg or 250 mg/Cap. Bot. 100s, 1000s.
Use: Laxative.

DUOTAL. (Approved) 1.5 gr: Secobarbital sodium 3/4 gr, amobarbital 3/4 gr/Cap. 3 gr: Secobarbital sodium 1.5 gr, amobarbital 1.5 gr/Cap. Bot. 100s, 500s, 1000s.
Use: Sedative/hypnotic.

DUOTAL.
See: Guaiacol Carbonate (Various Mfr.).

DUOTRATE 30. (Jones Medical) Pentaerythritol tetranitrate 30 mg/SR Cap. Bot. 100s.
Use: Antianginal.

DUOTRATE 45. (Jones Medical) Pentaerythritol tetranitrate 45 mg/SR Cap. Bot. 100s.
Use: Antianginal.

DUOTRONE. (Arnar-Stone; Dunhall) Estrone 2 mg, testosterone 25 mg/ml. Vial 10 ml.
Use: Estrogen, androgen combination.

DUOVIN-S. (Spanner) Estrone 2.5 mg, progesterone 25 mg/ml. Vial 10 ml.
Use: Estrogen, progestin combination.

DUO-WR, No. 1 & No. 2. (Whorton) **No. 1:** Salicylic acid, compound tincture benzoin. **No. 2:** Compound tincture benzoin, formaldehyde. Bot. 0.25 oz.
Use: Keratolytic.

DUPHALAC. (Solvay) Lactulose 10 Gm/15 ml (> 2.2 Gm galactose, > 1.2 Gm lactose, 1.2 Gm or less of other sugars). Syr. Bot. 240 ml, pt, qt, UD 30 ml.
Use: Laxative.

DUPLAST. (Beiersdorf) Adhesive coated elastic cloth. 8″×4″ Strip. Box 10s. 10″×5″ Strip. Box 8s, 10s.

DUPLEX SHAMPOO. (C & M Pharmacal) Sodium lauryl sulfate, lauramide DEA, purified water. Bot. pt, gal.
Use: Shampoo.

DUPLEX T SHAMPOO (C & M Pharmacal) Sodium lauryl sulfate, purified water, lauramide DEA, solution of coal tar, alcohol 8.3%. Bot. pt, gal.
Use: Antiseborrheic.

DUPONOL.
See: Gardinol-type detergents (Sodium Lauryl Sulfate) (Various Mfr.).

DURABOLIN. (Organon) Nandrolone phenpropionate 25 mg/ml in sesame oil, benzyl alcohol 5%. Inj. Vial 5 ml.
Use: Anabolic steroid.
See: Deca-Durabolin, Inj. (Organon).

DURABOLIN. (Organon) Nandrolone phenpropionate 50 mg/ml in sterile sesame oil, benzyl alcohol 10%. Inj. Vial 2 ml.
Use: Anabolic steroid.

DURACARE. (Blairex) Buffered hypertonic salt solution, non-ionic detergents with thimerosal 0.004%, EDTA 0.1%. Soln. Bot. 30 ml.
Use: Soft contact lens care.

DURACARE II. (Blairex Lab.) Buffered hypertonic salt solution, ethylene and propylene oxide, octylphenoxypolyethoxyethanol, lauryl sulfate salt of imidazoline, sodium bisulfite 0.1%, sorbic acid 0.1%, trisodium EDTA 0.25%.
Use: Contact lens care.

DURA-CHORION PLUS. (Pharmex) Estradiol valerate 10 mg/ml. Vial 10 ml.
Use: Estrogen.

DURACID. (Fielding) Antacid. Bot 100s.
Use: Antacid.

DURADYNE. (Forest) Aspirin 230 mg, acetaminophen 180 mg, caffeine 15 mg/Tab. Bot. 1000s.
Use: Analgesic combination.

DURADYNE DHC. (Forest) Hydrocodone bitartrate 5 mg, acetaminophen 500 mg/Tab. Bot. 100s, 1000s.
Use: Narcotic analgesic combination.

DURA-ESTRIN. (Hauck) Estradiol cypionate in oil 5 mg/ml. Inj. Vial 10 ml.
Use: Estrogen.

DURAGEN. (Hauck) Estradiol valerate in oil 10 mg, 20 mg or 40 mg/ml. Inj. Vial 10 ml.
Use: Estrogen.

•**DURAGESIC.** (Janssen) Fentanyl transdermal.
Use: Narcotic analgesic.

DURA-GEST. (Dura) Phenylpropanolamine HCl 45 mg, phenylephrine HCl 5 mg, guaifenesin 200 mg/Cap. Bot. 100s, 500s.
Use: Decongestant, expectorant.

DURA-KELLIN. (Pharmex) Estrone 2 mg, potassium estrone sulfate 1 mg, sodium phosphate buffer, sodium carboxymethylcellulose 0.2%, thimerosal 1:20,000, benzyl alcohol 1.5%/ml. Vial 10 ml.
Use: Estrogen combination.

DURALEX. (American Urologicals) Pseudoephedrine HCl 120 mg, chlorpheniramine maleate 8 mg/SR Cap. Bot. 100s, 1000s.
Use: Decongestant, antihistamine.

DURALONE INJECTION. (Hauck) Methylprednisolone acetate 40 mg or 80 mg/ml Susp. for Inj. **40 mg:** Vial 10 ml. **80 mg:** Vial 5 ml.
Use: Corticosteroid.

DURALUTIN INJECTION. (Hauck) Hydroxyprogesterone 250 mg/ml. Vial 5 ml.
Use: Progesterone.

DURA-METH. (Foy) Methylprednisolone 40 mg/ml. Vial 5 ml, 10 ml.
Use: Corticosteroid.

DURAMIST PLUS. (Pfeiffer) Oxymetazoline HCl 0.05%. Spray. 15 ml.
Use: Nasal decongestant.

DURAMORPH. (Elkins-Sinn) Morphine sulfate. Inj. 0.5 mg/ml or 1 mg/ml. Amp. 10 ml Box 10s. Preservative free.
Use: Narcotic analgesic.

DURANDROL. (Pharmex) Methandriol dipropionate 50 mg/ml. Vial 10 ml.

DURANEST HCl. (Astra) Etidocaine. **1%:** Vial 30 ml. **1% w/epinephrine 1:200,000:** Vial 30 ml. **1.5% w/epinephrine 1:200,000:** Amp. 20 ml.
Use: Local anesthetic.

DURAPAM. (Major) Flurazepam HCl 15 mg or 30 mg/Cap. Bot. 100s, 500s.
Use: Sedative/hypnotic.

•**DURAPATITE.** USAN.
Use: Prosthetic aid.

DURAQUIN. (Parke-Davis) Quinidine gluconate 330 mg/SR Tab. Bot. 100s, UD 100s.
Use: Cardiac depressant.

DURA-TAP/PD. (Dura) Pseudoephedrine HCl 60 mg, chlorpheniramine maleate 4 mg. Cap. Bot. 100s.
Use: Decongestant, antihistamine.

DURATEARS. (Alcon) White petroleum, anhydrous liquid lanolin, mineral oil. Oint. Tube 3.5 Gm.
Use: Lubricant, ophthalmic.

DURATEST-200/DURATEST-100. (Hauck) Testosterone cypionate in oil 100 mg or 200 mg/ml. Inj. Vial 10 ml.
Use: Androgen.

DURA-TESTOSTERONE. (Pharmex) Testosterone enthanate 200 mg/ml. Vial 10 ml.
Use: Androgen.

DURATESTRIN. (Hauck) Estradiol cypionate 2 mg, testosterone cypionate 50 mg/ml with chlorobutanol in cottonseed oil. Vial 10 ml.
Use: Estrogen, androgen combination.

DURA-TESTRONE. (Pharmex) Testosterone enthanate 90 mg, estradiol valerate 4 mg/ml.
Use: Androgen, estrogen combination.

DURA-TESTERONE FORTE. (Pharmex) Testosterone enthanate 180 mg, estradiol valerate 8 mg/ml. Vial 10 ml.
Use: Androgen, estrogen combination.

DURATHATE-200 INJECTION. (Hauck) Testosterone enanthate in oil 200 mg/ml. Vial 10 ml.
Use: Androgen.

DURATION MENTHOLATED VAPOR SPRAY. (Schering-Plough) Oxymetazoline HCl 0.05%, aromatics. Squeeze bot. 15 ml.
Use: Nasal decongestant.

DURATION MILD NASAL SPRAY. (Schering-Plough) Phenylephrine HCl 0.5%. Bot. 15 ml.
Use: Decongestant.

DURATION NASAL SPRAY. (Schering-Plough) Oxymetazoline HCl 0.05%. Aqueous soln. Squeeze bot. 15 ml, 30 ml.
Use: Nasal decongestant.

DURATESTRIN. (Hauck) Testosterone cypionate 50 mg, estradiol cypionate 2 mg/ml. Vial 10 ml.
Use: Androgen, estrogen combination.

DURA-VENT. (Dura) Phenylpropanolamine HCl 75 mg, guaifenesin 600 mg. SR Tab. Bot. 100s.
Use: Decongestant, expectorant.

DURA-VENT/A. (Dura) Phenylpropanolamine HCl 75 mg, chlorpheniramine maleate 10 mg. SR Cap. Bot. 100s.
Use: Decongestant, antihistamine.

DURA-VENT/DA. (Dura) Phenylephrine HCl 20 mg, chlorpheniramine maleate 8 mg, methscopolamine nitrate 2.5 mg. SR Tab. Bot. 100s.
Use: Decongestant, antihistamine, anticholinergic.

DURAZYME. (Blairex) Nonionic detergent preserved w/thimerosal 0.004%, EDTA 0.1% in sterile buffered hypertonic salt soln. Bot. 30 ml.
Use: Contact lens care.

DURICEF. (Mead Johnson) Cefadroxil. **Tab.:** 1 Gm. Bot. 100s. **Cap.:** 500 mg. Bot. 100s, 500s. **Susp.:** 125 mg/5 ml, 250 mg/5 ml or 500 mg/5 ml Bot. 50 ml, 100 ml.
Use: Antibacterial, cephalosporin.

DUROLENE OINTMENT. (Durel) Glyceryl monostearate, petrolatum, cholesterol, polyoxyethyl sorbitol monolaurate. Jar 1 lb, 6 lb.
Use: Ointment base.

DUROMANTEL CREAM. (Durel) Spermaceti, cetyl alcohol, stearyl alcohol, glycerine, alcohol sulfates, aluminum acetate solution, purified water, methyl and propyl parasepts. Jar 1 lb, 6 lb.

DUROSHAM. (Durel) Soapless shampoo concentrate. Bot. 6 oz, gal.
Use: Shampoo.

DUSOTAL. (Harvey) Sodium amobarbital ¾ gr, sodium secobarbital ¾ gr/Cap. Bot. 1000s. (3 gr) Bot. 1000s.
Use: Sedative/hypnotic.

•**DUSTING POWDER, ABSORBABLE,** U.S.P. XXII. Starch-derivative dusting pow.
Use: Surgical aid (glove lubricant).

DUSTING POWDER, SURGICAL.
See: B-F-I Powder (Calgon).

DUTCH DROPS. Oil of turpentine, sulfurated.

DUTCH OIL. Oil of turpentine, sulfurated.

DUVOID. (Norwich Eaton) Bethanechol Cl 10 mg, 25 mg or 50 mg/Tab. Bot. 100s, UD ctn. 100s.
Use: Urinary tract product.

D V CREAM. (Merrell Dow) Dienestrol 0.01% w/ lactose, propylene glycol, stearic acid, diglycol stearate, TEA, benzoic acid, butylated hydroxytoluene, disodium edetate, buffered w/lactic acid to an acid pH. Tube 3 oz, w/applicator.
Use: Estrogen, vaginal.

D-VASO-S. (Dunhall) Pentylenetetrazole 50 mg, niacin 50 mg, dimenhydrinate 25 mg, alcohol 18%, sherry wine vehicle. Bot. pt.

DWIATOL. (Kenyon) Hyoscyamine HBr 0.256 mg, hyoscine HBr 0.0144 mg, atropine sulfate 0.048 mg, phenobarbital 0.5 gr/Tab. Bot. 100s, 1000s.
Use: Anticholinergic/antispasmodic.

D-XYLOSE.
See: Xylo-Pfan. (Adria).

DYANTOIN CAPS. (Major) Phenytoin sodium 100 mg/Cap. Bot. 100s, 1000s.
Use: Anticonvulsant.

DX 114 FOOT POWDER. (Amlab) Zinc undecylenate 1%, salicylic acid 1%, benzoic acid 1%, ammonium alum 5%, boric acid 10.5% w/zinc stearate, chlorophyll, talc, kaolin, starch, calcium silicate, oil of wormwood. Cont. 2 oz.
Use: Antifungal, external.

DYAZIDE. (SmithKline Beecham) Triamterene 50 mg, hydrochlorothiazide 25 mg/Cap. Bot. 1000s, UD 100s, Patient Pack 100s.
Use: Diuretic, antihypertensive.

DYCILL. (Beecham Labs) Dicloxacillin sodium 250 mg or 500 mg/Cap. Bot. 100s.
Use: Antibacterial, penicillin.

DYCLONE. (Astra) Dyclonine HCl 0.5% or 1%. Soln. Bot. 30 ml.
Use: Local anesthetic, topical.

•**DYCLONINE HCl,** U.S.P. XXII. Gel, Topical Soln., U.S.P. XXII. 4′-Butoxy-3-piperidinopropiophenone.
HCl.
Use: Topical anesthetic.
See: Dyclone, Soln. (Astra).
W/Neomycinsulfate, polymyxin B sulfate, hydrocortisone acetate.
See: Neo-polycin HC, Oint. (Merrell Dow).

DYCOMENE. (Hance) Hydrocodone bitartrate ⅙ gr, pyrilamine maleate 1 1/7 gr/fl. oz. Bot. 3 oz, gal.
Use: Antitussive, sleep aid.

DYES.
See: Antiseptic, Dyes.
DYFLEX-200 TABLETS. (Econo Med) Dyphylline 200 mg/Tab. Bot. 100s, 1000s.
Use: Bronchodilator.
DYFLEX-400 TABLETS. (Econo Med) Dyphylline 400 mg/Tab. Bot. 100s, 500s.
Use: Bronchodilator.
DYFLEX-G TABLETS. (Econo Med) Dyphylline 200 mg, guaifenesin 200 mg/Tab. Bot. 100s, 1000s.
Use: Bronchodilator, expectorant.
DYFLOS. B.A.N. Di-isopropyl phosphorofluoridate. Di-isopropyl fluorophosphonate.
Use: Agent for glaucoma.
DYLATE. Clonitrate.
Use: Coronary vasodilator.
DYLINE-GG LIQUID. (Seatrace) Dyphylline 100 mg, guaifenesin 100 mg/5 ml. Bot. pt, gal.
Use: Bronchodilator, expectorant.
DYLINE-GG TABLETS. (Seatrace) Dyphylline 200 mg, guaifenesin 200 mg/Tab. Bot. 100s, 1000s.
Use: Bronchodilator, expectorant.
DYMANTHINE HYDROCHLORIDE. USAN. N,N-dimethyloctadecylamine hydrochloride.
Use: Anthelmintic.
DYMELOR. (Lilly) Acetohexamide 250 mg or 500 mg/Tab. Bot. 50s, 200s, 500s, Blister Pkg. 10 × 10s.
Use: Antidiabetic agent.
DYMENATE. (Keene) Dimenhydrinate 50 mg/ml. Vial 10 ml.
Use: Antiemetic/antivertigo.
DYNACIRC. (Sandoz) Isradipine.
Use: Calcium channel blocker.
DYNACORYL.
See: Nikethamide, Preps. (Various Mfr.).
DYNAPEN. (Bristol) Sodium dicloxacillin. **Cap.:** 125 mg, 250 mg or 500 mg. Bot. 24s, 50s, 100s. **Susp.:** 62.5 mg/5 ml. Bot. 80 ml, 100 ml, 200 ml.
Use: Antibacterial, penicillin.
DYNAPLEX. (Alton) Vitamin B complex. Bot. 100s, 1000s.
Use: Vitamin B supplement.
DYNARSAN.
See: Acetarsone, Tab.
DY-O-DERM. (Owen) Purified water, isopropyl alcohol, acetone, dihydroxyacetone, F D&C yellow No. 6, F D&C blue No. 1, D&C Red No. 33. Bot. 4 oz.
Use: Water-soluble vitiligo stain.
DY-PHYL-LIN. (Foy) Dyphylline 250 mg/ml with benzyl alcohol. Inj. Vial 10 ml.
Use: Bronchodilator.
DYPHYLLINE, U.S.P. XXII. Elixir, Inj., Tab., U.S.P. XXII. 7-(2,3-Dihydroxypropyl) Theophylline, Hyphylline.
Use: Vasodilator, bronchodilator.
See: Brophylline, Inj., Granucaps (Solvay).
Dilor, Preps. (Savage).
Emfabid TD, Tab. (Saron).
Lardet, Inj. (Standex).
Neothylline, Tab. (Lemmon).
Prophyllin, Oint., Pow. (Rystan).
W/Chlorpheniramine maleate, guaifenesin, dextromethorphan HBr, phenylephrine HCl.
See: Hycoff-A, Syr. (Saron).
W/Guaifenesin.
See: Bronkolate-G, Tab. (Parmed).
Dilor-G, Liq., Tab. (Savage).
Embron, Syr., Cap. (Amid).
Emfaseem, Cap., Elix., Inj. (Saron).
Neothylline GG, Liq. (Lemmon).
DYPHYLLINE GG ELIXIR. (Goldline) Bot. pt.
Use: Bronchodilator.
DYRENIUM. (SmithKline Beecham) Triamterene. **50 mg/Cap.:** Bot. 100s, UD 100s. **100 mg/Cap.:** Bot. 100s, 1000s, UD 100s.
Use: Diuretic.
DYRETIC. (Keene) Furosemide 10 mg/ml. Vial 10 ml.
Use: Diuretic.
DYSENAID JR. (Jenkins) Paregoric 5 min., bismuth subgallate 1 gr, kaolin 1 gr, pectin ⅛ gr/Tab. Bot. 1000s.
Use: Antidiarrheal.
DYREXAN-OD. (Trimen) Phendimetrazine tartrate 105 mg. SR Cap. Bot. 100s.
Use: Anorexiant.
DYSPEL. (Dover) Acetaminophen, ephedrine sulfate, atropine sulfate. Sugar, lactose and salt free. Tab. UD Box 500s.
Use: Analgesic.

E

EACA (Lederle) Epsilon aminocaproic acid.
Use: Antifibrinolytic agent.
See: Amicar (Lederle).
EARDRO. (Jenkins) Benzocaine 15 Gm, antipyrine 0.7 Gm, glycerol q.s./0.5 oz. Liq. Dropper Bot. 0.5 oz.
Use: Otic preparation.
EAR DROPS. (Weeks & Leo) Carbamide peroxide 6.5% in an anhydrous glycerin base. Bot. oz.
Use: Otic preparation.
EAR-DRY. (Scherer) Isopropyl alcohol, boric acid 2.75%. Dropper bot. 30 ml.
Use: Otic preparation.
EAREX EAR DROPS. (Approved) Benzocaine 0.15 Gm, antipyrine 0.7 Gm/0.5 oz. Bot. 0.5 oz.
Use: Otic prepartion.
EAR-EZE. (Hyrex) Hydrocortisone 1%, chloroxylenol 0.1%, pramoxine HCl 1%. Dropper bot. 15 ml.
Use: Corticosteroid, antibacterial, local anesthetic (otic).
EARLY DETECTOR KIT. (Warner-Lambert Prods) In-home self-test to detect hidden blood in the stool. Test kit 3s.

Use: Diagnostic aid.

EAROCOL EAR DROPS. (Mallard) Benzocaine 1.4%, antipyrine 5.4%, glycerin, oxyquinoline sulfate. Soln. Dropper bot. 15 ml.
Use: Otic preparation.

EARTHNUT OIL. Peanut Oil.

EASPRIN. (Parke-Davis) Aspirin 15 gr/EC Tab. Bot. 100s.
Use: Salicylate analgesic.

EAST-A. (Eastwood) Therapeutic lotion. Bot. 16 oz.
Use: Emollient.

EAST-GESIC. (Eastwood) Tab. Bot. 100s.

EASTINIC. (Eastwood) Tab. Bot. 100s.

EAST-IRON. (Eastwood) Tab. Bot. 100s.

EAST-NATA. (Eastwood) Tab. Bot. 100s.

EAST-SERPINE. (Eastwood) Tab. Bot. 100s.

EASTWOOD HEMATINIC. (Eastwood) Tab. Bot. 100s.

EASYCLEAN/GP DAILY CLEANER. (Allergan) Cocoamphocarboxyglycinate, sodium lauryl sulfate, sodium Cl, sodium phosphate, hexylene glycol, EDTA. Bot. 30 ml; preservative free.
Use: RGP contact lens care.

EASY EYES. (Eaton Medicals) Salt tablets for normal saline 250 mg. Bot. 27.7 ml. Tab. 90s, 180s.
Use: Soft contact lens care.

EASY-LAX. (Walgreen) Docusate sodium 100 mg/Cap. Bot. 60s.
Use: Laxative.

EASY-LAX PLUS. (Walgreen) Docusate sodium 100 mg, casanthranol 30 mg/Cap. Bot. 60s.
Use: Laxative.

EAZOL. (Mallard) Fructose, dextrose, orthophosphoric acid with controlled hydrogen ion concentration. Bot. 473 ml.
Use: Antinauseant.

•**EBASTINE.** USAN.
Use: Antihistamine.

EBV-VCA. (Wampole-Zeus) Epstein-Barr virus, viral capsid antigen antibody test. Qualitative and semi-quantitative detection of EBV antibody in human serum. Test 100s.
Use: Diagnostic aid.

EBV-VCA Ig. (Wampole-Zeus) Epstein-Barr virus, viral capsid antigen Ig antibody. Qualitative and semiqualitative detection of EBV-VCA Ig antibody in human serum. Test 50s.
Use: Diagnostic aid.

ECBOLINE. Ergotoxine.

ECEE PLUS. (Edwards) Vitamin E 165 mg, ascorbic acid 100 mg, magnesium sulfate 70 mg, zinc sulfate 80 mg/Tab. Bot. 100s.
Use: Vitamin/mineral supplement.

•**ECHOTHIOPHATE IODIDE,** U.S.P. XXII. Ophth. Soln. U.S.P. XXII. Ethanaminium, 2-[(diethoxyphosphinyl)-thio]-N,N,N-trimethyl-, iodide. (2-Mercaptoethyl)-trimethylammonium iodide S-ester with O,O-diethyl phosphorothioate. Bot. 100s.
Use: Glaucoma; cholinergic.
See: Echodide, Ophth. Soln. (Alcon).
Phospholine Iodide, Pow. (Wyeth-Ayerst).

•**ECLANAMINE MALEATE.** USAN.
Use: Antidepressant.

•**ECLAZOLAST.** USAN.
Use: Antiallergic, inhibitor.

ECLIPSE AFTER SUN. (Dorsey) Petrolatum, glycerin, oleth-3 phosphate, carbomer-934, imidazolidinyl urea, benzyl alcohol, cetyl esters wax. Lot. Bot. 180 ml.
Use: Emollient.

ECLIPSE LIP AND FACE PROTECTANT. (Dorsey) Padimate O, oxybenzone. Stick 4.5 Gm.
Use: Sunscreen for lips.

ECLIPSE ORIGINAL SUNSCREEN. (Dorsey) Padimate O, glyceryl PABA. Lot. Bot. 120 ml.
Use: Sunscreen.

ECLIPSE SUNTAN, PARTIAL. (Dorsey) Padimate O. Lot. Bot. 120 ml.
Use: Sunscreen.

•**ECONAZOLE.** USAN.
Use: Antifungal.

•**ECONAZOLE NITRATE.** USAN. U.S.P. XXII
Use: Antifungal.

ECONO B & C. (Vanguard) Vitamins B_1 15 mg, B_2 10.2 mg, B_3 50 mg, B_5 10 mg, B_6 5 mg, C 300 mg/Capl. Bot. 100s, 1000s, UD 100s.
Use: Vitamin B supplement.

ECONOPRED OPHTHALMIC. (Alcon) Prednisolone acetate 0.125%, benzalkonium Cl 0.01% w/hydroxymethyl cellulose. Susp. Droptainer 5 ml, 10 ml.
Use: Anti-inflammatory, ophthalmic.

ECONOPRED PLUS. (Alcon) Prednisolone acetate 1%, benzalkonium Cl 0.01%, w/hydroxymethyl cellulose. Susp. Droptainer 5 ml, 10 ml.
Use: Corticosteroid, ophthalmic.

ECOSONE CREAM. (Star) Hydrocortisone 0.5% in a water-soluble cream base. Tube oz.
Use: Corticosteroid.

ECOTHIOPATE IODIDE. B.A.N. S-2-Dimethylaminoethyl diethyl phosphorothioate methiodide.
Use: Agent for glaucoma.

ECOTRIN REGULAR STRENGTH TABLETS. (SmithKline Prods) Aspirin 325 mg/EC Tab. Bot. 100s, 250s, 1000s.
Use: Salicylate analgesic.

ECTOL. (Approved) Chlorpheniramine maleate, pyrilamine maleate, diperodon, hexachlorphene, benzalkonium, menthol, camphor. Tube oz.
Use: Antihistamine, antipruritic.

ECTYLUREA. B.A.N. (2-Ethylcrotonoyl) urea.
Use: Sedative.

EDATHAMIL. Edetate ethylenediaminetetraacetic acid.
See: Nullapons (General Aniline).

EDATHAMIL CALCIUM-DISODIUM. Calcium disodium ethylenediamine tetraacetate.
See: Calcium Disodium Versenate, Amp. & Tab. (Riker).

EDATHAMIL DISODIUM. Disodium salt of ethylene diamine tetraacetic acid.
See: Endrate, Amp. (Abbott).

•**EDATREXATE.** USAN.
Use: Antineoplastic.

EDECRIN. (Merck Sharp & Dohme) Ethacrynic acid 25 mg or 50 mg/Tab. Bot. 100s.
Use: Diuretic.

EDECRIN SODIUM INTRAVENOUS. (Merck Sharp & Dohme) Ethacrynate sodium equivalent to 50 mg ethacrynic acid w/mannitol 62.5 mg, thimerosal 0.1 mg/Vial. Vial 50 ml for reconstitution.
Use: Diuretic.

•**EDETATE CALCIUM DISODIUM,** U.S.P. XXII. Inj., U.S.P. XXII. Calciate (2-), [[N,N′-1,2-ethanediylbis[N-(carboxymethyl)-glycinato]](4-)-N,N′,O,O′,-O″,O‴]-, disodium, hydrate, (OC-6-21)-. Disodium (ethylenedinitrilo)tetraceto calciate (2-) hydrate.
Use: Pharmaceutic aid (Chelating agent).
See: Calcium Disodium Versenate, Amp., Tab. (Riker).

EDETATE DIPOTASSIUM. USAN.
Use: Chelating agent.

•**EDETATE DISODIUM,** U.S.P. XXII. Inj., U.S.P. XXII. Glycine, N,N′-1,2-ethanediylbis[N-(carboxymethyl)-, disodium salt, dihydrate. Disodium (ethylenedinitrilo)tetraacetate dihydrate.
Use: Chelating agent.
See: Disotate, Inj. (Fellows-Testagar).
Endrate, Amp. (Abbott).
Sodium Versenate (Riker).
W/Benzalkonium Cl, boric acid, potassium Cl, sodium carbonate anhydrous.
See: Swim-Eye Drops (Savage).
W/Phenylephrine HCl, methapyrilene HCl, benzalkonium Cl, sodium bisulfite.
See: Allerest Nasal Spray (Pharmacraft).
W/Phenylephrine HCl, benzalkonium Cl, sodium bisulfate.
See: Sinarest, Aerosol (Pharmacraft).
W/Potassium Cl, benzalkonium Cl, isotonic boric acid.
See: Dacriose (Smith, Miller & Patch).
W/Prednisolone sodium phosphate, niacinamide, sodium bisulfite, phenol.
See: P.S.P. IV. Inj. (Solvay).
Solu-Pred, Vial (Kenyon).
W/Sodium thiosulfate, salicylic acid, isopropyl alcohol, propylene glycol, menthol, colloidal alumina.
See: Tinver Lotion (Barnes-Hind).

EDETATE SODIUM. USAN. Tetrasodium (ethylenedinitrilo)-tetraacetate, or tetrasodium ethylenediaminetetraacetate.
Use: Chelating agent.
See: Disodium Versenate (Riker).
Vagisec, Liq. (Julius Schmid).

EDETATE TRISODIUM. USAN. Trisodium hydrogen (ethylenedinitrilo) tetraacetate, or trisodium hydrogen ethylenediaminetetraacetate.
Use: Chelating agent.

•**EDETIC ACID,** N.F. XVII. (Ethylenedinitrilo) tetraacetic acid.
Use: Pharmaceutic (Metal-complexing agent).

•**EDETOL.** USAN.
Use: Alkalinizing agent.

•**EDIFOLONE ACETATE.** USAN.
Use: Cardiac depressant (antiarrhythmic).

EDITHAMIL.
See: Edathamil.

EDOGESTRONE. B.A.N. 17-Acetoxy-3,3-ethylene-dioxy-6-methylpregn-5-en-20-one.
Use: Progestational steroid.

•**EDOXUDINE.** USAN.
Use: Antiviral.

EDROFURADENE. Name used for Nifurdazil.

•**EDROPHONIUM CHLORIDE,** U.S.P. XXII. Inj. U.S.P. XXII. Dimethylethyl (3-hydroxyphenyl) ammonium chloride. Ethyl (m-hydroxyphenyl)dimethyl- ammonium chloride. Benzenaminium, N-ethyl-3-hydroxy-N,N-dimethyl-chloride.
Use: Antidote to curare principles; dianogsitc aid (myathenia gravis).
See: Enlon, Inj. (Anaquest).
Tensilon Chloride, Vial (Roche).

EDTA.
See: Edathamil (Various Mfr.).

E.E.S. 400 FILMTAB. (Abbott) Erythromycin ethylsuccinate representing 400 mg erythromycin activity/Tab. Pkg. 100s, 500s, UD 100s.
Use: Anti-infective.

E.E.S. DROPS. (Abbott) Erythromycin ethylsuccinate representing erythromycin activity 100 mg/2.5 ml when reconstituted w/water. Dropper Bot. 50 ml.
Use: Anti-infective.

E.E.S. GRANULES. (Abbott) Erythromycin ethylsuccinate representing erythromycin activity 200 mg/5 ml oral susp. Gran. Bot. 60 ml, 100 ml, 200 ml, UD 5 ml.
Use: Anti-infective.

E.E.S. LIQUID-200 & 400. (Abbott) Erythromycin ethylsuccinate representing erythromycin activity 200 mg/5 ml. Bot. 100 ml, 480 ml; erythromycin activity 400 mg/5 ml. Bot. 100 ml, 480 ml.
Use: Anti-infective.

EFAMOL PMS. (Murdock) Vitamins B_6 21 mg, E 12 IU, C 100 mg, calcium 20 mg, magnesium 30 mg, zinc 3 mg, -linoleic acid 45 mg, cis-linoleic acid 115 mg, α-linolenic acid 35 mg, eicosapentanoeic acid 14 mg, decosahexanoeic acid 9 mg/cap. Bot. 30s, 90s.
Use: Vitamin/mineral supplement.

EFED-II. (Alto) Ephedrine sulfate 25 mg/Cap. Box 24s.
Use: Decongestant.

EFEDRON NASAL. (Hyrex) Ephedrine HCl 0.6%, chlorobutanol 0.5% w/sodium Cl, menthol and cinnamon oil in a water-soluble jelly base. Tube 20 Gm.
Use: Decongestant.

E-FEROL SPRAY. (Forest Pharm.) Alpha tocopherol equivalent to 30 IU Vitamin E/ml. Can 6 oz.

E-FEROL SUCCINATE. (Forest Pharm.) d-alpha Tocopherol acid succinate, equivalent to Vita-

min E. **100 or 400 IU/Cap.:** Bot. 100s, 500s, 1000s. **200** IU/Cap.: Bot. 50s, 100s, 500s, 1000s. **50 IU/Tab.:** Bot. 100s, 500s, 1000s.
Use: Vitamin E supplement.

E-FEROL VANISHING CREAM. (Forest Pharm.) Alpha tocopherol. Jar 2 oz.
Use: Emollient.

EFFECTIN TABLETS. (Winthrop Products) Bitolterol mesylate.
Use: Bronchodilator.

EFFER-K. (Nomax) Potassium 25 mEq. (as bicarbonate and citrate), saccharin. Effervescent tab. Box foil 30s, 250s.
Use: Mineral supplement.

EFFER-SYLLIUM. (Stuart) Psyllium hydrocolloid 3 Gm in rounded tsp. (7 Gm). Sodium free. Bot. 270 Gm, 480 Gm. Convenient packet 12s, 24s.
Use: Laxative.

EFFICOL COUGH WHIP, SUPPRESSANT, DECONGESTANT. (Block) Phenylpropanolamine HCl 6.25 mg, dextromethorphan HBr 2.5 mg/5 ml Bot. 8 oz.
Use: Decongestant, antitussive.

EFFICOL COUGH WHIP, SUPPRESSANT, DECONGESTANT, ANTIHISTAMINE. (Block) Dextromethorphan HBr 2.5 mg, phenylpropanolamine HCl 6.25 mg, chlorpheniramine maleate 1 mg/5 ml Bot. 8 oz.
Use: Antitussive, decongestant, antihistamine.

•**EFLORNITHINE HYDROCHLORIDE.** USAN.
Use: Antineoplastic, antiprotozoal.
See: Ornidyl (Marion Merrell Dow).

EFO-DINE OINTMENT. (Fougera) Povidone-iodine oint. Foilpac 1/32 oz, Tube oz. Jar lb.

EFRICON EXPECTORANT LIQUID. (Lannett) Phenylephrine HCl 5 mg, chlorpheniramine maleate 2 mg, codeine phosphate 11 mg, ammonium chloride 90 mg, potassium guaiacolsulfonate 90 mg, sodium citrate 60 mg/5 ml. Bot. pt, gal.
Use: Decongestant, antihistamine, antitussive, expectorant.

•**EFROTOMYCIN.** USAN.
Use: Growth stimulant (veterinary).

EFUDEX. (Roche) Fluorouracil. **Soln:** Fluorouracil 2% or 5%, w/propylene glycol, hydroxypropyl cellulose, parabens, disodium edetate. Drop Dispenser 10 ml. **Cream:** Fluorouracil 5%, in vanishing cream base w/white petrolatum, stearyl alcohol, propylene glycol, polysorbate 60, parabens. Tube 25 Gm.
Use: Antineoplastic agent.

EGRAINE. A protein binder from oats.

•**EGTAZIC ACID.** USAN.
Use: Pharmaceutic aid.

EHDP.
See: Etidronate Disodium.

EHRLICH 594.
See: Acetarsone, Tab.

EHRLICH 606.
See: Arspheramine (Various Mfr.).

•**ELANTRINE.** USAN.
Use: Anticholinergic.

ELASE-CHLOROMYCETIN OINTMENT. (Parke-Davis) Fibrinolysin 10 units, desoxyribonuclease 6666 units, chloramphenicol 100 mg. Tube 10 Gm. Fibrinolysin 30 units, desoxyribonuclease 20,000 units, chloramphenicol 300 mg and thimerosal. In 30 Gm.
Use: Topical enzyme preparation.

ELASE OINT. & PWD. FOR SOL. (Parke-Davis) **Pow.:** Fibrinolysin 25 units, desoxyribonuclease 15,000 units, thimerosal 0.1 mg/Vial as lyophilized powder. May be reconstituted with 10 ml of isotonic sodium Cl Soln. **Oint.:** Fibrinolysin 30 units, desoxyribonuclease 20,000 units, thimerosal 0.12 mg/30 Gm Tube. Fibrinolysin 10 units, desoxyribonuclease 6,666 units/10 Gm w/ thimerosal 0.04 mg as preservative. Ointment base of liquid petrolatum, polyethylene w/sucrose, sodium Cl. Tube 10 Gm, 30 Gm.
Use: Enzyme preparation, topical.

•**ELASTOFILCON A.** USAN.
Use: Contact lens material.

ELAVIL. (Merck Sharp & Dohme) Amitriptyline HCl. **Tab.: 10 mg:** Bot. 100s, 1000s; **25 mg:** Bot. 100s, 1000s; **50 mg:** Bot. 100s, 1000s; **75 mg, 100 mg:** Bot. 100s; **150 mg:** Bot. 30s, 100s. All strengths in UD 100s. **Inj.:** Vial 10 mg/ml w/dextrose 44 mg, methylparaben 1.5 mg, propylparaben 0.2 mg/ml w/water for injection. q.s. Vial 1 ml, 10 ml.
Use: Antidepressant.

ELDEC KAPSEALS. (Parke-Davis) Elemental iron 3.3 mg, Vitamins A 1667 IU, E 10 mg, B_1 10 mg, B_2 0.9 mg, B_3 17 mg, B_5 10 mg, B_6 0.7 mg, B_{12} 2 mcg, C 67 mg, folic acid 0.3 mg, calcium iodine/Cap. Bot. 100s.
Use: Vitamin/mineral supplement.

ELDEPRYL. (Somerset) Selegiline 5 mg. Tab. Bot. 60s.
Use: Antiparkinson agent.

ELDERCAPS. (Mayrand) Vitamins A 4000 IU, D-2 400 IU, E 25 mg, ascorbic acid 200 mg, thiamine mononitrate 10 mg, riboflavin 5 mg, pyridoxine HCl 2 mg, niacinamide 25 mg, d-calcium pantothenate 10 mg, zinc sulfate 25.3 mg, magnesium sulfate 70 mg, manganese sulfate 5 mg, folic acid 1 mg/Cap. Bot. 100s.
Use: Vitamin/mineral supplement.

ELDER'S RVP. Red Vet. Petrolatum.
Use: Dermatoses.

ELDERTONIC ELIXIR. (Mayrand) Vitamins B_1 0.17 mg, B_2 0.19 mg, B_3 2.22 mg, B_5 1.11 mg, B_6 0.22 mg, B_{12} 0.67 mcg, alcohol 13.5%, Mg, Mn, zinc 1.67 mg/5 ml. Bot. pt, gal, 240 ml.
Use: Vitamin/mineral supplement.

ELDISINE.
See: Vindesine sulfate.

ELDO-B & C. (Canright) Vitamins C 250 mg, B_1 25 mg, B_2 10 mg, niacinamide 150 mg, B_6 5 mg, d-calcium pantothenate 20 mg/Tab. Bot. 100s, 1000s.
Use: Vitamin supplement.

ELDOFE. (Canright) Ferrous fumarate 225 mg/Chew. tab. Bot. 100s, 1000s.
Use: Iron supplement.

ELDOFE-C. (Canright) Ferrous fumarate 225 mg, ascorbic acid 50 mg/Tab. Bot. 100s.
Use: Vitamin/mineral supplement.

ELDONAL. (Canright) Pentobarbital sodium 0.25 gr, hyoscyamine sulfate 0.1075 mg, atropine sulfate 0.0195 mg, hyoscine HBr 0.007 mg/Tab. or 5 ml. Tab. Bot. 100s, 1000s. Elix. Bot. pt.
Use: Sedative/hypnotic, anticholinergic/antispasmodic.

ELDONAL-L.A. (Canright) Hyoscyamine sulfate 0.3225 mg, atropine sulfate 0.0585 mg, hyoscine HBr 0.021 mg, pentobarbital sodium ¾ gr/Cap. Bot. 50s.
Use: Anticholinergic/antispasmodic, sedative/hypnotic.

ELDONAL-S. (Canright) Hyoscyamine sulfate 0.1075 mg, atropine sulfate 0.0195 mg, hyoscine HBr 0.007 mg, pentobarbital sodium 32.5 mg/Tab. Bot. 100s, 1000s.
Use: Anticholinergic/antispasmodic, sedative/hypnotic.

ELDOPAQUE. (Elder) Hydroquinone 2% in a tinted sunblocking cream base. Tube 15 Gm, 30 Gm.
Use: Skin bleaching agent.

ELDOPAQUE FORTE. (Elder) Hydroquinone 4% in a tinted sunblocking cream base. Tube 15 Gm, 30 Gm.
Use: Skin bleaching agent.

ELDOQUIN. (Elder) Hydroquinone 2% in a vanishing cream base. Tube 15 Gm, 30 Gm.
Use: Skin bleaching agent.

ELDOQUIN FORTE. (Elder) Hydroquinone 4% in vanishing cream base. Tube 15 Gm, 30 Gm.
Use: Skin bleaching agent.

ELDOQUIN LOTION. (Elder) Hydroquinone 2% in lotion base. Bot. 0.5 oz.
Use: Skin bleaching agent.

ELDOVITE. (Canright) Vitamin/mineral formula. Bot. 100s.
Use: Vitamin/mineral supplement.

ELECAL. (Western Research) Calcium 250 mg, magnesium 15 mg/Tab. Bot. 1000s.
Use: Mineral supplement.

ELECTROLYTE #48 INJECTION. Pediatric maintenance electrolyte solution. Dextrose 5% in electrolyte #48 w/sodium 25 mEq, potassium 20 mEq, magnesium 3 mEq, chloride 22 mEq, lactate 23 mEq, phosphate 3 mEq/L.
Use: Water, caloric, electrolyte supplement.

ELECTROLYTE #75 and 5% DEXTROSE.
See: 5% Dextrose and Electrolyte #75.

ELECTROLYTE THERAPY.
See: K.M.C., Amp. (Ingram).
Lytren, Ready-to-Use, Liq. (Mead Johnson).

ELEGEN-G. (Grafton) Amitriptyline 10 mg, 25 mg or 50 mg/Tab. Bot. 100s, 1000s.
Use: Antidepressant.

ELEVITES. (Barth's) Vitamins A 6000 IU, D 400 IU, B_1 1.5 mg, B_2 3 mg, C 60 mg, B_{12} 10 mcg, niacin 1 mg, E 10 IU, malt diastase 15 mg, iron 15 mg, calcium 381 mg, phosphorus 0.172 mg, citrus bioflavonoid complex 15 mg, rutin 15 mg, nucleic acid 3 mg, redbone marrow 30 mg, peppermint leaves 10 mg, wheat germ 30 mg/Tab. or Cap. Bot. 100s, 500s, 1000s.
Use: Vitamin/mineral supplement.

•**ELFAZEPAM.** USAN.
Use: Appetite stimulant.

ELIXICON. (Berlex) Theophylline 100 mg/5 ml with methyl and propyl parabens. Susp. Bot. 237 ml.
Use: Bronchodilator.

ELIXIRAL. (Vita Elixir) Phenobarbital 16.2 mg, hyoscyamine sulfate 0.1037 mg, atropine sulfate 0.194 mg, hyoscine HBr 0.0065 mg/5 ml. Liq. pt, gal.
Use: Sedative/hypnotic, anticholinergic/antispasmodic.

ELIXOMIN. (Cenci) Theophylline 80 mg, alcohol 20%/15 ml. Bot. pt, gal.
Use: Bronchodilator.

ELIXOPHYLLIN CAPSULES, DYE-FREE. (Forest) Anhydrous theophylline 100 mg or 200 mg/Cap. **100 mg:** Bot. 100s; **200 mg:** Bot. 100s, 500s, UD 100s.
Use: Bronchodilator.

ELIXOPHYLLIN ELIXIR. (Forest) Anhydrous theophylline 80 mg, alcohol 20%/15 ml. Bot. pt, qt, gal.
Use: Bronchodilator.

ELIXOPHYLLIN-GG ORAL LIQUID. (Forest) Theophylline 100 mg, guaifenesin 100 mg/15 ml. Alcohol free. Bot. 240, 480 ml.
Use: Antiasthmatic combination.

ELIXOPHYLLIN-KI ELIXIR. (Forest) Anhydrous theophylline 80 mg, potassium iodide 130 mg, alcohol 10%/15 ml. Bot. 237 ml.
Use: Antiasthmatic combination.

ELIXOPHYLLIN SR CAPSULES. (Forest) Anhydrous theophylline 125 mg or 250 mg/SR cap. Bot. 100s, 500s, UD 100s.
Use: Bronchodilator.

ELLESDINE. (Janssen) Pipenperone.
Use: Tranquilizer.

ELOCON CREAM. (Schering) Mometasone furoate 0.1%, hexylene glycol, phosphoric acid, propylene glycol stearate, stearyl alcohol, ceteareth-20, titanium dioxide, aluminum starch octenyl succinate, white wax, white petrolatum. 15 Gm, 45 Gm.
Use: Corticosteroid, topical.

ELOCON LOTION. (Schering) Mometasone furoate 0.1%. Bot. 30 ml, 60 ml.
Use: Corticosteroid, topical.

ELOCON OINTMENT. (Schering) Mometasone furoate 0.1%, hexylene glycol, propylene glycol stearate, white wax, white petrolatum. 15 Gm, 45 Gm.
Use: Corticosteroid, topical.

E-LOR. (UAD) Propoxyphene HCl 65 mg, acetaminophen 650 mg/Tab. Bot. 100s.
Use: Narcotic analgesic.

ELPHEMET. (Canright) Phendimetrazine tartrate 35 mg/Tab. Bot. 100s, 1000s.
Use: Anorexiant.

ELPRECAL. (Canright) Vitamins A 5000 IU, D 400 IU, B_1 3 mg, B_2 2 mg, B_6 0.1 mg, B_{12} 1 mcg, C 50 mg, E 2 IU, calcium pantothenate 2.5 mg, niacinamide 15 mg, inositol 5 mg, choline 5 mg, calcium lactate 500 mg, ferrous sulfate 50 mg, copper 1 mg, manganese 1 mg, magnesium 2 mg, potassium 2 mg, zinc 0.5 mg, sulfur 1 mg/Cap. Bot. 100s.
Use: Vitamin/mineral supplement.

•**ELSAMITRUCIN.** USAN.
Use: Antineoplastic.

ELSERPINE. (Canright) Reserpine 0.25 mg/Tab. Bot. 100s, 1000s.
Use: Antihypertensive.

ELSPAR. (Merck Sharp & Dohme) Asparaginase 10,000 IU, mannitol 80 mg/Vial 10 ml.
Use: Antineoplastic agent.

•**ELUCAINE.** USAN.
Use: Anticholinergic.

ELVANOL. (Du Pont) Polyvinyl alcohol.

EMAGRIN. (Otis Clapp) Salicylamide, caffeine, aspirin/Tab. Sugar, lactose and salt free. Bot. 100s.
Use: Salicylate analgesic.

EMAGRIN FORTE TABLETS. (Clapp) Phenylephrine 5 mg, acetaminophen 261 mg, guaifenesin 101 mg, caffeine 32 mg. Bot. 100s, 200s, 500s.
Use: Decongestant, analgesic, expectorant.

EMAGRIN PROFESSIONAL STRENGTH. (Otis Clapp) Aspirin, salicylamide, caffeine. Sugar, lactose and salt free. Safety pack 500s, Medipak 200s, Aidpak 100s, Unit box 10s, 20s. Bot. 1000s.
Use: Salicylate analgesic.

EMBECHINE. Aliphatic chloroethylamine.
Use: Antineoplastic.

EMBRAMINE. B.A.N. N-2-(4-Bromo-α-methylbenzhydryloxy)ethyldimethylamine.
Use: Antihistamine.

EMBUTRAMIDE. B.A.N. N-[2-Ethyl-2-(3-methoxyphenyl)butyl]-4-hydroxybutyramide.
Use: Narcotic analgesic.

EMCODEINE TABS. (Major) Aspirin with codeine as #2, #3 or #4. Bot. 100s, 500s.
Use: Narcotic analgesic combination.

EMCYT. (Pharmacia) Estramustine phosphate sodium equivalent to 140 mg estramustine phosphate/Cap. Bot. 100s.
Use: Antineoplastic agent.

EMDOL. (Approved) Salicylamide, para-aminobenzoic acid, sodium calcium succinate, vitamin D-1250. Bot. 100s, 1000s.
Use: Analgesic combination.

EMEPRONIUM BROMIDE. B.A.N. Ethyldimethyl-1-methyl-3,3-diphenylpropylammonium bromide.
Use: Anticholinergic.

EMERGENT-EZ. (Healthfirst Corp.) Adrenalin 2 amp., aminophylline 1 amp., ammonia inhalants (3), amyl nitrite inhalants (2), atropine 2 amp., Benadryl 2 amp., nitroglycerin 1 bottle, Solu-Cortef 1 mix-o-vial, Talwin 1 amp., Tigan 1 amp., Valium 2 amp., Wyamine 2 amp., plastic air way (1), disposable syringes, tracheotomy needle (1) and tourniquet (1)/kit.
Use: Emergency kit.

EMEROID. (Delta) Zinc oxide 5%, diperodon HCl 0.25%, bismuth subcarbonate 0.2%, pyrilamine maleate 0.1%, phenylephrine HCl 0.25%, in a petrolatum base containing cod liver oil. Tube 1.25 oz.
Use: Anorectal preparation.

EMERSAL. (Medco Lab) Ammoniated mercury 5%, salicylic acid 2.5%, castor oil 23%, liquid petrolatum, polyoxyl 40 stearate, polysorbate 80, water. Lot. Plastic bot. 120 ml.
Use: Antipsoriatic.

EMESIS. (Kenyon) Levulose and dextrose 57.6 Gm, orthophosphoric acid 0.5 Gm/100 ml. Bot. 4 oz, pt, gal.
Use: Antiemetic.

EMERSON 1% SODIUM FLUORIDE DENTAL GEL. (Emerson) Red and plain. Bot. 2 oz.
Use: Dental caries preventative.

EMETE-CON. (Roerig) Benzquinamide HCl 25 mg or 50 mg/ml, citric acid 1%. Vial 50 mg, 10s.
Use: Antiemetic.

EMETICS.
See: Apomorphine HCl.
Cupric Sulfate.
Ipecac Syr.

EMETINE BISMUTH IODIDE.
See: Emetine HCl.

•**EMETINE HYDROCHLORIDE,** U.S.P. XXII. Inj., U.S.P. XXII. Emetan, 6′, 7′, 10,11-tetramethoxy-,diHCl. (Lilly) Amp. 65 mg/1 ml.
Use: Antiamebic.

EMETROL. (Rorer Consumer) Oral soln. containing balanced amounts of levulose (fructose) and dextrose (glucose) with orthophosphoric acid, stabilized at an optimal pH. Bot. 90 ml, 480 ml.
Use: Antiemetic.

EMFASEEM. (Saron) **Liq.:** Dyphylline 100 mg, guaifenesin 50 mg/15 ml w/alcohol 5%. Bot. pt. **Cap.:** Dyphylline 200 mg, guaifenesin 100 mg/Cap. Bot. 100s, 1000s. Unident 100s. **Inj.:** Vial 10 ml.
Use: Antiasthmatic combination.

EM-GG. (Econo Med) Guaifenesin 100 mg/5 ml. Bot. pt.
Use: Expectorant.

•**EMILIUM TOSYLATE.** USAN.
Use: Cardiac depressant.

EMINASE. (Beecham) Anistreplase 30 units/vial.
Use: Thrombolytic enzyme.

EMITRIP TABS. (Major) Amitriptyline **10 mg or 25 mg/Tab.:** Bot. 100s, 250s, 1000s, UD 100s. **50 mg/Tab.:** Bot. 100s, 250s, 1000s, UD 100s. **75 mg/Tab.:** Bot. 100s, 250s, UD 100s. **100 mg/Tab.:** Bot. 100s, 250s, 1000s, UD 100s. **150 mg/Tab.:** Bot. 100s, 250s.
Use: Antidepressant.

EMKO BECAUSE CONTRACEPTOR. (Emko-Schering) Nonoxynol-9 (8% concentration). Contraceptor container w/applicator. Tube 10 Gm.

Use: Vaginal contraceptive.
EMKO PRE-FIL. (Schering) Nonoxynol-9 (8% concentration). Aerosol Can 30 Gm, Refill 60 Gm.
Use: Vaginal contraceptive.
EMKO VAGINAL FOAM. (Schering) Nonoxynol-9 (8% concentration). Kit Aerosol w/applicator 40 Gm, Refill 40 Gm, 90 Gm.
Use: Vaginal contraceptive.
EMOLLIA-CREME. (Gordon) Cetyl alcohol, lubricating oils in water-soluble base. Jar 4 oz, 5 lb.
Use: Emollient.
EMOLLIA-LOTION. (Gordon) Water-dispersable waxes, lubricating bland oils in a water-soluble lotion base. Bot. 1 oz, 4 oz, gal.
Use: Emollient.
EMPIRIN ASPIRIN TABLETS. (Burroughs Well come) Aspirin 325 mg/Tab. Bot. 50s, 100s, 250s.
Use: Analgesic.
EMPIRIN WITH CODEINE. (Burroughs Wellcome) Aspirin 325 mg with codeine phosphate 15 mg, 30 mg or 60 mg/Tab. **No. 2:** Codeine phosphate 15 mg (0.25 gr). Bot. 100s. **No. 3:** Codeine phosphate 30 mg (0.5 gr). Bot. 100s, 500s, 1000s, Dispenserpak 25s. **No. 4:** Codeine phosphate 60 mg (1 gr). Bot. 100s, 500s, 1000s, Dispenserpak 25s.
Use: Narcotic analgesic combination.
EMULAVE. (CooperCare)
See: Aveenobar Oilated (CooperCare).
EMUL-O-BALM. (Pennwalt) Menthol, camphor, methyl salicylate. Bot. 2 oz, 8 oz, gal.
Use: External analgesic.
EMULSOIL. (Paddock) Castor oil 95%. Bot. 60 ml.
Use: Laxative.
E-MYCIN. (Upjohn) Erythromycin. **250 mg**/EC Tab.: Bot. 100s, 500s, UD 100s, Unit-of-Use 40s. **333 mg**/EC Tab.: Bot. 100s, 500s, UD 100s.
Use: Anti-infective.
EMYLCAMATE. B.A.N. 1-Ethyl-1-methylpropyl carbamate.
Use: Tranquilizer, muscle relaxant.
ENALAPRIL MALEATE. USAN.
Use: Antihypertensive.
See: Vasotec, Tab. (Merck Sharp & Dohme).
W/Hydrochlorothiazide.
See: Vaseretic, Tab. (Merck Sharp & Dohme).
ENALAPRILAT. USAN.
Use: Antihypertensive.
ENALKIREN. USAN.
Use: Antihypertensive.
ENBUCRILATE. B.A.N. Butyl 2-cyanoacrylate.
Use: Surgical tissue adhesive.
ENCAINIDE HYDROCHLORIDE. USAN.
Use: Cardiac depressant.
See: Enkaid, Cap. (Bristol).
ENCARE. (Thompson Medical) Nonoxynol-9 (2.27%). Supp. 12s, 24s.
Use: Vaginal contraceptive.
ENCLOMIPHENE. USAN. Cisclomiphene is name previously used.
ENCYPRATE. USAN. Ethyl N-benzylcyclopropane-carbamate.
Use: Antidepressant.
ENDAL. (UAD Labs) Phenylephrine HCl 20 mg, guaifenesin 300 mg/TR tab., dye free. Bot. 100s.
Use: Decongestant, expectorant.
ENDAL EXPECTORANT. (UAD Labs) Codeine phosphate 10 mg, phenylpropanolamine HCl 12.5 mg, guaifenesin 100 mg/5 ml w/alcohol 5%. Bot. pt.
Use: Antitussive, decongestant, expectorant.
ENDECON. (DuPont) Phenylpropanolamine HCl 25 mg, acetaminophen 325 mg/Tab. Bot. 60s.
Use: Decongestant, analgesic.
ENDEP. (Roche) Amitriptyline HCl 10 mg, 25 mg, 50 mg, 75 mg, 100 mg or 150 mg/Tab. **10 mg:** Bot. 100s, Tel-E-Dose 100s. **25 mg:** Bot. 100s, 500s, Tel-E-Dose 100s. **50 mg:** Bot. 100s, 500s, Tel-E-Dose 100s. **75 mg:** Bot. 100s, Tel-E-Dose 100s. **100 mg:** Bot. 100s, Tel-E-Dose 100s. **150 mg:** Bot 100s.
Use: Antidepressant.
ENDOBENZILINE BROMIDE. N,N-(dimethyl)-aminoethyl-α-(bicyclo[2.2.1]-5-neptenyl) mandelate methyl bromide.
Use: Anticholinergic.
ENDOCAINE. Pyrrocaine.
Use: Local anesthetic.
ENDOJODIN.
See: Entodon.
ENDOLOR. (Keene) Butalbital 50 mg, caffeine 40 mg, acetaminophen 325 mg/Cap. Bot. 100s.
Use: Sedative/hypnotic, analgesic.
ENDOMYCIN. A new antibiotic obtained from cultures of *Streptomyces endus.* Under study.
ENDOPHENOLPHTHALEIN. (Roche) Diacetyldioxyphenylisatin-isacen-bisatin.
Use: Laxative.
See: Diacetylhydroxphenylisatin, Prep. (Various Mfr.)
•**ENDRALAZINE MESYLATE.** USAN.
Use: Antihypertensive.
ENDRATE. (Abbott Hospital Prods) Edetate disodium 150 mg/ml. Amp. 20 ml.
Use: Treatment of hypercalcemia, control of ventricular arrhythmias associated with digitalis toxicity.
•**ENDRYSONE.** USAN.
Use: Anti-inflammatory.
ENDURON. (Abbott) Methyclothiazide 2.5 mg or 5 mg/Tab. **2.5 mg:** Bot. 100s, 1000s. **5 mg:** Bot. 100s, 1000s, UD 100s.
Use: Diuretic.
ENDURONYL. (Abbott) Methyclothiazide 5 mg, deserpidine 0.25 mg/Tab. Bot. 100s, 1000s, UD 100s.
Use: Antihypertensive, diuretic.
ENDURONYL FORTE. (Abbott) Methyclothiazide 5 mg, deserpidine 0.5 mg/Tab. Bot. 100s, 1000s.
Use: Antihypertensive, diuretic.
ENEBAG 2. (Lafayette) Air contrast barium enema bag. Case 24s.
Use: Radiopaque agent.

ENEBAG XL. (Lafayette) Air contrast barium enema bag 3000 ml w/lumen tubing, enema tip and side clamp. Case 24s.
Use: Radiopaque agent.

ENECAT. (Lafayette) Barium sulfate suspension CT colon exam kit. Case 12s.
Use: Radiopaque agent.

ENEMARK. (Lafayette) Rectal marker. 85% w/v liquid barium. Case of 12 kits.
Use: Rectal marker during radiation therapy.

ENERJETS. (Chilton) Caffeine 65 mg/Loz. pkg. 10s.
Use: Analeptic.

ENESET 1. (Lafayette) Barium sulfate suspension 300 ml/air contrast examination kit. Unit-of-use kit. Case 12s.
Use: Radiopaque agent.

ENESET 2. (Lafayette) Barium sulfate suspension 450 ml/contrast examination kit. Unit-of-use kit. Case 12s.
Use: Radiopaque agent.

ENESET 600. (Lafayette) Barium sulfate suspension 600 ml/air contrast examination kit. Unit-of-use kit. Case 12s.
Use: Radiopaque agent.

ENFAMIL. (Mead Johnson Nutrition) Vitamins A 2000 IU, D 400 IU, E 20 IU, C 52 mg, B_1 0.5 mg, B_2 1 mg, B_6 0.4 mg, B_{12} 1.5 mcg, niacin 8 mg, calcium 440 mg, phosphorus 300 mg, folic acid 100 mcg, pantothenic acid 3 mg, inositol 30 mg, biotin 15 mcg, K-1 55 mcg, choline 100 mg, iron 1.4 mg, potassium 650 mg, chloride 400 mg, copper 0.6 mg, iodine 65 mcg, sodium 175 mg, magnesium 50 mg, zinc 5 mg, manganese 100 mg/Qt. Concentrated Liq. 13 fl oz, Instant Pow. lb.
Use: Enteral nutritional supplement.

ENFAMIL HUMAN MILK FORTIFIER. (Mead Johnson) Whey protein, casein, corn syrup solids, lactose, protein 0.7 Gm, carbohydrate 2.7 Gm, fat 0.04 Gm, calories 14. Pow. Packet 0.95 Gm, Box 100s.
Use: Enteral nutritional supplement.

ENFAMIL WITH IRON. (Mead Johnson Nutrition) Iron 12 mg/Qt. Pkg. Con. Liq. 13 fl oz. 24s. Pow. 1 lb. 6s.
Use: Enteral nutritional supplement.

ENFAMIL WITH IRON READY TO USE. (Mead Johnson Nutrition) Ready-to-use Enfamil with Iron infant formula 20 kcal/fl oz. Can 8 fl oz, 6-can pack; 32 fl oz, 6 cans per case.
Use: Enteral nutritional supplement.

ENFAMIL NURSETTE. (Mead Johnson Nutrition) Ready-to-feed Enfamil 20 kcal/fl oz, 4 fl oz, 6 fl oz and 8 fl oz. 4 bottles/sealed carton. W/Iron. Ready to use. Bot. 6 fl oz 4s, 24s.
Use: Enteral nutritional supplement.

ENFAMIL PREMATURE FORMULA. (Mead Johnson) Nonfat milk, whey protein concentrate, corn syrup solids, lactose, coconut oil, corn oil, medium chain triglycerides, soy lecithin. Protein 2.8 Gm, carbohydrate 10.7 Gm, fat 4.9 Gm, calories 96. Pow. Nursettes 120 ml.
Use: Enteral nutritional supplement.

ENFAMIL READY TO USE. (Mead Johnson Nutrition) Ready-to-use Enfamil infant formula 20 kcal/fl oz. Can 8 fl oz, 6-can pack; 32 fl oz, 6 cans per case.
Use: Enteral nutritional supplement.

•**ENFLURANE,** U.S.P. XXII. 2-Chloro-1,1,2-trifluoroethyl difluoromethyl ether. Ethrane (Ohio Medical).
Use: Anesthetic (inhalation).

ENGERIX-B. (SKF) Hepatitis B vaccine (recombinant). **Inj.:** 20 mcg hepatitis B surface antigen/ml. Single dose vial. **Pediatric Inj.:** 10 mcg hepatitis B surface antigen/ml. Single dose vial.
Use: Vaccine.

•**ENILCONAZOLE.** USAN.
Use: Antifungal.

•**ENISOPROST.** USAN.
Use: Antiulcerative.

ENISYL. (Person & Covey) L-Lysine monohydrochloride 334 mg or 500 mg/Tab. Bot. 100s, 250s.
Use: Dietary supplement.

ENKAID. (Bristol) Encainide HCl 25 mg, 35 mg or 50 mg/Cap. Bot. 100s, UD 100s.
Use: Antiarrhythmic.

ENLON INJECTION. (Anaquest) Edrophonium Cl 10 mg/ml, phenol 0.45%, sodium sulfite 0.2%. Vial 15 ml.
Use: Cholinergic muscle stimulant.

ENNEX OINTMENT. (Ennex) Aloe vera extract 37.5%. **Skin Oint.:** Zinc oxide 12.5%, coal tar 1.5%, alcohol 4.5%. Tube oz. **Hemorrhoidal Oint.:** Tube oz.
Use: Anti-inflammatory, astringent, antipruritic.

ENO. (Beecham Products) Sodium tartrate 1620 mg, sodium citrate 1172 mg. Bot. Pow. 105 Gm, 210 Gm.
Use: Antacid.

•**ENOLICAM SODIUM.** USAN.
Use: Anti-inflammatory, antirheumatic.

ENOMINE CAPSULES. (Major) Phenylpropanolamine 45 mg, phenylephrine 5 mg, guaifenesin 200 mg/Cap. Bot. 100s, 500s.
Use: Decongestant, expectorant.

ENOVID. (Searle) Norethynodrel, mestranol 5 mg or 10 mg/Tab. **5 mg:** Norethynodrel 5 mg, mestranol 75 mcg. Bot. 100s, 6 × 20s calendar-pak. **10 mg:** Norethynodrel 9.85 mg, mestranol 0.15 mg. Bot. 50s.
Use: Estrogen, progestin combination.

ENOVID-E 21. (Searle) Norethynodrel 2.5 mg, mestranol 0.1 mg/Tab. Compack disp. 21s, 6×21. Refill 21s, 12×21.
Use: Estrogen, progestin combination.

ENOVIL. (Hauck) Amtriptyline HCl 10 mg/ml. Vial 10 ml.
Use: Antidepressant.

•**ENOXACIN.** USAN.
Use: Antibacterial.

•**ENOXIMONE.** USAN.
Use: Cardiotonic.

ENOXOLONE. B.A.N. 3β-Hydroxy-11-oxo-olean-12-en-30-oic acid.
Use: Treatment of skin diseases.

ENPIPRAZOLE. B.A.N. 1-(2-Chlorophenyl)-4-[2-(1-methylpyrazol-4-yl)ethyl]piperazine.
Use: Psychotropic drug.

•**ENPIROLINE PHOSPHATE.** USAN.
Use: Antimalarial.

•**ENPROFYLLINE.** USAN.
Use: Bronchodilator.

•**ENPROMATE.** USAN.
Use: Antineoplastic.

•**ENPROSTIL.** USAN.
Use: Antisecretory, antiulcerative.

ENRICH. (Ross) Liquid food with fiber providing complete, balanced nutrition as a full liquid diet, liquid supplement, or tube feeding. One serving provides 5 Gm dietary fiber. 1100 calories/L. 1530 calories provides 100% US RDA for vitamins and minerals. Can Ready-to-Use 8 fl oz (vanilla, chocolate).
Use: Enteral nutritional supplement.

•**ENROFLOXACIN.** USAN.
Use: Antibacterial (Veterinary).

ENSIDON. (Geigy) Opipramol HCl.

ENSURE. (Ross) Liquid food providing 1.06 calories/ml. Can be used as a full liquid diet, liquid supplement or tube feeding. Two quarts (2000 calories) provides 100% US RDA for vitamins and minerals for adults and children over 4 yrs. **Ready-to-Use:** Bot. 8 fl oz (vanilla). Can 8 fl oz (chocolate, black walnut, coffee, strawberry, eggnog, vanilla), 32 fl oz (vanilla, chocolate). **Pow.:** Can 14 oz (400 Gm) (vanilla).
Use: Enteral nutritional supplement.

ENSURE HN. (Ross) High nitrogen low residue liquid food providing complete, balanced nutrition as tube feeding or oral supplement with 1.06 calories/ml. Provides 100% US RDA for vitamins and minerals for adults and children over 4 yrs. 1400 calories (1321 ml). Ready-to-Use: Can 8 fl oz (vanilla).
Use: Enteral nutritional supplement.

ENSURE OSMOLITE. (Ross).
See: Osmolite (Ross).

ENSURE PLUS. (Ross) High calorie liquid food w/caloric density of 1500 calories/L. Six servings (8 oz and 2130 calories each) provides 100% US RDA for vitamins and minerals for adults and children. Ready-to-Use: Bot. 8 fl oz (vanilla). Can 8 fl oz (chocolate, vanilla, eggnog, coffee, strawberry).
Use: Enteral nutritional supplement.

ENSURE PLUS HN. (Ross) High-calorie, high-nitrogen liquid food providing 1.5 calories/ml; 1420 calories provides 100% US RDA for vitamins and minerals for adults and children. Calorie/nitrogen ratio is 150:1. Can 8 fl oz (vanilla).
Use: Enteral nutritional supplement.

ENSURE PUDDING. (Ross) 17% US RDA vitamins and minerals for adults and children/5 oz. serving. Can 4s (chocolate, vanilla, tapioca, butterscotch).
Use: Nutritional supplement.

ENTAB 650. (Mayrand) Aspirin 650 mg/EC tab. Bot. 100s.
Use: Salicylate analgesic.

ENTERO-TEST. (HDC Corp.) Cap. To identify duodenal parasites; to diagnose and locate upper GI bleeding, pH disorders, achlorhydria and esophageal reflux. Bot. 10s, 25s.
Use: Diagnostic aid.

ENTERO-TEST PEDIATRIC. (HDC Corp.) To identify duodenal parasites; to diagnose and locate upper GI bleeding, pH disorders, achlorhydria and esophageal reflux. Cap. Bot. 10s, 25s.
Use: Diagnostic aid.

ENTEROTUBE. (Roche Diagnostics) Culture-identification method for enterobacteriaceae ACA. Test kit 25s.
Use: Diagnostic aid.

ENTEX. (Norwich Eaton) Phenylephrine HCl 5 mg, phenylpropanolamine HCl 45 mg, guaifenesin 200 mg/Cap. Bot. 100s, 500s.
Use: Decongestant, expectorant.

ENTEX LA. (Norwich Eaton) Phenylpropanolamine HCl 75 mg, guaifenesin 400 mg/T.R. Tab. Bot. 100s, 500s.
Use: Decongestant, expectorant.

ENTEX LIQUID. (Norwich Eaton) Phenylephrine HCl 5 mg, phenylpropanolamine HCl 20 mg, guaifenesin 100 mg/5 ml, alcohol 5%. Elix. Bot. 480 ml.
Use: Decongestant, expectorant.

ENTIRE B W/C. (Pharmex) Vitamin B complex with vitamin C. Cap. Bot. 100s, 1000s.
Use: Vitamin supplement.

ENTODON. Propiodal, Entoidoin, Endojodin, 2-Hydroxytrimethylene-bis-(trimethylammonium iodide).

ENTOIDOIN.
See: Entodon.

ENTOLASE HP. (Robins) Lipase 8,000 units, protease 50,000 units, amylase 40,000 units/Cap. (enteric coated microbeads). Bot. 100s, 250s.
Use: Digestive enzymes.

ENTOZYME. (Robins) Pepsin 250 mg in outer core, pancreatin 300 mg, bile salts 150 mg in enteric coated inner core/Tab. Bot. 100s, 500s.
Use: Digestive enzymes.

ENTRITION ENTRI-PAK. (Biosearch) Calcium caseinate, sodium caseinate, maltodextrin, corn oil, soy lecithin, mono and diglycerides. Protein 35 Gm, carbohydrate 136 Gm, fat 35 Gm, sodium 700 mg, potassium 1200 mg, calories 1/ml, osmolarity 300 mOsm/kg, water. Pouch 1 L.
Use: Enteral nutritional supplement.

ENTRITION HN ENTRI-PAK. (Biosearch). Sodium and calcium caseinates, soy protein isolate, maltodextrin, corn oil, soy lecithin, mono and diglycerides, vitamins A, B_1, B_2, B_3, B_5, B_6, B_{12}, C, D, E, K, folic acid, biotin, choline, Ca, Cl, Cu, Fe, I, Mg, Mn, P, Zn. Pouch 1 L.
Use: Enteral nutritional supplement.

ENTROBAG SET. (Lafayette) Enteroclysis set. Case 6 sets.
Use: Enteroclysis of the small intestine.

ENTROBAR. (Lafayette) Barium sulfate 50%w/v susp. Bot. 500 ml, case 12 Bot.
Use: Radiopaque agent.

ENTROKIT. (Lafayette) Barium sulfate susp. (Entrobar), methylcellulose (Entrolcel). Case 4 kits.
Use: Radiopaque agent.

ENTROKIT WITH MAGLINTE CATHETER. Entrokit complete with Magnite catheter.
Use: Radiopaque agent.

ENTROLCEL. (Lafayette) Methylcellulose 1.8% w/w concentrate for dilution at time of use. Bot. 500 ml, case 24 Bot.
Use: Diagnostic aid.

•**ENTSUFFEN SODIUM.** USAN.
Use: Detergent.

E.N.T. SYRUP. (Springbok) Brompheniramine maleate 4 mg, phenylephrine HCl 5 mg, phenylpropanolamine HCl 5 mg/5 ml. Bot. 16 oz.
Use: Antihistamine, decongestant.

E.N.T. TABLETS. (Springbok) Phenylephrine HCl 25 mg, phenylpropanolamine HCl 50 mg, chlorpheniramine maleate 8 mg/SA Tab. Bot. 100s, 500s.
Use: Decongestant, antihistamine.

ENTUSS. (Hauck) **Tab.:** Hydrocodone bitartrate 5 mg, guaifenesin 300 mg/Tab. Bot. 100s. **Syr.:** 5 mg hydrocodone bitartate, 300 mg potassium guaiacolsulfonate/5 ml. Alcohol free. Bot. 120 ml, 480 ml.
Use: Antitussive, expectorant.

ENTUSS-D LIQUID. (Hauck) Hydrocodone bitartrate 5 mg, pseudoephedrine 30 mg/5 ml. Sugar, alcohol, corn and dye free. Bot. 16 oz.
Use: Antitussive, decongestant.

ENTUSS-D TABLETS. (Hauck) Pseudoephedrine 30 mg, hydrocodone bitartrate 5 mg, guaifenesin 300 mg/Tab. Bot. 100s.
Use: Decongestant, antitussive, expectorant.

ENUCLENE. (Alcon Surgical) Tyloxapol 0.25%, benzalkonium Cl 0.02%, hydroxypropyl methylcellulose 0.85%. Soln. Drop-tainer 15 ml.
Use: Artificial eye care.

ENULOSE. (Barre-National) Lactulose 10 Gm, galactose $>$ 2.2 Gm, lactose $>$ 1.2 Gm, other sugars $\leq$ 1.2 Gm. Syr. pt, 2 qt.
Use: Laxative.

•**ENVIRADENE.** USAN.
Use: Antiviral.

ENVIRO-STRESS. (Vitaline) Vitamins B_1 50 mg, B_2 50 mg, B_3 100 mg, B_5 50 mg, B_6 50 mg, B_{12} 25 mcg, C 600 mg, E 30 IU, folic acid 0.4 mg, zinc 30 mg, Mg, Se, PABA. Tab. Bot. 90s, 1000s.
Use: Vitamin/mineral supplement.

•**ENVIROXIME.** USAN.
Use: Antiviral.

ENVISAN TREATMENT MULTIPACK. (Marion) Dextranomer with PEG 3000 and PEG 600. Paste 10 Gm packets with nylon net and semi-occlusive film.
Use: Wound debridement.

ENZEST. (Barth's) Seven natural enzymes, calcium carbonate 250 mg/Tab. Bot. 100s, 250s, 500s.
Use: Digestive enzymes, antacid.

ENZOBILE IMPROVED. (Mallard) Pancreatic enzyme concentrate 100 mg, ox bile extract 100 mg, cellulase 10 mg in inner core and pepsin 150 mg in outer layer. EC tab. Bot. 100s.
Use: Digestive enzymes.

ENZYME FORMULA #E-2. (Barth's) Amylase 30 mg, lipase 25 mg, bile salts 1 gr, wilzyme 10 mg, pepsin 2 gr, pancreatin 0.5 gr, calcium carbonate 4 gr/Tab. Bot. 100s, 250s.
Use: Digestive aid.

ENZYMES.
See: Alpha Chymar, Vial (Armour).
Ananase, Tab. (Rorer).
Cholinesterase (Various Mfr.).
Chymotrypsin.
Cotazym, Cap. (Organon).
Creon (Solvay)
Diastase (Various Mfr.).
Dornavac, Vial (Merck Sharp & Dohme).
Fibrinolysin.
Hyaluronidase (Various Mfr.).
Neutrapen, Vial (Riker).
Pancreatin (Various Mfr.).
Papain (Various Mfr.).
Papase, Tab. (Warner-Chilcott).
Penicillinase (Various Mfr.).
Pepsin (Various Mfr.).
Plasmin.
Rennin (Various Mfr.).
Taka-Diastase, Prep. (Parke-Davis).
Travase, Oint. (Flint).
Thrombolysin, I.V. Inj. (Merck Sharp & Dohme).
Varidase, Prep. (Lederle).

EPA CAPSULES. (Nature's Bounty) N-3 fat content (mg) EPA 180 mg, DHA 120 mg, vitamin E 1 IU. Bot. 50s, 100s.
Use: Nutritional supplement.

•**EPHEDRINE,** U.S.P. XXII. l-α-[1-(Methylamino)-ethyl]benzyl alcohol. (Various Mfr.) (−)-erythro-a-[1-(Methylamino)ethyl]benzyl Alcohol.
Use: Adrenergic (bronchodilator).
See: Bofedrol Inhalant (Bowman).
Racephedrine HCl (Various Mfr.).
W/Procaine.
See: Ephedrine and Procaine, Rx "A", Amp. (Lilly).
W/Pyrilamine maleate, guaifenesin, theophylline.
W/Theophylline, guaifenesin, phenobarbital.
See: Duovent, Tab. (Riker).

EPHEDRINE & AMYTAL. (Lilly) Ephedrine sulfate 25 mg, amobarbital 50 mg/Pulv. Bot. 100s.
Use: Decongestant, sedative/hypnotic.

EPHEDRINE HYDROCHLORIDE, U.S.P. XXII. l-a-[1-(Methylamino) ethyl]benzyl alcohol hydrochloride. (−)-erythro-α-[1-(Methylamino)ethyl]-benzyl Alcohol hydrochloride. (Various Mfr.); Cryst. Box ⅛ oz, 0.25 oz, 4 oz.
Use: Adrenergic (bronchodilator).

EPHEDRINE HCl W/COMBINATIONS.

See: Asma-lief, Tab., Susp. (Quality Generics).
Ceepa, Tab. (Geneva).
Co-Xan, Elix. (Central).
Derma Medicone (Medicone).
Derma Medicone HC, Oint. (Medicone).
Ectasule, Ectasule Minus, Cap. (Fleming).
Golacal, Syr. (Arcum).
Kie, Tab., Syr. (Laser).
Lardet Expectorant, Tab. (Standex).
Lardet, Tab. (Standex).
Mudrane GG, Tab. (Poythress).
Mudrane, Tab. (Poythress).
Panaphyllin, Susp. (Panamerican).
Pyrralan DM, Expectorant (Lannett).
Quadrinal, Tab., Susp. (Knoll).
Quelidrine, Syr. (Abbott).
Quibron Plus (Bristol).
Tedral-25, Tab. (Parke-Davis).
T-E-P Compound, Tab. (Stanlabs).
Theofedral, Tab. (Redford).
Theofenal, Susp., Tab. (Spencer-Mead).

EPHEDRINE HYDROCHLORIDE NASAL JELLY.
See: Efedron Nasal (Hyrex).

EPHEDRINE and PHENOBARBITAL. (Jenkins) Phenobarbital 0.25 gr, ephedrine HCl 3/8 gr/Tab. Bot. 1000s.
Use: Sedative/hypnotic, decongestant.

EPHEDRINE-RELATED COMPOUNDS.
See: Sympathomimetic Agents.

•**EPHEDRINE SULFATE,** U.S.P. XXII. Cap., Inj., Nasal Soln., Syr., Tab., U.S.P. XXII. (−)-erythro-α-[1-(Methylamino)ethyl]-benzyl Alcohol. Benzenemethanol, α-[1-(methylamino)ethyl]-, sulfate (2:1) (salt). (Various Mfr). (Abbott) Inj. 50 mg/1 ml amp.
Use: Adrenergic (bronchodilator, nasal decongestant).
See: Ectasule Minus Jr. and Sr., Cap. (Fleming).
Slo-Fedrin, Cap. (Dooner).

EPHEDRINE SULFATE W/COMBINATIONS
See: B.M.E., Elix. (Brothers).
Bronkaid, Tab. (Winthrop Consumer Products).
Bronkolixir, Elix. (Winthrop Pharm).
Bronkotabs (Winthrop Pharm).
Ectasule, Cap. (Fleming).
Ectasule Minus, Cap. (Fleming).
Eponal, Prep. (Cenci).
Marax DF, Syr. (Roerig).
Marax, Tab., Syr. (Roerig).
Neogen, Supp. (Premo).
Pazo, Oint., Supp. (Bristol-Myers).
Rectacort, Supp. (Century).
Va-Tro-Nol, Nose Drops (Vicks).
Wyanoids, Preps. (Wyeth-Ayerst).

EPHEDRINE SULFATE AND PHENOBARBITAL CAPSULES, U.S.P. XXII.
Use: Adrenergic (Bronchodilator).

1-EPHENAMINE PENICILLIN G. Compenamine.

EPHENYLLIN. (CMC) Theophylline 130 mg, ephedrine HCl 24 mg, phenobarbital 8 mg/Tab. Bot. 100s, 500s, 1000s.
Use: Bronchodilator, decongestant, sedative/hypnotic.

EPHRINE NASAL SPRAY. (Walgreen) Phenylephrine HCl 0.5%. Bot. 20 ml.
Use: Decongestant.

EPHRINITE NO. 1. (Kenyon) Phenylephrine HCl 5 mg, prophenpyridamine 12.5 mg/Tab. Bot. 100s.
Use: Decongestant.

•**EPICILLIN.** USAN. 6-(D-α-Aminocyclohexa-1,4-dien-1-ylacetamido)penicillanic acid.
Use: Antibiotic.
See: Dexacillin.

EPI-DERM BALM. (Pedinol) Methyl salicylate, menthol, propylene glycol, alcohol. Bot. gal.
Use: External analgesic.

EPIFOAM. (Reed & Carnrick) Hydrocortisone acetate 1%, pramoxine HCl 1% in base of propylene glycol, cetyl alcohol, PEG-100 stearate, glyceryl stearate, laureth-23, polyoxyl-40 stearate, methylparaben, propylparaben, trolamine, or hydrochloric acid to adjust pH, purified water, butane, propane inert propellant. Aerosol container 10 Gm.
Use: Corticosteroid, topical.

EPIFORM-HC. (Delta) Hydrocortisone 1%, iodohydroxyquin 3% in cream base. Tube 20 Gm.
Use: Corticosteroid, antifungal, topical.

EPIFRIN STERILE OPHTHALMIC SOLUTION. (Allergan) Levo-epinephrine HCl 0.25%, 0.5%, 1% or 2%, benzalkonium Cl, sodium metabisulfite, edetate disodium, purified water. 0.25% also contains sodium Cl. Bot. w/dropper 15 ml.
Use: Agent for glaucoma.

EPILEPSY.
See: Anticonvulsants.

E-PILO. (Iolab Pharm.) Pilocarpine HCl 1%, 2%, 3%, 4% or 6%, epinephrine bitartrate 1%, benzalkonium Cl 0.01%, edetate disodium 0.01%. Bot. 10 ml w/dropper-tip plastic vial.
Use: Agent for glaucoma.

•**EPIMESTROL.** USAN. 3-Methoxy-estra-1,3,5(10)-triene-16α, 17α-diol. Stimovul (Organon).
Use: Anterior pituitary activator.

EPIMYCIN A. (Delta) Polymyxin B sulfate 5000 units, bacitracin 400 units, neomycin sulfate 3.5 mg, diperodon HCl 10 mg/Gm. Oint. Tube 0.5 oz.
Use: Anti-infective, external.

EPINAL. (Alcon) Epinephrine 0.5%, 1% as borate complex, benzalkonium Cl 0.01%, ascorbic acid, acetylcysteine, boric acid, sodium carbonate. Dropper Bot. 7.5 ml
Use: Agent for glaucoma.

EPINEPHRAN.
See: Epinephrine, Preps. (Various Mfr.).

•**EPINEPHRINE,** U.S.P. XXII. Inh., Soln., Aerosol, Inj., Nasal Soln., Ophth. Soln., Sterile Oil Susp., U.S.P. XXII. (−)-3,4-Dihydroxy-alpha-[(methylamino)methyl]benzyl Alcohol. 1,2-Benzenediol,4-[1-hydroxy-2-(methylamino)ethyl]-Inhalation. Adnephrine, adrenal, adrenamine, adrenine, epinephran, eptreman, hemisine, hemostatin, nephridine, levorenine, paranephrin, ren-

aglandin, renalina, supra-capsulin, suprarenaline, suprarenin, renoform, renostypticin, renostyptin, styptirenal, supradin, supranephrane, surrenine, takamina, vasoconstrictine, vasotonin, hypernephrin, renaleptine, scurenaline, nieraline. **Pediatric Inj.:** (Abbott) Soln. 0.01 mg/ml; 5 ml single-dose Abboject Syringe.
Use: Asthma, hayfever, acute allergic states, cardiac arrest, acute hypersensitivity reactions.
See: Asthma Meter, Aerosol (Rexall).
Asmolin, Vial (Lincoln).
Emergency Ana-Kit (Hollister-Stier).
W/Lidocaine HCl.
See: Ardecaine 1%, 2%, Inj. (Burgin-Arden).

•**EPINEPHRINE BITARTRATE,** U.S.P. XXII. Inhalation Aerosol, Ophth. Soln., for Ophth. Soln., U.S.P. XXII.
Use: Adrenergic (ophthalmic).
See: Epitrate, Liq. (Ayerst).
W/Pilocarpine HCl.
See: E-Pilo, Liq. (Smith, Miller & Patch).

EPINEPHRINE HYDROCHLORIDE.
Use: Adrenergic, ophthalmic.
See: Adrenalin Cl, Soln. (Parke-Davis).
Epifrin, Ophth. Soln. (Allergan).
Epinal, Ophth. Soln. (Alcon).
Sus-Phrine, Amp., Vial (Berlex).
Vaponefrin Solution & Nebulizer, Vial (Fisons).
W/Benzalkonium Cl, sodium Cl, sodium metabisulfite.
See: Glaucon, Soln. (Alcon).
W/Pilocarpine HCl.
See: Epicar, Soln. (Barnes-Hind).

EPINEPHRINE, RACEMIC.
See: Asthmanefrin Solution (Norcliff-Thayer).

EPINEPHRINE-RELATED COMPOUNDS.
See: Sympathomimetic Agents.

•**EPINEPHRYL BORATE.** F.D.A. Cyclic (-)-4-[l-hydroxy-2-(methylamino)ethyl]-o-phenylene borate.

•**EPINEPHRYL BORATE OPHTHALMIC SOLUTION,** U.S.P. XXII. (−)-3,4-Dihydroxy-α-[(methyl-amino)methyl]benzyl alcohol, cyclic 3,4-ester w/boric acid.
Use: Adrenergic (ophthalmic).
See: Epinal (Alcon).
Eppy (Barnes-Hind).

EPIOSTRIOL. B.A.N. Estra-1,3,5(10)-triene-3,16β,17β-triol. 16-epiestriol.
Use: Estrogen.

EPIPEN AUTO-INJECTOR. (Center) Epinephrine injection 1:1000. Delivers dose of 0.3 mg. Pkg. 1s, 2s, 2 ml injectors.
Use: Emergency kit.

EPIPEN JR. AUTO-INJECTOR. (Center) Epinephrine injection 1:2000. Delivers dose of 0.15 mg. Pkg. 1s, 2s, 2 ml injectors.
Use: Emergency kit.

EPIPHENETHICILLIN. L-(a-phenoxy-propionamido) penicillanic acid.

•**EPIPROPIDINE.** USAN. 1,1′-Bis(2,3-epoxypropyl)-4,4′bipiperidine. Eponate.
Use: Antineoplastic.

EPIRENAN.
See: Epinephrine (Various Mfr.).

•**EPIRIZOLE.** USAN.
Use: Analgesic, anti-inflammatory.

•**EPIRUBICIN HYDROCHLORIDE.** USAN.
Use: Antineoplastic.

EPISONE. (Delta) Hydrocortisone 10 mg in a base containing steryl alcohol, white petrolatum, mineral oil, propylene glycol, polyoxyl 40 stearate, purified water, methyl and propyl parabens. Tube oz.
Use: Corticosteroid.

•**EPITETRACYCLINE HYDROCHLORIDE,** U.S.P.XXII.
Use: Antibiotic.

•**EPITHIAZIDE.** USAN. 3-[(2,2,2-Trifluoroethylthio)methyl]-6-chloro-3,4-dihydro-2H-1,2,4-benzothiadiazine-7-sulfonamide 1,1-dioxide.
Use: Hypotensive and diuretic.

EPITOL. (Lemmon) Carbamazepine 200 mg/Tab. Bot. 100s, 500s, 1000s.
Use: Anticonvulsant.

EPITRATE AYERST. (Wyeth-Ayerst) Epinephrine bitartrate ophthalmic solution 2%, equivalent to 1% base w/chlorobutanol (chloral derivative 0.6%), sodium bisulfite, sodium Cl, polyoxypropylene-polyoxyethylene-diol, disodium edetate. Drop. Bot. 7.5 ml.
Use: Agent for glaucoma.

E-PLUS. (Drug Industries) Vitamins E 73.5 mg, niacin 20 mg, lemon bioflavonoid complex 25 mg, C 50 mg, B_6 2 mg, B_1 5 mg/Tab. Bot. 100s, 500s.
Use: Vitamin supplement.

•**EPOETIN ALFA.** USAN.
Use: Recombinant human erythropoietin, antianemic.

•**EPOETIN BETA.** USAN.
Use: Recombinant human erythropoietin, antianemic.

EPOGEN. (Amgen) Epoetin Alfa (Erythropoietin; EPO) 2,000 units, 4,000 units, 10,000 units. Preservative free. 1 ml.
Use: Recombinant human erythropoietin.

EPONAL. (Cenci) Theophylline 2 gr, ephedrine sulfate ⅜ gr, phenobarbital ⅛ gr/Tab. Bot. 100s, 1000s.
Use: Bronchodilator, decongestant, sedative/hypnotic.

EPONAL-G. (Cenci) Theophylline 2 gr, ephedrine sulfate ⅜ gr, phenobarbital ⅛ gr, guaifenesin 1½ gr/Tab. Bot. 100s, 1000s.
Use: Bronchodilator, decongestant, sedative/hypnotic, expectorant.

•**EPOPROSTENOL.** USAN.
Use: Inhibitor (platelet).

•**EPOPROSTENOL SODIUM.** USAN.
Use: Inhibitor (platelet).

•**EPOSTANE.** USAN.
Use: Interceptive agent.

EPOXYTROPINE TROPATE METHYLBROMIDE.
See: Methscopolamine Bromide (Various Mfr.).

EPPY/N. (Barnes-Hind) Epinephryl borate ophthalmic soln. 0.5%, 1% or 2%. Bot. 7.5 ml.
Use: Agent for glaucoma.

EPROMATE. (Major) Aspirin 325 mg, meprobamate 200 mg Tab. Bot. 100s, 500s.
Use: Salicylate analgesic, antianxiety agent.

EPSAL. (Press) Saturated soln. of epsom salts 80% in ointment form. Jar 0.5 oz, 2 oz.
Use: Drawing ointment.

EPSIVITE 100. (Standex) Vitamin E 100 IU/Cap. Bot. 100s.
Use: Vitamin E supplement.

EPSIVITE 200. (Standex) Vitamin E 200 IU/Cap. Bot. 100s.
Use: Vitamin E supplement.

EPSIVITE 400. (Standex) Vitamin E 400 IU/Cap. Bot. 100s.
Use: Vitamin E supplement.

EPSIVITE FORTE. (Standex) Vitamin E 1000 IU/Cap. Bot. 100s.
Use: Vitamin E supplement.

EPSOM SALT.
See: Magnesium Sulfate.

EPT. (Parke-Davis Prods) In-home pregnancy test.
Use: Diagnostic aid.

E.P.T. PLUS. (Warner-Lambert) Reagent in-home kit for urine testing. Pregnancy test. Kit 1s.
Use: Diagnostic aid.

EPTOIN.
See: Phenytoin Sodium (Various Mfr.).

EQUAGESIC. (Wyeth-Ayerst) Meprobamate 200 mg, aspirin 325 mg/Tab. Bot. 100s, Redi-pak 100s.
Use: Antianxiety agent, salicylate analgesic.

EQUAL. (Nutrasweet) Aspartame. **Packet:** 0.035 oz. (1 Gm). Box 50s, 100s, 200s. **Tab.:** Bot. 100s.
Use: Artificial sweetener.

EQUALACTIN. (Pfizer) Polycarbophil 500 mg (as calcium polycarbophil)/Chew. tab.
Use: Antidiarrheal or laxative.

EQUANIL. (Wyeth-Ayerst) Meprobamate 200 mg or 400 mg/Tab. **200 mg:** Bot. 100s. **400 mg:** Bot. 100s, 500s, Redipak 25s.
Use: Antianxiety agent.

EQUAZINE M. (Rugby) Aspirin 325 mg, meprobamate 200 mg, tartrazine tab. Bot. 100s, 500s.
Use: Salicylate analgesic, antianxiety agent.

EQUILET. (Mission) Calcium carbonate 500 mg/Chew. tab. Strip packed in 100s.
Use: Antacid.

•**EQUILIN,** U.S.P. XXII. Estra-1, 3-5 (10), 7-tetraen-17 one, 3 hydroxy-3-Hydroxestra-1,3,5 (10), 7-tetraen-17-one.
Use: Estrogen.

EQUIPERTINE CAPSULES. (Winthrop Products) Oxypertine.
Use: Antianxiety agent, tranquilizer.

ERADACIL CAPSULES. (Winthrop Products) Rosoxacin.
Use: Antigonococcal agent.

ERAMYCIN. (Wesley) Erythromycin 250 mg (as stearate)/FC tab. Bot. 100s, 500s.
Use: Anti-infective.

ERCAF. (Geneva Marsam) Ergotamine tartrate 1 mg, caffeine 100 mg/Tab. Bot. 100s, 1000s.
Use: Agent for migraine.

ERGAMISOL. (Janssen) Levamisole (base) 50 mg/Tab. Blister pack 36s.
Use: Antineoplastic agent.

ERGOCAF. (Robinson) Ergotamine tartrate, caffeine. Bot. 100s, 500s, 1000s.
Use: Agent for migraine.

ERGO CAFF. (Rugby) Ergotamine tartrate 1 mg, caffeine 100 mg/Tab. Bot. 100s.
Use: Agent for migraine.

•**ERGOCALCIFEROL,** U.S.P. XXII. Cap., Tab., Oral Soln. U.S.P. XXII. 9, 10-Secoergosta-5,7,10(19),22-tetraen-3-ol, (3β-. Irradiated Ergosta-5,7,22-trien-3-beta-ol.
Use: Vitamin D (antirachitis).
See: Calciferol.
Drisdol, Liq., Cap. (Winthrop Pharm).
Geltabs, Cap. (Upjohn).

ERGOCORNINE. (Various Mfr.) Ergot alkaloid.
Use: Peripheral vascular disorders.

ERGOCRISTINE. (Various Mfr.) Ergot alkaloid.
Use: Vascular disorders.

ERGOCRYPTINE. (Various Mfr.) Ergot alkaloid.
Use: Peripheral vascular disorders.

•**ERGOLOID MESYLATES,** U.S.P. XXII. Oral Soln., Tab., U.S.P.XXII. (Lederle) **0.5 mg:** Dihydroergocornine 0.167 mg, dihydroergocristine 0.167 mg, dihydroergocryptine 0.167 mg/0.5 mg Sublingual Tab. **1 mg:** Dihydroergocornine 0.333 mg, dihydroergocristine 0.333 mg, dihydro-ergocryptine 0.333 mg/1 mg Tab. Bot. 100s, 1000s.
Use: Psychotherapeutic agent.
See: Deapril-ST, Tab. (Mead Johnson).
Hydergine Prods. (Sandoz).

ERGOMAR. (Fisons) Ergotamine tartrate 2 mg/Sublingual Tab. Pkg. 20s.
Use: Agent for migraine.

ERGOMETRINE MALEATE.
See: Ergonovine (Various Mfr.).

ERGONAL. (Vita Elixir) Ergot powder 259.2 mg, aloin 8.1 mg, apiol fluid green 290 mg, oil pennyroyal 28 mg/Cap. Bot. 24s.
Use: Oxytocic.

ERGONOVINE. (Various Mfr.) Ergobasine, erolklinine, ergometrine, ergostetrine, ergotocine.
Use: Oxytocic.
See: Ergonovine Maleate.

•**ERGONOVINE MALEATE,** U.S.P. XXII. Inj., Tab., U.S.P. XXII. 9,10-Didehydro-N-[(S)-2-hydroxy-1-methylethyl]-6-methylergoline-8β-carboxamide maleate.
Use: IV, IM, orally, oxytocic.
See: Ergotrate Maleate, Preps. (Lilly).

ERGOSTAT. (Parke-Davis) Ergotamine tartrate 2 mg/Sublingual Tab. Vial UD 24s.
Use: Agent for migraine.

ERGOSTEROL, ACTIVATED OR IRRADIATED.
See: Ergocalciferol, U.S.P. XXII.

ERGOSTETRINE.
See: Ergonovine (Various Mfr.).

•**ERGOTAMINE TARTRATE,** U.S.P. XXII. Inj., Inhalation Aerosol, Tab., U.S.P. XXII. Ergotaman-3′,6′,18-trione, 12′-hydroxy-2′-methyl-5′-(phenylmethyl)-2,3-dihydroxybutanedioate (2:1) (salt). Femergin.
Use: Analgesic (specific in migraine).
See: Ergomar, Tab. (Fisons).
Ergostat, Tab. (Parke-Davis).
Gynergen, Amp., Tab. (Sandoz).
Medihaler-Ergotamine, Vial (Riker).
W/Belladonna alkaloids, acetophenetidin, caffeine.
See: Wigraine, Tab., Supp. (Organon).
W/Belladonna alkaloids, pentobarbital.
See: Cafergot P-B, Supp., Tab. (Sandoz).
W/Belladonna alkaloids, phenobarbital.
See: Bellergal, Tab. (Dorsey).
W/Caffeine.
See: Cafergot, Tab., Supp. (Sandoz).
W/Caffeine, homatropine methylbromide.
See: Ergotatropin, Tab. (Cole).
W/Cyclizine HCl, caffeine.
See: Migral Tab. (Burroughs Wellcome).
W/1-Hyoscyamine sulfate, phenobarbital.
See: Ergkatal, Tab. (Gilbert).

•**ERGOTAMINE TARTRATE AND CAFFEINE SUPPOSITORIES,** U.S.P. XXII.
Use: Vascular headache.
See: Cafergot, Supp. (Sandoz).

•**ERGOTAMINE TARTRATE AND CAFFEINE TABLETS,** U.S.P. XXII.
Use: Vascular headache.
See: Cafergot, Tab. (Sandoz).
Ergocaf, Tab. (Robinson).
Lanatrate, Tab. (Lannett).

ERGOT, FLUID EXTRACT. (Various Mfr.) Ergot 1 Gm/ml Bot. 4 oz, pt.

ERGOTIDINE.
See: Histamine (Various Mfr.).

ERGOTOCINE.
See: Ergonovine (Various Mfr.).

ERGOTRATE.
See: Ergonovine (Various Mfr.).

ERGOTRATE-H.
See: Ergonovine (Various Mfr.).

ERGOTRATE MALEATE. (Lilly) Ergonovine maleate. **Amp.:** (0.2 mg) 1 ml, Pkg. 6s, 100s; **Tab.:** 0.2 mg. Bot. 100s, 1000s, Blister pkg. 10 × 10s.
Use: Oxytocic.

ERGOT-RELATED PRODUCTS.
See: Cafergot, Supp., Tab. (Sandoz).
Deapril-ST, Tab. (Mead Johnson).
Cafergot P-B, Tab., Supp. (Sandoz).
DHE-45, Amp. (Sandoz).
Ergonovine (Various Mfr.).
Ergotamine (Various Mfr.).
Ergotrate (Various Mfr.).
Gynergen, Amp., Tab. (Sandoz).
Hydergine, Sub. Tab. (Sandoz).
Hydro-Ergot, Tab. (Interstate).
Methergine, Amp., Tab. (Sandoz).
Trigot, Sublingual Tab. (Squibb).
Wigraine, Supp., Tab. (Organon).

ERGOZIDE. (Jenkins) Carbolic acid 2.25%, ergot extract 2.5%, zinc oxide 10%, balsam Peru 1.25%, oil cade 0.3%. Pkg. lb.

ERIDIONE. (Eric, Kirk & Gary) Phenindione 50 mg/Tab. Bot. 100s, 1000s.
Use: Anticoagulant.

ERIDIUM. (Hauck) Phenazopyridine HCl 100 mg/Tab. Bot. 32s, 1000s.
Use: Urinary analgesic.

ERIODICTIN.
See: Vitamin P & Rutin.

•**ERIODICTYON,** N.F. XVII. Flext., Aromatic Syrup, N.F. XVII.
Use: Pharmaceutic aid (flavor).
See: Vitamin P & Rutin.

E-R-O. (Scherer) Propylene glycol, glycerol. Bot. w/dropper tip 15 ml.
Use: Otic preparation.

ERTINE. (Approved) Hexachlorophene, benzocaine, cod liver oil, allantoin, boric acid, lanolin. Tube 1.5 oz.
Use: Burn and first aid remedy.

ERYCETTE. (Ortho Derm) Erythromycin 2% 20 mg/ml. Pkg. 60 pledgets.
Use: Anti-acne.

ERYDERM 2%. (Abbott) Erythromycin topical soln. 2%. Bot. 60 ml.
Use: Anti-acne.

ERYGEL. (Herbert) Erythromycin 2%. Gel Tube 30 Gm.
Use: Anti-infective, external.

ERYMAX TOPICAL SOLUTION. (Herbert) Erythromycin 2% Soln. 60 ml, 120 ml.
Use: Anti-acne.

ERYPAR. (Parke-Davis) Erythromycin stearate 250 mg or 500 mg/Filmseal. **250 mg:** Bot. 100s, 500s. **500 mg:** Bot. 100s.
Use: Anti-infective.

ERYPED. (Abbott) Erythromycin ethylsuccinate granules for oral susp. representing erythromycin activity of 400 mg/5 ml. Bot. 60 ml, 100 ml, 200 ml, UD 5 ml, 100s.
Use: Anti-infective.

ERY-TAB. (Abbott) Erythromycin enteric coated 250 mg, 333 mg or 500 mg/Tab. **250 mg:** Bot. 30s, 40s, 100s, 500s, UD 100s. **333 mg:** Bot. 100s, 500s, UD 100s. **500 mg:** Bot. 100s, UD 100s.
Use: Anti-infective.

•**ERYTHRITYL TETRANITRATE, DILUTED,** U.S.P. XXII.
Use: Coronary vasodilator.

•**ERYTHRITYL TETRANITRATE TABLETS,** U.S.P. XXII. (Various Mfr.) Erythritol, erythrol tetranitrate, nitroerythrite, tetranitrin, tetranitrol.
Use: Coronary vasodilator.
See: Anginar, Tab. (Pasadena Research Labs.).
Cardilate, Tab. (Burroughs Wellcome).
W/Phenobarbital.
See: Cardilate-P, Tab. (Burroughs Wellcome).

ERYTHROCIN LACTOBIONATE, I.V. (Abbott Hospital Prods) Erythromycin lactobionate. Pow.

500 mg/vial w/benzyl alcohol 90 mg; 1 Gm/vial w/benzyl alcohol 180 mg. Pkg. Vial 5s.
Use: Anti-infective.

ERYTHROCIN LACTOBIONATE PIGGYBACK. (Abbott Hospital Prods) Erythromycin lactobionate for injection, 500 mg/dispensing vial. 5 mg/ml of erythromycin after reconstitution w/90 mg benzyl alcohol. Pow. Pkg. 5×100 ml dispensing vials.
Use: Anti-infective.

ERYTHROCIN STEARATE. (Abbott) Erythromycin stearate 250 mg or 500 mg/Tab. **250 mg:** Bot. 40s, 100s, 500s, UD 100s; **500 mg:** Bot. 100s.
Use: Anti-infective.

•**ERYTHROMYCIN,** U.S.P. XXII. Delayed-release Cap., Oint., Ophth. Oint., Delayed-release Tab., Tab., Topical Soln., Topical Gel, U.S.P. XXII. An antibiotic from *Streptomyces erythreus.* (Upjohn) Tab. 100 mg. Bot. 100s; 250 mg. Bot. 25s, 100s.
Use: Antibiotic.
See: Dowmycin E, Tab. (Merrell Dow).
E-Mycin, Tab. (Upjohn).
Erymax, Soln. (Herbert).
EryDerm, Soln. (Abbott).
Erythrocin, Prep. (Abbott).
Erythromycin Base, Filmtab (Abbott).
Ilotycin, Prep. (Dista).
PCE, Tab. (Abbott).
Robimycin, Tab. (Robins).
RP-Mycin, Tab. (Solvay).

•**ERYTHROMYCIN ACISTRATE.** USAN.
Use: Antibiotic.

•**ERYTHROMYCIN AND BENZOYL PEROXIDE TOPICAL GEL,** U.S.P. XXII.
Use: Antibiotic, keratolytic.

ERYTHROMYCIN BASE FILMTAB. (Abbott) Erythromycin base 250 mg or 500 mg/Tab. **250 mg:** Bot. 100s, 500s, UD 100s. **500 mg:** Bot 100s.
Use: Anti-infective.

•**ERYTHROMYCIN ESTOLATE,** U.S.P. XXII. Cap., Oral Susp., for Oral Susp., Tab., U.S.P. XXII. Supp., Erythromycin 2′-propionate dodecyl sulfate. Lauryl sulfate salt of the propionic acid ester of erythromycin.
Use: Antibiotic.
See: Ilosone, Preps. (Dista).

•**ERYTHROMYCIN ETHYLSUCCINATE,** U.S.P. XXII. Inj., Tab., for Oral Susp., Oral Susp., Sterile, U.S.P. XXII. Erythromycin 2′-(Ethylsuccinate).
Use: Antibiotic.
See: E.E.S. Prods. (Abbott).
E-mycin E, Liq. (Upjohn).
Pediamycin Prods. (Ross).
Pediazole, Liq. (Ross).
Wyamycin-E, Liq. (Wyeth-Ayerst).

•**ERYTHROMYCIN ETHYLSUCCINATE AND SULFISOXAZOLE ACETYL FOR ORAL SUSPENSION,** U.S.P. XXII.
Use: Antibiotic, anti-infective.
See: Pediazole, Susp. (Ross).

•**ERYTHROMYCIN GLUCEPTATE, STERILE,** U.S.P. XXII.
Use: Antibacterial.
See: Ilotycin Gluceptate, Amp. (Lilly).

•**ERYTHROMYCIN GLUCOHEPTONATE.**
See: Erythromycin Gluceptate, U.S.P. XXII.
Ilotycin Glucoheptonate, Amp. (Dista).

•**ERYTHROMYCIN LACTOBIONATE FOR INJECTION,** U.S.P. XXII.
Use: Antibacterial.
See: Erythrocin Lactobionate, Vial (Abbott).

ERYTHROMYCIN 2′-PROPIONATE DODECYL SULFATE. Erythromycin Estolate, U.S.P. XXII.
Use: Antibacterial.

•**ERYTHROMYCIN PLEDGETS,** U.S.P. XXII.
Use: Antibiotic.

ERYTHROMYCIN PROPIONATE LAURYL SULFATE.
Use: Anti-infective.
See: Erthromycin Estolate.
Ilosone, Preps. (Dista).

•**ERYTHROMYCIN STEARATE,** U.S.P. XXII. Tab., for Oral Susp., U.S.P. XXII.
Use: Antibacterial.
See: Dowmycin-E, Tab. (Merrell Dow).
Erythrocin Stearate Prods. (Abbott).
Erypar Filmseal, Tab. (Parke-Davis).
Wyamycin-S, Tab. (Wyeth-Ayerst).

ERYTHROMYCIN SULFATE.
Use: Anti-infective.

•**ERYTHROSINE SODIUM, U.S.P. XXII. Topical Soln., Soluble Tab., U.S.P. XXII.**
Use: Diagnostic aid (dental disclosing agent).

ERYZOLE. (Alra) Erythromycin ethylsuccinate 200 mg, acetyl sulfisoxazole 600 mg/5 ml when reconstituted. Gran for Susp. 100 ml, 150 ml, 200 ml.
Use: Anti-infective.

ESCLABRON. Guaithylline.
Use: Antiasthmatic.

ESERDINE FORTE TABS. (Major) Methyclothiazide, reserpine 0.5 mg/Tab. Bot. 100s.
Use: Diuretic, antihypertensive.

ESERDINE TABS. (Major) Methyclothiazide, reserpine 0.25 mg/Tab. Bot. 100s, 250s.
Use: Diuretic, antihypertensive.

ESERINE. Physostigmine as alkaloid, salicylate or sulfate salt.
Use: Agent for glaucoma.

ESERINE SALICYLATE. (Alcon) Physostigmine 0.5%. Soln. 2 ml.
Use: Agent for glaucoma.

ESERINE SULFATE STERILE OPHTHALMIC OINTMENT. (CooperVision) Physostigmine sulfate 0.25%. Tube 3.5 Gm.
Use: Agent for glaucoma.

ESERINE SULFATE. (Robinson) Physostigmine sulfate 0.25%. Oint. Tube ⅛ oz.
Use: Agent for glaucoma.

ESGIC CAPSULES. (Forest) Butalbital 50 mg, caffeine 40 mg, acetaminophen 325 mg/Cap. Bot. 100s.
Use: Sedative/hypnotic, analgesic.

ESGIC TABLETS. (Forest) Butalbital 50 mg, caffeine 40 mg, acetaminophen 325 mg/Tab. Bot. 100s.
Use: Sedative/hypnotic, analgesic.

ESIDRIX. (Ciba) Hydrochlorothiazide 25 mg, 50 mg or 100 mg/Tab. **25 mg:** Bot. 100s, 1000s, UD 100s. **50 mg:** Bot. 100s, 360s, 720s, 1000s, UD 100s. **100 mg:** Bot. 100s.
Use: Diuretic, antihypertensive.
W/Apresoline.
See: Apresoline-Esidrix, Tab. (Ciba).

ESIMIL. (Ciba) Hydrochlorothiazide 25 mg, guanethidine monosulfate 10 mg/Tab. Bot. 100s, Consumer Pack 100s.
Use: Diuretic, antihypertensive.

ESKALITH. (SKF) Lithium carbonate. **Cap.:** 300 mg. Bot. 100s, 500s; **Tab.:** 300 mg. Bot. 100s.
Use: Antipsychotic agent.

ESKALITH CR. (SKF) Lithium carbonate 450 mg/CR tab. Bot. 100s.
Use: Antipsychotic agent.

•**ESMOLOL HYDROCHLORIDE.** USAN. (1) Benzenepropanoic acid, 4-[2-hydroxy-3-[(1-methylethyl)amino]propoxy]-, methyl ester, hydrochloride, (±)-; (2) (±)-Methyl *p*-[2-hydroxy-3-(isopropyl-amino)propoxy]hydrocinnamate hydrochloride.
Use: Short acting beta-adrenergic blocking agent.
See: Brevibloc, Inj. (DuPont).

E-SOLVE. (Syosset) Alcohol 75%, propylene glycol, diethanolamide, polysorbate 80, talc, titanium dioxide, iron oxides, povidone, water soluble cellulose gum. Lot. Bot. 50 ml.
Use: Lotion base.

E-SOLVE-2. (Syosset) Erythromycin 2%, alcohol 80%, propylene glycol, lauramide DEA, zinc acetate, hydroxypropyl cellulose, iron oxides. Topical soln. Bot. 60 ml.
Use: Anti-acne.

E-SON. (Eastwood) Bot. 100s.

•**ESORUBICIN HYDROCHLORIDE.** USAN.
Use: Antineoplastic.

ESOTERICA DRY SKIN TREATMENT LOTION. (Norcliff Thayer) Bot. 13 fl oz.
Use: Emollient.

ESOTERICA MEDICATED FADE CREAM, FACIAL. (Norcliff Thayer) Hydroquinone 2%, padimate O 3.3%, oxybenzone 2.5% in cream base. Jar 90 Gm.
Use: Skin bleaching agent.

ESOTERICA MEDICATED FADE CREAM. (Norcliff Thayer) Hydroquinone 2%, padimate O 3.3%, oxybenzone 2.5%. Cream. Jar 90 Gm, scented or unscented.
Use: Skin bleaching agent.

ESOTERICA MEDICATED FADE CREAM, REGULAR. (Norcliff Thayer) Hydroquinone 2%. Cream. Jar 90 Gm.
Use: Skin bleaching agent.

ESPOTABS. (Combe) Yellow phenolphthalein 97.2 mg/Tab. Bot. 12s, 30s, 60s.
Use: Laxative.

•**ESPROQUIN HYDROCHLORIDE.** USAN.
Use: Adrenergic.

ESSENTIAL-8. Liquid amino acid protein supplement.
Use: Protein supplement.
See: Vivonex Diets, Liq. (Norwich Eaton).

ESTAR. (Westwood) Tar equivalent to 5% coal tar, U.S.P. in a hydro-alcoholic gel w/alcohol 13.8%. Tube 3 oz.
Use: Antipsoriatic, antipruritic.

•**ESTAZOLAM.** USAN.
Use: Sedative/Hypnotic.
See: ProSom (Abbott).

•**ESTERIFILCON A.** USAN.
Use: Contact lens material.

ESTILBEN.
See: Diethylstilbestrol Dipropionate (Various Mfr.).

ESTINYL. (Schering) Ethinyl estradiol. **0.02 mg, 0.05 mg/Tab., coated:** Bot. 100s, 250s; **0.5 mg/Tab.:** Bot. 100s.
Use: Estrogen.

ESTIVIN II. (Alcon) Naphazoline 0.012%. Soln. 7.5 ml.
Use: Vasoconstrictor/mydriatic, ophthalmic.

ESTOLATE. Erythromycin.
See: Erythromycin Propionate Lauryl Sulfate.

ESTOPEN.
See: Benzylpenicillin 2-diethylaminoethyl ester HI.

ESTRACE. (Bristol-Myers) 17β-Estradiol micronized 1 mg or 2 mg/Tab. Bot. 100s.
Use: Estrogen.

ESTRACE VAGINAL CREAM. (Mead Johnson) 17β-Estradiol 0.1 mg/Gm. Tube 42.5 Gm.
Use: Estrogen.

ESTRACON. (Freeport) Conjugated estrogens 1.25 mg/Tab. Bot. 1000s.
Use: Estrogen.

ESTRA-D. (Seatrace) Estradiol cypionate in oil 5 mg/ml Inj. Vial 10 ml.
Use: Estrogen.

ESTRADERM TRANSDERMAL. (Ciba) Estradiol. **0.05:** Each 10 × 10 cm. system contains 4 mg of estradiol for nominal delivery of 0.05 mg estradiol/day. Patient calendar packs of 8 systems. Ctn 6s. **0.1:** Each 20 × 20 cm. system contains 8 mg estradiol for nominal delivery of 0.1 mg estradiol/day. Patient calendar packs of 8 systems. Ctn. 6s.
Use: Estrogen.

•**ESTRADIOL,** U.S.P. XXII. Pellets, Sterile Susp., Tab., U.S.P. XXII. Estra-1,3,5(10)-triene-3,17-β-diol. Beta-estradiol, agofollin, dihydroxyestrin, dihydrotheelin, gynergon, gynoestryl. The form now known to be physiologically active is the "beta" form rather than the "alpha" form.
Use: Estrogen-replacement therapy.
See: Aquagen, Vial, Aq. (Remsen).
Estrace, Tab., Vaginal Creme (Mead Johnson).
Estraderm, Transdermal (Ciba).
Femogen, Susp., Tab. (Fellows-Testagar).
Progynon, Pellets (Schering).
W/Estriol, estrone.
See: Estro Plus, Tab., Vial (Rocky Mtn.).
Hormonin No. 1 and 2, Tab. (Carnrick).

W/Estrone, estriol.
See: Sanestro, Tab. (Sandia).
W/Estrone, potassium estrone sulfate.
See: Tri-Estrin, Inj. (Keene).
W/Progesterone, testosterone, procaine HCl, procaine base.
See: Horm-Triad, Vial (Bell).
W/Testosterone and chlorobutanol in cottonseed oil.
See: Depo-Testadiol, Vial (Upjohn).
Transdermal.
See: Estraderm, Patch (Ciba).

ESTRADIOL CYCLOPENTYLPROPIONATE, Estradiol 17-beta(3-cyclopentyl)propionate. Estradiol Cypionate, U.S.P. XXII.
W/Testosterone cypionate.
See: Depo-Testadiol, Vial (Upjohn).

•**ESTRADIOL CYPIONATE,** U.S.P. XXII. Inj. U.S.P. XXII. Estradiol 17-β-(3-Cyclopentyl)propionate Estradiol 17-cyclopentanepropionate. Estra-1,3,5-(10)-triene-3,17-diol,(17 beta)-, 17-cyclopentane-propanoate.
Use: Estrogen.
See: Estradiol cyclopentylpropionate.
Dep-Estradiol, Inj. (Rocky Mtn.).
Depo-Estradiol Cypionate, Inj. (Upjohn).
Depogen, Inj. (Hyrex).
D-Est, Inj. (Burgin-Arden).
Estra-C, Inj. (Amfre-Grant).
Estro-Cyp, Vial (Keene).
Estroject-L.A., Vial (Mayrand).
Hormogen Depot, Inj. (Hauck).
Span-F, Inj. (Scrip).
W/Testosterone cypionate.
See: D-Diol, Inj. (Burgin-Arden).
Dep-Tesestro, Inj. (ICN).
Dep-Testradiol, Inj. (Rocky Mtn.).
Duo-Cyp, Vial (Keene).
Duracrine, Inj. (Ascher).
Estran-C, Inj. (Amfre-Grant).
Menoject, L.A., Vial (Mayrand).
T.E. Ionate P.A., Inj. (Solvay).
W/Testosterone cypionate, chlorobutanol.
See: Depo-Testadiol (Upjohn).
Span F.M., Inj. (Scrip).
T.E. Ionate P.A., Inj. (Solvay).

ESTRADIOL DIPROPIONATE. Estra-1,3,5(10)-triene-3,17 β-diol dipropionate. Ovocyclin Dipropionate.
Use: Estrogen.

•**ESTRADIOL ENANTHATE.** USAN. Estradiol 17-enanthate.
Use: Estrogen.

ESTRADIOL, ETHINYL.
See: Ethinyl Estradiol.

ESTRADIOL MONOBENZONATE.
See: Estradiol Benzoate.

ESTRADIOL PHOSPHATE.
See: Estradurin, Secule (Wyeth-Ayerst).

•**ESTRADIOL UNDECYLATE.** USAN. Estradiol 17-undecanoate.
Use: Estrogen.
See: Delestrec.

•**ESTRADIOL VAGINAL CREAM,** U.S.P. XXII.
Use: Estrogen.

•**ESTRADIOL VALERATE,** U.S.P. XXII. Inj., U.S.P. XXII. Estra-1,3,5(10)-triene-3,17-diol (17β)-,17-pentano-ate. Estradiol 17-valerate.
Use: Estrogen.
See: Ardefem 10, 20, Inj. (Burgin-Arden).
Delestrogen, Vial (Squibb Mark).
Depogen, Inj. (Sig).
Dioval, Preps. (Keene).
Duratrad, Inj. (Ascher).
Estate, Inj. (Savage).
Estra-L, Inj. (Pasadena Research).
Femogen, L.A., Inj. (Fellows-Testagar).
Retestrin, Inj. (Rocky Mtn.).
Span-Est, Inj. (Scrip).
Valergen, Inj. (Hyrex).
W/Benzyl alcohol.
See: Estate, Vial (Savage).
Reposo E-40, Vial (Paddock).
W/Hydroxyprogesterone caproate.
See: Hy-Gestradol, Inj. (Pasadena-Research).
Hylutin-Est, Inj. (Hyrex).
W/Testosterone cypionate.
See: Depo-Testadiol, Inj. (Upjohn).
W/Testosterone enanthate.
See: Ardiol 90/4, 180/8, Inj. (Burgin-Arden).
Deladumone, Vial (Squibb Mark).
Delatestadiol, Vial (Dunhall).
Duoval-P.A., I.M. (Solvay).
Estra-Testrin, Inj. (Pasadena Research).
Retadiamone, Inj. (Rocky Mtn.).
Span-Est-Test 4, Inj. (Scrip).
Teev, Inj. (Keene).
Tesogen L.A., Inj. (Sig).
Testanate, Vial (Kenyon).
Valertest, Inj. (Hyrex).
W/Testosterone enanthate, benzyl alcohol, sesame oil.
See: Repose-TE (Paddock).

ESTRADOL. (Kenyon) Ethinyl estradiol. **No. 1:** 0.02 mg/Tab. **No. 2:** 0.05 mg/Tab. Bot.
Use: Estrogen.

ESTRADURIN. (Wyeth-Ayerst) Polyestradiol phosphate. Amp. for injection 40 mg w/2 ml sterile diluent. W/polyestradiol phosphate 40 mg, phenylmercuric nitrate 0.02 mg, sodium phosphate 5.2 mg, niacinamide 25 mg, propylene glycol 4 mg.
Use: Estrogen.

ESTRA-L. (Pasadena Research) Estradiol valerate in castor oil. **20 mg/ml:** Vial 10 ml. **40 mg/ml:** Vial 10 ml.
Use: Estrogen.

ESTRALUTIN.
See: Relutin (Solvay).

•**ESTRAMUSTINE.** USAN. Estradiol 3-bis (2-chloroethyl) carbamate 17-(dihydrogen phosphate), disodium salt.
Use: Antineoplastic agent.
See: Emcyt, Cap. (Roche).

•**ESTRAMUSTINE PHOSPHATE SODIUM.** USAN.

Use: Antineoplastic agent.
ESTRATAB. (Solvay) **Tab.:** Esterified estrogens, principally sodium estrone sulfate 0.3 mg, 0.625 mg, 1.25 mg or 2.5 mg/Tab. Bot. 100s, 1000s.
Use: Estrogen.
ESTRATEST. (Solvay) Esterified estrogens 1.25 mg, methyltestosterone 2.5 mg/Tab. Bot. 100s, 1000s.
Use: Estrogen, androgen combination.
ESTRATEST H.S. (Solvay) Esterified estrogens 0.625 mg, methyltestosterone 1.25 mg/Tab. Bot. 100s.
Use: Estrogen, androgen combination.
ESTRA-TESTRIN. (Pasadena Research) Testosterone enanthate 90 mg, estradiol valerate 4 mg in oil/ml. Inj. Vial 10 ml.
Use: Androgen, estrogen combination.
•**ESTRAZINOL HYDROBROMIDE.** USAN. dl-trans-3-Methoxy-8-aza-19-nor-17a-pregna-1,3,5-trien-20-yn-17-ol hydrobromide.
Use: Estrogen.
ESTRIN.
See: Estrone.
•**ESTRIOL,** U.S.P. XXII.
Use: Estrogen.
W/Estrone, estradiol.
See: Estro Plus, Tab. (Rocky Mtn.).
ESTRITONE NO. 1. (Kenyon) Conjugated estrogens equine 0.625 mg, methyltestosterone 5 mg/Tab. Bot. 100s, 1000s.
Use: Estrogen, androgen combination.
ESTRITONE NO. 2. (Kenyon) Conjugated estrogens equine 1.25 mg, methyltestosterone 10 mg/Tab. Bot. 100s, 1000s.
Use: Estrogen, androgen combination.
ESTROBENE DP.
See: Diethylstilbestrol Dipropionate (Various Mfr.).
ESTRO-CYP. (Keene) Estradiol cypionate 5 mg/ml in oil. Inj. Vial 10 ml.
Use: Estrogen.
ESTROFEM. (Pasadena Research) Estradiol cypionate 5 mg/ml in oil. Inj. Vial 10 ml.
Use: Estrogen.
•**ESTROFURATE.** USAN. (1)21, 23-Epoxy-19-24-dinor-17α-chola-1,3,5(10),7,20,22-hexaene-3,17-diol-3-acetate; (2) 17-(3-furyl) estra-1,3,5-(10),7-tetraene-3,17β-diol-3-acetate.
Use: Estrogen.
ESTROGENIC SUBSTANCES, CONJUGATED. (Water-soluble) A mixture containing the sodium salts of the sulfate esters of the estrogenic substances, principally estrone and equilin that are of the type excreted by pregnant mares.
Cream.
See: Premarin Vaginal Cream (Wyeth-Ayerst).
Intravenous.
See: Estroject, Vial (Mayrand).
Premarin (Wyeth-Ayerst).
Tab.
See: Aquagen, Inj. (Remsen).
Ces (ICN).
Co-Estro, Tab. (Robinson).
Estroquin, Tab. (Sheryl).
Estrosan, Tab. (Recsei).
Evestrone, Tab. (Delta).
Femogen, Oil, Tab., Susp. (Fellows-Testegar).
Genisis, Tab. (Organon).
Menotabs, Tab. (Fleming).
Orapin (Standex).
Prelestrin, Tab. (Pasadena Research).
Premarin, Tab. (Wyeth-Ayerst).
Tag-39 H, Tab. (Solvay).
W/α-Estradiol.
See: Makrogen Aqueous Susp. (O'Neal).
W/Ethinyl estradiol.
See: Demulen, Tab. (Searle).
W/Meprobamate.
See: Milprem, Tab. (Wallace).
PMB 200, Tab. (Wyeth-Ayerst).
PMB 400, Tab. (Wyeth-Ayerst).
W/Methyltestosterone.
See: Menotab-M #1 and 2, Tab. (Fleming).
Premarin with Methyltestosterone, Tab. (Wyeth-Ayerst).
ESTROGENIC SUBSTANCES IN AQUEOUS SUSPENSION. (Wyeth-Ayerst) Sterile estrone suspension 2 mg/ml. Vial 10 ml.
Use: Estrogen.
ESTROGENIC SUBSTANCES MIXED. May be a crystalline or an amorphous mixture of the naturally occurring estrogens obtained from the urine of pregnant mares.
Aqueous Susp.
See: Gravigen Inj. (Bluco).
Lanestrin, Vial (Lannett).
Cap.
See: Urestrin, Cap. (Upjohn).
W/Androgen therapy, vitamins, iron, d-desoxyephedrine HCl.
See: Mediatric, Preps. (Wyeth-Ayerst).
W/Methyltestosterone.
See: Premarin w/methyltestosterone, Tab. (Wyeth-Ayerst).
W/Testosterone.
See: Andrestraq, Vial (Central).
ESTROGEN-ANDROGEN THERAPY.
See: Androgen-Estrogen Therapy.
•**ESTROGENS, CONJUGATED,** U.S.P. XXII. Inj. U.S.P. XXII.
Use: Estrogen.
See: Conest, Tab. (Century).
Congens, Tab. (Blaine).
Congesterone, Tab. (Kenyon).
Estrocon, Tab. (Savage).
Ganeake, Tab. (Geneva).
Menotab, Tab. (Fleming).
PMB, Tab. (Wyeth-Ayerst).
Premarin, Tab., I.V. (Wyeth-Ayerst).
Premarin Vaginal Cream (Wyeth-Ayerst).
Premarin with Methyltestosterone, Tab. (Wyeth-Ayerst).
Sodestrin and Sodestrin-H, Tab. (Solvay).
Tag-39, Tab. (Solvay).
Zeste, Tab. (Ascher).

ESTROGENS EQUINE.
See: Estrogen.
PMB, Tab. (Wyeth-Ayerst).
Premarin, Tab., I.V. (Wyeth-Ayerst).
Premarin Vaginal Cream (Wyeth-Ayerst).
Premarin with Methyltestosterone, Tab. (Wyeth-Ayerst).

ESTROGENS, ESTERIFIED, U.S.P. XXII. Tab., U.S.P. XXII.
Use: Estrogen.
See: Amnestrogen, Tab. (Squibb).
Estratab (Solvay).
Evex, Tab. (Syntex).
Menest, Tab. (Beecham Labs).
Ms-Med, Tab. (Dunhall).

ESTROGENS, ESTERIFIED & ANDROGENS.
Use: Estrogen & Androgen supplementation.
See: Estratest.

ESTROGENS, NATURAL.
Use: Estrogen.
See: Depogen, Vial (Hyrex).
Estradiol, Preps. (Various Mfr.).
Estrone, Preps. (Various Mfr.).
Estrogenic Substance (Various Mfr.).
PMB, Tab. (Wyeth-Ayerst).
Premarin, Tab., I.V. (Wyeth-Ayerst).
Premarin Vaginal Cream (Wyeth-Ayerst).
Premarin with Methyltestosterone, Tab. (Wyeth-Ayerst).

ESTROGENS, SYNTHETIC.
See: Dienestrol, Preps. (Various Mfr.).
Diethylstilbestrol, Preps. (Various Mfr.).
Hexestrol, Preps. (Various Mfr.).
Meprane, Tab. (Reed & Carnrick).
TACE, Cap. (Merrell Dow).
Vallestril, Tab. (Searle).

ESTROGESTIN A. (Harvey) Estrogenic substance 1 mg, progesterone 10 mg/ml in peanut oil. Vial 10 ml.
Use: Estrogen, progestin combination.

ESTROGESTIN C. (Harvey) Estrogenic substance 1 mg, progesterone 12.5 mg/ml in peanut oil. Vial 10 ml.
Use: Estrogen, progestin combination.

ESTROJECT. (Mayrand) Estrogenic substance. **2 mg/ml:** Vial 10 ml, 30 ml. **5 mg/ml:** Vial 10 ml.
Use: Estrogen.

ESTROJECT-2. (Mayrand) Estrogenic substance or estrogens, sodium carboxymethylcellulose, povidone, benzyl alcohol, methyl and propyl parabens. Aqueous susp. Inj. Vial 10 ml, 30 ml.
Use: Estrogen.

ESTROJECT-LA. (Mayrand) Estradiol cypionate in oil 5 mg/ml. Inj. Vial 10 ml.
Use: Estrogen.

ESTROLAN. (Lannett) Estrogenic substance natural in oil 10,000 IU/ml. Vial 30 ml.
Use: Estrogen.

ESTRONE, U.S.P. XXII. Inj., Sterile susp., U.S.P. XXII. 3-Hydroxy-estra-1,3,5(10)-trien-17-one. Oil Inj., Femidyn, follicular hormone, folliculin, follicunodis, cristallovar, glandubolin, hiestrone, ketohydroxy-estratriene, ketohydroxyestrin. 1 mg equals 10,000 IU.
Use: Estrogen.
See: Bestrone Suspension, Inj. (Bluco).
Estrogenic Substances in Aqueous Susp. (Wyeth-Ayerst).
Foygen, Vial (Foy).
Menagen, Cap. (Parke-Davis).
Menformon (A), Vial (Organon).
Par-Supp, Vag. Supp. (Parmed).
Propagon-S, Inj. (Spanner).
Theelin, Vial, Aqueous and Oil (Parke-Davis).
W/Hydrocortisone acetate.
See: Estro-V HC, Supp. (Webcon).
W/Estradiol, potassium estrone sulfate.
Tri-Orapin (Standex).
W/Estradiol, vitamin B_{12}.
See: Ovest, Tab. (Trimen).
Ovulin, Inj. (Sig).
W/Estriol, estradiol.
See: Estro Plus, Tab., Vial (Rocky Mtn.).
Hormonin, Tab. (Carnrick).
W/Estrogens.
See: Estrogenic Mixtures, Preps. (Various Mfr.).
Estrogenic Substances, Preps. (Various Mfr.).
W/Lactose.
See: Estrovag, Supp. (Fellows-Testagar).
W/Potassium estrone sulfate.
See: Dura-Keelin, Vial (Pharmex).
Estro Plus, Inj. (Rocky Mtn.).
Mer-Estrone, Inj. (Keene).
Sodestrin, Inj. (Solvay).
Spanestrin-P, Vial (Savage).
W/Progesterone.
See: Duovin-S, Inj. (Spanner).
W/Testosterone.
See: Andesterone, Vial (Lincoln).
Anestro, Inj. (Hauck).
Di-Hormone, Susp. (Paddock).
Di-Met Susp. (Organon).
Diorapin (Standex).
Dl-Steroid, Vial (Kremers-Urban).
Estratest, Tab. (Solvay).
Estrone-Testosterone, Vial (Maurry).
W/Testosterone, progesterone.
See: Tripole-F, Inj. (Spanner).
W/Testosterone, sodium carboxymethylcellulose, sodium Cl.
See: Tostestro, Inj. (Bowman).
W/Testosterone, vitamins.
See: Android-G, Vial (Brown).
Geratic Forte, Inj. (Keene Pharm.).
Geriamic, Tab. (Vortech).
Geritag, Inj., Cap. (Solvay).
W/Testosterone, vitamin and mineral formula, amino acids.
See: Geramine, Tab., Inj. (Brown).
W/Testosterone propionate.

ESTRONE "5". (Keene) Estrone 5 mg/ml, sodium carboxymethyl- cellulose, povidone, benzyl alcohol, methyl and propyl parabens. Inj. Vial 10 ml.

Use: Estrogen.
ESTRONE SULFATE, PIPERAZINE.
See: Ogen, Tab., Vaginal Cream (Abbott).
ESTRONE SULFATE, POTASSIUM.
See: Estrogen, Vial (Med. Chem.).
Kaytron, Inj. (Pasadena Research).
ESTRONE SULFATE POTASSIUM W/ESTRONE.
See: Dura-Keelin, Vial (Pharmex).
ESTRONOL AQUEOUS. (Central) Estrone 2 mg/ml w/preservatives and stabilizers. Inj. Vial 10 ml, 30 ml.
Use: Estrogen.
ESTRONOL-LA. (Central) Estradiol cypionate in oil 5 mg/ml w/chlorobutanol 0.5%. Inj. Vial 10 ml, Box 6s.
Use: Estrogen.
•**ESTROPIPITATE,** U.S.P. XXII. Vaginal Cream, Tab., U.S.P. XXII. Estrone hydrogen sulfate compound with piperazine (1:1). Piperazine estrone sulfate.
Use: Estrogen.
See: Ogen, Tab., Vaginal Cream (Abbott).
ESTRO PLUS. (Rocky Mtn.) **Inj.:** Estrone 2 mg, potassium estrone sulfate 1 mg/ml. Vial 10 ml. **Tab.:** Estrone 0.7 mg, estriol 0.135 mg, estradiol 0.3 mg/Tab. or estrone 1.4 mg, estriol 0.27 mg, estradiol 0.6 mg/#2 Tab. Bot. 100s.
Use: Estrogen.
ESTROQUIN TABLET. (Sheryl) Purified conjugated estrogens 1.25 mg/Tab. Bot. 100s.
Use: Estrogen.
ESTROVIS. (Parke-Davis) Quinestrol 100 mcg/Tab. Bot. 100s.
Use: Estrogen.
•**ETAFEDRINE HCL.** USAN.
Use: Bronchodilator.
See: Mercodol w/Decapryn, Liq. (Merrell Dow).
Nethamine (Merrell Dow).
•**ETAFILCON A.** USAN.
Use: Contact lens material.
ETALENT. (Roger) Ethaverine HCl 100 mg/Cap. Bot. 50s, 500s.
Use: Peripheral vasodilator.
ETAMIPHYLLINE. B.A.N. 7-(2-Diethylaminoethyl)- theophylline.
Use: Smooth muscle relaxant.
•**ETANIDAZOLE.** USAN.
Use: Antineoplastic (hypoxic cell radiosensitizer).
E-TAPP ELIXIR. (Edwards) Brompheniramine maleate 4 mg, phenylephrine HCl 5 mg, phenylpropanolamine HCl 5 mg/5 ml, alcohol 2.3%. Bot. gal.
Use: Antihistamine, decongestant.
•**ETAROTENE.** USAN.
Use: Keratolytic, topical.
•**ETAZOLATE HYDROCHLORIDE.** USAN.
Use: Antipsychotic.
ETENZAMIDE. B.A.N. 2-Ethoxybenzamide.
Use: Analgesic.
ETERNA 27 CREAM. (Revlon) Pregnenolone acetate 0.5% in cream base.
Use: Emollient.
•**ETEROBARB.** USAN.
Use: Anticonvulsant.
•**ETHACRYNATE SODIUM FOR INJECTION,** U.S.P. XXII. Sodium [2,3-dichloro-4-(2-methylenebutyryl)-phenoxy]acetate.
Use: Diuretic.
See: Edecrin Sodium I.V., Inj. (Merck Sharp & Dohme).
•**ETHACRYNIC ACID,** U.S.P. XXII. Tab., U.S.P. XXII. Acetic acid, [2,3-dichloro-4-(2-methylene-1-oxobutyl)phenoxy].
Use: Diuretic.
See: Edecrin, Tab. (Merck Sharp & Dohme).
•**ETHAMBUTOL HCl,** U.S.P. XXII. Tab., U.S.P. XXII. (+)-2,2′-(Ethylenediimino)-di-1-butanol Di HCl.
Use: Antitubercular.
See: Myambutol HCl (Lederle).
ETHAMICORT.
See: Hydrocortamate.
ETHAMIVAN. B.A.N. NN-Diethylvanillamide.
Use: Central nervous system stimulant.
•**ETHAMSYLATE.** USAN. Diethylammonium 2,5-dihydroxybenzenesulfonate. Dicynene.
Use: Hemostatic.
ETHANOL. (Various Mfr.) Alcohol, anhydrous. Alcohol, U.S.P. XXII.
ETHANOLAMINE. Olamine.
•**ETHANOLAMINE OLEATE.** USAN.
Use: Sclerosing agent.
ETHAQUIN. (Ascher) Ethaverine HCl 100 mg/Tab. Bot. 100s, 500s, 1000s.
Use: Peripheral vasodilator.
ETHASULFATE SODIUM. Sodium 2-Ethyl-1-hexanol sulfate.
ETHAVERINE HYDROCHLORIDE. The ethyl analog of papaverine HCl, 6,7-diethoxy-1-(3′,4′-diethoxybenzyl) isoquinoline HCl. Diquinol HCl, Preparin HCl, Perperine HCl. The tetraethyl homolog of papaverine is 2 to 4 times more active and less than half as toxic as the parent drug. (Lincoln) Tab. (0.5 gr) Bot. 100s, 300s.
Vial (15 mg/ml) 10 ml.
Use: Antispasmodic.
See: Etalent, Cap. (Roger).
Ethaquin, Tab. (Ascher).
Neopavrin, Tab., Elix. (Savage).
Roldiol, Tab. (Robinson).
Spasodil, Tab. (Rand).
(Pharmex) Vial 15 mg/ml, 20 mg/ml, 45 mg/ml, 75 mg/ml.
ETHAVEROL "75." (Pharmex) Ethaverine HCl 75 mg/ml. Vial 10 ml.
Use: Peripheral vasodilator.

ETHAVEX-100 TABLETS. (Econo Med) Ethaverine HCl 100 mg/Tab. Bot. 100s, 1000s.
Use: Peripheral vasodilator.

•**ETHCHLORVYNOL,** U.S.P. XXII. Cap., U.S.P. XXII. 1-Chloro-3-ethyl-1-penten-4 yn-3-ol.
Use: Hypnotic, sedative.
See: Placidyl, Cap. (Abbott).
Serensil, Prods. (Ciba).

ETHEBENECID. B.A.N. 4-Diethylsulamoyl benzoic acid.
Use: Uricosuric.

ETHENOL, HOMOPOLYMER. Polyvinyl Alcohol, U.S.P. XXII.

ETHENZAMIDE. o-Ethoxybenzamide.

•**ETHER,** U.S.P. XXII. Ethyl ether.
Use: General anesthetic.

ETHIAZIDE. B.A.N. 6-Chloro-3-ethyl-3,4-dihydro-1,2,4-benzothiadiazine-7-sulfonamide 1,1-dioxide.
Use: Diuretic.

•**ETHINYL ESTRADIOL,** U.S.P. XXII. Tab., U.S.P. XXII. 17-Ethinyl-3,17-estradiol. 19-Norpregna-1,3,5(10)-trien-20-yne-3,17-diol,(17α)-. 19-Nor-17α-pregna-1, 3,5-(10)-trien-20-yne-3,17-diol.
Use: Estrogen.
See: Estinyl, Tab. (Schering).
Feminone, Tab. (Upjohn).
Lynoral, Tab. (Organon).
Menolyn, Tab. (Arcum).
Ovogyn, Tab. (Pasadena Research).

ETHINYL ESTRADIOL W/COMBINATIONS
See: Ardiatric, Tab. (Burgin-Arden).
Brevicon, Tab. (Syntex).
Demulen, Tab. (Searle).
Halodrin, Tab. (Upjohn).
Loestrin 1/20, Tab. (Parke-Davis).
Loestrin 1.5/30, Tab. (Parke-Davis).
Lo/Ovral, Tab. (Wyeth-Ayerst).
Modicon 21 and 28, Tab. (Ortho).
Nordette, Tab. (Wyeth-Ayerst).
Norinyl, Prods. (Syntex).
Norlestrin, Tab. (Parke-Davis).
Norlestrin Fe, Tab. (Parke-Davis).
Ortho-Novum 1/35, 21 and 28 (Ortho).
Os-Cal-Mone, Tab. (Marion).
Ovcon-35, Tab. (Mead Johnson).
Ovcon-50, Tab. (Mead Johnson).
Ovlin, Vial (ICN).
Ovral, Tab. (Wyeth-Ayerst).
Triphasil, Tab. (Wyeth-Ayerst).

ETHINYL ESTRADIOL AND DIMETHISTERONE TABLETS.
Use: Estrogen, progestin combination.

ETHINYL ESTRENOL.
See: Lynestrenol (Organon).

•**ETHIODIZED OIL INJECTION,** U.S.P. XXII.
Use: Diagnostic aid (radiopaque medium).
See: Ethiodol, Inj. (Savage).

•**ETHIODIZED OIL I-131.** USAN. Radioactive iodine addition to ethyl ester of poppyseed oil. Ethiodal-131.
Use: Antineoplastic, radioactive agent.

ETHIODOL. (Savage) Ethiodized oil. Fatty acid ethyl ester of poppy-seed oil, iodine 37%. Inj. Amp. 10 ml, Box 2s.
Use: Diagnostic aid.

•**ETHIOFOS.** USAN.
Formerly gammaphos.
Use: Radioprotector.

•**ETHIONAMIDE,** U.S.P. XXII. Tab., U.S.P. XXII. 2-Ethylthioisonicotinamide. 4-Pyridinecarbothioamide, 2-ethyl.
Use: Tuberculostatic.
See: Trecator S.C., Tab. (Wyeth-Ayerst).

ETHISTERONE. 17-Hydroxy-17a-pregn-4-en-20-yn-3-one.
See: Anhydrohydroxyprogesterone (Various Mfr.).

ETHMOZINE. (DuPont) Moricizine HCl 200 mg, 250 mg or 300 mg/Tab. Bot. 21s, 100s, UD 100s.
Use: Antiarrhythmic.

ETHOCAINE.
See: Procaine HCl (Various Mfr.).

ETHOCYLORVYNOL. β-Chlorovinyl ethyl ethynyl carbinol. Ethchlorvynol, U.S.P. XXII.

ETHODRYL.
See: Diethylcarbamazine Citrate.

ETHOGLUCID. B.A.N. 1,2:15,16-Diepoxy-4,7,10,-13-tetraoxahexadecane.
Use: Antineoplastic agent.

ETHOHEPTAZINE. B.A.N. Ethyl hexahydro-1-methyl-4-phenylazepine-4-carboxylate.
Use: Analgesic.

ETHOHEPTAZINE CITRATE. Ethyl Hexahydro-1-methyl-4-phenylazepine-4-carboxylate Dihydrogen citrate. Ethyl Hexahydro-1-methyl-4-phenyl-1H-azepine-4-carboxylate Citrate (1:1).

ETHOHEXADIOL. Ethyl hexanediol, 2-ethylhexane-1,3-diol, Rutgers 612. Used in Comp. Dimethyl Phthalate.
Use: Insect repellent.

ETHOMOXANE. B.A.N. 2-Butylaminomethyl-8-ethoxy-1,4-benzodioxan.
Use: Adrenaline antagonist.

ETHON TABS. (Major) Methyclothiazide 2.5 mg or 5 mg/Tab. **2.5 mg:** Bot. 100s. **5 mg:** Bot. 100s, 1000s.
Use: Diuretic.

•**ETHONAM NITRATE.** USAN. Ethyl 1-(1,2,3-4-tetrahydro-1-naphthyl)imidazole-5-carboxylate nitrate.
Use: Fungicide.

•**ETHOPROPAZINE HYDROCHLORIDE,** U.S.P. XXII. Tab. U.S.P. XXII. 10H-Phenothiazine-10-ethanamine, N,N-diethyl-α-methyl-,monohydrochloride. 10-[2-(Diethylamino)propyl]-phenothiazine monohydrochloride. Lysivane.
Use: Antiparkinsonian.
See: Parsidol HCl, Tab. (Warner-Chilcott).

ETHOSALAMIDE. B.A.N. 2-(2-Ethoxyethoxy) benzamide.
Use: Analgesic; antipyretic.

•**ETHOSUXIMIDE,** U.S.P. XXII. Cap., U.S.P. XXII. 2-Ethyl-2-methyl-succinimide.

Use: Anticonvulsant.
See: Zarontin, Cap., Syr. (Parke-Davis).

ETHOTOIN. B.A.N. 3-Ethyl-5-phenylimidazoline-2,4-dione.
Use: Anticonvulsant.
See: Peganone, Tab. (Abbott).

ETHOVAN. Ethyl Vanillin.

ETHOXZOLAMIDE. 6-Ethoxy-2-benzothiazolesulfonamide.
Use: Carbonic anhydrase inhibitor.

ETHRANE. (Anaquest) Enflurane. Volatile Liq. Bot. 125 ml, 250 ml.
Use: General anesthetic.

•**ETHYBENZTROPINE.** USAN. 3-(diphenylmethoxy)-8-ethylnortropane. Panolid. Methylbenztropine.
Use: Anticholinergic.

•**ETHYL ACETATE,** N.F. XVII.
Use: Flavor.

ETHYL AMINOBENZOATE. Anesthesin, anesthrone, benzocaine, parathesin.
Use: Local anesthetic.
See: Benzocaine (Various Mfr.).

ETHYL BISCOUMACETATE. B.A.N. Ethyl di(4-hydroxycoumarin-3-yl)acetate.
Use: Anticoagulant.

ETHYL BISCOUMACETATE. 3,3′-(Carboxymethylene) bis (4-hydroxycoumarin) ethyl ester. Ethyl Bis (4-hydroxy-2-oxo-2H-1-benzopyran-3-yl) acetate.

ETHYL BROMIDE. (Various Mfr.) Bromoethane.
Use: General anesthetic.

ETHYL CARBAMATE.
See: Urethan (Various Mfr.).

•**ETHYLCELLULOSE,** N.F. XVII.
Use: Tablet binder.

•**ETHYLCELLULOSE AQUEOUS DISPERSION,** N.F. XVII.
Use: Tablet binder.

ETHYL CHAULMOOGRATE.
Use: Hansen's disease, sarcoidosis.

•**ETHYL CHLORIDE,** U.S.P. XXII. Chloroethane.
Use: Local anesthetic.
See: Gebauer-Spra-Pak.
Stratford-Cook-Spray, 100 Gm.

•**ETHYL DIBUNATE.** USAN. Ethyl 2,7-di-t-butylnaphthalene-1-sulfonate.
Use: Cough suppressant.

ETHYL DIIODOBRASSIDATE. Iodobrassid. Lipoiodine.

ETHYLDIMETHYLAMMONIUM BROMIDE.
See: Ambutonium Bromide.

ETHYLENE. (Various Mfr.) Ethene.
Use: General anesthetic.

•**ETHYLENEDIAMINE,** U.S.P. XXII.
Use: Component of aminophylline.

ETHYLENEDIAMINE SOLUTION. (67% w/v).
Use: Solvent (Aminophylline Inj.).

ETHYLENEDIAMINETETRAACETIC ACID.
See. Edathamil, EDTA (Various Mfr.).

ETHYLENEDIAMINE TETRAACETIC ACID DISODIUM SALT.
See: Endrate Disodium, Amp. (Abbott).

ETHYLESTRENOL. B.A.N. 17α-Ethylestr-4-en-17β-ol.
Use: Anabolic steroid.

ETHYLHYDROCUPREINE HCl. 0[6′] Ethylhydrocupreine monohydrochloride.
Use: Antiseptic.

ETHYLMETHYLTHIAMBUTENE. B.A.N. 3-Ethylmethylamino-1,1-di-(2-thienyl)but-1-ene.
Use: Narcotic analgesic.

ETHYLMORPHINE HYDROCHLORIDE. 7,8-Didehydro-4,5α-epoxy-3-ethoxy-17-methyl-morphinan-6α-ol Hydrochloride. Dionin.
Use: Narcotic.

ETHYL NITRITE SPIRIT. Ethyl nitrite. Sweet Spirit of Niter. Spirit of Nitrous Ether.

•**ETHYLNOREPINEPHRINE HCl,** U.S.P. XXII. Inj., U.S.P. XXII.
Use: Bronchodilator.
See: Bronkephrine, Amp. (Winthrop Pharm).

•**ETHYL OLEATE,** N.F. XVII.
Use: Pharmaceutic aid (vehicle).

ETHYL OXIDE; ETHYL ETHER,
Use: Solvent.

ETHYLPAPAVERINE HCl.
See: Ethaverine HCl (Various Mfr.).

•**ETHYLPARABEN,** N.F. XVII. Ethyl p-Hydroxybenzoate.
Use: Pharmaceutic aid (antifungal preservative).

ETHYL PYROPHOSPHATE. B.A.N. Tetraethyl pyrophosphate.
Use: Treatment of myasthenia gravis.

ETHYLSTIBAMINE. Astaril, neostibosan.
Use: Antimony therapy.

ETHYL VANILLATE. Ethyl-hydroxy-methoxy-benzoate.

•**ETHYL VANILLIN,** N.F. XVII. 3-Ethoxy-4-hydroxybenzaldehyde.
Use: Flavor.

•**ETHYNERONE.** USAN.
Use: Progestin.

•**ETHYNODIOL DIACETATE,** U.S.P. XXII. 19-Nor-17α-pregn-4-en-20-yne-3B,17-diol diacetate; 17α-ethynyl-4-estrene-3β,17β-diol diacetate.
Use: As progesterone, progestin.
See: Ovulen, Tab. (Searle).
W/Ethinyl estradiol.
See: Demulen, Preps. (Searle).
W/Mestranol.
See: Ovulen, Tab. (Searle).

•**ETHYNODIOL DIACETATE AND ETHINYL ESTRADIOL TABLETS,** U.S.P. XXII.
Use: Oral contraceptive.

•**ETHYNODIOL DIACETATE AND MESTRANOL TABLETS,** U.S.P. XXII.
Use: Oral contraceptive.

ETHYNYLESTRADIOL.
See: Ethinyl Estradiol, U.S.P. (Various Mfr.)
Mestranol (Various Mfr.).

ETHYNYLESTRADIOL 3-METHYL ETHER.

See: Enovid, Tab. (Searle).

•**ETIBENDAZOLE.** USAN.
Use: Anthelmintic.

ETICYLOL. (Ciba) Ethinyl estradiol.
Use: Estrogen.

•**ETIDOCAINE.** USAN. (±)-2-(N-Ethylpropylamino)-butyro-2′,6′-xylidide.
Use: Local anesthetic.
See: Duranest (base and hydrochloride).

•**ETIDRONATE DISODIUM,** U.S.P. XXII. Tab., U.S.P. XXII. The disodium salt of (1-Hydroxyethylidene) diphosphonic acid.
Use: Treatment of symptomatic Paget's disease of bone (osteitis deformans).
See: Didronel, Tab. (Procter & Gamble).

•**ETIDRONIC ACID.** USAN. (1-Hydroxy-ethylidene) diphosphonic acid.
Use: Bone calcium regulator.

ETIFENIN. USAN.
Use: Diagnostic aid.

ETIFOXINE. B.A.N. 6-Chloro-2-ethylamino-4-methyl-4-phenyl-4H-3,1-benzoxazine.
Use: Tranquilizer.

ETINTIDINE HYDROCHLORIDE. USAN.
Use: Antagonist.

ETISAZOLE. V.B.A.N. 3-Ethylamino-1,2-benzisothiazole.
Use: Fungicide, veterinary medicine.

ETOCRYLENE. USAN.
Use: Ultraviolet screen.

ETODOLAC. USAN.
Use: Anti-inflammatory.
See: Lodine (Wyeth-Ayerst).

ETOFENAMATE. USAN.
Use: Analgesic, anti-inflammatory.

ETOFORMIN HYDROCHLORIDE. USAN.
Use: Antidiabetic.

ETOMIDATE. USAN.
Use: Hypnotic.

ETOMIDE HYDROCHLORIDE. Bandol. Carbiphene HCl.

ETONITAZENE. B.A.N. 1-(2-Diethylaminoethyl)-2-(4-ethoxybenzyl)-5-nitrobenzimidazole.
Use: Narcotic analgesic.

ETOPOSIDE. USAN.
Use: Antineoplastic.
See: Vepesid, Inj., Cap. (Bristol).

ETOPRINE. USAN.
Use: Antineoplastic.

ETOQUINOL SODIUM. Name used for Actinoquinol sodium.

ETORPHINE. B.A.N. 7,8-Dihydro-7α-[1(R)-hydroxy-1-methylbutyl]-0[6]-methyl-6,14-endoethenomorphine.
Use: Narcotic analgesic.

ETOVAL.
See: Butethal, N.F. (Various Mfr.).

ETOXADROL HYDROCHLORIDE. USAN.
Use: Anesthetic.

ETOXERIDINE. B.A.N. Ethyl 1-[2-(2-hydroxyethoxy)ethyl]-4-phenylpiperidine-4-carboxylate.
Use: Narcotic analgesic.

•**ETOZOLIN.** USAN.
Use: Diuretic.

ETRAFON (2-10). (Schering) Perphenazine 2 mg, amitriptyline HCl 10 mg/Tab. Bot. 100s, 500s, UD 100s.
Use: Psychotherapeutic combination.

ETRAFON (2-25). (Schering) Perphenazine 2 mg, amitriptyline HCl 25 mg/Tab. Bot. 100s, 500s, UD 100s.
Use: Psychotherapeutic combination.

ETRAFON-A (4-10). (Schering) Perphenazine 4 mg, amitriptyline HCl 10 mg/Tab. Bot. 100s, UD 100s.
Use: Psychotherapeutic combination.

ETRAFON FORTE TABLETS (4-25). (Schering) Perphenazine 4 mg, amitriptyline HCl 25 mg/Tab. Bot. 100s, 500s, UD 100s.
Use: Psychotherapeutic combination.

•**ETRETINATE.** USAN.
Use: Antipsoriatic.
See: Tegison, Cap. (Roche).

ETRYNIT. Propatyl nitrate.
Use: Coronary agent.

•**ETRYPTAMINE ACETATE.** USAN. 3-(2-Aminobutyl)-indole Acetate.
Use: Central stimulant.
See: Monase (Upjohn).

ETS-2%. (Paddock) Erythromycin topical 2%. Soln. Bot. 60 ml.
Use: Anti-acne.

ETTRIOL TRINITRATE.
See: Propatyl nitrate.

ETYBENZATROPINE. Ethybenztropine.

ETYNODIOL ACETATE. Ethynodiol Diacetate.

EUBASIN.
See: Sulfapyridine (Various Mfr.).

EUCAINE HCl. 2,2,6-Trimethyl-4-piperidinol benzoate HCl.

EUCALYPTOL. 1,8-Epoxy-p-menthane.
Use: Pharmaceutic aid (flavor), antitussive, nasal decongestant.
See: Vicks Sinex, Nasal Spray (Vicks).
Vicks Va-Tro-Nol, Nose Drops (Vicks).
Vicks Prods. (Vicks).

•**EUCALYPTUS OIL,** N.F. XVII.
Use: Flavor, antitussive, nasal decongestant, expectorant, topical analgesic.
See: Vicks Prods. (Vicks).
Victors Regular, Cherry Loz. (Vicks).

EUCAPINE SYRUP. (Lannett) Ammonium Cl 10 gr, potassium guaiacol-sulfonate 8 gr. White pine and wild cherry syrup. Bot. pt, gal.
Use: Expectorant.

•**EUCATROPINE HYDROCHLORIDE,** U.S.P. XXII. Ophth. Soln., U.S.P. XXII. 1,2,2,6-Tetramethyl-4-piperidyl mandelate HCl. Benzeneacetic acid, alpha-hydroxy-, 1,2,2,6-tetramethyl-4-piperidinyl ester hydrochloride. (Glogau) Crystal, Bot. Gm.
Use: Pharmaceutical necessity for ophthalmic dosage form.

EUCERIN. (Beiersdorf) Unscented moisturizing formula. **Creme:** Jar 120 Gm, lb. **Lot.:** Bot. 240 ml, 480 ml.
Use: Emollient.
EUCODAL.
See: Oxycodone (No Mfr. currently lists).
EUCORAN.
See: Nikethamide (Various Mfr.).
EUCUPIN DIHYDROCHLORIDE. Isoamylhydrocupreine dihydrochloride.
EUFLAVINE.
See: Acriflavine (Various Mfr.).
•**EUGENOL,** U.S.P. XXII. (Various Mfr.) 4-Allyl-2-methoxy-phenol. Phenol, 2-methoxy-4-(2-propenyl)-.
Use: Dental analgesic, oral anesthetic.
See: Benzodent, Oint. (Vicks).
EUKADOL.
See: Dihydrohydroxycodeinone, Preps. (No Mfr. currently lists).
EULCIN. (Leeds) Methscopolamine bromide 2.5 mg, butabarbital sodium 10 mg, aluminum hydroxide gel, dried, 250 mg, magnesium trisilicate 250 mg/Tab. Bot. 100s.
Use: Anticholinergic/antispasmodic, sedative/hypnotic, antacid.
EULEXIN. (Schering) Flutamide 125 mg/Cap. 100s, 500s, UD 100s.
Use: Antineoplastic agent.
EUMYDRIN DROPS. (Winthrop Products) Atropine methonitrate.
Use: Anticholinergic/antispasmodic.
EUNERYL.
See: Phenobarbital (Various Mfr.).
EUPHORBIA COMPOUND. (Sherwood) Euphorbia pilulifera fluidextract 1.5 ml, iobelia tincture 2.2 ml, nitroglycerin spirit 0.29 ml, sodium iodide 1.04 Gm, sodium bromide 1.04 Gm, alcohol 24%/30 ml. Bot. pt, gal.
Use: Sedative/hypnotic, expectorant.
EUPHORBIA PILULIFERA.
W/Cocillana, squill, antimony potassium tartrate, senega.
See: Cylana, Syr. (Bowman).
W/Phenyl salicylate and various oils.
See: Rayderm, Oint. (Velvet Pharmacal).
EUPRACTONE. (Travenol) Dimethadione.
EUPRAX. Albution.
•**EUPROCIN HCl.** USAN. $O^{6'}$-Isopentylhydrocupreine dihydrochloride.
Use: Topical anesthetic.
See: Eucupin HCl.
EUQUININE. Quinine ethyl carbonate.
Use: Antimalarial, antipyretic.
EURAX CREAM. (Westwood) Crotamiton 10% in vanishing-cream base of glyceryl monostearate, anhydrous lanolin, PEG 6-32, glycerin, polysorbate 80, water, benzyl alcohol, mineral oil, white wax, quaternium-15, fragrance. Tube 60 Gm.
Use: Scabicide/pediculocide.
EURAX LOTION. (Westwood) Crotamiton 10% in emollient-lotion base of glyceryl monostearate, anhydrous lanolin, PEG 6-32, glycerin, polysorbate 80, water, benzyl alcohol, light mineral oil, carboxymethylcellulose, simethicone, quaternium-15, fragrance. Bot. 60 Gm, 454 Gm.
Use: Scabicide/pediculocide.
EUTHROID. (Parke-Davis) Liotrix (sodium levothyroxine and sodium liothyronine combined in T_4:T_3 4:1 ratio). Available as: **½:** T_4=30 mcg, T_3=7.5 mcg Bot. 100s. **1:** T_4=60 mcg, T_3=15 mcg Bot. 100s, 1000s. **2:** T_4=120 mcg, T_3=30 mcg Bot. 100s. **3:** T_4=180 mcg, T_3=45 mcg Bot. 100s.
Use: Thyroid hormone.
EUTONYL. (Abbott) Pargyline HCl 10 mg/Tab. Bot. 100s.
Use: Antihypertensive.
EVAC-Q-KIT. (Adria) Each kit contains: **Evac-Q-Mag:** Magnesium citrate 300 ml, citric acid, potassium citrate. **Evac-Q-Tabs:** 2 tab. phenolphthalein 130 mg/Tab. **Evac-Q-Sert:** 2 supp. containing potassium bitartrate, sodium bicarbonate/supp. in polyethylene glycol base. Patient instruction sheet.
Use: Bowel evacuant.
EVAC-Q-KWIK. (Adria) Each kit contains: **Evac-Q-Mag:** magnesium citrate 300 ml, citric acid, potassium citrate in cherry-flavored base. **Evac-Q-Tabs:** 2 tab. phenolphthalein 130 mg. **Evac-Q-Kwik Supp.:** bisacodyl 10 mg.
Use: Bowel evacuant.
EVAC SUPPOSITORIES. (Burgin-Arden) Sodium bicarbonate, sodium biphosphate, dioctyl sodium sulfosuccinate 50 mg/Supp.
Use: Laxative.
EVAC TABLETS. (Burgin-Arden) Guar gum 300 mg, danthron 50 mg, sodium 100 mg/Tab.
Use: Laxative.
EVACTOL. (Delta) Docusate sodium 100 mg, sodium carboxymethyl cellulose 200 mg/Cap. Pkg. 10s, Bot. 10s, 30s, 100s.
Use: Laxative.
EVAC-U-LAX. (Mallard) Yellow phenolphthalein 80 mg/Chew. tab. Bot. 100s.
Use: Laxative.
•**EVANS BLUE,** U.S.P. XXII. Inj., U.S.P. XXII. 1,3-Naphthalenedisulfonic acid, 6,6′-[(3,3′-dimethyl[1,1′-biphenyl]-4,4′-diyl)bis(azo)]bis[4-amino-5-hydroxy]-, tetrasodium salt. Azovan Blue, B.A.N. (Harvey) Pure diazo dye. Amp. (0.5%) 5 ml 12s, 25s, 100s.
Use: Diagnostic aid (blood volume determination).
EVERONE. (Hyrex) Testosterone enanthate in oil 100 mg or 200 mg/ml. Vial 10 ml.
Use: Androgen.
EVICYL TABLETS. (Winthrop Products) Inositol hexanicotinate.
Use: Hypolipidemic, peripheral vasodilator.
EVIRON. (Delta) Ferrous fumarate 160 mg, copper 1 mg, ascorbic acid 75 mg/Tab.
Use: Mineral supplement.

E-VISTA. (Seatrace) Hydroxyzine HCl 50 mg/ml Inj. Vial 10 ml.
Use: Antianxiety agent.
E-VITAL CREME. (Pasadena Research) Vitamins E 100 IU, A 250 IU, D 100 IU, d-panthenol 0.2%, allantoin 0.1%/Gm. Jar 2 oz, lb.
Use: Emollient.
EVITAMIN OINTMENT. (Forest) d-alpha tocoph erol acetate 30 IU/Gm. Tube 1.5 oz. Jar 2 oz, lb.
Use: Emollient.
EWIN NINOS TABLETS. (Winthrop Products) Aspirin.
Use: Salicylate analgesic.
EXAMETAZINE. USAN.
Use: Diagnostic aid, cerebrovascular disease.
EXAPROLOL HYDROCHLORIDE. USAN.
Use: Antiadrenergic.
EX-AQUA. (E.J. Moore) Extract of buchu, extract of uva ursi, extract of corn silk, extract of juniper, caffeine/Tab. Bot. 80s.
Use: Diuretic.
EX-CALORIC WAFERS. (Eastern Research) Carboxymethylcellulose 181 mg, methylcellulose 272 mg/Wafer. Bot. 100s, 500s, 5000s.
Use: Diet aid.
EXCEDRIN CAPLETS. (Bristol-Myers) Aspirin 250 mg, acetaminophen 250 mg, caffeine 65 mg/Capl. Bot. 24s, 50s, 80s.
Use: Analgesic combination.
EXCEDRIN P.M. ASPIRIN FREE. (Bristol-Myers) Acetaminophen 500 mg, diphenhydramine citrate 38 mg/Tab. Bot. 10s, 30s, 50s, 80s.
Use: Analgesic, sleep aid.
EXCEDRIN SINUS. (Bristol-Myers) Pseudoephedrine HCl 30 mg, acetaminophen 500 mg/Tab. Bot. 24s.
Use: Decongestant, analgesic.
EXCEDRIN SINUS CAPLET. (Bristol-Myers) Acetaminophen 500 mg, pseudoephedrine HCl 30 mg/Tab. Bot. 24s.
Use: Analgesic, decongestant.
EXCEDRIN TABLETS. (Bristol-Myers) Acetaminophen 250 mg, caffeine 65 mg, aspirin 250 mg/Tab. Bot. 12s, 30s, 60s, 100s, 165s, 225s.
Use: Analgesic combination.
EXCITA EXTRA. (Schmid) Nonoxynol 9 5.6% (Ribbed). Condom. Box 12s.
Use: Condom with spermicide.
EXELDERM. (Westwood) Sulconazole nitrate 1%. Soln. Bot. 30 ml.
Use: Antifungal, external.
EXIDINE SKIN CLEANSER. (Xttrium) Chlorhexidine gluconate 4%, isopropyl alcohol 4%. Bot. 120 ml, 240 ml, 16 oz, 32 oz, gal.
Use: Antiseptic, germicide.
EX-LAX. (Sandoz Consumer) Yellow phenolphthalein 90 mg/chocolate Chew. Tab. or unflavored pill. Chocolate Tab. 6s, 18s, 48s, 72s. Unflavored pill 8s, 30s, 60s.
Use: Laxative.
EX-LAX EXTRA GENTLE. (Sandoz Consumer) Phenolphthalein 65 mg, docusate sodium 75 mg/Tab. Pkg. 24s, 48s.
Use: Laxative.
EXNA. (Robins) Benzthiazide 50 mg/Tab. Bot. 100s.
Use: Diuretic, antihypertensive.
EXOCAINE. (Commerce) Methyl salicylate 25%. Tube 1.3 oz.
Use: External analgesic.
EXOCAINE ODOR FREE. (Commerce) Triethanolamine salicylate 10%. Tube 3 oz.
Use: External analgesic.
EXOCAINE PLUS. (Commerce) Methyl salicylate 30%. Jar 4 oz, Tube 1.3 oz.
Use: External analgesic.
EXOL. Di-isobutyl ethoxy ethyl dimethyl benzyl ammonium Cl.
W/Benzocaine, menthol, calamine, pyrilamine maleate.
EXONIC OT. Dioctyl Sodium Sulphosuccinate.
Use: Laxative.
EXORBIN. (Various Mfr.) Polyamine-methylene resin.
EXOSURF (Burroughs Wellcome) Dipalmitoylphosphatidylcholine (DPPC). Lyophilized pow. Vial 10 ml.
Use: Synthetic lung surfactant.
EXPECTORANT DM COUGH SYRUP. (Weeks & Leo) Dextromethorphan HBr 15 mg, guaifenesin 100 mg/5 ml, alcohol 7.125%. Bot. 6 oz.
Use: Antitussive, expectorant.
EXPENDABLE BLOOD COLLECTION UNIT—ACD. (Travenol) Citric acid 540 mg, sodium citrate 1.49 Gm, dextrose 1.65 Gm/67.5 ml.
Use: Anticoagulant.
EXSEL. (Herbert) Selenium sulfide 2.5% in shampoo/lotion base. Bot. 4 oz.
Use: Antiseborrheic.
EXTEN STRONE 10. (Schlicksup) Estradiol valerate 10 mg/ml. Vial 10 ml.
Use: Estrogen.
EXTEND. (E.J. Moore) Benzocaine, dibucaine. Tube oz.
Use: Local anesthetic.
EXTENDRYL CHEWABLE TABLETS. (Fleming) Chlorpheniramine maleate 2 mg, phenylephrine HCl 10 mg, methscopolamine nitrate 1.25 mg/Chew. tab. Bot. 100s, 1000s.
Use: Antihistamine, decongestant, anticholinergic/antispasmodic.
EXTENDRYL JUNIOR. (Fleming) Chlorpheniramine maleate 4 mg, phenylephrine HCl 10 mg, methscopolamine nitrate 1.25 mg/TD Cap. 100s, 1000s.
Use: Antihistamine, decongestant, anticholinergic/antispasmodic.
EXTENDRYL SENIOR. (Fleming) Chlorpheniramine maleate 8 mg, phenylephrine HCl 20 mg, methscopolamine nitrate 2.5 mg/TD Cap. Bot. 100s, 1000s.
Use: Antihistamine, decongestant, anticholinergic/antispasmodic.
EXTENDRYL SYRUP. (Fleming) Chlorpheniramine maleate 2 mg, phenylephrine HCl 10 mg,

methscopolamine nitrate 1.25 mg/5 ml. Bot. pt, gal.
Use: Antihistamine, decongestant, anticholinergic/antispasmodic.

EXTENZYME SOFLENS PROTEIN CLEANER. (Allergan) Papain, sodium Cl, sodium carbonate, sodium borate, edetate disodium. Vial w/ Tab. 24s. Refill 36s.
Use: Soft contact lens care.

EXTRA STRENGTH ASPIRIN CAPSULES. (Walgreen) Aspirin 500 mg/Cap. Bot. 80s.
Use: Salicylate analgesic.

EXTRA STRENGTH GAS-X. (Sandoz Consumer) Simethicone 125 mg/Tab. Pkg. 18s.
Use: Antiflatulent.

EXTREME COLD FORMULA. (Major) Pseudoephedrine HCl 30 mg, chlorpheniramine maleate 1 mg, dextromethorphan HBr 15 mg, acetaminophen 500 mg/Cap. Bot. 10s.
Use: Decongestant, antihistamine, antitussive, analgesic.

EXUL. (Yorktown Products Co.) Nupra (non-hormonic, nonsteridic extract of beef organs, liver, brain, adrenals) 2000 standard chick units, dehydrated milk (55% fat) 14 Gm, thiamine HCl 0.6 mg, niacinamide 1.2 mg, ferrous gluconate 8.7 mg, cocoa, coconut oil, casein, sucrose, ethyl vanillin malt extract/Wafer. Bot. 25s.
Use: Anti-ulcer agent.

EYE FACE AND BODY WASH STATION. (Lavoptik) Sodium Cl 0.49 Gm, sodium biphosphate 0.4 Gm, sodium phosphate 0.45 Gm/100 ml, benzalkonium Cl 0.005%. Bot. 32 oz.
Use: Emergency wash.

EYE MO. (Winthrop Products) Boric acid, benzalkonium Cl, phenylephrine HCl, zinc sulfate.
Use: Astringent, ophthalmic.

EYE-SED OPHTHALMIC SOLUTION. (Scherer) Boric acid 2.17%, zinc sulfate 0.217%, benzalkonium Cl 0.01% in purified water. Bot. 15 ml.
Use: Astringent, ophthalmic.

EYE-STREAM. (Alcon) Sodium Cl, potassium Cl, calcium Cl, magnesium Cl, benzalkonium Cl 0.013%, sodium citrate, sodium acetate. Bot. 30 ml, 120 ml.
Use: Irrigating agent, ophthalmic.

EYE WASH. (Bausch & Lomb) Sodium Cl Soln. Bot. 4 oz. w/eye cup.
Use: Irrigating agent, ophthalmic.

EZ-DETECT. (NMS) Occult blood screening test. Kit 3s.
Use: Diagnostic aid.

EZ DETECT STREP-A TEST. (NMS) Coated stick test for detection of group A streptococci taken directly from a throat swab.
Use: Diagnostic aid.

EZE PAIN. (Halsey) Acetaminophen 2.5 gr, salicylamide, caffeine/Cap. Bot. 21s.
Use: Analgesic.

EZOL. (Stewart-Jackson) Butalbital 50 mg, caffeine 40 mg, acetaminophen 325 mg. Bot. 100s.
Use: Sedative/hypnotic, analgesic.

EZOL #3. (Stewart-Jackson) Acetaminophen 650 mg, codeine 30 mg. Bot. 100s.
Use: Narcotic analgesic.

F

FACT HOME PREGNANCY TEST. (Advanced Care) Accurate test for pregnancy in 45 minutes, for use as early as 3 days after a missed period. 1 Test kit 1s.
Use: Diagnostic aid.

FACTOR VIII.
See: Antihemophilic Factor.

•**FACTOR IX COMPLEX,** U.S.P. XXII.
Use: Hemostatic.

FACTOR XIII.
See: Fibrogammin.

FACTREL. (Wyeth-Ayerst) Gonadorelin HCl 100 mcg or 500 mcg/Vial w/Amp. of 2 ml sterile diluent.
Use: Diagnostic aid.

•**FADROZOLE HYDROCHLORIDE.** USAN.
Use: Antineoplastic.

FALGOS TABLETS. (Winthrop Products) Acetylsalicylic acid.
Use: Salicylate analgesic.

FALMONOX. (Winthrop Products) Teclozan. Susp., Tab..
Use: Amebicide.

•**FAMOTIDINE.** USAN.
Use: Antagonist (to histamine hydrogen receptors).
See: Pepcid, Tab., Susp., Inj. (Merck Sharp & Dohme).

•**FAMOTIN HCl.** USAN. 1-[(p-Chlorophenoxy)-methyl] -3, 4-dihydroisoquinoline HCl.
Use: Antiviral.

FAMPROFAZONE. B.A.N. 4-Isopropyl-2-methyl-3-[N-methyl-N-(α-methyl-phenethyl)aminomethyl]-1-phenyl-5-pyrazolone.
Use: Analgesic; antipyretic.

•**FANETIZOLE MESYLATE.** USAN.
Use: Immunoregulator.

FANSIDAR. (Roche) Sulfadoxine 500 mg, pyrimethamine 25 mg/Tab. Box 25s.
Use: Antimalarial.

•**FANTRIDONE HCl.** USAN. 5-[3-(Dimethylamino)propyl]-6(5H)-phenanthridinone monohydrochloride monohydrate.
Use: Antidepressant.

FARA-GEL ANTACID TABLETS. (Faraday) Tab. Bot. 100s.
Use: Antacid.

FARAMALS. (Faraday) Vitamins A 10,000 IU, D 2000 IU, B_1 6 mg, B_2 4 mg, B_6 0.5 mg, folic acid 0.1 mg, C 100 mg, calcium pantothenate mg, niacinamide 30 mg, E 5 IU, B_{12} 3 mcg/Tab. Bot. 100s, 250s, 500s, 1000s.
Use: Vitamin/mineral supplement.

FARAMALS-M. (Faraday) Faramals plus calcium 103 mg, cobalt 0.1 mg, copper 1 mg, iodine

0.15 mg, iron 10 mg, magnesium 6 mg, molybdenum 0.2 mg, phosphorus 80 mg, potassium 5 mg, zinc 1.2 mg/Tab. Bot. 100s, 250s, 500s, 1000s.
Use: Vitamin/mineral supplement.

FARAMINS. (Faraday) Vitamins B_1 20 mg, B_2 6 mg, C 40 mg, niacinamide 20 mg, calcium pantothenate 3 mg, B_6 0.5 mg, powdered whole dried liver 125 mg, dried debittered yeast 125 mg, choline dihydrogen citrate 20 mg, inositol 20 mg, dl-methionine 20 mg, folic acid 0.1 mg, B_{12} 10 mcg, ferrous gluconate 30 mg, dicalcium phosphate 250 mg, copper sulfate 5 mg, magnesium sulfate 10 mg, manganese sulfate 5 mg, cobalt sulfate 0.2 mg, potassium Cl 2 mg, potassium iodide 0.15 mg/Tab. Bot. 100s, 250s, 500s, 1000s.
Use: Vitamin/mineral supplement.

FARA-SIN. (Faraday) Tab. Bot. 50s.
Use: Analgesic.

FARATAC. (Faraday) Flat 10 (contac). Cap. Flat 10.

FARATOL. (Faraday) Vitamins A 12,500 IU, D 1000 IU, B_1 20 mg, B_2 6 mg, B_6 0.5 mg, B_{12} 15 mcg, folic acid 0.1 mg, niacinamide 10 mg, calcium pantothenate 3 mg, C 60 mg, E 5 IU, choline dihydrogen citrate 20 mg, inositol 20 mg, dl-methionine 20 mg, whole dried liver 100 mg, dried debittered yeast 100 mg, dicalcium phosphate 200 mg, ferrous gluconate 30 mg, potassium iodide 0.2 mg, magnesium sulfate 7.2 mg, copper sulfate 5 mg, manganese sulfate 3.4 mg, cobalt sulfate 0.2 mg, potassium Cl 1.3 mg, zinc sulfate 2 mg, molybdenum 0.2 mg in a base of alfalfa/Tab. Bot. 100s, 250s, 500s, 1000s.
Use: Vitamin/mineral supplement.

FARATUSS. (Faraday) Coca-Cola base. Bot. 4 oz, 8 oz.
Use: Cough preparation.

FARATUSS JR. (Faraday) Coca-Cola base. Bot. 4 oz.
Use: Cough preparation.

FARBITAL COMPOUND CAPSULES. (Major) Butalbital, caffeine, aspirin. Bot. 100s.
Use: Sedative/hypnotic, salicylate analgesic.

FARBITAL COMPOUND WITH CODEINE #3. (Major) Butalbital, caffeine, aspirin, codeine 30 mg. Bot. 1000s.
Use: Sedative/hypnotic, salicylate analgesic.

FARBITAL TABS. (Major) Butalbital. Bot. 100s.
Use: Sedative/hypnotic.

FARNOQUINONE. 2-Difarnesyl-3-methyl-1, 4-naphthoquinone.

FASTIN. (Beecham Labs) Phentermine HCl 30 mg/Cap. Bot. 100s, 450s. Pack 150s. (5 × 30s).
Use: Anorexiant.

FAT EMULSION, INTRAVENOUS.
See: Liposyn 10% (Abbott).
Liposyn 20% (Abbott).
Travamulsion 10% (Travenol).
Travamulsion 20% (Travenol).
Intralipid 10% (Kabi Vitrum).
Intralipid 20% (Kabi Vitrum).
Soyacal 10% (Alpha Therapeutic).
Soyacal 20% (Alpha Therapeutic).
Liposyn II 10% (Abbott).
Liposyn II 20% (Abbott).

FATHER JOHN'S MEDICINE PLUS. (Oakhurst) Phenylephrine HCl 2.5 mg, chlorpheniramine maleate 1 mg, dextromethorphan HBr 7.5 mg, guaifenesin 30 mg, ammonium Cl 100 mg, sodium citrate/5 ml. Bot. 120 ml, 240 ml.
Use: Decongestant, antihistamine, antitussive, expectorant.

FATTIBASE. (Paddock) Preblended fatty acid suppository base composed of triglycerides of coconut oil and palm kernel oil. Jar 1 lb, 5 lb.
Use: Fatty acid suppository base.

FAT, UNSATURATED.
See: Arcofac, Emul. (Armour).
Lufa, Cap. (USV Pharm.).

FATTY ACIDS, UNSATURATED.
See: Fats, Unsaturated.
Undecylenic Acid (Various Mfr.).

FAZADINIUM BROMIDE. 1,1′-Azobis(3-methyl-2-phenylimidazo[1,2-α]pyridinium bromide).
Use: Neuromuscular blocking agent.

•**FAZARABINE.** USAN.
Use: Antineoplastic.

F.C.A.H. CAPSULES. (Scherer) Chlorpheniramine maleate 4 mg, acetaminophen 162 mg, salicylamide 162 mg/Cap. Bot. 100s, 500s.
Use: Antihistaminic, analgesic.

•**FEBANTEL.** USAN.
Use: Anthelmintic.

FEBERIN. (Arcum) Ferrous gluconate 3 gr, vitamins C 25 mg, B_1 2 mg, B_6 1 mg, B_2 1 mg, niacinamide 5 mg/Tab. Bot. 100s, 1000s.
Use: Vitamin/mineral supplement.

FEBREX ELIXIR. (Pan American) Acetaminophen 125 mg/5 ml. Bot. 16 oz.
Use: Analgesic.

FEBRILE ANTIGENS. (Laboratory Diagnostics) Group O antigens (somatic) are dyed blue and group H antigens (flagellars) are dyed red for clear identification for detection of bacterial agglutinins, bacterial infections. Vial 5 ml.
Use: Diagnostic aid.

FEBRIN. (Jenkins) Acetophenetidin 0.1 Gm, acetylsalicylic acid 0.12 Gm, caffeine 15 mg, camphor monobromated 60 mg/Tab. Bot. 1000s.
Use: Analgesic combination.

FEBRINOL. (Vitarine) Acetaminophen 325 mg/Tab. Bot. 100s, 1000s.
Use: Analgesic.

FE-BRONE. (Forest Pharm.) Vitamins B_{12} 1 IU, folic acid 1 mg, ferrous sulfate exsiccated (powdered) 200 mg, ferrous sulfate exsiccated (timed) 200 mg, C acid 100 mg, B_6 0.5 mg, B_1 2 mg, B_2 1 mg, copper 0.9 mg, zinc 0.5 mg, manganese 0.3 mg/Cap. Bot. 30s, 100s, 1000s.
Use: Vitamin/mineral supplement.

FEDAHIST DECONGEST. (Kremers-Urban) **Syr.:** Pseudoephedrine HCl 30 mg, chlorpheniramine maleate 2 mg/5 ml, saccharin, sorbitol. Alcohol

free. Bot. 120 ml. **Tab.:** Pseudoephedrine HCl 60 mg, chlorpheniramine maleate 4 mg. Bot. 100s.
Use: Decongestant, antihistamine.

FEDAHIST EXPECTORANT. (Kremers-Urban) **Drops:** Pseudoephedrine HCl 7.5 mg, guaifenesin 40 mg/ml. Bot. 30 ml. **Liq.:** Pseudoephedrine HCl 30 mg, guaifenesin 200 mg/5 ml. Bot. 120 ml. **Syr.:** Pseudoephedrine HCl 30 mg, chlorpheniramine maleate 2 mg, guaifenesin 100 mg/5 ml, saccharin, sorbitol. Alcohol free. Bot. 120 ml.
Use: Decongestant, expectorant, antihistamine.

FEDAHIST GYROCAPS. (Kremers-Urban) Pseudoephedrine HCl 65 mg, chlorpheniramine maleate 10 mg/SR Cap. Bot. 100s.
Use: Decongestant, antihistamine.

FEDAHIST TIMECAPS. (Kremers-Urban) Pseudoephedrine HCl 120 mg, chlorpheniramine maleate 8 mg/SR Cap. Bot. 100s.
Use: Decongestant, antihistamine.

FEDRAZIL. (Burroughs Wellcome) Pseudoephedrine HCl 30 mg, chlorcyclizine HCl 25 mg/Tab. Box 24s. Bot. 100s.
Use: Decongestant, antihistamine.

FEDRINAL. (H.L. Moore) Ephedrine HCl 12 mg, phenobarbital 12 mg, potassium iodide 160 mg, theophylline anhydrous 31.2 mg/5 ml. Bot. pt, gal.
Use: Decongestant, sedative/hypnotic, expectorant, bronchodilator.

FEEN-A-MINT DUAL FORMULA. (Plough) Docusate sodium 100 mg, yellow phenolphthalein 65 mg/Tab. Box 15s, 30s, 60s.
Use: Laxative.

FEEN-A-MINT GUM. (Plough) Yellow phenolphthalein 97.2 mg/Chewing gum Tab. Box 5s, 16s, 40s.
Use: Laxative.

FEEN-A-MINT MINT. (Plough) Yellow phenolphthalein 97.2 mg/Chewable mint tab. Box 20s.
Use: Laxative.

FEEN-A-MINT PILLS. (Plough) Docusate sodium 100 mg, yellow phenolphthalein 65 mg/Tab. Box 15s, 30s, 60s.
Use: Laxative.

FEG-L. (Western Research) Ferrous gluconate 300 mg/Tab. Handicount 28s (36 bags of 28 tab.).
Use: Iron supplement.

FEIBA VH IMMUNO. (Immuno-U.S.) Freeze-dried anti-inhibitor coagulant complex. Heparin free. Vapor heated. Inj. Vial with diluent and needle.
Use: Antihemophilic.

•**FELBINAC.** USAN.
Use: Anti-inflammatory.

FELDENE. (Pfizer Laboratories) Piroxicam 10 mg or 20 mg/Cap. **10 mg:** Bot 100s. **20 mg:** Bot. 100s, 500s, UD 100s.
Use: Nonsteroidal anti-inflammatory drug; analgesic.

FELLOBOLIC INJECTION. (Forest Pharm.) Methandriol dipropionate 50 mg/ml. Vial 10 ml.

•**FELODIPINE.** USAN.
Use: Vasodilator.

•**FELYPRESSIN.** USAN. 2-(Phenylalanine)-8-lysine vasopressin.
Use: Vasoconstrictor.

FEMAGENE. (Tennessee) Boric acid, sodium borate, lactic acid, menthol, methylbenzethonium Cl, parachlorometaxylenol, lactose, surface-active agents. Pow. 6 oz.
Use: Feminine hygiene.

FEMAZOLE TABS. (Major) Metronidazole 250 mg or 500 mg/Tab. **250 mg:** Bot. 100s, 250s, 500s. **500 mg:** Bot. 50s, 100s.
Use: Anti-infective.

FEMCAPS. (Buffington) Acetaminophen, caffeine, ephedrine sulfate, atropine sulfate/Tab. Sugar, lactose and salt free Dispens-a-Kit 500s, Aid-paks 100s.
Use: Analgesic, bronchodilator, anticholinergic/antispasmodic.

FEMERGIN.
See: Ergotamine Tartrate (Various Mfr.).

FEMID GREEN LABEL. (Cenci) Sodium bicarbonate, sodium borate, sodium Cl, sodium perborate, menthol. Pow. Bot. 7 oz, 15 oz.
Use: Vaginal cleansing and deodorant.

FEMID PINK LABEL. (Cenci) Sodium lauryl sulfate, aluminum ammonium sulfate, boric acid, citric acid, menthol. Pow. Bot. 7 oz.
Use: Vaginal cleansing and deodorant.

FEMIDINE. (A.V.P.) Povidone-iodine. Bot. 240 ml.
Use: Cleansing douche.

FEMIDYN.
See: Estrone (Various Mfr.).

FEMILAX. (G & W Labs) Docusate sodium 100 mg, phenolphthalein 65 mg/Tab. Bot. 30s, 60s, 90s.
Use: Laxative.

FEMINIQUE DISPOSABLE DOUCHE. (Schmid) Sodium benzoate, sorbic acid, lactic acid, octoxynol-9. Twin-pack Bot. 150 ml.
Use: Douche.

FEMINIQUE DISPOSABLE DOUCHE. (Schmid) Vinegar and water. Soln. Twin-packs. Bot. 150 ml
Use: Douche.

FEMINONE. (Upjohn) Ethinyl estradiol 0.05 mg/Tab. Bot. 100s.
Use: Estrogen.

FEMIRON. (Beecham Products) Iron 20 mg/Tab. Bot 40s, 120s.
Use: Iron supplement.

FEMIRON MULTI-VITAMINS AND IRON. (Beecham Products) Iron 20 mg, vitamins A 5,000 IU, D 400 IU, B_1 1.5 mg, riboflavin 1.7 mg, niacinamide 20 mg, C 60 mg, B_6 2 mg, B_{12} 6 mcg calcium pantothenate 10 mg, folic acid 0.4 mg, E 15 mg/Tab. Bot. 40s, 120s.
Use: Vitamin/mineral supplement.

FEMOTRONE. (Bluco) Progesterone in oil 50 mg/ml. Vial 10 ml.
Use: Progestin.

FEMSTAT VAGINAL CREAM. (Syntex) Butoconazole nitrate 2% in water-washable emollient cream. Tube 28 Gm w/applicators.

Use: Antifungal, vaginal.

ENALAMIDE. USAN. (1) Ethyl N-[2-(diethylamino)-ethyl]-2-ethyl-2-phenylmalonamate; (2) Phenylethylmalonic acid monoethyl ester diethylaminoethylamide.
Use: Smooth muscle relaxant.

ENAMISAL. Phenyl aminosalicylate.

ENAMOLE. USAN. 5-Amino-1-phenyl-1H-tetrazol.
Use: Anti-inflammatory agent.

ENAPRIN TABLETS. (Winthrop Products) Aspirin, chlormezanone.
Use: Salicylate analgesic, antianxiety agent.

ENAROL. (Winthrop Products) Chlormezanone 100 mg or 200 mg/Tab. Bot. 100s.
Use: Antianxiety agent.

ENARSONE.
See: Carbarsone (Various Mfr.).

ENBENDAZOLE. USAN.
Use: Anthelmintic.

ENBUFEN. USAN.
Use: Anti-inflammatory.

ENCAMFAMIN. B.A.N. N-Ethyl-3-phenylbicyclo-[2.2.1]hept-2-ylamine.
Use: Central nervous system stimulant; appetite suppressant.

ENCHLORPHOS. V.B.A.N. OO-Dimethyl O-(2,4,5-trichlorophenyl) phosphorothioate.
Use: Insecticide, veterinary medicine.

ENCILBUTIROL. USAN.
Use: Choleretic.

ENCLOFENAC. USAN. 2-(2,4-Dichlorophenoxy)-phenylacetic acid.
Use: Anti-inflammatory.

ENCLONINE. USAN. dl-3-(p-Chlorophenyl)-alanine. Under study by Pfizer.
Use: Serotonin biosynthesis inhibitor.

NCLORAC. USAN.
Use: Anti-inflammatory.

NCLOZIC ACID. B.A.N. 2-(4-Chlorophenyl)-thiazol-4-ylacetic acid.
Use: Anti-inflammatory.

ND. (Mine Safety Appliances).

A-2—Water soluble cream which forms a physical barrier to water insoluble irritants. Tube 3 oz, Jar lb.

E-2—This cream combines the functions of the water soluble Fend A-2 and water insoluble Fend I-2 creams. Tube 3 oz, Jar lb.

-2—Water insoluble cream which forms a physical barrier to water soluble irritants. Tube 3 oz, Jar lb.

-2—A silicone cream which forms a barrier against a combination of water soluble and water insoluble irritants. Tube 3 oz, Jar lb.

(—Industrial cold cream which rubs well into the skin and serves as a skin conditioner. Tube 3 oz, Jar lb.
se: Skin protectant.

NDOL. (Buffington) Salicylamide, caffeine, actaminophen, phenylephrine HCl/Tab. Sugar, lacose and salt free. Dispens-A-Kit 500s. Bot. 100s.
Use: Analgesic combination.

•**FENDOSAL.** USAN.
Use: Anti-inflammatory.

•**FENESTREL.** USAN. 5-Ethyl-6-methyl-4-phenyl-3-cyclohexene-1-carboxylic acid. Under study.
Use: Nonsteroid estrogen.

•**FENETHYLLINE HYDROCHLORIDE.** USAN. 7-[2-[(α-Methylphenethyl)-amino]-ethyl]theophylline hydrochloride.
Use: Stimulant center.

•**FENFLURAMINE HYDROCHLORIDE.** USAN. N-ethyl-α-methyl-m-(trifluoro-methyl)-phenethylamine hydrochloride.
Use: Sympathomimetic (anorexiant).
See: Pondimin, Tab. (Robins).

•**FENGABINE.** USAN.
Use: Mood regulator.

•**FENIMIDE.** USAN. 3-Ethyl-2-methyl-2-phenylsuccinimide.
Use: Tranquilizer.

•**FENISOREX.** USAN. (±)-cis-7-Fluoro-1-phenylisochroman-3-ylmethylamine.
Use: Anorexigenic.

•**FENMETOZOLE HYDROCHLORIDE.** USAN.
Use: Antidepressant antagonist.

•**FENMETRAMIDE.** USAN.
Use: Antidepressant.

•**FENNEL OIL,** N.F. XVII.
Use: Pharmaceutic aid (flavor).

•**FENOBAM.** USAN.
Use: Sedative.

•**FENOCTIMINE SULFATE.** USAN.
Use: Gastric antisecretory.

•**FENOLDOPAM MESYLATE.** USAN.
Use: Antihypertensive.

•**FENOPROFEN.** USAN. 2-(3-phenoxyphenyl)-propionic acid. (±)-m-Phenoxyhydratropic acid; (2) dl-2-(3-phenoxyphenyl)-propionic acid.
Use: Anti-inflammatory, analgesic.

•**FENOPROFEN CALCIUM,** U.S.P. XXII. Cap., Tab., U.S.P. XXII.
Use: Anti-inflammatory, analgesic.

•**FENOTEROL.** USAN. (1)3,5-Dihydroxy-α-[[(p-hydroxy-α-methylphenethyl) amino] methyl]-benzyl alcohol; (2) 1-(3,5-Dihydroxyphenyl)-2-[[1-(4-hydroxy-benzyl)ethyl]amino] ethanol.
Use: Bronchodilator.

•**FENPIPALONE.** USAN.
Use: Anti-inflammatory.

FENPIPRAMIDE. B.A.N. 2,2-Diphenyl-4-piperidonobutyramide.
Use: Spasmolytic.

FENPIPRANE. B.A.N. 1-(3,3-Diphenylpropyl)-piperidine.
Use: Spasmolytic.

•**FENPRINAST HYDROCHLORIDE.** USAN.
Use: Anti-allergic, bronchodilator.

•**FENPROSTALENE.** USAN.
Use: Luteolysin.

•**FENQUIZONE.** USAN.
Use: Diuretic.

•**FENRETINIDE.** USAN.

Use: Antineoplastic.

•**FENSPIRIDE HYDROCHLORIDE.** USAN.
Use: Bronchodilator, anti-adrenergic.

•**FENTANYL.**
Use: Narcotic analgesic.
See: Duragesic, Transdermal (Janssen).

•**FENTANYL CITRATE,** U.S.P. XXII. Inj. U.S.P. XXII. N-(1-phenethyl-4-piperidyl) propionanilide citrate. Propanamide, N-phenyl-N-[1-(2-phenylethyl)-4-piperidinyl]-,2-hydroxy-1,2,3-propanetricarboxylate (1:1).
Use: Narcotic analgesic.
See: Innovar, Inj. (Janssen).
Sublimaze, Inj. (Janssen).

•**FENTIAZAC.** USAN.
Use: Anti-inflammatory.

•**FENTICLOR.** USAN. Di-(5-chloro-2-hydroxyphenyl)-sulfide.
Use: Antiseptic, fungicide.

•**FENTICONAZOLE NITRATE.** USAN.
Use: Antifungal.

FENTON ELIXIR. (Winthrop Products) Ferrous gluconate.
Use: Iron supplement.

FENYLHIST. (Mallard) Diphenhydramine HCl 25 mg or 50 mg/Cap. Bot. 1000s.
Use: Antihistamine.

FENYRAMIDOL HCl. Phenyramidol HCl.

•**FENYRIPOL HYDROCHLORIDE.** USAN. α-(2-pyrimidinylaminomethyl) benzyl alcohol hydrochloride.
Use: Skeletal muscle relaxant.

FEOCYTE. (Dunhall) Iron 110 mg, vitamins C 100 mg, B_6 2 mg, B_{12} 50 mcg, copper sulfate 2 mg, folic acid 0.8 mg, desiccated liver/Prolonged Action Tab. Bot. 100s.
Use: Vitamin/mineral supplement.

FEOCYTE INJECTABLE. (Dunhall) Peptonized iron 15 mg, vitamin B_{12} 200 mcg, liver injection N.F. beef 10 units, sodium citrate 10 mg, benzyl alcohol 2%/ml. Vial 10 ml.
Use: Vitamin/mineral supplement.

FE-O.D. (Trimen) Iron 100 mg, ascorbic acid 500 mg/Tab. Bot. 100s.
Use: Vitamin/mineral supplement.

FEOSOL CAPSULES. (SmithKline Prods.) Dried ferrous sulfate 159 mg (50 mg iron)/SR Cap. Bot. 30s, 100s, 500s, UD 100s.
Use: Iron supplement.

FEOSOL ELIXIR. (SmithKline Prods.) Ferrous sulfate (44 mg iron) 220 mg/5 ml, alcohol 5%. Bot. 16 oz.
Use: Iron supplement.

FEOSOL TABLETS. (SmithKline Prods.) Dried ferrous sulfate 200 mg (65 mg iron)/Tab. Bot. 100s, 1000s, UD 100s.
Use: Iron supplement.

FEOSTAT. (Forest) **Tab.:** Ferrous fumarate 100 mg (33 mg iron)/Chew. tab. Bot. 100s, 1000s. **Drops:** Ferrous fumarate 45 mg (15 mg iron)/ 0.6 ml. Bot. 60 ml.
Use: Iron supplement.

FEOSTAT SUSPENSION. (Forest) Ferrous fumarate 100 mg (33 mg iron)/5 ml. Bot. 240 ml.
Use: Iron supplement.

FE-PLUS PROTEIN. (Miller) Iron (as an iron-protein complex) 50 mg/Tab. Bot. 100s.
Use: Iron supplement.

FEPRAZONE. B.A.N. 4-(3-Methylbut-2-enyl)-1,2-diphenylpyrazolidine-3,5-dione.
Use: Analgesic; anti-inflammatory.

FERANCEE. (Stuart) Elemental iron 67 mg (from 200 mg ferrous fumarate), ascorbic acid 49 mg, sodium ascorbate 114 mg/Tab. Bot. 100s.
Use: Vitamin/mineral supplement.

FERANCEE-HP. (Stuart) Elemental iron 110 mg (from 330 mg ferrous fumarate), ascorbic acid 350 mg, sodium ascorbate 281 mg/Tab. Bot. 60s.
Use: Vitamin/mineral supplement.

FERATE-C. (Vale) Ferrous fumarate 150 mg, ascorbic acid 200 mg, docusate sodium 25 mg/ Tab. Bot. 100s, 1000s.
Use: Vitamin/mineral supplement.

FER-GEN-SOL DROPS. (Goldline) Ferrous sulfate drops. Bot. 50 ml.
Use: Iron supplement.

FERGON. (Winthrop Consumer) Pure ferrous gluconate. **Tab.:** 320 mg equal to approximately 37 mg ferrous iron/Tab. Bot. 100s, 500s, 1000s. **Elix.:** 300 mg = 35 mg iron/5 ml. Bot. 16 fl. oz.
Use: Iron supplement.

FERGON IRON PLUS CALCIUM. (Winthrop) Calcium 600 mg, vitamin D 125 IU, iron 18 mg/ Capl. Bot. 60s.
Use: Vitamin/mineral supplement.

FERGON PLUS. (Winthrop) Iron 58 mg (from ferrous gluconate) vitamin B_{12} w/intrinsic factor concentrate 0.5 units, ascorbic acid 75 mg/Cap. Bot. 100s.
Use: Vitamin/mineral supplement.

FER-IN-SOL. (Mead Johnson Nutrition) **Drops:** Elemental iron 15 mg/0.6 ml, alcohol 0.02%. Bot. w/dropper 50 ml. **Syr.:** 18 mg/5 ml. Alcohol 5%. Bot. 16 fl oz. **Cap.:** 60 mg. Bot. 100s.
Use: Iron supplement.

FER-IRON. (Various Mfr.) Ferrous sulfate 125 mg (iron 25 mg)/ml. Drops. Bot. 50 ml.
Use: Iron supplement.

FERMALOX. (Rorer Consumer) Iron 40 mg (ferrous sulfate 200 mg) magnesium and aluminum hydroxides (Maalox) 200 mg/Tab. Bot. 100s.
Use: Iron supplement, antacid.

FERMETONE COMPOUND CAPSULES. (Winthrop Products) Pancreatin.
Use: Digestive enzyme.

FERNCORT LOTION. (Ferndale) Hydrocortisone acetate 0.5% in lotion base. Bot. 120 ml.
Use: Corticosteroid.

FEROCYL. (Hudson) Ferrous fumarate 150 mg (iron 50 mg), docusate sodium 100 mg/TR Cap. Bot. 100s.
Use: Iron supplement.

FERO-FOLIC 500. (Abbott) Ferrous sulfate controlled-release (equivalent to 105 mg iron), vita

min C 500 mg, folic acid 800 mcg/Filmtab. Bot. 100s, 500s.
Use: Vitamin/mineral supplement.

FERO-GRAD 500 FILMTAB. (Abbott) Sodium ascorbate 500 mg, ferrous sulfate equivalent to 105 mg iron/CR Filmtab. Bot. 30s, 100s, 500s, UD 100s.
Use: Iron supplement.

FERO-GRADUMET FILMTAB. (Abbott) Ferrous sulfate 525 mg controlled-release equivalent to 105 mg iron/Filmtab. Bot. 100s.
Use: Iron supplement.

FEROLIX. (Century) Ferrous sulfate 5 gr, alcohol 5%/10 ml Elix. Bot. 8 oz, pt, gal.
Use: Iron supplement.

FEROSAN FORTE. (Sandia) Ferrous fumarate 300 mg, liver-stomach concentrate 150 mg, vitamin B_{12} w/intrinsic factor concentrate 7.5 mcg, intrinsic factor concentrate 150 mg, B_{12} 7.5 mcg, ascorbic acid 75 mg, folic acid 1 mg, sorbitol 50 mg/Tab. Bot. 100s.
Use: Vitamin/mineral supplement.

FEROSAN SYRUP. (Sandia) Ferrous fumarate 91.2 mg, B_1 10 mg, B_6 3 mg, B_{12} 25 mcg/5 ml 16 oz, gal.
Use: Iron supplement.

FEROSPACE. (Hudson) Ferrous sulfate 250 mg (iron 50 mg)/TR Cap. Bot. 100s.
Use: Iron supplement.

FEROTRINSIC. (Rugby) Iron 36.3 mg (from ferrous fumarate), vitamins B_{12} 15 mcg, C 75 mg, intrinsic factor (as concentrate or from stomach preparations) 240 mg, folic acid 0.5 mg/Cap. 100s, 1000s.
Use: Vitamin/mineral supplement.

FEROWEET. (Barth's) Vitamins B_1 6 mg, B_2 12 mg, niacin 4 mg, iron 30 mg, B_{12} 10 mcg, B_6 95 mcg, pantothenic acid 50 mcg/3 Cap. Bot. 100s, 500s, 1000s.
Use: Vitamin/mineral supplement.

FERRACOMP. (Hauck) Liver 2 mcg, vitamins B_{12} 15 mcg, B_1 10 mg, B_2 5 mg, B_6 1 mg, calcium pantothenate 1 mg, niacinamide 10 mg, iron 31.3 mg/ml. Vial 30 ml.
Use: Vitamin/mineral supplement.

FERRALET. (Mission) Ferrous gluconate 320 mg (37 mg iron)/Tab. Bot. 100s.
Use: Iron supplement.

FERRALET PLUS. (Mission) Ferrous gluconate equivalent to 46 mg iron, ascorbic acid 400 mg, folic acid 0.8 mg, vitamin B_{12} 25 mcg/Tab. Bot. 100s.
Use: Vitamin/mineral supplement.

FERRALYN LANACAPS. (Lannett) Ferrous sulfate 250 mg (50 mg iron)/TR Cap. Bot. 100s, 500s, 1000s.
Use: Iron supplement.

FERRANOL. (Robinson) Ferrous fumarate 3 gr or 5 gr/Tab. Bot. 100s, 1000s.
Use: Iron supplement.

FERRA-TD. (Goldline) Ferrous sulfate 250 mg (iron 50 mg)/TR Cap. Bot. 100s, 1000s.
Use: Iron supplement.

FERRETS. (Pharmics) Ferrous fumarate 325 mg, iron 106 mg/Tab. Bot. 100s.
Use: Iron supplement.

FERRIC AMMONIUM CITRATE. Ammonium iron (Fe^{+++}) citrate.
Use: Iron supplement.

FERRIC AMMONIUM SULFATE. (Various Mfr.).
Use: Astringent.

FERRIC AMMONIUM TARTRATE. (Various Mfr.).
Use: Iron supplement.

FERRIC CACODYLATE. (Various Mfr.).
Use: Leukemias & iron deficiency.

FERRIC CHLORIDE. (Various Mfr.).
Use: Astringent.

•**FERRIC CHLORIDE Fe 59.** USAN.
Use: Radioactive agent.

FERRIC CITROCHLORIDE TINCTURE. Iron (3+) chloride citrate.
Use: Hematinic.

•**FERRIC FRUCTOSE.** USAN. Fructose iron complex with potassium (2:1).
Use: Hematinic.

FERRIC GLYCEROPHOSPHATE. Glycerol phosphate iron (3+) salt.
Use: Pharmaceutic necessity.

FERRIC HYPOPHOSPHITE. Iron (3+) phosphinate.
Use: Pharmaceutic necessity.

•**FERRICLATE CALCIUM SODIUM.** USAN.
Use: Hematinic.

•**FERRIC OXIDE, RED,** N.F. XVII.
Use: Pharmaceutic aid (color).

•**FERRIC OXIDE, YELLOW,** N.F. XVII.
Use: Pharmaceutic aid (color).

FERRIC "PEPTONATE." (Various Mfr.).
See: Iron Peptonized.

FERRIC PYROPHOSPHATE, SOLUBLE. Iron (3+) citrate pyrophosphate.

FERRIC QUININE CITRATE, "GREEN." (Various Mfr.).
Use: Iron supplement.

FERRIC SUBSULFATE SOLUTION. (Various Mfr.).
Use: Local use on the skin.

FERRINAL-C. (Cenci) Ferrous fumarate 3 gr, vitamin C 150 mg/Tab. Bot. 100s, 1000s.
Use: Iron supplement.

FERRINAL CHRONCAP. (Cenci) Ferrous fumarate 330 mg, thiamine Cl 5 mg/SR Cap. Bot. 30s, 100s.
Use: Vitamin/mineral supplement.

FERRINAL TABLETS. (Cenci) Ferrous fumarate 3 gr/Tab. Bot. 100s, 1000s.
Use: Iron supplement.

FERRIZYME. (Abbott Diagnostics) Enzyme immunoassay for qualitative determination of ferritin in human serum or plasma. Test kit 100s.
Use: Diagnostic aid.

FERROCHOLATE.
See: Ferrocholinate.

FERROCHOLINATE. Ferrocholate. Ferrocholine. A chelate prepared by reacting equimolar quan-

tities of freshly precipitated ferric hydroxide with choline dihydrogen citrate.
Use: Iron supplement.
See: Chel-Iron, Preps. (Kinney).

FERROCHOLINE.
See: Ferrocholinate.
Kelex, Tabseal. (Nutrition).

FERRO-CYTE. (Spanner) Iron peptonate 20 mg, liver injection (20 mg/ml) 0.25 ml, vitamins B_1 22 mg, B_2 0.5 mg, B_6 2.5 mg, B_{12} 30 mcg, niacinamide 25 mg, panthenol 1 mg/ml. Inj. Multiple dose vial 10 ml.
Use: Vitamin/mineral supplement.

FERRO-DOK TR. (Major) Ferrous fumarate 150 mg (iron 50 mg), docusate sodium 100 mg/TR Cap. Bot. 100s.
Use: Iron supplement.

FERRO-DSS. (Geneva Marsam) Ferrous fumarate 150 mg (iron 50 mg), docusate sodium 100 mg/TR Cap. Bot. 100s.
Use: Iron supplement.

FERRODYL CHEWABLE TABLETS. (Arcum) Ferrous fumarate 320 mg, vitamin C 200 mg/Tab. Bot. 100s, 1000s.
Use: Vitamin/mineral supplement.

FERROMAX (INTRAMUSCULAR IRON). (Kenyon) Iron peptonized 100 mg, copper gluconate 0.2 mg, cobalt Cl 4 mg, pectin 10 mg/ml. Vial 10 ml.
Use: Mineral supplement.

FERRONEED. (Hanlon) Ferrous gluconate 300 mg, ascorbic acid 60 mg/Cap. Bot. 100s.
Use: Vitamin/mineral supplement.

FERRONEED T-CAPS. (Hanlon) Ferrous fumarate 250 mg, thiamine HCl 5 mg, ascorbic acid 50 mg/TD Cap. Bot. 100s.
Use: Vitamin/mineral supplement.

FERRONEX. (Pasadena Research) Iron from ferrous gluconate 2.9 mg, Vitamins B_{12} equivalent 1 mcg, B_2 0.75 mg, B_3 50 mg, B_5 1.25 mg, B_{12} 15 mcg, procaine 2%/ml. Inj. Vial 30 ml.
Use: Vitamin/mineral supplement.

FERRO-SEQUELS. (Lederle) Ferrous fumarate 150 mg (equivalent to 50 mg elemental iron), dioctyl sodium sulfosuccinate 100 mg/TD Cap. Bot. 30s, 100s, 1000s, UD 10×10s.
Use: Iron supplement.

FERROSPAN CAPSULES. (Imperial Lab.) Ferrous fumarate 200 mg, ascorbic acid 100 mg/Tab. Bot. 100s, 1000s.
Use: Vitamin/mineral supplement.

FERROSYN INJECTION. (Standex) Cyanocobalamin 30 mcg, liver 2 mcg, ferrous gluconate 100 mg, riboflavin 1.5 mg, panthenol 2.5 mg, niacinamide 100 mg, procaine 2%. Vial 30 ml.
Use: Vitamin/mineral supplement.

FERROSYN S.C. (Standex) Iron 60 mg, vitamin B_{12} 5 mcg, magnesium 0.6 mg, copper 0.3 mg, manganese 0.1 mg, potassium 0.5 mg, zinc 0.15 mg/Tab. Bot. 100s, 1000s.
Use: Vitamin/mineral supplement.

FERROSYN SEE TABS. (Standex) Iron 34 mg, ascorbic acid 60 mg/Tab. Bot. 100s, 1000s.
Use: Vitamin/mineral supplement.

FERROSYN TAB. (Standex) Iron 60 mg, vitamin B_{12} 5 mcg, magnesium 0.6 mg, copper 0.3 mg, manganese 0.1 mg, potassium 0.5 mg, zinc 0.15 mg/Tab. Bot. 100s.
Use: Vitamin/mineral supplement.

FERROUS BROMIDE. (Various Mfr.).
Use: In chorea & tuberculous cervical adenitis.

FERROUS CARBONATE MASS. Vallet's mass. (Various Mfr.).
Use: Iron supplement.

FERROUS CARBONATE, SACCHARATED. (Various Mfr.).
Use: Iron supplement.

•**FERROUS CITRATE Fe-59 INJECTION,** U.S.P. XXII.
Use: Radioactive agent.

•**FERROUS FUMARATE,** U.S.P. XXII. Tab., U.S.P. XXII.
Use: Hematinic.
See: Childron, Susp. (Fleming).
Eldofe, Tab. (Canright).
El-Ped-Ron, Liq. (Elder).
Farbegen, Cap. (Hickam).
Feco-T, Cap. (Blaine).
Fumasorb, Tab. (Marion).
Fumerin, Tab. (Laser).
Ircon, Tab. (Key).
Laud-Iron, Tab., Susp. (Amfre-Grant).
Maniron, Meltab. (Bowman).
W/Ascorbic Acid.
See: C-Ron, Preps. (Solvay).
Cytoferin, Tab. (Wyeth-Ayerst).
Eldofe-C, Tab. (Canright).
Ferancee, Tab. (Stuart).
Ferancee-HP, Tab. (Stuart).
Ferrodyl Chewable Tab. (Arcum).
Min-Hema Chewable, Tab. (Scrip).
W/Ascorbic acid and folic acid.
See: C-Ron F.A., Tab. (Solvay).
W/Docusate sodium.
See: Fer-Regules, Cap. (Quality Generics).
Ferro-Sequels, Cap. (Lederle).
W/Norethindrone, mestranol.
See: Ortho Novum 1/80 Fe-28, 1/50 Fe-28, 1 mg Fe-28, Tab. (Ortho).
W/Vitamins and minerals.
See: Stuart Formula, Tab. (Stuart).
Stuart Prenatal, Tab. (Stuart).
Stuartnatal 1 + 1, Tab. (Stuart).
Theron, Tab. (Stuart).
Vitanate, Tab. (Century).

•**FERROUS GLUCONATE,** U.S.P. XXII. Cap., Elixir, Tab., U.S.P. XXII. Iron (2+) Gluconate.

Use: Iron deficiency.
See: Entron, Cap., Tab. (LaCrosse).
Fergon Prods. (Winthrop Consumer Products).
W/Ascorbic acid, desiccated liver, vitamin B complex.
See: I.L.X. w/B_{12}, Tab. (Kenwood).
Stuart Hematinic, Liq. (Stuart).
W/Polyoxyethylene glucitan monolaurate.
See: Simron, Cap. (Merrell Dow).
FERROUS IODIDE. (Various Mfr.).
Use: In chronic tuberculosis.
FERROUS IODIDE SYRUP. (Various Mfr.).
Use: In chronic tuberculosis.
FERROUS LACTATE. (Various Mfr.).
Use: Iron deficiency.
FERROUS SULFATE, U.S.P. XXII. Tab., Dried, Syr., Oral Soln., U.S.P. XXII.
Use: Iron deficiency.
See: Feosol, Spansule, Tab., Elix. (SmithKline Prods).
Ferralyn, Cap. (Lannett).
Fero-Gradumet, Tab. (Abbott).
Ferolix, Elix. (Century).
Ferrous Sulfate Filmseals, Tab. (Parke-Davis).
Fesotyme SR, Cap. (Elder).
Irospan, Cap., Tab. (Fielding).
Mol-Iron, Prods. (Schering).
Telefon, Cap. (Kenyon).
W/Ascorbic acid.
See: Fero-Grad-500, Tab. (Abbott).
Mol-Iron W/Vitamin C, Tab., Chronosules (Schering).
W/Ascorbic acid, folic acid.
See: Fero-Folic-500, Tab. (Abbott).
W/Cyanocobalamin, ascorbic acid, folic acid.
See: Intrin, Cap. (Merit).
W/Folic acid.
See: Folvron, Cap. (Lederle).
W/Maalox.
See: Fermalox, Tab. (Rorer Consumer).
FERROUS SULFATE FILMSEALS. (Parke-Davis) Ferrous sulfate 5 gr/DR Tab. Bot. 1000s, UD 100s.
Use: Iron supplement.
FERROUS SULFATE Fe 59. USAN.
Use: Radioisotope.
FERTILITY TAPE. (Weston Labs.) Regular, extrasensitive, less-sensitive. W/Fertility Testor, cervical glucose test. Pkg. test 60s.
Use: Diagnostic aid.
FERTIRELIN ACETATE. USAN.
Use: Hormone (gonadotropin-releasing).
FERUSAL. (Vitarine) Ferrous sulfate 325 mg/Tab.
Use: Iron supplement.
FESTAL II. (Hoechst) Lipase 6000 units, amylase 30,000 units, protease 20,000 units/Tab. Bot. 100s, 500s.
Use: Digestive enzyme.
FESTALAN. (Hoechst) Lipase 6000 units, amylase 30,000 units, protease 20,000 units, atropine methylnitrate 1 mg/EC Tab. Bot. 100s, 1000s.
Use: Digestive enzyme.
FETINIC. (Hauck) Iron 3.6 mg, vitamins B_{12} equivalent 2 mcg, B_1 10 mg, B_2 0.5 mg, B_3 10 mg, B_5 1 mg, B_6 1 mg, B_{12} 15 mcg, chlorobutanol 0.5%, benzyl alcohol 2%/ml. Vial 30 ml.
Use: Vitamin/mineral supplement.
FETINIC-MW. (Hauck) Iron 66 mg (from ferrous fumarate), vitamins B_{12} 5 mcg, C 60 mg/SR Cap. Bot. 100s.
Use: Vitamin/mineral supplement.
•**FETOXYLATE HYDROCHLORIDE.** USAN.
Use: Relaxant.
•**FEZOLAMINE FUMARATE.** USAN.
Use: Antidepressant.
FIBERALL NATURAL FLAVOR. (Ciba Consumer) **Pow.:** Psyllium hydrophilic mucilloid 3.4 Gm, wheat bran, sodium $>$ 10 mg, potassium $>$ 60 mg, calories 6/5.9 Gm, saccharin. Can 150 Gm, 300 Gm, 450 Gm. **Wafer:** Psyllium hydrophilic mucilloid 3.4 Gm, wheat bran, oats, sucrose. Box 14s.
Use: Laxative.
FIBERALL ORANGE FLAVOR. (Ciba Consumer) Psyllium hydrophilic mucilloid 3.4 Gm, wheat bran, sodium $>$ 10 mg, potassium $>$ 60 mg, calories 6/5.9 Gm Pow. Can 150 Gm, 300 Gm, 450 Gm.
Use: Laxative.
FIBERCON. (Lederle) Calcium polycarbophil 500 mg/Tab. Bot. 36s, 60s.
Use: Laxative.
FIBER GUARD. (Wyeth-Ayerst) All natural high fiber supplement 530 mg/Tab. Bot. 100s, 200s.
Use: Fiber supplement.
FIBERMED HIGH-FIBER SNACKS. (Purdue Frederick) One serving (15 snacks) contains 5 Gm dietary fiber. Box 8 oz. Packs of 24 × 1.3 oz.
Use: Fiber supplement.
FIBERMED HIGH-FIBER SUPPLEMENT. (Purdue Frederick) Each supplement contains 5 Gm dietary fiber. Box 14s. Institutional pack, Box 144s of two supplements.
Use: Fiber supplement.
FIBER RICH. (O'Connor) Phenylpropanolamine HCl 75 mg/Tab. Bot. 24s.
Use: Diet aid.
FIBRE TRIM TABLETS. (Schering) Grain and citrus fruit concentrated dietary fiber. Bot. 100s, 250s.
Use: Diet aid.
FIBRE TRIM w/CALCIUM TABLETS. (Schering) Grain and citrus fruit concentrated dietary fiber w/calcium. Bot. 90s, 225s.
Use: Diet aid.
FIBRIN HYDROLYSATE.
See: Aminosol, Soln. (Abbott).
FIBRINOGEN (HUMAN). Partially purified fibrinogen prepared by fractionation from normal human plasma.
Use: Coagulant (clotting factor).
•**FIBRINOGEN I-125.** USAN.
Use: Diagnostic aid.
FIBRINOLYSIN (HUMAN) WITH DESOXYRIBONUCLEASE. Plasmin. An enzyme prepared by

activating a human blood plasma fraction with streptokinase.
Use: Topical enzyme preparation.
See: Elase, Oint., Pow. (Parke-Davis).

FIBRINOLYSIS INHIBITOR.
See: Amicar Syr., Tab., Vial (Lederle).

FIBROGAMMIN. (Factor XIII) (Orphan Drug).
Use: Cogenital Factor XIII deficiency.
Sponsor: Hoechst-Roussel.

FILAXIS. (Amlab) Vitamins A 25,000 IU, D 1250 IU, C 150 mg, E 5 IU, B_1 12 mg, B_2 5 mg, B_6 0.5 mg, B_{12} 5 mcg, calcium pantothenate 5 mg, niacinamide 100 mg, iron 15 mg, iodine 0.15 mg, magnesium 10 mg, potassium 5 mg, calcium 75 mg, phosphorous 60 mg/Tab. Bot. 30s, 100s. Available w/B_{12}. Bot. 30s, 60s, 100s.
Use: Vitamin/mineral supplement.

•**FILGRASTIM (G-CSF).** USAN.
Use: Biological response modifier; antineoplastic adjunct.
See: Neupogen (Amgen).

FILIBON. (Lederle) Vitamins A 5000 IU, D 400 IU, B_1 1.5 mg, B_6 2 mg, niacinamide 20 mg, B_2 1.7 mg, B_{12} 6 mcg, E 30 mg, C 60 mg, folic acid 0.4 mg, elemental iron 18 mg, iodine 150 mcg, magnesium 100 mg, elemental calcium 125 mg/Tab. Bot 100s.
Use: Vitamin/mineral supplement.

FILIBON F.A. (Lederle) Elemental calcium 250 mg, elemental iron 45 mg, vitamins A 8000 IU, D 400 IU, E 30 mg, B_1 1.7 mg, B_2 2 mg, B_3 20 mg, B_6 4 mg, B_{12} 8 mcg, C 60 mg, folic acid 1 mg, I, Mg/Tab. Bot. 100s.
Use: Vitamin/mineral supplement.

FILIBON FORTE. (Lederle) Vitamins A 8000 IU, D 400 IU, E 45 mg, C 90 mg, niacinamide 30 mg, B_6 3 mg, B_1 2 mg, B_2 2.5 mg, folic acid 1 mg, B_{12} 12 mcg, calcium 300 mg, iron 45 mg, magnesium 100 mg, iodine 200 mcg/Tab. Bot. 100s.
Use: Vitamin/mineral supplement.

•**FILIPIN.** USAN.
Use: Antifungal.

FINAC. (C & M Pharmacal) Sulfur 2% in tinted lotion base. Bot. 60 ml.
Use: Anti-acne.

•**FINASTERIDE.** USAN.
Use: Benign prostatic hypertrophy therapy; antineoplastic.

FIOGESIC. (Sandoz) Phenylpropanolamine HCl 25 mg, pyrilamine maleate 12.5 mg, pheniramine maleate 12.5 mg, calcium carbaspirin 382 mg (equiv. to 300 mg ASA)/Tab. Bot. 100s.
Use: Decongestant, antihistamine, analgesic.

FIORGEN TABS PF. (Goldline) Butabarbital 50 mg, aspirin 325 mg, caffeine 40 mg/Tab. Bot. 100s, 1000s.
Use: Sedative/hypnotic, salicylate/analgesic.

FIORICET. (Sandoz) Acetaminophen 325 mg, butalbital 50 mg, caffeine 40 mg/Tab. Bot. 100s, 500s. SandoPak 100s.
Use: Analgesic, sedative/hypnotic.

FIORINAL. (Sandoz) Butalbital (Sandoptal) 50 mg, caffeine 40 mg, aspirin 325 mg/Tab. or Cap. **Tab.:** Bot. 100s, 1000s. Sandopak 100s. **Cap.:** Bot. 100s, 500s. Control Pak 25s.
Use: Sedative/hypnotic, salicylate analgesic.

FIORINAL WITH CODEINE NO. 3 CAPSULES. (Sandoz) Butalbital (Sandoptal) 50 mg, caffeine 40 mg, aspirin 325 mg, codeine phosphate 30 mg/Cap. Bot. 100s. Control Pak 25s.
Use: Sedative/hypnotic, analgesic combination.

FIRMDENT. (Moyco) Formerly Moy. Karaya gum 94.6%, sodium borate 5.36% Pkg. 3 oz.
Use: Denture adhesive.

FIRST AID CREAM. (Johnson & Johnson) Cetyl alcohol, glyceryl stearate, isopropyl palmitate, stearyl alcohol, synthetic beeswax. Tube 0.8 oz, 1.5 oz, 2.5 oz.
Use: Antiseptic, skin protectant.

FIRST AID CREAM. (Walgreen) Benzocaine 3%, allantoin 0.2%, benzyl alcohol 4%, phenol 0.25%. Tube 1.5 oz.
Use: Anesthetic, antiseptic.

FIRST RESPONSE OVULATION PREDICTOR. (Tambrands) Monoclonal antibody-based enzyme immunoassay test for hLH in urine. Test kit 1s.
Use: Diagnostic aid.

FIRST RESPONSE PREGNANCY TEST. (Tambrands) Reagent in-home kit for urine testing. Test kit 1s.
Use: Diagnostic aid.

FISH OIL CONCENTRATE, NATURAL. Natural fish oil concentrate containing EPA (Eicosapentaenoicacid) and DHA (Docosahexaenoic acid).
Use: Fish oil.
See: Comega, Cap. (Upsher-Smith).

FITACOL. (Standex) Atropine sulfate 0.2 mg, phenylpropanolamine 12.5 mg, chlorpheniramine maleate 0.5 mg, chlorobutanol 0.5 mg, water q.s./ml. Bot. pt.
Use: Anticholinergic/antispasmodic, decongestant, antihistamine.

FITACOL STANKAPS. (Standex) Belladonna alkaloidal salts 0.16 mg (atropine sulfate 0.024 mg, scopolamine HBr 0.014 mg, hyoscyamine sulfate 0.122 mg), phenylpropanolamine HCl 50 mg, chlorpheniramine maleate 1 mg, pheniramine maleate 12.5 mg/Cap. Bot. 100s.
Use: Anticholinergic/antispasmodic, decongestant, antihistamine.

5-FC.
See: Flucytosine.

5-FU.
See: Fluorouracil.

523 TABLETS. (Enzyme Process) Pancreatin 200 mg 4x/Tab. Tryspin, chymotrypsin, amylase, lipase enzymes from pancreatin, raw beef pancreas. Bot. 100s, 250s.
Use: Digestive enzyme.

FIXODENT. (Vicks Prods) Calcium sodium poly (vinyl methyl ether-maleate), carboxymethylcellulose sodium in a petrolatum base. Tube 0.75

oz, 1.5 oz, 2.5 oz.
Use: Denture adhesive cream.

FLAGYL. (Searle) Metronidazole 250 mg or 500 mg/Tab. **250 mg:** Bot. 50s, 100s, 250s, 1000s, 2500s, UD 100s; **500 mg:** Bot. 50s, 100s, 500s, UD 100s.
Use: Anti-infective.

FLAGYL I.V. (Searle) Metronidazole HCl sterile lyophilized powder in single-dose vials equivalent to 500 mg metronidazole. Carton 10s.
Use: Anti-infective.

FLAGYL I.V. RTU. (Searle) Metronidazole ready-to-use, premixed, 500 mg/100 ml Soln. Vial (glass), Box 6s; Container, (plastic), Box 24s.
Use: Anti-infective.

FLANDERS BUTTOCKS OINTMENT. (Flanders) Zinc oxide, castor oil, balsam peru, boric acid in an emollient base. 60 Gm.
Use: Minor skin irritations.

FLATULENCE TABLETS. (Vale) Nux vomica 16.2 mg, cascara sagrada extract 64.8 mg, ginger 48.6 mg, capsicum 16.2 mg/Tab. w/asafetida.
Use: Laxative, antiflatulent.

FLATULEX. (Dayton) **Tab.:** Simethicone 80 mg, activated charcoal 250 mg/Tab. Bot. 100s. **Drops:** Simethicone 40 mg/0.6 ml. Bot. 30 ml with calibrated dropper.
Use: Antiflatulent.

FLATUS (Foy) Nux vomica extract 0.25 gr, cascara extract 1 gr, ginger ¾ gr, capsicum ⅛ gr/Tab. w/asfetida qs. Bot. 1000s.
Use: Antiflatulent, laxative.

FLAV-A-D. (Kirkman) Vitamins A 5000 IU, D 1000 IU, C 100 mg/Tab. Bot. 100s, 1000s. Also w/fluoride. Bot. 100s, 1000s.
Use: Vitamin supplement.

FLAVINE.
See: Acriflavine Hydrochloride (Various Mfr.).

FLAVINOID-C. (Barth's) **Tab.:** Vitamin C 150 mg, hesperidin complex 10 mg, citrus bioflavonoid 50 mg, rutin 20 mg/Tab. Bot. 100s, 500s, 1000s. **Liq.:** Vitamin C 100 mg, bioflavonoid complex 100 mg/5 ml. Bot. 4 oz.
Use: Vitamin supplement.

•**FLAVODILOL MALEATE.** USAN.
Use: Antihypertensive.

FLAVOLUTAN.
See: Progesterone (Various Mfr.).

FLAVONOID COMPOUNDS.
See: Bio-Flavonoid Compounds Vitamin P.

FLAVONS-500. (Freeda) Citrus bioflavonoids complex 500 mg, hesperidin complex/Tab. Bot. 100s, 250s, 500s.
Use: Vitamin supplement.

FLAVORCEE. (Nature's Bounty) Ascorbic acid 100 mg or 250 mg/Chew. Tab. **100 mg:** Bot. 100s; **250 mg:** Bot. 250s.
Use: Vitamin C supplement.

FLAVORED DILUENT. (Roxane) Flavored vehicle for the immediate administration of crushed tablet or capsule product. Bot. 500 ml, UD 15 ml × 100.
Use: Flavored vehicle.

•**FLAVOXATE HCl.** USAN. 2-Piperidinoethyl-3-methyl-4-oxo-2-phenyl-4H-1-benzopyran-8-carboxylate HCl.
Use: Urinary antispasmodic.
See: Urispas, Tab. (SmithKline).

FLAVUROL. Merbromin.
Use: Antiseptic.

FLAXEDIL TRIETHIODIDE. Gallamine triethiodide soln.
Use: Skeletal muscle relaxant.

•**FLAZALONE.** USAN. p-Fluoro-phenyl 4-(p-fluorophenyl)-4-hydroxy-1-methyl-3-piperidyl ketone. 3-(4-Fluorobenzoyl)-4-(4-fluorophenyl)-1-methylpiperidin-4-ol.
Use: Anti-inflammatory.

•**FLECAINIDE ACETATE.** USAN.
Use: Cardiac depressant.

FLEET BABYLAX. (Fleet) Glycerin 4 ml in disposable pre-lubricated rectal applicator. Liq. pkg. 6s.
Use: Laxative.

FLEET BAGENEMA. (Fleet) Castile soap or Fleets bisacodyl prep.
Use: Laxative.

FLEET BISACODYL. (Fleet) Bisacodyl. **EC Tab.:** 5 mg/Tab. Bot. 24s, 100s, 1000s. **Supp.:** 10 mg. Box 4s, 50s, 100s. **Enema:** 10 mg/30 ml. Disposable enema 37 ml.
Use: Laxative.

FLEET BISACODYL PREP PACKETS. (Fleet) Bisacodyl 10 mg/10 ml packet. 36 packets/box.
Use: Laxative.

FLEET ENEMA. (Fleet) Sodium biphosphate 19 Gm, sodium phosphate 7 Gm/118 ml. Bot. w/rectal tube 4.5 oz. Pediatric size 67.5 ml, 135 ml.
Use: Laxative.

FLEET FLAVORED CASTOR OIL EMULSION. (Fleet) 1 oz delivers 30 ml castor oil. Bot. 1.5 oz, 3 oz.
Use: Laxative.

FLEET GLYCERIN SUPPOSITORIES. (Fleet) Adult: Jar 12s, 24s, 50s. Child Size: Jar 12s.
Use: Laxative.

FLEET MINERAL OIL ENEMA. (Fleet) Mineral oil 4.5 fl oz in an unbreakable vinyl squeeze bottle.
Use: Laxative.

FLEET PHOSPHO-SODA. (Fleet) Sodium phosphate 18 Gm, sodium biphosphate 48 Gm/100 ml (96.4 mEq sodium/20 ml). Bot. 45 ml, 90 ml, 240 ml.
Use: Laxative.

FLEET PREP KIT. (Fleet) A series of different laxative kits for use prior to barium enema, bowel surgery, proctoscopy, colonoscopy, etc. w/complete patient instruction form:
Prep Kit #1: Fleet® Phospho-Soda 45 ml, Fleet® Bisacodyl Tablets 4×5 mg, Fleet® Bisacodyl Suppository 1×10 mg.
Prep Kit #2: Fleet® Phospho-Soda 45 ml, Fleet® Bisacodyl Tablets 4×5 mg, 1 Fleet®

Bagenema set for large volume enema, including optional Castile Soap Packet. 20 ml.
Prep Kit #3: Fleet® Phospho-Soda 45 ml, Fleet® Bisacodyl Tablets 4×5 mg, Fleet® Bisacodyl Enema 1×30 ml. 10 mg.
Prep Kit #4: Fleet® Flavored Castor Oil Emulsion 45 ml, Fleet® Bisacodyl Tablets 4×5 mg, Fleet® Bisacodyl Suppository 1×10 mg.
Prep Kit #5: Fleet® Flavored Castor Oil Emulsion 45 ml, Fleet® Bisacodyl Tablets 4×5 mg, 1 Fleet® Bagenema set for large volume enema, including optional Castile Soap Packet. 20 ml.
Prep Kit #6: Fleet® Flavored Castor Oil Emulsion 45 ml, Fleet® Bisacodyl Tablets 4×5 mg, Fleet® Bisacodyl Enema 1×30 ml. 10 mg.
Use: Laxative.

FLEET RELIEF ANESTHETIC HEMORRHOIDAL OINTMENT. (Fleet) Pramoxine HCl 1%. Six disposable pre-filled applicators. Tube 30 Gm.
Use: Anorectal preparation.

•**FLEROXACIN.** USAN.
Use: Antibacterial.

•**FLESTOLOL SULFATE.** USAN.
Use: Anti-adrenergic.

•**FLETAZEPAM.** USAN.
Use: Relaxant.

FLETCHER'S CASTORIA for CHILDREN. (Mentholatum) Senna 6.5%, alcohol 3.5%. Liq. Bot. 75 ml, 150 ml.
Use: Laxative.

FLEX ANTI-DANDRUFF SHAMPOO. (Revlon) Zinc pyrithione 1% in liquid shampoo.
Use: Antiseborrheic.

FLEX ANTI-DANDRUFF STYLING MOUSSE. (Revlon) Zinc pyrithione 0.1%. Aerosol foam.
Use: Antiseborrheic.

FLEX-CARE FOR SENSITIVE EYES. (Alcon Lenscare) Sterile solution of chlorhexidine 0.005%, edetate disodium 0.1%. Bot. 120 ml, 237 ml, 355 ml.
Use: Soft contact lens care.

FLEXERIL. (Merck Sharp & Dohme) Cyclobenzaprine HCl 10 mg/Tab. Bot. 100s, UD 100s, Unit-of-Use 30s.
Use: Muscle relaxant.

FLEXOJECT. (Mayrand) Orphenadrine citrate 30 mg/ml. Inj. Vial 10 ml.
Use: Muscle relaxant.

FLEXON. (Keene) Orphenadrine citrate 30 mg/ml. Inj. Vial 10 ml.
Use: Muscle relaxant.

FLEXSOL. (Alcon Lenscare) Sterile, buffered, isotonic aqueous soln. of sodium Cl, sodium borate, boric acid, adsorbobase. Bot. 6 oz.
Use: Soft contact lens care.

FLINT SSD. (Flint) Silver sulfadiazine cream 1%. Jar 50 Gm, 400 Gm, 1000 Gm.
Use: Burn preparation.

FLINTSTONES. (Miles) Vitamin A 2500 IU, E 15 mg, C 60 mg, folic acid 0.3 mg, B_1 1.05 mg, B_2 1.2 mg, niacin 13.5 mg, B_6 1.05 mg, B_{12} 4.5 mcg, D 400 IU/Chew. Tab. Bot. 60s, 100s.
Use: Vitamin supplement.

FLINTSTONES COMPLETE. (Miles) Elemental iron 18 mg, vitamins A 5000 IU, D 400 IU, E 30 mg, B_1 1.5 mg, B_2 1.7 mg, B_3 20 mg, B_5 10 mg, B_6 2 mg, B_{12} 6 mcg, C 60 mg, folic acid 0.4 mg, biotin 40 mcg, Ca, Cu, I, Mg, P, zinc 15 mg/Chew. Tab. Bot. 60s, 100s.
Use: Vitamin/mineral supplement.

FLINTSTONES WITH EXTRA C. (Miles) Vitamins A 2500 IU, D 400 IU, E 15 mg, C 250 mg, folic acid 0.3 mg, B_1 1.05 mg, B_2 1.2 mg, niacin 13.5 mg, B_6 1.05 mg, B_{12} 4.5 mcg/Tab. Bot. 60s, 100s.
Use: Vitamin supplement.

FLINTSTONES WITH IRON. (Miles) Vitamins A 2500 IU, E 15 mg, C 60 mg, folic acid 0.3 mg, B_1 1.05 mg, B_2 1.2 mg, niacin 13.5 mg, B_6 1.05 mg, B_{12} 4.5 mcg, D 400 IU, iron 15 mg/Chew. Tab. Bot. 60s.
Use: Vitamin/mineral supplement.

•**FLOCTAFENINE.** USAN.
Use: Analgesic.

FLOLAN. Epoprostenol (Orphan Drug).
Use: Antihypertensive, replacement of heparin in some hemodialysis patients.
Sponsors: Burroughs Wellcome, Upjohn.

FLORAJEN. (Jenkins) Fluoride 0.5 mg, vitamins A 4000 IU, D 400 IU, ascorbic acid 75 mg, B_1 2 mg, B_2 2 mg, niacinamide 18 mg, B_6 1 mg, calcium pantothenate dextro 5 mg, cyanocobalamin 2 mcg/Tab. Bot. 100s, 500s, 1000s.
Use: Vitamin/mineral supplement.

FLORANTYRONE. B.A.N. 4-(Fluoranthen-8-yl)-4-oxobutyric acid.
Use: Stimulation of bile acid secretion.

FLOR-D CHEWABLE TAB. (Derm Pharm.) Fluoride 1 mg, vitamins A 4000 IU, D 400 IU, C 75 mg, B_1 1.5 mg, B_2 1.8 mg, niacinamide 15 mg, B_6 1 mg, B_{12} 3 mcg, calcium pantothenate 10 mg/Tab. Bot. 100s.
Use: Vitamin/mineral supplement.

FLOR-D DROPS. (Derm Pharm.) Fluoride 0.5 mg, vitamins A 3000 IU, D 400 IU, C 60 mg, B_1 1 mg, B_2 1.2 mg, niacinamide 8 mg/0.6 ml. Bot. 60 ml.
Use: Vitamin/mineral supplement.

•**FLORDIPINE.** USAN.
Use: Antihypertensive.

•**FLORFENICOL.** USAN.
Use: Antibacterial (veterinary).

FLORICAL. (Mericon) Sodium fluoride 8.3 mg, calcium carbonate 364 mg (equivalent to 145.6 mg calcium)/Cap. Bot. 100s, 500s.
Use: Mineral supplement.

FLORIDA FOAM. (Hill) Benzalkonium Cl, aluminum subacetate, boric acid 2%. Bot. 8 oz.
Use: Soap substitute, antiseborrheic, antifungal, anti-acne.

FLORINEF ACETATE TABLETS. (Squibb Mark) Fludrocortisone acetate, 0.1 mg/Tab. Bot. 100s.
Use: Mineralocorticoid.

FLORITAL. (Cenci) Butabital 50 mg, aspirin 200 mg, phenacetin 130 mg, caffeine 40 mg/Tab. Bot. 100s.
Use: Sedative/hypnotic, salicylate analgesic.

FLORONE CREAM. (Dermik) Diflorasone diacetate 0.5 mg/Gm (0.05%) w/stearic acid, sorbitan mono-oleate, polysorbate 60, sorbic acid, citric acid, propylene glycol, purified water. Tube 15 Gm, 30 Gm, 60 Gm.
Use: Corticosteroid.

FLORONE E. (Dermik) Diflorasone diacetate 0.5 mg. Tube 15 Gm, 30 Gm, 60 Gm.
Use: Corticosteroid.

FLORONE OINTMENT. (Dermik) Diflorasone diacetate 0.5 mg/Gm (0.05%) W/polyoxypropylene 15-stearyl ether, stearic acid, lanolin alcohol and white petrolatum. Tube 15 Gm, 30 Gm, 60 Gm.
Use: Corticosteroid.

FLOROPRYL. (Merck Sharp & Dohme) Isoflurophate 0.025% in sterile ophthalmic ointment in polyethylene-mineral oil gel. Tube 3.5 Gm.
Use: Agent for glaucoma.

FLORVITE CHEWABLE TABLETS. (Everett) Vitamins, fluoride 0.5 mg/Chew. tab. Bot 100s.
Use: Dental caries preventative.

FLORVITE & IRON DROPS. (Everett) Elemental fluorine. **0.25 mg:** Vitamins A 1500 IU, D 400 IU, E 5 mg, B_1 0.5 mg, B_2 0.6 mg, B_3 8 mg, B_6 0.4 mg, C 35 mg, iron 10 mg/ml. **0.5 mg:** Vitamins A 1500 IU, D 400 IU, E 5 mg, B_1 0.5 mg, B_2 0.6 mg, B_3 8 mg, B_6 0.4 mg, C 35 mg, iron 10 mg/ml. Bot. 50 ml.
Use: Vitamin/mineral supplement, dental caries preventative.

FLORVITE & IRON CHEWABLE. (Everett) Fluoride 1 mg, iron 12 mg, vitamins A 2500 IU, D 400 IU, E 15 mg, B_1 1.05 mg, B_2 1.2 mg, B_3 13.5 mg, B_6 1.05 mg, B_{12} 4.5 mcg, C 60 mg, folic acid 0.3 mg/Chew. tab. Bot. 100s.
Use: Vitamin/mineral supplement, dental caries preventative.

FLORVITE PEDIATRIC DROPS. (Everett) Elemental fluorine. **0.25 mg/ml:** vitamins A 1500 IU, D 400 IU, E 5 mg, B_1 0.5 mg, B_2 0.6 mg, B_3 8 mg, B_6 0.4 mg, B_{12} 2 mcg, C 35 mg/ml. **0.5 mg/ml:** vitamins A 1500 IU, D 400 IU, E 5 mg, B_1 0.5 mg, B_2 0.6 mg, B_3 8 mg, B_6 0.4 mg, B_{12} 2 mcg, C 35 mg, iron 10 mg/ml Bot. 50 ml.
Use: Vitamin/mineral supplement, dental caries preventative.

FLORVITE TABLETS-1 mg (Everett) Elemental fluorine 1 mg, vitamins A 2500 IU, D 400 IU, E 15 mg, B_1 1.05 mg, B_2 1.2 mg, B_3 13.5 mg, B_6 1.05 mg, B_{12} 4.5 mcg, C 60 mg, folic acid 0.3 mg/Chew. tab. Bot. 100s, 1000s.
Use: Vitamin/mineral supplement, dental caries preventative.

•**FLOXACILLIN.** USAN.
Use: Antibacterial.

•**FLOXIN.** (Ortho) Ofloxacin.
Use: Antibacterial, fluoroquinolone.

FLOXURIDINE, U.S.P. XXI. Sterile, U.S.P. XXI. 2′-Deoxy-5-fluorouridine.
Use: Antiviral agent.
See: FUDR, Vial (Roche).

FLUANISONE. B.A.N. 4-Fluoro--[4-(2-methoxyphenyl)piperazin-1-yl]butyrophenone.
Use: Neuroleptic.

•**FLUAZACORT.** USAN.
Use: Anti-inflammatory.

•**FLUBANILATE HYDROCHLORIDE.** USAN. Ethyl N-[2(dimethylamino)ethyl]-m-(trifluoromethyl) carbanilate HCl.
Use: Antidepressant.

•**FLUBENDAZOLE.** USAN.
Use: Antiprotozoal.

FLUCARBRIL. 1-Methyl-6-(trifluromethyl)carbostyril.
Use: Muscle relaxant, analgesic.

•**FLUCINDOLE.** USAN.
Use: Antipsychotic.

FLUCLOROLONE ACETONIDE. B.A.N. 9α,-11β-Dichloro-6α-fluoro-21-hydroxy-16α,17α-isopropylidenedioxypregna-1,4-diene-3,20-dione.
Use: Corticosteroid.

•**FLUCLORONIDE.** USAN. 9, 11β-Dichloro-6α-fluoro-16α, 17, 21-trihydroxypregna-1, 4-diene-3, 20-dione cyclic 16, 17-acetal with acetone.
Use: Glucocorticoid.

FLUCLOXACILLIN. B.A.N. 6-[3-(2-Chloro-6-fluorophenyl)-5-methylisoxazole-4-carboxamido]-penicillanic acid.
Use: Antibiotic.

•**FLUCONAZOLE.** USAN.
Use: Antifungal.
See: Diflucan (Roerig).

•**FLUCRYLATE.** USAN. 2,2,2-Trifluoro-1-methylethyl-2-cyanoacrylate.
Use: Surgical aid (tissue adhesive).

•**FLUCYTOSINE,** U.S.P. XXII. Cap. U.S.P. XXII. 5-Fluorocytosine.
Use: Antifungal.
See: Ancobon, Cap. (Roche).

•**FLUCYTOSINE.** USAN. 4-Amino-5-fluoro-1,2-dihydropyrimidin-2-one. 5-Fluorocytosine.
Use: Antifungal.
See: Alcobon.

•**FLUDARABINE PHOSPHATE.** USAN.
Use: Antineoplastic.

•**FLUDAZONIUM CHLORIDE.** USAN.
Use: Anti-infective, topical.

•**FLUDALANINE.** USAN.
Use: Antibacterial.

•**FLUDEOXYGLUCOSE F 18 INJECTION,** U.S.P. XXII. USAN.
Use: Diagnostic aid. For brain disorders, thyroid disorders, liver disorders, cardiac disease and neoplastic disease.

•**FLUDOREX.** USAN.
Use: Anorexic, anti-emetic.

•**FLUDROCORTISONE ACETATE,** U.S.P. XXII. Tab. U.S.P. XXII. 9-alpha-Fluorohydrocortisone. Pregn-4-ene-3,20-dione,21-(acetyloxy)-9-fluoro-11,-17-dihydroxy-, (11 beta)-.9-Fluoro-11 beta,

17,21-trihydroxypregn-4-ene-3,20-dione 21-acetate.
Use: Adrenocortical steroid (salt-regulation).
See: Florinef Acetate, Tab. (Squibb).

•**FLUFENAMIC ACID.** USAN. N-(α, α, α-Trifluoro-m-tolyl) anthranilic acid.
Use: Anti-inflammatory agent.

•**FLUFENSIAL.** USAN.
Use: Analgesic.

FLUGESTONE. B.A.N. 9α-Fluoro-11β,17-dihydroxy-pregn-4-ene-3,20-dione.
Use: Progesterone steroid.

FLUIDEX. (O'Connor) Natural botanical ingredients. Tab. Bot. 36s, 72s.
Use: Diuretic.

FLUIDEX WITH PAMABROM. (O'Connor) Pamabrom 50 mg/Cap. Pkg. 3s, 12s, 24s.
Use: Diuretic.

FLUITRAN. Trichlormethiazide.

•**FLUMAZENIL.** USAN.
Use: Antagonist (to benzodiazepine).

FLUMECINOL.
See: Zixoryn.

FLUMEDROXONE. B.A.N. 17α-Hydroxy-6α-trifluoromethylpregn-4-ene-3,20-dione.
Use: Agent for migraine.

•**FLUMEQUINE.** USAN.
Use: Antibacterial.

•**FLUMERIDONE.** USAN.
Use: Anti-emetic.

•**FLUMETHASONE.** USAN. 6α,9α-Difluoro-11β, 17α,21-trihydroxy-16α-methylpregna-1,4-diene-3,20- dione. 6α,9α-Difluoro-16α-methylprednisolone.
Use: Corticosteroid.
See: Locorten [21-pivalate] (Ciba).

FLUMETHIAZIDE. 6-Trifluoromethyl-7-sulfamyl-1,2,4-benzothiadiazine-1,1-dioxide.
Use: Diuretic.
See: Rautrax, Tab. (Squibb).

FLUMETHIAZIDE. B.A.N. 6-Trifluoromethyl-1,2,4-benzothiadiazine-7-sulphonamide 1,1-dioxide.
Use: Diuretic.

•**FLUMETRAMIDE.** USAN.
Use: Relaxant.

•**FLUMEZAPINE.** USAN.
Use: Antipsychotic, neuroleptic.

•**FLUMINOREX.** USAN.
Use: Anorexic.

• **FLUMIZOLE.** USAN.
Use: Anti-inflammatory.

•**FLUNARIZINE HCl.** USAN. (E)-1-[Bis-(p-fluorophenyl) methyl]-4-cinnamyl-piperazine dihydrochloride.
Use: Vasodilator.

•**FLUNIDAZOLE.** USAN.
Use: Antiprotozoal.

•**FLUNISOLIDE.**
See: AcroBid (Key Pharm.).
Nasalide (Syntex).

•**FLUNISOLIDE ACETATE.** USAN. Fluoxolonate.
Use: Anti-inflammatory.

•**FLUNITRAZEPAM.** USAN. 5-Fluorophenyl-1,3-dihydro-1-methyl-7-nitro-2H-1,4-benzodiazepin-2-one.
Use: Hynoptic.

•**FLUNIXIN.** USAN.
Use: Anti-inflammatory, analgesic.

FLUOCET. (NMC Labs) Fluocinolone acetonide cream 0.025% or 0.01%. Tube 15 Gm, 60 Gm.
Use: Corticosteroid.

FLUOCINOLIDE. Fluocinonide, U.S.P. XXII.

•**FLUOCINOLONE ACETONIDE,** U.S.P. XXII. Cream, Oint., Topical Soln. U.S.P. XXII. Pregna-1,4-diene-3,20-dione,6,9-difluoro-11,21-dihydroxy-16,17-[(1-methylethylidene)bis(oxy)], (6α,11β,-16α)-. 9a-Difluoro-16a-hydroxyprednisolone-16, 17-acetonide. 6α,9α-Difluoro-11β,16α,17,21-tetrahydroxypregna-1,4-diene-3,20-dione. Cyclic 16,-17-Acetal with Acetone.
Use: Adrenocortical steroid (topical anti-inflammatory).
See: Fluonid, Cream, Oint., Soln. (Herbert).
Synalar, Cream, Oint., Soln. (Syntex).
W/Neomycin sulfate.
See: Neo-Synalar (Syntex).

•**FLUOCINONIDE TOPICAL SOLUTION,** U.S.P. XXII.
Use: Corticosteroid.

•**FLUOCINONIDE,** U.S.P. XXII. Cream, Gel, Oint., U.S.P. XXII. F.D.A. 6α, 9α-Difluoro-11β-16α, 17α-21-tetrahydroxypregna-1,4-diene-3,20-dione, cyclic 16, 17-acetal with acetone, 21-acetate. B.A.N. 21-Acetoxy-6α,9α-difluoro-11β-hydroxy-16α, 17α-iso- propylidene-dioxypregna-1,4-diene-3,20-dione. Fluocinolone 16α, 17α-acetonide 21 acetate.
Use: Corticosteroid.
See: Lidex, Cream, Oint., Soln. (Syntex).
Lidex-E, Cream (Syntex).
Metosyn.
Topsyn, Gel (Syntex).

•**FLUOCORTIN BUTYL.** USAN. Butyl-6α-fluoro-11β-hydroxy-16α-methyl-3,20-dioxopregna-1,4-dien-21oate.
Use: Anti-inflammatory.

•**FLUOCORTOLONE.** USAN. 6α-Fluoro-11β,21-dihy- droxy-16α-methylpregna-1,4-diene-20-dione. (Berlin) 6α-Fluoro-11β, 21-dihydroxy-16α-methylpregna-1, 4-diene-3, 20-dione.
Use: Corticosteroid.
See: Ultralanum [21-hexanoate]

•**FLUOCORTOLONE CAPROATE.** USAN.
Use: Glucocorticoid.

FLUOGEN. (Parke-Davis) Influenza virus vaccine, trivalent—Immunizing antigen, ether extracted. Vial 5 ml, UD syringe 0.5 ml. The 5 ml vial contains sufficient product to deliver ten 0.5 ml doses.
Use: Vaccine, viral.

FLUONID. (Herbert) Fluocinolone Acetonide.
Soln.: 0.01%. Bot. 20 ml, 60 ml.
Use: Corticosteroid.

FLUOPROMAZINE. B.A.N. 10-(3-Dimethylaminopropyl)-2-trifluoromethylpiamothiazine. Triflupro-

mazine (I.N.N.).
Use: Tranquilizer.

•**FLUORESCEIN,** U.S.P. XXII. Inj. U.S.P. XXII.
Use: Diagnostic aid (corneal trauma indicator).

•**FLUORESCEIN SODIUM,** U.S.P. XXII. Ophth. Strip, U.S.P. XXII. Spiro[isoberzofuran-1(3H), 9-[9H]xanthene]-3-one, 3′6′-dihydroxy, disodium salt. (Various Mfr.) Soluble fluorescein. Bot. 1 oz.
Use: 2% soln. in diagnosis of eye conditions. (circulation time).
See: Fluor-I-Strip. (Wyeth-Ayerst).
Funduscein, Amp. (CooperVision).
Plak-Lite Soln. (Internat. Pharm.).

FLUORESCEIN SODIUM I.V.
See: Fluorescite, Amp. (Alcon).

FLUORESCEIN SODIUM 2% SOLUTION. (Alcon) Drop-Tainer 15 ml, Steri-Unit 2 ml 12s.
Use: Diagnostic aid, ophthalmic.

FLUORESCEIN SODIUM 2%. (CooperVision) A sterile aqueous solution containing fluorescein sodium 2%. Dropperette 1 ml, Box 12s.
Use: Diagnostic aid, ophthalmic.

FLUORESCITE. (Alcon) Fluorescein as sodium salt. Inj. Soln. **10%:** Amp. 5 ml, Box 12s, Disposable Syringe 5 ml, 12s; **25%:** Amp 2 ml. Box 12s.
Use: Diagnostic aid, ophthalmic.

FLUORESOFT. (Holles) Fluorexon 0.35%. Soln. Pipette 0.5 ml, Box 12s.
Use: Diagnostic aid, ophthalmic.

FLUORETS. (Akorn) Fluorescein sodium 1 mg. Strip. Box 100s.
Use: Diagnostic aid, ophthalmic.

FLUOREXON.
See: Fluoresoft (Holles).

FLUORIDE SODIUM.
See: Dentafluor Chewable, Tab. (Western Pharm.).
Karidium, Top. Soln., Tab. (Lorvic).
Karigel, Gel (Lorvic).

FLUORIDE THERAPY.
See: Adeflor Preps. (Upjohn).
Cari-Tab, Softab Tab. (Stuart).
Coral Prods. (Lorvic).
Fluorineed, Chew. Tab. (Hanlon).
Fluorinse, Liq. (Pacemaker).
Fluora, Loz. (Kirkman).
Gal-Kam, Preps. (Scherer).
Luride Preps. (Hoyt).
Mulvidren-F, Softab Tab. (Stuart).
Point Two, Rinse (Hoyt).
Poly-Vi-Flor, Drops, Tab. (Mead Johnson).
Soluvite-F, Drops (Pharmics).
Tri-Vi-Flor, Drops, Tab. (Mead Johnson).

FLUORIGARD. (Colgate-Palmolive) Fluoride 0.02% (from sodium fluoride 0.05%), alcohol 6%, tartrazine. Bot. 180 ml, 300 ml, 480 ml.
Use: Dental caries preventative.

FLUORI-METHANE SPRAY. (Gebauer) Dichlorodifluoromethane 15%, trichloromonofluoromethane 85%. Bot. 4 oz.
Use: "Painful motion" syndromes.

FLUORINEED. (Hanlon) Fluoride 1 mg/Chew. Tab. Bot. 100s, 1000s.
Use: Dental caries preventative.

FLUORINSE. (Oral-B) Fluoride 0.09% from sodium fluoride 0.2%. Bot. 480 ml.
Use: Dental caries preventative.

FLUORINSE. (Pacemaker) Fluoride mouthwash. Pack. Fluoride ion level 0.05% or 0.2%. UD Bot. 32 oz. Concentrate 1 oz, 4 oz, gal.
Use: Dental caries preventative.

FLUOR-I-STRIP. (Wyeth-Ayerst) Fluorescein sodium 9 mg/ophthalmic strip. Box. 300s.
Use: Diagnostic aid, ophthalmic.

FLUOR-I-STRIP-A.T. (Wyeth-Ayerst) Fluorescein sodium 1 mg/ophthalmic strip. Box 300s (150 × 2).
Use: Diagnostic aid, ophthalmic.

FLUORITAB. (Fluoritab) Sodium fluoride 2.2 mg equivalent to 1 mg of fluorine (as fluoride ion) w/inert organic filler 75.8 mg/Tab. Bot. 100s; Liq. dropper bot. (fluorine 0.25 mg from 0.55 mg sodium fluoride/Drop) 19 ml.
Use: Dental caries preventative.

FLUORACAINE. (Akorn) Proparacaine HCl 0.5%, fluorescein sodium 0.25%, glycerin, povidone, thimerosal 0.01%. Dropper bot. 2 ml, 5 ml.
Use: Local anesthetic, ophthalmic.

5-FLUOROCYTOSINE.
See: Ancobon, Cap. (Roche).

•**FLUORODOPA F 18.** USAN.
Use: Diagnostic radiopharmaceutical.

FLUOROGESTONE ACETATE. 9-Fluoro-11β, 17-dihydroxypregn-4-ene-3, 20-dione, 17-acetate.
Use: Progestin.

FLUOROHYDROCORTISONE ACETATE. 9-α-Fluorohydrocortisone.
See: Fludrocortisone Acetate (Various Mfr.).

•**FLUOROMETHOLONE,** U.S.P. XXII. Cream, Ophth. Susp., U.S.P. XXII. Pregna-1,4-diene-3,20-diene, 9-fluoro-11,17-dihydroxy-6-methyl-,(6α,11β)-. 6α-Methyl-9α-fluoro-21-desoxyprednisolone. 9-Fluoro-11β, 17-dihydroxy-6α-methylpregna-1, 4-diene-3, 20-dione. B.A.N. 9α-Fluoro-11β-17α-dihydroxy-6α-methylpregna-1,4-diene-3,20-dione.
Use: Glucocorticoid.
See: Fluor-Op, Susp. (CooperVision).
FML, Liquifilm, Ophth. Susp., Oint. (Allergan).
Oxylone, Cream Ophth. Susp. (Upjohn).
W/Neomycin sulfate.
See: Neo-Oxylone, Oint. (Upjohn).

•**FLUOROMETHOLONE ACETATE.** USAN.
Use: Glucocorticoid, anti-inflammatory.

FLUOR-OP. (Iolab Pharm.) Fluorometholone 0.1% (1 mg/ml) susp. Bot. 5 ml, 10 ml, 15 ml w/ dropper.
Use: Corticosteroid.

FLUOROPHENE.
Use: Antiseptic.

FLUOROPLEX TOPICAL SOLUTION AND TOPICAL CREAM. (Herbert) **Soln.:** Fluorouracil 1%

in a propylene glycol base. Plastic bot. w/dropper 30 ml. **Cream:** Fluorouracil 1% in emulsion base w/benzyl alcohol 0.5%, emulsifying wax, mineral oil, isopropyl myristate, sodium hydroxide, purified water. Tube 30 Gm.
Use: Topical treatment of multiple actinic (solar) keratoses.

FLUOROQUINOLONES.
Use: Anti-infective.
See: Floxin (Ortho).
Ciloxan (Alcon).
Noroxin (Merck Sharp and Dohme).
Cipro (Miles).
Cipro I.V. (Miles).

•**FLUOROSALAN.** USAN. 3, 5-dibromo-3′-trifluoromethyl salicylanilide. Fluorophene.
Use: Antiseptic.

FLUOR-O-SOL. (Hoyt) Fluoride 1.2% with silicon dioxide abrasive. Jar 50 Gm, Carton 6s.
Use: Dental caries preventative.

FLUOROTHYL. Bis (2, 2, 2-trifluoroethyl) ether.
See: Flurothyl.

•**FLUOROURACIL,** U.S.P. XXII. Cream, Inj., Topical Soln., U.S.P. XXII. 5-Fluorouracil. (Roche) Amp. 10 ml, 500 mg, Box 10s.
Use: Malignancies, antineoplastic.
See: Adrucil, Inj. (Adria).
Efudex, Soln., Cream (Roche).
Fluoroplex, Soln., Cream (Herbert Labs.).

FLUOSOL. (Alpha Therapeutic) Perfluorochemicals 20%. Emulsion in 400 ml flexible plastic bag. Additive solutions 1 and 2 supplied in a separate continuous oxygenation kit.
Use: Perfluorochemical emulsion.

FLUOTHANE. (Wyeth-Ayerst) Halothane. Bot. 125 ml, 250 ml.
Use: Inhalation anesthetic.

•**FLUOTRACEN HYDROCHLORIDE.** USAN.
Use: Antipsychotic, antidepressant.

•**FLUOXETINE.** USAN.
Use: Antidepressant.

•**FLUOXYMESTERONE,** U.S.P. XXII. Tab., U.S.P. XXII. 9-α-Fluoro-11-β-hydroxy-17-α-methyltestosterone. 9-Fluoro-11β, 17β-dihydroxy-17-methylandrost-4-en-3-one.
Use: Androgen.
See: Android-F, Tab. (Brown).
Halotestin, Tab. (Upjohn).
Ora-Testryl, Tab. (Squibb Mark).
W/Ethinyl estradiol.
See: Halodrin, Tab. (Upjohn).

FLUOXYMESTERONE. B.A.N. 9α-Fluoro-11β, 17 b-dihy 17α-methylandrost-4-en-3-one. 9α-Fluoro-11 β-hydroxymethyltestosterone.
Use: Androgen, anabolic steroid.

FLUPENTHIXOL. B.A.N. 9-3-[4-(2-Hydroxyethel)-piperazin-1-yl]propylidene-2-trifluoromethylthioxanthene.
Use: Tranquilizer.

•**FLUPERAMIDE.** USAN.
Use: Antiperistaltic.

•**FLUPEROLONE ACETATE.** USAN. 9α-Fluoro-21-methylprednisolone, 9α-Fluoro-11β,17α,21-trihy-droxy-21-methylpregna-1:4-diene-3:20-dione acetate. Methral.
Use: Corticosteroid.

FLUPHENAZINE DECANOATE.
See: Prolixin Decanoate, Soln. (Princeton).
Use: Antipsychotic.

•**FLUPHENAZINE ENANTHATE,** U.S.P. XXII. Inj., U.S.P. XXII. 4-(3-(2-(Trifluoromethyl)phenothiazine-10-yl)-propyl)-1-piperazine-ethanol.
Use: Tranquilizer.
See: Prolixin Enanthate Prods. (Princeton).

•**FLUPHENAZINE HYDROCHLORIDE,** U.S.P. XXII. Elixir, Inj., Oral Soln., Tab., U.S.P. XXII. 1-(2-Hydroxyethyl)-4-[3-(2-trifluoromethyl)-10H-Phenothiazinyl-propyl]-piperazine diHCl. 4-(3-(2-(Trifluoromethyl) phenothiazine-10-yl) propyl)-1-piperazine-ethanol Dihydrochloride.
Use: Tranquilizer.
See: Permitil, Preps. (Schering).
Prolixin, Tab., Elix., Vial (Princeton).

•**FLUPIRTINE MALEATE.** USAN.
Use: Analgesic.

FLUPREDNIDENE. B.A.N. 9α-Fluoro-11β-17 a,21-trihydroxy-16-methylenepregna-1,4-diene-3, 20-dione.
Use: Glucocorticosteroid.

•**FLUPREDNISOLONE VALERATE.** USAN. 6-Fluoro-11β, 17, 21-trihydroxypregna-1, 4-diene-3,20-dione 17-valerate.
Use: Glucocorticoid.

FLUPROFEN. B.A.N. 2-(2′-Fluorobiphenyl-4-yl)-propionic acid.
Use: Anti-inflammatory, analgesic.

•**FLUPROQUAZONE.** USAN.
Use: Analgesic.

FLUPROSTENOL. B.A.N. (±)-7-(1R,2R,3R,5S)-3,5- Dihydroxy-2-[(3R)-3-hydroxy-4-(3-trifluoromethylphenoxy)but-1-(E)-enyl]cyclopent-1-yl hept-5-(Z)-enoic acid.
Use: Infertility (veterinary).
See: Equimate (sodium salt).

•**FLUPROSTENOL SODIUM.** USAN.
Use: Prostaglandin.

•**FLUQUAZONE.** USAN.
Use: Anti-inflammatory.

•**FLURADOLINE HYDROCHLORIDE.** USAN.
Use: Analgesic.

FLURA DROPS. (Kirkman) Fluoride. **Drops:** 0.25 mg (from 0.55 mg sodium fluoride). Bot. 24 ml. **Rinse:** 0.02% (from 0.05% sodium fluoride). Bot. 480 ml.
Use: Dental caries preventative.

FLURA-LOZ. (Kirkman) Sodium fluoride 2.2 mg providing 1 mg fluoride/Loz. Bot. 100s, 1000s.
Use: Dental caries preventative.

•**FLURANDRENOLIDE,** U.S.P. XXII. Cream, Oint., Lotion, Tape, U.S.P. XXII.
Use: Adrenocortical steroid (topical anti-inflammatory).
See: Cordran, Preps.(Dista).

FLURANDRENOLONE. 6α-Fluoro-16α-hydroxy-hydrocortisone 16, 17-acetonide.
Use: Corticosteroid.

FLURANDRENOLONE. B.A.N. 6α-Fluoro-11β,-21-dihydroxy-16α, 17α-isopropylidenedioxy-pregn-4-ene-3,20-dione. 6α-Fluoro-16α, 17α-isopropylidenedioxyhydrocortisone. Fludroxycortide (I.N.N.).
Use: Corticosteroid.

FLURA-TABLETS. (Kirkman) Sodium fluoride 2.21 mg, equivalent to 1 mg fluoride ion/Tab. Bot. 100s, 1000s.
Use: Dental caries preventative.

•**FLURAZEPAM HYDROCHLORIDE,** U.S.P. XXII. Cap., U.S.P. XXII. 7-Chloro-1-[2-(diethylamino)ethyl]-5-(o-fluorophenyl)-3,-dihydro-2H-1,4-benzodiazepin-2-one dihydrochloride. B.A.N. 7-Chloro-1-(2-diethylamino-ethyl)-5-(2-fluorophenyl)-1,3-dihydro-2H-1,4-benzodiazepin-2-one.
Use: Hypnotic.
See: Dalmane, Cap. (Roche).

•**FLURBIPROFEN SODIUM,** U.S.P. XXII, Ophth., USAN. 2-(2-Fluorobiphenyl-4-yl)propionic acid.
Use: Anti-inflammatory; analgesic.
See: Ocufen, Drops (Allergan).

FLURESS. (Barnes-Hind) Fluorescein sodium 0.25%, benoxinate HCl 0.4% in isotonic boric acid soln., chlorobutanol 1%. Bot. 5 ml.
Use: Local anesthetic, diagnostic aid.

•**FLURETOFEN.** USAN.
Use: Anti-inflammatory, antithrombotic.

•**FLURFAMIDE.** USAN.
Use: Enzyme inhibitor.

•**FLUROCITABINE.** USAN.
Use: Antineoplastic.

FLURO-ETHYL. (Gebauer) Ethyl Cl 25%, dichlorotetrafluoroethane 75%. Aerosol can 255 Gm.
Use: Topical anesthetic.

•**FLUROGESTONE ACETATE.** USAN.
Use: Progestin.

FLUROSYN. (Rugby) **Cream:** Fluocinolone acetonide 0.01% or 0.025%. Tube 15 Gm, 60 Gm, 425 Gm. **Oint:** Fluocinolone acetonide 0.025% in a white petrolatum base. Tube 15 Gm, 60 Gm.
Use: Corticosteroid topical.

FLUROTHYL, U.S.P. XXI. Bis (2,2,2-trifluoroethyl) ether. Hexafluorodiethyl ether. B.A.N. Di-(2,2,2-trifluoroethyl) ether. Bis(2,2,2-trifluoroethyl)ether.
Use: Central nervous system stimulant, shock inducing agent (convulsant).
See: Indoklon.

•**FLUROXENE.** USAN. 2,2,2-Trifluoroethyl vinyl ether. Fluoromar.
Use: General inhalation anesthetic.

•**FLUSPIPERONE.** USAN.
Use: Antipsychotic.

•**FLUSPIRILENE.** USAN. 8-[4, 4-bis(p-Fluorophenyl)butyl]-1-phenyl-1,3,8-triazaspiro-[4.5] decan-4-one.
Use: Tranquilizer, antipsychotic.
See: Imap (McNeil).

•**FLUTAMIDE.** USAN.
Use: Antiandrogen.

FLUTEX. (Syosset) Triamcinolone acetonide. **0.025%:** Tube 30 Gm, 60 Gm. **0.1%:** Tube 30 Gm, 60 Gm, 120 Gm. **0.5%:** Tube 30 Gm.
Use: Corticosteroid, topical.

•**FLUTIAZIN.** USAN.
Use: Anti-inflammatory.

•**FLUTICASONE PROPIONATE.** USAN.
Use: Anti-inflammatory.
See: Cutivate (Glaxo).

FLUTRA. Trichlormethiazide.
Use: Diuretic.

•**FLUTROLINE.** USAN.
Use: Antipsychotic.

•**FLUVASTATIN SODIUM.** USAN
Use: Antihyperlipidemic.

•**FLUZINAMIDE.** USAN.
Use: Anticonvulsant.

FLUZONE. (Squibb) Influenza virus vaccine. Vial 5 ml (10 doses) (Whole-virus); Vial 5 ml, UD syringes 0.5 ml (Split-virus).
Use: Agent for immunization.

FML. (Allergan) Fluorometholone 0.1% Oint. Tube 3.5 Gm.
Use: Corticosteroid, ophthalmic.

FML FORTE. (Allergan) Fluorometholone 0.25%, benzalkonium Cl 0.005%, EDTA, polysorbate 80, polyvinyl alcohol 1.4%. Susp. Dropper bot. 2 ml, 5 ml, 10 ml, 15 ml.
Use: Corticosteroid, ophthalmic.

FML LIQUIFILM. (Allergan) Fluorometholone 0.1%, polyvinyl alcohol 1.4%, benzalkonium Cl, edetate disodium, sodium Cl, sodium phosphate monobasic, monohydrate, sodium phosphate dibasic (anhydrous), polysorbate 80, purified water, sodium hydroxide to adjust pH. Dropper bot. 1 ml, 5 ml, 10 ml, 15 ml.
Use: Corticosteroid, ophthalmic.

•**FOCOFILCON A.** USAN.
Use: Contact lens material.

FOILLE. (Blistex) Benzocaine 2%, benzyl alcohol 4% in a bland vegetable oil base. Oint. Tube 30 Gm.
Use: Local anesthetic.

FOILLECORT. (Blistex) Hydrocortisone acetate 0.5%. Cream. Tube 3.5 Gm.
Use: Corticosteroid, topical.

FOILLE MEDICATED FIRST AID. (Blistex) **Aerosol:** Benzocaine 5% with chloroxylenol 0.1% in a bland vegetable oil base with benzyl alcohol. Spray 92 Gm. **Oint.:** Benzocaine 5%, chloroxylenol 0.1% in a bland vegetable oil base. Tube 30 Gm. **Lot.:** Benzocaine 5%, chloroxylenol 0.1% in a bland vegetable oil base with benzyl alcohol 30 ml.
Use: Local anesthetic.

FOILLE PLUS. (Blistex) **Cream:** Benzocaine 5%, benzyl alcohol 4% in a nonstaining washable base. Tube 3.5 Gm. **Soln.:** Benzocaine 5%, benzyl alcohol, alcohol 77.8%. Aerosol spray 105 Gm.

Use: Local anesthetic.

FOLABEE. (Vortech) Liver inj. B_{12} equivalent to 10 mcg, crystalline B_{12} 100 mcg, folic acid 0.4 mg. Inj. Vial 10 ml.
Use: Vitamin supplement.

FOLACIN.
See: Folic acid.

FOLACINE.
See: Folic acid. (Various Mfr.).

FOLATE, SODIUM.
See: Folvite, Soln. (Lederle).

FOLEX. (Adria) Methotrexate sodium 25 mg, 50 mg, 100 mg or 250 mg/Vial. Pow. for injection. UD vials.
Use: Antineoplastic agent.

FOLEX PFS INJECTION. (Adria) Methotrexate sodium 25 mg/ml. Preservative free. Inj. Vial. 2 ml, 4 ml, 8 ml.
Use: Antineoplastic agent.

•**FOLIC ACID,** U.S.P. XXII. Inj., Tab. U.S.P. XXII. Pteroylglutamic acid. N-[p-[[(2-Amino-4-hydroxy-6-pteridinyl)-methyl]-amino] benzoyl]-L-glutamic acid. L-Glutamic acid, N-[4-[[(2-amino-1,4-dihydro-4-oxo-6-pteridinyl)methyl]-amino]benzoyl]-. Vitamin Bc.
Use: Vitamin therapy.
See: Folvite, Tab., Soln. (Lederle).

FOLIC ACID ANTAGONISTS.
See: Methotrexate Inj., Tab. (Lederle).

FOLIC ACID SALTS.
See: Folvite, Tab., Soln. (Lederle).

FOLINIC ACID. Leucovorin Calcium, U.S.P. XXII. (Various Mfr.)

FOLIVER "12." (Pharmex) Vitamin B_{12} activity from liver inj. equivalent to cyanocobalamin 10 mcg, folic acid 1 mg, B_{12} 100 mcg/ml. Vial 10 ml, Univial 10 ml.
Use: Vitamin supplement.

FOL-LI-BEE. (Foy) Liver inj. equivalent to cyanocobalamin 10 mcg, folic acid 1 mg, cyanocobalamin 100 mcg/ml, phenol 0.5% pH adjusted w/ sodium hydroxide and/or HCl. Vial 10 ml multidose, Monovials.
Use: Vitamin supplement.

FOLLICLE STIMULATING HORMONE, HUMAN. Menotropins, Pergonal.

FOLLICORMON.
See: Estradiol Benzoate. (Various Mfr.).

FOLLICULAR HORMONES.
See: Estrone (Various Mfr.).

FOLLICULIN.
See: Estrone (Various Mfr.).

FOLLUTEIN. (Squibb Mark) Chorionic gonadotropin (HCG). Pow. with 10 ml diluent. 10,000 units (W/Sodium Cl 83 mg, sodium hydroxide, phenol 0.5%). Pow. for inj.
Use: Chorionic gonadotropin.

FOLTRIN. (Vitarine) Liver and stomach concentrate 240 mg, B_{12} 15 mcg, iron 110 mg, C 75 mg, folic acid 0.5 mg/Cap. Bot. 100s, 1000s.
Use: Vitamin/mineral supplement.

FOLVITE. (Lederle) Folic acid (as sodium folate). **Soln.:** (Sequestrene sodium 0.2%, water for injection, sodium hydroxide, benzyl alcohol 1.5%) 5 mg/ml. Vial 10 ml. **Tab.:** 1 mg. Bot. 100s, 1000s, UD 10 × 10s.
Use: Megaloblastic anemias of folate deficiency.

•**FOMEPIZOLE.** USAN.
Use: Antidote (alcohol dehydrogenase inhibitor).

FOMOCAINE. B.A.N. 4-(3-Morpholinopropyl)-benzyl phenyl ether.
Use: Local anesthetic.

FONATOL.
See: Diethylstilbestrol (Various Mfr.).

•**FONAZINE.** USAN. Dimethothiazine.
Use: Serotonin inhibitor.

FONAZINE MESYLATE. 10-[2-Dimethylamino)propyl]-N, N-dimethylphenothiazine-2-sulfonamide methanesulfonate.
Use: Antihistamine, antiserotonin, antibradykinin.

FONTARSOL.
See: Dichlorophenarsine Hydrochloride.

FORALICON PLUS ELIXIR. (Forbes) Vitamins B_{12} 16.7 mcg, B_6 4 mg, iron 200 mg (equivalent to elemental iron 24 mg), niacinamide 40 mg, folic acid 0.8 mg, sorbitol soln. q.s./15 ml. Bot. 8 oz, 16 oz.
Use: Vitamin/mineral supplement.

FORANE. (Anaquest) Isoflurane. Gas. Volume 100 ml.
Use: General anesthetic.

FORDUSTIN. (Sween) Cornstarch based powder with deodorizing action. Bot. 3 oz, 8 oz.
Use: Baby powder.

FORMADON SOLUTION.(Gordon) Formalin solution 3.7% to 4% (10% of U.S.P. strength) in an aqueous perfumed base. Bot. 1 oz, 4 oz, 0.5 gal, gal.
Use: Bromidrosis, hyperhidrosis.

FORMADRIN. (Kenyon) Chlorpheniramine maleate 12 mg, potassium guaiacol sulfonate 8 gr, ammonium Cl 8 gr, tartar emetic 1/12 gr, dl-desoxyephedrine HCl 2 mg/oz. Bot. 4 oz.
Use: Antihistamine, expectorant.

•**FORMALDEHYDE SOLUTION,** U.S.P. XXII. A 37% aqueous solution.
Use: For poison ivy, fungus infections of the skin, hyperhidrosis and as an astringent disinfectant.

FORMALIN.
See: Formaldehyde Solution (Various Mfr.).

FORMA-RAY SOLUTION. (Gordon) Formalin 7.4% to 8% (20% of USP strength) in aqueous, scented, tinted solution. Bot. 1.5 oz, 4 oz.
Use: Drying agent following laser treatment for verrucae, excessive perspiration and odor.

FORMEBOLONE. B.A.N. 2-Formyl-11α, 17β-dihydroxy-17α-methylandrosta-1,4-dien-3-one.

Use: Anabolic steroid.

FORMIC ACID.
W/Silicic acid.
See: Nyloxin, Inj. (Hyson, Westcott & Dunning).

FORMINITRAZOLE. B.A.N. 2-Formamido-5-nitrothiazole.
Use: Treatment of trichomoniasis.

•**FORMOCORTAL.** USAN. 3-(2-Chloroethoxy)-9-fluoro-11β, 16α, 17, 21-tetrahydroxy-20-oxopregna-3, 5-diene-6-carboxaldehyde, cyclic 16, 17-acetal with acetone, 21-acetate.
Use: Glucocorticoid.

FORMULA "K." (Pharmex) Calcium gluconate 1.5 Gm, potassium Cl 4.47 Gm, magnesium sulfate 60 mg/ml. Vial 30 ml.
Use: Mineral supplement.

FORMULA 44 COUGH CONTROL DISCS. (Vicks).
See: Vicks Formula 44 Cough Discs (Vicks).

FORMULA 44 COUGH MIXTURE. (Vicks) Chlorpheniramine maleate 2 mg, dextromethorphan HBr 15 mg, alcohol 10%/5 ml. Liq. Bot. 120 ml, 240 ml.
Use: Antihistamine, antitussive.

FORMULA 44D DECONGESTANT COUGH MIXTURE. (Vicks) Pseudoephedrine HCl 20 mg, dextromethorphan HBr 10 mg, guaifenesin 67 mg, alcohol 10%/5 ml. Liq. Bot. 120 ml, 240 ml.
Use: Decongestant, antitussive, expectorant.

FORMULA 44M. (Vicks Health Care) Pseudoephedrine HCl 15 mg, dextromethorphan HBr 7.5 mg, guaifenesin 50 mg, acetaminophen 125 mg/5 ml, alcohol 20%, saccharin. Liq. Bot. 120 ml, 240 ml.
Use: Decongestant, antitussive, expectorant, analgesic.

FORMULA NO. 81. (Fellows) Liver (beef) for inj. 1 mcg, ferrous gluconate 100 mg, niacinamide 100 mg, B_2 1.5 mg, panthenol 2.5 mg, B_{12} 3 mcg, procaine HCl 25 mg/2 ml. Vial 30 ml.
Use: Vitamin/mineral supplement.

FORMULA 1207. (Thurston) Iodine, liver fraction No. 2, caseinates/Tab. Bot. 100s, 250s.
Use: Mineral supplement.

FORMYL TETRAHYDROPTEROYLGLUTAMIC ACID. Leucovorin Calcium, U.S.P. XXII.

FORTA CEREAL MIX. (Ross) Milk protein isolate, instant oats, oat bran, corn bran, vitamins A, B_1, B_2, B_3, B_5, B_6, B_{12}, C, D, E, folic acid, biotin, Ca, Fe, P, I, Mg, Zn, Cu, Mn. Can 673 Gm.
Use: Enteral nutritional supplement.

FORTA DRINK POWDER. (Ross) Whey protein concentrate, sucrose, vitamins A, B_1, B_2, B_3, B_5, B_6, B_{12}, C, D, E, folic acid, biotin, Ca, Cu, Fe, I, Mg, Mn, P, Zn. Can. 805 Gm.
Use: Enteral nutritional supplement.

FORTA-FLORA. (Barth's) Whey-lactose 90%, pectin. **Pow.:** Jar lb. **Wafer:** Bot. 100s.

FORTAGESIC TABLETS. (Winthrop Products) Paracetamol, pentazocine.
Use: Narcotic analgesic.

FORTA INSTANT CEREAL. (Ross) Lactose-free oat or bran cereal provides 6.25 Gm dietary fiber/serving. Can 1 lb 1 oz.
Use: Enteral nutritional supplement.

FORTA INSTANT PUDDING. (Ross) Lactose-free in pudding base. Can 1 lb 12 oz. Vanilla, chocolate, butterscotch flavors.
Use: Enteral nutritional supplement.

FORTA PUDDING MIX. (Ross) Milk protein isolate, sucrose, hydrolyzed cornstarch, modified tapioca starch, partially hydrogenated soybean oil, vitamins A, B_1, B_2, B_3, B_5, B_6, B_{12}, C, D, E, folic acid, biotin, Ca, Fe, P, I, Mg, Zn, Cu, Mn, tartrazine. Can 794 Gm.
Use: Enteral nutritional supplement.

FORTA SHAKE POWDER. (Ross) Nonfat dry milk, sucrose, vitamins A, B_1, B_2, B_3, B_5, B_6, B_{12}, C, D, E, folic acid, biotin, Ca, Cu, Fe, I, Mg, Mn, P, Zn, tartrazine. Can lb, pkt. 1.4 oz. Can 1 lb 2.7 oz, pkt. 1.6 oz.
Use: Enteral nutritional supplement.

FORTA SOUP MIX. (Ross) Milk protein isolate, sodium and calcium caseinate, hydrolyzed cornstarch, modified tapioca starch, powdered shortening (partially hydrogenated coconut oil), vitamins A, B_1, B_2, B_3, B_5, B_6, B_{12}, C, D, E, folic acid, biotin, Ca, Cu, Fe, I, Mg, Mn, P, Zn. Chicken flavor. Can. 454 Gm.
Use: Enteral nutritional supplement.

FORTAZ. (Glaxo) Ceftazidime powder for parenteral administration 500 mg, 1 Gm, 2 Gm, or 6 Gm Vial. **500 mg:** Tray 25s. **1 Gm:** Tray 25s, Infusion Pack Tray 10s. **2 Gm:** Tray 10s, Infusion Pack Tray 10s. **6 Gm:** Pharmacy Bulk Pkg. Tray 6s.
Use: Antibacterial, cephalosporin.

FORTE L.I.V. (Foy) Cyanocobalamin 15 mcg liver injection equivalent to vitamin B_{12} activity 1 mcg, ferrous gluconate 50 mg, B_2 0.75 mg, panthenol 1.25 mg, niacinamide 50 mg, citric acid 8.2 mg, sodium citrate 118 mg/ml, procaine HCl 2%. Bot. 30 ml.
Use: Vitamin supplement.

FORTEL OVULATION. (NMS) Monoclonal antibody-based home test to predict ovulation. Kit 1s.
Use: Diagnostic aid.

FORTRAL. (Winthrop Products) Pentazocine as solution and tablets.
Use: Narcotic analgesic.

FORTRAMIN. (Thurston) Vitamins E 200 IU, A 6000 IU, D 600 IU, B_1 4.5 mg, B_2 4.5 mg, B_6 4.5 mg, B_{12} 5 mcg, C 2.75 mg, rutin 8 mg, hesperidin complex 10 mg, lemon bioflavonoids 15 mg, d-calcium pantothenate 50 mg, para-aminobenzoic acid 7.5 mg, biotin 10 mg, folic acid 24 mcg, niacinamide 20 mg, desiccated liver 25 mg, iron 3 mg, calcium 75 mg, phosphorous 34 mg, manganese 10 mg, copper 0.5 mg, zinc 0.5 mg, iodine 0.375 mg, potassium 500 mg, magnesium 5 mg/Tab. Bot. 100s, 250s.

Use: Vitamin/mineral supplement.
•**FOSARILATE.** USAN.
Use: Antiviral.
•**FOSAZEPAM.** USAN. 7-Chloro-1-dimethylphosphinylmethyl-1,3-dihydro-5-phenyl-2H-1,4-benzodiazepin-2-one.
Use: Hypnotic.
•**FOSCARNET SODIUM.** USAN.
Use: Antiviral.
•**FOSENOPRIL SODIUM.** USAN.
Use: Antihypertensive, enzyme inhibitor.
FOSFESTROL. B.A.N. trans-αα′-Diethylstilbene-4,4′-diol bis(dihydrogen phosphate).
Use: Treatment of carcinoma of the prostate.
•**FOSFOMYCIN.** USAN.
Use: Antibacterial.
•**FOSFONET SODIUM.** USAN.
Use: Antiviral.
•**FOSPIRATE.** USAN.
Use: Anthelmintic.
FOSFREE. (Mission) Calcium lactate 250 mg, calcium gluconate 250 mg, calcium carbonate 300 mg, calcium 175.7 mg, ferrous gluconate 125 mg (iron 14.5 mg), vitamins A 1500 IU, B_1 5 mg, B_2 2 mg, B_3 10 mg, B_5 1 mg, B_6 3 mg, B_{12} 2 mcg, C 50 mg, D 150 IU/Tab. Bot. 100s.
Use: Vitamin/mineral supplement.
•**FOSINOPRIL.**
Use: Angiotensin converting enzyme inhibitor, antihypertensive.
See: Monopril (Mead Johnson).
•**FOSINOPRILAT.** USAN.
Use: Antihypertensive.
•**FOSQUIDONE.** USAN.
Use: Antineoplastic.
•**FOSTEDIL.** USAN.
Use: Vasodilator.
FOSTEX MEDICATED COVER-UP. (Westwood) Sulfur 2% in a flesh-tinted greasless base. Cream Tube 30 Gm.
Use: Anti-acne.
FOSTEX MEDICATED CLEANSING. (Westwood) Sulfur 2%, salicylic acid 2% w/soapless cleansers and wetting agents. Shampoo Tube 120 Gm.
Use: Anti-acne.
FOSTEX MEDICATED CLEANSING BAR. (Westwood) Sulfur 2%, salicylic acid 2% in base of soapless cleansers and wetting agents. Bar 112.5 Gm.
Use: Anti-acne.
FOSTEX 5% BPO. (Westwood) Benzyl peroxide 5% in Laureth-4 base. Gel 45 Gm.
Use: Anti-acne.
FOSTEX 10% BPO CLEANSING BAR. (Westwood) Benzoyl peroxide 10%. Bar 3.75 oz.
Use: Anti-acne.
FOSTEX 10% BPO WASH. (Westwood) Benzoyl peroxide 10% with water base. Liq. Bot. 150 ml.
Use: Anti-acne.
•**FOSTRIECIN SODIUM.** USAN.
Use: Antineoplastic.
FOSTRIL. (Westwood) Sulfur 2% in greaseless base. Lot. Tube 30 ml.
Use: Anti-acne.
FOTOTAR CREAM. (Elder) Coal tar 1.6% (from 2% coal tar extract) in emollient moisturizing cream base. Tube 90 Gm, 480 Gm.
Use: Chronic skin disorders.
FOURSALCO. (Jenkins) Salicylic acid 0.5 gr, sodium bicarbonate 3 gr, magnesium salicylate 2 gr, strontium salicylate 2 gr, acetophenetidin 0.25 gr, methyl salicylate, pancreatin 1/40 gr, diastase 1/40 gr/Tab. Bot. 1000s.
Use: Analgesic.
4-WAY COLD TABLETS. (Bristol-Myers) Aspirin 324 mg, phenylpropanolamine HCl 12.5 mg, chlorpheniramine maleate 2 mg/Tab. Bot. 36s, 60s, Card 15s.
Use: Analgesic, decongestant, antihistamine.
4-WAY NASAL SPRAY. (Bristol-Myers) Phenylephrine HCl 0.5%, naphazoline HCl 0.05%, pyrilamine maleate 0.2%, buffered isotonic aqueous soln., thimerosal 0.005%. Atomizer 15 ml, 30 ml.
Use: Decongestant, antihistamine.
4-WAY LONG ACTING NASAL SPRAY. (Bristol-Myers) Oxymetazoline HCl 0.05% in isotonic buffered soln., thimerosal 0.005%. Spray Bot. 15 ml.
Use: Nasal decongestant.
FOWLER'S SOLUTION. Potassium Arsenite Solution (Various Mfr.).
FOXALIN. (Standex) Digitoxin 0.1 mg, sodium carboxymethylcellulose/Cap. Bot. 100s.
Use: Cardiac glycoside.
FOXGLOVE.
See: Digitalis (Various Mfr.).
FOYGEN AQUEOUS. (Foy) Estrogenic substance or estrogens 2 mg/ml with sodium carboxymethylcellulose, povidone, benzyl alcohol, methyl and propyl parabens. Inj. Vial 10 ml.
Use: Estrogen.
FOYPLEX INJECTION. (Foy) Sterile injectable soln. of nine water-soluble vitamins. Packaged as 2 separate solutions for extemporaneous combination.
Use: Parenteral nutritional supplement.
FRAMYCETIN. B.A.N. An antibiotic produced by *Streptomyces decaris*.
Use: Antibiotic.
FRANODIL. (Winthrop) Ephedrine sulfate, theophylline, anhydrous, chlormezanone.
Use: Bronchodilator.
FRANOL. (Winthrop) Theophylline anhydrous, ephedrine sulfate, phenobarbital, thenyldiamine HCl.
Use: Bronchodilator.
FREAMINE III. (Kendall McGaw) Amino acid 8.5% or 10%. Bot. 500 ml, 1000 ml.
Use: Parenteral nutritional supplement.
FREAMINE III W/ELECTROLYTES. (Kendall McGaw) Amino acid 3% with electrolytes. Bot. 1000 ml.

Use: Parenteral nutritional supplement.
FREAMINE 8.5% III W/ELECTROLYTES. (Kendall McGraw) Sodium 60 mEq/L, potassium 60 mEq/L, magnesium 10 mEq/L, Cl 60 mEq/L, phosphate 40 mEq/L, acetate 125 mEq/L. Soln. Bot. 500 ml, 1000 ml.
Use: Parenteral nutritional supplement.
FREAMINE HBC. (American McGaw) High branched 6.9% amino acid formulation for hypercatabolic patients. Bot. 1000 ml.
Use: Parenteral nutritional supplement.
FREEDAVITE. (Freeda) Iron 30 mg (from ferrous fumarate), vitamins A 5000 IU, D 400 IU, E 3 IU, B_1 5 mg, B_2 3 mg, B_3 25 mg, B_5 5 mg, B_6 0.5 mg, B_{12} 2 mcg, C 60 mg, choline, inositol, Ca, Cu, K, Mg, Mn, Zn. Bot. 100s, 250s, 500s.
Use: Vitamin/mineral supplement.
FREEZONE. (Whitehall) Salicylic acid 13.6%, alcohol 20.5%, ether 64.8% in flexible collodion base. Bot. 9.3 ml 13 oz.
Use: Keratolytic.
•**FRENTIZOLE.** USAN.
Use: Immunoregulator.
FRESH n' FEMININE. (Walgreen) Benzethonium Cl 0.2% Bot. 8 oz.
Use: Vaginal preparation.
•**FRUCTOSE,** U.S.P. XXII. Inj., U.S.P. XXII. (Abbott) (Cutter) Soln. 10%. Bot. 1000 ml.
Use: Nutrient.
See: Frutabs, Tab. (Pfanstiehl).
•**FRUCTOSE AND SODIUM CHLORIDE INJECTION,** U.S.P. XXII.
Use: Fluid, nutrient and electrolyte replenisher.
FRUITY CHEWS. (Goldline) Vitamins A 2500 IU, D 400 IU, E 15 mg, B_1 1.05 mg, B_2 1.2 mg, B_3 13.5 mg, B_6 1.05 mg, B_{12} 4.5 mcg, C (as sodium ascorbate and ascorbic acid) 60 mg, folic acid 0.3 mg/Chew. Tab. Bot. 100s.
Use: Vitamin/mineral supplement.
FRUITY CHEWS WITH IRON. (Goldline) Elemental iron 12 mg, vitamins A 2500 IU, D 400 IU, E 15 mg, B_1 1.05 mg, B_2 1.2 mg, B_3 13.5 mg, B_6 1.05 mg, B_{12} 4.5 mg, C (as sodium ascorbate and ascorbic acid) 60 mg, folic acid 0.3 mg, zinc 8 mg/Chew. Tab. Bot. 100s.
Use: Vitamin/mineral supplement.
FRUSEMIDE. 4-Chloro-N-furfuryl-5-sulfamoylanthranilic acid. Lasix.
FRUSEMIDE. B.A.N. 4-Chloro-N-furfuryl-5-sulphamoylanthranilic acid. Furosemide (I.N.N.).
Use: Diuretic.
FRUTABS. (Pfanstiehl) Fructose 2 Gm. Tab. Bot. 100s.
Use: Carbohydrate.
FTA-ABS. (Wampole-Zeus) Fluorescent treponemal antibody-absorbed test *in vitro* for confirming a positive reagin test for syphillis. Test 100s.
Use: Diagnostic aid.
FTA-ABS/DS. (Wampole-Zeus) Fluorescent treponemal antibody-absorbed test *in vitro* for confirming a positive reagin test for syphilis. Test 100s.
Use: Diagnostic aid.
•**FUCHSIN, BASIC,** U.S.P. XXII. Basic Fuchsin is a mixture of rosaniline and pararosaniline HCl. Basic Magenta.
Use: Ingredient in Carbo-Fuchsin Solution anti-infective (topical).
FUDR. (Roche) Floxuridine 500 mg sterile pow. for inj. Vial 5 ml.
Use: Antineoplastic agent.
FUL-GLO. (Barnes-Hind) Fluorescein sodium 0.6 mg/Strip. Box 300s.
Use: Diagnostic aid, ophthalmic.
FULLER. (Birchwood) Pkg. 1 shield.
Use: Anorectal protective garment.
FULVICIN P/G. (Schering) Griseofulvin ultramicrosize 125 mg, 165 mg, 250 mg or 330 mg/Tab. Bot. 100s.
Use: Antifungal.
FULVICIN-U/F. (Schering) Griseofulvin microsize 250 mg or 500 mg/Tab. Bot. 60s, 250s.
Use: Antifungal.
FUMAGILLIN. B.A.N. A crystalline antibiotic produced during the growth of a strain of *Aspergillus fumigatus*.
•**FUMARIC ACID.** N.F. XVII. 2-Butenedioic acid.
Use: Acidifier.
FUMASORB. (Milance) Ferrous fumarate 200 mg (iron 66 mg)/Tab. Bot. 30s, 60s.
Use: Iron supplement.
FUMATINIC CAPSULES. (Laser) Iron 90 mg (from ferrous fumarate), vitamins C 100 mg, B_{12} 15 mcg, folic acid 1 mg/SR Cap. Bot. 100s, 1000s.
Use: Vitamin/mineral supplement.
FUMERIN. (Laser) Ferrous fumarate 195 mg equivalent to iron 64 mg/Tab. Bot. 100s, 1000s.
Use: Iron supplement.
FUMERON. (Vitarine) Ferrous fumarate 330 mg, vitamin B_1 5 mg/TR Cap.
Use: Vitamin/mineral supplement.
FUMIDE. (Everett) Furosemide 40 mg/Tab. Bot. 100s, 1000s.
Use: Diuretic.
•**FUMOXICILLIN.** USAN.
Use: Antibacterial.
FUNDUSCEIN. (Iolab) Sodium fluorescein. Inj. **10%:** Amp. 5 ml. 12s. **25%:** Amp. 3 ml. 12s.
Use: Diagnostic aid, ophthalmic.
FUNGACETIN OINTMENT. (Blair) Triacetin (glyceryl triacetate) 25% in a water-miscible ointment base. Tube 30 Gm.
Use: Antifungal, external.
FUNGATIN. (Major) Tolnaftate 1%. Cream Tube 15 Gm.
Use: Antifungal, external.
FUNGICIDES.
See: Aftate, Prods. (Plough).
Arcum, Preps. (Arcum).
Asterol.
Basic Fuchsin (Various Mfr.).
Desenex, Prods. (Pharmacraft).
Dichlorophene.

Nifuroxime (Various Mfr.).
Nitrofurfuryl Methyl Ether (Various Mfr.).
Phenylmercuric Preps. (Various Mfr.).
Propionate, Sodium (Various Mfr.).
Propionic Acid (Various Mfr.).
Undecylenic Acid (Various Mfr.).

•**FUNGIMYCIN.** USAN.
Use: Antifungal.

FUNGINAIL. (Kramer) Resorcinol 1%, salicyclic acid 2%, parachlorometaxylenol 2%, benzocaine 0.5%, acetic acid 2.5%, propylene glycol, hydroxypropyl methylcellulose, alcohol 0.5%. Bot. 30 ml.
Use: Antifungal, external.

FUNGIZONE. (Squibb) Amphotericin B 3%, thimerosal, titanium dioxide. **Lot.:** Plastic bot. 30 ml. **Cream, Oint:** Tube 20 Gm.
Use: Antifungal, external.

FUNGIZONE INTRAVENOUS. (Squibb) Amphotericin B 50 mg, sodium desoxycholate 41 mg, sodium phosphate 25.2 mg/Vial (lyophilized).
Use: Antifungal.

FUNGIZONE FOR LABORATORY USE IN TISSUE CULTURE. (Squibb) Amphotericin B 50 mg, sodium desoxycholate 41 mg/Vial 20 ml.
Use: Laboratory.

FUNGOID CREME. (Pedinol) Cetylpyridinium Cl, triacetin, chloroxylenol in vanishing cream base. Tube 30 Gm.
Use: Antifungal, external.

FUNGOID SOLUTION. (Pedinol) Cetylpyridinium Cl, triacetin, chloroxylenol. Plastic dropper bot. 15 ml.
Use: Antifungal, external.

FUNGOID TINCTURE. (Pedinol) Cetylpyridinium Cl, triacetin, chloroxylenol, glacial acetic acid, sodium propionate, propionic acid, isopropyl alcohol, benzyl alcohol, acetone, propylene glycol, eucalyptol. Bot. 30 ml, pt. w/brush applicator.
Use: Antifungal, external.

FURACIN SOLUBLE DRESSING. (Norwich Eaton) Nitrofurazone 0.2% in a water-soluble, nondrying, ointment-like base of polyethylene glycols. Jar 454 Gm, Tube 28 Gm, 56 Gm.
Use: Burn preparation.

FURACIN TOPICAL CREAM. (Norwich Eaton) Furacin 0.2% in a water miscible, self-emulsifying cream w/glycerin, cetyl alcohol, mineral oil, ethoxylated fatty alcohol, methylparaben, propylparaben, water. Tube 28 Gm.
Use: Burn preparation.

FURADANTIN. (Norwich Eaton) Nitrofurantoin 50 mg or 100 mg/Tab. Bot. 100s, 500s, UD 100s.
Use: Urinary anti-infective.

FURADANTIN ORAL SUSPENSION. (Norwich Eaton) Nitrofurantoin 5 mg/ml. Bot. 60 ml, 470 ml.
Use: Urinary anti-infective.

FURALAN. (Lannett) Nitrofurantoin 50 mg or 100 mg/Tab. Bot. 100s, 500s, 1000s.
Use: Urinary anti-infective.

FURALAZINE HYDROCHLORIDE. 3-Amino-6-[2-(5-nitro-2-furyl)vinyl]-as-triazine HCl.
Use: Antimicrobial compound.

FURALTADONE. (±)-5-Morpholinomethyl-3-[(5-ni-trofurfurylidene)amino]-2-oxazolidinone.

FURAN. (American Urologicals) Nitrofurantoin 50 mg. Tab. Bot. 100s, 1000s.
Use: Urinary anti-infective.

FURANITE TABS. (Major) Nitrofurantoin 50 mg or 100 mg/Tab. Bot. 100s.
Use: Urinary anti-infective.

•**FURAPROFEN.** USAN.
Use: Anti-inflammatory.

•**FURAZOLIDONE,** U.S.P. XXII. Oral Susp., Tab., U.S.P. XXII. 2-Oxazolidone, 3-(((5-nitro-2 furanyl) methyl-ene)amino). 3[(5-Nitrofurfurylidene)-amino]-2-oxazolidinone.
Use: Antimicrobial agent.
See: Furoxone Tab., Susp. (Norwich Eaton).

•**FURAZOLIUM CHLORIDE.** USAN.
Use: Antibacterial.

•**FURAZOLIUM TARTRATE.** USAN.
Use: Antibacterial.

FURAZOSIN HCl. 1-(4-Amino-6, 7-dimethoxy-2-quin-azolinyl)-4-(2-furoyl)piperazine monohydrochloride. Under study.
Use: Antihypertensive.

•**FUREGRELATE SODIUM.** USAN.
Use: Inhibitor (thromboxene synthetase).

FURETHIDINE. 1-(2-Tetrahydrofurfuryloxyethyl)-4-phenylpiperidine-4-carboxylic acid ethyl ester.

FURETHIDINE. B.A.N. Ethyl 4-phenyl-1-[2-(tetrahydrofurfuryloxy)ethyl]piperidine-4-carboxylate.
Use: Narcotic analgesic.

•**FURODAZOLE.** USAN.
Use: Anthelmintic.

FUROMIDE M.D. INJECTION. (Hyrex) Furosemide 10 mg/ml. Inj. Vial 10 ml.
Use: Diuretic.

FURONATAL FA. (Metro Med) Vitamins A 8000 IU, D 400 IU, E 30 IU, C 60 mg, folic acid 1 mg, B_1 2 mg, B_2 2.8 mg, B_6 2.5 mg, B_{12} 8 mcg, niacinamide 20 mg, iron 65 mg, calcium 125 mg/Tab. Bot. 100s, 1000s.
Use: Vitamin/mineral supplement.

•**FUROSEMIDE,** U.S.P. XXII. Inj., Tab., U.S.P. XXII. 4-Chloro-N-(furfuryl-)-5-sulfamoylanthranilic acid. Benzoic acid, 5-(aminosulfonyl)-4-chloro-2[(2-furanylmethyl)amino]. (Abbott) 10 mg/ml. Inj. Single dose syringe 2 ml, 5 ml, 10 ml, single dose vial 2 ml, 10 ml, partial fill single dose vial 4 ml.
Use: Diuretic.
See: Fumide, Tab. (Everett).
Furomide, Vial (Hyrex).
Lasix, Tab., Inj. (Hoechst-Roussel).

FUROSEMIDE. (Roxane) Furosemide. **10 mg/ml:** Soln. Dropper bot. 60 ml. **40 mg/5 ml:** Soln. Bot. 5 ml, 10 ml, 500 ml.
Use: Diuretic.

FUROXONE. (Norwich Eaton) Furazolidone. **Tab.:** 100 mg. Bot. 20s, 100s. **Liq.:** 50 mg/15 ml. Bot. 60 ml, 473 ml.
Use: Antibacterial.

•**FURSALAN.** USAN. 3, 5-Dibromo-N-(tetrahydrofurfuryl)- salicylamide. Under study.
Use: Germicide.

FUSAFUNGINE. B.A.N. An antibiotic produced by *Fusarium lateritium*.

•**FUSIDATE SODIUM.** USAN. (I) Sodium 3α, 11α, 16β-trihydroxy-29-nor-8α,9β,13α,14β-dammara-17(20),24-dien-21-oate 16-acetate. Fucidine (Squibb).
Use: Antibacterial.
See: Fucidine (Squibb).

•**FUSIDIC ACID.** USAN. An antibiotic produced by a strain of Fusidium. cis-16β-Acetoxy-3α,-11 α-dihydroxy-4α,8, 14-trimethyl-18-nor-5α,-8α,9β,13α,14β-cholesta-17(20),24-dien-21-oic acid.
Use: Antibacterial.

G

G-1. (Hauck) Acetaminophen 500 mg, butalbital 50 mg, caffeine 40 mg/Cap. Bot. 100s. UD 1000s.
Use: Analgesic, sedative/hypnotic.

G-4.
See: Dichlorophene.

G-11. (Givaudan) Hexachlorophene Pow. for mfg.
See: Hexachlorophene, U.S.P. XXII.

GACID TAB. (Arcum) Magnesium trisilicate 500 mg, aluminum hydroxide 250 mg/Tab. Bot. 100s, 1000s.
Use: Antacid.

•**GADODIAMIDE.** USAN.
Use: Diagnostic aid, paramagnetic.

•**GADOTERIDOL.** USAN.
Use: Diagnostic aid, paramagnetic.

•**GALLAMINE TRIETHIODIDE,** U.S.P. XXII. Inj. U.S.P. XXII. [v-Phenenyltris(oxyethylene)] tris[triethylam-monium] Triiodide. Ethanaminium, 2,2′,2″-[1,2,3-benzenetriyltris(oxy)]tris-[N,N,N-triethyl]-,triiodide.
Use: Skeletal muscle relaxant.
See: Flaxedil (Davis & Geck).

•**GALLIUM CITRATE Ga-67 INJECTION,** U.S.P. XXII.
Use: Diagnostic aid (radiopaque medium).

•**GALLIUM NITRATE.**
Use: Treatment of cancer-related hypercalcemia.
See: Ganite (Fujisawa).

GALLOCHROME.
See: Merbromin (Various Mfr.).

GALLOTANNIC ACID.
See: Tannic Acid, Preps. (Various Mfr.).

GAMASTAN. (Cutter) Immune serum globulin (human) U.S.P. Vial 2 ml, 10 ml.
Use: Immune serum.

GAMAZOLE TABS. (Major) Sulfamethoxazole 500 mg/Tab. Bot. 100s, 500s, 1000s.
Use: Antibacterial, sulfonamide.

•**GAMFEXINE.** USAN. N,N-Dimethyl--phenyl-cyclohexanepropylamine.
Use: Antidepressant.

GAMIMUNE N. (Cutter Biologicals) Immune globulin IV (human) 5% in maltose 10%. Inj. Vial 10 ml, 50 ml, 100 ml.
Use: Immune serum.

GAMMA BENZENE HEXACHLORIDE. B.A.N.-1,2,3,4,5,6-Hexachlorocyclohexane. Lindane, U.S.P. XXII.
Use: Antiparaasitic.

GAMMAGARD. (Hyland) Immune globulin intravenous (human) 2.5 Gm or 5 Gm/Vial. Inj. Dried concentrate w/diluent.
Use: Immune serum.

GAMMA GLOBULIN.
See: Immune Globulin Intramuscular.

GAMMA HYDROXYBUTYRATE (GBA). (Orphan Drug)
Use: Narcolepsy and auxiliary symptoms of cataplexy, sleep paralysis, hypnagogic hallucinations and automatic behavior.
Sponsor: Sigma Chemical.

GAMMAR. (Armour) Immune globulin, (human) U.S.P. Vial 2 ml, 10 ml.

GAMOLENIC ACID. B.A.N. cis, cis, cis-Octadeca-6,9,12-trienoic acid.
Use: Treatment of hypercholesterolemia.

G.A.M.P.A.K. (Fellows) Gastric mucin 10 gr, aminoacetic acid 4.5 gr, magnesium trisilicate 30 gr, aluminum hydroxide gel 31.21 gr, colloidal kaolin 194.5 gr/oz. Bot. 4 oz, 8 oz.
Use: Antacid.

GAMULIN Rh. (Armour) Rho (D) Immune globulin (Human). Vial, syringe 1 dose.
Use: Rh-negative mothers after delivery of an Rh-positive infant.

•**GANCICLOVIR.** USAN.
Use: Antiviral.
See: Cytovene (Syntex).

•**GANCICLOVIR SODIUM.** USAN.
Use: Antiviral.
See: Cytovene (Syntex).

G AND W PRODUCTS. (G & W) G and W markets the following products under the G & W brand name:
Aminophylline Rectal Supp., 250 mg, 500 mg.
Aspirin Rectal Supp., 125 mg, 300 mg, 600 mg.
Bisacodyl Supp., 10 mg.
Glycerin Supp., Adult and Infant Sizes.
Hemorrhoidal Rectal Ointment.
Hemorrhoidal Rectal Supp., Formula C-116 and Formula C-119.
Hemorrhoidal Rectal Supp. w/Hydrocortisone Acetate 10 mg or 25 mg/Supp.
Vaginal Sulfa Cream.

GANEAKE. (Geneva) Conjugated Estrogens, 0.625 mg, 1.25 mg or 2.5 mg/Tab. Bot. 100s, 1000s.

Use: Estrogen.

GANGLIONIC BLOCKING AGENTS.
See: Arfonad, Amp. (Roche).
Dibenzyline HCl, Cap. (SmithKline).
Hexamethonium Cl and Bromide (Various Mfr.).
Hydergine, Amp., Tab. (Sandoz).
Inversine, Tab. (Merck Sharp & Dohme).
Priscoline HCl, Tab., Vial (Ciba).
Regitine, Amp., Tab. (Ciba).

GANITE. (Fujisawa) Gallium nitrate.
Use: Treatment of cancer-related hypercalcemia.

GANTANOL. (Roche) Sulfamethoxazole. **Tab.:** 0.5 Gm/Tab. Bot. 100s, 500s, Tel-E-Dose 100s. **Susp:** 0.5 Gm/5 ml (cherry flavor) Bot. 1 pt.
Use: Antibacterial, sulfonamide.

GANTANOL DS. (Roche) Sulfamethoxazole 1 Gm/Tab. Bot. 100s.
Use: Antibacterial, sulfonamide.

GANTRISIN, AZO. (Roche)
See: Azo Gantrisin, Tab. (Roche).

GANTRISIN INJECTABLE. (Roche) Sulfisoxazole diolamine 4 mg/ml.
W/sodium metabisulfite 2 mg. Pkg. 10s.
Use: Antibacterial, sulfonamide.

GANTRISIN, LIPO. (Roche) Acetyl Sulfisoxazole.
Use: Antibacterial, sulfonamide.
See: Lipo Gantrisin, Susp. (Roche).

GANTRISIN OPHTHALMIC SOLUTION & OINTMENT. (Roche) Sulfisoxazole 4% as the diolamine salt. **Ophth. Oint.:** Tube 3.75 Gm; Soln. Dropper Bot. 15 ml.
Use: Antibacterial, sulfonamide.

GANTRISIN PEDIATRIC SUSPENSION. (Roche) Acetyl sulfisoxazole 0.5 Gm/5 ml. Bot. 120 ml, 480 ml.
Use: Antibacterial, sulfonamide.

GANTRISIN SYRUP. (Roche) Acetyl Sulfisoxazole 0.5 Gm/5 ml. Syr. Bot. pt.
Use: Antibacterial, sulfonamide.

GANTRISIN TABLETS. (Roche) Sulfisoxazole 0.5 Gm/Tab. Tel-E-Dose Pkg. 100s (10 strips of 10), Bot. 100s, 500s.
Use: Antibacterial, sulfonamide.W/Phenylazo-diamino-pyridine HCl.
See: Azo Gantrisin, Tab. (Roche).

GARAMYCIN. (Schering) **Cream:** Gentamicin sulfate 1.7 mg (equivalent to gentamicin base 1 mg). Methylparaben 1 mg, butylparaben 4 mg as preservatives, stearic acid, propylene glycol monostearate, isopropyl myristate, propylene glycol, polysorbate 40, sorbitol soln., water/Gm. Tube 15 Gm. **Oint.:** Gentamicin sulfate 1.7 mg (equivalent to gentamicin base 1 mg), methylparaben 0.5 mg, propylparaben 0.1 mg in petrolatum base/Gm. Tube 15 Gm.
Use: Anti-infective, external.

GARAMYCIN INJECTABLE. (Schering) Gentamicin sulfate. Inj. equivalent to 40 mg gentamicin base, methylparaben 1.8 mg, propylparaben 0.2 mg, as preservatives, sodium bisulfite 3.2 mg, disodium edetate 0.1 mg/ml Vial 2 ml (80 mg), 20 ml (800 mg); Syringe 1.5 ml (60 mg), 2 ml (80 mg); **Pediatric Inj.:** 10 mg/ml w/methylparaben 1.3 mg, propylparaben 0.2 mg, sodium bisulfite 3.2 mg, edetate disodium 0.1 mg/ml. Vial 2 ml (20 mg).
Use: Antibacterial, aminoglycoside.

GARAMYCIN INTRATHECAL INJECTION. (Schering) Gentamicin sulfate equivalent to 2 mg/ml gentamicin base, 8.5 mg sodium Cl/ml. Amp. 2 ml.
Use: Antibacterial, aminoglycoside.

GARAMYCIN I.V. PIGGYBACK. (Schering) Gentamicin sulfate equivalent to 1 mg gentamicin base, 8.9 mg sodium Cl, (no preservatives). Inj. Bot. 60 ml (60 mg), 80 ml (80 mg).
Use: Antibacterial, aminoglycoside.

GARAMYCIN OPHTHALMIC OINTMENT-STERILE. (Schering) Gentamicin sulfate equivalent to 3 mg, gentamicin, methylparaben and propylparaben as preservatives/Gm in petrolatum base. Tube 3.75 Gm
Use: Anti-infective, ophthalmic.

GARAMYCIN OPHTHALMIC SOLUTION, STERILE. (Schering) Gentamicin sulfate equivalent to 3 mg gentamicin, disodium phosphate, monosodium phosphate, sodium Cl, benzalkonium Cl/ml. Plastic dropper bot. 5 ml.
Use: Anti-infective, ophthalmic.

GARDAN. (Winthrop Products) Dipyrone.
Use: Analgesic, antipyretic, anti-inflammatory.

GARDENAL.
See: Phenobarbital. (Various Mfr.).

GARDINOL TYPE DETERGENTS. Aurinol, Cyclopon, Dreft, Drene, Duponol, Lissapol, Maprofix, Modinal, Orvus, Sandopan, Sadipan.
Use: Detergents.

GARDOL. Sodium Lauryl Sarcosinate.

GARFIELDS TEA. (Last) Senna leaf powder 68.3%. Bot. 2 oz.
Use: Laxative.

GARITABS. (Blue Cross) Iron 50 mg, vitamins B_1 5 mg, B_2 5 mg, C 75 mg, niacinamide 30 mg, B_5 2 mg, B_6 0.5 mg, B_{12} 3 mcg Bot. 1000s.
Use: Vitamin/mineral supplement.

GARITONE. (Halsey) Bot. 16 oz.
Use: Dietary supplement.

GARI-TONIC HEMATINIC. (Blue Cross) Vitamins B_1 5 mg, niacinamide 100 mg, B_2 5 mg, pantothenic acid 4 mg, B_6 1 mg, B_{12} 6 mcg, choline bitartrate 100 mg, iron 100 mg/30 ml Bot. 16 oz.
Use: Vitamin/mineral supplement.

GARLIC. Allium.
Use: Intestinal antispasmodic.
See: Allimin, Tab. (Mosso).

GARLIC CAPSULES. (Miller) Garlic 166 mg/Cap. Bot. 100s.
Use: Intestinal antispasmodic.

GARLIC CONCENTRATE.
W/Parsley Concentrate.
See: Allimin, Tab. (Mosso).

GARLIC OIL.
See: Natural Garlic Oil, Cap. (Spirt).
GARLIC OIL CAPSULES. (Kirkman) Bot. 100s.
GAS-EZE. (E.J. Moore) Aluminum hydroxide, magnesium hydroxide, calcium carbonate, glycine, mannitol, oil peppermint/Tab. Bot. 50s, Pak 36s.
Use: Antacid.
GAS PERMEABLE DAILY CLEANER. (Barnes-Hind) Nonionic aqueous solution cleaning agents in alkaline buffered medium w/edetate disodium 2%, thimerosal 0.004%. Bot. 30 ml.
Use: Gas permeable contact lens care.
GAS PERMEABLE LENS STARTER SYSTEM. (Barnes-Hind) Daily cleanser, Bot. 3 ml, Wetting and soaking soln., Bot. 60 ml, Hydra-Mat II spin cleansing unit. Kit.
Use: Gas permeable contact lens care.
GAS PERMEABLE WETTING & SOAKING SOLUTION. (Barnes-Hind) Sterile aqueous, isotonic soln. of low viscosity, buffered to physiological pH. Bot. 60 ml, 120 ml.
Use: Gas permeable contact lens care.
GASTRIC MUCIN.
(Wilson) Granules 8 oz., 1 lb.
Use: Anti-ulcer.
W/Magnesium glycinate, aluminum hydroxide gel.
See: Mucogel, Tab. (Inwood).
GASTROCCULT. (SmithKline Diagnostics) Occult blood screening test. In 40s.
Use: Diagnostic aid.
GASTROCROM. (Fisons) Cromolyn sodium 100 mg/Cap. Bot. 100s.
Use: Respiratory inhalant.
GASTROGRAFIN. (Squibb) Diatrizoate methylglucamine 66%, sodium diatrizoate 10%. Soln. Bot. 120 ml.
Use: Radiopaque agent.
GASTROLYTE. (Rorer) Dextrose 4000 mg, sodium 18 mEq, chloride 16 mEq, citrate 6 mEq, potassium 4 mEq/Packet. Box 6s (single dose).
Use: Fluid/electrolyte replacement.
GASTRON. (Winthrop Products) Pancreatin.
Use: Digestive enzyme.
GASTRO-TEST. (HDC Corp.) To determine stomach pH and to diagnose and locate gastric bleeding. Test 25s.
Use: Diagnostic aid.
GAS-X. (Sandoz Consumer) Simethicone 80 mg/ Chew. Tab. Pkg. 12s, 30s.
Use: Antiflatulent.
GAS-X, EXTRA STRENGTH. (Sandoz Consumer) Simethicone 125 mg. Chew. Tab. Box 18s.
Use: Antiflatulent.
•**GAUZE, ABSORBENT,** U.S.P. XXII.
Use: Surgical aid.
•**GAUZE, PETROLATUM,** U.S.P. XXII.
Use: Surgical aid.
GAVISCON. (Marion) Aluminum hydroxide gel, dried, 80 mg, magnesium trisilicate 20 mg/ Chew. Tab. Bot. 100s, Box 30s.
Use: Antacid.
GAVISCON-2. (Marion) Aluminum hydroxide gel, dried, 160 mg, magnesium trisilicate 40 mg/ Chew. Tab. Box 48s.
Use: Antacid.
GAVISCON LIQUID. (Marion) Aluminum hydroxide 95 mg, magnesium carbonate 411 mg/15 ml Bot. 180 ml, 360 ml.
Use: Antacid.
GBA.
See: Gamma hydroxybutyrate.
G.B.H. LOTION. (Century) Gamma benzene hexachloride 1%. Bot. 2 oz, pt, gal.
Use: Scabicide/pediculicide.
G.B.S. (Forest) Dehydrocholic acid 125 mg, phenobarbital 8 mg, homatropine methylbromide 2.5 mg/Tab. 100s, 1000s.
Use: Hydrocholeretic.
GEBAUER'S 114. (Gebauer) Dichlorotetrafluoroethane 100%. Can 8 oz.
Use: Local anesthetic.
GEBAUER ETHYL CHLORIDE. (Gebauer) Ethyl Cl. Bot. 4 oz, metal tube 100 Gm.
Use: Local anesthetic.
GEE-GEE. (Bowman) Guaifenesin 200 mg/Tab. Bot. 1000s.
Use: Expectorant.
GEFARNATE. B.A.N. A mixture of steroisomers of 3,7-dimethylocta-2,6-dienyl 5,9,13-trimethyltet-radeca-4,8,12-trienoate. Geranyl farnesylacetate. Gefarnil.
Use: Treatment of peptic ulcer.
GEL II. (Oral-B) Fluoride 0.5% (from sodium flouride 1.1%). Tube 60 Gm.
Use: Dental caries preventative.
GEL II TOPICAL GEL. (Oral-B) Fluoride ion 1.23% from sodium fluoride and hydrofluoric acid (acidulated phosphate fluoride). Bot. 480 Gm.
Use: Dental caries preventative.
GEL-A-CAP. (Kenyon) Gelatin 10 gr/Cap. Bot. 100s, 1000s.
GELADINE. (Barth's) Gelatin, protein, vitamin D/ Cap. Bot. 100s, 500s.
GELAMAL. (Halsey) Magnesium-aluminum hydroxide gel. Bot. 12 oz.
Use: Antacid.
•**GELATIN,** N.F. XVII.
Use: Pharmaceutic aid.
•**GELATIN FILM, ABSORBABLE,** U.S.P. XXII.
Use: Local hemostatic.
See: Gelfilm (Upjohn).
GELATIN POWDER, STERILE.
See: Gelfoam Powder (Upjohn).
•**GELATIN SPONGE, ABSORBABLE,** U.S.P. XXII.
Use: Local hemostatic.
See: Gelfoam, Paks (Upjohn).
GELATIN, ZINC.
See: Zinc gelatin. (Various Mfr.).
GEL-CLEAN. (Barnes-Hind) Gel formulated with nonionic surfactant. Tube 30 Gm.

Use: Hard contact lens care.

GELFILM. (Upjohn) Sterile, absorbable gelatin film. Envelope 1s. 100 mm × 125 mm. Also available as Ophth. Sterile 25 × 50 mm. Box 6s.
Use: Hemostatic.

GELFOAM. (Upjohn)
STERILE SPONGES:
Size 12-3mm 20 × 60 mm (12 sq. cm) × 3 mm.
Box 4 sponges in individual envelopes.
Size 12-7mm. 20 × 60 mm (12 sq. cm.) × 7 mm.
Box 12 sponges in individual envelopes, jar 4 sponges.
Size 50-10mm. 62.5 × 80 mm (50 sq. cm.) × 10 mm. Box 4 sponges in individual envelopes.
Size 100-10mm. 80 × 125 mm (100 sq. cm.) × 10 mm.
Box 6 sponges in individual envelopes.
Size 200-10mm. 80 × 250 mm (200 sq. cm.) × 10 mm.
Box 6 sponges in individual envelopes.
Compressed size 100 (intended primarily for application in the dry state). 80 × 125 mm. Boxes of 6 sponges in individual envelopes.
PACKS:
Packs size 2 cm. (Designed particularly for nasal packing). 2 × 40 cm. Single jar. (Packing cavities).
Size 6 cm. 6 × 40 cm. Box 6 sponges in individual envelopes.
Use: Hemostatic, topical.

GELFOAM COMPRESSED. (Upjohn) Size 100 (80 × 125 mm.) Box 6s.
Use: Hemostatic, topical.

GELFOAM DENTAL PACK. (Upjohn) Size 4, 20 mm × 20 mm × 7 mm. Jar 15 sponges. Size 2, 10 mm × 20 mm (2 sq. cm.) × 7 mm. Jar 15 sponges.
Use: Hemostatic, topical.

GELFOAM POWDER. (Upjohn) Sterile Jar 1 Gm.
Use: Hemostatic.

GELFOAM PROSTATECTOMY CONES. (Upjohn) Prostatectomy cones (for use with Foley catheter). 13 cm, 18 cm in diameter. Box 6s.
Use: Hemostatic.

GEL JET GELATIN CAPSULES. (Kirkman) Bot. 100s, 250s.

GEL-KAM. (Scherer) Fluoride 0.1% (stannous fluoride 0.4%). Cinnamon flavor. Gel. Bot. w/applicator tip 69 Gm, 105 Gm, 129 Gm.
Use: Dental caries preventative.

GELOCAST. (Beiersdorf) Unna's Boot medicated bandage: Semi-rigid cast impregnated with zinc oxide mixtures. Box 4 inches × 10 yd, 3 inches × 10 yd.
Use: Unna's cast dressing.

GELPIRIN TABLETS. (Alra) Aspirin 240 mg, acetaminophen 125 mg, caffeine 32 mg, gelsinate 50 mg/Tab. Bot. 100s, 1000s, Packet 2s.
Use: Analgesic.

GELPIRIN CCF. (Atra) Acetaminophen 325 mg, guaifenesin 25 mg, phenylpropanolamine maleate 12.5 mg/Tab. Bot. 50s, 200s, 500s.
Use: Analgesic, expectorant, decongestant.

GELSAF SUPER. (Robinson) Safflower oil 750 mg/Cap. Bot. 100s, 1000s, Pkg. 30s, Bulk pkg. 5000s.
Use: Enteral nutritional supplement.

GELSAF SUPER W/B_6. (Robinson) Safflower oil 912 mg, vitamin B_6 0.5 mg/Cap. or Safflower oil 1150 mg, B_6 3 mg/Cap. Bot. 100s, 250s, 1000s.
Use: Enteral nutritional supplement.

GELSEMIUM. (Various Mfr.) Pkg. oz.
Use: For neuralgia.
W/APC.
See: APC Combinations.

GELSEMIUM W/COMBINATIONS.
See: Briacel, Tab. (Briar).
Bricor, Tab. (Briar).
Cystitol, Tab. (Briar).
Lanased, Tab. (Lannett).
Ricor, Tab. (Vortech).
Sodadide, Tab. (Scrip).
UB, Tab. (Scrip).
Urisan-P, Tab. (Sandia).
Uriseptic w/Gelsemium, Tab. (Spencer-Mead).
Uritol, Tab. (Kenyon).
Urothyn Improved, Tab. (Solvay).
Urseptic, Tab. (Century).
U-Tract, Tab. (Bowman).

GEL-TIN. (Young Dental) Fluoride 0.1% (from stannous flouride 0.4%) Gel Bot. 57 Gm, 623 Gm.
Use: Dental caries preventative.

GELUSIL. (Parke-Davis) Magnesium hydroxide 200 mg, aluminum hydroxide 200 mg, simethicone 25 mg/5 ml or Chew. Tab. **Susp.** Bot. 180 ml, 360 ml. **Tab.** Bot. 165s, Strip box 50s, 100s, 1000s.
Use: Antacid.

GELUSIL II. (Parke-Davis) Magnesium hydroxide 400 mg, aluminum hydroxide 400 mg, simethicone 30 mg/5 ml or Chew. Tab. **Liq.** Bot. 360 ml. **Tab.** Strip 80s.
Use: Antacid.

•**GEMCADIOL.** USAN.
Use: Antihyperlipoproteinemic.

•**GEMCITABINE.** USAN.
Use: Antineoplastic.

•**GEMCITABINE** HYDROCHLORIDE. USAN.
Use: Antineoplastic.

•**GEMEPROST.** USAN.
Use: Prostaglandin.

•**GEMFIBROZIL,** U.S.P. XXII. Cap. U.S.P. XXII. 2,2-Dimethyl-5-(2,5-xyly-loxy) valeric acid.
Use: Treatment of hypercholesterolemia.
See: Lopid, Cap. (Parke-Davis).

GEMNISYN. (Kremers-Urban) Acetaminophen 325 mg, aspirin 325 mg. Tab. Bot. 100s.
Use: Analgesic combination.

GENABID T.D. CAPS. (Goldline) Papaverine HCl 150 mg/Cap. Bot. 100s, 1000s.
Use: Peripheral vasodilator.

GENAC TABLETS. (Goldline) Triprolidine HCl 2.5 mg, pseudoephedrine HCl 60 mg/Tab. Bot. 24s, 100s.
Use: Antihistamine, decongestant.

GENACED TABLETS. (Goldline) Bot. 100s.
Use: Analgesic.

GENACOL TABLETS. (Goldline) Bot. 50s.
Use: Analgesic, decongestant.

GENACOTE TABLETS. (Goldline) 5 gr/Tab. Bot. 100s.
Use: Anti-inflammatory agent.

GENAGESIC TABS. (Goldline) Propoxyphene HCl 165 mg, acetaminophen 650 mg/Tab. Bot. 100s, 500s.
Use: Narcotic analgesic combination.

GENAHIST. (Goldline) Diphenhydramine HCl 25 mg/Cap or Tab. Bot. 24s.
Use: Antihistamine.

GENAHIST LIQUID. (Goldline) Diphenhydramine 12.5 mg/5 ml. Elix. 120 ml.
Use: Antihistamine.

GENALAC TABS. (Goldline) Calcium carbonate 420 mg, glycerin. Bot. 100s, 1000s.
Use: Antacid.

GENALG CREME LINIMENT. (Goldline) Bot. 2 oz.
Use: External analgesic.

GENALLERATE TABLETS. (Goldline) Chlorpheniramine maleate 4 mg/Tab. Bot. 24s.
Use: Antihistamine.

GENAMIN COLD SYRUP. (Goldline) Phenylpropanolamine HCl 12.5 mg, chlorpheniramine maleate 2 mg. Alcohol free. In 120 ml.
Use: Decongestant, antihistamine.

GENAMIN EXPECTORANT. (Goldline) Phenylpropanolamine 12.5 mg, guaifenesin 100 mg, alcohol 5%. In 120 ml.
Use: Decongestant, expectorant.

GENAPAP CHILDREN'S CHEWABLE TABS. (Goldline) Acetaminophen 80 mg/Tab. Bot. 30s.
Use: Analgesic.

GENAPAP CHILDREN'S ELIXIR. (Goldline) Acetaminophen 160 mg/5 ml. Cherry flavor. Bot. 120 ml.
Use: Analgesic.

GENAPAP-C TABLETS. (Goldline) Bot. 100s.
Use: Analgesic.

GENAPAP EXTRA STRENGTH CAPLETS. (Goldline) Acetaminophen 500 mg/Cap. Bot. 50s, 100s.
Use: Analgesic.

GENAPAP INFANTS' DROPS. (Goldline) Acetaminophen 100 mg/ml, alcohol 7%. Soln. Dropper bot. 15 ml.
Use: Analgesic.

GENAPAP TABLETS. (Goldline) Acetaminophen 325 mg/Tab. Bot. 100s.
Use: Analgesic.

GENAPAX. (Key) Gentian violet 5 mg/tampon. Box 12s.
Use: Antifungal, vaginal.

GENAPHED PLUS TABLETS. (Goldline) Bot. 24s.
Use: Decongestant.

GENAPHED TABLETS. (Goldline) Pseudoephedrine HCl 30 mg/Tab. Bot. 24s, 100s.
Use: Decongestant.

GENAREG TABLETS. (Goldline) Bot. 30s.
Use: Laxative.

GENASAL. (Goldline) Oxymetazoline 0.05%. Soln. 15 ml, 30 ml.
Use: Decongestant.

GENASEC TABLETS. (Goldline) Bot. 24s, 90s.
Use: Analgesic.

GENASOFT CAPSULES. (Goldline) Docusate sodium 100 mg/Cap. Bot. 60s.
Use: Laxative.

GENASOFT PLUS CAPSULES. (Goldline) Docusate sodium 100 mg, casanthranol 30 mg/Cap. Bot. 60s.
Use: Laxative.

GENASONE CREAM. (Goldline) Tube 0.5 oz.
Use: Anti-inflammatory, antipruritic.

GENASPOR ANTIFUNGAL CREAM. (Goldline) Tolnaftate 1%. Bot. 15 Gm.
Use: Antifungal, external.

GENASYME TABLETS. (Goldline) Simethicone 80 mg/Tab. Bot. 100s.
Use: Antiflatulent.

GENATAP ELIXIR. (Goldline) Brompheniramine maleate 2 mg, phenylpropanolamine HCl 12.5 mg, alcohol 2.3%/5 ml. Bot. 120 ml.
Use: Antihistamine, decongestant.

GENATON LIQUID. (Goldline) Bot. 12 oz.
Use: Antacid.

GENATROPINE HCl. Atropine-N-oxide HCl. Aminoxytropine Tropate HCl.
See: X-tro, Cap. (Xttrium).

GENATUSS DM SYRUP. (Goldline) Dextromethorphan HBr 15 mg, guaifenesin 100 mg, alcohol 1.4%. Bot. 120 ml.
Use: Antitussive, expectorant.

GENATUSS SYRUP. (Goldline) Guaifenesin 100 mg/5 ml, alcohol 3.5%. Bot. 120 ml.
Use: Expectorant.

GEN-BEE WITH C. (Goldline) Vitamins B_1 15 mg, B_2 10.2 mg, B_3 50 mg, B_5 10 mg, B_6 5 mg, C 300 mg, tartrazine. Cap. Bot. 130s, 1000s.
Use: Vitamin supplement.

GENCALC 600 TABLETS. (Goldline) Calcium 600 mg (from calcium carbonate 1.5 Gm)/Tab. Bot. 60s.
Use: Calcium supplement.

GENCOLD CAPSULES. (Goldline) Phenylpropanolamine HCl 75 mg, chlorpheniramine maleate 8 mg/SR Tab. Bot. 10s.
Use: Decongestant, antihistamine.

GENDECON TABLETS. (Goldline) Bot. 24s, 50s.
Use: Analgesic, decongestant.

GEN-D-PHEN. (Goldline) Diphenhydramine 12.5 mg. Syr. 120 ml.
Use: Antihistamine.

GENEBS EXTRA STRENGTH CAPLETS. (Goldline) Acetaminophen 500 mg/Cap. Bot. 100s, 1000s.
Use: Analgesic.

GENEBS EXTRA STRENGTH TABLETS. (Goldline) Acetaminophen 500 mg/Tab. Bot. 100s, 1000s.
Use: Analgesic.

GENEBS TABLETS. (Goldline) Acetaminophen 325 mg/Tab. Bot. 100s, 1000s.
Use: Analgesic.

GENERBON LIQUID. (Goldline) Bot. pt, gal.
Use: Dietary supplement.

GENERET-500. (Goldline) Iron 105 mg, Vitamins B_1 6mg, B_2 6 mg, B_3 30 mg, B_5 10 mg, B_6 5 mg, B_{12} 25 mcg, C (as sodium ascorbate) 500 mg. TR Tab. Bot. 60s.
Use: Vitamin/mineral supplement.

GENERIX-T. (Goldline) Elemental iron 15 mg, vitamins A 10,000 IU, D 400 IU, E 5.5 mg, B_1 15 mg, B_2 10 mg, B_3 100 mg, B_5 10 mg, B_6 2 mg, B_{12} 7.5 mcg, C 150 mg, Cu, I, Mg, Mn, zinc 1.5 mg. Tab. Bot. 100s, 1000s.
Use: Vitamin/mineral supplement.

GENEYES DROPS. (Goldline) Bot. 0.5 oz.
Use: Eye irritations.

GENEX CAPS. (Goldline) Phenylpropanolamine HCl 18 mg, acetaminophen 325 mg/Cap. Bot. 100s, 1000s.
Use: Decongestant, analgesic.

GENFIBER. (Goldline) Bot. 14 oz.
Use: Laxative.

GENITAL HERPES TREATMENT.
See: Acyclovir.
Zovirax Cap., Oint. (Burroughs Wellcome).

GENITE. (Goldline) Pseudoephedrine HCl 10 mg, doxylamine succinate 1.25 mg, dextromethorphan HBr 5 mg, acetaminophen 167 mg, alcohol 25%/5 ml. Bot. 177 ml.
Use: Decongestant, antihistamine, antitussive, analgesic.

GEN-K POWDER. (Goldline) Potassium Cl. Pow. 20 mEq/packet. Box 30s.
Use: Potassium supplement.

GEN-K TABS. (Goldline) Effervescent potassium. Bot. 30s.
Use: Potassium supplement.

GENNA TABLETS. (Goldline) Senna concentrate 217 mg/Tab. Bot. 100s, 1000s.
Use: Laxative.

GENNIN TABLETS. (Goldline) Buffered aspirin 5 gr. Bot. 100s.
Use: Salicylate analgesic.

GENOPHYLLIN.
See: Aminophylline (Various Mfr.).

GENOPTIC LIQUIFILM STERILE OPHTHALMIC SOLUTION. (Allergan) Gentamicin sulfate equivalent to 3 mg gentamicin/ml w/polyvinyl alcohol 1.4%, edetate disodium, HCl, benzalkonium Cl. Bot. 1 ml, 5 ml.
Use: Anti-infective, ophthalmic.

GENOPTIC S.O.P. STERILE OPHTHALMIC OINTMENT. (Allergan) Gentamicin sulfate equivalent to 3 mg gentamicin/Gm w/white petrolatum, methylparaben, propylparaben. Oint. Tube 3.5 Gm.
Use: Anti-infective, ophthalmic.

GENORA 1/35-21 TABLETS. (Rugby) Norethindrone 1 mg, ethinylestradiol 0.035 mg/Tab. Pkg. 126s (6-pak).
Use: Oral contraceptive.

GENORA 1/35-28 TABLETS. (Rugby) Norethindrone 1 mg, ethinylestradiol 0.035 mg/Tab., 7 inert tab. Pkg. 168s (6-pak).
Use: Oral contraceptive.

GENORA 1/50-21 TABLETS. (Rugby) Norethindrone 1 mg, mestranol 0.05 mg/Tab. Pkg. 126s (6-pak).
Use: Oral contraceptive.

GENORA 1/50-28 TABLETS. (Rugby) Norethindrone 1 mg, mestranol 0.05 mg/Tab., 7 inert tab. Pkg. 168s (6-pak).
Use: Oral contraceptive.

GENPREP OINTMENT. (Goldline) Live yeast cell derivative supplying 2000 units skin respiratory factor/oz of ointment w/shark liver oil 3%, phenylmercuric nitrate 1:10,000. Tube 2 oz.
Use: Anorectal preparation.

GENPRIL. (Goldline) Ibuprofen 200 mg. Tab. 50s, 100s.
Use: Nonsteroidal anti-inflammatory agent.

GENPRIN. (Goldline) Aspirin 325 mg. Tab. 100s.
Use: Salicylate analgesic.

GENSALATE SODIUM. Sodium gentisate. (Sodium salt of 2,5-dihydroxybenzoic acid).
Use: Analgesic.

GENSAN TABLETS. (Goldline) Aspirin 400 mg, caffeine 32 mg/Tab. Bot. 100s.
Use: Analgesic combination.

GENSLIM C/F CAPSULES. (Goldline) Bot. 28s.
Use: Appetite suppressant.

GENSLIM EXTRA STRENGTH CAPSULES. (Goldline) Bot. 20s.
Use: Appetite suppressant.

GENTACIDIN OPHTHALMIC OINTMENT. (Iolab) Gentamicin 3 mg/Gm. Oint. Tube 3.5 Gm.
Use: Anti-infective, ophthalmic.

GENTACIDIN OPHTHALMIC SOLUTION. (Iolab) Gentamicin sulfate 3 mg/ml. Soln. Bot. 5 ml.
Use: Anti-infective, ophthalmic.

GENTAFAIR. (Pharmafair) **Oint.:** Gentamicin 3 mg/Gm with liquid lanolin, white petrolatum, mineral oil, parabens. Tube 3.75 Gm, 15 Gm. **Soln.:** Gentamicin 3 mg/ml, polyoxyl 40 stearate, polyethylene glycol. Dropper bot. 5 ml, 15 ml.
Use: Anti-infective, ophthalmic.

GENTAK. (Akorn) **Oint.:** Gentamicin 3 mg/Gm with liquid lanolin, white petrolatum, mineral oil, parabens. Tube 3.5 Gm, 5 Gm, 15 Gm. **Soln.:**

Gentamicin 3 mg/ml with polyoxyl 40 stearate, polyethylene glycol. Bot. 5 ml, 15 ml.
Use: Anti-infective, ophthalmic.

•**GENTAMICIN SULFATE,** U.S.P. XXII. Cream, Oint., Inj., Ophth. Oint., Ophth. Soln., Sterile, U.S.P. XXII. (Schering) Produced by *Micromonospora purpurea.*
Use: Antibacterial.
See: Apogen, Inj. (Beecham Labs).
Garamycin, Preps. (Schering).
Genoptic, Preps. (Allergan).

•**GENTAMICIN AND PREDNISOLONE ACETATE OPHTHALMIC SUSPENSION,** U.S.P. XXII.
Use: Antibiotic, anti-inflammatory.

•**GENTIAN VIOLET,** U.S.P. XXII. Topical Soln., Cream, U.S.P. XXII. Methylrosaniline Cl. Bismuth Violet.
Use: Topical anti-infective.
See: Genapax, tampon. (Key).
GVS, Vaginal cream and inserts. (Savage).
W/Surfactants.
See: Hyva, Vaginal Tab. (Holland-Rantos).

GENTISATE SODIUM. 5-Hydroxysalicylate sodium, 2,5-Dihydroxy benzoate sodium.

•**GENTISIC ACID ETHANOLAMIDE,** N.F. XVII.
Use: Pharmaceutic aid.

GENTLAX S TABLETS. (Blair) Standardized senna concentrate 187 mg, docusate sodium 50 mg. Tab. Bot. 30s, 60s.
Use: Laxative.

GENTLE NATURE NATURAL VEGETABLE LAXATIVE.(Sandoz Consumer) Sennosides A and B as calcium salts. 20 mg/Tab. Box 16s, 32s.
Use: Laxative.

GENTLE SHAMPOO. (Ulmer) Bot. 4 oz, gal.
Use: Mild, neutral shampoo.

GENTRAN. (Baxter) **Inj.:** Dextran-70 6%, sodium Cl 0.9%. Plastic Bot. 500 ml; Dextran-40 10% in saline. Plastic Bot. 500 ml. Dextran-40 10% w/ Dextrose 5%. Plastic bot. 500 ml.
Use: Plasma expander.

GENTRAN 75. (Baxter) Dextran 75 6% in sodium Cl 0.9%. Inj. Bot. 500 ml.
Use: Plasma expander.

GENTRASUL. (Bausch & Lomb) Gentamicin 3 mg. **Oint.:** 3.5 Gm. **Soln.:** Dropper bot. 5 ml.
Use: Anti-infective, ophthalmic.

GENTRIM. (Goldline) Bot. 16 oz.
Use: Meal replacement.

GENTZ RECTAL WIPES. (Roxane) Pramoxine HCl 1%, alcloxa 0.2%, witch hazel 50%, propylene glycol 10%. Box 100s, 120s (individually wrapped disposable wipes).
Use: Anorectal preparation.

GENUINE BAYER ASPIRIN. (Glenbrook) Aspirin 325 mg/FC Tab. Bot. 12s, 24s, 50s, 200s, 300s.
Use: Salicylate analgesic.

GENVITE. (Goldline) Bot. 130s.
Use: Vitamin supplement.

GEOCILLIN. (Roerig) Carbenicillin indanyl sodium 382 mg/Tab. Bot. 100s, UD 100s.
Use: Antibacterial, penicillin.

GEOPEN. (Roerig) Carbenicillin Disodium. Inj. **Vial:** 1 Gm, 2 Gm, 5 Gm. Pkg. 10s. **Piggyback Vial:** 2 Gm, 5 Gm, 10 Gm. **Bulk Pharmacy Pack:** 30 Gm.
Use: Antibacterial, penicillin.

•**GEPIRONE HYDROCHLORIDE.** USAN. Marketed by Mead Johnson.
Use: Antianxiety, antidepressant.

GERA PLUS. (Towne) Iron 50 mg, vitamins B_1 5 mg, B_2 5 mg, C 75 mg, niacinamide 30 mg, calcium pantothenate 2 mg, B_6 0.5 mg, B_{12} 3 mcg/ Tab. Bot. 100s.
Use: Vitamin/mineral supplement.

GERAVITE ELIXIR. (Hauck) Lysine monohydrochloride 150 mg, vitamins B_1 1 mg, B_2 1.2 mg, niacinamide 100 mg, B_{12} 10 mcg/15 ml w/ alcohol 15%. Bot. 16 oz, gal.
Use: Vitamin/mineral supplement.

GERI-ALL-D. (Barth's) Vitamins A 10,000 IU, D 400 IU, B_1 7 mg, B_2 14 mg, C 200 mg, niacin 4.17 mg, B_{12} 25 mcg, E 50 IU, B_6 0.35 mg, pantothenic acid 0.63 mg, trace minerals and other factors. 2 Cap. Bot. 1 mo., 3 mo. and 6 mo. supply of Geri-All regular and Geri-All-D.
Use: Vitamin/mineral supplement.

GERIATRAZOLE. (Kenyon) Vitamins B_{12} 50 mg, B_2 2 mg, liver-painless 2 mcg, dl-methionine 10 mg, inositol 20 mg, d-panthenol 20 mg, B_1 20 mg, B_6 5 mg, niacinamide 75 mg, pentylenetetrazole 10 mg/ml. Vial 30 ml.
Use: Vitamin/mineral supplement.

GERIATROPLEX. (Morton) Cyanocobalamin 30 mcg, liver inj. 0.1 ml vitamins B_{12} activity 2 mcg, ferrous gluconate 50 mg, B_2 1.5 mg, calcium pantothenate 2.5 mg, niacinamide 100 mg, citric acid 16.4 mg, sodium citrate 23.6 mg/2 ml. Vial 30 ml.
Use: Vitamin/mineral supplement.

GERIDEN. (Kenyon) Methyltestosterone 2 mg, ethinyl estradiol 0.01 mg, rutin 10 mg, vitamins C 30 mg, B_{12} 2 mcg, A 5000 IU, D 500 IU, E 2 IU, calcium pantothenate 3 mg, B_1 2.5 mg, B_6 0.5 mg, niacinamide 15 mg, iron 5 mg, copper 0.2 mg, manganese 1 mg, magnesium 5 mg, potassium 2 mg, choline bitartrate 40 mg, PABA 10 mg, inositol 20 mg/Cap. Bot. 100s, 1000s.
Use: Vitamin/mineral supplement.

GERI-DERM. (Barth's) Vitamins A 400,000 IU, D 40,000 IU, E 200 IU, panthenol 800 mg/4 oz. Jar 4 oz.
Use: Skin supplement.

GERIDIUM TABLETS. (Goldline) Phenazopyridine HCl 100 mg or 200 mg/Tab. Bot. 100s, 1000s.
Use: Urinary analgesic, anti-infective.

GERIFORT PLUS. (A.P.C.) Vitamins A 10,000 IU, B_1 5 mg, B_2 6 mg, B_6 2 mg, C 75 mg, D-2 1000 IU, niacinamide 60 mg, iron 10 mg, cal-

cium 115 mg, phosphorous 83 mg, iodine 0.1 mg, calcium pantothenate 10 mg, d-alpha tocopheryl acid succinate 3 IU, cobalamin concentrate 3 mcg, choline bitartrate 70 mg, inositol 35 mg, biotin 15 mcg, Zn 0.2 mg, magnesium 2 mg, manganese 0.5 mg, potassium 0.15 mg/ Amcap. Bot. 100s.
Use: Vitamin/mineral supplement.

GERIJEN IMPROVED. (Jenkins) Testosterone 10 mg, estrone 1 mg, cyanocobalamin 50 mcg, niacinamide 50 mg, inositol 5 mg, methionine 5 mg, choline Cl 5 mg/ml, pectin 0.25%. Vial 10 ml.

GERILETS. (Abbott) Vitamins A 5000 IU, D 400 IU, E 45 IU, C 90 mg (from sodium ascorbate), folic acid 0.4 mg, B_1 2.25 mg, B_2 2.6 mg, niacin 30 mg, B_6 3 mg, B_{12} 9 mcg, biotin 0.45 mg, pantothenic acid 15 mg, iron 27 mg (from ferrous sulfate)/Tab. Bot. 100s.
Use: Vitamin/mineral supplement.

GERIMED. (Fielding) Vitamins A 5000 IU, D 400 IU, E 30 mg, B_1 3 mg, B_2 3 mg, B_3 25 mg, B_6 2 mg, B_{12} 6 mcg, C 120 mg, calcium 370 mg, zinc 15 mg, Mg, phosphorous 130 mg/Tab. Bot. 60s.
Use: Vitamin/mineral supplement.

GERINEED. (Hanlon) Vitamins A 5000 IU, B_1 20 mg, B_2 5 mg, niacinamide 20 mg, B_6 0.5 mg, calcium pantothenate 5 mg, B_{12} 5 mcg, rutin 25 mg, C 50 mg, E 10 IU, choline 50 mg, inositol 50 mg, calcium lactate 1.64 mg, iron sulfate 10 mg, copper 1 mg, iodine 0.5 mg, manganese 1 mg, magnesium sulfate 1 mg, potassium sulfate 5 mg, zinc sulfate 0.5 mg/Cap. Bot. 100s.
Use: Vitamin/mineral supplement.

GERIOT. (Goldline) Iron 50 mg (from ferrous sulfate), vitamins B_1 5 mg, B_2 5 mg, B_3 30 mg, B_5 2 mg, B_6 0.5 mg, B_{12} 3 mcg, C 75 mg Tab. Bot. 100s.
Use: Vitamin/mineral supplement.

GERIPLEX-FS. (Parke-Davis) Vitamins A 5000 IU, B_1 5 mg, B_2 5 mg, B_{12} 2 mcg, nicotinamide 15 mg, C 50 mg, choline dihydrogen citrate 20 mg, E 5 mg, iron 6 mg, copper sulfate 4 mg, manganese sulfate 4 mg, zinc sulfate 0.5 mg, calcium 59 mg, docusate sodium 100 mg, aspergillus oryzea enzymes 162.5 mg/Kapseal Bot. 100s.
Use: Vitamin/mineral supplement.

GERI-PLUS. (Approved) Vitamins A 12,500 IU, D 1200 IU, B_1 15 mg, B_2 10 mg, C 75 mg, niacinamide 30 mg, calcium pantothenate 2 mg, B_6 0.5 mg, E 5 IU, Brewer's yeast 10 mg, B_{12} 15 mcg, iron 11.58 mg, desiccated liver 15 mg, choline bitartrate 30 mg, inositol 30 mg, calcium 59 mg, phosphorous 45 mg, zinc 0.68 mg, francium dicalcium phosphate 200 mg, Mn, enzymatic factors, amino acids/Cap. Bot. 50s, 100s, 1000s.
Use: Vitamin/mineral supplement.

GERI-PLUS ELIXIR. (Approved) Vitamins B_1 25 mg, B_2 10 mg, B_6 1 mg, niacinamide 100 mg, calcium pantothenate 5 mg, B_{12} 20 mcg, iron ammonium citrate 100 mg, choline 200 mg, inositol 100 mg, magnesium Cl 2 mg, manganese citrate 2 mg, zinc acetate 2 mg, amino acids/fl oz. Bot. pt.
Use: Vitamin/mineral supplement.

GERISPAN. (Robinson) Vitamins A 12,500 IU, D 1000 IU, B_1 5 mg, B_2 2.5 mg, niacinamide 40 mg, B_6 1 mg, calcium pantothenate 4 mg, B_{12} 2 mcg, C 75 mg, E 2 IU, choline bitartrate 31.4 mg, inositol 15 mg, calcium 75 mg, phosphorus 58 mg, iron 30 mg, magnesium 3 mg, manganese 0.5 mg, potassium 2 mg, zinc 0.5 mg/ Cap. Bot. 100s, 1000s, Bulk Pack 5000s.
Use: Vitamin/mineral supplement.

GERITOL COMPLETE TABLETS. (Beecham Products) Vitamins A 5000 IU, E 30 IU, C 60 mg, folic acid 400 mcg, B_1 1.5 mg, B_2 1.7 mg, niacinamide 20 mg, B_6 2 mg, B_{12} 6 mcg, D 400 IU, K 50 mcg, biotin 300 mcg, pantothenic acid 10 mg, calcium 162 mg, phosphorous 125 mg, iodine 150 mcg, iron (as ferrous fumarate) 50 mg, magnesium 100 mg, copper 2 mg, manganese 7.5 mg, potassium 37.5 mg, chloride 34.1 mg, cromium 15 mcg, molybdenum 15 mcg, selenium 15 mcg, zinc 15 mg, nickel 5 mcg, silicon 80 mcg, Sn. V/Tab. Bot. 14s, 40s, 100s, 180s, 300s.
Use: Vitamin/mineral supplement.

GERITOL TONIC LIQUID. (Beecham Products) Iron 50 mg (from iron ammonium citrate), Vitamins B_1 2.5 mg, B_2 2.5 mg, niacinamide 50 mg, panthenol 2 mg, pyridoxine 0.5 mg, B_{12} 0.75 mcg, methionine 25 mg, choline bitartrate 50 mg/15 ml. Alcohol 12%. Bot. 120 ml, 360 ml, 720 ml.
Use: Vitamin/mineral supplement.

GERIVITES. (Various Mfr.) Iron (from ferrous sulfate) 50 mg, vitamins B_1 5 mg, B_2 5 mg, B_3 30 mg, B_5 2 mg, B_6 0.5 mg, B_{12} 3 mcg, C 75 mg/ Tab. Bot. 40s, 100s, 1000s.
Use: Vitamin/mineral supplement.

GERIX ELIXIR. (Abbott) Vitamins B_1 6 mg, B_2 6 mg, niacin 100 mg, iron 15 mg, B_6 1.6 mg, cyanocobalamin 6 mcg, alcohol 20%/30 ml. Bot. 480 ml.
Use: Vitamin/mineral supplement.

GERLIPO. (Kenyon) Choline bitartrate 250 mg, methionine 150 mg, inositol 100 mg, desiccated whole liver 100 mg, B-cotrate 100 mg, vitamins B_1 1.5 mg, B_2 1 mg, B_6 0.1 mg, d-calcium pantothenate 2 mg, niacinamide 15 mg/3 Tab. Bot. 100s, 1000s.
Use: Vitamin/mineral supplement.

GERMANIN. (CDC)
Use: Anti-infective.
See: Suramin sodium (Naphuride sodium).

GER-O-FOAM. (Geriatric) Methylsalicylate 30%, benzocaine 3%, volatile oils. Aerosol can 4 oz.
Use: Analgesic, anesthetic.

GERTEROL DEPO. (Fellows) Medroxyprogesterone acetate 50 mg or 100 mg/ml. Vial 5 ml.

Use: Progestin.

GESIC. (Lexalabs) Aspirin 226.8 mg, caffeine 32.4 mg, codeine 32.4 mg/Tab. Bot. 100s.
Use: Narcotic analgesic combination.

•**GESTACLONE.** USAN. (1) 17β-Acetyl-6-chloro-1β, 1a,2β,8β,9α,10,11,12,13,14α-,15,16β,16a,17-tetradecahydro-10β,13β-dimethyl-3H-dicyclopropa[1,2:16,17]cyclopenta-[a]-phenanthren-3-one.
Use: Progestin.

GESTEROL L.A. 250 (Forest) Hydroxyprogesterone caproate 250 mg/ml. Vial 5 ml.
Use: Progestin.

GESTIN. (Dalin) Formerly G.I. 8. Bot. 4 oz, 8 oz.

•**GESTODENE.** USAN.
Use: Progestin.

GESTONEED. (Hanlon) Calcium lactate 1069 mg, vitamins C 100 mg, nicotinic acid 18 mg, B_2 2.4 mg, B_1 1.8 mg, B_6 9 mg, D 500 IU, A 6000 IU/Cap. Bot. 100s.
Use: Vitamin/mineral supplement.

•**GESTONORONE CAPROATE.** USAN. 17-Hydroxy-19-norpregn-4-ene-3,20-dione hexanoate.
Use: Progestin.

•**GESTRINONE.** USAN.
Use: Progestin.

•**GESTRONOL,** B.A.N. 17-Hydroxy-19-norpregn-4-ene-3,20-dione.
Use: Progesterone steroid.

GETS-IT. (Oakhurst) Salicyclic acid, zinc Cl, collodion in ether ≈ 35%, alcohol ≈ 28%. Liq. Bot. 12 ml.
Use: Keratolytic.

•**GEVOTROLINE HYDROCHLORIDE.** USAN.
Use: Antipsychotic.

GEVRABON. (Lederle) Vitamins B_1 5 mg, B_2 2.5 mg, B_{12} 1 mcg, niacinamide 50 mg, B_6 1 mg, pantothenic acid 10 mg, choline 100 mg, zinc 2 mg, iodine 100 mg, magnesium 2 mg, manganese 2 mg, iron 15 mg/30 ml w/alcohol 18%. Bot. 480 ml.
Use: Vitamin/mineral supplement.

GEVRAL. (Lederle) Vitamins A 5000 IU, B_1 1.5 mg, B_2 1.7 mg, B_6 2 mg, B_{12} 6 mcg, folic acid 0.4 mg, C 60 mg, E 30 mg, niacinamide 20 mg, calcium 162 mg, phosphorous 125 mg, elemental iron 18 mg, magnesium 100 mg, iodine 150 mcg/Tab. Bot. 100s.
Use: Vitamin/mineral supplement.

GEVRAL PROTEIN. (Lederle) Calcium caseinate, sucrose, protein 15.6 Gm, carbohydrate 7.05 Gm, fat 0.52 Gm, sodium 50 mg, potassium 13 mg, calories 95.3/26 Gm. Pow. Can. 8 oz, 5 lb.
Use: Enteral nutritional supplement.

GEVRAL T. (Lederle) Vitamins A 5000 IU, D 400 IU, B_1 2.25 mg, B_2 2.6 mg, B_6 3 mg, B_{12} 9 mcg, C 90 mg, E 45 IU, niacinamide 30 mg, calcium 162 mg, folic acid 0.4 mg, phosphorous 125 mg, elemental iron (from ferrous fumarate) 27 mg, magnesium 100 mg, iodine 225 mcg, copper 1.5 mg, zinc 22.5 mg/Tab. Bot. 100s.
Use: Vitamin/mineral supplement.

GG-CEN CAPSULES. (Central) Guaifenesin 200 mg/Cap. Bot. 24s, 100s.
Use: Expectorant.

GL-2 SKIN ADHERENT. (Gordon) Ready to use. Bot. pt, qt, gal.

G L-7 SKIN ADHERENT. (Gordon) Plastic material which may be used full strength or diluted with 3 to 10 parts 99% isopropyl alcohol, acetone or naphtha. Pkg. pt, qt, gal.

GLANDUBOLIN.
See: Estrone (Various Mfr.).

GLAUBER'S SALT.
See: Sodium Sulfate (Various Mfr.).

GLAUCON SOLUTION. (Alcon) Epinephrine HCl 1% or 2% w/benzalkonium Cl, sodium Cl 0.01%, sodium metabisulfite, EDTA. Dropper bot. 10 ml.
Use: Agent for glaucoma.

•**GLAZE, PHARMACEUTICAL,** N.F. XVII.
Use: Pharmaceutic aid (tablet coating).

•**GLEPTOFERRON.** USAN.
Use: Hematinic.

•**GLIAMILIDE.** USAN.
Use: Antidiabetic.

GLIBENCLAMIDE. B.A.N. 1- 4-[2-(5-Chloro-2-methoxybenzamido)ethyl]benzenesulphonyl-3-cyclohexylurea glyburide.
Use: Oral hypoglycemic agent.

•**GLIBORNURIDE.** USAN. endo-1-[(IR)-(2-Hydroxy-3-bornyl)]-3-(p-tolysulfonyl) urea. Glutril.
Use: Oral hypoglycemic agent.

•**GLICETANILE SODIUM.** USAN.
Use: Antidiabetic.

•**GLIFLUMIDE.** USAN.
Use: Antidiabetic.

GLIM.
See: Gardinol Type Detergents (Various Mfr.).

•**GLIPIZIDE.** USAN.
Use: Antidiabetic.

GLIQUIDONE. B.A.N. 1-Cyclohexyl-3-p-[2-(3,4-dihydro-7-methoxy-4,4-dimethyl-1,3-dioxo-2(1H)-isoquinolyl)ethyl]phenylsulfonylurea.
Use: Oral hypoglycemic agent.

GLISOXEPIDE. B.A.N. 3-[4-(Perhydroazepin-1-ylure-idosulfonyl)phenethylcarbamoyl]-5-methylis-oxazole.
Use: Oral hypoglycemic agent.

GLOBULIN, GAMMA.
See: Gamma Globulin (Various Mfr.).
Poliomyelitis Immune Globulin, Human, Vial. (Various Mfr.).

GLOBULIN, HEPATITIS B IMMUNE.
See: H-BIG, Vial (Abbott).

•**GLOBULIN, IMMUNE,** U.S.P. XXII.
Use: I.M., measles prophylactic and polio; passive immunizing agent.
See: Gammagee, Vial (Merck, Sharp & Dohme).
Generic, Vial 2 ml, 10 ml (Cutter).
Generic, Vial 2 ml (Lederle).

•**GLOBULIN, Rho(D) IMMUNE,** U.S.P. XXII.
Use: Immunosuppressive.

GLOBULIN, POLIOMYELITIS IMMUNE. Human.
See: Poliomyelitis Immune Globulin (Various Mfr.).

•**GLOXAZONE.** USAN. 3-Ethoxybutane-1,2-dione bis(thiosemicarbazone).
Use: Antiprotozoan (veterinary).
See: Contrapar.

•**GLOXIMONAM.** USAN.
Use: Antibacterial.

GLUBIONATE CALCIUM.
See: Neo-Calglucon, Syrup (Dorsey).

•**GLUCAGON,** U.S.P. XXII. Inj., U.S.P. XXII. (Lilly) 1 unit/ml w/diluent. 10 units w/10 ml diluent. Glucagon HCl 1 mg or 10 mg w/diluent; soln. contains lactose, glycerin 1.6% w/phenol 0.2% as a preservative. Vial.
Use: Hypoglycemic shock.

GLUCAMIDE. (Lemmon) Chlorpropamide 100 mg or 250 mg/Tab. Bot. 100s, 250s, 500s, 1000s, UD 100s.
Use: Antidiabetic.

•**GLUCEPTATE SODIUM.** USAN.
Use: Pharmaceutic aid.

d-GLUCITOL (d-Sorbitol)/Homatropine methylbromide.
See: ProBilagol, Liq. (Purdue Frederick).

GLUCOCORTICOIDS.
See: Cortical Hormone Products.

GLUCOLET AUTOMATIC LANCING DEVICE. (Ames) To obtain sample for blood glucose testing. Automatic spring loaded lancing device.
Use: Diagnostic aid.

GLUCOLET ENDCAPS. (Ames) To obtain sample for blood glucose testing. Controls depth of lancet penetration. Regular or super puncture.
Use: Diagnostic aid.

GLUCOMETER II BLOOD GLUCOSE METER. (Ames) Electronic meter for blood glucose testing.
Use: Diagnostic aid.

D-GLUCONIC ACID, CALCIUM SALT. Calcium Gluconate, U.S.P. XXII.

GLUCONIC ACID SALTS.
See: Calcium Gluconate.
Ferrous Gluconate.
Magnesium Gluconate.
Potassium Gluconate.

•**GLUCOSAMINE.** USAN. 2-Amino-2-deoxy-β-D-glucopyranose.
Use: Pharmaceutic aid.
W/Nystatin, oxytetracycline.
See: Terrastatin, Cap., Soln. (Pfizer).
W/Tetracycline HCl, nystatin.
See: Tetrastatin Cap., Susp. (Pfizer).
W/Tetracycline.
See: Tetracyn, Cap., Syr. (Roerig).
W/Oxytetracycline.
See: Terramycin, Prep (Pfizer).

GLUCOSE.
See: Pal-A-Dex, Pow. (Baker).

•**GLUCOSE ENZYMATIC TEST STRIP,** U.S.P. XXII.
Use: Diagnostic aid (in vitro, reducing sugars in urine).

GLUCOSE (HK) REAGENT STRIPS. Reagent strip test for detection of glucose in serum or plasma. Bot. 50s.
Use: Diagnostic aid.

•**GLUCOSE, LIQUID,** N.F. XVII. (Various Mfr.) Cerelose, Dextrose.
Use: As a 5% to 50% solution as nutrient; for acute hepatitis and dehydration; to increase blood volume; pharmaceutic aid (tablet binder, coating agent).

D-GLUCOSE, MONOHYDRATE. Dextrose, U.S.P. XXII.

GLUCOSE-40 OPHTHALMIC OINTMENT. (CooperVision) Liquid glucose 40% in white petrolatum, anhydrous lanolin with parabens. Tube 3.75 Gm.
Use: Hyperosmolar preparation.

GLUCOSE OXIDASE. W/peroxidase, potassium iodide.
See: Diastix, Vial, Tab. (Ames).

GLUCOSE POLYMERS.
See: Polycose, Pow., Liq. (Ross).

GLUCOSE REAGENT STRIPS. (Ames) A quantitative strip test for glucose in serum or plasma. Seralyzer reagent strips. Bot. 50s.
Use: Diagnostic aid.

GLUCOSE TEST.
See: Combistix (Ames).
Glucose Reagent Strips (Ames).

GLUCOSE TOLERANCE TEST PREPARATION
See: Glucola (Ames).

GLUCOSTIX REAGENT STRIPS. (Ames) Cellulose strip containing glucose oxidase and indicator system. Bot. 50s, 100s, UD 25s.
Use: Diagnostic aid.

GLUCOSULFONE SODIUM, INJ. *See:* Sodium Glucosulfone Injection.

GLUCO SYSTEM LANCETS. (Ames) Disposable lancets for use in Ames Autolet or Glucolet.
Use: Diagnostic aid.

GLUCOTROL. (Roerig) Glipizide 5 mg or 10 mg. Tab. Bot. 100s, UD 100s.
Use: Antidiabetic.

GLUCOVITE. (Vale) Ferrous gluconate 260 mg, vitamins B_1 1 mg, B_2 0.5 mg, C 10 mg/Tab. Bot. 1000s, 5000s.
Use: Vitamin/mineral supplement.

GLUCUROLACTONE. Gamma lactone of glucofuranuronic acid.
See: Preltron-Oral, Tab. (Pasadena Research).

GLUCURONATE SODIUM.
See: Preltron, Inj. (Pasadena Research).

GLU-K. (Western Research) Potassium glucona[te] 486 mg/Tab. Bot. 1000s.
Use: Potassium supplement.

GLUKOR. (Hyrex) Chorionic gonadotropin 200 IU/ml when reconstituted. Pow. for inj. Vial 10 ml, 25 ml w/diluent.

Use: Chorionic gonadotropin.
GLUSIDE.
See: Saccharin (Various Mfr.).
GLUTAMATE SODIUM.
W/Niacin, vitamins, minerals.
See: L-Glutavite, Cap. (Cooper).
GLUTAMIC ACID HYDROCHLORIDE. Acidogen, aciglumin, glutasin.
Use: Gastric acidifier.
See: Acidulin, Pulv. (Lilly).
W/Cellulase, pepsin, pancreatin, ox bile extract.
See: Kanulase, Tab. (Dorsey).
GLUTAMIC ACID SALTS.
See: Calcium Glutamate (Various Mfr.).
GLUTARAL CONCENTRATE, U.S.P. XXII.
Use: Disinfectant.
See: Cidex (Surgikos).
GLUTARALDEHYDE. (City Chem.) Glutaraldehyde 25% in water. Pkg. 3 kg; (Wyeth-Ayerst) Sonacide Soln., Gal, 5 Gal.
Use: Germicide.
GLUTETHIMIDE. B.A.N. 2-Ethyl-2-phenylglutatimide.
Use: Non-barbiturate hypnotic.
GLUTETHIMIDE, U.S.P. XXII. Cap., Tab., U.S.P. XXII. Alpha-ethyl-alpha-phenyl-glutarimide. 2-Ethyl-2-phenylglutarimide.
Use: Non-barbiturate hypnotic.
See: Dorimide, Tab. (Cenci).
Doriden, Cap. (Rorer).
Rolathimide, Tab. (Robinson).
GLUTOFAC. (Kenwood) Vitamins C 300 mg, B_1 15 mg, B_2 10 mg, niacinamide 50 mg, B_6 50 mg, calcium pantothenate 20 mg, magnesium 133 mg, selenium 25 mcg, GTF chromium complex 25 mcg/Tab. Trace amounts of Mg, K, Fe, Cu, P. Bot. 90s.
Use: Vitamin/mineral supplement.
GLUTOL. (Paddock) Dextrose 100 Gm/180 ml. Bot. 180 ml.
Use: Diagnostic aid.
GLUTOSE. (Paddock) Liquid glucose (40% dextrose). Concentrated glucose for insulin reactions. Gel. Bot. 60 Gm.
Use: Glucose elevating agent.
GLYATE. (Geneva Marsam) Guaifenesin 100 mg/5 ml, alcohol 3.5%. Syr. Bot. 118 ml, 480 ml.
Use: Expectorant.
GLYBURIDE. USAN.
Use: Antidiabetic.
See: Diabeta (Hoechst).
Micronase, Tab. (Upjohn).
GLYCALOX. B.A.N. A polymerized complex of glycerol and aluminum hydroxide. Glucalox (I.N.N.).
Use: Treatment of gastric hyperacidity.
GLYCARNINE IRON.
See: Ferronord, Tab. (Cooper).
GLYCATE CHEWABLES. (Forest) Glycine 150 mg, calcium carbonate 300 mg/Tab. Bot. 1000s.
Use: Antacid.
•**GLYCERIN,** U.S.P. XXII. Ophth. Soln., Oral Soln., U.S.P. XXII. 1,2,3-Propanetriol.
Use: Pharmaceutic aid (humectant, solvent).
See: Corn Huskers Lot. (Warner-Lambert).
Osmoglyn (Alcon).
W/Urea.
See: Kerid Ear Drops (Blair).
•**GLYCERIN SUPPOSITORIES,** U.S.P. XXII. (Various Mfr.) Glycerin, sodium stearate.
Use: Rectal evacuant, cathartic.
•**GLYCEROL, IODINATED.** USAN.
Use: Expectorant.
•**GLYCERYL BEHENATE,** N.F. XVII.
Use: Pharmaceutic aid.
GLYCERYL GUAIACOLATE.
Use: Expectorant.
See: Guaifenesin, U.S.P. XXII.
GLYCERYL GUAIACOLATE CARBAMATE. Methocarbamol.
See: Robaxin, Tab., Inj. (Robins).
Robaxin 750, Tab. (Robins).
GLYCERYL GUAIACOLETHER.
See: Guaifenesin.
•**GLYCERYL MONOSTEARATE,** N.F. XVII. (Various Mfr.) Monostearin.
Use: Pharmaceutic aid (emulsifying agent).
GLYCERYL-T. (Rugby) Theophylline 150 mg, guaifenesin 90 mg/Cap. Bot. 100s, 1000s.
Use: Bronchodilator, expectorant.
GLYCERYL TRIACETATE.
See: Triacetin.
GLYCERYL TRIACETIN. (Various Mfr.) Triacetin.
See: Enzactin, Aerosal, Pow., Cream (Wyeth-Ayerst).
Fungacetin, Oint, Liq. (Blair Labs.).
GLYCERYL TRINITRATE OINTMENT.
See: Nitrol, Oint. (Kremers-Urban).
GLYCERYL TRINITRATE TABLETS.
See: Nitroglycerin (Various Mfr.).
Nitroglyn, Tab. (Key Corp.).
GLYCETS-ANTACID TABLETS. (Weeks & Leo) Calcium carbonate 350 mg, simethicone 25 mg/Chew. Tab. Bot. 100s.
Use: Antacid/antiflatulent.
GLYCINATO DIHYDROXYALUMINUM HYDRATE.
See: Dihydroxyaluminum Aminoacetate, U.S.P. XXII.
•**GLYCINE,** U.S.P. XXII. Irrigation, U.S.P. XXI. Aminoacetic Acid.
Use: Myasthenia gravis treatment, irrigating solution.
W/Aluminum hydroxide-magnesium carbonate coprecipitated gel.
See: Glycogel, Tab., Susp. (Central).
W/Aluminum, magnesium hydroxide, magnesium trisilicate, belladonna extract, mannitol, peppermint oil.
See: Gas-Eze, Tab. (E.J. Moore).
W/Calcium Carbonate.
See: Antacid No. 6, Tab. (Bowman).
Glycate Chewables, Tab. (O'Neal).

P.H. Tab. (Scrip).
Titralac, Liq., Tab. (Riker).
W/Calcium carbonate, amylolytic, proteolytic cellulolytic enzymes.
See: Co-gel, Tab. (Arco).
W/Chlortrimeton, sodium salicylate.
See: Corilin, Liq. (Schering).
W/Glutamic acid, alanine.
See: Prostall, Cap. (Metabolic Prods.).
W/Magnesium trisilicate, calcium carbonate.
See: P.H. Tab., Chewable, Mix (Scrip).

GLYCINE, ALUMINUM SALT.
See: Dihydroxyaluminum Aminoacetate, U.S.P. XXII.

GLYCINE HYDROCHLORIDE. (Various Mfr.).
Use: Gastric acidifier.

GLYCOBIARSOL, U.S.P. XXI. Tab., U.S.P. XXI. Bismuthyl-N-Glycolylarsanilate, Chemo Puro, Pow. for Mfr. (Hydrogen N-glycoloylarsanilato) oxobismuth.
Use: Amebiasis, Trichomonas vaginalis, Monilia albicans.

GLYCOBIARSOL. (I.N.N.) Bismuth Glycollylarsanilate, B.A.N.

GLYCOCOLL. Glycine.
See: Aminoacetic Acid (Various Mfr.).

GLYCOCYAMINE. Guanidoacetic acid.

GLYCOFED TABLETS. (Pal-Pak) Pseudoephedrine 30 mg, guaifenesin 100 mg. Bot. 1000s.
Use: Decongestant, expectorant.

GLYCO IOPHEN SOLUTION. (Wade) Tincture of iodine, phenol 2%, glycerine q.s., peppermint oil. Bot. 2 oz, 4 oz, pt, gal.
Use: Antiseptic.

•**GLYCOL DISTERATE.** USAN.
Use: Pharmaceutic aid.

GLYCOL MONOSALICYLATE.
W/Oil of mustard, camphor, menthol, methyl salicylate.
See: Musterole, Oint., Cream (Plough).

GLYCOPHENYLATE BROMIDE.
See: Mepenzolate Methylbromide.

•**GLYCOPYRROLATE,** U.S.P. XXII. Inj., Tab., U.S.P. XXII. 1-Methyl-3-pyrrolidyl a-phenylcyclopentaneglycolate methobromide. 3-Hydroxy-1,1-dimethylpyrrolidinium bromideα-cyclopentylmandelate.
Use: Anticholinergic.
See: Robinul, Tab., Inj. (Robins).
Robinul Forte, Tab. (Robins).

GLYCOPYRRONIUM BROMIDE. B.A.N. 3-α-Cyclo-pentylmandeloyloxy-1,1-dimethylpyrrolidinium bromide.
Use: Anticholinergic.

GLYCOTUSS. (Vale) Guaifenesin 100 mg/Tab. Bot. 100s, 1000s.
Use: Expectorant.

GLYCOTUSS-dM. (Vale) Guaifenesin 100 mg, dextromethorphan HBr 10 mg/Tab. Bot. 100s, 1000s.
Use: Expectorant, antitussive.

•**GLYCYRRHIZA,** U.S.P. XXII. Pure extract, Fluidextract, U.S.P. XXII. Licorice root.
Use: Flavoring agent.

•**GLYCYRRHIZA** EXTRACT, PURE, U.S.P. XXII.
Use: Flavoring agent.

•**GLYCYRRHIZA** FLUIDEXTRACT, N.F. XVII.
Use: Flavoring agent.
W/Camphorated opium tincture, tartar emetic, glycerin.
See: Brown Mixture. (Bowman).
W/Pepsin-papain complex, pancreas, malt diastase, charcoal, ox bile.
See: Pepsocoll, Tab. (Western Research Labs.).

GLYDANILE SODIUM. (1)5′-Chloro-2-[p-[(5-isobutyl-2-pyrimidinyl)sulfamoyl]-phenyl]-o-acetanilidide monosodium salt; (2) 4-[N-(5-isobutyl-2-pyrimidinyl)-sulfamoyl] phenylacetic acid-5-chloro-2-methoxyanilide sodium salt.
Use: Antidiabetic.

•**GLYHEXAMIDE.** USAN.
Use: Antidiabetic.

•**GLYMIDINE SODIUM.** USAN. [N-[5-(2-Methoxyethoxy)-2-idinyl] benzene-sulfonamido]-sodium.
Use: Oral hypoglycemic agent.

GLYMOL.
See: Petrolatum Liquid (Various Mfr.).

GLYNAZAN EXPECTORANT. (Scherer) Theophylline sodium glycinate 60 mg (equivalent to theophylline 30 mg), guaifenesin 50 mg, sodium citrate 100 mg/5 ml. Bot. pt.
Use: Bronchodilator, expectorant.

•**GLYOCTAMIDE.** USAN. 1-Cyclooctyl-3(p-tolylsulfonyl) urea.
Use: Hypoglycemic agent.

GLY-OXIDE. (Marion) Carbamide peroxide 10% in flavored anhydrous glycerol. Liq. bot. 15 ml, 60 ml w/applicator.
Use: Mouth and throat product.

GLYOXYLDIUREIDE.
See: Allantoin (Various Mfr.).

•**GLYPARAMIDE.** USAN. 1-(p-Chlorophenylsulfonyl)-3-(p-dimethylaminophenyl) urea.
Use: Oral hypoglycemic agent.

GLYTUSS. (Mayrand) Guaifenesin 200 mg/Tab. Bot. 100s.
Use: Expectorant.

GLYVENOL. (Ciba) Tribenoside. Not available in U.S.
Use: Venoprotective agent.

G-MYTICIN CREME AND OINTMENT. (Pedinol) Gentamicin sulfate equivalent to gentamicin base 1 mg. Tube 15 Gm.
Use: Anti-infective.

GOLACOL. (Arcum) Codeine sulfate 30 mg, papaverine HCl 30 mg, emetine HCl 2 mg, ephedrine HCl 15 mg, q.s./30 ml. Alcohol 6.25%. Syr Bot. 4 oz, 16 oz, gal. Orange flavor.
Use: Antitussive.

GOLD (Au^{198}) Colloid Radio.
Use: Antineoplastic agent.

See: Radio Gold (Au^{198}).
GOLD Au 198 INJECTION.
Use: Antineoplastic; diagnostic for liver scanning.
GOLD COMPOUNDS.
See: Aurocein-10, Vial (Christina).
Gold Sodium Thiosulfate (Various Mfr.).
Myochrysine, Amp. (Merck, Sharp &Dohme).
Solganal, Vial (Schering).
GOLD SODIUM THIOMALATE, U.S.P. XXI. Inj., U.S.P. XXI. Gold, mercaptobutanedioato(1-)-, disodium salt, monohydrate. (Disodium mercaptosuccinato) gold monohydrate.
Use: Rheumatoid arthritis.
See: Myochrysine, Amp. (Merck, Sharp & Dohme).
GOLD SODIUM THIOSULFATE. Sterile, Auricidine, Aurocidin, Aurolin, Auropin, Aurosan, Novacrysin, Solfocrisol and Thiochrysine.
Use: Antirheumatic agent.
GOLD THIOGLUCOSE.
See: Aurothioglucose, U.S.P. XXII.
GOLDEN BALM. (Jenkins) Methyl salicylate, menthol, camphor/fl oz. Bot. 3 oz, pt, gal.
Use: External analgesic.
GOLDEN-WEST COMPOUND. (Golden-West) Gentian root, licorice root, cascara sagrada, damiana leaves, senna leaves, psyllium seed, buchu leaves, crude pepsin. Box 1.5 oz.
Use: Laxative.
GOLDICIDE CONCENTRATE. (Pedinol) N-Alkyldimethylbenzylammonium chloride, cetyl dimethyl ammonium Cl. Bot. (Conc.) oz. Ctn. 10s.
Use: Chemical disinfection of surgical and podiatry instruments.
GOLD SEAL CALCIUM 600. (Walgreen) Calcium 1200 mg/Tab. Bot. 60s.
Use: Calcium supplement.
GOLD SEAL CALCIUM 600 WITH VITAMIN D. (Walgreen) Calcium 1200 mg, vitamin D/Tab. Bot. 60s.
Use: Calcium supplement.
GOLD SEAL CHEWABLE VITAMIN C. (Walgreen) Ascorbic acid 250 mg or 500 mg/Tab. Bot. 100s.
Use: Vitamin C supplement.
GOLD SEAL FERROUS GLUCONATE. (Walgreen) Iron 37 mg/Tab. Bot. 100s.
Use: Iron supplement.
GOLD SEAL FERROUS SULFATE TABLETS. (Walgreen) Ferrous sulfate 325 mg/Tab. Bot. 100s, 1000s.
Use: Iron supplement.
GOLD SEAL TIME RELEASE FERROUS SULFATE. (Walgreen) Iron 50 mg/Tab. Bot. 100s.
Use: Iron supplement.
GOLYTELY. (Braintree) Pow. for oral soln. after reconstitution containing PEG-3350 236 Gm, sodium sulfate 22.74 Gm, sodium bicarbonate 6.74 Gm, sodium Cl 5.86 Gm, potassium Cl 2.97 Gm when made up to 4 L. Disposable container 4800 ml.
Use: Laxative.
GONACRINE.
See: Acriflavine (Various Mfr.).
•**GONADORELIN ACETATE.** USAN.
Use: Gonad-stimulating principle.
See: Cryptolin Prods. (Hoechst).
•**GONADORELIN HYDROCHLORIDE.** USAN.
Use: Gonad-stimulating principle.
GONADOTROPIC SUBSTANCE.
See: Gonadotropin Chorionic.
•**GONADOTROPIN, CHORIONIC,** U.S.P. XXII. For Inj., U.S.P. XXII. Human Pregnancy Urine.
Use: In the female: Chronic cystic mastitis, functional sterility, dysmenorrhea, premenstrual tension, threatened abortion. In the male: Cryptorchidism, hypogenitalism, dwarfism, impotency, enuresis.
See: Android HCG, Inj. (Brown).
Antuitrin "S", Vial (Parke-Davis).
A.P.L., Secules (Wyeth-Ayerst).
Chopion-Plus, Vial (Pharmex).
Corgonject, Vial (Mayrand).
Dura-Chroion Plus, Vial (Pharmex).
Follutein Pow. (Squibb).
Gonadamine 5000, Vial (Torigian).
Harvatropin, Vial (Harvey).
Libigen, Vial (Savage).
Pregnyl, Amp. (Organon).
W/Vitamin B_1, glutamic acid, procaine HCl.
See: Glukor, Vial (Brown).
GONADOTROPIN, PITUITARY ANT. LOBE. Extracted from anterior lobe of equine pituitaries (not pregnant mare urine) (rat unit = 1 Fevold-Hisaw unit).
GONADOTROPIN SERUM. Pregnant mare's serum.
GONADOTROPIN SPECIAL DILUENT. (Kenyon) Sodium succinate 0.5%, sodium nicotinate 1%, glutamic acid 52.5 ppm, propylparaben 0.02%, chlorobutanol 0.5%. Vial 10 ml.
GONAK. (Akorn) Hydroxypropyl methylcellulose 2.5%, boric acid, EDTA, benzalkonium Cl 0.01%, sodium borate. Soln. Bot. 15 ml.
Use: Ophthalmic preparation.
GONIC. (Hauck) Chorionic gonadotropin 10,000 units/vial. Pow. for inj. Vial 10 ml w/diluent.
Use: Chorionic gonadotropin.
GONIOSCOPIC HYDROXYPROPYL METHYLCELLULOSE.
See: Goniosol Lacrivial, Soln. (Smith, Miller & Patch).
GONIOSCOPIC PRISM SOLUTION. (Alcon) Hydroxyethyl cellulose preserved with thimerosal 0.004%, edetate sodium 0.1%. Soln. Plastic dispenser 15 ml.
Use: Ophthalmic preparation.
GONIOSOL. (Iolab) Gonioscopic hydroxypropylmethylcellulose 2.5%. Bot. 15 ml.
Use: Ophthalmic preparation.
GONOZYME. (Abbott Diagnostics) Enzyme immunoassay for detection of *neisseria gonorr-*

hoeae in urogenital swab specimens. Test kit 100s.
Use: Diagnostic aid.

GOOD SAMARITAN OINTMENT. (Good Samaritan) Tube 1.25 oz.
Use: Counter-irritant.

GO PAIN. (DePree) **Cream:** Methyl salicylate, chlorobutanol, menthol, camphor, thymol. Tube 1.5 oz, 4 oz. **Oral Gel:** Benzocaine, eugenol. Tube ⅜ oz. **Throat spray:** 4 oz.
Use: External analgesic.

GO PAIN EXTRA STRENGTH BALM. (DePree) Methyl salicylate. Jar 3¾ oz.
Use: External analgesic.

GORDOBALM. (Gordon) Chloroxylenol, methyl salicylate, menthol, camphor, thymol, eucalyptus oil, isopropyl alcohol 16%, fast-drying gum base. Bot. 4 oz, gal.
Use: External analgesic.

GORDOCHOM. (Gordon) Undecylenic acid 25%, chloroxylenol 3%, penetrating oil base. Liq. Bot. 15 ml, 30 ml w/applicator.
Use: Antifungal, external.

GORDOFILM. (Gordon) Salicylic acid 16.7%, lactic acid 16.7% in flexible collodian. Bot. 15 ml.
Use: Keratolytic.

GORDOGESIC CREAM. (Gordon) Methyl salicylate 10% in absorption base. Jar 2.5 oz, 1 lb.
Use: External analgesic.

GORDOMATIC CRYSTALS. (Gordon) Sodium borate, sodium bicarbonate, sodium Cl, thymol, menthol, eucalyptus oil. Jar 8 oz, 7 lb.
Use: Counter-irritant.

GORDOMATIC LOTION. (Gordon) Menthol, camphor, propylene glycol, isopropyl alcohol. Bot. 1 oz, 4 oz, gal.
Use: Counter-irritant.

GORDOMATIC POWDER. (Gordon) Menthol, thymol camphor, eucalyptus oil, salicylic acid, alum bentonite, talc. Shaker can 3.5 oz. Can 1 lb, 5 lb.
Use: Counter-irritant.

GORDOPHENE. (Gordon) Neutral coconut oil soap 15%, glycerin with Septi-Chlor (trichlorohydroxy diphenyl ether) broad spectrum antimicrobial and bacteriostatic agent. Bot. 4 oz, gal.
Use: Surgical soap.

GORDO-POOL WHIRLPOOL CONCENTRATE. (Gordon) Bot. pt.
Use: Water softener, cleanser.

GORDO-VITE A CREME. (Gordon) Vitamin A 100,000 IU/oz. in water soluble base. Jar 0.5 oz, 2.5 oz, 4 oz, lb, 5 lb.
Use: Emollient.

GORDO-VITE A LOTION. (Gordon) Vitamin A 100,000 IU/oz. Plastic bot. 4 oz, gal.
Use: Emollient.

GORDO-VITE E CREME. (Gordon) Vitamin E 1500 IU/oz in water soluble base. Jar 2.5 oz, lb.
Use: Emollient.

GORD-UREA. (Gordon) Urea 22% or 40% in petrolatum base. Jar oz.
Use: Emollient.

GORMEL CREAM. (Gordon) Urea 20% in emollient base. Jar 0.5 oz, 2.5 oz, 4 oz, 1 lb, 5 lb.
Use: Emollient.

•**GOSERELIN.** USAN.
Use: LHRH agonist.
See: Zoladex (Stuart).

GOTAMINE. (Vita Elixir) Ergotamine tartrate 1 mg, caffeine 100 mg/Tab.
Use: Agent for migraine.

•**GRAMICIDIN,** U.S.P. XXII.
Use: Antibacterial.
W/Neomycin.
See: Spectrocin Oint. (Squibb).
W/Neomycin sulfate, polymyxin B sulfate, thimerosal.
See: Neo-Polycin Ophthalmic Soln. (Merrell Dow).
W/Neomycin sulfate, polymyxin B sulfate, benzocaine.
See: Tricidin, Oint. (Amlab).
W/Neomycin, triamcinolone, nystatin.
See: Mycolog Cream, Oint. (Squibb).
W/Polymyxin B sulfate, neomycin sulfate.
See: Neosporin, Ophthalmic Soln. (Burroughs Wellcome).
Neosporin-G Cream (Burroughs Wellcome).
W/Polymyxin B sulfate, neomycin sulfate, hydrocortisone acetate.
See: Cortisporin, Cream (Burroughs Wellcome).

GRAMINEAE POLLENS.
See: Allergenic Extracts, Timothy and Related Pollens (Parke-Davis).

GRANULEX. (Hickam) Trypsin 0.1 mg, balsam Peru 72.5 mg, castor oil 650 mg w/emulsifier/ 0.82 ml. Spray can 2 oz, 4 oz.
Use: Wound-healing agent.

GRAPEFRUIT DIET PLAN with DIADAX CAPSULES. (O'Connor) Natural grapefruit extract 50 mg, phenylpropanolamine HCl 30 mg/Cap. and Capl. Bot. 20s, 50s.
Use: Diet aid.

GRAPEFRUIT DIET PLAN with DIADAX EXTRA STRENGTH CAPSULES. (O'Connor) Natural grapefruit extract 100 mg, phenylpropanolamine HCl 75 mg/Cap. and Capl. Bot. 10s, 24s.
Use: Diet aid.

GRAPEFRUIT DIET PLAN with DIADAX TABLETS. (O'Connor) Natural grapefruit extract, phenylpropanolamine HCl 12.5 mg/Chew. tab. Bot. 42s, 90s.
Use: Diet aid.

GRATUS STROPHANTHIN.
See: Ouabain (Various Mfr.).

GRAVINEED. (Hanlon) Vitamins C 100 mg, E 10 IU, B_1 3 mg, B_2 2 mg, B_6 10 mg, B_{12} 5 mcg, A 4000 IU, D 400 IU, niacin 10 mg, folic acid 0.1 mg, iron fumarate 40 mg, calcium 67 mg/Cap. Bot. 100s.
Use: Vitamin/mineral supplement.

GREEN MINT. (Block) Urea, glycine, polysorbate 60, sorbitol, alcohol 12.2%, peppermint oil, menthol, chlorophyllin-copper complex. Bot. 7 oz, 12 oz.
Use: Mouth and throat product.
GREEN SOAP, U.S.P. XXII.
Use: Detergent.
GRIFULVIN V. (Ortho Derm) Griseofulvin microsize. **Tab:** 250 mg. Bot. 100s; 500 mg. Bot. 100s, 500s. **Susp:** 125 mg/5 ml. Bot. 120 ml.
Use: Antifungal.
GRILLODYNE TABLETS. (Forest Pharm.) Aspirin 3.5 gr, phenacetin 2.5 gr, caffeine alkaloid 0.5 gr, phenobarbital 0.25 gr/Tab. Bot. 1000s.
Use: Salicylate analgesic, sedative/hypnotic.
GRISACTIN. (Wyeth-Ayerst) Griseofulvin microsize. **Cap.: 125 mg:** Bot. 100s; **250 mg:** Bot. 100s, 500s. **Tab.: 500 mg:** Bot. 60s.
Use: Antifungal.
GRISACTIN ULTRA. (Wyeth-Ayerst) Griseofulvin ultramicrosize 125 mg, 250 mg or 330 mg/Tab. Bot. 100s.
Use: Antifungal.
•**GRISEOFULVIN,** U.S.P. XXII. Cap., Oral Susp., Tab., Ultramicrosized Tab., U.S.P. XXII. An antibiotic. 7-Chloro-4,6-dimethoxy-coumaran-3-one-2-spiro-1′-(2′-methoxy-6′-methylcyclohex-2′-en-4′-one). 7-Chloro-2′,4,6-trimethoxy-6′-methylspiro[benzofuran-2(3H), 1′[2]-cyclohexene]-3,4′-dione. Spiro[benzofuran-2(3H)-1′-[2]cyclohexene]-3,4′-dione,7-chloro-2′,4,6-trimethoxy-6′-methyl-, (1′s-trans)-. Fulcin, Grisovin.
Use: Antifungal (antibiotic).
See: Fulvicin P/G, Tab. (Schering).
Fulvicin-U/F, Tab. (Schering).
Grifulvin V, Tab., Susp. (Ortho).
Grisactin, Cap., Tab. (Wyeth-Ayerst).
Grisactin Ultra, Tab. (Wyeth-Ayerst).
GRISEOFULVIN MICROCRYSTALLINE.
Use: Antifungal.
See: Fulvicin U/F, Tab. (Schering).
Grifulvin V, Tab., Susp. (Ortho).
Grisactin, Cap., Tab. (Wyeth-Ayerst).
GRISEOFULVIN ULTRAMICROSIZE.
Use: Antifungal.
See: Fulvicin P/G, Tab.(Schering).
Gris-Peg, Tab. (Dorsey).
GRIS-PEG TABLETS. (Herbert) Griseofulvin ultramicrosize 125 mg or 250 mg/Tab. **125 mg:** Bot. 100s, 500s. **250 mg:** Bot. 100s, 250s, 500s.
Use: Antifungal.
GROWTH HORMONE. Extract of human pituitaries containing predominantly growth hormone.
See: Crescormon.
G-STROPHANTHIN.
See: Ouabain. (Various Mfr.).
GUAIACOHIST. (Pharmex) Potassium guaiacolsulfonate 40 mg, sodium iodide 50 mg, chlorpheniramine maleate 5 mg/ml. Vial 30 ml.
Use: Expectorant, antihistamine.
GUAIACOL. (Various Mfr.) Methylcatechol.
Use: Expectorant.
GUAIACOL. (Jenkins) Guaiacol 0.1 Gm, eucalyptol 0.08 Gm, iodoform 0.02 Gm, camphor 0.05 Gm, sesame oil q.s./2 ml. Vial 10 ml.
Use: Expectorant.
W/Methyl salicylate, menthol.
See: Guaiamen, Cream (Lannett).
GUAIACOL CARBONATE. (Various Mfr.) (Duotal).
Use: Expectorant.
GUAIACOL GLYCERYL ETHER.
See: Guaifenesin.
GUAIACOL POTASSIUM SULFONATE.
See: Bronchial, Syr. (DePree).
W/Ammonium Cl, sodium citrate, benzyl alcohol, carbinoxamine maleate.
See: Clistin Expectorant, Syr. (McNeil).
W/Dextromethorphan HBr.
Bronchial DM, Syr. (DePree).
W/Dextromethorphan HBr, chlorpheniramine maleate, ammonium Cl, tartar emetic.
See: Duomine, Syr. (Kenyon).
W/Pheniramine maleate, pyrilamine maleate, codeine phosphate.
See: Tritussin, Syr. (Towne).
GUAIADOL. (Medwick) Aqueous. Vial 30 ml.
GUAIADOL COMPOUND. (Medical Chem.) Naiouli oil 100 mg, eucalyptol 80 mg, guaiacol 100 mg, iodoform 20 mg, camphor 50 mg/2 ml. Aqueous or in oil. Vial 30 ml.
GUAIADOL COMPOUND. (Medwick) Oil. Vial 30 ml.
GUAIAMEN. (Lannett) Methyl salicylate, guaiacol, menthol in greaseless base. 4 oz, 1 lb.
Use: Analgesic, expectorant.
GUAIANESIN.
See: Guaifenesin.
Use: Expectorant.
•**GUAIAPATE.** USAN.
Use: Antitussive.
GUAIFED CAPSULES. (Muro) Guaifenesin 250 mg, pseudoephedrine HCl 120 mg/TR Cap. Bot. 100s, 500s.
Use: Expectorant, decongestant.
GUAIFED PD CAPSULES. (Muro) Pseudoephedrine HCl 60 mg, guaifenesin 300 mg/TR Cap. Bot. 100s, 500s.
Use: Decogestant, expectorant.
•**GUAIFENESIN,** U.S.P. XXII. Cap., Syr., Tab., U.S.P. XXII. Methphenoxydiol. 3-(o-methoxyphenoxy)-1,2-propanediol.
Synonyms:
Glyceryl Guaiacolate.
Glyceryl Guaiacol Ether.
Guaianesin.
Guaifylline.
Guayanesin.
Use: Expectorant.
See: Anti-tuss, Liq. (Century).
Consin-GG, Syr. (Wisconsin).
Dilyn, Liq., Tab. (Elder).
2/G, Liq. (Merrell Dow).

G-100, Syr. (Bock).
GG-Cen, Syr. (Central).
Glycotuss, Tab., Syr. (Vale).
Glytuss, Tab. (Mayrand).
G-Tussin, Syr. (Quality Generics).
Humibid L.A., Tab. (Adams).
Hytuss, Tab., Cap. (Hyrex).
Robitussin, Syr. (Robins).
Tursen, Tab. (Wren).
Wal-Tussin, Syr. (Walgreen).

W/Combinations.

See: Actified C Expectorant, Liq. (Burroughs Wellcome).
Actol Exp., Syr., Tab. (Beecham Labs).
Airet G.G., Cap., Elix. (Baylor Labs).
Ambenyl-D, Liq. (Marion).
Anti-tuss D.M., Liq. (Century).
Antitussive Guaiacolate, Syr. (Med. Chem.).
Asbron G, Tab., Elix. (Dorsey).
Bur-Tuss Expectorant (Burlington).
Brexin, Cap., Liq. (Savage).
Bri-stan, Liq. (Briar).
Broncholate, Cap., Elix. (Bock).
Bronchovent, Tab. (Mills).
Bronkolate-G, Tab. (Parmed).
Bronkolixir, Elix. (Winthrop Pharm).
Bronkotabs, Tab. (Winthrop Pharm).
Bro-Tane, Expectorant (Scrip).
C.D.M., Expectorant (Lannett).
Cerylin, Liq. (Spencer-Mead).
Cheracol-D, Syr. (Upjohn).
Chlor-Trimeton, Expectorant (Schering).
Colrex, Expectorant (Solvay).
Conar-A, Susp., Tab. (Beecham Labs).
Conar Expectorant, Liq. (Beecham Labs).
Congestac, Tab. (SmithKline Prods).
Consin-DM, Syr. (Wisconsin).
Coricidin Children's Cough Syr. (Schering).
Cortane D.C., Exp. (Standex).
Dextro-Tuss GG, Liq. (Ulmer).
Dilaudid, Syr. (Knoll).
Dilor-G, Tab., Liq. (Savage).
Dilyn, Liq. (Elder).
Dimacol, Cap. (Robins).
Dimetane Expectorant, Liq. (Robins).
Dimetane Expectorant-DC, Liq. (Robins).
DM Plus, Liq. (West-Ward).
Donatussin, Syr. (Laser).
Duovent, Tab. (Riker).
Emfaseem, Liq., Tab. (Saron).
Entex, Cap., Liq. (Norwich Eaton).
Formula 44D Decongestant Cough Mixture, Syr. (Vicks).
G-100/DM, Syr. (Bock).
G-Bron Elix. (Laser).
2G/DM, Liq. (Merrell Dow).
Glycotuss-DM, Tab. (Vale).
Guiatussin w/Codeine, Liq. (Spencer-Mead).
Guistrey Fortis, Tab. (Bowman).
Gylanphen, Tab. (Lannett).
Histussinol, Syr. (Bock).
Hycoff-A, Syr. (Saron).
Hycotuss Expectorant, Liq. (Du Pont).
Hylate, Tab., Syr. (Hyrex).
Isoclor Expectorant (American Critical Care).
Lanatuss, Expectorant (Lannett).
Lardet Expectorant, Tab. (Standex).
Mudrane GG, Tab., Elix. (Poythress).
Neospect, Tab. (Lemmon).
Novahistine Cough Formula, Liq. (Merrell Dow).
Novahistine DMX, Liq. (Merrell Dow).
Novahistine, Expectorant (Merrell Dow).
Panaphyllin, Susp. (Panamerican).
Partuss-A, Tab. (Parmed).
Partuss AC (Parmed).
Phenatuss, Liq. (Dalin).
PMP, Expectorant, Syr. (Schlicksup).
Polaramine Expectorant (Schering).
Poly-Histine Expectorant (Bock).
Polytuss-DM, Liq. (Rhode).
P.R. Syrup, Liq. (Fleming).
Queltuss, Syr., Tab. (Westerfield).
Quibron, Cap., Liq. (Bristol).
Quibron-300, Cap. (Bristol).
Quibron Plus, Cap., Elix. (Bristol).
Rentuss, Cap., Syr. (Wren).
Rhinex DM (Lemmon).
Robitussin AC, CF, DAC, DM, PE (Robins).
Robitussin-DM Cough Calmers, Loz. (Robins).
Rondec-DM, Syr. (Ross).
Rymed, Prods. (Edwards).
Santussin, Cap. (Sandia).
Scotcof, Liq. (Scott/Cord).
Silexin, Cough Syr. (Clapp).
Slo-Phyllin GG, Cap., Syr. (Dooner).
Sorbase Cough Syr. (Fort David).
Sorbase II Cough Syr. (Fort David).
Spen-Histine Expectorant (Spencer-Mead).
Sudafed Cough Syr. (Burroughs Wellcome).
Tolu-Sed, Liq. (Scherer).
Tolu-Sed DM, Liq. (Scherer).
Triaminic Expectorant (Sandoz Consumer).
Trihista-Phen, Liq. (Recsei).
Tri-Histin Expectorant (Recsei).
Tri-Mine, Expectorant (Spencer-Mead).
Trind-DM, Liq. (Mead Johnson).
Trind, Liq. (Mead Johnson).
Tussafed, Expectorant (Calvital).
Tussar-2, Syr. (Rorer).
Tussar SF, Liq. (Rorer).
Tussend, Liq. (Merrell Dow).
Verequad, Tab., Susp. (Knoll).
Vicks Cough Syr. (Vicks).
Vicks Formula 44D Decongestant Cough Mixture, Syr. (Vicks).
Wal-Tussin DM, Syr. (Walgreen).

GUAIODOL AQUEOUS. (Kenyon) Potassium guaiacolsulfonate 40 mg, sodium iodide 50 mg in saturated aqueous naiouli, guaiacol, eucalyptol, menthol/ml. Vial 30 ml.
Use: Expectorant.

GUAIODOL COMPOUND. (Kenyon) Naiouli oil 0.1 Gm, eucalyptol 0.08 Gm, guaiacol 0.1 Gm,

iodoform 0.02 Gm, camphor 0.05 Gm/2 ml. Vial 30 ml.
Use: Expectorant.

GUAIPHENESIN. B.A.N. 3- -Methoxyphenoxy-propane-1:2-diol. Guaiacol glycerol ether.
Use: Cough suppressant.

GUAIPHOTOL. (Foy) Iodine 1/30 gr, calcium cresoate 4 gr/Tab. Bot. 1000s.
Use: Expectorant.

GUAITHYLLINE. USAN. 3-(o-Methoxy-phenoxy)-1,2- propanediol w/theophylline.
Use: Antiasthmatic.

GUAMECYCLINE. B.A.N. N-(4-Guanidinoformimidoylpiperazin-1-ylmethyl)tetracycline.
Use: Antibiotic.

GUAMIDE.
See: Sulfaguanidine (Various Mfr.).

GUANABENZ. USAN.[(2,6-Dichlorobenzylidene)-amino] guanidine.
Use: Antihypertensive.
See: Wytensin, Tab. (Wyeth-Ayerst).

GUANABENZ ACETATE, U.S.P. XXII. Tab., U.S.P. XXII.
Use: Antihypertensive.

GUANACLINE. B.A.N. 1-(2-Guanidinoethyl)-1,-2,3,6-tetrahydro-4-picoline.
Use: Hypotensive.

GUANADREL SULFATE, U.S.P. XXII. Tab., U.S.P. XXII. (1,4-Dioxaspiro[4.5] dec-2-ylmethyl)guanidine sulfate (2:1).
Use: Antihypertensive.
See: Hylorel, Tab. (Pennwalt).

GUANCYDINE. USAN.
Use: Antihypertensive.

GUANETHIDINE MONOSULFATE, U.S.P. XXII. Tab., U.S.P. XXII. [2-(Hex-ahydro-1(2H)-azocinyl)-ethyl]guanidine sulfate (2:1), or [2-(hexahydro-1(2H)-azocinyl)-ethyl] guanidine hydrogen sulfate.
Use: Antihypertensive.
W/Hydrochlorothiazide.
See: Esimil, Tab. (Ciba).

GUANETHIDINE SULFATE, U.S.P. XXI. Tab. U.S.P. XXI. Guanidine, 2-(hexahydro-1(2H)-azocinyl)ethyl-, sulfate (2:1). [2-(Hexahydro-1-(2H)-azocinyl)ethyl] guanidine sulfate.
Use: Antihypertensive.
See: Ismelin, Tab. (Ciba).
W/Hydrochlorothiazide.
See: Esimil, Tab. (Ciba).

GUANFACINE HYDROCHLORIDE. USAN.
Use: Antihypertensive.
See: Tenex, Tab. (Robins).

GUANIDINE HCl. (Key) Guanidine HCl 125 mg/Tab. Bot. 100s.
Use: Cholinergic muscle stimulant.

GUANISOQUIN. 7-Bromo- 3,4-dihydro-2-(1H)-isoquinoline carboxamidine sulfate (2:1).
Use: Antihypertensive.

GUANISOQUIN SULFATE. USAN.
Use: Antihypertensive.

•**GUANOCLOR SULFATE.** USAN.[[2-(2,6-Di-chlorophenoxy)-ethyl]amino] guanidine sulfate.
Use: Antihypertensive.
See: Vatensoln.

•**GUANOCTINE HYDROCHLORIDE.** USAN.
Use: Antihypertensive.

•**GUANOXABENZ.** USAN.
Use: Antihypertensive.

GUANOXAN. B.A.N. 2-Guanidinomethyl-1,4-benzodioxan.
Use: Hypotensive.

•**GUANOXAN SULFATE.** USAN. (1,4-Benzodioxane-2-ylmethyl)-guanidinesulfate. Envacar.
Use: Antihypertensive.

•**GUANOXYFEN SULFATE.** USAN. (3-Phenoxy-propyl) guanidine sulfate.
Use: Antihypertensive, antidepressant.

GUARDAL. (Morton) Vitamins A 10,000 IU, B_1 20 mg, B_2 8 mg, C 50 mg, niacinamide 10 mg, calcium d-pantothenate 5 mg, iron 10 mg, dried whole liver 100 mg, yeast 100 mg, choline bitartrate 30 mg, B_6 0.5 mg, B_{12} 8 mcg, mixed tocopherols 5 mg, dicalcium phosphate anhydrous 150 mg, magnesium sulfate dried 7.2 mg, sodium 1 mg, potassium Cl 1.3 mg/Tab. Bot. 100s.
Use: Vitamin/mineral supplement.

GUARDEX. (Archer-Taylor) Tube 4 oz, 1 lb, 4.5 lb.
Use: Emollient.

•**GUAR GUM,** N.F. XVII.
Use: Pharmaceutic aid (tablet binder; tablet disintegrant).
W/Danthron, docusate sodium.
See: Guarsol, Tab. (Western Research).
W/Standardized senna concentrate.
See: GentlaxB, Granules, Tab. (Blair).

GUAYANESIN.
Use: Expectorant.
See: Guaifenesin (Various Mfr.).

GUIAMID EXPECTORANT. (Vangard) Guaifenesin 100 mg/5 ml, alcohol 3.5%. Bot. pt, gal.
Use: Expectorant.

GUIAPHED ELIXIR. (Various Mfr.) Theophylline 45 mg, ephedrine sulfate 36 mg, guaifenesin 150 mg, phenobarbital 12 mg, alcohol 19%/15 ml Liq. Bot. 480 ml.
Use: Antiasthmatic combination.

GUIATUSS A.C. SYRUP. (Various Mfr.) Codeine phosphate 10 mg, guaifenesin 100 mg, alcohol 3.5%/5 ml. Syr. Bot. 120 ml, pt, gal.
Use: Antitussive, expectorant.

GUIATUSS BERTUSS COUGH SYRUP. (Alton) Bot. 4 oz, 8 oz, 16 oz, gal.
Use: Cough preparation.

GUIATUSS DAC SYRUP. (Various Mfr.) Pseudoephedrine HCl 30 mg, codeine phosphate 10 mg, guaifenesin 100 mg, alcohol 1.4%/5 ml. Syr. Bot. 120 ml, 240 ml, 480 ml.
Use: Decongestant, antitussive, expectorant.

GUIATUSS DM BERTUSS COUGH SYRUP. (Alton) Bot. 4 oz, 8 oz, 16 oz, gal.

Use: Cough preparation.

GUIATUSS D.M. SYRUP. (Various Mfr.) Dextromethorphan HBr 15 mg, guaifenesin 100 mg, alcohol 1.4%. Syr. Bot. 120 ml, 240 ml, pt, gal.
Use: Antitussive, expectorant.

GUIATUSS SYRUP. (Various Mfr.) Guaifenesin 100 mg/5 ml. Syr. Bot. 120 ml, 240 ml, pt, gal.
Use: Expectorant.

GUIATUSSIN W/CODEINE EXPECTORANT. (Rugby) Codeine phosphate 10 mg, guaifenesin 100 mg/5 ml, alcohol 3.5%. Syr. Bot. 120 ml, pt, gal.
Use: Antitussive, expectorant.

GUIDO. (Rocky Mtn.) Camphor 0.025 Gm, guaiacol 0.05 Gm, iodoform 0.01 Gm, eucalyptol 0.04 Gm. Vial 30 ml.
Use: Expectorant.

GUISTREY FORTIS. (Bowman) Guaifenesin 100 mg, phenylephrine HCl 10 mg, chlorpheniramine maleate 1 mg/Tab. Bot. 1000s.
Use: Expectorant, decongestant, antihistamine.

GULFASIN TABS. (Major) Sulfisoxazole 500 mg/Tab. Bot. 100s, 250s, 1000s.
Use: Antibacterial, sulfonamide.

GUNCOTTON, SOLUBLE. Pyroxylin.

GUSTALAC. (Geriatric) Calcium carbonate 300 mg, defatted skim milk pow. 200 mg/Tab. Bot. 100s, 250s, 1000s.
Use: Antacid/calcium supplement.

GUSTASE. (Geriatric) Gerilase (standard amylolytic enzyme) 30 Gm, geriprotase (standard proteolytic enzyme) 6 mg, gericellulase (standard cellulolytic enzyme) 2 mg/Tab. Bot. 42s, 100s, 500s.
Use: Digestive aid.

GUSTASE PLUS. (Geriatric) Phenobarbital 8 mg, homatropine methylbromide 2.5 mg, gerilase 30 mg, geriprotase 6 mg, gericellulase 2 mg/Tab. Bot. 42s, 100s, 500s.
Use: Sedative/hypnotic, anticholinergic/antispasmodic, digestive aid.

•**GUTTA PERCHA,** U.S.P. XXII.
Use: Dental restoration agent.

G-VITAMIN.
See: Riboflavin (Various Mfr.).

GLYNAPHEN TABLETS. (Lannett) Phenobarbital ⅛ gr, hyoscyamus extract 1/10 gr, terpin hydrate 2 gr, guaifenesin 1 gr, calcium lactate 1 gr/Tab. Bot. 1000s.

G-WELL LOTION. (Goldline) Bot. 2 oz, pt.
Use: Scabicide.

G-WELL SHAMPOO. (Goldline) Bot. 2 oz, pt, gal.
Use: Pediculicide.

GYNECORT. (Combe) Hydrocortisone acetate 0.5%. Cream Tube 15 Gm.
Use: Corticosteroid, topical.

GYNE-LOTRIMIN VAGINAL CREAM 1%. (Schering) Clotrimazole ≈ 5 Gm/applicatorful. Tube 45 Gm, 45 Gm twin-packs w/applicator.
Use: Antifungal, vaginal.

GYNE-LOTRIMIN VAGINAL TABLETS. (Schering) Clotrimazole 100 mg/Tab. Box 7 Tab. w/applicator, Box 6s; 500 mg/Tab. in 1s w/applicator
Use: Antifungal, vaginal.

GYNERGON.
See: Estradiol (Various Mfr.).

GYNE-SULF. (G & W) Sulfathiazole 3.42%, sulfacetamide 2.86%, sulfabenzamide 3.7%, urea 0.64%. Cream Tube with applicator 82.5 Gm.
Use: Anti-infective, vaginal.

GYNOGEN. (Forest) Estrogenic substance 2 mg/ml. Inj. Vial 30 ml.
Use: Estrogen.

GYNOGEN L.A. 10. (Forest) Estradiol valerate in sesame oil 10 mg/ml. Vial 10 ml.
Use: Estrogen.

GYNOGEN L.A. 20. (Forest) Estradiol valerate in castor oil 20 mg/ml. Vial 10 ml.
Use: Estrogen.

GYNOL II CONTRACEPTIVE VAGINAL JELLY. (Ortho) Nonoxynol-9 in 2% concentration. Starter 75 Gm tube w/applicator. Refill 75 Gm, 114 Gm/Tube.
Use: Contraceptive.

GYNO-PETRARYL. (Janssen) Econazole nitrate.
Use: Antifungal, vaginal.

H

HACHIMYCIN. B.A.N. An antibiotic produced by *Streptomyces hachijoensis.*
Use: Antibiotic used in the treatment of trichomoniasis.
See: Trichomycin.

•**HALAZEPAM,** U.S.P. XXII.
Use: Sedative.
See: Paxipam, Tab. (Schering).

•**HALAZONE,** U.S.P. XXII Tab. for Soln., U.S.P. XXII. p-(Dichlorosulfamoyl) benzoic acid. (Abbott) Tab. 4 mg. Bot. 100s.
Use: Disinfectant.

•**HALCINONIDE,** U.S.P. XXII. Cream, Oint., Topical Soln., U.S.P. XXII. Corticosteroid halcinonide. 21-Chloro-9-fluoro-11,16,17-trihydroxypregna-4-ene-3,20-dione, cyclic 16,17 acetal.
Use: Anti-inflammatory.
See: Halog Cream, Oint., Soln. (Princeton).

HALCION. (Upjohn) Triazolam 0.125 mg or 0.25 mg/Tab. **0.125 mg**: Bot. 100s, Visipak 100s. (4 × 25s). **0.25 mg:** Bot. 100s, UD 100s, Visipak 100s. (4 × 25s).
Use: Sedative/hypnotic.

HALDOL. (McNeil Pharm) Haloperidol. **Tab.:** 0.5 mg, 1 mg, 2 mg, 5 mg or 10 mg/Tab. Bot. 100s, 1000s, UD blisterpacks 10 × 10s. 20 mg/Tab. Bot. 100s, UD blisterpacks 10 × 10s. **Conc. Soln.:** 2 mg/ml. Bot. 15 ml, 120 ml, 240 ml. **Inj.:** (w/methylparaben 1.8 mg, propylparaben 0.2 mg, lactic acid) amp. 5 mg/ml. Box 10×1 ml, multidose vial of 10 ml Prefilled Syringe 10×1 ml.

Use: Antipsychotic.

HALDOL DECANOATE. (McNeil Pharm) Haloperidol 70.5 mg/ml to provide Haldol 50 mg/ml. Inj. Amp. 1 ml. Box 3s, 10s.
Use: Antipsychotic.

HALDRONE. (Lilly) Paramethasone acetate 1 mg or 2 mg/Tab. Bot. 100s.
Use: Corticosteroid.

HALENOL. (Halsey) Acetaminophen 325 mg/Tab. Bot. 100s, 1000s.
Use: Analgesic.

HALENOL, CHILDREN'S. (Halsey) Acetaminophen 160 mg/5 ml. Elix. Bot. 120 ml, 240 ml, pt, gal.
Use: Analgesic.

HALENOL ELIXIR. (Blue Cross) Acetaminophen 120 mg/5 ml, alcohol 7%. Bot. 4 oz.
Use: Analgesic.

HALENOL EXTRA STRENGTH CAPLETS. (Halsey) Acetaminophen 500 mg/Cap. Bot. 1000s.
Use: Analgesic.

HALENOL EXTRA STRENGTH TABLETS. (Halsey) Acetaminophen 500 mg/Tab. Bot. 100s, 1000s.
Use: Analgesic.

HALERCOL. (Mallard) Vitamins A 5000 IU, D 400 IU, E 1.36 mg, B_1 1.5 mg, B_2 2 mg, B_3 20 mg, B_5 1 mg, B_6 0.1 mg, B_{12} 1 mcg, C 37.5 mg/Cap. Bot. 100s.
Use: Vitamin supplement.

HALETHAZOLE. B.A.N. 5-Chloro-2-[4-(2-diethylaminoethoxy)phenyl]benzothiazole.
Use: Antifungal agent.

HALEY'S M-O. (Winthrop-Breon) Mineral oil 25%, milk of magnesia in emulsion base. Flavored or regular. Bot. 240 ml, 480 ml, 960 ml.
Use: Laxative.

HALFORT-T. (Blue Cross) Vitamins C 300 mg, B_1 15 mg, B_2 10 mg, niacin 100 mg, B_6 5 mg, B_{12} 4 mcg, pantothenic acid 20 mg/Tab. Bot. 100s.
Use: Vitamin supplement.

HALI-BEST. (Barth's) Vitamins A 10,000 IU, D 400 IU/Cap. Bot. 100s, 500s.
Use: Vitamin supplement.

HALIBUT LIVER OIL.
Use: Vitamin supplement.

HALIVER OIL.
See: Halibut Liver Oil (Various Mfr.).

HALIVER OIL WITH VIOSTEROL.
See: Halibut Liver Oil with Viosterol.

HALLS MENTHO-LYPTUS DECONGESTANT LIQUID. (Warner-Lambert Prods) Dextromethorphan HBr 15 mg, phenylpropanolamine HCl 37.5 mg, menthol 14 mg, eucalyptus oil 12.7 mg/10 ml, alcohol 22%. Bot. 90 ml.
Use: Antitussive, decongestant.

HALL'S MENTHO-LYPTUS COUGH LOZENGES. (Warner-Lambert Prods) Menthol and eucalyptus oil in varying amounts and flavors. Stick-Pack 9s. Bag 30s.
Use: Mouth and throat product.

HALOBEX T. (Halsey) Dietary supplement.

•**HALOBETASOL PROPIONATE.**
Use: Corticosteroid, topical.
See: Ultravate (Westwood Squibb).

HALODRIN. (Upjohn) Fluoxymesterone 1 mg, ethinyl estradiol 0.02 mg/Tab. Bot. 100s.
Use: Androgen, estrogen combination.

•**HALOFANTRINE HYDROCHLORIDE.** USAN.
Use: Antimalarial.

HALOFED. (Halsey) **Tab.:** Pseudoephedrine HCl 30 mg or 60 mg. Bot. 100s, 1000s. **Syr.:** Pseudoephedrine HCl 30 mg/5 ml. Bot. 120 ml, 240 ml, pt, gal.
Use: Decongestant.

•**HALOFENATE.** USAN. 2-Acetamidoethyl (4-chlorophenyl) (3-trifluoromethylphenoxy)-acetate.
Use: Hypolipemic agent.
See: Livipas (Merck, Sharp & Dohme).

•**HALOFUGINONE HYDROBROMIDE.** USAN.
Use: Anti-protozoal (veterinary).

HALOGAN. (Blue Cross) Chloroxylenol, acetic acid, glycerin, benzalkonium Cl. Bot. 0.5 oz.
Use: Otic preparation.

HALOG CREAM. (Princeton) Halcinonide 0.025% or 0.1%, in specially formulated cream base consisting of glyceryl monostearate, cetyl alcohol, myristyl stearate, isopropyl palmitate, polysorbate 60, propylene glycol, purified water. **0.1%:** Tube 15 Gm, 30 Gm, 60 Gm, Jar 240 Gm. **0.025%:** Tube 15 Gm, 60 Gm.
Use: Corticosteroid, topical.

HALOG E CREAM. (Princeton) Halcinonide 0.1% in hydrophilic vanishing cream base consisting of propylene glycol dimethicone 350, castor oil, cetearyl alcohol, ceteareth-20, propylene glycol stearate, white petrolatum, water. Tube 15 Gm, 30 Gm, 60 Gm.
Use: Corticosteroid, topical.

HALOG OINTMENT. (Princeton) Halcinonide 0.1%, in Plastibase (plasicized hydrocarbon gel), PEG 400, PEG 6000 distearate, PEG 300, PEG 1540, butylated hydroxy toluene. Tube 15 Gm, 30 Gm, 60 Gm, Jar 240 Gm.
Use: Corticosteroid, topical.

HALOG SOLUTION. (Princeton) Halcinonide 0.1%, edetate disodium, PEG 300, purified water, butylated hydroxy toluene as preservative. Bot. 20 ml, 60 ml.
Use: Corticosteroid, topical.

•**HALOPEMIDE.** USAN.
Use: Antipsychotic.

HALOPENIUM CHLORIDE. B.A.N. 4-Bromo-benzyl-3-(4-chloro-2-isopropyl-5-methyl-phenoxy)-propyldimethylammonium chloride.
Use: Antiseptic.

•**HALOPERIDOL,** U.S.P. XXII. Tab., Inj., Oral Soln. U.S.P. XXII. 4[-4-p-Chlorophenyl-4-hydroxy-piperidino]-4′-fluorobutyrophenone. Serenace Soln.
Use: Antipsychotic, tranquilizer.
See: Haldol, Tab., Conc., Inj. (McNeil).

•**HALOPERIDOL DECANOATE.** USAN.

Use: Antipsychotic.

•**HALOPREDONE ACETATE.** USAN.
Use: Anti-inflammatory.

•**HALOPROGESTERONE.** USAN. 6α-Fluoro-17α-bromo-progesterone.
Use: Progestin.

•**HALOPROGIN,** U.S.P. XXII. Cream, Top. Soln., U.S.P. XXII. 3-Iodo-2-propynyl-2, 4, 5-trichlorophenyl ether.
Use: Antimicrobic.
See: Halotex, Cream, Soln. (Westwood).

HALOPYRAMINE. B.A.N. 2-(4-Chloro-N-2-pyridylbenzylamino)ethyldimethylamine. Chloropyramine (I.N.N.).
Use: Antihistamine.

HALOTESTIN. (Upjohn) Fluoxymesterone 2 mg, 5 mg or 10 mg. **2 mg:** Bot. 100s; **5 mg:** Bot. 100s; **10 mg:** Bot. 30s, 100s.
Use: Androgen.
W/Ethinyl estradiol.
See: Halodrin, Tab. (Upjohn).

HALOTEX CREAM. (Westwood) Haloprogin 1% in water dispersible base composed of PEG-400, PEG-4000, diethyl sebacate, polyvinylpyrrolidone. Tube 15 Gm, 30 Gm.
Use: Antifungal, topical.

HALOTEX SOLUTION. (Westwood) Haloprogin 1% in a clear colorless vehicle of diethyl sebacate w/alcohol 75%. Bot. 10 ml, 30 ml.
Use: Antifungal, topical.

•**HALOTHANE,** U.S.P. XXII. 2-Bromo-2-chloro-1-1,1-trifluoroethane. Fluothane.
Use: General anesthetic (inhalation).
See: Fluothane, Liq. (Wyeth-Ayerst).
Halothane, 250 ml Liq. (Abbott).

HALOTUSSIN. (Blue Cross) Guaifenesin 100 mg/5 ml. Bot. 4 oz.
Use: Expectorant.

HALOTUSSIN-DM. (Various Mfr.) Dextromethorphan HBr 15 mg, guaifenesin 100 mg, alcohol 1.4%. In 120 ml, 240 ml, pt, gal.
Use: Antitussive, expectorant.

HALOXON. V.B.A.N. Bis(2-chloroethyl)3-chloro-4-methylcoumarin-7-yl-phosphate.
Use: Anthelmintic (veterinary medicine).

HALQUINOL. B.A.N. A mixture of the chlorinated products of 8-hydroxyquinoline containing about 65% of 5,7-dichloro-8-hydroxyquinoline.
Use: Anti-infective.

•**HALQUINOLS.** USAN. 5, 7-Dichloro-8-quinolinol; 5-chloro-8-quinolinol and 7-chloro-8-quinolinol in proportions resulting naturally from chlorination of 8-quinolinol.
Use: Antimicrobial, topical.
See: Quinolor (Squibb).
Tarquinor (Squibb).

HALTRAN TABLETS. (Upjohn) Ibuprofen 200 mg/Tab. Bot. 30s, 50s. Blister pkg. 12s.
Use: Nonsteroidal anti-inflammatory drug analgesic.

HAMA. Hydroxy-aluminum magnesium aminoacetate.

HAMAMELIS WATER.
See: Witch hazel (Various Mfr.).
Tucks (Parke-Davis).

•**HAMYCIN.** USAN.
Use: Antifungal.

HANG-OVER-CURE. (Silvers) Calcium carbonate, glycine, thiamine HCl, pyridoxine HCl, aspirin. Cont. Tab. 6 Gm.
Use: Antacid, analgesic combination.

HANIFORM. (Hanlon) Vitamins A 25,000 IU, D 1,000 IU, B_1 10 mg, B_2 5 mg, C 150 mg, niacinamide 150 mg/Cap. Bot. 100s.
Use: Vitamin supplement.

HANIPLEX. (Hanlon) Vitamins B_1 20 mg, B_2 10 mg, B_6 1 mg, calcium pantothenate 10 mg, B_{12} 5 mcg, niacin 20 mg, liver concentrate 50 mg, C 150 mg/Cap. Bot. 100s.
Use: Vitamin supplement.

HANSEN'S DISEASE. Leprosy.
See: Diasone, Sodium, Tab. (Abbott).
Ethyl Chaulmoograte (Various Mfr.).
Isoniazid (Various Mfr.).

HAPONAL. (Kenyon) Atropine sulfate 0.0195 mg, hyoscine HBr 0.0065 mg, hyoscyamine sulfate 0.1040 mg, phenobarbital 0.25 gr./Tab. Bot. 100s, 1000s.
Use: Anticholinergic/antispasmodic, sedative/hypnotic.

HARBOLIN. (Arcum) Hydralazine HCl 25 mg, hydrochlorothiazide 15 mg, reserpine 0.1 mg/Tab. Bot. 100s, 1000s.
Use: Antihypertensive combination.

HARCYTE. (Harvey) Estradiol benzoate 2.5 mg, progesterone 25 mg/ml sesame oil. Vial 10 ml.
Use: Estrogen, progestin combination.

•**HARD FAT,** N.F. XVII.
Use: Pharmaceutic necessity.

HARMONYL. (Abbott) Deserpidine 0.25 mg/Tab. Bot. 100s.
Use: Antihypertensive.

HARTSHORN. Ammonium Carbonate.

HARVADEN. (Harvey) Adenosine-5-monophosphoric acid 25 mg, vitamin B_{12} 60 mcg/ml. Vial 10 ml.
Use: Antineuritic, antipruritic.
W/Phenobarbital. (Durst) Atropine methyl nitrate 1/60 gr, phenobarbital 0.25 gr/Tab. Bot. 100s, 1000s, 5000s.
Use: Antispasmodic, sedative/hypnotic.

HARVATROPIN. (Harvey) Chorionic gonadotropin 1000 IU/ml when diluted. Vial 10 ml w/diluent.
Use: Chorionic gonadotropin.

HAUGASE. (Madland) Trypsin, chymotrypsin. Bot. 50s, 250s.
Use: Enzyme preparation.

HAUTOSONE. (Forest Pharm.) Hydrocortisone 0.5% in Triusol (three polyols) 15 Gm. Box 6s.
Use: Corticosteroid, topical.

HAVAB. (Abbott Diagnostics) Radioimmunoassay or enzyme immunoassay for detection of antibody to hepatitis A virus. Test kit 100s.

Use: Diagnostic aid.

HAVAB EIA. (Abbott Diagnostics) Enzyme Immunoassay for the detection of antibody to hepatitis A virus.
Use: Diagnostic aid.

HAVAB-M. (Abbott Diagnostics) Radioimmunoassay for the detection of specific IgM antibody to hepatitis A virus. Test kit 100s.
Use: Diagnostic aid.

HAVAB-M EIA. (Abbott Diagnostics) Enzyme immunoassay for the detection of IgM antibody to hepatitis A virus.
Use: Diagnostic aid.

HAWAIIAN TROPIC ALOE PABA SUNSCREEN. (Tanning Research) Padimate 0, oxybenzone. Cream Bot. 120 Gm.
Use: Sunscreen.

HAWAIIAN TROPIC BABY FACES SUNBLOCK. (Tanning Research) Padimate 0, oxybenzone, octyl methoxycinnamate. Lot. Bot. 120 ml.
Use: Sunscreen.

HAWAIIAN TROPIC DARK TANNING WITH SUNSCREEN. (Tanning Research) Padimate 0, ethylhexl p-methoxycinnamate. Oil Bot. 240 ml.
Use: Sunscreen.

HAWAIIAN TROPIC LIP BALM SUNBLOCK. (Tanning Research) Padimate 0, oxybenzone. Stick 4 Gm.
Use: Sunscreen.

HAWAIIAN TROPIC 15 PLUS SUNBLOCK. (Tanning Research) Padimate 0 7%, oxybenzone 3%. Lot. Bot. 120 ml.
Use: Suncreen.

HAWAIIAN TROPIC PROTECTIVE TANNING. (Tanning Research) Padimate 0, oxybenzone. Lot. Bot. 240 ml.
Use: Sunscreen.

HAWAIIAN TROPIC SWIM 'N' SUN. (Tanning Research) Padimate 0, oxybenzone. Lot. Bot. 120 ml.
Use: Sunscreen.

HAZOGEL BODY AND FOOT RUB. (Nortech) Witch hazel 70%, isopropanol 20% in a neutralized resin vehicle. Bot. 4 oz.
Use: Astringent, antipruritic.

H-BIG HEPATITIS B IMMUNE GLOBULIN (HUMAN). (Abbott Diagnostics) Hepatitis B immune globulin (human). Vial 4 ml, 5 ml.
Use: Immune serum.

HC DERMA-PAX. (Recsei) Hydrocortisone 0.5% in liquid base. Dropper Bot. 2 oz.
Use: Corticosteroid, topical.

HCG.
See: Chorionic Gonadotropin.

H-CORT. (Torch) Hydrocortisone micronized pow. Bot. 5 Gm, 10 Gm, 100 Gm.
Use: Extemporaneous prescription compounding.

HCV CREME. (Saron) Hydrocortisone alcohol 1%, clioquinol 3%. Tube 15 Gm, 45 Gm.
Use: Corticosteroid, antifungal (topical).

HD 85. (Lafayette) High density barium suspension 85% w/v. Bot. 4 x 2000 ml.
Use: Radiopaque agent.

HEAD & SHOULDERS CONDITIONER. (Procter & Gamble) Pyrithione zinc 0.3%. Bot. 4 oz, 11 oz.
Use: Antiseborrheic.

HEAD & SHOULDERS SHAMPOO. (Procter & Gamble) Pyrithione zinc 1%. **Cream:** Tube 51 Gm, 75 Gm, 120 Gm, 210 Gm. **Lot:** 120 ml, 210 ml, 330 ml, 450 ml.
Use: Antiseborrheic.

HEALON. (Pharmacia) Sodium hyaluronate 10 mg/ml. Inj. Syringe 0.4 ml, 0.75 ml, 2 ml.
Use: Surgical aid, ophthalmic.

HEALTHBREAK. (Lemar Labs) Silver acetate 6 mg. Chewing gum. Pack 24s.
Use: Smoking deterrent.

HEARTBURN ANTACID. (Walgreen) Aluminum hydroxide dried gel 80 mg, magnesium trisilicate 60 mg/Tab. Bot. 100s.
Use: Antacid.

HEART MUSCLE DEPRESSANT.
See: Pronestyl HCl, Cap., Vial (Squibb).

HEART MUSCLE EXTRACTS. Adenosine-5-Mono-phosphate sodium.**HEATROL.** (Otis Clapp) **Tab.:** Sodium Cl 635 mg, potassium Cl 40.6 mg, calcium phosphate 31.5 mg, magnesium carbonate 9.1 mg/Tab. Safety pk. 1000s, Medipak 200s, Aidpak 100s, Dispenser 350s.
Use: Fluid/electrolyte replacement.

HEAVY METAL POISONING, ANTIDOTE.
See: BAL., Amp. (Hynson, Westcott & Dunning).
Calcium Disodium Versenate, Amp., Tab. (Riker).

HEB CREAM BASE. (Barnes-Hind) Washable, hypoallergenic, odorless base. Jar lb.
Use: Extemporaneous prescription compounding.

HEDAQUINIUM CHLORIDE. B.A.N. Hexadecamethylenedi-(2-isoquinolinium chloride).
Use: Antifungal.

HEDEX CAPLETS. (Winthrop Products) Paracetamol.
Use: Analgesic.

HEET LINIMENT. (Whitehall) Methyl salicylate 15%, camphor 3.6%, oloeoresin capsicum 0.025%, alcohol 70%. Bot. 2⅓ oz, 5 oz.
Use: External analgesic.

•**HEFILCON A.** USAN.
Use: Contact lens material.

•**HELFILCON B.** USAN.
Use: Contact lens material.

•**HELIUM,** U.S.P. XXII.
Use: Diluent for gases.

HEMABATE. (Upjohn) Carboprost tromethamine equivalent to 250 mcg carboprost, tromethamine 83 mcg/ml. Inj. Amp 1 ml.
Use: Abortifacient.

HEMA-CHEK SLIDES. (Ames) Fecal occult blood test containing slide tests, developer and applicators. Pkg. 100s, 300s, 1000s.
Use: Diagnostic aid.

HEMA-COMBISTIX REAGENT STRIPS. (Ames) Four-way strip test for urinary pH, glucose, protein and occult blood. Strip. Bot. 100s.
Use: Diagnostic aid.

HEMAFATE T.D. CAPSULES. (Knight) Bot. 60s.
Use: Hematinic.

HEMAFERRIN TABLETS. (Western Research) Ferrous fumarate 150 mg, desiccated liver 50 mg, docusate sodium 25 mg, betaine HCl 100 mg, folic acid 0.4 mg, vitamins C 50 mg, B_6 2 mg, manganese 2 mg, B_{12} 5 mcg, copper 1 mg, zinc 2 mg, molybdenum 0.4 mg/Tab. 28 Pack 1000s.
Use: Vitamin/mineral supplement.

HEMAFOLATE. (Canright) Ferrous gluconate 293 mg, liver fraction II 250 mg, gastric substance 100 mg, vitamins C 50 mg, B_{12} 10 mcg/Tab. Bot. 100s, 1000s.
Use: Vitamin/mineral supplement.

HEMA-FORTE. (Stayner) Vitamins B_1 5 mg, B_2 5 mg, B_6 1 mg, calcium pantothenate 2 mg, niacinamide 25 mg, desiccated liver 300 mg, iron 25 mg, inositol 25 mg, choline bitartrate 25 mg, B_{12} 5 mcg, C 50 mg/Tab. Bot. 100s, 1000s.
Use: Vitamin/mineral supplement.

HEMIN.
Use: Acute intermittent porphyria.
See: Panhematin, Inj. (Abbott).

HEMOGLOBIN REAGENT STRIPS. (Ames) Seralyzer reagent strips. Bot. 50s. Quantitive strip test for hemoglobin in whole blood.
Use: Diagnostic aid.

HEMALIVE LIQUID. (Barth's) Vitamins B_1 3.15 mg, B_2 3.33 mg, niacin 22.5 mg, B_6 0.81 mg, B_{12} 6 mcg, biotin 3.6 mcg, iron 60 mg, choline, inositol, liver fraction No. 1, pantothenic acid/15 ml. Bot. 8 oz, 24 oz.
Use: Vitamin/mineral supplement.

HEMALIVE TABLETS. (Barth's) Vitamins B_{12} 25 mcg, iron 75 mg, B_1 2.5 mg, B_2 5 mg, niacin 1.4 mg, C 30 mg, liver 240 mg, B_6, pantothenic acid, aminobenzoic acid, choline, inositol, biotin, Mg, Mn, Cu/3 Tab. Bot. 100s, 500s, 1000s.
Use: Vitamin/mineral supplement.

HEMANEED. (Hanlon) Hematinic B_{12}, intrinsic factor, Fe/Cap. Bot. 100s.
Use: Vitamin/mineral supplement.

HEMAPOIETIC AGENTS.
See: Iron products.
Lipotropic Preparations.
Liver Products.
Vitamins.

HEMASPAN TABLETS. (Bock) Iron 110 mg (from ferrous fumarate), ascorbic acid 200 mg, docusate sodium 20 mg/Tab. Bot. 100s, 1000s.
Use: Iron supplement.

HEMASTIX REAGENT STRIPS. (Ames) Cellulose strip, impregnated with a peroxide and orthotolidine for detection of hematuria and hemoglobinuria. Strip Bot. 50s.
Use: Diagnostic aid.

HEMAT. (Kenyon) Iron 57.4 mg, vitamins B_1 3 mg, B_2 2 mg, B_{12} 1 mcg, niacinamide 5 mg, desiccated liver 2 gr, stomach substance 50 mg/Tab. Bot. 100s, 1000s.
Use: Vitamin/mineral supplement.

HEMATEST REAGENT TABLETS. (Ames) Reagent Tab. for blood in the feces. Bot. 100s.
Use: Diagnostic aid.

HEMATINIC. (Canright) Ferrous gluconate 180 mg, desiccated liver 200 mg, vitamins B_{12} 1 mcg, C 25 mg, B_1 3.3 mg, copper gluconate 0.3 mg/Tab. Bot. 100s, 1000s.
Use: Vitamin/mineral supplement.

HEMATINIC CAPSULES. (Robinson) Vitamins B_1 1 mg, B_2 2 mg, B_{12} 1 mcg, iron 40 mg, desiccated liver 200 mg/Cap. Bot. 100s, 1000s.
Use: Vitamin/mineral supplement.

HEMATINICS.
See: Iron Products.
Ferric Compounds.
Ferrous Compounds.
Liver Products.
Vitamin B_{12}.
Vitamin Products.

HEMATRIN. (Towne) Iron 50 mg, vitamins B_{12} 10 mcg, B_1 10 mg, B_2 10 mg, B_6 2 mg, C 150 mg, copper 2 mg, niacinamide 50 mg, calcium pantothenate 5 mg, desiccated liver 200 mg/Captab. Bot. 60s, 100s.
Use: Vitamin/mineral supplement.

HEMATRIN NO. 1. (Kenyon) Ferrous sulfate extract 200 mg, desiccated liver N.F. 200 mg, stomach substance 100 mg, vitamin C 50 mg, folic acid 1 mg, B_{12} w/intrinsic factor concentrate 0.25 IU, B_{12} N.F. (from cobalamin concentrate) 6.26 mcg/Tab. Bot. 1000s.
Use: Vitamin/mineral supplement.

HEMATRIN NO. 2. (Kenyon) Intrinsic factor w/vitamin B_{12} 0.5 IU, liver stomach concentrate 175 mg, vitamins B_{12} concentrate 10 mcg, folic acid 0.2 mg, ferrous sulfate exsiccate 400 mg, C 75 mg/Cap. Bot. 100s, 1000s.
Use: Vitamin/mineral supplement.

HEMEX. (Vogarell) Oint. Tube 1.25 oz. Supp. Box 12s.
Use: Anorectal preparation.

HEMISINE.
See: Epinephrine (Various Mfr.).

HEMISUCCINOXYPREGNENOLONE, DELTA-5-Panzalone.

HEMOCAINE OINTMENT. (Mallard) Diperodon HCl 0.25%, pyrilamine maleate 0.1%, phenylephrine HCl 0.25%, bismuth subcarbonate 0.2%, zinc oxide 5% in a cod liver oil and petrolatum base. Oint. 37.5 Gm.
Use: Local anesthetic, anorectal.

HEMOCCULT SLIDES. (SmithKline Diagnostics) Occult blood detection (fecal). In 100s, 1000s and tape dispensers (test 100s).

Use: Diagnostic aid.

HEMOCCULT II. (SmithKline Diagnostics) Occult blood detection (fecal). In 102s, kit 100s.
Use: Diagnostic aid.

HEMOCYTE. (U.S. Pharm) Ferrous fumarate 324 mg (Fe 106 mg)/Tab. Bot. 100s.
Use: Iron supplement.

HEMOCYTE-F. (U.S. Pharm) Iron 106 mg (from ferrous fumarate), folic acid 1 mg/Tab. 100s.
Use: Iron supplement.

HEMOCYTE PLUS. (U.S. Pharm) Iron 106 mg (from ferrous fumarate), sodium ascorbate 200 mg, vitamins B_1 10 mg, B_2 6 mg, B_6 5 mg, B_{12} 15 mcg, folic acid 1 mg, niacinamide 30 mg, calcium pantothenate 10 mg, zinc sulfate 80 mg, magnesium sulfate 70 mg, manganese sulfate 4 mg, copper sulfate 2 mg/Tabule. Bot. 100s.
Use: Vitamin/mineral supplement.

HEMOFIL T. (Hyland) Antihemophilia Factor (Human), method four, dried, heat-treated 225-375 IU/10 ml; 450-650 IU/20 ml; 675-999 IU/30ml; 1000-1600 IU/30 ml.
Use: Treatment of Hemophilia A, for prevention and control of hemorrhagic episodes.

HEMOGEST. (Mills) Betaine HCl 50 mg, ferrous fumarate 100 mg, folic acid 0.05 mg, zinc gluconate 5 mg, copper gluconate 10 mg, manganese gluconate 5 mg, vitamins B_1 1 mg, B_2 1 mg, B_6 0.5 mg, B_{12} 1 mcg, niacinamide 10 mg/Tab. Bot. 100s.
Use: Vitamin/mineral supplement.

HEMORRHOIDAL OINTMENT. (Goldline) Live yeast cell derivative supplying skin respiratory factor 2000 units/oz of ointment w/shark liver oil 3%, phenyl mercuric nitrate 1:10,000.
Use: Anorectal preparation.

HEMORRHOIDAL HC. (Various Mfr.) Hydrocortisone acetate 10 mg, bismuth subgallate 2.25%, bismuth resorcin compound 1.75%, benzyl benzoate 1.2%, balsam Peru 1.8%, zinc oxide 11%/Supp. Bot. 12s, 50s, 100s, UD 12s.
Use: Anorectal preparation.

HEMORRHOIDAL SUPPOSITORIES. (Goldline) Bismuth subgallate 2.25%, bismuth resorcin compound 1.75%, benzyl benzoate 1.2%, balsam Peru 1.8%, zinc oxide 11%/Supp. Box 12s.
Use: Anorectal preparation.

HEMORRHOIDAL UNISERTS. (Upsher-Smith) Bismuth subgallate 2.25%, bismuth resorcin compound 1.75%, benzyl benzoate 1.2%, balsam Peru 1.8%, zinc oxide 11%/Supp. Carton 12s, 50s.
Use: Anorectal preparation.

HEMOSTATICS, LOCAL.
See: Absorbable Gelatin Sponge (Upjohn).
Gelfilm (Upjohn).
Gelfoam, Preps.(Upjohn).
Oxidized Cellulose.
Thrombin (Various Mfr.).

HEMOSTATICS, SYSTEMIC.
See: Adrenosem Salicylate, Preps. (Beecham-Massengill).
Aquamephyton, Inj. (Merck, Sharp & Dohme).
Carbazochrome Salicylate.
Mephyton, Tab. (Merck, Sharp & Dohme).

HEMOSTATIN.
See: Epinephrine (Various Mfr.).

HEMO-VITE. (Drug Industries) Ferrous fumarate to equal iron 79 mg, copper sulfate 1 mg, vitamins C 150 mg, B_1 5 mg, B_2 5 mg, B_6 1 mg, calcium pantothenate 10 mg, niacinamide 50 mg, folic acid 2 mg, intrinsic factor, B_{12} 0.5 NF unit/Tab. Bot. 100s, 500s.
Use: Vitamin/mineral supplement.

HEMOVITE LIQUID. (Drug Industries) Vitamin B_{12} crystallin 8.34 mcg, B_6 2 mg, ferric pyrophosphate soluble to equal iron 100 mg, folic acid 0.25 mg, niacinamide 13.3 mg/5 ml. Bot. 473 ml.
Use: Vitamin/mineral supplement.

HEM-PREP. (G & W) Shark liver oil, phenylmercuric nitrate 1:10,000, bismuth subgallate, zinc oxide, benzocaine/Supp. Bot. 12s, 24s.
Use: Anorectal preparation.

HEMOZYME ELIXIR. (Barrows) Vitamins B_1 5 mg, B_2 5 mg, B_6 1 mg, panthenol 4 mg, niacinamide 100 mg, B_{12} 3 mcg, iron 100 mg, choline bitartrate 100 mg, dl-methionine 100 mg, yeast extract, alcohol 12%/fl oz. Bot. 12 oz.
Use: Vitamin/mineral supplement.

HEMRIL UNISERTS. (Upsher-Smith) Bismuth subgallate 2.25%, bismuth resorcin compound 1.75%, benzyl benzoate 1.2%, balsam Peru 1.8%, zinc oxide 11%/Supp. 12s, 50s.
Use: Anorectal preparation.

HEMRIL-HC UNISERTS. (Upsher-Smith) Hydrocortisone acetate 25 mg/Supp. 12s.
Use: Anorectal preparation.

HENBANE.
See: Hyoscyamus (Various Mfr.).

HENYDIN-M. (Arcum) Thyroid desiccated pow. 0.5 gr, vitamins B_1 1 mg, B_2 0.5 mg, B_6 0.5 mg, niacinamide 2.5 mg/Tab. Bot. 100s, 1000s.
Use: Vitamin supplement.

HENYDIN-R. (Arcum) Thyroid desiccated pow. 1 gr, vitamins B_1 2 mg, B_2 1 mg, B_6 1 mg, niacinamide 5 mg/Tab. Bot. 100s, 1000s.
Use: Vitamin supplement.

HEPANE-LS EXTRA. (Kenyon) Vitamin B_{12} activity 40 mcg/ml. Vial 10 ml.
Use: Vitamin supplement.

HEPARIN SODIUM AND 0.45% SODIUM CHLORIDE. (Abbott) 12,500, 25,000 units in 250 ml Inj.
Use: Anticoagulant.

HEPARIN ANTAGONIST.
See: Protamine Sulfate (Various Mfr.).

HEPARIN CALCIUM.
Use: Anticoagulant.
See: Calciparine, Inj. (American Critical Care).

•**HEPARIN CALCIUM,** U.S.P. XXII. Inj., U.S.P. XXII.

Use: Anticoagulant.

HEPARIN LOCK FLUSH SOLUTION. (Winthrop Pharm) **10 USP units/1 ml:** Cartridge 2 ml HEP-PAK containing 1 cartridge heparin lock flush Soln. (1 ml) and 2 cartridges sodium Cl Inj. HEP-PAK-2 containing 1 cartridge heparin lock flush soln. (1 ml) and 1 cartridge sodium Cl Inj. **10 USP units/2 ml:** Cartridge 2 ml. **100 USP units/1 ml:** Cartridge 2 ml HEP-PAK containing 1 cartridge heparin lock flush soln (1 ml) and 2 cartridges sodium Cl Inj. HEP-PAK-2 containing 1 cartridge of heparin lock flush soln (1 ml) and 1 cartridge sodium Cl Inj. **100 USP units/2 ml:** Cartridge 2 ml.
Use: Maintaining patency of indwelling IV catheter.

HEPARIN LOCK FLUSH SOLUTION. (Wyeth-Ayerst) Heparin sodium 10 units or 100 units/1 ml vial. Pkg. 50 Tubex 1 ml, 2 ml.
Use: Clearing intermittent infusion sets.

•**HEPARIN SODIUM.** U.S.P. XXII. Inj., Lock Flush Soln., U.S.P. XXII. (Upjohn) 1000 units/ml. Vial 10 ml, 30 ml 5000 units/ml. Vial 1 ml, 10 ml 10,000 units/ml. Vial 1 ml, 4 ml (Winthrop Pharm) 5000 USP units/1 ml. Carpuject 1 ml fill in 2 ml cartridge.
Use: I.M., I.V. or S.C., anticoagulant in prevention and treatment of thrombosis or embolism. Note: Protamine sulfate is antidote.
See: Hepathrom, Amp., Vial (Fellows-Testagar).
Heprinar, Inj. (Armour).
Lipo-Hepin, Amp., Vial (Riker).
Lipo-Hepin/BL, Amp., Vial (Riker).
Liquaemin, Vial (Organon).
W/Choline Cl, Vitamin B_{12}, folic acid, niacinamide.
Hep-Plex, Vial (Kenyon).
W/Vit. B_{12}, folic acid, niacinamide, choline Cl.
See: Heparin-B, Vial (Medical Chem.).

HEPARIN SODIUM AND 0.9% SODIUM CHLORIDE. (Travenol) Inj.: 1000 units in 500 ml Viaflex. 2000, 5000 units in 1000 ml Viaflex.
Use: Anticoagulant.

HEPATAMINE. (Kendall McGaw) Amino acid 8%. Inj. Bot. 500 ml.
Use: Parenteral nutritional supplement.

HEPATIC-AID II INSTANT DRINK POWDER. (Kendall McGaw) Amino acids (high BCAA, low AAA), maltodextrin, sucrose, partially hydrogenated soybean oil, lecithin, mono and diglycerides. In 3 oz packet of 12s.
Use: Enteral nutritional supplement.

•**HEPATITIS B IMMUNE GLOBULIN,** U.S.P. XXII.
Use: Passive immunizing agent.
See: Hep-B-Gammagee, Inj. (Merck, Sharp & Dohme).

HEPATITIS B VACCINE, RECOMBINANT.
Use: Agent for immunization.
See: Recombivax-HB, Inj. (Merck, Sharp & Dohme).

•**HEPATITIS B VIRUS VACCINE INACTIVATED,** U.S.P. XXII.
Use: Active immunizing agent.
See: Heptavax-B (Merck, Sharp & Dohme).

HEP-B-GAMMAGEE. (Merck, Sharp & Dohme) Hepatitis B Immune Globulin. Vial 5 ml.
Use: Agent for immunization.

HEPFOMIN R INJECTION. (Keene) Liver inj. equivalent to cyanocobalamin 10 mcg, folic acid 0.4 mg, cyanocobalamin 100 mcg. Vial 10 ml.
Use: Parenteral nutritional supplement.

HEP-FORTE. (Marlyn) Vitamins A 1200 IU, E 6.7 mg, B_1 1 mg, B_2 1 mg, B_3 10 mg, B_5 2 mg, B_6 0.5 mg, B_{12} 1 mcg, C 10 mg, folic acid 0.06 mg, zinc 2 mg, choline 21 mg, inositol 10 mg, biotin 3.3 mg, dl-methionine 10 mg, dried yeast 64.8 mg, desiccated liver 194.4 mg, liver concentrate 64.8 mg, liver fraction number 2 64.8 mg, lecithin/Cap. Bot. 100s, 300s, 500s.
Use: Vitamin/liver supplement.

HEP-LOCK. (Elkins-Sinn) Sterile heparin sodium soln. in saline 10 units or 100 units/ml. Dosette 1 ml, 2 ml, multiple dose vial 10 ml, 30 ml.
Use: Maintenance of patency of heparin lock catheters.

HEP-LOCK PF. (Elkins-Sinn) Preservative-free heparin flush soln. 10 units/ml or 100 units/ml. Vial 1 ml.
Use: Maintenance of patency of heparin lock catheters.

HEP-PLEX. (Kenyon) Heparin sodium 2500 units, vitamin B_{12} 50 mcg, choline Cl 100 mg, folic acid 2 mg, niacinamide 50 mg in isotonic saline/ml. Vial 10 ml.
Use:

HEPROFAX.
See: Mucoplex (Stuart).

HEPTABARBITONE. B.A.N. 5-(Cyclohept-1-enyl)-5-ethylbarbituric acid.
Use: Sedative/hypnotic.

HEPTAMINOL. B.A.N. 6-Amino-2-methylheptan-2-ol.
Use: Coronary vasodilator.

HEPTAVAX-B. (Merck, Sharp & Dohme) Hepatitis B surface antigen. **Adult:** 20 mcg/ml. Vial 3 ml. **Pediatric:** 10 mcg/0.5 ml. Vial 0.5 ml.
Use: Agent for immunization.

HEPTUNA PLUS. (Roerig) Vitamins B_1 3.1 mg, B_2 2 mg, B_6 1.6 mg, niacinamide 15 mg, calcium pantothenate 0.9 mg, B_{12} 5 mcg, with intrinsic factor concentrate 25 mg, C 150 mg from sodium ascorbate, desiccated liver 50 mg, iron 100 mg (from ferrous sulfate), copper 1 mg, molybdenum 0.2 mg, calcium 37.4 mg, iodine 0.05 mg, manganese 0.033 mg, magnesium 2 mg, phosphorus 29 mg, potassium 1.7 mg/Cap. Bot. 100s.
Use: Vitamin/mineral supplement.

HERMAL BATH OIL. (Hermal) Soybean oil-based bath oil. Bot. 8 oz, 32 oz.
Use: Emollient.

HEROIN. Forbidden in U.S.A. by Federal statute because of its addiction-causing nature.
See: Diacetylmorphine.

HERPECIN-L. (Campbell) Allantoin, octylp-(dimethylamino)-benzoate (Padimate O), titanium

dioxide, pyridoxine HCl in a balanced, acidic lipid system. Lip balm. Tube 2.5 Gm.
Use: Cold sore treatment.

HERPETROL. (Alva) L-lysine, vitamin A, E, B_2, ascorbic acid, Zn/Tab. Bot. 42s, 84s.
Use: Nutritional supplement.

HERPLEX LIQUIFILM. (Allergan) Idoxuridine 0.1%, polyvinyl alcohol 1.4%. Soln. Bot. w/dropper 15 ml.
Use: Antiviral.

HESACORB. (Jenkins) Citrus bioflavonoids compound 100 mg, vitamin C 100 mg/Cap. Bot. 1000s.
Use: Vitamin supplement.

HES-BIC. (Kenyon) **Cap.:** Purified hesperidin 100 mg, ascorbic acid 100 mg. **Tab.:** Purified hesperidin 200 mg, ascorbic acid 200 mg. Bot. 100s, 1000s.
Use: Vitamin supplement.

HESPAN INJECTION. (DuPont Critical Care) Hetastarch 6 Gm, sodium Cl 0.9%/100 ml. Bot. 500 ml.
Use: Plasma volume expander.

HESPERIDIN.
Use: Capillary fragility and permeability, hemorrhage.
See: Vitamin P; also Rutin.
W/Combinations.
See: A.C.N., Tab. (Person & Covey).
Acna-Vite, Cap. (Cenci).
Ceebec, Tab. (Person & Covey).
HesBic, Cap., Tab. (Kenyon).
Hesper Bitabs, Tab. (Merrell Dow).
Nialex, Tab. (Mallard).
Norimex-Plus, Cap. (Vortech).
Pregent, Tab. (Beutlich).
Vita Cebus, Tab. (Cenci).

HESPERIDIN W/C. (Various Mfr.).
Use: Vitamin supplement.
See: Min-Hest, Cap. (Scrip).

HESPERIDIN METHYL CHALCONE.
Use: Vitamin P supplement.

•**HETACILLIN POTASSIUM,** U.S.P. XXII. Cap., Intramammary Inf., Oral Susp., Tab., Sterile, U.S.P. XXII.
Use: Antibacterial.

•**HETAFLUR.** USAN.
Use: Dental caries prophylactic.

•**HETASTARCH.** USAN.
Use: Plasma volume extender.
See: Hespan, Inj. (American Critical Care).

•**HETERONIUM BROMIDE.** USAN. (±)-3-Hydroxy-1, 1-dimethypyrrolidinium bromide, α-phenyl-2-thiopheneglycolate. Hetrum Cl.
Use: Anticholinergic.

HEXABAMATE #1. (Rugby) Tridihexethyl Cl 25 mg, meprobamate 200 mg/Tab. Bot. 100s, 500s.
Use: Anticholinergic combination.

HEXABAMATE #2. (Rugby) Tridihexethyl Cl 25 mg, meprobamate 400 mg/Tab. Bot. 100s, 500s.
Use: Anticholinergic combination.

HEXABAX. (Kirkman) Skin cleanser. Bot. pt.
Use: Antibacterial, topical.

HEXA-BETALIN. (Lilly) Pyridoxine HCl. Inj. Vial 100 mg/ml. Ctn. 10s, vial 10 ml.
Use: Vitamin B_6 supplement.

HEXABRIX SOLUTION. (Mallinckrodt) Ioxaglate meglumine 39.3%, ioxaglate sodium 19.6% (32% iodine). Vial 20 ml, 30 ml, 50 ml, 100 ml fill in bot. 150 ml, 200 ml fill in bot. 250 ml, bot. 150 ml.
Use: Radiopaque agent.

HEXACHLORCYCLOHEXANE.
See: Benzene Hexachloride, Gamma.

•**HEXACHLOROPHENE,** U.S.P. XXII. Phenol, 2,2′-methylenebis[3,4,6-trichloro-. 2.2′-Methylenebis (3,4,6-trichlorophenol). Di-(3,5,6-trichloro-2-hydroxy- phenyl)methane. Hexachlorophene (I.N.N.).
Use: Antiseptic.
See: Derl.
Gamophen, Leaves, Bar (Arbrook).
pHisoHex Prods. (Winthrop Pharm).
W/Soya protein complex.
See: Soy-Dome Cleanser, Liq. (Miles Pharm).

•**HEXACHLOROPHENE CLEANSING EMULSION,** U.S.P. XXII.
Use: Anti-infective, topical detergent.

•**HEXACHLOROPHENE LIQUID SOAP, DETERGENT LIQUID,** U.S.P. XXII.
See: pHisoHex Liq. Prods. (Winthrop Pharm).
Use: Anti-infective, topical detergent.

HEXACOSE. Mixture of C-6 alcohols derived from oxidation of tetracosane—$C_{24}H_{50}$.
See: Hexathricin, Aerospra (Lincoln).

HEXACREST. (Nutrition) Vitamin B_6 100 mg/ml, benzyl alcohol 1.5%. Vial 10 ml.
Use: Vitamin B_6 supplement.

HEXADECADROL.
See: Dexamethasone.

HEXADIENOL. Hexacose.

HEXADIMETHRINE BROMIDE. B.A.N. Poly-(NNN′N′-tetra-methyl-N-trimethylenehexamethylenediammonium dibromide). Polybrene.
Use: Heparin antagonist.

HEXADROL. (Organon) Dexamethasone. **Tab.:** 4 mg. Bot. 100s, UD 100s, Strip 10 X 10s. **Elix.:** 0.5 mg/5 ml, alcohol 5%. Bot. 120 ml.
Use: Corticosteroid.

HEXADROL PHOSPHATE. (Organon) Dexamethasone sodium phosphate 4 mg/ml, 10 mg/ml or 20 mg/ml, benzyl alcohol. **4 mg/ml:** Vial 1 ml, 5 ml, disposable syringe 1 ml. **10 mg/ml:** Vial 10 ml, disposable syringe 1 ml. **20 mg/ml:** Vial 5 ml, disposable syringe 5 ml.
Use: Corticosteroid.

•**HEXAFLUORENIUM.** F.D.A. Hexamethylene bis-[9-fluorenyldimethylammonium ion]
Use: Muscle relaxant.

HEXAFLUORENIUM BROMIDE, U.S.P. XXI. Inj., U.S.P. XXI. Hexamethyl-enebis-[fluoren-9-yldimethyl-ammonium] dibromide.

Use: Muscle relaxant; potentiator (succinylcholine).
HEXAFLUORODIETHYL ETHER. Name used for Flurothyl.
HEXAHYDROXYCYCLOHEXANE.
See: Inositol, Preps. (Various Mfr.).
HEXAKOSE. Mixture of tetracosanes and oxidation products.
See: Hexathricin, Aerospra (Lincoln).
W/Benzethonium Cl, p-chloro-m-xylenol, ethyl p-aminobenzoate and tyrothricin.
See: Hexathricin, Aeropak (Lincoln).
HEXALEN. (US Bioscience) Altretamine.
Use: Antineoplastic.
HEXALOL. (Central) Atropine sulfate 0.03 mg, hyoscyamine 0.03 mg, methenamine 40.8 mg, phenyl salicylate 18.1 mg, benzoic acid 4.5 mg, methylene blue 5.4 mg/Tab. Bot. 100s.
Use: Urinary anti-infective.
HEXAMARIUM BROMIDE. (Hexamethylene bis(3-pyridyl N-methylcarbamate) dimethyl bromide.
HEXAMETHONIUM.
W/Rauwiloid.
See: Rauwiloid w/hexamethonium, Tab. (Riker).
HEXAMETHONIUM BROMIDE. B.A.N. Vegolysen. Hexamethylene (bistrimethyl ammonium) bromide.
Use: Hypotensive.
HEXAMETHONIUM CHLORIDE. (Various Mfr.) Hexamethylene (bistrimethylammonium) Cl.
HEXAMETHONIUM IODIDE. B.A.N. Hexamethylenedi(trimethylammonium iodide).
Use: Hypotensive.
HEXAMETHONIUM TARTRATE. B.A.N. Hexamethylenedi(trimethylammonium hydrogen tartrate).
Use: Hypotensive.
HEXAMETHYLENAMINE.
See: Methenamine (Various Mfr.).
HEXAMETHYLENETETRAMINE.
See: Methenamine, U.S.P. XXII. Hexamethylenetetramine Mandelate.
HEXAMETHYLAMINE.
See: Hexastat.
HEXAMETHYLPARAROSANILINE CHLORIDE.
See: Bismuth Violet, Soln. (Table Rock).
HEXAMETHYLROSANILINE CHLORIDE.
See: Gentian Violet.
HEXAMINE HIPPURATE. B.A.N. A 1:1 complex of hexamine and hippuric acid.
Use: Antiseptic.
HEXAMINE.
See: Methenamine (Various Mfr.).
HEXAPRADOL HCl. a-(1-Aminohexyl)benzhydrol HCl.
Use: CNS stimulant.
HEXAPROFEN. B.A.N. 2-(4-Cychlohexylphenyl)-propionic acid.
Use: Anti-inflammatory, antipyretic, analgesic.
HEXAPROPYMATE. B.A.N. 1-(2-Propynyl)cyclohexanol carbamate. Merinax.
Use: Sedative/hypnotic.
HEXASTAT. Hexamethylmelamine (Orphan Drug).
Use: Advanced ovarian adenocarcinoma.
Sponsor: Ives.
HEXATE. (Davis & Sly) Atropine sulfate 1/2000 gr, extract of hyoscyamus 0.25 gr, methylene blue 1/10 gr, methanamine 0.5 gr, benzoic acid 0.5 gr, salol 0.5 gr./Tab. Bot. 1000s.
Use: Urinary anti-infective.
HEXATHRICIN AEROSPRA. (Lincoln) Hexadienol 8 Gm, benzethonium Cl 80 mg, p-chloro m-xylenol 800 mg, tyrothricin 40 mg, ethyl-p-aminobenzoate 1.6 Gm/6 oz. Aeropak 3 oz.
Use: Counterirritant, antifungal (topical).
HEXATHRICIN EPISIOTOMY AEROSPRA. (Lincoln) Hexakose (hexadienol) 4.2 Gm, p-chloro-m-xylenol 420 mg, benzethonium Cl 55 mg, ethyl-p-aminobenzoate 2.77 Gm/3 oz. can. Aerospra can 3 oz.
HEXAVITAMIN. (A.V.P.) Vitamins A 5000 IU, D 400 IU, C 75 mg, B_1 2 mg, B_2 3 mg, niacin 20 mg/Tab. Bot. 500s.
Use: Vitamin supplement.
HEXAVITAMIN. (Upsher-Smith) Tab. Bot. 100s, 1000s, UD 100s.
Use: Vitamin supplement.
HEXAVITAMIN CAPSULES and TABLETS, U.S.P. XXI. Vitamins A 5000 IU, B_1 2 mg, B_2 3 mg, C 75 mg, D 400 IU, nicotinamide 20 mg/Tab. or Cap. Bot. 100s, 500s, 1000s, UD 100s. (Various Mfr.).
Use: Multivitamin.
See: Hepicebrin, Tab. (Lilly).
HEXAVITAMINS SC. (Halsey).
Use: Vitamin supplement.
HEXAVITAMIN TABLETS. (A.V.P.) Vitamins A 5000 IU, D 400 IU, C 75 mg, B_1 2 mg, B_2 3 mg, niacin 20 mg/Tab. Bot. 500s.
Use: Vitamin supplement.
HEXAVITAMIN TABLETS, N.F. (Forest Pharm.) Vitamin A 1.5 mg, D 10 mcg, C 75 mg, B_1 2 mg, B_2 3 mg, nicotinamide 20 mg/SC Tab. Bot. 1000s.
Use: Vitamin supplement.
HEXAZOLE. B.A.N. 4-Cyclohexyl-3-ethyl-1,2,4-triazole.
Use: Central nervous system stimulant.
HEXCARBACHOLINE BROMIDE (I.N.N.). Carbolinium Bromide. B.A.N.
HEXCARBACHOLINE BROMIDE. 1,6-Hexamethylenebiscarbaminoylcholine bromide.
•**HEXEDINE.** USAN. 2,6-bis(2-Ethylhexyl)hexahydro-7a-methyl-1H imidasol[1,5c]imidazole.
Use: Antibacterial.
HEXENE-OL. Hexacose.
HEXENOL. Hexacose.
HEXETHAL SODIUM. (Hebaral) Sodium ethylhexylbarbiturate.
Use: Sedative/hypnotic.
HEXETIDINE. B.A.N. 5-Amino-1,3-bis(beta-ethylhexyl)-5-methylhexahydropyrimide. Triocil.

Use: Bactericide, fungicide.
HEXOBARBITAL, U.S.P. XXI.
See: Sombulex, Tab. (Riker).
W/Acetaminophen, salicylamide, d-amphetamine sulfate, secobarbital sodium, butabarbital sodium, phenobarbital.
See: Sedragesic, Tab. (Lannett).
W/Dihydrohydroxycodeinone HCl, dihydrohydroxycodeinone terephthalate, homatropine terephthalate, aspirin, phenacetin, caffeine.
See: Percobarb, Cap. (Du Pont).
W/Dihydrohydroxycodeinone terephthalate, dihydrohydroxycodeinone HCl, homatropine terephthalate, aspirin, phenacetin, caffeine.
See: Percobarb-Demi, Cap. (Du Pont).
•**HEXOBENDINE.** USAN. Hexobendine HCl. 1,2-Di-[N-methyl-3-(3,4,5-trimethoxybenzoyloxy)propylamino]ethane.
Use: Coronary vasodilator.
HEXOCYCLIUM METHYLSULFATE. B.A.N. N-β-Cyclohexyl-β-hydroxy-β-phenylethyl)-N′-methylpiperazine dimethylsulfate.
Use: Anticholinergic.
HEXOESTROL.
See: Hexestrol (Various Mfr.).
HEXOPAL. (Winthrop Products) Inositol hexanicotinate.
Use: Hypolipidemic, peripheral vasodilator.
HEXOPRENALINE. B.A.N. NN′-Di-[2-(3,4-dihydroxyphenyl)-2-hydroxyethyl]hexamethylenediamine.
Use: Bronchodilator.
•**HEXYLENE GLYCOL,** N.F. XVII.
Use: Pharmaceutic aid (humectant, solvent).
HEXYLRESORCINOL, U.S.P. XXII. Pil, U.S.P. XXI. 4-Hexylresorcinol. (Various Mfr.).
Use: Anthelmintic (intestinal roundworms and trematodes), minor throat irritations.
See: Jayne's P.W., Tab. (Glenbrook).
Listerine Antiseptic Throat Loz. (Warner-Lambert).
Sucrets Sore Throat Loz. (Calgon).
HEXYPHEN-2. (Robinson) Trihexyphenidyl HCl 2 mg/Tab. Bot. 100s.
Use: Antiparkinson agent.
HEXYPHEN-5. (Robinson) Trihexyphenidyl HCl 5 mg/Tab. Bot. 100s, 1000s.
Use: Antiparkinson agent.
H.H.R. (Geneva Generics) Hydralazine HCl 25 mg, hydrochlorothiazide 15 mg, reserpine 0.1 mg/Tab. Bot. 100s, 1000s.
Use: Antihypertensive.
HI B WITH C. (Towne) Vitamin C 300 mg, B_1 15 mg, B_2 10.2 mg, niacin 50 mg, B_6 5 mg, pantothenic acid 10 mg/Cap. Bot. 100s.
Use: Vitamin supplement.
HIBICLENS. (Stuart) Chlorhexidine gluconate 4%, isopropyl alcohol 4%, in a non-alkaline base. Bot. 4 oz, 8 oz, 16 oz, 32 oz, gal. Packette 15 ml.
Use: Antiseptic, germicide.
HIBICLENS SPONGE BRUSH. (Stuart) Chlorhexidine gluconate impregnated sponge brush. Unit-of-use 22 ml sponge brushes.
Use: Antiseptic, germicide.
HIB-IMUNE. (Lederle) Haemophilus b polysaccharide 25 mcg, sucrose 4 mg/0.5 ml dose. Pow. for inj. Vial 5×0.5 ml w/diluent.
Use: Agent for immunization.
HIBISCRUB. Chlorhexidine gluconate. B.A.N.
Use: Surgical hand scrub.
HIBISTAT. (Stuart) Chlorhexidine gluconate 0.5%. **Liq.:** Isopropyl alcohol 70%, emollients. Bot. 4 oz, 8 oz. **Towelettes**: Unit-of-use pocket-size towelette impregnated with 5 ml Hibistat.
Use: Antiseptic, germicide.
HIBPLEX. (Standex) Vitamins B_1 100 mg, B_2 2 mg, B_3 100 mg, panthenol 2 mg/ml. Vial 30 ml.
Use: Vitamin supplement.
HibTITER VACCINE. (Praxis Biologics) Purified Hemophilus b saccharide 10 mcg, diphtheria CRM_{197} protein ≈ 25 mcg. Inj. single-dose vials.
Use: Agent for immunization.
HI-COR 1.0. (C & M Pharmacal) Hydrocortisone 1% in a nonionic, ester-free, salt-free, paraben-free washable base. Tube 30 Gm, Jar 60 Gm, lb.
Use: Corticosteroid, topical.
HI-COR 2.5. (C & M Pharmacal) Hydrocortisone 2.5% in a nonionic, ester-free, salt-free, paraben-free washable base. Tube 30 Gm. Jar 60 Gm.
Use: Corticosteroid, topical.
HIESTRONE.
See: Estrone (Various Mfr.).
HIGH B12. (Barth's) Vitamin B_{12}, desiccated liver. Cap. Bot. 100s, 500s.
Use: Vitamin/liver supplement.
HIGH POTENCY COLD CAP. (Weeks & Leo) Salicylamide 325 mg, chlorpheniramine maleate 4 mg, dextromethorphan HBr 15 mg, caffeine 16.2 mg/Tab. Bot. 18s.
Use: Salicylate analgesic, antihistamine, antitussive.
HIGH POTENCY PAIN RELIEVERS. (Weeks & Leo) Acetaminophen 300 mg, salicylamide 300 mg/Cap. Bot. 20s, 40s.
Use: Analgesic.
HIGH POTENCY VITAMINS AND MINERALS. (Burgin-Arden) Vitamins A 25,000 IU, D 400 IU, B_1 10 mg, B_2 5 mg, C 150 mg, niacinamide 100 mg, calcium 103 mg, phosphorous 80 mg, iron 10 mg, B_6 1 mg, B_{12} 5 mcg, magnesium 5.5 mg, manganese 1 mg, potassium 5 mg, zinc 1.4 mg/Tab. Bot. 100s.
Use: Vitamin/mineral supplement.
HILL-SHADE LOTION. (Hill) Para-aminobenzoic acid, alcohol 65%. SPF 22.
Use: Sunscreen.
HI-PO-VITES TABLETS. (Nature's Bounty) Iron 5.8 mg, vitamins A 25,000 IU, D 400 IU, E 15 mg, B_1 25 mg, B_2 25 mg, B_3 50 mg, B_5 12.5 mg, B_6 15 mg, B_{12} 50 mcg, C 150 mg, folic acid

0.4 mg, Ca, Cu, I, K, Mg, Mn, P, Zn, biotin 1 mcg, PABA, choline bitartrate, betaine, rutin, inositol, citrus bioflavanoids, desiccated liver, bone meal, lecithin. Tab. Bot. 100s.
Use: Vitamin/mineral supplement.

HI-POTENCY B-COMPLEX. (Kenyon) Vitamins B_1 20 mg, B_2 12 mg, B_6 2 mg, B_{12} 3 mcg, C 50 mg, calcium pantothenate 5 mg, folic acid 0.1 mg, niacinamide 25 mg, liver fraction II 30 mg, yeast 175 mg, iron gluconate 30 mg, iron reduced 10 mg, choline bitartrate 20 mg, inositol 20 mg, dl-methionine 20 mg/Tab. Bot. 100s, 1000s.
Use: Vitamin/mineral supplement.

HIPPRAMINE.
See: Methenamine hippurate.

HIPPUTOPE. (Squibb) Radio-iodinated sodium iodohippurate (^{131}I) Inj. Bot. 1 m Ci, 2 m Ci.
Use: Diagnostic aid.

HIPREX. (Merrell Dow) Methenamine hippurate 1 Gm/Tab. Bot. 100s.
Use: Urinary anti-infective.

HI-PRO WAFERS. (Mills) Casein-lactalbumin fusion 13.3 gr, dl-methionine 5 mg, l-lysine monohydrochloride 16.7 mg, l-cystine 5 mg/Tab. Bot. 336s.

HI-RIBO. (Kenyon) Vitamin B_2 riboflavin-5-phos, 50 mg/ml. Vial 10 ml.
Use: Vitamin supplement.

HISMANAL. (Janssen) Astemizole 10 mg/Tab. 100s, UD 100s.
Use: Antihistamine.

HISTACHLOR. (Kenyon) Chlorpheniramine maleate 4 mg/Tab. Bot. 100s, 1000s.
Use: Antihistamine.

HISTACHLOR D-8, D-12. (Kenyon) Chlorpheniramine maleate 8 mg, 12 mg/DA Tab. Bot. 1000s.
Use: Antihistamine.

HISTACHLOR T-8, T-12. (Kenyon) Chlorpheniramine maleate 8 mg or 12 mg/TR Cap. Bot. 100s, 1000s.
Use: Antihistamine.

HISTACHLOR W/A.P.C. (Kenyon) Chlorpheniramine maleate 2 mg, salicylamide 3.5 gr, phenacetin 2.5 gr, caffeine 0.5 gr./Tab. Bot. 100s, 1000s.
Use: Antihistamine, analgesic.

HISTACOMP SYRUP. (Approved) Thenylpyramine HCl 80 mg, ammonium Cl 10 gr, sodium citrate 5 gr, antimony potassium tartrate 1/24 gr, menthol, aromatics q.s./fl oz. Syr. Bot. 4 oz, 8 oz. Also available w/dextromethorphan. Bot. 4 oz.
Use: Cough preparation.

HISTACOMP TABLETS. (Approved) Pyrilamine maleate 25 mg, aspirin 3.5 gr, phenacetin 2.5 gr, caffeine 0.5 gr./Tab. Bot. 30s, 100s, 1000s.
Use: Antihistamine, analgesic.

HISTACON. (Marsh Labs) Chlorpheniramine maleate 12 mg, ephedrine HCl 15 mg/SR Tab. Bot. 100s, 1000s.
Use: Antihistamine, decongestant.

HISTACON SYRUP. (Marsh Labs) Chlorpheniramine maleate 3 mg, ephedrine HCl 4 mg/5 ml, alcohol 5%. Bot. pt.
Use: Antihistamine, decongestant.

HISTA-DERFULE. (Forest) Chlorpheniramine maleate 4 mg, acetaminophen 325 mg, phenylpropanolamine HCl 25 mg, powdered opium 2 mg/ Cap. Bot. 100s, 1000s.
Use: Antihistamine, analgesic, decongestant.

HISTAFED C COUGH SYRUP. (Life Labs) Pseudoephedrine 30 mg, triprolidine 1.25 mg, codeine phosphate 10 mg, alcohol 4.3%. In 120 ml, pt, gal.
Use: Decongestant, antihistamine, antitussive.

HISTAGESIC D.M. (Bowman) Phenylpropanolamine HCl 25 mg, chlorpheniramine maleate 4 mg, dextromethorphan HBr 10 mg, acetaminophen 324 mg/Tab. Bot. 100s, 1000s.
Use: Decongestant, antihistamine, antitussive, analgesic.

HISTAGESIC MODIFIED. (Bowman) Acetaminophen 324 mg, phenylephrine HCl 10 mg, chlorpheniramine maleate 4 mg/Tab.
Use: Analgesic, decongestant, antihistamine.

HISTAGESIC MODIFIED TABLETS. (Jones Medical) Phenylephrine HCl 10 mg, chlorpheniramine maleate 4 mg, acetaminophen 324 mg/ Tab. Bot. 1000s.
Use: Decongestant, antihistamine, analgesic.

HISTAJECT. (Mayrand) Brompheniramine maleate 10 mg/ml, methyl and propyl parabens. Inj. Vial 10 ml.
Use: Antihistamine.

HISTAJEN. (Jenkins) Codeine phosphate 10 mg, pyrilamine maleate 12 mg, ammonium Cl 175 mg, potassium citrate 131 mg, alcohol 2%/5 ml. Syr. Bot. 3 oz, 4 oz, gal.
Use: Antitussive, antihistamine, expectorant.

HISTAJEN JR. (Jenkins) Chlorpheniramine maleate 1 mg, acetophenetidin 75 mg, caffeine 15 mg, salicylamide 105 mg/Tab. Bot. 1000s.
Use: Antihistamine, analgesic.

HISTALET. (Solvay) **Syr.:** Pseudoephedrine HCl 45 mg, chlorpheniramine maleate 3 mg/5 ml. Bot. 480 ml. **Forte:** Phenylephrine HCl 10 mg, pyrilamine maleate 25 mg, chlorpheniramine maleate 4 mg, phenylpropanolamine HCl 50 mg/SR Tab. Bot. 100s, 250s.
Use: Decongestant, antihistamine.

HISTALET X. (Solvay) **Syr.:** Pseudoephedrine HCl 45 mg, guaifenesin 200 mg/5 ml, alcohol 15%. Bot. 480 ml. **Tab.:** Pseudoephedrine HCl 120 mg, guaifenesin 400 mg/Tab. Bot. 100s.
Use: Decongestant, expectorant.

HISTAMIC CAPSULES. (Metro Med) Phenylpropanolamine HCl 50 mg, phenylephrine HCl 25 mg, phenyltoloxamine citrate 30 mg, chlorpheniramine maleate 12 mg/SR Cap. Bot. 100s, 1000s.
Use: Decongestant, antihistamine.

HISTAMIC TABLETS. (Metro Med) Phenylpropanolamine HCl 40 mg, phenylephrine HCl 10 mg, phenyltoloxamine citrate 15 mg, chlorpheniramine maleate 5 mg/Tab. Bot. 100s, 1000s.
Use: Decongestant, antihistamine.

HISTAMINE. 2-(4-Imidazolyl) ethylamine.
Use: Diagnostic aid.

HISTAMINE ACID PHOSPHATE.
See: Histamine Phosphate, U.S.P. XXII.

HISTAMINE DIHYDROCHLORIDE.
W/Methyl nicotinate, oleoresincapicum, glycomonosalicylate.
Use: External analgesic.
See: Akes-N-Pain Rub, Oint. (E.J. Moore).
W/Menthol, thymol, methyl salicylate.
See: Imahist Unction (Gordon).

•**HISTAMINE PHOSPHATE,** U.S.P. XXII. Inj, U.S.P. XXII. 1H-Imidazole-4-ethanamine, phosphate (1:2). 4-(2-Aminoethyl) imidazole Bis (Dihydrogen Phosphate).
Use: S.C., I.V., allergy therapy, diagnostic aid.

HISTAPCO. (Apco) Chlorpheniramine maleate 4 mg, ipecac and opium pow. 0.25 gr, (contains opium 0.025 gr), camphor monobromated 1/8 gr, salicylamide 2 gr, phenacetin 1.5 gr, caffeine alkaloid 1/8 gr, atropine sulfate 1/500 gr/Tab.
Use: Antihistamine, analgesic, anticholinergic combination.

HISTAQUAD. (Richlyn) Phenylpropanolamine HCl 25 mg, pyrilamine maleate 12.5 mg, pheniramine maleate 12.5 mg, phenylephrine HCl 2.5 mg/Cap. Bot. 1000s.
Use: Decongestant, antihistamine.

HISTAQUAD. (Richlyn) Pyrilamine maleate 6.25 mg, phenyltoloxamine dihydrogen citrate 6.25 mg, prophenpyridamine maleate 6.25 mg/Tab. Bot. 1000s.
Use: Antihistamine.

HISTARON-4. (Approved) Chloroprophenpyridamine maleate 4 mg/Tab. Bot. 100s, 500s, 1000s.
Use: Antihistamine.

HISTARON-12. (Approved) Chloroprophenpyridamine maleate 12 mg/Cap. Bot. 100s, 500s, 1000s.
Use: Antihistamine.

HISTASPAN-D. (USV) Chlorpheniramine maleate 8 mg, phenylephrine HCl 20 mg, methscopolamine nitrate 2.5 mg/Cap. in sustained-release micro-dialysis cells. Bot. 100s, 1000s.
Use: Antihistamine, decongestant, anticholinergic.

HISTATAB PLUS. (Century) Chlorpheniramine maleate 2 mg, phenylephrine HCl 5 mg/Tab. Bot. 100s, 1000s.
Use: Antihistamine, decongestant.

HISTATROL. (Center) Histamine phosphate control 1:1000 and 1:10,000. Dropper vial 2 ml 1:1000 or vial 1:100,000 intradermal.
Use: Skin test control.

HISTA-VADRIN SYRUP. (Scherer) Phenylpropanolamine HCl 20 mg, chlorpheniramine maleate 2 mg, phenylephrino HCl 2.5 mg, alcohol 2%/5 ml. Bot. pt.
Use: Decongestant, antihistamine.

HISTA-VADRIN TABLETS. (Scherer) Phenylpropanolamine HCl 40 mg, chlorpheniramine maleate 6 mg, phenylephrine HCl 5 mg/Tab. Bot. 100s.
Use: Decongestant, antihistamine.

HISTA-VADRIN T.D. CAPSULES. (Scherer) Phenylpropanolamine HCl 50 mg, chlorpheniramine maleate 4 mg, belladonna alkaloids 0.2 mg/Cap. Bot. 50s, 250s.
Use: Decongestant, antihistamine combination.

HISTERONE INJECTION. (Hauck) Testosterone aqueous susp. 50 mg or 100 mg/ml. Vial 10 ml.
Use: Androgen.

•**HISTIDINE,** U.S.P. XXII. $C_6H_9N_3O_2$. L-histidine.
Use: Amino acid.

HISTIDINE MONOHYDROCHLORIDE. Beta-4-Imidazolyl-1-amino propionic acid HCl.
Use: I.M., peptic and jejunal ulcers.

HISTINE-1. (Freeport) Diphenhydramine HCl 10 mg, alcohol 12% to 14%/4 ml. Bot. 4 oz.
Use: Antihistamine with anticholinergic, antitussive, antiemetic and sedative effects.

HISTINE-2. (Freeport) Diphenhydramine HCl 12.5 mg/5 ml w/alcohol 5%. Bot. 4 oz.
Use: Antihistamine with anticholinergic, antitussive, antiemetic and sedative effects.

HISTINE-4. (Freeport) Chlorpheniramine maleate 4 mg/Tab. Bot. 1000s.
Use: Antihistamine.

HISTINE-8. (Freeport) Chlorpheniramine maleate 8 mg/TR Tab. Bot. 1000s.
Use: Antihistamine.

HISTINE-12. (Freeport) Chlorpheniramine maleate 12 mg/TR Tab. Bot. 1000s.
Use: Antihistamine.

HISTINE-25. (Freeport) Diphenhydramine HCl 25 mg/Cap. Bot. 1000s.
Use: Antihistamine with anticholinergic, antitussive, antiemetic and sedative effects.

HISTINE-50. (Freeport) Diphenhydramine HCl 50 mg/Cap. Bot. 1000s.
Use: Antihistamine with anticholinergic, antitussive, antiemetic and sedative effects.

HISTJEN CAPSULE. (Jenkins) Phenylpropanolamine HCl 25 mg, pyrilamine maleate 12.5 mg, prophenpyridamine maleate 12.5 mg, phenylephrine HCl 2.5 mg/Cap. Bot. 1000s.
Use: Decongestant, antihistamine.

HISTOGESIC. (Century) Phenylpropanolamine HCl 25 mg, pyrilamine maleate 10 mg, chlorpheniramine maleate 2 mg, terpin hydrate 2.5 gr, acetaminophen 5 gr/Tab. Bot. 100s, 1000s.
Use: Decongestant, antihistamine, expectorant, analgesic.

HISTOLYN-CYL. (Berkeley Biologicals) Histoplasmin sterile filtrate from yeast cells of *Histoplasma capsulatum.* Vial 1.3 ml.
Use: Skin test.

•**HISTOPLASMIN.** Diluted, U.S.P. XXII. (Parke-Davis) An aqueous solution containing standardized sterile culture filtrate of *Histoplasma capsulatum* grown on liquid synthetic medium. Vial 1 ml to give 10 tests.
Use: Diagnostic aid in testing for histoplasmosis.

HISTOR-D. (Hauck) **Timecelle:** Chlorpheniramine maleate 8 mg, phenylephrine HCl 20 mg, methscopolamine 2.5 mg. Bot. 100s, 500s. **Syr.:** Chlorpheniramine maleate 2 mg, phenylephrine HCl 5 mg/5 ml w/alcohol 2%. Bot. 16 oz.
Use: Antihistamine, decongestant combination.

HISTOSAL. (Ferndale) Pyrilamine maleate 12.5 mg, phenylpropanolamine HCl 20 mg, acetaminophen 324 mg, caffeine 30 mg/Tab. Bot. 100s.
Use: Antihistamine, decongestant, analgesic.

•**HISTRELIN.** USAN.
Use: LHRH agonist.

HIST-SPAN. (Kenyon) Pyrilamine maleate 25 mg, phenylpropanolamine HCl 25 mg, prophenpyridamine maleate 10 mg/TR Cap. Bot. 100s, 1000s.
Use: Antihistamine, decongestant.

HIST-SPAN NO. 2. (Kenyon) Pyrilamine maleate 25 mg, phenylpropanolamine HCl 25 mg, prophenpyridamine maleate 10 mg, phenylephrine HCl 10 mg/TR Cap. Bot. 100s, 1000s.
Use: Antihistamine, decongestant.

HISTUSSIN-HC SYRUP. (Bock) Phenylephrine HCl 5 mg, chlorpheniramine maleate 2 mg, hydrocodone bitartrate 2.5 mg. In 480 ml.
Use: Decongestant, antihistamine, narcotic analgesic.

HITONE. (Lafayette) Barium sulfate suspension 125% w/v. Bot. 2000 ml Case 4s.
Use: Radiopaque agent.

HI-TOR. (Barth's) Vitamins B_{12} 15 mcg, niacin 1.5 mg, B_1 6 mg, B_2 12 mg, B_6 54 mcg, pantothenic acid 150 mcg, choline 3.75 mg, inositol 5.25 mg/Tab. Bot. 100s, 500s, 1000s.
Use: Vitamin supplement.

HI-TOR 900. (Barth's) Vitamins B_1 13.5 mg, B_2 5.2 mg, niacin 15 mg, B_6 0.6 mg, pantothenic acid 1.2 mg, biotin, B_{12} 2.5 mcg, iron 0.9 mg, protein 7.5 Gm, inositol 50 mg, choline 40 mg, aminobenzoic acid 0.15 to 2.4 mg/15 Gm. Bot. 1 lb, 3 lb.
Use: Vitamin/mineral supplement.

HI-VEGI-LIP TABLETS. (Freeda) Pancreatin 2400 mg, lipase 12,000 units, protease 60,000 units, amylase 60,000 units/Tab. Bot. 100s, 250s.
Use: Digestive aid.

HIWOLFIA. (Bowman) Rauwolfia 25 mg, 50 mg or 100 mg/Tab. Bot. 100s, 1000s.
Use: Antihypertensive.

HMS LIQUIFILM. (Allergan) Medrysone 1%, Liquifilm (polyvinyl alcohol) 1.4%, benzalkonium Cl, edetate disodium, sodium Cl, potassium Cl, sodium phosphate monobasic monohydrate, sodium phosphate dibasic anhydrous, hydroxypropyl methylcellulose, purified water, sodium hydroxide or hydrochloric acid. Ophth. Susp. Dropper Bot. 5 ml, 10 ml.
Use: Anti-inflammatory, ophthalmic.

H_2OEX. (Fellows) Benzthiazide 50 mg/Tab. Bot. 100s, 1000s.
Use: Diuretic.

HOLD. (Beecham Products) Dextromethorphan HBr 5 mg/Loz. Plastic tube 10 Loz.
Use: Antitussive.

HOLD LOZENGES (CHILDREN'S FORMULA). (Beecham) Phenylpropanolamine HCl 6.25 mg, dextromethorphan HBr 3.75 mg/Loz. Roll 10s.
Use: Decongestant, antitussive.

HOLOCAINE HYDROCHLORIDE. (Various Mfr.) Phenacaine HCl.
Use: Local anesthetic.

HOMARYLAMINE HYDROCHLORIDE. N-Methyl-3,4-methylenedioxyphenethylamine HCl.

•**HOMATROPINE HYDROBROMIDE,** U.S.P. XXII. Ophth. Soln., U.S.P. XXII. Benzeneacetic acid, a-hydroxy-, 8-methyl-β-azabicyclo-[3.2.1]-oct-3-yl ester, HBr, endo-(±)-. 1αH, 3αH-Tropan-3α-ol mandelate (ester) HBr.
Use: Mydriatic/cycloplegic.
See: Murocoll, Liq. (Muro).

HOMATROPINE HYDROCHLORIDE.
Use: Topically, mydriatic/cyclopegic; anticholinergic.

HOMATROPINE METHYLBROMIDE W/COMBINATIONS
See: Dranochol, Tab. (Marin).
Homapin, Tab. (Mission).
Hycodan, Tab., Pow., Syr. (Du Pont).
Obe-Slim, Tab. (Jenkins).
Panitol H.M.B., Tab. (Wesley).
Spasmatol, Tab. (Pharmed).
Tapuline, Tab. (Wesley).

HOMATROPINE METHYLBROMIDE AND PHENOBARBITAL COMBINATIONS
See: Gustase-Plus, Tab. (Geriatric).
Lanokalin, Tab. (Lannett).
Spasmed Jr., Tab. (Jenkins).

HOMICEBRIN. (Lilly) Vitamin A 2500 U.S.P. units, B_1 1 mg, B_2 1.2 mg, B_6 0.8 mg, niacinamide 10 mg, B_{12} 3 mcg, C 60 mg, D 400 U.S.P. units/5 ml w/alcohol 5%. Liq. Bot. 473 ml.
Use: Vitamin supplement.

HOMOCHLORCYCLIZINE. B.A.N. 1-(p-Chlorobenzhydryl)-4-methylhomopiperazine. 1-(4-Chlorobenzhydrylhexahydro-4-methyl-1,4-diazepine.
Use: Antihistamine.

HOMOGENE-S. (Spanner) Testosterone 25 mg, 50 mg or 100 mg/ml. Vial 10 ml.
Use: Androgen.

•**HOMOSALATE.** USAN.
Use: Ultraviolet sunscreen.
W/Combinations.
See: Coppertone, Prods. (Plough).

HOMPRENORPHINE. B.A.N. N-Cyclopropylmethyl-7,8-dihydro-7α-[1(R)-hydroxy-1-methylpropyl]-$0^3 0^6$-dimethyl-endoethenonormorphine.

Use: Analgesic.
•**HOQUIZIL HCl.** USAN. 2-Hydroxy-2-methylpropyl 4-(6,7-dimethoxy-4-quinazolinyl)-1-piperazine-carboxylate monohydrochloride.
Use: Bronchodilator.
HORMOFOLLIN.
See: Estrone (Various Mfr.).
HORMOPLETE. (Key) Conjugated estrogenic substance 0.25 mg, methyltestosterone 2.5 mg, vitamins A 12,500 IU, D 1000 IU, B_1 10 mg, B_2 3 mg, B_6 2 mg, niacinamide 25 mg, nicotinic acid 5 mg, calcium pantothenate 5 mg, C 75 mg, E 2 IU, B_{12} 2 mcg, ferrous sulfate 50 mg, pancreatin 100 mg, dl-methionine 15 mg, inositol 20 mg, choline bitartrate 40 mg, calcium 60 mg, phosphorus 30 mg, copper 0.45 mg, manganese 0.5 mg, potassium 2 mg, zinc 0.5 mg, magnesium 3 mg/Tab. Bot. 50s, 500s.
Use: Vitamin/mineral/hormone supplement.
Homosalate w/combinations.
See: Coppertone, Liq. (Plough).
HOSPITAL FOAM CLEANER. (Health & Medical Techniques) 0-phenylphenol 0.1%, 4-chloro-2-cyclopentyl-phenol 0.08%, lauric diethanolamide 0.2%, triethanolamine dodecylbenzenesulfonate 0.3%. Aerosol spray 19 oz.
Use: Germicidal, disinfectant.
HOSPITAL LOTION. (Paddock) Diisobutylcresoxyethoxy-ethyl dimethyl benzyl ammonium Cl, menthol, lanolin, mineral and vegetable oils. Bot. 4 oz, 8 oz, gal.
Use: Emollient.
HPA-23. (antimoniotungstate) An experimental compound developed at the Pasteur Institute in Paris to stop or slow the reproduction of the Acquired Immune Deficiency Syndrone (AIDS) virus, at least temporarily.
H.P. ACTHAR GEL. (Armour) Repository corticotropin injection highly purified 40 U.S.P. units/1 ml. Vial 1 ml, 5 ml; 80 U.S.P. units/1 ml. Vial 1 ml, 5 ml.
Use: Corticosteroid.
H-R LUBRICATING JELLY. (Holland-Rantos) Tube 5 oz.
Use: Lubricating agent.
HRC-PRENATAL TABLETS. (Cenci) Comprehensive, well-balanced, vitamin-mineral formula. Tab. Bot. 90s, 500s.
Use: Vitamin/mineral supplement.
HRC-TYLAPRIN ELIXIR. (Cenci) Acetaminophen 120 mg, alcohol 7%/5 ml. Bot. 2 oz, 4 oz.
Use: Analgesic.
H.S. NEED. (Hanlon) Chloral hydrate 3¾ gr, 7.5 gr/Cap. Bot. 100s.
Use: Sedative.
HSV-1. (Wampole-Zeus) Herpes simplex virus type I test system. For the qualitative and semi-quantitative detection of HSV-1 antibody in human serum. Test 100s.
Use: Diagnostic aid.
HSV-2. (Wampole-Zeus) Herpes simplex virus type II antibody test. For the qualitative and semi-quantitative detection of HSV-2 antibody in human serum. Test 100s.
Use: Diagnostic aid.
H.T. FACTORATE. (Armour) Antihemophilic factor (human) dried, heat treated for I.V. administration only. Single-dose vial w/diluent and needles.
Use: Classical hemophilia treatment.
H.T. FACTORATE GENERATION II. (Armour) Antihemophilic factor (human) dried, heat treated for I.V. administration only. Single dose vial w/diluent and needles.
Use: Classical hemophilia treatment.
HTSH EIA. (Abbott Diagnostics) Enzyme immunoassay for the quantitative determination of human thyroid stimulating hormone (HTSH) in human serum or plasma.
Use: Diagnostic aid.
HTSH RIABEAD. (Abbott Diagnostics) Immunoradiometric assay for the quantitative measurement of human thyroid stimulating hormone (HTSH) in serum.
Use: Diagnostic aid.
HUMAN ANTIHEMOPHILIC FACTOR.
See: Antihemophilic factor
HUMAN COAGULATION. Fraction II, IX and X. B.A.N. A preparation of human blood containing coagulating factors II, IX and X.
Use: Treatment of hemophilia B deficiency.
HUMAN INSULIN. Insulin Human, U.S.P. XXII.
Use: Hypoglycemic.
See: Humulin Prods. (Lilly).
HUMAN MEASLES IMMUNE SERUM.
See: Immune Globulin, U.S.P. XXII.
HUMAN SERUM ALBUMIN.
See: Albumotope (Squibb).
HUMATE-P. (Armour). Pasteurized, purified lyophilized concentrate of antihemophilic factor (human). Inj. single dose vial.
Use: Antihemophilic.
HUMATIN CAPSULES. (Parke-Davis) Paromycin sulfate 250 mg/Cap. Bot. 16s.
Use: Amebicide.
HUMATROPE. (Lilly) Somatropin (recombinant DNA origin). Inj. 5 mg/vial.
Use: Growth hormone.
HUMIBID L.A. (Adams Labs) Guaifenesin 600 mg/SR Tab. Bot. 100s.
Use: Expectorant.
HUMIST. (Scherer) Sodium Cl 0.65%, chlorobutanol 0.35%. Soln. Bot. 45 ml.
Use: Nasal decongestant combination.
HUMORSOL. (Merck, Sharp & Dohme) Demecarium bromide 0.125% or 0.25% ophthalmic soln. w/benzalkonium Cl 1:5000. Soln. 5 ml Ocumeter.
Use: Agent for glaucoma.
HUMULIN BR. (Lilly) Buffered regular insulin (recombinant DNA origin) 100 units/ml. Inj. Vial 10 ml. Box 1s. Only in external insulin pumps.
Use: Antidiabetic agent.

HUMULIN L. (Lilly) Lente human insulin (recombinant DNA origin) 100 units/ml. Vial 10 ml.
Use: Antidiabetic agent.

HUMULIN N. (Lilly) NPH human insulin (recombinant DNA origin) 100 units/ml. Vial 10 ml.
Use: Antidiabetic agent.

HUMULIN R. (Lilly) Regular human insulin (recombinant DNA origin) 100 units/ml. Vial 10 ml.
Use: Antidiabetic agent.

HUMULIN U. (Lilly) Ultralente human insulin (recombinant DNA origin) 100 units/ml. Inj. Vial 10 ml.
Use: Antidiabetic agent.

HURRICAINE. (Beutlich) Benzocaine 20%. Liq. or Gel Bot. 30 ml.
Use: Anesthetic, topical.

HURRICAINE GEL. (Beutlich) Benzocaine 20%. Gel Bot. 30 ml.
Use: Anesthetic, topical.

HURRICAINE LIQUID. (Beutlich) Benzocaine 20%. Liq. Bot. 30 ml.
Use: Anesthetic, topical.

HURRICAINE LIQUID PACK. (Beutlich) Benzocaine 20%. Packet UD 0.25 ml. Box 50s.
Use: Anesthetic, topical.

HURRICAINE TOPICAL ANESTHETIC SPRAY. (Beutlich) Benzocaine 20%. Aerosol 60 Gm.
Use: Anesthetic, topical.

HURRICAINE TOPICAL ANESTHETIC SPRAY KIT. (Beutlich) Benzocaine 20%. Kit: Aerosol 60 Gm plus 200 disposable extension tubes.
Use: Anesthetic, topical.

HU-TET. (Hyland) Tetanus immune globulin (human) sterile soln. 16.5%, gamma globulin fraction of the plasma of persons who have been immunized w/tetanus toxoid. Vial syringe 250 units.
Use: Agent for immunization.

HVS 1 & 2. (Chemi-Tech) Benzalkonium Cl in a specially formulated base. Soln. Bot. 15 ml.
Use: Cold sores, fever blisters, herpes virus.

HYACIDE. (Niltig) Benzethonium Cl 0.1%, sodium nitrite 0.55%. Soln. Bot. oz.
Use: Antiseptic.

HYALEX. (Miller) Magnesium salicylate 260 mg, magnesium p-aminobenzoate 163 mg, vitamins A 1500 IU, C 30 mg, D 100 IU, E 3 IU, B_{12} 2 mcg, pantothenic acid 5 mg, zinc 0.7 mg/Tab. Bot. 100s.
Use: Vitamin/mineral supplement.

HYALIDASE.
See: Hyaluronidase (Various Mfr.).

•**HYALURONATE SODIUM.** USAN.
Use: Synovitis agent (veterinary).

•**HYALURONIDASE INJECTION,** U.S.P. XXII. Hyalidase, Hydase Enzymes which depolymerize hyaluronic acid. Hyalase, Rondase.
Use: Hypodermoclyses, promotion of diffusion.
See: Alidase, Vial (Searle).
Wydase, Vial (Wyeth-Ayerst).

•**HYALURONIDASE FOR INJECTION,** U.S.P. XXII.
Use: Spreading factor.

HYAMAGNATE. Hydroxy-Aluminum-Magnesium-Aminoacetate, Sodium-free.

HYBEC FORTE. (Amlab) Vitamins B_1 100 mg, B_2 20 mg, B_6 2.5 mg, niacinamide 25 mg, C 200 mg, B_{12} 10 mcg, calcium pantothenate 5 mg, iron 10 mg, choline bitartrate 24 mg, inositol 10 mg, biotin 5 mcg, liver 50 mg, yeast 100 mg/Tab. Bot. 30s, 100s.
Use: Vitamin/mineral supplement.

HYBOLIN DECANOATE. (Hyrex) Nandrolone decanoate 50 mg or 100 mg/ml in oil. Vial 2 ml.
Use: Anabolic steroid.

HYBOLIN IMPROVED. (Hyrex) Nandrolone phenpropionate 25 mg or 50 mg/ml in oil. Vial 2 ml.
Use: Anabolic steroid.

•**HYCANTHONE.** USAN. 1-[(2-(Diethylamino)-ethyl)-amino]-4-(hydroxymethyl)thioxanthen-9-one.
Use: Schistosomacide.

HYCLORITE. Sodium Hypochlorite soln., U.S.P. XXII.

HYCODAN. (Du Pont) Hydrocodone bitartrate 5 mg, homatropine methylbromide 1.5 mg/5 ml or Tab. **Syr.:** Bot. pt, gal. **Tab.:** Bot. 100s, 500s.
Use: Antitussive combination.

HYCOFF-A-NN LIQUID. (Saron) Dextromethorphan HBr 15 mg, pseudoephedrine HCl 45 mg, dyphylline 100 mg/15 ml. Alcohol free. Bot. pt.
Use: Antitussive, decongestant, bronchodilator.

HYCOFF X-NN. (Saron) Dextromethorphan HBr 10 mg, pseudoephedrine HCl 30 mg/5 ml. Alcohol and sugar free. Bot. pt.
Use: Antitussive, decongestant.

HYCOMINE COMPOUND TABLETS. (Du Pont) Hydrocodone bitartrate 5 mg, chlorpheniramine maleate 2 mg, phenylephrine HCl 10 mg, acetaminophen 250 mg, caffeine (anhydrous) 30 mg/Tab. Bot. 100s, 500s.
Use: Antitussive, antihistamine, decongestant, analgesic.

HYCOMINE PEDIATRIC SYRUP. (Du Pont) Hydrocodone bitartrate 2.5 mg, phenylpropanolamine HCl 12.5 mg/5 ml. Bot. 480 ml.
Use: Antitussive, decongestant.

HYCOMINE SYRUP. (Du Pont) Hydrocodone bitartrate 5 mg, phenylpropanolamine HCl 25 mg/5 ml. Syr. Bot. pt, gal.
Use: Antitussive, decongestant.

HYCORT CREAM. (Everett) Hydrocortisone 1% in a cream base. Tube oz.
Use: Corticosteroid, topical.

HYCORT OINTMENT. (Everett) Hydrocortisone 1% in ointment base. Tube oz.
Use: Corticosteroid, topical.

HYCORTOLE. (Premo) Hydrocortisone. **Cream:** 0.5%: 5 Gm, 20 Gm; 1%: 5 Gm, 20 Gm, 4 oz; 2.5%: Tube 5 Gm, 20 Gm; **Oint.:** 1% or 2.5%. Tube 5 Gm, 20 Gm.
Use: Corticosteroid, topical.

HYCOTUSS EXPECTORANT. (Du Pont) Hydrocodone bitartrate 5 mg, guaifenesin 100 mg, alcohol 10%(v/v)/5 ml. Bot. 480 ml.
Use: Antitussive, expectorant.

HYDANTOIN DERIVATIVES.
Use: Anticonvulsant.
See: Dilantin, Preps. (Parke-Davis).
Diphenylhydantoin Sodium, U.S.P.
Ethotoin.
Mesantoin, Tab. (Sandoz).
Phenantoin.

HYDASE.
Use: Hypodermoclyses, promotion of diffusion.
See: Hyaluronidase (Various Mfr.).

HYDELTRASOL INJECTION. (Merck, Sharp & Dohme) Prednisolone sodium phosphate 20 mg/ml w/niacinamide 25 mg, sodium hydroxide to adjust pH, disodium edetate 0.5 mg, sodium bisulfite 1 mg, phenol 5 mg, water for injection q.s. 1 ml. Vial 2 ml, 5 ml.
Use: Corticosteroid.

HYDELTRA-T.B.A. (Merck, Sharp & Dohme) Prednisolone tebutate 20 mg/ml w/sodium citrate 1 mg, polysorbate 80 1 mg, sorbitol soln. 0.5 ml (equivalent to 450 mg d-sorbitol), benzyl alcohol 9 mg, water for injection q.s. 1 ml. Vial 1 ml, 5 ml.
Use: Corticosteroid.

HYDERGINE LC LIQUID CAPSULES. (Sandoz) Ergoloid mesylates 1 mg/Cap. Bot. 100s, 500s. SandoPak 100s, 500s.
Use: Psychotherapeutic agent.

HYDERGINE LIQUID. (Sandoz) Equal parts of dihydroergocornine, dihydroergocristine, dihydroergocryptine. (Ergoloid Mesylates). 1 mg/ml. Bot. 100 ml w/dropper.
Use: Psychotherapeutic agent.

HYDERGINE, ORAL. (Sandoz) Equal parts of dihydroergocornine, dihydroergocristine, dihydroergocryptine (Ergoloid Mesylates). 1 mg/Tab. Bot. 100s, 500s. SandoPak (UD) 100s, 500s.
Use: Psychotherapeutic agent.

HYDERGINE, SUBLINGUAL. (Sandoz) Equal parts of dihydroergocornine, dihydroergocristine, dihydroergocryptine (Ergoloid Mesylates). 0.5 mg or 1 mg/Tab. Bot. 100s, 1000s, SandoPak (UD) 100s.
Use: Psychotherapeutic agent.

HYDEX. (Moore Kirk) Methamphetamine HCl 5 mg or 10 mg/Tab. Bot. 1000s.
Use: CNS stimulant.

HYDORIL. (Cenci) Hydrochlorthiazide 25 mg or 50 mg/Tab. Bot. 100s, 1000s.
Use: Diuretic.

HYDRABAMINE PHENOXYMETHYL PENICILLIN.
See: Penicillin V Hydrabamine.

HYDRACRYLIC ACID BETA LACTONE.
See: Propiolactone.

•**HYDRALAZINE HCl,** U.S.P. XXII. Inj., Tab., U.S.P. XXII. 1-Hydrazinophthalazine HCl. Phthalazine, 1-hydrazino-, HCl.
Use: Antihypertensive.
See: Apresoline, Amp., Tab. (Ciba).
Dralzine, Tab. (Lemmon).
Hydralyn, Tab. (Kenyon).
W/Hydrochlorothiazide.
See: Apresazide, Cap. (Ciba).
Apresoline-Esidrix, Tab. (Ciba).
Hydralazide, Tab. (Zenith).
Hydroserpine Plus, Tab. (Zenith).
W/Reserpine.
See: Dralserp, Tab. (Lemmon).
Serpasil-Apresoline, Tab. (Ciba).
W/Reserpine, hydrochlorothiazide (Esidrix).
See: Harbolin, Tab. (Arcum).
Ser-Ap-Es, Tab. (Ciba).
Serapine, Tab. (Cenci).
Thia-Serpa-Zine, Tab. (Robinson).
Unipres, Tab. (Solvay).

•**HYDRALAZINE POLISTIREX.** USAN.
Use: Antihypertensive.

HYDRALYN. (Kenyon) Hydralazine HCl 25 mg, 50 mg/Tab. Bot. 100s, 1000s.
Use: Antihypertensive.

HYDRA MAG TABLETS. (Vale) Aluminum hydroxide gel, dried, 195 mg, magnesium trisilicate 195 mg, kaolin 162 mg/Tab. Bot. 1000s.
Use: Antacid.

HYDRAMINE. (Goldline). Diphenhydramine 12.5 mg/5 ml. **Elix.:** 120 ml, pt, gal. **Syr.:** 5% alcohol. 120 ml, 240 ml, pt, gal.
Use: Antihistamine.

HYDRARGAPHEN. B.A.N. 2,2′-(Binaphthalene-3-sulfonyloxyphenylmercury). Phenylmercury 2:2′-dinaphthylmethane-3:3′-disulfonate.
Use: Antiparasitic; anti-infective.

HYDRASERP. (Geneva) Hydrochlorothiazide 25 mg or 50 mg, reserpine 0.1 mg/Tab. Bot. 100s, 1000s.
Use: Antihypertensive combination.

HYDRASTINE. (Penick) Alkaloid. Bot. oz.

HYDRASTINE HYDROCHLORIDE. (Penick) Pow. Bot. oz.
Use: Uterine hemostatic.

HYDRATE. (Hyrex) Dimenhydrinate 50 mg/ml w/ propylene glycol 50%, benzyl alcohol 5%. Amp. 1 ml. Box 25s, 100s; Vial 10 ml.
Use: Antiemetic/antivertigo, antihistamine.

HYDRAZIDE CAPSULES. (Goldline) **25/25:** Hydrochlorothiazide 25 mg, hydralazine 25 mg/ Cap. **50/50:** Hydrochlorothiazide 50 mg, hydralazine 50 mg/Cap. Bot. 100s.
Use: Antihypertensive.

HYDRA-ZIDE CAPSULES. (Par Pharm.) 50/50: Hydralazine HCl 50 mg, hydrochlorothiazide 50 mg/Cap. Bot. 100s, 500s, 1000s.
Use: Antihypertensive.

HYDRAZONE. 3-(4-Methyl-piperazinyliminomethyl)rifamycin SV.
Use: Pulmonary tuberculosis.
See: Rimactane, Cap. (Ciba).

HYDREA. (Squibb Mark) Hydroxyurea. 500 mg/ Cap. Bot. 100s.

Use: Antineoplastic agent.

HYDRIODIC ACID. (Various Mfr.).
Use: Expectorant.

HYDRIODIC ACID THERAPY.
See: Aminoacetic Acid HI.

HYDRISALIC GEL. (Pedinol) Salicylic acid 6%, isopropranolol, propylene glycol, hydroxypropyl cellulose. Tube 30 Gm.
Use: Keratolytic.

HYDRISEA LOTION. (Pedinol) Dead sea salts concentrate 8%, sodium, potassium, calcium magnesium Cl, propylene glycol stearate, polysorbate 40, silicone oil, coloring agent. Bot. 4 oz.
Use: Hyperkeratotic, emollient.

HYDRISINOL CREME AND LOTION. (Pedinol) Sulfonated hydrogenated castor oil. **Cream:** Spout Cap Jar 4 oz, lb. **Lot.:** Bot. 8 oz.
Use: Emollient.

HYDRO-12. (Table Rock) Crystalline hydroxocobalamin 1000 mcg/ml Pkg. 10 ml.
Use: Vitamin B_{12} supplement.

HYDRO-BAN CAPSULES. (Whiteworth) Juniper oil 10 mg, uva ursi 50 mg, buchu extract 50 mg, parsley piert extract 50 mg, iron 6 mg/Cap. Bot. 42s.
Use: Diuretic with iron.

HYDROBEXAN. (Keene) Hydroxocobalamin 1000 mcg/ml. Inj. Vial 10 ml.
Use: Vitamin B_{12} supplement.

HYDROCET. (Carnrick) Hydrocodone bitartrate 5 mg, acetaminophen 500 mg/Cap. Bot. 100s, UD Box 4 × 25s.
Use: Narcotic analgesic combination.

HYDROCHLORATE. Same as Hydrochloride.

•**HYDROCHLORIC ACID,** N.F XVII. Diluted, N.F. XVII. (Various Mfr.) Muriatic Acid, Absolute 38%. Diluted 10%.
Use: Well diluted, achlorhydria; pharmaceutic aid (acidifying agent).

HYDROCHLORIC ACID THERAPY.
Use: Gastric acidifier.
See: Betaine HCl (Various Mfr.).
Glutamic Acid HCl (Various Mfr.).
Glycine HCl (Various Mfr.).

HYDROCHLOROSERPINE. (Freeport) Hydralazine HCl 25 mg, hydrochlorthiazide 15 mg, reserpine 0.1 mg/Tab. Bot. 1000s.
Use: Antihypertensive combination.

•**HYDROCHLOROTHIAZIDE,** U.S.P. XXII. Tab. U.S.P. XXII. 2H-1,2,4-Benzothiadiazine-7-sulfonamide, 6-chloro-3,4-dihydro-,1,1-dioxide. 6-Chloro-3,4-dihydro-2H-1,2,4-Benzothiadiazene-7-sulfonamide 1, 1-dioxide.
Use: Diuretic.
See: Chlorzide, Tab. (Foy).
Delco-Retic, Tab. (Delco).
Diu-Scrip, Cap. (Scrip).
Esidrix, Tab. (Ciba).
Hydromal, Tab. (Mallard).
HydroDiuril, Tab. (Merck, Sharp & Dohme).
Hydrozide-50, Tab. (Mayrand).
Kenazide-E,-H, Tab. (Kenyon).
Oretic, Tab. (Abbott).
Ro-Hydrazide, Tab. (Robinson).
Thiuretic, Tab. (Parke-Davis).
Zide, Tab. (Solvay).
W/Deserpidine.
See: Oreticyl, Tab. (Abbott).
W/Enalapril.
See: Vaseretic, Tab. (Merck, Sharp & Dohme).
W/Guanethidine monosulfate.
See: Esimil, Tab. (Ciba).
W/Hydralazine HCl.
See: Apresazide, Cap. (Ciba).
Apresoline-Esidrix, Tab. (Ciba).
Hydralazide, Tab. (Zenith).
W/Labetalol.
See: Trandate HCT, Tab. (Allen & H).
W/Methyldopa.
See: Aldoril, Tab. (Merck, Sharp & Dohme).
W/Propranolol.
See: Inderide, Tab. (Wyeth-Ayerst).
W/Reserpine.
See: Aquapres-R, Tab. (Castal).
Hydropres, Tab. (Merck, Sharp & Dohme).
Hydroserp, Tab. (Zenith).
Hydroserpine, Tab. (Geneva).
Hydrotensin-50, Tab. (Mayrand).
Hyperserp, Tab. (Elder).
Mallopress, Tab. (Mallard).
Serpasil-Esidrix, Tab. (Ciba).
Thia-Serp-25, Tab. (Robinson).
Thia-Serp-50, Tab. (Robinson).
W/Reserpine, Hydralazine HCl.
See: Harbolin, Tab. (Arcum).
Hydroserpine Plus, Tab. (Zenith).
SER-AP-ES, Tab. (Ciba).
Serapine, Tab. (Cenci).
Thia-Serpa-Zine, Tab. (Robinson).
Unipres, Tab. (Solvay).
W/Spironolactone.
See: Aldactazide, Tab. (Searle).
W/Timolol maleate.
See: Timolide, Tab. (Merck, Sharp & Dohme).
W/Triamterene.
See: Dyazide, Cap. (SmithKline).

HYDROCHOLERETICS.
See: Bile Salts (Various Mfr.).
Dehydrocholic Acid (Various Mfr.).
Desoxycholic Acid (Various Mfr.).
Ox Bile Extract (Various Mfr.).

HYDROCIL INSTANT. (Solvay) Blond psyllium coating containing psyllium 3.5 Gm/3.7 Gm dose. Tan granular, instant mix, sugar-free, low sodium, low potassium powder. UD packets. 3.7 Gm in 30s, 500s, Jar 250 Gm.
Use: Laxative.

HYDRO COBEX. (Pasadena Research) Hydroxocobalamin 1000 mcg/Vial 10 ml.
Use: Vitamin B_{12} supplement.

•**HYDROCODONE BITARTRATE,** U.S.P. XXII. Tab., U.S.P. XXII. Dihydrocodeinone bitartrate.

4,5α-Epoxy-3-methoxy-17-methylmorphinan-6-one tartrate (1:1) hydrate (2:5).
Use: Antitussive.
See: Dicodethal, Elix. (Lannett).
W/Combinations.
See: Hydrocet, Cap. (Carnrick) Vicodin, Tab. (Knoll).

HYDROCODONE COMP. SYRUP. (Goldline) Hydrocodone bitartrate w/homatropine methylbromide, Bot. pt, gal.
Use: Antitussive.

•**HYDROCODONE POLISTIREX.** USAN.
Use: Antitussive.

HYDROCODONE RESIN COMPLEX.
Use: Antitussive.
W/Phenyltoloxamine resin complex.
See: Tussionex, Prods. (Pennwalt).

HYDROCORT. (Kenyon) Hydrocortisone 1%, clioquinol 3%, pramoxine HCl 0.5% in a cream base. Jar 20 Gm.
Use: Corticosteroid combination, topical.

HYDROCORTAMATE HCl. 17-Hydroxycorticoster-one-21-diethylaminoaceate HCl.
Use: Anti-inflammatory, topical.
See: Ulcortar, Oint. (Ulmer).

HYDROCORTEX. (Kenyon) Hydrocortisone 1% in cream base. Jar 20 Gm.
Use: Corticosteroid, topical.

•**HYDROCORTISONE,** U.S.P. XXII. Cream, Sterile, Susp., Oint., Gel, Tab., Lot., Enema, U.S.P. XXII. Pregn-4-ene-3,20-dione, 11,17,21-trihydroxy- (11β)- Hydrocortisone. 11β, 17, 21-Trihydroxypregn-4-ene-3, 20-Dione. Compound F. Cortisoln. (Upjohn) Micronized non-sterile powder for prescription compounding.
Use: Anti-inflammatory, topical.
See: Acticort Lotion 100. (Cummins).
Aeroseb-HC, Aerosol (Herbert).
Alphaderm, Cream (Norwich Eaton).
Caldecort Spray (Pharmacraft).
Cetacort, Lot. (Owen).
Cort-Dome, Cream, Lot., Supp. (Miles Pharm).
Cortef, Tab., Cream, Oint. (Upjohn).
Cortenema, Enema (Solvay).
Cortinal, Tube (Kenyon).
Cortril, Oint. (Pfizer).
Cremesone, Cream (Dalin).
Delacort, Lot. (Mericon).
Dermacort, Cream, Lot. (Solvay).
Dermolate, Prods. (Schering).
Durel-Cort, Creme, Oint., Lot. (Durel).
Ecosone, Cream (Star).
HC Derma-Pax, Liq. (Recsei).
HI-COR-1.0, Cream, (C & M Pharmacal).
HI-COR-2.5, Cream (C & M Pharmacal).
Hycort, Cream, Oint. (Everett).
Hycortole,Cream, Oint. (Premo).
Hydrocortex, Tube (Kenyon).
Hydrocortone, Tab. (Merck, Sharp & Dohme).
Hytone, Cream, Oint., Lot. (Dermik).
Lexocort, Pow., Lot. (Lexington).
Lipo-Adrenal Cortex, Vial (Upjohn).
Maso-Cort, Lot. (Mason).
Microcort, Lot. (Alto Pharm.).
My Cort, Cream (Scrip).
Optef, Soln. (Upjohn).
Proctocort, Oint. (Solvay).
Rocort, Lot. (Rocky Mtn.).
Signef, Supp. (Forest Pharm.).
Synacort, Cream (Syntex).
Tarcortin, Cream (Reed & Carnrick).
Texacort 25, 50, Lot. (Cooper).
Ulcort, Cream, Lot. (Ulmer).

HYDROCORTISONE W/COMBINATIONS
See: Achromycin W/Hydrocortisone, Oint., Ophth. Oint. (Lederle).
Acrisan w/Hydrocortisone, Liq. (Recsei).
Aural Acute, Ear Drops (Saron).
Bafil, Cream. (Scruggs).
Barseb HC, Scalp Lot. (Barnes-Hind).
Barseb Thera-spray, Aerosol (Barnes-Hind).
Biscolan HC, Supp. (Lannett).
Bro-Parin, Otic Susp. (Riker).
Calmurid HC, Cream (Pharmacia).
Caquin, Cream (O'Neal, Jones, Feldman).
Carmol HC, Cream (Ingram).
Coidocort, Cream (Coast).
Cor-Tar-Quin, Cream, Lot. (Miles Pharm).
Cortef, Preps. (Upjohn).
Corticoid, Cream (Jenkins).
Cortin, Cream (C & M Pharm.).
Cortisporin, Prep. (Burroughs Wellcome).
Derma-Cover-HC, Liq., Oint. (Scrip).
Dermarex, Cream (Hyrex-Key).
Dicort, Cream, Supp. (Hickam).
Doak Oil Forte, Liq. (Doak).
Drotic No. 2, Drops (Ascher).
Durel-Cort "V,' Cream, Oint., Lot. (Durel).
Fostril HC, Lot. (Westwood).
HC-Form, Jelly (Recsei).
HC-Jel, Jelly (Recsei).
Heb-Cort., Cream, Lot. (Barnes-Hind).
Heb-Cort MC, Lot. (Barnes-Hind).
Heb-Cort. V, Cream, Lot. (Barnes-Hind).
Hi-Cort N Cream (Blaine).
Hill-Cortac, Cream, Lot. (Hill).
Hydrocort, Tube (Kenyon).
Hydroquin, Cream, Oint. (Robinson).
Hysone, Oint. (Mallard).
Kencort, Cream (Kenyon).
Kleer, Spray (Scrip).
Lanvisone, Cream (Lannett).
Loroxide-HC, Lot. (Dermik).
Maso-Form, Cream (Mason).
Mity-quin, Cream (Solvay).
Myci-Cort, Liq., Spray (Misemer).
My-Cort, Drops, Lot., Oint., Spray (Scrip).
Neocort, Oint. (H.V.P.).
Neo-Cort Dome, Cream, Lot., Drops (Miles Pharm).
Neo Cort Top, Oint. (Standex).
Neo-Domeform-HC, Cream, Lot., Susp. (Miles Pharm).

Nutracort, Cream, Gel, Lot.(Owen).
1 + 1 Creme, 1 + 1-F Creme (Dunhall).
Ophthel, Liq. (Elder).
Ophthocort, Oint. (Parke Davis).
Orlex HC Otic (Baylor).
Oto, Drops (Solvay).
Otobiotic, Soln. (Schering).
Otocalm-H Ear Drops (Parmed).
Otostan H.C. (Standex).
Panhydrosone, Tab., Pow. (Panray).
Pyocidin-Otic, Soln. (Berlex).
Racet Forte, Cream (Lemmon).
Racet LCD, Cream (Lemmon).
Rectal Medicone-HC (Medicone).
Sherform-HC, Creme (Sheryl).
Stera-Form, Creme (Mayrand).
Steramine Otic, Drops (Mayrand).
Syntar HC Cream, Oint. (Elder).
Tarcortin, Cream (Reed & Carnrick).
Tar-Quin-HC, Oint. (Jenkins).
Tenda HC, Cream (Dermik).
Terra-Cortril, Preps. (Pfipharmecs).
Theracort, Lot. (C & M Pharm.).
T-Spray, Spray (Saron).
Vanoxide-HC, Lot. (Dermik).
V-Cort, Cream (Scrip).
Vioform-Hydrocortisone, Preps. (Ciba).
Vio-Hydrocort, Oint., Cream (Quality Generics).
Vytone, Cream, (Dermik).

•**HYDROCORTISONE ACETATE,** U.S.P. XXII. Sterile Susp., Lot., Ophth. Oint., Ophth. Susp., Oint., Cream, U.S.P. XXII. Pregn-4-ene-3,20-dione, 21-(acetyloxy)-11,17-dihydroxy-, (11β)-. Hydrocortisone 21-acetate. 17-Hydroxycorticosterone-21-acetate,comp.F. (Upjohn) Micronized non-sterile powder for prescription compounding.
Use: Adrenocortical steroid (topical anti-inflammatory).
See: Anusol-HC, Supp. (Warner-Chilcott).
Caldecort, Cream (Pharmacraft).
Caldecort Light, Cream (Pharmacraft).
Cortef Acetate, Ophth. Oint., Inj. (Upjohn).
Cortifoam, Aerosol (Reed & Carnrick).
Cortiprel, Cream (Pasadena Research).
Cortril Acetate, Aqueous Susp., Oint. (Pfipharmecs).
Ferncort, Lot. (Ferndale).
Fernisone Inj., Vial (Ferndale).
Gynecort, Oint. (Combe).
Hydro-Can (Paddock).
Hydrocort, Vial (Dunhall).
Hydrocortone Acetate, Inj. (Merck, Sharp & Dohme).
Hydrosone, Inj. (Sig).
My-Cort, Lot. (Scrip).
Pramosone Cream, Lot. (Ferndale).
Span-Ster, Inj. (Scrip).
Tucks-HC (Parke-Davis).

HYDROCORTISONE ACETATE W/COMBINATIONS
See: Anusol-HC, Cream, Supp. (Warner-Chilcott).
Biotic-Opth W/HC, Oint. (Scrip).
Biotres HC, Cream (Central).
Biscolan HC, Supp. (Lannett).
Carmol HC, Cream (Ingram).
Chloromycetin-Hydrocortisone Ophth. Susp. (Parke-Davis).
Coly-Mycin-S Otic, Soln. (Warner-Chilcott).
Cor-Oticin, Liq. (Maurry).
Cortaid, Cream, Lot., Oint. (Upjohn).
Cortef Acetate, Inj., Oint., Susp. (Upjohn).
Corticaine Cream (Whitby).
Derma Medicone-HC, Oint. (Medicone).
Dicort, Supp. (Hickam).
Doctient HC, Supp. (Suppositoria).
Epifoam, Aerosol (Reed & Carnrick).
Estro-V HC, Supp. (Webcon).
Eye-Cort, Soln. (Mallard).
Furacin-HC Otic (Eaton).
Furacin HC Urethral Inserts (Eaton).
Furacort Cream (Eaton).
Komed HC, Lot. (Barnes-Hind).
Lida-Mantle HC, Cream (Miles Pharm).
Mantadil, Cream (Burroughs Wellcome).
Neo-Cortef, Preps. (Upjohn).
Neo-Hytone Cream (Dermik).
Neopolycin-HC, Oint., Ophth. Oint. (Merrell Dow).
Ophthocort, Oint. (Parke-Davis).
Proctofoam-HC, Aerosol (Reid and Carnrick).
Pyracort, Liq. (Lemmon).
Racet Forte, Cream (Lemmon).
Rectacort, Supp. (Century).
Rectal Medicone-HC, Supp. (Medicone).
Wyanoids HC, Supp. (Wyeth-Ayerst).

•**HYDROCORTISONE AND ACETIC ACID OTIC SOLUTION,** U.S.P. XXII.
Use: Anti-inflammatory.

•**HYDROCORTISONE BUTEPRATE,** USAN.
Use: Anti-inflammatory.

•**HYDROCORTISONE BUTYRATE,** U.S.P. XXII.
Use: Glucocorticoid.

•**HYDROCORTISONE CYPIONATE,** U.S.P. XXII. Oral Susp., U.S.P. XXII. Hydrocortisone 21-cyclopentanepropionate. Hydrocortisone Cypionate.
Use: Glucocorticoid.

HYDROCORTISONE DIETHYLAMINOACETATE HCl.
See: Hydrocortamate.

HYDROCORTISONE DYPROPIONATE.
See: Cortef, Fluid (Upjohn).

•**HYDROCORTISONE HEMISUCCINATE,** U.S.P. XXII.

HYDROCORTISONE I.V.
See: A-Hydro Cort, Vial (Abbott).
Solu-Cortef, Vial (Upjohn).

HYDROCORTISONE/IODOCHLORHYDROXYQUIN. (Various Mfr.) **Cream:** Hydrocortisone 0.5% or 3%, iodochlorhydroxyquin 3%. 15 Gm,

30 Gm, 480 Gm. **Oint.:** Hydrocortisone 1%, iodochlorhydroxyquin 3%. 20 Gm, 30 Gm.
Use: Corticosteroid, topical.

HYDROCORTISONE/NEOMYCIN. (Various Mfr.) Hydrocortisone 1%, neomycin sulfate 0.5%. Oint. 20 Gm.
Use: Corticosteroid, topical.

HYDROCORTISONE PHOSPHATE.
See: Hydrocortone Phosphate, Inj. (Merck, Sharp & Dohme).

•**HYDROCORTISONE SODIUM PHOSPHATE,** U.S.P. XXII. Inj., U.S.P. XXII. Pregn-4-ene-3,20-dione, 11,17-dihydroxy-21-(phosphonoxy)-, disodium salt, (11β)-. Hydrocortisone 21-(disodium phosphate). Hydrocortisone Sodium Phosphate.
Use: Adrenocortical steroid (anti-inflammatory).

•**HYDROCORTISONE SODIUM SUCCINATE,** U.S.P. XXII. Inj., U.S.P. XXII. Pregn-4-ene-3,20-dione, 31-(3-carboxy-l-oxopropoxy)-11,17-dihydroxy-, (11β)-. Hydrocortisone 21-(sodium succinate). Hydrocortisone Sodium Succinate.
Use: Adrenocortical steroid (anti-inflammatory).
See: A-hydroCort, Vial (Abbott).
Solu-Cortef, Vial (Upjohn).

•**HYDROCORTISONE VALERATE,** U.S.P. XXII. Cream, U.S.P. XXII.
Use: Glucocorticoid.
See: Westcort Cream (Westwood).

HYDROCORTONE ACETATE SALINE SUSPENSION. (Merck, Sharp & Dohme) Hydrocortisone acetate 25 mg or 50 mg/ml, sodium Cl 9 mg, polysorbate 80 4 mg, sodium carboxymethylcellulose 5 mg/ml, benzyl alcohol 9 mg q.s. water for injection to 1 ml. Vial 5 ml.
Use: Corticosteroid.

HYDROCORTONE PHOSPHATE INJECTION. (Merck, Sharp & Dohme) Hydrocortisone sodium phosphate equivalent to hydrocortisone 50 mg/ml, creatinine 8 mg, sodium citrate 10 mg/ml, sodium hydroxide to adjust pH, sodium bisulfite 3.2 mg, methylparaben 1.5 mg, propylparaben 0.2 mg, water for injection q.s./ml. Vial 2 ml multiple dose, 10 ml multiple dose. Disposable syringe 2 ml single dose.
Use: Corticosteroid.

HYDROCORTONE TABLETS. (Merck, Sharp & Dohme) Hydrocortisone 10 mg or 20 mg/Tab. Bot. 100s.
Use: Corticosteroid.

HYDRO-CRYSTI 12. (Hauck) Hydroxocobalamin, crystalline (vitamin B_{12}) 1000 mcg/ml Inj. Vial 10 ml.
Use: Vitamin B_{12} supplement.

HYDRO-D TABLETS. (Blue Cross) Hydrochlorothiazide. 25 mg or 50 mg/Tab. Bot. 1000s.
Use: Diuretic.

HYDRODIURIL. (Merck, Sharp & Dohme) Hydrochlorothiazide. **25 mg/Tab.:** Bot. 100s, 1000s, UD 100s; **50 mg/Tab.:** Bot. 100s, 1000s, UD 100s; **100 mg/Tab.:** Bot. 100s.
Use: Diuretic.

HYDRO-ERGOT. (Interstate) Hydrogenated ergot alkaloids 0.5 mg or 1 mg/Tab. Bot. 100s.
Use: Psychotherapeutic agent.

•**HYDROFILCON A.** USAN.
Use: Contact lens material.

•**HYDROFLUMETHIAZIDE,** U.S.P. XXII. Tab., U.S.P. XXII. 3,4-Dihydro-6-tri-fluoromethyl-7-sulfamoylbenzo-1,2,4-thiadiazine1,1 dioxide,3,4-Dihydro-6-(tri- fluoromethyl)-2H-1,2,4-benzo-thiadiazine-7-sulfonamide-1,1-Dioxide. Di-Ademil; Hydrenox; Naclex; Rontyl.
Use: Edema, hypertension.
See: Diucardin, Tab. (Wyeth-Ayerst).
Saluron, Tab. (Bristol).
W/Reserpine.
See: Salutensin, Tab. (Bristol).
Salutensin-Demi, Tab. (Bristol).

HYDROGEN DIOXIDE.
See: Hydrogen Peroxide.

HYDROGEN IODIDE.
Use: Expectorant.
See: Hydriodic acid.

•**HYDROGEN PEROXIDE CONCENTRATE,** U.S.P. XXII.
Use: Anti-infective (topical) when diluted.

•**HYDROGEN PEROXIDE TOPICAL SOLUTION,** U.S.P. XXII. (Various Mfr.) (3%). 4 oz, 8 oz, pt.
Use: Anti-infective, topical.

HYDROGEN PEROXIDE SOLUTION 30%. Perhydrol, hydrogen pioxide. Bot. 0.25 lb, 0.5 lb, 1 lb.
Use: Dentistry, preparing the 3% solution.

HYDROGESIC. (Edwards) Hydrocodone bitartrate 5 mg, acetaminophen 500 mg/Cap. Bot. 100s.
Use: Narcotic analgesic combination.

HYDROLOID-G SUBLINGUAL. (Major) Ergoloid mesylates. **0.5 mg/Tab.:** Bot. 100s, 250s, 500s, UD 100s. **1 mg/Tab.:** Bot. 100s, 250s, 1000s, UD 100s.
Use: Psychotherapeutic agent.

HYDROLOID-G TABS. (Major) Ergoloid mesylates 1 mg/Tab. Bot. 100s, 250s, 1000s, UD 100s.
Use: Psychotherapeutic agent.

HYDROMAL. (Mallard) Hydrochlorothiazide 50 mg/Tab. Bot. 1000s.
Use: Diuretic.

HYDROMAX SYRUP. (Blue Cross) Ephedrine sulfate 6.25 mg, theophylline 32.5 mg, hydroxyzine HCl 2.5 mg/5 ml. Bot. 16 oz.
Use: Bronchodilator.

HYDROMORPHINOL. B.A.N. 7,8-Dihydro-14-hydroxymorphine. Numorphan Oral.
Use: Narcotic analgesic.

HYDROMORPHONE. B.A.N. 7,8-Dihydromorphinone. Dilaudid hydrochloride.
Use: Narcotic analgesic.

HYDROMORPHONE. 4,5-Epoxy-3-hydroxy-17-methylmorphinan-6-one.
Use: Narcotic analgesic.

•**HYDROMORPHONE HYDROCHLORIDE,** U.S.P. XXII. Inj., Tab., U.S.P. XXII. Dihydromorphinone

HCl. 4,5α-Epoxy-3-hydroxy-17-methylmorphinan-6-one HCl.
Use: Analgesic; narcotic.
See: Dilaudid Prods. (Knoll).
W/sodium citrate, antimony potassium tartrate and chloroform. Inj.
See: Dilocol, Liq. (Table Rock).
HYDROMORPHONE SULFATE. 4,5-Epoxy 3-hydroxy-17-methylmorphinan-6-one sulfate (2:1).
Use: Narcotic analgesic.
HYDROMOX. (Lederle) Quinethazone 50 mg/Tab. Bot. 100s, 500s.
Use: Diuretic.
HYDROMOX-R. (Lederle) Quinethazone 50 mg, reserpine 0.125 mg/Tab. Bot. 100s, 500s.
Use: Antihypertensive combination.
HYDROPANE. (Halsey) Hydrocodone bitartrate 5 mg, homatropine methylbromide 1.5 mg. Pt, gal.
Use: Antitussive combination.
HYDROPEL. (C & M Pharmacal) Silicone 30%, hydrophobic starch derivative 10%, petrolatum. Jar. 2 oz, lb.
Use: Emollient.
HYDROPHED TABLETS. (Rugby) Theophylline 130 mg, ephedrine sulfate 25 mg, hydroxyzine HCl 10 mg/Tab. Bot. 100s, 500s, 1000s.
Use: Antiasthmatic combination.
HYDROPHEN SYRUP. (Rugby) Phenylpropanolamine HCl 25 mg, hydrocodone bitartrate 5 mg/5 ml. Bot. pt, gal.
Use: Decongestant, antitussive.
HYDROPHEN PEDIATRIC SYRUP. (Rugby) Phenylpropanolamine HCl 12.5 mg, hydrocodone bitartrate 2.5 mg/5 ml. Bot. 480 ml.
Use: Decongestant, antitussive.
HYDROPHILIC OINTMENT, U.S.P. XXII. Stearyl alcohol, white petrolatum, propylene glycol, sodium lauryl sulfate, water. Jar lb. (Fougera).
Use: Ointment base.
HYDROPHILIC OINTMENT BASE. Oil in water emulsion bases. (Emerson) 1 lb.
Use: Ointment base.
See: Aquaphilic Ointment (Medco).
Cetaphil, Cream, Lot. (Texas Pharmacal).
Dermovan, Cream (Texas Pharmacal).
Lanaphilic Ointment (Medco).
Monobase, Oint. (Torch).
Polysorb, Oint. (Savage).
Unibase, Oint. (Parke-Davis).
HYDROPINE. (Rugby) Hydroflumethiazide 25 mg, reserpine 0.125 mg/Tab. Bot. 100s.
Use: Antihypertensive combination.
HYDROPINE H.P. TABLETS. (Rugby) Hydroflumethiazide 50 mg, reserpine 0.125 mg/Tab. Bot. 100s, 500s, 1000s.
Use: Antihypertensive combination.
HYDROPRES-25 & 50. (Merck, Sharp & Dohme) **25:** Hydrochlorothiazide 25 mg, reserpine 0.125 mg/Tab. **50:** Hydrochlorothiazide 50 mg, reserpine 0.125 mg/Tab. Bot. 100s, 1000s.
Use: Antihypertensive combination.
HYDROPRIN. (Cenci) Hydrochlorothiazide 25 mg or 50 mg, reserpine 0.125 mg/Tab. Bot. 100s, 1000s.
Use: Antihypertensive combination.
HYDROQUIN. (Robinson) Hydrocortisone 1%, clioquinol 3%. Cream: Tube 5 Gm, 20 Gm, Jar 4 oz, 8 oz, lb. **Oint.:** Jar 4 oz, lb.
Use: Corticosteroid, topical.
HYDROQUIN W/COAL TAR SOLUTION. (Robinson) Hydrocortisone 0.5%, clioquinol 1%, coal tar soln. 3%. Tube 0.5 oz.
Use: Corticosteroid combination, topical.
•**HYDROQUINONE,** U.S.P. XXII. Cream, Topical Soln., U.S.P. XXII. 1,4-Benzenediol.
Use: Depigmenting agent.
See: Artra Skin Tone Cream (Plough).
Black and White Bleaching Cream (Plough).
Derma-Blanch, Cream (Chattem).
Eldopaque Cream, Oint. (Elder).
Eldopaque Forte Cream, Oint. (Elder).
Eldoquin, Cream, Lot. (Elder).
Esoterica Medicated Cream Prods. (Norcliff Thayer).
HYDROQUINONE MONOBENZYL ETHER.
See: Benoquin, Oint., Lot. (Elder).
HYDROSAL. (Hydrosal Co.) Aluminum acetate 5%. **Susp.:** Bot. 16 oz, gal. **Oint.:** 54 Gm, 113.4 Gm, Jar 54 Gm, 454 Gm.
HYDROSERP. (Zenith) Hydrochlorothiazide 25 mg or 50 mg, reserpine 0.125 mg or 0.1 mg/Tab. Bot. 100s, 1000s.
Use: Antihypertensive combination.
HYDROSERP-50. (Freeport) Hydrochlorothiazide 50 mg, reserpine 0.125 mg/Tab. Bot. 1000s.
Use: Antihypertensive combination.
HYDROSERPINE. (Geneva) Hydrochlorothiazide 25 mg or 50 mg, reserpine 0.125 mg/Tab. Bot. 100s.
Use: Antihypertensive combination.
HYDROSERPINE 25. (Goldline) Hydrochlorothiazide 25 mg, reserpine. Bot. 100s, 1000s.
Use: Antihypertensive combination.
HYDROSERPINE 50. (Goldline) Hydrochlorothiazide 50 mg, reserpine. Bot. 100s, 1000s.
Use: Antihypertensive combination.
HYDROSINE 25 TABLETS. (Major) Hydrochlorothiazide 25 mg, reserpine 0.125 mg/Tab. Bot. 100s. Tartrazine.
Use: Antihypertensive combination.
HYDROSINE 50 TABLETS. (Major) Hydrochlorothiazide 50 mg, reserpine 0.125 mg/Tab. Bot. 100s.
Use: Antihypertensive combination.
HYDROSOL. (Rocky Mtn.) Prednisolone 21 phosphate 20 mg/ml. Vial 10 ml.
Use: Corticosteroid.
HYDROSONE. (Sig) Hydrocortisone acetate 25 mg or 50 mg/ml. Vial 5 ml.
Use: Corticosteroid.
HYDRO-T TABS. (Major) Hydrochlorothiazide. **25 mg/Tab:** Bot. 100s, 1000s, UD 100s; **50 mg/**

Tab: Bot. 100s, 1000s, UD 100s; **100 mg/Tab:** Bot. 100s, 250s, 1000s, UD 100s.
Use: Diuretic.

HYDROTALCITE. B.A.N. Aluminum magnesium hydroxide carbonate hydrate. Altacite.
Use: Antacid.

HYDROTENSIN-50. (Mayrand) Hydrochlorothiazide 50 mg, reserpine 0.125 mg/Tab. Bot. 100s, 1000s.
Use: Antihypertensive combination.

HYDRO-TEX CREAM. (Syosset) Hydrocortisone 0.5% or 1%. Greaseless base. Cream 30 Gm, 60 Gm, 120 Gm.
Use: Corticosteroid, topical.

HYDROTOIN CREAM. (Knight) Hydrocortisone 0.5%. Tube 0.5 oz.
Use: Corticosteroid, topical.

HYDROXACEN. (Central) Hydroxyzine HCl 50 mg/ml, benzyl alcohol. Vial 10 ml.
Use: Antianxiety agent.

HYDROX B_{12}. (Rocky Mtn.) Hydroxocobalamin 1000 mcg/ml. Vial 10 ml.
Use: Vitamin B_{12} supplement.

HYDROXAMETHOCAINE. B.A.N. 2-Dimethylaminoethyl 4-butylaminosalicylate. Hydroxytetracaine (I.N.N.).
Use: Local anesthetic.

HYDROXINDASOL HCl. 5-Hydroxy-1-(p-methoxy-benzyl)-2-methyltryptamine HCl.

HYDROXOCOBALAMIN, U.S.P. XXII. Inj., U.S.P. XXII. α-(5,6-Dimethylbenzimidazolyl) hydroxocobamide. Vitamin B 12a and B 12b. Hydrovit; Neo-Cytamen.
Use: Treatment of megaloblastic anemia.
See: AlphaRedisol, Inj. (Merck, Sharp & Dohme).
Alpha-Ruvite, Vial (Savage).
Cobavite L.A., Vial (Lemmon).
Droxomin, Inj. (Solvay).
Hydrobexan, Vial (Keene).
Rubesol-L.A. 1000, Inj. (Central).
Span-12, Inj. (Scrip).
Sytobex-H, Vial (Parke-Davis).
Twelve-Span, Vial (Foy).

HYDROXY BIS(ACETATO)ALUMINUM. Aluminum Subacetate Topical Soln, U.S.P. XXII.

2-HYDROXYBENZAMIDE.
See: Salicylamide.

HYDROXYBIS (SALICYLATO) ALUMINUM DIACETATE.
See: Aluminum aspirin.

HYDROXYCHOLECALCIFEROL. (D_3).
Use: Vitamin D supplement.
See: Calcifediol.

HYDROXYCHLOROQUINE SULFATE, U.S.P. XXII. Tab., U.S.P. XXII. Ethanol, 2-4-(7-chloro-4-quinolinyl)-amino pentyl ethylamino-, sulfate (1:1) salt. 7-Chloro-4- 4-[ethyl(2-hydroxyethyl)-amino]-1-methyl- butylamino quinoline sulfate. 2-[[4-[(7chloro-4-quinolyl)amino]-pentyl]ethylamino]ethanol Sulfate (1:1).
Use: Antimalarial, lupus erythematosus suppressant.

HYDROXYDIONE SODIUM. 21-Hydroxy-pregnane- dione sodium succinate.

HYDROXYDIONE SODIUM SUCCINATE. B.A.N. Sodium 21-hydroxypregnane-3,20-dione succinate.
Use: Anesthetic.

•**HYDROXYETHYL CELLULOSE,** N.F. XVII.
Use: Topical protectant, thickening agent.

HYDROXYETHYL STARCH. (HES).
Use: Plasma volume expander.
See: Hespan, Inj. (DuPont Critical Care).

HYDROXYISOINDOLIN. Under study.
Use: Antihypertensive.

HYDROXYMAGNESIUM ALUMINATE.
Use: Antacid.
See: Magaldrate.

HYDROXYMYCIN. An antibiotic substance obtained from cultures of *Streptomyces paucisporogenes.*

HYDROXYPETHIDINE. B.A.N. Ethyl 4-(3-hydroxy-phenyl)-1-methylpiperidine-4-carboxylate.
Use: Narcotic analgesic.

•**HYDROXYPHENAMATE.** USAN. 2-Hydroxy-2-phenyl-butyl carbamate.
Use: Tranquilizer.

HYDROXYPROCAINE. B.A.N. 2-Diethylaminoethyl 4-aminosalicylate.
Use: Local anesthetic.

•**HYDROXYPROGESTERONE CAPROATE,** U.S.P. XXII. Inj., U.S.P. XXII. 17α-Hydrogypregn-4-ene-3,20-dione. Pregn-4-ene-3,20-dione,17-[(l)oxohexyl)-oxy]-.
Use: Progestin.
See: Delalutin, Vial (Squibb).
Hy-Gestrone, Vial (Pasadena Research).
Hylutin, Inj. (Hyrex).
Hyprogest 250, Inj. (Keene).
W/Estradiol valerate.
See: Hy-Gestradol, Inj. (Pasadena Research).
Hylutin-Est., Inj. (Hyrex).

•**HYDROXYPROPYL CELLULOSE, LOW-SUBSTITUTED,** N.F. XVII.
Use: Topical protectant, tablet coating agent.

•**HYDROXYPROPYL METHYLCELLULOSE,** U.S.P. XXII. Ophth. soln. U.S.P. XXII. Cellulose, 2-hydroxypropyl methyl ether. Cellulose hydroxypropyl methyl ether. The propylene glycol ether of methylcellulose available in the 2208, 2906 and 2910 forms.
Use: Suspending agent, topical protectant (ophthalmic).
See: Anestacon (Alcon).
Econopred, Susp. (Alcon).
W/benzalkonium Cl.
See: Goniosol (Smith, Miller & Patch).
Isopto Tears (Alcon).
Ultra Tears, Soln. (Alcon).

•**HYDROXYPROPYL METHYLCELLULOSE PHTHALATE 200731,** N.F. XVII.
Use: Pharmaceutic aid, tablet coating agent.

•**HYDROXYPROPYL METHYLCELLULOSE PHTHALATE 200824,** N.F. XVII.
Use: Pharmaceutic aid, tablet coating agent.

•**HYROXYPROPYL METHYLCELLULOSE PHTHALATE,** N.F. XVII.
Use: Pharmaceutic aid, tablet coating agent.

HYDROXYSTEARIN SULFATE. Sulfonate hydrogenated castor oil.

HYDROXYSTILBAMIDINE. B.A.N. 4,4′-Diamidino-2-hydroxystilbene.
Use: Treatment of leishmaniasis and trypanosomiasis.

HYDROXYTOLUIC ACID. B.A.N. 2-Hydroxy-m-toluic acid. 3-Methylsalicylic acid.
Use: Analgesic.

•**HYDROXYUREA,** U.S.P. XXII. Cap., U.S.P. XXII. Hydroxycarbamide (I.N.N.).
Use: Antineoplastic agent.
See: Hydrea, Cap. (Squibb Mark).

HYDRO-Z-50 TABLETS. (Mayrand) Hydrochlorothiazide 50 mg/Tab. Bot. 100s, 1000s.
Use: Diuretic.

•**HYDROXYZINE HCl,** U.S.P. XXII. Inj., Syr., Tab., U.S.P. XXII. 2-[2-[-4-(p-Chloro-α-phenylbenzyl-)-1- piperazinyl]ethoxy]ethanol dihydrochloride. Inj.: (Abbott) 100 mg/2 ml amp. or Abboject syringe, 500 mg/10 ml vial.
Use: Tranquilizer, antihistamine.
See: Atarax, Syr., Tab. (Roerig).
Hyzine-50, Inj. (Hyrex).
Vistazine 25, Inj. (Keene).
Vistazine 50, Inj. (Keene).
Vistaril Isoject. (Roerig).
Vistaril, Cap., Susp. (Pfizer Laboratories).
W/Ephedrine sulf., theophylline.
See: Marax DF, Syr. (Roerig).
Marax Tab. (Roerig).
Theo-Drox, Tab. (Quality Generics).
W/Pentaerythritol tetranitrate.
See: Cartrax 10, 20, Tab. (Roerig).

•**HYDROXYZINEPAMOATE,** U.S.P. XXII. Cap., Oral Susp., U.S.P. XXII. 1,1′-Methylene bis(2-hydroxy-3-naphthalene-carboxylic acid salt of 1-p-chlorobenzhydryl)-4-[2-2-hydroxy-ethoxyethyl]piperazine. 2-(2-(4-(piperazine. 2-(2-(4-(p-Chloro-α-phenyl-benzyl)-1-piperazinyl)ethoxy)ethanol 4,4′-Methylenebis-(3-hydroxy-2-napthoate) (1:1).
Use: Tranquilizer; antihistamine.
See: Hy-Pam 25 Cap. (Lemmon).
Vistaril, Cap., Susp. (Pfizer Laboratories).

HY-E-PLEX. (Nutrition) Vitamin E 400 IU/Cap. Vial. Bot. 100s.
Use: Vitamin E supplement.

Hy-FLOW SOLUTION. (CooperVision) Polyvinyl alcohol with hydroxyethylcellulose, benzalkonium Cl, EDTA. Bot. 60 ml.
Use: Hard contact lens care.

HY-GESTRONE. (Pasadena Research) Hydroxyprogesterone caproate. **125 mg/ml.:** Vial 10 ml. **250 mg/ml.:** Vial 5 ml.
Use: Progestin.

HYGIENIC POWDER.
See: Bo-Car-Al, Pow. (Calgon).

HYGROTON. (Rorer) Chlorthalidone 25 mg, 50 mg or 100 mg/Tab. Bot. 100s, 1000s, UD 100s.
Use: Diuretic.

HYLIDONE TABS. (Major) Chlorthalidone. **25 mg or 50 mg/Tab:** Bot. 100s, 250s, 1000s, UD 100s. **100 mg/Tab:** Bot. 100s, 250s, 500s, 1000s.
Use: Diuretic.

HYLIVER PLUS. (Hyrex) Folic acid 0.4 mg, liver 10 mcg, vitamin B_{12} 100 mcg/ml. Vial 10 ml with phenol.
Use: Vitamin supplement.

HYLOREL TABLETS. (Pennwalt) Guanadrel sulfate 10 mg or 25 mg/Tab. Bot. 100s.
Use: Antihypertensive.

HYLUTIN INJECTABLE. (Hyrex) Hydroxyprogesterone caproate in oil 250 mg/ml. Vial 5 ml.
Use: Progestin.

HYMAC CREAM. (NMC Labs) Hydrocortisone 0.5% or 1% in cream base. Tube oz.
Use: Corticosteroid, topical.

HYMAC OINTMENT. (NMC Labs) Hydrocortisone 0.5% or 1% in ointment base. Tube oz.
Use: Corticosteroid, topical.

•**HYMECROMONE.** USAN.
Use: Choleretic.

HY-N.B.P. OINTMENT. (Bowman) Bacitracin zinc 400 units, neomycin sulfate 5 mg, polymixin B sulfate 10,000 units/Gm. Tube ⅛ oz.
Use: Anti-infective, topical.

HYOSCINE HYDROBROMIDE. Scopolamine HBr, U.S.P. XXII.
Use: Intestinal antispasmodic.

HYOSCINE-HYOSCYAMINE-ATROPINE.
Use: Anticholinergic.
See: Atropine w/hyoscyamine w/hyoscine.

HYOSCINE METHOBROMIDE. B.A.N.
Use: Treatment of peptic ulcer.

•**HYOSCYAMINE,** U.S.P. XXII. Tab., U.S.P. XXII. 1αH,5αH-Tropan-3α-ol(−)-tropate (ester). Levo form of atropine.
Use: Anticholinergic.
See: Bellafoline, Amp., Tab. (Sandoz).
Cysto-Spaz, Tab. (Webcon).

HYOSCYAMINE-ATROPINE-HYOSCINE.
Use: Anticholinergic.
See: Atropine w/hyoscyamine w/hyoscine.

•**HYOSCYAMINE HYDROBROMIDE,** U.S.P. XXII. 1αH,5αH-Tropan-3α-ol(−)-tropate HBr. Daturine HBr. (Various Mfr.).
Use: Anticholinergic.
W/Physostigmine salicylate.
See: Pyatromine-H Inj. (Kremers-Urban).

HYOSCYAMINE HYDROCHLORIDE. (Various Mfr.).

HYOSCYAMINE MALEATE.
See: Bellafoline, Amp., Tab. (Sandoz).

HYOSCYAMINE SALTS.
Use: Anticholinergic.
W/Atropine salts.

See: Atropine W/Hyoscyamine.
HYOSCYAMINE SULFATE, U.S.P. XXII. Elix., Inj., Oral Soln., Tab., U.S.P. XXII. 1αH,5αH-Tropan-3α-ol-(−)-tropate (ester) sulfate (2:1) dihydrate.
Use: Anticholinergic.
See: Anaspaz, Tab. (Ascher).
Cystospaz-M, Cap. (Webcon).
W/Atropine sulfate, hyoscine HBr, phenobarbital.
See: DeTal, Elix., Tab. (DeLeon).
Donnatal, Prods.(Robins).
Hyatal, Elix., Liq. (Kenyon).
Hyonal C.T., Tab. (Paddock).
Maso-Donna, Elix., Tab. (Mason).
Peece, Tab. (Scrip).
Sedamine, Tab. (Dunhall).
Spasaid, Cap. (Century).
Spasmolin, Tab. (Kenyon).
Spasquid, Elix. (Geneva).
W/Atropine sulfate, hyoscine HBr, phenobarbital, pepsin, pancreatin, bile salts.
See: Donnazyme, Tab. (Robins).
W/Atropine sulfate. Scopolamine HCl, phenobarbital.
See: Ultabs, Tab. (Burlington).
W/Belladonna Alkaloids.
See: Belladonna Prods.
W/Butabarbital.
See: Cystospaz-SR, Cap. (Webcon).
W/Methenamine, atropine sulfate, methylene blue, salol, benzoic acid, gelsemium.
See: Uriprel, Tab. (Pasadena Research).
W/Phenobarbital, simethicone, atropine sulfate, scopolamine HBr.
See: Kinesed, Tab. (Stuart).
HYOSCYAMUS EXTRACT.
W/A.P.C.
See: Valacet Junior, Tab. (Vale).
W/A.P.C., gelsemium extract.
See: Valacet, Tab. (Vale).
HYOSCYAMUS PRODUCTS AND PHENOBARBITAL COMBINATIONS.
Use: Anticholinergic, sedative.
See: Anaspaz PB, Tab. (Pasadena Research).
Donnacin, Elix., Tab. (Pharmex).
Donnatal, Preps. (Robins).
Elixiral, Elix. (Vita Elixir).
Floramine, Tab. (Lemmon).
Gylanphen, Tab. (Lannett).
Kinesed, Tab. (Stuart).
Neoquess, Tab. (O'Neal).
Nevrotose, Cap. (Vale).
Sedajen, Tab. (Jenkins).
HYOSOPHEN TABLETS. (Rugby). Atropine sulfate 0.0194 mg, scopolamine HBr 0.0065 mg, hyoscyamine HBr or SO_4 0.1037 mg, phenobarbital 16.2 mg. In 1000s.
Use: Anticholinergic combination.
HYPAQUE-76. (Winthrop Pharm.) Diatrizoate meglumine 66%, diatrizoate sodium 10%, iodine 37%, EDTA. Vial 30 ml, 50 ml, 100 ml.
Use: Radiopaque agent.
HYPAQUE-CYSTO. (Winthrop Pharm) Diatrizoate meglumine 30% soln., iodine 14.1%. 250 ml in 500 ml dilution bottle. Pediatric 100 ml in 300 ml dilution bottle.
Use: Radiopaque agent.
HYPAQUE-M 75%. (Winthrop Pharm) Diatrizoate meglumine 50%, diatrizoate sodium 25%, iodine 38.5%, EDTA. Vial 20 ml, 50 ml.
Use: Radiopaque agent.
HYPAQUE-M 90%. (Winthrop Pharm) Diatrizoate meglumine 60%, diatrizoate sodium 30%, EDTA. Vial 50 ml.
Use: Radiopaque agent.
HYPAQUE MEGLUMINE 30%. (Winthrop Pharm) Diatrizoate meglumine 30%, iodine 14.1%. Bot. 100 ml, 300 ml w/and w/o I.V. infusion set.
Use: Radiopaque agent.
HYPAQUE MEGLUMINE 60%. (Winthrop Pharm) Diatrizoate meglumine 60%, iodine 28%, EDTA. Vial 20 ml, 30 ml, 50 ml, 100 ml.
Use: Radiopaque agent.
HYPAQUE ORAL. (Winthrop Pharm) **Pow.:** Diatrizoate sodium oral pow. containing iodine 600 mg/Gm. Can 250 Gm, Bot. 10 Gm. **Liq.:** Soln. 41.66%. Bot. 120 ml.
Use: Radiopaque agent.
HYPAQUE SODIUM 20%. (Winthrop Pharm) Diatrizoate sodium 20%, iodine 12%, EDTA. Vial 100 ml.
Use: Radiopaque agent.
HYPAQUE SODIUM 25%. (Winthrop Pharm) Diatrizoate sodium 25%, iodine 15%. Bot. 300 ml, w/and w/out I.V. infusion set.
Use: Radiopaque agent.
HYPAQUE SODIUM 50%. (Winthrop Pharm) Diatrizoate sodium 50%, iodine 30%. **Vial:** 20 ml, 30 ml, 50 ml. **Dilution Bottle:** 200 ml with EDTA.
Use: Radiopaque agent.
HYPERAB. (Cutter) Rabies immune globulin (Human) 150 IU/ml. **Pediatric:** Vial 2 ml. **Adult:** Vial 10 ml.
Use: Agent for immunization.
HYPERHEP. (Cutter) Hepatitis B immune globulin (Human). Vial 250 unit, prefilled syringe 250 unit.
Use: Agent for immunization.
HYPERLYTE. (American McGaw) Sodium 25 mEq, potassium 40.5 mEq, calcium 5 mEq, magnesium 8 mEq, chloride 33.5 mEq, acetate 40.6 mEq, gluconate 5 mEq, 6050 mOsm/L. Inj. Vial 25 ml fill in 50 ml.
Use: Parenteral nutritional supplement.
HYPERLYTE CR. (American McGaw) Sodium 25 mEq, potassium 20 mEq, calcium 5 mEq, magnesium 5 mEq, chloride 30 mEq, acetate 30 mEq, 5500 mOsm/L. Inj. Super-vial 150 ml, 250 ml fill.
Use: Parenteral nutritional supplement.
HYPERLYTE R. (American McGaw) Sodium 25 mEq, potassium 20 mEq, calcium 5 mEq, mag-

nesium 5 mEq, chloride 30 mEq, acetate 25 mEq, 4200 mOsm/L. Inj. Vial 25 ml fill in 50 ml.
Use: Parenteral nutritional supplement.

HYPEROPTO 5%. (Professional Pharmacal) Sodium Cl 5%. Oint. Tube 3.5 Gm.
Use: Ophthalmic preparation.

HYPEROPTO OINTMENT. (Professional Pharmacal) Sodium HCl 50 mg, D.I. water 150 mg, anhydrous lanolin 150 mg, liquid petrolatum 50 mg, white petrolatum 599 mg, methylparaben 7 mg, propylparaben 3 mg/Gm. Tube 3.5 Gm.
Use: Ophthalmic preparation.

HYPERSTAT I.V. INJECTION. (Schering) Diazoxide 300 mg, pH adjusted to approximately 11.6 with sodium hydroxide/20 ml Amp.
Use: Antihypertensive.

HYPERTEN. (Kenyon) Phenobarbital 0.25 gr, nitroglycerin 1/300 gr, sodium nitrate 1 gr, veratrum viride 3/4 gr/Tab. Bot. 100s, 1000s.
Use: Antihypertensive.

HYPERTENSION DIAGNOSIS.
See: Regitine, Amp., Tab. (Ciba).

HYPERTENSION THERAPY.
See: Aldoclor, Tab. (Merck, Sharp & Dohme).
Aldomet, Tab. (Merck, Sharp & Dohme).
Aldomet Ester HCl, Amp. (Merck, Sharp & Dohme).
Aldoril, Tab. (Merck, Sharp & Dohme).
Alkavervir.
Alseroxylon.
Apresoline, Amp., Tab. (Ciba).
Apresoline, Apresoline Esidrix, Amp., Tab. (Ciba).
Arfonad, Amp. (Roche).
Blocadren, Tab. (Merck, Sharp & Dohme).
Corgard, Tab. (Squibb).
Deserpidine.
Dibenzyline HCl, Cap. (SmithKline).
Diupres, Tab. (Merck, Sharp & Dohme).
Diutensen and Diutensen-R, Tab. (Wallace).
Dyazide, Cap. (SmithKline).
Enduron, Tab. (Abbott).
Enduronyl, Tab. (Abbott).
Enduronyl Forte, Tab. (Abbott).
Esidrix, Tab. (Ciba).
Eutonyl, Tab. (Abbott).
Eutron, Tab. (Abbott).
Exna and Exna-R, Tab. (Robins).
Hesperidin Methyl Chalcone (Various Mfr.).
Hexamethonium Cl and Bromide (Various Mfr.).
HydroDiuril, Tab. (Merck, Sharp & Dohme).
Hydropres, Tab. (Merck, Sharp & Dohme).
Hygroton, Tab. (USV).
Hyperstat, I.V. Inj. (Schering).
Inversine, Tab. (Merck, Sharp & Dohme).
Lopressor, Tab. (Geigy).
Metatensin, Tab. (Merrell Dow).
Midamor, Tab. (Merck, Sharp & Dohme).
Moderil, Tab. (Pfizer).
Moduretic, Tab. (Merck, Sharp & Dohme).
Naturetin, Tab. (Squibb).
Naquival, Tab. (Schering).
Oretic, Tab. (Abbott).
Oreticyl, Tab. (Abbott).
Priscoline HCl, Preps. (Ciba).
Protoveratrines A & B.
Raudixin, Tab. (Squibb).
Rauwolfia Serpentina (Various Mfr.).
Rauzide, Tab. (Squibb).
Regroton, Tab. (USV).
Renese-R, Tab. (Pfizer).
Rescinnamine, Tab. (Various Mfr.).
Reserpine (Various Mfr.).
Rutin, Tab. (Various Mfr.).
Sectral, Cap. (Wyeth-Ayerst).
Tetraethylammonium Chloride (Various Mfr.).
Timolide, Tab. (Merck, Sharp & Dohme).
Trandate Products (Allen & Hanburys).
Vasodilators.
Vasotec, Tab. (Merck, Sharp & Dohme).
Veratrum Alba.
Veratrum Viride.
Wytensin, Tab. (Wyeth-Ayerst).
Zaroxolyn, Tab. (Pennwalt).

HYPER-TET. (Cutter) Tetanus immune globulin (Human) U.S.P. Vial 250 units, Disp. Syringe 250 units.
Use: Immune serum.

HYPERTHYROIDISM.
See: Antithyroid agents.

HY-PHEN TABLETS. (Ascher) Hydrocodone bitartrate 5 mg, acetaminophen 500 mg. Bot. 100s, 500s.
Use: Antitussive, analgesic.

HYPHYLLINE. Dyphylline. (7-Dihydroxy-propyltheophylline).
See: Neothylline, Elix., Amp., Tab. (Lemmon).

HYPNOGENE.
See: Barbital (Various Mfr.).

HYPNOMIDATE. (Janssen) Etomidate.
Use: General anesthetic.

HYPNO-SED. (Jenkins) Bromisovalum 1 gr, carbromal 3 gr, thiamine mononitrate 9 mg/Tab. Bot. 1000s.

HYPNOTICS.
See: Sedatives.

"HYPO".
See: Sodium Thiosulfate (Various Mfr.).

HYPO-BEE. (Towne) Vitamins B_1 50 mg, B_2 20 mg, B_6 5 mg, B_{12} 15 mcg, niacinamide 25 mg, calcium pantothenate 5 mg, C 300 mg, E 200 IU, iron 10 mg/Tab. Bot. 30s, 100s.
Use: Vitamin/mineral supplement.

HYPOCHLORITE PREPS.
See: Antiformin.
Dakin's Soln.
Hyclorite.

HYPOCLEAR. (Bausch & Lomb) Isotonic soln. with sodium Cl 0.9%. Aerosol soln. 240 ml, 30 ml.
Use: Soft contact lens care.

HYPOGLYCEMIC AGENTS.

See: Chlorpropamide.
Diabinese, Tab. (Pfizer).
Dymelor, Tab. (Lilly).
Orinase, Tab., Vial (Upjohn).
Phenformin HCl.
Tolbutamide.
Tolinase, Tab. (Upjohn).

α-HYPOPHAMINE. Oxytocin.

HYPOPHYOSPHOROUS ACID, N.F. XVII.
Use: Antioxidant.

HYPOTEARS OPHTHALMIC LIQUID. (Iolab Pharm.) Polyvinyl alcohol 1%, PEG-8000, dextrose, benzalkonium Cl, EDTA. Bot. 15 ml, 30 ml.
Use: Ophthalmic lubricant.

HYPOTEARS OPHTHALMIC OINTMENT. (Iolab Pharm.) White petrolatum, light mineral oil. Tube 3.5 Gm.
Use: Ophthalmic lubricant.

HYPOTENSIVE AGENTS.
See: Hypertension Therapy.

HYPRHO-D. (Cutter) Rho (D) Immune globulin (Human). Pre-filled single dose syringe. Single dose vial. Pkg. 10s.
Use: Immune serum.

HYPRHO-D MINI-DOSE. (Cutter Biological) RH_O (D) Immune Globulin Micro-Dose. Each package contains a single dose syringe.
Use: Immune serum.

HYPROGEST 250. (Keene) Hydroxyprogesterone caproate 250 mg/ml. Inj. Vial 5 ml.
Use: Progestin.

HYPROMELLOSE. B.A.N. A partial mixed methyl and hydroxypropyl ether of cellulose.
Use: Surface active agent.

HYREXIN. (Hyrex) Diphenhydramine HCl 50 mg/ml. Vial 10 ml.
Use: Antihistamine.

HYRUNAL. (Kenyon) Rutin 20 mg, mannitol hexanitrate 0.5 gr, phenobarbital 0.25 gr/Tab. Bot. 100s, 1000s.
Use: Antihypertensive combination.

HYRUNAL W/VERATRUM VIRIDE. (Kenyon) Phenobarbital 0.25 gr, mannitol hexanitrate 0.5 gr, rutin 10 mg, veratrum viride 100 mg/Tab. Bot. 100s, 1000s.
Use: Antihypertensive combination.

HYSCORBIC PLUS TABLETS. (Bock) Vitamins E 45 IU, C 600 mg, folic acid 400 mcg, B_1 20 mg, B_2 10 mg, niacinamide 100 mg, B_6 10 mg, B_{12} 25 mcg, pantothenic acid 25 mg, copper 3 mg, zinc 23.9 mg/Tab. Bot. 60s.
Use: Vitamin/mineral supplement.

HYSERP. (Freeport) Reserpine alkaloid 0.25 mg/Tab. Bot. 1000s.
Use: Antihypertensive.

HYSKON. (Pharmacia) Dextran 70 32% in 10% w/v dextrose. Bot. 100 ml, 250 ml.
Use: Diagnostic aid. For distending the uterine cavity and in irrigating and visualizing its surfaces.

HYSONE. (Mallard) Iodochlorhydroxquin 3%, hydrocortisone 0.5%. Tube 15 Gm.
Use: Antifungal, corticosteroid, topical.

HYSTERONE TABS. (Major) Fluoxymesterone 10 mg/Tab. Bot. 100s.
Use: Androgen.

HYTAKEROL. (Winthrop Pharm) Dihydrotachysterol. **Cap.:** 0.125 mg. Bot. 50s. **Soln.:** 0.25 mg/ml in oil. Bot. 15 ml.
Use: Treatment of tetany and hypoparathyroidism.

HYTINIC. (Hyrex) Polysaccharide-iron complex 150 mg/Cap. Bot. 50s, 500s.
Use: Iron supplement.

HYTINIC INJECTION. (Hyrex) Ferrous gluconate 2.9 mg, liver equivalent to vitamins B_{12} 15 mcg, vitamins B_2 0.75 mg, B_5 1.25 mg, B_{12} equivalent 1 mcg. Vial 30 ml.
Use: Vitamin/mineral supplement.

HYTONE CREAM. (Dermik) Hydrocortisone in cream base. **1%:** Tube 1 oz, Jar 4 oz. **2.5%:** Tube 1 oz, 2 oz.
Use: Corticosteroid, topical.

HYTONE LOTION 1%. (Dermik) Hydrocortisone 1% (10 mg/ml). Bot. 120 ml.
Use: Corticosteroid, topical.

HYTONE LOTION 2.5%. (Dermik) Hydrocortisone 2 1/2% (25 mg/ml) in lotion base. Bot. 60 ml.
Use: Corticosteroid, topical.

HYTONE OINTMENT. (Dermik) Hydrocortisone in ointment base. **1%:** Tube 28.3 Gm, 113.4 Gm. **2.5%:** Tube 28.3 Gm.
Use: Corticosteroid, topical.

HYTRIN. (Abbott/Burroughs Wellcome) Terazosin HCl 1 mg, 2 mg or 5 mg/Tab. Bot. 100s, 500s, UD 100s.
Use: Antihypertensive.

HYTUSS TABLETS. (Hyrex) Guaifenesin 100 mg/Tab. Bot. 100s, 1000s.
Use: Expectorant.

HYTUSS-2X. (Hyrex) Guaifenesin 200 mg/Cap. Bot. 100s, 1000s.
Use: Expectorant.

HYZINE-50. (Hyrex) Hydroxyzine HCl 50 mg as HCl/ml. Vial 10 ml.
Use: Antianxiety agent.

I

IBENZMETHYZIN. Name used for Procarbazine Hydrochloride.

IBERET. (Abbott) Ferrous sulfate 105 mg, ascorbic acid 150 mg, vitamins B_{12} 25 mcg, B_1 6 mg, B_2 6 mg, niacinamide 30 mg, B_6 5 mg/CR Filmtab. Bot. 60s, 500s.
Use: Vitamin/mineral supplement.

IBERET-500. (Abbott) Ascorbic acid 500 mg, ferrous sulfate 105 mg, vitamins B_1 6 mg, B_2 6 mg, B_3 30 mg, B_5 10 mg, B_6 5 mg, B_{12} 25 mcg/CR Filmtab. Bot. 30s, 60s, 500s, UD 100s.
Use: Vitamin/mineral supplement.

IBERET-FOLIC-500 FILMTAB. (Abbott) Ferrous sulfate 105 mg, vitamin C 500 mg, niacinamide 30 mg, calcium pantothenate 10 mg, thiamine mononitrate 6 mg, B_2 6 mg, B_6 5 mg, folic acid 0.8 mg/CR Filmtab. Bot. 100s, 500s.
Use: Vitamin/mineral supplement.

IBERET LIQUID. (Abbott) Ferrous sulfate 78.75 mg, vitamins C 375 mg, B_{12} 18.75 mcg, B_1 4.5 mg, B_2 4.5 mg, B_3 22.5 mg, B_5 7.5 mg, B_6 3.75 mg sorbitol, parabens, alcohol 1%, dexpanthenol 2.5 mg/5 ml. Bot. 240 ml.
Use: Vitamin/mineral supplement.

IBERET-500 LIQUID, ORAL SOLUTION. (Abbott) Ferrous sulfate 78.75 mg, vitamins B_1 4.5 mg, B_2 4.5 mg, B_3 22.5 mg, B_5 7.5 mg, B_6 3.75 mg, B_{12} 18.75 mcg, C 112.5 mg, sorbitol, parabens/5 ml. Bot. 240 ml.
Use: Vitamin/mineral supplement.

IBEROL. (Abbott) Vitamins B_{12} 12.5 mcg, iron (as ferrous sulfate) 105 mg, C 75 mg (as sodium ascorbate), B_1 3 mg, B_2 3 mg, niacinamide 15 mg, B_6 1.5 mg, B_5 3 mg/Filmtab. Bot. 100s.
Use: Vitamin/mineral supplement.

IBEROL-F. (Abbott) Vitamins B_{12} 12.5 mcg, elemental iron (as 525 mg ferrous sulfate) 105 mg, folic acid 0.2 mg, C 75 mg, B_1 3 mg, B_2 3 mg, niacinamide 15 mg, B_6 1.5 mg, calcium pantothenate 3 mg/Filmtab. Bot. 100s.
Use: Vitamin/mineral supplement.

•**IBOPAMINE.** USAN.
Use: Dopaminergic agent (peripheral).

•**IBUFENAC.** USAN. (p-Isobutylphenyl-acetic acid).
Use: Antirheumatic (anti-inflammatory, analgesic and antipyretic).
See: Dytransin.

•**IBUPROFEN.**
Use: Nonsteroidal anti-inflammatory drug; analgesic.
See: Haltran, Tab. (Upjohn).
Ifen, Tab. (Everett).
Medipren, Tab., Capl. (McNeil Prods).
Motrin, Tab. (Upjohn).
Nuprin, Tab. (Bristol-Myers).
Rufen, Tab. (Boots).

•**IBUPROFEN ALUMINUM.** USAN.
Use: Anti-inflammatory.

•**IBUPROFEN PICONOL.** USAN.
Use: Topical anti-inflammatory.

IBU-TAB. (Alra) Ibuprofen 400 mg, 600 mg or 800 mg/Tab. Bot. 100s, 500s, 1000s, UD 100s.
Use: Nonsteroidal anti-inflammatory drug; analgesic.

•**IBUTILIDE FUMARATE.** USAN.
Use: Cardiac depressant.

ICE MINT. (Westwood) Stearic acid, synthetic cocoa butter, lanolin oil, camphor, menthol, beeswax, mineral oil, sodium borate, aromatic oils, emulsifiers, water. Jar 4 oz.
Use: Emollient, counterirritant.

I-CHLOR 0.5%. (Americal) Chloramphenicol 5 mg/ml. Bot. 7.5 ml, 15 ml.
Use: Anti-infective, ophthalmic.

•**ICHTHAMMOL,** U.S.P. XXII. Oint., U.S.P. XXII. Ichthynate. Isarol Oint. (Lilly) 10% and 20% ointment.
Use: Mild antiseptic in skin disorders.
W/Aluminum acetate, phenol, zinc oxide, boric acid, eucalyptol.
See: Lanaburn, Oint. (Lannett).
W/Aluminum hydroxide, phenol, zinc oxide, camphor, eucalyptol.
See: Almophen, Oint. (Bowman).
W/Benzocaine, resin cerate, carbolic acid, thymol, camphor, juniper tar, hexachlorophene.
See: Boil-Ease Anesthetic Drawing Salve (Commerce).
W/Benzocaine, tetracaine, resin cerate, thymol iodide.
See: Boilaid, Oint. (E. J. Moore).
W/Hydrocortisone acetate, benzocaine, oxyquinoline sulfate, ephedrine HCl.
See: Derma Medicone-HC (Medicone).
W/Naftalan, calamine, amber pet.
See: Naftalan, Oint. (Paddock).
W/Phenol, benzocaine, balsam peru, aluminum exsiccated, cade oil, eucalyptus oil, carbolic acid.
See: Alucaine, Oint. (Jenkins).

ICHTHYNATE.
See: Ichthammol.

•**ICOTIDINE.** USAN.
Use: Antagonist (to histamine H_2 and H_1 receptors).

•**ICTASOL.** USAN.
Use: Disinfectant.

ICTOTEST REAGENT TABLETS. (Ames) Reagent Tab. For urinary bilirubin. Bot. 100s.
Use: Diagnostic aid.

ICY HOT BALM. (Vicks) Methyl salicylate 29%, menthol 7.6%. Jar 3.5 oz, 7 oz.
Use: External analgesic.

ICY HOT CREAM. (Vicks) Methyl salicylate 30%, menthol 10%. Tube 0.25 oz, 1.25 oz, 3 oz.
Use: External analgesic.

ICY HOT STICK. (Vicks) Methyl salicylate 15%, menthol 8%. Stick 1.75 oz.
Use: External analgesic.

I.D.A. CAPSULES. (Goldline) Isometheptene mucate 65 mg, dichloralphenazone 100 mg, acetaminophen 324 mg/Cap. Bot. 100s.
Use: Analgesic.

IDAMYCIN. (Adria) Idarubicin HCl. Vial 5 mg, 10 mg.
Use: Antineoplastic agent.

•**IDARUBICIN HYDROCHLORIDE.** USAN.
Use: Antineoplastic.
See: Idamycin (Adria).

•**IDOXURIDINE,** U.S.P. XXII. Ophth. Oint., Soln., U.S.P. XXII. 5-Iodo-2′-deoxyuridine. Uridine; Dendroid; Kerecid; Ophthalmidine.
Use: Treatment of herpes simplex; antiviral.
See: Herplex, Ophthalmic Soln. (Allergan).
Stoxil, Ophthalmic Soln., Oint. (SmithKline).

I-DROPS. (Americal) Tetrahydrozoline HCl 0.5%. Ophthalmic soln. Bot. 0.5 oz
Use: Ophthalmic vasoconstrictor/mydriatic.

IFEN. (Everett) Ibuprofen 400 mg or 600 mg/Tab. Bot. 100s, 500s.
Use: Nonsteroidal anti-inflammatory drug; analgesic.

IFEX. (Mead Johnson Oncology) Ifosfamide 1 Gm or 3 Gm. Pow. for Inj. Vial single dose.
Use: Antineoplastic agent.

•**IFOSFAMIDE.** USAN.
Use: Investigative: Antineoplastic.

I-GENT. (Americal) Gentamicin sulfate 3 mg/ml. Ophthalmic soln. Bot. 5 ml.
Use: Anti-infective, ophthalmic.

IGEPAL Co-430. (General Aniline & Film) Nonoxynol 4.

IGEPAL Co-730. (General Aniline & Film) Nonoxynol 15.

IGEPAL Co-880. (General Aniline & Film) Nonoxynol 30.

I-HOMATRINE 5%. (Americal) Homatropine hydrobromide 5%. Ophthalmic soln. Bot. 5 ml.
Use: Cycloplegic mydriatic.

ILETIN I. (Lilly) Regular and modified insulin products from beef and pork.
Protamine Zinc: 40 units or 100 units/ml. Vial 10 ml.
Regular: 40 units or 100 units/ml. Vial 10 ml
Lente: 40 units or 100 units/ml. Vial 10 ml.
Semilente: 40 units or 100 units/ml. Vial 10 ml.
Ultralente: 40 units or 100 units/ml. Vial 10 ml.
NPH: 40 units or 100 units/ml. Vial 10 ml.
Use: Antidiabetic agent.

ILETIN II. (Lilly) Special insulin products prepared from purified beef or purified pork.
Regular: 100 units/ml. Vial 10 ml.
Lente: 100 units/ml. Vial 10 ml.
NPH: 100 units/ml. Vial 10 ml.
Protamine Zinc: 100 units/ml. Vial 10 ml.
Use: Antidiabetic agent.

ILETIN II CONCENTRATED. (Lilly) Purified pork regular insulin 500 units/ml. Vial 20 ml.
Use: Antidiabetic agent.

I-LIQUI-TEARS. (Americal) Artificial tear soln. w/ polyvinyl alcohol 1%, hydroxyethyl cellulose 0.5%, BAC 0.01%, EDTA, sodium Cl. Bot. 15 ml.
Use: Ophthalmic lubricant.

ILMOFOSINE. USAN.
Use: Antineoplastic.

ILOPAN. (Adria) Dexpanthenol 250 mg/ml. Amp. 2 ml, Disp. Syringe 2 ml.
Use: GI stimulant.

ILOPAN- CHOLINE. (Adria) Ilopan 50 mg, choline bitartrate 25 mg/Tab. Bot. 100s, 500s.
Use: GI stimulant.

ILOSONE. (Dista) Erythromycin estolate. **Cap.:** (Erythromycin base) 250 mg/Pulv. Bot. 24s, 100s, UD 100s, Blister pkg. 10 × 10s. **Liq.:** 125 mg or 250 mg/5 ml. Bot. 100 ml, 16 fl oz. **Tab.:** 500 mg. Bot. 50s. **Susp.:** 125 mg or 250 mg/5 ml. Bot. 10 ml.
Use: Anti-infective.

ILOSONE CHEWABLE. (Dista) Erythromycin estolate 125 mg or 250 mg/Tab. Bot. 50s.
Use: Anti-infective.

ILOTYCIN GLUCEPTATE I.V. (Dista) Erythromycin gluceptate. Vial. I.V. 1 Gm, vial 30 ml. Box 1s.
Use: Anti-infective.

ILOTYCIN OPHTHALMIC OINTMENT. (Dista) Erythromycin 5 mg/Gm. Tube 3.75 Gm, UD 1 Gm/dose tube. Box 24s.
Use: Anti-infective.

ILOZYME. (Adria) Pancrelipase equivalent to lipase 11,000 units, protease 30,000 units, amylase 30,000 units/Tab. Bot. 250s.
Use: Digestive enzymes.

I-LUBE. (Americal) Petrolatum ophthalmic ointment. Tube 0.125 oz
Use: Ophthalmic lubricant.

I.L.X. B12 ELIXIR. (Kenwood) Liver fraction 98 mg, iron 102 mg, vitamins B_1 5 mg, B_2 2 mg, nicotinamide 10 mg, B_{12} 10 mcg/15 ml, alcohol 8%. Bot. 12 oz
Use: Vitamin/mineral supplement.

I.L.X. B12 TABLETS. (Kenwood) Iron 37.5 mg, vitamins C 120 mg, B_{12} 12 mcg, desiccated liver 130 mg, B_1 2 mg, B_2 2 mg/Tab. Bot. 100s.
Use: Vitamin/mineral supplement.

I.L.X. ELIXIR. (Kenwood) Iron 70 mg, liver concentrate 98 mg, vitamins B_1 5 mg, B_2 2 mg, nicotinamide 10 mg/15 ml, alcohol 8%. Bot. 12 oz.
Use: Vitamin/mineral supplement.

•**IMAFEN HYDROCHLORIDE.** USAN.
Use: Antidepressant.

•**IMAZODAN HYDROCHLORIDE.** USAN.
Use: Cardiotonic.

•**IMCARBOFOS.** USAN.
Use: Anthelmintic.

IMENOL. (Sig) Guaiacol 0.1 Gm, eucalyptol 0.08 Gm, iodoform 0.02 Gm, camphor 0.05 Gm/ml. Vial 30 ml.
Use: Expectorant.

I-METHASONE 0.1%. (American) Dexamethasone sodium phosphate 0.1%. Ophthalmic soln. Bot. 5 ml.
Use: Corticosteroid.

IMFERON. (Fisons) An iron-dextran complex containing iron 50 mg/ml. Amp. 2 ml. Box 10s. Vial (w/phenol 0.5%) 10 ml. Box 2s.
Use: Iron supplement.

•**IMIDECYL IODINE.** USAN. 1-Carboxymethylene-1-(2-ethanol)-2-alkyl(C_7 to C_{17})-2-imidazolinium chloride-tridecyl polyoxyethylene-ethanol-iodine complex.
Use: Anti-infective (topical).

•**IMIDOCARB HCl.** USAN. 3,3′-Di-2-imidazolin-2-ylcarbanilidedihydrochloride.
Use: Veterinary antiprotozoal.

•**IMIDOLINE HYDROCHLORIDE.** USAN. 1-(m-

Chlorophenyl)-3-(2-(dimethylamino)ethyl)-2-imidazolidinone hydrochloride.
Use: Tranquilizer.

•**IMIDUREA,** N.F. XVII.
Use: Antimicrobial.

•**IMILOXAN HYDROCHLORIDE.** USAN.
Use: Antidepressant.

IMIPEMIDE.
Use: Anti-infective.
See: Imipenem, USAN.

•**IMIPENEM.** USAN.
Use: Antibacterial.
W/Cilastatin sodium.
See: Primaxin, Inj (Merck, Sharp & Dohme).

•**IMIPRAMINE HCl,** U.S.P. XXII. Inj., Tab., U.S.P. XXII. 5H-Dibenz [b,f] azepine-5-propanamine, 10,11-dihydro-N,N-dimethyl-, HCl. 5-(3-Dimethyl-aminopropyl)-10,11,dihydro-5H-dibenz-(b,f) azepine HCl. Praminil. Berkomine, IA-Pram, Impamin, Iprogen, Norpramine, & Tofranil HCl salts.
Use: Antidepressant.
See: Janimine, Tab. (Abbott).
Presamine, Tab. (USV).
Tofranil, Tab., Amp. (Geigy).
W.D.D., Tab. (Solvay).

IMIPRAMINE PAMOATE. bis 5-[3-(Di-methyl-amino) propyl]-10,11-dihydro-5H-dibenz [b,f] azapine compound (2:1)with 4,4-methylenebis-[3-hydroxy-2-naphthoic acid].
Use: Antidepressant.
See: Tofranil-PM, Cap. (Geigy).

•**IMMUNE GLOBULIN,** U.S.P. XXII. Immune Serum Globulin Human. Gamma-globulin fraction of normal human plasma. Vial 10 ml. Tubex 1 ml, 2 ml w/thimerosal 1:10,000.
Use: Modification of active measles, prophylaxis of hepatitis, treatment of immune deficiencies.
See: Gamastan, Vial (Cutter).
Gamimune, Vial (Cutter).
Gammar, Vial (Armour).
Immuglobin, Vial (Savage).

IMMUNE GLOBULIN, Rh_0 (D).
See: Gamulin Rh (Parke-Davis).
HypRho-D (Cutter).
RhoGAM (Ortho Diagnostics).

IMMUNE SERUMS.
See: Cytomegalovirus Immune Globulin Intravenous (Human) (Massachusetts Public Health Biologic Laboratories).
Human Measles Immune Serum (Various Mfr.).
Immune Serum Globulin (Human).

IMMUNE SERUM (ANIMAL).
See: Botulism Antitoxin, Vial (Lederle).
Diphtheria Antitoxin.
Gas Gangrene Antitoxin.
Tetanus Antitoxin.
Tetanus Antitoxin—Gas Gangrene Combined.

IMMUNE SERUM (HUMAN).
See: Hypertussis, Vial (Cutter).
Poliomyelitis Immune Globulin (Various Mfr.).

IMMUNEX CRP. (Wampole) Two-minute latex agglutination slide test for the qualitative detection of C-Reactive protein in serum. Kit 100s.
Use: Diagnostic aid.

IMODIUM CAPSULES. (Janssen) Loperamide 2 mg/Cap. Bot. 100s, 500s, UD 100s.
Use: Antidiarrheal.

IMODIUM LIQUID. (Janssen) Loperamide 0.2 mg/ml. Bot. 120 ml.
Use: Antidiarrheal.

IMODIUM A-D. (McNeil) Loperamide 1 mg/5 ml, alcohol 5.25%.
Use: Antidiarrheal.

IMOGAM RABIES IMMUNE GLOBULIN. (Merieux Institute) Rabies immune globulin (human) 150 IU/ml. Vials 2 ml, 10 ml in tamper proof box.
Use: Rabies prophylaxis agent.

IMOLAMINE. B.A.N. 4-(2-Diethylaminoethyl)-5-imino-3-phenyl-1,2,4-oxadiazoline.
Use: Treatment of angina pectoris.

IMOVAX RABIES I.D. (Merieux Institute) Rabies vaccine 0.25 IU/0.1 ml for I.D. administration for pre-exposure treatment only. Wistar rabies virus strain PM-1503-3M grown in human diploid cell culture. Vaccine is lypholized inside an ID syringe sealed in vaccum tube. In single dose syringe w/1 vial diluent.
Use: Rabies prophylaxis agent.

IMOVAX RABIES VACCINE. (Merieux Institute) Merieux rabies vaccine, Wistar rabies virus strain PM-1503-3M grown in human diploid cell cultures. Tamper proof box w/1 ml vaccine, syringe, needles, and 1 vial diluent.
Use: Rabies prophylaxis agent.

IMPACT. (Approved) Belladonna alkaloids 0.16 mg, phenylpropanolamine HCl 50 mg, chlorpheniramine maleate 1 mg, pheniramine maleate 12.5 mg/Cap. Pack 12s, 24s. Vial 15s, 30s, Bot. 1000s.
Use: Anticholinergic/antispasmodic, decongestant, antihistamine.

IMPROMEN. (Janssen) Bromperidol decanoate.
Use: Antipsychotic.

IMPROMEN DECANOAS. (Janssen) Bromperidol decanoate.
Use: Antipsychotic.

•**IMPROMIDINE HYDROCHLORIDE.** USAN.
Use: Diagnostic aid.

IMURAN. (Burroughs Wellcome) **Tab.:** Azathioprine 50 mg/Tab. Bot. 100s. **Inj.:** Azathioprine 100 mg/20 ml. Vial.
Use: Immunosuppressive agent.

INACTIVATED DIAGNOSTIC DIPHTHERIA TOXIN.
See: Diphtheria Toxin for Schick Test, U.S.P. XXII.

I-NAPHLINE 0.1%. (American) Naphazoline HCl 0.1%. Ophthalmic soln. Bot. 15 ml.
Use: Vasoconstrictor/mydriatic.

INAPSINE. (Janssen) Droperidol 2.5 mg/ml. Amp. 2 ml, 5 ml, 10 ml. Box 10s. Multi-dose Vial w/

methylparaben 1.8 mg, propylparaben 0.2 mg, lactic acid/10 ml. Box 10s.
Use: General anesthetic.
W/Fentanyl citrate.
See: Innovar, Inj. (Janssen).

INCREMIN W/IRON. (Lederle) l-Lysine HCl 300 mg, vitamins B_{12} 25 mcg, B_1 10 mg, B_6 5 mg, ferric pyrophosphate soluble 30 mg, sorbitol 3.5 Gm, alcohol 0.75%/5 ml. Syr. Bot. 4 fl oz, 16 fl oz.
Use: Vitamin/mineral supplement.

•**INDACRINONE.** USAN.
Use: Antihypertensive, diuretic.

INDALONE.
See: Butopyronoxyl (Various Mfr.).

•**INDAPAMIDE.** USAN.
Use: Antihypertensive, diuretic.
See: Lozol, Tab. (Rorer).

•**INDECAINIDE HYDROCHLORIDE.** USAN.
Use: Cardiac depressant.
See: Decabid (Lilly).

•**INDELOXAZINE HYDROCHLORIDE.** USAN.
Use: Antidepressant.

INDERAL INJECTION. (Wyeth-Ayerst) Propranolol HCl 1 mg/ml. Amp. 1 ml. Box 10s.
Use: Beta-adrenergic blocking agent.

INDERAL TABLETS. (Wyeth-Ayerst) Propranolol HCl 10 mg, 20 mg, 40 mg, 60 mg or 80 mg/Tab. Bot. 100s, 1000s, UD 100s.
Use: Beta-adrenergic blocking agent.

INDERAL-LA. (Wyeth-Ayerst) Propranolol HCl 80 mg, 120 mg or 160 mg/SR Cap. Bot. 100s, 1000s, UD 100s.
Use: Beta-adrenergic blocking agent.

•**INDERIDE.** (Wyeth-Ayerst) Propranolol HCl 40 mg, hydrochlorothiazide 25 mg/Tab. Bot. 100s, 1000s, UD 100s. Propranolol HCl 80 mg, hydrochlorothiazide 25 mg/Tab. Bot. 100s, 1000s, UD 100s.
Use: Antihypertensive combination.

•**INDERIDE LA CAPSULES.** (Wyeth-Ayerst) Propranolol HCl/hydrochlorothiazide Long Acting Caps: 80 mg/50 mg, 120 mg/50 mg or 160 mg/50 mg. Bot. 100s.
Use: Antihypertensive combination.

INDIAN GUM.
See: Karaya Gum.

INDIGO CARMINE. (Hynson, Westcott & Dunning) Sodium indigotindisulfonate 8 mg/ml. Amp. 5 ml. Box 10s, 100s.
Use: Diagnostic aid.
See: Sodium indigotindisulfonate.

INDIGO CARMINE SOLUTION. (Hynson, Westcott & Dunning) Indigotindisulfonate sodium inj. (0.8% aqueous soln. sodium salt of indigotindisulfonic acid) 40 mg/5 ml. Amp. 5 ml, 10s.
Use: Diagnostic aid.

•**INDIGOTINDISULFONATE SODIUM,** U.S.P. XXII. Inj., U.S.P. XXII. 1H-Indole-5-sulfonic acid, 2-(1,3-dihydro-4-oxo-5-sulfo-2H-indol-2-ylidene)-2,3-dihydro-3-oxo-, sodium salt. Indigo Carmine, Amp. (Various Mfr.).
Use: Diagnostic aid (cystoscopy).
See: Sodium Indigotindisulfonate.

•**INDIUM In III OXYQUINOLINE.** USAN.
Use: Radioactive agent, diagnostic aid.

•**INDIUM In 111 PENTETRATE INJECTION,** U.S.P. XXII.
Use: Diagnostic aid for cardiac output determination.

INDOCIN. (Merck, Sharp & Dohme) Indomethacin. **Cap.:** 25 mg. Bot. 100s, 1000s, UD 100s. Unit-of-use 100s; 50 mg. Bot. 100s, UD 100s. **Supp.:** 50 mg. Pkg. 30s. **Oral Susp.:** 25 mg/5 ml, alcohol 1%, sorbitol 0.1%. Bot. 237 ml.
Use: Nonsteroidal anti-inflammatory drug; analgesic.

INDOCIN I.V. (Merck, Sharp & Dohme) Indomethacin sodium trihydrate equivalent to 1 mg indomethacin/Vial. Vial single dose.
Use: Agent for patent ductus arteriosus.

INDOCIN SR. (Merck, Sharp & Dohme) Indomethacin 75 mg/SR Cap. Unit-of-Use 30s, 60s.
Use: Nonsteroidal anti-inflammatory drug; analgesic.

•**INDOCYANINE GREEN,** U.S.P. XXII. Sterile, U.S.P. XXII. A tricarbocyanine dye. 1H-Benz [e] indolium, 2-[7-[1,3-dihydro-1,1-dimethyl-3-(4-sulfobutyl)-2H-benz [e] indol-2-ylidene]-1,3,5-heptatrienyl]-1,1-dimethyl-3-(4-sulfobutyl)-, hydroxide, inner salt, sodium salt.
Use: Diagnostic aid (cardiac output determination, hepatic function determination).
See: Cardio-Green, Inj. (Hynson, Westcott & Dunning).

INDOGESIC. (Century) Acetaminophen 32.5 mg, butalbital 50 mg/Tab. Bot. 100s, 1000s.
Use: Analgesic, sedative/hypnotic.

INDOKLON. Hexafluorodiethyl ether. Flurothyl. Bis-(2,2,2-trifluorethyl)ether.
Use: Shock inducing agent (convulsant).

•**INDOLAPRIL HYDROCHLORIDE.** USAN.
Use: Antihypertensive.

INDO-LEMMON. (Lemmon) Indomethacin 25 mg or 50 mg/Cap. Bot. 100s, 500s, 1000s.
Use: Nonsteroidal anti-inflammatory drug; analgesic.

•**INDOLIDAN.** USAN.
Use: Cardiotonic.

INDOMETH CAPS. (Major) Indomethacin 25 mg or 50 mg/Tab. **25 mg:** Bot. 100s, 1000s. **50 mg:** Bot. 100s, 500s.
Use: Nonsteroidal anti-inflammatory drug; analgesic.

•**INDOMETHACIN,** U.S.P. XXII. Cap., Supp., Extended-release Cap., Suspension. 1-(p-Chlorobenzoyl)-5-methoxy-2-methyl-indole-3-acetic acid.
Use: Anti-inflammatory agent (nonsteroid).
See: Indocin, Cap., S.R. Cap., I.V., Oral Susp., Supp. (Merck, Sharp & Dohme).
Indo-Lemmon, Cap. (Lemmon).

•**INDOMETHACIN SODIUM.** USAN.
Use: Anti-inflammatory.

•**INDOPROFEN.** USAN.
Use: Analgesic, anti-inflammatory.

•**INDORAMIN.** USAN. N-[1-(2-Indol-3-ylethyl)-4-piperidyl]benzamide. 3-[2-(4-Benzamidopiperidino)ethyl]indole.
Use: Antihypertensive.

•**INDORAMIN HYDROCHLORIDE.** USAN.
Use: Antihypertensive.

•**INDORENATE HYDROCHLORIDE.** USAN.
Use: Antihypertensive.

•**INDOXOLE.** USAN.
Use: Antipyretic, anti-inflammatory.

•**INDRILINE HYDROCHLORIDE.** USAN.
Use: Stimulant.

I-NEOCORT. (American) Neomycin sulfate 5 mg, hydrocortisone acetate 15 mg/5 ml. Ophthalmic susp. Bot. 5 ml.
Use: Anti-infective, corticosteroid.

I-NEOSPOR. (American) Polymixin B sulfate, gramicidin, neomycin sulfate ophthalmic soln. Bot. 10 ml.
Use: Anti-infective.

INFACAPS A & D. (Lannett) Vitamins A 3000 IU, D 800 IU/Cap. Bot. 1000s, 5000s.
Use: Vitamin supplement.

INFANTOL PINK. (Scherer) Paregoric (equivalent) contains opium 15 mg/fl oz, bismuth subsalicylate, calcium carageenan, pectin, zinc phenolsulfonate, alcohol 2%. Susp. Bot. 4 oz, 8 oz, pt.
Use: Antidiarrheal.

INFANT'S NO-ASPIRIN DROPS. (Walgreen) Acetaminophen 80 mg/0.8 ml. Non-alcoholic. Bot. 15 ml.
Use: Analgesic.

INFARUB CREAM. (Whitehall) Methyl salicylate 35%, menthol 10% in vanishing cream base. Tube 1.25 oz, 3.5 oz.
Use: External analgesic.

INFATUSS. (Scott/Cord) Dextromethorphan HBr 7.2 mg, chlorpheniramine maleate 1.1 mg, phenylpropanolamine HCl 4.8 mg, ammonium Cl 50 mg/5 ml. Bot. 4 oz, pt, gal.
Use: Antitussive, antihistamine, decongestant, expectorant.

INFLAMASE MILD 1/8% OPHTHALMIC SOLUTION. (CooperVision) Prednisolone sodium phosphate 0.125% (equivalent to prednisolone phosphate 0.11%). Bot. 5 ml, 10 ml w/dropper.
Use: Corticosteroid, ophthalmic.

INFLAMASE FORTE 1% OPHTHALMIC SOLUTION. (CooperVision) Prednisolone sodium phosphate 1% (equivalent to prednisolone phosphate 0.91%). Bot. 5 ml, 10 ml.
Use: Corticoisteroid, ophthalmic.

•**INFLUENZA VIRUS VACCINE,** U.S.P. XXII.
Use: Active immunizing agent.
See: Fluzone, Inj. (Squibb/Connaught).

INFLUENZAE TYPE B SERUM (RABBIT) ANTI-HEMOPHILUS. (Various Mfr.) The sterile suspension of formaldehyde-killed influenza virus, type A, Asian strain grown in the extra-embryonic fluid of chick eggs.
Use: Agent for immunization.

INFLUENZA VIRUS VACCINE.
Lederle—Bivalent types A and B. A/Port Chalmers/1/73 (h3n2)-700 CCA units, B/Hong-Kong/5/72-500 CCA units. Vial 5 ml.
Wyeth—Types A and B Tubex Cartridge-Needle Unit 0.5 ml, 10s. Vial 5 ml.
Use: Agent for immunization.
See: Fluzone, Inj. (Squibb/Connaught).

INGADINE TABS. (Major) Guanethidine sulfate 10 mg or 25 mg/Tab. Bot. 100s, 1000s.
Use: Antihypertensive.

INH. (Ciba) Isoniazid 300 mg/Tab.
Use: Antituberculous agent.
See: Rimactane/INH, Dual Pack (Ciba).

INHAL-AID. (Key)
Use: Drug delivery system for metered dose inhalers.

INNERCLEAN HERBAL LAXATIVE. (Last) Senna leaf powder, psyllium seed, buckthorne, anise seed, fennel seed. Bot. 1 oz, 2 oz.
Use: Laxative.

INNERTABS. (Last) Senna leaf powder and psyllium seed tablets. Bot. 80s, 200s.
Use: Laxative.

INNOVAR INJECTION. (Janssen) Fentanyl citrate 0.05 mg, droperidol 2.5 mg/ml. Amp. 2 ml, 5 ml. Box of 10s.
Use: Narcotic analgesic, general anesthetic.

INOCOR LACTATE. (Winthrop Products) Amrinone lactate (base equivalent) 5 mg/ml, sodium metabisulfite 0.25 mg. Amp. 20 ml. Box 5s.
Use: Short-term management of congestive heart failure.

INOPHYLLINE.
See: Aminophylline (Various Mfr.).

INOSIT.
See: Inositol (Various Mfr.).

INOSITOL. 1,2,3,5/4,6-Cyclohexanehexol. Commercial solvents (Bios 1,Hexahydroxycyclohexane, Inosit, Dambose).
Use: Lipotropic.
W/Choline bitartrate, vitamins, minerals.
W/Choline Cl, dl-methionine, vitamin B_{12}.
See: Cho-Meth, Vial (Kenyon).
See: Lypo-B, Vial (Rocky Mtn.).
W/Methionine, choline bitartrate, liver desiccated, vitamin B_{12}.
See: Limvic, Tab. (Briar).
W/Panthenol, choline Cl, vitamins, minerals, estrone, testosterone.
See: Geramine, Inj. (Brown).
W/Panthenol, choline Cl, vitamins, minerals, estrone, testosterone, polydigestase.
See: Geramine, Tab. (Brown).

•**INOSITOL NIACINATE.** USAN. Myo-Inositol hexanicotinate. Meso-inositol hexanicotinate, hexanicotinate. Meso-inositol hexanicotinate. Hexopal; Mesonex.

Use: Peripheral vasodilator.
INOSITOL NICOTINATE. Inositol Niacinate.
INPERSOL W/DEXTROSE. (Abbott Hospital Prods) Dextrose 1.5%, 2.5% or 4.25%, sodium Cl 140.5 mEq, calcium Cl 3.5 mEq, magnesium Cl 1.5 mEq, sodium lactate 445 mEq/100 ml. **1.5% Dextrose:** 1000 ml, 2000 ml. **2.5% Dextrose:** 1000 ml, 2000 ml. **4.25% Dextrose:** 2000 ml.
Use: Peritoneal dialysis solution.
INPERSOL-LM W/DEXTROSE. (Abbott Hospital Prods) Inpersol-LM w/dextrose 1.5%, 2.5% or 4.25%. **1.5% Dextrose:** 1000 ml, 2000 ml flexible container. **2.5% Dextrose:** 1000 ml, 2000 ml flexible container. **4.25% Dextrose:** 2000 ml flexible container.
Use: Peritoneal dialysis solution.
INPROQUONE. B.A.N. 2,5-Di(aziridin-1-yl)-3,6-dipropoxy-1,4-benzoquinone.
Use: Antineoplastic agent.
INSPIREASE. (Key).
Use: Drug delivery system for metered-dose inhalers.
INSTA-CHAR. (Kerr) **Regular:** Aqueous suspension activated charcoal 50 Gm/8 oz. **Pediatric:** Aqueous suspension activated charcoal 15 Gm/4 oz.
Use: Antidote.
INSTA-GLUCOSE. (ICN) Undiluted USP glucose. UD tube containing liquid glucose 31 Gm.
Use: Glucose elevating agent.
INST-E-VITE. (Barth's) Vitamin E 100 IU or 200 IU/Cap. **100 IU:** Bot. 100s, 500s, 1000s. **200 IU:** Bot. 100s, 250s, 500s.
Use: Vitamin E supplement.
INSULATARD NPH. (Nordisk) Isophane purified pork insulin suspension 100 IU/ml. Vial 10 ml.
Use: Antidiabetic agent.
INSULATARD NPH HUMAN. (Nordisk-USA) Human insulin isophane suspension 100 IU/ml.
Use: Antidiabetic agent.
INSULIN. U.S.P. XXII. Inj., U.S.P. XXII.
Use: Antidiabetic.
See: Iletin Prods. (Lilly).
Insulin Prods. (Squibb).
INSULIN. (Nordisk) Insulatard NPH Mixtard Velosulin.
Use: Antidiabetic agent.
INSULIN, DALANATED. USAN.
Use: Antidiabetic.
INSULIN, GLOBIN ZINC INJECTION.
Use: Antidiabetic agent.
INSULIN HUMAN, U.S.P. XXII. Inj., U.S.P. XXII.
Use: Antidiabetic.
INSULIN I-125. USAN.
Use: Radioactive agent.
INSULIN I-131. USAN.
Use: Radioactive agent.
INSULIN INJECTION, U.S.P. XXII. Insulin, insulin HCl.
Use: Antidiabetic.
INSULIN, NEUTRAL. USAN.
Use: Antidiabetic.
INSULIN NOVO RAPITARD. Biphasic Insulin Injection, B.A.N.
•**INSULIN, PROTAMINE ZINC SUSPENSION,** U.S.P. XXII. 40 or 100 units/ml. Vials 10 ml.
Use: Antidiabetic.
•**INSULIN ZINC SUSPENSION,** U.S.P. XXII.
Use: Antidiabetic.
See: Lente Insulin, Vial (Lilly).
•**INSULIN ZINC SUSPENSION, EXTENDED,** U.S.P. XXII.
Use: Antidiabetic.
•**INSULIN ZINC SUSPENSION, PROMPT,** U.S.P. XXII.
Use: Antidiabetic, hypoglycemic.
INTAL CAPSULES. (Fisons) Cromolyn sodium 20 mg, lactose powder 20 mg/Cap. Box 60s, 120s.
Use: Respiratory inhalant product.
INTAL INHALER. (Fisons) Cromolyn sodium inhalation aerosol 800 mcg/actuation. Canister 8.1 Gm, 14.2 Gm.
Use: Respiratory inhalant product.
INTAL NEBULIZER SOLUTION. (Fisons) Cromolyn sodium 20 mg in 2 ml distilled water for use with a power operated nebulizer unit. Box 60s, 120s, Amp. 2 ml.
Use: Respiratory inhalant product.
INTENSOL. (Roxane) A system of concentrated solutions of drugs w/calibrated dropper:
Chlorpromazine HCl 30 mg or 100 mg/ml.
Dexamethasone 1 mg/ml.
Dihydrotachysterol 0.2 mg/ml.
Hydrochlorothiazide 100 mg/ml.
Prednisone 5 mg/ml.
Thioridazine HCl 30 mg or 100 mg/ml.
INTERCEPT CONTRACEPTIVE INSERTS. (Advanced Care) Nonoxynol-9 5.56% at pH 4.5. Starter 12 inserts w/applicator. Refill 12 inserts.
Use: Contraceptive insert.
INTEGRIN CAPS. (Winthrop Products) Oxypertine.
Use: Anxiolytic, tranquilizer.
•**INTERFERON.** USAN. A family of naturally occurring, small protein molecules with molecular weights of approximately 15,000 to 21,000 daltons. They are formed by the interaction of animal cells with viruses capable of conferring on animal cells resistance to virus infection. Three major classes of interferons have been identified: alpha, beta, and gamma. Interferon was first derived from human white blood cells and originally used in Finland.
Use: Antineoplastic, antiviral. Treatment of breast cancer lymphoma, multiple melanoma and malignant melanoma.
See: Intron-A, Inj. (Schering).
•**INTERFERON ALFA-2A.** USAN.
Use: Antineoplastic, antiviral.
See: Roferon-A (Roche).
•**INTERFERON ALFA-2B.** USAN.
Use: Antineoplastic, antiviral.

See: Intron-A (Schering).
•**INTERFERON ALFA-N1.** USAN.
Use: Antiviral, antineoplastic.
See: Wellferon (Burroughs Wellcome).
•**INTEFERON ALFA-N3.** Formerly Leukocyte Interferon.
Use: Antiviral, antineoplastic.
•**INTERFERON GAMMA-1B.** USAN.
Use: Antineoplastic, antiviral, immunoregulator.
See: Actimmune (Genentech).
INTESTINAL ANTI-INFLAMMATORY AGENTS.
Use: Ulcerative colitis.
See: Dipentum (Pharmacia).
Rowasa (Solvay).
INTRALIPID 10% I.V. FAT EMULSION. (KabiVitrum) I.V. fat emulsion containing soybean oil 10%, egg yolk phospholipids 1.2%, glycerin 2.25% and water for injection. I.V. Flask 50 ml, 100 ml, 250 ml, 500 ml.
Use: Parenteral nutritional supplement.
INTRALIPID 20% I.V. FAT EMULSION. (KabiVitrum) I.V. fat emulsion containing soybean oil 20%, egg yolk phospholipids 1.2%, glycerin 2.25% and water for injection. I.V. Flask 50 ml, 100 ml, 250 ml, 500 ml.
Use: Parenteral nutritional supplement.
INTRA-SUL. (Torigian) Sodium thiosulfate, sodium sulfide, sulfur. Amp. 2 ml. 6s, 25s, 100s.
INTRAVAL SODIUM.
See: Pentothal Sodium, Preps. (Abbott).
•**INTRAZOLE.** USAN. 1-(p-Chlorobenzoyl)-3-(1H-tetrazol-5-ylmethyl) indole.
Use: Anti-inflammatory.
•**INTRIPTYLINE HYDROCHLORIDE.** USAN.
Use: Antidepressant.
INTRON-A FOR INJECTION. (Schering) Interferon alfa-2b (IFN-alpha 2; rIFN-α2; α-2-interferon) recombinant as 3 million, 5 million, 10 million, 20 million or 50 million IU/Vial. Subcutaneous or intramuscular injection. Vial 1s w/diluent.
Use: Antineoplastic agent.
INTROPAQUE LIQUID. (Lafayette) Barium sulfate 60% w/v suspension. Bot. gal. Case 4 Bot.
Use: Radiopaque agent.
INTROPIN 200 mg. (DuPont Critical Care) Dopamine HCl 40 mg/ml, sodium bisulfite 1% as an antioxidant. Vial 5 ml. Box 20s; Amp. 5 ml. Box 20s; Prefilled additive Syr. 5 ml. Box 5s.
Use: Vasopressor used in shock.
INTROPIN 400 mg. (DuPont Critical Care) Dopamine HCl 80 mg/ml, sodium bisulfite 1% as an antioxidant. Vial 5 ml. Box 20s.; Prefilled additive Syringe 5 ml. Box 5s.
Use: Vasopressor used in shock.
INTROPIN 800 mg. (DuPont Critical Care) Dopamine HCl 160 mg/ml, sodium bisulfite 1% as an antioxidant. Vial 5 ml. Box 20s.; Prefilled additive syringe 5 ml. Box 5s.
Use: Vasopressor used in shock.
INULIN. (American Critical Care) Purified inulin 5 Gm/50 ml sodium Cl 0.9%, sodium hydroxide to adjust pH. Amp. 50 ml.
Use: Diagnostic aid.
•**INULIN IN SODIUM CHLORIDE INJECTION,** U.S.P. XXII.
Use: Diagnostic aid.
INVERSINE. (Merck, Sharp & Dohme) Mecamylamine HCl 2.5 mg/Tab. Bot. 100s.
Use: Antihypertensive.
INVERT SUGAR. (Abbott) 10% soln. Bot. 1000 ml.
Use: Parenteral nutritional supplement.
See: Emetrol, Liq. (Rorer).
Travert, Soln. (Travenol).
•**INVERT SUGAR INJECTION,** U.S.P. XXII.
Use: Replenisher (fluid and nutrient).
•**IOBENZAMIC ACID.** USAN. N-3-(3-Amino-2,4,6-triiodobenzoyl)-N-phenyl-β-alanine. Osbil. (Mallinkcrodt).
Use: Contrast medium for cholecystography.
•**IOCARMATE MEGLUMINE.** USAN.
Use: Diagnostic aid.
•**IOCARMIC ACID.** USAN. 5,5′-(Adipoyldiamino)-bis-(2,4,6-tri-iodo-N-methylisophthalamic acid). Dimer X is a sterile solution of the meglumine salt.
Use: Radiopaque substance.
•**IOCETAMIC ACID,** U.S.P. XXII. Tab., U.S.P. XXII. N-Acetyl-N-(3-amino-2,4,6-triiodophenyl)-2-methylalanine. 3-(N-3-Amino-2,4,6-tri-iodophenyl)acetamido-2-methylpropionic acid.
Use: Diagnostic aid (radiopaque medium).
IOCON GEL. (Owen) Polyoxyethylene ethers, coal tar solution, lopol (a cationic polymer), alcohol 1%, benzalkonium Cl in a non-ionic/amphoteric base. Tube 3.5 oz
Use: Antiseborrheic.
•**IODAMIDE.** USAN. 3-Acetamido-5-(acetamidomethyl)-2,4,6-triiodobenzoic acid. α,5-Di(acetamido)-2,4,6-tri-iodo-m-toluic acid.
Use: Radiopaque, diagnostic aid.
•**IODAMIDE MEGLUMIDE.** USAN.
Use: Radiopaque, diagnostic aid.
W/Combinations:
See: Renovue-65, Vial (Squibb).
Renovue-Dip, Vial (Squibb).
IODEX. (Medtech) Iodine 4.7% in petrolatum ointment base. Jar 1 oz, 14 oz.
Use: Antiseptic, germicide.
IODEX W/METHYL SALICYLATE. (Medtech) Iodine 4.7%, methyl salicylate 4.8% in petrolatum ointment base.
Use: Antiseptic, external analgesic.
•**IODIDE,SODIUM, I-123 CAPSULES,** U.S.P. XXII.
Use: Diagnostic aid (thyroid function determination).
•**IODIDE, SODIUM, I-123 TABLETS,** U.S.P. XXII.
Use: Diagnostic aid (thyroid function determination).
•**IODIDE, SODIUM, I-125 CAPSULES,** U.S.P. XXII.

Use: Diagnostic aid (thyroid function determination), radioactive agent.

IODIDE, SODIUM, I-125 SOLUTION, U.S.P. XXII.
Use: Diagnostic aid (thyroid function determination), radioactive agent.

IODIDE, SODIUM, I-131 CAPSULES, U.S.P. XXII.
Use: Antineoplastic, diagnostic aid (thyroid function determination), radioactive agent.

IODIDE, SODIUM, I-131 SOLUTION, U.S.P. XXII.
Use: Antineoplastic, diagnostic aid (thyroid function determination), radioactive agent.

IODINATED GLYCEROL. B.A.N. A mixture of iodinated dimers of glycerol.
Use: Mucolytic expectorant.
See: Organidin, Elix., Soln., Tab. (Wallace).

IODINATED I-125 ALBUMIN INJECTION, U.S.P. XXII.
Use: Diagnostic aid (blood volume determination), radioactive agent.

IODINATED I-131 ALBUMIN AGGREGATED INJECTION, U.S.P. XXII.
Use: Radioactive agent.

IODINATED I-131 ALBUMIN INJECTION, U.S.P. XXII.
Use: Diagnostic aid (blood volume determination and intrathecal imaging), radioactive agent.

IODINATED HUMAN SERUM ALBUMIN.
See: Albumotope (Squibb).

IODINE, U.S.P. XXII. Topical Soln., Strong Soln., Tincture, U.S.P. XXII.
Use: Topical anti-infective; source of iodine.
See: Kelp, Tab. (Quality Generics).

IODINE 131: CAPSULES DIAGNOSTIC-CAPSULES THERAPEUTIC-SOLUTION THERAPEUTIC ORAL.
See: Iodotope (Squibb).

IODINE CACODYLATE, COLLOIDAL. Cacodyne Iodine.

IODINE COMBINATION.
See: Calcidrine, Syr. (Abbott).

IODINE-IODOPHOR.
See: Betadine, Preps. (Purdue Frederick).
Isodine, Preps. (Blair).

IODINE POVIDONE.
See: Efodine, Oint. (Fougera).
Iodophor.
Mallsol, Liq. (Hauck).

IODINE PRODUCTS, ANTI-INFECTIVE.
See: Anayodin.
Betadine, Preps. (Purdue Frederick).
Chiniofon.
Diodoquin, Tab. (Searle).
Diiodo-Hydroxyquinoline (Various Mfr.).
Isodine, Preps. (Blair).
Prepodyne, Soln., Scrub (West).
Quinoxyl.
Surgidine, Liq. (Continental).
Vioform, Preps. (Ciba).

IODINE PRODUCTS, DIAGNOSTIC.
See: Chloriodized Oil (Various Mfr.).
Ethyl Iodophenylundecylate (Various Mfr.).
Iodized Oil.
Iodoalphionic Acid (Various Mfr.).
Iodobrassid.
Iodohippurate Sodium (Various Mfr.).
Iodopanoic Acid (Various Mfr.).
Iodophthalein Sodium (Various Mfr.).
Iodopyracet, Preps. (Various Mfr.).
Lipiodol Lafay, Amp., Vial (Savage).
Methiodal Sodium (Various Mfr.).
Pantopaque, Amp. (Lafayette).
Sodium Acetrizoate (Various Mfr.).
Sodium Iodomethamate (Various Mfr.).
Telepaque, Tab. (Winthrop Pharm).

IODINE PRODUCTS, NUTRITIONAL.
See: Calcium Iodobehenate (Various Mfr.).
Entodon.
Hydriodic Acid (Various Mfr.).
Iodobrassid (Various Mfr.).
Potassium Iodide (Various Mfr.).

IODINE RATION, (Barth's) Iodine (from kelp) 0.15 mg, trace minerals/Tab. Bot. 90s, 180s, 360s.
Use: Mineral supplement.

IODINE RATION. (Nion) Iodine (from kelp) 0.15 mg/3 Tab. Bot. 175s, 500s.
Use: Iodine supplement.

IODINE SOLUBLE.
See: Burnham Soluble Iodine, Soln. (Burnham).

IODINE SURFACE ACTIVE COMPLEX.
See: Ioprep, Soln. (Arbrook).

•**IODINE TINCTURE, STRONG,** U.S.P. XXII.
Use: Anti-infective (topical).

•**IODIPAMIDE,** U.S.P. XXII. Benzoic acid, 3,3′-[(1,6-dioxo-1,6-hexanediyl)diimino]bis[2,4,6-triiodo-. NN′-Di-(3-carboxy-2,4,6-tri-iodophenyl)-adipamide. Adipiodone (I.N.N.).
Use: Pharmaceutic necessity for Iodipamide Meglumine Injection.

•**IODIPAMIDE MEGLUMINE INJECTION,** U.S.P. XXII. Benzoic acid, 3,3′-[(1,6-dioxo-1,6-hexanediyl)diimino] bis [2,4,6-triiodo-, compound with 1-deoxy-1-(methylamino)-d-glucitol (1:2).
Use: Diagnostic aid (radiopaque medium).

IODIPAMIDE METHYLGLUCAMINE. N,N′-Adipyl-bis(3-amino-2,4,6-triiodobenzoic acid). Also sodium salt inj.
W/Diatrizoate methylglucamine.
See: Sinografin, Vial (Squibb).

•**IODIPAMIDE SODIUM I-131.** USAN.
Use: Radioactive agent.

IODIPAMIDE SODIUM INJECTION.
See: Cholografin Sodium, Soln. (Various Mfr.).

•**IODIXANOL.** USAN
Use: Diagnostic aid (radiopaque medium).

IODIZED OIL. A vegetable oil containing not less than 38% and not more than 42% of organically combined iodine.
Use: Diagnostic aid.
See: Lipiodol Lafay, Amp., Vial (Savage).

IODIZED POPPY-SEED OIL.
See: Lipiodol Lafay, Amp., Vial (Savage).

IODOALPHIONIC ACID. 3-(4-Hydroxy-3,5-Diiodophenyl)-2-phenylpropionic acid. Biliselectan dikol, pheniodol.

•**IODOANTIPYRINE I-131.** USAN.
Use: Radioactive agent.

IODOBEHENATE CALCIUM. Calcium iododocosanoate.
Use: Antigoitrogenic.

IODOBRASSID. Ethyl Diiodobrassidate. Lipoiodine.

•**IODOCETYLIC ACID I-123.** USAN.
Use: Diagnostic aid.

•**IODOCHOLESTEROL I-131.** USAN.
Use: Radioactive agent.

IODOCHLORHYDROXYQUIN. Clioquinol, U.S.P. XXII.

IODO CREAM. (Day-Baldwin) Clioquinol 3%. Tube 1 oz, Jar 1 lb.
Use: Antifungal, external.

IODOFORM.(Various Mfr.) Triiodomethane. Pow., Bot. 1/8 oz, 1 oz, 0.25 lb, 1 lb.
Use: Wound dressing agent.
W/Guaiacol, eucalyptol, camphor.
See: Camusol, Vial (Central).
Guaiphoto, Vial (Foy).
Guido, Vial (Rocky Mtn.).
Imenol, Inj. (Sig).
Kleer, Vial (Scrip).
Respirex, Vial (Savage).

IODO H-C. (Day-Baldwin) Clioquinol 3%, hydrocortisone 1%. **Oint.:** Tube 20 Gm, Jar 1 lb. **Cream:** Tube 20 Gm, Jar 1 lb.
Use: Antifungal, corticosteroid.

•**IODOHIPPURATE SODIUM I-123 INJECTION,** U.S.P. XXII.
Use: Radioactive agent.

•**IODOHIPPURATE SODIUM I-125.** USAN.
Use: Radioactive agent.
See: Hipputope I 125 (Squibb).

•**IODOHIPPURATE, SODIUM I-131 INJECTION,** U.S.P. XXII. Glycine, N-(2-iodo-^{131}1-benzoyl)-, sodium salt.
Use: Diagnostic aid (renal function determination).
See: Hipputope (Squibb).

IODO-HIPPURIC ACID.
See: Hipputope (Squibb).

IODOL. 2,3,4,5-Tetraiodopyrrole.

IODO-NIACIN TABLETS. (Forest) Potassium iodide 135 mg, niacinamide HCl 25 mg/Tab. Bot. 100s, 500s.
Use: Expectortant.

IODO OINTMENT. (Day-Baldwin) Clioquinol 3%. Tube oz, Jar lb.
Use: Antifungal, external.

IODO-PAK. (SoloPak) Iodine 100 mcg/ml. Inj. Vial 10 ml.
Use: Parenteral nutritional supplement.

IODOPANOIC ACID.
Use: Diagnostic aid (radiopaque medium).

IODOPEN. (Lyphomed) Sodium iodide 118 mcg/ml. Vial 3 ml, 10 ml.
Use: Parenteral nutritional supplement.

IODOPHENE. Iodophthalein.

IODOPHENE SODIUM.
See: Iodophthalein Sodium. (Various Mfr.).

IODOPHOR.
See: Betadine, Preps. (Purdue Frederick).
Isodine, Preps. (Blair).

IODOPHTHALEIN SODIUM. Tetraiodophenolphthalein Sodium, Tetraiodophthalein Sodium, Tetiothalein Sodium (Antinosin, Cholepulvis, Cholumbrin, Foriod, Iodophene, Iodorayoral, Nosophene Sodium, Opacin, Photobiline, Piliophen, Radiotetrane).
Use: Radiopaque agent.

IODO-PRO. (Fellows) Sodium iodide 40 mg, peptone 20 mg/ml. Vial 30 ml.

IODOPROPYLIDENE GLYCEROL.
See: Organidin, Elix., Tab., Soln. (Wampole).

•**IODOPYRACET I-125.** USAN.
Use: Radioactive agent.

•**IODOPYRACET I-131.** USAN.
Use: Radioactive agent.
See: Diodrast (R)-131

IODOPYRACET INJ. (Diatrast, Diodone, Iopyracil, Neo-Methiodal, NeoSkiodan) 3,5-Diiodo-4-oxo-1(4H)-pyridineacetic Acid 2,2-Iminodiethanol (1:1) Compound.
Use: Radiopaque medium.

IODOPYRACET COMPOUND. Diodrast.

IODOPYRACET CONCENTRATED. Diodrast.

IODOPYRINE. Antipyrine "iodide."
Use: Iodides, analgesic.

•**IODOQUINOL,** U.S.P. XXII. Tab., U.S.P. XXII. 8-Quinolinol-5,7-diiodo. Diiodohydroxyquinoline, (Embequin, Enterosept)5,7-Diiodo-8-quinolinol.
Use: Anti-amebic.
See: Floraquin (Searle).
Sebaquin, Shampoo (Summers Labs.).
W/9-Aminoacridine HCl.
See: Vagitric, Cream (Elder).
Yodoxin, Tab., Pow. (Glenwood).
W/Hydrocortisone alcohol.
See: Vytone, Cream (Dermik).
W/Hydrocortisone, coal tar solution.
See: Cor-Tar-Quin, Cream, Lot. (Miles Pharm).
W/Stilbestrol, sulfadiazine, tartaric acid, boric acid etc.
See: Gynben, Vag. Insert, Cream (I. C. N).
Gynben Insufflate, Pow. (I. C. N).
W/Surfactants.
See: Lycinate, Supp. (Hoechst).
W/Sulfanilamide, diethylstilbestrol.
See: Amide V/S, Vaginal Insert. (Scrip).
D.I.T.I. Creme (Dunhall).

IODOTHIOURACIL. B.A.N. 1,2-Dihydro-5-iodo-2-thioxopyrimidin-4-one. 5-Iodo-2-thiouracil.
Use: Antithyroid substance.

IODOTOPE (Diagnostic). (Squibb) Sodium iodide I-131 for oral use. 7, 14, 28, 70, 106 units Ci/Vial of 5, 10, 15, 20 Cap.
Use: Diagnostic aid.

IODOTOPE (Therapeutic). (Squibb) Sodium iodide I-131. 1 to 50 mCi Cap./7, 14, 28, 70, 106 mCi solution.
Use: Antithyroid agent.

•**IODOXAMIC ACID.** USAN. NN′-(1,16-Dioxo-4,-7,10,13-tetraoxahexadecane-1,16-diyl)di-(3-amino-2,4,6-tri-iodobenzoic acid).
Use: Contrast medium.

IODOXYL.
See: Sodium Iodomethamate (Various Mfr.).

•**IOFETAMINE HYDROCHLORIDE I 123.** USAN.
Use: Diagnostic aid, radioactive agent.

•**IOGLICIC ACID.** USAN.
Use: Diagnostic aid (radiopaque medium).

•**IOGLUCOL.** USAN.
Use: Diagnostic aid (radiopaque medium).

•**IOGLUCOMIDE.** USAN.
Use: Diagnostic aid.

•**IOGLYCAMIC ACID.** USAN. 3,3-(Diglycoloyl-diimino)-bis-[2,4,6-triiodobenzoic acid]. Biligram, Bilivistan.
Use: Radiopaque (cholecystographic and cholangiographic).

•**IOGULAMIDE.** USAN.
Use: Diagnostic aid (radiopaque medium).

•**IOHEXOL.** USAN.
Use: Diagnostic aid (radiopaque medium).

IOHYDRO CREAM. (Freeport) Hydrocortisone 1%, clioquinol 3%, pramoxine HCl 0.5%/0.5 oz. Tube 0.5 oz.
Use: Corticosteroid, antifungal, local anesthetic.

•**IOMEPROL.** USAN
Use: Diagnostic agent, radiopaque.

•**IOMETHIN I-125.** USAN. 4-[[3-(Dimethylamino)propyl]amino]-7-iodo-^{125} I-quinoline.
Use: Diagnostic aid (neoplasm).

•**IOMETHIN I-131.** USAN. 4-[[3-Dimethylamino)propyl]amino]-7-iodo-^{131} I-quinoline.
Use: Diagnostic aid (neoplasm).

•**IONAMIN.** (Pennwalt) Phentermine. Phenyl-tertiary-butylamine as resin complex 15 mg or 30 mg/Cap. Bot. 100s, 400s.
Use: Anorexiant.

•**IONAX ASTRINGENT CLEANSER.** (Owen) Isopropyl alcohol 48%, Owenethers, (polyoxyethylene ethers), acetone, salicylic acid, allantoin. Bot. 8 oz.
Use: Anti-acne.

•**IONAX FOAM.** (Owen) Polyoxyethylene ethers, benzalkonium Cl 0.2%, purified water, isobutane, propylene glycol, myristamide, DEA, PEG 1000, D&C No. 5. Aerosol can 2.5 oz, 5 oz.
Use: Anti-acne.

•**IONAX SCRUB.** (Owen) Polyethylene granules, polyoxyethylene ethers, alcohol 10%, benzalkonium Cl. Tube 2 oz, 4 oz.
Use: Anti-acne.

•**IONAZE.**
See: Propazolamide.

•**ION-EXCHANGE RESINS.**
See: Polyamine Methylene Resin.
Resins, Sodium Removing.

IONIL PLUS SHAMPOO. (Owen) Salicylic acid 2%, water, sodium laureth sulfate, lauramide dea, quaternium-22, talloweth-60 myristyl glycol, laureth-23, tea lauryl sulfate, glycol disterate, laureth-4, tea-abietoyl hydrolyzed collagen, DMDM hydantoin, tetrasodium EDTA, sodium hydroxide, fragrance, FD&C blue no. 1. Bot. 4 oz, 8 oz.
Use: Antiseborrheic.

IONIL RINSE. (Owen) Conditioners with benzalkonium Cl in water base. Bot. 16 oz.
Use: Hair rinse.

IONIL SHAMPOO. (Owen) Salicylic acid, benzalkonium Cl, alcohol 12%, polyoxyethylene ethers. Plasic bot. w/dispenser cap 4 oz, 8 oz, 16 oz, 32 oz.
Use: Antiseborrheic.

IONIL T. (Owen) A nonionic/cationic foaming shampoo w/coal tar, salicylic acid, benzalkonium Cl, alcohol 12%, polyoxyethylene ethers. Plastic bot. 4 oz, 8 oz, 16 oz, 32 oz.
Use: Antiseborrheic.

IONIL T PLUS SHAMPOO. (Owen) Owentar II (equivalent to 2% coal tar), water, sodium laureth sulfate, lauramide dea, quaternium-22, laureth-23, talloweth-60 myristyl glycol, tea lauryl sulfate, glycol distearate, laureth-4, tea abietoyl hydrolyzed collagen, DMDM hydantoin, disodium EDTA, fragrance, FD&C blue #1, D&C yellow no. 70. Bot. 4 oz, 8 oz.
Use: Antiseborrheic.

IONOSOL D-CM. (Abbott Hospital Prods) Sodium Cl 516 mg, potassium Cl 89.4 mg, calcium Cl anhydrous 27.8 mg, magnesium Cl anhydrous 14.2 mg, sodium lactate 560 mg/100 ml. Bot. 1000 ml.
Use: Parenteral nutrient.

•**IOPAMIDOL,** U.S.P. XXII.
Use: Diagnostic aid (radiopaque medium).
See: Isovue-300, Inj. (Squibb).
Isovue-370, Inj. (Squibb).
Isovue-M 200, Inj. (Squibb).
Isovue-M 300, Inj. (Squibb).

•**IOPANOIC ACID,** U.S.P. XXII. Tabs. U.S.P. XXII. Benzenepropanoic acid, 3-amino-α-ethyl-2,4,6-triiodo-. 2-(3-Amino-2,4,6-tri-iodobenzyl)-butyric acid. 3-Amino-a-ethyl-2,4,6 Triiodohydrocinnamic acid.
Use: Diagnostic aid (radiopaque medium).
See: Telepaque, Tab. (Winthrop Pharm).

•**IOPENTOL.** USAN.
Use: Diagnostic aid (radiopaque medium).

IOPHEN. (Various Mfr.) Iodinated glycerol 60 mg (30 mg organically bound iodine)/5 ml. Elix. Bot. pt.
Use: Expectorant.

IOPHEN-C. (Various Mfr.) Codeine phosphate 10 mg, iodinated glycerol 30 mg/5 ml. Liq. Bot. 120 ml, pt, gal.
Use: Antitussive, expectorant.

IOPHEN DM ELIXIR. (Various Mfr.) Dextromethorphan HBr 10 mg, iodinated glycerol 30 mg/5 ml Elix. Bot. 120 ml, 480 ml, 760 ml.
Use: Antitussive, expectorant.

•**IOPHENDYLATE,** U.S.P. XXII. Benzenedecanoic acid, iodo-t-methyl-, ethyl ester.
Use: Diagnostic aid (radiopaque medium).

•**IOPHENDYLATE INJECTION,** U.S.P. XXII. Ethiodan, Myodil. Ethyl Iodophenylundecylate.
Use: Diagnostic aid (radiopaque medium).
See: Pantopaque, Amp. (LaFayette).

IOPHENOXIC ACID. Tab. a-(2-4,6-Triiodo-3-hydroxybenxyl) butyric acid.

IOPIDINE. (Alcon) Apraclonidine 1%, benzalkonium Cl 0.01%. Dispenser bot. 0.25 ml.
Use: Agent for glaucoma.

IOPODATE SODIUM.
See Ipodate Sodium.

IOPREP. (Surgikos) Nonylphenoxypolyethylenoxy (4) ethanol and nonylphenoxypolyethyleneoxy (15) ethanol iodine complex 5.5%, nonylphenoxypolyethyleneoxy (30) ethanol 10%. Solution provides 1% available iodine. Plastic bot. gal.
Use: Antiseptic.

•**IOPROCEMIC ACID.** USAN.
Use: Diagnostic aid.

•**IOPRONIC ACID.** USAN.
Use: Diagnostic aid.

•**IOPYDOL.** USAN. 1-(2,3-Dihydroxypropyl)-3,5-diiodo-4(1H)-pyridone.
Use: X-ray contrast medium for bronchography.

•**IOPYDONE.** USAN. 3,5-Diiodo-4-(1H)-pyridone.
Use: X-ray contrast medium for bronchography.

•**IOSEFAMIC ACID.** USAN. 5,5′-(Sebacoyldiimino) bis[2,4,6-triiodo-N-methylisophthalamic acid]
Use: Contrast medium.

•**IOSERIC ACID.** USAN.
Use: Diagnostic aid.

•**IOSULAMIDE MEGLUMINE.** USAN.
Use: Diagnostic aid.

•**IOSUMETIC ACID.** USAN.
Use: Diagnostic aid.

•**IOTASUL.** USAN.
Use: Diagnostic aid.

•**IOTETRIC ACID.** USAN.
Use: Diagnostic aid.

•**IOTHALAMATE MEGLUMIDE AND IOTHALMATE SODIUM INJECTION,** U.S.P. XXII.
Use: Diagnostic aid (radiopaque medium).

•**IOTHALAMATE MEGLUMINE INJECTION,** U.S.P. XXII. Benzoic acid, 3-(acetylamino)-2,4,6-triiodo-5-[(methylamino)carbonyl]-, compound with 1-deoxy-1-(methylamino)-d-glucitol (1:1).
Use: Diagnostic aid (radiopaque medium).

•**IOTHALAMATE SODIUM I-125.** USAN.
Use: Radioactive agent.

•**IOTHALAMATE SODIUM I-131.** USAN.
Use: Radioactive agent.

•**IOTHALAMATE SODIUM INJECTION,** U.S.P. XXII. Benzoic acid, 3-(acetylamino)-2,4,6-triiodo-5-[(methylamino)carbonyl]-, sodium salt. 5-Acetamido-2,4,6-triiodo-N-methylisophthalamic acid, sodium salt. Sodium Iothalamate.
Use: Diagnostic aid (radiopaque medium).

•**IOTHALAMIC ACID,** 3-(acetylamino)-2,4,6-triiodo-5-[(methylamino)carbonyl]-. 5-Acetamino-2,4,6-triiodo-N-methylisophthalamic acid.
Use: Radiopaque; pharmaceutic necessity for Iothalamate Meglumine Injection, Iothalamate Meglumine and Iothalamate Sodium Injection, and Iothalamate Sodium Injection.

IOTHIOURACIL SODIUM. Sodium salt of 5-iodo-2-thiouracil.

•**IOTROL.** USAN.
Use: Radiopaque medium.

•**IOTROXIC ACID.** USAN.
Use: Diagnostic aid (radiopaque medium).

•**IOTYROSINE 1-131.** USAN.
Use: Radioactive agent.

•**IOVERSOL.** USAN.
Use: Diagnostic aid (radiopaque medium).

•**IOXAGLATE MEGLUMINE.** USAN.
Use: Diagnostic agent (radiopaque medium).
See: Hexabrix, Inj. (Wallace).

•**IOXAGLATE SODIUM.** USAN.
Use: Diagnostic agent (radiopaque medium).

•**IOXAGLIC ACID.** USAN.
Use: Diagnostic agent (radiopaque medium).

•**IOXILAN.** USAN
Use: Diagnostic agent.

•**IOXOTRIZOIC ACID.** USAN.
Use: Diagnostic aid.

I-PARACAINE. (Akorn) Proparacaine HCl 0.5%. Bot. 15 ml.
Use: Local anesthetic.

I-PARESCEIN. (Akorn) Fluorescein 0.25%, proparacaine HCl 0.5%. Ophthalmic soln. Bot. 5 ml.
Use: Diagnostic aid, local anesthetic.

IPATERP. (Fellows) Terpin hydrate 2 gr, ammonium Cl 1 gr, licorice extract 0.5 gr, ipecac 1/10 gr/Tab. Bot. 1000s.
Use: Expectorant, antitussive.

•**IPAZOLIDE FUMARATE.** USAN
Use: Antiarrhythmic.

•**IPECAC,** U.S.P. XXII. Pow., Syr. U.S.P. XXII.
Use: Emetic.

W/Combinations.
See: Balmial Cough Syrup, Syr. (Clapp).
Creozets, Loz. (Creomulsion Co.).
Derfort, Cap. (Cole).
Diatrol, Tab. (Otis Clapp).
Ipsatol/DM, Cough Syr. (Key).
Ipsatol, Syr. (Key).
Mallergan, Liq. (Hauck).
Neo-Bronchoid, Tab. (Moore-Kirk).
Phenatrocaps, Cap. (O'Neal).
Phenatrohist, Cap. (O'Neal).
Polyectin, Liq. (Amid).
Proclan, Preps. (Cenci).
Romilar, CF, Syr. (Block).
Rubacac, Tab. (Scrip).

Spenlaxo, Tab. (Spencer-Mead).
Terpium, Tab. (Scrip).

I-PENTOLATE 1%. (Akorn) Cyclopentolate HCl 1%. Ophthalmic soln. Bot. 2 ml, 15 ml.
Use: Cycloplegic.

•**IPEXIDINE MESYLATE.** USAN.
Use: Dental caries prophylactic.

I-PHRINE. (Akorn) Phenylephrine HCl 2.5% or 10%. Ophthalmic soln. Bot. 2 ml, 5 ml, 15 ml.
Use: Vasoconstrictor/mydriatic.

I-PICAMIDE 1%. (Akorn) Tropicamide 1%. Ophthalmic soln. Bot. 2 ml, 15 ml.
Use: Mydriatic.

I-PILOPINE. (Akorn) Pilocarpine HCl 1%, 2% or 4%. Ophthalmic soln. Bot. 15 ml.
Use: Miotic.

•**IPODATE CALCIUM,** U.S.P. XXII. Oral Susp., U.S.P. XXII. Benzenepropanoic acid, 3-[[(dimethylamino)methylene]amino]-2,4,6-triiodo-, calcium salt.
Use: Diagnostic aid (radiopaque medium).
See: Oragrafin calcium, Granules (Squibb).

•**IPODATE SODIUM,** U.S.P. XXII. Cap., U.S.P. XXII. Benzenepropanoic acid, 3-[[(dimethylamino)-methylene] amino]-2,4,6-triiodo-, sodium salt.
Use: Diagnostic aid (radiopaque medium).
See: Bilivist, Cap. (Berlex).
Oragrafin sodium, Cap., Vial (Squibb).

IPRAN. (Major) Propranolol HCl 10 mg, 20 mg, 40 mg, 60 mg, 80 mg, 90 mg/Tab. **10 mg, 20 mg, 40 mg:** Bot. 100s, 250s, 1000s, UD 100s; **60 mg:** Bot. 100s, 500s; **80 mg:** Bot. 100s, 500s, 1000s, UD 100s; **90 mg:** Bot. 100s, 500s.
Use: Beta-adrenergic blocking agent.

IPRATROPIUM BROMIDE. USAN. 8-Isopropyl-3-(±)-tropoyloxy-1αH,5αH-tropanium bromide. N-Isopro-pylatropinium bromide.
Use: Bronchodilator.
See: Atrovent, Aerosol (Boehringer Ingelheim).

I-PRED. (Akorn) Prednisolone sodium phosphate 0.5% or 1%. Ophthalmic soln. Bot. 5 ml.
Use: Corticosteroid.

I-PREDNICET. (Akorn) Prednisolone acetate 1%. Ophthalmic soln. Bot. 5 ml, 10 ml.
Use: Corticosteroid.

•**IPRINDOLE.** USAN. 5-[3-(Dimethylamino)-propyl]-6,7,8,9,10,11-hexahydro-5H-cyclo-oct[β]-indole. 5-(3-Dimethylaminopropyl)-6,7,8,9,10-11-hexahydrocyclooct[β]indole. Prondol hydrochloride.
Use: Antidepressant.

•**IPROCINODINE HYDROCHLORIDE.** USAN.
Use: Antibacterial.

IPROCLOZIDE. B.A.N. 4-Chlorophenoxy-2′-iso-pro-pylacetohydrazide.
Use: Monoamine oxidase inhibitor.

•**IPROFENIN.** USAN.
Use: Diagnostic aid.

IPRONIAZID. B.A.N. l-isonicotinyl-2-isopropylhydrazinephosphate. 2′-Isopropylisonicotinohydrazide.
Use: Monoamine oxidase inhibitor.

•**IPRONIDAZOLE.** USAN. 2-Isopropyl-1-methyl-5-nitroimidazole. Ipropran (Hoffman-LaRoche).
Use: Antiprotozoal (Histomonas).

•**IPROPLATIN.** USAN.
Use: Antineoplastic.

IPROVERATRIL. Name used for verapamil.

•**IPROXAMINE HYDROCHLORIDE.** USAN.
Use: Vasodilator.

•**IPSAPIRONE HYDROCHLORIDE.** USAN.
Use: Anxiolytic.

IPSATOL. (Kenwood) Guaifenesin 100 mg, dextromethorphan HBr 10 mg, phenylpropanolamine HCl 9 mg/5 ml. Bot. 118 ml.
Use: Expectorant, antitussive, decongestant.

IPV.
Use: Poliomyelitis immunization.
See: Polio Virus Vaccine, Inactivated.

IRCON. (Key) Ferrous fumarate 200 mg/Tab. Bot. 100s.
Use: Iron supplement.

IRCON-FA. (Key) Ferrous fumarate 250 mg, folic acid 1 mg/Tab. Bot. 100s.
Use: Iron supplement.

I-RESCEIN. (Akorn) Fluorescein sodium 10% or 25%. Soln. Amp. 2 ml, 5 ml.
Use: Diagnostic aid.

IRGASAN CF3. Cloflucarban. Under study.
Use: Antiseptic.

•**IRIDIUM IR-192.** USAN.
Use: Radioactive agent.
See: Iriditope (Squibb).

IRIGATE. (Ketchum) Bot. 4 oz
Use: Eyewash.

I-RINSE. (Akorn) Balanced salt solution. Bot. 1 oz, 4 oz
Use: Ophthalmic irrigation solution.

IRISIN. A polysaccharide found in several species of iris.

IROCAINE.
See: Procaine HCl (Various Mfr.).

IRODEX. (Keene) Iron dextran complex 50 mg/ml. Vial 10 ml.
Use: Iron supplement.

IROMIN-G. (Mission) Ferrous gluconate 260 mg (iron 30 mg), vitamins B_{12} (crystalline on resin) 2 mcg, C 100 mg, A acetate 4000 IU, D-2 400 IU, B_1 5 mg, B_2 2 mg, B_6 25 mg, niacinamide 10 mg, calcium pantothenate 1 mg, folic acid 0.8 mg, calcium gluconate 100 mg, calcium lactate 100 mg, calcium carbonate 70 mg (calcium 50 mg)/Tab. Bot. 100s.
Use: Vitamin/mineral supplement.

IRON BILE SALTS.
See: Bilron, Pulvules (Lilly).

IRON CACODYLATE. (Torigian) Metallic iron 12%, organically combined arsenic as ferric salt of dimethylarsonate. Amp. 0.5 gr 1 ml, 25s, 100s. 1 gr 2 ml 5 ml, 25s, 100s.

IRON CARBONATE COMPLEX.
See: Polyferose.

IRON CHOLINE CITRATE COMPLEX.

See: Chel-Iron, Tab. (Kinney).
Kelex, Tabseals (Nutrition Control).

IRONCO-B. (Vale) Ferrous sulfate 120.4 mg, manganese sulfate 21.6 mg, dicalcium phosphate 129.6 mg, vitamins B_1 1 mg, B_2 1 mg, niacin 6 mg, D 100 IU/Tab. Bot. 100s, 1000s.
Use: Vitamin/mineral supplement.

•**IRON-DEXTRAN INJECTION,** U.S.P. XXII.
Use: Hematinic.
See: Ferrodex, Inj. (Keene Pharm.).
Hydextran, Inj. (Hyrex).
Imferon, Amp., Vial (Merrell Dow).

IRON-FOLIC ACID-LIVER. (Medwick) Vial 30 ml.

"IRON FOR WOMEN". (Pharmex) Ferrous fumarate 5 gr/Tab. Bot. 90s.
Use: Iron supplement.

IRON (2+) FUMARATE. Ferrous Fumarate, U.S.P. XXII.

IRON (2+) GLUCONATE.
See: Ferrous Gluconate, U.S.P. XXII.

IRON OXIDE MIXTUREWITH ZINC OXIDE. Calamine, U.S.P. XXII.

IRON PEPTONIZED.
See: Saferon, Tab. (Elder).

IRON PROTEIN COMPLEX.

•**IRON SORBITEX.** USAN. A sterile, colloidal solution of a complex of trivalent iron, sorbitol, and citric acid, stabilized with dextrin and sorbitol.
Use: Hematinic.

•**IRON SORBITEX INJECTION,** U.S.P. XXII. (Formerly iron sorbitol).
Use: Iron supplement.
See: Jectofer, Amp. (Astra).

IRON SULFATE. W/Maalox.
See: Fermalox, Tab. (Rorer).

IROPHOS D. (Lannett) Dicalcium phosphate anhydrous 330 mg, ferrous sulfate 30 mg, vitamin D 333 IU/Cap. Bot. 500s, 1000s.
Use: Vitamin/mineral supplement.

IROSPAN. (Fielding) Ferrous sulfate 200 mg, vitamin C 150 mg/Cap. Bot. 60s. Tab. Bot. 100s.
Use: Vitamin/mineral supplement.

IRRADIATED ERGOSTEROL.
See: Calciferol.

IRRIGATE. (Professional Pharmacal) Boric acid 1.2%, potassium Cl 0.38%, sodium carbonate 0.014%, benzalkonium Cl 0.01%, disodium edetate 0.05%. Bot. 0.5 oz, 4 oz.
Use: Ocular cleanser.

ISACEN.
See: Oxyphenisatin, Preps. (Various Mfr.).

•**ISAMOXOLE.** USAN.
Use: Antiasthmatic.

•**ISEPAMICIN.** USAN.
Use: Antibacterial.

ISMELIN. (Ciba) Guanethidine monosulfate 10 mg or 25 mg/Tab. Bot. 100s, 1000s.
Use: Antihypertensive.

ISMOTIC. (Alcon Surgical) Isosorbide solution. W/ sodium 4.6 mEq, potassium 0.9 mEq/220 ml, alcohol, saccharin, sorbitol. In 220 ml.
Use: Osmotic diuretic.

ISO-ALCOHOLIC ELIXIR.
Use: Vehicle.

ISOAMINILE. B.A.N. (Robins) 4-Dimethylamino-2-isopropyl-2-phenylvaleronitrile. Dimyril citrate.
Use: Antitussive.

ISOAMYLHYDROCUPREINE DIHYDROCHLORIDE.
See: Eucupin Dihydrochloride.

ISOAMYL NITRATE.
See: Amyl Nitrite, U.S.P. XXII.

ISOAMYNE.
See: Amphetamine (Various Mfr.).

ISO-BID. (Geriatric) Isosorbide dinitrate 40 mg/ Cap. Bot. 30s, 100s, 500s.
Use: Antianginal agent.

ISOBORNYL THIOCYANOACETATE, TECHNICAL.
Use: Pediculicide.
See: Barc, Liq. (Commerce).
W/Anhydrous soap.
W/Docusate sodium and related terpenes.
See: Barc, Cream (Commerce).

ISOBUCAINE HYDROCHLORIDE, U.S.P. XXI. 2-Isobutylamino-2-methylpropyl benzoate HCl. 2- (Isobutylamino)-2-methyl-1-propanol benzoate (ester) HCl.
Use: Local anesthetic (dental).

ISOBUCAINE HCl & EPINEPHRINE INJECTION, U.S.P. XXI.
Use: Local anesthetic (dental).

•**ISOBUTAMBEN.** USAN. Isobutyl p-aminobenzoate. Isocaine. Cycloform.
Use: As a surface anesthetic.

•**ISOBUTANE,** N.F. XVII.
Use: Aerosol propellant.

ISOBUTYLALLYLBARBITURIC ACID.
W/Aspirin, phenacetin, caffeine.
See: Buff-A-Comp, Tab., Cap. (Mayrand).
Fiorinal, Tab., Cap. (Sandoz).
Lanorinal, Cap. (Lannett).
Palgesic, Tab., Cap. (Pan Amer.).
Tenstan, Tab. (Standex).
W/Aspirin, phenacetin, caffeine, codeine phosphate.
See: Fiorinal w/codeine, Cap. (Sandoz).

ISOBUTYL p-AMINOBENZOATE. Isobutamben, U.S.A.N.

ISOBUZOLE. B.A.N. 5-Isobutyl-2-(4-methoxybenzenesulphonamido)-1,3,4-thiadiazole. Glysobuzole (I.N.N.).
Use: Oral hypoglycemic agent.

ISOCAINE. Isobutamben, USAN.

ISOCAINE HCl. (Novocal) Mepivacaine 2% with 1:20,000 levonordefrin. Inj. Dental cartridge 1.8 ml.
Use: Local anesthetic.

ISOCAL. (Mead Johnson Nutrition) Lactose-free isotonic liquid containing as a percentage of the calories protein 13% as caseinate and soy protein; fat 37% as soy oil and medium chain triglycerides; carbohydrate 50% as corn syrup

solids w/vitamins and minerals for the tube fed patient. Bot. 8 fl oz, 12 fl oz, 32 fl oz.
Use: Enteral nutritional supplement.

ISOCAL HCN. (Mead Johnson Nutrition) High calorie, nitrogen nutritionally complete food. Protein 15%, fat 45%, carbohydrate 40%. Can 8 fl oz.
Use: Enteral nutritional supplement.

ISOCAL HN. (Mead Johnson) ≈ 1 Kcal/ml with protein 44 Gm, fat 45 Gm, carbohydrates 124 Gm/L. In 237 ml.
Use: Enteral nutritional supplement.

•**ISOCARBOXAZID,** U.S.P. XXII. Tab., U.S.P. XXII. 1-Benzyl[-2-(5-methyl-3-isoxazolyl-carbonyl)hydra- zine. 5-Methyl-3-isoxazolecarboxylic acid 2-benzyl- hydrazide. 3-(2-Benzylhydrazinocarbonyl)-5-meth- ylisoxazole. 2′-Benzyl-5-methylisoxazole-3-carbohy- drazide.
Use: Antidepressant.
See: Marplan, Tab. (Roche).

ISOCLOR EXPECTORANT. (Fisons) Codeine phosphate 10 mg, pseudoephedrine HCl 30 mg, guaifenesin 100 mg/5 ml, alcohol 5%. Bot. pt.
Use: Antitussive, decongestant, expectorant.

ISOCLOR LIQUID. (Fisons) Chlorpheniramine maleate 2 mg, pseudoephedrine HCl 30 mg/5 ml, sorbitol. Bot. pt.
Use: Antihistamine, decongestant.

ISOCLOR TABLETS. (Fisons) Chlorpheniramine maleate 4 mg, pseudoephedrine HCl 60 mg/Tab. Bot. 100s.
Use: Antihistamine, decongestant.

ISOCLOR TIMESULE CAPSULES. (Fisons) Chlorpheniramine maleate 8 mg, pseudoephedrine HCl 120 mg/Cap. Bot. 100s, 500s.
Use: Antihistamine, decongestant.

ISOCOCAINE. Pseudococaine.

ISOCOM. (Nutripharm) Isometheptene mucate 65 mg, dichloralphenazone 100 mg, acetaminophen 325 mg/Cap. Bot. 50s, 100s, 250s.
Use: Agent for migraine.

ISOCONAZOLE. USAN.
Use: Antibacterial, antifungal.

ISO D. (Dunhall) Isosorbide dinitrate. **Cap.:** 40 mg. Bot. 100s, 1000s. **Tab.:** 5 mg (sublingual). Bot. 100s.
Use: Antianginal agent.

ISOEPHEDRINE HCl. d-Isoephedrine HCl.
See: Pseudoephedrine HCl.
W/Chlorpheniramine maleate.
See: Isoclor, Tab., Expectorant Timesule, Liq. (Arnar-Stone).
W/Chlorprophenpyridamine maleate.
See: Isoclor, Tab. (Arnar-Stone).
W/Theophylline sodium glycinate, guaifenesin.
See: Iso-Tabs 60 Tab. (Solvay).

D-ISOEPHEDRINE SULFATE.
See: Pseudoephedrine Sulfate.

•**ISOETHARINE.** USAN. 3,4-Dihydroxy α-(l-isopropylamino-propyl)benzyl alcohol. 1-(3,4-Dihy- droxy- phenyl)-2-isopropylaminobutan-1-ol. Numotac hydrochloride.
Use: Bronchodilator.

•**ISOETHARINE HYDROCHLORIDE,** U.S.P. XXII.
Use: Bronchodilator.
See: Bronkosol, Soln. (Winthrop Pharm).

•**ISOETHARINE INHALATION SOLUTION,** U.S.P. XXII.
Use: Bronchodilator.

•**ISOETHARINE MESYLATE,** U.S.P. XXII. Inhalation Aerosol, U.S.P. XXII.
Use: Bronchodilator.
See: Bronkometer, Aerosol (Winthrop Pharm).

•**ISOFLUPREDONE ACETATE.** USAN.
Use: Anti-inflammatory.

•**ISOFLURANE,** U.S.P. XXII.
Use: Anesthetic.

ISOGREGNENONE. Dydrogesterone.
See: Duphaston, Tab. (Philips Roxane).

ISO-IODEIKON.
See: Phentetiothalein Sodium (No Mfr. currently lists).

ISOJECT. (Roerig) A purified, sterile, disposable injection system.
Permapen (benzathine pencillin G) aqueous soln. 1,200,000 units/2 ml. 10s.
Terramycin (oxytetracycline) intramuscular soln. 250 mg/2 ml. 10s.
Use: Injection system.

I-SOL SOLUTION. (DeyLabs) Sodium Cl 0.64%, potassium Cl 0.075%, calcium Cl 0.048%, magnesium Cl 0.03%, sodium acetate 0.39%, sodium citrate 0.17%, sodium hydroxide or hydrochloric acid. Soln. Bot. 20 ml, 200 ml.
Use: Ophthalmic irrigation solution.

ISOLATE COMPOUND ELIXIR. (Various Mfr.) Theophylline 45 mg, ephedrine sulfate 12 mg, isoproterenol HCl 2.5 mg, potassium iodide 150 mg, phenobarbital 6 mg/15 ml, alcohol 19%. Elix. Bot. pt, gal.
Use: Antiasmatic combination.

•**ISOLEUCINE,** U.S.P. XXII. $C_6H_{13}NO_2$, L-isoleucine. DL-Isoleucine. (Pfaltz & Bauer)—Pow. 10 Gm.
Use: Nutrient.

ISOLLYL IMPROVED. (Rugby) Aspirin 325 mg, caffeine 40 mg, butalbital 50 mg/Tab. or Cap. Bot. 100s, 1000s.
Use: Salicylate analgesic, sedative/hypnotic.

ISOLYTE E. (American McGaw) Sodium 140 mEq, potassium 10 mEq, calcium 5 mEq, magnesium 3 mEq, chloride 103 mEq, acetate 49 mEq, citrate 8 mEq, 315 mOsm/L. Inj. Soln. 1000 ml.
Use: Parenteral nutritional supplement.

ISOLYTE E WITH 5% DEXTROSE. (American McGaw) Sodium 141 mEq, potassium 10 mEq, calcium 5 mEq, magnesium 3 mEq, chloride 103 mEq, citrate 8 mEq, acetate 49 mEq, dextrose 50 Gm, 180 Cal, 570 mOsm/L. Inj. Soln. 1000 ml.
Use: Parenteral nutritional supplement.

ISOLYTE G WITH DEXTROSE. (American McGaw) Sodium 65 mEq, potassium 17 mEq, chloride 150 mEq, NH_4 70 mEq, dextrose 50 Gm, 170 Cal, 555 mOsm/L. Bot. 1000 ml.
Use: Parenteral nutritional supplement.

ISOLYTE H WITH 5% DEXTROSE. (American McGaw) Sodium 70 mEq, potassium 13 mEq, magnesium 3 mEq, chloride 40 mEq, acetate 16 mEq, dextrose 50 Gm, 170 Cal, 370 mOsm/L. Inj. Soln. 1000 ml.
Use: Parenteral nutritional supplement.

ISOLYTE M WITH 5% DEXTROSE. (American McGaw) Sodium 38 mEq, potassium 35 mEq, chloride 44 mEq, phosphate 15 mEq, acetate 20 mEq, dextrose 50 Gm, 175 Cal, 405 mOsm/L. Inj. Soln. 1000 ml.
Use: Parenteral nutritional supplement.

ISOLYTE P WITH 5% DEXTROSE. (American McGaw) Sodium 25 mEq, potassium 19 mEq, magnesium 3 mEq, chloride 23 mEq, phosphate 3 mEq, acetate 23 mEq, dextrose 50 Gm, 175 Cal, 350 mOsm/L. Inj. Soln. 250 ml, 500 ml, 1000 ml.
Use: Parenteral nutritional therapy.

ISOLYTE R WITH 5% DEXTROSE. (American McGaw) Sodium 41 mEq, potassium 16 mEq, calcium 5 mEq, magnesium 3 mEq, chloride 40 mEq, acetate 24 mEq, dextrose 50 Gm, 175 Cal, 380 mOsm/L. Inj. Soln. 1000 ml.
Use: Parenteral nutritional supplement.

ISOLYTE S pH 7.4. (American McGaw) Sodium 140 mEq, potassium 5 mEq, magnesium 3 mEq, chloride 98 mEq, acetate 27 mEq, gluconate 23 mEq, 295 mOsm/L. Inj. Soln. 500 ml, 1000 ml.
Use: Parenteral nutritional supplement.

ISOLYTE S WITH 5% DEXTROSE. (American McGaw) Sodium 140 mEq, potassium 5 mEq, magnesium 3 mEq, chloride 98 mEq, acetate 27 mEq, gluconate 23 mEq, dextrose 50 Gm, 185 Cal, 550 mOsm/L. Inj. Soln. 1000 ml.
Use: Parenteral nutritional supplement.

•**ISOMAZOLE HYDROCHLORIDE.** USAN.
Use: Cardiotonic.

ISOMEPROBAMATE.
See: Carisoprodol (Various Mfr.).

•**ISOMEROL.** USAN.
Use: Antiseptic.

ISOMETHADONE. B.A.N. 6-Dimethylamino-5-methyl-4,4-diphenylhexan-3-one.
Use: Narcotic analgesic.

ISOMETAMIDIUM. B.A.N. 8-m-Amidinophenyl- diazoamino-3-amino-5-ethyl-6-phenylphenanthridinium chloride.
Use: Antiprotozoan, veterinary medicine.

ISOMETHEPTENE MUCATE.
See: Midrin, Cap. (Carnick).
Octinum, Tab. (Knoll).

ISOMETHEPTENE TARTRATE.
See: Tri-Grain, Vial (Pharmex).

ISOMIL. (Ross) Soy protein isolate infant formula containing 20 calories/fl oz. **Pow.:** Can 14 oz. **Concentrated Liq.:** Can 13 fl oz. **Ready-to-feed:** Can 32 fl oz. **Nursing Bottles:** Hospital use. Bot. 8 fl oz.
Use: Enteral nutritional supplement.

ISOMIL SF. (Ross) Low osmolar sucrose-free soy protein isolate infant formula containing 20 calories/fl oz. **Concentrated Liq.:** Can 13 fl oz. **Ready-to-feed:** Can 32 fl oz. **Nursing Bottles:** Hospital use. Bot. 8 fl oz.
Use: Enteral nutritional supplement.

ISOMUNE-CK. (Roche Diagnostics) Rapid immunochemical separation method of the heart specific CK-MB isoenzyme for quantitation when used with an appropriate CK substrate reagent. Test kit 100s, 250s.
Use: Diagnostic aid.

ISOMUNE-LD. (Roche Diagnostics) Rapid immunochemical separation method of the heart specific LD-1 isoenzyme for quantitation when used with an appropriate LD substrate reagent. Test kit 40s, 100s.
Use: Diagnostic aid.

•**ISOMYLAMINE HCl.** USAN. 2-(Diethylamino)ethyl 1-isopentylcyclohexanecarboxylate HCl.
Use: Smooth muscle relaxant.

ISOMYN.
See: Amphetamine (Various Mfr.).

ISONATE SUBLINGUAL. (Major) Isosorbide 2.5 mg or 5 mg/Sublingual Tab. Bot. 100s, 1000s, UD 100s.
Use: Antianginal agent.

ISONATE TABLETS. (Major) Isosorbide 5 mg, 10 mg, 20 mg or 30 mg/Tab. **5 mg or 10 mg:** Bot. 100s, 1000s, UD 100s. **20 mg or 30 mg:** Bot. 100s, 1000s.
Use: Antianginal agent.

ISONATE TD-CAPS. (Major) Isosorbide 40 mg/TD Cap. Bot. 100s, 1000s.
Use: Antianginal agent.

ISONATE T.R. TABS. (Major) Isosorbide 40 mg/TD Tab. Bot. 100s, 1000s.
Use: Antianginal agent.

ISONIAZID. (Carolina Medical Products) Isoniazid 50 mg/5 ml. Syr. Bot. pt.
Use: Antituberculous agent.

•**ISONIAZID,** U.S.P. XXII. Inj., Syr., Tab. U.S.P. XXII. Isonicotinic acid hydrazide, isonicotinyl hydrazide. Cotinazin; I.N.H.; Mybasan; Neumandin; Nicetal; Nydrazid; Pycazide; Rimifon; Tubomel; Vazadrine.
Use: Antibacterial (tuberculostatic).
See: Dow-Isoniazid, Tab. (Merrell Dow).
INH, Tab. (Ciba).
Laniazid, Tab. (Lannett).
Niconyl, Tab. (Parke-Davis).
Nydrazid, Inj. (Squibb Mark).
Nydrazid, Tab. (Squibb Marsam).
Rolazid, Tab. (Robinson).
Teebaconin, Tab., Pow. (Consoln. Mid.).
Triniad, Tab. (Kasar).

Uniad, Tab. (Kasar).
W/Calcium paraminosalicylate.
See: Calpas-INH, Tab. (American Chem. & Drug).
W/Calcium p-aminosalicylate, vitamin B_6.
See: Calpas Isoxine, Tab. (American Chem. & Drug).
Calpas-INAH-6, Tab. (American Chem. & Drug).
W/Pyridoxine HCl. (vitamin B_6).
See: Niadox, Tab.(Barnes-Hind).
P-I-N Forte, Syr., Tab. (Lannett).
Teebaconin w/B_6 (Consoln. Mid.).
Triniad Plus 30, Tab. (Kasar).
Uniad-Plus, Tab. (Kasar).
W/Pyridoxine HCl, sodium aminosalicylate.
See: Pasna, Tri-Pack 300, Granules (Barnes-Hind).
W/Rifampin.
See: Rimactane/INH DuoPack (Ciba).
W/Sodium aminosalicylate, pyridoxine.
See: Pasna Tri-Pack, Granules (Barnes-Hind).

ISONICOTINIC ACID HYDRAZIDE.
See: Isoniazid, U.S.P. XXII. (Various Mfr.).

ISONICOTINYL HYDRAZIDE.
See: Isoniazid, U.S.P. XXII. (Various Mfr.).

ISONIPECAINE HYDROCHLORIDE.
See: Meperidine Hydrochloride, U.S.P. XXII. (Various Mfr.).

ISOPENTAQUINE.
Use: Antimalarial.

•**ISOPHANE INSULIN SUSPENSION,** U.S.P. XXII.
Use: Hypoglycemic agent.
See: NPH Iletin, Vial (Lilly).

ISOPREDNIDENE. B.A.N. 11β,17α,21-Trihydroxy-16-methylenepregna-4,6-diene-3,20-dione.
Use: ACTH inhibitor.

ISOPREGNENONE.
See: Duphaston, Tab. (Philips Roxane).
Dydrogesterone.

ISOPRENALINE. B.A.N. ($\pm$)-1-(3,4-Dihydroxyphenyl)-2-isopropylaminoethanol. Isopropylnoradrenaline.
Use: Sympathomimetic.

•**ISOPROPAMIDE IODIDE,** U.S.P. XXII. Tab., U.S.P. XXII. (3-Carbamoyl-3,3-diphenylpropyl) diisopropyl-methylammonium iodide. Tyrimide.
Use: Anticholinergic.
See: Darbid, Tab. (SmithKline).
W/Prochlorperazine maleate.
See: Iso-Perazine, Cap. (Lemmon).

ISOPROPHENAMINE HCl. Name used for Clorprenaline HCl.

ISOPROPICILLIN POTASSIUM. Potassium 3,3-dimethyl-6-(2-methyl-2-phenoxypropionamido)-7-oxo-4-thia-1-azabicyclo [3.2.0]heptane-2-carboyxlate.
Use: Anti-infective.

•**ISOPROPYL ALCOHOL,** U.S.P. XXII.
Use: Local anti-infective; pharmaceutic aid (solvent).

•**ISOPROPYL ALCOHOL, AZEOTROPIC,** U.S.P. XXII.

ISOPROPYL ALCOHOL SPRAY. (Morton) Isopropyl alcohol w/propellant. Aerosol Can 6 oz.
Use: Isopropyl alcohol.

ISOPROPYLARTERENOL HYDROCHLORIDE.
Use: Asthma, vasoconstrictor and allergic states.

ISOPROPYLARTERENOL SULFATE.
See: Isoproterenol Sulfate.

•**ISOPROPYL MYRISTATE,** N.F. XVII.
Use: Pharmaceutic aid (emollient).

ISOPROPYL-NORADRENALINE HCl.
See: Isoproterenol HCl, U.S.P. XXII.

•**ISOPROPYL PALMITATE,** N.F. XVII.
Use: Pharmaceutic aid (oleaginous vehicle).

ISOPROPYL PHENAZONE. 4-Isopropyl antipyrine. Larodon.

•**ISOPROPYL RUBBING ALCOHOL,** U.S.P. XXII.
Use: Rubefacient, solvent.

ISOPROTERENOL.
See: Norisidrine (Abbott).
W/Butabarbital, theophylline, ephedrine HCl.
See: Medihaler-Iso, Vial (Riker).

•**ISOPROTERENOL HYDROCHLORIDE,** U.S.P. XXII. Inhalation, Tab. Inj.; U.S.P. XXII. 1,2-Benzenediol,4-[1-hydroxy-2-[(1-methylethyl)-amino]ethyl]-, HCl. 3,4-Dihydroxy-α-[(isopropylamino)methylbenzyl alcohol hydrochloride. Oleudrin-Proternol. 1:5,000 5 ml and 10 ml in Univ. Add. Syr.; 1:5,000 1 mg and 2 mg pintop vials; 1:50,000 10 ml with Abboject Syr. (21G X 1 0.5″).
Use: Adrenergic (bronchodilator).
See: Isuprel HCl, Prods. (Winthrop Pharm).
Norisodrine, Aerotrol, Syr. (Abbott).
Proternol, Tab. (Key Pharm.).
Vapo-Iso, Soln. (Fisons).
W/Aminophylline, ephedrine sulfate, phenobarbital.
See: Asminorel, Tab. (Solvay).
W/Clopane (clopentamine) HCl, propylene glycol, ascorbic acid.
See: Aerolone Compound, Soln. (Lilly).
W/Phenobarbital, ephedrine sulfate, theophylline, potassium iodide.
See: Isophed, Tab. (Jamieson-McKames).
W/Phenobarbital sodium, ephedrine sulfate, theophylline hydrous.
See: Iso-asminyl, Tab. (Cole).
W/Phenylephrine bitartrate.
See: Duo-Medihaler, Vial (Riker).

•**ISOPROTERENOL INHALATION SOLUTION,** U.S.P. XXII.
Use: Bronchodilator.

•**ISOPROTERENOL HYDROCHLORIDE AND PHENYLEPHRINE BITARTRATE INHALATION AEROSOL,** U.S.P. XXII.
Use: Adrenergic (bronchodilator).
See: Duo-Medihaler, Vial (Riker).

•**ISOPROTERENOL SULFATE,** U.S.P. XXII. Inhal. Aerosol, Inhal. Soln., U.S.P. XXII.
Use: Adrenergic (bronchodilator).
See: Medihaler-Iso, Vial (Riker).
W/Calcium iodide (anhydrous), alcohol.
See: Norisodrine, Syr. (Abbott).

ISOPTIN. (Knoll) Verapamil HCl 10 mg/4 ml. Amp. 4 ml.
Use: Calcium channel blocking agent.

ISOPTIN SR TABLETS. (Knoll) Verapamil HCl 240 mg/SR Tab. Bot. 100s.
Use: Calcium channel blocking agent.

ISOPTIN I.V. (Knoll) Verapamil HCl. **Single Dose Vial:** 5 mg/2 ml or 10 mg/4 ml. **Pre-filled Syringe:** 5 mg/2 ml or 10 mg/4 ml.
Use: Calcium channel blocking agent.

ISOPTIN TABLETS. (Knoll) Verapamil HCl 80 mg or 120 mg/Tab. Bot. 100s, 500s, 1000s, UD 10 X 10s.
Use: Calcium channel blocking agent.

ISOPTO ALKALINE. (Alcon) Methylcellulose 1%, benzalkonium Cl 0.01%. Sterile ophthalmic soln. Dropper bot. 15 ml.
Use: Artificial tear solution.

ISOPTO ATROPINE. (Alcon) Atropine sulfate 0.5%, 1% or 3% in methylcellulose solution. **0.5% or 3%:** Drop-Tainer 5 ml. **1%:** Drop-Tainer 5 ml, 15 ml.
Use: Cycloplegic mydriatic.

ISOPTO CARBACHOL. (Alcon) Carbachol U.S.P. 0.75%, 1.5%, 2.25% or 3%, in a sterile buffered solution of methylcellulose 1%. **2.25%:** Drop-Tainer 15 ml. **0.75%, 1.5% or 3%:** Drop-Tainer 15 ml, 30 ml.
Use: Agent for glaucoma.

ISOPTO CARPINE. (Alcon) Pilocarpine HCl in stable sterile 0.5% methylcellulose soln. w/isotonicity of lacrimal fluid. **0.25%, 0.5%, 1%, 2%, 3%, 4%, 5%, 6%, 8% or 10%:** Bot. Drop-Tainer 15 ml; **0.5%, 1%, 2%, 3%, 4% or 6%:** Bot. Drop-Tainer 30 ml.
Use: Agent for glaucoma.

ISOPTO CETAMIDE. (Alcon) Sodium sulfacetamide 15% in buffered pH 7.4, methylcellulose 0.5%. Soln. Drop-Tainer 5 ml, 15 ml.
Use: Anti-infective, ophthalmic.

ISOPTO CETAPRED. (Alcon) Sulfacetamide sodium U.S.P. 10%, prednisolone U.S.P. 0.25%, methylcellulose 0.5% in a sterile, buffered and stable suspension. Drop-Tainer 5 ml, 15 ml.
Use: Anti-infective, ophthalmic.

ISOPTO ESERINE. (Alcon) Eserine salicylate 0.25% or 0.5% in stable sterile 0.5% methylcellulose soln. Drop-Tainer 15 ml.
Use: Agent for glaucoma.

ISOPTO FRIN. (Alcon) Phenylephrine HCl 0.12% in a methylcellulose soln. Drop-Tainer 15 ml.
Use: Ophthalmic vasoconstrictor/mydriatic.

ISOPTO HOMATROPINE. (Alcon) Homatropine HBr 2% or 5% in methylcellulose soln. Drop-Tainer 5 ml, 15 ml.
Use: Cycloplegic mydriatic.

ISOPTO HYOSCINE. (Alcon) Hyoscine HBr 0.25% in a methylcellulose soln. Drop-Tainer 5 ml, 15 ml.
Use: Cycloplegic mydriatic.

ISOPTO P-ES. (Alcon) Pilocarpine 2%, eserine salicylate 0.25%, sterile buffered, isotonic vehicle containing methylcellulose 0.5%. Plastic Drop-Tainer 15 ml.
Use: Agent for glaucoma.

ISOPTO PLAIN. (Alcon) Hydroxypropyl methylcellulose 0.5%, benzalkonium Cl 0.01%. Drop-Tainer 15 ml.
Use: Artificial tear solution.

ISOPTO TEARS. (Alcon) Hydroxypropyl methylcellulose 0.5%, benzalkonium Cl 0.01%. Bot. Drop-Tainer 15 ml, 30 ml.
Use: Artificial tear solution.

ISORDIL SUBLINGUAL. (Wyeth-Ayerst) Isosorbide dinitrate 2.5 mg, 5 mg or 10 mg/Tab. **2.5 mg:** Bot. 100s, 500s, Clinipak 100s. **5 mg:** Bot. 100s, 250s, 500s, Clinipak 100s. **10 mg:** Bot. 100s.
Use: Antianginal agent.

ISORDIL TEMBIDS. (Wyeth-Ayerst) Isosorbide dinitrate 40 mg/Tab. or Cap. **Tab.:** Bot. 100s, 500s, 1000s. **Cap.:** Bot. 100s, 500s.
Use: Antianginal agent.

ISORDIL TITRADOSE TABLETS. (Wyeth-Ayerst) Isosorbide dinitrate 5 mg, 10 mg, 20 mg, 30 mg or 40 mg/Tab. **5 mg.:** Bot. 100s, 500s, 1000s, Clinipak 100s. **10 mg:** Bot. 100s, 500s, 1000s, Clinipak 100s. **20 mg:** Bot. 100s, 500s, Clinipak 100s. **30 mg:** Bot. 100s, 500s. Clinipak 100s. **40 mg:** Bot. 100s, Clinipak 100s.
Use: Antianginal agent.

ISORGEN-G. (Grafton) Isosorbide 5 mg or 10 mg/Tab. Bot. 1000s.
Use: Antianginal agent.

ISOSORB5. (Robinson) Isosorbide dinitrate oral 10 mg/Tab. Bot. 100s, 1000s.
Use: Antianginal agent.

ISOSORB10. (Robinson) Isosorbide dinitrate 10 mg/Tab. Bot. 100s, 1000s.
Use: Antianginal agent.

•**ISOSORBIDE.** USAN.
Use: Diuretic.

•**ISOSORBIDE CONCENTRATE,** U.S.P. XXII.
Use: Diuretic.

•**ISOSORBIDE ORAL SOLUTION,** U.S.P. XXII.
Use: Diuretic.

•**ISOSORBIDE DINITRATE,** U.S.P. XXII. Extended-release Cap., Chewable Tab., Extended-release Tab., Sublingual Tab., Tab., U.S.P. XXII. D-Glucitol, 1,4:3,6-dianhydro-, dinitrate.
Use: Coronary vasodilator; antianginal.
See: Dilatrate-SR, Cap. (Reed & Carnrick).
Iso-Bid, Cap. (Geriatric).

Iso-D, Tab., Cap. (Dunhall).
Isordil, Tab. (Wyeth-Ayerst).
Isordil Tembids Cap., Tab. (Wyeth-Ayerst).
Isosorb, Prods. (Robinson).
Nitromed, Tab. (U.S. Ethicals).
Onset, Tab. (Bock).
Sorbitrate, Tab. (Stuart).
Sorquad, Tab. (Solvay).
W/Phenobarbital.
See: Sorbitrate w/Phenobarbital, Tab. (Stuart).

•**ISOSORBIDE MONONITRATE.** USAN.
Use: Coronary vasodilator.

•**ISOSTERYL ALCOHOL.** USAN.
Use: Pharmaceutic aid.

•**ISOSULFAN BLUE.** USAN.
Use: Diagnostic aid.

ISOTEIN HN. (Sandoz Nutrition) Vanilla Flavor. Maltodextrin, delactosed lactalbumin, partially hydrogenated soy oil with BHA, fructose, medium chain triglycerides, artificial flavor, sodium caseinate, mono and diglycerides, sodium Cl, vitamins, minerals. Pow. Packet 2.75 oz.
Use: Enteral nutritional supplement.

ISOTHIPENDYL. B.A.N. 10-(2-Dimethylamino-propyl)-10H-pyrido[3,2-b]-[1,4]benzothiazine.
Use: Antihistamine.

•**ISOTIQUIMIDE.** USAN.
Use: Antiulcerative.

ISOTRATE. (Hauck) Isosorbide dinitrate 40 mg/Timecelle. Bot. 100s, 500s, UD 50s.
Use: Antianginal agent.

•**ISOTRETINOIN.** USAN.
Use: Keratolytic.

ISOTRETINOIN, U.S.P. XXII. 13-cis-retinoic acid.
Use: Treatment of severe recalcitrant cystic acne.
See: Accutane, Cap. (Roche).

ISOVEX. (U.S. Chemical) Ethaverine HCl 100 mg/Cap. Bot. 100s, 1000s.
Use: Peripheral vasodilator.

ISOVUE 300 INJECTION. (Squibb) Iopamidol 612 mg, tromethamine 1 mg, edetate calcium disodium 0.39 mg/ml. Vial 50 ml, Box 10s. Bot. 100 ml, Box 10s.
Use: Radiopaque agent.

ISOVUE 370 INJECTION. (Squibb) Iopamidol 755 mg, tromethamine 1 mg, edetate calcium disodium 0.48 mg/ml. Vial 50 ml, Box 10s; Bot. 100 ml, Box 10s; 150 ml, Box 10s; 200 ml, Box 10s.
Use: Radiopaque agent.

ISOVUE-M 200 INJECTION. (Squibb) Iopamidol 408 mg, tromethamine 1 mg, edetate calcium disodium 0.26 mg/ml. Vial 20 ml, Box 10s.
Use: Radiopaque agent.

ISOVUE-M 300 INJECTION. (Squibb) Iopamidol 612 mg, tromethamine 1 mg, edetate calcium disodium 0.39 mg/ml. Vial 20 ml, Box 10s.
Use: Radiopaque agent.

•**ISOXEPAC.** USAN.
Use: Anti-inflammatory.

•**ISOXICAM.** USAN.
Use: Anti-inflammatory.

•**ISOXSUPRINE HCl,** U.S.P. XXII. Inj., Tab., U.S.P. XXII. 1-(p-Hydroxy-phenyl)-2-(1′-methyl-2′-phenoxy ethylamino) propanol-1 HCl. p-Hydroxy-α-[1-[(1-methyl-2-phenoxyethyl)amino ethyl benzyl alcohol HCl.
Use: Vasodilator.
See: Rolisox-10, Tab. (Robinson).
Rolisox-20, Tab. (Robinson).
Vasodilan, Tab. (Mead Johnson).

I-SOYALAC. (Loma Linda) P-soy protein isolate, l-methionine, CHO-sucrose, tapioca dextrin. F-soy oil, soy lecithin. Corn free. Protein 20.2 Gm, carbohydrate 63.4 Gm, fat 35.5 Gm, iron 12 mg, 640 Cal/serving (1 qt). Concentrate 390 ml, ready to use 1 qt.
Use: Enteral nutritional supplement.

•**ISRADIPINE.** USAN.
Use: Antagonist (calcium channel).
See: DynaCirc (Sandoz).

I-SULFACET. (American) Sulfacetamide sodium 10%, 15% or 30% ophthalmic soln. Bot. 2 ml, 5 ml, 15 ml.
Use: Anti-infective, ophthalmic.

I-SULFALONE SUSPENSION. (American) Sulfacetamide sodium 100 mg, prednisolone acetate 5 mg. Ophthalmic susp. Bot. 5 ml, 15 ml.
Use: Anti-infective, ophthalmic.

ISUPREL GLOSSETS. (Winthrop Pharm) Isoproterenol HCl 10 mg or 15 mg/Tab. Bot. 50s.
Use: Bronchodilator.

ISUPREL INHALATION SOLUTION. (Winthrop Pharm) Isoproterenol HCl inhalation soln. 1:200 or 1:100. Bot. 10 ml, 60 ml.
Use: Bronchodilator.

ISUPREL MISTOMETER. (Winthrop Pharm) Isoproterenol HCl. Complete nebulizing unit of aerosol soln. containing 10 ml or 15 ml of isoproterenol HCl w/inert propellants, alcohol 33%, ascorbic acid. Measured dose of approximately 131 mcg. Aerosol Unit. Bot. 15 ml, 22.5 ml. Refill 15 ml, 22.5 ml.
Use: Bronchodilator.

ISUPREL STERILE INJECTION. (Winthrop Pharm) Isoproterenol HCl 0.2 mg, lactic acid 0.12 mg, sodium lactate 1.8 mg, sodium Cl 7 mg and not more than 1 mg sodium metabisulfite as preservative/ml of 1:5000 soln. Amp. 1 ml Box 25s; 5 ml Box 10s.
Use: Adjunct treatment of shock, cardiac standstill, etc.

ISUPRENE.
See: Isoproterenol (Various Mfr.).

•**ITAZIGREL.** USAN.
Use: Platelet anti-aggregatory agent.

ITCHAWAY. (Moyco) Zinc undecylenate 20%, undecylenic acid 2%. Pow. Can 1.5 oz.
Use: Antifungal, external.

ITOBARBITAL.
W/Acetaminophen.
See: Panitol, Tab. (Wesley).
•**ITRACONAZOLE.** USAN, B.A.N..
Use: Antifungal.
ITRAMIN TOSYLATE. B.A.N. 2-Nitratoethylamine toluene-p-sulfonate.
Use: Angina pectoris; vasodilator.
I-TROL. (Akorn) Neomycin sulfate-polymyxin B sulfate-dexamethasone 0.1%. Ophthalmic susp. Bot. 5 ml.
Use: Anti-infective, ophthalmic.
I-TROPINE. (Akorn) Atropine sulfate 1%. Ophthalmic soln. Bot. 2 ml, 5 ml, 15 ml.
Use: Cycloplegic mydriatic.
IVAREST. (Blistex) Calamine 14%, benzocaine 5%. **Cream:** 60 Gm. **Lot.:** 120 ml.
Use: Topical treatment of poison ivy, oak, sumac.
I.V. ESTRO. (Rocky Mtn.) Potassium estrone sulfate 4 mg/ml. Vial 10 ml Amp. 5 ml. Box 6s.
Use: Estrogen.
IVOCORT. (Hauck) Micronized hydrocortisone alcohol 0.5% or 1%. Bot. 4 oz.
Use: Corticosteroid.
IVY-CHEX. (Bowman) Polyvinyl pyrrolidone-vinyl acetate, benzalkonium Cl 1:1000 in alcohol acetone base. Aerosol can 4 oz.
Use: Treatment or prevention of poison ivy, poison oak, poison sumac dermatitis.
IVY DRY. (Ivy) Tannic acid 10%, isopropyl alcohol 12.5% Liq. 4 oz, Cream 1 oz, Super 6 oz.
Use: Relief of itching.
IVY-RID. (Mallard) Polyvinyl pyrrolidone-vinyl acetate, benzalkonium Cl. Spray can 2.75 oz.
Use: Relief of itching and discomfort of poison ivy, poison oak and poison sumac.
I-WASH. (Akorn) Phosphate buffered saline soln. Bot. 4 oz, 8 oz.
Use: Eye wash.
I-WHITE. (Akorn) Phenylephrine 0.12%, polyvinyl alcohol, hydroxyethyl cellulose. Soln. Bot. 15 ml.
Use: Ophthalmic vasoconstrictor/mydriatic.
IZONID TABLETS. (Major) Isoniazid 300 mg/Tab. Bot. 100s.
Use: Antituberculous agent.

J

JALOVIS.
See: Hyaluronidase (Various Mfr.).
JANIMINE. (Abbott) Imipramine HCl 10 mg, 25 mg or 50 mg/Tab. Bot. 100s, 1000s.
Use: Antidepressant.
JAPAN AGAR.
See: Agar (Various Mfr.).
JAPAN GELATIN.
See: Agar (Various Mfr.).
JAPAN ISINGLASS.
See: Agar (Various Mfr.).
JENAMICIN. (Hauck) Gentamicin sulfate 40 mg/ml. Vial 2 ml.
Use: Antibacterial, aminoglycoside.
JENSENEX. (Jenkins) Nicotinic acid 50 mg, salicylamide 0.3 Gm, vitamins B_{12} activity 3 mcg, C 15 mg/Tab. Bot. 1000s.
Use: Vitamin supplement, analgesic.
JEN-VITE. (Jenkins) Vitamins A 5000 IU, D 1000 IU, B_1 2.5 mg, B_2 2.5 mg, nicotinamide 20 mg, B_6 1 mg, calcium pantothenate 5 mg, B_{12} 2 mcg, C 40 mg, E 2 IU/Cap. Bot. 100s, 1000s.
Use: Vitamin supplement.
JERI-BATH. (Dermik) Concentrated moisturizing bath oil. Plastic Bot. 8 oz.
Use: Bath dermatological.
JETS. (Freeda) Lysine 300 mg, vitamins C 25 mg, B_{12} 25 mcg, B_6 5 mg, B_1 10 mg/Chew. tab. Bot. 30s, 250s, 500s.
Use: Vitamin supplement.
JEVITY LIQUID. (Ross) Calcium and sodium caseinates, soy fiber, hydrolyzed cornstarch, MCT (fractionated coconut oil) soy oil, corn oil, soy lecithin, vitamins A, B_1, B_2, B_3, B_5 B_6, B_{12}, C, D, E, K, folic acid, biotin, choline, Ca, P, Mg, Fe, Mn, Cu, Zn, I, Cl. In 240 ml.
Use: Enteral nutritional supplement.
JIFFY. (Block) Benzocaine, menthol, eugenol in glycerin-water base with SD alcohol 38-B 76%. Bot. 0.125 oz.
Use: Local anesthetic.
J-LIBERTY. (J Pharmacal) Chlordiazepoxide HCl 5 mg, 10 mg or 25 mg/Cap.
Use: Antianxiety agent.
JOHNSON'S BABY CREAM. (Johnson & Johnson) Dimethicone 2%. Jar 4 oz, 6 oz, Tube 2 oz.
Use: Skin protectant.
JOHNSON'S MEDICATED POWDER. (Johnson & Johnson) Bentonite, kaolin, talc, zinc oxide. Pow. Small, Medium, Large.
Use: Diaper rash product.
•**JOSAMYCIN.** USAN.
Use: Antibacterial.
JUNICOID. (Jenkins) Dextromethorphan HBr 5 mg, cocillana compound 88 mg, potassium guaiacolsulfonate 66 mg, citric acid 22 mg/5 ml. Syr. Bot. 3 oz, 4 oz, gal.
Use: Antitussive, expectorant.
•**JUNIPER TAR,** U.S.P. XXII. Oil of cade.
Use: Local anti-eczematic.
JUNYER-ALL. (Barth's) Vitamins A 6000 IU, D 400 IU, B_1 3 mg, B_2 6 mg, C 120 mg, niacin 1 mg, E 12 IU, B_{12} 10 mcg, calcium 217 mg, phosphorus 97.5 mg, red bone marrow 10 mg, organic iron 15 mg, iodine 0.1 mg, beef peptone 20 mg/2 Cap. Bot. 10 month, 3 month, 6 month supply.
Use: Vitamin supplement.

JUVOCAINE.
See: Procaine HCl (Various Mfr.).

K

K+10. (Alra) Potassium Cl 10 mEq/Tab. Bot. 100s, 500s, 1000s.
Use: Potassium supplement.

K-10 SOLUTION. (Cenci) Potassium Cl 10% in a sugarless nonalcoholic solution (20 mEq/15 ml). Bot. pt, gal.
Use: Potassium supplement.

K 34. Hexachlorophene.

KABIKINASE. (SKF) Streptokinase 250,000 IU, 600,000 IU or 750,000 IU/Vial. Pow. for inj. Vial 5 ml.
Use: Thrombolytic enzyme.

KAERGONA.
See: Menadione (Various Mfr.).

KAINAIR. (Pharmafair) Proparacaine HCl 0.5%. Ophthalmic soln. Bot. 2 ml, 15 ml.
Use: Local anesthetic, ophthalmic.

•**KALAFUNGIN.** USAN.
Use: Antifungal.

KALLIDINOGENASE. B.A.N. An enzyme that splits kinin and kallidin from kininogen.
Use: Vasodilator.

KALOL. (Jenkins) Boric acid, sodium biborate, sodium Cl, menthol, thymol, oil of eucalyptus, methyl salicylate (synthetic), carbolic acid/Tab. Bot. 1000s.

KALORY-PLUS. (Tyler) Thyroid 3 gr, amphetamine sulfate 15 mg, atropine sulfate 1/180 gr, aloin 0.25 gr, phenobarbital 0.25 gr/TR cap. Bot. 100s, 1000s.
Use: Anorexiant.

KAMAGEL. (Towne) Opium 15 mg, colloidal kaolin 6 Gm, pectin 300 mg, milk of bismuth 5 ml/fl oz. Bot. 4 oz.
Use: Antidiarrheal.

KAMFOLENE. (Wade) Camphor, menthol, methyl salicylate, oils turpentine and eucalyptus, carbolic acid 2%, calamine, zinc oxide in lanolin base. Jar 2 oz, lb.
Use: Antiseptic.

KANALKA TABLETS. (Lannett) Phenobarbital sodium 0.25 gr, benzocaine 0.25 gr, magnesium carbonate 2 gr, calcium carbonate 3 gr/Tab. Bot. 100s, 1000s.
Use: Sedative/hypnotic, antacid.

•**KANAMYCIN SULFATE,** U.S.P. XXII. Caps., Inj., Sterile, U.S.P. XXII. D-Streptamine, 0-3-amino-3-deoxy-α-d-glucopyranosyl-(1→6)-0-6-amino-6-deoxy-α-d-gluco-pyranosyl-(1→4)-2-deoxy-, sulfate (1:1). An antibiotic obtained from *Streptomycin kanamyceticus.*
Use: Antibacterial.
See: Kantrex, Cap., Vial (Bristol).
Klebcil, Inj. (Beecham).

KANKEX. (EJ Moore) Benzocaine, tannic acid, benzyl alcohol, diisobutyl-crosoxy-ethoxy-ethyl-dimethyl-benzyl-ammonium Cl, in propylene base. Bot. 0.5 oz w/applicator.
Use: Local anesthetic, topical.

KANTREX. (Bristol) Kanamycin sulfate. **Cap.:** 0.5 Gm. Bot. 20s, 100s. **Vial:** 0.5 Gm/2 ml or 1 Gm/3 ml. **Pediatric Inj.:** 75 mg/2 ml. **Disposable Syringe:** 500 mg/2 ml.
Use: Aminoglycoside.

KAOCASIL. (Jenkins) Kaolin colloidal 60 mg, calcium carbonate 0.1 Gm, magnesium trisilicate 60 mg, bismuth subgallate 15 mg, papain 8 mg, atropine sulfate 1/2000 gr/Tab. Bot. 1000s.
Use: Antacid, antidiarrheal, digestive aid, anticholinergic/antispasmodic.

KAOCHLOR 10% LIQUID. (Adria) Potassium and chloride 20 mEq/15 ml (potassium Cl 10%), alcohol 5%, saccharin, FD&C Yellow No. 5. Bot. pt.
Use: Potassium supplement.

KAOCHLOR-EFF. (Adria) Elemental potassium 20 mEq, chloride 20 mEq/Tab. Supplied by: Potassium Cl 0.6 Gm, potassium citrate 0.22 Gm, potassium bicarbonate 1 Gm, betaine HCl 1.84 Gm, saccharin 20 mg, artificial fruit flavor, tartrazine (color)/Tab. Sugar free. Carton 60s.
Use: Potassium supplement.

KAOCHLOR S-F 10% LIQUID. (Adria) Potassium 20 mEq, chloride 20 mEq/15 ml, saccharin, flavoring, alcohol 5%. Sugar free. Bot. 4 oz, pt.
Use: Potassium supplement.

KAODENE NON-NARCOTIC. (Pfeiffer) Kaolin 3.9 Gm, pectin 194.4 mg, sodium carboxymethylcellulose, bismuth subsalicylate/30 ml. Alcohol free. Susp. Bot. 120 ml.
Use: Antidiarrheal.

KAODENE WITH CODEINE. (Pfeiffer) Codeine phosphate 32.4 mg, kaolin 3.9 Gm, pectin 194.4 mg, sodium carboxymethylcellulose, bismuth subsalicylate/30 ml. Susp. Bot. 120 ml.
Use: Antidiarrheal.

KAODENE WITH PAREGORIC. (Pfeiffer) Anhydrous morphine 1.5 mg (paregoric ≈ 3.75 ml), kaolin 3.9 Gm, pectin 194.4 mg, sodium carboxymethylcellulose, bismuth subsalicylate/30 ml. Alcohol free. Susp. Bot. 120 ml.
Use: Antidiarrheal.

•**KAOLIN,** U.S.P. XXII. (Various Mfr.).
Use: Adsorbent for diarrhea.
W/Atropine sulfate, phenobarbital.
W/Belladonna, phenobarbital.
See: Bellkata, Tab. (Ferndale).
W/Bismuth compound.
See: Kaomine, Pow. (Lilly).
W/Bismuth subgallate.
See: Diastop, Liq. (Elder).
W/Bismuth subgallate, pectin, zinc phenolsulfonate, opium pow.
See: Diastay, Tab. (Elder).
W/Bismuth subsalicylate, salol, methyl salicylate, benzocaine, pectin.
W/Calcium carbonate, magnesium trisilicate, bismuth subgallate, papain, atropine sulphate.

See: Kaocasil, Tab. (Jenkins).
W/Cornstarch, camphor, zinc oxide, eucalyptus oil.
See: Mexsana, Pow. (Plough).
W/Furazolidone, pectin.
See: Furoxone, Liq. (Eaton).
W/Hyoscyamine sulfate, sodium benzoate, atropine sulfate, hyoscine HBR, pectin.
See: Donnagel, Susp. (Robins).
W/Neomycin sulfate, pectin.
See: Pecto-Kalin, Liq. (Harvey).
W/Opium pow., bismuth subgallate, pectin, zinc phenolsulfonate.
See: Bismuth, Pectin & Paregoric (Lemmon).
W/Opium pow., pectin, hyoscyamine sulfate, atropine sulfate, hyoscine HBr, alcohol.
See: Donnagel P.G., Susp. (Robins).
W/Paregoric, aluminum hydroxide, bismuth subcarbonate, pectin.
See: Kapinal, Tab. (Jenkins).
W/Pectin.
See: Kaopectate, Liq. (Upjohn).
Kapectin, Liq. (Approved).
Pecto-Kalin, Susp. (Lemmon).
Pectokay Mixture (Bowman).
W/Pectin, belladonna alkaloids.
See: Kapectolin, Liq. (GMC).
W/Pectin, bismuth subcarbonate.
See: B-K-P Mixture, Liq. (Sutliff & Case).
W/Pectin, bismuth subcarbonate, belladonna.
See: Kay-Pec, Liq. (Case).
W/Pectin, bismuth subcarbonate, opium pow.
See: KBP/O, Cap. (Cole).
W/Pectin, bismuth subsalicylate.
W/Pectin, bismuth subsalicylate, paregoric, zinc sulfocarbolate.
W/Pectin, hyoscyamine sulfate, atropine sulfate, hyoscine HBr.
See: Kapigam, Liq. (Reid-Rowell).
Palsorb Improved, Liq. (Hauck).
W/Pectin, pow. opium extract.
See: Pecto-Kalin, Susp. (Lemmon).
W/Pectin, opium pow., bismuth subgallate, zinc phenolsulfonate.
See: Cholactabs, Tab. (Philips Roxane).
B.P.P., Tab. (Lemmon).
W/Pectin, paregoric (equivalent).
See: Duosorb, Liq. (Reid-Rowell).
Kaoparin, Liq. (McKesson).
Kapectin, Liq. (Approved).
Ka-Pek w/Paregoric, Liq. (APC).
Parepectolin, Susp. (Rorer).
W/Pectin, zinc phenolsulfonate.
See: Pectocel, Susp. (Lilly).
Pectocomp, Liq. (Lannett).
W/Phenobarbital, atropine sulfate, aluminum hydroxide gel.
See: Kao-Lumin, Tab. (Philips Roxane).
W/Salol, zinc sulfocarbolate, aluminum hydroxide, bismuth subsalicylate, pectin.
See: Wescola Antidiarrheal-Stomach Upset (Western Research).

KAOLIN COLLOIDAL.
W/Bismuth subcarbonate.
See: Bisilad, Susp. (Central).
W/Magnesium trisilicate, aluminum hydroxide dried gel.
See: Kamadrox, Tab. (Elder).
Kathmagel, Tab. (Mason).
W/Opium, pectin, milk of bismuth.
See: Kamagel Liq. (Towne).
W/Paregoric, pectin.
See: Parepectolin, Susp. (Rorer Consumer).
W/Paregoric, pectin, milk of bismuth, methyl parahydroxybenzoate, alcohol.
See: Mul-Sed, Susp. (Webcon).
W/Pectin, aromatics.
See: Paocin, Susp. (Beecham-Massengill).
W/Pectin, belladonna alkaloids.
See: Kamabel, Liq. (Towne).
W/Phenobarbital, homatropine methylbromide.
See: Lanokalin, Tab. (Lannett).

KAON CL CONTROLLED RELEASE TABLETS. (Adria) Potassium Cl 500 mg/Tab., FD&C Yellow No. 5. Bot. 100s, 250s, 1000s.
Use: Potassium supplement.

KAON CL-10 CONTROLLED RELEASE TABLETS. (Adria) Potassium Cl 750 mg/Tab. Bot. 100s, 500s, 1000s. Stat-Pak 100s.
Use: Potassium supplement.

KAON CL 20%. (Adria) Potassium and chloride 40 mEq (to potassium Cl 3 Gm)/15 ml, saccharin, flavoring, alcohol 5%. Bot. pt.
Use: Potassium supplement.

KAON ELIXIR. (Adria) Elemental potassium 20 mEq (as potassium gluconate 4.68 Gm)/15 ml, aromatics, grape and lemon-lime flavors, alcohol 5%, saccharin. Unit pkg. pt, gal.
Use: Potassium supplement.

KAON TABLETS. (Adria) Elemental potassium 5 mEq obtained from potassium gluconate 1.17 Gm/SC Tab. Bot. 100s, 500s.
Use: Potassium supplement.

KAOPECTATE. (Upjohn) Kaolin 5.85 Gm, pectin 130 mg/oz. Bot. 8 oz, 12 oz, 16 oz, 1 gal, UD pkg. 3 oz.
Use: Antidiarrheal.

KAOPECTATE TABLET FORMULA. (Upjohn) Attapulgite 750 mg/Tab. Blister pak 12s, 20s.
Use: Antidiarrheal.

KAOPHEN TABLETS. (Vale) Phenobarbital 6.5 mg, belladonna extract 0.1 mg, kaolin 388.8 mg/Tab. Bot. 100s, 1000s.
Use: Antidiarrheal.

KAO-TIN. (Major) Kaolin 5.85 Gm, pectin 130 mg/30 ml. Susp. Bot. 120 ml, 240 ml, pt, gal.
Use: Antidiarrheal.

KAPECTIN. (Approved) Kaolin 90 gr, pectin 2 gr/oz. Bot. gal.
W/Paregoric Liq. 4 oz.
Use: Antidiarrheal.

KAPECTOLIN. (Goldline) Kaolin 5.85 Gm, pectin 130 mg/30 ml. Susp. Bot. gal.
Use: Antidiarrheal.

KAPECTOLIN-PG LIQUID. (Goldline) Bot. 6 oz, pt, gal.
Use: Antidiarrheal.

KAPECTOLIN P.G. (Century) Powdered opium 24 mg, kaolin 6 mg, pectin 142.8 mg, hyoscyamine sulfate 0.1037 mg, atropine sulfate 0.0194 mg, hyoscine hydrobromide 0.0065 mg, sodium benzoate preservative 65 mg Bot. 120 ml, 180 ml, pt, gal.
Use: Antidiarrheal.

KA-PEK. (APC) Kaolin 90 gr, pectin 4.5 gr/fl oz. Bot. 6 oz, gal.
Use: Antidiarrheal.

KA-PEK WITH PAREGORIC. (APC) Paregoric 60 min, kaolin 90 gr, pectin 4.5 gr/fl oz. Bot. 4 oz.
Use: Antidiarrheal.

KAPILIN.
See: Menadione (Various Mfr.).

KARAYA GUM. (Penick) Indian Gum. Sterculia gum,
See: Tri-Costivin (Prof. Lab.).
W/Frangula.
See: Saraka, Gran. (Plough).
W/Psyllium seed, plantago ovata, brewers yeast.
See: Plantamucin Gran. (Elder).
W/Cortex rhamni frangulae.
See: Movicol (Norgine).
W/Refined psyllium mucilloid.
See: Hydrocil regular (Reid-Rowell).

KARAYA POWDER. (Sween) Bot. 3 oz.
Use: Ostomy care product.

KAREON.
See: Menadione (Various Mfr.).

KARIDIUM. (Lorvic) **Tab.:** Sodium fluoride 2.21 mg, sodium Cl 94.49 mg, disintegrant 0.5 mg. Bot. 180s, 1000s. **Liq.:** Sodium fluoride 2.21 mg, sodium Cl 10 mg, purified water q.s./8 drops. Bot. 30 ml, 60 ml.
Use: Dental caries preventative.

KARIGEL. (Lorvic) Fluoride ion 0.5%, pH 5.6. Gel. Bot. 30 ml, 130 ml, 250 ml.
Use: Dental caries preventative.

KARIGEL-N. (Lorvic) Fluoride ion 0.5% in neutral pH gel. Bot. 24 ml, 125 ml.
Use: Dental caries preventative.

•**KASAL.** USAN. Approximately $Na_8AP_2(OH_2(PO_4)_4$ with about 30% of dibasic sodium phosphate; sodium aluminum phosphate, basic.
Use: Food additive.

KASDENOL. (E.J. Moore) Clorpactin WCS-60. Jar 10 Gm.
Use: Germicidal for bleeding gums.

KASOF. (Stuart) Docusate potassium 240 mg/Cap. Bot. 30s, 60s.
Use: Laxative.

KASUGAMYCIN. Under study.
Use: Antibiotic.

KATO. (ICN) Potassium Cl for oral soln. potassium 20 mEq. Carton 30s, 120s.
Use: Potassium supplement.

KAVITON.
See: Menadione, U.S.P. XXII. (Various Mfr.).

KAY CIEL ELIXIR. (Forest) Potassium Cl 1.5 Gm/15 ml. (20 mEq/15 ml), alcohol 4%. Bot. 120 ml, 473 ml, gal.
Use: Potassium supplement.

KAY CIEL POWDER. (Forest) Potassium chloride 1.5 Gm/Packette. (20 mEq/Packet), 4% alcohol. Box 30s, 100s, 500s.
Use: Potassium supplement.

KAYEXALATE. (Winthrop Pharm.) Sodium polystyrene sulfonate. Jar lb.
Use: Potassium removing resin.

KAYLIXIR. (Lannett) Potassium (as potassium gluconate) 20 mEq/15 ml, alcohol 5%, saccharin. Elix. Bot. pt, gal.
Use: Potassium supplement.

KBP/O. (Forest) Kaolin 350 mg, pectin 60 mg, powdered opium 3 mg, bismuth subcarbonate 60 mg/Cap. Bot. 100s, 1000s.
Use: Antidiarrheal.

K+CARE ET. (Alra) Potassium bicarbonate 25 mEq/Effervescent tab. Bot. 30s, 100s, 1000s.
Use: Potassium supplement.

K-C LIQUID. (Century) Kaolin 5.2 Gm, pectin 260 mg, bismuth subcarbonate 260 mg/oz. Bot. 4 oz, pt, gal.
Use: Antidiarrheal.

K-C SUSPENSION. (Century Pharm.) Kaolin 5.2 Gm, pectin 260 mg, bismuth subcarbonate 260 mg/30 ml. Bot. 120 ml, pt, gal.
Use: Antidiarrheal.

KC-20 ELIXIR. (Scruggs) Bot. pt, gal.

KCL-20. (Western Research) Potassium Cl 1.5 Gm (potassium 20 mEq, chloride 20 mEq)/Packet. Box 30s.
Use: Potassium supplement.

K.D.C. VAGINAL CREAM. (Kenyon) Sulfanilamide 15%, 9-aminoacridine HCl 0.2%, allantoin 2% in a dispersible base containing stearic acid, diglycol, stearate, triethanolamine, propylene glycol, lactic acid, water.
Use: Anti-infective, vaginal.

K-DEC TABLETS. (Schein) Iron 27 mg, vitamins A 5000 IU, D 400 IU, E 30 IU, B_1 2.25 mg, B_2 2.6 mg, B_3 20 mg, B_5 10 mg, B_6 3 mg, B_{12} 9 mcg, C 90 mg, folic acid 0.4 mg, biotin 45 mcg, Ca, Cl, Cr, Cu, I, K, Mg, Mn, P, Se, Zn/Tab. Bot. 100s.
Use: Vitamin/mineral supplement.

K-DUR 10 & 20. (Key) **10:** Potassium Cl 750 mg (10 mEq)/SR Tab. **20:** Potassium Cl 1500 mg (20 mEq)/SR Tab. Bot. 100s.
Use: Potassium supplement.

KE.
See: Cortisone Acetate (Various Mfr.).

KEDRIN TABLET. (Dolcin) Analgesic compound. Bot. 100s.
Use: Analgesic.

KEELAMIN. (Mericon) Zinc 20 mg, manganese 5 mg, copper 3 mg/Tab. Bot. 100s.
Use: Mineral supplement.

KEEP-A-WAKE. (Stayner) Vitamins B_1 5 mg, B_2 2 mg, B_{12} activity (cobalamin concentrate 1.5 mcg), niacinamide 10 mg, caffeine citrate 2.5 gr/Tab. Bot. 24s.
Use: CNS stimulant.

KEFLET TABLETS. (Dista) Cephalexin 250 mg, 500 mg or 1 Gm/Tab. **250 mg or 500 mg:** Bot. 20s, 100s. **1 Gm:** Bot. 24s, UD 100s.
Use: Antibacterial, cephalosporin.

KEFLEX. (Dista) Cephalexin. **Pulvule:** 250 mg or 500 mg. Bot. 20s, 100s. Blister pkg. 10 × 10s; **Tab.:** 1 Gm. Bot. 24s. Blister pkg. 100s. **For Oral Susp.:** 125 mg/5 ml. Bot. 60 ml, 100 ml, 200 ml, UD 5 ml × 100s; 250 mg/5 ml. Bot. 100 ml, 200 ml, UD 5 ml × 100s.
Use: Antibacterial, cephalosporin.

KEFLEX FOR PEDIATRIC DROPS. (Dista) Cephalexin 100 mg/ml. Dropper bot. 10 ml.
Use: Antibacterial, cephalosporin.

KEFTAB. (Dista) Cephalexin HCl monohydrate 250 mg or 500 mg/Tab. Bot. 100s.
Use: Antibacterial, cephalosporin.

KEFUROX. (Lilly) Cefuroxime sodium 750 mg or 1.5 Gm/Vial. ADD-VANTAGE **750 mg:** Vial 10 ml, Box 25s. Vial 100 ml, Box 10s. **1.5 Gm:** Vial 100 ml, Box 10s. 1.5 Gm Vial, 10s.
Use: Antibacterial, cephalosporin.

KEFZOL. (Lilly) Cefazolin sodium 250 mg, 500 mg or 1 Gm/10 ml and 500 mg, 1 Gm or 10 Gm/100 ml. **250 mg/10 ml:** Vial 1s; **500 mg/10 ml:** Vial 1s. Traypak 25s; **500 mg/100 ml:** Vial. Traypak 10s; **1 Gm/10 ml:** Vial 1s. Traypak 25s; **1 Gm/100 ml:** Vial. Traypak 10s; **10 Gm/100 ml:** Vial. Traypak 6s; **Redi Vial 500 mg:** 1s, Traypak 10s; **Redi Vial 1 Gm:** 1s. Traypak 10s; **Faspak 500 mg or 1 Gm:** Box 96s. **Add-Vantage Vial 500 mg or 1 Gm:** 25s.
Use: Antibacterial, cephalosporin.

KELEX. (Nutrition) Iron choline citrate 360 mg providing approximately 40 mg of elemental iron/Tabseal. Bot. 90s.
Use: Iron supplement.

KELGIN. Algin.

KELL E. (Canright) di-α Tocopheryl 100 IU, 200 IU or 400 IU. Bot. 100s.
Use: Vitamin E supplement.

KELLOGG'S TASTELESS CASTOR OIL. (Beecham Products) Castor oil 100%. Bot. 2 oz.
Use: Laxative.

KELP. (Arcum) Tab. Bot. 100s, 1000s.

KELP TABLETS. (Faraday) Iodine from kelp 0.15 mg/Tab. Bot. 100s.

KELP PLUS. (Barth's) Iodine from kelp plus 16 trace minerals/Tab. Bot. 100s, 500s, 1000s.

KEMADRIN. (Burroughs Wellcome) Procyclidine HCl 5 mg/Tab. Bot. 100s.
Use: Antiparkinson agent.

KEMITHAL. Thialbarbital. 5-Allyl-5-cyclohex-2-enyl-2-thiobarbituric acid.

KENAC CREAM. (NMC Labs) Triamcinolone acetonide cream 0.025% or 0.1%. Tube 15 Gm, 60 Gm, 80 Gm, Jar 240 Gm.
Use: Corticosteroid, topical.

KENAC OINTMENT. (NMC Labs) Triamcinolone acetonide ointment 0.1%. Tube 15 Gm, 80 Gm.
Use: Corticosteroid, topical.

KENACORT DIACETATE. (Squibb Mark) Triamcinolone diacetate equivalent to triamcinolone 4 mg, buffered with sodium citrate, sodium phosphate/5 ml. Bot. 120 ml.
Use: Corticosteroid.

KENAHIST-S.A. (Kenyon) Phenylpropanolamine HCl 50 mg, pheniramine maleate 25 mg, pyrilamine maleate 25 mg/Tab. Bot. 100s, 1000s.
Use: Decongestant, antihistamine.

KENAJECT. (Mayrand) Triamcinolone acetonide 4 mg/ml. Vial 5 ml.
Use: Corticosteroid.

KENAKION. (Harriett Lane Home of Johns Hopkins Hospital) Vitamin K-1 oxide.
Use: Vitamin K-induced kernicterus.

KENALOG. (Squibb Mark) Triamcinolone acetonide. **0.1% Cream:** Tube 15 Gm, 60 Gm, 80 Gm, Jar 240 Gm, in aqueous lotion base w/propylene glycol, cetyl and stearyl alcohols, glyceryl monostearate, sorbitan monopalmitate, polyoxyethylene sorbitan monolaurate, methylparaben, propylparaben, polyethylene glycol monostearate, simethicone, sorbic acid. **0.5% Cream:** Tube 20 Gm. **0.1% Oint.:** (w/base of polyethylene, mineral oil) Tube 15 Gm, 60 Gm, 80 Gm; Jar 240 Gm, **0.5% Oint.:** Tube 20 Gm. **Spray:** 6.6 mg/100 Gm, alcohol 10.3%. Can 23 Gm, 63 Gm.
Use: Corticosteroid, topical.

KENALOG 0.025%. (Squibb Mark) Triamcinolone acetonide. **Cream:** Tube 15 Gm, 80 Gm, Jar 240 Gm. **Lot.:** In aqueous lotion base w/ propylene glycol, cetyl and stearyl alcohols, glyceryl monostearate, sorbitan monopalmitate, polyoxyethylene sorbitan monolaurate, methylparaben, propylparaben, polyethylene glycol monostearate, simethicone, sorbic acid, tinted in an isopropyl palmitate vehicle with alcohol (4.7%). Bot. 60 ml. **Oint.:** Plastibase (w/base of polyethylene and mineral oil gel). 15 Gm, 80 Gm, 240 Gm.
Use: Corticosteroid, topical.

KENALOG H. (Squibb Mark) Triamcinolone acetonide cream USP 0.1%. Each Gm of cream provides 1 mg of triamcinolone acetonide in a specially formulated hydrophilic vanishing cream base containing propylene glycol, dimethicone 350, castor oil, cetearyl alcohol and ceteareth-20, propylene glycol stearate, white petrolatum, purified water. Tube 15 Gm, 60 Gm.
Use: Corticosteroid, topical.

KENALOG-10 INJECTION. (Squibb Mark) Sterile triamcinolone acetonide suspension 10 mg/ml, sodium Cl for isotonicity, benzyl alcohol 0.9% (w/v) as a preservative, sodium carboxymethylcellulose 0.75%, polysorbate 80 0.04%. Sodium hydroxide or HCl acid may be present to adjust

pH to 5 to 7.5. Nitrogen packed at the time of manufacture. Vial 5 ml.
Use: Corticosteroid.

KENALOG-40 INJECTION. (Squibb Mark) Sterile triamcinolone acetonide suspension 40 mg/ml, sodium chloride for isotonicity, benzyl alcohol 0.9% (w/v) as a preservative, sodium carboxymethylcellulose 0.75%, polysorbate 80 0.04%. Sodium hydroxide or HCl acid may be present to adjust pH to 5 to 7.5. Nitrogen packed at the time of manufacture. Vial 1 ml, 5 ml, 10 ml.
Use: Corticosteroid.

KENALOG IN ORABASE. (Squibb Mark) Triamcinolone acetonide 0.1% in Orabase. Triamcinolone acetonide 1 mg/Gm. Tube 5 Gm.
Use: Corticosteroid.

KENAZIDE-E. (Kenyon) Hydrochlorothiazide 50 mg/Tab. Bot. 100s, 1000s.
Use: Antihypertensive.

KENAZIDE-H. (Kenyon) Hydrochlorothiazide 50 mg/Tab. Bot. 100s, 1000s.
Use: Antihypertensive.

KENCORT. (Kenyon) Hydrocortisone 1%, clioquinol 3% in bland, water washable base. Jar lb.
Use: Corticosteroid, antifungal.

KENDALL'S "COMPOUND B."
See: Corticosterone (Various Mfr.).

KENDALL'S "COMPOUND E."
See: Cortisone Acetate (Various Mfr.).

KENDALL'S "COMPOUND F."
See: 17-Hydroxycorticosterone (Various Mfr.).

KENDALL'S "DESOXY COMPOUND B."
See: Desoxycorticosterone Acetate (Various Mfr.).

KENISONE DROPS. (Kenyon) Neomycin sulfate 6 mg, hydrocortisone 5 mg, parachlorometaxylenol 0.05%, pramoxine HCl 1%, alcohol 4.8%/ml. Bot. 15 ml.
Use: Anti-infective, corticosteroid, otic.

KENTONIC. (Kenyon) Vitamins A 25,000 IU, D 1000 IU, B_1 10 mg, B_2 10 mg, B_6 5 mg, B_{12} 5 mg, C 200 mg, niacinamide 100 mg, calcium pantothenate 20 mg/Cap. Bot. 1000s.
Use: Vitamin supplement.

KEN-TUSS. (Kenyon) Dextromethorphan HBr 10 mg, phenylephrine HCl 5 mg, chlorpheniramine maleate 2 mg, salicylamide 227 mg, phenacetin 100 mg, caffeine alkaloid 10 mg, ascorbic acid 20 mg/Tab. Bot. 100s, 1000s.
Use: Antitussive, decongestant, antihistamine, analgesic.

KENWOOD THERAPEUTIC LIQUID. (Kenwood) Vitamins A 10,000 IU, D 400 IU, E 4.5 IU, C 150 mg, B_1 6 mg, B_2 3 mg, niacinamide 60 mg, B_6 1 mg, calcium pantothenate 6 mg, calcium 38 mg, phosphorus 29 mg, magnesium 6 mg, manganese 1 mg, potassium 5 mg/15 ml. Bot. 12 oz.
Use: Vitamin/mineral supplement.

KERALYT GEL. (Westwood) Salicylic acid 6% in a gel base of propylene glycol w/alcohol 19.4%, hydroxypropyl cellulose, water. Tube 1 oz.
Use: Keratolytic.

KERATOLYTICS.
See: Condylox (Oclassen).

KERI CREME. (Westwood) Cream containing water, mineral oil, talc, sorbitol, ceresin, lanolin alcohol, magnesium stearate, glyceryl oleate/propylene glycol, isopropyl myristate, methylparaben, propylparaben, fragrance, quaternium-15. Tube 2.5 oz.
Use: Emollient.

KERI FACIAL CLEANSER. (Westwood) Water, glycerin, squalane, propylene glycol, glyceryl stearate, PEG-100 stearate, stearic acid, steareth-20, lanolin alcohol, magnesium aluminium silicate, cetyl alcohol, beeswax, PEG-20 sorbitan, beeswax, methylparaben, propylparaben, quaternium-15, fragrance. Bot. 4 oz.
Use: Therapeutic skin cleanser.

KERI FACIAL SOAP. (Westwood) Sodium tallowate, sodium cocoate, water, mineral oil, octyl hydroxystearate, fragrance, glycerin, titanium dioxide, PEG-75, lanolin oil, docusate sodium, PEG-4 dilaurate, propylparaben, PEG-40 stearate, glyceryl monostearate, PEG-100 stearate, sodium Cl, BHT, EDTA. Bar 3.25 oz.
Use: Therapeutic skin cleanser.

KERI LIGHT LOTION. (Westwood) Water, stearyl alcohol, ceteareath-20, cetearyl octaneoate, glycerin, stearyl heptanoate, stearyl alcohol, Carbomer 934, sodium hydroxide, squalane, methylparaben, propylparaben, fragrance. Bot. 6.5 oz, 13 oz.
Use: Emollient.

KERI LOTION. (Westwood) Mineral oil, lanolin oil, water, propylene glycol, glyceryl stearate, PEG-100 stearate, PEG 40 stearate, PEG-4 dilaurate, laureth-4, parabens, docusate sodium, triethanolamine, quaternium 15, carbomer 934, fragrance. Bot. 6.5 oz, 13 oz, 20 oz.
Use: Emollient.

KERID EAR DROPS. (Blair) Urea, glycerin in propylene glycol. Bot. w/dropper 8 ml.
Use: Otic preparation.

KERLONE. (Searle) Betaxolol HCl 10 mg or 25 mg/Tab. Bot. 100s, UD 100s.
Use: Beta-adrenergic blocking agent.

KEROCAINE.
See: Procaine HCl (Various Mfr.).

KERODEX. (Wyeth-Ayerst)
No. 51: Water-miscible. Tube 4 oz, Jar lb.
No. 71: Water-repellent. Tube 4 oz, Jar lb.
Use: Emollient.

KEROHYDRIC. A de-waxed, oil-soluble fraction of lanolin.
Use: Emollient, cleanser.
See: Alpha-Keri, Soap, Spray (Westwood).
Keri, Cream, Lot. (Westwood).

W/Docusate sodium, sodium alkyl polyether sulfonate, sodium sulfoacetate, sulfur, salicylic acid, hexachlorophene.
See: Sebulex, Cream, Liq. (Westwood).

KERR INSTA-CHAR. (Kerr) **Regular:** Aqueous suspension activated charcoal 50 Gm/8 oz. **Pediatric:** Aqueous suspension activated charcoal 15 Gm/4 oz.
Use: Antidote.

KERR TRIPLE DYE. (Kerr) Gentian violet, proflavine hemisulfate, brilliant green in water. Dispensing bot. 15 ml. Single Use Dispos-A-Swab 0.65 ml, Box 10s, Case 10 × 50 Box.
Use: Antiseptic.

KESSADROX. (McKesson) Magnesium-aluminum hydroxide gel. Bot. 12 oz.
Use: Antacid.

KESSOTAPP ELIXIR. (McKesson) Brompheniramine maleate, phenylephrine HCl, phenylpropanolamine HCl/5 ml. Bot. pt, gal.
Use: Antihistamine, decongestant.

KESSO-TETRA. (McKesson) Tetracycline HCl 250 mg or 500 mg/Cap. Bot. 100s, 1000s, 5000s.
Use: Anti-infective.

KESTRIN AQUEOUS. (Hyrex) Conjugated estrogens 20,000 units. (2 mg/ml) in aqueous soln. Vial 10 ml.
Use: Estrogen.

KESTRONE 5. (Hyrex) Estrone 50,000 units (5 mg/ml) in aqueous soln. Vial 10 ml.
Use: Estrogen.

KETALAR. (Parke-Davis) Ketamine HCl, sodium Cl, benzethonium Cl. **10 mg/ml:** Vial 20 ml, 25 ml and 50 ml. Pkg. 10s; **50 mg/ml:** Vial 10 ml. **100 mg/ml:** Vial 5 ml. Pkg. 10s.
Use: General anesthetic.

•**KETAMINE HCl,** U.S.P. XXII. Inj., U.S.P. XXII. (±)-2-(o-Chlorophenyl)-2-(methylamino) cyclohexanone HCl.
Use: Anesthetic.
See: Ketaject, Vial (Bristol).
Ketalar, Inj. (Parke-Davis).

•**KETANSERIN.** USAN.
Use: Serotonin antagonist.

•**KETAZOCINE.** USAN.
Use: Analgesic.

•**KETAZOLAM.** USAN.
Use: Tranquilizer.

•**KETHOXAL.** USAN.
Use: Antiviral.

•**KETIPRAMINE FUMARATE.** USAN. 5-[3-Diethylamino)propyl]-5,11-dihydro-10H-dibenz[b, f]-azepin-10-one fumarate (1:1).
Use: Antidepressant.

KETOBEMIDONE. B.A.N. 4-(3-Hydroxyphenyl)-1-methyl-4-propionylpiperidine. Cliradon.
Use: Narcotic analgesic.

•**KETOCONAZOLE.** USAN.
Use: Antifungal.

•**KETOCONAZOLE,** U.S.P. XXII. Tab., U.S.P. XXII. 1-acetyl-4 (4-((2-2(2,4 dichlorophenyl)-2-(1-H-imidazol-1-yimethyl)-1,3-dioxolan-4-yl)methoxy) phenyl) piperazine.
Use: Broad spectrum antifungal.
See: Nizoral, Tab. (Janssen).

KETODESTRIN.
See: Estrone (Various Mfr.).

KETO-DIASTIX REAGENT STRIPS. (Ames) Dip and read reagent strip test for glucose and ketones in urine. Two test areas: glucose levels from 30 mg to 5000 mg/dL; Ketone test (acetoacetic acid) negative 5 mg, 40 mg, 80 mg, 160 mg/dL. Strip Bot. 50s, 100s.
Use: Diagnostic aid.

KETOHEXAZINE. 4, 6-Diethyl-3(2H)-pyridazinono (Lederle).
Use: Hypnotic.

KETOHYDROXYESTRATRIENE.
See: Estrone.

KETOHYDROXYESTRIN.
See: Estrone (Various Mfr.).

•**KETOPROFEN.** USAN.
Use: Anti-inflammatory.
See: Orudis, Cap. (Wyeth-Ayerst).

•**KETORFANOL.** USAN.
Use: Analgesic.

•**KETOROLAC TROMETHAMINE.** USAN.
Use: Analgesic.
See: Toradol (Syntex).

KETOSTIX REAGENT STRIPS. (Ames) Sodium nitroprusside, sodium phosphate, glycine. Stick test for ketones in urine (measures acetoacetic acid). Bot. 50s, 100s, UD 20s.
Use: Diagnostic aid.

•**KETOTIFEN FUMARATE.** USAN.
Use: Antiasthmatic.

KEY-PLEX UNIVIAL. (Hyrex) Vitamins B_1 50 mg, B_2 5 mg, B_{12} 1000 mcg, pyridoxine HCl 5 mg, d-panthenol 6 mg, niacinamide 125 mg, ascorbic acid 50 mg/ml. Vial 10 ml.
Use: Parenteral nutritional supplement.

KEY-PRED. (Hyrex) Prednisolone. **25 mg/ml:** Vial 10 ml, 30 ml; **50 mg/ml:** Vial 10 ml.
Use: Corticosteroid.

KEY-PRED-SP. (Hyrex) Prednisolone sodium phosphate 20 mg/ml. Vial 10 ml.
Use: Corticosteroid.

K-FORTE. (O'Connor) Potassium 39 mg (from potassium gluconate, potassium citrate, potassium Cl), Vitamin C 10 mg/Tab. Bot. 90s.
Use: Potassium supplement.

K-FORTE MAXIMUM STRENGTH. (O'Connor) Potassium 99 mg, Vitamin C 25 mg/Tab. Bot. 60s.
Use: Potassium supplement.

K-G ELIXIR. (Geneva Marsam) Potassium (as potassium gluconate) 20 mEq/15 ml, alcohol 5%. Elix. Bot. pt.
Use: Potassium replacement.

KHAROPHEN.
See: Acetarsone (Various Mfr.).

KHELLIN. 5,8-dimethoxy-2-methyl-4′,5′-furano-6,7-chromone.
Use: Coronary vasodilator.

KIDDIE POWDER. (Gordon) Pure fine Italian talc. Can 3.5 oz.
Use: Antifungal.

KIDDIES SIALCO. (Foy) Chlorpheniramine maleate 2 mg, phenylephrine HCl 2.5 mg, acetaminophen 62.5 mg, salicylamide 75 mg/Tab. Bot. 1000s.
Use: Antihistamine, decongestant, analgesic.

KIDDI-VITES, Improved. (Geneva Marsam) Vitamins A 5000 IU, D 500 IU, B_1 1 mg, B_2 1.5 mg, B_{12} 2 mcg, C 50 mg, B_6 1 mg, pantothenate 2 mg, niacinamide 10 mg/Tab. Bot. 100s, 1000s.
Use: Vitamin supplement.

KIDNEY FUNCTION AGENTS.
See: Indigo Carmine Soln. (Various Mfr.).
Inulin, Amp. (Arnar-Stone).
Iodohippurate, Sodium.
Mannitol Soln., Amp. (Merck Sharp & Dohme).
Methylene Blue (Various Mfr.).
Phenolsulfonphthalein (Various Mfr.).

KIE SYRUP. (Laser) Potassium iodide 150 mg, ephedrine HCl 8 mg/5 ml. Syr. Bot. pt, gal.
Use: Expectorant, decongestant.

KINATE. Hexahydrotetra hydroxybenzoate salt, quinic acid salt.

KINESED. (Stuart) Phenobarbital 16 mg, hyoscyamine sulfate, atropine sulfate 0.12 mg, scopolamine hydrobromide 0.007 mg/Tab. Bot. 100s.
Use: Anticholinergic combination.

KINEVAC. (Squibb) Sincalide 5 mcg/vial. For gallbladder, pancreatic secretion and cholecystography.
Use: Diagnostic aid.

KIN WHITE. (Whiteworth) Triamcinolone acetonide. **Cream:** 0.025% or 1%. Tube 15 Gm, 80 Gm. **Oint.:** 1%. Tube 15 Gm, 80 Gm.
Use: Corticosteroid, topical.

•**KITASAMYCIN.** USAN. An antibiotic substance obtained from cultures of *Streptomyces kitasatoensis.* Under study.
Use: Antibiotic.

KLAVIKORDAL. (U.S. Ethicals) Nitroglycerin 2.6 mg/SR Tab. Bot. 100s, 1000s.
Use: Antihypertensive.

KLEBSIELLA PNEUMONIAE.
W/*Haemophilus influenzae, Neisseria catarrhalis, streptococci, staphylococci, pneumococci,* killed.
See: Mixed Vaccine No. 4 W/H. Influenzae (Lilly).

KLEER COMPOUND. (Scrip) Acetaminophen 300 mg, phenylpropanolamine HCl 35 mg, guaifenesin. Tab. Bot. 100s.
Use: Analgesic, decongestant, expectorant.

KLEER IMPROVED. (Scrip) Atropine sulfate 0.2 mg, chlorpheniramine maleate 5 mg/ml.
Use: Anticholinergic, antihistamine.

KLEER MILD. (Scrip) Phenylpropanolamine HCl 75 mg/Cap. Bot. 100s.
Use: Decongestant.

KLERIST-D. (Nutripharm) **Cap.:** Pseudoephedrine HCl 120 mg, chlorpheniramine maleate 8 mg. Bot. 100s, **Tab.:** Pseudoephedrine HCl 60 mg, chlorpheniramine maleate 4 mg. Bot. 100s.
Use: Decongestant, antihistamine.

KLER-RO LIQUID. (Ulmer) Surgical cleanser and laboratory detergent. Bot. gal.
Use: Antiseptic.

KLER-RO POWDER. (Ulmer) Surgical cleanser and laboratory detergent. Can 2 lb, Bot. 6 lb.
Use: Antiseptic.

KLONOPIN. (Roche) Clonazepam 0.5 mg, 1 mg or 2 mg/Tab. Prescription Pak 100s.
Use: Anticonvulsant.

K-LOR. (Abbott) Potassium Cl equivalent to potassium 20 mEq and Cl 20 mEq/2.6 Gm for oral soln. w/saccharin. Pkg. 30s, 100s. 15 mEq/2 Gm Pkg. 100s.
Use: Potassium supplement.

KLOR-CON 8. (Upsher-Smith) Potassium Cl 8 mEq/ER Tab. Bot. 100s, 500s.
Use: Potassium supplement.

KLOR-CON 10. (Upsher-Smith) Potassium Cl 10 mEq/ER Tab. Bot. 100s, 500s.
Use: Potassium supplement.

KLOR-CON/25 POWDER. (Upsher-Smith) Potassium Cl for oral soln 25 mEq/Pkt. Carton 30s, 100s, 250s.
Use: Potassium supplement.

KLOR-CON/EF. (Upsher-Smith) Potassium bicarbonate 25 mEq/Tab. Carton 30s, 100s.
Use: Potassium supplement.

KLOR-CON POWDER. (Upsher-Smith) Potassium Cl for oral soln. 20 mEq/Packet. w/saccharin. Packet 1.5 Gm. Box 30s, 100s.
Use: Potassium supplement.

KLORLYPTUS. (High) Eucalyptus oil, chlorine in a petroleum ointment and light oil base. **Oint.:** Jar oz, lb. **Oil:** Bot. 30 ml, pt.
Use: Topical dressing.

KLORVESS EFFERVESCENT GRANULES. (Sandoz) Potassium 20 mEq, Cl 20 mEq supplied by potassium Cl 1.125 Gm, potassium bicarbonate 0.5 Gm, L-lysine monohydrochloride 0.913 Gm/Packet. w/saccharin. Box 30s.
Use: Potassium supplement.

KLORVESS EFFERVESCENT TABLETS. (Sandoz) Potassium Cl 1.125 Gm, potassium bicarbonate 0.5 Gm, L-lysine HCl 0.913 Gm/Effervescent Tab. Sodium and sugar free. w/saccharin. Pkg. 60s, 1000s.
Use: Potassium supplement.

KLORVESS LIQUID. (Sandoz) Potassium Cl 1.5 Gm (20 mEq)/15 ml, alcohol 0.75%. Bot. pt.
Use: Potassium supplement.

KLOTRIX. (Mead Johnson) Potassium Cl 10 mEq/SR Tab. Bot. 100s, 1000s, UD 100s.
Use: Potassium supplement.

K-LYTE. (Bristol) Potassium bicarbonate and citrate 25 mEq, saccharin. Lime and orange flavors. Effervescent Tab. Pkg. 30s, 100s, 250s.
Use: Potassium supplement.

K-LYTE/CL. (Bristol) Potassium Cl 25 mEq, saccharin. Citrus and fruit punch flavor. Effervescent Tab. Pkg. 30s, 100s, 250s. Bulk powder 225 Gm/Can.

Use: Potassium supplement.

K-LYTE/CL 50. (Bristol) Potassium Cl 50 mEq, saccharin. Citrus and fruit punch flavors. Pkg. 30s, 100s.
Use: Potassium supplement.

K-LYTE DS. (Bristol) Potassium bicarbonate and citrate 50 mEq, saccharin. Lime and orange flavor. Effervescent Tab. Pkg. 30s, 100s.
Use: Potassium supplement.

K-NORM. (Pennwalt) Potassium Cl 10 mEq/CR Cap. Bot. 100s, 500s.
Use: Potassium supplement.

KOATE-HS. (Cutter) Antihemophilic factor heated in aqueous soln. Vial. Single dose with diluent.
Use: Antihemophilic factor for Hemophilia A.

KODONYL EXPECTORANT. (Blue Cross) Bromodiphenhydramine HCl 3.75 mg, diphenhydramine HCl 8.75 mg, ammonium Cl 80 mg, potassium guaiacolsulfonate 80 mg, menthol 0.5 mg/5 ml. Bot. 16 oz.
Use: Antihistamine, expectorant.

KOLEPHRIN CAPLETS. (Pfeiffer) Pseudoephedrine HCl 30 mg, chlorpheniramine maleate 2 mg, acetaminophen 325 mg/Capl. Bot. 36s.
Use: Decongestant, antihistamine, analgesic.

KOLEPHRIN/DM CAPLETS. (Pfeiffer) Pseudoephedrine HCl 30 mg, chlorpheniramine maleate 2 mg, dextromethorphan HBr 10 mg, acetaminophen 325 mg/Capl. Bot. 30s.
Use: Decongestant, antihistamine, antitussive, analgesic.

KOLEPHRIN GG/DM EXPECTORANT. (Pfeiffer) Dextromethorphan HBr 10 mg, guaifenesin 150 mg/5 ml. Alcohol free. Bot. 120 ml.
Use: Antitussive, expectorant.

KOLEPHRIN NN LIQUID. (Pfeiffer) Phenylpropanolamine HCl 12.5 mg, pyrilamine maleate 10 mg, dextromethorphan HBr 7.5 mg/5 ml. Alcohol free. Bot. 120 ml.
Use: Decongestant, antihistamine, antitussive.

•**KOLFOCON A.** USAN.
Use: Contact lens material (hydrophobic).

•**KOLFOCON B.** USAN.
Use: Contact lens material (hydrophobic).

•**KOLFOCON C.** USAN.
Use: Contact lens material (hydrophobic).

•**KOLFOCON D.** USAN.
Use: Contact lens material (hydrophobic).

KOLYUM LIQUID AND POWDER. (Pennwalt) Potassium ion 20 mEq, chloride ion 3.4 mEq from potassium gluconate 3.9 Gm, potassium Cl 0.25 Gm/15 ml or 5 Gm/15 ml. w/saccharin, sorbitol. **Liq.:** Bot. pt, gal. **Pow.:** Packet 5 Gm, 30s.
Use: Potassium supplement.

KOMED LOTION. (Barnes-Hind) Sodium thiosulfate 8%, salicylic acid 2%, isopropyl alcohol 25%, menthol, camphor, colloidal alumina. Squeeze bot. 1.75 oz.
Use: Anti-acne.

KOMEX. (Barnes-Hind) Sodium tetraborate decahydrate. Jar 75 Gm.
Use: Anti-acne.

KONAKION. (Roche) Phytonadione-synthetic vitamin K_1, polysorbate 80, phenol, propylene glycol, sodium acetate, glacial acetic acid. Amp. 2 mg/0.5 ml or 10 mg/1 ml. Box 10s.
Use: Prevention and treatment of hypoprothrombinemia.

KONDON'S NASAL JELLY. (Kondon) Tube 20 Gm w/ephedrine alkaloid. Tube 20 Gm.
Use: Nasal decongestant.

KONDREMUL. (Fisons) Mineral oil 55%, Irish moss. Emulsion Bot. pt.
Use: Laxative.
W/Phenolphthalein 2.2 gr/Tbsp. Bot. pt.
W/Cascara 0.66 Gm/15 ml. Bot. 14 oz.

KONSTO. (Freeport) Docusate sodium 100 mg/ Cap. Bot. 1000s.
Use: Laxative.

KONSYL POWDER. (Boots) Psyllium hydrophyllic mucilloid. Canister 300 Gm, 450 Gm, Packet 6 Gm, Ctn. 25s.
Use: Laxative.

KONSYL-D POWDER. (Boots) Psyllium hydrophilic mucilloid, dextrose. Canister 325 Gm, 500 Gm, Packet 6.5 Gm, Ctn. 25s.
Use: Laxative.

KONYNE-HT. (Cutter) Factor IX complex, human heat treated. Vial 500 units or 1000 units w/diluent.
Use: Antihemophilic.

KOPHANE COUGH AND COLD FORMULA SYRUP. (Pfeiffer) Phenylpropanolamine HCl 5 mg, chlorpheniramine maleate 0.5 mg, dextromethorphan HBr 10 mg, ammonium Cl 90 mg/5 ml, sodium citrate. Alcohol free. Bot. 120 ml.
Use: Decongestant, antihistamine, antitussive, expectorant.

KORIGESIC TABLETS. (Trimen) Phenylephrine HCl 5 mg, chlorpheniramine maleate 4 mg, acetaminophen 325 mg, caffeine 30 mg/Tab. Bot. 100s.
Use: Decongestant, antihistamine, analgesic.

KORO-FLEX. (Holland-Rantos) Improved contouring spring natural latex diaphragm 60 mm-95 mm.
Use: Contraceptive.

KOROMEX. (Holland-Rantos) **Cream:** Octoxynol 3%, base of purified water, propylene glycol, stearic acid, sorbitan stearate, polysorbate 60, boric acid, fragrance, pH buffered and adjusted to 4.5. Tube 115 Gm w/applicator. **Jelly:** Nonoxynol-9 3% in base of purified water, propylene glycol, cellulose gum, boric acid, sorbitol, starch, simethicone, fragrance, pH buffered and adjusted to 4.5. Tube 126 Gm. **Foam:** Nonoxynol-9 12.5%. Aerosol can 40 Gm.
Use: Spermicide.

KOROMEX COIL SPRING DIAPHRAGM. (Holland-Rantos) Diaphragm made of pure latex rubber, cadmium plated coil spring. Koromex Jelly and Cream/kit. 50 mm-95 mm at graduations of 5 mm.

Use: Contraceptive.

KOROMEX COMBINATION. (Holland-Rantos) Diaphragm 50 mm-95 mm, Koromex Jelly and Cream/Kit.
Use: Contraceptive.

KOROMEX CRYSTAL CLEAR GEL. (Holland-Rantos) Nonoxynol-9 2% in base of purified water, propylene glycol, cellulose gum, boric acid, sorbitol, simethicone w/pH 4.5. Tube 126 Gm w/applicator.
Use: Contraceptive.

KORUM. (Geneva) Acetaminophen 5 gr/Tab. Bot. 1000s.
Use: Analgesic.

KOTABARB. (Wesley) Phenobarbital 1/4 gr/Tab. Bot. 1000s.
Use: Sedative/hypnotic.

KOVITONIC LIQUID. (Freeda) Iron 350 mg, vitamins B_1 5 mg, B_6 10 mg, B_{12} 30 mcg, folic acid 0.1 mg, l-Lysine 10 mg/15 ml, sorbitol. Liq. Bot. 120 ml, 240 ml, pt, gal.
Use: Vitamin/mineral supplement.

K-PEK. (Rugby) Kaolin 5.85 Gm, pectin 130 mg/ 30 ml. Bot. 360 ml, pt, gal.
Use: Antidiarrheal.

K-PHOS M.F. (Beach) Potassium acid phosphate 155 mg, sodium acid phosphate 350 mg/Tab. Bot. 100s, 500s.
Use: Urinary acidifier.

K-PHOS NEUTRAL. (Beach) Dibasic sodium phosphate 852 mg, potassium acid phosphate 155 mg, sodium acid phosphate 130 mg/Tab. Bot. 100s, 500s.
Use: Phosphorus supplement.

K-PHOS NO. 2 (Beach) Potassium acid phosphate 305 mg, sodium acid phosphate, anhydrous 700 mg/Tab. Bot. 100s, 500s.
Use: Urinary acidifier.

K-PHOS ORIGINAL. (Beach) Potassium acid phosphate 500 mg/Tab. Bot. 100s, 500s.
Use: Urinary acidifier, phosphorus supplement.

K-P SUSPENSION. (Century) Kaolin 5.2 Gm, pectin 260 mg/oz. Bot. gal.
Use: Antidiarrheal.

KRONOFED-A-JR. (Ferndale) Pseudoephedrine HCl 60 mg, chlorpheniramine maleate 4 mg/ Cap. Bot. 100s, 500s.
Use: Decongestant, antihistamine.

KRONOFED-A KRONOCAPS. (Ferndale) Pseudoephedrine HCl 120 mg, chlorpheniramine maleate 8 mg/Cap. Bot. 100s, 500s.
Use: Decongestant, antihistamine.

KRONOHIST KRONOCAPS. (Ferndale) Chlorpheniramine maleate 4 mg, pyrilamine maleate 25 mg, phenylpropanolamine HCl 50 mg/Cap. Bot. 100s, 1000s.
Use: Antihistamine, decongestant.

KRYPTON CLATHRATE Kr 85. USAN.
Use: Radioactive agent.

KRYPTON Kr 81m, U.S.P. XXII.
Use: Radioactive agent.

K-TAB. (Abbott) Potassium Cl (10 mEq) 750 mg/ ER Tab. Bot. 100s, 1000s, UD 100s.
Use: Potassium supplement.

K.T.V. TABLETS. (Knight) Vitamin B_{12}, minerals. Bot. 50s.
Use: Vitamin/mineral supplement.

KUDROX DOUBLE STRENGTH LIQUID. (Kremers-Urban) Aluminum hydroxide 565 mg, magnesium hydroxide 180 mg/5 ml, sodium $\leq$ 15 mg. Bot. 360 ml.
Use: Antacid.

KUTAPRESSIN. (Kremers-Urban) Liver derivative complex composed of peptides and amino acids. Inj. Vial 20 ml.
Use: Liver derivative complex.

KUTRASE. (Kremers-Urban) Amylase 30 mg, protease 6 mg, lipase 25 mg, cellulase 2 mg, l-hyoscyamine sulfate 0.0625 mg, phenyltoloxamine citrate 15 mg/Cap. Bot. 100s, 500s.
Use: Digestive aid.

KU-ZYME. (Kremers-Urban) Amylase 30 mg, protease 6 mg, lipase 75 mg, cellulase 2 mg/Cap. Bot. 100s, 500s.
Use: Digestive aid.

KU-ZYME HP. (Kremers-Urban) Lipase 8000 units, protease 30,000 units, amylase 30,000 units/Cap. Bot. 100s.
Use: Digestive aid.

KWELCOF. (Ascher) Hydrocodone bitartrate 5 mg, guaifenesin 100 mg/5 ml. Bot. pt, UD 5 ml. Pkg. 10s, 100s. Alcohol, dye, sugar, and corn free.
Use: Antitussive, expectorant.

KWELL. (Reed & Carnrick) Lindane 1%. **Lot.:** W/ Glyceryl monostearate, cetyl alcohol, stearic acid, trolamine, 2-amino-2-methyl-1-propanol, methyl p-hydroxybenzoate, butyl p-hydroxybenzoate, carrageenan. Bot. 2 oz, 16 oz. **Shampoo:** W/Polyethylene sorbitan monostearate, TEA-lauryl sulfate, acetone, purified water. Bot. 2 oz, pt, gal. **Cream:** W/Stearic acid, lanolin, glycerin, 2-amino-2-methyl-1-propanol, perfume, purified water. Tube 2 oz, Jar lb.
Use: Scabicide, pediculicide.

KWIKDERM CREAM. (NMC Labs) Tolnaftate 1%. Cream. Tube 15 Gm.
Use: Antifungal, external.

KWIKDERM SOLUTION. (NMC Labs) Tolnaftate 1%. Soln. Bot. 10 ml.
Use: Antifungal, external.

KWILDANE SHAMPOO. (Major) Gamma benzene hexachloride 1%. Bot. 60 ml, pt, gal.
Use: Pediculicide.

K-Y. (Johnson & Johnson) Glucono delta lactate, sodium hydroxide, glycerin, chlorhexidine gluconate, hydroxyethylcellulose. Jelly Tube 2.7 Gm, 5 Gm (single use), 5 Gm, 60 Gm.
Use: Vaginal and rectal lubricant.

KYODEX REAGENT STRIPS. (Kyoto) A disposable plastic reagent strip for determination of glucose in whole blood. Vial 25s.
Use: Diagnostic aid.

KYOTEST UG REAGENT STRIPS. (Kyoto) Reagent strips for glucose and ketones in urine.
Use: Diagnostic aid.
KYOTEST UGK REAGENT STRIP. (Kyoto) Disposable reagent strip for measurement of glucose and ketones in the urine. Vial 50s, 100s.
Use: Diagnostic aid.
KYOTEST UK REAGENT STRIPS. (Kyoto) Reagent strip for ketones in urine. Vial 50s.
Use: Diagnostic aid.

L

LA-12. (Hyrex) Hydroxocobalamin 1000 mcg/ml. Vial 10 ml.
Use: Vitamin B_{12} supplement.
•**LABETALOL HYDROCHLORIDE,** U.S.P. XXII, Inj., Tab, U.S.P. XXII, USAN.
Use: Antihypertensive.
See: Trandate Inj., Tab. (Glaxo).
W/Hydrochlorothiazide.
See: Trandate HCT, Tab. (Allen & H).
LABSTIX REAGENT STRIPS. (Ames) Urine screening test. Bot 100s.
Use: Diagnostic aid.
LAC-HYDRIN LOTION. (Westwood) Lactic acid 12% neutralized w/ammonium hydroxide. Tube 5 oz.
Use: Emollient.
LACLEDE CLEANER. (Laclede) Container. 2 lb.
Use: Detergent for instruments and trays.
LACLEDE DISCLOSING SWAB. (Laclede) Swabs 6″. 100s, 500s, 1000s.
Use: Dental swab.
LACLEDE TOPI-FLUOR A.P.F. TOPICAL CREAM. (Laclede) Fluoride ion 1.23% (from sodium fluoride) in orthophosphoric acid 0.98%. Jar 50 ml, 500 ml, 1000 ml, 2000 ml.
Use: Dental caries preventative.
LACOTEIN. (Christina) Protein digest 5% w/preservatives. Vial 30 ml (w/iodochin), Vial 30 ml.
Use: Protein supplement.
LACRIL ARTIFICAL TEARS. (Allergan) Hydroxypropyl methylcellulose, gelatin A, chlorobutanol 0.5%. Soln. Dropper bot. 15 ml.
Use: Lubricant, ophthalmic.
LACRI-LUBE NP. (Allergan) White petrolatum 55.5%, mineral oil 42.5%, petrolatum/lanolin alcohol 2%. Oint. 0.7 Gm.
Use: Lubricant, ophthalmic.
LACRI-LUBE S.O.P. (Allergan) White petrolatum, mineral oil, nonionic lanolin derivatives, chlorobutanol. UD 0.7 Gm, Tube 3.5 Gm, 7 Gm.
Use: Lubricant, ophthalmic.
LACRISERT. (Merck Sharp & Dohme) Hydroxypropyl cellulose 5 mg/insert. Pkg. 60 UDs, 2 reusable applicators and storage container.
Use: Artificial tear insert, ophthalmic.
LACTAID. (LactAid Inc.) **Liq.:** Beta-D-galactosidase derived from Kluyveromyces lactis yeast (1000 Neutral Lactase units/5 drop dosage) in carrier of glycerol 50%, water 30%, inert yeast dry matter 20%. Units of 4, 12, 30 and 75 one-quart dosages at 5 drops/dose. **Tab.:** Beta-D-galactosidase from Aspergillis oryzae (3300 FCC lactase units/Tab.) In 12s, 100s.
Use: Enteral nutritional supplement.
LACTALBUMIN HYDROLYSATE.
See: Aminonat.
•**LACTATED RINGER'S INJECTION,** U.S.P. XXII.
Use: Electrolyte and fluid replenisher, systemic alkalizer.
•**LACTIC ACID,** U.S.P. XXII. Propanoic acid, 2-hydroxy.
Use: Pharmaceutic necessity for Sodium Lactate Injection, U.S.P. XXII.
W/Sodium pyrrolidone carboxylate.
See: LactiCare (Stiefel).
LACTICARE-HC LOTION. (Stiefel) Hydrocortisone lotion 1% or 2.5%. **1%:** Bot 4 oz. **2.5%:** Bot. 2 oz.
Use: Corticosteroid, topical.
LACTICARE LOTION. (Stiefel) Lactic acid 5%, sodium pyrrolidone carboxylate 2.5% in an emollient lotion base. Bot. 8 oz, 12 oz, w/pump dispenser.
Use: Emollient.
LACTINEX. (Hynson, Westcott & Dunning) *Lactobacillus acidophilus & Lactobacillus bulgaricus* mixed culture. Tab. 250 mg, Bot. 50s. Gran. 1 Gm pk. Box 12s.
Use: Antidiarrheal.
LACTISOL. (C & M Pharmacal) Salicylic acid 16.7%, lactic acid 16.7% in film forming vehicle. Bot. 0.5 oz, w/brush applicator.
Use: Keratolytic.
LACTOBACILLUS ACIDOPHILUS. Preparation made from acid-producing bacterium.
Use: Antidiarrheal.
See: Bacid (Fisons).
DoFUS (Miller).
LACTOBACILLUS ACIDOPHILUS & BULGARICUS MIXED CULTURE.
See: Lactinex, Tab., Gran. (Hynson, Westcott & Dunning).
LACTOBACILLUS ACIDOPHILUS, VIABLE CULTURE.
See: DoFus, Tab. (Miller)
Lactinex Granules, Tab. (Hynson, Westcott & Dunning).
LACTOCAL-F. (Laser) Vitamin A 8000 IU, D 400 IU, E 30 IU, C 100 mg, folic acid 1 mg, B_1 3 mg, B_2 3.4 mg, nicotinamide 20 mg, B_6 5 mg, B_{12} 12 mcg, calcium 200 mg, iodine 0.15 mg, iron 65 mg, magnesium 10 mg, copper 2 mg, zinc 15 mg/Tab. Bot. 100s, 1000s.
Use: Vitamin/mineral supplement.
LACTOFLAVIN.
See: Riboflavin, U.S.P. XXII. (Various Mfr.).
•**LACTOSE,** N.F. XVII. Milk sugar.
Use: Pharmaceutic aid (tablet and capsule diluent).
See: Natur-Aid, pow. (Scott/Cord).

LACTRASE. (Rorer) Standardized enzyme lactase (β-D-galactosidase) 125 mg dispersed in maltodextrins. Cap. Bot. 100s.
Use: Enteral nutritional supplement.

•**LACTULOSE,** U.S.P. XXII. Concentrate, Syr., U.S.P. XXII. 4-0-β-D-Galactopyranosyl-D-fructose. Duphalac.
Use: Treatment of hepatic coma and chronic constipation.
See: Cephulac, Syr. (Merrell Dow).
Chronulac, Liq. (Merrell Dow).

LADOGAL. (Winthrop Products) Danazol.
Use: Androgen.

LADOGAR. (Winthrop Products) Danazol.
Use: Androgen.

L.A.E.20. (Seatrace) Estradiol valerate 20 mg/ml. Vial 10 ml.
Use: Estrogen.

L.A.E. 40. (Seatrace) Estradiol valerate 40 mg/ml. Vial 10 ml.
Use: Estrogen.

LAGOL OIL. (Last) 8 Hydroxyquinoline 0.038% in oil base. Bot. 1 oz, 2 oz, 4 oz, 16 oz.
Use: Cleanser.

LAGOL OINTMENT. (Last) Allantoin 1%, benzocaine 5%. Jar 1 oz, 8 oz, 16 oz, 5 lb.
Use: Topical dressing, local anesthetic.

LAIDLOMYCIN PROPIONATE POTASSIUM. USAN.
Use: Growth promoter, coccidiostat (veterinary).

LAKTOMOL. (Durel) Whole milk, dewaxed lanolin esters. Bot. pt, gal.
Use: Skin conditioner.

LAMOTANE-X. (Myers) Trichlorethylamino-glycolbenzoate (ethylaminobenzoate-chloralhydrate derivative). Bot. 4 oz, 6 oz, 8 oz, pt, qt, gal.
Use: Antiseptic, anesthetic, antipruritic.

LAMOTRIGINE. USAN.
Use: Anticonvulsant.

LAMPRENE. (Geigy) Clofazimine 50 mg or 100 mg/Cap. Bot. 100s.
Use: Leprostatic.

LANABAC. (Lannett) Aspirin 0.3 gr, caffeine 15 mg, potassium bromide 15 mg, sodium bromide 15 mg/Tab. Bot. 1000s.
Use: Analgesic combination.

LANABARB. (Lannett) **No. 1:** Sodium amobarbital ¾ gr, sodium secobarbital ¾ gr/Cap. Bot. 500s, 1000s. **No. 2:** Sodium amobarbital 1.5 gr, sodium secobarbital 1.5 gr/Cap. Bot. 500s, 1000s.
Use: Sedative/hypnotic.

LANABIOTIC. (Combe) Polymyxin B sulfate 5000 units, neomycin (as sulfate) 3.5 mg, bacitracin 500 units, lidocaine 40 mg/Gm. Oint. 15 Gm, 30 Gm.
Use: Anti-infective, local anesthetic.

LANABROM ELIXIR. (Lannett) 60 gr of combined bromides of sodium, potassium, strontium, ammonium/fl oz, Bot. pt, gal.

LANABURN OINT. (Lannett) Aluminum basic acetate, phenol, zinc oxide, boric acid, ichthammol, eucalyptol. Jar lb.

LANACANE CREME. (Combe) Benzocaine, chlorothymol, resorcin. Tube 1.25 oz, 2.5 oz, Spray can 3 oz.
Use: Local anesthetic.

LANACILLIN. (Lannett) Penicillin G potassium **200,000 units/5 ml:** Bot. 100 ml. **400,000 units/5 ml:** Bot. 100 ml, 150 ml.
Use: Antibacterial, penicillin.

LANACILLIN VK TABLETS. (Lannett) Potassium phenoxymethyl penicillin 400,000 units (250 mg), 800,000 units (500 mg)/Tab. Bot. 100s.
Use: Antibacterial, penicillin.

LANACILLIN VK POWDER. (Lannett) Potassium phenoxymethyl penicillin. **125 mg/5 ml** (200,000 units), **250 mg/5 ml** (400,000 units). Bot. 100 ml.
Use: Antibacterial, penicillin.

LANACORT CREAM. (Combe) Hydrocortisone acetate 0.5%. Tube 0.5 oz, 1 oz.
Use: Corticosteroid, topical.

LANAMINS. (Lannett) Vitamin combination. Cap. Bot. 100s, 1000s.
Use: Vitamin supplement.

LANAPHILIC OINTMENT. (Medco Lab) Sorbitol, isopropyl palmitate, stearyl alcohol, white petrolatum, lanolin oil, sodium lauryl sulfate, propylene glycol, methylparaben, propylparaben. Jar 16 oz. Also available w/urea 10% or 20%.
Use: Emollient.

LANAPHILIC W/UREA 10%. (Medco Labs) Urea, stearyl alcohol, white petrolatum, isopropyl palmitate, propylene glycol, sorbitol, sodium lauryl sulfate, lactic acid, parabens. Oint. Jar lb.
Use: Emollient.

LANASED. (Lannett) Atropine sulfate 0.03 mg, hyoscyamine 0.03 mg, methenamine 408 mg, methylene blue 5.4 mg, phenyl salicylate 18.1 mg, gelsemium 6.1 mg, benzoic acid 4.5 mg/Tab. Bot. 1000s.
Use: Anticholineric combination.

LANATOSIDE C. B.A.N. 3-(3″-Acetyl-4″-β -glucosyltridigitoxosido)-digoxogenin.
Use: Myocardial stimulant.

LANATRATE. (Lannett) Ergotamine tartrate 1 mg, caffeine alkaloid 100 mg/Tab. Bot. 100s, 500s, 1000s.
Use: Agent for migraine.

LANATUSS. (Lannett) Guaifenesin 100 mg, phenylpropanolamine HCl 5 mg, chlorpheniramine maleate 2 mg, sodium citrate 197 mg, citric acid 60 mg/5 ml. Bot. 120 ml, pt, gal.
Use: Expectorant, decongestant, antihistamine.

LANAURINE. (Lannett) Antipyrine, benzocaine in glycerin. Bot. 0.5 oz, 4 oz.
Use: Otic preparation.

LANAVITE. (Lannett) Vitamins A 5000 IU, D 1000 IU, E 1 IU, B_1 1.5 mg, B_2 2 mg, B_6 0.1 mg, C 37.5 mg, B_{12} 1 mcg, niacinamide 20 mg,

calcium pantothenate 1 mg. Cap. Bot. 500s, 1000s.
Use: Vitamin/mineral supplement.

LANAVITE DROPS. (Lannett) Vitamins A 3000 IU, D 400 IU, B_1 1 mg, B_2 1.2 mg, niacinamide 8 mg, C 60 mg/0.6 ml. Dropper bot. 15 ml, 60 ml.
Use: Vitamin supplement.

LANAZETS. (Lannett) Cetylpyridinium 1 mg, benzocaine 5 mg/Loz. Bot. 500s, 1000s.
Use: Mouth and throat preparation.

LANESTRIN. (Lannett) Estrogenic substance natural in aqueus susp. 20,000 units/ml. Vial 30 ml.
Use: Estrogen.

LANIAZID TABLETS. (Lannett) Isoniazid 50 mg or 100 mg. **50 mg:** Tab. Bot. 100s, 500s. **100 mg:** Tab. Bot. 100s, 500s, 1000s.
Use: Antituberculous agent.

LANIAZID C.T. (Lannett) Isoniazid 300 mg/Tab. Bot. 100s, 1000s.
Use: Antituberculous agent.

LANNATES ELIXIR. (Lannett) Sodium glycerophosphate 2 gr, calcium glycerophosphate 2 gr, phosphoric acid 1.5 min, wine base/fl oz. Bot. pt, gal.

LANOKALIN. (Lannett) Phenobarbital 15 mg, homatropine methylbromide 5 mg, colloidal kaolin 300 mg/Tab. Bot. 1000s.
Use: Antacid combination.

•**LANOLIN,** U.S.P. XXII. Anhydrous, U.S.P. XXII.
Use: Water-in-oil emulsion ointment base; absorbent ointment base.
See: Kerohydric (Westwood).
W/Coconut oil, pine oil, castor oil, cholesterols, lecithin and parachlorometaxylenol.
See: Sebacide, Liq. (Paddock).
W/Diiosbutylcresoxyethoxyethyl, dimethyl benzyl ammonium Cl, menthol.
See: Hospital Lot. (Paddock).

•**LANOLIN ALCOHOLS,** N.F. XVII.
Use: Pharmaceutic aid (ointment base ingredient).

LANOLINE. (Burroughs Wellcome) Perfumed emollient. Oint. Tube 1.75 oz.
Use: Emollient.

LANO-LO BATH OIL. (Whorton) 8 oz.

LANOLOR. (Squibb) Cream. Jar 8 oz, tube 2 oz.

LANOPHYLLIN ELIXIR. (Lannett) Anhydrous theophylline 80 mg, alcohol 20%/15 ml. Bot. pt, gal.
Use: Bronchodilator.

LANOPHYLLIN-GG CAPSULES. (Lannett) Theophylline 150 mg, guaifenesin 90 mg. Cap. Bot. 100s, 500s.
Use: Bronchodilator, expectorant.

LANOPHYLLIN INJ. (Lannett) Theophylline 250 mg/ml. Inj. Vial 10 ml.
Use: Bronchodilator.

LANOPLEX ELIXIR. (Lannett) Vitamins B_1 4 mg, nicotinamide 40 mg, B_6 2 mg/fl oz. Bot. pt, gal.
Use: Vitamin supplement.

LANOPLEX FORTE CAPSULES. (Lannett) Vitamins B_1 25 mg, B_2 12.5 mg, nicotinamide 50 mg, C 250 mg, B_6 3 mg, B_{12} 5 mcg, calcium pantothenate 10 mg/Cap. Bot. 100s, 500s, 1000s.
Use: Vitamin supplement.

LANOPLEX INJECTION. (Lannett) Vitamins B_1 100 mg, B_2 1 mg, B_6 2 mg, niacinamide 50 mg, calcium pantothenate 10 mg, benzyl alcohol 1%, urea 10%, chlorobutanol 0.5%/ml. Vial 30 ml.
Use: Parenteral nutritional supplement.

LANORINAL. (Lannett) Isobutylallybarbituric acid 50 mg, caffeine 40 mg, aspirin 200 mg, phenacetin 130 mg/Cap. or Tab. **Cap.** Bot. 100s, 1000s. **Tab.** Bot. 1000s.
Use: Analgesic combination.

LANOTHAL PILLS. (Lannett) Phenolphthalein 0.5 gr, aloin 0.25 gr, ipecac 1/15 gr, belladonna extract 1/12 gr/Pill. Bot. 1000s.

LANOXICAPS. (Burroughs Wellcome) Digoxin 0.05 mg, 0.1 mg, 0.2 mg. Soln. in cap. Bot. 100s.
Use: Cardiac glycoside.

LANOXIN. (Burroughs Wellcome) Digoxin. **Tab. 0.125 mg:** Bot. 100s, 1000s, Unit-of-use 30s, UD 100s. **0.25 mg:** Bot. 100s, 1000s, 5000s, UD 100s, Unit-of-use 30s. **0.5 mg:** Bot. 100s. **Pediatric Elix.:** 0.05 mg/ml, alcohol 10%. Bot. 60 ml. **Inj.:** (w/propylene glycol 40%, alcohol 10%, sodium phosphate 0.3%, anhydrous citric acid 0.08%) Amp. 0.5 mg/2 ml. Amp. 10s, 50s. **Pediatric Inj.:** 0.1 mg/ml. Amp. 1 ml 10s.
Use: Cardiac glycoside.

•**LANSOPRAZOLE.** USAN.
Use: Gastric acid pump inhibitor; antiulcer agent.

LANTRISUL. (Lannett) Sulfamerazine 2.5 gr, sulfadiazine 2.5 gr, sulfamethazine 2.5 gr. **Tab.:** Bot. 100s, 500s, 1000s. **Susp.:** Bot. pt, gal.
Use: Sulfonamide combination.

LANTURIL. (Winthrop Products) Oxypertine.
Use: Anxiolytic, tranquilizer.

LANUM. (Various Mfr.) Lanolin.

LANVISONE CREAM. (Lannett) Hydrocortisone 1%, clioquinol 3%. Tube 20 Gm.
Use: Corticosteroid, antifungal (external).

•**LAPYRIUM CHLORIDE.** USAN.
Use: Pharmaceutic aid (surfactant).

LARDET. (Standex) Phenobarbital 8 mg, theophylline 130 mg, ephedrine HCl 24 mg/Tab. Bot. 100s.
Use: Antiasthmatic combination.

LARDET EXPECTORANT. (Standex) Phenobarbital 8 mg, theophylline 130 mg, ephedrine HCl 24 mg, guaifenesin 100 mg/Tab. Bot. 100s.
Use: Antiasthamatic combination.

LARGON. (Wyeth-Ayerst) Propiomazine HCl 20 mg/ml w/sodium formaldehyde sulfoxylate, sodium acetate buffer. Amp. 1 ml, 2 ml. Pkg. 25s, Tubex syringe 1 ml.
Use: Sedative/hypnotic.

LARIAM. (Roche) Mefloquine HCl 250 mg/Tab. UD 25s.
Use: Antimalarial.
LAROBEC. (Roche) Vitamins B_1 15 mg, B_2 15 mg, niacinamide 100 mg, calcium pantothenate 18 mg, B_{12} 5 mcg, folic acid 0.5 mg, C 500 mg/ Tab. Bot. 100s.
Use: Vitamin/mineral supplement.
LARODOPA CAPSULES. (Roche) Levodopa 100 mg, 250 mg or 500 mg/Cap. **100 mg:** Bot. 100s. **250 mg:** Bot. 100s, 500s. **500 mg:** Bot. 100s, 500s.
Use: Antiparkinson agent.
LARODOPA TABLETS. (Roche) Levodopa 100 mg, 250 mg or 500 mg. **100 mg:** Bot. 100s. **250 mg and 500 mg:** Bot. 100s, 500s.
Use: Antiparkinson agent.
LAROTID. (Beecham Labs) Amoxicillin. **Cap.: 250 mg:** Bot. 100s, 500s, UD 100s, unit-of-use 18s. **500 mg:** Bot. 50s, 500s. **Oral Susp.:** 125 mg or 250 mg (as trihydrate)/5 ml. Bot. 80 ml, 100 ml, 150 ml. **Pediatric drops:** 50 mg (as trihydrate)/ml. Bot. 15 ml.
Use: Antibacterial, penicillin.
LARYLGAN THROAT SPRAY. (Wyeth-Ayerst) Antipyrine 0.3%, pyrilamine maleate 0.05%, sodium caprylate 0.50%, w/alcohol 1%, methyl salicylate, benzyl alcohol 0.05%, methylparaben, propylparaben, gentian violet, menthol, isobornyl acetate, aromatics, glycerin, sodium saccharin. Bot. 28 ml (0.94 fl oz.).
Use: Throat preparation.
LARYNEX. (Dover) Benzocaine. Sugar, lactose and salt free. Loz. UD Box 500s.
Use: Local anesthetic.
•**LASALOCID.** USAN.
Use: Coccidiostat.
LASAN NASAL SPRAY. (Eastwood) Bot. 2/3 oz.
LASAN OINTMENT. (Stiefel) Anthralin 0.4% in ointment base. Tube 60 Gm.
Use: Antipsoriatic.
LASIX. (Hoechst) Furosemide. **Tab.:** 20 mg or 40 mg/Tab. Bot. 100s, 500s, 1000s, UD 100s; 40 mg/Tab. 30s, 60s; 80 mg/Tab. Bot. 50s. **Inj.:** 2 ml/Amp. Box 5s, 50s; 4 ml/Amp. Box 5s, 25s; 10 ml/Amp. Box 5s, 25s; Syringe 2 ml, 4 ml, 10 ml. Box 5s. Single Use Vial 2 ml, 4 ml, 10 ml. **Oral Soln.:** Alcohol 11.5%. Dropper Bot 60 ml, Bot. 120 ml.
Use: Diuretic.
LASSAR'S PASTE.
See: Zinc Oxide Paste, U.S.P. XXII. (Various Mfr.).
LATEST-CRP KIT. (Fisher) Measures C-reactive protein in serum. Kit 1s.
Use: Diagnostic aid.
LAUDEXIUM METHYLSULFATE. B.A.N. Decamethylene-α, ο-bis-(1-(3′, 4′-dimethoxybenzyl)-1,-2,3,4-tetrahydro-6,7-dimethoxy-2-methylisoquinolinium methosulfate. Laudolissin.
Use: Neuromuscular blocking agent.
•**LAURETH 4.** USAN.
Use: Pharmaceutic aid.
•**LAURETH 9.** USAN. Mixture of polyoxyethylene lauryl ethers having a statistical average of 9 ethylene oxide groups per molecule.
Use: Surfactant, emulsifier, spermaticide.
•**LAURETH 10S.** USAN.
Use: Spermaticide.
•**LAUROCAPRAM.** USAN.
Use: Pharmaceutic aid.
LAURO EYE WASH. (Otis Clapp) Boric acid, sodium Cl. Bot. 0.5 oz, 4 oz.
Use: Ophthalmic preparation.
LAUROLINIUM ACETATE. B.A.N. 4-Amino-1-dodecylquinaldinium acetate. Laurodin.
Use: Surface-active agent.
LAUROMACROGOL 400. Laureth 9.
•**LAURYL ISOQUINOLINIUM BROMIDE.** USAN.
Use: Anti-infective.
LAURYL SOLUTION. (Knight) Bot. pt.
Use: Vaginal preparation.
LAURYL SULFOACETATE.
See: Lowila, Cake, Liq., Oint. (Westwood).
LAVACOL. (Parke-Davis Prods) Ethyl alcohol 70%. Bot. pt.
LAVATAR. (Doak) Coal tar distillate 25.5% in a bath oil base. Liq. Bot. 4 oz, pt.
Use: Antipsoriatic, antipruritic.
•**LAVENDER OIL,** N.F. XVII.
Use: Perfume.
•**LAVOLTIDINE SUCCINATE.** USAN.
Use: Histamine H_2-receptor blocker.
LAVOPTIK EMERGENCY WASH. (Lavoptik) Eye, face, body wash. 32 oz/Emergency station.
Use: Emergency wash.
LAVOPTIK EYE WASH. (Lavoptik) Sodium Cl 0.49%, sodium biphosphate 0.4%, sodium phosphate 0.45%/100 ml w/benzalkonium Cl 0.005%. Bot. 6 oz.
Use: Irrigating agent, ophthalmic.
LAVORIS. (Procter & Gamble) Zinc Cl, glycerin, poloxamer 407, saccharin, polysorbate 80, flavors, clove oil, alcohol, citric acid, water. Bot. 6 oz, 12 oz, 18 oz, 24 oz.
Use: Mouthwash.
LAXATAB. (Freeport) Danthron 75 mg, docusate sodium 100 mg, D-calcium pantothenate 25 mg/Tab. Bot. 1000s.
Use: Laxative.
LAXATIVE CAPS. (Weeks & Leo) Docusate sodium 100 mg, casanthranol 30 mg/Cap. Bot. 30s, 60s.
Use: Laxative.
LAXATIVES.
See: Agar-Gel (Various Mfr.).
Aloe (Various Mfr.).
Aloin (Various Mfr.).
Bile Salts (Various Mfr.).
Bisacodyl, Tab., Supp. (Various Mfr.).
Bisacodyl Tannex (Barnes-Hind).
Carboxymethylcellulose Sodium (Various Mfr.).

Casanthranol, Cap., Tab. (Various Mfr.).
Cascara Sagrada (Various Mfr.).
Cascara Sagrada Fluidextract, Liq. (Parke-Davis).
Cascara Tab. (Various Mfr.).
Castor Oil (Various Mfr.).
Correctol, Tab. (Plough).
Docusate Sodium (Various Mfr.).
Ex-Lax, Tab., Pow. (Ex-Lax. Inc.).
Feen-a-Mint, Gum, Mints (Plough).
Karaya Gum (Penick).
Liquid Petrolatum, Liq. (Various Mfr.).
Magnesia Magma (Various Mfr.).
Maltsupex (Wallace).
Methylcellulose (Various Mfr.).
Mucilloid of Psyllium Seed W/Dextrose (Searle).
Natures Remedy (Norcliff Thayer).
Nujol, Liq. (Plough).
Oxyphenisatin Acetate (Various Mfr.).
Petrolatum, Liq. (Various Mfr.).
Petrolatum, Liq., Emulsion (Various Mfr.).
Phenolphthalein (Various Mfr.).
Plantago ovata, Coating (Various Mfr.).
Poloxalkol, Cap., Soln. (Various Mfr.).
Prune Concentrate, Tab., Cap. (Various Mfr.).
Prune Preps. (Various Mfr.).
Psyllium Granules W/Dextrose (Med. Chem.).
Psyllium Husk Pow. (Upjohn).
Psyllium Hydrocolloid, Pow. (Stuart).
Psyllium Hydrophilic Mucilloid (Various Mfr.).
Psyllium Seed, Gel, Gran. (Various Mfr.).
Regutol, Tab. (Plough).
Sakara, Gran. (Plough).
Senna, Alexandrian, Liq., Tab. (Various Mfr.).
Senna, Cassia angustifolia, Tab. (Brayten).
Senna Conc., Standardized, Gran., Tab., Pow.,
Supp. (Various Mfr.).
Senna Fruit Extract, Liq. (Various Mfr.).
Sennosides A&B, Tab. (Dorsey).
Sodium Biphosphate (Various Mfr.).
Sodium Phosphate (Various Mfr.).

LAXINATE 100. (Mallard) Dioctyl sodium sulfosuccinate 100 mg/Cap. Bot. 100s, 1000s.
Use: Laxative.

LAX-PILLS. (G & W) Yellow phenolphthalein 90 mg/Tab. Bot. 30s, 60s.
Use: Laxative.

LAYOR CARANG.
See: Agar (Various Mfr.).

LAZER CREME. (Pedinol) Vitamins E 3500 units, A 100,000 units/oz. Jar 2 oz.
Use: Emollient.

LAZERFORMALYDE SOLUTION. (Pedinol) Formaldehyde 10%, polysorbate 20, hydroxyethyl cellulose. Bot. 3 oz.
Use: Antiperspirant drying agent for presurgical removal of warts or nonsurgical laser treatment of warts.

LAZERSPORIN-C SOLUTION. (Pedinol) Neomycin sulfate 3.5 mg, polymyxin B sulfate 10,000 units, hydrocortisone 1%. Bot. 10 ml.
Use: Anti-infective combination, topical.

LC-65 DAILY CONTACT LENS CLEANER. (Allergan) Daily cleaning solution for all hard, soft (hydrophilic), Polycon and Paraperm oxygen gas permeable contact lenses. Dropper Bot. 0.5 oz, 2 oz.
Use: Contact lens care.

L-CAINE. (Century) Lidocaine HCl. **Inj.:** 1%, 50 ml. **Topical Liq.:** 4%, 50 ml.
Use: Local anesthetic.

L-CAINE E. (Century) Lidocaine HCl 1% or 2%, epinephrine 1:100,000/ml. Inj. 20 ml, 50 ml.
Use: Local anesthetic.

L-CAINE VISCOUS. (Century) Lidocaine HCl 2% with sodium carboxymethylcellulose. Soln. Bot. 100 ml.
Use: Local anesthetic.

L-CARNITINE. Amino acid derivative 250 mg/Cap. Bot. 60s.
Use: Vitamin supplement.
See: Vitacarn.
Carnitor (Sigma-Tau).

L.C.D. (Almay) Alcohol extractions of crude coal tar. Cream, soln. Bot. 4 oz, pt.
Use: Antipsoriatic, antipruritic.
See: Coal Tar Topical Soln., U.S.P. XXII.

LCR.
Use: Antineoplastic.
See: Vincristine sulfate.

LDH REAGENT STRIP. (Ames) A quantitative strip test for LDH in serum or plasma. Seralyzer reagent strip. Bot. 25s.
Use: Diagnostic aid.

LEBER TABULAE. (Paddock) Aloe 0.09 Gm, extract of rhei 0.03 Gm, myrrh 0.01 Gm, frangula 5 mg, galbanum 2 mg, olibanum 3 mg/Tab. Bot. 100s, 500s, 1000s.

LEBER TAURINE. (Paddock) Sodium salicylate 8 gr, ox bile 2.25 gr, extract of cascara 1:4 4.5 gr, pancreatin 1.25 gr, pepsin 1:10,000 3/10 gr/fl oz. Bot. pt, gal.

LEC-E-PLEX. (Barth's) Vitamin E 100 IU, 200 IU or 400 IU/Cap. w/lecithin. Bot. 100s, 500s, 1000s.
Use: Vitamin E supplement.

LECITHIN. (Various Mfr.) Lecithin. **Cap.:** 520 mg. Bot. 100s, 250s, 1000s; 650 mg. Bot. 90s, 100s, 250s, 500s. **Pow.:** 120 Gm, kg, lb.
Use: Nutritional supplement.

•**LECITHIN,** N.F. XVII.
Use: Pharmaceutic aid (emulsifying agent).
(Arcum) 1200 mg/Cap. Bot. 100s, 1000s; Gran. Bot. 8 oz; Pow. Bot. 4 oz.
(Barth's) 8 gr/Cap. Bot. 100s, 500s, 1000s; Gran. Can 8 oz, 16 oz; Pow. Can 10 oz.
(Cavendish) Tab. (0.5 gr) Bot. 500s.
(Quality Generics) 1200 mg, Cap. 100s.
(De Pree) Cap. Bot. 100s.
(Pfanstiehl) 25 Gm, 100 Gm, 500 Gm/Pkg.

W/Choline base, cephalin, lipositol.
See: Alcolec Cap., Gran. (American Lecithin).
W/Coconut oil, pine oil, castor oil, lanolin, cholesterols, parachlorometaxylenol.
See: Sebacide, Liq. (Paddock).
W/Vitamins.
See: Acletin, Cap. (Associated Concentrates). Lec-E-Plex, Cap. (Barth's).

LEDERCILLIN VK. (Lederle) Penicillin V potassium, saccharin. **Soln.:** 125 mg or 250 mg/5 ml in 100 ml, 150 ml, 200 ml. **Tab.:** 250 mg. Bot. 100s, 1000s, UD 10s, Unit of issue 480s; 500 mg. Bot. 100s, 500s, UD 100s.
Use: Antibacterial, penicillin.

LEDERPLEX CAPSULES. (Lederle) Vitamins B_1 2.25 mg, B_2 2.6 mg, niacinamide 30 mg, B_6 3 mg, calcium pantothenate 15 mg, B_{12} 9 mcg/Cap. Bot. 100s.
Use: Vitamin/mineral supplement.

LEDERPLEX LIQUID. (Lederle) Vitamins B_1 2.25 mg, B_2 2.6 mg, niacinamide 30 mg, pantothenic acid 15 mg, B_6 3 mg, B_{12} 9 mcg/10 ml. Bot. 12 oz.
Use: Vitamin/mineral supplement.

LEGATRIN NIGHT LEG CRAMP RELIEF TABLETS. (Scholl) Quinine sulfate 130 mg/Cap. Bot. 30s.
Use: Antimalarial; treatment of night leg cramps.

LEGIONELLA. (Wampole-Zeus) Direct fluorescent test for legionella organisms. Identification of various legionella bacteria in tissue specimens, sputum, cultures.
Use: Diagnostic aid.

LEGIONELLA, INDIRECT. (Wampole-Zeus) Indirect fluorescent antibody test for *Legionella pneumophila*.
Use: Diagnostic aid.

LEMON OIL, N.F. XVII.
Use: Pharmaceutic aid (flavor).

LENATE. (American) Topical analgesic. Bot. 1 oz, 4 oz, 8 oz, 16 oz.
Use: Throat preparation.

LENETRAN. Mephenoxalone.
Use: Tranquilizer.

LENICET.
See: Aluminum Acetate, Basic (Various Mfr.).

LENIQUINSIN. USAN. 6,7-Dimethoxy-4-(vera-trylideneamino) quinoline. Under study.
Use: Antihypertensive.

LENIUM MEDICATED SHAMPOO. (Winthrop Products) Selenium sulfide.
Use: Antiseborrheic.

LENPERONE. USAN.
Use: Antipsychotic.

LENS CLEAR. (Allergan) Sterile, isotonic solution surfactant cleaner w/sorbic acid 0.1%, edetate disodium 0.2%. Bot. 15 ml.
Use: Soft contact lens care.

LENSEN. (Geneva) Diphenhydramine HCl 25 mg or 50 mg/Cap. Bot. 1000s.

LENSFRESH. (Allergan) Sterile, buffered, isotonic aqueous soln. W/hydroxyethyl cellulose, sodium Cl, boric acid, sodium borate, white sorbic acid 0.1%, edetate disodium 0.2%. Bot. 0.5 oz.
Use: Contact lens care.

LENSINE EXTRA STRENGTH. (CooperVision) Cleaning agent with benzalkonium Cl 0.01%, EDTA 0.1%. Soln. Bot. 45 ml.
Use: Hard contact lens care.

LENS PLUS. (Allergan) Isotonic soln. w/sodium Cl 0.9%. Aerosol 3 oz, 8 oz, 12 oz. Preservative free.
Use: Soft contact lens care.

LENS PLUS REWETTING DROPS. (Allergan) Sterile, non-preserved isotonic solution w/sodium Cl, boric acid. UD 0.01 oz (30s).
Use: Soft contact lens care.

LENSRINS. (Allergan) Sterile preserved saline for heat disinfection, rinsing and storage of soft (hydrophilic) contact lenses; rinsing solution for chemical disinfection. Soln. Bot. 8 oz.
Use: Soft contact lens care.

LENS-WET. (Allergan) Isotonic, buffered soln. of polyvinyl alcohol, thimerosal 0.002%, EDTA 0.01%. Bot. 0.5 fl oz.
Use: Contact lens care.

LENTE INSULIN. Susp. of zinc insulin crystals.
See: Iletin Lente, Vial (Lilly).

LENTE INSULIN. (Squibb/Novo) Insulin zinc susp. U-40 (40 units/ml), U-80 (80 units/ml), and U-100 (100 units/ml). Vial 10 ml.
Use: Antidiabetic agent.

LEPROSY THERAPY.
See: Hansen's disease.

LEPTAZOL.
See: Pentylenetetrazol.

•**LERGOTRILE MESYLATE.** USAN.
Use: Enzyme inhibitor.

LERTON OVULES. (Vita Elixir) Caffeine 250 mg/Cap.
Use: Analeptic.

LESTEROL. (Dram) Nicotinic acid 500 mg/Tab. Bot. 250s.
Use: Antihyperlipidemic.

LETHOPHEROL. (Nutrition) Vitamin E 100 IU/Kapule. Bot. 100s.
Use: Vitamin E supplement.

•**LETIMIDE HCl.** USAN. 3-[2-(Diethylamino)-ethyl]-2H-1,3-benzoxazine-2,4-(3H)-dione monohydrochloride.
Use: Analgesic.

LETUSIN. Naphthalene-2-sulfonate ester of levopropoxyphene. Levopropoxyphene (Lilly).

•**LEUCINE,** U.S.P. XXII. $C_6H_13NO_2$. L-leucine.
Use: Amino acid.

LEUCOVORIN CALCIUM. (Lederle) Leucovorin calcium 10 mg. In 12s, 24s.
Use: Folic acid antagonist overdosage.

•**LEUCOVORIN CALCIUM,** U.S.P. XXII. Inj., U.S.P. XXII. L-Glutamic acid, N-[(2-amino-5-formyl-1,4,5,6,7,8-hexahydro-4-oxo-6-pteridinyl)-methyl]amino]benzoyl]-, calcium salt (1:1), pentahydrate. Folinic acid-S.F. Formyl tetrahydropteroylglutamic acid, a derivative of folic acid as

calcium salt. (Lederle) **Inj.:** Amp. 3 mg/1 ml. Box 6s. Vial 10 mg/ml after reconstitution w/5 ml sterile water for inj. **Tab.:** 5 mg. Bot. 30s, 100s.
Use: Antagonist of aminopterin and other folic-acid antagonists. Anti-anemic (folate-deficiency); antidote to folic acid antagonists.

LEUKEMIA AGENTS.
See: Antineoplastics.

LEUKERAN. (Burroughs Wellcome) Chlorambucil 2 mg/Tab. Bot. 50s.
Use: Antineoplastic agent.

LEUKINE. (Immunex) Sargramostim (GM-CSF).
Use: Adjunct in bone marrow transplantation.

•**LEUPROLIDE ACETATE.** USAN.
Use: Antineoplastic agent.

LEUROCRISTINE.
See: Vincristine Sulfate (Lilly).

LEUROCRISTINE SULFATE (1:1) (SALT). Vincristine Sulfate, U.S.P. XXII.

LEVALLORPHAN. B.A.N. 1-3-Hydroxy-N-allylmorphinan.(—)-N-Allyl-3-hydroxymorphinan.
Use: Narcotic antagonist.

LEVAMFETAMINE. F.D.A. (—)-α-Methylphenethylamine.

LEVAMFETAMINE.
See: Levamphetamine succinate.

•**LEVAMISOLE HYDROCHLORIDE.** USAN.
Use: Antineoplastic.

•**LEVAMPHETAMINE SUCCINATE.** USAN. (l-isomer), 1-phenyl-2-amino propane succinate. Amphetamine, levo. 1-a-methylphenethylamine succinate.
Use: Anorexiant.
See: Amodril, Cap. (North Amer. Pharmacal).

LEVARTERENOL BITARTRATE.
See: Norepinephrine Bitartate, U.S.P. XXII.

•**LEVCYCLOSERINE.** USAN.
Use: Enzyme inhibitor (Gaucher's disease).

LEVIRON. (Approved) Desiccated liver 7 gr, iron and ammonium citrate 3 gr, vitamins B_1 1 mg, B_2 0.5 mg, B_6 0.5 mg, calcium pantothenate 0.3 mg, niacinamide 2.5 mg, B_{12} 1 mcg/Cap. Bot. 100s, 1000s.
Use: Vitamin/mineral supplement.

LEVLEN 21 TABLETS. (Berlex) Levonorgestrel 0.15 mg, ethinyl estradiol 0.03 mg/Tab. Slidecase 21s, Box 3s.
Use: Oral contraceptive.

LEVLEN 28 TABLETS. (Berlex) Levonorgestrel 0.15 mg, ethinyl estradiol 0.03 mg/Tab. (21 active, 7 inert). Slidecase 28s, Box 3s.
Use: Oral contraceptive.

LEVO-AMPHETAMINE. Alginate (l-isomer) alpha-2-phenylaminopropane succinate.
See: Levamphetamine.

LEVO-AMPHETAMINE SUCCINATE.
See: Pedestal, Cap., Tab. (Len-Tag).

LEVOBUNOLOL HYDROCHLORIDE, U.S.P. XXII, Ophth.
See: Betagan, Ophth. Soln. (Allergan).

•**LEVOCABASTINE HYDROCHLORIDE.** USAN.
Use: Antihistamine.

•**LEVOCARNITINE,** U.S.P. XXII, Oral, USAN.
Use: Carnitine deficiency.
See: Carnitor, Liq., Tab. (Sigma Tau).
L-Carnitine, Cap. (R & D Labs).
Vitacarn, Liq. (Kendall McGaw).

•**LEVODOPA,** U.S.P. XXII. Cap., Tab., U.S.P. XXII. L-Tyrosine, 3-hydroxy-. (—)-3-(3,4-Dihydroxyphenyl)-L-alanine. Berkdopa; Brocadopa; Veldopa.
Use: Treatment of the Parkinsonian syndrome.
See: Bio Dopa, Cap. (Bio-Deriv.).
Dopar, Cap. (Norwich Eaton).
Larodopa, Tab. or Cap. (Roche).
Levopa, Cap. (ICN).
Parda, Cap. (Parke-Davis).
W/Carbidopa.
See: Sinemet, Tab. (Merck Sharp & Dohme).

LEVO-DROMORAN. (Roche) Levorphanol tartrate. **Amp.:** 2 mg/ml w/methyl and propyl parabens, sodium hydroxide to adjust pH. Amp. 1 ml, Box 10s. **Vial:** 2 mg/ml w/phenol 0.45%, sodium hydroxide to adjust pH. Vial 10 ml. **Tab.:** 2 mg. Bot. 100s.
Use: Narcotic analgesic.

LEVO-EPINEPHRINE BITARTRATE.
See: Lyophrin, Soln. (Alcon).

•**LEVOFURALTADONE.** USAN. 1-5-Morpholinomethyl-3-[(5-nitrofurfurylidene)amino]-2-oxazolidinone.
Use: Antibacterial, antiprotozoal.

LEVOID. (Nutrition) Levothyroxine sodium. **Tab.:** 0.1 mg or 0.2 mg. Bot. 90s, 500s. **Inj.:** 0.1 mg/ml w/sodium formaldehyde sulfoxylate 0.1%, phenol 0.5%, sodium hydroxide, glycine buffer. Vial 10 ml.
Use: Thyroid hormone.

•**LEVOBUNOLOL HYDROCHLORIDE.** USAN.
Use: Antiadrenergic.

•**LEVOMETHADYL ACETATE.** USAN.
Use: Narcotic analgesic.

LEVOMETHORPHAN. B.A.N. (—)-3-Methoxy-N-methylmorphinan.
Use: Cough suppressant.

LEVOMORAMIDE. B.A.N. (—)-1-(3-Methyl-4-mor-pholino-2,2-diphenylbutyryl)pyrrolidine.
Use: Narcotic analgesic.

•**LEVONANTRADOL HYDROCHLORIDE.** USAN.
Use: Analgesic.

•**LEVONORGESTREL,** U.S.P. XXII.
Use: Progestin.
See: Norplant (Wyeth-Ayerst).

•**LEVONORGESTREL AND ETHINYL ESTRADIOL TABLETS,** U.S.P. XXII.
Use: Oral contraceptive.
See: Nordette, Tab. (Wyeth-Ayerst).

•**LEVONORDEFRIN,** U.S.P. XXII. l-1-(1-Aminoethyl)3,4-Dihydroxy benzyl alcohol. Levonordefrin. (-)-α-(1-Aminoethyl)-3,4-dihydroxybenzyl Alcohol.
Use: Adrenergic (vasoconstrictor).

LEVOPHED. (Breon) Norepinephrine bitartrate 1 mg/ml Amp. 4 ml.
Use: Vasopressor used in shock.

LEVOPHED BITARTRATE. (Winthrop Pharm) Norepinephrine bitartrate w/sodium Cl, sodium metabisulfite 1 mg or 2 mg/ml. Amp. 4 ml. Box 10s.
Use: Vasopressor used in shock.

LEVOPHENACYLMORPHAN. B.A.N. (—)-3-Hydroxy-N-phenacylmorphinan.
Use: Narcotic analgesic.

LEVOPROME. (Lederle) Methotrimeprazine 20 mg/ml w/benzyl alcohol 0.9% w/v, disodium edetate 0.065% w/v, sodium metabisulfite 0.3% w/v. Vial 10 ml.
Use: CNS analgesic.

LEVOPROPOXYPHENE NAPSYLATE, U.S.P. XXII. Cap., Oral susp., U.S.P. XXII. 2-Naphthalenesulfonic acid compound with (—)-α-[2-(dimethylamino)-1-methylethyl]-α-phenylphenethyl propionate (1:1) monohydrate. α-1-4-Dimethylamino-1,2-diphenyl-3-methyl-2-butanol propionate 2-naphthalene-sulfonate hydrate. (—)-α-4-(Dimethylamino)-3-methyl-1,2-diphenyl-2-butanol Propionate (ester) 2-Naphthalensulfonate (salt).
Use: Antitussive.

LEVOPROPYLCILLIN POTASSIUM. USAN. (1) Potassium 3,3-Dimethyl-7-oxo-6-(—)-(2-phenoxybutyramido)-4-thia-1-azabicyclo[3.2.0]-heptane-2-carboxylate; (2) Potassium 6-(—)-(2-phenoxybutyramido) penicillinate.
Use: Antibacterial.

LEVORENINE.
See: Epinephrine, U.S.P. XXII. (Various Mfr.).

LEVOROXINE. (Bariatric) Sodium levothyroxine 0.05 mg, 0.1 mg, 0.2 mg or 0.3 mg/Tab. Bot. 100s, 500s.
Use: Thyroid hormone.

LEVORPHAN TARTRATE.

LEVORPHANOL TARTRATE, U.S.P. XXII. Inj., Tab., U.S.P. XXII. 1-3-Hydroxy-N-methyl-morphinan bitartrate. 17-Methylmorphinan-3-ol Tartrate (1:1).
Use: Narcotic analgesic.
See: Levo-Dromoran, Amp., Tab., Vial (Roche).

LEVOTHROID. (Rorer) Levothyroxine sodium. **Tab.:** 25 mcg, 50 mcg, 75 mcg, 100 mcg, 125 mcg, 150 mcg, 175 mcg, 200 mcg or 300 mcg/Tab. Bot. 100s, 1000s, UD 100s (except for 25 mcg). **Inj.:** 200 mcg or 500 mcg. Vial 6 ml.
Use: Thyroid hormone.

LEVOTHYROXINE SODIUM. (McGuff) Levothyroxine sodium 500 mcg/Vial (100 mcg/ml reconstituted). Pow. for Inj.
Use: Thyroid hormone.

LEVOTHYROXINE SODIUM, U.S.P. XXII. Tab., U.S.P. XXII. L-Tyrosine, 0-(4-hydroxy-3,5-diiodophenyl)-3,5-diiodo-, monosodium salt, hydrate. Sodium L-3-[4-(4-Hydroxy-3,5-diiodophenoxy)-3,5-di-iodopheny]-alanine.
Use: Thyroid hormone.
See: Cytolen, Tab. (Len-Tag).
Levoid, Tab., Vial (Nutrition Control Products).
Levothroid, Tab., Inj. (Rorer).
Synthroid, Tab., Inj. (Flint).
W/Mannitol.
See: Synthroid, Inj. (Flint).
W/Sodium liothyronine.
Use: Thyroid hormone.
See: Thyrolar, Tab. (Rorer).

•**LEVOXADROL HYDROCHLORIDE.** USAN. l-2(2,2-Diphenyl-1,3-dioxolan-4-yl) piperidine hydrochloride levo form of dioxadrol HCl.
Use: Local anesthetic.

LEVOXINE. (Daniels) Levothyroxine sodium 25 mcg, 50 mcg, 75 mcg, 100 mcg, 125 mcg, 150 mcg, 175 mcg, 200 mcg or 300 mcg/Tab. Bot. 100s, 1000s.
Use: Thyroid hormone.

LEVSIN. (Kremers-Urban) L-hyoscyamine sulfate. **Tab.:** 0.125 mg. Bot. 100s, 500s. **Soln.:** 0.125 mg/ml, alcohol 5%. Bot. 15 ml. **Elix.:** 0.125 mg/5 ml, alcohol 20%. Bot. pt. **Inj.:** 0.5 mg/ml. Vial 1 ml, 10 ml.
Use: Anticholinergic/antispasmodic.

LEVSIN-PB DROPS. (Kremers-Urban) Hyoscyamine sulfate 0.125 mg, phenobarbital 15 mg/ml, alcohol 5%. Liq. Bot. 15 ml.
Use: Anticholinergic/antispasmodic, sedative/hypnotic.

LEVSIN W/PHENOBARBITAL ELIXIR. (Kremers-Urban) Hyoscyamine sulfate 0.125 mg, phenobarbital 15 mg/5 ml, alcohol 20%. Elix. Bot. pt.
Use: Anticholinergic/antispasmodic, sedative/hypnotic.

LEVSINEX TIMECAPS. (Kremers-Urban) L-hyoscyamine sulfate 0.375 mg/TR Cap. Bot. 100s, 500s.
Use: Anticholinergic/antispasmodic.

LEVSINEX W/PHENOBARBITAL TIMECAPS. (Kremers-Urban) Hyoscyamine sulfate 0.375 mg, phenobarbital 45 mg/TR Cap. Bot. 100s.
Use: Anticholinergic/antispasmodic, sedative/hypnotic.

LEVULOSE. Fructose.

LEVULOSE-DEXTROSE.
See: Invert Sugar.

LEXOCORT POWDER. (Lexington) Hydrocortisone 0.1% in a talc base. Pkg. 20 Gm.
Use: Corticosteroid, topical.

LEXTRON. (Lilly) Liver-stomach concentrate 50 mg, iron 30 mg, vitamins B_{12} (activity equivalent) 2 mcg, B_1 1 mg, B_2 0.25 mg w/other factors of vitamin B complex present in the liver-stomach concentrate/Pulv. Bot. 84s.
Use: Vitamin supplement.

L'HOMME. (Geneva) Vitamins A 4000 IU, D 400 IU, B_1 1 mg, B_2 1.2 mg, B_{12} 2 mcg, calcium pantothenate 5 mg, B_3 10 mg, C 30 mg, calcium 100 mg, phosphorus 76 mg, iron 10 mg, manganese 1 mg, magnesium 1 mg, zinc 1 mg. Bot. 100s.
Use: Vitamin/mineral supplement.

LI BAN SPRAY. (Leeming) Synthetic pyrethroid 0.5%, related compounds 0.065%, aromatic petroleum hydrocarbons 0.664%. Bot. 5 oz, Box 6s.
Use: Control of lice, fleas on bedding, furniture, etc. (Not to be used on humans or animals).

•**LIBENZAPRIL.** USAN.
Use: ACE inhibitor.

LIBRAX. (Roche) Clidinium bromide (Quarzan) 2.5 mg, chlordiazepoxide HCl (Librium) 5 mg/Cap. Bot. 100s, 500s, Teledose 100s (10 strips of 10).
Use: Anticholinergic combination.

LIBRITABS. (Roche) Chlordiazepoxide 5 mg, 10 mg or 25 mg/Tab. **5 mg:** Bot. 100s, 500s; **10 mg:** Bot. 100s, 500s; **25 mg:** Bot. 100s.
Use: Antianxiety agent.

LIBRIUM. (Roche) Chlordiazepoxide HCl 5 mg, 10 mg or 25 mg/Cap. Bot. 100s, 500s, Tel-E-Dose (10 strips of 10; 4 cards of 25) in RNP (Reverse Numbered Package).
Use: Antianxiety agent.

LIBRIUM INJECTABLE. (Roche) Chlordiazepoxide HCl 100 mg/dry filled amp. plus special I.M. diluent, 2 ml for I.M. administration/compound w/benzyl alcohol 1.5%, polysorbate 80 4%, propylene glycol 20%, w/maleic acid and sodium hydroxide to adjust pH to approx. 3. Amp. 5 ml w/2 ml diluent, Box 10s.
Use: Antianxiety agent.

LICETROL LIQUID. (Republic) Pyrethrins 0.2%, piperonyl butoxide technical 2%, petroleum distillate 0.8%. Bot. 60 ml, 120 ml.
Use: Pediculicide.

LICOPLEX DS. (Keene) Iron 2.9 mg, vitamins B_{12} equivalent 1 mcg, B_2 0.75 mg, B_3 50 mg, B_5 1.25 mg, B_{12} 15 mcg/ml, procaine 2%. Inj. Vial 30 ml.
Use: Parenteral nutritional supplement.

LICOPLEX. (Mills) Desiccated whole bile 2 gr, dried whole pancreatic substance ¾ gr, dl-methionine 2 gr, choline bitartrate 3 gr/Tab. Bot. 100s.
Use: Bile laxative, cholagogue.

LICOPLEX DS. (Keene) Cyanocobalamin 15 mcg, liver inj. equivalent to cyanocobalamin activity 1 mcg, ferrous gluconate 25 mg, riboflavin 0.75 mg, calcium pantothenate 1.25 mg, niacinamide 50 mg. Vial 30 ml.
Use: Vitamin/mineral supplement.

•**LICRYFILCON A.** USAN.
Use: Contact lens material.

•**LICRYFILCON B.** USAN.
Use: Contact lens material.

LIDA-MANTLE-HC CREME. (Miles Pharm) Lidocaine 3%, hydrocortisone acetate 0.5% in cream base. Tube oz.
Use: Corticosteroid combination, topical.

•**LIDAMIDINE HYDROCHLORIDE.** USAN.
Use: Antiperistaltic.

LIDEX CREAM. (Syntex) Fluocinonide 0.05%. Cream. In 15 Gm, 30 Gm, 60 Gm, 120 Gm.
Use: Corticosteroid, topical.

LIDEX-E. (Syntex) Fluocinonide 0.05% in aqueous emollient base. Tube 15 Gm, 30 Gm, 60 Gm, 120 Gm.
Use: Corticosteroid, topical.

LIDEX GEL. (Syntex) Fluocinonide 0.05% in gel base. Tube 15 Gm, 30 Gm, 60 Gm, 120 Gm.
Use: Corticosteroid, topical.

LIDEX OINTMENT. (Syntex) Fluocinonide 0.05% in ointment base. Tube 15 Gm, 30 Gm, 60 Gm, 120 Gm.
Use: Corticosteroid, topical.

LIDEX TOPICAL SOLUTION. (Syntex) Fluocinonide 0.05%. Soln. Bot. 20 ml, 60 ml.
Use: Corticosteroid, topical.

•**LIDOCAINE,** U.S.P. XXII. Oint., Oral topical soln., Sterile, Topical aerosol, U.S.P. XXII. 2-Diethylamino-2′,6′-acetoxylidide. Acetamide, 2-(diethylamino)-N-(2,6-dimethylphenyl)-
Use: Local anesthetic.

•**LIDOCAINE AND EPINEPHRINE INJECTION,** U.S.P. XXII.
Use: Local anesthetic.
See: L-Caine E, Vial (Century).
Norocaine 1%, 2% w/Epinephrine. (Vortech).
Xylocaine W/Epinephrine, Soln. (Astra).

•**LIDOCAINE HYDROCHLORIDE,** U.S.P. XXII. Inj., Jelly, Topical Soln., U.S.P. XXII. Acetamide, 2-(diethylamino)-N-(2,6-dimethylphenyl)-, HCl. 2-Die- thylamino-2′,6′-acetoxylidide HCl.
Use: Cardiac depressant (antiarrhythmic), local anesthetic.
(Abbott) **0.2%, 0.4%, 0.8%:** w/5% Dextrose. 250 ml single-dose container; **1%, 2%.** Abboject syringe 5 ml; Vial 1 Gm, 2 Gm. Premixed: 0.2%, 0.4% in 5% dextrose. Inj. containers (flexible or glass) 500 ml. **1%:** 2 ml, 5 ml single-dose amp. **1.5%:** 20 ml single-dose amp. **2%:** 10 ml/20 ml vial (for dilution to prepare I.V. drip soln.) **5%:** w/7.5% Dextrose amp. 2 ml.
(Maurry) 2%. Vial.
(Pharmex) 1%, 2%. Vial 50 ml.
Use: Injection for infiltration block anesthesia and I.V. drip for cardiac arrhythmias.
See: Anestacon, Liq. (Webcon).
Ardecaine 1%, 2%, Inj. (Burgin-Arden).
Dolicaine, I.M. (Reid-Rowell).
L-Caine, Inj., Liq. (Century).
Nervocaine, Inj. (Keene).
Norocaine, Inj. (Vortech).
Rocaine, Inj. (Rocky Mtn.).
Stanacaine (Standex).
Xylocaine HCl, Preps. (Astra).

W/Benzalkonium Cl.
See: Medi-Quik, Aerosol (Lehn & Fink).
Medi-Quick Pump Spray (Lehn & Fink).

W/Benzalkonium Cl, phenol, menthol, eugenol, thyme oil, eucalyptus oil.
See: Unguentine Spray (Norwich).

W/Cetyltrimethylammonium bromide, hexachlorophene.
See: Aerosept, Aerosol (Dalin).

W/Hydrocortisone, clioquinol.
See: Bafil, Lot. (Scruggs).
Hil-20 Lot. (Reid-Rowell).
W/Dextrose.
W/Methylparaben, sodium Cl.
W/Methyl parasept.
See: L-Caine, Inj. (Century).
W/Methyl parasept, epinephrine.
See: L-Caine-E, Inj. (Century).
W/Orthohydroxyphenyl mercuric Cl, menthol, camphor, allantoin.
See: Kip First Aid preps. (Youngs Drug).
W/Parachlorometaxylenol, phenol, zinc oxide.
See: Unguentine Plus, Cream (Norwich).
W/Polymyxin B sulfate.
See: Lidosporin, Otic soln. (Burroughs-Wellcome).
W/Testosterone, estrone, liver inj., niacinamide, panthenol, Vitamin B complex.

LIDOCAINE HYDROCHLORIDE AND DEXTROSE INJECTION, U.S.P. XXII.

LIDOCAINE HYDROCHLORIDE AND EPINEPHRINE BITARTRATE. INJECTION, U.S.P. XXII.

LIDOCAINE HYDROCHLORIDE AND EPINEPHRINE INJECTION, U.S.P. XXII.

LIDOFENIN. USAN.
Use: Diagnostic aid.

LIDOFILCON A. USAN.
Use: Contact lens material.

LIDOFILCON B. USAN.
Use: Contact lens material.

LIDOFLAZINE. USAN. 4-[4,4-bis(p-Fluro-phenyl)-butyl]-1-piperazineaceto-2′,6′-xylidide. 4-[3-(4,4′-Di- fluorobenzhydryl)propyl]piperazin-1-ylacet-2′,6′- xylidide.
Use: Cardiovascular agent.

LIDOJECT-1. (Mayrand) Lidocaine HCl 1%. Vial 50 ml.
Use: Local anesthetic.

LIDOJECT-2. (Mayrand) Lidocaine HCl 2%. Vial 50 ml.
Use: Local anesthetic.

LIDOPEN AUTO-INJECTOR. (Survival Technology) Lidocaine HCl 300 mg/3 ml. Auto-injection device.
Use: Antiarrhythmic.

LIDOX CAPS. (Major) Chlordiazepoxide HCl 10 mg, clidinium bromide 2.5 mg. Cap. Bot. 100s, 500s, 1000s, UD 100s.
Use: Anticholinergic combination.

LIDOXIDE. (Interstate) Chlordiazepoxide HCl 5 mg, clidinium bromide 2.5 mg/Tab. Bot. 100s, 500s.
Use: Anticholinergic combination.

LIFER-B. (Burgin-Arden) Cyanocobalamin 30 mcg, liver inj. 0.1 ml, ferrous gluconate 100 mg, riboflavin 1.5 mg, panthenol 2.5 mg, niacinamide 100 mg, citric acid 16.4 mg, sodium citrate 23.6 mg/ml. Vial 30 ml.
Use: Vitamin/mineral supplement.

LIFE SAVER KIT. (Whiteworth) Ipecac syrup two 1 oz bottles, activated charcoal pow. 1 oz, poison treatment instruction booklet.
Use: Antidote kit.

LIFE SPANNER. (Spanner) Vitamins A 12,500 IU, D 400 IU, E 5 IU, B_1 10 mg, B_2 5 mg, B_6 2 mg, B_{12} 5 mcg, niacinamide 50 mg, calcium pantothenate 10 mg, biotin 10 mcg, C 100 mg, hesperidin complex 10 mg, rutin 20 mg, choline bitartrate 40 mg, inositol 30 mg, betaine anhydrous 15 mg, l-lysine monohydrochloride 25 mg, iron 30 mg, copper 1 mg, manganese 1 mg, potassium 5 mg, calcium 105 mg, phosphorus 82 mg, magnesium 5.56 mg, zinc 1 mg/Cap. Bot. 100s.
Use: Vitamin/mineral supplement.

•**LIFIBRATE.** USAN.
Use: Antihyperlipoproteinemic.

LIFOJECT. (Mayrand) Liver, folic acid, Vitamin B_{12}. Vial 10 ml.
Use: Nutritional supplement.

LIFOL-B. (Burgin-Arden) Liver inj. 10 mcg, folic acid 1 mg, cyanocobalamin 100 mcg, phenol 0.5%/ml. Inj. Vial 10 ml.
Use: Nutritional supplement.

LIFOLBEX. (Central) Cyanocobalamin 100 mcg, folic acid 0.4 mg, liver 0.5 mcg/ml w/phenol 0.5%. Inj. Vial 10 ml, Box 12s.
Use: Parenteral liver combination.

LIFOLEX. (Pasadena Research) Liver 10 mcg, cyanocobalamin 100 mcg, folic acid 5 mg/ml. Inj. Vial 10 ml.
Use: Nutritional supplement.

LIGNOCAINE. B.A.N. N-(Diethylaminoacetyl)-2,6-xylidine. Duncaine; Lidothesin; Lignostab; Xylocaine; Xylotox.
Use: Local anesthetic.

LILLY BULK PRODUCTS. (Lilly) The following products are supplied by Eli Lilly under the U.S.P., N.F. or chemical name as a service to the health professions:
Ammoniated Mercury Oint.
Amyl Nitrite.
Analgesic Balm.
Apomorphine HCl.
Aromatic Elix.
Aromatic Ammonia.
Atropine Sulfate.
Bacitracin Oint.
Belladonna Tincture.
Benzoin.
Boric Acid.
Calcium Gluceptate.
Calcium Gluconate.
Calcium Gluconate with Vitamin D.
Calcium Hydroxide.
Calcium Lactate.
Carbarsone.
Cascara, Aromatic, fluidextract.
Cascara Sagrada fluidextract.
Citrated Caffeine.
Cocaine HCl.

Codeine Phosphate.
Codeine Sulfate.
Colchicine.
Compound Benzoin.
Dibasic Calcium Phosphate.
Diethylstilbestrol.
Ephedrine Sulfate.
Ferrous Gluconate.
Ferrous Sulfate.
Folic Acid.
Glucagon for Inj.
Green Soap Tincture.
Heparin Sodium.
Histamine Phosphate.
Ipecac.
Isoniazid.
Isopropyl Alcohol, 91%.
Liver, Vial for Inj.
Magnesium Sulfate.
Mercuric Oxide, Yellow.
Methadone HCl.
Methenamine for Timed Burning.
Methyltestosterone.
Milk of Bismuth.
Morphine Sulfate.
Myrrh.
Neomycin Sulfate.
Niacin.
Niacinamide.
Nitroglycerin.
Opium (Deodorized).
Ox Bile Extract.
Pancreatin.
Papaverine HCl.
Paregoric.
Penicillin G Potassium.
Phenobarbital.
Phenobarbital Sodium.
Potassium Cl.
Potassium Iodide.
Powder Papers (Glassine).
Progesterone.
Propylthiouracil.
Protamine Sulfate.
Pyridoxine HCl.
Quinidine Gluconate.
Quinidine Sulfate.
Quinine Sulfate.
Riboflavin.
Silver Nitrate.
Sodium Bicarbonate.
Sodium Chloride.
Sodium Salicylate.
Streptomycin Sulfate.
Sulfadiazine.
Sulfapyridine.
Sulfur.
Terpin Hydrate.
Terpin Hydrate and Codeine.
Testosterone Propionate.
Thiamine HCl.
Thyroid.
Tubocurarine HCl.
Tylosterone.
Whitfield's Oint.
Wild Cherry Syrup.
Zinc Oxide.
Zinc Oxide Paste.

LIMARSOL.
See: Acetarsone. (City Chemical).

LIMBITROL. (Roche) Chlordiazepoxide 5 mg, amitriptyline HCl 12.5 mg/Tab. Bot. 100s, 500s, Tel-E-Dose 100s, Prescription pak 50s.
Use: Psychotherapeutic agent.

LIMBITROL DS. (Roche) Chlordiazepoxide 10 mg, amitriptyline HCl 25 mg/Tab. Bot. 100s, 500s, Tel-E-Dose 100s, Prescription pak 50s.
Use: Psychotherapeutic agent.

•**LIME,** U.S.P. XXII.
Use: Pharmaceutical necessity.

LIME SOLUTION, SULFURATED, U.S.P. XXI.
Use: Scabicide.

LIME SULFUR SOLUTION. Calcium polysulfide, calcium thiosulfate.
Use: Wet dressing.
See: Vlem-Dome, Liq. Concentrate (Miles Pharm).

LINCOCIN. (Upjohn) Lincomycin HCl 500 mg/Cap. Bot. 24s, 100s. **Pediatric:** 250 mg/Cap. Bot. 24s.
Use: Anti-infective.

LINCOCIN STERILE SOLUTION. (Upjohn) Lincomycin HCl equivalent to 300 mg or 600 mg lincomycin base, benzyl alcohol 9.45 mg/ml. Vial 2 ml in 5s, 25s, 100s; 10 ml U-Ject.
Use: Anti-infective.

•**LINCOMYCIN.** USAN. Antibiotic produced by *Streptomyces lincolnensis.* Methyl 6,8-Di-deoxy-6-(1-methyl-4-propyl-L-2-pyrrolidine-carboxamido)-1-thio-D-Erythro-α-D-galacto-octopyranoside.
Use: Antibiotic, infections due to gram-positive organisms.

•**LINCOMYCIN HYDROCHLORIDE,** U.S.P. XXII. Inj., Cap., Sterile, Syr., U.S.P. XXII. D-erythro-α-D-galacto-Octopyranoside, methyl-6,8-dideoxy-6-[[1-methyl-4-propyl-2-pyrrolidinyl)carbonyl]amino]-1-thio, HCl.
Use: Antibacterial.
See: Lincocin, Cap., Soln., Syr. (Upjohn).

•**LINDANE,** U.S.P. XXII. Cream, Lot., Shampoo, U.S.P. XXII. Gamma-benzene-hexachloride, hexachlorocyclohexane.
Fidelity Lab.—Pow. 50%, Pkg. 1 lb, 5 lb.
Imperial—Pow. 50%, Pkg. 1 lb, 4 lb; 12%, Pkg. 1 lb, 4 lb.
Use: Pediculicide, scabicide.
See: Kwell, Cream, Lot., Shampoo (Reed & Carnrick).

LINDORA. (Westwood) Sodium laureth sulfate, water, cocamide DEA, sodium Cl, lactic acid, tetra sodium EDTA, benzophenone-4, FD&C Blue #1, fragrance. Bot. 8 oz.
Use: Skin cleanser.

LINIMENTO NO. 1. (D'Franssia).
Use: External analgesic.
LINODIL CAPSULES. (Winthrop Products) Inositol hexanicotinate.
Use: Hyperlipidemic, peripheral vasodilator.
•**LINOGLIRIDE.** USAN.
Use: Antidiabetic agent.
•**LINOGLIRIDE FUMARATE.** USAN.
Use: Antidiabetic agent.
LINOLENIC ACID W/VIT. E.
See: Petropin, Cap. (Lannett).
LINUCEE TABLETS. (Fellows) Vitamins B_1 15 mg, B_2 10 mg, B_6 10 mg, nicotinic acid 100 mg, pantholate 25 mg, B_{12} 10 mcg, biotin 50 mcg/Tab. Bot. 100s.
Use: Vitamin/mineral supplement.
LIORESAL. (Geigy) Baclofen 10 mg or 20 mg/Tab. Bot. 100s, UD 100s.
Use: Muscle relaxant.
LIOTHYRONINE. B.A.N. 3-[4-(4-Hydroxy-3-iodophenoxy)-3,5-di-iodophenyl]-alanine.(—)-Tri-iodothyronine. Cynomel and Tertroxin sodium derivative.
Use: Thyroid hormone.
•**LIOTHYRONINE I-125.** USAN.
Use: Radioactive agent.
•**LIOTHYRONINE I-131.** USAN.
Use: Radioactive agent.
LIOTHYRONINE RESIN.
•**LIOTHYRONINE** SODIUM, U.S.P. XXII., Tab. U.S.P. XXII. L-Tyrosine, 0-(4-hydroxy-3-iodophenyl)-3,5-diiodo-, sodium salt. Sodium L-triiodo-thyronine. Sodium L-4-(3-iodo-4-hydroxphenoxy)-3,5-diiodo-phenylalanine.
Use: Thyroid hormone.
See: Cytomel, Tab. (SmithKline).
LIOTRIX, U.S.P. XXII. A combination of sodium levothyroxine and sodium 1-triiodothyronine in a ratio of 4 to 1 by weight.
Use: Thyroid hormone.
See: Euthroid, Tab. (Parke-Davis).
Thyrolar, Tab. (Rorer).
LIPASE. W/Amylase, Protease.
Use: Digestive enzyme.
W/Amylase, bile salts, wilzyme, pepsin, pancreatin, calcium.
See: Enzyme, Tab. (Barth's).
W/Alpha-amylase W-100, proteinase W-300, cellase W-100, estrone, testosterone, vitamins, minerals.
See: Geramine, Tab. (Brown).
W/Alpha-Amylase, proteinasa, cellase.
See: Kutrase (Kremers-Urban).
Ku-Zyme (Kremers-Urban).
W/Amylolytic, proteolytic, cellulolytic enzymes.
See: Arco-Lase, Tab. (Arco).
W/Amylolytic, proteolytic, cellulolytic enzymes, phenobarbital, hyoscyamine sulfate, atropine sulfate.
See: Arco-Lase Plus, Tab. (Arco).
W/Pancreatin, protease, amylase.
See: Dizymes, Cap. (Recsei).
W/Pepsin, homatropine methylbromide, amylase, protease, bile salts.
See: Digesplen, Tab., Elix., Drops (Med. Prod.).
LIPKOTE BY COPPERTONE. (Plough) Padimate O, oxybenzone. SPF 15. Lip balm 4.2 Gm.
Use: Sunscreen.
LIPKOTE SPF 15 ULTRA SUNSCREEN LIPBALM. (Plough) Tube 0.15 oz,
Use: Sunscreen.
LIP MEDEX. (Blistex) Petrolatum, camphor 1%, phenol 0.54%, cocoa butter, dimethyl oxazolidine, lanolin, mixed waxes. Oint. 210 Gm.
Use: Treatment of fever blisters and sore, dry cracked lips.
LIPOCHOLINE. *See:* Choline dihydrogen citrate. (Various Mfr.).
LIPODERM. (Spirt) Pancreas (porcine) 500 mg, vitamin B_6 3 mg. Cap. Bot. 180s, 500s.
Use: Antipsoriatic.
LIPOFLAVONOID CAPSULES. (Numark) Choline 111 mg, inositol 111 mg, vitamins B_1 0.3 mg, B_2 0.3 mg, B_3 3.3 mg, B_5 1.7 mg, B_6 0.3 mg, B_{12} 1.7 mcg, C 100 mg, lemon bioflavonoid complex. Cap. Bot. 100s, 500s.
Use: Vitamin supplement.
LIPOGEN CAPSULES. (Various Mfr.) Choline 111 mg, inositol 111 mg, Vitamins B_1 0.3 mg, B_2 0.3 mg, B_3 3.3 mg, B_5 1.7 mg, B_6 0.3 mg, B_{12} 1.7 mcg, C 100 mg/Cap. Bot. 60s, 100s.
Use: Vitamin supplement.
LIPO-K CAPSULES. (Marcen) Epinephrine-neutralizing factor 25 units, pancreatic lipotropic factor 1.2 mg, Cy-mucopolysaccharides 2.5 mg, choline bitartrate 100 mg, dl-methionine 50 mg, inositol 25 mg, bile extract 5 mg/Cap. Bot. 100s, 500s, 1000s.
Use: Treatment of circulatory disturbances.
LIPO-K INJECTABLE. (Marcen) Pancreatic lipotropic factor 1.2 mg, epinephrine-neutralizing factor 25 units, Cy-mucopolysaccharides 0.5 mg, sodium citrate 10 mg, inositol 5 mg, phenol 0.5%/ml. Multi-dose Vial 10 ml, 30 ml.
Use: Treatment of circulatory disturbances.
LIPOLYTIC ENZYME.
W/Proteolytic enzyme, amylolytic enzyme, cellulolytic enzyme, methyl polysiloxane, ox bile, betaine HCl.
See: Zymme, Cap. (Scrip).
LIPOMUL. (Upjohn) Corn oil 10 Gm/15 ml w/d-Alpha tocopheryl acetate, butylated hydroxy-anisole, polysorbate 80, glyceride phosphates, sodium saccharin, sodium benzoate 0.05%, benzoic acid 0.05%, sorbic acid 0.07%. Bot. pt.
Use: Enteral nutritional supplement.
LIPO-NIACIN. (Brown) Niacin 300 mg, vitamin C 150 mg, B_1 25 mg, B_2 2 mg, B_6 10 mg/TR Cap. 100s.
Use: Peripheral vasodilator.
LIPO-NICIN 100 mg. (Brown) Nicotinic acid 100 mg, niacinamide 75 mg, vitamins C 150 mg, B_1 25 mg, B_2 2 mg, B_6 10 mg/Tab. Bot. 100s, 500s.

Use: Peripheral vasodilator combination.

LIPO-NICIN 250 mg. (Brown) Nicotinic acid 250 mg, niacinamide 75 mg, vitamins C 150 mg, B_{12} 5 mg, B_2 2 mg, B_6 10 mg/Tab. Bot. 100s, 500s.
Use: Peripheral vasodilator combination.

LIPO-NICIN 300 mg TIMED CAPS. (Brown) Nicotinic acid 300 mg, vitamins C 150 mg, B_1 25 mg, B_2 2 mg, B_6 10 mg/TR Cap. Bot. 100s, 500s.
Use: Peripheral vasodilator combination.

LIPONOL CAPSULES. (Rugby) Choline 115 mg, inositol 83 mg, methionine 110 mg, vitamins B_1 3 mg, B_2 3 mg, B_3 10 mg, B_5 2 mg, B_6 2 mg, B_{12} 2 mcg, desiccated liver 56 mg, liver concentrate 30 mg/Cap. Bot. 100s, 500s.
Use: Nutritional supplement.

LIPOSYN. (Abbott Hospital Prods) Intravenous fat emulsion containing safflower oil 10%, egg phosphatides 1.2%, glycerin 2.5% in water for inj. **10%:** Single-dose container 50 ml, 100 ml, 200 ml, 500 ml; Syringe Pump Unit 50 ml single-dose. **20%:** Single-dose container 200 ml, 500 ml Syringe Pump Unit 25 ml or 50 ml single-dose.
Use: Parenteral nutritional supplement.

LIPOSYN II. (Abbott Hospital Prods) Intravenous fat emulsion: **10%:** Safflower oil 5%, soybean oil 5%. Bot. 100 ml, 200 ml, 500 ml. **20%:** Safflower oil 10%, soybean oil 10% w/egg phosphatides 1.2%, glycerin 2.5%. 200 ml, 500 ml. Bot. Syringe pump unit 25 ml, 50 ml.
Use: Parenteral nutritional supplement.

LIPOSYN III. (Abbott) Oil, soybean, egg yolk phospholipids. **10%:** 100, 200, 500 ml. **20%:** 100, 500 ml.
Use: Parenteral nutritional supplement.

LIPOTRIAD CAPSULES. (Numark) Vitamins B_1, B_2, B_6, B_{12}, niacin, choline, pantothenic acid, inositol. Bot. 100s, 1000s.
Use: Vitamin supplement.

LIPOTRIAD LIQUID. (Numark) Vitamins B_1, B_2, B_6, B_{12}, niacin, choline, pantothenic acid, inositol, saccharin. Bot. 16 fl oz.
Use: Vitamin supplement.

LIPOTROPIC AGENTS.
See: Betaine Prods. (Various Mfr.).
Choline Prods. (Various Mfr.).
Cho-Meth, Vial (Med. Chem.).
Cytellin, Susp. (Lilly).
Inositol Prods. (Various Mfr.).
Lecithin Prods. (Various Mfr.).
Methionine Prods. (Various Mfr.).

LIPOVITE CAPSULES. (Rugby) Vitamins B_1 0.3 mg, B_2 0.3 mg, B_3 3.3 mg, B_5 1.67 mg, B_6 0.3 mg, B_{12} 1.67 mcg, choline bitartrate 111 mg/Cap. Bot. 100s, 1000s.
Use: Vitamin B supplement.

LIPOXIDE CAPS. (Major) Chlordiazepoxide HCl 5 mg, 10 mg or 25 mg/Cap. Bot. 100s, 500s, 1000s.
Use: Antianxiety agent.

LIQUAEMIN SODIUM. (Organon) Heparin sodium aqueous soln., benzyl alcohol 1%. **1,000 units/ml:** Vial 10 ml, 30 ml. Box 25s. **5,000 units/ml:** Vial 1 ml, 10 ml. Box 25s. **10,000 units/ml:** Vial 1 ml, 4 ml, Box 25s. **20,000 units/ml:** Vial 1 ml, 2 ml, Box 25s. 5 ml Box 1s. **40,000 units/ml:** Vial 1 ml, Box 25s.
Use: Anticoagulant.

LIQUAEMIN SODIUM-PRESERVATIVE FREE. (Organon) Heparin sodium, preservative free. **1,000 units/ml:** Amp. 1 ml Box 50s. **5,000 units/ml:** Amp. 1 ml Box 50s. **10,000 units/ml:** Amp. 1 ml Box 50s.
Use: Anticoagulant.

LIQUA-GEL. (Paddock) Boric acid, glycerine, propylene glycol, methylparaben, propylparaben, Irish moss extract, methylcellulose. Bot. 4 oz, 16 oz.

LIQUI-CHAR. (Jones Medical) Acitvated charcoal. **Liq. Bot.:** 12.5 Gm/60 ml, 15 Gm/75 ml. **Squeeze container.:** 25 Gm/120 ml, 50 Gm/240 ml, 30 Gm/120 ml.
Use: Antidote.

LIQUI-DOSS. (Ferndale) Docusate sodium 60 mg, mineral oil. Bot. pt.
Use: Laxative.

LIQUID LATHER. (Ulmer) Gentle wash for hands, body, face, hair. Bot. 8 oz, gal.
Use: Cleanser.

LIQUID PETROLATUM EMULSION.
See: Mineral Oil Emulsion, U.S.P. XXII.

LIQUID PRED SYRUP. (Muro) Prednisone 5 mg/5 ml in syrup base. Alcohol 5%, saccharin, sorbitol. Bot. 120 ml, 240 ml.
Use: Corticosteorid.

LIQUIFILM FORTE. (Allergan) Enhanced artificial tears w/polyvinyl alcohol 3%, thimerosal 0.002%, edetate disodium in a buffered sterile, isotonic soln. Bot. 0.5 fl oz, 1 fl oz.
Use: Artificial tears.

LIQUIFILM TEARS. (Allergan) Polyvinyl alcohol 1.4%, chlorobutanol 0.5%, sodium Cl, purified water. Bot. 15 ml, 30 ml.
Use: Artificial tears.

LIQUIFILM WETTING SOLUTION. (Allergan) Polyvinyl alcohol, hydroxypropyl methylcellulose, edetate disodium, sodium Cl, potassium Cl, benzalkonium Cl. Bot. 20 ml, 60 ml.
Use: Hard contact lens care.

LIQUIMAT. (Owen) Sulfur 5%, alcohol 22%, in drying makeup base. Plastic Bot. 1.5 oz.
Use: Anti-acne.

LIQUI-NOX. (Alconox) qt, gal.
Use: Anionic and nonionic detergents and wetting agents.

LIQUIPAKE. (Lafayette) Barium sulfate suspension 100% w/v for dilution. Bot. 1850 ml, Case 4s.
Use: Radiopaque agent.

LIQUIPRIN. (Norcliff Thayer) Acetaminophen 80 mg/1.66 ml, saccharin. Soln. Bot. 35 ml w/dropper.

Use: Analgesic.

LIQUOR CARBONIS DETERGENS.
See: Coal Tar Topical Soln., U.S.P. XXII. (Various Mfr.).

LIRON B12 1000. (Kenyon) Vitamin B_{12} 1000 mcg, vitamins B_1 10 mg, B_6 1 mg, B_2 1 mg, liver 2 mcg, iron peptonate 20 mg, cobalt Cl 0.2 mg/ml. Vial 10 ml.
Use: Vitamin/mineral supplement.

LIRON B12 50. (Kenyon) Same formula as Liron B_{12} 1000, except B_{12} 50 mg/ml. Vial 10 ml.
Use: Vitamin/mineral supplement.

LISADIMATE. USAN.
Use: Sunscreen.

LISINOPRIL. USAN.
Use: Antihypertensive.

LISTEREX SCRUB MEDICATED LOTION. (Warner-Lambert Prods) Salicylic acid 2% Lot. Bot. 4 oz, 8 oz.
Use: Anti-acne.

LISTERINE ANTISEPTIC. (Warner-Lambert Prods) Thymol, eucalyptol, methyl salicylate, menthol. Alcohol 26.9%. Bot. 3 oz, 6 oz, 12 oz, 18 oz, 24 oz, 32 oz.
Use: Mouthwash.

LISTERINE ANTISEPTIC THROAT LOZENGES. (Warner-Lambert Prods) Hexylresorcinol 2.4 mg/Loz. Box 24s.
Use: Throat preparation.

LISTERINE MAXIMUM STRENGTH ANTISEPTIC THROAT LOZENGES. (Warner-Lambert Prods) Hexylresorcinol 4 mg/Loz. Box 24s.
Use: Throat preparation.

LISTERMINT WITH FLUORIDE. (Warner-Lambert Prods) Sodium fluoride 0.02% w/water, alcohol 6.65%, glycerin, poloxamer 407, sodium lauryl sulfate, sodium citrate, sodium saccharin, zinc Cl, citric acid, flavors, colors. Bot. 6 oz, 12 oz, 18 oz, 24 oz, 32 oz.
Use: Mouth preparation, dental caries preventative.

LITE PRED. (Horizon) Prednisolone sodium phosphate 0.125%. Soln. Bot. 5 ml.
Use: Corticosteroid, ophthalmic.

LITHANE. (Miles Pharm) Lithium carbonate 300 mg, tartrazine. Tab. Bot. 100s.
Use: Antipsychotic agent.

LITHIUM CARBONATE, U.S.P. XXII. ER Cap., Cap., Tab., U.S.P. XXII. Carbonic acid, dilithium salt.
Use: Antidepressant.
See: Eskalith, Cap., Tab. (SmithKline).
Lithane, Tab. (Miles Pharm).
Lithobid, Tab. (Ciba).
Lithotabs, Tab. (Reid-Rowell).

LITHIUM CARBONATE CAPSULES AND TABLETS. (Roxane) Lithium carbonate. **Tab.:** 300 mg. Bot. 100s, 1000s, UD 100s. **Cap.:** 150 mg, 300 mg or 600 mg. Bot. 100s, 1000s, UD 100s.
Use: Antipsychotic agent.

•**LITHIUM CITRATE,** U.S.P. XXII. Syr. U.S.P. XXII. CH_2 (COO Li) C (OH)(COOLi) CH_2 COO Li.x. $H_2O.C_6H_5Li_3O_7$ (Roxane) 8 mEq/5 ml.
Use: Manic-depressive states.
See: Cibalith-Si, Liq. (Ciba).
Lithonate-S, Liq. (Reid-Rowell).

•**LITHIUM HYDROXIDE,** U.S.P. XXII. LiOH.x.H_2O. Lithium hydroxide monohydrate.
Use: Manic-depressive states.

LITHOBID. (Ciba) Lithium carbonate 300 mg/SR Tab. Bot. 100s, 1000s, UD 100s.
Use: Antipsychotic agent.

LITHONATE. (Reid-Rowell) Lithium carbonate 300 mg/Cap. Bot. 100s, 1000s, Unit-of-use 90s, 100s, 120s, UD 100s.
Use: Antipsychotic agent.

LITHOSTAT. (Mission) Acetohydroxamic acid 250 mg/Tab. Bot. 120s.
Use: Urinary anti-infective.

LITHOTABS. (Reid-Rowell) Lithium carbonate 300 mg/Tab. Bot. 100s, 1000s, UD 100s.
Use: Antipsychotic agent.

LIVEC. (Enzyme Process) Vitamins A 5000 IU, B_1 1.5 mg, B_2 1.7 mg, niacin 20 mg, C 60 mg, B_6 2 mg, pantothenic acid 10 mg, E 30 IU, B_{12} 6 mcg, calcium 250 mg, iron 5 mg, D 400 IU, folacin 0.075 mg/3 Tab. Bot. 100s, 300s.
Use: Vitamin/mineral supplement.

LIVERBEX. (Spanner) Liver 2 mcg, vitamins B_1, B_2, B_6, B_{12}, niacinamide, pantothenate/ml. Vial 30 ml.
Use: Nutritional supplement.

LIVER, B12 AND FOLIC ACID. (Lincoln) Vitamin B_{12} activity 5 mcg, cyanocobalamin 35 mcg, cyanocobalamin 5 mg, folic acid, w/phenol 0.5%, sodium citrate 0.25%, disodium sequestrene 0.01%, sodium bisulfite 0.025%/ml. Vial 15 ml.
Use: Nutritional supplement.

LIVER COMBO NO. 5. (Rugby) Liver vitamin B_{12} equivalent 10 mcg, crystalline B_{12} 100 mcg, folic acid 0.4 mg/ml. Inj. Vial 10 ml.
Use: Parenteral liver supplement.

LIVER DESICCATED. Desiccated liver substance.

LIVER EXTRACT. Dry liver extract w/Vitamin B_{12}, folic acid.

LIVER FUNCTION AGENTS.
See: Bromsulphalein, Amp. (Hynson, Westcott & Dunning).
Iodophthalein (Various Mfr.).
Sulfobromophthalein Sodium U.S.P. XXII (Gotham).

LIVERGRAN. (Rawl) Desiccated whole liver 9 Gm, vitamins B_1 18 mg, B_2 36 mg, niacinamide 90 mg, choline bitartrate 216 mg, B_6 3.6 mg, calcium pantothenate 3.6 mg, inositol 90 mg, biotin 6 mcg, vitamins B_{12} 5.4 mcg, methionine 198 mg, arginine 242 mg, cystine 72 mg, glutamic acid 675 mg, histidine 99 mg, isoleucine 333 mg, leucine 495 mg, lysine 297 mg, phenylalanine 189 mg, threonine 333 mg, trypto-

phan 45 mg, tyrosine 180 mg, valine 306 mg/3 Tsp. Bot. 15 oz.
Use: Nutritional supplement.

LIVER INJECTION. (Various Mfr.). Liver extract for parenteral use.
Use: Parenteral liver supplement.

LIVER INJECTION. (Arcum; Lederle) Vitamin B_{12} 20 mcg/ml. Vial 10 ml.
Use: Nutritional supplement.

LIVER INJECTION, CRUDE. (Lilly) 2 mcg/ml. Vial 30 ml; (Medwick) 2 mcg/ml. Vial 30 ml.
Use: Liver supplement.

LIVER-IRON-B COMPLEX WITH VITAMIN B12. (Maurry) Liver 2 mcg, vitamins B_{12} 15 mcg, ferrous gluconate 31.1 mg, B_1 10 mg, B_2 0.5 mg, B_6 1 mg, calcium pantothenate 1 mg, niacinamide 10 mg, d-Glucose 1%, chlorobutanol 0.5%, benzyl alcohol 2%/Inj.
Use: Nutritional supplement.

LIVER, IRON, FOLIC & COBALT. (Kenyon) Liver refined (B_{12} equivalent) 10 mcg, iron peptonate 59 mg, cobalt gluconate 9 mg, folic acid 5 mg, procaine HCl 1%/2 ml. Vial 30 ml.
Use: Nutritional supplement.

LIVER IRON VITAMINS INJ. (Arcum) Liver inj. (10 mcg B_{12} activity/ml) 0.1 ml, crude liver inj. (2 mcg B_{12} activity/ml) 0.125 ml, green ferric ammonium citrate 20 mg, niacinamide 50 mg, vitamin B_6 0.3 mg, B_2 0.3 mg, procaine HCl 0.5%, phenol 0.5%/2 ml. Vial 30 ml.
Use: Nutritional supplement.

LIVER, IRON, VITAMINS. (Kenyon) Liver (B_{12} equivalent) 1 mcg, iron gluconate 59 mg, niacinamide 50 mg, vitamin B_2 (as 5-phos.) 0.3 mg, B_6 0.3 mg, sodium dicitrate 10 mg/2 ml, procaine HCl 1%. Vial 30 ml.
Use: Nutritional supplement.

LIVER, IRON & VITAMINS. (Pharmex) Liver (equivalent to vitamin B_{12} 1 mcg) 100 mg, vitamin B_{12} 5 mcg, B_2 0.3 mg, B_6 0.3 mg, niacinamide 50 mg, iron peptonate 19.5 mg, sodium citrate 1%, phenol 0.5%/3 ml. Vial 30 ml.
Use: Nutritional supplement.

LIVER, IRON, VITAMINS AND AMINO ACIDS. (Kenyon) Liver B_{12} equivalent, 1 mcg, ferrous gluconate 50 mg, B_2 (as 5-phos.) 0.5 mg, d-panthenol 2.5 mg, niacinamide 100 mg, dl-methionine 10 mg, choline Cl 5 mg/2 ml. Vial 30 ml.
Use: Nutritional supplement.

LIVER, IRON, VITAMINS WITH B12. (Kenyon) Liver (B_{12} equivalent) 2 mcg, vitamin B_{12} 15 mcg, ferrous lactate 20 mg, B_1 10 mg, B_2 (as 5-phos.) 9.5 mg, B_6 1 mg, d-panthenol 1 mg, niacinamide 10 mg, choline Cl 0.5 mg/ml. Vial 30 ml.
Use: Nutritional supplement.

LIVER, REFINED. (Medwick) 20 mcg/ml. Vial 10 ml, 30 ml.
Use: Nutritional supplement.

LIVER VASOCONSTRICTOR.
See: Kutapressin, Vial, Amp. (Kremers-Urban).

LIVIFOL. (Dunhall) Vitamin B_{12} activity from liver inj. equivalent to cyanocobalamin 10 mcg, folic acid 1 mg, cyanocobalamin 100 mcg/ml. Vial 10 ml.
Use: Vitamin/mineral supplement.

LIVI-PLEX FORTIFIED. (Rocky Mtn.) Vitamin B_{12} 30 mcg, liver inj. 1 ml, ferrous gluconate 50 mg, riboflavin 1.5 mg, calcium pantothenate 2.5 mg, niacinamide 100 mg, citric acid 16.4 mg, sodium citrate 23.6 mg, benzyl alcohol 2%, procaine HCl 2%/2 ml. Vial 30 ml.
Use: Nutritional supplement.

LIVITAMIN. (Beecham Labs) Ferrous fumarate 100 mg, Vitamins B_1 3 mg, B_2 3 mg, B_6 3 mg, C 100 mg, niacinamide 10 mg, calcium pantothenate 2 mg, B_{12} 5 mcg, copper 0.66 mg, desiccated liver 150 mg/Cap. Bot. 100s.
Use: Vitamin/mineral supplement.

LIVITAMIN CHEWABLE TABLETS. (Beecham Labs) Ferrous fumarate 50 mg, Vitamins C 100 mg, B_1 3 mg, B_2 3 mg, niacinamide 10 mg, B_6 3 mg, calcium pantothenate 2 mg, cyanocobalamin 5 mcg, copper 0.33 mg/Tab. Bot. 100s.
Use: Vitamin/mineral supplement.

LIVITAMIN W/INTRINSIC FACTOR. (Beecham Labs) Desiccated liver 150 mg, ferrous fumarate 100 mg, Vitamins B_1 3 mg, C 100 mg, B_2 3 mg, niacinamide 10 mg, B_{12} 5 mcg, B_6 3 mg, calcium pantothenate 2 mg, copper 0.66 mg, B_{12} w/intrinsic factor ⅓ units/Cap. Bot. 100s.
Use: Vitamin/mineral supplement.

LIVITAMIN LIQUID. (Beecham Labs) Iron peptonized N.F. 210 mg, liver fraction No. 1 0.5 Gm, Vitamins B_1 3 mg, B_2 3 mg, niacinamide 10 mg, B_6 HCl 3 mg, pantothenic acid 2 mg, B_{12} 5 mcg, copper 0.66 mg/15 ml. Bot. 8 oz, pt, gal.
Use: Vitamin/mineral supplement.

LIVITRINSIC-F CAPSULES. (Goldline) Iron 36.3 mg, vitamins B_{12} 15 mcg, C 75 mg, intrinsic factor concentrate 240 mg, folic acid 0.5 mg/Cap. Bot. 100s, 1000s.
Use: Vitamin/mineral supplement.

LIV-O-VITE. (Jenkins) Ferrous fumarate 3 gr (elemental iron 1 gr), desiccated liver 2 gr, thiamine HCl 3 mg, riboflavin 3 mg, cyanocobalamin 3 mcg/Tab. Bot. 1000s.
Use: Vitamin/mineral supplement.

LIV-O-REX. (Nutrition) Desiccated liver 1.4 gr, green iron, ammonium citrate 3 gr, Vitamins B_1 1.5 mg, B_2 0.5 mg, calcium pantothenate 0.25 mg, B_6 0.15 mg, niacinamide 10 mg/Cap. Bot. 100s, 1000s.
Use: Vitamin/mineral supplement.

LIVROBEN. (Forest) Liver 10 mcg, folic acid 0.4 mg, cyanocobalamin 100 mcg/ml. Vial 10 ml.
Use: Nutritional supplement.

•**LIXAZINONE SULFATE.** USAN.
Use: Cardiotonic (phosphodiesterase inhibitor).

LIXOIL. (Lixoil Labs.) Sulfonated fatty oils and one or more esters of higher fatty acids. Bot. 16 oz.
Use: Dermatologic.

LKV-DROPS. (Freeda) Vitamins A 5000 IU, D 400 IU, E 2 mg, B_1 1.5 mg, B_2 1.5 mg, B_3 10 mg, B_5 2 mg, B_6 2 mg, B_{12} 6 mcg, C 50 mg, biotin 50 mcg/0.6 ml. Bot. 60 ml.
Use: Vitamin supplement.

LLD FACTOR.
See: Vitamin B_{12}, Preps. (Various Mfr.).

LMD. (Abbott Hospital Prods) Low molecular weight dextran. LMD 10% w/v in D5-W and LMD 10% w/v in saline 0.9%, 500 ml each.
Use: Plasma volume expander.

LMWD-DEXTRAN 40. (Pharmachem) Normal saline 0.9%, dextrose 10%.
Use: Plasma volume expander.

LOBAC. (Seatrace) Chlorzoxazone 250 mg, acetaminophen 300 mg/Cap. Bot. 40s, 100s, 1000s.
Use: Muscle relaxant, analgesic.

LOBAK TABLETS. (Winthrop Products) Chlormezanone 250 mg, acetaminophen 300 mg/Tab. In 40s, 100s, 1000s.
Use: Antianxiety agent, analgesic.

LOBANA BODY SHAMPOO. (Ulmer) Bot. 8 oz, gal.
Use: Hair & body cleanser.

LOBANA CONDITIONING SHAMPOO. (Ulmer) Bot. 8 oz, gal.
Use: Shampoo for hair and scalp.

LOBANA DERM-ADE CREAM. (Ulmer) Vitamin A, D, E cream. Jar 2 oz, 8 oz.
Use: Minor skin irritations.

LOBANA LIQUID HAND SOAP. (Ulmer) Dispenser 14 oz, refill 24 oz. Bot. gal.
Use: Cleanser.

LOBANA PERI-GARD. (Ulmer) Water-resistant ointment containing vitamin A & D. Jar 2 oz, 8 oz.
Use: Skin protectant.

LOBANA PERINEAL CLEANSER. (Ulmer) Sprayer 4 oz, 8 oz. Bot. gal.
Use: Urine and fecal cleanser.

LOBELIA FLUIDEXTRACT.
W/Hyoscyamus fluidextract, grindelia fluidextract, potassium iodide.
See: L.S. Mixture, Liq. (Paddock).

LOBELINE SULFATE.
See: Lobidram, Tab. (Dram).
Nikoban, Loz., Gum. (Thompson).

•**LOBENDAZOLE.** USAN.
Use: Anthelmintic.

•**LOBENZARIT SODIUM.** USAN.
Use: Antirheumatic.

LOBIDRAM. (Dram) Lobeline sulfate 2 mg/Tab. Pkg. 15s, 30s.
Use: Withdrawal symptoms of smoking.

LOCOID. (Owen) **Cream:** Hydrocortisone butyrate 0.1%. Tube 15 Gm, 45 Gm. **Oint.:** Hydrocortisone butyrate 0.1%. Tube 15 Gm, 45 Gm.
Use: Corticosteroid, topical.

LODINE. (Wyeth-Ayerst) Etodolac.
Use: Anti-inflammatory.

LODOSYN. (MSD) Carbidopa 25 mg/Tab. Bot. 100s.
Use: Antiparkinson agent.

•**LODOXAMIDE ETHYL.** USAN.
Use: Antiasthmatic, anti-allergic.

•**LODOXAMIDE TROMETHAMINE.** USAN.
Use: Antiasthmatic, anti-allergic.

LODRANE CR. (Poythress) Theophylline anhydrous 100 mg, 200 mg or 300 mg/CR Tab. Bot. 100s, 500s, 1000s, UD 100s, 500s, 1000s.
Use: Bronchodialtor.

LOESTRIN 21 1/20. (Parke-Davis) Norethindrone acetate 1 mg, ethinyl estradiol 20 mcg Tab. Petipac compact 21 Tab. Ctn. 5 compacts or Ctn. 5 refills.
Use: Oral contraceptive.

LOESTRIN 21 1.5/30. (Parke-Davis) Norethindrone acetate 1.5 mg, ethinyl estradiol 30 mcg/Tab. Petipac compact. Ctn. 5 compacts or Ctn. 5 refills.
Use: Oral contraceptive.

LOESTRIN Fe 1/20. (Parke-Davis) White Tab.: Norethindrone acetate 1 mg, ethinyl estradiol 20 mcg/Tab.; **Brown Tab.:** Ferrous fumarate 75 mg (7 tabs.) Carton 5 petipac compacts 28 Tab., carton of 5 refills 28 Tab.
Use: Oral contraceptive.

LOESTRIN Fe 1.5/30. (Parke-Davis) Green Tab.: Norethindrone acetate 1.5 mg, ethinyl estradiol 30 mcg. **Brown Tab.:** Ferrous fumarate 75 mg (7 tabs.). Carton 5 petipac compacts 28 Tab., carton of 5 refills 28 Tab.
Use: Oral contraceptive.

•**LOFEMIZOLE HYDROCHLORIDE.** USAN.
Use: Anti-inflammatory.

LOFENALAC. (Mead Johnson Nutrition) Corn syrup solids 49.2%, casein hydrolysate 18.7% (enzymic digest of casein containing amino acids and small peptides), corn oil 18%, modified tapioca starch 9.57%, protein equivalent 15%, fat 18%, carbohydrate 60%, minerals (ash) 3.6%, phenylalanine 75 mg/100 Gm pow., Vitamins A 1600 IU, D 400 IU, E 10 IU, C 52 mg, folic acid 100 mcg, B_1 0.5 mg, B_2 0.6 mg, niacin 8 mg, B_6 0.4 mg, B_{12} 2 mcg, biotin 0.05 mg, pantothenic acid 3 mg, Vitamin K-1 100 mcg, choline 85 mg, inositol 30 mg, calcium 600 mg, phosphorus 450 mg, iodine 45 mcg, iron 12 mg, magnesium 70 mg, copper 0.6 mg, zinc 4 mg, manganese 1 mg, chloride 450 mg, potassium 650 mg, sodium 300 mg/qt. at normal dilution of 20 k cal/fl oz, Can 2 1/2 lb.
Use: Enteral nutritional supplement.

LOFENE. (Lannett) Diphenoxylate HCl 2.5 mg, atropine sulfate 0.025 mg Bot. 100s, 500s, 1000s.
Use: Antidiarrheal.

•**LOFENTANIL OXALATE.** USAN.
Use: Analgesic, narcotic.

LOFEPRAMINE. B.A.N. 5-3-[N-(4-Chlorophenacyl)methylamino]-propyl-10, 11-dihydrobenz[b,f]azepine. Lopramine (I.N.N.).
Use: Antidepressant.

•**LOFEPRAMINE HYDROCHLORIDE.** USAN.

Use: Antidepressant.
•**LOFEXIDINE HYDROCHLORIDE.** USAN.
Use: Antihypertensive.
LOGEN LIQUID. (Goldline) Diphenoxylate HCl w/ atropine sulfate. Bot. 2 oz.
Use: Antidiarrheal.
LOGEN TABLETS. (Goldline) Diphenoxylate HCl, atropine sulfate. Bot. 100s, 500s, 1000s.
Use: Antidiarrheal.
L.O.L. LOTION. (O'Leary) Bot 8 oz, 16 oz.
Use: Anti-acne.
LOMANATE. (Various Mfr.) Diphenoxylate HCl 2.5 mg, atropine sulfate 0.025 mg/5 ml. Bot. 60 ml.
Use: Antidiarrheal.
•**LOMETRALINE HYDROCHLORIDE.** USAN.
Use: Antipsychotic, antiparkinson agent.
•**LOMETREXOL SODIUM.** USAN.
Use: Antineoplastic.
•**LOMOFUNGIN.** USAN.
Use: Antifungal.
LOMOTIL. (Searle) Diphenoxylate HCl 2.5 mg, atropine sulfate 0.025 mg/Tab. or 5 ml. **Tab.:** Bot. 100s, 500s, 1000s, 2500s, UD 100s. **Liq.:** Bot. w/dropper 2 oz.
Use: Antidiarrheal.
•**LOMUSTINE.** USAN. CCNU; NSC-79037. 1-(2-Chloroethyl)-3-cyclohexyl-1-nitrosourea.
Use: Antineoplastic agent.
See: CeeNu, Cap. (Bristol).
LONALAC. (Mead Johnson Nutrition) Protein as casein 21%, fat as coconut oil 49%, carbohydrate as lactose 30%, vitamins A 1440 IU, B_1 0.6 mg, B_2 2.6 mg, niacin 1.2 mg, calcium 1.69 Gm, phosphorous 1.5 Gm, chloride 750 mg, potassium 1.88 Gm, sodium 38 mg, magnesium 135 mg/qt. Pow. Can 16 oz.
Use: Enteral nutritional supplement.
•**LONAPALENE.** USAN.
Use: Antipsoriatic.
LONG ACTING NEO-SYNEPHRINE II NOSE DROPS AND NASAL SPRAY. (Winthrop Consumer Products) Xylometazoline HCl 0.1% (adult strength) or 0.05% (child strength). Bot. 1 oz, Spray 0.5 oz (adult strength).
Use: Nasal decongestant.
LONG ACTING NEO-SYNEPHRINE II VAPOR SPRAY. (Winthrop Consumer Products) Xylometazoline HCl 0.1%. Mentholated. Spray Bot. 0.5 fl oz.
Use: Nasal decongestant.
LONG ACTING NASAL SPRAY. (Weeks & Leo) Oxymetazoline HCl 0.05%. Soln. Bot. 0.75 oz.
Use: Nasal decongestant.
LONITEN. (Upjohn) Minoxidil 2.5 mg or 10 mg/ Tab. 2.5 mg: Unit-of-Use Bot. 100s. 10 mg: Bot. 500s, Unit-of-Use Bot. 100s.
Use: Antihypertensive.
Note: FDA approval pending for use in treating male-pattern baldness.
LONOX. (Geneva Generics) Diphenoxylate HCl 2.5 mg, atropine sulfate 0.025 mg/Tab. Bot. 100s, 500s, 1000s, UD 100s.
Use: Antidiarrheal.
LO/OVRAL. (Wyeth-Ayerst) Norgestrel 0.3 mg, ethinyl estradiol 0.03 mg/Tab. Pilpak dispenser 6s, Tab. 21s.
Use: Oral contraceptive.
LO/OVRAL-28. (Wyeth-Ayerst) Tab. 21s, each containing norgestrel 0.03 mg, ethinyl estradiol 0.03 mg, 7 pink inert. Tab. Pilpak dispenser 6s, Tab 28s.
Use: Oral contraceptive.
•**LOPERAMIDE HCL,** U.S.P. XXII. Cap., U.S.P. XXII.
Use: Antiperistaltic.
See: Imodium, Cap. (Ortho).
LOPID. (Parke-Davis) Gemfibrozil. **300 mg:** Cap. Bot. 100s, 500s. **600 mg:** Tab. Bot. 60s.
Use: Antihyperlipidemic agent.
LOPRESSOR. (Geigy) Metoprolol tartrate. **Tab.:** 50 mg or 100 mg. Bot. 100s, 1000s, UD 100s, Gy-Pak 60s, 100s. **Amp.:** 5 mg/5 ml.
Use: Beta-adrenergic blocking agent.
LOPRESSOR HCT. (Geigy) Metoprolol tartrate, hydrochlorothiazide. **Tab.:** 50/25 mg, 100/25 mg or 100/50 mg. Bot. 100s.
Use: Beta-adrenergic blocking agent.
LOPROX. (Hoechst) Ciclopirox olamine 1% in cream base. Tube 15 Gm, 30 Gm, 90 Gm.
Use: Antifungal, external.
LOPURIN. (Boots) Allopurinol 100 mg or 300 mg/ Tab. Bot. 100s, 1000s, UD 100s.
Use: Agent for gout.
•**LORACARBEF.** USAN.
Use: Antibacterial.
•**LORAJMINE HYDROCHLORIDE.** USAN.
Use: Cardiac depressant.
•**LORATADINE.** USAN.
Use: Antihistamine.
LORAZEPAM, U.S.P. XXII, Tab., Inj. 7-Chloro-5-(o-chlorophenyl)-1,3-dihydro-3-hydroxy-2H-1,4-benzodiazepin-2-one.
Use: Minor tranquilizer.
See: Alzapam, Tab. (Ultra).
Ativan, Tab., Inj. (Wyeth-Ayerst).
LORAZEPAM. (Purepac) Lorazepam. **Tab.:** 0.5 mg Bot. 100s, 500s. 1 mg, 2 mg Bot. 100s, 500s, 1000s.
Use: Antianxiety, sedative/hypnotic.
•**LORBAMATE.** USAN.
Use: Muscle relaxant.
•**LORCAINIDE HYDROCHLORIDE.** USAN.
Use: Cardiac depressant.
LORCET. (UAD Labs) Hydrocodone bitartrate 5 mg, acetaminophen 500 mg/Tab. Bot. 100s.
Use: Narcotic analgesic combination.
LORCET HD. (UAD Labs) Hydrocodone bitartrate 5 mg, acetaminophen 500 mg/Cap. Bot. 100s.
Use: Narcotic analgesic combination.

LORCET PLUS. (UAD Labs) Hydrocodone bitartrate 7.5 mg, acetaminophen 650 mg/Tab. Bot. 100s.
Use: Narcotic analgesic combination.

LORELCO. (Merrell Dow) Probucol 250 mg/Tab. Bot. 120s.
Use: Antihyperlipidemic.

•**LORMETAZEPAM.** USAN.
Use: Sedative/hypnotic.

LOROXIDE. (Dermik) Benzoyl peroxide 5.5%, propylene glycol, cetyl alcohol, hydroxyethylcellulose, kaolin, caramel, talc, cholesterol and related sterols, propylene glycolstearate, polysorbate 20, lanolin alcohol, propylparaben, methylparaben, tetrasodium EDTA, pH buffers, antioxidants, silicone emulsion, silica, decyl oleate, vegetable oil, purcelline oil syn., titanium dioxide, cyclohexanediamine tetraacetic acid, calcium phosphate. Lot. Bot. 25 Gm.
Use: Anti-acne.

LORPHEN. (Geneva) **Cap.:** Chlorpheniramine maleate 8 mg or 12 mg. Bot. 100s. **Tab.:** 4 mg. Bot. 100s.
Use: Antihistamine.

LORPRN. (Russ) Aspirin 325 mg, caffeine 40 mg, butalbital 50 mg/Cap. Bot. 100s.
Use: Narcotic analgesic combination.

LORTAB. (Russ) Hydrocodone 2.5 mg, acetaminophen 325 mg/Tab. Bot. 100s, UD 100s.
Use: Narcotic analgesic combination.

LORTAB 5. (Russ) Hydrocodone 5 mg, acetaminophen 500 mg/Tab. Bot. 100s, 500s, UD 100s.
Use: Narcotic analgesic combination.

LORTAB 7. (Russ) Hydrocodone 7.5 mg, acetaminophen 500 mg/Tab. Bot. 100s, UD 100s.
Use: Narcotic analgesic combination.

LORTAB ASA. (Russ) Hydrocodone bitartrate 5 mg, aspirin 500 mg/Tab. Bot. 100s.
Use: Narcotic analgesic combination.

LORTAB LIQUID. (Russ) Hydrocodone 2.5 mg, acetaminophen 120 mg/5 ml w/alcohol 7%. Bot. 1 oz, 4 oz, pt.
Use: Narcotic analgesic combination.

•**LORTALAMINE.** USAN.
Use: Antidepressant.

•**LORZAFONE.** USAN.
Use: Minor tranquilizer.

LOSEC. (Merck, Sharpe and Dohme) Omeprazole 20 mg/Cap. Bot. 30s, UD 100s.
Use: Gastric acid suppressant.

LOSOPAN LIQUID. (Goldline) Magaldrate 540 mg/5 ml. Bot. 12 oz.
Use: Antacid.

LOSOPAN PLUS LIQUID. (Goldline) Magaldrate 540 mg, simethicone 20 mg/5 ml. Bot. 12 oz.
Use: Antacid, antiflatulent.

•**LOSULAZINE HYDROCHLORIDE.** USAN.
Use: Antihypertensive.

LOTALBA CREAM. (Durel) Lotalba 30%, zinc oxide 10%, sulfur potassium 5%, greaseless ointment base 55%. Jar 3 oz, lb.
Use: Anti-acne.

LOTALBA OINTMENT. (Durel) Stabilized white lotion (lotio alba), glycerine, mineral gums. Jar 3 oz, lb.
Use: Anti-acne.

LOTAWIN CAPSULES. (Winthrop Products) Oxypertine.
Use: Anxiolytic, tranquilizer.

•**LOTEPREDNOL ETABONATE.** USAN.
Use: Anti-inflammatory (topical).

LOTIO ALBA. White lotion.
Use: Anti-acne, antiseborrheic.
W/Sulfur, calamine, alcohol.
See: Sulfa-Lo, Lot. (Whorton).

LOTIO ALSULFA. (Doak) Colloidal sulfur 5%. Bot. 4 oz.
Use: Anti-acne, antiseborrheic.

LOTOCREME. (C.S. Dent) Bot. 8 oz.
Use: Body rub.

LOTION-JEL. (C.S. Dent) Benzocaine in gel base. Tube 0.2 oz.
Use: Local anesthetic.

LOTRIMIN. (Schering) Clotrimazole 1%. **Cream:** Tube 15 Gm, 30 Gm, 45 Gm, 90 Gm. **Lot.:** Bot. 30 ml. **Soln.:** 1%. Bot. 10 ml, 30 ml.
Use: Antifungal, external.

LOTRISONE. (Schering) Clotrimazole 1%, betamethasone dipropionate 0.05%/Gm. Tube 15 Gm, 45 Gm.
Use: Antifungal, external.

LOSOTRON PLUS LIQUID. (Various Mfr.) Magaldrate 540 mg, simethicone 20 mg/5 ml. Bot. 360 ml.
Use: Antacid, antiflatulent.

LO-TROP. (Vangard) Diphenoxylate HCl 2.5 mg, atropine sulfate 0.025 mg/Tab. Bot. 100s, 1000s.
Use: Antidiarrheal.

LOUCEVERIN CALCIUM. Calcium 5-formyl-5, 6, 7, 8-tetrahydroteroylglutamate.

•**LOVASTATIN.** USAN. Butanoic acid, 2-methyl-, 1,2,3,7,8,8a-hexahydro-3,7-di-methyl-8-[2-(tetrahydro-4-hydroxy-6-oxo-2*H*-pyran-2-yl)-ethyl]-1-naphthalenyl ester, [1*S*-[1α(*R**),3α,7β,8β(2*S*-*,-4*S**),8aβ]]-; (2) (*S*)-2-Methylbutyric acid, 8-ester with (4*R*,-6*R*)-6-[2-[(1*S*,2*S*,6*R*,8*S*,8a*R*)-1,2,6,7,8,8a-hexahydro-8-hydroxy-2,6-dimethyl-1-naphthyl]ethyl]tetrahydro-4-hydroxy-2*H*-pyran-2-one.
Use: Antihypercholesteremic.
See: Mevacor, Tab. (Merck Sharp & Dohme).

LOVE LONGER. (Youngs Drug) Benzocaine 7.5% in water-soluble lubricant base. Tube 0.5 oz.
Use: Local anesthetic.

LOWILA CAKE. (Westwood) Sodium lauryl sulfoacetate, dextrin, boric acid, urea, sorbitol, mineral oil, PEG 14 M, lactic acid, cellulose gum, docusate sodium, water, fragrance. Cake 3¾ oz.
Use: Skin cleanser.

LOW-QUEL. (Blue Cross) Diphenoxylate HCl 2.5 mg, atropine sulfate 0.025 mg/Tab. Bot. 100s.
Use: Antidiarrheal.

LOWSIUM. (Rugby) Magaldrate 540 mg/5 ml. Susp. Bot. 360 ml.
Use: Antacid.

LOWSIUM PLUS. (Rugby) **Tab.:** Magaldrate 480 mg, simethicone 20 mg. Bot. 60s. **Susp.:** Magaldrate 540 mg, simethicone 20 mg/5 ml. Bot. 360 ml.
Use: Antacid, antiflatulent.

•**LOXAPINE.** USAN. 2-Chloro-11-(4-methyl-1-piperazinyl) dibenz [b,f] [1,4] oxazepine.
Use: Tranquilizer.

LOXAPINE HYDROCHLORIDE.
Use: Tranquilizer.
See: Daxolin Concentrate, Liq. (Miles Pharm).
Loxitane-C Oral Concentrate (Lederle).
Loxitane, Inj. (Lederle).

•**LOXAPINE SUCCINATE.** USAN. (1)2-Chloro-11-(4-methyl-1-piperazinyl) dibenz-[b,f] [1,4]-oxazepine succinate; (2) Succinic acid compound with 2-chloro-11-(4-methyl-1-piperazinyl) dibenz-[b,f] [1,4] oxazepine.
Use: Tranquilizer.
See: Loxitane, Cap. (Lederle).

LOXITANE-C. (Lederle) Loxapine HCl oral concentrate 25 mg/ml. Bot. 120 ml w/dropper.
Use: Antipsychotic agent.

LOXITANE CAPSULES. (Lederle) Loxapine succinate. **5 mg/Cap.:** Bot. 100s, UD 10 × 10s. **10 mg, 25 mg or 50 mg/Cap.:** Bot. 100s, 1000s, UD 10 × 10s.
Use: Antipsychotic agent.

LOXITANE IM. (Lederle) Loxitane HCl (base equivalent) 50 mg/ml. Amp 1 ml. Box 10s.
Use: Antipsychotic agent.

•**LOXORIBINE.** USAN.
Use: Immunostimulant; vaccine adjuvant.

LOZOL. (Rorer) Indapamide 2.5 mg/Tab. Bot. 100s, 1000s, 2500s, Strip dispenser 100s.
Use: Diuretic, antihypertensive.

L-PAM. p-Di(2-chloroethyl) amino-L-phenylalamine.
Use: An alkylating antineoplastic agent. Under study.

L-SARCOLYSIN.
See: Alkeran, Tab. (Burroughs Wellcome).

LUBAFAX. (Burroughs Wellcome) Surgical lubricant, sterile; water soluble, non-staining. Foil wrapper 2.7 Gm, 5 Gm. Box 144s.
Use: Surgical lubricant.

LUBATH. (Warner-Lambert Prods) Mineral oil, PPG-15, stearyl ether, oleth-2, nonoxynol-5, fragrance, D&C Green No. 6. Bot. 4 oz, 8 oz, 16 oz.
Use: Emollient.

LUBINOL. (Purepac) Light, heavy and extra heavy mineral oil. Bot. pt, qt, gal. (Extra heavy Bot.) 8 oz, pt, qt, gal.
Use: Emollient.

LUBRASEPTIC JELLY. (Guardian) Water-soluble amyl phenyl phenol complex 0.12%, phenylmercuric nitrate, 0.007%. Bellows-type tube 10 Gm, 24s.
Use: Urethral instillation, urologic and proctologic exams.

LUBRASOL BATH OIL. (Pharmaceutical Specialties) Mineral oil, lanolin oil, PEG-200 dilaurate, oxybenzone. Bot. 240 ml, 480 ml, gal.
Use: Emollient.

LUBRIDERM CREAM. (Warner-Lambert Prods) Water, mineral oil, petrolatum, glycerin, glyceryl stearate, PEG-100 stearate, squalane, lanolin, lanolin alcohol, lanolin oil, cetyl alcohol, sorbitan laurate, fragrance (if scented), methylparaben, butylparaben, propylparaben, quaternium-15. Tube: (scented) 1.5 oz, 4 oz,; (unscented) 4 oz.
Use: Emollient.

LUBRIDERM LOTION. (Warner-Lambert Prods) Water, mineral oil, petrolatum, sorbitol, lanolin, lanolin alcohol, stearic acid, TEA, cetyl alcohol, fragrance (if scented), butylparaben, methylparaben, propylparaben, sodium Cl. Bot. (scented), 4 oz, 8 oz, 16 oz; (unscented) 8 oz, 16 oz.
Use: Emollient.

LUBRIDERM LUBATH OIL. (Warner-Lambert) Mineral oil, PPG-15 stearyl ether, oleth-2, nonoxynol-5. Lanolin free. Bot. 240 ml, pt.
Use: Emollient.

LUBRIN. (Upsher-Smith) Glycerin, laureth-23, PEG 40 stearate, PEG-6-32, PEG-20, caprylic/capric triglyceride. Pkg. 5 inserts.
Use: Vaginal lubricant.

•**LUCANTHONE HYDROCHLORIDE.** USAN. 1-[[2-(Diethylamino)ethyl] amino]-4-methylthioxanthen-9-one Monohydrochloride.
Use: Antischistosomal.

LUDENS COUGH DROPS. (Luden's) Honey lemon, honey licorice, menthol, strong flavor menthol, strong flavor eucalyptus or wild cherry flavored loz. Square-pack. Box, bag.
Use: Cough suppressant.

LUDIOMIL. (Ciba) Maprotiline 25 mg, 50 mg or 75 mg/Tab. Bot. 100s, Accu-Pak 100s.
Use: Antidepressant.

LUFYLLIN. (Wallace) Dyphylline. Inj. **Amp.:** (500 mg/2 ml) Box 25s. **Elix.:** 100 mg/15 ml; alcohol 20%. Bot. pt, gal. **Tab.:** 200 mg. Bot. 100s, 1000s, UD 100s.
Use: Bronchodilator.

LUFYLLIN-EPG. (Wallace) Ephedrine HCl 16 mg, dyphylline 100 mg, phenobarbital 16 mg, guaifenesin 200 mg/Tab. or 10 ml. **Tab.:** Bot. 100s. **Elix.:** (alcohol 5.5%) Bot. pt.
Use: Antiasthmatic combination.

LUFYLLIN-400. (Wallace) Dyphylline 400 mg/Tab. Bot. 100s, 1000s.
Use: Bronchodilator.

LUFYLLIN-GG. (Wallace) **Tab.:** Dyphylline 200 mg, guaifenesin 200 mg/Tab. Bot. 100s, 1000s.

Elix.: Dyphylline 100 mg, guaifenesin 100 mg, alcohol 17%/15 ml. Elix. Bot. pt, gal.
Use: Bronchodilator, expectorant.

LUGOL'S SOLUTION. Strong iodine soln, U.S.P. XXII. (Lyne). Iodine 5 Gm, potassium iodide 10 Gm, in purified water to make 100 ml. Bot. 15 ml.
(Wisconsin) Bot. pt.

LUMINAL INJECTION. (Winthrop Pharm) Phenobarbital 1 ml. 130 mg/Amp. Box 100s.
Use: Sedative/hypnotic.

LUMOPAQUE CAPSULES. (Winthrop Products) Tyropanoate sodium.
Use: Radiopaque agent.

LUNG SURFACTANTS.
Use: Surfactant replacement therapy in neonatal respiratory distress syndrome.
See: Exosurf (Burroughs Wellcome).
Survanta (Ross).

LUPITIDINE HYDROCHLORIDE. USAN.
Use: Antegonist (to histamine hydrogen receptors, veterinary).

LUPRON INJECTION. (TAP) Leuprolide acetate 1 mg/0.2 ml. Vial 2.8 ml.
Use: Antineoplastic agent.

LURAMIDE TABS. (Major) Furosemide 20 mg, 40 mg or 80 mg/Tab. Bot. 100s, 1000s.
Use: Diuretic.

LURIDE DROPS. (Hoyt) Sodium fluoride equivalent to 0.125 mg of fluoride/Drop. Plastic dropper bot. 30 ml.
Use: Dental caries preventative.

LURIDE-F LOZI TABLETS. (Hoyt) Sodium fluoride in Lozi base tab. available as fluoride. **0.25 mg:** Bot. 120s; **0.5 mg:** Bot. 120s, 1200s; **1 mg:** Bot. 120s, 1000s, 5000s.
Use: Dental caries preventative.

LURIDE PROPHYLAXIS PASTE. (Hoyt) Acidulated phosphate sodium fluoride containing 0.4% fluoride ion w/silicon dioxide abrasive. UD 3 Gm, Jar 50 Gm.
Use: Teeth cleaner.

LURIDE-SF LOZI TABLETS. (Hoyt) Sodium fluoride 1 mg fluoride/Tab. Bot. 120s.
Use: Dental caries preventative.

LURIDE TOPICAL GEL. (Hoyt) Acidulated phosphate sodium fluoride containing fluoride ion 1.2% at pH 3.0 to 4.0 in gel base. Bot. 32 oz, 250 ml.
Use: Dental caries preventative.

LURIDE TOPICAL SOLUTION. (Hoyt) Acidulated phosphate sodium fluoride w/pH 3.2. Bot. 250 ml.
Use: Dental caries preventative.

LUROTIN CAPS. (BASF Wyandotte) Beta-carotene 25 mg/Cap. Bot. 100s.
Use: Nutritional supplement.

LUSTOZYME. (Kenyon) Lucelzyme (cellulolytic enzyme) 1 mg, lumylzyme (amylolytic enzyme) 25 mg, luprozyme (proteolytic enzyme) 10 mg, dehydrocholic acid 100 mg, hyoscyamine HBr 0.1 mg, hyoscine HBr 0.0065 mg, atropine sulfate 0.02 mg/Tab. Bot. 100s, 1000s.
Use: Antiflatulent.

LUTEOGAN.
See: Progesterone (Various Mfr.).

LUTEOSAN.
See: Progesterone (Various Mfr.).

LUTOCYLOL. (Ciba) Ethisterone.

LUTOLIN-F. (Spanner) Progesterone 25 mg or 50 mg/ml. Vial 10 ml.
Use: Progestin.

LUTOLIN-S. (Spanner) Progesterone 25 mg/ml. Vial 10 ml.
Use: Progestin.

•**LUTRELIN ACETATE.** USAN.
Use: Agonist.

LUTREN.
See: Progesterone (Various Mfr.).

LUTREPULSE. (Ortho) Gonadorelin acetate 0.8 mg or 3.2 mg/vial. Pow. for reconstitution (lyophilized). Vial 10 ml.
Use: Gonadotropin-releasing hormone.

LUTUTRIN.
See: Lutrexin, Tab. (Hynson, Westcott & Dunning).

•**LYAPOLATE SODIUM.** USAN. Sodium ethenesulfonate polymer. Peson (Hoechst).
Use: Anticoagulant.

•**LYCETAMINE.** USAN.
Use: Antimicrobial.

LYCINE HYDROCHLORIDE.
See: Betaine HCl (Various Mfr.).

LYCOLAN ELIXIR. (Lannett) Glycocoll 28 gr, lysine 100 mg in Tokay wine base/15 ml. Bot. pt.
Use: Vitamin supplement.

LYDIA E. PINKHAM TABLETS. (Numark) 72s, 250s.

LYDIA E. PINKHAM VEGETABLE COMPOUND. (Numark) Bot. 8 fl oz, 16 fl oz.

•**LYDIMYCIN.** USAN.
Use: Antifungal.

LYMECYCLINE. B.A.N. A water-soluble combination of tetracycline, lysine and formaldehyde. Armyl; Mucomycin; Tetralysal.
Use: Antibiotic.

LYMPHAZURIN. (Hirsch) Isosulfan blue 10 mg, sodium monohydrogen phosphate 6.6 mg, potassium dihydrogen phosphate 2.7 mg/ml. Vial 5 ml.
Use: Radiopaque agent.

LYMPHOCYTE IMMUNE GLOBULIN.
Use: Management of rejection in renal transplant.
See: Atgam, Inj. (Upjohn).

LYMPHOGRANULOMA VENEREUM ANTIGEN, U.S.P. XXI. Lymphogranuloma venereum skin test antigen.
Use: Diagnostic aid (dermal reactivity indicator).

•**LYNESTRENOL.** USAN.(1) 19-Nor-17α-pregn-4-en-20-yn-17-ol; (2) 17α-Ethinyl-17β-hydroxyestr-4-ene. Orgametril.
Use: Progestin.

LYNOESTRENOL. Lynestrenol.

LYPHOCIN P. (Lyphomed) Vancomycin HCl 500 mg. Vial 10 ml.
Use: Anti-infective.

LYPHOLYTE. (Lyphomed) Multiple electrolye concentrate. Vial 20 ml, 40 ml, Maxivial 100 ml, 200 ml.
Use: Electrolyte replacement.

LYPHOLYTE II. (Lyphomed) Na^+ 35 mEq/L, K^+ 20 mEq/L, Ca^{++} 4.5 mEq/L, Mg^{++} 5 mEq/L, Cl^- 35 mEq/L, acetate 29.5 mEq/L. Single dose flip-top vial 20 ml, 40 ml; flip-top vial 100 ml, 200 ml.
Use: Parenteral nutritional supplement.

LYPO-B. (Rocky Mtn.) Choline Cl 200 mg, dl-methionine 50 mg, inositol 100 mg, B_{12} crystalline 20 mcg/2 ml. Vial 30 ml.
Use: Nutritional supplement.

•**LYPRESSIN NASAL SOLUTION,** U.S.P. XXII. 8-Lysine vasopressin. Syntopressin.
Use: Antidiuretic.
See: Diapid Nasal Spray (Sandoz).

LYSERGIDE. B.A.N. NN-Diethyl-lysergamide. Lysergic acid diethylamide LSD, Delysid.
Use: Psychotomimetic.

LYSIDIN. Methyl glyoxalidin.

LYSINE. USAN.
Use: Nutrient, rapid weight gain.

•**LYSINE ACETATE,** U.S.P. XXII. $C_6H_14N_2O_2$-$C_2H_4O_2$
Use: Amino acid.

•**LYSINE MONOHYDROCHLORIDE,** U.S.P. XXII. $C_6H_{14}N_2O_2$-HCl
Use: Amino acid.
See: Enisyl, Tab. (Person & Covey).

LYSITONE. (Jenkins) l-Lysine HCl 300 mg, iron peptonate 200 mg, cobalamine concentrate 10 mcg, vitamins B_1 10 mg, niacinamide 20 mg, B_2 2.5 mg, B_6 2 mg, panthenol 2 mg, d-sorbitol 1.83 Gm, alcohol 11%/fl oz. Bot. 3 oz, 8 oz, gal.
Use: Vitamin/mineral supplement.

LYSIVANE.
See: Parsidol, Tab. (Warner-Chilcott).

LYSODREN. (Bristol-Myers/Bristol Oncology) Mitotane 500 mg/Tab. Bot. 100s.
Use: Antineoplastic agent.

•**LYSOSTAPHIN.** USAN. Antibiotic derived from *Staphylococcus staphylolyticus.*
Use: Antibiotic.

LYSURIDE. B.A.N. 9-(3,3-Diethylureido)-4,6,-6a,7,8,9-hexahydro-7-methylindolo[4,3-f,g]-quinoline.
Use: Prophylaxis of migraine.

LYTEERS. (Barnes-Hind) Isotonic, viscous liquid adjusted to pH of tears. Balanced amounts of sodium and potassium ions, cellulose derivative, benzalkonium Cl 0.01%, disodium edetate 0.05%. Bot. 15 ml.
Use: Lubricant, ophthalmic.

LYTREN. (Mead Johnson Nutrition) Water, dextrose, sodium citrate, citric acid, sodium Cl, potassium citrate. Ready-To-Use Bot. 8 fl. oz.
Use: Fluid/electrolyte replacement.

M

MAAGEL. (Approved) Aluminum and magnesium hydroxide. Bot. 12 oz, gal.
Use: Antacid.

MAALOX EXTRA STRENGTH PLUS SUSPENSION. (Rorer) Magnesium hydroxide 450 mg, aluminum hydroxide 500 mg, simethicone 40 mg/5 ml, sodium (0.05 mEq) 1.2 mg/5 ml. Susp. Bot. 6 oz, 12 oz, UD 15 ml, 30 ml.
Use: Antacid, antiflatulent.

MAALOX EXTRA STRENGTH TABLETS. (Rorer) Magnesium hydroxide 400 mg, dried aluminum hydroxide gel 400 mg/Tab., sodium (0.06 mEq) 1.4 mg/Tab. Bot. 50s, Strip 24s, 100s.
Use: Antacid.

MAALOX EXTRA STRENGTH WHIP. (Rorer) Edible aerosol foam of magnesium hydroxide 480 mg, aluminum hydroxide 525 mg/4 Gm, sodium 5 mg/4 Gm. Can 2 oz, 8 oz.
Use: Antacid.

MAALOX NO. 1 TABLETS. (Rorer) Aluminum hydroxide 200 mg, magnesium hydroxide 200 mg, sodium 0.7 mg/Chew. Tab., Saccharin, sorbitol. Bot. 100s.
Use: Antacid.

MAALOX PLUS TABLETS. (Rorer) Magnesium hydroxide 200 mg, dried aluminum hydroxide gel 200 mg, simethicone 25 mg/Tab. Sodium content (0.03 mEq) 0.8 mg/Tab. Bot. 50s. Strip 100s, Pocket Pack 12s, Roll Pack 12s.
Use: Antacid, antiflatulent.

MAALOX SUSPENSION. (Rorer) Magnesium hydroxide 200 mg, aluminum hydroxide 225 mg/5 ml, sodium (0.06 mEq) 1.4 mg/5 ml. Susp. Bot. 5 oz, 6 oz, 12 oz, 26 oz, UD 15 ml, 30 ml.
Use: Antacid.

MAALOX TABLETS. (Rorer) Magnesium hydroxide 200 mg, dried aluminum hydroxide gel 200 mg/Tab, sodium (0.03 mEq) 0.7 mg/Tab. Bot. 100s.
Use: Antacid.

MAALOX TC (THERAPEUTIC CONCENTRATE) SUSPENSION. (Rorer) Magnesium hydroxide 300 mg, aluminum hydroxide 600 mg/5 ml, sodium (0.03 mEq) 0.8 mg/5 ml. Susp. Bot. 6 oz, 12 oz, UD 15 ml, 30 ml.
Use: Antacid.

MAALOX TC (THERAPEUTIC CONCENTRATE) TABLETS. (Rorer) Magnesium hydroxide 300 mg, aluminum hydroxide 600 mg, sodium (0.02 mEq) 0.5 mg/Tab. Bot. 48s.
Use: Antacid.

MACPAC. (Norwich Eaton) Nitrofurantoin macrocrystals 50 mg or 100 mg/Cap. UD 28s.
Use: Urinary anti-infective.

MACRISALB (^{131}I) INJECTION. B.A.N. Macroaggregated iodinated (^{131}I) human albumin injection.

Use: Examination of pulmonary perfusion.
MACROAGGREGATED ALBUMIN.
See: Albumotope-LS. (Squibb).
MACRODANTIN. (Norwich Eaton) Nitrofurantoin macrocrystals **25 mg/Cap.:** Bot. 100s. **50 mg or 100 mg/Cap.:** Bot. 100s, 500s, 1000s, Hospital UD 100s.
Use: Urinary anti-infective.
MACRODEX. (Pharmacia) Dextran 6% w/v in normal saline, 6% w/v in dextrose 5% in water. Bot. 500 ml.
Use: Plasma volume expander.
MACROGOL 400. B.A.N. Polyoxyl stearate.
Use: Surface-active agent.
See: Polyethylene glycol 400.
MACROGOL 4000. B.A.N.
Use: Surface-active agent.
See: Polyethylene glycol 4000.
MACROGOL STEARATE 2000. Polyoxyl 40 Stearate.
MACROTEC. (Squibb) Technetium Tc99m Medronate kit. Vial Kit 10s.
Use: Radiopaque agent.
MACROTIN W/Phenobarbital, hyoscyamus extract, caulophyllin, helonin, pulsatilla extract.
See: Tranquilans, Tab. (Noyes).
•**MADURAMICIN.** USAN.
Use: Anticoccidal.
•**MAFENIDE.** USAN. α-Aminotoluene-p-sulfonamide. Marfanil [HCl], Sulfomyl [propionate], Sulfamylon [acetate].
Use: Antibacterial.
•**MAFENIDE ACETATE,** U.S.P. XXII. Cream, U.S.P. XXII. α-Aminotoluene-p-sulfonamide monoacetate.
See: Sulfamylon Cream (Winthrop Pharm).
•**MAFILCON A.** USAN.
Use: Contact lens material.
MAFYLON CREAM. (Winthrop Products) Mafenide acetate.
Use: Burn preparation.
•**MAGALDRATE,** U.S.P. XXII. Oral Susp., Tab., U.S.P. XXII. (Wyeth-Ayerst) Monalium Hydrate. Aluminum Magnesium Hydroxide.
Use: Antacid.
See: Monalium Hydrate.
Riopan, Tab., Susp. (Wyeth-Ayerst).
•**MAGALDRATE AND SIMETHICONE.** U.S.P. XXII, Oral Susp, Tabs., U.S.P. XXII.
Use: Antacid, antiflatulant.
See: Lowsium. (Rugby).
Lowsium Plus. (Rugby).
Riopan Plus. (Wyeth-Ayerst).
MAGAN. (Adria) Magnesium salicylate (anhydrous) 545 mg/Tab. Bot. 100s, 500s.
Use: Salicylate analgesic.
MAGDROX. (Vita Elixir) Magnesium hydroxide, aluminum hydroxide.
Use: Antacid.
MAGLAGEL. (Kenyon) Magnesium-aluminum hydroxide gel. Bot. 12 oz, pt, gal.
Use: Antacid.
MAG-LUM. (Kenyon) Magnesium trisilicate 7.5 gr, dried aluminum hydroxide gel 4 gr. Tab. Bot. 100s, 1000s.
Use: Antacid.
MAGMA ALBA. (Durel) Sulfurated lime solution (Vleminckx's) 60%, saturated zinc sulfate solution 40%. Jar 3 oz, lb.
Use: Anti-acne.
MAGMALIN LOZENGE. (Vale) Magnesium hydroxide 0.2 Gm, aluminum hydroxide gel, dried 0.2 Gm/Loz. Bot. 1000s.
Use: Antacid.
MAGNACAL LIQUID. (Biosearch) Protein-calcium, sodium caseinate, carbohydrate-maltodextrin, sucrose, fat (partially hydrogenated), soy oil, lecithin, mono- and diglycerides. 1.5 Cal/ml, 590 mOsm/kg H_2O. Protein 70 Gm, CHO 250 Gm, fat 80 Gm, sodium 1000 mg, potassium 1250 mg/L. Can 120 ml, 240 ml.
Use: Enteral nutritional supplement.
MAGNAGEL. (Hauck) Aluminum hydroxide-magnesium carbonate 325 mg/Tab. Bot. 100s, 500s.
Use: Antacid.
MAGNALUM. (Richlyn) Magnesium hydroxide 3.75 gr, aluminum hydroxide 2 gr/Tab. Bot. 1000s.
Use: Antacid.
MAGNAPRIN ARTHRITIS STRENGTH TABLETS. (Rugby) Aspirin 325 mg, dried aluminum hydroxide gel 150 mg, magnesium hydroxide 150 mg/Tab. Bot. 100s, 500s.
Use: Analgesic.
MAGNAPRIN TABLETS. (Rugby) Aspirin 325 mg, dried aluminum hydroxide gel 75 mg, magnesium hydroxide 75 mg/Tab. Bot. 100s, 500s.
Use: Analgesic.
MAGNATE TABLETS. (Mission) Magnesium gluconate 500 mg (25 mg magnesium)/Tab. Bot. 100s.
Use: Magnesium supplement.
MAGNATRIL. (Lannett) Dried aluminum hydroxide gel 4 gr, magnesium trisilicate 7 gr, magnesium hydroxide 2 gr/Tab. Bot. 50s, 100s.
Use: Antacid.
MAGNATRIL SUSPENSION. (Lannett) Magnesium trisilicate 4 gr, colloidal susp. of magnesium and aluminum hydroxides/5 ml. Bot. 12 fl oz.
Use: Antacid.
•**MAGNESIA TABLETS,** U.S.P. XXII.
Use: Antacid.
•**MAGNESIA & ALUMINA ORAL SUSPENSION,** U.S.P. XXII. (Philips Roxane) Oral Susp. 6 fl oz. 25s.
Use: Antacid.
See: Maalox, Liq. (Rorer).
•**MAGNESIA & ALUMINA TABLETS,** U.S.P. XXII.
Use: Antacid.
See: Maalox, Tab. (Rorer).
MAGNESIA MAGMA. Milk of Magnesia, U.S.P. XXII.

Use: Antacid, cathartic.
See: Magnesium Hydroxide, Preps.
MAGNESIUM ACETYLSALICYLATE. Apyron, Magnespirin, Magisal, Novacetyl.
Use: Salicylate analgesic.
MAGNESIUM ALUMINATE HYDRATED.
Use: Antacid.
See: Riopan, Susp., Tab. (Wyeth-Ayerst).
MAGNESIUM ALUMINUM HYDROXIDE.
Use: Antacid.
See: Maalox, Susp. (Rorer).
Maglagel (Kenyon).
Malogel, Gel (Quality Generics).
Medalox, Gel (Med. Chem.).
W/APC.
See: Buffadyne, Tab. (Lemmon).
W/Calcium carbonate.
See: Camalox, Susp. (Rorer).
W/Magnesium trisilicate.
See: Magnatril Susp. (Lannett).
W/Simethicone.
See: Maalox Plus, Susp. (Rorer).
•**MAGNESIUM ALUMINUM SILICATE,** U.S.P. XXII.
Use: Suspending agent.
•**MAGNESIUM CARBONATE,** U.S.P. XXII. (Baker, J. T.) Pow. 4 oz, 1 lb, 5 lb.
Use: Antacid.
•**MAGNESIUM CARBONATE AND SODIUM BICARBONATE FOR ORAL SUSPENSION,** U.S.P. XXII.
Use: Antacid.
MAGNESIUM CARBONATE W/COMBINATIONS.
Use: Antacid.
See: Algicon, Tab. (Rorer).
Alkets, Tab. (Upjohn).
Antacid No. 2, Tab. (Bowman).
Bismatesia, Can (Noyes).
Bufferin, Tab. (Bristol-Myers).
Di-Gel, Tab., Liq. (Schering-Plough).
Dimacid, Tab. (Otis Clapp).
Kanalka, Tab. (Lannett).
Magnagel, Liq., Tab. (Hauck).
Marblen, Susp., Tab. (Fleming).
Panacarb, Tab. (Lannett).
•**MAGNESIUM CHLORIDE,** U.S.P. XXII. Magnesium Cl hexahydrate.
Use: Electrolyte replenisher, pharmaceutical necessity for hemodialysis and peritoneal dialysis.
W/Potassium Cl, calcium Cl, red phenol.
See: Electrolytic replenisher, Vial (Invenex).
•**MAGNESIUM CITRATE ORAL SOLUTION,** U.S.P. XXII. 1,2,3-Propanetricarboxylic acid, hydroxymagnesium salt (2:3).
Use: Cathartic.
•**MAGNESIUM GLUCONATE,** U.S.P. XXII. Tab., U.S.P. XXII.
Use: Magnesium supplement.
See: Almora, Tab. (Forest Pharm.).
MAGNESIUM GLUCONATE. (Western Research) Magnesium gluconate 500 mg/Tab. Bot. 1000s.
Use: Magnesium supplement.
MAGNESIUM GLYCINATE.
W/Aspirin, magnesium carbonate.
See: Buffinol, Tab. (Otis Clapp).
W/Gastric mucin, aluminum hydroxide gel.
See: Mucogel, Tab. (Inwood).
•**MAGNESIUM HYDROXIDE,** U.S.P. XXII.
Use: Antacid, cathartic.
See: Magnesia Magma.
Milk of Magnesia.
MAGNESIUM HYDROXIDE W/COMBINATIONS.
See: Aludrox, Susp., Tab., Vial (Wyeth-Ayerst).
Ascriptin, Tab. (Rorer).
Ascriptin A/D, Tab. (Rorer).
Ascriptin Extra Strength, Tab. (Rorer).
Ascriptin w/Codeine, Tab. (Rorer).
Banacid, Tab. (Buffington).
Camalox, Susp., Tab.(Rorer).
Delcid, Susp. (Merrell Dow).
Fermalox, Tab. (Rorer).
Gas-Eze, Tab. (E.J. Moore).
Kolantyl, Gel, Wafer (Merrell Dow).
Laxsil Liquid, Liq. (Reed & Carnrick).
Maalox, Susp., Tab. (Rorer).
Maalox Plus, Susp., Tab. (Rorer).
Magnatril, Susp., Tab. (Lannett).
Mylanta, Mylanta II, Liq., Tab. (Stuart).
Simeco, Liq. (Wyeth-Ayerst).
WinGel, Liq., Tab. (Winthrop Consumer Products).
MAGNESIUM OROTATE. (Nutrition) 500 mg/Tab. Bot. 100s.
See: Magora, Tab. (Miller).
•**MAGNESIUM OXIDE,** U.S.P. XXII. Cap., Tab., U.S.P. XXII.
Use: Pharmaceutic aid (sorbent).
(Manne) 420 mg/Tab. Bot. 250s, 1000s.
(Stanlabs) 10 gr/Tab. Bot. 100s, 1000s.
Use: Pharm. aid (sorbant).
See: Mag-Ox, Tab.(Blaine).
Mag-Ox 400, Tab. (Blaine).
Niko-Mag, Cap. (Scruggs).
Oxabid, Cap. (Jamieson-McKames).
Par-Mag, Cap. (Parmed).
Uro-Mag, Cap. (Blaine).
W/Calcium, Vitamin D.
See: Elekap, Cap. (Western Research).
W/Glutamic acid magnesium complex, N-acetyl-P-aminophenol, ascorbic acid, dl-methionine, lemon bioflavonoid complex, dl-α-tocopheryl acetate, glycine, soybean flour.
See: Ulcimins, Tab. (Miller).
W/Magnesium carbonate, calcium carbonate.
See: Alkets, Tab. (Upjohn).
W/Ox bile (desiccated), hog bile (desiccated.).
See: Hyper-Cholate, Tab. (Hauck).
W/Phenobarbital, atropine sulfate.
See: Magnox, Tab. (Bowman).
•**MAGNESIUM PHOSPHATE,** U.S.P. XXII.

Use: Antacid.
•**MAGNESIUM SALICYLATE,** U.S.P. XXII. Tab. U.S.P. XXII.
Use: Analgesic, antipyretic, antirheumatic.
See: Analate, Tab. (Winston).
Efficin, Tab. (Adria).
Magan, Tab. (Adria).
W/Phenyltoloxamine citrate.
See: Mobigesic, Tab. (Ascher).
•**MAGNESIUM SILICATE,** N.F. XVII.
Use: Pharmaceutic aid (tablet excipient).
•**MAGNESIUM STEARATE,** N.F. XVII.
Use: Pharmaceutic aid (lubricant).
•**MAGNESIUM SULFATE,** U.S.P. XXII. Inj. U.S.P. XXII. Epsom salt.
Use: Pow. or crystals cathartic: Inj. anticonvulsant, electrolyte replenisher.
(Abbott)—50% Amp. 2 ml Box 25s, 100s. Abboject Syringe (20 G X 2.5″) 5 ml, 10 ml; 12.5% in Pintop Vial, 8 ml, 20 ml.
(Atlas)—10% Amp. 10 ml Box 100s; 1 Gm/2 ml. Box 100s.
(Baxter)—10%. Vial 10 ml, 20 ml.
(CMC)—1 Gm/2 ml, 10% Amp. 10 ml, 20 ml; 25% Amp. 10 ml 50%. Vial 30 ml.
(Quality Generics)—50% Amp. 2 ml, 100s.
(Lilly)—10% Amp 20 ml Box 6s, 25s; 50% 1 Gm Amp. 2 ml, Box 12s, 100s.
(Parke-Davis)—50% Amp. 2 ml, 10s.
(Torigian)—50% Amp. 2 ml 12s, 25s, 100s.
(Trent)—50% Amp. 2 ml, 10 ml.
•**MAGNESIUM TRISILICATE,** U.S.P. XXII. Tab., U.S.P. XXII. Magnesium silicate hydrate.
Use: Antacid.
See: Trisomin, Tab. (Lilly).
MAGNESIUM TRISILICATE W/COMBINATIONS.
See: Alsorb Gel C.T., Gel (Standex).
Arcodex Tablets, Tab. (Arcum).
Banacid, Tab. (Buffington).
Gacid, Tab. (Arcum).
Gaviscon, Tab. (Marion).
Kaocasil, Tab. (Jenkins).
Magnatril, Susp., Tab. (Lannett).
Maracid 2, Tab. (Marin).
Silmagel, Tab. (Lannett).
MAGNESIUM ZINC SHAKE LOTION. (Durel) Magnesium carbonate, zinc oxide, lime water, menthol, phenol 0.5%. Bot. 8 oz, gal.
Use: Antipruritic, counter-irritant.
MAGNEVIST. (Berlex) Gadopentetate dimeglumine 469.01 mg, meglumine 0.39 mg, diethylenetriamine pentaacetic acid 0.15 mg. Inj. Vial 20 ml.
Use: Radiopaque agent.
MAGONATE. (Fleming) Magnesium gluconate 500 mg/Tab. Bot. 100s, 1000s.
Use: Magnesium supplement.
MAG-OX. (Blaine) Magnesium oxide 400 mg/Tab. Bot. 100s, 1000s.
Use: Antacid.
MAGSAL. (U.S. Chemical) Magnesium salicylate 600 mg, phenyltoloxamine citrate 25 mg/Tab. Bot. 100s.
Use: Analgesic combination.
MAINTENANCE VITAMIN FORMULA W/MINERALS. (Towne) Vitamins A palmitate 10,000 IU, D 400 IU, B_1 5 mg, B_2 2.5 mg, C 75 mg, niacinamide 40 mg, B_6 1 mg, calcium pantothenate 4 mg, B_{12} 2 mcg, E 2 IU, choline bitartrate 31.4 mg, inositol 15 mg, calcium 75 mg, phosphorous 58 mg, iron 30 mg, magnesium 3 mg, manganese 0.5 mg, potassium 2 mg, zinc 0.5 mg/Cap. Bot. 100s.
Use: Vitamin/mineral supplement.
MAJEPTIL. Thioproperazine. Psychopharmacologic agent; pending release.
MALAGRIDE.
See: Acetarsone.
MALARAQUIN. (Winthrop Products) Chloroquine phosphate.
Use: Antimalarial.
MALATAL TABLETS. (Hauck) Atropine sulfate 0.0194 mg, scopolamine HBr 0.0065 mg, hyoscyamine HBr, SO_4 0.1037 mg, phenobarbital 16.2 mg/Tab. Bot. 1000s.
Use: Anticholinergic/antispasmodic, sedative/hypnotic.
•**MALATHION,** U.S.P. XXII. Lot., U.S.P. XXII.
Use: Pediculicide.
•**MALETHAMER.** USAN. Maleic anhydride ethylene polymer.
Use: Antidiarrheal, antiperistaltic.
•**MALIC ACID,** N.F. XVII.
Use: Pharmaceutic aid (acidifying agent).
MALIC ACID WITH PECTIN.
See: Mallo-Pectin, Liq. (Hauck).
MALLAMINT. (Hauck) Calcium carbonate 420 mg/Tab. Bot. 100s.
Use: Antacid.
MALLAZINE DROPS. (Hauck) Tetrahydrozoline 0.05%. Soln. 15 ml.
Use: Ophthalmic vasoconstrictor/mydriatic.
MALLERGAN-VC W/CODEINE SYRUP. (Hauck) Phenylephrine HCl 5 mg, promethazine HCl 6.25 mg, codeine phosphate 10 mg/5 ml, alcohol 7%. Syr. Bot. 120 ml.
Use: Decongestant, antihistamine, antitussive.
MALLISOL. (Hauck) Povidone-iodine.
Use: Germicidal, antiseptic surgical scrub.
MALOGEN INJECTION AQUEOUS. (Forest Pharm.) Testosterone. **25 mg/ml:** 10 ml, 30 ml; **50 mg/ml:** 10 ml; **100 mg/ml:** 10 ml.
Use: Androgen.
MALOGEN 100 L.A. IN OIL INJ. (Forest Pharm.) Testosterone enanthate 100 mg/ml. 10 ml.
Use: Androgen.
MALOGEN 200 L.A. IN OIL INJ. (Forest Pharm.) Testosterone enanthate 200 mg/ml. 10 ml.
Use: Androgen.
MALOGEN CYP. (Forest Pharm.) Testosterone cypionate in oil 100 mg or 200 mg/ml. Vial 10 ml.

Use: Androgen.
MALONAL.
See: Barbital (Various Mfr.).
•**MALOTILATE.** USAN.
Use: Liver disorder treatment.
MALOTRONE AQUEOUS INJECTION. (Bluco) Testosterone, USP 25 mg or 50 mg/ml in aqueous susp. Vial 10 ml.
Use: Androgen.
MALOTUSS. (Hauck) Guaifenesin 100 mg/5 ml. Bot. 3 oz.
Use: Expectorant.
MALTSUPEX. (Wallace) Laxative derived from natural barley malt extract for relief of constipation in children and adults. **Liq.:** Bot. 8 oz, pt. **Pow.:** Jar 8 oz, lb. **Tab.:** Malt soup extract 750 mg/Tab. Bot. 100s.
W/Psyllium seed husks.
Use: Laxative.
See: Syllamalt, Pow. (Wallace).
MAMMOL OINTMENT. (Abbott) Bismuth subnitrate 40%, castor oil 30%, anhydrous lanolin 22%, ceresin wax 7%, balsam Peru 1%. Tube ⅞ oz. Ctn. 12s.
Use: Skin protectant, emollient.
MANCHANIL. (D'Franssia)
Use: Skin bleaching agent.
MANDAMETH. (Major) Methenamine mandelate 0.5 Gm/EC Tab. Bot. 1000s.
Use: Urinary anti-infective.
MANDELAMINE. (Parke-Davis) **Susp.:** 250 mg/5 ml. Bot. pt. **Gran.:** 1 Gm/Packet. Box 56s.
Use: Urinary anti-infective.
MANDELAMINE "HAFGRAMS." (Parke-Davis) Methenamine mandelate 0.5 Gm/Tab. Bot. 100s, 1000s, UD 100s.
Use: Urinary anti-infective.
MANDELAMINE 1 GM. (Parke-Davis) Methenamine mandelate 1 Gm/Tab. Bot. 100s, 1000s, UD 100s.
Use: Urinary anti-infective.
MANDELAMINE SUSPENSION FORTE. (Parke-Davis) Methenamine mandelate 500 mg/5 ml. Susp. Bot. 8 oz, pt.
Use: Urinary anti-infective.
MANDELIC ACID.
Use: Urinary anti-infective.
MANDELIC ACID SALTS.
See: Calcium mandelate (Various Mfr.).
MANDELYLTROPEINE.
See: Homatropine Salts (Various Mfr.).
MANDOL. (Lilly) Cefamandole nafate. Vial: **500 mg/10 ml or 1 Gm/10 ml:** Traypak 25s; **1 Gm/100 ml or 2 Gm/20 ml:** Traypak 10s; **2 Gm/100 ml:** Traypak 10s; **10 Gm/100 ml:** Traypak 6s; Faspak: 1 Gm or 2 Gm, Pkg 96s. ADD-VANTAGE Vial 1 Gm 25s, 2 Gm 10s.
Use: Antibacterial, cephalosporin.
•**MANGANESE CHLORIDE,** U.S.P. XXII. Inj., U.S.P. XXII.
Use: Manganese deficiency treatment.
•**MANGANESE GLUCONATE.** U.S.P. XXII.
Use: Manganese deficiency.
MANGANESE GLYCEROPHOSPHATE. Glycerol phosphate manganese salt.
Use: Pharmaceutical necessity.
MANGANESE HYPOPHOSPHITE. Manganese (2+) phosphinate.
Use: Pharmaceutical necessity.
•**MANGANESE SULFATE,** U.S.P. XXII. Inj., U.S.P. XXII.
Use: Supplement (trace mineral).
W/Thyroid, ferrous sulfate, ferrous gluconate, sodium ferric pyrophosphate, extract of nux vomica.
See: Hemocrine, Tab. (Hauck).
MANGANESE TRACE METAL ADDITIVE. (IMS) Manganese 0.5 mg. Inj. Vial 10 ml.
Use: Parenteral nutritional supplement.
MANGA-PAK. (SoloPak) Manganese 0.1 mg/ml. Inj. Vial 10 ml, 30 ml.
Use: Parenteral nutritional supplement.
MANIRON. (Bowman) Ferrous fumarate 3 mg/Tab. Bot. 100s, 1000s, 5000s.
Use: Iron supplement.
MANN A.R.P. SOLUTION. (Mann) Bot. pt, qt, 0.5 gal, gal.
Use: Rust preventative, sterilizers.
MANN ASTRINGENT MOUTH WASH CONCENTRATE. (Mann) Bot. 4 oz, qt, 0.5 gal, gal. Also mint flavored. Bot. 4 oz, qt, 0.5 gal, gal.
Use: Mouthwash.
MANNA SUGAR.
See: Mannitol (Various Mfr.).
MANNAN. (Rugby) Purified glucomannan 500 mg/Cap. Bot. 90s.
Use: Nutritional supplement.
MANN BODY DEODORANT. (Mann) Bot. 4 oz, 8 oz, pt, qt.
MANN BREATH DEODORANT. (Mann) Bot. 1 oz, 4 oz, 8 oz, pt, qt, 0.5 gal.
MANN EMOLLIENT. (Mann) Jar. 100 Gm.
Use: Emollient.
MANN EUGENOL U.S.P. EXTRA. (Mann) 0.06 lb, 0.13 lb, 0.25 lb, 0.5 lb, 1 lb.
Use: With zinc oxide as protective pack.
MANN GERMICIDAL SOLUTION. (Mann) **Regular:** Bot. gal, 4 gal. **Conc.:** 12.8%. Bot. pt, qt, 0.5 gal, gal.
Use: Germicide.
MANN HAND LOTION. (Mann) Twin pack, gal.
Use: Emollient.
MANN HEMOSTATIC. (Mann) Bot. 1 oz, 4 oz, 8 oz, pt, qt.
Use: Hemostatic.
MANN LIQUID SOAP. (Mann) Concentrated cocastile. Bot. qt, 0.5 gal, gal.
Use: Emollient.
MANN LUBRICANT AND CLEANSER. (Mann) Bot. pt, qt.
Use: Emollient.
MANN SUPERFATTED BAR SOAP. (Mann) Rich in lanolin. Cake. 12s.
Use: Emollient.

MANN TALBOT'S IODINE. (Mann) Glycerin base. Bot. 1 oz, 4 oz, 8 oz, pt, qt.
Use: Antiseptic.

MANN TOPICAL ANESTHETIC. (Mann) Bot. 1 oz, 4 oz, 8 oz, pt. W/stain to indicate area treated. Bot. 1 oz, 4 oz, 8 oz.
Use: Local anesthetic, topical.

MANNITE.
See: Mannitol, U.S.P. XXII.

•**MANNITOL,** U.S.P. XXII. Inj. U.S.P. XXII. Manna Sugar, D-Mannitol, Mannite.
Use: Diagnostic aid (renal function determination), diuretic.
See: Osmitrol (Travenol).
W/Aluminum hydroxide, magnesium hydroxide, glycine, calcium carbonate, peppermint oil.
See: Gas-Eze, Tab. (E.J. Moore).
W/Sorbitol.
See: Cystosol, Liq. (Travenol).
Cytal, Liq. (Cutter).

•**MANNITOL INJECTION,** U.S.P. XXII. (Abbott) 15% or 20%. Abbo-Vac Single dose container 500 ml.
Use: Diagnostic aid (renal function determination), diuretic.
See: Mannitol Solution, Amp. (Merck Sharp & Dohme).

MANNITOL HEXANITRATE.
Use: Coronary vasodilator.
See: Vascunitol, Tab. (Apco).
W/Reserpine, rutin, ascorbic acid.
See: Ruhexatal W/Reserpine, Tab. (Lemmon).

MANNITOL HEXANITRATE & PHENOBARBITAL TAB. (Bowman; Quality Generics; Jenkins; Kenyon) Mannitol hexanitrate 0.5 gr, phenobarbital 0.25 gr/Tab. Bot. 1000s. (Kenyon): Bot. 100s, 1000s.
Use: Vasodilator.

MANNITOL HEXANITRATE WITH PHENOBARBITAL COMBINATIONS.
See: Hyrunal, Tab. (Kenyon).
Manotensin,Tab. (Dunhall).
Ruhexatal, Tab. (Lemmon).
Vascused, Tab. (Apco).
Vermantin, Tab. (Trout).

•**MANNITOL IN SODIUM CHLORIDE INJECTION.** U.S.P. XXII.
Use: Diuretic.

MANNOMUSTINE. B.A.N. 1,6-Di-(2-chloroethylamino)-1,6-dideoxy-D-mannitol. Degranol dihydrochloride.
Use: Antineoplastic agent.

MANOTENSIN. (Dunhall) Mannitol hexanitrate 32 mg, phenobarbital 16 mg/Tab. Bot. 100s, 1000s.
Use: Vasodilator combination.

MANTADIL. (Burroughs Wellcome) Chlorocyclizine HCl 2%, hydrocortisone acetate 0.5%, liquid and white petrolatum, wax, methylparaben 0.25%. Cream Tube 15 Gm.
Use: Antipruritic, anti-inflammatory, anesthetic.

MANTOUX TEST.
See: Tuberculin, U.S.P. XXII. Test (Parke-Davis).

MANVENE. 3-Methoxy-16a-methyl-1,3,5: 10-estra-triene-16B,17B-diol.
Use: Antineoplastic agent.

MAOLATE TABLETS. (Upjohn) Chlorphenesin carbamate 400 mg/Tab. Bot. 50s, 500s, UD 100s.
Use: Muscle relaxant, mild tranquilizer.

MAOX. (Kenneth Manne) Magnesium oxide 420 mg/Tab. Bot. 250s, 1000s.
Use: Antacid.

MAPHENIDE. p-Sulphamoylbenzylamine HCl.
See: Sulfbenzamine HCl.

MAPROFIX.
See: Gardinol Type Detergents (Various Mfr.).

•**MAPROTILINE.** USAN. N-Methyl-9, 10-ethanoanthracene-9(10H)-propylamine. 3-(9, 10-Dihydro-9, 10-ethanoanthracen-9-yl)propylmethylamine.
Use: Antidepressant.
See: Ludiomil, Tab. (Ciba).

•**MAPROTILINE HYDROCHLORIDE,** U.S.P. XXII. Tab., U.S.P. XXII. 9,10-Ethanoathracene-9(10H)- propanamine, N-methyl-, hydrochloride.
Use: Antidepressant.

MARACID 2. (Marin) Magnesium trisilicate 150 mg, aluminum hydroxide dried gel 90 mg, aminoacetic acid 75 mg/Tab. Bot.
Use: Antacid, adsorbant.

MARANOX. (C.S. Dent) Acetaminophen 325 mg/ Tab. Bot. 8s.
Use: Analgesic.

MARAX DF SYRUP. (Roerig) Hydroxyzine HCl 2.5 mg, ephedrine sulfate 6.25 mg, theophylline 32.5 mg, alcohol 5%/5 ml. Color free, dye free. Bot. pt, gal.
Use: Antiasthmatic combination.

MARAX TAB. (Roerig) Hydroxyzine HCl 10 mg, ephedrine sulfate 25 mg, theophylline 130 mg/ Tab. Bot. 100s, 500s.
Use: Antiasthmatic combination.

MARBEC. (Marlyn) High potency B and C vitamins. Tab. Bot. 100s, 1000s.
Use: Vitamin supplement.

MARBLEN LIQUID. (Fleming) Magnesium carbonate 400 mg, calcium carbonate 520 mg/5 ml. Bot. pt, gal.
Use: Antacid.

MARBLEN TABLETS. (Fleming) Magnesium and calcium carbonate 21 gr/Tab. Bot. 100s, 1000s.
Use: Antacid.

MARCAINE. (Winthrop Pharm) Bupivacaine in sterile isotonic soln. containing sodium Cl pH adjusted 4.0 to 6.5 w/sodium hydroxide or hydrochloric acid. Multiple-dose vial also contains methylparaben 1 mg/ml as preservative. **0.25%:** Amp. 50 ml. Box 5s. Vial: Single dose 10 ml, 30 ml. Box 10s; multiple dose 50 ml. Box 1s. **0.5%:** Amp. 30 ml. Box 1s. Vial: Single dose 10 ml, 30 ml. Box 10s; multiple dose 50 ml. Box 1s. **0.75%:** Amp. 30 ml. Box 5s. Vial (single dose) 10 ml, 30 ml. Box 10s.

Use: Local anesthetic.

MARCAINE WITH EPINEPHRINE (1:200,000). (Winthrop Pharm) **Bupivacaine 0.25%:** with epinephrine 1:200,000 in sterile isotonic soln. containing sodium Cl. Each 1 ml contains bupivacaine HCl 2.5 mg, epinephrine bitartrate 0.0091 mg, sodium metabisulfite 0.5 mg, monothioglycerol 0.001 ml, ascorbic acid 2 mg and edetate calcium disodium 0.1 mg. In Multiple Dose Vial, each 1 ml also contains methylparaben 1 mg as antiseptic preservative. pH adjusted to between 3.4 and 4.5 with sodium hydroxide or hydrochloric acid. Amp. 50 ml, 5s, Single Dose Vial 10 ml, 30 ml. 10s, Multiple Dose Vial 50 ml 1s. **Bupivacaine 0.5%:** with epinephrine 1:200,000 in sterile isotonic soln. containing sodium Cl. Each 1 ml contains bupivacaine HCl 5 mg and epinephrine bitartrate 0.0091 mg, with sodium metabisulfite 0.5 mg, monothioglycerol 0.001 ml and ascorbic acid 2 mg, edetate calcium disodium 0.1 mg. In Multiple Dose Vial, each 1 ml also contains methylparaben 1 mg antiseptic preservative. pH adjusted to between 3.4 and 4.5 with sodium hydroxide or hydrochloric acid. Amp. 3 ml 10s, 30 ml 5s. Single Dose Vial 10 ml, 30 ml 10s. Multiple Dose Vial 50 ml 1s. **Bupivacaine 0.75%:** with epinephrine 1:200,000 in sterile isotonic soln. containing sodium Cl. Each 1 ml contains bupivacaine HCl 7.5 mg, epinephrine bitartrate 0.0091 mg with sodium metabisulfite 0.5 mg, monothioglycerol 0.001 ml, ascorbic acid 2 mg as antioxidants, edetate calcium disodium 0.1 mg. pH adjusted to between 3.4 and 4.5 with sodium hydroxide or hydrochloric acid. Amp 30 ml in 5s.
Use: Local anesthetic.

MARCAINE SPINAL. (Winthrop Pharm) Bupivacaine HCl 15 mg/2 ml (0.75%) and dextrose 165 mg/2 ml (8.25%). Amp. 2 ml, UD pak 10s.
Use: Local anesthetic.

MARDON. (Geneva Marsam) Propoxyphene HCl. **32 mg Cap.:** Bot. 100s, 1000s. **65 mg Cap:** Bot. 100s, 500s, 1000s.
Use: Narcotic analgesic.

MARDON COMPOUND. (Geneva) Propoxyphene compound 65 mg, aspirin 3.5 gr, phenacetin 2.5 gr, caffeine 0.5 gr/Cap. Bot. 100s, 500s, 1000s.
Use: Narcotic analgesic combination.

MAREZINE INJECTION. (Burroughs Wellcome) Cyclizine lactate. Amp. (50 mg/ml) 1 ml. Box 10s.
Use: Anticholinergic.

MAREZINE TABLETS. (Burroughs Wellcome) Cyclizine HCl 50 mg/Tab. Bot. 100s. Box 12s.
Use: Anticholinergic.

W/Ergotamine tartrate, caffeine.
See: Migral, Tab. (Burroughs Wellcome).

MARFANIL.
See: Sulfbenzamine HCl (Various Mfr.).

MARHIST. (Marlop) Chlorpheniramine maleate 20 mg, phenylephrine HCl 2.5 mg, methscopolamine nitrate in special base/Cap. Bot. 30s, 100s. Expectorant Bot. 4 oz, pt, gal.
Use: Antihistamine, decongestant, anticholinergic.

MARINE 500 CAPSULES. (Murdock) Omega-3 polyunsaturated fatty acids 500 mg/Cap. containing EPA 90 mg, DHA 60 mg, vitamin E 13 IU/Cap. Bot. 90s.
Use: Nutritional supplement.

MARINE 1000 CAPSULES. (Murdock) Omega-3 polyunsaturated fatty acids 1000 mg/Cap. containing EPA 180 mg, DHA 120 mg, vitamin E 1 IU/Cap. Bot. 60s, 90s, 180s, 300s.
Use: Nutritional supplement.

MARINOL CAPSULES. (Roxane) Dronabinol 2.5 mg, 5 mg or 10 mg/Cap. Bot. 25s.
Use: Antiemetic.

MARLIN SALT SYSTEM II. (Marlin) Salt tablets for normal saline 250 mg/Tab. Bot. 200s with bot. 27.7 ml.
Use: Soft contact lens care.

MARLIPIDS III CAPSULES. (Fibertone) N-3 fat content, EPA, 180, DHA, 120, vitamin E[1] 5 IU. 100s.
Use: Fish Oil.

MARLYN FORMULA 50. (Marlyn) Vitamin B_6 w/ 18 amino acids/Cap. Bot. 100s, 250s, 1000s.
Use: Nutritional supplement.

MARPLAN. (Roche) Isocarboxazid 10 mg/Tab. Bot. 100s.
Use: Monoamine oxidase inhibitor, antidepressant.

•**MASOPROCOL.** USAN.
Use: Antineoplastic.

MASSE BREAST CREAM. (Advanced Care) Water, glyceryl monostearate, glycerin, cetyl alcohol, lanolin, peanut oil, Span-60, stearic acid, Tween-60, sodium benzoate, propylparaben, methylparaben, potassium hydroxide. Tube 2 oz.
Use: Emollient.

MASSENGILL FEMININE DEODORANT SPRAY. (Beecham Products) Aerosol Bot. 3 oz.
Use: Vaginal preparation.

MASSENGILL DISPOSABLE DOUCHE. (Beecham Products) Water, S.D. alcohol 40, lactic acid, sodium lactate, octoxymol-9, cetylpyridium Cl, diazolidinyl urea, disodium EDTA, methyl and propyl paraben, fragrance, color. Bot. 6 oz.
Use: Vaginal preparation.

MASSENGILL LIQUID. (Beecham Products) Lactic acid, S.D. alcohol 40, octoxynol-9, water, sodium lacate. Bot. 4 oz, 8 oz.
Use: Vaginal preparation.

MASSENGILL MEDICATED. (Beecham Products) Povidone iodine 0.3% when added to sanitized fluid. Bot. 6 oz.
Use: Vaginal preparation.

MASSENGILL POWDER. (Beecham Products) Sodium Cl, ammonium alum, PEG-8, phenol, methyl salicylate, eucalyptus oil, menthol, thy-

mol, phenol. Jar 4 oz, 8 oz, 16 oz, 22 oz. Packette 10s, 12s.
Use: Vaginal preparation.

MASSENGILL VINEGAR-WATER DISPOSABLE DOUCHE. (Beecham Products) Water and vinegar solution. Bot. 6 oz.
Use: Vaginal preparation.

MASTER FORMULA. (Barth's) Vitamins A 10,000 IU, D 400 IU, C 180 mg, B_1 7 mg, B_2 14 mg, niacin 4.6 mg, B_6 292 mcg, pantothenic acid 210 mcg, B_{12} 25 mcg, biotin 2.9 mcg, E 50 IU, calcium 800 mg, phosphorus 387 mg, iron 10 mg, iodine 0.1 mg, choline 7.78 mg, inositol 11.6 mg, aminobenzoic acid 35 mcg, rutin 30 mg, citrus bioflavonoid complex 30 mg/4 Tab. Bot. 120s, 600s, 1200s.
Use: Vitamin/mineral supplement.

MASTISOL. (Ferndale) Nonirritating medical adhesive. Bot. 4 oz.
Use: Skin dressing adhesive.

MATERNA. (Lederle) Vitamins A 8000 IU, D 400 IU, E 30 IU, C 100 mg, folic acid 1 mg, B_1 3 mg, B_2 3.4 mg, B_6 4 mg, niacinamide 20 mg, B_{12} 12 mcg, calcium 250 mg, iodine 0.3 mg, magnesium 25 mg, iron 60 mg, copper 2 mg, zinc 25 mg/Tab. Bot. 100s.
Use: Vitamin/mineral supplement.

MATULANE. (Roche) Procarbazine HCl 50 mg/Cap. Bot. 100s.
Use: Antineoplastic agent.

MAURRY'S FUNGICIDE. (Maurry) Nitromersol 37 mg, alcohol 70% - 74%/oz. Bot. oz, pt.
Use: Antifungal, external.

MAXAFIL CREAM. (Rydelle) Cinoxate 4%, methyl anthranilate 5% in cream base. Tube oz.
Use: Sunscreen.

MAXAIR. (Riker) Pirbuterol acetate aerosol 0.2 mg pirbuterol/actuation. Metered dose inhaler 25.6 Gm ($\approx$ 300 inhalations).
Use: Sympathomimetic bronchodilator.

MAX-CARO. (Marlyn) Beta-carotene 15 mg, lecithin. Cap. Bot. 250s.
Use: To reduce severity of photosensitivity reactions in patients with erythropoietic protoporphyria.

MAX EPA CAPSULES. (Various Mfr.) Omega-3 polyunsaturated fatty acids 1000 mg/Cap. containing EPA 180 mg, DHA 60 mg/Cap. Bot. 50s, 60s, 100s.
Use: Fish oil.

MAXIDEX. (Alcon) Dexamethasone 0.1% in a 0.5% soln., methylcellulose vehicle/5 ml. Bot. 5 ml, 15 ml.
Use: Corticosteroid, ophthalmic.

MAXIFLOR CREAM & OINTMENT. (Herbert) Diflorasone diacetate 0.05%. Tubes 15 Gm, 30 Gm, 60 Gm.
Use: Corticosteroid, topical.

MAXIMUM BAYER ASPIRIN TABLETS AND CAPSULES. (Glenbrook) Aspirin (Acetylsalicylic Acid; ASA) 500 mg. **Tab.:** 10s, 30s, 60s, 100s. **Capl.:** 60s.
Use: Salicylate analgesic.

MAXIMUM STRENGTH NO-ASPIRIN SINUS MEDICATION. (Walgreen) Acetaminophen 500 mg, pseudoephedrine HCl 30 mg/Tab. Bot. 50s.
Use: Analgesic, decongestant.

MAXIMUM STRENGTH SINUTAB NIGHTTIME. (Parke-Davis Consumer) Pseudoephedrine HCl 10 mg, diphenhydramine HCl 8.33 mg, acetaminophen 167 mg/5 ml. Alcohol free. In 120 ml.
Use: Decongestant, antihistamine, analgesic.

MAXITON.
See: Amphetamine (Various Mfr.).

MAXITROL OINTMENT. (Alcon) Dexamethasone 0.1%, neomycin 3.5 mg, polymyxin B sulfate 10,000 units/Gm. Tube 3.5 Gm.
Use: Anti-infective, ophthalmic.

MAXITROL OPHTHALMIC SUSPENSION. (Alcon) Dexamethasone 0.1%, neomycin (as sulfate) 3.5 mg, polymyxin B sulfate 10,000 units/ml. Bot. 5 ml drop-tainer.
Use: Anti-infective, ophthalmic.

MAXIVATE. (Westwood) Betamethasone dipropionate 0.05%. Cream, Oint. Tube 15 Gm, 45 Gm.
Use: Corticosteroid, topical.

MAXOLON TABLETS. (Beecham Labs) Metoclopramide HCl 10 mg/Tab. Bot. 100s.
Use: GI stimulant.

MAXZIDE. (Lederle) Hydrochlorothiazide 50 mg, triamterene 75 mg/Tab. Bot. 100s, 500s, UD 10 $\times$ 10s.
Use: Diuretic, antihypertensive.

MAYASEN. (Janssen) Astemizole.
Use: Anti-allergenic, antihistamine.

•**MAYTANSINE.** USAN.
Use: Antineoplastic.

MAY-VITA ELIXIR. (Mayrand) Dexpanthenol 10 mg, niacinamide 40 mg, B_6 4 mg, B_{12} 12 mcg, folic acid 1 mg, iron 36 mg, zinc 15 mg, manganese 4 mg/45 ml w/alcohol 13%. Bot. pt.
Use: Vitamin/mineral supplement.

MAZANOR. (Wyeth-Ayerst) Mazindol 1 mg/Tab. Bot. 30s.
Use: Anorexiant.

•**MAZINDOL,** U.S.P. XXII. Tab., U.S.P. XXII. 5-(p-Chlorophenyl)-2,3-dihydro-5,H-imidazo [2,1-a]isoindol-5-ol.
Use: Anorexic, appetite suppressant.
See: Mazanor, Tab. (Wyeth-Ayerst).
Sanorex, Tab. (Sandoz).

M-CAPS. (Mill-Mark) Methionine 200 mg/Cap. Bot. 50s, 1000s.
Use: Diaper rash product.

MCT OIL. (Mead Johnson) Triglycerides of medium chain fatty acids. Lipid fraction of coconut oil; fatty acid shorter than C-8 >6%, C_8(octanoic) 67%, $C_1$0(decanoic) 23%, longer than $C_1$0>4%. Bot. qt.
Use: Enteral nutritional supplement.

MD-GASTROVIEW. (Mallinckrodt) Diatrizoate meglumine 66%, diatrizoate sodium 10%. Soln. 120 ml, 240 ml.
Use: Radiopaque agent.

MD-60. (Mallinckrodt) Diatrizoate meglumine 52%, diatrizoate sodium 8% (29.2% iodine). Inj. Vial 30 ml, 50 ml.
Use: Radiopaque agent.

MD-76. (Mallinckrodt) Diatrizoate meglumine 66%, diatrizoate sodium 10% (37% iodine). Inj. Vial 50 ml, 100 ml, 150 ml, 200 ml.
Use: Radiopaque agent.

MDP-SQUIBB. (Squibb) Technetium Tc 99 medronate. Reaction vial pkg. 10s.
Use: Radiopaque agent.

MEADININ. Mixture of Amoidin & Amidin alk. of Ammi Majus Linn.

MEASLES CONVALESCENT SERUM.
See: Measles Immune Human Serum.

MEASLES IMMUNE GLOBULIN (HUMAN). Sterile soln. of gamma globulin derived from pooled normal human plasma.
Use: Immune serum.

MEASLES PROPHYLACTIC SERUM.
See: Immune Serum Globulin (Human).

•**MEASLES & MUMPS VIRUS VACCINE LIVE,** U.S.P. XXII.
Use: Immunizing agent (active).

MEASLES, MUMPS AND RUBELLA VIRUS VACCINE LIVE, U.S.P. XXII.

MEASLES AND RUBELLA VIRUS VACCINE LIVE, U.S.P. XXII.
See: M-R-Vax, Inj. (Merck Sharp & Dohme).

•**MEASLES VIRUS VACCINE, LIVE,** U.S.P. XXII. Modified live-virus measles vaccine (Schwarz strain).
Use: One-shot vaccine for common measles (rubeola).
Use: Active immunizing agent.
See: Attenuvax, Inj. (Merck Sharp & Dohme).
Lirugen, Inj. (Merrell Dow).
M-Vac, Inj. (Lederle).
W/Mumps virus vaccine, rubella virus vaccine.
See: Lirutrin, Vial (Merrell Dow).
W/Rubella virus vaccine.
See: Lirubel, Vial (Merrell Dow).
M-R-Vax, Inj. (Merck Sharp & Dohme).

MEASLES VIRUS VACCINE, LIVE ATTENUATED. Moraten line derived from Enders' attenuated Edmonston strain grown in cell cultures of chick embryos.
See: Attenuvax, Inj. (Merck Sharp & Dohme).
W/Mumps virus vaccine, rubella virus vaccine.
See: M-M-R., Vial (Merck Sharp & Dohme).
W/Rubella virus vaccine.
See: M-R-Vax, Inj. (Merck Sharp & Dohme).

MEASURIN. (Winthrop Pharm) Aspirin 10 gr./SR Tab. Bot. 60s.
Use: Analgesic.

MEBANAZINE. B.A.N. α-Methylbenzylhydrazine. Actomol.
Use: Monoamine oxidase inhibitor.

MEBARAL. (Winthrop Pharm) Mephobarbital. Tab. **0.5 gr:** Bot. 250s, 1000s. **0.75 gr or 1.5 gr:** Bot. 250s.
Use: Sedative, anticonvulsant.

•**MEBENDAZOLE,** U.S.P. XXII. Tab., U.S.P. XXII. Methyl 5-benzoyl-2-benzimidazolecarbanate.
Use: Anthelmintic.
See: Vermox, Tab. (Janssen).

•**MEBEVERINE HYDROCHLORIDE.** USAN. 4-[Ethyl (p-methoxy-α-methyl-phenethyl) amino] butyl veratrate hydrochloride.
Use: Spasmolytic agent.

MEBEZONIUM IODIDE. B.A.N. 4,4′-Methylenedi-(cy- clohexyltrimethylammonium iodide).
Use: Neuromuscular blocking agent.

MEBHYDROLIN. B.A.N. 5-Benzyl-1,2,3,4-tetrahydro-2-methyl--carboline. Fabahistin napadisylate.
Use: Antihistamine.

•**MEBROFENIN.** USAN.
Use: Diagnostic aid (hepatobiliary function determination).

•**MEBUTAMATE.** USAN. 2-Carbamoyloxymethyl-2,3-dimethyl carbamate. Capla.
Use: Hypotensive.

MECAMYLAMINE HYDROCHLORIDE, U.S.P. XXI. Tab., U.S.P. XXI. N, 2, 3, 3-Tetramethyl-2-norbornanamine HCl. 3-Methylaminoiso-camphane HCl. N-Methyl-di-isobornylamine HCl.
Use: Antihypertensive.
See: Inversine, Tab. (Merck Sharp & Dohme).

•**MECETRONIUM ETHYLSULFATE.** USAN.
Use: Antiseptic.

•**MECHLORETHAMINE HYDROCHLORIDE,** U.S.P. XXII. Inj. U.S.P. XXII. 2,2′-Dichloro-n-methyl-diethylamine HCl. Trituration. Dichloren.
Use: Antineoplastic.
See: Mustargen, Vial (Merck Sharp & Dohme).

MECHOL TABS. (Manne) dl B_6 5 mg, soy protein 100 mg, vitamins B_1 5 mg, B_2 2 mg, C 75 mg, niacinamide 20 mg, pantothenic acid 2 mg, Brewer's yeast 2.5 gr/Tab. Bot. 120s, 1000s.
Use: Vitamin supplement.

MECHOLIN HCl.
See: Methacholine Cl, U.S.P. XXII.

MECHOLYL OINTMENT. (Gordon) Methacholine Cl 0.25%, methyl salicylate 10% in ointment base. Jar 4 oz, 1 lb, 5 lb.
Use: External analgesic.

MECILLINAM. B.A.N. (2S,5R,6R)-6-(Perhydroazepin-1-ylmethyleneamino)penicillanic acid.
Use: Antibiotic.

MECLAN. (Ortho Derm) Meclocycline sulfosalicylate 1%. Cream Tube 20 Gm, 45 Gm.
Use: Anti-acne.

MECLASTINE. Clemastine.

•**MECLIZINE HYDROCHLORIDE,** U.S.P. XXII. Tab., U.S.P. XXII. 1(p-Chloro-α-phenylbenzyl)-4-m-(methylbenzyl)piperazine 2 HCl.
Use: Antinauseant.
See: Antivert, Chew. Tab. (Roerig).
Bonine, Tab. (Roerig).

•**MECLOCYCLINE.** USAN. 7-Chloro-4-(di-me- thylamino)-1, 4, 4a, 5, 5a, 6, 11, 12a-octahydro-3, 5,10, 12, 12a-pentahydroxy-6-methylene-1, 11-dioxo-2-naphthacenecarboxamide.
Use: Antibiotic.

•**MECLOCYCLINE SULFOSALICYLATE,** U.S.P. XXII. Cream, U.S.P. XXII.
Use: Antibiotic.
See: Meclan, Cream (Ortho).

•**MECLOFENAMATE SODIUM,** U.S.P. XXII. Cap., U.S.P. XXII. Benjoic acid, 2-(2, 6-dichloro-3-methylphenyl) amino)-, monosodium salt, monohydrate.
Use: Nonsteroidal anti-inflammatory agent.

MECLOFENAMATE SODIUM. (Mylan) Meclofenamate sodium 50 mg or 100 mg/Cap. Bot. 100s, 500s.
Use: Nonsteroidal anti-inflammatory agent.

•**MECLOFENAMIC ACID.** USAN. N-(2,6-Dichloro-m-tolyl)-anthranilic acid.
Use: Anti-inflammatory.

MECLOFENOXATE. B.A.N. 2-Dimethylaminoethyl 4-chlorophenoxyacetate. Lucidril hydrochloride.
Use: Cerebral stimulant.

MECLOMEN. (Parke-Davis) Meclofenamate sodium monohydrate equivalent to 50 mg or 100 mg meclofenamic acid/Cap. Bot. 100s, 500s (100 mg), UD 100s.
Use: Non-steroidal anti-inflammatory agent.

•**MECLOQUALONE.** USAN. 3-(o-Chlorophenyl)-2-methyl-4 (3 H)-quinazolinone.
Use: Sedative/hypnotic.

•**MECLORISONE DIBUTYRATE.** USAN.
Use: Anti-inflammatory.

•**MECOBALAMIN.** USAN.
Use: Vitamin.

MECLOZINE. B.A.N. 1-(4-Chlorobenzhydryl)-4-(3-methylbenzyl)piperazine. Ancolan dihydrochloride.
Use: Antihistamine.

MECOBALAMIN. B.A.N. α-(5,6-Dimethylbenzimidazol-1-yl)cobamide methyl.
Use: Treatment of vitamin B_{12} deficiency.

MECODRIN.
See: Amphetamine (Various Mfr.).

•**MECRYLATE.** USAN. Methyl 2-cyanoacrylate.
Use: Surgical aid (tissue adhesive).

MECYSTEINE. Methyl Cysteine.

MEDA-HIST ELIXIR. (Medwick) Bot. 4 oz, pt, gal.
Use: Decongestant.

MEDA-HIST EXPECTORANT. (Medwick) Bot. 4 oz, pt, gal.
Use: Decongestant, antitussive.

MEDA-HIST DH. (Medwick) Bot. 4 oz, pt, gal.
Use: Decongestant, antitussive.

MEDALOX GEL. (Med. Chem.) Magnesium aluminum hydroxide gel. Bot. 12 oz, pt, gal.
Use: Antacid.

MED-APAP ELIXIR. (Medwick) Bot. 4 oz, pt, gal.

MEDA CAP. (Circle) Acetaminophen 500 mg/Cap. Bot. 100s.
Use: Analgesic.

MEDA TAB. (Circle) Acetaminophen 325 mg/Tab. Bot. 100s.
Use: Analgesic.

MEDA-TUSS. (Medwick) Bot. 4 oz, pt, gal.

MEDA-TUSS A-C. (Medwick) Bot. 4 oz, pt, gal.

MEDA-TUSS DM. (Medwick) Bot. 4 oz, pt, gal.

MEDA-TUSS PE. (Medwick) Bot. 4 oz, pt, gal.

MEDAZEPAM. B.A.N. 7-Chloro-2,3-dihydro-1-methyl-5-phenyl-1H-1,4-benzodiazepine. Nobrium.
Use: Tranquilizer.

•**MEDAZEPAM HCl.** USAN. 7-Chloro-2, 3-dihydro-1-methyl-5-phenyl-lH-1, 4-benzodiazepine mono-HCl. Under study.
Use: Tranquilizer.

MEDENT. (Stewart-Jackson) Pseudoephedrine HCl 120 mg, guaifenesin 500 mg/Tab. Bot. 100s.
Use: Decongestant, expectorant.

•**MEDETOMIDINE HYDROCHLORIDE.** USAN.
Use: Analgesic (veterinary), sedative (veterinary).

MEDICAINE CREAM. (Walgreen) Benzocaine 3%, resorcinol 2%. Tube 1.25 oz.
Use: Antipruritic.

MEDICATED HEALER. (Walgreen) Strong ammonia soln. 10%, camphor 2.6%. Bot. 6 oz.
Use: Emollient.

MEDICATED POWDER. (Johnson & Johnson) Zinc oxide, talc, fragrance, menthol. Plastic container 3 oz, 6 oz, 11 oz.
Use: Antipruritic.

MEDICONE DRESSING. (Medicone) Cod liver oil 125 mg, zinc oxide 125 mg, 8-hydroxyquinoline-sulfate 0.5 mg, benzocaine 5 mg, menthol 1.8 mg/Gm w/petrolatum, lanolin, talcum, paraffin, perfume. Tube 1 oz, 3 oz, Jar lb.
Use: Local anesthetic.

MEDICONE RECTAL. (Medicone) Benzocaine 130 mg, hydroxyquinoline sulfate 16 mg, zinc oxide 195 mg, menthol 9 mg, balsam Peru 65 mg. In a vegetable and petroleum oil base. Supp. 12s, 24s.
Use: Anorectal preparation.

MEDICONE-HC RECTAL. (Medicone) Hydrocortisone acetate 10 mg, benzocaine 2 gr, oxyquinoline sulfate 0.25 gr, zinc oxide 3 gr, menthol 1/7 gr, balsam Peru 1 gr, in a cocoa butter base/Supp. Box 12s.
Use: Anorectal preparation.

MEDICONET. (Medicone) Benzalkonium Cl 0.02%, ethoxylated lanolin 0.5%, methylparaben 0.15%, hamamelis water 50%, glycerin 10%. Cloth wipe Box 20s.
Use: Anorectal preparation.

MEDIGESIC PLUS. (U.S. Pharm. Corp.) Acetaminophen 325 mg, caffeine 40 mg, butalbital 50 mg/Cap. Bot. 100s.
Use: Analgesic, sedative/hypnotic.

MEDIHALER-DUO. Now Duo-Medihaler.(Riker).

MEDIHALER-EPI. (Riker) Epinephrine bitartrate 7 mg/ml. Soln. Pkg. Medihaler in inert propellant. Oral adapter w/15 ml. Vial. Refill vial 15 ml.
Use: Antiasthmatic.

MEDIHALER-ERGOTAMINE. (Riker) Ergotamine tartrate 9 mg/ml, 0.36 mg delivered with each inhalation. Oral adapter w/2.5 ml. Vial.
Use: Agent for migraine.

MEDIHALER-ISO. (Riker) Isoproterenol sulfate 2 mg/ml. Soln. Oral adapter w/15 ml. Oral adapter w/22.5 ml vial. Refill vial 15 ml and 22.5 ml.
Use: Antiasthmatic.

MEDI-JECT UD VIALS. (Century) Tamper-proof rubber stoppered vial containing 1 ml sterile soln. Single dose use.
See: Ulti-ject disposable syringe prods.
Atropine sulfate 0.4 mg/ml.
Atropine sulfate 1.2 mg/ml.
Scopolamine HBr 400 mcg/ml.

MEDIPAK. (Geneva) First-aid kit.

MEDI-PHITE. (Shionagi) Vitamins B_1 and B_{12}. Syr. Bot. 4 oz, pt, gal.
Use: Vitamin supplement.

MEDIPLAST. (Beiersdorf) Salicylic acid plaster 40%. Box 25s.
Use: Keratolytic.

MEDIPLEX TABULES. (U.S. Chemical) B-complex, vitamin C, E, trace minerals, zinc/Tab. Bot. 100s.
Use: Vitamin/mineral supplement.

MEDIPREN. (McNeil Prods) Ibuprofen 200 mg/Capl. or Tab. Bot. 6s, 24s, 50s, 100s.
Use: Nonsteroidal anti-inflammatory agent.

MEDIQUE EAR DROPS. (E.J. Moore) Carbamide peroxide in anhydrous glycerol.
Use: Antiseptic, otic.

MEDIQUELL. (Parke-Davis Prods) Dextromethorphan HBr 15 mg/Chewy square. Pkg. 12s, 24s.
Use: Antitussive.

MEDI-QUIK AEROSOL. (Mentholatum) Lidocaine 2.5%, benzalkonium Cl 0.1%, ethanol 38%. Aerosol 3 oz.
Use: Antiseptic, local anesthetic.

MEDI-QUICK ANTIBIOTIC OINTMENT. (Mentholatum) Bacitracin neomycin, polymyxin in ointment base. Tube 0.5 oz.
Use: Anti-infective, topical.

MEDI-SPAS ELIXIR. (Medical Chemicals) Phenobarbital 16.2 mg, hyoscyamine sulfate 0.1037 mg, atropine sulfate 0.0194 mg, hyoscine hydrobromide 0.0065 mg, alcohol 23%/5 ml. Bot. 4 oz, pt, gal.
Use: Anticholinergic/antispasmodic, sedative/hypnotic.

MEDI-TAL. (Medi-Rx) Phenobarbital 16 mg, hyoscyamine sulfate 0.1037 mg, atropine sulfate 0.0194 mg, scopolamine HBr 0.0065 mg, alcohol 23%/5 ml. Bot. pt, gal. Tab. Bot. 100s, 1000s.
Use: Anticholinergic/antispasmodic, sedative/hypnotic.

MEDITUSSIN-X LIQUID. (Hauck) Codeine phosphate 50 mg, ammonium Cl 520 mg, potassium guaiacolsulfonate 520 mg, pyrilamine maleate 50 mg, phenylpropanolamine HCl 50 mg, dl-desoxyephedrine HCl 2 mg, tartar emetic 5 mg, phenyltoloxamine dihydrogen citrate 30 mg/30 ml. Bot. pt, gal.
Use: Antitussive, expectorant, antihistamine.

•**MEDORINONE.** USAN.
Use: Cardiotonic.

MEDOTAR. (Medco Lab) Coal tar 1%, polysorbate 80 0.5%, octoxynol 5, zinc oxide, starch, white petrolatum. Jar lb.
Use: Antipsoriatic, antipruritic.

MEDOTOPES. (Squibb) Radiopharmaceuticals.
See: A-C-D Solution Modified (Squibb).
Acid Citrate Dextrose Anticoagulant Solution Modified (Squibb).
Aggregated Albumin (Squibb).
Albumotope (Squibb).
Angiotensin Immutope Kit (Squibb).
Cobalt-Labeled Vitamin B_{12} (Squibb).
Cobalt Standards for Vitamin B_{12} (Squibb).
Cobatope (Squibb).
Digoxin (^{125}I) Immutope Kit (Squibb).
Gastrin (^{125}I) Immutope Kit (Squibb).
Gold-198 (Squibb).
Hipputope (Squibb).
Human Serum Albumin (Squibb).
Iodine 131: Capsules Diagnostic-Capsules Therapeutic-Solution Therapeutic Oral (Squibb).
Iodinated Human Serum Albumin (Squibb).
Iodo-hippuric Acid (Squibb).
Macroaggregated Albumin (Squibb).
Macrotec (Squibb).
Minitec (Squibb).
Phosphorus-32: Solution Oral, Therapeutic-Sodium Phosphate Solution U.S.P. for oral or IV use therapeutic or diagnostic (Squibb).
Red Cell Tagging Solution (Squibb).
Renotec (Squibb).
Rose Bengal (Squibb).
Rubratope-57: Diagnostic Capsules-Diagnostic Kit (Squibb).
Rubratope-60: Diagnostic Capsules-Diagnostic Kit (Squibb).
Selenomethionine (Squibb).
Sethotope (Squibb).
Technetium 99m (Squibb).
Technetium 99m-Iron-Ascorbate (DTPA) (Squibb).
Technetium 99m Sulfur Colloid Kit (Squibb).
Tesuloid (Squibb).
Thyrostat-FTI (Squibb).
Thyrostat-3 (Squibb).
Thyrostat-4 FTI (Squibb).

MEDRALONE 40. (Keene) Methylprednisolone acetate 40 mg/ml. Vial 5 ml.
Use: Corticosteroid.

MEDRALONE 80. (Keene) Methylprednisolone acetate 80 mg/ml. Vial 5 ml.

Use: Corticosteroid.
•**MEDROGESTONE.** USAN. Formerly Metrogestone. Dimethyl pregna-4, 6 diene-3, 20-dione.
Use: Oral progestin.
See: Colprone (Wyeth-Ayerst).
MEDROL. (Upjohn) Methylprednisolone. **Tab.:** 2 mg. Bot. 100s; 4 mg Bot. 30s, 100s, 500s, UD 100s; 8 mg Bot. 25s; 16 mg Bot. 50s; 24 mg Bot. 25s; 32 mg Bot. 25s. **Dosepak:** 4 mg Pkg. 21s. **Alternate Daypak:** 16 mg Pkg. 14s.
Use: Corticosteroid.
MEDROL ACETATE TOPICAL. (Upjohn) Methylprednisolone acetate 0.25% or 1%, methylparaben 4 mg, butylparaben 3 mg/Gm. Tube 30 Gm.
Use: Corticosteroid, topical.
•**MEDRONATE DISODIUM.** USAN.
Use: Pharmaceutic aid.
•**MEDRONIC ACID.** USAN.
Use: Pharmaceutic aid.
MEDROSPHOL Hg-197. 1-(Hydroxymercuri-197 Hg)-2-propanol.
See: Merprane.
•**MEDROXALOL.** USAN.
Use: Antihypertensive.
MEDROXALOL HYDROCHLORIDE. USAN.
Use: Antihypertensive.
MEDROXYPROGESTERONE ACETATE. (Lederle) Medroxyprogesterone acetate 10 mg/Tab. Bot. 50s, 250s.
Use: Progestin.
•**MEDROXYPROGESTERONE ACETATE,** U.S.P. XXII. Sterile Susp., Tab., U.S.P. XXII. 17-Hydroxy-6α-methylpregn-4-ene-3, 20-dione 17-Acetate. (CMC) 50 mg, 100 mg/ml. Vial 5 ml.
Use: Progestin.
See: Amen, Tab. (Carnrick).
Curretab, Tab. (Solvay).
depCorlutin (Forest).
Depo-Provera, Vial (Upjohn).
P-Medrate-P.A., Inj. (Solvay).
Provera, Tab. (Upjohn).
•**MEDRYSONE,** U.S.P. XXII. Ophthalmic Susp. U.S.P. XXII. 11 β-Hydroxy-6α-methylpregn-4-ene-3,20-dione.
Use: Topical anti-inflammatory agent.
See: HMS Liquifilm, Ophth. Soln. (Allergan).
MED-TANE ELIXIR. (Medwick) Brompheniramine maleate. Bot. 4 oz, pt, gal.
Use: Antihistamine.
MED-TANE EXPECTORANT DC. (Medwick) Brompheniramine maleate. Bot. 4 oz, pt, gal.
Use: Antihistamine.
MED-TAPP ELIXIR. (Medwick) Bot. 4 oz, pt, gal.
•**MEFENAMIC ACID.** USAN. U.S.P. XXII. Cap. N-(2,3-Xylyl) anthranilic acid. Ponstan.
Use: Anti-inflammatory agent.
See: Ponstel, Kapseal (Parke-Davis).
•**MEFENIDIL.** USAN.
Use: Cerebral vasodilator.
•**MEFENIDIL FUMARATE.** USAN.
Use: Cerebral vasodilator.
MEFENOREX HCl. USAN. N-(3-chloropropyl)-α-methylphenethylamineHCl. Under study.
Use: Anorexiant.
•**MEFEXAMIDE.** USAN.
Use: Stimulant.
•**MEFLOQUINE.** USAN.
Use: Antimalarial.
•**MEFLOQUINE HYDROCHLORIDE.** USAN.
Use: Antimalarial.
See: Lariam (Roche).
MEFOXIN. (Merck Sharp & Dohme) Sterile cefoxitin sodium 1 Gm or 2 Gm/Vial. **1 Gm:** Vial 10 ml. 10s, 25s, ADD-Vantage Vial Tray 25s. Infusion bottle 100 ml, Tray 10s. Premixed I.V. Soln. in 50 ml. D5W, 24s. **2 Gm:** Vial 20 ml. 10s, 25s, ADD-Vantage Vial, Tray 25s, Infusion bottle 100 ml, Tray 10s. Premixed I.V. Soln. in 50 ml. D5W, 24s. Bulk pkg. 10 Gm/100 ml. Bot.
Use: Antibacterial, cephalosporin.
MEFOXIN IN 5% DEXTROSE. (Merck Sharp & Dohme) Cefoxitin sodium 1 Gm or 2 Gm in Dextrose in Water 5%. Inj. Viaflex plus containers 50 ml.
Use: Antibacterial, cephalosporin.
MEFRUSIDE. USAN. (FBA) 4-Chloro-N′-methyl-N′-(tetrahydro-2-methylfurfuryl)-m-benzenedisulfonamide. Baycaron.
Use: Diuretic.
MEGA-B. (Arco) Vitamins B_1 100 mg, B_2 60 mg, B_6 100 mg, B_{12} 100 mcg, niacinamide 100 mg, folic acid 100 mcg, pantothenic acid 100 mg, d-biotin 100 mcg, PABA 100 mg/Tab. Bot. 30s, 100s, 500s.
Use: Vitamin B supplement.
MEGACE. (Bristol-Myers/Mead Johnson Oncology) Megestrol acetate 20 mg or 40 mg/Tab. **20 mg/Tab.:** Bot. 100s; **40 mg/Tab.:** Bot. 100s, 250s, 500s.
Use: Antineoplastic agent.
MEGADOSE. (Arco) Vitamins A 25,000 USP units, D 1000 USP units, C 250 mg, E 100 IU, folic acid 400 mcg, B_1 80 mg, B_2 80 mg, niacinamide 80 mg, B_6 80 mg, B_{12} 80 mcg, biotin 80 mcg, pantothenic acid 80 mg, choline bitartrate 80 mg, inositol 80 mg, para-aminobenzoic acid 80 mg, rutin 30 mg, citrus bioflavonoids 30 mg, betaine HCl 30 mg, glutamic acid 30 mg, hesperidin complex 5 mg, iodine 0.15 mg, calcium gluconate 10 mg, ferrous gluconate 10 mg, magnesium gluconate 7 mg, manganese gluconate 6 mg, copper gluconate 0.5 mg/Cap. Bot. 100s, 250s.
Use: Vitamin/nutritional supplement.
•**MEGALOMICIN POTASSIUM PHOSPHATE.** USAN.
Use: Antibacterial.
MEGATON. (Hyrex) Dexpanthenol 10 mg, niacinamide 40 mg, vitamins B_6 4 mg, B_{12} 12 mcg, folic acid 1 mg, iron 36 mg, zinc 15 mg, manganese 4 mg, alcohol 13%. Bot. 16 oz.
Use: Vitamin/mineral supplement.

MEGA-VITA. (Saron) Vitamins C 500 mg, niacinamide 500 mg, B_6 50 mg, B_1 25 mg, B_2 10 mg, B_{12} 50 mcg, folic acid 150 mcg, E 200 IU, pantothenic acid 10 mg, A 2500 IU, D 333 IU, magnesium oxide 50 mg, zinc sulfate 50 mg/3 Tab. Bot. 100s.
Use: Vitamin/mineral supplement.

MEGA-VITA HEMATINIC. (Saron) Mega-Vita formula with iron 50 mg, vitamin A 1000 IU, copper 2 mg, manganese 1.8 mg, iodine 0.1 mg, potassium 10 mg/3 Tab.
Use: Vitamin/mineral supplement.

MEGA-VITA TONIC. (Saron) Vitamins B_{12} 25 mcg, B_6 6 mg, niacin 25 mg, aminoacetic acid 750 mg/15 ml, alcohol 17%.
Use: Vitamin supplement.

•**MEGESTROL ACETATE,** U.S.P. XXII. Tab., U.S.P. XXII. 17 α-acetoxy-6-methylpregna-4,6-diene-3, 20-dione.
Use: Palliative treatment of advanced carcinoma of the breast or endometrium.
See: Megace (Bristol Oncology).
Pallace, Tab. (Bristol).

MEGLUMINE, U.S.P. XXII. 1-Deoxy-1-methylamino glucitol. 1-Methylamino-1-deoxy-D-glucitol.
Use: Pharmaceutical aid.

•**MEGLUMINE, DIATRIZOATE INJ.,** U.S.P. XXII. N-Meglumine salt of 3, 5 diacetamido-2, 4, 6-triiodo-benzoic acid. Methylglucamine Diatrizoate. D-Glucitol, 1-deoxy-1-(methylamino).
Use: Radiopaque medium.
See: Cardiografin, Vial (Squibb).
Cystografin, Vial (Squibb).
Gastrografin, Soln. (Squibb).
Hypaque-76, Inj. (Winthrop Pharm).
Hypaque-M 75%, Inj. (Winthrop Pharm).
Hypaque-M 90%, Inj. (Winthrop Pharm).
Hypaque Meglumine, Vial (Winthrop Pharm).
Reno-M-30, -60, Vial (Squibb).
Reno-M-Dip, Vial (Squibb).
W/Meglumine iodipamide.
See: Sinografin, Soln. (Squibb).
W/Sodium diatrizoate.
See: Gastrografin, Soln. (Squibb).
Renografin-60, Inj. (Squibb).
Renografin-76, Inj. (Squibb).
Renovist II, Inj. (Squibb).

•**MEGLUMINE, IODIPAMIDE INJ.,** U.S.P. XXII. 1-Deoxy-1-(Methyl amino) glucitol, D glucitol, 1-deoxy-1-(methylamino).
Use: Radiopaque medium.
See: Cholografin, Vial (Squibb).
W/Meglumine diatrizoate.
See: Sinografin, Soln. (Squibb).

•**MEGLUMINE, IOTHALAMATE INJ.,** U.S.P. XXII. 5-Acetamido-2,4,6-triiodo-N-methylisophthalamic acid, N-methylglucamine.
Use: Radiopaque medium.

•**MEGLUTOL.** USAN.
Use: Antihyperlipoproteinemic.

MEJEPTIL.
See: Thioperazine (SmithKline).

MELADRAZINE. B.A.N. 2,4-Di(diethylamino)-6-hydrazino-1,3,5-triazine. Lisidonil (+)-tartrate.
Use: Polysynaptic inhibitor.

•**MELAFOCON A.** USAN.
Use: Contact lens material (hydrophilic).

MELANEX. (Neutrogena) Hydroquinone 3% in solution containing alcohol 47.3%. Bot. 1 oz w/ Appliderm applicator and pinpoint rod applicator.
Use: Skln bleaching agent.

MELARSONYL POTASSIUM. B.A.N. Dipotassium 2-[4-(4,6-diamino-1,3,5-triazin-2-ylamino)phenyl]-1,3,2-dithiarsolan-4,5-dicarboxylate. Trimelarsan.
Use: Treatment of trypanosomiasis.

MELARSOPROL. B.A.N. 2-[4-(4,6-Diamino-1,3,5-triazin-2-ylamino)phenyl]-4-hydroxymethyl-1,3,2-dithiarsolan. Mel B.
Use: Treatment of trypanosomiasis.

•**MELENGESTROL ACETATE.** USAN.
Use: Antineoplastic, progestin.

MELFIAT (Solvay) Phendimetrazine tartrate 105 mg/Cap. Bot. 100s.
Use: Anorexiant.

MELHORAL CHILD TABLET. (Winthrop Products) Acetylsalicylic acid.
Use: Salicylate analgesic.

MELITOXIN.
See: Dicumarol (Various Mfr.).

•**MELITRACEN HYDROCHLORIDE.** USAN.
Use: Antidepressant.

•**MELIZAME.** USAN.
Use: Sweetener.

MELLARIL CONCENTRATE. (Sandoz) Thioridazine HCl 30 mg/ml, alcohol 3%. Soln. Bot. 4 oz. Concentrate 100 mg/ml. Pk. 4 oz.
Use: Antipsychotic agent.

MELLARIL S. (Sandoz) Thioridazine 25 mg/5 ml or 100 mg/5 ml. Susp. Bot. pt.
Use: Antipsychotic agent.

MELLARIL TABLETS. (Sandoz) Thioridazine HCl 10 mg, 15 mg, 25 mg, 50 mg, 100 mg, 150 mg or 200 mg/Tab. Bot. 100s, 1000s. Sando-Pak pkg. 100s (except 150 mg).
Use: Antipsychotic agent.

MELLOSE. Methylcellulose.

MELONEX. Metahexamide.
Use: Oral antidiabetic.

•**MELPHALAN,** U.S.P. XXII. Tab., U.S.P. XXII. L-3- {p[bis(2-Chloroethyl)amino]phenyl} alanine. Previously Sarcolysin.
Use: Antineoplastic.
See: Alkeran, Tab. (Burroughs Wellcome).

•**MEMOTINE HCl.** USAN. 3, 4-Dihydro-1-[(p-methoxyphen-oxy)methyl]isoquinoline HCl.
Use: Antiviral.

•**MEMOTINE HYDROCHLORIDE.** USAN.
Use: Antiviral.

•**MENABITAN HYDROCHLORIDE.** USAN.
Use: Analgesic.

•**MENADIOL SODIUM DIPHOSPHATE,** U.S.P. XXII. Inj., Tab., U.S.P. XXII. 1,4-Naphtha-lene-diol,2- methyl-,bis(dihydrogen phosphate), tetrasodium salt, hexahydrate.
Use: Vitamin K therapy (Orally or I.M. 4 to 75 mg).
See: Kappadione, Amp. (Lilly).
Synkayvite, Amp., Tab. (Roche).

•**MENADIONE,** U.S.P. XXII. Inj., U.S.P. XXII. 2-Methyl-1,4-naphthoquinone (Menaphthone, Danitamon K, Aquinone, Aquaday, Menaquinone).
Use: Orally & I.M., Vitamin K therapy.
W/Ascorbic acid.
See: Rependo, Cap. (Scruggs).
W/Ascorbic acid, hesperidin.
See: Hescor-K, Tab. (Madland).
W/Bioflavonoid citrus compound, ascorbic acid.
See: C.V.P. W/Vitamin K, Syr., Tab. (USV Pharm.).

MENADIONE DIPHOSPHATE SODIUM.
See: Menadiol Sodium Diphosphate.

MENADOXIME. B.A.N. Ammonium salt of 2-methylnaphthaquinone-4-oxime O-carboxymethyl ether. Kapilon Soluble.
Use: Treatment of hypoprothrombinemia.

MENAPHTHENE OR MENAPHTHONE.
See: Menadione (Various Mfr.).

MENAQUINONE.
See: Menadione (Various Mfr.).

MENEST. (Beecham Labs) Esterified estrogens, conjugated estrogens (equine) **0.3 mg or 0.625 mg/Tab.:** Bot. 100s. **1.25 mg/Tab.:** Bot. 100s, 1000s; **2.5 mg/Tab.:** Bot. 50s.
Use: Estrogen combination.

MENI-D. (Seatrace) Meclizine 25 mg/Cap. Bot. 100s.
Use: Antiemetic/antivertigo.

MENINGOCOCCAL POLYSACCHARIDE VACCINE GROUP A, U.S.P. XXII.
Use: Immunizing agent (active).

MENINGOCOCCAL POLYSACCHARIDE VACCINE GROUPS A AND C COMBINED}, U.S.P. XXI.
Use: Immunizing agent (active).
W/Groups A, C, Y, W-135 Combined.
See: Menomune, Inj. (Squibb/Connaught).

MENINGOCOCCAL POLYSACCHARIDE VACCINE GROUP C, U.S.P. XXII.
Use: Immunizing agent (active).

MENOCTONE. USAN. 2-(8-Cyclohexyl-octyl)-3-hydroxy-1, 4-naphthoquinone. Under study.
Use: Antimalarial.

MENOGARIL. USAN.
Use: Antineoplastic.

MENOJECT L.A. (Mayrand) Testosterone cypionate, estradiol cypionate. Vial 10 ml.
Use: Androgen, estrogen combination.

MENOLYN. (Arcum) Ethinyl estradiol 0.05 mg/Tab. Bot. 100s, 1000s.
Use: Estrogen.

MENOMUNE. (Squibb/Connaught) Meningococcal polysaccharide vaccine, Groups A, C, Y, W-135. Vial 10 or 50 dose w/diluent.
Use: Agent for immunization. **MENOMUNE-C VACCINE.** Group-specific polysaccharide antigen from Neisseria meningitis, Group C. Bot. 10 and 50 dose vial.
Use: Agent for immunization.

MENOPLEX TABLETS. (Fiske) Acetaminophen 325 mg, phenyltoloxamine citrate 30 mg/Tab. Bot. 20s.
Use: Analgesic.

•**MENOTROPINS,** U.S.P. XXII. For Inj., U.S.P. XXII.
Use: Gonadotropin.
See: Pergonal.

MENRIUM. (Roche) **Menrium 5-2:** Chlordiazepoxide 5 mg, water-soluble esterified estrogens 0.2 mg/Tab. **Menrium 5-4:** Chlordiazepoxide 5 mg, water-soluble esterified estrogens 0.4 mg/Tab. **Menrium 10-4:** Chlordiazepoxide 10 mg, water-soluble esterified estrogens 0.4 mg/Tab. Bot. 100s.
Use: Estrogen.

MENSTRESS CAPS. (Pharmex) Cap. Bot. 15s.
Use: Cramps.

MENTHOL, U.S.P. XXII. Cyclohexanol, 5-methyl-2-(1-methylethyl). p-Menthan-3-ol.
Use: Topical antipruritic, local analgesic, nasal decongestant, antitussive.
See: Benzedrex Inhaler (SmithKline).
Vicks Cough Silencers, Loz. (Vicks).
Vicks Formula 44 Cough Control Discs, Loz. (Vicks).
Vicks Inhaler (Vicks).
Vicks Blue Mint, Lemon, Regular and Wild Cherry Medicated Cough Drops (Vicks).
Vicks Medi-Trating Throat Loz. (Vicks).
Vicks Oracin Regular and Cherry, Loz. (Vicks).
Vicks Sinex, Nasal Spray (Vicks).
Vicks Vaporub, Oint. (Vicks).
Vicks Vaposteam, Liq. (Vicks).
Vicks Va-Tro-Nol, Nose Drops (Vicks).
Victors Regular and Cherry, Loz. (Vicks).
W/Combinations.
See: Halls Mentho-Lyptus, Prods. (Warner-Lambert).
Listerine Antiseptic, Liq. (Warner-Lambert).

MENTHOLATUM. (Mentholatum) Menthol 1.35%, camphor 9%, titanium dioxide and fragrance in ointment base of petrolatum. Tube 0.4 oz, 1 oz. Jar 1 oz, 3 oz.
Use: External analgesic.

MENTHOLATUM DEEP HEATING LOTION. (Mentholatum) Menthol 6%, methyl salicylate 20%, lanolin derivative in lotion base. Bot. 2 oz, 4 oz.
Use: External analgesic.

MENTHOLATUM DEEP HEATING RUB. (Mentholatum) Menthol 5.8%, methyl salicylate 12.7%, eucalyptus oil, turpentine oil, anhydrous

lanolin, vehicle and fragrance. Tube 1.25 oz, 3.33 oz, 5 oz.
Use: External analgesic.

MENTHOLIN. (Apco) Methyl salicylate 30%, chloroform 20%, hard soap 3%, camphor gum 2.2%, menthol 0.8%, alcohol 35%. Bot. 2 oz.
Use: External analgesic.

MENTHYL VALERATE. Validol.
Use: Sedative.

MENTROLZ. (Mayer) Mayercin (Homatropine methylbromide 0.5 mg and ammonium Cl 300 mg), caffeine alkaline 32 mg, acetophenetidin 150 mg, salicylamide 225 mg/Tab. Bot. 16s.
Use: Analgesic combination.

•**MEOBENTINE SULFATE.** USAN.
Use: Cardiac depressant.

MEPACRINE HYDROCHLORIDE.
Use: Anthelmintic, antimalarial.
See: Quinacrine HCl, U.S.P. XXII.

MEPARFYNOL. 2-Ethinylbutanol-2. Methylparafynol, methylpentynol.

•**MEPARTRICIN.** USAN.
Use: Antifungal, antiprotozoal.

MEPAVLON.
See: Meprobamate, U.S.P. XXII.

MEPAZINE ACETATE & HCl. 10-[1-Methyl-3-(piperidyl)methyl] phenothiazine acetate or HCl.

MEPENZOLATE BROMIDE, U.S.P. XXI. Syr., Tab., U.S.P. XXI. N-methyl-3-hydroxypiperidine benzilate methobromide.
Use: Anticholinergic.
See: Cantil, Tab., Liq. (Merrell Dow).
W/Phenobarbital.
See: Cantil w/phenobarbital (Merrell Dow).

MEPENZOLATE METHYL BROMIDE. Mepenzolate bromide.
Use: Anticholinergic.

MEPERGAN. (Wyeth-Ayerst) Promethazine HCl 25 mg, meperidine HCl 25 mg/ml. Inj. Vial 10 ml, Tubex 2 ml. Box 10s.
Use: Narcotic analgesic combination.

MEPERGAN FORTIS. (Wyeth-Ayerst) Meperidine HCl 50 mg, promethazine HCl 25 mg/Cap. Bot. 100s.
Use: Narcotic analgesic combination.

•**MEPERIDINE HYDROCHLORIDE,** U.S.P. XXII. Inj., Syr., Tab., U.S.P. XXII. (Various Mfr.) Ethyl-1-methyl-4-phenylisonipecotate HCl. (Parke-Davis) 50 mg/ml, 75 mg/ml or 100 mg/ml as 1 ml fill in 2 ml Steri-dose syringe. (Dolantal, Dolantin, Dolosal, Dolvanol, Endolate, Isonipecaine, Pethidine).
Use: Analgesic (narcotic).
See: Demerol HCl, Prods. (Winthrop Pharm).
W/Acetaminophen.
See: Demerol APAP, Tab. (Winthrop Pharm).
W/Promethazine HCl.
See: Mepergan, Preps. (Wyeth-Ayerst).

MEPERIDINE HCl AND ATROPINE SULFATE.
Use: General anesthetic.
See: Atropine and Demerol, Inj.(Winthrop Pharm.).

MEPHENESIN. 3-o-Tolyloxypropane-1,2-diol. Lissephen; Myanesin; Tolseram carbamate.
Use: Skeletal muscle relaxant.
See: Mervaldin, Tab. (Lannett).
Myanesin.
W/Acetaminophen, Vitamin C, butabarbital.
See: T-Caps, Cap. (Burlington).
W/Mephobarbital, hyoscine HBr.
See: Tranquil, Tab. (Kenyon).
W/Pentobarbital.
See: Nebralin, Tab. (Dorsey).
W/Salicylamide, butabarbital sodium.
See: Metrogesic, Tab. (Metro Med).

MEPHENESIN CARBAMATE.
See: Methoxydone.

MEPHENOXALONE. 5-(o-Methoxyphenoxymethyl-)-2-oxazolidinone.

•**MEPHENTERMINE SULFATE,** U.S.P. XXII. Inj., U.S.P. XXII. N,α,α-Trimethyl-phenethylamine sulfate. Mephine.
Use: Vasoconstrictor and nasal decongestant. Also I.V. or I.M.
See: Wyamine Sulfate Inj. (Wyeth-Ayerst).
W/Phenacetin, aspirin, promethazine HCl.

•**MEPHENYTOIN,** U.S.P. XXII. Tab., U.S.P. XXII. 5-Ethyl-3-methyl-5-phenylhydantoin.
Use: Anticonvulsant.
See: Mesantoin, Tab. (Sandoz).

MEP-40. (Parnell) Methylprednisolone acetate 40 mg/ml. Inj. Susp. Vial. 5 ml.
Use: Corticosteroid.

•**MEPHOBARBITAL,** U.S.P. XXII. Tab., U.S.P. XXII. 5-Ethyl-5-phenyl N-methyl-barbituric acid. 5-Ethyl-1-methyl-5-phenylbarbituric Acid.
Use: Anticonvulsant, sedative.
See: Mebaral, Tab. (Winthrop Pharm).
W/Acetaminophen.
See: Koly-Tabs (Scrip).
W/Homatropine methylbromide, atropine methylnitrate and hyoscine HBr.
W/Mephenesin, hyoscine HBr.
See: Tranquil, Tab. (Kenyon).

MEPHONE.
See: Mephentermine.

MEPHYTON. (Merck Sharp & Dohme) Phytonadione (vitamin K-1) 5 mg/Tab. Bot. 100s.
Use: Anticoagulant.

MEPIBEN. (Schen Labs.) Methylpiperidyl benzhydryl ether.
Use: Antihistamine.

MEPIPERPHENIDOL BROMIDE. 1-(3 Hydroxy-5-methyl-4-phenylexyl)-1-methyl piperidium bromide.
Use: Anticholinergic.

MEPIPRAZOLE. B.A.N. 1-(3-Chlorophenyl)-4-[2-(5-methylpyrazol-3-yl)ethyl]piperazine.
Use: Psychotropic agent.

•**MEPIVACAINE HCl,** U.S.P. XXII. Inj., U.S.P. XXII. dl-1-Methyl-2′,6′-pipecoloxylidide monohydrochloride.(±)-1-Methyl-2′,6′-pipecoloxylidide Hydrochloride.
Use: Local anesthetic.

See: Carbocaine, Cartridge, Vial (Cook-Waite).
Carbocaine, Vial (Winthrop Pharm).
Cavacaine, Vial (Graham).
Polocaine, Vial (Astra).

•**MEPIVACAINE HYDROCHLORIDE AND LEVONORDEFRIN INJ.,** U.S.P. XXII.
Use: Local anesthetic.
See: Carbocaine, Cartridge, Vial (Cook-Waite).

•**MEPREDNISONE,** U.S.P. XXII. 17,21-Dihydroxy-16β-methylpregna-1,4-diene-3,11,20-trione. Betaspred.
Use: Glucocorticoid.

•**MEPROBAMATE,** U.S.P. XXII. Oral Susp., Tab., U.S.P. XXII. 2-Methyl-2-n-propyl-1,3-propanediol di-carbamate. 2,2-Di(carbamoyloxymethyl)pentane. 2-Carbamoyloxymethyl-2-methylpentyl carbamate. Me-pavlon.
Use: Minor tranquilizer, sedative.
See: Arcoban Tab. (Arcum).
Bamate, Tab. (Century).
Equanil Tab., Cap., (Wyeth-Ayerst).
Meprospan, Cap. (Wallace).
Miltown, Tab. (Wallace).
Pax-400,Tab. (Kenyon).
Tranmep, Tab. (Solvay).
W/Acetylsalicylic acid.
See: Equagesic, Tab. (Wyeth-Ayerst).
W/Benactyzine HCl.
See: Deprol, Tab. (Wallace).
W/Estrogens conjugated.
See: Milprem, Tab. (Wallace).
W/Pentaerythritol tetranitrate.
See: Miltrate, Tab. (Wallace).
Robam-Petn, Tab. (Robinson).
W/Premarin.
See: PMB 200, Tab. (Wyeth-Ayerst).
W/Tridihexethyl Cl.
See: Milpath, Tab. (Wallace).
Pathibamate—200, 400, Tab. (Lederle).

MEPROBAMATE, N-ISOPROPYL.
See: Carisoprodol.

MEPROCHOL. B.A.N. (2-Methoxyprop-2-enyl)-trime-thylammonium bromide. Esmodil.
Use: Parasympathomimetic.

MEPROLONE TABS. (Major) Methylprednisolone 4 mg/Tab. Bot. 25s, 100s.
Use: Corticosteroid.

MEPROSPAN. (Wallace) Meprobamate in form of coated pellets which release drug continuously for 10 - 12 hours. 200 mg or 400 mg/Cap. Bot. 100s.
Use: Antianxiety agent.

MEPROTHIXOL. B.A.N. 9-(3-Dimethylamino-propyl)-9-hydroxy-2-methoxythiaxanthen.
Use: Analgesic, anti-inflammatory.

•**MEPRYLCAINE HYDROCHLORIDE,** U.S.P. XXII. 2-Methyl-2-propylaminopropyl Benzoate HCl. 2-Methyl-2-(propylamino)-1-propanol benzoate (Ester) Hydrochloride.
Use: Local anesthetic (dental).

•**MEPRYLCAINE HYDROCHLORIDE AND EPINEPHRINE INJ.,** U.S.P. XXII.
Use: Local anesthetic.

•**MEPTAZINOL HYDROCHLORIDE.** USAN.
Use: Analgesic.

MEPYRAMINE. B.A.N. N-4-Methoxybenzyl-N′N′-di-methyl-N-2-pyridylethylenediamine. 2-(N-p-Anisyl-N-2-pyridylamino)ethyldimethylamine. Anthical; Anthisan; Flavelix; Neo-antergan hydrogen maleate.
Use: Antihistamine.

MEPYRAPONE. 2-Methyl-1,2-dl-3-pyridyl-1-propane.
See: Metopirone, Tab., Amp. (Ciba).

•**MEQUIDOX.** USAN. 3-Methyl-2-quinozaline-methanol 1,4-dioxide. Under study.
Use: Antibacterial.

MEQUINOLATE. Name used for Proquinolate.

MERAGIDONE SODIUM. The sodium salt of anhydro-N-(beta-methoxy-gamma-hydroxymercuripropyl)-2-pyridone-5-carboxylic acid-theophylline.

•**MERALEIN SODIUM.** USAN.
Use: Topical anti-infective.
See: Sodium Meralein.

MERALLURIDE. B.A.N. Equal amts. of theophylline and methoxyhydroxymercuripropyl succinylurea. [3-[3-(3-Carboxypropionyl)ureido]-2-methoxypropyl]hydroxy-mercury mixture with theophylline.
Use: Diuretic.

MERBAPHEN. 2-(Carboxymethoxy)-3-chlorophenyl (5,5-diethylbarbiturato)mercury.

MERBROMIN. Disodium 2,7-dibrom-4-hydroxymercurifluorescein. (Asceptichrome, Chromargyre, Cynochrome, Flavurol, Gallochrome Mercurocol, Mercurophage, Mercurome, Planochrome).
Use: Topical antiseptic.

•**MERCAPTOPURINE,** U.S.P. XXII. Tab., U.S.P. XXII. 6-Mercaptopurine. Purine-6-thiol. monohydrate; 6H-purine-6-thione, monohydrate.
Use: Antineoplastic.
See: Purinethol, Tab. (Burroughs Wellcome).

MERCARBOLID. o-Hydroxy-phenylmercuric Cl.

MERCAZOLE.
See: Methimazole, U.S.P. XXII.

MERCOCRESOLS.
See: Mercresin, Tr. (Upjohn).

•**MERCUFENOL CHLORIDE.** USAN.
Use: Anti-infective.

MERCUPURIN.
See: Mercurophylline Inj. (Various Mfr.).

MERCURANINE.
See: Merbromin (City Chem.).

MERCURIAL, ANTISYPHILITICS. Mercuric Oleate Mercuric Salicylate.

MERCURIC OLEATE. Oleate of mercury.
Use: Parasitic and fungal skin diseases.
W/Coal tar crude, salicylic acid, phenol & p-nitrophenol.
See: Prosol, Emulsion (Torch).
Estercol, Emulsion (less p-Nitrophenol) (Torch).

MERCURIC OXIDE OPHTHALMIC OINTMENT, YELLOW.
Use: Local anti-infective.

MERCURIC SALICYLATE. Mercury subsalicylate.
Use: Parasitic and fungal skin diseases.

MERCURIC SUCCINIMIDE. BisSuccinimidatomercury.

MERCURIC SULFIDE, RED. W/Colloidal sulfur, urea.
See: Teenac Cream, Oint. (Elder).

MERCURIN. Sodium salt of β-methoxy-hydroxymercuri propylamide of camphoramic acid. Trimethylcyclopentanedicarboxylic acid. Combined with theophyline is mercurophylline sodium.

MERCUROCAL.
See: Merbromin Soln. (Premo).

MERCUROCHROME. (Various Mfr.) Merbromin 2%. Soln. Bot. 15 ml, 30 ml.
Use: Topical antiseptic.

MERCUROCHROME II. (Becton Dickinson) Lidocaine HCl, benzalkonium Cl, menthol, isopropyl alcohol 5%. Liq. 30 ml; Spray 60 ml, 120 ml.
Use: Local anesthetic.

MERCUROL. (Durel) Oleate of mercury 0.5%, phenol 0.5%, salicylic acid 3%, coal tar solution 1.2% in Moisturizing hand and body lotion. Bot. 4 oz, pt, gal.
Use: Antipsoriatic, antiseborrheic.

MERCUROME.
See: Merbromin Soln. (City Chem.).

MERCUROPHYLLINE SODIUM. B.A.N. Sodium salt of (beta-methoxygamma-hydroxy-mercuripropylamide of camphoramic acid) trimethylcyclopentanedicarboxylic acid and theophylline. Mercuzanthin Inj. Amp. 2 ml, Box 6s, 25s, 100s. Tab. Bot. 50s, 100s, 1000s.
Use: Diuretic.

•**MERCURY, AMMONIATED,** U.S.P. XXII. Oint., Ophth. Oint., U.S.P. XXII.
Use: Topical anti-infective.

MERCURY BICHLORIDE.
See: Diamond, Tab. (Lilly).

MERCURY COMPOUNDS.
See: Antiseptics, Mercurials.

MERCURY-197-203.
See: Chlormerodrin (Squibb).

MERCURY OLEATE. Mercury (2+) oleate. Pharmaceutic aid.

MERDEX. (Faraday) Docusate sodium 100 mg/Tab. Vial 60 ml.
Use: Laxative.

•**MERISOPROL ACETATE Hg 197.** USAN.
Use: Radioactive agent.

•**MERISOPROL ACETATE Hg 203.** USAN.
Use: Radioactive agent.

•**MERISOPROL Hg 197.** USAN.
Use: Diagnostic aid.

MERITENE LIQUID. (Sandoz Nutrition) Vanilla Flavor: Concentrated sweet skim milk, corn syrup solids, corn oil, sodium caseinate, sucrose, artificial flavor, cellulose flour, mono and diglycerides, salt, cellulose gum, carrageenan, vitamins and minerals. Ready-to-serve 250 ml cans. Vanilla, chocolate, eggnog, vanilla supreme flavor.
Use: Enteral nutritional supplement.

MERITENE POWDER. (Sandoz Nutrition) Vanilla flavor: Specially processed nonfat dry milk, corn syrup solids, sucrose, fructose, calcium caseinate, sodium Cl, natural and artificial flavors, lecithin, vitamins and minerals. Can 1 lb, 4.5 lb, 25 lb. Packet 1.14 oz. Vanilla, chocolate, eggnog, milk chocolate, plain flavors.
Use: Enteral nutritional supplement.

MERODICEIN. Sodium meralein.
W/Saligenin.
See: Thantis, Loz. (Hynson, Westcott & Dunning).

MERPRANE. 1-(Hydroxymercuri-197 Hg)-2-propanol.
Use: Diagnostic aid.

MERSOL. (Century) Thimerosal tincture, N.F. 1/1000. 1 oz, 4 oz, pt, gal.
Use: Antiseptic.

MERTHIOLATE. (Lilly) Thimerosal.
Soln: 1:1000: 4 fl. oz, 16 fl oz, gal.
Tincture: 1:1000: alcohol 50%, 0.75 oz, 4 fl oz, 16 fl oz, gal.
Use: Antiseptic.

MERUVAX II. (Merck Sharp & Dohme) Lyophilized, live attenuated rubella virus of the Wistar Institute RA 27/3 strain. Each dose contains approximately 25 mcg of neomycin. Single dose Vial w/diluent. Pkg. 1s, 10s.
Use: Agent for immunization.
W/Attenuvax.
See: M-R-Vax II, Vial (Merck Sharp & Dohme).
W/Attenuvax, Mumpsvax.
See: M-M-R II, Vial (Merck Sharp & Dohme).
W/Mumpsvax.
See: Biavax II, Vial (Merck Sharp & Dohme)).

MERVALDIN. (Lannett) Formerly Proloxin. Mephenesin. 0.5 Gm/Tab. Bot. 500s, 1000s.
Use: Muscle relaxant.

•**MESALAMINE.** USAN.
Use: Anti-infammatory.

MESALAMINE. (Solvay)
See: Rowasa-enema and suppositories.

MESANTOIN. (Sandoz) (Mephenytoin) Phenantoin, 3-Methyl 5,5-phenylethylhydantoin 100 mg/Tab. Bot. 100s.
Use: Anticonvulsant.

MESCOMINE.
See: Methscopolamine bromide (Various Mfr.).

•**MESECLAZONE.** USAN.
Use: Anti-inflammatory.

•**MESIFILCON A.** USAN.
Use: Contact lens material.

•**MESNA.** USAN.
Use: Hemorrhagic cystitis prophylactic.

MESNEX. (Mead Johnson Oncology) Mesna 100 mg. Inj. Amp. 2 ml, 4 ml, 10 ml.
Use: Antidote.

•**MESORIDAZINE.** USAN. 10-[-2-(1-Methyl-2-piperidyl)ethyl]-2-(methylsulfinyl)phenothiazine. Lidanil.
Use: Tranquilizer.

•**MESORIDAZINE BESYLATE,** U.S.P. XXII. Inj., Oral Soln., Tab., U.S.P. XXII. 10-2-(1-methyl-2-piperidyl)-ethyl-2-(methylsulfinyl)phenothiazine monobenzenesulfonate.
Use: Antipsychotic agent.
See: Serentil, Amp., Liq., Tab. (Boehringer-Ingelheim).

MESTANOLONE. B.A.N. 17 β-Hydroxy-17αmethyl-5αandrostan-3-one. Androstalone.
Use: Anabolic steroid.

•**MESTEROLONE.** USAN.
Use: Androgen.

MESTIBOL. Monomestrol.

MESTINON. (Roche) Pyridostigmine bromide 60 mg/Tab. Bot. 100s, 500s. Timespan 180 mg/Tab. Bot. 100s, 500s.
Use: Cholinergic muscle stimulant.

MESTINON INJECTABLE. (Roche) Pyridostigmine bromide 5 mg/ml, w/methyl and propyl parabens 0.2%, sodium citrate 0.02%, pH adjusted to approximately 5 w/citric acid, sodium hydroxide. Amp. 2 ml. Box 10s.
Use: Cholinergic muscle stimulant.

MESTINON SYRUP. (Roche) Pyridostigmine bromide 60 mg/5 ml, alcohol 5%. Bot. pt.
Use: Cholinergic muscle stimulant.

MESTINON TIMESPAN. (Roche) Pyridostigmine bromide 180 mg/Timespan Tab. Bot. 100s.
Use: Cholinergic muscle stimulant.

•**MESTRANOL,** U.S.P. XXII. 17 αEthynylestradiol 3-methyl ether. 3-Methoxy-19-nor-17-alpha-pregna-1,3,5(10)-trien-20-yn-17-ol. 19 Nor-pregna-1,3,5(10)trien-20-yn-17-ol,3-methoxy-, (17α)-.
Use: Estrogenic compound.
W/Ethynodiol Diacetate.
See: Ovulen, Tab. (Searle).
Ovulen-21, Tab. (Searle).
Ovulen-28, Tab. (Searle).
W/Norethindrone.
See: Norinyl, Tab. (Syntex).
Norinyl-1 Fe 28 (Syntex).
Ortho-Novum, Tab. (Ortho).
W/Norethindrone, ferrous fumarate.
See: Ortho Novum 1/80 Fe-28, 1/50 Fe-28, 1 mg Fe-28, Tab. (Ortho).
W/Norethynodrel.
See: Enovid, Tab. (Searle).
Enovid-E, Tab. (Searle).
Enovid-E 21, Tab. (Searle).

MESULPHEN. B.A.N. 2,7-Dimethylthianthren. Mitigal; Sudermo.
Use: Treatment of skin infections.

•**MESUPRINE HYDROCHLORIDE.** USAN.
Use: Vasodilator, smooth muscle relaxant.

METABALM. (Noyes) Menthol, camphor, thymol, methyl salicylate, clove and cassia oil in a non-staining vanishing base. Tube oz.
Use: Antipruritic, counter-irritant.

METABOLIN. (Thurston) Vitamins A 833 IU, D 66 IU, B_1 833 mcg, B_2 500 mcg, B_6 0.083 mcg, calcium pantothenate 833 mcg, niacinamide 5 mg, folic acid 0.066 mcg, niacinamide 5 mg, p-aminobenzoic acid 0.416 mcg, inositol 833 mcg, B_{12} 500 mcg, C 5 mg, calcium 33.1 mg, phosphorus 14.6 mg, iron 2.5 mg, iodine 0.15 mg/Tab. Bot. 100s, 500s, 1000s.
Use: Vitamin/mineral supplement.

•**METABROMSALEN.** USAN. 3,5-Dibromosalicylanilide.
Use: Germicide, disinfectant.

METABUTETHAMINE HYDROCHLORIDE. 2-Isobutylaminoethyl m-aminobenzoid HCl. 2-(Isobutylamino)ethanol m-Aminobenzoate (Ester) Monohydrochloride.
Use: Local anesthetic.

METABUTOXYCAINE HYDROCHLORIDE. 2′-Diethylaminoethyl 3-Amino-2-butoxybenzoate Hydro- Cl.
Use: Local anesthetic.

METACARAPHEN HYDROCHLORIDE. Netrin.

METACETAMOL. B.A.N. 3-Acetamidophenol.
Use: Analgesic.

METACORDRALONE.
See: Prednisolone. (Various Mfr.).

METACORTALONE.
See: Meticortelone, Susp. (Schering).

METACORTANDRACIN.
See: Prednisone, Tab. (Various Mfr.).

METACORTIN.
See: Meticorten, Tab. (Schering).

META-DELPHENE. Diethyltoluamide U.S.P. XXII.

METAGLYCODOL. 2-m-Chlorophenyl-3-methyl-2,3-butanediol.
Use: Central nervous system depressant.

METAHEXAMIDE. B.A.N. N-Cyclohexyl-N′-(3-amino-4-methylbenzene Sulfonyl) urea. Euglycin. Melanex.
Use: Hypoglycemic agent.

METAHYDRIN. (Merrell Dow) Trichlormethiazide 2 mg or 4 mg/Tab. Bot. 100s.
Use: Diuretic.

•**METALOL HYDROCHLORIDE.** USAN. 4′-[Hydroxy-2-(methylamino)-propyl methanesulfonanilide hydrochloride. Under study.
Use: Adrenergic β receptor antagonist.

METALONE T.B.A. (Foy) Prednisolone tertiary butylacetate 20 mg, sodium citrate 1 mg, polysorbate 80 1 mg, d-sorbitol 450 mg/ml, benzyl alcohol 0.9%, water for inj. Vial 10 ml.
Use: Corticosteroid.

METAMFEPRAMONE (I.N.N.). Dimepropion, B.A.N.

METAMUCIL. (Procter & Gamble) Psyllium hydrophilic mucilloid, sodium 1 mg, potassium 31 mg/Dose. **Regular Flavor:** w/dextrose. Jar 7 oz, 14 oz, 21 oz. Packette 5.4 Gm. Box 100s. **Orange and Strawberry Flavors:** w/flavoring, sucrose and coloring. Jar 7 oz, 14 oz, 21 oz.
Use: Laxative.

METAMUCIL INSTANT MIX. (Procter & Gamble) Psyllium hydrophilic mucilloid with citric acid, sucrose, potassium bicarbonate, sodium bicarbonate. Powder when combined with water forms an effervescent, flavored liquid. **Lemon Lime Flavor:** w/calcium carbonate. Cartons of 16, 30 or 100 packets of 3.4 Gm **Orange Flavor:** w/ flavoring and coloring. Ctn. 16 or 30 packets of 3.4 Gm.
Use: Laxative.

METAMUCIL, SUGAR FREE. (Procter & Gamble) Psyllium hydrophilic mucilloid in sugar-free formula. **Regular Flavor:** Jar 3.7 oz, 7.4 oz, 11.1 oz. Packet 3.4 Gm. Box 100s. **Orange Flavor:** Jar 3.7 oz, 7.4 oz, 11.1 oz.
Use: Laxative.

METANDREN. (Ciba) Methyltestosterone. **Linguet:** 5 mg or 10 mg Bot. 100s. **Tab.:** 10 mg or 25 mg Bot. 100s.
Use: Androgen.

METAPHENYLBARBITURIC ACID.
See: Mephobarbital.

METAPHYLLIN.
See: Aminophylline (Various Mfr.).

METAPREL INHALENT SOLUTION 5%. (Sandoz) Metaproterenol sulfate 50 mg/ml. Bot. 10 ml w/dropper.
Use: Bronchodilator.

METAPREL METERED DOSE INHALER. (Sandoz) Metaproterenol sulfate 225 mg, micronized powder in inert propellant/15 ml. Metered dose inhaler. (Approx. 0.65 mg/inhalation).
Use: Bronchodilator.

METAPREL SYRUP. (Sandoz) Metaproterenol sulfate 10 mg/5 ml. Bot. pt.
Use: Bronchodilator.

METAPREL TABLETS. (Sandoz) Metaproterenol sulfate 10 mg or 20 mg/Tab. Bot. 100s.
Use: Bronchodilator.

•**METAPROTERENOL SULFATE,** U.S.P. XXII. Inhalation Aerosol, Inhalation Soln., Syrup, Tab., U.S.P. XXII. 1,-(3,5-Dihydroxyphenyl)-2-isopropyl-amino-ethanol sulfate, Alupent.
Use: Bronchodilator.
See: Alupent Inhalation (Geigy).
Metaprel, Tab., Inhalation, Syr. (Sandoz).

METARAMINOL BITARTRATE, U.S.P. XXI. Inj., U.S.P. XXI. 1-α-(1-Aminoethyl)-m-hydroxybenzyl alcohol bitartrate. Benzenemethanol, a-(1 aminoethyl)-3-hydroxy-R-(R*,R*)-2,3-dihydroxybutandioate (1:1) (salt).
Use: Sympathomimetic amine (vasopressor).
See: Aramine, Amp., Vial (Merck Sharp & Dohme).

METASEP. (MiLance) Parachlorometaxylenol 2%, isopropyl alcohol 9%. Shampoo 120 ml.
Use: Antiseborrheic.

METATENSIN. (Merrell Dow) Trichlormethiazide 2 mg or 4 mg, each containing reserpine 0.1 mg/Tab. Bot. 100s.
Use: Antihypertensive.

METAZOCINE. B.A.N. 1,2,3,4,5,6-Hexahydro-8-hydroxy-3,6, 11-trimethyl-2,6-methano-3-benzazocine.
Use: Narcotic analgesic.

METCARAPHEN HYDROCHLORIDE. 2-Diethylaminoethyl-1-(3′,4′dimethylphenyl) cyclopentanecarboxylate HCl.

•**METENEPROST.** USAN.
Use: Oxytocic, prostaglandin.

METETHOHEPTAZINE. Ethyl hexahydro-1,3-dimethyl-4-phenyl-1H-azepine-4-carboxylate.
Use: Analgesic.

•**METFORMIN.** USAN. 1,1-Dimethylbiguanide. Diguanil; Glucophage; Metiguanide; Obin [HCl].
Use: Oral hypoglycemic.

METHACHOLINE BROMIDE. Mecholin bromide. (2-Hydroxypropyl)-trimethylammonium bromide acetate. Mecholyl Bromide.
Use: Cholinergic.

•**METHACHOLINE CHLORIDE,** U.S.P. XXII. (2-Hydroxypropyl)-trimethylammonium Cl acetate. Methylacetyl choline. Amechol.
Use: Cholinergic.
See: Mecholyl Cl, Amp. (J.T. Baker).
Provocholine, Amp. (Roche).
W/Camphor, menthol and methyl salicylate.
See: Surin, Oint. (McKesson).

METHACHOLINE CHLORIDE.
Use: Diagnostic aid.
See: Provocholine, pow. for reconstitution. (Roche).

•**METHACRYLIC ACID COPOLYMER,** N.F. XVII.
Use: Pharmaceutic aid (tablet coating agent).

•**METHACYCLINE.** USAN. 6-Deoxy-6-demethyl-6-methylene-5-oxytetracycline.
Use: Antibiotic.
See: Rondomycin, Cap., Syr. (Wallace).

•**METHACYCLINE HYDROCHLORIDE,** U.S.P. XXII. Cap., Oral Susp., U.S.P. XXII.
Use: Antibacterial.
See: Rondomycin, Cap., Syr. (Wallace).

•**METHADONE HYDROCHLORIDE,** U.S.P. XXII. Inj., Oral Concentrate, Tab., U.S.P. XXII. 6-Dimethylamino-4,4-diphenyl-3-heptanone hydrochloride. 3 Heptanone, 6-(dimethylamino)-4,4-diphenyl hydrochloride. Amidon HCl, Butalgin, Diaminon HCl, Hoechst 10820, Miadone, Physeptone HCl, Polamidon HCl.
Use: Narcotic analgesic, narcotic abstinence syndrome suppressant.
See: Dolophine HCl, Preps. (Lilly).
W/Aspirin, phenacetin, caffeine.
See: Nodalin, Tab. (Table Rock).

•**METHADYLACETATE.** USAN. 6-(Dimethylamino)-4,4-diphenyl-3-heptanol acetate (ester). 1-Ethyl-4-dimethylamino-2,2-diphenylpentyl acetate. Acetyl- methadol (I.N.N.).
Use: Narcotic analgesic.

•**METHAFILCON B.** USAN.
Use: Contact lens material.

METHAGUAL. (Gordon) Guaiacol 2%, methyl salicylate 8% in petrolatum. Oint. 2 oz, lb.

Use: External analgesic.

METHALAMIC ACID. Name used for Iothalamic acid, U.S.P. XXII.

METHALGEN. (Alra) Camphor, menthol, mustard oil, methyl salicylate in non-greasy cream base. Bot. 2 oz, Jar 4 oz, lb.
Use: External analgesic.

METHALLATAL. 5-Ethyl-5-(2-methylallyl)-2-thiobarbituric acid.

METHALLENESTRIL. B.A.N. 3-(6-Methoxy-2-naphthyl)-2,2-dimethylpentanoic acid.
Use: Estrogen.

•**METHALLIBURE.** USAN. 1-Methyl-6-(1-methylallyl)-2,5-dithiobiurea.
Use: Suppression of pituitary, ovarian, and adrenal function.

•**METHALTHIAZIDE.** USAN. 3-[(Allylthio)-methyl]-6-chloro-3,4-dihydro-2-methyl-2H-1,2,4-benzothiadiazine-7-sulfonamide 1,1-dioxide.
Use: Hypotensive, diuretic.

METHAMINODIAZEPOXIDE. Chlordiazepoxide HCl, U.S.P. XXII.
See: Librium, Cap., Amp. (Roche).

METHAMOCTOL. 2-Methyl-6-(methylamino)-2-heptanol.
Use: Adrenergic.

METHAMPHAZONE. B.A.N. 4-Amino-6-methyl-2-phenyl-3((2H)-pyridazone.
Use: Analgesic, antirheumatic.

•**METHAMPHETAMINE HYDROCHLORIDE,** U.S.P. XXII Deoxyephedrine hydrochloride; N-α-Dimethyl-phenethylamine hydrochloride.
Use: Central nervous system stimulant.
See: Desoxyn, Gradumets, Tab. (Abbott).
Methampex, Tab. (Lemmon).
Methamphetamine HCl, Tab. (Various Mfr.).
W/Amobarbital; homatropine methylbromide.
See: Obe-Slim, Tab. (Jenkins).
W/dl-Methamphetamine HCl, butabarbital.
See: Span-RD, Tab. (Metro Med).
W/Pamabrom, pyrilamine maleate, homatropine methylbromide, hyoscyamine sulfate, scopolamine HBr.
See: Aridol, Tab. (MPL).
W/Pentobarbital sodium, vitamins, minerals.
See: Fetamin, Tab. (Mission).

dl-METHAMPHETAMINE HCl. dl-Desoxyephedrine HCl.
See: Oxydess, Tab. (North American).
Roxyn, Tab. (Rocky Mtn.).
W/d-Methamphetamine HCl, butabarbital.
See: Span-RD, Span RD-12, Tab. (Metro Med).
W/Pyrilamine maleate, phenyltoloxamine dihydrogen citrate, didesoxyephedrine HCl, codeine phosphate, ammonium Cl, potassium guaiacolsulfonate, chloroform, phenylpropanolamine tartar emetic.
See: Meditussin-X Liquid (Hauck).

METHAMPYRONE.
See: Dipyrone.

METHANDIENONE. B.A.N. 17 β-Hydroxy-17 α-methylandrosta-1,4-dien-3-one. Dianabol.
Use: Anabolic steroid.

METHANDRIOL. Methylandrostenediol. (Various Mfr.) 17-alpha-methyl-Δ^5-androstene-3-beta, 17 beta-diol. Diolostene, Mestenediol, Methanabol, Spenbolic.
See: Anabol, Inj. (Keene Pharm.).

METHANDRIOL DIPROPIONATE.
See: Andriol Inj. (Solvay).
Arbolic, Inj. (Burgin-Arden).
Crestabolic, Vial (Nutrition).
Durandrol, Vial (Pharmex).
Fellobolic, Vial (Fellows-Testagar).
Probolik (Hickam).
Robolic, Vial (Rocky Mtn.).

METHANDROSTENOLONE. Δ^1-17 α-methyltestosterone. 17 α-Methyl-17 β-hydroxyandrosta-1,4-dien-3one. 17 β-Hydroxy-17-methylandrosta-1,4-dien-3-one.
See: Dianabol, Tab. (Ciba).

METHANTHELINIUM BROMIDE. B.A.N. 2-Diethyl- aminoethyl xanthen-9-carboxylate methobromide. Banthine Bromide.
Use: Anticholinergic.

•**METHANTHELINE BROMIDE,** U.S.P. XXII. Sterile, Tab., U.S.P. XXII. Diethyl (2-hydroxyethyl)methyl-ammonium bromide xanthene-9-carboxylate.
Use: Parasympatholytic, anticholinergic.
See: Banthine, Vial, Tab. (Searle).
W/Phenobarbital.
See: Banthine w/Phenobarbital, Tab. (Searle).

METHAPHENILENE. B.A.N. 2-(N-Phenyl-N-2-thenylamino)ethyldimethylamine. Diatrin [hydrochloride].
Use: Antihistamine.

METHAPHOR. (Borden) Protein hydrolysate (l-leucine, l-isoleucine, l-methionine, l-phenylalanine, l-tyrosine); methionine, camphor, benzethonium Cl, in Dermabase vehicle/Oint. Tube 1.5 oz.
Use: Dermatologic, amino acid preparation.

METHAPYRILENE FUMARATE. 2-[[2-(Dimethylami-no)-ethyl]-2-thenylamino pyridine fumarate (2:3).
NOTE: Due to recent legislation many products are being reformulated to exclude oral use of this drug. This drug is no longer official in the U.S.P.
Use: Antihistamine.

METHAPYRILENE HYDROCHLORIDE, 2-[[2-Diemthylamino)-ethyl]-2-thenylamino] pyridine hydrochloride. (Thenylpyramine, Teralin). Blue Line—Elixir 200 mg/fl oz. Bot. pt, gal. Kenyon-Vial 20 mg/ml.
NOTE: Due to recent legislation many products are being reformulated to exclude oral use of this drug. This drug is no longer official in the U.S.P.
Use: Antihistamine.

METHAPYRILENE HYDROCHLORIDE W/COMBINATIONS.
NOTE: Due to recent legislation many prod-

ucts are being reformulated to exclude oral use of this drug.

•**METHARBITAL,** U.S.P. XXII. Tab., U.S.P. XXII. 5,5′-Diethyl-1-methylbarbituric acid.
Use: Anticonvulsant.
See: Gemonil, Tab. (Abbott).

METHARBITONE. B.A.N. 5,5-Diethyl-1-methylbarbituric acid.
Use: Anticonvulsant.

METHATROPIC CAPSULES. (Goldline) Choline 115 mg, inositol 83 mg, methionine 110 mg, vitamins B_1 3 mg, B_2 3 mg, B_3 10 mg, B_5 2 mg, B_6 2 mg, B_{12} 2 mcg, desiccated liver 56 mg, liver concentrate 30 mg/Cap. Bot. 100s, 1000s.
Use: Nutritional supplement.

METHAZINE. (Pharmex) Promethazine HCl 50 mg/ml. Vial 10 ml.
Use: Antihistamine.

•**METHAZOLAMIDE,** U.S.P. XXII. Tab. U.S.P. XXII. N-(4-Methyl-2-sulfamoyl-Δ^2-1,3,4-thiadiazolin-5-ylidene)acetamide. Acetamide, N-5-(aminosulfonyl)-3-methyl-1,3,4-thiadiazol-2(3H)-ylidene-. 5-Acetylimino-4-meth-yl-1,3,4-thiadiazoline-2-sulfonamide.
Use: Carbonic anhydrase inhibitor.
See: Neptazane.
Neptazane, Tab. (Lederle).

METH-CHOLINE CAPSULES. (Schein) Choline 115 mg, inositol 83 mg, methionine 110 mg, vitamins B_1 3 mg, B_2 3 mg, B_3 10 mg, B_5 2 mg, B_6 2 mg, B_{12} 2 mcg, desiccated liver 56 mg, liver concentrate 30 mg/Cap. Bot. 100s, 250s, 1000s.
Use: Nutritional supplement.

METH-DIA-MER SULFA TABLETS. Trisulfapyrimidines Tab., U.S.P. XXII.
Use: Triple sulfonamide therapy.
See: Chemozine, Tab. (Tennessee Pharm.).
Neotrizine, Tab. (Lilly).
Terfonyl, Susp., (Squibb).
Triple Sulfa, Tab. (Various Mfr.).

METH-DIA-MER SULFONAMIDES.
Use: Triple sulfonamide therapy.
W/Sulfacetamide.
See: Sulfa-Plex Vaginal Cream (Solvay).
W/Sulfacetamide, hexestrol.
See: Vagi-Plex, Cream (Solvay).

METH-DIA-MER SULFONAMIDES SUSPENSION, Trisulfapyrimidines Oral Suspension, U.S.P. XXII.
Use: Triple sulfonamide therapy.
See: Chemozine, Susp. (Tennessee Pharm.).
Neotrizine, Susp. (Lilly).
Terfonyl, Susp. (Squibb).
Triple Sulfa, Susp. (CMC).

METHDILAZINE, U.S.P. XXII. Tab., U.S.P. XXII. 10-(1-Methylpyrrolidin-3-ylmethyl)phenothiazine. Dilosyn (hydrochloride).
See: Tacaryl Chew. Tab. (Westwood).

•**METHDILAZINE HCl,** U.S.P. XXII. Syrup, Tab., U.S.P. XXII. 10-(1-Methyl-pyrrolidinyl)phenothiazine HCl.
Use: Antipruritic.
See: Tacaryl, Tab. (Westwood).

•**METHENAMINE,** U.S.P. XXII. Elix., Tab., U.S.P. XXII. (Hexamethyleneamine, Cystamin, Cystogen, Hexamine, Hexamethylenetetramine.).
Use: Antibacterial (urinary).

METHENAMINE W/COMBINATIONS.
Use: Urinary anti-infective.
See: Cystamine, Tab. (Tennessee Pharm.).
Cystised, Tab. (Jenkins).
Cystitol, Tab. (Briar).
Cysto, Tab. (Freeport).
Cystrea, Tab. (Moore Kirk).
Hexalol, Tab. (Central).
Lanased, Tab. (Lannett).
Urelief, Tab. (Rocky Mtn.).
Urisan-P, Tab. (Sandia).
Urised, Tab. (Webcon).
Uritrol, Tab. (Kenyon).
Uro Phosphate, Tab. (Poythress).
UTA, Tab. (Bentex).
U-Tract, Tab. (Bowman).
U-Tran, Tab. (Scruggs).

METHENAMINE AND MONOBASIC SODIUM PHOSPHATE TABLETS, U.S.P. XXII.
Use: Antibacterial (urinary).

METHENAMINE ANHYDROMETHYLENE CITRATE. Formanol, Uropurgol, Urotropin.

•**METHENAMINE HIPPURATE,** U.S.P. XXII. Tab., U.S.P. XXII. A 1:1 complex of methenamine and hippuric acid.
Use: Urinary antiseptic.
See: Hiprex, Tab. (Merrell Dow).
Urex, Tab.(Riker).

•**METHENAMINE MANDELATE,** U.S.P. XXII. Tab., For Oral Soln., Oral Susp.; U.S.P. XXII.
Use: Urinary antibacterial.
See: Mandacon, Tab. (Webcon).
Mandalay, Tab. (Beutlich).
Mandelamine, Tab., Susp. (Parke-Davis).
Mandelamine "Hafgram" Tab. (Parke-Davis).
Mandelets, Tab. (Quality Generics).
Methavin, Tab. (Star).
Renelate, Tab. (Forest Pharm.).

METHENAMINE MANDELATE W/COMBINATIONS.
Use: Antibacterial (urinary).
See: Mandex, Tab. (Vale).
Pyrisul Plus, Tab. (Kenyon).
Thiacide, Tab. (Beach).
Urisedamine, Tab. (Webcon).

•**METHENOLONE ACETATE.** USAN. 17 β-Hydroxy-1-methyl-5 α-androst-1-en-3-one acetate. Primobolan.
Use: Anabolic agent.

•**METHENOLONE ENANTHATE.** USAN. 17β-Hydroxy-1-methyl-5αandrost-1-en-3-one heptanoate. Nibal injection. Primobolan.
Use: Anabolic.

METHEPONEX. (Rawl) Choline 0.54 Gm, dl-methionine 1.80 Gm, inositol 0.27 Gm, whole desiccated liver 8.10 Gm, vitamins B_1 18 mg, B_2 36

mg, niacinamide 90 mg, B_6 3.6 mg, calcium pantothenate 3.6 mg, biotin 10.8 mcg, B_{12} 5.4 mcg and amino acid/daily therapeutic dose. Cap. Bot. 100s, 500s.
Use: Antidiabetic, nutritional supplement.

METHEPTAZINE. Methyl hexahydro-1, 2-dimethyl-4-phenyl-1H-azepine-4-carboxylate.
Use: Analgesic.

METHERGINE. (Sandoz) Methylergonovine maleate. **Amp.:** 0.2 mg/ml, tartaric acid 0.25 mg, sodium Cl 3 mg/ml. SandoPak 20s, 100s. **Tab.:** 0.2 mg. Bot. 100s, 1000s, SandoPak pkgs. 100s.
Use: Hormone.

METHESTROL.
See: Promethestrol (Various Mfr.).

METHETHARIMIDE BEMEGRIDE. 3-Methyl-3-ethyl glutarimide.

METHETOIN. USAN. 5-Ethyl-1-methyl-5- phenylimidazoline-2,4-dione. Deltoin.
Use: Anticonvulsant.

METHIBON CAPSULES. (Barrows) Choline dihydrogen citrate 278 mg, dl-methionine 111 mg, inositol 83.3 mg, vitamin B_{12} 2 mcg, liver concentrate, desiccated liver 86.6 mg/Cap. Bot. 100s.
Use: Antidiabetic, nutritional supplement.

METHICILLIN SODIUM, STERILE, U.S.P. XXII., Inj., U.S.P. XXII. Sodium 2,6-Dimethoxyphenyl penicillin. Dimethoxyphenyl pencillin sodium
Use: Antibiotic.
See: Celbenin, Vial (Beecham Labs).
Staphcillin, Vial (Bristol).

METHIMAZOLE, U.S.P. XXII. Tab., U.S.P. XXII. 1-Methylimidazole-2-thiol. Mercazole. 2H-imidazole-2-thione, 1,3-dihydro-1-methyl.
Use: Thyroid inhibitor (5 mg to 20 mg).
See: Tapazole, Tab. (Lilly).
Thiamazole (I.N.N.).

METHINDIZATE. V.B.A.N. 2-(1-Methyloctahydroindol-3-yl)ethyl benzilate. Present in Isaverine HCl.
Use: Spasmolytic (veterinary).

METHIODAL SODIUM, U.S.P. XXI. Inj., U.S.P. XXII. Sodium monoiodomethanesulfonate. Abrodil, Radiographol, Diagnorenol.
Use: Radiopaque.

METHIOKAPS. (Vale) dl-methionine 200 mg/Cap. Bot. 1000s.
Use: Diaper rash product.

METHIOMEPRAZINE HCl. dl-10-(3-Dimethylamino-2-methylpropyl)-2-methylthiophenothiazine HCl. (SmithKline).
Use: Antiemetic.

METHIONINE, U.S.P. XXII. **Note:** Also see Racemethionine, U.S.P. XXII.
Use: Amino acid.

METHIOPLEX. (Lincoln) Methionine 25 mg, vitamins B_1 50 mg, niacinamide 100 mg, B_2 2 mg, choline 50 mg, B_6 2 mg, panthenol 2 mg, benzyl alcohol 1%, distilled water q.s./ml. Vial 30 ml.
Use: Nutritional supplement.

•**METHISAZONE.** USAN. N-methylisatin-β-thiosemicarbazone. 1-Methylindoline-2,3-dione 3-thiosemicarbazone. Marboran.
Use: Antiviral drug.

METHITURAL SODIUM. 5-(1-Methylbutyl)-5-[2-(methylthio)ethyl]-2-thiobarbituric acid sodium salt.
Use: Hypnotic; sedative.

METHIXENE. B.A.N. 9-(1-Methyl-3-piperidylmethyl)- thiaxanthen. Tremonil (hydrochloride).
Use: Treatment of the Parkinsonian syndrome.

METHNITE. (Kenyon) Methscopolamine nitrate 2.5 mg/Tab. Bot. 100s, 1000s.
Use: Antispasmodic.

•**METHOCARBAMOL,** U.S.P. XXII. Cap., Tab., U.S.P. XXII. 1,2-Propanediol, 3-(2-methoxy phenoxy)-, 1-carbamate. (2-Hydroxy-3-o-methoxyphenoxypropyl) carbamate. 3-(o-Methoxyphenoxy)-1,2-propanediol1-carbamate.
Use: Skeletal muscle relaxant.
See: Delaxin, Tab. (Ferndale).
Robaxin, Tab., Inj. (Robins).
Romethocarb, Tab. (Robinson).
W/Aspirin.
See: Robaxisal, Tab. (Robins).

METHOCEL. Methylcellulose.

•**METHOHEXITAL,** U.S.P. XXII.
Use: Pharmaceutical necessity for Methohexital Sodium for Injection.

•**METHOHEXITAL SODIUM FOR INJECTION,** U.S.P. XXII. Alpha-(dl)-5-allyl-1-methyl-5-(1-methyl-2-pentynyl) barbituric sodium 2,4,6(IH,-3H,5H)-pyrimidinetrione,. 1-methyl-5-(1-methyl-2-pentynyl)-5-(2-propenyl)-, (±) monosodium salt.
Use: General anesthetic (intravenous).
See: Brevital, Amp., Pow. (Lilly).

METHOHEXITONE. B.A.N. α-5-Allyl-1-methyl-5-(1-methylpent-2-ynyl)barbituric acid.
Use: Anesthetic.

METHOIN. B.A.N. 5-Ethyl-3-methyl-5-phenylhydantoin. 5-Ethyl-3-methyl-5-phenylimidazoline-2,4-dione. Mephenytoin (I.N.N.).
Use: Anticonvulsant.

•**METHOPHOLINE HCl.** USAN. 1-(p-Chlorophenethyl)-2-methyl-6, 7-dimethoxy-1,2,3,4-tetrahydroisoquinoline HCl.
Use: Analgesic.
See: Versidyne.

METHOPTO 0.25%. (Professional Pharmacal) Methylcellulose pow. 2.5 mg (0.25% soln.), boric acid 12 mg, potassium Cl 7.3 mg, benzalkonium Cl 0.04 mg, glycerin 12 mg/ml w/sodium carbonate to adjust pH and purified water. Bot. 15 ml, 30 ml.
Use: Artificial tear solution.

METHOPTO FORTE 0.5%. (Professional Pharmacal) Methylcellulose pow. 5 mg (0.5% soln.), boric acid 12 mg, potassium Cl 7.3 mg, benzalkonium Cl 0.4 mg, glycerin 12 mg/ml w/sodium

carbonate to adjust pH and purified water. Bot. 15 ml.
Use: Artificial tear solution.
METHOPTO FORTE 1%. (Professional Pharmacal) Methylcellulose pow. 10 mg (1% soln.), boric acid 12 mg, potassium Cl 7.3 mg, benzalkonium Cl 0.04 mg, glycerin 12 mg/ml w/sodium carbonate to adjust pH and purified water. Bot. 15 ml.
Use: Artificial tear solution.
METHOPYRAPHONE.
See: Metopirone, Tab., Amp. (Ciba).
METHORATE.
See: Dextromethorphan HBr.
METHORBATE S.C. (Standex) Methenamine 40.8 mg, atropine sulfate 0.03 mg, hyoscyamine sulfate 0.03 mg, salol 18.1 mg, benzoic acid 4.5 mg, methylene blue 5.4 mg/Tab. Bot. 100s.
Use: Urinary anti-infective.
d-METHORPHAN HBr.
See: Dextromethorphan HBr (Various Mfr.).
METHORPHINAN. •Racemorphan HBr. Dromoran.
l-METHORPHINAN LEVORPHANOL.
See: Levo-Dromoran, Amp., Tab., Vial (Roche).
METHOSERPIDINE. B.A.N. 10-Methoxydeserpidine.
Use: Hypotensive.
•**METHOTREXATE,** U.S.P. XXII. Tab., U.S.P. XXII. Amethopterin. 4-Amino-10-methylfolic acid. N-[p-[[(2,4-Diamino-6-pteridinyl)-methyl]-methylamino]benzoyl] glutamic acid. L-glutamic acid, N-[4-[[(2,4-diamino-6-pteridinyl)methyl] -me-thylamino]benzoyl]. (Lederle) Tab. 2.5 mg. Bot. 100s.
Use: Leukemia in children, antineoplastic, antipsoriatic.
•**METHOTREXATE SODIUM FOR INJECTION.** U.S.P. XXII. 4-Amino-N^{10}-methyl-pteroylglutamic acid sodium. (Lederle) 2.5 mg/ml Vial 2 ml; 25 mg/ml. Vial 2 ml w/preservatives; 20 mg, 50 mg, 100 mg Vial cryodesiccated, preservative free; 50 mg, 100 mg, 200 mg Vial; 25 mg/ml solution preservative free.
Use: Leukemia therapy, psoriasis.
See: Folex, Inj. (Adria) Folex PFS. Inj. (Adria) Methotrexate, Inj., Pow. (Lederle).
Mexate, Inj. (Bristol).
•**METHOTRIMEPRAZINE,** U.S.P. XXII. Inj., U.S.P. XXII. 2-Methoxy-10-(3-dimethylamino-2-methylpropyl)phenothiazine. (—)-10-(3-(Dimethylamino)-2-methyl-propyl)-2-methoxyphenothiazine. Levomepromazine (I.N.N.) Veractil.
Use: Tranquilizer, non-addicting analgesic.
See: Levoprome, Amp., Vial (Lederle).
•**METHOXSALEN,** U.S.P. XXII. Cap., U.S.P. XXII.
Use: Topical pigmenting agent.
See: Meloxine, (Upjohn).
Oxsoralen, Cap., Lot. (Elder).
Oxsoralen-Ultra, Cap. (Elder).
•**METHOXSALEN TOPICAL SOLUTION,** U.S.P. XXII. 8-Methoxypsoralen. 8-Hydroxy-4′,5′,6,7-furocoumarin, ammoidin, xanthotoxin. 7H-Furo[3,2-g][1] benzopyran-7-one,2-methoxy-9-methoxy-7H-Furo[3,2-g][1]benzopyran-7-one.
Use: Topical pigmenting agent.
METHOXYDONE.
See: Mephenoxalone (Various Mfr.).
•**METHOXYFLURANE,** U.S.P. XXII. 2,2-Dichloro-1,1-difluoroethyl methyl ether.
Use: General inhalation anesthetic.
See: Penthrane, Liq. (Abbott).
METHOXYPHENAMINE HYDROCHLORIDE, U.S.P. XXI. o-Methoxy-N, α-dimethylphenethylamino HCl.
Use: Adrenergic (bronchodilator).
W/Chlorpheniramine maleate, acetophenetidin, acetylsalicylic acid, caffeine.
See: Pyrroxate, Cap., Tab. (Upjohn).
W/Dextromethorphan HCl, orthoxine, sodium citrate.
See: Orthoxicol, Syr. (Upjohn).
W/Dextromethorphan HBr, phenylephrine HCl, chlorpheniramine maleate.
See: Statuss, Syr., Cap. (Elder).
W/Medrol.
See: Medrol, Tab. (Upjohn).
METHOXYPROMAZINE MALEATE. 10-[3-(Dimethylamino)propyl]-2-methoxyphenothiazine maleate. Tentone.
Use: CNS depressant.
•**METHSCOPOLAMINE BROMIDE,** U.S.P. XXII. Tab., U.S.P. XXII. Inj. U.S.P. XXI. Epoxytropine tropate methylbromide, scopolamine methylbromide, hyoscine methylbromide. 6β, 7β-Epoxy-3α-hydroxy-8-methyl-1αH, 5αH-tropanium bromide(−)-Tropate.
Use: Anticholinergic.
See: Pamine, Tab., Vial (Upjohn).
Scoline, Tab.(Westerfield).
W/Amobarbital.
See: Scoline-Amobarbital, Tab. (Westerfield).
W/Butabarbital Sodium, dried aluminum hydroxide gel and magnesium trisilicate.
See: Eulcin, Tab. (Leeds Pharmacal).
W/Phenobarbital.
See: Pamine PB, Preps. (Upjohn).
Synt-PB, Tab. (Scrip).
W/Phenylpropanolamine HCl, chlorpheniramine maleate.
See: Bobid, Cap. (Boyd).
Symptrol, Cap. (Saron).
METHSCOPOLAMINE NITRATE. Scopolamine Methyl Nitrate, Preps. (Various Mfr.) Mescomine.
See: Cenahist, Cap. (Century).
Conalsyn Chroncap, Cap. (Cenci).
Dallergy, Cap., Tab., Syr. (Laser).
Extendryl, Cap., Tab., Syr. (Fleming).
Histaspan-D, Cap. (Rorer).
Sanhist T.D. 12, Tab. (Sandia).
Scotnord, Tab. (Scott/Cord).
Sinovan, Timed Cap. (Drug Ind.).

Spasmid, Elix., Tab. (Dalin).

METHSUXIMIDE, U.S.P. XXII. Cap., U.S.P. XXII. N,2-Dimethyl-2-phenylsuccinamide Mesuximide (I.N.N.).
Use: Anticonvulsant.
See: Celontin Kapseal (Parke-Davis).

METHYCLODINE. (Rugby) Methyclothiazide 5 mg, deserpidine 0.25 mg/Tab. Bot. 100s.
Use: Antihypertensive, diuretic.

METHYCLOTHIAZIDE, U.S.P. XXII. Tab., U.S.P. XXII. 6-Chloro-3-chloro-methyl-2-methyl-7-sulfamyl-3,4-dihydro-1,2,4-benzothiadiazine-1,1-dioxide. 6-Chloro-3-(chloromethyl)-3,4-dihydro-2-methyl-2H-1,2,4-benzothiadiazine-7-sulfonamide 1,1-Dioxide.
Use: Diuretic, antihypertensive.
See: Enduron, Tab. (Abbott) Methyclodine, Tab. (Rugby).
W/Deserpidine.
See: Enduronyl, Tab. (Abbott).
Enduronyl Forte, Tab. (Abbott).
W/Pargyline HCl.
See: Eutron, Tab. (Abbott).

METHYLACETYLCHOLINE.
See: Methacholine.

METHYL ALCOHOL, N.F. XVII.
Use: Pharmaceutic acid (solvent).

METHYLAMPHETAMINE HYDROCHLORIDE & SULFATE.
See: Desoxyephedrine HCl (Various Mfr.).

METHYLANDROSTENEDIOL.
See: Hybolin, Vial (Hyrex).
Methandriol.
Methyldiol, Preps. (North American Pharm).
W/Adrenal cortex extract, Vitamin B_{12}.
See: Geri-Ace, Inj. (Brown).
W/Carboxymethylcellulose sodium, thimerosal.
See: Cenabolic, Vial (Century).
W/Pentylenetetrazol, nicotinic acid, l-lysine, dl-methionine, ethinyl estradiol, thiamine, pyridoxine, riboflavin, vitamins B_{12}, A, D, ascorbic acid.
See: Ardiatric, Tab. (Burgin-Arden).

METHYLBENZETHONIUM CHLORIDE, U.S.P. XXII. Lotion, Oint., Pow., U.S.P. XXII. Benzyl-dimethyl-2[2-(p-1,1,3-tetramethyl-butyl-cresoxy)ethoxy]-ethyl ammonium Cl. (p-Tertiary octyl cresoxy ethoxy ethyl dimethyl-benzyl ammonium Cl). Benzyldimethyl[2[2-[[4-(1,1,3,3-tetramethylbutyl)tolyl]oxy]ethoxy]-ethyl]ammonium Cl.
Use: Bactericide, local anti-infective.
See: Ammorid, Oint. (Kinney).
Benephen, Prods. (Halsted).
Cuticura Acne Cream (Purex).
Cuticura Medicated First Aid Cream (Purex).
Diaparene Prods. (Glenbrook).
Fordustin, Pow. (Sween).
Surgi-Kleen, Liq. (Sween).
W/Cod liver oil.
See: Benephen, Prods. (Halsted).
Sween Cream (Sween).
W/Magnesium stearate.
See: Mennen Baby Pow. (Mennen).
W/Phenol, acetanilid, zinc oxide, calamine and eucalyptol.
See: Taloin, Oint. (Warren-Teed).
W/Phenylmercuric acetate, methylparaben.
See: Lorophyn, Supp. (Eaton).
Norforms, Aerosal, Supp. (Norwich).
W/Zinc oxide, calamine, eucalyptol.
See: Taloin, Tube (Warren-Teed).

METHYL BENZOQUATE. V.B.A.N. Methyl 7-benzyloxy-6-butyl-1,4-dihydro-4-oxoquinoline-3-carboxylate. Nequinate (I.N.N.) Statyl.
Use: Antiprotozoan, veterinary medicine.

METHYLBENZTROPINE.
See: Ethybenztropine (Sandoz).

METHYLBROMTROPIN MANDELATE.
See: Homatropine Methylbromide, U.S.P. XXII.

•**METHYLCELLULOSE,** U.S.P. XXII. Ophth. Soln., Oral Soln., Tab., U.S.P. XXII. Cellulose methylether. Mellose.
Use: Suspending agent.
See: Cellothyl, Tab. (International Drug).
Cologel, Soln. (Lilly).
Isopto-Plain, Liq. (Alcon).
Melozets, Wafer (Calgon).
Tearisol, Soln. (Smith, Miller & Patch).
W/Benzocaine, vitamins, minerals, niacinamide.
See: Rite-Diet, Cap. (E.J. Moore).
W/Boric acid, glycerine, propylene glycol, methylparaben, propylparaben, irish moss extract.
See: Canfield Lubricating Jelly (Paddock).
W/Carboxymethylcellulose.
See: Ex-Caloric, Wafer (Eastern Research).
W/Dicyclomine HCl, magnesium trisilicate, aluminum hydroxide-magnesium carbonate, dried.
See: Triactin Tab. (Norwich).
W/Dicyclomine HCl, aluminum hydroxide and magnesium hydroxide.
See: Triactin Liq. (Norwich).
W/Phenylephrine HCl.
See: Vernacel (Professional Pharmacal).
W/Phenylephrine HCl, benzalkonium Cl.
See: Efricel ⅛% (Professional Pharmacal).
W/Polysorbate 80, boric acid.
See: Lacril Artificial Tears (Allergan).

METHYLCHROMONE. B.A.N. 3-Methyl-(4H)-chromen-4-one.
Use: Coronary vasodilator.

METHYLCYSTEINE. B.A.N. Methyl 2-amino-3-mercaptoproprionate. Mecysteine (I.N.N.) Acdrile; Visclair [hydrochloride]
Use: Vasoconstrictor.

METHYL CYSTEINE HYDROCHLORIDE. Cysteine methyl ester hydrochloride.
Use: Mucolytic agent.

METHYLDESORPHINE. B.A.N. 6-Methyl-Δ^6-deoxymorphine.
Use: Narcotic analgesic.

•**METHYLDOPA,** U.S.P. XXII. Oral Susp., Tab. U.S.P. XXII. Levo-3-(3,4-dihydroxyphenyl)-2-methylalanine.
Use: Antihypertensive.
See: Aldomet, Tab. (Merck Sharp & Dohme).

•**METHYLDOPA AND CHLOROTHIAZIDE TABLETS,** U.S.P. XXII.
Use: Antihypertensive.
See: Aldoclor, Tab. (Merck Sharp & Dohme).

•**METHYLDOPA AND HYDROCHLOROTHIAZIDE TABLETS,** U.S.P. XXII.
Use: Antihypertensive.
See: Aldoril, Tab. (Merck Sharp & Dohme).

METHYLDOPA/HYDROCHLOROTHIAZIDE. (Mylan) Methyldopa 250 mg, hydrochlorothiazide 15 mg or 25 mg/Tab. Bot. 100s, 1000s.
Use: Antihypertensive.

METHYLDOPA/HYDROCHLOROTHIAZIDE. (Rugby) Methyldopa 500 mg, hydrochlorothiazide 50 mg/Tab. Bot. 100s.
Use: Antihypertensive.

•**METHYLDOPATE HCl,** U.S.P. XXII. Inj. U.S.P. XXII. (Merck Sharp & Dohme) Ethyl ester of levo-3-(3,4-dihydroxyphenyl)-2-methylalanine HCl. l-Tyrosine, 3-hydroxy-α-methyl-,ethyl ester hydrochloride-.
Use: Antihypertensive agent.
See: Aldomet Ester HCl, Inj. (Merck Sharp & Dohme).

METHYLDOPATE HCl. (Lyphomed) Methyldopate HCl 250 mg/5 ml. Inj. Vial. 6 ml.
Use: Antihypertensive.

•**METHYLENE BLUE,** U.S.P. XXII. Inj. U.S.P. XXII. (Various Mfr.) Methylthionine Cl. 3,7-Bix-(Dimethyl-amino)phenzathionium Cl.
Use: Antimethemoglobinemic, antidote to cyanide poisoning.
See: Urolene Blue, Tab. (Star).
Wright's Stain, Liq. (Hynson, Westcott & Dunning).

METHYLENE BLUE W/COMBINATIONS.
See: Cystrea, Tab. (Moore Kirk).
Hexalol, Tab. (Central).
Lanased, Tab. (Lannett).
Urised, Tab. (Webcon).
U-Tract, Tab. (Bowman).

•**METHYLENE CHLORIDE,** N.F. XVII.
Use: Pharmaceutic aid (solvent).

METHYLERGOMETRINE. B.A.N. N-(+)-1-(Hydroxymethyl)propyl-(+)-lysergamide.
Use: Uterine stimulant.

•**METHYLERGONOVINE MALEATE,** U.S.P. XXII. Inj., Tab., U.S.P. XXII. 9,10-Didehydro-N-[(S)-1-(hydroxymethyl) propyl]-6-methylergoline-8-carboxamide maleate (1:1).
Use: Oxytocic.
See: Methergine, Amp., Tab. (Sandoz).

METHYLETHYLAMINO-PHENYLPROPANOL HCl.
See: Nethamine HCl. (Various Mfr.).

METHYLGLUCAMINE DIATRIZOATE, INJ., A water-soluble radiopaque iodine cpd. N-methylglucamine salt of Diatrizoate.
See: Diatrizoate (Various Mfr.).
Diatrizoate Meglumine Inj., U.S.P. XXII.

METHULGLUCAMINE IODIPAMIDE, INJ.
See: Meglumine Iodipamide, Inj., U.S.P. XXII. (Various Mfr.).
W/Diatrizoate methylglucamine.
See: Sinografin, Vial (Squibb).

METHYLGLYOXAL-BIS-GUANYLHYDRAZONE. Methyl GAG.

N-METHYLHYDRAZINE.
Use: Antineoplastic.
See: Procarbazine.

N-METHYLISATIN BETA-THIOSEMICARBAZONE. Under study.
Use: Smallpox protection.

•**METHYL ISOBUTYL KETONE,** N.F. XVII. 4-Methyl-2-pentanone.
Use: Pharmaceutic aid (alcohol denaturant).

METHYLISO-OCTENYLAMINE.
See: Isometheptene HCl (Various Mfr.).

METHYLMERCADONE. Name used for Nifuratel.

METHYL NICOTINATE.
W/Histamine dihydrochloride, oleoresin capsicum, glycomonosalicylate.
See: Akes-N-Pain Rub, Oint. (Moore).
W/methyl salicylate, menthol.
See: Musterole Deep Strength Oint. (Schering-Plough).
W/Methyl salicylate, menthol, camphor, dipropylene glycol salicylate, cassia oil, oleoresins capsicum, ginger.
See: Arthaderm, Lot. (Paddock).
Scrip-Gesic, Oint. (Scrip).

METHYLONE. (Paddock) Methylprednisolone acetate 40 mg/ml. Vial 5 ml.
Use: Corticosteroid.

•**METHYL PALMOXIRATE.** USAN.
Use: Antidiabetic.
See: Antidiabetic.

•**METHYLPARABEN,** N.F. XVII. (Various Mfr.) Methyl p-hydroxybenzoate. Methyl Chemosept.
Use: Pharmaceutic aid (antifungal preservative).

•**METHYLPARABEN SODIUM.** USAN. N.F. XVII.
Use: Antifungal preservative (Pharmaceutic aid).

METHYLPARAFYNOL. 3-Methyl-pentyne-1-ol-3. Oblivon, Somnesin.

METHYLPENTYNOL. B.A.N. 3-Methylpent-1-yn-3-ol. Atempol, Insomnol, Meparfynol, Methylparafynol, Oblivon, Somnesin and Oblivon-C Carbamate.
Use: Tranquilizer.

METHYLPHENETHYLAMINE. 1-alpha-Methylphenethylamine.
See: Amphetamine HCl (Various Mfr.).

•**METHYLPHENIDATE HCl,** U.S.P. XXII. Tab., Extended-release Tab., U.S.P. XXII. Methyl a-phenyl-2-piperidine-acetate hydrochloride.
Use: CNS stimulant.
See: Ritalin HCl, Tab., Vial (Ciba).

METHYLPHENIDYLACETATE HCl. Methyl 1-phenyl-2-piperidylacetate.
See: Methylphenidate HCl (Various Mfr.).

METHYLPHENOBARBITAL. N-Methyl-5-ethyl-5-phenylbarbituric Acid.
See: Mephobarbital.

d-METHYLPHENYLAMINE SULFATE.
See: Dextroamphetamine Sulfate, U.S.P. XXII. (Various Mfr.).
METHYL PHENYLETHYLHYDANTOIN.
See: Mesantoin, Tab. (Sandoz).
METHYLPHENYLSUCCINIMIDE.
See: Milontin, Kapseal, Susp. (Parke-Davis).
METHYLPHYTYL NAPHTHOQUINONE.
Use: Vitamin K supplement.
See: Phytonadione.
METHYL POLYSILOXANE.
See: Mylicon, Tab., Drops (Stuart).
Phasil, Tab. (Reed & Carnrick).
Silain, Tab. (Robins).
Simethicone.
METHYLPRED-40. (Seatrace) Methylprednisolone acetate 40 mg/ml. Vial 5 ml, 10 ml.
Use: Corticosteroid.
•**METHYLPREDNISOLONE,** U.S.P. XXII. Tab., U.S.P. XXII. 11 α,17,21-Trihydroxy-6-α-methylpregna-1,4-diene-3,20-dione. Medrone, Metastab.
Use: Glucocorticoid.
See: A-Methapred, Inj. (Abbott).
Dura-Meth, Inj. (Foy).
Medralone 40, Inj. (Keene).
Medralone 80, Inj. (Keene).
Medrol, Tab. (Upjohn).
W/Neomycin sulfate.
See: Neo-Medrol, Oint. (Upjohn).
W/Sodium succinate.
See: Solu-Medrol, Vial (Upjohn).
•**METHYLPREDNISOLONE ACETATE,** U.S.P. XXII. Cream, for Enema, Sterile Susp., U.S.P. XXII. 6-α-methylprednisolone-21-acetate.
Use: Glucocorticoid.
See: Depo-Medrol, Inj., Rectal (Upjohn).
Depo-Pred., Vial (Hyrex).
Medrol Preps., Cream (Upjohn).
Mepred-40, Susp. (Savage).
Mepred-80, Susp. (Savage).
Neo-Medrol, Preps. (Upjohn).
Rep-Pred, Vial (Central).
METHYLPREDNISOLONE ACETATE FOR ENEMA, U.S.P. XXII.
Use: Glucocorticoid.
•**METHYLPREDNISOLONE HEMISUCCINATE,** U.S.P. XXII.
Use: Adrenocortical steroid.
METHYLPREDNISOLONE SODIUM PHOSPHATE. USAN.
Use: Glucocorticoid.
•**METHYLPREDNISOLONE SODIUM SUCCINATE,** U.S.P. XXII. For Inj., U.S.P. XXII. Methylprednisolone 21-(Hydrogen Succinate) sodium salt.
Use: Adrenocorticoid steroid.
See: Solu-Medrol, Mix-O-Vial (Upjohn).
•**METHYLPREDNISOLONE SULEPTANATE.** USAN.
Use: Adrenocortical steroid, anti-inflammatory.
METHYLPROMAZINE. 10-(3-Dimethylaminopropyl)-2-methylphenothiazine.
METHYLPYRIMAL.
See: Sulfamerazine (Various Mfr.).
METHYLROSANILINE CHLORIDE.
Use: Anthelmintic, anti-infective.
See: Gentian Violet, U.S.P. XXII. (Various Mfr.).
•**METHYL SALICYLATE,** N.F. XVII. (Various Mfr.) Oil of wintergreen.
Use: Pharmaceutic aid (flavor).
METHYL SALICYLATE W/COMBINATIONS.
Use: Rubefacient rub (external).
See: Analbalm, Liq. (Central).
Analgesic Balm (Various Mfr.).
Analgesic Ointment "Lannett," Oint. (Lannett).
Banalg, Liniment (Forest).
Chloral-Methylol, Oint. (Ulmer).
Cydonol, Lot. (Gordon).
Emul-o-balm, Liq. (Pennwalt).
Gordobalm, Oint. (Gordon).
Guaiamen, Cream (Lannett).
Listerine Antiseptic, Liq. (Warner-Lambert).
Musterole, Oint. (Schering-Plough).
Sloan's Liniment, Liq. (Warner-Lambert).
Stimurub, Cream (Otis Clapp).
METHYL SULFANIL AMIDOISOXAZOLE. Sulfamethoxazole.
See: Gantanol, Tab., Susp. (Roche Lab.).
•**METHYLTESTOSTERONE,** U.S.P. XXII. Tab., Cap., U.S.P. XXII. Buccal, Tab. 17-Methyltestosterone. 17β-Hydroxy-17-methylandrost-4-en-3-one. (Anertan, Glasso-Sterandryl, Testoviron).
Use: Androgen.
See: Android-5, 10 or 25, Tab. (Brown).
Arcosterone, Tab. (Arcum).
Metandren, Linguet, Tab. (Ciba).
Neo-Hombreol-M, Tab. (Organon).
Oreton-M, Tab., Buccal Tab. (Schering).
Ostone, Tab. (Solvay).
Testred, Cap. (ICN).
METHYLTESTOSTERONE W/COMBINATIONS.
Use: Androgen.
See: Android-5, 10 or 25, Tab. (Brown).
Estritone, Tab. (Kenyon).
Mediatric, Cap., Liq., Tab. (Wyeth-Ayerst).
Premarin w/Methyltestosterone, Tab. (Wyeth-Ayerst).
Virilon, Cap. (Star).
METHYLTHIONINE CHLORIDE. Name used for Methylene Blue.
METHYLTHIONINE HCl. Name used for Methylene Blue.
METHYLTHIOURACIL, U.S.P. XXI. 6-Methyl-2-thi-ouracil. 4-Methyl-2-thiouracil. Antibason, Methiocil.
Use: Thyroid inhibition.
METHYL VIOLET.
See: Gentian Violet, Crystal Violet, Methylrosaniline Cl.
METHYNDAMINE. Name used for Tetrydamine.
•**METHYNODIOL DIACETATE.** USAN.
Use: Oral progestin.

•**METHYPRYLON,** U.S.P. XXII. Cap., Tab., U.S.P. XXII. 3,3-Diethyl-5-methyl-2,4-piperidinedione.
Use: Hypnotic.
See: Noludar, Cap., Tab. (Roche).
METHYRIDINE. V.B.A.N. 2-(2-Methoxyethyl)pyridine. Promintic.
Use: Anthelmintic, (veterinary).
•**METHYSERGIDE.** USAN.
Use: Vasoconstrictor.
•**METHYSERGIDE MALEATE,** U.S.P. XXII. Tab., U.S.P. XXII. N-[1-(Hydroxymethyl)propyl]-1-methyl-D-lysergamide bimaleate. 1-Methyl-D-lysergic acid butanolamide. (+)-9,10-Didehydro-N-[1-(hydroxymethyl)-propyl]-1,6-dimethylergoline-8β-carboxamide Maleate (1:1).
Use: Analgesic (specific in migraine).
See: Sansert, Tab. (Sandoz).
•**METIAMIDE.** USAN. Histamine H_2 antagonist. 1-Methyl-3-[2-(5-methylimidazol-4-ylmethylthio)ethyl]thiourea.
Use: Treatment for peptic ulcer.
•**METIAPINE.** USAN.
Use: Antipsychotic.
METICLOPINDOL. Name used for Clopidol.
METICORTEN. (Schering) Prednisone 1 mg/Tab. Bot. 100s.
Use: Corticosteroid.
METIMYD OPHTHALMIC OINT. STERILE. (Schering) Prednisolone acetate 0.5% (5 mg), sulfacetamide sodium 10%. Tube 0.125 oz.
Use: Corticosteroid, sulfonamide (topical).
METIMYD OPHTHALMIC SUSP. STERILE. (Schering) Prednisolone acetate 5 mg, sulfacetamide sodium 100 mg/ml. Bot. dropper 5 ml.
Use: Corticosteroid, sulfonamide (topical).
•**METIOPRIM.** USAN.
Use: Antibacterial.
•**METIPRANOLOL HCl.** USAN.
Use: Antibacterial.
•**METIZOLINE.** F.D.A. 2-[(2-Methylbenzo[b]-thien-3-yl)methyl]-2-imidazoline.
Use: Nasal decongestant.
See: Benazoline.
•**METIZOLINE HYDROCHLORIDE.** USAN.
Use: Adrengeric.
•**METKEPHAMID ACETATE.** USAN.
Use: Analgesic.
METOCLOPRAMIDE. 4-Amino-5-chloro-N-(2-diethylaminoethyl)-2-methoxybenzamide. Primperan is the hydrochloride.
•**METOCLOPRAMIDE HYDROCHLORIDE,** U.S.P. XXII, Tab., Inj., U.S.P. XXII. 4-Amino-5-chloro-n-[2-(diethyl-amino)-ethyl]-o-anisamide dihydrochloride hydrate. 4-amino-5-chloro-N-[2-(diethylamino) ethyl]-2-methoxybenzamide monohydrochloride monohydrate.
Use: Antiemetic.
See: Reclomide, Tab. (Ultra).
Reglan, Amp. (Robins).
•**METOCURINE IODIDE,** U.S.P. XXII. Inj., U.S.P. XXII. (+)-O,O′-Dimethylchondro-curarine di-iodide.
Use: Skeletal muscle relaxant.
See: Metubine Iodid, Vial (Lilly).
METOFOLINE. B.A.N. 1-(4-Chlorophenethyl)-1,2,3,4-tetrahydro-6,7-dimethoxy-2-methylisoquinoline.
Use: Analgesic.
METOFURONE. Name used for Nifurmerone.
•**METOGEST.** USAN.
Use: Hormone.
•**METOLAZONE.** USAN. 7-Chloro-1,2,3,4-tetrahydro-2-methyl-4-oxo-3-o-tolyl-6-quinazolinesulfonamide.
Use: Diuretic, antihypertensive.
See: Diulo, Tab. (Searle).
Mykrox, Tab. (Fisons).
Zaroxolyn, Tab. (Pennwalt).
•**METOPIMAZINE.** USAN. 10-[3-(4-Carbamoyl-piperidino)propyl]-2-methanesulfonylphenothiazine.
Use: Antiemetic.
METOPIRONE. (Ciba) Metyrapone 250 mg/Tab. For pituitary function determination. Bot. 18s.
Use: Diagnostic aid.
METOPON. B.A.N. Methyldihydromorphinone 7,8-Dihydro-5-methylmorphinone.
Use: Analgesic.
•**METOPRINE.** USAN.
Use: Antineoplastic agent.
•**METOPROLOL.** USAN. (±)-1-Isopropylamino-3-p-(2-methoxyethyl)phenoxypropan-2-ol.
Use: Beta-adrenergic blocking agent.
•**METOPROLOL FUMARATE.** USAN.
Use: Antihypertensive.
•**METOPROLOL TARTRATE,** U.S.P. XXII. Inj., Tab., U.S.P. XXII.
Use: Beta-adrenergic blocking agent.
See: Lopressor, Tab. (Geigy).
•**METOPROLOL TARTRATE AND HYDROCHLOROTHIAZIDE,** U.S.P. XXII, Tab., U.S.P. XXII.
Use: Antihypertensive.
See: Lopressor HCT 100/50, Tab. (Geigy).
Lopressor HCT 100/25, Tab. (Geigy).
Lopressor HCT 50/25, Tab. (Geigy).
METOQUINE.
Use: Antimalarial.
See: Quinacrine HCl.
•**METOQUIZINE.** USAN. 4,7-Dimethyl-9-(3,5-dimethyl-pyrazole-1-carboxamido)-4,6,6a,7,8,9,10,-10a-octahydroindolo-[4,3-fg]quinoline.
Use: Anti-ulcer agent, anticholinergic.
•**METOSERPATE HYDROCHLORIDE.** USAN.
Use: Sedative.
METRA. (Forest) Phendimetrazine 35 mg/Tab. Bot. 1000s.
Use: Anorexiant.
METRETON OPHTHALMIC SOLUTION. (Schering) Prednisolone sodium phosphate 5.5 mg/ml. Bot. 5 ml.
Use: Corticosteroid, ophthalmic.

METRIC 21. (Fielding) Metronidazole 250 mg/ Tab. Bot. 100s.
Use: Anti-infective.

METRIFONATE. V.B.A.N. Dimethyl 2,2,2-trichloro-1-hydroxyethylphosphonate. Trichlorphon. Dipterex; Dyvon; Neguvon; Tugon.
Use: Insecticide; anthelmintic, veterinary medicine.

•**METRIZAMIDE.** USAN. 2-[3-Acetamido-2, 4, 6-triiodo-5-(N-methylacetamido) benzamido]-2-deoxy-D- glucopyranose.
Use: Myelography, diagnostic aid (radiopaque medium).
See: Amipaque, Inj. (Winthrop Pharm).

•**METRIZOATE SODIUM.** USAN.
Use: Diagnostic aid (radiopaque medium).
See: Sodium metrizoate.

METRODIN. (Serono) Urofollitropin 0.83 mg containing 75 IU follicle stimulating hormone activity/Amp; and 2.2 ml sodium Cl injection/Amp.
Use: Ovulation stimulant.

METROGEL. (Curatek) Metronidazole 0.75%. Gel Tube 30 Gm.
Use: Anti-acne.

METROGESIC. (Metro Med) Salicylamide 325 mg, acetaminophen 162 mg, phenacetin 65 mg/ Tab. Bot. 100s.
Use: Analgesic.

METROGESTONE. 6,17-Dimethylpregna-4,6-diene-3, 20-dione.
Use: Progestin.

METROJEN. (Jenkins) Metrate 1 mg, triple barb 12 mg (representing 33⅓% each, pentobarbital, sodium butabarbital, sodium phenobarbital)/Tab. Bot. 1000s.
Use: Sedative/hypnotic.

•**METRONIDAZOLE,** U.S.P. XXII. Inj., Tab., U.S.P. XXII. 1-(2-Hydroxethyl)-2-methyl-5-nitromidazole. 2-Methyl-5-nitromidazole-1-ethanol.
Use: Antitrichomonal.
See: Flagyl, Tab. (Searle).
Flagyl I.V., Vial (Searle).
Flagyl I.V. RTU, Vial (Searle).
Metronid, Tab. (Ascher).
Metryl, Tab., Vial (Lemmon).

•**METRONIDAZOLE HYDROCHLORIDE.** USAN.
Use: Antibacterial.
See: Flagyl I.V. (Searle).

•**METRONIDAZOLE PHOSPHATE.** USAN.
Use: Antibacterial, antiprotozoal.

METRONIDAZOLE REDI-INFUSION. (Elkins-Sinn) Metronidazole 500 mg/100 ml Vial.
Use: Amebicide.

METROZOLE. (Metro Med) Metronidazole 250 mg or 500 mg/Tab. **250 mg:** Bot. 100s, 250s; **500 mg:** Bot. 100s.
Use: Anti-infective, amebicide.

METRYL. (Lemmon) Metronidazole 250 mg/Tab. Bot. 100s, 250s, 500s, UD 100s.
Use: Anti-infective, amebicide.

METRYL 500. (Lemmon) Metronidazole 500 mg/ Tab. Bot. 100s, 500s.
Use: Anti-infective, amebicide.

METUBINE IODIDE. (Lilly) Metocurine iodide 2 mg/ml. Vial 20 ml.
Use: Skeletal muscle relaxant.

•**METUREDEPA.** USAN. Formerly Dimethyl urethimine. Ethyl [bis(2,2-dimethyl-aziridinyl)-phosphinyl]-carbamate. Turloc.
Use: Antineoplastic.

METUSSIN. (Faraday) Dextromethorphan. Bot. 4 oz.
Use: Antitussive.

METUSSIN JR. (Faraday) Dextromethorphan. Bot. 4 oz.
Use: Antitussive.

•**METYRAPONE,** U.S.P. XXII. Tab., U.S.P. XXII. 2-Methyl-1,2-di-3-pyridyl-1-propanone.
Use: Diagnostic aid (pituitary function determination).
See: Metopirone, Tab. (Ciba).

METYRAPONE DITARTRATE. 2-Methyl-1,2-di-3-pyridyl-1-propanone ditartrate. Methopyrapone.
Use: Diagnostic aid.
Adrenocortical enzyme inhibitor.
See: Metopirone, Amp. (Ciba).

•**METYRAPONE TARTRATE.** USAN.
Use: Diagnostic aid.

METYRAPONE TARTRATE INJECTION. 2-methyl-1,2-di-3-pyridyl-1-propanone tartrate (1:2).
Use: Diagnostic aid.

•**METYROSINE,** U.S.P. XXII. Cap., U.S.P. XXII. L-Tyrosine, a-methyl-,(-)-.
Use: Antihypertensive.
See: Demser (Merck, Sharp & Dohme).

METYZOLINE. B.A.N. 3-(2-Imidazolin-2-ylmethyl)-2-methylbenzo[b]thiophene. Eunasin [hydrochloride.]
Use: Vasoconstrictor.

MEVACOR. (Merck, Sharp & Dohme) Lovastatin 20 mg/Tab. In UD 60s, 100s.
Use: Antihyperlipidemic.

MEVANIN-C. (Beutlich) Vitamin C 200 mg, hesperidin complex 30 mg, calcium lactate 300 mg, cyanocobalamin 1 mcg, ferrous sulfate 65 mg, folic acid 0.1 mg, vitamins A 3000 IU, D 300 IU, B_1 2 mg, B_2 2 mg, B_6 0.5 mg, niacin 5 mg, copper 0.33 mg, zinc 0.4 mg, manganese 0.33 mg, magnesium 1 mg, potassium 1.5 mg, iodine 0.03 mg/Cap. Bot. 90s, 450s.
Use: Vitamin/mineral supplement.

MEVINOLIN.
See: Lovastatin.

MEXATE-AQ. (Bristol-Myers/Bristol Oncology) Preservative-free liquid. Methotrexate 50 mg, 100 mg or 250 mg/Vial.
Use: Antineoplastic agent.

MEXENONE. B.A.N. 2-Hydroxy-4-methoxy-4′-methylbenzophenone. Uvistat.
Use: Protection of skin from sunlight.

•**MEXILETINE HYDROCHLORIDE,** U.S.P. XXII, Cap., U.S.P. XXII.
Use: Cardiac depressant (antiarrhythmic).

See: Mexitil, Cap. (Boehringer Ingelheim).

MEXITIL. (Boehringer Ingelheim) Mexiletine HCl 150 mg, 200 mg or 250 mg/Cap. Bot. 100s, UD 100s.
Use: Antiarrhythmic agent.

•**MEXRENOATE POTASSIUM.** USAN.
Use: Aldosterone antagonist.

MEXSANA MEDICATED POWDER. (Schering-Plough) Corn starch, kaolin, triclosan, zinc oxide. Can 3 oz, 6.25 oz, 11 oz.
Use: Diaper rash product.

MEXTRA. (Kenyon) Prednisolone 0.5 mg, acetylsalicylic acid 5 gr/Tab. Bot. 100s, 1000s.
Use: Corticosteroid, analgesic.

MEXTRAFOR. (Kenyon) Acetylsalicylic acid 5 gr, prednisolone 1.5 mg/Cap. Bot. 100s, 1000s.
Use: Corticosteroid, analgesic.

MEYENBERG GOAT MILK. (Jackson-Mitchell) Evaporated and powdered cans of goat milk. Foil pack 4 oz. (makes one quart).
Use: Cows' milk allergies.

MEZLIN. (Miles Pharm) Mezlocillin sodium. Vial 1 Gm, 2 Gm 3 Gm, 4 Gm. Infusion Bot. 2 Gm, 3 Gm, 4 Gm.
Use: Antibacterial, penicillin.

•**MEZLOCILLIN.** USAN. 6-[D2-(Methylsulfonyl-2-oxoimidazolin-1-ylcarboxamido)-2-phenylacetamido]penicillanic acid.
Use: Antibiotic.

•**MEZLOCILLIN SODIUM, STERILE,** U.S.P. XXII.
Use: Antibiotic.
See: Mezlin, Inj. (Miles Pharm).

MG-OROATE. (Miller) Magnesium (as magnesium orotate) 33 mg/Tab. Bot. 100s.
Use: Magnesium supplement.

MG 217 MEDICATED FORMULA. (Outdoor Recreations) Coal tar solution 5%, colloidal sulfur 2%, salicylic acid 2% in a special base of cleansers, wetting agents and lanolin. Oint. 120 Gm, 480 Gm. Shampoo 240 ml.
Use: Antiseborrheic, antipruritic.

Mg-PLUS PROTEIN. (Miller) Magnesium-protein complex made w/specially isolated soy protein 133 mg/Tab. Bot. 100s.
Use: Magnesium supplement.

MIACALCIN. (Sandoz) Calcitonin salmon 100 IU/ml. Inj. Amp. 1 ml.
Use: Hormone.

MI-ACID LIQUID. (Major) Aluminum hydroxide 200 mg, magnesium hydroxide 200 mg, simethicone 20 mg/5 ml. Bot. 360 ml, gal.
Use: Antacid, antiflatulent.

MIADONE.
See: Methadone HCl. (Various Mfr.).

•**MIANSERIN HCl.** USAN. 1,2,3,4,10,14b-Hexahydro-2-methyldibenzo[c,f]pyrazino-[1,2-a]-azepine monohydrochloride. Under study.
Use: Antiserotonin, antihistamine.

MIAQUIN.
See: Camoquin, Tab. (Parke-Davis).

•**MIBOLERONE.** USAN.
Use: Anabolic, androgen.

See: Cheque (Upjohn).

MICASORB. W/Red Veterinary Petrolatum.
See: RV Plus, Oint. (Elder).

MICATIN. (Advanced Care) Miconazole nitrate 2%. **Cream:** Tube 0.5 oz, 1 oz. **Spray powder:** Aerosol 3 oz. **Spray Liquid Aerosol:** Bot. 3.5 oz.
Use: Antifungal, topical.

MI-CEBRIN. (Dista) Vitamins B_1 10 mg, B_2 5 mg, B_6 1.7 mg, pantothenic acid 10 mg, niacinamide 30 mg, B_{12} (activity equiv.) 3 mcg, C 100 mg, E 5.5 IU, A 10,000 IU, D 400 IU, iron 15 mg, copper 1 mg, iodine 0.15 mg, manganese 1 mg, magnesium 5 mg, zinc 1.5 mg/Tab. Pkg. 60s, 100s, 1000s, Blister pkg. 10 × 10s.
Use: Vitamin/mineral supplement.

MI-CEBRIN T. (Dista) Vitamins B_1 15 mg, B_2 10 mg, B_6 2 mg, pantothenic acid 10 mg, niacinamide 100 mg, B_{12} 7.5 mcg, C 150 mg, E 5.5 IU, A 10,000 IU, D 400 IU, iron 15 mg, copper 1 mg, iodine 0.15 mg, manganese 1 mg, magnesium 5 mg, zinc 1.5 mg/Tab. Bot. 30s, 100s, 1000s, Blister pkg. 10 × 10s.
Use: Vitamin/mineral supplement.

MICOFUR. Anti 5-Nitro-2-Furaldoxime, Nifuroxime.
Use: Antifungal, antibacterial (topical).
See: Tricofuron, Vaginal Pow., Supp. (Eaton).

•**MICONAZOLE,** U.S.P. XXII. Inj., U.S.P. XXII. 1-[2,4-Dichloro-β-(2,4-dichlorobenzyloxy)phenethyl]imidazole.
Use: Antifungal agent.
See: Monistat IV, Inj. (Janssen).

•**MICONAZOLE NITRATE,** U.S.P. XXII. Cream, Vaginal Supp., Pow., U.S.P. XXII. 1-[2,4-Dichloro-β-[(2,4-dichlorobenzyl)-oxy]-phenylmethyl]imidazole mononitrate.
Use: Antifungal.
See: Monistat, Cream, (Ortho).
Monistat-Derm, Prods. (Ortho).
Nibustat Prods. (Ortho).

MICOREN. (Geigy) n-Crotonyl α-Ethylaminobutyric acid diethylamine and n-crotonyl α-propylaminobutyric acid diethylamide in aqueous soln. A respiratory stimulant; pending release.

MICRAININ. (Wallace) Meprobamate 200 mg, aspirin 325 mg/Tab. Bot. 100s.
Use: Analgesic combination.

MICRhoGAM. (Ortho Diagnostic) Rh_0 (D) immune globulin (Human) micro dose. Single-dose prefilled syringe. Pkg. 5s, 25s.
Use: Agent for immunization.

MICRIDIUM. (Johnson & Johnson) Phenacridane (9-(p-hexyloxphenyl)-10-methyl-acridinium Cl).
Use: Skin disorders in infants and children.

MICRIN PLUS. (Johnson & Johnson) Water, S.D. alcohol 38-B, glycerin, poloxamer 407, flavor, sodium saccharin, glutamic acid buffer, cetylpyridinium Cl, FD & C Yellow #5, Blue #1. Bot. 12 oz, 24 oz.
Use: Mouth preparation.

MICROCULT-GC TEST. (Ames) Miniaturized culture test for the detection of *Neisseria Gonorrhoeae.* Test Kit 25s.
Use: Diagnostic aid.

MICROFIBRILLAR COLLAGEN HEMOSTAT.
Use: Hemostatic, topical.
See: Avitene (Alcon).

MICRO-GUARD. (Sween) Antimicrobial skin cream. Tube 0.5 oz, Jar 2 oz.
Use: Antifungal, external.

MICRO-K EXTENCAPS. (Robins) Potassium Cl (8 mEq) 600 mg/Cap. Bot. 100s, 500s, Dis-Co pack 100s.
Use: Potassium supplement.

MICRO-K 10 EXTENTABS. (Robins) Potassium Cl 750 mg (10 mEq)/Cap. Bot. 100s, 500s, Dis-co UD 100s.
Use: Potassium supplement.

MICRO-K LS. (Robins) Potassium Cl 20 mEq (1500 mg). Extended release Susp. Packet 30s, 100s.
Use: Potassium supplement.

MICROLIPID. (Biosearch) Fat emulsion 50%, safflower oil, polyglycerol esters of fatty acids, soy lecithin, xanthan gum, ascorbic acid. Cal 4500, fat 500 Gm/L, 80 mOsm/Kg. H_2O. 120 ml.
Use: Enteral nutritional supplement.

MICRONASE TABLETS. (Upjohn) Glyburide 1.25, 2.5 or 5 mg/Tab. **1.25 mg:** Bot. 100s. **2.5 mg:** Bot. 100s, UD 100s. **5 mg:** Bot. 100s, 500s, 1000s, Box 100s, Unit-of-Use Bot. 30s.
Use: Antidiabetic.

MICRONEFRIN. (Bird) Racemic methylaminoethanol catechol HCl 2.25 Gm, sodium Cl, sodium bisulfite, potassium metabisulfite 0.99 Gm, chlorobutanol 0.5 Gm, benzoic acid 0.5 Gm, propylene glycol 8 mg/100 ml. Bot 15 ml, 30 ml.
Use: Antiasthmatic.

MICRONOR. (Ortho) Norethindrone 0.35 mg/Tab. Dialpak 28s.
Use: Oral contraceptive.

MICROSOL. (Star) Sulfamethizole 0.5 Gm or 1 Gm/Tab. Bot. 100s, 1000s.
Use: Urinary anti-infective.

MICROSOL-A. (Star) Phenazopyridine 50 mg, sulfamethizole 0.5 Gm/Tab. Bot. 100s, 1000s.
Use: Urinary anti-infective.

MICROSTIX CANDIDA. (Ames) Test for *candida* species in vaginal specimens. Box 25s.
Use: Diagnostic aid.

MICROSTIX-3 REAGENT STRIPS. (Ames) For recognition of nitrite in urine and for semi-quantitation of bacterial growth. Bot. 25s w/25 incubation pouches.
Use: Diagnostic aid.

MICROTRAK CHLAMYDIA TRACHOMATIS DIRECT SPECIMEN TEST. (Syva) To detect and identify chlamydia trachomatis. Slide test 60s.
Use: Diagnostic aid.

MICROTRAK HSV 1/HSV 2 CULTURE CONFIRMATION/TYPING TEST. (Syva) For identification and typing of herpes simplex in tissue culture. Test kit 1s.
Use: Diagnostic aid.

MICROTRAK NEISSERIA GONORRHEA CULTURE TEST. (Syva) For endocervical, urethral, rectal and pharyngeal cultures. Test kit 85s.
Use: Diganostic aid.

MICRURUS FULVIUS ANTIVENIN. (Wyeth-Ayerst) Inj. Combination package: One vial antivenin, one vial diluent (Bacteriostatic Water for Injection 10 ml.).
Use: Antivenin.

MICTONE 25. (Kenyon) Bethanechol Cl 25 mg/Tab. Bot. 100s, 1000s.
Use: Cholinergic stimulant.

MICTRIN. (Econo Med) Hydrochlorothiazide 50 mg/Tab. Bot. 100s, 1000s.
Use: Diuretic.

•**MIDAFLUR.** USAN. 4-Amino-2,2,5,5-tetrakis-(trifluoromethyl)-3-imidazoline.
Use: Sedative.

MIDAHIST EXPECTORANT. (Vangard) Codeine phosphate 10 mg, phenylpropanolamine HCl 18.75 mg, guaifenesin 100 mg/5 ml, alcohol 7.5%. Bot. pt, gal.
Use: Antitussive, decongestant, expectorant.

MIDAMALINE HCl. N-(5-chloro-2-benzimidazolylmethyl)-N-phenyl-N′N′-dimethyl-ethylene-diamine HCl.
Use: Local anesthetic.

MIDAMOR. (Merck Sharp & Dohme) Amiloride 5 mg/Tab. Bot. 100s.
Use: Diuretic, antihypertensive.

MIDANEED. (Hanlon) Vitamins A 5000 IU, D 500 IU, B_1 5 mg, B_2 3 mg, B_6 0.5 mcg, B_{12} 5 mcg, C 100 mg, niacinamide 10 mg, calcium pantothenate 5 mg/Cap. Bot. 100s.
Use: Vitamin supplement.

MIDATANE DC EXPECTORANT. (Vangard) Brompheniramine maleate 2 mg, guaifenesin 100 mg, phenylephrine HCl 5 mg, phenylpropanolamine HCl 5 mg, codeine phosphate 10 mg/5 ml, alcohol 3.5% Bot. pt, gal.
Use: Antihistamine, expectorant, decongestant, antitussive.

MIDATAPP TR TABLETS. (Vangard) Brompheniramine maleate 12 mg, phenylephrine HCl 15 mg, phenylpropanolamine HCl 15 mg/Tab. Bot. 100s, 500s, 1000s.
Use: Antihistamine, decongestant.

•**MIDAZOLAM HYDROCHLORIDE.** USAN.
Use: Injectable anesthetic.
See: Versed, Inj. (Roche).

•**MIDAZOLAM MALEATE.** USAN.
Use: Anesthetic.

•**MIDODRINE HYDROCHLORIDE.** USAN.
Use: Antihypertensive, vasoconstrictor.

MIDOL 200. (Glenbrook) Ibuprofen 200 mg/Tab. Bot. 8s, 16s, 32s.
Use: Nonsteroidal anti-inflammatory drug; analgesic.

MIDOL FOR CRAMPS CAPLETS. (Glenbrook) Aspirin 500 mg, caffeine 32.4 mg, cinnamedrine HCl 14.9 mg/Tab. In 8s, 16s, 32s.
Use: Analgesic combination.

MIDOL MAXIMUM STRENGTH. (Glenbrook) Cinnamedrine HCl 14.9 mg, aspirin 500 mg, caffeine 32.4 mg/Tab. Bot. 12s, 30s, 60s.
Use: Analgesic combination.

MIDOL ORIGINAL FORMULA. (Glenbrook) Cinnamedrine HCl 14.9 mg, aspirin 454 mg, caffeine 32.4 mg/Tab. Bot. 30s, 60s. Strip pack 12s.
Use: Analgesic combination.

MIDOL PMS. (Glenbrook) Acetaminophen 500 mg, pamabrom 25 mg, pyrilamine maleate 15 mg/Capl. Bot. 16s, 32s.
Use: Analgesic combination.

MIDRIN. (Carnrick) Isometheptene mucate 65 mg, acetaminophen 325 mg, dichloralphenazone 100 mg/Cap. Bot. 50s, 100s.
Use: Agent for migraine.

•**MIFOBATE.** USAN.
Use: Antiatherosclerotic.

•**MIGLITOL.** USAN.
Use: Antidiabetic.

MIH.
Use: Antineoplastic agent.
See: Procarbazine HCl.

MIKAMYCIN. B.A.N. An antibiotic produced by *Streptomyces mitakoensis.* Mikamycin B is Ostreogrycin B.

•**MILACEMIDE HYDROCHLORIDE.** USAN.
Use: Anticonvulsant, antidepressant.

MILD SILVER PROTEIN.
See: Silver Protein, Mild.

•**MILENPERONE.** USAN.
Use: Antipyschotic.

MILES NERVINE. (Miles) Diphenhydramine 25 mg/Tab. Pkg. 12s, Bot. 30s, 50s.
Use: Sleep aid.

•**MILIPERTINE.** USAN. 5,6-Dimethoxy-3-[2-[4(o-methoxy-phenyl)-1-piperazinyl]ethyl]-2-methyl-indole.
Use: Tranquilizer.

MILKINOL. (Kremers-Urban) Mineral oil in an emulsifying base. Bot. 240 ml.
Use: Laxative.

•**MILK OF BISMUTH,** U.S.P. XXII. (Various Mfr.) Bismuth hydroxide, bismuth subcarb.
Use: Orally, intestinal disturbances.
W/Paregoric, kaolin & pectin, methyl parahydroxybenzoate.
See: Mul-Sed, Liq. (Webcon).

•**MILK OF MAGNESIA,** U.S.P. XXII. (Various Mfr.). Magnesia (Magnesium hydroxide) 325 mg, 390 mg. **Tab.:** 250s, 1000s; **Liq.:** 120 ml, 360 ml, 720 ml, pt, qt, gal, UD 10 ml, 15 ml, 20 ml, 30 ml, 100 ml, 180 ml, 400 ml. **Susp.:** Pt, qt, gal, UD 15 and 30 ml.
Use: Antacid.
See: Magnesium hydroxide.

MILK OF MAGNESIA-CONCENTRATED. (Roxane) Magnesium hydroxide. Liq. Bot. 100 ml, 180 ml, 400 ml, UD 10 ml, 15 ml, 20 ml, 30 ml.
Use: Antacid.

MILLAZINE. (Major) Thioridazine. **10 mg or 15 mg/Tab.:** Bot. 100s; **25 mg/Tab.:** Bot. 100s, 1000s; **100 mg, 150 mg or 200 mg/Tab.:** Bot. 100s, 500s.
Use: Antipsychotic agent.

MILONTIN. (Parke-Davis) Phensuximide 0.5 Gm/Kapseal. Bot. 100s.
Use: Anticonvulsant.

MILOPHENE. (Milex) Clomiphene citrate 50 mg/Tab. 30s, UD 30s.
Use: Ovulation stimulant.

MILPAR. (Winthrop Products) Magnesium hydroxide, mineral oil.
Use: Antacid, laxative.

MILPREM. (Wallace) Meprobamate 400 mg, conjugated estrogens (equine) 0.45 mg/Tab. Bot. 100s.
Use: Antianxiety agent, estrogen.

•**MILRINONE.** USAN.
Use: Cardiotonic.

MILROY ARTIFICIAL TEARS. (Milton Roy) Bot. 22 ml.
Use: Artificial tear solution.

MILTOWN. (Wallace) Meprobamate. **200 mg/Tab.** Bot. 100s. **400 mg/Tab.** Bot. 100s, 500s, 1000s. **600 mg/Tab.** Bot. 100s.
Use: Antianxiety agent.
See: Meprospan (Wallace).

MILTOWN 600. (Wallace) Meprobamate 600 mg/Tab. Bot. 100s.
Use: Antianxiety agent.

•**MIMBANE HYDROCHLORIDE.** USAN. 1-Methylyohimbane HCl.
Use: Analgesic.

•**MINAPRINE.** USAN.
Use: Psychotropic.

•**MINAPRINE HYDROCHLORIDE.** USAN.
Use: Antidepressant.

•**MINAXOLONE.** USAN.
Use: Anesthetic.

MINCARD. Aminometradine. 1-Allyl-3-ethyl-6-aminotetrahydropyrimidinedione.
Use: Diuretic.

MINEPENTATE. B.A.N. 2-(2-Dimethylamino- ethoxy)ethyl 1-phenylcyclopentanecarboxylate.
Use: Treatment of the Parkinsonian syndrome.

MINERAL-CORTICOIDS.
See: Desoxycorticosterone salts (Various Mfr.).

•**MINERAL OIL,** U.S.P. XXII.
Use: Cathartic, pharmaceutic aid (solvent, oleaginous vehicle).
See: Petrolatum, Liq.

•**MINERAL OIL EMULSION,** U.S.P. XXII.
Use: Cathartic.

•**MINERAL OIL ENEMA,** U.S.P. XXII.
Use: Cathartic.

•**MINERAL OIL, LIGHT,** N.F. XVII.
Use: Vehicle.

•**MINERAL OIL, LIGHT, TOPICAL,** U.S.P. XXII.

MINIBEX. (Faraday) Vitamins B_1 6 mg, B_2 3 mg, B_6 0.5 mg, C 50 mg, niacinamide 10 mg, calcium pantothenate 3 mg, B_{12} 2 mcg, folic acid 0.1 mg/Cap. Bot. 100s, 250s, 1000s.
Use: Vitamin supplement.

MINI-GAMULIN Rh. (Armour) Rho (D) Immune Globulin (Human) in one-sixth the quantity contained in a standard dose.
Use: Agent for immunization.

MINIPRESS. (Pfizer Laboratories) Prazosin HCl 1 mg, 2 mg or 5 mg/Cap. **1 mg, 2 mg**: Bot. 250s, 1000s, UD 100s; **5 mg:** Bot. 250s, 500s, UD 100s.
Use: Antihypertensive.

MINITEC. (Squibb) Sodium pertechnetate Tc 99 m generator.
Use: Radiopaque agent.

MINITEC GENERATOR (COMPLETE WITH COMPONENTS). (Squibb) Medotopes Kit.
Use: Diagnostic aid.

MINITRAN TRANSDERMAL DELIVERY SYSTEM. (Riker) Nitroglycerin 9 mg. Patch 33s.
Use: Antianginal.

MINIT-RUB. (Bristol-Myers) Methyl salicylate 15%, methol 3.5%, camphor 2.3% in anhydrous base. Tube 1.5 oz, 3 oz.
Use: External analgesic.

MINIZIDE. (Pfizer Laboratories) Prazosin HCl and polythiazide. **Minizide 1:** Prazosin 1 mg, polythiazide 0.5 mg/Cap. **Minizide 2:** Prazosin 2 mg, polythiazide 0.5 mg/Cap. **Minizide 5:** Prazosin 5 mg, polythiazide 0.5 mg/Cap. Bot. 100s.
Use: Antihypertensive.

MINOCIN. (Lederle) Minocycline HCl. **Cap. 50 mg:** Bot. 100s, UD 10 × 10s; **100 mg:** Bot. 50s, 100s, UD 10 × 10s. **I.V.:** 100 mg/Vial. **Oral Susp.:** 50 mg/5 ml, propylparaben 0.1%, butylparaben 0.06%, alcohol 5% v/v. Bot. 2 oz. **Tab.:** 50 mg Bot. 100s; 100 mg Bot. 50s.
Use: Antibacterial, tetracycline.

•**MINOCROMIL.** USAN.
Use: Antiallergic.

•**MINOCYCLINE.** USAN.
Use: Antibacterial.
See: Minocyn (Lederle).

•**MINOCYCLINE HYDROCHLORIDE,** U.S.P. XXII. Cap., Oral Susp., Sterile, Tab., U.S.P. XXII. 4,7-bis-(Dimethylamino)-1,4,4a,5,5a,6,11,12a-octahydro-3,10, 12,12a,tetrahydroxy-1,11-dioxo-2-naph- thacenecarboxamide.
Use: Antibiotic.
See: Minocin, Cap., Syr., Vial (Lederle).

MINOXIDIL. (Danbury) Minoxidil 2.5 mg/Tab. Bot. 100s, 500s, 1000s.
Use: Antihypertensive.

MINOXIDIL. (Rugby) Minoxidil 10 mg/Tab. Bot. 500s.
Use: Antihypertensive.

•**MINOXIDIL,** U.S.P. XXII. Tab., U.S.P. XXII. 2,4-diamino-6-piperidinopyrimide-3-oxide.
Use: Antihypertensive peripheral vasodilator.
See: Loniten, Tab. (Upjohn).

MINOXIDIL, TOPICAL.
Use: Treatment of male pattern baldness.
See: Rogaine, Soln. (Upjohn).

MINTEZOL. (Merck Sharp & Dohme) Thiabendazole. **Susp.:** 500 mg/5 ml. Bot. 120 ml. **Chew. Tab.:** 500 mg. Pkg. 36s.
Use: Anthelmintic.

MINTO-CHLOR SYRUP. (Vale) Codeine sulfate 10 mg, potassium citrate 219 mg, alcohol 2%. Gal.
Use: Antitussive, expectorant.

MINT-O-FECTANT. (Lannett) Mint odor, phenol coefficient 5. Bot. pt, gal, 5 gal, 55 gal drum.
Use: Laxative.

MINTOX. (Major) Aluminum hydroxide 225 mg, magnesium hydroxide 200 mg/5 ml. Susp. Bot. 360 ml, 480 ml, gal.
Use: Antacid.

MINTOX PLUS LIQUID. (Major) Aluminim hydroxide 225 mg, magnesium hydroxide 200 mg, simethicone 25 mg/5 ml. Bot. 360 ml.
Use: Antacid, antiflatulent.

MINUTE-GEL. (Oral-B) Acidulated phosphate fluoride 1.23% Gel. Bot. 16 oz.
Use: Dental caries preventative.

MIOCHOL. (CooperVision) Acetylcholine Cl 20 mg, mannitol 60 mg, Sterile Water for Inj. 2 ml/ 2 ml univial. 1:100 intraocular.
Use: Agent for glaucoma.

•**MIOFLAZINE HYDROCHLORIDE.** USAN.
Use: Vasodilator.

MIOSTAT INTRAOCULAR SOLUTION. (Alcon Surgical) Carbochol 0.01%. Vial 1.5 ml. Pkg. 12s.
Use: Agent for glaucoma.

MIRAFLOW EXTRA STRENGTH. (CooperVision) Isopropyl alcohol 20%, poloxamer 407, amphoteric 10. Thimerosal free. Soln. Bot. 25 ml.
Use: Hard contact lens care.

MIRAL. (Geneva) Dexamethasone 0.75 mg/Tab. Bot. 100s, 1000s.
Use: Corticosteroid.

MIRASEPT. (CooperVision) Mirasept disinfecting solution, Mirasept rinsing, neutralizing solution w/lens case.
Use: Soft contact lens care.

•**MIRFENTANIL HYDROCHLORIDE.** USAN.
Use: Analgesic.

•**MIRINCAMYCIN HYDROCHLORIDE.** USAN.
Use: Antibacterial, antimalarial.

•**MIRTAZAPINE.** USAN.
Use: Antidepressant.

•**MISONIDAZOLE.** USAN.
Use: Antiprotozoal *(trichomonas).*

•**MISOPROSTOL.** USAN.
Use: Anti-ulcerative.

MISSION PRENATAL. (Mission) Ferrous gluconate 260 mg (iron 30 mg), vitamins C 100 mg, B_1 5 mg, B_6 3 mg, B_2 2 mg, niacinamide 10 mg, d-calcium pantothenate 1 mg, B_{12} 2 mcg, A (acetate) 4000 IU, D-2 400 IU, calcium carbon-

ate 70 mg, calcium gluconate 100 mg, calcium lactate 100 mg (calcium 50 mg), zinc 15 mg/Tab. Bot. 100s.
Use: Vitamin/mineral supplement.

MISSION PRENATAL F.A. (Mission) Ferrous gluconate 260 mg (iron 30 mg), vitamins C 100 mg, B_1 5 mg, B_6 10 mg, B_2 2 mg, niacinamide 10 mg, B_{12} 2 mcg, folic acid 0.8 mg, A acetate 4000 IU, D2 400 IU, calcium carbonate 70 mg, calcium gluconate 100 mg, calcium lactate 100 mg, (calcium 50 mg), d-calcium pantothenate 1 mg/Tab. Bot. 100s.
Use: Vitamin/mineral supplement.

MISSION PRENATAL H.P. (Mission) Ferrous gluconate 260 mg (iron 30 mg), vitamins C 100 mg, B_1 5 mg, B_6 25 mg, B_2 2 mg, niacinamide 10 mg, calcium pantothenate 1 mg, B_{12} 2 mcg, folic acid 1 mg, A 4000 IU, D 400 IU, calcium carbonate 70 mg, calcium gluconate 100 mg, calcium lactate 100 mg/Tab. Bot. 100s.
Use: Vitamin/mineral supplement.

MISSION PRENATAL-RX. (Mission) Vitamins A 8000 IU, D 400 IU, C 240 mg, B_1 4 mg, B_2 2 mg, B_3 20 mg, B_5 10 mg, B_6 20 mg, B_{12} 8 mcg, folic acid 1 mg, iron 60 mg, calcium 175 mg, iodine 0.3 mg, zinc 15 mg, copper 2 mg/Tab. Bot. 100s.
Use: Vitamin/mineral supplement.

MISSION PRESURGICAL. (Mission) Vitamins C 500 mg, B_1 2.5 mg, B_2 2.6 mg, B_3 30 mg, B_5 16.3 mg, B_6 3.6 mg, B_{12} 9 mcg, A 5000 USP units, D-2 400 USP units, E 45 IU, ferrous gluconate 233 mg, zinc 22.5 mg/Tab. Bot. 100s.
Use: Vitamin/mineral supplement.

MITHRACIN. (Miles Pharm) Plicamycin 2500 mcg/Vial. Unit vial 10s.
Use: Antineoplastic agent, antihypercalcemic.

MITHRAMYCIN.
Use: Antineoplastic agent.
See: Plicamycin.

•**MITINDOMIDE.** USAN.
Use: Antineoplastic agent.

MITOBRONITOL. B.A.N. 1,6-Dibromo-1,6-dideoxy-D-mannitol. Myelobromol.
Use: Antineoplastic agent.

•**MITOCARCIN.** USAN. Antibiotic derived from *Streptomyces* species.
Use: Antineoplastic agent.

MITOCLOMINE. B.A.N. NN-Di-(2-chloroethyl)-4-me-thoxy-3-methyl-1-naphthylamine.
Use: Antineoplastic agent.

•**MITOCROMIN.** USAN. Produced by *Streptomyces virdochromogenes.*
Use: Antineoplastic agent.

•**MITOGILLIN.** USAN. An antibiotic obtained from a "unique strain" of *Aspergillus restrictus.*
Use: Antitumorigenic antibiotic.

•**MITOMALCIN.** USAN. Produced by *Streptomyces malayensis.* Under study.
Use: Antineoplastic.

•**MITOMYCIN,** U.S.P. XXII. For Inj., U.S.P. XXII. In literature as Mitomycin C. Antibiotic isolated from *Streptomyces caespitosis.*
Use: Antibiotic.
See: Mutamycin, Inj. (Bristol).

MITOPODOZIDE. B.A.N. 2′-Ethylpodophyllohydrazide.
Use: Antineoplastic agent.

•**MITOSPER.** USAN. Substance derived from *Aspergillus* of the *glaucus* group.
Use: Antineoplastic.

•**MITOTANE,** U.S.P. XXII. Tab. U.S.P. XXII. 1,1-Di-chloro-2-(o-chlorophenyl)-2-(p-chlorophenyl)-ethane. Lysodren. Benzene,1-chloro-2-[2,2-dichloro-l-(4-chlorophenyl)ethyl]-.
Use: Antineoplastic agent.
See: Lysodren, Tab. (Bristol).

MITOTENAMINE. B.A.N. 5-Bromo-3-[N-(2-chloroethyl)ethylaminomethyl]benzo[b]thiophen.
Use: Antineoplastic agent.

•**MITOXANTRONE HYDROCHLORIDE.** USAN.
Use: Antineoplastic agent.
See: Novantrone (Lederle).

MITRAN. (Hauck) Chlordiazepoxide HCl 10 mg/Cap. Bot. 100s.
Use: Antianxiety agent.

MITROLAN. (Robins) Calcium polycarbophil equivalent to polycarbophil 500 mg/Tab. Blister Pak 36s, 100s.
Use: Laxative.

•**MIVACURIUM CHLORIDE.** USAN.
Use: Blocking agent (neuromuscular).

•**MIXIDINE.** USAN.
Use: Vasodilator (coronary).

MIXTARD. (Nordisk) Isophane purified pork insulin suspension 70% and purified pork insulin injection 30%, 100 units/ml.
Use: Antidiabetic.

MIXTURE 612. Dimethyl Phthalate Solution, Compound.

MLT-ASPIRIN. (Kenyon) Acetylsalicylic acid 7.5 gr/multi-layered Tab. Bot. 100s, 1000s.
Use: Salicylate analgesic.

M-M-R II. (Merck Sharp & Dohme) Lyophilized preparation of live attenuated measles virus vaccine (Attenuvax), live attenuated mumps virus vaccine (Mumpsvax), live attenuated rubella virus vaccine (Meruvax II). See details under Attenuvax, Mumpsvax and Meruvax II. Single dose vial w/diluent. Pkg. 1s, 10s.
Use: Agent for immunization.

MOBAN. (DuPont) Molindone HCl. **Liq.:** 20 mg/ml concentrate. Bot. 4 oz/w dropper. **Tab.:** 5 mg, 10 mg, 25 mg, 50 mg or 100 mg/Tab. Bot. 100s.
Use: Antipsychotic agent.

MOBENOL.
See: Tolbutamide, U.S.P. XXII.

MOBIDIN. (Ascher) Magnesium salicylate, anhydrous 600 mg/Tab. Bot. 100s, 500s.
Use: Antiarthritic agent.

MOBIGESIC. (Ascher) Magnesium salicylate 325 mg, phenyltoloxamine citrate 30 mg/Tab. Bot. 50s, 100s, Pkg. 18s.
Use: Analgesic combination.
MOBISYL CREME. (Ascher) Trolamine salicylate in vanishing creme base. Tubes 100 Gm.
Use: External analgesic.
MOCCASIN BITE.
See: Antivenin, Snake, Polyvalent (Wyeth-Ayerst).
•**MOCLOBEMIDE.** USAN.
Use: Antidepressant.
MOCTANIN. (Ascot) Synthetic esterfied glycerol. Bot. 120 ml.
Use: Gallstone-solubilizing agent.
•**MODALINE SULFATE.** USAN. 2-Methyl-3-piperidinopyrazine monosulfate.
Use: Antidepressant.
MODANE. (Adria) Phenolphthalein 130 mg/Tab. Pkg. 10s, 30s. Bot. 100s.
Use: Laxative.
MODANE BULK. (Adria) Powdered mixture of equal parts of psyllium and dextrose. Container 14 oz.
Use: Laxative.
MODANE MILD. (Adria) Phenolphthalein 60 mg/Tab. Bot. 10s, 30s, 100s.
Use: Laxative.
MODANE PLUS. (Adria) Phenolphthalein 60 mg, docusate sodium 100 mg/Tab. Bot. 100s, Box 10s, 30s.
Use: Laxative.
MODANE SOFT. (Adria) Docusate sodium 100 mg/Cap. UD Pkg. 30s.
Use: Laxative.
MODANE VERSABRAN. (Adria) Psyllium hydrophilic mucilloid in wheat bran base. Dose 3.4 Gm, Bot. 10 oz.
Use: Laxative.
•**MODECAINIDE.** USAN.
Use: Cardiac depressant.
MODERIL. (Pfizer Laboratories) Rescinnamine 0.25 mg or 0.5 mg Tab. Bot. 100s.
Use: Antihypertensive.
MODICON 21. (Ortho) Norethindrone 0.5 mg, ethinyl estradiol 35 mcg/Tab. Dialpak 21s.
Use: Oral contraceptive.
MODICON 28. (Ortho) Norethindrone 0.5 mg, ethinyl estradiol 35 mcg/Tab., 7 inert Tab. Dialpak 28s.
Use: Oral contraceptive.
MODINAL.
See: Gardinol Type Detergents (Various Mfr.).
MODRASTANE. (Winthrop Pharm) Trilostane 30 mg or 60 mg/Cap. Bot. 100s.
Use: Adrenal steroid inhibitor.
MODUCAL. (Mead Johnson Nutrition) Maltodextrin. Pow. Can 13 oz.
Use: Enteral nutritional supplement.
MODURETIC. (Merck Sharp & Dohme) Hydrochlorothiazide 50 mg, amiloride 5 mg/Tab. Bot. 100s, UD 100s.
Use: Diuretic, antihypertensive.
MOENOMYCIN. Phosphorus-containing glycolipide antibiotic. Active against gram-positive organisms. Under study.
M.O., HALEY'S. (Winthrop Consumer Products).
See: Haley's M.O., Liq. (Winthrop Products).
MOI-STIR. (Kingswood Lab) Dibasic sodium phosphate, magnesium Cl, calcium Cl, sodium Cl, potassium Cl, sorbitol, sodium carboxymethylcellulose, methyl and propyl parabens. Soln. 120 ml with pump spray.
Use: Saliva substitute.
MOI-STIR 10. (Kingswood Lab) Sodium carboxymethylcellulose, potassium Cl, dibasic sodium phosphate, methyl and propyl parabens. Soln. 60 ml with pump spray.
Use: Saliva substitute.
MOISTURE DROPS. (Bausch & Lomb) Hydroxypropyl methylcellulose, dextran 40. Soln. Bot. 0.5 oz, 1 oz.
Use: Artificial tear solution.
MOISTUREL LOTION. (Westwood) Petrolatum, glycerin, dimethicone steareth-2, cetyl alcohol, benzyl alcohol, laureth-23, carbomer-934, magnesium aluminum silicate, quaternium-15. Lot. Bot. 240 ml.
Use: Emollient.
MOLAR PHOSPHATE.
W/Fluoride ion.
See: Coral Prods. (Lorvic).
Karigel, Gel. (Lorvic).
•**MOLINAZONE.** USAN. 3-Morpholino-1,2,3-benzotriazin-4(3H)-one.
Use: Analgesic.
•**MOLINDONE HYDROCHLORIDE.** USAN.
Use: Antipsychotic.
See: Lidone, Cap. (Abbott).
Lidone Concentrate, Liq. (Abbott).
Moban, Tab. (Du Pont).
MOL-IRON TABLETS. (Schering) Ferrous sulfate 195 mg, (equivalent 39 mg elemental iron)/Tab. Bot. 100s.
Use: Iron supplement.
W/Vitamin C (Schering) Ferrous sulfate 195 mg, ascorbic acid 75 mg/Tab. Bot. 100s.
MOLLIFENE EAR DROPS. (Pfeiffer) Glycerin, camphor, cajaput oil, eucalyptus oil, thyme oil. Soln. Bot. 24 ml.
Use: Otic preparation.
•**MOLSIDOMINE.** USAN.
Use: Antianginal, vasodilator.
MOLYBDENUM SOLUTION. (American Quinine) Molybdenum 25 mcg/ml (as 46 mcg/ml ammonium molybdate tetrahydrate). Inj. Vial 10 ml.
Use: Parenteral nutritional supplement.
MOLYCU. (Burns) Meprobamate 400 mg, copper 60 mg/ml.
Use: Antidote.
MOLY-PAK. (SoloPak) Molybdenum 25 mcg. Inj. Vial 10 ml.
Use: Parenteral nutritional supplement.

MOLYPEN. (Lyphomed) Ammonium molybdate tetrahydrate 46 mcg/ml. Vial 10 ml.
Use: Parenteral nutritional supplement.

MOMENTUM. (Whitehall) Aspirin 500 mg, phenyltoloxamine citrate 15 mg/Tab. Bot. 24s, 48s.
Use: Analgesic.

•**MOMETASONE FUROATE.** USAN. (1) Pregna-1,4-diene-3,20-dione, 9,21-dichloro-17-[(2-furanylcarbonyl)oxy]-11-hydroxy-16-methyl-, (11β,16α)-; (2) 9,21-Dichloro-11β,17-dihydroxy-16α-methylpregna-1,4-diene-3,20-dione 17-(2-furoate).
Use: Topical corticosteroid.
See: Elocon Cream, Oint. (Schering).

MONACETYL PYROGALLOL. Eugallol. Pyrogallol Monoacetate.
Use: Keratolytic.

MONALIUM HYDRATE. Hydrated magnesium aluminate. Magalorate.
See: Riopan, Tab., Susp. (Wyeth-Ayerst).

•**MONENSIN.** USAN. (1) 2-[5-Ethyltetrahydro-5-[tetrahydro-3-methyl-5-[tetrahydro-6-hydroxy-6-(hydroxymethyl)-3,5-dimethyl-2H-pyran-2-yl]-2-furyl]-2-furyl]-9-hydroxy-β-methoxy-α,,2,8,-tetramethyl-1,6-dioxaspiro[4,5]decane-7-butyric acid. Coban (as sodium salt)(Lilly).
Use: Antiprotozoal, antibacterial, antifungal.

MONISTAT DUAL-PAK. (Ortho) Miconazole nitrate suppositories and cream. **200 mg/Supp.:** Pkg. 3s w/applicator; **Cream 2%.:** Tube 15 Gm.
Use: Antifungal, vaginal.

MONISTAT 3 VAGINAL SUPPOSITORIES. (Ortho) Miconazole nitrate 200 mg/Supp. Pkg. 3s w/applicator.
Use: Antifungal, vaginal.

MONISTAT IV. (Janssen) Miconazole 10 mg/ml, PEG 40, castor oil, lactate, methylparaben, propylparaben, water. Amp. 20 ml.
Use: Antifungal.

MONISTAT 7 VAGINAL CREAM. (Ortho) Miconazole nitrate 2% in water-miscible cream. Tube 45 Gm w/dose applicator.
Use: Antifungal, vaginal.

MONISTAT 7 VAGINAL SUPPOSITORIES. (Ortho) Miconazole nitrate 100 mg/Supp. Pkg. 7s w/applicator.
Use: Antifungal, vaginal.

MONISTAT-DERM CREAM. (Ortho Derm) Miconazole nitrate 2%, pegoxol 7 stearate, peglicol 5 oleate, mineral oil, benzoic acid, butylated hydroxyanisole. Tube oz, 15 Gm, 85 Gm.
Use: Antifungal, external.

MONISTAT-DERM LOTION. (Ortho Derm) Miconazole nitrate 2%, pegoxol 7 stearate, peglicol 5 oleate, mineral oil, benzoic acid, butylated hydroxyanisole. Squeeze bot. 30 ml, 60 ml.
Use: Antifungal, external.

MONOAMINE OXIDASE INHIBITORS.
See: Eutonyl Filmtabs (Abbott).
Marplan, Tab. (Roche).
Nardil, Tab. (Parke-Davis).
Parnate, Tab. (SKF).

•**MONO AND DI-ACETYLATED MONOGLYCERIDES,** N.F. XVII. A mixture of glycerin esterfied mono- and di-esters of edible fatty acids followed by direct acetylation.
Use: Plasticizer.

•**MONO AND DI-GLYCERIDES,** N.F. XVII. A mixture of mono- and di-esters of fatty acids from edible oils.
Use: Fatty acids, emulsifying agent.

MONOBASE. (Torch) Water-washable emulsion vehicle of fatty alcohols, natural wax, PEG. Consistency maintained over wide temperature range. Jar lb.
Use: Emollient.

•**MONOBENZONE,** U.S.P. XXII. Oint., U.S.P. XXI. Cream, U.S.P. XXII. p-(Benzyloxy)phenol.
Use: Depigmenting agent.
See: Benoquin, Oint., Lot. (Elder).

MONOBENZYL ETHER OF HYDROQUINONE.
See: Benoquin, Oint., Lot. (Elder).

MONOBROMISOVALERYLUREA.
See: Bromisovalum. (Various Mfr.).

MONO-CALAFORMULA. (Eric, Kirk & Gary) Calcium carbonate 500 mg, ferrous fumarate 90 mg, vitamins A 5000 IU, D 400 IU, B_1 1 mg, B_6 1 mg, B_{12} 3 mcg, C 50 mg, niacinamide 10 mg, B_2 1 mg, iodine 0.1 mg, manganese 1.5 mg, cobalt 0.1 mg, copper 1 mg, zinc 1.4 mg, magnesium 1 mg, potassium 5 mg/Tab. Bot. 30s, 100s, 180s, 1000s.
Use: Vitamin/mineral supplement.

MONOCAPS TABLETS. (Freeda) Iron 41 mg, vitamins A 10,000 IU, D 400 IU, E 15 IU, B_1 15 mg, B_2 15 mg, B_3 41 mg, B_5 15 mg, B_6 15 mcg, B_{12} 15 mcg, C 125 mg, folic acid 0.1 mg, biotin 15 mg, PABA, lysine, linoleic acid, Ca, Cu, I, K, Mg, Mn, Se, Zn/Tab. Bot. 100s, 250s, 500s.
Use: Vitamin/mineral supplement.

MONOCETE SOLUTION. (Pedinol) Monochloracetic acid 80% w/color. Bot. 15 ml.
Use: Cauterizing agent.

MONO-CHLOR. (Gordon) Monochloroacetic acid 80%. Bot. 15 ml.
Use: Cauterizing agent.

MONOCHLOROACETIC ACID.
Use: Cauterizing agent.
See: Monocete, Soln. (Pedinol).
Mono-Chlor, Soln. (Gordon).

MONOCID. (SmithKline) Cefonicid sodium 500 mg or 1 Gm/10 ml. Vial 1 Gm/100 ml piggyback. Pharmacy Bulk Vial equivalent to 10 Gm.
Use: Antibacterial, cephalosporin.

MONOCLATE. (Armour) Monoclonal antibody derived stable lyophilized concentrate of Factor VIII: R heat-treated. With albumin (human) 1% to 2%, mannitol 0.8%, histadine 1.2 mM. Inj. Vial 1 ml single dose with diluent.
Use: Antihemophilic.

MONOCLONAL ANTIBODIES (MURINE OR HUMAN) RECOGNIZING β-CELL LYMPHOMA IDIOTYPES. (Orphan Drug).
Use: β-cell lymphoma.

Sponsor: Damon Biotech, Inc.

MONOCTANOIN.
Use: Gallstone solubilizing agent.
See: Moctanin, Inf. (Ethiteck).

MONOCYCLINE HYDROCHLORIDE.
See: Minocin I.V., Syr., Cap. (Lederle).

MONODRAL. (Winthrop Products) Penthienate.
Use: Anticholinergic.

•**MONOETHANOLAMINE,** N.F. XVII. 2-Aminoethanol.
Use: Pharmaceutic aid (surfactant).

MONO-GESIC TABLETS. (Central) Salsalate (salicylsalicylic acid) 750 mg/Tab. Bot. 100s, 500s.
Use: Salicylate analgesic.

MONOIODOMETHANESULFONATE SODIUM.
See: Methiodal Sodium, U.S.P. XXII.

MONOJECT. (Sherwood) Liquid glucose (dextrose 40%). Gel. Tube UD 25 Gm.
Use: Glucose-elevating agent.

MONOJEL. (Sherwood) Glucose 40% in UD 25 Gm.
Use: Glucose-elevating agent.

MONO-LATEX. (Wampole) Two minute latex agglutination slide test for the qualitative or semiquantitative detection of infectious mononucleosis heterophile antibodies in serum or plasma. Test kit 50s.
Use: Diagnostic aid.

MONOPAR. Stilbazium Iodide.
Use: Anthelmintic.

MONOPHEN. 2-(4-Hydroxy-3,5-diiodobenzyl)-cyclohexane carboxylic acid.
Use: Orally, cholecystography.

•**MONOPRIL.** (Mead Johnson) Fosinopril.
Use: Antihypertensive.

•**MONOSODIUM GLUTAMATE,** N.F. XVII.

MONOSODIUM PHOSPHATE.
See: Sodium Biphosphate, U.S.P. XXII.

MONOSPOT. (Ortho Diagnostics) Diagnosis of infectious mononucleosis. Test kit 20s.
Use: Diagnostic aid.

MONOSTEARIN. (Various Mfr.) Glyceryl monostearate.

MONOSTICON DRI DOT. (Organon Technica) Diagnosis of infectious mononucleosis. Test kit 40s, 100s.
Use: Diagnostic aid.

MONO-SURE TEST. (Wampole) One-minute hemagglutination slide test for the differential qualitative detection and quantitative determination of infectious mononucleosis heterophile antibodies in serum or plasma. Kit 20s.
Use: Diagnostic aid.

MONOSYL. (Arcum) Secobarbital sodium 1 gr, butabarbital 0.5 gr/Tab. Bot. 100s, 1000s.
Use: Sedative/hypnotic.

MONOTARD HUMAN INSULIN. (Squibb/Novo) Human insulin zinc 100 units/ml. Susp. Vial 10 ml.
Use: Antidiabetic.

•**MONOTHIOGLYCEROL,** N.F. XVII. 3-Mercapto-1,2-propanediol.
Use: Pharmaceutic aid (preservative).

MONO-VACC. (Lincoln) Device used for vaccination against smallpox. Box 12 without vaccine or 20 sterile units with vaccine.
Use: Diagnostic biological.

MONO-VACC TEST O.T. (Merieux Institute) 5 tuberculin units by the mantoux method. Multiple puncture disposable device. Box 25s (tamperproof).
Use: Tuberculin test.

MONOXYCHLOROSENE. A stabilized, buffered, organic hypochlorous acid derivative.
See: Oxychlorosene (Guardian Chem.).

MONSEL SOLUTION. (Wade) Bot. 2 oz, 4 oz.
Use: Styptic solution.

MORANTEL. V.B.A.N. (E)-1,4,5,6-Tetrahydro-1-methyl-2-[2-(3-methyl-2-thienyl)vinyl]-pyrimidine.
Use: Anthelmintic (veterinary).

•**MORANTEL TARTRATE.** USAN. (E)-1,4,5,6-Tetrahydro-1-methyl-2-[2(3)methyl-2-thienyl-vinyl]pyrimidine tartrate.
Use: Anthelmintic.

MORANYL.
See: Suramin Sodium.

MORAZONE. B.A.N. 2:3-Dimethyl-4-(3-methyl-2-phenylmorpholinomethyl)-1-phenylpyrazol-5-one.
Use: Analgesic.

MORCO. (Archer-Taylor) Cod liver oil ointment, zinc oxide, benzethonium Cl, benzocaine 1%. 1.5 oz, lb.
Use: Antiseptic, antipruritic.

MORE-DOPHILUS. (Freeda) Acidophilus-carrot derivative 4 billion units/Gm Pow. 120 Gm.
Use: Antidiarrheal.

MORICIZINE. USAN.
Use: Antiarrhythmic.
See: Ethmozine (DuPont).

•**MORNIFLUMATE.** USAN.
Use: Anti-inflammatory.

MOROLINE. (Schering-Plough) Petrolatum. Jar 1.75 oz, 3.75 oz, 15 oz.
Use: Skin protectant, lubricant.

MOROXYDINE. B.A.N. 4-Morpholine-carboxymidoyl guanidine. N-(Guanidinoformimidoyl)-morpholine.
Use: Antiviral.

MORPEN TABS. (Major) Ibuprofen 400 mg or 600 mg/Tab. Bot. 500s.
Use: Nonsteroidal anti-inflammatory drug; analgesic.

MORPHERIDINE. B.A.N. Ethyl1-(2-morpholinoethyl)-4-phenylpiperidine-4-carboxylate. Morpholino-ethylnorpethidine.
Use: Narcotic analgesic.

MORPHINE ACETATE.
W/Terpin hydrate, ammonium hypophosphite, potassium guaiacol-sulfonate.
See: Broncho-Tussin Soln. (First Texas).

MORPHINE AND ATROPINE SULFATES TABLETS.

Use: Analgesic, parasympatholytic.

MORPHINE HYDROCHLORIDE. (Various Mfr.) Pow. Bot. 1 oz, 5 oz.
Use: Analgesic.

•**MORPHINE SULFATE,** U.S.P. XXII. Inj., U.S.P. XXII. (Various Mfr.) Flake or Pow. Bot. 1/8 oz, 1 oz, 5 oz, H.T. 1/8 gr, 1/6 gr, 0.25 gr, 0.5 gr, 1 gr.
Use: Narcotic analgesic, sedative.
W/Tartar emetic, bloodroot, ipecac, squill, wild cherry.
See: Pectoral, Preps. (Noyes).

•**MORRHUATE SODIUM INJECTION,** U.S.P. XXII.
Use: Sclerosing agent.

MORTON SALT SUBSTITUTE. (Morton Salt) Potassium Cl, fumaric acid, tricalcium phosphate, monocalcium phosphate. Sodium: > 0.5 mg/5 Gm (> 0.02 mEq/5 Gm), potassium 2800 mg/5 Gm (72 mEq/5 Gm) 88.6 Gm.
Use: Salt substitute.

MOSCO. (Medtech) Salicylic acid. Jar 0.4 oz, 0.8 oz.
Use: Keratolytic.

MOTILIUM. (Janssen) Domperidone maleate.
Use: Antiemetic.

MOTION AID TABLETS. (Vangard) Dimenhydrinate 50 mg/Tab. Bot. 100s, 1000s, UD 10×10s.
Use: Antiemetic/antivertigo.

MOTION CURE. (Wisconsin Pharm.) Meclizine 25 mg/Chew. Tab. 12s.
Use: Antiemetic/antivertigo.

MOTION SICKNESS AGENTS.
See: Antinauseants.
Bucladin, Softab Tab. (Stuart).
Dramamine, Preps. (Searle).
Emetrol, Liq. (Rorer).
Marezine, Tab., Amp. (Burroughs Wellcome).
Scopolamine HBr (Various Mfr.).

MOTOFEN. (Carnrick) Difenoxin HCl 1 mg, atropine sulfate 0.025 mg/Tab. Bot. 100s.
Use: Antidiarrheal.

•**MOTRETINIDE.** USAN.
Use: Keratolytic.

MOTRIN. (Upjohn) Ibuprofen. **Tab: 300 mg** Bot. 500s, Unit-Of-Use 60s; **400 mg** Bot. 500s, Unit-of-Use 100s, UD 100s; **600 mg** Bot. 500s, Unit-of-Use 100s, UD 100s; **800 mg** Bot. 500s, Unit-of-Use 100s, UD 100s.
Use: Nonsteroidal anti-inflammatory drug; analgesic.

•**MOXALACTAM DISODIUM.** USAN.
Use: Antibiotic.
See: Moxam, Inj. (Lilly).

•**MOXALACTAM DISODIUM FOR INJECTION,** U.S.P. XXII.
Use: Anti-infective.

MOXAM. (Lilly) Moxalactam disodium. Vial 1 Gm/10 ml Traypak 10s; Vial 2 Gm/20 ml Traypak 10s; Vial 10 Gm/100 ml Traypak 6s.
Use: Antibacterial, cephalosporin.

•**MOXAZOCINE.** USAN.
Use: Analgesic, antitussive.

•**MOXIDECTIN.** USAN.
Use: Parasiticide (veterinary).

MOXIPRAQUINE. B.A.N. 8- {6-[4-(3-Hydroxy-butyl)piperazin-1-yl]hexylamino} -6-methoxy-quinoline.
Use: Protozoacide.

•**MOXNIDAZOLE.** USAN.
Use: Antiprotozoal.

MOYCO FLUORIDE RINSE. (Moyco) Fluoride 2%. Flavor. Bot. 128 oz. with pump.
Use: Dental caries preventative.

M-PREDNISOL-40. (Pasadena) Methylprednisolone acetate 40 mg/ml. Inj. Susp. Vial 5 ml.
Use: Corticosteroid.

M-PREDNISOL-80. (Pasadena) Methylprednisolone acetate 80 mg/ml. Inj. Susp. Vial 5 ml.
Use: Corticosteroid.

MRV. (Hollister-Stier) 2000 million organisms/ml from Staphylococcus aureus (1200 million), Streptococcus, viradens and non-hemolytic (200 million), Streptococcus pneumoniae (150 million), Branhamella catarrhalis (150 million), Klebsiella pneumoniae (150 million), Hemophilus influenzae (150 million). Inj. Vial 20 ml.
Use: Agent for immunization.

M-R-VAX II. (Merck Sharp & Dohme) Live attenuated measles virus vaccine (ATTENUVAX) and live attenuated rubella virus vaccine (MERUVAX II). See details under Attenuvax and Meruvax II. Single dose vial w/diluent. Pkg. 1s, 10s.
Use: Agent for immunization.

MS CONTIN. (Purdue Frederick) Morphine. **CR Tab.: 30 mg** Bot. 50s, 100s, 250s, Card 25s. **60 mg** 100s, UD 25s.
Use: Narcotic analgesic.

MSIR TABLETS. (Purdue Frederick) Morphine 15 mg or 30 mg/IR Tab. Bot. 50s.
Use: Narcotic analgesic.

MSTA. (Squibb/Connaught) Mumps skin test antigen. Vial 1 ml.
Use: Diagnostic aid.

M.T.E.-4. (Lyphomed) Zinc 1 mg, copper 0.4 mg, chromium 4 mcg, manganese 0.1 mg/ml. Vial 3 ml, 10 ml, MD Vial 30 ml.
Use: Mineral supplement.

M.T.E.-4 CONCENTRATED. (Lyphomed) Zinc 5 mg, copper 1 mg, chromium 10 mcg, manganese 0.5 mg/ml. Vial 1 ml, MD Vial 10 ml.
Use: Mineral supplement.

M.T.E.-5. (Lyphomed) Zinc 1 mg, copper 0.4 mg, chromium 4 mcg, manganese 0.1 mg, selenium 20 mcg/ml. Vial 10 ml.
Use: Mineral supplement.

M.T.E.-5 CONCENTRATED. (Lyphomed) Zinc 5 mg, copper 1 mg, chromium 10 mcg, manganese 0.5 mg, selenium 60 mcg/ml. Vial 1 ml, MD vial 10 ml.
Use: Mineral supplement.

M.T.E.-6. (Lyphomed) Zinc 1 mg, copper 0.4 mg, chromium 4 mcg, manganese 0.1 mg, selenium 20 mcg, iodide 25 mcg/ml. Vial 10 ml.
Use: Mineral supplement.

M.T.E.-6 CONCENTRATE. (LyphoMed) Zinc 5 mg, copper 1 mg, chromium 10 mcg, manganese 0.5 mg, selenium 60 mcg, iodide 75 mcg/ml. Vial 1 ml. MD vial 10 ml.
Use: Mineral supplement.

M.T.E.-7. (LyphoMed) Zinc 1 mg copper 0.4 mg, manganese 0.1 mg, chromium 4 mcg, selenium 20 mcg, iodide 25 mcg, molybdenum 25 mcg/ml. Vial 10 ml.
Use: Mineral supplement.

MTX.
Use: Antineoplastic, antipsoriatic.
See: Methotrexate.

MUCILLIUM. (Robinson) Refined psyllium mucilloid, dextrose. Bot. 8 oz.
Use: Laxative.

MUCILLOID OF PSYLLIUM SEED.
W/Dextrose.
See: Metamucil, Liq. (Searle).

MUCIN.
See: Gastric Mucin (Wilson).

MUCIN, VEGETABLE.
W/Yeast or alkalized.
See: Plantamucin, Granules (Elder).

MUCOMYST. (Bristol) A sterile 20% solution of acetylcysteine for nebulization or direct instillation into the lung as a mucolytic agent. Approved as antidote for acetaminophen overdose. Vial. **4 ml:** Ctn. 12s; **10 ml:** Ctn. 3s with dropper; **30 ml:** Ctn. 3s.
Use: Respiratory inhalant.

MUCOMYST-10. (Bristol) A sterile 10% solution of acetylcysteine for nebulization or direct instillation into the lung as a mucolytic agent. Approved as antidote for acetaminophen overdose. Vial. **4 ml:** Ctn. 12s; **10 ml:** Ctn. 3s with dropper; **30 ml:** Ctn. 3s.
Use: Respiratory inhalant.

MUCOSAL 10 & 20 SOLUTION. (Dey) Acetylcysteine sodium salt 10% or 20%. Soln. Vial 4 ml Box 12s.
Use: Respiratory inhalant.

MUDD. (Chattem) Natural hydrated magnesium aluminum silicate. Topical preparation.
Use: Cleansing agent.

MUDRANE. (Poythress) Aminophylline (anhydrous) 130 mg, phenobarbital 8 mg, ephedrine HCl 16 mg, potassium iodide 195 mg/Tab. Bot. 100s, 1000s.
Use: Antiasthmatic combination.

MUDRANE-2. (Poythress) Potassium iodide 195 mg, aminophylline (anhydrous) 130 mg/Tab. Bot. 100s.
Use: Antiasthmatic combination.

MUDRANE GG. (Poythress) Aminophylline (anhydrous) 130 mg, ephedrine HCl 16 mg, guaifenesin 100 mg, phenobarbital 8 mg/Tab. Bot. 100s, 1000s.
Use: Antiasthmatic combination.

MUDRANE GG-2. (Poythress) Guaifenesin 100 mg, aminophylline (anhydrous) 130 mg/Tab. Bot. 100s.
Use: Antiasthmatic combination.

MUDRANE GG ELIXIR. (Poythress) Theophylline 20 mg, ephedrine HCl 4 mg, guaifenesin 26 mg, phenobarbital 2.5 mg/5 ml, alcohol 20%. Bot. pt, 0.5 gal.
Use: Antiasthmatic combination.

MULTABOLIC. (Kenyon) Adrenal cortex extract 50 mg, vitamin B_{12} 30 mcg, methylandrostenediol 10 mg, liver "pink", B_{12} equivalent. 10 mcg/ml. Vial 10 ml.
Use: Nutritional supplement.

MULTA-GEN 12 +E. (Bowman) Vitamin A 5000 IU, D 400 IU, B_1 2 mg, B_2 2 mg, B_6 0.5 mg, B_{12} 3 mcg, C 37.5 mg, E 15 IU, folic acid 0.2 mg, nicotinamide 20 mg/Cap. Bot. 60s, 500s, 1000s.
Use: Vitamin supplement.

MULTALAN. (Lannett) Vitamin A 5000 IU, D 400 IU, B_1 2.5 mg, B_2 2.5 mg, B_6 0.5 mg, B_{12} 2 mcg, C 50 mg, niacinamide 20 mg, calcium pantothenate 5 mg/Cap. Bot. 500s, 1000s.
Use: Vitamin supplement.

MULTE-PAK-4. (SoloPak) Zinc 1 mg, copper 0.4 mg, manganese 0.1 mg, chromium 4 mg/ml. Vial 3 ml, 10 ml, 30 ml.
Use: Mineral supplement.

MULTE-PAK-5. (SoloPak) Zinc 1 mg, copper 0.4 mg, manganese 0.1 mg, chromium 4 mg, selenium 20 mcg/ml. Vial 3 ml, 10 ml.
Use: Mineral supplement.

MULTI-B-PLEX. (Forest) Vitamins B_1 100 mg, B_2 1 mg, nicotinamide 100 mg, pantothenic acid 10 mg, B_6 10 mg/ml. Vial 10 ml, 30 ml.
Use: Vitamin supplement.

MULTI-B-PLEX CAPSULES. (Forest) Vitamins B_1 50 mg, B_2 5 mg, niacinamide 50 mg, calcium pantothenate 5.4 mg, B_6 0.2 mg, C 150 mg, B_{12} 1 mcg/Cap. Bot. 100s, 1000s.
Use: Vitamin supplement.

MULTI-GERM OIL. (Viobin) Corn, sunflower and wheat germ oils. Bot. 4 oz, 8 oz, pt, qt.
Use: Enteral nutritional supplement.

MULTI-JETS. (Kirkman) Vitamins A 10,000 IU, D_2 400 IU, B_1 20 mg, B_2 8 mg, C 120 mg, niacinamide 10 mg, calcium pantothenate 5 mg, B_6 0.5 mg, E 50 IU, desiccated liver 100 mg, dried debittered yeast 100 mg, choline bitartrate 62 mg, inositol 30 mg, dl methionine 30 mg, B_{12} 7 mcg, iron 2.6 mg, calcium (dical phosphate) 58 mg, phosphorus (dical phosphate) 45 mg, iodine (potassium iodide) 0.114 mg, magnesium sulfate 1 mg, copper sulfate 1.99 mg, manganese sulfate 1.11 mg, potassium Cl iodide 79 mg/Tab. Bot. 100s.
Use: Vitamin/mineral supplement.

MULTILEX TABLETS. (Rugby) Iron 15 mg, vitamins A 10,000 IU, D 400 IU, E 5.5 mg, B_1 10 mg, B_2 5 mg, B_3 30 mg, B_5 10 mg, B_6 1.7 mg, B_{12} 3 mcg, C 100 mg, zinc 1.5 mg, Cu, I, Mg, Mn/Tab. Bot. 100s, 1000s.
Use: Vitamin/mineral supplement.

MULTILEX T/M TABLETS. (Rugby) Iron 15 mg, vitamins A 10,000 IU, D 400 IU, E 5.5 mg, B_1

15 mg, B_2 10 mg, B_3 100 mg, B_5 10 mg, B_6 2 mg, B_{12} 7.5 mcg, C 150 mg, Cu, I, Mg, Mn, Zn/Tab. Bot. 100s, 500s, 1000s.
Use: Vitamin/mineral supplement.

MULTILYTE-20. (Lyphomed) Sodium$^+$ 25 mEq/L, potassium$^+$ 20 mEq/L, calcium^{++} 5 mEq/L, magnesium^{++} 5 mEq/L, chloride$^-$ 30 mEq/L, acetate 25 mEq/L, gluconate 5 mEq/L. Vial 25 ml fill in 50 ml.
Use: Fluid/electrolyte replacement.

MULTILYTE-40. (Lyphomed) Sodium$^+$ 25 mEq/L, potassium$^+$ 40.5 mEq/L, calcium^{++} 5 mEq/L, magnesium^{++} 8 mEq/L, chloride$^-$ 33.5 mEq/L, acetate 40.6 mEq/L, gluconate 5 mEq/L. Vial 25 ml fill in 50 ml.
Use: Fluid/electrolyte replacement.

MULTIPALS. (Faraday) Vitamins A 5000 IU, D 400 IU, C 50 mg, B_1 3 mg, B_6 0.5 mg, B_2 3 mg, calcium pantothenate 5 mg, niacinamide 20 mg, B_{12} 2 mcg/Tab. Bot. 100s, 250s, 1000s.
Use: Vitamin supplement.

MULTIPALS-M. (Faraday) Vitamins A 6000 IU, D 400 IU, B_1 3 mg, B_2 3 mg, B_6 0.5 mg, B_{12} 5 mcg, C 60 mg, E 2 IU, niacinamide 20 mg, calcium pantothenate 5 mg, iron 10 mg, iodine 0.15 mg, copper 1 mg, magnesium 6 mg, manganese 1 mg, potassium 5 mg/Tab. Bot. 100s, 250s, 1000s.
Use: Vitamin/mineral supplement.

MULTIPLE TRACE ELEMENT. (American Regent) Zinc sulfate 1 mg, copper sulfate 0.4 mg, manganese sulfate 0.1 mg, chromium Cl 4 mg/ml. Inj. Soln. Vial 10 ml.
Use: Mineral supplement.

MULTIPLE TRACE ELEMENT CONCENTRATED. (American Regent) Zinc sulfate 5 mg, copper sulfate 1 mg, manganese sulfate 0.5 mg, chromium Cl 10 mcg/ml. Inj. Soln. Vial 10 ml.
Use: Mineral supplement.

MULTIPLE TRACE ELEMENT PEDIATRIC. (American Regent) Zinc sulfate 0.5 mg, copper sulfate 0.1 mg, manganese sulfate 0.03 mg, chromium Cl 1 mcg/ml. Inj. Soln. Vial 10 ml.
Use: Mineral supplement.

MULTIPLE VITAMIN MINERAL FORMULA. (Kirkman) Vitamins A 5000 IU, D_2 400 IU, C 50 mg, B_1 2.5 mg, B_2 2.5 mg, B_6 0.5 mg, B_{12} 1 mcg, niacinamide 15 mg, calcium pantothenate 5 mg, E 0.1 IU, calcium 100 mg, iron 7.5 mg, magnesium 2.5 mg, potassium 2.5 mg, zinc 0.15 mg, manganese 0.5 mg, iodine 0.07 mg/Tab. Bot. 100s.
Use: Vitamin/mineral supplement.

MULTIPLE VITAMINS CHEWABLE. (Kirkman) Vitamins A 5000 IU, D 400 IU, C 50 mg, B_1 3 mg, B_2 2.5 mg, B_6 1 mg, B_{12} 1 mcg, niacinamide 20 mg/Tab. Bot. 100s.
Use: Vitamin supplement.

MULTIPLE VITAMINS W/IRON. (Kirkman) Vitamins A 5000 IU, D 400 IU, C 50 mg, B_1 3 mg, B_2 2.5 mg, B_6 1 mg, B_{12} 1 mcg, niacinamide 20 mg, iron 10 mg/Tab. Bot. 100s.
Use: Vitamin/mineral supplement.

MULTISTIX REAGENT STRIPS. (Ames) Urinalysis reagent strip test for pH, protein, glucose, ketone, bilirubin and blood. Box 100s.
Use: Diagnostic aid.

MULTISTIX SG REAGENT STRIPS. (Ames) Urinalysis reagent strip test for pH, glucose, protein, ketones, bilirubin, blood and urobilinogen. Box. 100s.
Use: Diagnostic aid.

MULTISTIX 2 REAGENT STRIPS. (Ames) Urinalysis reagent strip test for nitrite and leukocytes. Bot. 100s.
Use: Diagnostic aid.

MULTISTIX 7. (Ames) Urinalysis reagent strip test for glucose ketone, blood, pH, protein, nitrite and leukocytes. Box 100s.
Use: Diagnostic aid.

MULTISTIX 8. (Ames) Urinalysis reagent strip test for detecting glucose, ketone, blood, pH, protein, nitrite, bilirubin and leukocytes. Box. 100s.
Use: Diagnostic aid.

MULTISTIX 8 SG REAGENT STRIPS. (Ames) Urinalysis reagent strip test for glucose, ketone, specific gravity, blood, pH, protein nitrite, leukocytes. Box 100s.
Use: Diagnostic aid.

MULTISTIX 9 REAGENT STRIPS. (Ames) Urinalysis reagent strip test for glucose, bilirubin, ketone, blood, pH, protein, urobilinogen, nitrite, leukocytes. Box 100s.
Use: Diagnostic aid.

MULTISTIX 9 SG REAGENT STRIPS. (Ames) Urinalysis reagent strip test for glucose, bilirubin, ketone, specific gravity, blood, pH, protein, nitrite and leukocytes. Box 100s.
Use: Diagnostic aid.

MULTISTIX 10 SG REAGENT STRIPS. (Ames) Reagent strip test for glucose, bilirubin, ketone, specific gravity, blood, pH, protein, urobilinogen, nitrite and leukocytes in urine. Box 100s.
Use: Diagnostic aid.

MULTITEST CMI. (Merieux Institute) One disposable applicator pre-loaded with seven glycerinated liquid antigens and glycerin negative control. 10 units/box.
Use: Diagnostic aid.

MULTI-THERA TABLETS. (Nature's Bounty) Vitamins A 5500 IU, D 400 IU, E 30 mg, B_1 3 mg, B_2 3.4 mg, B_3 30 mg, B_5 10 mg, B_6 3 mg, B_{12} 9 mcg, C 120 mg, folic acid 0.4 mg, biotin 15 mcg/Tab. Bot. 100s.
Use: Vitamin supplement.

MULTI-THERA-M. (Nature's Bounty) Iron 27 mg, vitamins A 5500 IU, D 400 IU, E 30 mg, B_1 3 mg, B_2 3.4 mg, B_3 30 mg, B_5 10 mg, B_6 3 mg, B_{12} 9 mcg, C 120 mg, folic acid 0.4 mg, biotin 15 mcg, zinc 15 mg, Ca, Cl, Cr, Cu, I, K, Mg, Mn, Mo, Se/Tab. Bot. 130s.

Use: Vitamin/mineral supplement.

MULTI-VIT DROPS. (Barre) Vitamins A 500 IU, D 400 IU, E 5 mg, B_1 0.5 mg, B_2 0.6 mg, B_3 8 mg, B_6 0.4 mg, B_{12} 2 mcg, C 35 mg/ml. Bot. 50 ml.
Use: Vitamin supplement.

MULTI-VITA DROPS. (My-K Labs) Vitamins A 1500 IU, D 400 IU, E 5 mg, B_1 0.5 mg, B_2 0.6 mg, B_3 8 mg, B_6 0.4 mg, B_{12} 2 mcg, C 35 mg/ml. Alcohol free. Bot. 50 ml.
Use: Vitamin/mineral supplement.

MULTI-VITA DROPS W/FLOURIDE. (My-K Labs) Flouride 0.5 mg, vitamins A 1500 IU, D 400 IU, E 5 mg, B_1 0.5 mg, B_2 0.6 mg, B_3 8 mg, B_6 0.4 mg, B_{12} 2 mcg, C 35 mg/ml. Alcohol free. Bot. 50 ml.
Use: Vitamin supplement; dental caries preventative.

MULTI-VITA DROPS W/IRON. (My-K Labs) Iron 10 mg, vitamins A 1500 IU, D 400 IU, E 5 mg, B_1 0.5 mg, B_2 0.6 mg, B_3 8 mg, B_6 0.4 mg, C 35 mg/ml. Alcohol free. Bot. 50 ml.
Use: Vitamin/mineral supplement.

MULTI-VITAMINS CAPSULES. (Forest) Vitamins A 5000 IU, D 400 IU, B_1 1.5 mg, B_2 2 mg, B_6 0.1 mg, C 37.5 mg, calcium pantothenate 1 mg, niacinamide 20 mg/Cap. Bot. 100s, 1000s, 5000s.
Use: Vitamin supplement.

MULTIVITAMINS ROWELL. (Solvay) Vitamins A 5000 IU, D 400 IU, B_1 2.5 mg, B_2 2.5 mg, C 50 mg, niacinamide 20 mg, B_6 0.5 mg, calcium pantothenate 5 mg, B_{12} 2 mcg, E 10 IU/Cap. Bot. 100s, UD 100s.
Use: Vitamin supplement.

MULTIZINE.
See: Trisulfapyrimidines Tab., U.S.P. XXII.

MULTOREX. (Approved) Vitamins A 6000 IU, D 1250 IU, C 50 mg, E 5 IU, B_1 3 mg, B_2 3 mg, B_6 0.5 mg, niacinamide 20 mg, calcium pantothenate 5 mg, B_{12} 5 mcg, calcium 59 mg, phosphorus 45 mg/Cap. Bot. 100s, 250s, 1000s.
Use: Vitamin/mineral supplement.

MULVIDREN-F. (Stuart) Fluoride 1 mg, vitamins A 4000 units, D 400 units, C 75 mg, B_1 2 mg, B_2 2 mg, B_6 1.2 mg, B_{12} 3 mcg, calcium pantothenate 3 mg, niacinamide 10 mg/Softab Tab. Bot. 100s.
Use: Vitamin supplement, dental caries preventative.

MUMPS SKIN TEST ANTIGEN. (Connaught) Suspension of killed mumps virus, 40 complement fixing units/ml. Vial 1 ml. (test 10s).
Use: Diagnostic aid.

•**MUMPS SKIN TEST ANTIGEN,** U.S.P. XXII. (Lilly). Antigen made from allantoic fluid of chick embryos. Vial 1 ml (test 10s).
Use: Diagnostic aid (dermal reactivity indicator).

MUMPSVAX. (Merck Sharp & Dohme) Live mumps virus vaccine, Jeryl Lynn strain. Single-dose vial w/diluent Pkg. 1s, 10s.
Use: Agent for immunization.
W/Attenuvax, Meruvax II.
See: M-M-R II, Inj. (Merck Sharp & Dohme).
W/Meruvax II.
See: Biavax II (Merck Sharp & Dohme).

•**MUMPS VIRUS VACCINELIVE,** U.S.P. XXII.
Use: Active immunizing agent.
See: Mumpsvax, Inj. (Merck Sharp & Dohme).

MUMPS VIRUS VACCINE, LIVE ATTENUATED. Jeryl Lynn (B Level) strain.
W/Measles virus vaccine, rubella virus vaccine.
See: Lirutrin, Vial (Merrell Dow).
M-M-R, Inj. (Merck Sharp & Dohme).

•**MUPIROCIN.** USAN.
Use: Topical antibacterial.
See: Bactroban, Oint. (Beecham).

MURIATIC ACID.
See: Hydrochloric Acid, N.F. XVII.

MURI-LUBE. (Lyphomed) Mineral Oil "Light." Vial 2 ml, 10 ml.
Use: Lubricant for surgery.

MURINE EAR DROPS. (Ross) Carbamide peroxide 6.5% in anhydrous glycerin. Bot. 0.5 oz.
Use: Otic preparation.

MURINE EAR WAX REMOVAL SYSTEM. (Ross) Carbamide peroxide 6.5% in anhydrous glycerin w/ear washing syringe. Bot. 0.5 oz. and ear washer 1 oz.
Use: Otic preparation.

MURINE EYE DROPS. (Ross) Potassium Cl, sodium Cl, sodium phosphate, (monobasic and dibasic), water, glycerin, edetate disodium 0.05%, benzalkonium Cl 0.01%. Plastic dropper bot. 0.5 oz, 1 oz.
Use: Artificial tear solution.

MURINE PLUS EYE DROPS. (Ross) Tetrahydrozoline HCl 0.05%, boric acid, sodium borate, edetate disodium 0.1%, benzalkonium Cl 0.01%. Bot. 0.5 oz, 1 oz.
Use: Vasoconstrictor, ophthalmic.

MURO #128 OINTMENT. (Bausch & Lomb) Sodium Cl 5% in sterile ointment base. Tube 3.5 Gm.
Use: Hyperosmolar agent.

MURO #128 SOLUTION. (Bausch & Lomb) Sodium Cl 5%. Soln. Bot. 15 ml, 30 ml.
Use: Hyperosmolar agent.

MURO #128 2% SOLUTION. (Bausch & Lomb) Sodium Cl 2%. Soln. Dropper bot. 15 ml.
Use: Hyperosmolar agent.

MUROCEL SOLUTION. (Bausch & Lomb) Methylcellulose 1%. Soln. Bot. 15 ml.
Use: Artificial tear solution.

MUROCOLL-2. (Bausch & Lomb) Phenylephrine HCl 10%, scopolamine HBR 0.3% Bot. 5 ml.
Use: Mydriatic, cycloplegic.

MUROMONAB-CD3.
Use: Immunosuppressive agent.
See: Orthoclone OKT3, Inj. (Ortho).

MURO'S OPCON A SOLUTION. (Bausch & Lomb) Naphazoline HCl 0.025%, pheniramine maleate 0.3%. Bot. 15 ml.
Use: Decongestant, antihistamine (ophthalmic).

MURO'S OPCON SOLUTION. (Bausch & Lomb) Naphazoline HCl 0.1%. Bot. 15 ml.
Use: Decongestant, ophthalmic.

MURO TEARS SOLUTION. (Bausch & Lomb) Hydroxypropyl methylcellulose, dextran 40. Soln. Bot. 15 ml.
Use: Artificial tear solution.

MUSCLE ADENYLIC ACID. (Various Mfr.) Active form of adenosine 5-monophosphate.
See: Adenosine 5-monophosphate, Preps. (Various Mfr.).

MUSCLE RELAXANTS.
See: Arduan (Organon).
Curare (Various Mfr.).
Flaxedil Triethiodide, Vial (Davis & Geck).
Flexeril, Tab. (Merck, Sharp & Dohme).
Lioresal, Tab. (Geigy)
Mephenesin (Various Mfr.).
Meprobamate (Various Mfr.).
Metubine Iodine, Vial (Lilly).
Neostig, Tab. (Freeport).
Norflex, Tab., Inj. (Riker).
Nuromax (Burroughs Wellcome).
Parafon Forte, Tab. (McNeil).
P-A-V, Cap. (Amid).
Rela, Tab. (Schering).
Robaxin, Tab., Inj. (Robins).
Soma, Tab., Cap. (Wallace).
Succinylcholine Cl (Various Mfr.).
d-Tubocurarine Cl (Various Mfr.).

MUSTARAL OIL.
See: Allyl Isothiocyanate.

MUSTARGEN. (Merck Sharp & Dohme) Mechlorethamine HCl 10 mg/Vial, sodium Cl q.s. 100 mg/Vial. Treatment set vial 4s.
Use: Nitrogen mustard.

MUSTEROLE. (Schering-Plough) **Regular:** Camphor 4%, menthol 2%. Jar 0.9 oz. **Extra Strength:** Camphor 5%, menthol 3%. Jar 0.9 oz., Tube 1 oz, 2.25 oz.
Use: External analgesic.

MUSTEROLE DEEP STRENGTH. (Schering-Plough) Methyl salicylate 30%, menthol 3%, methyl nicotinate 0.5%. Jar 1.25 oz, Tube 3 oz.
Use: External analgesic.

MUSTIN.
See: Mechlorethamine HCl, Sterile, U.S.P.

MUSTINE. B.A.N. NN-Di-(2-chloroethyl) methylamine. Chlormethine (I.N.N.).
Use: Antineoplastic agent.

MUTALIN. (Spanner) Protein and iodine. Vial 30 ml.

MUTAMYCIN. (Bristol-Myers/Bristol Oncology) Mitomycin 5 mg, 20 mg or 40 mg/Vial.
Use: Antineoplastic agent.

•**MUZOLIMINE.** USAN.
Use: Diuretic, antihypertensive.

M.V.C. 9 + 3. (Lyphomed) Multivitamin injection for IV infusion. Vial 5 ml, 10 ml, 50 ml.
Use: Vitamin supplement.

M.V.I.-12. (Armour) **Vial 1:** Vitamins A 1 mg, D 5 mcg, E 10 mg, C 100 mg, B_1 3 mg, B_2 3.6 mg, B_6 4 mg, niacinamide 40 mg, dexpanthenol 15 mg/5 ml. **Vial 2:** Biotin 60 mcg, folic acid 400 mcg, Vitamin B_{12} 5 mcg/5 ml. Vials 1 and 2 used together. Box 25s, Ctn. 100s. Vial.
Use: Parenteral nutritional supplement.

M.V.I. PEDIATRIC. (Armour) Vitamin A 0.7 mg, D 10 mcg, E 7 mg, C 80 mcg, B_1 1.2 mg, B_2 1.4 mg, B_6 1 mg, B_{12} 1 mcg, potassium 200 mcg, niacinamide 17 mg, dexpanthenol 5 mg, biotin 20 mcg, folic acid 140 mcg/Vial. Box 25s, 5 dose multiple-dose vial, Box 5s.
Use: Parenteral nutritional supplement.

MYAGEN. Bolasterone.
Use: Anabolic agent.

MYAMBUTOL. (Lederle) Ethambutol HCl. Tab. **100 mg:** Bot. 100s. **400 mg:** Bot. 100s, 1000s, UD 10 × 10s.
Use: Antituberculous agent.

MYANESIN.
See: Mephenesin (Various Mfr.).

MYAPAP DROPS. (My-K) Acetaminophen 80 mg/0.8 ml. Bot. 15 ml w/dropper.
Use: Analgesic.

MYAPAP ELIXIR. (My-K) Acetaminophen 160 mg/5 ml. Bot. 4 oz, pt, gal.
Use: Analgesic.

MYAPAP WITH CODEINE ELIXIR. (My-K) Acetaminophen 120 mg, codeine phosphate 12 mg/5 ml. Bot. 4 oz, pt, gal.
Use: Analgesic, antitussive.

MYBANIL. (My-K) Codeine phosphate 10 mg, bromodiphenhydramine HCl 12.5 mg/5 ml, alcohol 5%. Bot. 4 oz, pt, gal.
Use: Antitussive, antihistamine.

MYCADEC DM DROPS. (My-K) Pseudoephedrine 25 mg, carbonoxamine maleate 2 mg, dextromethorphan HBr 4 mg. Bot. 30 ml.
Use: Decongestant, antihistamine, antitussive.

MYCADEC DM SYRUP. (My-K) Carbinoxamine maleate 4 mg, pseudoephedrine HCl 60 mg, dextromethorphan HBr 15 mg/5 ml, alcohol 0.6%. Bot. 4 oz, pt, gal.
Use: Antihistamine, decongestant, antitussive.

MYCADEC DROPS. (My-K) Pseudoephedrine HCl 25 mg, dextromethorphan HBr 4 mg, carbinoxamine maleate 2 mg/ml. Bot. 30 ml.
Use: Decongestant, antitussive, antihistamine.

MYCELEX. (Miles Pharm) Clotrimazole. **Topical Cream:** 1%. Tube 15 Gm, 30 Gm, 90 Gm (2 × 45 Gm). **Topical Soln.:** 1%. Bot. 10 ml, 30 ml.
Use: Antifungal, external.

MYCELEX-G. (Miles Pharm) Clotrimazole. **Vaginal Tab.:** 100 mg. Pkg. 7s w/applicator. **Cream:** 1%. Tube 45 Gm, 90 Gm.
Use: Antifungal, vaginal.

MYCELEX-G 500. (Miles Pharm) Clotrimazole 500 mg/Vaginal Tab. w/applicator.
Use: Antifungal, vaginal.

MYCELEX TWIN PACK. (Miles Pharm) Clotrimazole 500 mg/Vaginal Tab. w/applicator. Topical cream 1%. Tube 7 Gm.
Use: Antifungal, vaginal.

MYCHEL-S. (Rachelle) Sterile chloramphenicol sodium succinate. Vial 1 Gm/15 ml. Box 5s.
Use: Anti-infective.

MYCIFRADIN. (Upjohn) Neomycin sulfate 125 mg/5 ml (equivalent to 87.5 mg neomycin). Oral soln. Bot. pt.
Use: Anti-infective.

MYCIGUENT. (Upjohn) Neomycin sulfate. **Cream:** 5 mg/Gm. Tube 0.5 oz. **Oint.:** 5 mg/Gm. Tube 0.5 oz, 1 oz, 4 oz.
Use: Anti-infective, topical.

MYCINETTES. (Pfeiffer) Benzocaine 15 mg, cetylpyridinium Cl, terpin hydrate, sodium citrate, sorbitol in a demulcent base. Loz. 12s.
Use: Local anesthetic, antiseptic, expectorant.

MYCI-SPRAY. (Misemer) Phenylephrine HCl 0.25%, pyrilamine maleate 0.15%/ml. Bot. 20 ml.
Use: Decongestant, antihistamine.

MYCITRACIN. (Upjohn) Bacitracin 500 units, neomycin sulfate 5 mg, polymyxin B sulfate 5000 units/Gm. Oint.: Tube 0.5 oz. Box 36s; 1 oz; UD 1/32 oz Box 144s.
Use: Anti-infective, topical.

MYCODONE SYRUP. (My-K) Hydrocodone bitartrate 5 mg, homatropine MBr 1.5 mg/5 ml. Bot. 4 oz, pt, gal.
Use: Antitussive.

MYCOGEN II CREAM. (Goldline) Nystatin 100,000 units, triamcinolone acetonide 1 mg/Gm. Cream Tube 15 Gm, 30 Gm, 60 Gm, 120 Gm, lb.
Use: Antifungal, corticosteroid combination.

MYCOGEN II OINTMENT. (Goldline) Nystatin 100,000 units, triamcinolone acetonide 1 mg/Gm. Oint. Tube 15 Gm, 30 Gm, 60 Gm.
Use: Antifungal, corticosteroid combination.

MYCOLOG II CREAM AND OINTMENT. (Squibb) Triamcinolone acetonide 1 mg, nystatin 100,000 units/Gm. Ointment base w/Plastibase (polyethylene, mineral oil). Tube 15 Gm, 30 Gm, 60 Gm, Jar 120 Gm.
Use: Antifungal, corticosteroid combination.

MYCOMIST. (Gordon) Chlorophyll, formalin, benzalkonium Cl. Bot. 4 oz, plastic Bot. 1 oz.
Use: Antifungal for clothing.

MYCOPHENOLATE MOFETIL. USAN.
Use: Immunomodulator.

MYCOPHENOLIC ACID. USAN. (E)-6-(4-Hydroxy-6-methoxy-7-methyl-3-oxo-5-phthalanyl)-4-methyl-4-hexenoic acid.
Use: Antineoplastic agent.

MYCOPLASMA PNEUMONIA IFA IgM TEST. (Wampole-Zeus) Indirect fluorescent assay for IgM antibodies to *Mycoplasma pneumoniae.* Box test 100s.
Use: Diagnostic aid.

MYCOPLASMA PNEUMONIA IFA TEST. (Wampole-Zeus) Indirect fluorescent assay for antibodies to *Mycoplasma pneumoniae.* Box test 100s.
Use: Diagnostic aid.

MYCOSTATIN. (Squibb) Nystatin. **Tab.:** 500,000 units. Bot. 100s. **Cream:** 100,000 units/Gm in aqueous base. Tube 15 Gm, 30 Gm. **Oint.:** 100,000 units/Gm in Plastibase (polyethylene and mineral oil). Tube 15 Gm, 30 Gm. **Susp.:** 100,000 units/ml. In vehicle containing sucrose 50%, saccharin, > alcohol 1%. Bot. w/dropper 60 ml, Unimatic 5 ml. **Troche:** 200,000 units. 30s. **Vaginal Tab:** 100,000 units, lactose 0.95 Gm, ethyl cellulose, stearic acid, starch. Pkg. 15s, 30s, Unimatic Carton 50s. **Pow.:** (topical) 100,000 units/Gm in talc. Shaker bot. 15 Gm.
Use: Antifungal.

MYCOSTATIN PASTILLES. (Squibb) Nystatin, 200,000 units/Troche. 30s.
Use: Antifungal.

MYCO TRIACET. (Various Mfr.) Triamcinolone acetonide 0.1%, neomycin sulfate 0.25%, gramicidin 0.25 mg, nystatin 100,000 units/Gm. **Cream:** 15 Gm, 30 Gm, 60 Gm, 480 Gm. **Oint.:** 15 Gm, 30 Gm, 60 Gm.
Use: Corticosteroid, antifungal.

MYCO TRIACET II CREAM & OINTMENT. (Lemmon) Nystatin 100,000 units, triamcinolone acetonide 1 mg/Gm. **Cream:** White petrolatum and mineral oil. Tube 15 Gm, 30 Gm, 60 Gm. **Oint.:** Tube 15 Gm, 30 Gm, 60 Gm.
Use: Antifungal, corticosteroid.

MYCOTUSSIN EXPECTORANT. (My-K) Pseudoephedrine HCl 60 mg, hydrocodone bitartrate 5 mg, guaifenesin 200 mg/5 ml, alcohol 12.5%. Bot. 4 oz, pt, gal.
Use: Decongestant, antitussive, expectorant.

MYCOTUSSIN LIQUID. (My-K) Pseudoephedrine HCl 60 mg, hydrocodone bitartrate 5 mg/5 ml, alcohol 5%. Bot. 4 oz, pt, gal.
Use: Decongestant, antitussive.

MYDACOL. (My-K) Vitamins B_1 5 mg, B_2 2.5 mg, niacinamide 50 mg, B_6 1 mg, B_{12} 1 mcg, pantothenic acid 10 mg, iodine 100 mcg, iron 15 mg, magnesium 2 mg, zinc 2 mg, choline 100 mg, manganese 2 mg/30 ml. Bot. pt, gal.
Use: Vitamin/mineral supplement.

MYDFRIN OPHTHALMIC 2.5%. (Alcon) Phenylephrine HCl 2.5%, benzalkonium Cl 0.01%, EDTA, sodium bisulfite. Bot. 5 ml.
Use: Mydriatic.

MYDRAPRED. (Alcon) Prednisolone acetate 0.25%, atropine sulfate 1%, benzalkonium Cl 0.01% in a sterile, buffered, isotonic susp. Plastic Bot. 5 ml Drop-tainers.
Use: Corticosteroid/mydriatic combination.

MYDRIACYL. (Alcon) N-Ethyl-2-phenyl-N-(4-pyridyl-methyl) hydracrylamide. Tropicamide 0.5% or 1%, benzalkonium Cl 0.01%, EDTA. Sterile aqueous soln. 15 ml Drop-Tainer.
Use: Cycloplegic mydriatic.

MYDRIATICS.

Parasympatholytic Types

Atropine Salts (Various Mfr.).
Homatropine Hydrobromide (Various Mfr.).
Scopolamine Salts (Various Mfr.).

Sympathomimetic Types
Amphetamine Sulfate 3% (Various Mfr.).
Clopane HCl, Liq. (Lilly).
Ephedrine Sulfate (Various Mfr.).
Epinephrine HCl (Various Mfr.).
Neo-Synephrine HCl, Preps. (Winthrop Pharm).
Phenylephrine HCl. (Various Mfr.).

MYELO-KIT. (Winthrop Pharm) Omnipaque 180 or 240 in various sizes and one sterile myelogram tray.
Use: Radiopaque agent.

MYFEDRINE. (Pharmaceutical Basics) Pseudoephedrine 30 mg/5 ml. Liq. Bot. 473 ml.
Use: Decongestant.

MYFEDRINE PLUS SYRUP. (My-K) Pseudoephedrine HCl 30 mg, chlorpheniramine maleate 2 mg/5 ml. Bot. 4 oz, pt, gal.
Use: Decongestant, antihistamine.

MYGEL LIQUID. (Geneva Generics) Aluminum hydroxide 200 mg, magnesium hydroxide 200 mg, simethicone 20 mg, sodium 1.38 mg/5 ml. Liq. Bot. 360 ml.
Use: Antacid, antiflatulent.

MYGEL II LIQUID. (Geneva Generics) Aluminum hydroxide 400 mg, magnesium hydroxide 400 mg, sodium 1.3 mg/5 ml. Liq. Bot. 360 ml.
Use: Antacid, antiflatulent.

MYFED SYRUP. (My-K) Triprolidine HCl 1.25 mg, pseudoephedrine HCl 30 mg/5 ml. Bot. 4 oz, pt, gal.
Use: Antihistamine, decongestant.

MYHISTINE DH. (My-K) Codeine phosphate 10 mg, chlorpheniramine maleate 2 mg, pseudoephedrine HCl 30 mg/5 ml. Liq. Bot. 4 oz, pt, gal.
Use: Antitussive, antihistamine, decongestant.

MYHISTINE ELIXIR. (My-K) Chlorpheniramine maleate 2 mg, phenylephrine HCl 5 mg/5 ml, alcohol 5%. Liq. Bot. 4 oz, pt, gal.
Use: Antihistamine, decongestant.

MYHISTINE EXPECTORANT. (My-K) Codeine phosphate 10 mg, guaifenesin 100 mg, pseudoephedrine HCl 30 mg/5 ml, alcohol 7.5%. Liq. Bot. 4 oz, pt, gal.
Use: Antitussive, expectorant, decongestant.

MYHYDROMINE PEDIATRIC. (My-K) Phenylpropanolamine HCl 12.5 mg, hydrocodone bitartrate 2.5 mg/5 ml. Bot. pt, gal.
Use: Decongestant, antitussive.

MYHYDROMINE SYRUP. (My-K) Phenylpropanolamine HCl 25 mg, hydrocodone bitartrate 5 mg/5 ml. Bot. 4 oz, pt, gal.
Use: Decongestive, antitussive.

MYIDONE TABS. (Major) Primidone 250 mg/Tab. Bot. 100s, 1000s.
Use: Anticonvulsant.

MYIDIL. (My-K) Triprolidine HCl 1.25 mg/5 ml, alcohol 4%. Syr. Bot. 120 ml, pt, gal.
Use: Antihistamine.

MYIDYL SYRUP. (My-K) Triprolidine HCl 1.25 mg/5 ml, alcohol 4%. Bot. 4 oz, pt, gal.
Use: Antihistamine.

MYKACET CREAM. (NMC Labs) Nystatin 100,000 units, triamcinolone acetonide 0.1%/Gm. Tube 15 Gm, 30 Gm, 60 Gm.
Use: Antifungal, corticosteroid.

MY-K ELIXIR. (My-K) Potassium 20 mEq/15 ml, alcohol 5%, saccharin. Bot. pt, gal.
Use: Potassium supplement.

MY-K FORMULA 77 LIQUID. (My-K) Doxylamine succinate 3.75 mg, dextromethorphan HBr 7.5 mg/5 ml, alcohol 10%. Liq. Bot. 180 ml.
Use: Antihistamine, antitussive.

MY-K FORMULA 77D. (My-K) Phenylpropanolamine HCl 12.5 mg, dextromethorphan HBr 10 mg, guaifenesin 100 mg/5 ml, alcohol 10%. Liq. Bot. 180 ml.
Use: Decongestant, antitussive, expectorant.

MYKINAC CREAM. (NMC Labs) Nystatin 100,000 units/Gm in cream base. Tube 15 Gm, 30 Gm.
Use: Antifungal.

MY-K NASAL SPRAY. (My-K) Oxymetazoline HCl 0.05%. Bot. 0.5 oz.
Use: Nasal decongestant.

MYKROX. (Fisons) Metolazone 0.5 mg/Tab. Bot. 100s, 500s, 1000s.
Use: Diuretic.

MYLAGEN LIQUID. (Goldline) Magnesium hydroxide 400 mg, simethicone 40 mg/5 ml. Bot. 12 oz, gal.
Use: Antacid, antiflatulent.

MYLAGEN II SUSPENSION. (Goldline) Aluminum hydroxide 400 mg, magnesium hydroxide 400 mg, simethicone 40 mg/5 ml. Bot. 12 oz.
Use: Antacid, antiflatulent.

MYLANTA LIQUID. (Stuart) Magnesium hydroxide 200 mg, aluminum hydroxide 200 mg, simethicone 20 mg, sodium 0.68 mg/5 ml. Bot. 5 oz, 12 oz, UD 30 ml. 100s.
Use: Antacid, antiflatulent.

MYLANTA TABLETS. (Stuart) Magnesium hydroxide 200 mg, aluminum hydroxide 200 mg, simethicone 20 mg, sodium 0.77 mg, sorbitol/Chew. Tab. Box 40s, 100s, Bot. 180s, Convenience pack 48s.
Use: Antacid, antiflatulent.

MYLANTA-II LIQUID. (Stuart) Magnesium hydroxide 400 mg, aluminum hydroxide 400 mg, simethicone 40 mg, sodium 1.14 mg, sorbitol/5 ml. Bot. 0.5 oz, 12 oz, UD 30 ml, 100s.
Use: Antacid, antiflatulent.

MYLANTA-II TABLETS. (Stuart) Magnesium hydroxide 400 mg, aluminum hydroxide 400 mg, simethicone 40 mg, sodium 1.3 mg/Chew. Tab. Box 24s, 60s.
Use: Antacid, antiflatulent.

MYLASE 100. Alpha-amylase.
See: Diastase.
W/Prolase, cellulase, calcium carbonate, magnesium glycinate.
See: Zylase Tab. (Vitarine).

MYLERAN. (Burroughs Wellcome) Busulfan 2 mg/Tab. Bot. 25s.

Use: Alkylating agent.

MYLICON. (Stuart) Simethicone 40 mg. **Chew. Tab.:** Bot. 100s, 500s, UD 100s. **Drops:** 40 mg/0.6 ml. Bot. 30 ml.
Use: Antiflatulent.

MYLICON-80. (Stuart) Simethicone 80 mg/Chew. Tab. Bot. 100s, Box 12s, 48s, UD 100s.
Use: Antiflatulent.

MYLICON-125. (Stuart) Simethicone 125 mg/ Chew. Tab. In 12s, 50s.
Use: Antiflatulent.

MYLOCAINE 2% VISCOUS SOLUTION. (My-K) Lidocaine HCl 2%. Bot. 100 ml.
Use: Local anesthetic.

MYLOCAINE 4% SOLUTION. (My-K) Lidocaine HCl 4%. Bot. 50 ml, 100 ml.
Use: Local anesthetic.

MYMETHASONE ELIXIR. (My-K) Dexamethasone 0.5 mg/5 ml, alcohol 5%. Bot. 100 ml, 240 ml.
Use: Corticosteroid.

MYMINIC EXPECTORANT. (My-K) Phenylpropanolamine HCl 12.5 mg, guaifenesin 100 mg/5 ml, alcohol 5%. Bot. 4 oz, pt, gal.
Use: Decongestant, expectorant.

MYMINIC PEDIATRIC. (My-K) Phenylpropanolamine HCl 12.5 mg, guaifenesin 100 mg/5 ml, alcohol 5%. Liq. Bot. 4 oz, pt, gal.
Use: Decongestant, expectorant.

MYMINIC SYRUP. (My-K) Phenylpropanolamine HCl 12.5 mg, chlorpheniramine maleate 2 mg/5 ml. Alcohol free. Bot. 4 oz, pt, gal.
Use: Decongestant, antihistamine.

MYMINICOL LIQUID. (My-K) Phenylpropanolamine HCl 12.5 mg, chlorpheniramine maleate 2 mg, dextromethorphan HBr 10 mg/5 ml. Liq. Bot. 4 oz, pt, gal.
Use: Decongestant, antihistamine, antitussive.

MYO-B. (Sig) Adenosine-5-monophosphoric acid, vitamin B_{12}. Vial 10 ml.

MYOCALM. (Parmed) Acetaminophen 8 gr, salicylamide 2 gr, phenyltoloxamine citrate 40 mg/ Tab. Bot. 100s, 1000s.
Use: Analgesic, antihistamine.

MYOCHRYSINE. (Merck Sharp & Dohme) Sterile aqueous soln. of gold sodium thiomalate 25 mg or 50 mg/ml, benzyl alcohol 0.5%. Amp. 1 ml, Vial 50 mg/ml, 10 ml.
Use: Antirheumatic agent.

MYODIL.
See: Iophendylate Inj., U.S.P. XXII.

MYODINE C LIQUID. (My-K) Iodinated glycerol 30 mg, codeine phosphate 10 mg/5 ml. Bot. pt, gal.
Use: Expectorant, antitussive.

MYODINE DM LIQUID. (My-K) Iodinated glycerol 30 mg, dextromethorphan HBr 10 mg/5 ml. Bot. pt, gal.
Use: Expectorant, antitussive,

MYODINE LIQUID. (My-K) Iodinated glycerol 60 mg/5 ml. Bot. pt, gal.
Use: Expectorant.

MYOFLEX CREME. (Rorer) Trolamine salicylate 10% in a vanishing cream base. Tube 2 oz, 4 oz, Jar 8 oz, lb, Pump dispenser 3 oz.
Use: External analgesic.

MYOLIN. (Hauck) Orphenadrine citrate 30 mg/ml. Vial 10 ml.
Use: Skeletal muscle relaxant.

MYORGAL. Mysuran. Ambenonium Cl.
Use: Cholinergic.

MYOTALIS. (Vita Elixir) Digitalis 1.5 gr/EC Tab.
Use: Digitalis therapy.

MYOTONACHOL. (Glenwood) Bethanechol Cl 10 mg or 25 mg/Tab. Bot. 100s.
Use: Urinary tract product.

MYOTOXIN. (Vita Elixir) **#1:** Digitoxin 0.1 mg/ Tab. **#2:** Digitoxin 0.2 mg/Tab.
Use: Cardiac glycoside.

MYPHENTOL ELIXIR. (My-K) Phenobarbital 16.2 mg, hyoscyamine SO_4 or HBr 0.1037 mg, atropine sulfate 0.0194 mg, scopolamine HBr 0.0065 mg/5 ml, alcohol 23%. Bot. 4 oz, pt, gal.
Use: Anticholinergic/antispasmodic, sedative/ hypnotic.

MYPHETANE DC COUGH SYRUP. (My-K) Codeine phosphate 10 mg, brompheniramine maleate 2 mg, phenylpropanolamine HCl 12.5 mg/ 5 ml, alcohol 0.95%. Bot. 4 oz, pt, gal.
Use: Antitussive, antihistamine, decongestant.

MYPHETANE DX COUGH SYRUP. (Various Mfr.) Brompheniramine maleate 2 mg, pseudoephedrine HCl 30 mg, dextromethorphan HBr 10 mg/5 ml, alcohol 0.95%. Bot. 4 oz, pt, gal.
Use: Antihistamine, decongestant, antitussive.

MYPHETANE ELIXIR. (My-K) Brompheniramine maleate 2 mg/5 ml, alcohol 3%.
Use: Antihistamine.

MYPHETAPP ELIXER. (My-K) Brompheniramine maleate 2 mg, phenylpropanolamine HCl 12.5 mg/5 ml, alcohol 2.3%. Bot. 4 oz, pt.
Use: Antihistamine, decongestant.

MYPROIC ACID SYRUP. (My-K) Valproic acid 250 mg (as sodium valproate)/5 ml. Bot. pt.
Use: Anticonvulsant.

MYRALACT. B.A.N. N-(2-Hydroxyethyl)tetradecylammonium lactate.
Use: Antiseptic.

MYRIATIN DROPS. (Winthrop Products) Atropine methonitrate BP.
Use: Antispasmodic.

MYRISTICA OIL.
Use: Flavor.

•**MYRISTYL ALCOHOL., N.F. XVII.**

MYRISTYL–PICOLINIUM CHLORIDE.
See: Wet Tone, Soln. (Riker).

MYRJ 45. (ICI Americas) Mixture of free polyoxyethylene glycol and its mono- and di-stearates. *Polyoxyl 8 stearate.
Use: Surface-active agent.

MYRJ 52 and 52S. (ICI Americas) Polyoxyethylene 40 stearate. Mixture of free polyoxyethylene glycol and its mono-and di-stearates.

Use: Surface-active agent.

MYRJ 53. (ICI Americas) Polyoxyl 50 stearate.
Use: Surface-active agent.

MYROPHINE. B.A.N. 0^3-Benzyl-0^6-tetradecanoylmorphine.
Use: Narcotic analgesic.

MYSOLINE. (Wyeth-Ayerst) Primidone, saccharin. **Tab.:** 50 mg Bot. 100s, 500s; 250 mg Bot. 100s, 1000s, UD 100s. **Susp.:** 250 mg/5 ml. Bot. 8 oz.
Use: Anticonvulsant.

MYSTECLIN-F. (Squibb) Tetracycline 250 mg, amphotericin B 50 mg/Cap. Bot. 16s, 100s, Unimatic 100s.
Use: Antibacterial, tetracycline.

MYSTECLIN-F SYRUP. (Squibb) Tetracycline 125 mg, potassium metaphosphate, amphotericin B 25 mg/5 ml. Bot. 240 ml.
Use: Antibacterial, tetracycline.

MYSURAN. Ambenonium Cl.
Use: Cholinergic muscle stimulant.
See: Mytelase Cl, Cap. (Winthrop-Breon).

MYTELASE. (Winthrop Pharm) Ambenonium Cl 10 mg/Cap. Bot. 100s.
Use: Cholinergic muscle stimulant.

MYTREX. (Savage) Triamcinolone acetonide 0.1%, nystatin 100,000 units/Gm. Cream, Oint. 15 Gm, 30 Gm, 60 Gm, 120 Gm.
Use: Topical corticosteroid, antifungal.

MYTUSSIN AC EXPECTORANT. (My-K) Guaifenesin 100 mg, codeine phosphate 10 mg/5 ml, alcohol 3.5%. Bot. 4 oz, pt, gal.
Use: Expectorant, antitussive.

MYTUSSIN DM EXPECTORANT. (My-K) Guaifenesin 100 mg, dextromethorphan HBr 15 mg/5 ml, alcohol 1.4%. Bot. 4 oz, pt, gal.
Use: Expectorant, antitussive.

MYTUSSIN DAC SYRUP. (My-K) Guaifenesin 100 mg, pseudoephedrine HCl 30 mg, codeine phosphate 10 mg/5 ml. Bot. 4 oz, pt, gal.
Use: Expectorant, decongestant, antitussive.

MYTUSSIN SYRUP. (My-K) Guaifenesin 100 mg/5 ml, alcohol 3.5%. Bot. 4 oz, pt, gal.
Use: Expectorant.

MYVEROL. (Eastman) Glyceryl monostearate.

N

NA-ANA-TAL. (Churchill) Phenobarbital 0.25 gr, phenacetin 2 gr, aspirin 3 gr, nicotinic acid 50 mg/Tab. Bot. 100s, Liq. Bot. 16 oz.
Use: Sedative/hypnotic, analgesic.

•**NABAZENIL.** USAN.
Use: Anticonvulsant.

•**NABITAN HYDROCHLORIDE.** USAN.
Use: Analgesic.

•**NABOCTATE HYDROCHLORIDE.** USAN.
Use: Antiglaucoma agent.

•**NABUMETONE.** USAN.
Use: Anti-inflammatory.

NACREM. (Jenkins) Ammonium Cl 1.5%, menthol, methyl salicylate, camphor, eucalyptus oil. Tube 0.25 oz.
Use: Sinus congestion, hay fever.

•**NADIDE.** USAN. 3-Carbamoyl-1-β-D-ribofuranosylpyridinium hydroxide. Nicotinamide adenine dinucleotide. 1-(3-Carbamoylpyridinio)-βD-ribofuranoside 5-(adenosine-5′-pyrophosphate). Ensopride. Codehydrogenase I.
Use: Treat alcoholism and drug addiction.

NADINOLA FOR DRY SKIN. (Strickland) Hydroquinone 2%. Bot. 1.25 oz, 2.25 oz.
Use: Skin bleaching agent.

NADINOLA (DELUXE) FOR OILY SKIN. (Strickland) Hydroquinone 2%. Bot. 1.25 oz, 2.25 oz.
Use: Skin bleaching agent.

NADINOLA (ULTRA) FOR NORMAL SKIN. (Strickland) Hydroquinone 2%. Bot. 1.25 oz, 3.75 oz, Tube 1.85 oz.
Use: Skin bleaching agent.

•**NADOLOL,** U.S.P. XXII. Tab., U.S.P. XXII.
Use: Antihypertensive and antianginal beta-blocker.
See: Corgard, Tab. (Princeton).

•**NADOLOL AND BENDROFLUMETHIAZIDE,** U.S.P. XXII. Tab.
Use: Antihypertensive and antianginal beta-blocker.

NAEPAINE HYDROCHLORIDE. 2-(Pentylamino)-ethanol-p-aminobenzoate HCl.
Use: Local anesthetic.

•**NAFARELIN ACETATE.** USAN.
Use: Agonist.
See: Synarel (Syntex).

NAFCIL. (Bristol) Nafcillin sodium pow. for inj. Sodium 2.9 mEq/Gm. Vial 500 mg, 1 Gm, 2 Gm; Bulk vial 10 Gm; Piggyback vial 1 Gm, 2 Gm.
Use: Anti-bacterial, penicillin.

•**NAFCILLIN, SODIUM,** U.S.P. XXII. Cap., Inj., Oral Soln, Sterile, Tab., U.S.P. XXII. 4-Thia-1-azabicyclo[3.2.0]-heptane-2-carboxylic acid, 6-[[(2-ethoxy-1-naph-thalenyl)carbonyl]amino]-3,3-dimethyl-7-oxo-monosodium salt, monohydrate,[2S-(2α,5α,6β)]. Monosodium 6-(2-ethoxy-1-naphthamido)-3,3-di- methyl-7-oxo-4-thia-1-azabicyclo [3.2.0.] heptane-2-carboxylate monohydrate. Sodium 6-(2-ethoxy-1-naphthamido)-penicillanate.
Use: Antibiotic.
See: Nafcil, Inj. (Bristol).
Unipen, Vial, Cap., Pow., Tab. (Wyeth-Ayerst).

NA-FEEN. (Pacemaker) Fluoride 1 mg/Dose. Tab. Bot. 100s, 500s, 1000s; Liq. 2 oz.
Use: Dental caries preventative.

•**NAFENOPIN.** USAN. 2-Methyl-2-[p-1,2,3,4-tetrahydro-1-naphthyl)phenoxy]propionic acid.
Use: Hypolipidemic.

•**NAFIMIDONE HYDROCHLORIDE.** USAN.
Use: Anticonvulsant.

•**NAFLOCORT.** USAN.

Use: Adrenocortical steroid.

NAFOMINE MALATE. USAN.
Use: Muscle relaxant.

NAFOXIDINE HYDROCHLORIDE. USAN.
Use: Anti-estrogen.

NAFRONYL OXALATE. USAN. 2-(Diethylaminoethyl tetrahydro-α-(1-naphthyl-methyl)2-furanpropionate oxalate. Dusodril.
Use: Vasodilator.

NAFTALAN
W/Ichthyol, calamine, amber petrolatum.
See: Nagtalan, Oint. (Paddock).

NAFTALOFOS. USAN.
Use: Anthelmintic.

NAFTAZONE. B.A.N. 1,2-Naphthaquinone 2-semicarbazone. Haemostop.
Use: Hemostatic.

NAFTIDROFURYL. B.A.N. 2-Diethylaminoethyl 2-(1-naphthylmethyl)-3-(tetrahydro-2-furyl)propionate. Praxilene [oxalate]
Use: Vasodilator.

NAFTIFINE HYDROCHLORIDE. USAN.
Use: Antifungal.
See: Naftin, Cream (Herbert).

NAFTIN. (Herbert) Naftifine HCl 1%. Cream. 2 Gm, 15 Gm, 30 Gm.
Use: Antifungal, external.

NAGANOL.
See: Suramin Sodium. Naphuride Sodium.

NAGEST Times Tabs. (Leeds) Phenylpropanolamine HCl 40 mg, phenylephrine HCl 10 mg, phenyltoloxamine dihydrogen citrate 15 mg, chlorpheniramine maleate 5 mg/SA Tab. Bot. 50s, 100s.
Use: Decongestant, antihistamine.

NAILICURE. (Purepac) Denatonium benzoate in a clear nail polish base. Bot. 0.33 oz.
Use: Nail biting deterrent.

NAIL PLUS. (Faraday) Gelatin Cap. Bot. 100s, 200s.

NALBUPHINE HYDROCHLORIDE. USAN. (−)-17-(cyclobutylmethyl)-4, 5a-epoxymorphinan-3, 6a, 14-triol, hydrochloride.
Use: Analgesic.
See: Nubain, Vial (DuPont).

NALDECON-CX ADULT LIQUID. (Bristol) Phenylpropanolamine 18 mg, guaifenesin 200 mg, codeine phosphate 10 mg/5 ml. Alcohol free. Bot. 4 oz, pt.
Use: Decongestant, expectorant, antitussive.

NALDECON-DX ADULT LIQUID. (Bristol) Phenylpropanolamine HCl 18 mg, guaifenesin 200 mg, dextromethorphan HBr 15 mg/5 ml, saccharin, sorbitol. Alcohol free. Bot. 4 oz, pt.
Use: Decongestant, expectorant, antitussive.

NALDECON-DX CHILDREN'S SYRUP. (Bristol) Phenylpropanolamine HCl 9 mg, dextromethorphan HBr 7.5 mg, guaifenesin 100 mg/5 ml, alcohol 5%. Bot. 4 oz, 16 oz.
Use: Decongestant, antitussive, expectorant.

NALDECON-DX PEDIATRIC DROPS. (Bristol) Phenylpropanolamine HCl 9 mg, guaifenesin 30 mg, dextromethorphan HBr 7.5 mg/ml, alcohol 0.6%, saccharin, sorbitol. Bot. 30 ml.
Use: Decongestant, expectorant, antitussive.

NALDECON-EX CHILDREN'S SYRUP. (Bristol) Phenylpropanolamine HCl 9 mg, guaifenesin 100 mg/5 ml, alcohol 5%, saccharin, sorbitol. Bot. 4 oz, pt.
Use: Decongestant, expectorant.

NALDECON-EX PEDIATRIC DROPS. (Bristol) Phenylpropanolamine 9 mg, guaifenesin 30 mg/ml, alcohol 0.6%. Bot. 30 ml. w/dropper.
Use: Decongestant, expectorant.

NALDECON PEDIATRIC DROPS. (Bristol) Chlorpheniramine maleate 0.5 mg, phenyltoloxamine citrate 2 mg, phenylpropanolamine HCl 5 mg, phenylephrine HCl 1.25 mg/ml. Bot. 30 ml.
Use: Antihistamine, decongestant.

NALDECON PEDIATRIC SYRUP. (Bristol) Chlorpheniramine maleate 0.5 mg, phenyltoloxamine citrate 2 mg, phenylpropanolamine HCl 5 mg, phenylephrine HCl 1.25 mg/5 ml, sorbitol. Bot. 16 oz.
Use: Antihistamine, decongestant.

NALDECON SYRUP. (Bristol) Chlorpheniramine maleate 2.5 mg, phenyltoloxamine citrate 7.5 mg, phenylpropanolamine HCl 20 mg, phenylephrine HCl 5 mg/5 ml, sorbitol. Bot. pt.
Use: Antihistamine, decongestant.

NALDECON TABLETS. (Bristol) Phenylephrine HCl 10 mg, phenylpropanolamine HCl 40 mg, phenyltoloxamine citrate 15 mg, chlorpheniramine maleate 5 mg/SR Tab. w/half each ingredient in inner and half in outer layer. Bot. 100s, 500s.
Use: Decongestant, antihistamine.

NALDEGESIC TABLETS. (Bristol) Pseudoephedrine HCl 15 mg, acetaminophen 325 mg/Tab. Bot. 100s.
Use: Decongestant, analgesic.

NALDELATE PEDIATRIC SYRUP. (Various Mfr.). Phenylpropanolamine 5 mg, phenylephrine 1.25 mg, chlorpheniramine maleate 0.5 mg, phenyltoloxamine citrate 2 mg. 120 ml, pt, gal.
Use: Decongestant, antihistamine.

NALDELATE SYRUP. (Various Mfr.) Phenylpropanolamine HCl 20 mg, phenylephrine HCl 5 mg, chlorpheniramine maleate 2.5 mg, phenyltoloxamine citrate 7.5 mg/5 ml, sorbitol. Syr. Bot. pt.
Use: Decongestant, antihistamine.

NALFON. (Dista) Fenoprofen calcium. **Cap.: 200 mg.** Rx Pak 100s. **300 mg.** Rx Pak 100s, Bot. 500s.; **Tab: 600 mg.** Rx Pak 100s, Bot. 500s.
Use: Nonsteroidal anti-inflammatory drug; analgesic.

NALGEST. (Major) Phenylpropanolamine HCl 40 mg, phenylephrine HCl 10 mg, chlorpheniramine maleate 5 mg, phenyltoloxamine citrate 15 mg/Tab. Bot. 100s, 250s, 1000s.
Use: Decongestant, antihistamine.

•**NALIDIXATE SODIUM.** USAN. Sodium 1-ethyl-

1,4-dihydro-7-methyl-4-oxo-1,8-naphthyridine-3-carboxylate monohydrate. Under study.
Use: Antibacterial.

•**NALIDIXIC ACID,** U.S.P. XXII. Oral Susp., Tab., U.S.P. XXII. 1-Ethyl-7-methyl-1,8-naphthyridin-4-one-3-carboxylic acid, 1-Ethyl-1,4-dihydro-7-methyl-4-oxo-1,8-naphthyridine-3-carboxylic Acid.
Use: Antibacterial.
See: NegGram, Capl., Susp. (Winthrop Pharm).

NALLPEN. (Beecham Labs) Nafcillin sodium monohydrate 500 mg, 1 Gm, 2 Gm/Vial. Inj. Piggyback 1 Gm, 2 Gm, Bulk 10 Gm.
Use: Antibacterial, penicillin.

•**NALMETRENE.** USAN.
Use: Antagonist to narcotics.

NALORPHINE. B.A.N. N-Allylnormorphine. Lethidrone [hydrobromide]
Use: Narcotic analgesic.

NALOXONE. B.A.N. (−)-17-Allyl-4,5α-epoxy-3,14-dihydroxymorphinan-6-one.
Use: Narcotic antagonist.
See: Narcan (Du Pont).

•**NALOXONE HYDROCHLORIDE,** U.S.P. XXII. Inj. U.S.P. XXII. Morphinan-6-one, 4,5-epoxy-3,14-dihy- droxy-17-(2-propenyl)-,hydrochloride.
Use: Narcotic antagonist.
See: Narcan, Amp. (Du Pont).

NALSA SPRAY. (Jenkins) Methapyrilene HCl 0.2%, naphazoline HCl 0.05%, cetylpyridinium Cl 0.02%, thimerosal 0.005%. Spray Bot. 20 ml.
Use: Antihistamine, decongestant.

•**NALTREXONE.** USAN.
Use: Antagonist to narcotics.
See: Trexal Tab. (Du Pont).

NAMAZENE. Phenothiazine.

NAMOL XENYRATE. 2-(4-Biphenylyl) butyric acid, compound with 2-dimethyl-amino- ethanol.
See: Namoxyrate.

•**NAMOXYRATE.** USAN. 2-[4-Biphenylyl]butyric acid cpd. w/2-dimethylaminoethanol. Namol Xenyrate-previous name.
Use: Analgesic.
See: Namol Xenyrate (Warner-Chilcott).

NAMURON.
See: Cyclobarbital Calcium (Various Mfr.).

NANDROBOLIC. (Forest) Nandrolone phenpropionate 25 mg/ml. Vial 5 ml.
Use: Anabolic steroid.

NANDROBOLIC L.A. (Forest) Nandrolone decanoate 100 mg/ml. Vial 2 ml, Box 5s.
Use: Anabolic steroid.

NANDROLONE. B.A.N. 17β-Hydroxyestr-4-en-3-one. 17β-Hydroxy-19-norandrost-4-en-3-one. Nortesterone (I.N.N.).
Use: Anabolic steroid.

•**NANDROLONE CYCLOTATE.** USAN.
Use: Anabolic.

•**NANDROLONE DECANOATE,** U.S.P. XXII. Inj., U.S.P. XXII. 17β-Hydroxy-estr-4-en-3-one-decanoate.
Use: Androgen.
See: Anabolin LA-100, Vial (Alto).
Androlone-D, Inj. (Keene).
Androlone-D 50, Inj. (Keene).
Deca-Durabolin, Amp., Vial (Organon).
Hybolin Decanoate, Inj. (Hyrex).

NANDROLONE PHENPROPIONATE, U.S.P. XXI. Inj. U.S.P. XXI. 19-nor-17-beta-Hydroxy-3-ketoandrost-4-ene-17-phenylpropionate. Norandrostenolone phenylpropionate. 17β-Hydroxy-estr-4-en-3-one Hydrocinnamate.
Use: Androgen.
See: Anabolin IM, Vial (Alto).
Androlone, Inj. (Keene).
Androlone 50, Inj. (Keene).
Durabolin Inj. (Organon).
Hybolin Improved, Vial (Hyrex).
Nandrolin, Inj. (Solvay).

•**NANTRADOL HCL.** USAN.
Use: Analgesic.

NAOTIN. (Drug Products) Sodium nicotinate. Amp. (equivalent to 10 mg nicotinic acid/ml) 10 ml, Box 25s, 100s.
Use: Vitamin B_3 supplement.

•**NAPACTADINE HYDROCHLORIDE.** USAN.
Use: Antidepressant.

•**NAPAMEZOLE HYDROCHLORIDE.** USAN.
Use: Antidepressant.

NAPAMIDE CAPS. (Major) Disopyramide phosphate 100 mg or 150 mg/Cap. Bot. 100s, 500s, UD 100s.
Use: Antiarrhythmic.

•**NAPHAZOLINE HYDROCHLORIDE,** U.S.P. XXII. Nasal Soln., Ophthalmic Soln., U.S.P. XXII. lH-Imidazole, 4,5-dihydro-2-(1-naphthalenylmethyl)-,monohydrochloride, 2-(1-Naphthylmethyl)-2-imidazoline HCl.
Use: Adrenergic.
See: Allerest Eye Drops, Soln. (Pharmacraft).
Clear Eyes, Drops (Abbott).
Naphcon, Drops (Alcon).
Privine HCl Soln., Spray (Ciba).
Vasocon Regular, Liq. (CooperVision).

W/Antazoline phosphate, boric acid, phenylmercuric acetate, sodium Cl, sodium carbonate anhydrous.
See: Vasocon-A Ophthalmic, Soln. (CooperVision).

W/Antazoline phosphate, polyvinyl alcohol.
See: Albalon-A Liquifilm, Ophth. (Allergan).

W/Methapyrilene HCl, cetylpyridinum Cl, thimerosal.
See: Vapocyn II Nasal Spray (Solvay).

W/Pheniramine maleate.
See: Naphcon A, Liq. (Alcon).

W/Phenylephrine HCl, pyrilamine maleate, phenylpropanolamine HCl.
See: 4-Way Nasal Spray (Bristol-Myers).

W/Polyvinyl alcohol.
See: Albalon, Ophth. Soln. (Allergan).
Albalon Liquifilm, Ophth. Soln. (Allergan).

NAPHCON. (Alcon) Naphazoline HCl 0.012%, benzalkonium Cl 0.01%. Drop-Tainer Bot. 15 ml.
Use: Ophthalmic vasoconstrictor/mydriatic.

NAPHCON A. (Alcon) Naphazoline HCl 0.025%, pheniramine maleate 0.3%. Bot. 15 ml.
Use: Ophthalmic decongestant combination.

NAPHCON FORTE. (Alcon) Naphazoline HCl 0.1%, benzalkonium Cl 0.01%, disodium edetate/ml. Drop-Tainer Bot. 15 ml.
Use: Ophthalmic vasoconstrictor/mydriatic.

NAPHOLINE. (Horizon) Naphazoline HCl 0.1%. Soln. Bot. 15 ml.
Use: Ophthalmic vasoconstrictor/mydriatic.

NAPHTHALOPHOS. N. N-(Diethoxyphosphinyloxy)naphthalimide. Rametin.
Use: Anthelmintic, veterinary medicine.

b-NAPHTHYL SALICYLATE. Betol, Naphthosalol, Salinaphthol.
Use: G.I. & G.U., antiseptic.

NAPHURIDE SODIUM. Suramin Sodium.

NAPRIL TABLETS. (Milance) Pseudoephedrine HCl 60 mg, chlorpheniramine maleate 4 mg/Tab. Bot. 30s.
Use: Decongestant, antihistamine.

NAPROSYN. (Syntex) Naproxen. **Oral susp.:** 125 mg/5 ml, sorbitol. In pt. **250 mg/Tab:** Bot. 100s, 500s, Blister pkg. 100s; **375 mg/Tab.** Bot. 100s, 500s, Blister pkg. 100s; **500 mg/Tab:** Bot. 100s, 500s.
Use: Nonsteroidal anti-inflammatory drug; analgesic.

NAPROXEN, U.S.P. XXII. Tab., U.S.P. XXII. (+)-6- Methoxy-αmethyl-2-naphthaleneacetic acid. (+)-2-(6 Methoxy-2-naphthyl)propionic acid.
Use: Anti-inflammatory, analgesic, antipyretic.
See: Naprosyn, Tab. (Syntex).

NAPROXEN SODIUM, U.S.P. XXII. Tab., U.S.P. XXII.
Use: Anti-inflammatory, analgesic, antipyretic.
See: Anaprox, Tab. (Syntex).
Anaprox DS, Tab. (Syntex).

NAPROXOL. USAN. (−)-6-Methoxy-β-methyl-2-naphthaleneethanol.
Use: Anti-inflammatory; analgesic; antipyretic.

NAQUA. (Schering) Trichlormethiazide 2 mg or 4 mg/Tab. Bot. 100s, 1000s.
Use: Diuretic.

N/Reserpine.
See: Naquival, Tab. (Schering).

NARANOL HCl. USAN. 8,9,10,11,11α,-12-Hexahydro-8,10-dimethyl-7 αH-naphtho[1′,2′:5,-6]pyrano-[3,2-c]pyridin-7-α-ol HCl.
Use: Tranquilizer.

NARASIN. USAN.
Use: Growth stimulant.

NARCAN. (DuPont) Naloxone HCl. **0.02 mg/ml:** Amp. 2 ml. **0.4 mg/ml:** Amp. 1 ml, Box 10s. Prefilled syringe 1 ml, Tray 10s; Multiple dose vials 10 ml, Box 1s. **1 mg/ml:** Amp. 2 ml, Box 10s; Multiple dose vial 10 ml, Box 1s.
Use: Narcotic antagonist.

NARCOTIC ANAQLGESICS.
See: Dalgan (Astra).
Duragesic (Janssen).

NARDIL. (Parke-Davis) Phenelzine sulfate 15 mg/Tab. Bot. 100s.
Use: Antidepressant.

NASADENT. (Scherer) Sodium metaphosphate, glycerin, distilled water, dicalcium phosphate dihydrate, sodium carboxymethylcellulose, oil of spearmint, sodium benzoate, saccharin.
Use: Ingestible dentifrice.

NASAHIST B INJECTABLE. (Keene) Brompheniramine maleate 10 ml. Vial 10 ml. For IM, IV and SC administration.
Use: Antihistamine.

NASAHIST CAPSULES. (Keene) Phenylpropanolamine HCl 40 mg, phenylephrine HCl 10 mg, chlorpheniramine maleate 12 mg/Cap. Bot. 100s.
Use: Decongestant, antihistamine.

NaSal SALINE NASAL. (Winthrop Pharm.) Sodium Cl 0.65%. Drops, Spray. Bot. 15 ml.
Use: Nasal moisturizer.

NASALCROM NASAL SOLUTION. (Fisons) Cromolyn sodium 40 mg/ml, benzalkonium Cl 0.01%, EDTA 0.01%. Metered dose spray. Delivers 5.2 mg/spray. Complete pkg. 13 ml. Refill 13 ml.
Use: Nasal antiallergic.

NASALIDE. (Syntex) Flunisolide 0.025% soln. Pump. Bot. 25 ml.
Use: Intranasal steroid.

NASAL SALINE. (Winthrop Consumer Products) Nasal spray and drops. Sodium Cl 0.65% buffered w/phosphates, preservatives. Bot. 15 ml. Spray Bot. 15 ml.
Use: Nasal moisturizer.

NASOPHEN. (Premo) Phenylephrine HCl 0.25%, 1%. Bot. pt.
Use: Decongestant.

NATABEC. (Parke-Davis) Vitamins A 4,000 IU, D 400 IU, B_1 3 mg, B_2 2 mg, B_6 3 mg, C 50 mg, B_{12} 5 mcg, B_3 10 mg, elemental calcium 240 mg, elemental iron 30 mg/Kapseal. Bot. 100s.
Use: Prenatal vitamin/mineral supplement.

NATABEC-F.A. (Parke-Davis) Same as Natabec, plus folic acid 0.1 mg/Kapseal, magnesium, bisulfites. Bot. 100s.
Use: Prenatal vitamin/mineral supplement.

NATABEC Rx. (Parke-Davis) Same as Natabec, plus folic acid 1 mg/Kapseal. Bot. 100s.
Use: Prenatal vitamin/mineral supplement.

NATABEC WITH FLUORIDE. (Parke-Davis) Same formula as Natabec, plus elemental fluoride 1 mg/Kapseal. Bot. 100s.
Use: Prenatal vitamin supplement, dental caries preventative.

NATACOMP-FA TABLETS. (Trimen) Calcium 250 mg, iron 60 mg, vitamins A 8000 IU, D 400 IU, E 30 mg, B_1 3 mg, B_2 3.4 mg, B_3 20 mg, B_5 10 mg, B_6 12 mg, B_{12} 12 mcg, C 120 mg, folic

acid 1 mg, Cu, I, Mg, zinc 15 mg/Tab. Bot. 100s, 500s.
Use: Prenatal vitamin/mineral supplement.

NATACYN. (Alcon) Natamycin (5%) 50 mg/ml. Bot. 15 ml.
Use: Antifungal agent, ophthalmic.

NATAFORT FILMSEAL. (Parke-Davis) Vitamins A 6000 IU, D 400 IU, C 120 mg, B_1 3 mg, B_2 2 mg, B_6 15 mg, B_{12} 6 mcg, niacin 20 mg, folic acid 1 mg, E 30 IU, calcium 350 mg, magnesium 100 mg, zinc 25 mg, iodine 0.15 mg, iron 65 mg/Tab. Bot. 100s.
Use: Prenatal vitamin/mineral supplement.

NATALINS. (Mead Johnson Nutrition) Vitamins A 5000 IU, D 400 IU, E 30 IU, C 90 mg, B_1 1.7 mg, B_2 2 mg, B_6 4 mg, B_{12} 8 mcg, niacin 20 mg, folic acid 0.8 mg, iodine 150 mcg, calcium 200 mg, iron 45 mg, magnesium 100 mg/Tab. Bot. 100s, 1000s Drum 36,000.
Use: Vitamin/mineral supplement.

NATALINS RX. (Mead Johnson Nutrition) Vitamins A 8000 IU, D 400 IU, E 30 IU, C 90 mg, B_1 2.55 mg, B_2 3 mg, B_6 10 mg, B_{12} 8 mcg, niacin 20 mg, folic acid 1 mg, pantothenic acid 15 mg, biotin 0.05 mg, calcium 200 mg, iron 60 mg, magnesium 100 mg, copper 2 mg, zinc 15 mg, iodine 150 mcg/Tab. Bot. 100s, 1000s.
Use: Prenatal vitamin/mineral supplement.

•**NATAMYCIN,** U.S.P. XXII. Ophth. Susp., U.S.P. XXII. An antibiotic produced by *Streptomyces natalensis.* Pimafucin.
Use: Antibiotic.

NATA-SAN. (Sandia) Vitamins A 4000 IU, D 400 IU, B_1 5 mg, B_2 4 mg, B_6 10 mg, nicotinic acid 10 mg, C 100 mg, B_{12} activity 5 mcg, ferrous fumarate 200 mg (elemental iron 65 mg), calcium carbonate 500 mg (calcium 196 mg), copper (sulfate) 0.5 mg, magnesium (sulfate) 0.1 mg, manganese (sulfate) 0.1 mg, potassium (sulfate) 0.1 mg, zinc (sulfate) 0.5 mg/Tab. Bot. 100s, 1000s.
Use: Vitamin/mineral supplement.

NATA-SAN F.A. (Sandia) Vitamins A 4000 IU, D 400 IU, B_1 5 mg, B_2 4 mg, B_6 10 mg, nicotinic acid 10 mg, C 100 mg, B_{12} activity 5 mcg, folic acid 1 mg, iron 65 mg, calcium 200 mg, copper (sulfate) 0.5 mg, magnesium (sulfate) 0.1 mg, manganese (sulfate) 0.1 mg, potassium (sulfate) 0.1 mg, zinc (sulfate) 0.5 mg/Tab. Bot. 100s, 1000s.
Use: Vitamin/mineral supplement.

NATODINE. (Faraday) Iodine in organic form as found in kelp 1 mg/Tab. Bot. 100s, 250s.

NATRAPEL. (Tender) Citronella 10% in 15% Aloe Vera base.
Use: Insect repellent.

NATRICO. (Drug Products) Potassium nitrate 2 gr, sodium nitrite 1 gr, nitroglycerin 0.25 gr, crataegus oxycantha 0.25 gr/Pulvoid. Bot. 100s, 1000s.
Use: Antihypertensive.

NATURACIL. (Mead Johnson Nutrition) Psyllium seed husks 3.4 Gm, carbohydrate 9.6 Gm, sodium 11 mg, 54 cal./2 pieces. Carton 24s, 40s.
Use: Laxative.

NATUR-AID. (Scott/Cord) Lactose, pectin-and Carob-lemon juice. Pow. 90%. Bot. 8 oz.
Use: Increase in normal intestinal flora.

NATURAL DIURETIC WATER TABLET. (Amlab) Buchu leaves 1 gr, uva ursi 1 gr, trilicum 1 gr, parsley 1 gr, juniper berries 1 gr, asparagus 1 gr, alfalfa powder 1 gr/Tab. Bot. 100s.
Use: Diuretic.

NATURAL VEGETABLE POWDER. (Various Mfr.) Psyllium hydrophilic mucilloid 3.4 Gm, dextrose, sodium $>$ 10 mg, 14 Cal/dose. Pow. 210 Gm, 420 Gm, 630 Gm.
Use: Laxative.

NATURAL VITAMIN A IN OIL.
See: Oleovitamin A, U.S.P.

NATURE'S AID LAXATIVE TABS. (Walgreen) Docusate sodium 100 mg, yellow phenolphthalein 65 mg/Tab. Bot. 60s.
Use: Laxative.

NATURE'S REMEDY TABLETS. (Norcliff Thayer) Aloe 100 mg, cascara sagrada 150 mg/FC Tab. Foil backed blister pkg. Box 12s, 30s, 60s.
Use: Laxative.

NATURETIN. (Princeton) Bendroflumethiazide. **5 mg/Tab.:** Bot. 100s, 1000s. **10 mg/Tab.:** Bot. 100s.
Use: Diuretic.

NATURIL. (Kenyon) Pow. uva ursi extract 0.5 gr, pow. buchu leaves extract 0.5 gr, pow. corn silk extract 0.5 gr, pow. juniper extract 0.25 gr, caffeine 0.25 gr/Tab. Bot. 100s, 1000s.

NATUR-LAX TABLETS. (Faraday) Rhubarb root, cape aloes, cascara sagrada extract, mandrake root, parsley, carrot. Protein coated tab. Bot. 100s.
Use: Laxative.

NAUS-A-TORIES. (Table Rock) Pyrilamine maleate 25 mg, secobarbital 30 mg/Supp. Box 12s.
Use: Antiemetic.

NAUSETROL. (Various Mfr.) Fructose, dextrose, orthophosphoric acid with controlled hydrogen ion concentration. Soln. Bot. 4 oz, pt, gal.
Use: Antiemetic.

NAVANE. (Roerig) Thiothixene. **Cap.:** 1 mg, 2 mg, 5 mg, 10 mg or 20 mg. Bot. 100s, 1000s, UD 100s. **Liq.:** 5 mg/ml. Bot. 1 oz, 4 oz. **IM soln.:** 2 mg/ml. Vial 2 ml. Pkg. 10s.
Use: Antipsychotic agent.

NAVANE CONCENTRATE. (Roerig) Thiothixene HCl 5 mg/ml, alcohol 7%. Soln. Bot. 30 ml, 120 ml with dropper.
Use: Antipsychotic agent.

NAVANE INTRAMUSCULAR FOR INJECTION. (Roerig) Thiothixene HCl 5 mg/ml. Lyophilized for reconstitution with 2.2 ml sterile water. Vial 2 ml. Pkg. vial 10s.
Use: Antipsychotic agent.

NAVIDRIX (NAVIDREX, CYCLOPENTHIAZIDE). Cyclopenthiazide. 3-Cyclopentylmethyl derivative of hydrochlorothiazide.
Use: Diuretic.

NAVSEAST. (Eastwood) Tab. Bot. 100s.

NAZAFAIR. (Various Mfr.) Naphazoline HCl 0.1%. Soln. Bot. 15 ml.
Use: Ophthalmic vasoconstrictor/mydriatic.

N.B.P. OINTMENT. (Bowman) Bacitracin zinc 400 units, neomycin sulfate 5 mg, polymyxin B sulfate 10,000 units/Gm Tube ⅛ oz, 0.5 oz.
Use: Anti-infective, external.

N.B.P. OINTMENT. (Forest) Neomycin, bacitracin, polymyxin ointment. Tube ⅛ oz, 0.5 oz.
Use: Anti-infective, external.

N-CHLORO COMPOUND ANTISEPTICS.
See: Antiseptic, N-Chloro Compounds.

N D CLEAR. (Seatrace) Chlorpheniramine maleate 8 mg, pseudoephedrine HCl 120 mg/T.D. Cap. Bot. 100s, 1000s.
Use: Antihistamine, decongestant.

N-DIETHYL META-TOLUAMIDE.
W/Red Veterinary Petrolatum.
See: RV Pellent, Oint. (Elder).

ND-GESIC. (Hyrex) Acetaminophen 300 mg, pyrilamine maleate 12.5 mg, chlorpheniramine maleate 2 mg, phenylephrine HCl 5 mg/Tab. Bot. 100s, 1000s.
Use: Analgesic, antihistamine, decongestant.

nDNA. (Wampole-Zeus) Anti-native DNA test by IFA. Confirmatory test for active SLE. Test 48s.
Use: Diagnostic aid.

ND-STAT. (Hyrex) Brompheniramine maleate 10 mg/ml. Vial 10 ml.
Use: Antihistamine.

NEALBARBITONE. B.A.N. 5-Allyl-5-neopentylbarbituric acid. Censedal; Nevental.
Use: Hypnotic; sedative.

NEBCIN. (Lilly) Tobramycin sulfate. **Inj.:** 80 mg/2 ml. Vial 2 ml. **Pow. (after reconstitution):** 30 mg/ml or 40 mg/ml. Vial 1.2 Gm. **Pediatric Inj.:** 20 mg/2 ml. Vial 2 ml. **Hyporets:** 60 mg/1.5 ml or 80 mg/2 ml.
Use: Antibacterial, aminoglycoside.

•**NEBIVOLOL.** USAN.
Use: Antihypertensive (beta-blocker).

•**NEBRAMYCIN.** USAN. A complex of antibiotic substances produced by *Streptomyces tenebrarius*.
Use: Antibacterial.

•**NEBUPENT.** (Lyphomed) Pentamidine isethionate 300 mg. Aerosol single dose vial.
Use: Anti-infective.

•**NEBU-PREL.** (Mahon) Isoproterenol sulfate 0.4%, phenylephrine HCl 2%, propylene glycol 10%. Liq. Vial 10 ml.
Use: Bronchodilator.

•**NECHLORIN.** (Interstate) Chlorpheniramine 5 mg, phenylpropanolamine 40 mg, phenylephrine 20 mg, phenyltoloxamine 15 mg/Tab. Bot. 100s.
Use: Antihistamine, decongestant.

•**NEDOCROMIL.** USAN.
Use: Antiallergic (prophylactic).

•**NEDOCROMIL CALCIUM.** USAN.
Use: Antiallergic (prophylactic).

•**NEDOCROMIL SODIUM.** USAN.
Use: Antiallergic (prophylactic).

•**NEFAZODONE HYDROCHLORIDE.** USAN. A Bristol Myers investigative drug.
Use: Antidepressant.

•**NEFLUMOZIDE HYDROCHLORIDE.** USAN.
Use: Antipsychotic.

•**NEFOCON A.** USAN.
Use: Hydrophobic contact lens material.

•**NEFOPAM HCl.** USAN. 3,4,5,6-Tetrahydro-5-methyl-1-phenyl-1H-2,5-benzoxazocine HCl.
Use: Muscle relaxant.

NEGACIDE. (Winthrop Products) Nalidixic acid.
Use: Urinary anti-infective.

NEGGRAM. (Winthrop-Breon) Nalidixic acid. **1 Gm/Capl.:** Bot. 100s, UD Pack 100s; **250 mg/Capl.:** Bot. 56s. **500 mg/Capl.:** Bot. 56s, 500s, 1000s, UD Pack 100s; Susp. **250 mg/5 ml:** Bot. pt.
Use: Urinary anti-infective.

•**NELEZAPRINE MALEATE.** USAN.
Use: Muscle relaxant.

NELOVA 1/35E. (Warner Chilcott) Norethindrone 1 mg, ethinyl estradiol 35 mcg/Tab. 21 day and 28 day (with 7 inert tabs.).
Use: Oral contraceptive.

NELOVA 1/50 M. (Warner-Chilcott) Norethindrone 1 mg, mestranol 50 mcg/Tab. 21 day (with 7 inert tabs).
Use: Oral contraceptive.

NELOVA 10/11. (Warner Chilcott) **Phase 1-** Norethindrone 0.5 mg, ethinyl estradiol 35 mcg/Tab., 10 tabs.; **Phase 2-** Norethindrone 1 mg, ethinyl estradiol 35 mcg/Tab., 11 tabs. 21 day and 28 day (with 7 inert tabs.).
Use: Oral contraceptive.

•**NEMADECTIN.** USAN.
Use: Parasiticide (veterinary).

NEMAZINE. 3-(p-Chlorophenyl)-4-imino-2-oxo-1-imidazolidine acetonitrile. Under study.
Use: Anti-inflammatory.

NEMBUTAL ELIXIR. (Abbott) Pentobarbital 18.2 mg/5 ml, alcohol 18% Bot. pt, gal.
Use: Sedative/hypnotic.

NEMBUTAL SODIUM. (Abbott) Pentobarbital sodium. **Inj. Vial:** 50 mg/ml. Vial 20 ml, 50 ml. Box 5s. **Cap.:** 50 mg: Bot. 100s, 500s, 1000s; 100 mg: Bot. 100s, 500s, 1000s, UD 100s (10 × 10s). Display pack 500s. **Supp.:** 30 mg, 60 mg, 120 mg or 200 mg. Box 12s.
Use: Sedative/hypnotic.

NEOARSPHENAMINE. Sodium 3,3′-diamino-4,4′-dihy-droxyarsenobenzene-N-methanal sulfoxylate. (Neosalvarsan, Neoarsenobenzol).

NEO-BENZ-ALL. (Xttrium) Benzalkonium Cl 20.1%. Packet 25 ml 15s. To make gal of 1:750 soln. Also Aqueous Neo-Benz-All 1:750 soln. Packet 20 ml, 50s.
Use: Antiseptic, germicidal.

NEO BESEROL. (Winthrop Products) Aspirin, methocarbamol.
Use: Salicylate analgesic, skeletal muscle relaxant.

NEOCALAMINE. (Various Mfr.) Red ferric oxide 30 Gm, yellow ferric oxide 40 Gm, zinc oxide 930 Gm.
Use: Astringent, antiseptic.

NEO-CALGLUCON. (Sandoz) Glubionate calcium 1.8 Gm/5 ml. Syr. Bot. pt.
Use: Calcium supplement.

NEO-CASTADERM. (Lannett) Resorcin, boric acid, acetone, phenol, alcohol 9%. Liq. Bot. 1 oz, 4 oz, 16 oz.
Use: Antifungal, external.

NEO-CHOLEX. (Lafayette) Fat emulsion containing 40%/w/v pure vegetable oil. Bot. 60 ml.
Use: Produce maximum cholecystokinetic activity in roentgen study.

NEOCIDIN. (Major) Polymyxin B sulfate 10,000 units, neomycin sulfate 1.75 mg, gramicidin 0.025 mg/ml. Soln. Bot. 10 ml.
Use: Anti-infective, ophthalmic.

NEOCINCHOPHEN. B.A.N. Ethyl 6-methyl-2-phenylquinolin-4-carboxylate. Novatophan.
Use: Analgesic, antipyretic and in gout.

NEO-COBEFRIN. levo-Nordefrin. 1-2,4-dihydroxyphenyl-3-hydroxy-2-isopropylamine.
Use: Vasoconstrictor.

NEO-CORTEF CREAM. (Upjohn) Hydrocortisone acetate 10 mg (1%), neomycin sulfate 5 mg (0.5%), methylparaben 1 mg, butylparaben 4 mg, polysorbate 80, propylene glycol, cetyl palmitate, glyceryl monostearate, emulsifier/Gm. When necessary, pH adjusted with sulfuric acid. Tube 20 Gm.
Use: Corticosteroid, anti-infective, external.

NEO-CORTEF OINTMENT. (Upjohn) **0.5%:** Hydrocortisone acetate 5 mg, neomycin sulfate 5 mg, methylparaben 0.2 mg, butylparaben 1.8 mg in a bland base of white petrolatum, microcrystalline wax, mineral oil, cholesterol/Gm. Tube 20 Gm. **1%:** Hydrocortisone acetate 10 mg, neomycin sulfate 5 mg/Gm Oint. Tube 5 Gm, 20 Gm.
Use: Corticosteroid, anti-infective.

NEO-CORT TOP OINTMENT. (Standex) Neomycin sulfate 0.5%, hydrocortisone 1%. Tube 0.5 oz.
Use: Anti-infective, corticosteroid.

NEO-CULTOL. (Fisons) Refined mineral oil jelly. Chocolate flavored. Bot. 6 oz.
Use: Laxative.

NEOCURB. (Pasadena Research) Phendimetrazine tartrate 35 mg/Tab. Bot. 100s, 1000s.
Use: Anorexient.

NEOCYLATE. (Central) Potassium salicylate 280 mg, aminobenzoic acid 250 mg/Tab. Bot. 100s, 1000s.
Use: Salicylate analgesic.

NeoDECADRON OPHTHALMIC SOLUTION. (Merck Sharp & Dohme) Dexamethasone sodium phosphate equivalent to 1 mg dexamethasone phosphate, neomycin sulfate equivalent to 3.5 mg neomycin base/ml, polysorbate 80, sodium bisulfite 0.1%, benzalkonium Cl 0.02%. Ocumeter ophthalmic dispenser 5 ml.
Use: Anti-infective.

NeoDECADRON OPHTHALMIC OINTMENT. (Merck Sharp & Dohme) Dexamethasone sodium phosphate equivalent to 0.5 mg dexamethasone phosphate, neomycin sulfate equivalent to 3.5 mg neomycin base/Gm, white petrolatum, mineral oil. Tube 3.5 Gm.
Use: Corticosteroid, anti-infective.

NeoDECADRON TOPICAL CREAM. (Merck Sharp & Dohme) Dexamethasone sodium phosphate equivalent to 1 mg dexamethasone phosphate, neomycin sulfate equivalent to 3.5 mg neomycin base/Gm, stearyl alcohol, cetyl alcohol, mineral oil, polyoxyl 40 stearate, sorbitol soln, methyl polysilicone emulsion, creatinine, disodium edetate, sodium citrate, sodium hydroxide to adjust pH, purified water, methylparaben 0.15%, sodium bisulfite 0.25%, sorbic acid 0.1%. Tube 15 Gm, 30 Gm.
Use: Corticosteroid, anti-infective.

NEODECYLLIN. (Penick) Neomycin undecylenate.
Use: Anti-infective.

NEODRENAL.
See: Isoproterenol.

NEO-DURABOLIC. (Hauck) Nandrolone decanoate injection. **50 mg/ml** or **100 mg/ml:** Vial 2 ml. **200 mg/ml:** Vial 1 ml.
Use: Anabolic steroid.

NEO FRANOL. (Winthrop Products) Theophylline monohydrate.
Use: Bronchodilator.

NEOGEN. (Premo) Theophylline 3 gr, aminophylline 4 gr, ephedrine sulfate 3/8 gr, pentobarbital 1 gr, benzocaine 3 gr/Supp. Also available 0.5 strength. Box 12s.
Use: Bronchodilator, sedative/hypnotic, local anesthetic.

NEO-GERASTAN. (Standex) Pentylenetetrazol 100 mg, nicotinic acid (niacin) 50 mg, glutamic acid 100 mg/Tab. Bot. 100s.
Use: CNS stimulant.

NEOGESIC TABLETS. (Vale) Aspirin 194.4 mg, acetaminophen 129.6 mg, caffeine 32.4 mg/Tab. Bot. 1000s.
Use: Analgesic combination.

NEOLOID. (Lederle) Castor oil 36.4% (emulsified) (w/w). Bot. 4 oz.
Use: Laxative.

NEOMAC OINTMENT. (NMC Labs) Triple antibiotic ointment. Tube 0.5 oz, 1 oz.
Use: Anti-infective, external.

NEO-MEDROL ACETATE TOPICAL. (Upjohn) Methylprednisolone acetate 2.5 mg or 10 mg, neomycin sulfate 5 mg, methylparaben 4 mg, butylparaben 3 mg/Gm. Tube 7.5 Gm, 30 Gm.

Use: Corticosteroid, anti-infective.

NEO-MIST NASAL SPRAY. (A.P.C.) Phenylephrine HCl 0.5%, cetalkonium Cl 0.02%. Spray Bot. 20 ml.
Use: Decongestant, antiseptic.

NEO-MIST PEDIATRIC 0.25% NASAL SPRAY. (A.P.C.) Phenylephrine HCl 0.25%, cetalkonium Cl 0.02%. Squeeze Bot. 20 ml.
Use: Decongestant, antiseptic.

NEOMIXIN. (Mallard) Bacitracin zinc 400 units, neomycin sulfate 3.5 mg, polymyxin B sulfate 5000 units in petrolatum base/Gm. Tube 15 Gm.
Use: Anti-infective, external.

NEOMYCIN. B.A.N. An antibiotic produced by a strain of *Streptomyces fradiae.* Expedil, Mycifradin, Myciguent, Neomin, Nivemycin [sulfate].
Use: Anti-infective.

NEOMYCIN BASE.
Use: Antibiotic.
W/Combinations.
See: Maxitrol, Oint., Susp. (Alcon).
Neo-Cort-Dome, Cream, Lot. (Miles Pharm).
Neotal, Oint. (Mallard).

NEOMYCIN-HYDROCORTISONE CREAM. (Day-Baldwin) Neomycin 5 mg/Gm, hydrocortisone 0.5% or 1% Tube 0.5 oz, 1 oz.
Use: Anti-infective, corticosteroid.

NEOMYCIN-HYDROCORTISONE OINTMENT. (Day-Baldwin) Neomycin 5 mg/Gm, hydrocortisone 0.5%. Tube 1 oz; w/hydrocortisone 1%: 20 Gm, 1 oz.
Use: Anti-infective, corticosteroid.

NEOMYCIN PALMITATE. USAN.
Use: Antibiotic.
See: Biozyme, Oint. (Armour).

NEOMYCIN AND POLYMYXIN B SULFATES, BACITRACIN, AND HYDROCORTISONE ACETATE OINTMENT, U.S.P. XXII.
Use: Antibiotic, antifungal.

NEOMYCIN AND POLYMYXIN B SULFATES, BACITRACIN, AND HYDROCORTISONE ACETATE OPHTHALMIC OINTMENT, U.S.P. XXII.
Use: Antibiotic, antifungal.

NEOMYCIN AND POLYMYXIN B SULFATES AND BACITRACIN OINTMENT, U.S.P. XXII.
Use: Antibiotic.

NEOMYCIN AND POLYMYXIN B SULFATES AND BACITRACIN OPHTHALMIC OINTMENT, U.S.P. XXII.
Use: Antibiotic.

NEOMYCIN AND POLYMYXIN B SULFATES, BACITRACIN ZINC, AND HYDROCORTISONE ACETATE OPHTHALMIC OINTMENT, U.S.P. XXII.
Use: Antibiotic, anti-inflammatory.

NEOMYCIN AND POLYMYXIN B SULFATES, BACITRACIN ZINC, AND HYDROCORTISONE OINTMENT, U.S.P. XXII.
Use: Antibiotic, anti-inflammatory.

•**NEOMYCIN AND POLYMYXIN B SULFATES, BACITRACIN ZINC, AND HYDROCORTISONE OPHTHALMIC OINTMENT,** U.S.P. XXII.
Use: Antibiotic, anti-inflammatory.

•**NEOMYCIN AND POLYMYXIN B SULFATES, BACITRACIN ZINC, AND LIDOCAINE OINTMENT,** U.S.P. XXII.
Use: Antibiotic, anesthetic.
See: Lanabiotic, Oint. (Combe).

•**NEOMYCIN AND POLYMYXIN B SULFATES AND BACITRACIN ZINC OINTMENT,** U.S.P. XXII.
Use: Local anti-infective.

•**NEOMYCIN AND POLYMYXIN B SULFATES AND BACITRACIN ZINC OPHTHALMIC OINTMENT,** U.S.P. XXII.
Use: Ophthalmic antibiotic.

NEOMYCIN AND POLYMYXIN B SULFATES AND BACITRACIN ZINC TOPICAL AEROSOL, U.S.P. XXI.
Use: Antibiotic.

NEOMYCIN AND POLYMYXIN B SULFATES AND BACITRACIN ZINC TOPICAL POWDER, U.S.P. XXI.
Use: Antibiotic.

•**NEOMYCIN AND POLYMYXIN B SULFATES CREAM,** U.S.P. XXII.
Use: Antibiotic.

•**NEOMYCIN AND POLYMYXIN B SULFATES AND DEXAMETHASONE OPHTHALMIC OINTMENT,** U.S.P. XXII.
Use: Antibiotic, anti-inflammatory.

•**NEOMYCIN AND POLYMYXIN B SULFATES AND DEXAMETHASONE OPHTHALMIC SUSPENSION,** U.S.P. XXII.
Use: Antibiotic, anti-inflammatory.

•**NEOMYCIN AND POLYMYXIN B SULFATES AND GRAMICIDIN CREAM,** U.S.P. XXII.
Use: Antibiotic.

•**NEOMYCIN AND POLYMYXIN B SULFATES, GRAMICIDIN, AND HYDROCORTISONE ACETATE CREAM,** U.S.P. XXII.
Use: Antibiotic, anti-inflammatory.

•**NEOMYCIN AND POLYMYXIN B SULFATES AND GRAMICIDIN OPHTHALMIC SOLUTION,** U.S.P. XXII.
Use: Antibiotic.

•**NEOMYCIN AND POLYMYXIN B SULFATES AND HYDROCORTISONE ACETATE CREAM,** U.S.P. XXII.
Use: Antibiotic, anti-inflammatory.

•**NEOMYCIN AND POLYMYXIN B SULFATES AND HYDROCORTISONE ACETATE OPHTHALMIC SUSPENSION,** U.S.P. XXII.
Use: Antibiotic, anti-inflammatory.

•**NEOMYCIN AND POLYMYXIN B SULFATES AND HYDROCORTISONE OPHTHALMIC** SUSPENSION, U.S.P. XXII.
Use: Antibiotic, anti-inflammatory.

•**NEOMYCIN AND POLYMYXIN B SULFATES AND HYDROCORTISONE OTIC SOLUTION,** U.S.P. XXII.

Use: Antibiotic, anti-inflammatory.

•**NEOMYCIN AND POLYMYXIN B SULFATES AND HYDROCORTISONE OTIC SUSPENSION,** U.S.P. XXII.
Use: Antibiotic, anti-inflammatory.

•**NEOMYCIN AND POLYMYXIN B SULFATES OPHTHALMIC OINTMENT,** U.S.P. XXII.
Use: Antibiotic.

•**NEOMYCIN AND POLYMYXIN B SULFATES AND PREDNISOLONE ACETATE OPHTHALMIC SUSPENSION,** U.S.P. XXII.
Use: Antibiotic, anti-inflammatory.

•**NEOMYCIN AND POLYMYXIN B SULFATES SOLUTION FOR IRRIGATION,** U.S.P. XXII.
Use: Irrigating solution, topical antibacterial.

•**NEOMYCIN AND POLYMYXIN B SULFATES OPHTHALMIC SOLUTION,** U.S.P. XXII.
Use: Ophthalmic antibiotic.

•**NEOMYCIN SULFATE,** U.S.P. XXII. Cream, Oint., Ophth. Oint., Oral Soln., Sterile, Tab., U.S.P. XXII. An antibiotic from *Streptomyces fradiae:* (Upjohn) Pow. micronized for compounding. Bot. 100 Gm.
Use: Antibacterial.
See: Mycifradin Sulfate, Tab., Soln. (Upjohn).
Myciguent, Oint., Ophth. Oint., Cream (Upjohn).
W/Combinations.
See: Aural Acute (Saron).
Bacitracin Neomycin, Oint. (Various Mfr.).
Baximin, Oint. (Quality Generics).
Biotic, Oint. (Scrip).
Biotres HC, Oint. (Central).
B.N.P. Ophthalmic Oint. (Solvay).
B.P.N., Oint. (Norwich).
Bro-Parin, Otic Susp. (Riker).
Coracin, Oint. (Mallard).
Cordran-N, Oint., Lot. (Dista).
Cor-Oticin, Liq. (Maurry).
Cortisporin, Preps. (Burroughs Wellcome).
Duo-Aqua-Drin, Loz. (McKesson).
Epimycin A, Oint. (Delta).
Hi-Cort N, Cream (Blaine).
Hysoquen Oint. (Solvay).
Maxitrol, Ophth., Oint., Susp. (Alcon).
Mity-Mycin Oint. (Solvay).
Mycifradin Sulfate Sterile, Vial (Upjohn).
Mycitracin, Oint., Ophth. Oint. (Upjohn).
My-Cort, Oint., Cream, Soln. (Scrip).
Necort, Oint. (A.V.P.).
Neo-Cort Dome, Otic Soln. (Miles Pharm).
Neo-Cortef, Preps. (Upjohn).
Neo Cort Top, Oint. (Standex).
Neo-Decadron, Ophth., Topical (Merck Sharp & Dohme).
Neo-Delta-Cortef, Preps. (Upjohn).
Neo-Hydeltrasol, Oint., Soln. (Merck Sharp & Dohme).
Neo-Hytone, Cream (Dermik).
Neo-Medrol, Preps. (Upjohn).
Neo-Nysta-Cort, Oint. (Miles Pharm).
Neo-Oxylone, Oint. (Upjohn).
Neosone, Ophth. Oint. (Upjohn).
Neosporin, Preps. (Burroughs Wellcome).
Neo-Thrycex, Oint. (Commerce).
Otobione Soln. (Schering).
Otoreid-HC, Liq. (Solvay).
P.B.N., Oint. (Jenkins).
Spectrocin, Oint. (Squibb Mark).
Statrol Sterile Ophthalmic Oint. (Alcon).
Tigo, Oint. (Burlington).
Tri-Bow Oint. (Bowman).
Tricidin, Oint. (Amlab).
Trimixin, Oint. (Hance).
Triple Antibiotic Oint. (Kenyon).

•**NEOMYCIN SULFATE AND BACITRACIN OINTMENT,** U.S.P. XXII.
Use: Antibiotic.

•**NEOMYCIN SULFATE AND BACITRACIN ZINC OINTMENT,** U.S.P. XXII.
Use: Antibiotic.

•**NEOMYCIN SULFATE AND DEXAMETHASONE SODIUM PHOSPHATE CREAM,** U.S.P. XXII.
Use: Antibiotic, anti-inflammatory.

•**NEOMYCIN SULFATE AND DEXAMETHASONE SODIUM PHOSPHATE OPHTHALMIC OINTMENT,** U.S.P. XXII.
Use: Antibiotic, anti-inflammatory.

•**NEOMYCIN SULFATE AND DEXAMETHASONE SODIUM PHOSPHATE OPHTHALMIC SOLUTION,** U.S.P. XXII.
Use: Antibiotic, anti-inflammatory.

•**NEOMYCIN SULFATE AND FLUOCINOLONE ACETONIDE CREAM,** U.S.P. XXII.
Use: Antibiotic, anti-inflammatory.

• **NEOMYCIN SULFATE AND FLUOROMETHOLONE OINTMENT,** U.S.P. XXII.
Use: Antibiotic, anti-inflammatory.

•**NEOMYCIN SULFATE AND FLURANDRENOLIDE,** U.S.P. XXII. Cream, Lot., Oint., U.S.P. XXII.
Use: Antibiotic, anti-inflammatory.
See: Cordran Prods. (Dista).

•**NEOMYCIN SULFATE AND GRAMICIDIN OINTMENT,** U.S.P. XXII.
Use: Antibiotic.

•**NEOMYCIN SULFATE AND HYDROCORTISONE,** U.S.P. XXII. Cream, Oint., U.S.P. XXII.
Use: Antibiotic, anti-inflammatory.

•**NEOMYCIN SULFATE AND HYDROCORTISONE ACETATE,** U.S.P. XXII. Cream, Lot., Oint., Ophth. Oint., Ophth. Susp., U.S.P. XXII.
Use: Antibiotic, anti-inflammatory.

•**NEOMYCIN SULFATE AND METHYLPREDNISOLONE ACETATE CREAM,** U.S.P. XXII.
Use: Antibiotic, anti-inflammatory.

•**NEOMYCIN SULFATE AND PREDNISOLONE ACETATE OINTMENT,** U.S.P. XXII.
Use: Antibiotic, anti-inflammatory.

•**NEOMYCIN SULFATE AND PREDNISOLONE ACETATE OPHTHALMIC OINTMENT,** U.S.P. XXII.
Use: Antibiotic, anti-inflammatory.

NEOMYCIN SULFATE AND PREDNISOLONE ACETATE OPHTHALMIC SUSPENSION, U.S.P. XXII.
Use: Antibiotic, anti-inflammatory.

NEOMYCIN SULFATE AND PREDNISOLONE SODIUM PHOSPHATE OPHTHALMIC OINTMENT, U.S.P. XXII.
Use: Antibiotic, anti-inflammatory.

NEOMYCIN SULFATE, SULFACETAMIDE SODIUM, AND PREDNISOLONE ACETATE OPHTHALMIC OINTMENT, U.S.P. XXII.
Use: Antibiotic, anti-inflammatory.

NEOMYCIN SULFATE AND TRIAMCINOLONE ACETONIDE CREAM, U.S.P. XXII.
Use: Antibiotic, anti-inflammatory.

NEOMYCIN SULFATE AND TRIAMCINOLONE ACETONIDE OPHTHALMIC OINTMENT, U.S.P. XXII.
Use: Antibiotic, anti-inflammatory.

NEOMYCIN UNDECYLENATE. USAN.
Use: Antibacterial.
See: Neodecyllin (Penick).

NEOMYCORSONE.
See: Neosone, Oint. (Upjohn).

NEO NOVALDIN. (Winthrop Products) Dipyrone.
Use: Analgesic.

NEOPAP. (Webcon) Acetaminophen 125 mg/Supp. In 12s.
Use: Analgesic.

NEOPHAM 6.4%. (KabiVitrum) Essential and non-essential amino acids 6.4%. Inj. 250 ml, 500 ml.
Use: Parenteral nutritional supplement.

NEO PHYRIN DROPS. (Winthrop Products) Phenylephrine HCl.
Use: Decongestant.
See: Phenylephrine HCl.

NEO PICATYL. (Winthrop Products) Glycobiarsoln.
Use: Amebicide.

NEOPLASTIC AGENTS.
See: Folic acid antagonists. Leukemia agents.

NEOQUESS INJECTION. (Forest) Dicyclomine HCl 10 mg/ml. Vial 10 ml.
Use: Anticholinergic/antispasmodic.

NEOQUESS TABLETS. (Forest) L-Hyoscyamine sulfate 0.125 mg/Tab. Bot. 1000s.
Use: Anticholinergic/antispasmodic.

NEOQUINOPHAN.
See: Neocinchophen (Various Mfr.).

NEO QUIPENYL. (Winthrop Products) Primaquine phosphate.
Use: Antimalarial.

NEOSAR. (Adria) Cyclophosphamide. For inj. **100 mg:** Cyclophosphamide 100 mg, sodium Cl 45 mg/Vial. Pkg. 12s. **200 mg:** Cyclophosphamide 200 mg, sodium Cl 90 mg/Vial. Pkg. 12s. **500 mg:** Cyclophosphamide 500 mg, sodium Cl 225 mg/Vial. Pkg 12s.
Use: Antineoplastic agent.

NEO-SKIODAN.
Iodopyracet, Diodrast.

NEOSPORIN CREAM. (Burroughs Wellcome) Polymyxin B sulfate, neomycin sulfate. Tube 0.5 oz, foil packet 1/32 oz. Ctn. 144s.
Use: Anti-infective, external.

NEOSPORIN G.U. IRRIGANT. (Burroughs Wellcome) Neomycin sulfate 40 mg, polymyxin B sulfate 200,000 units/ml. Amp. 1 ml. Box 10s, 50s, Multiple dose vial 20 ml.
Use: Genitourinary irrigant.

NEOSPORIN OINTMENT. (Burroughs Wellcome) Polymyxin B sulfate 5000 units, bacitracin zinc 400 units, neomycin sulfate 5 mg/Gm. Tube 0.5 oz, 1 oz. Foil packet 1/32 oz. Box 144s.
Use: Anti-infective, external.

NEOSPORIN OPHTHALMIC OINTMENT, STERILE. (Burroughs Wellcome) Polymyxin B sulfate 10,000 units, bacitracin zinc 400 units, neomycin sulfate 3.5 mg/Gm, special white petrolatum base. Tube 3.75 Gm.
Use: Anti-infective, ophthalmic.

NEOSPORIN OPHTHALMIC SOLUTION, STERILE. (Burroughs Wellcome) Polymyxin B sulfate 10,000 units, neomycin sulfate 1.75 mg, gramicidin 0.025 mg/ml, alcohol 0.5%, thimerosal 0.001%, propylene glycol, polyoxyethylene-polyoxypropylene compound, sodium Cl. Bot 10 ml. Drop-dose.
Use: Anti-infective, ophthalmic.

NEOSTIBOSAN. Ethylstibamine.

NEOSTIGMINE BROMIDE, U.S.P. XXI. Tab., U.S.P. XXI. Benzenaminium, 3-[[(dimethylamino)-carbonyl]oxy]-N,N,N-trimethyl-, bromide. (m-Hydroxyphenyl)trimethylammonium bromide dimethylcarbamate.
Use: Cholinergic.
See: Prostigmin Bromide, Tab. (Roche).

NEOSTIGMINE METHYLSULFATE, U.S.P. XXI. Inj., U.S.P. XXI. Benzenaminium, 3-[[(dimethylamino)carbonyl]-oxy]-N,N,N-trimethyl-, methyl sulfate. (m-Hydroxyphenyl) trimethylammonium methylsulfate dimethylcarbamate.
Use: Parasympathomimetic agent, cholinergic.
See: Prostigmin methylsulfate, Vial (Roche Lab.).

NEO-STREPSAN.
See: Sulfathiazole (Various Mfr.).

NEO-SYNALAR CREAM. (Syntex) Fluocinolone acetonide 0.025%, neomycin sulfate 0.5%, in a water-washable aqueous base, methylparaben and propylparaben as preservatives. Cream Tube 15 Gm, 30 Gm, 60 Gm.
Use: Corticosteroid, anti-infective.

NEO-SYNEPHRINE 12 HOUR. (Winthrop Pharm) Oxymetazoline HCl 0.05%. Drops Bot. 1 oz. Spray 0.5 oz.
Use: Nasal decongestant.

NEO-SYNEPHRINE HYDROCHLORIDE. (Winthrop Pharm) Phenylephrine HCl. **Spray:** 0.25% children and adult, 0.5% adult. **Regular:** Squeeze bot. 0.5 oz. **0.5% mentholated:** Squeeze bot. 0.5 oz. **Drops:** 0.125% infant; 0.25% children and adult; 0.5% adult; 1% adult

extra strength. Bot. 1 oz; 0.25% and 1% also bot. 16 oz. **Jelly:** 0.5%. Tube 18.75 Gm.
Use: Nasal decongestant.

NEO-SYNEPHRINE HYDROCHLORIDE. (Winthrop Pharm) Phenylephrine HCl. **Amp.:** 1%, Carpuject sterile cartridge-needle unit 10 mg/ml. (1 ml fill in 2 ml cartridge) w/22 gauge, 1.25 inch needle. Dispensing Bin 50s; Vial 1 ml Box 25s. **Ophthalmic:** 2.5%, Mono-Drop Bot. 15 ml; 10% Mono-Drop Bot. 5 ml.; 10% viscous soln., Mono-Drop Bot. 5 ml.
Use: **Amp.:** Vasopressor used in shock; **Ophth.:** Vasoconstrictor/mydriatic.

NEO-SYNEPHRINE VISCOUS OPHTHALMIC. (Winthrop Pharm) Phenylephrine HCl 10%. Soln. Bot. 5 ml.
Use: Ophthalmic vasoconstrictor/mydriatic.

NEOTAL. (Hauck) Zinc bacitracin 400 units, polymyxin B sulfate 5000 units, neomycin sulfate 5 mg, petrolatum and mineral oil base/Gm. Tube 3.75 Gm.
Use: Anti-infective, ophthalmic.

NEO-TEARS. (Barnes-Hind) Sterile, isotonic soln. containing polyvinyl alcohol, hydroxyethylcellulose, sodium Cl, PEG-300, thimerosal $\leq$ 0.004%, EDTA 0.02%. Bot. 15 ml.
Use: Artificial tear solution.

NEO-THRYCEX OINT. (Commerce) Bacitracin, neomycin sulfate, polymyxin B sulfate. Tube 0.5 oz.
Use: Anti-infective, external.

NEOTHYLLINE. (Lemmon) Dyphylline. **200 mg/Tab.:** Bot. 100s, 1000s. **400 mg/Tab.:** Bot. 100s, 500s.
Use: Bronchodilator.

NEOTHYLLINE-GG. (Lemmon) Dyphylline 200 mg, guaifenesin 200 mg/Tab. Bot. 100s, 1000s.
Use: Bronchodilator, expectorant.

NEOTRACE-4. (Lyphomed) Zinc 1.5 mg, copper 0.1 mg, chromium 0.85 mcg, manganese 25 mcg/ml. Vial 2 ml.
Use: Mineral supplement.

NEOTRICIN OPHTHALMIC OINTMENT. (Bausch & Lomb) Polymyxin B sulfate 10,000 units, neomycin sulfate 3.5 mg, bacitracin 400 units/Gm. In 3.5 Gm.
Use: Anti-infective, ophthalmic.

NEOTRICIN OPHTHALMIC SOLUTION. (Bausch and Lomb) Polymyxin B sulfate 10,000 units, neomycin sulfate 1.75 mg, gramicidin 0.025 mg/ml. Dropper bot. 10 ml.
Use: Anti-infective, ophthalmic.

NEO-TROBEX INJECTION. (Forest) Vitamins B_1 150 mg, B_6 10 mg, riboflavin 5-phosphate sodium 2 mg, niacinamide 150 mg, panthenol 10 mg, choline Cl 20 mg, inositol 20 mg/ml. Vial 30 ml.

NEOTROL. (Horizon) Phenylephrine HCl 0.25%, pyrilamine maleate 0.2%, cetalkonium Cl 0.05%, tyrothricin 0.03%, phenylmercuric acetate 1:50,000. Soln. Squeeze Bot. 20 ml.
Use: Decongestant, antihistamine.

NEOVADRIN CENTURION TABLETS. (Scherer) Iron 27 mg, vitamins A 5000 IU, D 400 IU, E 30 IU, B_1 2.25 mg, B_2 2.6 mg, B_3 20 mg, B_5 10 mg, B_6 3 mg, B_{12} 9 mcg, C 90 mg, folic acid 0.4 mg, biotin 45 mcg, Ca, Cr, Cu, I, K, Mg, Mn, Mo, Se, P, Zn/Tab. Bot. 100s.
Use: Vitamin/mineral supplement.

NEOVADRIN CHILDREN'S CHEWABLE TABLETS. (Scherer) Vitamins A 2500 IU, D 400 IU, E 15 mg, B_1 1.05 mg, B_2 1.2 mg, B_3 13.5 mg, B_6 1.05 mg, B_{12} 4.5 mcg, C 60 mg, folic acid 0.3 mg/Tab., tartrazine. Bot. 100s.
Use: Vitamin/mineral supplement.

NEOVADRIN CHILDREN'S WITH IRON. (Scherer) Iron 15 mg, vitamins A 2500 IU, D 400 IU, E 15 mg, B_1 1.05 mg, B_2 1.2 mg, B_3 13.5 mg, B_6 1.05 mg, B_{12} 4.5 mcg, C 60 mg, folic acid 0.3 mg/Tab., tartrazine. Bot. 100s.
Use: Vitamin/mineral supplement.

NEO-VADRIN STRESS FORMULA VITAMINS PLUS ZINC. (Scherer) Vitamins E 45 IU, C 600 mg, folic acid 400 mcg, B_1 20 mg, B_2 10 mg, B_{12} 25 mcg, biotin 45 mcg, pantothenic acid 25 mg, copper 3 mg, zinc 23.9 mg/Tab. Bot. 60s.
Use: Vitamin/mineral supplement.

NEO-VADRIN TIME RELEASE VIT. C. (Scherer) Vitamin C 500 mg/Cap. Bot. 50s, 100s.
Use: Vitamin C supplement.

NEO-VADRIN VITAMIN B_6 TR. (Scherer) Vitamin B_6 100 mg/Cap. Bot. 100s.
Use: Vitamin B_6 supplement.

NEOVAL. (Blue Cross) Vitamins A 10,000 IU, D 400 IU, B_1 10 mg, B_2 5 mg, B_6 2 mg, B_{12} 3 mcg, C 100 mg, E 5 mg, pantothenic acid 10 mg, niacinamide 30 mg, iron 15 mg, copper 1 mg, magnesium 5 mg, manganese 1 mg, zinc 1.5 mg, iodine 0.15 mg/Tab. Bot. 100s.
Use: Vitamin/mineral supplement.

NEOVAL T. (Blue Cross) Vitamins A 10,000 IU, D 400 IU, B_1 15 mg, B_2 10 mg, B_6 2 mg, C 150 mg, B_{12} 7.5 mcg, E 5 mg, pantothenic acid 10 mg, E 5 mg, niacinamide 100 mg, iron 15 mg, magnesium 5 mg, manganese 1 mg, zinc 1.5 mg, copper 1 mg/Tab. Bot. 1000s.
Use: Vitamin/mineral supplement.

NEOVICAPS. (Scherer) Vitamins B_1 15 mg, B_2 10 mg, B_6 5 mg, B_3 50 mg, C 300 mg, zinc 15 mg/TR Cap. Bot. 50s, 100s.
Use: Vitamin/mineral supplement.

NEO WHITE OINTMENT. (Whiteworth) Triple antibiotic ointment. Tube 0.5 oz, 1 oz.
Use: Anti-infective, external.

NEPHRAMINE. (Kendall-McGaw) Amino acid concentration 5.4%, nitrogen 0.65 Gm/100 ml. **Essential amino acids:** Isoleucine 560 mg, leucine 880 mg, lysine 640 mg, methionine 880 mg, phenylalanine 880 mg, threonine 400 mg, tryptophan 200 mg, valine 640 mg, histidine 250 mg/100 ml. **Nonessential amino acids:** Cysteine $>$20 mg/100 ml, sodium 5 mEq, acetate 44 mEq, chloride $>$3 mEq/L, sodium bisulfite. Inj. 250 ml.

Use: Parenteral nutritional supplement.
NEPHRIDINE.
See: Epinephrine (Various Mfr.).
NEPHRO-CALCI. (R & D) Calcium carbonate 1.5 Gm/Chew. Tab. (600 mg calcium). Bot. 100s, 200s, 500s, 1000s.
Use: Calcium supplement.
NEPHROCAPS CAPSULES. (Fleming) Vitamins B_1 1.5 mg, B_2 1.7 mg, B_3 20 mg, B_5 5 mg, B_6 10 mg, B_{12} 6 mcg, C 100 mg, folic acid 1 mg, biotin 150 mcg/Cap. Bot. 100s.
Use: Vitamin supplement.
NEPHRO-MAG. (R & D) Magnesium carbonate 250 mg/Cap. Bot. 100s, 1000s.
Use: Magnesium supplement.
NEPHRON INHALANT AND VAPORIZER. (Nephron) Racemic epinephrine HCl 2.25%. Bot. 0.25 oz, 0.5 oz, 1 oz.
Use: Bronchodilator.
NEPHROX. (Fleming) Aluminum hydroxide 320 mg, mineral oil 10%/5 ml. Bot. pt, gal.
Use: Antacid.
NEPTAZANE. (Lederle) Methazolamide 25 mg or 50 mg/Tab. Bot. 100s.
Use: Carbonic anhydrase inhibitor.
NEQUINATE. USAN.
Use: Coccidiostat.
NEQUINATE (I.N.N.). Methyl Benzoquate. B.A.N.
NERAVAL. Methitural Sodium 5-(1-Methylbutyl)-5-[2-(methylthio)ethyl]-2-thiobarbiturate.
Use: General anesthetic.
NERVINE NIGHTTIME SLEEP-AID. (Miles Labs) Diphenhydramine HCl 25 mg/Tab. Bot. 12s, 30s, 50s.
Use: Sleep aid.
NERVOCAINE. (Keene) Lidocaine HCl 1% or 2%. Inj. Vial 50 ml.
Use: Local anesthetic.
NESACAINE. (Astra) Chloroprocaine HCl 1% or 2%, methylparaben, EDTA. Inj. Vial 30 ml.
Use: Local anesthetic.
NESACAINE-CE. (Astra) **Conc. 2%:** Chloroprocaine HCl 20 mg/ml in a sterile soln containing sodium bisulfite, sodium Cl, HCl. Vial 30 ml. **Conc. 3%:** Chloroprocaine HCl 30 mg/ml in a sterile soln containing sodium bisulfite, sodium Cl, HCl. Vial 30 ml.
Use: Local anesthetic.
NESACAINE-MPF. (Astra) Chloroprocaine HCl 2% or 3%. EDTA or preservative-free. Inj. Vial 30 ml.
Use: Local anesthetic.
NESA NINE CAP. (Standex) Vitamins A 5000 IU, D 400 IU, C 37.5 mg, B_1 1.5 mg, B_2 2 mg, niacinamide 20 mg, B_6 0.1 mg, calcium pantothenate 1 mg, E 2 IU/Cap. Bot. 100s.
Use: Vitamin supplement.
NESDONAL SODIUM.
See: Thiopental Sodium U.S.P. XXII.
Pentothal Sodium, Prods. (Abbott).
NESTABS. (Fielding) Vitamins A 8000 IU, D 400 IU, E 30 mg, C 120 mg, B_1 3 mg, B_2 3 mg, B_3 20 mg, B_6 3 mg, B_{12} 8 mcg, calcium 200 mg, iron 36 mg, folic acid 0.8 mg, zinc 15 mg, I/Tab. Bot. 100s.
Use: Vitamin/mineral supplement.
NESTABS FA TABLETS. (Fielding) Vitamins A 8000 IU, D 400 IU, E 30 mg, C 120 mg, B_1 3 mg, B_2 3 mg, B_3 20 mg, B_6 3 mg, B_{12} 8 mcg, calcium 200 mg, iron (as elemental iron) 36 mg, folic acid 1 mg, zinc 15 mg, I/Tab. Bot. 100s.
Use: Vitamin/mineral supplement.
NESTREX. (Fielding) Pyridoxine 25 mg/Tab., dextrose. Bot. 100s.
Use: Vitamin B_6 supplement.
NETHAMINE. Etafedrine HCl. 1-N-ethylephedrine HCl, 2-methylethylamino-1-phenylpropanol-1 HCl.
W/Codeine phosphate, phenylephrine HCl, sodium citrate, doxylamine succinate.
See: Mercodol with Decapryn Syr. (Merrell Dow).
•**NETILMICIN SULATE,** U.S.P. XXII. Inj., U.S.P. XXII.
Use: Antibacterial.
See: Netromycin (Schering).
•**NETOBIMIN.** USAN.
Use: Anthelmintic (veterinary).
•**NETRAFILCON A.** USAN.
Use: Contact lens material (hydrophilic).
NETRIN. Under Study.
Use: Anticholinergic.
See: Metcaraphen HCl.
NETROMYCIN. (Schering) Netilmicin 100 mg/ml. Inj. Vial 1.5 ml Box 10s, 25s. Multi-dose vial 15 ml Box 5s. Disposable Syringe 1.5 ml Box 10s.
Use: Antibacterial, aminoglycoside.
NEULACTIL.
See: Pericyazine.
NEUPOGEN. (Amgen). Filgrastim (G-CSF).
Use: Colony stimulating factor.
NEUROSIN.
See: Calcium glycerophosphate (Various Mfr.).
NEUT [SODIUM BICARBONATE 4% ADDITIVE SOLUTION]. (Abbott) Sodium bicarbonate 4%. Vial (2.4 mEq each of sodium and bicarbonate), disodium edetate anhydrous 0.05% as stabilizer. Pintop Vial 5 ml, 10 ml. Box 25s, 100s.
Use: Parenteral nutritional supplement.
NEUTRAL ACRIFLAVIN.
See: Acriflavin (Various Mfr.).
NEUTRALIN. (Dover) Calcium carbonate, magnesium oxide/Tab. Sugar, lactose and salt free. UD Box 500s.
Use: Antacid.
NEUTRAL INSULIN INJECTION. B.A.N. A solution of insulin buffered at pH 7 Insulin Novo Actrapid; Nuso.
Use: Hypoglycemic agent.
NEUTRAL PROTAMINE HAGEDORN-INSULIN.
See: Insulin, N.P.H. Iletin (Lilly).
•**NEUTRAMYCIN.** USAN. A neutral macrolide antibiotic produced by a variant strain of *Streptomyces rimosus*.

Use: Antibacterial, antibiotic.
NEUTRA-PHOS. (Willen) Phosphorus 250 mg, potassium 7.125 mEq, sodium 7.125 mEq/dose. **Cap.:** Bot. 48s, 100s. **Pow.:** Bot. 64 Gm.
Use: Mineral supplement.
NEUTRA-PHOS-K. (Willen) Phosphorus 250 mg, potassium 14.25 mEq/dose. **Cap.:** Bot. 48s, 100s. **Pow.:** Bot. 71 Gm.
Use: Mineral supplement.
NEUTROFLAVIN.
See: Acriflavine (Various Mfr.).
NEUTROGENA ACNE CLEANSING SOAP. (Neutrogena) Triethanolamine, glycerin, stearic acid, tallow, coconut oil, castor oil, sodium hydroxide, oleic acid, acetylated lanolin alcohol, cocamide DEA, alcohol, TEA lauryl sulfate. Bar 105 Gm.
Use: Anti-acne.
NEUTROGENA ACNE DRYING GEL. (Neutrogena) Witch hazel, alcohol. Tube 0.75 oz.
Use: Anti-acne.
NEUTROGENA ACNE MASK. (Neutrogena) Benzoyl peroxide 5% in sebum absorbing facial mask vehicle. Tube 2 oz.
Use: Anti-acne.
NEUTROGENA BABY CLEANSING FORMULA SOAP. (Neutrogena) Triethanolamine, glycerin, stearic acid, tallow, coconut oil, castor oil, sodium hydroxide, oleic acid, laneth-10 acetate, cocamide DEA, nonoxynol 14, PEG-4 octoate. Bar 105 Gm.
Use: Skin cleanser.
NEUTROGENA BODY LOTION. (Neutrogena) Glyceryl stearate, isopropyl myristate, PEG-100 stearate, butylene glycol, imidazolidinyl urea, carbomer-934, parabens, sodium lauryl sulfate, triethanolamine, cetyl alcohol. Lot. Bot. 240 ml.
Use: Emollient.
NEUTROGENA BODY OIL. (Neutrogena) Isopropyl myristate, sesame oil, PEG-40 sorbitan peroleate, parabens. Bot. 240 ml.
Use: Emollient.
NEUTROGENA DRY SKIN SOAP. (Neutrogena) Triethanolamine, stearic acid, tallow, glycerin, coconut oil, castor oil, sodium hydroxide, oleic acid, laneth-10 acetate, cocamide DEA, nonoxynol 14, PEG-14 octoate, BHT, O-tolyl biguanide. Bar 105 Gm, 165 Gm. Scented or unscented.
Use: Skin cleanser.
NEUTROGENA NORWEGIAN FORMULA EMULSION. (Neutrogena) Glycerin base 2%. Pump dispenser 5.25 oz.
Use: Emollient.
NEUTROGENA NORWEGIAN FORMULA HAND CREAM. (Neutrogena) Glycerin base 41%. Tube 2 oz.
Use: Emollient.
NEUTROGENA SOAP. (Neutrogena) Triethanolamine, glycerin, stearic acid, tallow, coconut oil, castor oil, sodium hydroxide, oleic acid, cocamide DEA. Bar 105 Gm, 165 Gm.
Use: Skin cleanser.
NEUTROGENA OILY SKIN FORMULA SOAP. (Neutrogena) Triethanolamine, glycerin, fatty acids. Bar 3.5 oz.
Use: Skin cleanser.
NEUTROGENA ORIGINAL FORMULA SOAP. (Neutrogena) Triethanolamine, glycerin, fatty acids. Bar 3.5 oz, 5.5 oz.
Use: Skin cleanser.
NEUTROGENA SUNSCREEN. (Neutrogena) Ethylhexyl p-methoxycinnamate 7%, oxybenzone 4%, titanium dioxide 2%. Tube 3 oz.
Use: Sunscreen.
NEUTROGENA T/GEL. (Neutrogena) Coal tar extract 2%. Shampoo. Bot. 132 ml.
Use: Antiseborrheic.
NEW-DECONGEST. (Goldline) **Syr.:** Phenylpropanolamine HCl 20 mg, phenylephrine HCl 5 mg, chlorpheniramine maleate 2.5 mg, phenyltoloxamine citrate 7.5 mg/5 ml. Bot. pt, gal. **TR Tab.:** Phenylpropanolamine HCl 40 mg, phenylephrine HCl 10 mg, chlorpheniramine maleate 5 mg, phenyltoloxamine citrate 15 mg. Bot. 100s, 500s, 1000s.
Use: Decongestant, antihistamine.
NEW-DECONGEST PEDIATRIC SYRUP. (Goldline) Phenylpropanolamine HCl 5 mg, phenylephrine HCl 1.25 mg, chlorpheniramine maleate 0.5 mg, phenyltoloxamine citrate 2 mg/5 ml. Syr. Bot. pt, gal.
Use: Decongestant, antihistamine.
•**NEXERIDINE HYDROCHLORIDE.** USAN.
Use: Analgesic.
N.G.T. (Geneva Generics) Triamcinolone acetonide 0.1%, nystatin 100,000 units/Gm. Cream Tube 15 Gm.
Use: Topical corticosteroid, antifungal.
NIAC. (Forest) Nicotinic acid 300 mg/SR Cap. Bot. 100s.
Use: Vitamin B_3 supplement.
NIACAL. (Bowman) Calcium lactate 324 mg, niacin 25 mg/Tab. Peppermint flavor. Bot. 100s, 1000s.
Use: Vasodilator, vitamin supplement.
NIACAMIDE.
See: Nikethamide (Various Mfr.).
NIACELS. (Hauck) Niacin 400 mg/TR Cap. Bot. 100s.
Use: Vitamin B_3 supplement.
•**NIACIN,** U.S.P. XXII. Inj., Tab., U.S.P. XXII. 3-Pyridinecarboxylic acid.
Use: Vitamin B-complex component.
See: Efacin, Tab. (Person & Covey).
Niac, Cap. (Cole).
Nicobid, Cap. (Rorer).
Nicolar, Tab. (Rorer).
Nico-400 (Marion).
Ni Cord XL, Cap. (Scott/Cord).
Nicotinex, Elix.(Fleming).
Span Niacin 300, Tab. (Scrip).
Vasotherm, Inj. (Nutrition Control Products).
Wampocap, Cap. (Wallace).

NIACIN W/COMBINATIONS.
See: Adenocrest, Vial (Pharmex).
Lipo-Nicin, Tab., Cap. (Brown).
Vasostim, Cap. (Dunhall).
NIACINAMIDE, U.S.P. XXII. Inj., Tab., U.S.P. XXII. 3-Pyridinecarboxamide. Nicotinic acid amide. Nicotinamide.
Use: Enzyme co-factor vitamin.
See: Niacinamide (Various Mfr.).
W/Pentylenetetrazol, thiamine HCl, cyanocobalamin, alcohol.
See: Cenalene, Tab., Elix. (Central).
W/Potassium iodide.
See: Iodo-Niacin, Tab. (Cole).
W/Riboflavin.
See: Riboflavin and Niacinamide, Amp. (Lilly).
NIACINAMIDE HI.
W/Potassium iodide.
See: Iodo-Niacin, Tab. (Cole).
NIALAMIDE. B.A.N. N-Benzyl-α(isonicotinoyl hydrazine)propionamide. Isonicotinic Acid 2-[2-(Benzylcarbamoyl)ethyl]hydrazide.
Use: Monoamine oxidase inhibitor, antidepressant.
NIALEXO-C. (Mallard) Niacin 50 mg, vitamin C 30 mg/Tab. Bot. 100s.
Use: Vitamin supplement.
NIARB SUPER. (Miller) Magnesium 100 mg, vitamin C 200 mg, niacinamide 200 mg (as ascorbate)/Tab. Bot. 100s.
Use: Vitamin/mineral supplement.
NIAZIDE. (Major) Trichlormethiazide 4 mg/Tab. Bot. 100s, 1000s.
Use: Diuretic.
NIAZO. Neotropin.
Use: Urinary antiseptic.
NIB BASE. (Cenci) Washable self-emulsifying base especially developed for incorporation of many of the therapeutic agents used in dermatology. Pkg. 1 lb, 5 lb.
Use: Dermatological base.
NIBROXANE. USAN.
Use: Antimicrobial.
NICAMETATE. B.A.N. 2-Diethylaminoethyl nicotinate. Euclidan. [dihydrogen citrate].
Use: Peripheral vasodilator.
NICAMINDON.
See: Nicotinamide (Various Mfr.).
NICARDIPINE HYDROCHLORIDE. USAN.
Use: Vasodilator.
N' ICE. (Beecham Products) Menthol 5 mg/Loz. in sugarless sorbitol base. Pkg. 8s, 16s.
Use: Local anesthetic.
NICERGOLINE. USAN. 8β-(5-Bromonicotinoyl-oxy-methyl)-10-methoxy-1,6-dimethylergoline.
Use: Vasodilator.
NICERITROL. B.A.N. Pentaerythritol tetranicotinate.
Use: Treatment of hypercholesterolemia.
NICHOLS SYPHON POWDER. (Last) Sodium bicarbonate, sodium Cl, sodium borate. Pouch 12.2 Gm (add to 32 oz. water to yield isotonic soln.).
NICLOCIDE. (Miles Pharm) Niclosamide 500 mg/Chew. Tab. Box 4s.
Use: Anthelmintic.
NICLOFOLAN. 2,2′-Bis(4-chloro-6-nitrophenol). Bilevon.
Use: Anthelmintic, (veterinary).
•**NICLOSAMIDE.** USAN. 2′,5-Dichloro-4′-nitro-salicylanilide. Yomesan.
Use: Anthelmintic.
See: Niclocide, Tab. (Miles).
NICO-400. (Jones Medical) Niacin 400 mg/Cap. Bot. 100s.
Use: Vitamin B_3 supplement.
NICOBID. (Rorer) Nicotinic acid 125 mg, 250 mg or 500 mg/Tempule TR cap. Bot. 100s, 500s.
Use: Vitamin B_3 supplement.
NICOBION.
See: Nicotinamide (Various Mfr.).
NICOCODINE. B.A.N. O^3-Methyl-O^6-nicotinoylmorphine.
Use: Narcotic analgesic.
NICODICODINE. B.A.N. 7,8-Dihydro-0^3-methyl-O^6-nicotinoylmorphine.
Use: Antitussive.
NICODUOZIDE. A mixture of nicothazone and isoniazid.
NICOLAR. (Rorer) Niacin 500 mg/Tab. Bot. 100s.
Use: Vitamin B_3 supplement.
NICOMORPHINE. B.A.N. 3,6-Dinicotinoylmorphine.
Use: Narcotic analgesic.
•**NICORANDIL.** USAN.
Use: Coronary vasodilator.
NI CORD XL CAPS. (Scott/Cord) Nicotinic acid 400 mg/Cap. Bot. 100s, 500s.
Use: Vitamin B_3 supplement.
NICORETTE. (Lakeside) Nicotine polacrilex 2 mg/Chew. piece. Box 96s.
Use: Smoking deterrent.
NICOTAMIDE.
See: Nicotinamide (Various Mfr.).
NICOTHAZONE. Nicotinaldehyde thiosemicarbazone.
NICOTILAMIDE.
See: Nicotinamide (Various Mfr.).
NICOTINAMIDE. Niacinamide, U.S.P. XXII. Vitamin B_3, Aminicotin, Dipegyl, Nicamindon, Nicotamide, Nicotilamide, Nicotinic Acid Amide.
NICOTINAMIDE ADENINE DINUCLEOTIDE.
Name used for Nadide.
•**NICOTINE POLACRILEX.** USAN.
Use: Smoking deterrent.
See: Nicorette (Merrell Dow).
NICOTINEX ELIXIR. (Fleming) Niacin 50 mg/5 ml, alcohol 14%. Bot. pt, gal.
Use: Vitamin B_3 supplement.
NICOTINIC ACID. Niacin, U.S.P. XXII.
NICOTINIC ACID W/COMBINATIONS.
See: Niacin w/Combinations (Various Mfr.).

NICOTINIC ACID AMIDE. Niacinamide, U.S.P. XXII.
See: Niacinamide (Various Mfr.).

•**NICOTINYL ALCOHOL.** USAN. 3-Pyridine-methanol. beta-Pyridylcarbinol.
Use: Vasodilator.

NICOTINYL TARTRATE. 3-Pyridinemethanol tartrate.
See: Roniacol Timespan, Tab. (Roche).

NICOUMALONE. B.A.N. 3-[2-Acetyl-1-(4-nitrophenyl)ethyl]-4-hydroxycoumarin. Acenocoumarol (I.N.N.) Sinthrome.
Use: Anticoagulant.

NICO-VERT. (Edwards) Niacin 50 mg, dimenhydrinate 25 mg/Cap. Bot. 100s.
Use: Antiemetic/antivertigo.

NICOZIDE. (Premo) Isonicotinic acid hydrazide. (Isoniazid). Tab. 100 mg Bot. 100s, 1000s.
Use: Antituberculous agent.

NIDROXYZONE. 5-Nitro-2-furaldehyde-2-(2-hydroxy-ethyl)semicarbazone.

NIDRYL. (Geneva Generics) Diphenhydramine 12.5 mg/5 ml. Elix. Bot. 120 ml.
Use: Antihistamine.

NIERALINE.
See: Epinephrine (Various Mfr.).

•**NIFEDIPINE,** U.S.P. XXII. Cap., U.S.P. XXII. Dimethyl1,4-dihydro-2,6-dimethyl-4-(2-nitrophenyl)pyridine-3,5-dicarboxylate.
Use: Coronary vasodilator.
See: Adalat, Cap. (Miles Pharm).
Procardia, Cap. (Pfizer).

NIFENAZONE. B.A.N. 2,3-Dimethyl-4-nicotinamido-1-phenyl-5-pyrazolone. Thylin.
Use: Anti-inflammatory, analgesic.

NIFEREX. (Central) **Elix.:** Iron 100 mg/5 ml polysaccharide-iron complex, alcohol 10%. Sugar and dye free. Bot. 8 oz. **Tab.:** Iron 50 mg. Bot. 100s.
Use: Iron supplement.

NIFEREX-150. (Central) Polysaccharide iron complex equivalent to iron 150 mg/Cap. Bot. 100s, 1000s.
Use: Iron supplement.

NIFEREX FORTE ELIXIR. (Central) Iron 100 mg, folic acid 1 mg, vitamin B_{12} 25 mcg/5 ml. Bot. 4 oz.
Use: Iron supplement.

NIFEREX-150 FORTE CAPSULES. (Central) Elemental iron as polysaccharide-iron complex 150 mg, folic acid 1 mg, vitamin B_{12} 25 mcg/Cap. Bot. 100s, 1000s.
Use: Iron supplement.

NIFEREX-PN. (Central) Iron 60 mg, folic acid 1 mg, vitamins C 50 mg, B_{12} 3 mcg, A 4000 IU, D 400 IU, B_1 3 mg, B_2 3 mg, B_6 2 mg, B_3 10 mg, zinc sulfate 80 mg, calcium carbonate 312 mg/Tab, sorbitol. Bot. 100s, 1000s.
Use: Vitamin/mineral supplement.

NIFEREX-PN FORTE TABLETS. (Central) Calcium 250 mg, iron 60 mg, vitamins A 5000 IU, D 400 IU, E 30 mg, B_1 3 mg, B_2 3.4 mg, B_3 20 mg, B_6 4 mg, B_{12} 12 mcg, C 80 mg, folic acid 1 mg, Cu, I, Mg, zinc 25 mg/Tab. Bot. 100s.
Use: Vitamin/mineral supplement.

NIFEREX W/VITAMIN C. (Central) Iron 50 mg, vitamin C 269 mg (as ascorbic acid 100 mg, as sodium ascorbate 169 mg)/Tab. Bot. 50s.
Use: Vitamin/mineral supplement.

•**NIFLURIDIDE.** USAN.
Use: Ectoparasiticide.

•**NIFUNGIN.** USAN. Substance derived from *Aspergillus giganteus.*

•**NIFURADENE.** USAN. 1-[(5-Nitrofurfurylidene)-amino]-2-imidazolidinone.
Use: Antibacterial.

•**NIFURALDEZONE.** USAN. 5-Nitro-2-furaldehyde semioxamazone. Furamazone (Eaton).
Use: Antibacterial.

•**NIFURATEL.** USAN. 5-[(Methylthio)methyl]-3-[(5-nitro furfurylidene)-amino]-2-oxazolidinone. Macmiror, Magmilor, Polmiror. Under study.
Use: Antibacterial, antifungal, trichomonacidal.

•**NIFURATRONE.** USAN. N-(2-Hydroxy-ethyl)-α-(5-nitro-2-furyl)nitrone.
Use: Antibacterial.

•**NIFURDAZIL.** USAN. 1-(2-Hydroxyethyl)-3-[(5-nitrofurfurylidene)-amino]-2-imidazolidinone.
Use: Antibacterial.

NIFURETHAZONE. 5-Nitro-2-furaldehyde-2-[2-(dimethylamino)ethyl] semicarbazone.
Use: Antibacterial.

•**NIFURIMIDE.** USAN. (±-4-Methyl-1-[(5-nitro-furfurylidene)amino]-2-imidazolidinone.
Use: Antibacterial.

•**NIFURMERONE.** USAN. Chloromethyl 5-nitro-2-fufryl ketone. Metofurone.
Use: Antimycotic agent.

NIFUROXIME. 5-Nitro-2-fural-doxime. (Z)-5-Nitro-2-furaldehyde Oxime.
Use: Antifungal, antibacterial (topical), antiprotozoal.
See: Micofur.
W/Furazolidone.
See: Tricofuron, Pow., Supp. (Eaton).

•**NIFURPIRINOL.** USAN.
Use: Antibacterial.

•**NIFURQUINAZOL.** USAN. 2,2′-[[2-(5-Nitro-2-furyl)-4-quinazolinyl]imino]diethanol. Under study.
Use: Antibacterial.

•**NIFURSEMIZONE.** USAN. 5-Nitro-2-furaldehyde-2-ethyl-semicarbazone.
Use: Poultry histomonostat.

•**NIFURSOL.** USAN. 3,5-Dinitrosalicylic acid (5-nitrofurfurylidene) hydrazide.
Use: Histomonocide, vet. growth stimulant.

•**NIFURTHIAZOLE.** USAN. Formic acid 2-[4-(5-nitro-2-furyl)-2-thiazolyl]hydrazide.
Use: Antibacterial (veterinary).

NIFURTIMOX. B.A.N. Tetrahydro-3-methyl-4-(5-ni-trofurfurylideneamino)-1,4-thiazine 1,1-dioxide.
Use: Treatment of trypanosomiasis.

NIGHTTIME COLD MEDICINE. (McKesson) Bot. 6 oz
Use: Relief of cold symptoms.

NIGRIN. Streptonigrin.
Use: Antineoplastic.

NIHYDRAZONE. Acetic acid (5-nitrofurfurylidene) hydrazide. Veterinary.

NIKO-MAG. (Scruggs) Magnesium oxide 500 mg/Cap. Bot. 100s, 1000s.
Use: Antacid.

NIKOTIME TD CAPS. (Major) Niacin 125 mg or 250 mg/TD Cap. Bot. 100s, 1000s.
Use: Vitamin B_3 supplement.

NIL. (Century Pharm.) Sulfanilamide 15%, aminacrine HCl 0.2%, allantoin 1.5%. Vaginal Cream Tube 120 Gm w/applicator.
Use: Anti-infective, vaginal.

NILAIN. (A.V.P.) Aspirin 227 mg, acetaminophen 227 mg, caffeine 32.4 mg/Cap. Bot. 100s.
Use: Analgesic combination.

NILCOL ELIXIR. (Health Care Industries) Phenylpropanolamine 25 mg, chlorpheniramine maleate 2 mg, guaifenesin 100 mg, dextromethorphan HBr 15 mg/15 ml.
Use: Decongestant, antihistamine, expectorant, antitussive.

NILCOL TABLETS. (Health Care Industries) Phenylpropanolamine 50 mg, chlorpheniramine maleate 4 mg, guaifenesin 200 mg, dextromethorphan HBr 30 mg/Tab. Bot. 100s.
Use: Decongestant, antihistamine, expectorant, antitussive.

NILSPASM. (Parmed) Phenobarbital 50 mg, hyoscyamine sulfate 0.31 mg, atropine sulfate 0.06 mg, scopolamine hydrobromide 0.0195 mg/Tab. Bot. 100s, 1000s.
Use: Sedative/hypnotic, anticholinergic/antispasmodic.

NILSTAT OINTMENT & CREAM. (Lederle) Nystatin 100,000 units/Gm. **Cream base** w/Emulsifying wax, isopropyl myristate, glycerin, lactic acid, sodium hydroxide, sorbic acid 0.2%. Tube 15 Gm, Jar 240 Gm. **Oint. base:** w/light mineral oil, Plastibase 50 W. Tube 15 Gm.
Use: Antifungal, external.

NILSTAT ORAL. (Lederle) Nystatin 500,000 units/FC Tab. Bot. 100s, UD 10 × 10s.
Use: Antifungal.

NILSTAT ORAL SUSPENSION. (Lederle) Nystatin 100,000 units/ml, methylparaben 0.12%, propylparaben 0.03%, cherry flavor. Bot. 60 ml w/dropper, 16 fl oz.
Use: Antifungal.

NILSTAT POWDER. (Lederle) Nystatin pow. 150 million, 1 billion or 2 billion units/Bot.
Use: Antifungal.

NILSTAT VAGINAL TABLETS. (Lederle) Nystatin 100,000 units, starch, lactose, polyvinyl pyrrolidone, sorbitol, magnesium stearate/Tab. Pkg. 15s, 30s w/applicator.
Use: Antifungal, vaginal.

NIL TUSS. (Minnesota Pharm.) Dextromethorphan HBr 10 mg, chlorpheniramine maleate 1.25 mg, phenylephrine HCl 5 mg, ammonium Cl 83 mg/tsp. Syr. Bot. pt.
Use: Antitussive, antihistamine, decongestant, expectorant.

NIL VAGINAL CREAM. (Century) Sulfanilamide 15%, 9-aminoacridine HCl 0.2%, allantoin 1.5%. Bot. 4 oz. w/applicator.
Use: Anti-infective, vaginal.

•**NILVADIPINE.** USAN.
Use: Antagonist (calcium channel).

•**NIMAZONE.** USAN. 3-(p-Chlorophenyl)-4-imino-2-oxo-1-imidazolidineacetonitrile.
Use: Anti-inflammatory.

NIMBUS. (NMS Pharm.) Monoclonal antibody-based enzyme immunoassay. Screens for urinary chorionic gonadotropin. In 10s, 25s, 50s.
Use: Diagnostic aid.

NIMBUS II. (NMS Pharm.) Monoclonal antibody-based enzyme immunoassay. Screens for urinary chorionic gonadotropin. In 25s.
Use: Diagnostic aid.

•**NIMIDANE.** USAN.
Use: Acaricide.

•**NIMODIPINE.** USAN.
Use: Vasodilator.

NIMORAZOLE. B.A.N. 4-[2-(5-Nitroimidazol-1-yl)-ethyl]morpholine. Nitrimidazine. Naxogin; Nulogyl.
Use: Treatment of trichomoniasis.

NIMOTOP. (Miles Pharm.) Nimodipine 30 mg. Cap., liq. UD 100s.
Use: Calcium channel blocker.

NINE-VITA. (Robinson) Vitamins A 5000 IU, D 1000 IU, B_1 1.5 mg, B_2 2 mg, niacinamide 20 mg, B_6 0.1 mg, calcium pantothenate 1 mg, C 37.5 mg, E 2 IU/Cap. Bot. 100s, 1000s, Bulk Pack 5000s.
Use: Vitamin supplement.

NIONG. (U.S. Ethicals) Nitroglycerin 2.6 mg or 6.5 mg/CR Tab. Bot. 100s.
Use: Antianginal.

NIPRIDE. (Roche) Nitroprusside sodium 50 mg/5 ml. Vial 5 ml.
Use: Antihypertensive.

NIRATRON. (Progress) Chlorpheniramine maleate 4 mg/Tsp. Bot. pt.
Use: Antihistamine.

•**NIRIDAZOLE.** USAN. 1-(5-Nitrothiazol-2-yl)-imidazolidin-2-one. Ambilhar.
Use: Treatment of schistosomiasis.

NIRON. (Mills) Niacinamide 150 mg, vitamins B_1 10 mg, B_2 6 mg, B_{12} 25 mcg, iron 30 mg/PA Tab. Bot. 100s.
Use: Vitamin/mineral supplement.

NISAVAL. (Vale) Pyrilamine maleate 25 mg/Tab. Bot. 1000s.
Use: Antihistamine.

•**NISBUTEROL MESYLATE.** USAN.
Use: Bronchodilator.

•**NISOBAMATE.** USAN. (1) 2-(Hydroxymethyl)-2,3-dimethylpentyl isopropylcarbamate carbamate

(ester); (2)2-sec-Butyl-2-methyl-1,3-propanediol carbamate isopropylcarbamate.
Use: Minor tranquilizer, sedative, hypnotic.

•**NISOLDIPINE.** USAN.
Use: Vasodilator.

•**NISOXETINE.** USAN.
Use: Antidepressant.

•**NISTERIME ACETATE.** USAN.
Use: Androgen.

•**NITARSONE.** USAN. p-Nitrobenzenearsonic acid.
Use: Veterinary histomonastat.

•**NITHIAMIDE.** USAN.
Use: Antibacterial.

•**NITRAFUDAM HYDROCHLORIDE.** USAN.
Use: Antidepressant.

•**NITRALAMINE HYDROCHLORIDE.** USAN. 2-[[o-Chloro-α-(nitromethyl)benzyl]-thio] ethyl-amine HCl.
Use: Fungicide.

•**NITRAMISOLE HYDROCHLORIDE.** USAN.
Use: Anthelmintic.

•**NITRAZEPAM.** USAN. 1,3-Dihydro-7-nitro-5-phenyl-2H-1,4-benzodiazepin-2-one. Mogadon.
Use: Hypnotic, sedative.

NITRAZINE PAPER. (Squibb) Phenaphthazine. Sodium dinitrophenyl-azo-naphthol disulfonate. Determines pH of a solution, in pH 4.5-7.5 range. 15 ft. roll with dispenser and color chart.
Use: Diagnostic aid.

NITRAZONE. (Kenyon) Nitrofurazone. **Cream:** 2% in a water soluble base. Tube oz. **Soluble Dressing:** 0.2% in a water soluble base of polyethylene glycol.
Use: Burn preparation.

•**NITRENDIPINE.** USAN.
Use: Antihypertensive.

•**NITRIC ACID,** N.F. XVII.
Use: Pharmaceutic aid (acidifying agent).

NITRIC ACID SILVER. Silver Nitrate, U.S.P. XXII.

NITRO-BID. (Marion) Nitroglycerin 2.5 mg, 6.5 mg or 9 mg/TR Cap. Bot. 60s, 100s.
Use: Antianginal.

NITRO-BID IV. (Marion) Nitroglycerin 5 mg/ml. Vial 1 ml box 10s; 5 ml Box 10s; 10 ml Box 5s.
Use: Antianginal.

NITRO-BID OINTMENT. (Marion) Nitroglycerin (glyceryl trinitrate) 2%, lactose in lanolin and petrolatum base. Tube 20 Gm, 60 Gm, UD pak 100s.
Use: Antianginal.

NITRO-BID PLATEAU CAPS. (Marion) Nitroglycerin 2.5 mg, 6.5 mg or 9 mg/SR Cap. Bot. 60s, 100s.
Use: Antianginal.

NITROCAP. (Freeport) Nitroglycerin 2.5 mg/TR Cap. Bot. 100s.
Use: Antianginal.

NITROCINE TIMECAPS. (Kremers-Urban) Nitroglycerin 2.5 mg, 6.5 mg or 9 mg/SR Cap. Bot. 100s.
Use: Antianginal.

•**NITROCYCLINE.** USAN. 4-(Dimethylamino)-1-4,4α, 5,5α,6,11,12α-octahydro-3,10,12,12α-tetrahydroxy-7-nitro-1,11-dioxo-2-naphthacenecarboxamide.
Use: Antibiotic.

•**NITRODAN.** USAN.
Use: Anthelmintic.

NITRO-DIAL. (Rocky Mtn.) Nitroglycerin 2.5 mg/TD Cap. Bot. 50s, 250s.
Use: Antianginal.

NITRODISC. (Searle) Nitroglycerin. Transcutaneous nitroglycerin discs releasing 5 mg/24 hr, 7.5 mg/24 hr or 10 mg/24 hr. Carton 30s, 100s (7.5 mg/24 hr).
Use: Antianginal.

NITRO-DUR. (Key Pharm) Nitroglycerin. Transdermal system releasing 2.5 mg, 5 mg, 7.5 mg, 10 mg or 15 mg/24 hours. Carton 30s.
Use: Antianginal.

NITROFAN CAPS. (Major) Nitrofurantoin 50 mg or 100 mg/Cap. Bot. 100s, 500s.
Use: Urinary anti-infective.

NITROFOR-50. (Kenyon) Nitrofurantoin 50 mg/Tab. Bot. 100s, 1000s.
Use: Urinary anti-infective.

NITROFOR-100. (Kenyon) Nitrofurantoin 100 mg/Tab. Bot. 100s, 1000s.
Use: Urinary anti-infective.

•**NITROFURANTOIN,** U.S.P. XXII. Tab., Cap., Inj., U.S.P. XXII. 2,4-Imidazolidinedione, 1-[[(5-nitro-2-fura- nyl)methylene]-amino]-. 1-[(5-Nitrofur- furylidene)amino]hydantoin. 1-(5-Nitro-furfur- lyideneamino)imidazoline-2,4-dione. Berkfurin; Furadantin; Urantoin.
Use: Antibacterial for urinary tract infections.
See: Furadantin, Preps. (Norwich Eaton).
Furalan, Tab. (Lannett).
Nitrex, Tab. (Star).
Nitrofor-50, Tab. (Kenyon).
Nitrofor-100, Tab. (Kenyon).
Nitrofurantoin sodium, Vial (Norwich Eaton).
Sarodant (Saron).
Trantoin, Tab. (McKesson).
Urotoin, Tab. (Scruggs).

NITROFURANTOIN MACROCRYSTALS.
Use: Urinary anti-infective.
See: Macrodantin, Cap. (Norwich Eaton).

•**NITROFURAZONE,** U.S.P. XXII. Cream, Oint., Topical Soln., U.S.P. XXII. 5-Nitro-2-furaldehyde semicarbazone.
Use: Bacteriostatic for surface wounds.
See: Furacin, Preps. (Norwich Eaton).
Nitrazone, Cream, Soln., Dressing (Kenyon).
Nitrofurastan, Oint. (Standex).
Nitrozone, Oint. (Century).
W/Allantoin, stearic acid.
See: Eldezol, Oint. (Elder).

NITROFURFURYL METHYL ETHER. 2-(Methyloxymethyl)-5-nitrofuran.
Use: Antifungal (veterinary).

NITROGARD. (Parke-Davis) Transmucosal controlled-released nitroglycerin 1 mg, 2 mg or 3 mg/Tab. Bot. 100s.
Use: Antianginal.

•**NITROGEN,** N.F. XVII.
Use: Pharmaceutic aid (air displacement).

NITROGEN MONOXIDE. Laughing Gas, Nitrous Oxide.
Use: Inhalation anesthetic, analgesic.

NITROGEN MUSTARD.
See: Mustargen, Vial (Merck Sharp & Dohme).

NITROGEN MUSTARD DERIVATIVES.
See: Leukemia Agents.
Leukeran, Tab. (Burroughs-Wellcome).
Mustargen HCl, Vial (Merck Sharp & Dohme).
Triethylene Melamine, Tab. (Lederle).

•**NITROGLYCERIN, DILUTED,** U.S.P. XXII.
Use: Vasodilator.

•**NITROGLYCERIN INJECTION,** U.S.P. XXII. (Abbott) 25 mg/ml. Vial 5 ml, 10 ml.
Use: Vasodilator, treatment of angina.
See: Tridil, Inj. (American Critical Care).

•**NITROGLYCERIN OINTMENT,** U.S.P. XXII.
Use: Vasodilator.

•**NITROGLYCERIN TABLETS,** U.S.P. XXII. 1,2,3-Propanetriol, trinitrate. (Various Mfr.) Glyceryl Trinitrate, Glonoin, Nitroglycerol, Trinitrin, Trinitroglycerol Tab.
Use: Vasodilator.
See: Ang-O-Span, Cap. (Scrip).
Cardabid (Saron).
Niglycon, Tab. (Consoln. Midland).
Niong, Tab. (U.S. Ethicals).
Nitrobid, Cap. (Marion).
Nitrocels, Cap. (Winston).
Nitro-Dial, TD Cap. (Rocky Mtn.).
Nitrodyl, Cap. (Bock).
Nitrogard (Parke-Davis).
Nitroglyn, Tab. (Key Pharm.).
Nitrol Oint. (Kremers-Urban).
Nitro-Lyn, Cap. (Lynwood).
Nitrong, Tab. (Wharton).
Nitrospan, Cap. (Rorer).
Nitrotym, Cap. (Kenyon).
Nitro, TD Cap. (Fleming).
Trates, Cap. (Solvay).
Vasoglyn, Unicelles (Solvay).
W/Butabarbital.
See: Nitrodyl-B, Cap. (Bock).
Nitrotym-Plus, Cap. (Kenyon).
W/Nicotinic acid.
See: Nitrovas, Tab. (Amfre-Grant).
W/Veratrum viride, sodium nitrite, potassium nitrate, aconite root.
See: Nyomin, Tab. (Elder).

NITROGLYCERIN TRANSDERMAL.
Use: Vasodilator.
See: Deponit 5 and 10 (Wyeth-Ayerst).
Nitrodisc (Searle).
NTS (Bolar).
Transderm-Nitro (Ciba).

NITROGLYCEROL.
See: Nitroglycerin (Various Mfr.).

NITROGLYN. (Key) Nitroglycerin 2.5 mg, 6.5 mg or 9 mg/SR Cap. Bot. 100s.
Use: Antianginal.

NITROL IV. (Rorer) Nitroglycerin 0.8 mg/ml. Amp. 1 ml Box 25s; 10 ml Box 10s; 30 ml Box 5s.
Use: Antianginal.

NITROL IV CONCENTRATE. (Rorer) Nitroglycerin for infusion 50 mg/10 ml. Amp Box 10s.
Use: Antianginal.

NITROLIN. (Schein) Nitroglycerin 2.5 mg or 9 mg/SR Cap. **2.5 mg:** Bot. 100s. **9 mg:** Bot. 60s.
Use: Antianginal.

NITROLINGUAL SPRAY. (Rorer) Nitroglycerin lingual aerosol 0.4 mg/metered dose. Canister 13.8 Gm containing 200 metered doses.
Use: Antianginal.

NITROL OINTMENT. (Adria) Nitroglycerin 2% in lanolin and petrolatum base. Tube 30 Gm, 60 Gm, Pack 6s.
Use: Antianginal.

NITRO-LYN. (Lynwood) Nitroglycerin 2.5 mg/Cap. Bot. 100s.
Use: Antianginal.

NITROMANNITE.
See: Mannitol Hexanitrate (Various Mfr.).

NITROMANNITOL.
See: Mannitol Hexanitrate (Various Mfr.).

NITROMED. (U.S. Ethicals) Nitroglycerin 2.6 mg or 6.5 mg/CR Tab. Bot. 100s.
Use: Antianginal.

•**NITROMERSOL,** U.S.P. XXII. Topical Soln., U.S.P. XXII. Tincture, U.S.P. XXI. 4-Nitro-3-hydroxy mercuri-o-cresol anhydride. 5-Methyl-2-nitro-7-oxa-8-mercurabicyclo (4.2.0) octa-1,3,5-triene. Metaphen.
Use: Local anti-infective.

•**NITROMIDE.** USAN. 3,5-Dinitrobenzamide.
Use: Coccidiostat, antibacterial.

•**NITROMIFENE CITRATE.** USAN.
Use: Anti-estrogen.

NITRONET. (U.S. Ethicals) Nitroglycerin 2.6 mg or 6.5 mg/CR Tab. Bot. 100s.
Use: Antianginal.

NITRONG OINTMENT. (Wharton) Nitroglycerin 2%. Oint. Tube 30 Gm, 60 Gm with dose applicator.
Use: Antianginal.

NITRONG TABLETS. (Wharton) Nitroglycerin 2.6 mg, 6.5 mg or 9 mg/CR Tab. Bot. 30s, 60s (9 mg), 100s.
Use: Antianginal.

p-NITROPHENOL.
See: Niphen, Liq. (Torch).

NITROPRESS. (Abbott Hospital Prods.) Sodium nitroprusside 50 mg/2 ml. Vial.
Use: Antihypertensive.

NITROPRUSSIDE SODIUM.
Use: Antihypertensive.
See: Nipride, Pow. for Inj. (Roche).
Nitropress, Pow. for Inj. (Abbott).

Sodium Nitroprusside, Pow. for Inj. (Various Mfr.).

•**NITROSCANATE.** USAN.
Use: Anthelmintic.

NITROSTAT. (Parke-Davis) Nitroglycerin 0.15 mg, 0.3 mg, 0.4 mg or 0.6 mg/Tab. Bot. 25s, 100s, UD 100s.
Use: Antianginal.

NITROSTAT IV. (Parke-Davis) Nitroglycerin for infusion. **0.8 mg/ml:** Amp. 10 ml. **5 mg/ml:** Amp. 10 ml, Vial 10 ml. **10 mg/ml:** Vial 10 ml.
Use: Antianginal.

p-NITROSULFATHIAZOLE. 2-(p-Nitrophenylsulfonamide) thiazole.

NITROUS ACID, SODIUM SALT. Sodium Nitrite, U.S.P. XXII.

•**NITROUS OXIDE,** U.S.P. XXII. Laughing Gas. Nitrogen Monoxide.
Use: General anesthetic (inhalation).

NITROVIN. B.A.N. 1,5-Bis(5-nitro-2-furyl)penta-1,4-dien-3-one amidinohydrazone. Payzone and Panazon [hydrochloride]
Use: Growth promoter, veterinary medicine.

NITROXOLINE. B.A.N. 8-Hydroxy-5-nitroquinoline. Nibiol.
Use: Antibacterial.

NITROXYNIL. .B.A.N. 4-Hydroxy-3-iodo-5-nitrobenzonitrile. Trodax [meglumine salt].
Use: Anthelmintic, veterinary medicine.

•**NIVAZOL.** USAN. 2′-(p-Fluorophenyl-2′H-17α-pregna-2,4-dien-20-yno [3,2-c]pyrazol-17-ol.
Use: Glucocorticoid.

NIVEA MOISTURIZING. (Beiersdorf) **Cream:** Mineral oil, petrolatum, lanolin alcohol, glycerin, microcrystalline wax, paraffin, magnesium sulfate, decyloleate, octyl dodecanol, aluminum stearate, citric acid, magnesium stearate. In 120 Gm, 180 Gm, 300 Gm, 480 Gm. **Lot.:** Mineral oil, lanolin, isopropyl myristate, cetearyl alcohol, glyceryl stearate, acrylamide/sodium acrylate copolymer, simethicone, methychloroisothiazolinone, methylisothiazolinone. In 180 ml, 300 ml, 450 ml.
Use: Emollient.

NIVEA OIL. (Beiersdorf) Emulsion of neutral aliphatic hydrocarbons. **Liq.:** Bot. 2 oz, 4 fl oz, pt, qt. **Cream:** Tube 1 oz, 2⅓ oz, Jar 4 oz, 6 oz, 1 lb, 5 lb. tin. **Soap:** Bath or toilet size.
Use: Emollient.
See: Basic soap (Beiersdorf).

•**NIVIMEDONE SODIUM.** USAN.
Use: Anti-allergic.

NIX CREME RINSE. (Burroughs Wellcome) Permethrin 1%. Bot. 2 oz.
Use: Pediculicide.

•**NIZATIDINE.** USAN.
Use: Anti-ulcerative (Histamine H_2-receptor antagonist).
See: Axid, Cap. (Lilly).

NIZORAL CREAM. (Janssen) Ketoconazole 2% cream. Tube 15 Gm, 30 Gm.
Use: Antifungal, external.

NIZORAL SUSPENSION. (Janssen) Ketoconazole 20 mg/ml. Saccharin. Bot. 4 oz.
Use: Antifungal.

NIZORAL TABLETS. (Janssen) Ketoconazole 200 mg/Tab. Bot. 100s. Box of 10 strips of 10 tablets.
Use: Antifungal.

N-MULTISTIX S. G. REAGENT STRIPS. (Ames) Urinalysis reagent strip test for pH, protein, glucose, ketones, bilirubin, blood, nitrite, urobilinogen and specific gravity. Bot. 100s.
Use: Diagnostic aid.

NO-ASPIRIN. (Walgreen) Acetaminophen 325 mg/Tab. Bot. 100s.
Use: Analgesic.

NO-ASPIRIN EXTRA STRENGTH. (Walgreen) Acetaminophen 500 mg/Tab. or Cap. **Tab.:** Bot. 60s, 100s. **Cap.:** Bot. 50s, 100s.
Use: Analgesic.

•**NOCODAZOLE.** USAN.
Use: Antineoplastic.

NOCTEC. (Squibb) Chloral hydrate. **Syr.:** 500 mg/5 ml, saccharin. Bot. pt, gal. **Cap.:** 250 mg or 500 mg. Bot. 100s. Unimatic 25s, 100s.
Use: Sedative/hypnotic.

NO DOZ. (Bristol-Myers) Caffeine 100 mg/Tab. Bot. 60s. Card 15s, 36s.
Use: Analeptic.

•**NOGALAMYCIN.** USAN.
Use: Antineoplastic.

NO-HIST CAPSULES. (Dunhall) Phenylephrine HCl 5 mg, phenylpropanolamine HCl 40 mg, pseudoephedrine HCl 40 mg/Cap. Bot. 100s.
Use: Decongestant.

NO-HIST-S SYRUP. (Dunhall) Phenylephrine HCl 5 mg, phenylpropanolamine HCl 40 mg, pseudoephedrine HCl 40 mg/5 ml. Bot. pt.
Use: Decongestant.

NOKANE. (Wren) Salicylamide 4 gr, N-acetyl-p-aminophenol 4 gr, caffeine 0.5 gr/Tab. Bot. 40s.
Use: Analgesic combination.

NOLAHIST. (Carnrick) Phenindamine tartrate 25 mg/Tab. Bot. 100s.
Use: Antihistamine.

NOLAMINE. (Carnrick) Chlorpheniramine maleate 4 mg, phenindamine tartrate 24 mg, phenylpropanolamine HCl 50 mg/Tab. Bot. 100s, 250s.
Use: Antihistamine, decongestant.

NOLEX LA. (Carnrick). Phenylpropanolamine 75 mg, guaifenesin 400 mg/SR Tab. Bot. 100s.
Use: Decongestant, expectorant.

•**NOLINIUM BROMIDE.** USAN.
Use: Anti-ulcerative, antisecretory.

NOLVADEX. (ICI Pharma) Tamoxifen citrate equivalent to 10 mg tamoxifen/Tab. Bot. 60s, 250s.
Use: Antineoplastic agent.

NOMETIC. Diphenidol.
Use: Antiemetic.

NOMIFENSINE. B.A.N. 8-Amino-1,2,3,4-tetrahydro-2-methyl-4-phenylisoquinoline.

Use: Thymoleptic and central nervous system stimulant.
Note: Some products withdrawn from market due to incidence of hemolytic anemia.

NONAMIN. (Western Research) Calcium 100 mg, chloride 90 mg, magnesium 50 mg, zinc 3.75 mg, iron 4.5 mg, copper 0.5 mg, iodine 37.5 mcg, potassium 49 mg, phosphorus 100 mg/Tab. Bot. 1000s.
Use: Mineral supplement.

NONE. (Forest) Heparin sodium 1000 units/ml. No preservatives. Amps 5 ml. Box 25s.
Use: Anticoagulant.

NONOXYNOL. (Ortho) Nonylphenoxypolyethoxyethanol.
Use: Spermicide.
See: Emko, Preps. (Emko).

NONOXYNOL 4. USAN. Nonylphenoxy-poly-ethyleneoxyethanol. Igepal CO-430. Under study.
Use: Nonionic surfactant.

NONOXYNOL 9, U.S.P. XXII. Poly (ethylene glycol) p-nonylphenyl ether. Igepal CO-630.
Use: Spermatocide.
See: Conceptrol, Cream, Gel (Ortho).
Delfen, Foam (Ortho).
Emko Prods. (Emko-Schering).
Encare, Insert (Eaton-Merz).
Gynol II, Jelly (Ortho).
Intercept, Inserts (Ortho).
Ortho-Creme, Cream (Ortho).
Ortho-Gynol, Jelly (Ortho).

NONOXYNOL 10, U.S.P. XXII.
Use: Spermatocide.

NONOXYNOL 15. USAN. Nonylphenoxy-poly-ethyleneoxyethanol. Igepal CO-880. Under study.
Use: Nonionic surfactant.

NONOXYNOL 30. USAN. Nonylphenoxy-poly-ethyleneoxyethanol. Under study.
Use: Nonionic surfactant.

NONSPECIFIC PROTEIN THERAPY.
See: Protein, Nonspecific Therapy.

NONYLPHENOXYPOLYETHOXY ETHANOL. Nonoxynol.
Use: Spermicide.
See: Delfen Vaginal Foam (Ortho).
W/Benzethonium Cl.

NORACYMETHADOL HCl. USAN. α-4, 4-Diphenyl-6-methylamino-3-heptanol acetate HCl.
Use: Analgesic agent.

NORADEX TABS. (Major) Orphenadrine citrate 100 mg/Tab. Bot. 100s, 500s.
Use: Skeletal muscle relaxant.

NORADRENALINE. B.A.N. (−)-2-Amino-1-(3,4-dihydroxyphenyl)ethanol. Levarterenol (I.N.N.).
Use: Hypertensive.

NORBOLETHONE. USAN. 13-Ethyl-17-hydroxy-18, 19-dinor-17αa-pregn-4-en-3-one.
Use: Anabolic.

NORBUTRINE. B.A.N. 2-Cyclobutylamino-1-(3,4-dihydroxyphenyl) ethanol.
Use: Bronchodilator.

NORCET TABLETS. (Holloway) Hydrocodone bitartrate 5 mg, acetaminophen 500 mg/Tab. Bot. 100s.
Use: Narcotic analgesic combination.

NORCODEINE. B.A.N. N-Demethyl-O^3-methylmor-phine.
Use: Narcotic analgesic.

NORCURON. (Organon) Vecuronium bromide 10 mg/5 ml. **With diluent:** Vial 5 ml lyophilized powder and 5 ml ampul of sterile water for injection. Box 10s. **Without diluent:** Vial 5 ml lyophilized powder. Box 10s. **Prefilled syringe:** Vial 10 ml lyophilized powder and 10 ml syringe w/bacteriostatic water for injection. Box 10s.
Use: Muscle relaxant, adjunct to anesthesia.

NORCYCLINE. 6-Demethyl-6-deoxytetracycline. Bonomycin. Sancycline.
Use: Anti-infective.

NORDETTE-21. (Wyeth-Ayerst) Levonorgestrel 0.15 mg, ethinyl estradiol 0.03 mg/Tab. 6 Pilpak dispensers, 21 Tabs.
Use: Oral contraceptive.

NORDETTE-28. (Wyeth-Ayerst) Levonorgestrel 0.15 mg, ethinyl estradiol 0.03 mg/Orange Tab. (21) and pink inert tablets (7). 6 Pilpak dispensers, 28 tab.
Use: Oral contraceptive.

NOREL PLUS CAPSULES. (U.S. Pharmaceutical Corp.) Chlorpheniramine maleate 4 mg, phenyltoloxamine dihydrogen citrate 25 mg, phenylpropanolamine HCl 25 mg, acetaminophen 325 mg/Cap. Bot. 100s.
Use: Antihistamine, decongestant, analgesic.

dl-NOREPHEDRINE HYDROCHLORIDE. alpha-Hydroxy-beta-aminopropylbenzene HCl.
Use: See: Phenylpropanolamine Hydrochloride (Various Mfr.).
Propadrine, Cap., Elix. (Merck Sharp & Dohme).

•**NOREPINEPHRINE BITARTRATE,** U.S.P. XXII. Inj., U.S.P. XXII. 1,2-Benzenediol, 4-(2-amino-1-hydroxyethyl)-, 2,3-dihydroxybutanedioate (1:1) (Salt), monohydrate l-a-(Aminomethyl)3,4-dihydroxybenzyl alcohol bitartrate.
Use: Adrenergic (vasopressor).
See: Levophed Bitartrate, Soln., Amp. (Winthrop Pharm).

NORETHANDROLONE, B.A.N. 17-Alphaethyl-17-hydroxynorandrostenone, 17-Hydroxy-19-nor-17α- pregn-4-en-3-one. Nileyar.
Use: Anabolic steroid.

NORETHIN 1/50 M. (Searle) Norethindrone 1 mg, mestranol 50 mcg/Tab. 21 day and 28 day (with 7 inert tabs.).
Use: Oral contraceptive.

NORETHIN 1/35 E. (Searle) Norethindrone 1 mg, ethinyl estradiol 35 mg/Tab. 21 day and 28 day (with 7 inert tabs.).
Use: Oral contraceptive.

•**NORETHINDRONE,** U.S.P. XXII. Tab., U.S.P. XXII. 19-Norpregn-4-en-20-yn-3-one, 17-hy-

droxy-, (17α)-. 17-Hydroxy-19-nor-17-alpha-pregn-4-en-20-yn-3- one.
Use: Progestin.
See: Micronor, Tab. (Ortho).
Norlutin, Tab. (Parke-Davis).
Nor-Qd, Tab. (Syntex).
W/Ethinyl estradiol.
See: Brevicon 21 and 28, Tab. (Syntex).
Modicon 21 and 28, Tab. (Ortho).
Ortho-Novum 21 and 28, Prods. (Ortho).
Ovcon-35, Tab. (Mead Johnson).
Ovcon-50, Tab. (Mead Johnson).
W/Mestranol.
See: Norinyl, Prods. (Syntex).
Ortho-Novum, Prods. (Ortho).
W/Mestranol, ferrous fumarate.
See: Norinyl-l Fe 28, Prods. (Syntex).

•**NORETHINDRONE ACETATE,** U.S.P. XXII. Tab., U.S.P. XXII. 19-Norpregn-4-en-20-yn-3-one, 17-(acetyloxy)-, (17α)-, 17α-Ethinyl-19-nortestosterone. 17-Hydroxy-19-nor-17α-pregn-4-en-20-yn-3-one Acetate.
Use: Progestin.
See: Norlutate, Tab. (Parke-Davis).

•**NORETHINDRONE ACETATE AND ETHINYL ESTRADIOL TABLETS,** U.S.P. XXII.
Use: Oral contraceptive.
See: Brevicon, Tab. (Syntex).
Gestest, Tab. (Squibb).
Loestrin, Prods. (Parke-Davis).
Norinyl, Prods. (Syntex).
Norlestrin, Prods. (Parke-Davis).

•**NORETHINDRONE AND ETHINYL ESTRADIOL TABLETS,** U.S.P. XXII.
Use: Oral contraceptive.

•**NORETHINDRONE AND MESTRANOL TABLETS,** U.S.P. XXII.
Use: Oral contraceptive.

NORETHISTERONE. B.A.N. 17β-Hydroxy-19-norpregn-4-en-20-yn-3-one. 17α-Ethynyl-17β-hydroxyoestr-4-en-3-one. 17α-Ethynyl-19-nor-testosterone. Micronor; Noriday; Primolut N; Norlutin-A [acetate].
Use: Progestin.

•**NORETHYNODREL,** U.S.P. XXII. 17-Hydroxy-19-nor-17α-pregn-5(10)-en-20-yn-3-one.
Use: Progesterone agent.
See: Enovid, Prods (Searle).

NORFLEX. (Riker) Orphenadrine citrate 100 mg/SR Tab. Bot. 100s, 500s.
Use: Skeletal muscle relaxant.

NORFLEX INJECTABLE. (Riker) Orphenadrine citrate 60 mg, sodium bisulfite 2 mg, sodium Cl 5.8 mg, water for injection qs 2 ml. Amp. 2 ml 6s, 50s.
Use: Skeletal muscle relaxant.

•**NORFLOXACIN.** USAN.
Use: Quinolone antibacterial.
See: Noroxin, Tab. (Merck Sharp & Dohme).

•**NORFLURANE.** USAN. 1,1,1,2-Tetrafluoroethane. Under study.
Use: Inhalation anesthetic.

NORFORMS. (Fleet) PEG 20, PEG 6, PEG 20 palmitate, lactic acid, methylbenzethonium Cl/Supp. Unscented and herbal scent. Box 6s, 12s, 24s.
Use: Vaginal preparation.

NORGESIC FORTE TABLETS. (Riker) Orphenadrine citrate 50 mg, aspirin 770 mg, caffeine 60 mg/Tab. Bot. 100s, 500s, UD 100s.
Use: Skeletal muscle relaxant, salicylate analgesic.

NORGESIC TABLETS. (Riker) Orphenadrine citrate 25 mg, aspirin 385 mg, caffeine 30 mg/Tab. Bot. 100s, 500s, UD 100s.
Use: Skeletal muscle relaxant, salicylate analgesic.

•**NORGESTIMATE.** USAN.
Use: Progestin.

•**NORGESTOMET.** USAN.
Use: Progestin.

•**NORGESTREL,** U.S.P. XXII. Tab., U.S.P. XXII. 18,19-Dinorpregn-4-en-20-yn-3-one, 13-ethyl-17-hydroxy,-(17 α)-(+)-. (±)-13-Ethyl-17-hydroxy-18, 19-dinor-17α-pregn-4-en-20-yn-3-one. (±)-13-Ethyl-17α-ethynyl-17-hydroxygon-4-en-3-one.
Use: Oral contraceptive.
See: Ovrette, Tab. (Wyeth-Ayerst).

•**NORGESTREL AND ETHINYL ESTRADIOL TABLETS,** U.S.P. XXII.
Use: Oral contraceptive.
See: Lo/Ovral, Tab. (Wyeth-Ayerst).
Ovral-Prep. (Wyeth-Ayerst).

NORINYL 1 + 35. (Syntex) Norethindrone 1 mg, ethinyl estradiol 0.035 mg/Tab. Wallette 21 and 28 day (7 inert tabs).
Use: Oral contraceptive.

NORINYL 1 + 50. (Syntex) Norethindrone1 mg, mestranol 0.05 mg/Tab. Wallette 21 and 28 day (7 inert tabs).
Use: Oral contraceptive.

NORINYL 2 MG. (Syntex) Norethindrone 2 mg, mestranol 0.1 mg/Tab. Memorette Disp. of 20s. Refill folders of 20s.
Use: Oral contraceptive.

NORISODRINE AEROTROL. (Abbott) Norisodrine HCl (isoproterenol HCl) 0.25% (2.8 mg/ml) in inert chlorofluorohydrocarbon propellants, alcohol 33%, ascorbic acid 0.1% as preservative. Aerotrol 15 ml. Box 12s.
Use: Bronchodilator.

NORISODRINE WITH CALCIUM IODIDE SYRUP. (Abbott) Isoproterenol sulfate 3 mg, calcium iodide, anhydrous 150 mg/5 ml, alcohol 6%. Bot. pt.
Use: Bronchodilator.

NORLAC RX. (Solvay) Calcium 200 mg, iron 60 mg, vitamins A 8000 IU, D 400 IU, E 30 mg, B_1 2 mg, B_2 2 mg, B_3 20 mg, B_6 4 mg, B_{12} 8 mcg, C 90 mg, folic acid 1 mg, Cu, I, Mg, zinc 15 mg/Tab. Bot. 100s, Unit-of-use 100s.
Use: Vitamin/mineral supplement.

NORLESTRIN-21 1/50 TABLETS. (Parke-Davis) Norethindrone acetate 1 mg, ethinyl estradiol 50 mcg/tab. (yellow). Compact 21s. Pkg. 5 compacts. Pkg. 5 refills; Ctn. 10×5 refills.
Use: Oral contraceptive.

NORLESTRIN-28 1/50 TABLET. (Parke-Davis) Norethindrone acetate 1 mg, ethinyl estradiol 50 mcg/tab. (yellow). Compact 21 yellow, 7 white (inert) tablets. Pkg. 5 compacts. Pkg. 5 refills; Ctn. 10×5 refills.
Use: Oral contraceptive.

NORLESTRIN-21 2.5/50 TABLETS. (Parke-Davis) Norethindrone acetate 2.5 mg, ethinyl estradiol 50 mcg/tab. (pink). Compact 21s. Pkg. 5 compacts. Pkg. 5 refills; Ctn. 10×5 refills.
Use: Oral contraceptive.

NORLESTRIN Fe 1/50 TABLETS. (Parke-Davis) Norethindrone acetate 1 mg, ethinyl estradiol 50 mcg/tab. (yellow). Compact 21 yellow tab., 7 brown 75 mg ferrous fumarate tab. Pkg. 5 compacts. Pkg. 5 refills; ctn. 10×5 refills.
Use: Oral contraceptive.

NORLESTRIN Fe 2.5/50 TABLETS. (Parke-Davis) Norethindrone acetate 2.5 mg, ethinyl estradiol 50 mcg/tab. (pink). Compact 21 pink tab., 7 brown 75 mg ferrous fumarate tab. Pkg. 5 compacts. Pkg. 5 refills; Ctn. 10×5 refills.
Use: Oral contraceptive.

NORLEVORPHANOL. B.A.N. (−)-3-hydroxymorphinan.
Use: Narcotic analgesic.

NORLUTATE. (Parke-Davis) Norethindrone acetate 5 mg/Tab. Bot. 50s.
Use: Progestin.

NORLUTIN. (Parke-Davis) Norethindrone 5 mg/Tab. Bot. 50s.
Use: Progestin.

NORMADERM CREAM & LOTION. (Doak) Buffered lactic acid in vanishing bases. **Cream:** Jar 3¾ oz, 16 oz. **Lot.:** Bot. 4 oz, 16 oz, 128 oz.
Use: Emollient, acid restorer for skin.

NORMAL HUMAN SERUM ALBUMIN. Albumin Human, U.S.P. XXII.

NORMALINE KIT. (Apothecary Products) Salt tablets for normal saline 250 mg/Tab. Preservative free. 200s with Bot. 27.7 ml.
Use: Ophthalmic preparation.

NORMETHADONE. B.A.N. 6-Dimethylamino-4,4-di-phenylhexan-3-one.
Use: Narcotic analgesic.

NORMETHANDRONE. (Parke-Davis) 17-α-methyl-19-nortestoster-one. 17β-Hydroxy-17-methylestr-4-en-3-one. Methalutin.

NORMODYNE. (Schering) Labetalol HCl. **Inj.:** 5 mg/ml. Amp. 20 ml, 40 ml, 60 ml. **Tab.:** 100 mg, 200 mg or 300 mg. Bot. 100s, 500s, UD 100s. Calendar pak 56s.
Use: Antihypertensive.

NORMOL. (Alcon Lenscare) Sterile, isotonic solution of thimerosal 0.004%, chlorhexidine gluconate 0.005%, edetate disodium 0.1%. Bot. 8 oz.
Use: Soft contact lens care.

NORMORPHINE. B.A.N. N-Demethylmorphine.
Use: Narcotic analgesic.

NORMOSOL-M in D5-W. (Abbott Hospital Prods) Dextrose 5 Gm, sodium Cl 234 mg, potassium acetate 128 mg, magnesium acetate 21 mg, sodium bisulfite 30 mg/100 ml. Bot. 500 ml, 1000 ml in Abbo-Vac (glass) or Life Care (flexible) containers.
Use: Parenteral nutritional supplement.

NORMOSOL-R; NORMOSOL-R pH 7.4; 500 ml., 1000 ml. NORMOSOL-R D5-W. (Abbott Hospital Prods) Sodium Cl 526 mg, sodium acetate 222 mg, sodium gluconate 502 mg, potassium Cl 37 mg, magnesium Cl 14 mg pH of Normosol-R and Normosol R in D5-W adjusted with HCl/100 ml. Bot. 1,000 ml, 500 ml. in Life Care (flexible) containers.
Use: Parenteral nutritional supplement.

NORMOTENSIN. (Marcen) I.M. soln. for inj. Mucopolysaccharide 20 mg, sodium nucleate 25 mg, epinephrine-neutralizing factor 25 units, sodium citrate 10 mg, inositol 5 mg, phenol 0.5%/ml. Multi-dose vial 10 ml, 30 ml.
Use: Antihypertensive.

NORMOZIDE. (Schering) Labetalol HCl 100 mg, 200 mg or 300 mg, hydrochlorothiazide 25 mg/Tab. Bot. 100s.
Use: Antihypertensive.

NOROLON. (Winthrop Products) Chloroquine phosphate.
Use: Antimalarial.

NOROXIN. (Merck Sharp & Dohme) Norfloxacin 400 mg/Tab. Bot. 100s, UD 20s, UD 100s.
Use: Urinary anti-infective.

NORPACE. (Searle) Disopyramide phosphate 100 mg or 150 mg/Cap. Bot. 100s, 500s, 1000s, UD 100s.
Use: Antiarrhythmic.

NORPACE CR. (Searle) Disopyramide phosphate 100 mg or 150 mg/CR Cap. Bot. 100s, 500s, UD 100s.
Use: Antiarrhythmic.

NORPHYL. (Vita Elixir) Aminophylline 100 mg/Tab.
Use: Bronchodilator.

NORPIPANONE. B.A.N. 4,4-Diphenyl-6-piperidinohexan-3-one.
Use: Analgesic.

NORPLANT. (Wyeth-Ayerst) Levonorgestrel implants.
Use: Progestin.

NORPRAMIN. (Merrell Dow) Desipramine HCl 10 mg, 25 mg, 50 mg, 75 mg, 100 mg or 150 mg/Tab. **10 mg:** Bot. 100s; **25 mg:** Bot. 100s, 1000s, UD 100s; **50 mg:** Bot. 100s, 1000s, UD 100s; **75 mg:** Bot. 100s; **100 mg:** Bot. 100s. **150 mg:** Bot. 50s.
Use: Antidepressant.

NOR-Q.D. (Syntex) Norethindrone 0.35 mg/Tab. Dispenser 42s.
Use: Oral contraceptive.

NORTESTERIONATE. 19-Nortestosterone cyclopentylpropionate.

•**NORTRIPTYLINE HCl,** U.S.P. XXII. Oral Soln., Cap. U.S.P. XXII. 5-(3-Methyl-aminopropylidene)-10,11- dihydro-5H-dibenzo [a,d] cycloheptene HCl. 10,11-Dihydro-N-methyl-5H-dibenzo(a,d)cycloheptene-Δ^5, propylamine Hydrochloride.
Use: Antidepressant.
See: Aventyl HCl, Liq., Pulvule (Lilly). Pamelor, Cap., Liq. (Sandoz).

NORVAL. Docusate sodium.
Use: Laxative.

NORWICH ASPIRIN. (Vicks) Aspirin 325 mg/Tab. Bot. 100s, 250s, 500s.
Use: Salicylate analgesic.

NO SALT. (Norcliff-Thayer) Potassium Cl, potassium bitartrate, adipic acid, mineral oil, fumaric acid. Sodium $>$10 mg/5 Gm ($>$0.43 mEq/5 Gm), potassium 2502 mg/5 Gm(64 mEq/5 Gm). Pkg. 330 Gm.
Use: Salt substitute.

NOSALT SEASONED. (Norcliff Thayer) Potassium Cl, dextrose, onion and garlic, spices, lactose, cream of tartar, paprika, silica, disodium inosinate, disodium guanylate, turmeric. Sodium $>$ 5 mg/5 Gm ($>$ 0.2 mEq/5 Gm), potassium 1328 mg/5 Gm (34 mEq/5 Gm). Pkg. 240 Gm.
Use: Salt substitute.

NOSCAPINE HCl. l-Narcotine hydrochloride.
Use: Antitussive.
See: Conar Prods. (Beecham Labs).
W/Chlorpheniramine maleate, phenylephrine HCl, N-acetyl-p-aminophenol, salicylamide, vitamin C.
See: Noscaps, Cap. (Table Rock).
W/Phenylephrine HCl.
See: Conar Liq. (Beecham Labs).
W/Phenylephrine HCl, guaifensin.
See: Conar, Expectorant (Beecham Labs).

NOSCAPS. (Table Rock) Noscapine 7.5 mg, chlorpheniramine maleate 1 mg, phenylephrine HCl 5 mg, N-acetyl-p-aminophenol 150 mg, salicylamide 150 mg, vitamin C 20 mg/Cap. Bot. 100s, 500s.
Use: Antihistamine, decongestant, analgesic, vitamin C.

•**NOSIHEPTIDE.** USAN.
Use: Growth stimulant.

NOSKOTE. (Schering-Plough) Oxybenzone 3%, homosalate 8%. SPF 8. Cream 13.2 Gm, 30 Gm.
Use: Sunscreen.

NOSKOTE SUNBLOCK. (Schering-Plough) Padimate O 8%, oxybenzone 3%, benzyl alcohol. SPF 15. Cream. Tube 30 Gm.
Use: Sunscreen.

NOSTRIL. (Boehringer I) Phenylephrine HCl 0.25% or 0.5%, benzalkonium Cl 0.004% in buffered aqueous soln. Bot. 15 ml, pump spray.
Use: Decongestant.

NOSTRILLA. (Boehringer I) Oxymetazoline HCl 0.05%, benzalkonium Cl. 0.02% Bot. 15 ml, pump spray.
Use: Decongestant.

NOVA-DEC. (Rugby) Iron 20 mg, vitamins A 10,000 IU, D 400 IU, E 30 mg, B_1 10 mg, B_2 10 mg, B_3 100 mg, B_5 20 mg, B_6 5 mg, B_{12} 6 mcg, C 250 mg, folic acid 0.4 mg, Cu, I, Mg, Mn, zinc 20 mg/Tab. Bot. 100s.
Use: Vitamin/mineral supplement.

NOVADYNE EXPECTORANT. (Various Mfr.) Pseudoephedrine 30 mg, codeine phosphate 10 mg, guaifenesin 100 mg, alcohol 7.5%. Bot. 120 ml, pt, gal.
Use: Decongestant, antitussive, expectorant.

NOVAFED A CAPSULES (Merrell Dow) Pseudoephedrine HCl 120 mg, chlorpheniramine maleate 8 mg/CR Cap. Bot. 100s.
Use: Decongestant, antihistamine.

NOVAFED CAPSULES. (Merrell Dow) Pseudoephedrine HCl 120 mg/CR Cap. Bot. 100s.
Use: Decongestant.

NOVAHISTINE DH. (Lakeside) Pseudoephedrine HCl 30 mg, codeine phosphate 10 mg, chlorpheniramine maleate 2 mg/5 ml, alcohol 5%, saccharin, sorbitol. Bot. 4 oz, pt.
Use: Decongestant, antitussive, antihistamine.

NOVAHISTINE DMX. (Lakeside) Pseudoephedrine HCl 30 mg, dextromethorphan HBr 10 mg, guaifenesin 100 mg/5 ml, alcohol 10%, saccharin, sorbitol. Bot. 4 oz.
Use: Decongestant, antitussive, expectorant.

NOVAHISTINE ELIXIR. (Lakeside) Phenylephrine HCl 5 mg, chlorpheniramine maleate 2 mg/5 ml, alcohol 5%, sorbitol. Bot. 4 oz, 8 oz.
Use: Decongestant, antihistamine.

NOVAHISTINE EXPECTORANT. (Lakeside) Pseudoephedrine HCl 30 mg, codeine phosphate 10 mg, guaifenesin 100 mg/5 ml, alcohol 7.5%, saccharin, sorbitol. Bot. 4 oz, pt.
Use: Decongestant, antitussive, expectorant.

NOVALDIN. (Winthrop Products) Dipyrone. Available as Tab., Amp., Drops.
Use: Analgesic.

NOVAMIDON.
See: Aminopyrine (Various Mfr.).

NOVAMINE. (Clintec Nutrition) Amino acid concentration 11.4%, for infusion. Nitrogen 1.8 Gm/100 ml. Essential amino acids (mg/100 ml): Isoleucine 570, leucine 790, lysine 900, methionine 570, phenylalanine 790, threonine 570, tryptophan 190, valine 730. Nonessential amino acids (mg/100 ml): Alanine 1650, arginine 1120, histidine 680, proline 680, serine 450, tyrosine 30, glycine 790, glutamic acid 570, aspartic acid 330, acetate 114 mEq/L, sodium metabisulfite 30 mg/100 ml. In 250 ml, 500 ml, 1 L.
Use: Parenteral nutritional supplement.

NOVAMINE 15%. (Clintec Nutrition) Amino acids 15%: Lysine 1.18 Gm, leucine 1.04 Gm, phenylalanine 1.04 Gm, valine 960 mg, isoleucine 749 mg, methionine 749 mg, threonine 749 mg,

tryptophan 250 mg, alanine 2.17 Gm, arginine 1.47 Gm, glycine 1.04 Gm, histidine 894 mg, proline 894 mg, glutamic acid 749 mg, serine 592 mg, aspartic acid 434 mg, tyrosine 39 mg, nitrogen 2.37 Gm/100 ml. Inj. 500 ml, 1000 ml.
Use: Parenteral nutritional supplement.

NOVAMINE WITHOUT ELECTROLYTES. (Clintec Nutrition) Amino acid concentration 8.5%, for infusion. Nitrogen 1.35 Gm/100 ml. Essential amino acids (mg/100 ml): Isoleucine 420, leucine 590, lysine 673, methionine 420, phenylalanine 590, threonine 420, tryptophan 140, valine 550. Nonessential amino acids (mg/100 ml): Alanine 1240, arginine 840, histidine 500, proline 500, serine 340, tyrosine 20, glycine 590, glutamic acid 420, aspartic acid 250, acetate 88 mEq/L, sodium bisulfite 30 mg/100 ml. In 500 ml, 1 L.
Use: Parenteral nutritional supplement.

NOVANTRONE. (Lederle) Mitoxantrone HCl 2 mg base/ml. Inj. Vial 10 ml, 12.5 ml, 15 ml.
Use: Antineoplastic agent.

NOVATOPHAN.
See: Neocinchophen (Various Mfr.).

NOVATROPINE.
See: Homatropine Methylbromide (Various Mfr.).

•**NOVOBIOCIN CALCIUM,** U.S.P. XXII. Oral Susp., U.S.P. XXII.
Use: Antibacterial.
See: Cathomycin Calcium.

NOVOBIOCIN MONOSODIUM SALT.
Use: Antibacterial.
See: Sodium Novobiocin.

•**NOVOBIOCIN SODIUM,** U.S.P. XXII. Cap., U.S.P. XXII.
Use: Antibacterial.
See: Albamycin, Cap. (Upjohn).
Cathomycin Sodium.

NOVOCAIN. (Winthrop Pharm) Procaine HCl soln. **1%:** Amp. 2 ml, Box 25s. 6 ml, Box 50s; Vial 30 ml, Box 10s. **2%:** Vial 30 ml, Box 10s.
Use: Local anesthetic.

NOVOCAIN FOR SPINAL ANESTHESIA. (Winthrop Pharm) Procaine HCl 10% soln. Amp. 2 ml. Box 25s.
Use: Spinal anesthesia.

NOVOLIN 70/30. (Squibb-Novo) Isophane susp. 70% (human), regular insulin 30% (human, semi-synthetic). 100 units/ml. Inj. Vial 10 ml.
Use: Antidiabetic agent.

NOVOLIN L. (Squibb-Novo) Human insulin (semisynthetic) 100 units/ml. An insulin-zinc suspension (Lente). Inj. Vial 10 ml.
Use: Anti-diabetic agent.

NOVOLIN N. (Squibb-Novo) Human insulin NPH (semisynthetic) 100 units/ml. Isophane insulin suspension (insulin w/protamine and zinc). Inj. Vial 10 ml.
Use: Antidiabetic agent.

NOVOLIN R. (Squibb-Novo) Human insulin, regular (semisynthetic) 100 units/ml. Inj. Vial 10 ml.
Use: Antidiabetic agent.

NOVOLIN R PENFILL. (Squibb-Novo) Semisynthetic human regular insulin. 100 units/ml. Inj. 1.5 ml cartridges.
Use: Antidiabetic agent.

NOXIPTYLINE, B.A.N. 3-(2-Dimethylaminoethyloxy-imino)dibenzo[a,d]cyclohepta-1,4-diene.
Use: Antidepressant.

NOXYTHIOLIN. B.A.N. N-Hydroxymethyl-N′-methylthiourea. Noxyflex.
Use: Antifungal agent.

NOXZEMA ANTISEPTIC CLEANSER SENSITIVE SKIN FORMULA. (Noxell) Benzalkonium Cl 0.13%. Bot. 4 oz, 8 oz.
Use: Skin cleanser.

NOXZEMA ANTISEPTIC SKIN CLEANSER. (Noxell) SD-40 alcohol 63%. Bot. 4 oz, 8 oz.
Use: Skin cleanser.

NOXZEMA ANTISEPTIC SKIN CLEANSER EXTRA STRENGTH FORMULA. (Noxell) SD-40 alcohol 36%, isopropyl alcohol 34%. Bot. 4 oz, 8 oz.
Use: Skin cleanser.

NOXZEMA CLEAR-UPS. (Noxell) Salicylic acid 0.5% on pads. Jar 50s.
Use: Anti-acne.

NOXZEMA CLEAR UPS ACNE MEDICINE MAXIMUM STRENGTH LOTION. (Noxell) Benzoyl peroxide 10%. Bot. 1 oz. Vanishing formula.
Use: Anti-acne.

NOXZEMA CLEAR UPS MAXIMUM STRENGTH (Noxell) Salicylic acid 2% on pads. Jar 50s.
Use: Anti-acne.

NOXZEMA MEDICATED SKIN CREAM. (Noxell) Menthol, camphor, clove oil, eucalyptus oil, phenol. Jar 2.5 oz, 4 oz, 6 oz, 10 oz. Tube 4.5 oz. Bot. 6 oz., 14 oz. Pump Bottle 10.5 oz.
Use: Counterirritant.

NOXZEMA ON-THE-SPOT. (Noxell) Benzoyl peroxide 10% in vanishing and tinted lotion. Bot. 0.25 oz.
Use: Anti-acne.

NP-27 AEROSOL. (Thompson Medical) Tolnaftate 1%, alcohol 14.9%. Spray Can 100 ml.
Use: Antifungal, external.

NP-27 CREAM. (Thompson Medical) Tolnaftate 1% in cream base. Tube 45 Gm.
Use: Antifungal, external.

NP-27 LIQUID. (Thompson Medical) Tolnaftate 1%. Plastic bot. 2 oz.
Use: Antifungal, external.

NPH ILETIN I. (Lilly) Insulin from beef and pork, 40 units or 100 units/ml. Inj. Vial 10 ml.
Use: Antidiabetic agent.

NPH PURIFIED PORK. (Squibb-Novo) Purified pork insulin 100 units/ml in isophane insulin suspension (insulin w/protamine and zinc). Inj. Vial 10 ml.
Use: Antidiabetic agent.

NTS TRANSDERMAL SYSTEM. (Bolar) Nitroglycerin transdermal system 5 mg/24 hours or 15 mg/24 hours. Box 30s.
Use: Antianginal agent.

NTZ LONG-ACTING. (Winthrop Pharm.) Oxymetazoline HCl 0.05% benzalkonium Cl and phenylmercuric acetate 0.002% as preservatives. Drops Bot. 1 oz. Spray Bot. 1 oz.
Use: Decongestant.

NUBAIN. (Du Pont) Nalbuphine HCl, sodium metabisulfite 0.1%. **10 mg/ml:** Amp 1 ml. Vial 10 ml. Box 1s. **20 mg/ml:** Amp 1 ml. Syringe 1 ml calibrated. Vial 10 ml.
Use: Narcotic analgesic.

NU-BOLIC. (Seatrace) Nandrolone phenpropionate 25 mg/ml. Vial 5 ml.
Use: Anabolic steroid.

NUCITE.
See: Inositol (Various Mfr.).

NUCLEIC ACID ANTAGONISTS.
Use: Antineoplastic agent.
See: Leukeran, Tab. (Burroughs Wellcome).
Mustargen, Vial (Merck Sharp & Dohme).
Myleran, Tab. (Burroughs Wellcome).
Purinethol, Tab. (Burroughs Wellcome).
Triethylene Melamine, Tab. (Lederle).

NUCOFED. (Beecham Labs) Codeine phosphate 20 mg, pseudoephedrine HCl 60 mg/5 ml or Cap. Syrup is alcohol-free. **Liq.:** Bot. pt. **Cap.:** Bot. 60s.
Use: Antitussive, decongestant.

NUCOFED EXPECTORANT. (Beecham Labs) Codeine phosphate 20 mg, pseudoephedrine HCl 60 mg, guaifenesin 200 mg/5 ml, alcohol 12.5%, saccharin. Bot. pt.
Use: Antitussive, decongestant, expectorant.

NUCOFED PEDIATRIC EXPECTORANT. (Beecham Labs) Codeine phosphate 10 mg, pseudoephedrine HCl 30 mg, guaifenesin 100 mg/5 ml, alcohol 6%. Bot. pt.
Use: Antitussive, decongestant, expectorant.

•**NUFENOXOLE.** USAN.
Use: Antiperistaltic.

NU-IRON. (Mayrand) Polysaccharide-iron complex. **Cap.:** Elemental iron 150 mg. Bot. 100s. **Elix.:** Elemental iron 100 mg/5 ml. Bot. 8 oz.
Use: Iron supplement.

NU-IRON PLUS ELIXIR. (Mayrand) Polysaccharide iron complex 100 mg, folic acid 1 mg, vitamin B_{12} 25 mcg/5 ml, alcohol 10%. Bot. 8 oz.
Use: Vitamin/mineral supplement.

NU-IRON-V. (Mayrand) Polysaccharide iron 60 mg, folic acid 1 mg, ascorbic acid 50 mg, vitamins B_{12} 3 mcg, A 4000 IU, D 400 IU, B_1 3 mg, B_2 3 mg, niacinamide 10 mg, B_6 2 mg/Tab, calcium carbonate. Bot. 100s.
Use: Vitamin/mineral supplement.

NULLAPONS. (General Aniline & Film) The whole group of chelating agents related to ethylenediaminetetraacetic acid. Pkg. according to demand.
Use: Sequestering agent.

NULLO. (Chattem Consumer) Water-soluble chlorophyllin copper complex 33.3 mg/Tab. Bot. 30s, 60s, 135s.
Use: Systemic deodorizer.

NUL-TACH. (Davis & Sly) Potassium 16 mg, magnesium 13 mg, ascorbic acid 250 mg/Tab. Bot. 100s.
Use: Paroxysmal tachycardia.

NUMORPHAN. (Du Pont) Oxymorphone HCl. **1 mg/ml.:** Amp. 1 ml. Box 10s. **1.5 mg/ml.:** Amp. 1 ml, Box 10s. Vial 10 ml, Box 1s. **Rectal Supp.:** 5 mg. Box 6s.
Use: Narcotic analgesic.

NUMOTIZINE CATAPLASM. (Hobart) Guaiacol 0.26 Gm, beechwood creosote 1.302 Gm, methyl salicylate 0.26 Gm/100 Gm. Jar 4 oz.
Use: External analgesic.

NUMOTIZINE COUGH SYRUP. (Hobart) Guaifenesin 5 gr, ammonium Cl 5 gr, sodium citrate 20 gr, menthol 0.04 gr/fl oz. Bot. 3 oz, pt, gal.
Use: Expectorant.

NUMZIDENT. (Purepac) Benzocaine, clove oil, peppermint oil. Gel 0.5 oz.
Use: Topical anesthetic for mouth.

NUM-ZIT. (Purepac) Benzocaine, menthol, glycerin, methylparaben, alcohol 12%. Liq. Bot. 22.5 ml.
Use: Topical anesthetic for mouth.

NUM-ZIT GEL. (Purepac) Benzocaine, menthol. Tube 10 Gm.
Use: Topical anesthetic for mouth.

NUNOL.
See: Phenobarbital (Various Mfr.).

NUPERCAINAL. (Ciba) **Cream:** Dibucaine 0.5%, acetone, sodium bisulfite 37%. Tube 1.5 oz. **Oint.:** Dibucaine 1%, sodium bisulfite 0.5%. Tube 1 oz, 2 oz.
Use: Topical anesthetic.

NUPERCAINAL. (Ciba Consumer) Cocoa butter 2.4 Gm, zinc oxide 0.25 Gm, bismuth subgallate 0.25 Gm, sodium bisulfite 0.25 Gm/Supp. Box 12s, 24s.
Use: Anorectal preparation.

NUPRIN CAPLETS. (Bristol-Myers) Ibuprofen 200 mg/Capl. Bot. 100s.
Use: Nonsteroidal anti-inflammatory drug; analgesic.

NUPRIN TABLETS. (Bristol-Myers) Ibuprofen 200 mg/Tab. Blister Pak 8s. Bot. 24s, 50s, 200s.
Use: Nonsteroidal anti-inflammatory drug; analgesic.

NUROMAX. (Burroughs Wellcome) Doxacurium chloride.
Use: Neuromuscular blocking agent.

NURSOY. (Wyeth-Ayerst) Vitamins A 2500 IU, D-3 400 IU, C 55 mg, B_1 0.67 mg, B_2 1 mg, E 9 IU, niacin 9.5 mEq, B_6 0.4 mg, B_{12} 2 mcg, pantothenic acid 3 mg, K-1 0.1 mg, folic acid 50

mcg, choline 85 mg, inositol 26 mg, I, biotin, Ca, P, Na, K, Mg, Mn, Cl, Cu, Zn/qt of formula. Concentrated liq. Can 13 oz. Ready to feed Can 32 oz. Ready to feed Hospital Bot. 4 oz. Pow. Can 1 lb.
Use: Enteral nutritional supplement.

NU-SALT. (Cumberland Pkg.) Potassium Cl, potassium bitartrate, calcium silicate, natural flavor derived from yeast. Sodium 0.85 mg/5 Gm (> 0.04 mEq/5 Gm), potassium 2640 mg/5 Gm (68 mEq/5 Gm). Pkg. 90 Gm.
Use: Salt substitute.

NU-THERA. (Kirkman) Vitamins A 10,000 IU, D 400 IU, B_1 10 mg, B_2 5 mg, niacinamide 100 mg, B_6 1 mg, B_{12} 5 mcg, C 150 mg, calcium 103 mg, phosphorus 80 mg, iron 10 mg, magnesium 5.5 mg, manganese 1 mg, potassium 5 mg, zinc 1.4 mg/Cap. Bot. 100s.
Use: Vitamin/mineral supplement.

•**NUTMEG OIL,** N.F. XVII.
Use: Pharmaceutic aid (flavor).

NUTRACORT. (Owen/Galderma) Hydrocortisone 1%. **Cream:** Jar 4 oz. Tube 30 Gm, 60 Gm. **Lot.:** Bot. 2 oz, 4 oz.
Use: Corticosteroid, topical.

NUTRADERM. (Owen/Galderma) Oil-in-water emulsion. **Lot.:** Plastic bot. 8 oz, 16 oz. **Cream:** Tube 1.5 oz, 3 oz, Jar lb.
Use: Emollient.

NUTRADERM BATH OIL. (Owen/Galderma) Mineral oil, PEG-4 dilaurate, lanolin oil, butylparaben, benzophenone-3, fragrance, D & C Green No. 6. Bot. 8 oz.
Use: Emollient.

NUTRAJEL. (Cenci) Aluminum hydroxide 5 gr/5 ml. Bot. 12 oz.
Use: Antacid.

NUTRAMAG. (Cenci) Colloidalized gel of aluminum and magnesium hydroxide. Bot. 12 oz.
Use: Antacid.

NUTRAMENT DRINK BOX. (Drackett) Protein 10 Gm, fat 7 Gm, carbohydrate 35 Gm, vitamins, minerals/240 calories/8 oz. Drink Box.
Use: Enteral nutritional supplement.

NUTRAMENT LIQUID. (Drackett) Protein 16 Gm, fat 10 Gm, carbohydrates 52 Gm, vitamins, minerals/360 calories/12 oz. Can.
Use: Enteral nutritional supplement.

NUTRAMIGEN. (Mead Johnson Nutrition) Hypoallergenic formula that supplies 640 calories/qt. Protein 18 Gm, fat 25 Gm, carbohydrates 86 Gm, vitamins A 2000 IU, D 400 IU, E 20 IU, C 52 mg, folic acid 100 mcg, B_1 0.5 mg, B_2 0.6 mg, niacin 8 mg, B_6 0.4 mg, B_{12} 2 mcg, biotin 50 mcg, pantothenic acid 3 mg, K-1 100 mcg, choline 85 mg, inositol 30 mg, calcium 600 mg, phosphorus 400 mg, iodine 45 mcg, iron 12 mg, magnesium 70 mg, copper 0.6 mg, zinc 5 mg, manganese 200 mcg, chloride 550 mg, potassium 700 mg, sodium 300 mg/qt of formula (4.9 oz pow.). Can 16 oz.
Use: Enteral nutritional supplement.

NUTRAMIN. (Thurston) Vitamins A 666 IU, D 66 IU, B_1 666 mcg, B_2 333 mcg, niacinamide 2 mg, folic acid 0.0444 mcg, calcium 16.6 mg, phosphorus 8.33 mg, iron 1.33 mg, iodine 0.15 mg/Tab. Bot. 200s, 500s, 1000s.
Use: Vitamin/mineral supplement.

NUTRAMIN GRANULAR. (Thurston) Vitamins A 333 IU, D 333 IU, B_1 3.3 mg, B_2 1.6 mg, niacinamide 10 mg, folic acid 0.133 mg, calcium 250 mg, phosphorus 115 mg, iron 6.6 mg, iodine 0.15 mg/5 Gm. Bot. 10 oz, 32 oz.
Use: Vitamin/mineral supplement.

NUTRAPLUS. (Owen) Urea 10% in emollient cream base or lotion base with preservatives. **Cream:** Tube 3 oz, Jar lb. **Lot.:** Bot. 8 oz, 16 oz.
Use: Emollient.

NUTRAVIMS. (Approved) Vitamins A 6000 IU, D 1250 IU, C 50 mg, E 5 IU, B_{12} 5 mcg, B_1 3 mg, B_2 3 mg, B_6 0.5 mg, niacinamide 20 mg, calcium pantothenate 5 mg, zinc 1.5 mg, manganese 1 mg, iodine 0.15 mg, potassium 5 mg, magnesium 4 mg, iron 15 mg, calcium 59 mg, phosphorus 45 mg/Cap. Bot. 100s, 250s, 1000s.
Use: Vitamin/mineral supplement.

NUTREN 1.0 LIQUID. (Clintec Nutrition) Potassium and sodium caseinate, maltodextrin, sucrose, MCT, corn oil, lecithin, vitamins A, B_1, B_2, B_3, B_5, B_6, B_{12}, C, D, E, K, folic acid, biotin, choline, Ca, Cl, Cu, Fe, I, Mg, Mn, P, Zn. 250 ml.
Use: Enteral nutritional supplement.

NUTREN 1.5 LIQUID. (Clintec Nutrition) Casein, maltodextrin, corn syrup, sucrose, MCT, corn oil, vitamins A, B_1, B_2, B_3, B_5, B_6, B_{12}, C, D, E, K, folic acid, biotin, choline, Ca, Cl, Cu, Fe, I, Mg, Mn, P, Zn. 250 ml.
Use: Enteral nutritional supplement.

NUTREN 2.0 LIQUID. (Clintec Nutrition) Casein, maltodextrin, corn syrup, sucrose, MCT, corn oil, vitamins A, B_1, B_2, B_3, B_5, B_6, B_{12}, C, D, E, K, folic acid, biotin, choline, Ca, Cl, Cu, Fe, I, Mg, Mn, P, Zn. 250 ml.
Use: Enteral nutritional supplement.

NUTREX. (Holloway) Calcium 162 mg, iron 27 mg, vitamins A 5000 IU, D 400 IU, E 30 mg, B_1 2.25 mg, B_2 2.6 mg, B_3 20 mg, B_5 10 mg, B_6 3 mg, B_{12} 9 mcg, C 90 mg, folic acid 0.4 mg, Cu, I, K, Mg, Mn, P, zinc 22.5 mg, biotin 45 mcg/Tab. Bot. 100s.
Use: Vitamin/mineral supplement.

NUTRICOL. (Nutrition Control) Safflower oil 1530 mg, choline bitartrate 500 mg, soybean lecithin 600 mg, inositol 100 mg, natural tocopherols 20 mg, B_6 10 mg, B_{12} 5 mcg, panthenol 5 mg/Cap. Bot. 90s.
Use: Vitamin/mineral supplement.

NUTRICON TABLETS. (Pasadena) Calcium 200 mg, iron 20 mg, vitamins A 2500 IU, D 200 IU,

E 11 mg, B_1 1.5 mg, B_2 1.5 mg, B_3 10 mg, B_5 5 mg, B_6 2 mg, B_{12} 5 mcg, C 50 mg, folic acid 0.4 mg, Cu, I, Mg, zinc 3.75 mg, biotin/Tab. Bot. 120s.
Use: Vitamin/mineral supplement.

NUTRI-E. (Nutri Lab.) Vitamin E. **Cream:** 200 IU/Gm. Jar 1 oz, 2 oz. **Oil:** 1 oz. **Oint.:** 200 IU/Gm. Tube 1 oz, 1.5 oz. **Cap.:** 200 IU. Bot. 80s; 400 IU. Bot. 60s, 100s; 800 IU. Bot. 55s.
Use: Vitamin E supplement.

NUTRIGANIC. (Commerce) Multi-vitamin with minerals and amino acids. Tab. Bot. 50s.
Use: Vitamin/mineral supplement.

NUTRILIPID. (Kendall McGaw) Soybean oil intravenous fat emulsion. **10%:** Calories 1.1/ml. In 250 ml, 500 ml. **20%:** Calories 2/ml. In 250 ml, 500 ml.
Use: Parenteral nutritional supplement.

NUTRI-PLEX TABLETS. (Faraday) Vitamins B_1 5 mg, B_2 5 mg, B_6 5 mg, pantothenic acid 25 mg, B_{12} 12.5 mcg, niacinamide 50 mg, iron gluconate 30 mg, choline bitartrate 50 mg, inositol 50 mg, PABA 15 mg, C 150 mg/2 Tab. Bot. 100s, 250s.
Use: Vitamin/mineral supplement.

NUTRISOURCE MODULAR SYSTEM. (Sandoz Nutrition) Individual Nutrisource modules available: protein, amino acids, amino acids-high branched chain, carbohydrate, lipid-medium chain triglycerides, lipid-long branched chain triglycerides, vitamins, minerals. Cans of liquid. Packets of powder.
Use: Enteral nutritional supplement.

NUTRI-VAL. (Marcen) Vitamins A 5000 IU, D 500 IU, B_1 10 mg, B_2 5 mg, B_{12} activity 5 mcg, B_6 5 mcg, C 50 mg, hesperidin 5 mg, niacinamide 15 mg, folic acid 0.2 mg, calcium pantothenate 50 mg, choline bitartrate 50 mg, betaine HCl 25 mg, lipo-K 0.4 mg, duodenum substance 50 mg, pancreas substance 50 mg, inositol 25 mg, Cy-yeast hydrolysates 50 mg, rutin 5 mg, 1-lysine HCl 5 mg, E 5 IU, Ossonate (glucuronic complex) 8 mg, glutamic acid 30 mg, lecithin 5 mg, iron 20 mg, iodine 0.15 mg, calcium 50 mg, phosphorus 40 mg, boron 0.1 mg, copper 1 mg, manganese 1 mg, magnesium 1 mg, potassium 5 mg, zinc 0.5 mg, biotin 0.02 mg/Cap. Bot. 100s, 500s, 1000s.
Use: Vitamin/mineral supplement.

NUTRI-VITE NATURAL MULTIPLE VITAMIN AND MINERALS. (Faraday) Vitamins A 15,000 IU, D 400 IU, B_1 1.5 mg, B_2 3 mg, B_{12} 15 mcg, niacin 500 mcg, B_6 20 mcg, choline 1.75 mg, folic acid 13 mcg, pantothenic acid 50 mcg, p-aminobenzoic acid 12 mcg, inositol 1.72 mg, C 60 mg, citrus bioflavonoids 15 mg, E 50 IU, iron gluconate 15 mg, calcium 192 mg, phosphorus 85 mg, iodine 0.15 mg, red bone marrow 30 mg/3 Tab. Protein coated Tab. Bot. 100s, 250s.
Use: Vitamin/mineral supplement.

NUTRIZYME. (Enzyme Process) Vitamins A 5000 IU, D 400 IU, C 60 mg, B_1 1.5 mg, B_2 1.7 mg, niacinamide 20 mg, B_6 2 mg, pantothenate 10 mg, B_{12} 6 mcg, E 30 IU, iron 10 mg, copper 1 mg, zinc 1 mg, Folacin 0.025 mg/Tab. Bot. 90s, 250s.
Use: Vitamin/mineral supplement.

NUTROFEM-II. (Life's Finest) Calcium 250 mg, iron 9 mg, vitamins A 2500 IU, D 200 IU, E 10 mg, B_1 0.75 mg, B_2 0.85 mg, B_3 10 mg, B_5 5 mg, B_6 1 mg, B_{12} 3 mcg, C 30 mg, folic acid 0.2 mg, Cu, Mg, zinc 7.5 mg, biotin/Tab. Bot. 60s, 90s, 180s.
Use: Vitamin/mineral supplement.

NUX VOMICA EXTRACT. W/Iron oxide, cinchona, vitamin B_1, alcohol.
See: Briatonic, Liq. (Briar).
W/Methyl testosterone, yohimbine HCl.
See: Climactic, Tab. (Burgin-Arden).

NUZINE OINTMENT. (Hobart) Guaiacol 1.66 Gm, oxyquinoline sulfate 0.42 Gm, zinc oxide 2.5 Gm, glycerine 1.66 Gm, lanum (anhydrous) 43.76 Gm, petrolatum 50 Gm/100 Gm. Tube 1 oz.
Use: Anorectal preparation.

NYCOFF. (Dover) Dextromethorphan HBr/Tab. UD Box 500s. Sugar, lactose and salt free.
Use: Antitussive.

NYCO-WHITE. (Whiteworth) Nystatin, neomycin, gramcidin, triamcinolone. Cream. Tube 15 Gm, 30 Gm, 60 Gm.
Use: Anti-infective, external.

NYCO-WORTH. (Whiteworth) Nystatin. Cream Tube 15 Gm.
Use: Anti-infective, external.

NYCRALAN. (Lannett) Vitamin B_1 10 mg, calcium lactate 10 gr/Tab. Bot. 100s.
Use: Vitamin/mineral supplement.

NYDRAZID INJECTION. (Squibb) Isoniazid 100 mg/ml, chlorobutanol 0.25%, sodium hydroxide or hydrochloric acid to adjust pH. Vial 10 ml.
Use: Antituberculous agent.

•**NYLESTRIOL.** USAN. 3-Cyclopentyloxy-19-nor-17 α-pregna-1,3,5(10)-trien-20-yne-16, 17β-diol.
Use: Estrogen.

NYLIDRIN HYDROCHLORIDE, U.S.P. XXII. Inj., Tab., U.S.P. XXII. p-Hydroxy-a-[1-[(1-methyl-3-phenyl-propyl)-amino]ethyl]benzyl alcohol HCl.
Use: Peripheral vasodilator.
See: Arlidin, Tab. (Rorer).
Rolidrin-6, Tab. (Robinson).
Rolidrin-12, Tab. (Robinson).

NYQUIL NIGHT TIME COLDS MEDICINE LIQUID. (Vicks Health Care) Dextromethorphan HBr 30 mg, pseudoephedrine HCl 60 mg, doxylamine succinate 7.5 mg, acetaminophen 1000 mg/oz, alcohol 25%. Regular and cherry flavors. Regular flavor contains FDC Yellow #5 tartrazine. Bot. 6 oz, 10 oz, 14 oz.
Use: Antitussive, decongestant, antihistamine, analgesic.

NYRAL. (Vale) Cetylpyridinium Cl 0.5 mg, benzocaine 5 mg/Loz. w/parabens. Pkg. 100s, 1000s.
Use: Antiseptic.

NYSACETOL. (Kenyon) N-Acetyl-p-aminophenol 5 gr/Tab. Bot. 100s, 1000s.
Use: Analgesic.

•**NYSTATIN,** U.S.P. XXII. Cream, For Oral Susp., Lot., Oint., Topical Pow., Oral Susp., Tab., Vaginal Supp., Vaginal Tab., U.S.P. XXII. An antifungal antibiotic derived from cultures of *Streptomyces noursei.*
Use: Antifungal.
See: Mycostatin Preps. (Squibb).
Nilstat, Tab., Cream, Oint. (Lederle).
Nilstat Oral Drops (Lederle).
Nilstat Vaginal Tab. (Lederle).
Nystex, Cream, Oint. (Savage).
O-V Statin, Tab. (Squibb Mark).
W/Clioquinol.
See: Nystaform, Oint. (Miles Pharm).
W/Demethylchlortetracycline.
See: Declostatin, Tab., Cap. (Lederle).
W/Gramicidin, neomycin, triamcinolone.
See: Mycolog, Cream, Oint. (Squibb).
W/Neomycin base, gramicidin, triamcinolone acetonide.
See: Mycolog, Cream, Oint. (Squibb).
W/Tetracycline phosphate buffered.
See: Achrostatin-V, Cap. (Lederle).
W/Tetracycline phosphate complex.
See: Tetrex-F, Cap. (Bristol).

•**NYSTATIN AND CLOROQUINOL OINTMENT,** U.S.P. XXII.
Use: Antifungal.
See: Nystaform, Oint. (Miles Pharm).

•**NYSTATIN AND TRIAMCINOLONE ACETONIDE CREAM,** U.S.P. XXII.
Use: Antifungal, anti-inflammatory.

•**NYSTATIN AND TRIAMCINOLONE ACETONIDE OINTMENT,** U.S.P. XXII.
Use: Antifungal, anti-inflammatory.

•**NYSTATIN, NEOMYCIN SULFATE, GRAMICIDIN AND TRIAMCINOLONE ACETONIDE,** U.S.P. XXII. Cream, Oint., U.S.P. XXII.
Use: Antifungal, antibacterial, anti-inflammatory.
See: Mycolog, Prods. (Squibb).

NYSTEX CREAM & OINTMENT. (Savage) Nystatin 100,000 units/Gm. Tube 15 Gm, 30 Gm.
Use: Anti-infective, external.

NYSTEX ORAL SUSPENSION. (Savage) Nystatin 100,000 units/ml in suspension w/alcohol >1%, sucrose 50%. Bot. 60 ml.
Use: Anti-infective.

NYTIME COLD MEDICINE. (Rugby) Acetaminophen 1000 mg, doxylamine succinate 7.5 mg, pseudoephedrine HCl 60 mg, dextromethorphan HBr 30 mg/30 ml, alcohol 25%. Bot. 6 oz, 10 oz.
Use: Analgesic, antihistamine, decongestant, antitussive.

NYTOL. (Block) Diphenhydramine HCl 25 mg/Tab. Bot. 16s, 32s, 72s.
Use: Sleep aid.

O

O.A.D. (Sween) Ostomy deodorant. Bot. 1.25 oz, 4 oz, 8 oz.
Use: Ostomy appliance deodorant.

OASIS. (Zitar) Artificial saliva. Bot. 6 oz.
Use: To relieve xerostomia.

OATMEAL, GUM FRACTION.
See: Aveeno, Preps. (Cooper).

OBACIN. (Kenyon) Phendimetrazine tartrate 35 mg/Tab. Bot. 100s, 1000s.
Use: Anorexiant.

OBALAN. (Lannett) Phendimetrazine tartrate 35 mg/Tab. Bot. 100s, 1000s.
Use: Anorexiant.

OBE-NIX. (Holloway) Phentermine HCl 30 mg/Cap. (equivalent to 24 mg base) Bot. 100s.
Use: Anorexiant.

OBEPAR. (Tyler) Vitamins A 3000 IU, D 300 IU, B_1 3 mg, B_2 2 mg, nicotinamide 10 mg, B_6 3 mg, calcium pantothenate 2 mg, B_{12} 3 mcg, C 37.5 mg, calcium 150 mg, iron 5 mg, magnesium 1 mg, manganese 0.1 mg, potassium 1 mg, zinc 0.15 mg/Cap. Bot. 100s.
Use: Vitamin/mineral supplement.

OBEPHEN. (Mallard) Phentermine HCl 30 mg (equivalent to 24 mg base) Cap. Bot. 1000s.
Use: Anorexiant.

OBERMINE. (Forest) Phentermine HCl 30 mg/Cap. Bot. 1000s.
Use: Anorexiant.

OBESITY AGENTS.
See: Anti-Obesity Agents (Various Mfr.).

OBESTIN-30. (Ferndale) Phentermine HCl 30 mg/Cap. Bot. 100s, 1000s.
Use: Anorexiant.

OBE-TITE. (Scott/Cord) Phendimetrazine tartrate 35 mg/Tab. Bot. 100s, 500s.
Use: Anorexiant.

OBETROL. (Obetrol) Dextroamphetamine saccharate, amphetamine aspartate, amphetamine sulfate, dextroamphetamine sulfate in equal parts. 10 mg or 20 mg tab. Bot. 100s, 500s, 1000s.*Use:* Diet aid.

OBETROL-10 TABS. (Obetrol) Dextroamphetamine saccharate 2.5 mg, amphetamine asparate 2.5 mg, amphetamine sulfate 2.5 mg, dextroamphetamine sulfate 2.5 mg/Tab. Bot. 100s, 500s, 1000s.
Use: Diet aid.

OBETROL-20 TABS. (Obetrol) Methamphetamine saccharate 5 mg, amphetamine asparate 5 mg, amphetamine sulfate 5 mg, dextroamphetamine sulfate 5 mg/Tab. Bot. 100s, 500s, 1000s.
Use: Diet aid.

OBEZINE. (Western Research) Phendimetrazine tartrate 35 mg/Tab. Handicount 28 (36 bags of 28s).

Use: Anorexiant.

•**OBIDOXIME CHLORIDE.** USAN. 1,1′-(Oxydimethylene)-bis-[4-formylpyridinium]dichloride dioxime.
Use: Cholinesterase reactivator.

OB-NATAL. (Geneva) Prenatal vitamins and minerals/TR Tab. Bot. 100s.
Use: Vitamin/mineral supplement.

OB-NATAL PLUS. (Geneva) Prenatal vitamins and minerals. Tab. Bot. 100s.
Use: Vitamin/mineral supplement.

OBRICAL. (Canright) Calcium lactate 500 mg, vitamins D 400 IU, ferrous sulfate exsiccated 35 mg, B_1 1 mg, B_2 1 mg, C 10 mg/Tab. Bot. 100s, 1000s.
Use: Vitamin/mineral supplement.

OBRICAL-F. (Canright) Ferrous sulfate 50 mg, calcium lactate 500 mg, vitamins D 400 IU, B_1 1 mg, B_2 1 mg, C 10 mg, folic acid 0.67 mg/Tab. Bot. 100s, 1000s.
Use: Vitamin/mineral supplement.

OBRITE. (Milton Roy) Contact lens and eye glass cleaner. Plastic spray Bot. 30 ml, 55 ml.
Use: Contact lens and eye glass care.

OB-TINIC. (Hauck) Iron 65 mg, vitamins A 6000 IU, D 400 IU, E 30 IU, B_1 1.1 mg, B_2 1.8 mg, B_3 15 mg, B_6 2.5 mg, B_{12} 5 mcg, C 60 mg, folic acid 1 mg, Ca/Tab. Bot. 100s.
Use: Vitamin/mineral supplement.

OBTUNDIA CALAMINE CREAM. (Otis Clapp) Zinc oxide, calamine, camphorated meta-cresoln. Tube 2 oz. Aid pak 0.11 oz, Foil pak 36s. Unit box 0.11 oz, foil pak 6s.
Use: Antipruritic, skin protectant.

OBTUNDIA FIRST AID SPRAY. (Otis Clapp) Camphorated meta-cresoln. Aerosol can 2.5 oz.
Use: Antiseptic.

OBTUNDIA SURGICAL DRESSING. (Otis Clapp) Camphorated meta-cresoln. Bot. 0.5 oz, 4 oz. Swab pad Box 10s, Aid pak 100s.
Use: Antiseptic.

OBY-TRIM. (Rexar) Phentermine HCl 30 mg/Cap. Bot. 1000s.
Use: Anorexiant.

O-CAL F.A. (Pharmics) Iron 66 mg, calcium 200 mg, vitamins A 5000 IU, C 90 mg, D 400 IU, B_6 4 mg, B_1 3 mg, B_2 3 mg, niacinamide 20 mg, B_{12} 12 mcg, folic acid 1 mg, sodium fluoride 1.1 mg, iodine 0.15 mg, magnesium 100 mg, copper 2 mg, zinc 15 mg/Tab. Bot. 100s.
Use: Vitamin/mineral supplement.

OCCLUSAL. (GenDerm) Salicylic acid 17% in polyacrylic vehicle. Bot. 0.5 oz.
Use: Keratolytic.

OCCUCOAT. (Storz) Hydroxypropyl methylcellulose 2%. Soln. Syringe 1 ml with cannula.
Use: Ophthalmic preparation.

OCEAN. (Fleming) Sodium Cl 0.65%, benzyl alcohol. Bot. 45 ml, pt.
Use: Nasal membrane moisturizer.

OCEAN PLUS. (Fleming) Caffeine 2.5%, benzyl alcohol. Bot. 15 ml.

OCL SOLUTION. (Abbott Hospital Prods) Oral colonic lavage soln. Sodium Cl 146 mg, sodium bicarbonate 168 mg, sodium sulfate decahydrate 1.29 Gm, potassium Cl 75 mg, PEG-3350 6 Gm, polysorbate-80 30 ml/100 ml. 1.35 L 3-pack units.
Use: Laxative.

•**OCRYLATE.** USAN. Octyl 2-cyano-acrylate.
Use: Surgical aid (tissue adhesive).

•**OCTABENZONE.** USAN. 2-Hydroxy-4-(octyloxy) benzophenone. Spectra-Sorb UV 531. Under study.
Use: Sunscreen agent.

OCTACOSACTRIN. B.A.N. α^- Corticotrophin.
Use: Corticotrophic peptide.

OCTADECANOIC ACID.
See: Stearic Acid, N.F. XVII.

OCTADECANOIC ACID, SODIUM SALT.
See: Sodium Stearate, N.F. XVII.

OCTADECANOIC ACID, ZINC SALT.
See: Zinc Stearate, N.F. XVII.

l-OCTADECANOL.
See: Stearyl Alcohol, N.F. XVII.

OCTAMIDE. (Adria) Metoclopramide 10 mg/Tab. Bot. 100s, 500s.
Use: GI stimulant.

•**OCTANOIC ACID.** USAN.
Use: Antifungal.

OCTAPHONIUM CHLORIDE. B.A.N. Benzyldiethyl-2-[4-(1,1,3,3-tetramethylbutyl)phenoxy]-ethylammonium Cl. Octaphen; Phenoctide.
Use: Antiseptic.

OCTAREX. (Approved) Vitamins A 5000 IU, D 1000 IU, B_1 1.5 mg, B_2 2 mg, B_6 0.1 mg, calcium pantothenate 1 mg, niacinamide 20 mg, C 37.5 mg, E 1 IU, B_{12} 1 mcg/Cap. Bot. 100s, 1000s.
Use: Vitamin/mineral supplement.

OCTATROPINE METHYLBROMIDE. B.A.N. Anisotropine methylbromide. 2-Propyl-pentanoylmethyltropinium bromide. 8-Methyl-O-(2-propylvaleryl)tropinium bromide.
Use: Anticholinergic.

OCTAVERINE. B.A.N. 6,7-Dimethoxy-1-(3,4,5-triethoxyphenyl)isoquinoline.
Use: Antispasmodic.

OCTAVIMS. (Approved) Vitamins A 6000 IU, D 1250 IU, C 50 mg, E 5 IU, B_1 3 mg, B_2 3 mg, B_6 0.5 mg, niacinamide 20 mg, calcium pantothenate 5 mg, B_{12} 5 mcg, calcium 59 mg, phosphorus 45 mg/Cap. Bot. 100s, 250s, 1000s.
Use: Vitamin/mineral supplement.

•**OCTAZAMIDE.** USAN.
Use: Analgesic.

•**OCTENIDINE HYDROCHLORIDE.** USAN.
Use: Anti-infective, topical.

•**OCTENIDINE SACCHARIN.** USAN.
Use: Dental plaque inhibitor.

•**OCTICIZER.** USAN. 2-Ethylhexyl diphenyl phosphate. Santicizer 141 (Monsanto). SCAN Spray-On. (Johnson & Johnson).
Use: Pharmaceutic aid (plasticizer).

OCTOCAINE HCl. (Novocol) Lidocaine HCl 2%, epinephrine 1:50,000 or 1:100,000. Inj. Dent. Cartridge 1.8 ml.
Use: Local anesthetic.

•**OCTOCRYLENE.** USAN.
Use: Ultraviolet screen.

•**OCTODRINE.** USAN. 1,5-Dimethylhexylamine. Under study.
Use: Vasoconstrictor, local anesthetic.

OCTOFOLLIN.
See: Benzestrol, U.S.P. XXII.

•**OCTOXYNOL 9,** N.F. XVII.
Use: Surfactant.

•**OCTREOTIDE.** USAN.
Use: Antisecretory (gastric).

•**OCTREOTIDE ACETATE.** USAN.
Use: Antidiarrheal, gastrointestinal tumor; antihypotensive, carcinoid crisis; growth hormone suppressant, acromegaly.

•**OCTRIPTYLINE PHOSPHATE.** USAN.
Use: Antidepressant.

•**OCTRIZOLE.** USAN.
Use: Ultraviolet screen.

N-OCTYL BICYALOHEPTENE DICARBOSIMIDE. W/N-N-diethyl-m-toluamide, 2,3,4,5-bis-(delta-2-butylene) tetrahydrofurfural, Di-n-propyl isocinchomeronate, other isomers, isopropanol.
See: Bansum, Bot. (Summers).

•**OCTYLDODECANOL,** N.F. XVII.
Use: Pharmaceutic aid (oleaginous vehicle).

OCTYLPHENOXY POLYETHOXYETHANOL. A mono-ether of a polyethylene glycol. Igepal CA 630 (Antara).
W/Phenylmercuric acetate, methylparaben, sodium borate.
See: Lorophyn jelly, Supp. (Eaton).
W/Lactic acid, sodium lactate.
See: Jeneen premeasured liquid douche (Norwich).

OCU-BATH EYE LOTION. (Commerce Drug) Sodium Cl, sodium propionate, sodium borate, boric acid, glycerin, rose and camphor water, extract of witch hazel, berberine bisulfate, BAC. Bot. 4 oz w/eyecup.
Use: Ophthalmic irrigant.

OCUCLEAR EYE. (Schering) Oxymetazoline HCl 0.025%. Bot. 15 ml, 30 ml.
Use: Vasoconstrictor/mydriatric, ophthalmic.

OCU-DROP. (Commerce) Tetrahydrozoline HCl 0.05%, sodium Cl, sodium borate, boric acid, benzalkonium Cl 0.01%, EDTA 0.01%. Bot. 0.5 oz.
Use: Ophthalmic irrigant.

OCUFEN. (Allergan) Flurbiprofen sodium 0.03%. Bot. 2.5 ml, 5 ml, 10 ml w/dropper.
Use: Topical nonsteroidal anti-inflammatory drug, ophthalmic.

•**OCUFILCON A.** USAN.
Use: Contact lens material.

•**OCUFILCON B.** USAN.
Use: Contact lens material.

•**OCUFILCON C.** USAN.
Use: Contact lens material.

OCULINUM. (Allergan) Botulinum toxin type A 100 units, albumin 0.05 mg/vial. Pow. for inj. (lyophilized).
Use: Ophthalmic preparation.

OCU-LUBE. (Bausch & Lomb) Petrolatum sterile, preservative and lanolin free. Tube 3.5 Gm.
Use: Ophthalmic lubricant.

OCUMETER.
See: Decadron Phosphate, Preps. (Merck Sharp & Dohme).
Humorsol, Ophth. Soln. (Merck Sharp & Dohme).
Neo-Decadron, Preps. (Merck Sharp & Dohme).

OCUSERT. (Ciba) Pilocarpine ocular therapeutic system.
Pilo-20: Releases 20 mcg pilocarpine/hour for one week. Pkg. 8s.
Pilo-40: Releases 40 mcg pilocarpine/hour for one week. Pkg. 8s.
Use: Agent for glaucoma.

ODALATE. (Kenyon) Chlorpheniramine maleate 8 mg, phenylpropanolamine HCl 50 mg, atropine sulfate 0.36 mg/Cap. Bot. 100s, 1000s.
Use: Antihistamine, decongestant, anticholinergic/antispasmodic.

ODARA. (Lorvic) Alcohol 48%, carbolic acid less than 2%, zinc Cl, potassium iodide, glycerin, methyl salicylate, oil eucalyptus, tincture myrrh. Concentrated Liq. Bot. 8 oz.
Use: Mouthwash, gargle.

ODONIL. (Kenyon) dl-Methionine 200 mg/Cap. Bot. 100s, 1000s.
Use: Diaper rash product.

OESTERGON.
See: Estradiol (Various Mfr.).

OESTRADIOL.
See: Estradiol (Various Mfr.).

OESTRASID.
See: Dienestrol (Various Mfr.).

OESTRIN.
See: Estrone (Various Mfr.).

OESTRIOL SUCCINATE. B.A.N. Oestra-1,3,5-(10)-triene-3,16α,17β-triol 16,17-di(hydrogen succinate).
Use: Treatment of thrombocytopenic hemorrhage.

OESTRIOL SODIUM SUCCINATE. B.A.N. Oestra-1,3,5(10)-triene-3,16α,17β-di(sodium succinate).
Use: Treatment of thrombocytopenic hemorrhage.

OESTROFORM.
See: Estrone (Various Mfr.).

OESTROMENIN.
See: Diethylstilbestrol (Various Mfr.).

OESTROMON.
See: Diethylstilbestrol (Various Mfr.).

OFF-EZY CORN REMOVER. (Commerce) Salicylic acid 13.57% in flexible collodion base, ether 65%, alcohol 21%. Bot. 0.45 oz.

Use: Keratolytic.

OFF-EZY WART REMOVER. (Commerce) Salicylic acid 17% in flexible collodion base, ether 65%, alcohol 21%. Bot. 13.5 ml.
Use: Keratolytic.

O-FLEX. (Seatrace) Orphenadrine citrate 30 mg/ml. Inj. Vial 10 ml.
Use: Skeletal muscle relaxant.

•**OFLOXACIN.** USAN.
Use: Antibacterial.
See: Floxin (Ortho).

•**OFORNINE.** USAN.
Use: Antihypertensive.

OGEN. (Abbott) Estropipate. **Tab. 0.625:** Estropipate 0.75 mg/Tab. Bot. 100s. **Tab. 1.25:** Estropipate 1.5 mg/Tab. Bot. 100s. **Tab. 2.5:** Estropipate 3 mg/Tab. Bot. 100s. **Tab 5.:** Estropipate 6 mg/Tab. Bot. 100s.
Use: Estrogen.

OGEN VAGINAL CREAM. (Abbott) Estropipate 1.5 mg/Gm. Tube 1.5 oz w/applicator.
Use: Estrogen, vaginal.

OILATUM SOAP. (Stiefel) Polyunsaturated vegetable oil 7.5%. Bar 112 Gm.
Use: Skin cleanser.

OIL OF CAMPHOR W/COMBINATIONS.
See: Sloan's Liniment, Liq. (Warner-Lambert).

OIL OF CLOVES W/ALCOHOL.
See: Buckley "Z.O.", Liq. (Crosby).

OIL OF PINE W/COMBINATIONS.
See: Sloan's Liniment, Liq. (Warner-Lambert).

OIL-O-SOL. (Health Care Industries) Corn oil 52%, castor oil 40.8%, camphor 6.8%, hexylresorcinol 0.1%. Bot. 1 oz, 2 oz, 4 oz.
Use: Antiseptic.

OINTMENT BASE, WASHABLE.
See: Absorbent Base (Upsher-Smith).
Cetaphil, Cream, Lot. (Owen).
Velvachol, Cream (Owen).

•**OINTMENT, HYDROPHILIC,** U.S.P. XXII.
Use: Pharmaceutical aid (oil-in-water emulsion ointment base).

•**OINTMENT, WHITE,** U.S.P. XXII.
Use: Pharmaceutical aid (oleaginous ointment base).

•**OINTMENT, YELLOW,** U.S.P. XXII.
Use: Ointment base.

•**OLAFLUR.** USAN.
Use: Dental caries prophylactic.

OLAMINE.
See: Ethanolamine.

OLAQUINDOX. B.A.N. 2-(2-Hydroxyethylcarbamoyl)-3-methylquinoxaline 1,4-dioxide.
Use: Growth promoter, bactericide, veterinary medicine.

OLDEROL. (Doral) Vitamins B_1 15 mg, B_2 10 mg, niacinamide 100 mg, B_6 5 mg, B_{12} 4 mcg, calcium pantothenate 20 mg, folic acid 150 mcg, C 750 mg, E 30 IU/Cap. Bot. 60s.
Use: Vitamin/mineral supplement.

OLEANDOMYCIN. B.A.N. An antibiotic from *Streptomyces antibioticus.*
Use: Antibiotic.

OLEANDOMYCIN PHOSPHATE. Phosphate of an antibacterial substance produced by *Streptomyces antibioticus.*
Use: Anti-infective.

OLEANDOMYCIN SALT OF PENICILLIN.
See: Pen-M (Pfizer) Under study.

OLEANDOMYCIN, TRIACETYL. Troleandomycin, U.S.P. XX.

•**OLEIC ACID,** N.F. XVII. 9-Octadecanoic acid.
Use: Pharmaceutical aid (emulsion adjunct).

•**OLEIC ACID I-131.** USAN.
Use: Radioactive agent.

•**OLEIC ACID I-125.** USAN.
Use: Radioactive agent.

OLEOVITAMIN A, Vitamin A, U.S.P. XXII.

•**OLEOVITAMIN A & D,** U.S.P. XXII. Cap., U.S.P. XXII.
Use: Vitamin A & D therapy.
See: Super-D, Perles, Liq. (Upjohn).

•**OLEOVITAMIN D, SYNTHETIC.**
Use: Vitamin D supplement.
See: Viosterol in Oil.

•**OLEYL ALCOHOL,** N.F. XVII. (Z)-9-Octadecen-1-ol.
Use: Emulsifying agent, emollient.

•**OLIVE OIL,** N.F. XVII.
Use: Emollient, pharmaceutical aid (setting retardant for dental cements).

•**OLSALAZINE SODIUM.** USAN.
Use: Anti-inflammatory (gastrointestinal).
See: Dipentum (Pharmacia).

•**OLVANIL.** USAN.
Use: Analgesic.

OMBRE EXTRA STRENGTH. (E.J. Moore) Vitamins A palmitate, D, B_1, B_2, B_6, B_{12}, niacinamide, calcium pantothenate, ascorbic acid/Tab. Bot. 50s, 100s.
Use: Vitamin/mineral supplement.

OMEGA-3 (N-3) POLYUNSATURATED FATTY ACIDS. From cold water fish oils.
Use: Dietary supplement to reduce risk of coronary artery disease.
See: Cardi-Omega 3, Cap. (Thompson Medical).
Marine 500, 1000, Cap. (Murdock).
Max EPA, Cap. (Various Mfr.).
Promega, Cap. (Parke-Davis).
Proto-Chol, Cap. (Squibb).
Sea-Omega 50, Cap. (Rugby).

OMEGA OIL. (Block) Methyl nicotinate, methyl salicylate, capsicum oleoresin, histamine dihydrochloride, isopropyl alcohol 44%. Bot. 2.5 oz, 4.85 oz.
Use: External analgesic.

•**OMEPRAZOLE.** USAN.
*Use:*Inhibitor of gastric acid secretion.
See: Prilosec (Merck, Sharp & Dohme)

OMNICOL. (Delta) Dextromethorphan HBr 15 mg, chlorpheniramine maleate 4 mg, phenylephrine HCl 5 mg, phenindamine tartrate 4 mg, salicylamide 227 mg, acetaminophen 100 mg, caffeine alkaloid 10 mg, ascorbic acid 25 mg/Tab. Bot. 100s. Bot. pt.
Use: Antitussive, antihistamine, decongestant, analgesic.

OMNIHEMIN. (Delta) Iron 110 mg, vitamins C 150 mg, B_{12} 7.5 mcg, folic acid 1 mg, zinc 1 mg, copper 1 mg, manganese 1 mg, magnesium 1 mg/Tab. or 5 ml. **Cap.:** Bot. 100s; **Soln.:** Bot. pt.
Use: Vitamin/mineral supplement.

OMNI-M TABLETS. (Blue Cross) Vitamins, minerals. Bot. 100s.
Use: Vitamin/mineral supplement.

OMNINATAL. (Delta) Iron 60 mg, copper 2 mg, zinc 15 mg, vitamins A 8000 IU, D 400 IU, C 90 mg, calcium 200 mg, folic acid 1.5 mg, B_1 2.5 mg, B_2 3 mg, niacinamide 20 mg, pyridoxine HCl 10 mg, pantothenic acid 15 mg, B_{12} 8 mcg/Tab. Bot. 100s.
Use: Vitamin/mineral supplement.

OMNIPAQUE. (Winthrop Pharm) Iohexol (46.4% iodine). Nonionic contrast medium. **180 mg/ml:** Vial 10 ml, 20 ml. **240 mg/ml:** Vial 10 ml, 100 ml. Bot. 200 ml. **300 mg/ml:** Vial 10 ml, 30 ml, 50 ml, 100 ml. **350 mg/ml:** Vial 50 ml, 100 ml. Bot. 200 ml.
Use: Radiopaque agent.

OMNIPEN. (Wyeth-Ayerst) Ampicillin, anhydrous 250 mg or 500 mg/Cap. Bot. 100s, 500s.
Use: Antibacterial, penicillin.

OMNIPEN. (Wyeth-Ayerst) Ampicillin trihydrate 125 mg or 250 mg/5 ml when reconstituted. Pow. for oral susp. **125 mg/5 ml:** Bot. 100 ml, 150 ml, 200 ml. **250 mg/5 ml:** Bot. 100 ml, 150 ml, 200 ml, UD 5 ml × 20.
Use: Antibacterial, penicillin.

OMNIPEN-N. (Wyeth-Ayerst) Ampicillin sodium pow. for inj. 125 mg, 250 mg, 500 mg, 1 Gm or 2 Gm/Vial. Pkg. 10s. Piggyback units 500 mg, 1 Gm, 2 Gm, Bulk 10 Gm/Vial. Pkg. 1s.
Use: Antibacterial, penicillin.

OMNITABS. (Blue Cross) Vitamins A 5000 IU, D 400 IU, C 50 mg, B_1 3 mg, B_2 2.5 mg, niacin 20 mg, B_6 1 mg, B_{12} 1 mcg, pantothenic acid 0.9 mg/Tab. Bot. 100s.
Use: Vitamin supplement.

OMNITABS WITH IRON. (Blue Cross) Vitamins A 5000 IU, D 400 IU, B_1 3 mg, B_2 2.5 mg, B_6 1 mg, B_{12} 1 mcg, C 50 mg, niacinamide 20 mg, calcium pantothenate 1 mg, iron 15 mg/Tab. Bot. 100s.
Use: Vitamin/iron supplement.

OMNITRATE. (Kenyon) Vitamins A 6000 IU, D 600 IU, E 0.1 mg, B_1 1 mg, B_2 0.1 mg, B_6 0.1 mg, C 37.5 mg, B_{12} 1 mcg, niacinamide 15 mg, folic acid 0.067 mg, hesperidin 50 mg, calcium carbonate 400 mg, iron-ferrous iodide dried 20 mg, magnesium 15 mg, iodine 0.15 mg, manganese 3 mg, zinc 3 mg/3 Cap. Bot. 1000s.
Use: Vitamin/mineral supplement.

ONCOVIN SOLUTION. (Lilly) Vincristine sulfate for inj. 1 mg/ml, 2 mg/2 ml or 5 mg/5 ml. Ctn. 10s. Hyporets 1 mg/Pkg 3s; 2 mg/Pkg 3s.
Use: Antineoplastic agent.

•**ONDANSETRON HCl.** USAN.
Use: Antiemetic (cancer chemotherapy).
See: Zofran (Glaxo).

ONE-A-DAY ESSENTIAL. (Miles) Vitamins A 5000 IU, E 30 IU, C 60 mg, folic acid 0.4 mg, B_1 1.5 mg, B_2 1.7 mg, niacin 20 mg, B_6 2 mg, B_{12} 6 mcg, pantothenic acid 10 mg, D 400 IU/Tab. Sodium free. Bot. 100s.
Use: Vitamin supplement.

ONE-A-DAY MAXIMUM FORMULA. (Miles) Vitamins A 5000 IU, E 30 IU, C 60 mg, folic acid 0.4 mg, B_1 1.5 mg, B_2 1.7 mg, niacin 20 mg, B_6 2 mg, B_{12} 6 mcg, K 50 mcg, D 400 IU, pantothenic acid 10 mg, iron 18 mg, calcium 129.6 mg, phosphorus 100 mg, iodine 150 mcg, magnesium 100 mg, copper 2 mg, cromium 10 mcg, selenium 10 mcg, molybdenum 10 mcg, manganese 2.5 mg, potassium 37.5 mg, biotin 30 mcg, chloride 34 mg, zinc 15 mg/Tab. Bot. 30s, 60s, 100s.
Use: Vitamin/mineral supplement.

ONE-A-DAY PLUS EXTRA C. (Miles) Vitamins A 5000 IU, E 30 IU, C 300 mg, folic acid 0.4 mg, B_1 1.5 mg, B_2 1.7 mg, niacin 20 mg, B_6 2 mg, B_{12} 6 mcg, pantothenic acid 10 mg, D 400 IU/Tab. Sodium free. Bot. 60s.
Use: Vitamin supplement.

ONE-A-DAY STRESSGARD. (Miles) Vitamins A 5000 IU, C 600 mg, B_1 15 mg, B_2 10 mg, niacin 100 mg, D 400 IU, E 30 IU, B_6 5 mg, folic acid 400 mcg, B_{12} 12 mcg, pantothenic acid 20 mg, iron 18 mg, zinc 15 mg, copper 2 mg/Tab. Sodium free. Bot. 60s.
Use: Vitamin/mineral supplement.

ONE ONLY VITAMIN TABLETS. (Robinson) Vitamins A 5000 IU, D 400 IU, B_1 2 mg, B_2 2.5 mg, B_6 1 mg, B_{12} 1 mcg, niacinamide 20 mg, panthenol 1 mg/Tab. Bot. 100s, 250s, 1000s.
Use: Vitamin supplement.

ONE ONLY VITAMIN TABLETS WITH IRON. (Robinson) Vitamins A 5000 IU, D 400 IU, B_1 2 mg, B_2 2.5 mg, C 50 mg, B_6 1 mg, B_{12} 1 mcg, niacinamide 20 mg, calcium pantothenate 1 mg, iron 15 mg/Tab. Bot. 100s, 250s, 1000s.
Use: Vitamin/mineral supplement.

1000-BC, IM OR IV. (Solvay) Vitamins B_1 25 mg, B_2 2.5 mg, B_6 5 mg, panthenol 5 mg, B_{12} 500 mcg, niacinamide 75 mg, C 100 mg/ml. Vial 10 ml.
Use: Vitamin supplement.

1+1-F CREME. (Dunhall) Hydrocortisone 1%, pramoxine HCl 1%, iodochlorhydroxyquin 3%. Tube 30 Gm.
Use: Corticosteroid, local anesthetic, antifungal.

1-2-3 OINTMENT NO. 20. (Durel) Burow's solution, lanolin, zinc oxide (Lassar's paste). Jar oz, 1 lb, 6 lb.
Use: Anti-inflammatory agent, topical.

1-2-3 OINTMENT NO. 21. (Durel) Burow's solution 1 part, lanolin 2, zinc oxide (Lassar's paste) 1.5, cold cream 1.5. Jar oz, 1 lb, 6 lb.
Use: Anti-inflammatory agent, topical.

ONE TABLET DAILY. (Various Mfr.) Vitamins A 5000 IU, D 400 IU, E 30 mg, B_1 1.5 mg, B_2 1.7 mg, B_3 20 mg, B_5 10 mg, B_6 2 mg, B_{12} 6 mcg, C 60 mg, folic acid 0.4 mg/Tab. Bot. 100s, 250s, 365s.
Use: Vitamin supplement.

ONE TABLET DAILY PLUS IRON. (Various Mfr.) Iron 18 mg, vitamins A 5000 IU, D 400 IU, E 15 mg, B_1 1.5 mg, B_2 1.7 mg, B_3 20 mg, B_6 2 mg, B_{12} 6 mcg, C 60 mg, folic acid 0.4 mg/Tab. Bot. 100s, 250s, 365s.
Use: Vitamin/mineral supplement.

ONOTON TABLETS. (Winthrop Products) Pancreatin, hemicellulose, ox bile extracts.
Use: Digestive aid.

ONTOSEIN.
See: Orgotein (Diagnostic Data).

OPCON. (Bausch & Lomb) Naphazoline HCl 0.1%. Bot. 15 ml.
Use: Vasoconstrictor/mydriatic, (ophthalmic).

OPCON-A. (Bausch & Lomb) Naphazoline HCl 0.025%, pheniramine maleate 0.3%. Bot. 15 ml.
Use: Vasoconstrictor/mydriatic, antihistamine (ophthalmic).

OPERAND. (Redi-Products) **Aerosal:** Iodine 0.5%. 90 ml. **Skin cleanser:** Iodine 1%. 90 ml. **Oint.:** Iodine 1%. 30 Gm, lb, packette 1.2 Gm and 2.7 Gm. **Perineal wash conc.:** Iodine 1%. 240 ml. **Prep soln.:** Iodine 1%. 60 ml, 120 ml, 240 ml, pt, qt. **Soln:** Prep pad 100s, swab stick 25s. **Surgical scrub:** Povidone-iodine 7.5%. 60 ml, 120 ml, 240 ml, pt, qt, gal, packette 22.5 ml. **Whirlpool conc.:** Iodine 1%. gal.
Use: Antiseptic, germicide.

OPERAND DOUCHE. (Redi-Products) Povidone-iodine. Soln. 60 ml, 240 ml, UD 15 ml.
Use: Vaginal preparation.

OPHTHA P/S OPHTHALMIC SUSPENSION. (Misemer) Sodium sulfacetamide 10%, prednisolone acetate 0.5%. Bot. 5 ml w/dropper.
Use: Steroid/sulfonamide combination, ophthalmic.

OPHTHAINE HCl. (Squibb) Proparacaine HCl 0.5%, glycerin 2.45%, chlorobutanol 0.2%, benzalkonium Cl, sodium hydroxide or hydrochloric acid to adjust pH. Soln. Bot. w/dropper 15 ml.
Use: Local anesthetic, ophthalmic.

OPHTHALGAN. (Wyeth-Ayerst) Glycerin ophthalmic soln. w/chlorobutanol (chloral derivative 0.55%) as preservative. Bot. 7.5 ml w/dropper screw cap.
Use: Hyperosmolar preparation.

OPHTHETIC STERILE OPHTHALMIC SOLUTION. (Allergan) Proparacaine HCl 0.5%, benzalkonium Cl, glycerin, sodium Cl, purified water. Dropper bot. 15 ml.
Use: Local anesthetic, ophthalmic.

OPHTHOCHLOR. (Parke-Davis) Chloramphenicol 5 mg/ml in a boric acid-sodium borate buffer soln., with sodium hydroxide to adjust pH. Plastic drop. Bot. 15 ml.
Use: Anti-infective, ophthalmic.

OPHTHOCORT. (Parke-Davis) Hydrocortisone acetate 0.5%, chloramphenicol 1%, polymyxin B sulfate 10,000 units/Gm Oint. Tube 3.75 Gm.
Use: Corticosteroid, anti-infective (ophthalmic).

OPIPRAMOL. B.A.N. 5- 3-[4-(2-Hydroxyethyl)-piperazin-1-yl]propyl -dibenz[b,f]azepine.
Use: Antidepressant.

•**OPIPRAMOL HYDROCHLORIDE.** USAN. 4-[3-(5H-Dibenz[b,f]azepin-5yl)-propyl]-1-piperazine-ethanol dihydrochloride.
Use: Antidepressant, tranquilizer.

•**OPIUM,** U.S.P. XXII.
Use: Pharmaceutical necessity for powdered opium.

OPIUM ALKALOIDS, TOTAL, ASTHE HYDROCHLORIDE SALT.
See: Pantopon, Amp. (Roche).

OPIUM AND BELLADONNA. (Wyeth-Ayerst) Powdered opium 60 mg, extract of belladonna 0.25 gr/Supp. Box 20s.
Use: Narcotic analgesic, anticholinergic/antispasmodic.

•**OPIUM POWDER,** U.S.P. XXII.
Use: Pharmaceutical necessity for Paregoric.
W/Albumin tannate, colloidal kaolin, pectin.
See: Ekrised, Tab. (Mallard).
W/Atropine sulfate, alcohol.
See: Stopit Liq. (Scrip).
W/Belladonna extract.
See: B & O, Supp. (Webcon).
W/Bismuth subgallate, kaolin, pectin, zinc phenolsulfonate.
See: Diastay, Tab. (Elder).
W/Kaolin, pectin, bismuth subcarbonate.
See: KBP/O, Cap. (Cole).
W/Kaolin, pectin, hyoscyamine sulfate, atropine sulfate, hyoscine HBr.
See: Donnagel-PG, Susp. (Robins).
W/Ipecac powder, phenacetin, aspirin, camphor monobromated, caffeine, anhydrous, atropine sulfate.
See: Phenatrocaps, Cap. (O'Neal).
W/Ipecac powdered, phenacetin, atropine sulfate, monobromated camphor, methapyrilene HCl, salicylamide, caffeine.
See: Phenatrohist, Cap. (O'Neal).

•**OPIUM TINCTURE,** U.S.P. XXII.
W/Homatropine MBr, Pectin.
See: Dia-Quel, Liq. (I.P.C.).
W/Pectin.
See: Opecto, Elix. (Bowman).
Parelixir, Liq. (Purdue Frederick).

OPIUM TINCTURE, CAMPHORATED.
Use: Antidiarrheal.
See: Paregoric, U.S.P. XXII.
W/Glycyrrhiza fluid extract, tartar emetic, glycerin.
See: Brown Mixture.

OPTI-BON EYE DROPS. (Barrows) Phenylephrine HCl, berberine sulfate, boric acid, sodium Cl, sodium bisulfite, glycerine, camphor water, peppermint water, thimerosal 0.004%. Bot. 1 oz.
Use: Ophthalmic preparation.

OPTICAPS. (Approved) Vitamins A 32,500 IU, D 3250 IU, B_1 15 mg, B_2 5 mg, B_6 0.5 mg, C 150 mg, E 5 IU, calcium pantothenate 3 mg, niacinamide 150 mg, B_{12} 20 mcg, iron 11.26 mg, choline bitartrate 30 mg, inositol 30 mg, pepsin 32.5 mg, diastase 32.5 mg, calcium 30 mg, phosphorus 25 mg, magnesium 0.7 mg, Fr. dicalcium phosphate 110 mg, manganese 1.3 mg, potassium 0.68 mg, zinc 0.45 mg, hesperidin compound 25 mg, biotin 20 mcg, Brewer's yeast 50 mg, wheat germ oil 20 mg, hydrolized yeast 81.25 mg, protein digest. 47.04 mg, amino acids 34.21 mg/Cap. Bot. 30s, 60s, 90s, 1000s.
Use: Vitamin/mineral supplement.

OPTI-CLEAN. (Alcon) Polysorbate 21, polymeric cleaning beads, thimerosal 0.004%, EDTA 0.1%. Bot 12 ml, 20 ml.
Use: Contact lens care.

OPTI-CLEAN II. (Alcon) Isotonic polymeric cleaning agent, hydroxyethylcellulose, polysorbate 21, EDTA 0.1%, polyquaternium-1 0.01%. Thimerosal free. Bot. 12 ml, 20 ml.
Use: Contact lens care.

OPTICROM 4%. (Fisons) Cromolyn sodium 4% ophthalmic solution. Pkg. 10 ml w/dropper.
Use: Antiallergic, ophthalmic.

OPTIGENE 3. (Pfeiffer) Tetrahydrozoline HCl 0.05%. Soln. Bot. 15 ml.
Use: Vasoconstrictor/mydriatic, ophthalmic.

OPTILETS-500. (Abbott) Vitamins B_1 15 mg, B_2 10 mg, niacinamide 100 mg, calcium pantothenate 20 mg, B_6 5 mg, C 500 mg, A 10,000 IU, D 400 IU, E 30 IU, B_{12} 12 mcg/Filmtab. Bot. 100s, 130s.
Use: Vitamin/mineral supplement.

OPTILETS-M-500. (Abbott) Vitamins C 500 mg, niacinamide 100 mg, calcium pantothenate 20 mg, B_1 15 mg, A 10,000 IU, B_2 10 mg, B_6 5 mg, D 400 IU, B_{12} 12 mcg, E 30 IU, iron 20 mg, magnesium 80 mg, zinc 1.5 mg, copper 2 mg, manganese 1 mg, iodine 0.15 mg/Filmtab. Bot. 100s.
Use: Vitamin/mineral supplement.

OPTIMINE. (Schering) Azatadine maleate 1 mg/Tab. Bot. 100s.
Use: Antihistamine.

OPTIMYD. (Schering) Prednisolone phosphate 0.5%, sodium sulfacetamide 10%, sodium thiosulfate. Soln-Sterile. Drop bot. 5 ml.
Use: Steroid/sulfonamide combination, ophthalmic.

OPTIPRANOLOL. (Bausch & Lomb) Metipranolol HCl 0.3%. Bot. 5 ml, 10 ml.
Use: Agent for glaucoma.

OPTIRAY. (Mallinckrodt) Ioversoln.
Use: Diagnostic aid.

OPTISED SOLN. (Ketchum) Zinc sulfate 0.025%, phenylephrine HCl 0.12%. Bot. 15 ml.
Use: Decongestant combination, ophthalmic.

OPTI-SOFT. (Alcon) Isotonic soln of sodium Cl, borate buffer, EDTA 0.1%, polyquaternium-1 0.001%. Thimerosal free. Soln. Bot. 237 ml, 355 ml.
Use: Soft contact lens care.

OPTI-TEARS. (Alcon) Isotonic solution with dextran, sodium Cl, potassium Cl, hydroxypropyl methylcellulose, EDTA 0.1%, polyquaternium-1 0.01%. Thimerosal free. Soln. Bot. 15 ml.
Use: Soft contact lens care.

OPTIVITE FOR WOMEN. (Optimox) Vitamins A 2083 IU, D 16.7 IU, E 14 mg, B_1 4.2 mg, B_2 4.2 mg, B_3 4.2 mg, B_5 4.2 mg, B_6 50 mg, B_{12} 10.4 mcg, C 250 mg, iron 2.5 mg, folic acid 0.03 mg, zinc 4.2 mg, choline 52 mg, inositol 10 mg, Cr, Cu, I, K, Mg, Mn, Se, citrus bioflavonoids, PABA, rutin, pancreatin, biotin/Tab. Bot. 180s.
Use: Vitamin/mineral supplement.

OPTI-ZYME ENZYMATIC CLEANER FOR SENSITIVE EYES. (Alcon Lenscare) Pork pancreatin tablets. Pak 8s, 24s, 36s.
Use: Contact lens care.

OPTO-MIST. (Ketchum) Sodium propionate, sodium Cl, camphor, peppermint oil. Bot. 0.5 oz.

ORA5. (McHenry) Copper sulfate, iodine, potassium iodide, alcohol 1.5%. Liq. Bot. 3.75 ml, 30 ml.
Use: Mouth preparation.

ORABASE. (Colgate-Hoyt) Gelatin, pectin, sodium carboxymethylcellulose in hydrocarbon gel w/polyethylene and mineral oil. 0.75 gm Packet Box 100s. Tube 5 Gm, 15 Gm.
Use: Mouth preparation.

ORABASE HCA. (Colgate-Hoyt) Hydrocortisone acetate 0.5% in paste base. Packet 0.75 Gm Box 100s. Tube 5 Gm.
Use: Corticosteroid mouth preparation.

ORABASE-O. (Colgate-Hoyt) Benzocaine 20% in a polyethylene, mineral oil base. Gel. In 15 Gm.
Use: Local anesthetic.

ORABASE WITH BENZOCAINE. (Colgate-Hoyt) Benzocaine 20% in gel base. Packet 0.75 Gm, Box 100s. Tube 5 Gm, 15 Gm.
Use: Local anesthetic.

ORACAP CAPSULES. (Vangard) Phenylpropanolamine HCl 75 mg, chlorpheniramine maleate 12 mg/Cap. Bot. 100s, 1000s.
Use: Decongestant, antihistamine.

ORACIN. (Vicks) **Regular:** Benzocaine 6.25 mg, menthol 0.1%/Regular Loz. w/FDC Yellow #5 (tartrazine). **Cherry:** Benzocaine 6.25 mg, men-

thol 0.08%/Cherry Loz. in sorbitol base. Pkg. 18s.
Use: Local anesthetic.
ORACIT. (Carolina Medical Prod.) Sodium citrate 490 mg, citric acid 640 mg/5 ml, (sodium 1 mEq/ml equivalent to 1 mEq bicarbonate), alcohol 0.25%. Soln. Bot. pt, UD 15, 30 ml.
Use: Systemic alkalinizer.
ORADERM LIP BALM. (Schattner) Sodium phenolate, sodium tetraborate, phenol, base containing an anionic emulsifier. ⅛ oz.
Use: Local anesthetic, antiseptic.
ORADEX-C. (Commerce) Cetylpyridinium Cl 2.5 mg, benzocaine 10 mg/Troche. Bot. 10s.
Use: Antiseptic, local anesthetic.
ORAFIX MEDICATED. (Norcliff Thayer) Allantoin 0.2%, benzocaine 2%. Tube 0.75 oz.
Use: Local anesthetic, denture adhesive.
ORAFIX ORIGINAL. (Norcliff Thayer) Tube 1.5 oz, 2.5 oz, 4 oz.
Use: Denture adhesive.
ORAFIX SPECIAL. (Norcliff Thayer) Tube 1.4 oz, 2.4 oz.
Use: Denture adhesive.
ORA-FRESH. (A.V.P.) Sugar-free, non-alcoholic, nontoxic, flavored mouthwash. UD cup 1 oz, Bot. 4 oz, 16 oz.
Use: Mouth preparation.
ORAGEST S.R. (Major) Phenylpropanolamine HCl 75 mg, chlorpheniramine maleate 12 mg/SR Cap. Bot. 100s, 250s, 1000s, UD 100s.
Use: Decongestant, antihistamine.
ORAGRAFIN CALCIUM GRANULES. (Squibb) Ipodate calcium (61.7% iodine) 3 Gm/8 Gm Pkg. 25 × 1 dose pkg.
Use: Radiopaque agent.
ORAGRAFIN SODIUM CAPSULES. (Squibb) Ipodate sodium (61.4% iodine) 0.5 Gm/Cap. Bot. 100s, 144s. Unimatic pkg. 100s. Card 6s. Box 25s.
Use: Radiopaque agent.
ORAHESIVE POWDER. (Hoyt) Gelatin, pectin, sodium carboxymethylcellulose. Bot. 25 Gm.
Use: Denture adhesive.
ORAHIST TR. (Vangard) Chlorpheniramine maleate 8 mg, phenylpropanolamine HCl 50 mg, isopropamide iodide 2.5 mg/TR Cap. Bot. 100s, 1000s.
Use: Antihistamine, decongestant.
ORAJEL. (Commerce) Benzocaine 10% in a special base. Tube 0.2 oz, 0.5 oz.
Use: Local anesthetic.
ORAJEL BABY. (Commerce) Benzocaine 7.5% in a special base. Tube 0.5 oz.
Use: Local anesthetic.
ORAJEL BRACE-AID ORAL ANESTHETIC GEL. (Commerce) Benzocaine 20% in sugarless gel base. Tube 0.5 oz.
Use: Local anesthetic.
ORAJEL BRACE-AID ORAL HYGIENIC RINSE. (Commerce) Carbamide peroxide 10% in anhydrous glycerin. Tube oz.
Use: Mouth preparation.
ORAJEL D. (Commerce) Benzocaine in a special anti-irritant base. Tube 0.5 oz.
Use: Local anesthetic.
ORAJEL MAXIMUM STRENGTH. (Commerce) Benzocaine 20% in special base. Tube 1/3 oz, 3/16 oz.
Use: Local anesthetic.
ORAJEL MOUTH-AID. (Commerce) Benzocaine 20%, benzalkonium Cl 0.12%, zinc Cl 0.1% in special emollient base. Tube 0.33 oz.
Use: Local anesthetic, antibacterial.
ORAL-B MUPPETS FLUORIDE TOOTHPASTE. (Oral-B) Fluoride 0.22%. Pump 4.3 oz.
Use: Dental caries preventative.
ORALCID.
See: Acetarsone.
ORAL CONTRACEPTIVES.
See: Demulen, Tab. (Searle).
Enovid-E, Tab. (Searle).
Loestrin, Prods. (Parke-Davis).
Lo/Ovral, Prods. (Wyeth-Ayerst).
Miconor, Tab. (Ortho).
Modicon, Prods. (Ortho).
Nordette, Tab. (Wyeth-Ayerst).
Norinyl, Prods. (Syntex).
Norlestrin, Prods. (Parke-Davis).
Norquen, Tab. (Syntex).
Ortho-Novum, Prods. (Ortho).
Ovcon-35, Tab. (Mead Johnson).
Ovcon-50, Tab. (Mead Johnson).
Ovral, Tab. (Wyeth-Ayerst).
Ovrette, Tab. (Wyeth-Ayerst).
Ovulen, Tab. (Searle).
Triphasil, Tab. (Wyeth-Ayerst).
ORAL DROPS/CANKER SORE RELIEF. (Weeks & Leo) Carbamide peroxide 10% in anhydrous glycerin base. Bot. 30 ml.
Use: Mouth preparation.
ORALONE DENTAL. (Thames) Triamcinolone acetonide 0.1%. Paste 5 Gm.
Use: Corticosteroid, topical.
•**ORAL REHYDRATION SALTS,** U.S.P. XXII.
ORAMIDE. (Major) Tolbutamide 0.5 Gm/Tab. Bot. 100s, 1000s.
Use: Antidiabetic agent.
•**ORANGE FLOWER OIL,** N.F. XVII.
Use: Flavor, perfume, vehicle.
•**ORANGE FLOWER WATER,** N.F. XVII.
Use: Flavor, perfume.
•**ORANGE OIL,** N.F. XVII.
Use: Flavor.
•**ORANGE PEEL TINCTURE, SWEET,** N.F. XVII.
Use: Flavor.
•**ORANGE SPIRIT, COMPOUND,** N.F. XVII.
Use: Flavor.
•**ORANGE SYRUP,** N.F. XVII.
Use: Flavored vehicle.
ORANYL. (Otis Clapp) Pseudoephedrine HCl 30 mg/Tab. Sugar, caffeine, lactose and salt free. Safety pack 500s.
Use: Decongestant.

ORANYL PLUS. (Otis Clapp) Acetaminophen, pseudoephedrine HCl/Tab. Caffeine, sugar, lactose and salt free.
Use: Analgesic, decongestant.

ORAP. (McNeil Pharm) Pimozide 2 mg/Tab. Bot. 100s.
Use: Antipsychotic agent.

ORAPIN. (Standex) Conjugated estrogen 0.625 mg or 1.25 mg/Tab. Bot. 100s.
Use: Estrogen.

ORAPIN INJ. (Standex) Estrogenic substance 20,000 units/30 ml. Susp. aqueous or oil.
Use: Estrogen.

ORARSAN.
See: Acetarsone.

ORASEPT. (Pharmakon Labs) Tannic acid 114.9 mg, methylbenzethonium HCl 14.4 mg, benzocaine 14.4 mg, ethyl alcohol 61%/ml, camphor, menthol, benzyl alcohol, spearmint oil, cassia oil. Liq. Bot. 15 ml.
Use: Mouth and throat preparation.

ORASONE. (Solvay) Prednisone **1 mg, 5 mg, 10 mg** or **20 mg/Tab.:** Bot. 100s, 1000s, UD 100s. **50 mg/Tab.:** Bot. 100s, UD 100s.
Use: Corticosteroid.

ORATUSS TR. (Vangard) Caramiphen edisylate 20 mg, chlorpheniramine maleate 8 mg, phenylpropanolamine HCl 50 mg, isopropamide iodide 2.5 mg/TR Cap. Bot. 100s, 500s.
Use: Antitussive, antihistamine, decongestant, anticholinergic/antispasmodic.

ORAZINC. (Mericon) Zinc sulfate 220 mg/Cap. Bot. 100s, 1000s.
Use: Mineral supplement.

ORBENIN. Sodium cloxacillin.
Use: Antibiotic.

ORBETIC. (Cenci) Tolbutamide 0.5 Gm/Tab. Bot. 200s, 1000s.
Use: Antidiabetic agent.

ORBIFERROUS. (Orbit) Ferrous fumarate 300 mg, vitamins B_{12} 12 mcg, C 50 mg, B_1 3 mg, defatted desiccated liver 50 mg/Tab. Bot. 60s, 500s.
Use: Vitamin/mineral supplement.

ORBIT. (Spanner) Vitamins A 6250 IU, D 400 IU, B_1 3 mg, B_2 3 mg, B_6 2 mg, B_{12} 5 mcg, C 75 mg, niacinamide 20 mg, calcium pantothenate 10 mg, E 15 IU, biotin 15 mcg, iron 20 mg/Tab. Bot. 100s.
Use: Vitamin/mineral supplement.

•**ORCIPRENALINE.** B.A.N. 1-(3,5-Dihydroxyphenyl)-2-isopropylaminoethanol.
Use: Bronchodilator.

•**ORCONAZOLE NITRATE.** USAN.
Use: Antifungal.

ORDRINE. (Vitarine) Chlorpheniramine maleate 12 mg, phenylpropanolamine HCl 75 mg/SR Cap. Bot. 100s, 1000s.
Use: Antihistamine, decongestant.

ORETIC. (Abbott) Hydrochlorothiazide 25 mg or 50 mg/Tab. Bot. 100s, 1000s, UD 100s.
Use: Diuretic.

ORETICYL 25 and 50. (Abbott) **25:** Hydrochlorothiazide 25 mg, deserpidine 0.125 mg/Tab. Bot. 100s. **50:** Hydrochlorothiazide 50 mg, deserpidine 0.125 mg/Tab. Bot. 100s.
Use: Antihypertensive combination.

ORETICYL FORTE. (Abbott) Hydrochlorothiazide 25 mg, deserpidine 0.25 mg/Tab. Bot. 100s.
Use: Antihypertensive combination.

ORETON METHYL. (Schering) Methyltestosterone. **Buccal Tab.:** 10 mg, Bot. 100s. **Tab.:** 10 mg or 25 mg. Bot. 100s.
Use: Androgen.

OREX. (Young Dental) Monobasic and dibasic potassium phosphates, magnesium, potassium, calcium and sodium Cl, sodium flouride, sorbitol solution, sodium carboxymethylcellulose, methylparaben. Soln. Bot. 180 ml.
Use: Saliva substitute.

OREXIN. (Stuart) Vitamins B_1 10 mg, B_6 5 mg, B_{12} 25 mcg/Softab Tab. Bot. 100s.
Use: Vitamin supplement.

ORGANIDIN. (Wallace) Iodinated glycerol. **Elix.:** 1.2%, 60 mg/5 ml, alcohol 21.75%. Bot. pt, gal. **Soln.:** 50 mg/ml. Dropper bot 30 ml. **Tab.:** 30 mg. Bot. 100s.
Use: Expectorant.
W/Codeine phosphate.
See: Tussi-Organidin, Liq. (Wallace).
W/Dextromethorphan HBr.
See: Tussi-Organidin DM, Liq. (Wallace).

ORGLAGEN TABLETS. (Goldline) Orphenidrine citrate 100 mg/Tab. Bot. 100s, 1000s.
Use: Skeletal muscle relaxant.

•**ORGOTEIN.** USAN. A group of soluble metalloproteins isolated from liver, red blood cells, and other mammalian tissues.
Use: Anti-inflammatory.

ORGOTEIN. (Diagnostic Data) Pure water soluble protein with a compact conformation maintained by 4 Gm atoms of chelated divalent metals, produced from bovine liver as a Cu-Zn mixed chelate having superoxide dismutase activity. Ontosein, Palosein.

ORIMUNE TRIVALENT. (Lederle) Poliovirus vaccine. Live, Oral, Trivalent. Sabin strains Types 1, 2, and 3. Dose of 0.5 ml Dispette disposable pipette 1 dose. 10s. Pkg. 5s, 20s, 50s.
Use: Agent for immunization.

ORINASE. (Upjohn) Tolbutamide 250 mg or 500 mg/Tab. **250 mg:** Bot. 100s; **500 mg:** Bot. 200s, 500s, 1000s, UD Box 100s, Unit-of-Use Bot. 50s, 100s.
Use: Antidiabetic agent.

ORINASE DIAGNOSTIC. (Upjohn) Tolbutamide sodium 1 Gm/Vial. Pow. for inj. Vial with 20 ml amp diluent.
Use: Diagnostic aid.

ORISUL. (Ciba) Sulfaphenazole. A sulfonamide under study.

•**ORMAPLATIN.** USAN.
Use: Antineoplastic.

ORMAZINE. (Hauck) Chlorpromazine HCl 25 mg/ml. Vial 10 ml.
Use: Antipsychotic agent.

•**ORMETROPRIM.** USAN. (1)2,4-Diamino-5-(6-methylveratryl)pyrimidine; (2)2,4-diamino-5-(4,5-dimethoxy-2-methylbenzyl)pyrimidine.
Use: Antibacterial.

ORNADE. (SmithKline) Phenylpropanolamine HCl 75 mg, chlorpheniramine maleate 12 mg/Spansule. Bot. 50s, 500s, UD 100s.
Use: Decongestant, antihistamine.

ORNEX. (SmithKline Prods) Acetaminophen 325 mg, phenylpropanolamine HCl 12.5 mg/Capl. Blister Pak 24s, 48s. Bot. 100s. Dispensary pak 792s.
Use: Analgesic, decongestant.

•**ORNIDAZOLE.** USAN.
Use: Anti-infective.

ORNIDYL. (Marion Merrell Dow) Eflornithine HCl.
Use: Antineoplastic, antiprotozoal.

•**ORPANOXIN.** USAN.
Use: Anti-inflammatory.

ORPENEED VK. (Hanlon) Penicillin, buffered 400,000 units/Tab. Bot. 100s.
Use: Antibacterial, penicillin.

•**ORPHENADRINE CITRATE,** U.S.P. XXII. Inj., U.S.P. XXII. N,N-Dimethyl-2-(0-methyl-α-phenylbenzyloxy)-ethylamine. N,N-Dimethyl-2-((o-methyl-α-phenylbenzyl)oxy)-ethylamine Citrate (1:1).
Use: Skeletal muscle relaxant, antihistamine.
See: Flexon, Inj. (Keene).
Norflex, Tab., Amp. (Riker).
Orphanate, Inj. (Hyrex).
W/Aspirin, phenacetin, caffeine.
See: Norgesic, Tab. (Riker).
Norgesic Forte, Tab. (Riker).

ORPHENADRINE HYDROCHLORIDE. N,N-Dimethyl-2-(o-methyl-α-phenylbenzyloxy)ethylamine.
See: Disipal, Tab. (Riker).
W/Comb.
See: Estomul, Liq., Tab. (Riker).

ORPHENATE INJECTION. (Hyrex) Orphenadrine citrate 30 mg/ml. Inj. Vial 10 ml.
Use: Skeletal muscle relaxant.

ORPHENGESIC. (Various Mfr.) Orphenadrine citrate 25 mg, aspirin 385 mg, caffeine 30 mg/Tab. Bot. 100s, 500s, UD 100s.
Use: Skeletal muscle relaxant, salicylate analgesic.

ORPHENGESIC FORTE. (Various Mfr.) Orphenadrine citrate 50 mg, aspirin 770 mg, caffeine 60 mg/Tab. Bot. 100s, 500s.
Use: Skeletal muscle relaxant, salicylate analgesic.

ORTAC-DM LIQUID. (Ion) Dextromethorphan 10 mg, phenylephrine HCl 5 mg, guaifenesin 100 mg/5 ml. Bot. 4 oz.
Use: Antitussive, decongestant, expectorant.

ORTAL SODIUM. Sodium 5-ethyl-5-hexylbarbiturate. Hexethal sodium.

ORTEDRINE.
See: Amphetamine (Various Mfr.).

ORTHESIN.
See: Benzocaine.

ORTHO ALL-FLEX DIAPHRAGM. (Ortho) Diaphragm kit (all flex arcing spring) in plastic compact, sizes 55, 60, 65, 70, 75, 80, 85, 90, 95 mm.
Use: Contraceptive.

ORTHO DIAPHRAGM. (Ortho) Diaphragm kit, coil spring sizes 50, 55, 60, 65, 70, 75, 80, 85, 90, 95, 100, 105 mm.
Use: Contraceptive.

ORTHOCAINE.
See: Orthoform (No mfr. listed).

ORTHOCLONE OKT3 STERILE SOLUTION. (Ortho) Orthoclone OKT3 is murine monoclonal antibody to the T3 antigen of human T cells which function as immunosuppressant. Amp. 5 ml.
Use: Immunosuppressive agent.

ORTHO-CREME CONTRACEPTIVE CREAM. (Advanced Care) Nonoxynol-9 2% in nonfatty acid cream base. Tube 70 Gm w/measured dose applicator. Refill tube 70 Gm, 115 Gm.
Use: Contraceptive.

ORTHO DIAPHRAGM-WHITE. (Ortho) Diaphragm kit, flat spring sizes 55, 60, 65, 70, 75, 80, 85, 90, 95 mm.
Use: Contraceptive.

ORTHO DIENESTROL CREAM. (Ortho) Dienestrol 0.01%. Tube 78 Gm with or without applicator.
Use: Estrogen.

ORTHOFLAVIN. (Enzyme Process) Vitamins C 150 mg, E 25 mg/Tab. Bot. 100s, 250s.
Use: Vitamin supplement.

ORTHOFORM. (No mfr. listed.) Menthyl 3-amino-4-hydroxybenzoate.
Use: Local anesthetic.
W/Tyrothricin. (Columbus) Tyrothricin 0.5 mg, tetracaine HCl 0.5%, epinephrine 1/1000 Soln. 2%/Gm. Oint., Tube ⅛ oz.
Use: Anti-infective, ophthalmic.

ORTHO-GYNOL CONTRACEPTIVE JELLY. (Advanced Care) p-diisobutyl-phenoxy-polyethoxy-ethanol 1%, in water-dispersible jelly at pH 4.5. Tube 81 Gm w/measured-dose applicator. Tube 81 Gm, 126 Gm.
Use: Contraceptive.

ORTHO-HYDROXYBENZOIC ACID, Salicylic Acid, U.S.P. XXII.

ORTHOHYDROXYPHENYLMERCURIC CHLORIDE. (O-chloromercuriphenol).
Use: Antiseptic.
W/Benzocaine, ephedrine HCl.
See: Myrimgacaine, Liq. (Upjohn).
W/Benzocaine, parachlorometaxylenol, benzalkonium Cl, phenol.
See: Unguentine Aerosol (Norwich).
W/Benzoic acid, salicylic acid.
See: NP-27 Liq. (Norwich).

ORTHOHYDROXYPHENYLMERCURIC CHLORIDE.
W/Benzoic acid, salicylic acid, sec.-amyltricresols.
See: Salicresin, Liq.(Upjohn).
W/Zinc acetate, salicylic acid, phenol.
See: Zemacol, Medicated Skin Lotion (Norwich).

ORTHO-NOVUM 1/35-21. (Ortho) Norethindrone 1 mg, ethinyl estradiol 0.035 mg/Tab. Dialpak 21s.
Use: Oral contraceptive.

ORTHO-NOVUM 1/35-28. (Ortho) Norethindrone 1 mg, ethinyl estradiol 0.035 mg/Tab. w/7 inert Tab. Dialpak 28s.
Use: Oral contraceptive.

ORTHO-NOVUM 1/50-21. (Ortho) Norethindrone 1 mg, mestranol 50 mcg/Tab. Dialpak 21s.
Use: Oral contraceptive.

ORTHO-NOVUM 1/50-28. (Ortho) Norethindrone 1 mg, mestranol 50 mcg/Tab. w/7 inert Tab. Dialpak 28s.
Use: Oral contraceptive.

ORTHO-NOVUM 7/7/7/-21 TABLETS. (Ortho) Norethindrone 0.5 mg, ethinyl estradiol 0.035 mg/Tab.; norethindrone 0.75 mg, ethinyl estradiol 0.035 mg/Tab.; norethindrone 1 mg, ethinyl estradiol 0.035 mg/Tab. Dialpak 21s.
Use: Oral contraceptive.

ORTHO-NOVUM 7/7/7/-28 TABLETS. (Ortho) Same as Ortho-Novum 7/7/7/-21 w/7 inert tab. Dialpak 28s.
Use: Oral contraceptive.

ORTHO-NOVUM 10/11-21 TABLETS. (Ortho) Norethindrone 0.5 mg, ethinyl estradiol 0.035 mg/Tab; norethindrone 1 mg, ethinyl estradiol 0.035 mg/Tab. Dialpak 21s.
Use: Oral contraceptive.

ORTHO-NOVUM 10/11-28 TABLETS. (Ortho) Norethindrone 0.5 mg, ethinyl estradiol 0.035 mg/Tab; norethindrone 1 mg, ethinyl estradiol 0.035 mg/Tab; w/inert tab. Dialpak 28s.
Use: Oral contraceptive.

ORTHO PERSONAL LUBRICANT. (Advanced Care) Greaseless, water soluble and non-staining aqueous hydrocolloid gel. Acid buffered to vaginal pH. Tube 2 oz, 4 oz.
Use: Lubricant.

ORTHOXICOL. (Upjohn) Dextromethorphan HBr 10 mg, methoxyphenamine HCl 17 mg/5 ml. Bot. 2 oz, 4 oz, pt.
Use: Antitussive combination.

ORTHOXINE. Methoxyphenamine.

ORTICALM.
Use: Hypotensive, tranquilizer.
See: Serpasil, Prod. (Squibb).

ORUDIS. (Wyeth-Ayerst) Ketoprofen 25 mg, 50 mg or 75 mg/Cap. Bot. 100s, 500s.
Use: Nonsteroidal anti-inflammatory drug; analgesic.

ORVUS.
See: Gardinol Type Detergents (Various Mfr.).

OSARSAL.
See: Acetarsone.

OS-CAL 250. (Marion) Oyster shell powder as calcium 250 mg, vitamin D 125 IU and trace minerals (Cu, Fe, Mg, Mn, Zn, silica)/Tab. Bot. 100s, 240s, 500s, 1000s.
Use: Calcium/vitamin D supplement.

OS-CAL 500. (Marion) Calcium 500 mg/Tab. Bot. 60s, 120s.
Use: Calcium supplement.

OS-CAL + D. (Marion) Calcium carbonate 625 mg, vitamin D 125 units/Tab. Bot. 100s.
Use: Calcium/vitamin D supplement.

OS-CAL 500 + D. (Marion) Calcium carbonate 1250 mg, vitamin D 125 units/Tab. Bot. 60s.
Use: Calcium/vitamin D supplement.

OS-CAL 500 CHEWABLE TABLETS. (Marion) Calcium 500 mg/Tab. Bot. 60s.
Use: Calcium supplement.

OS-CAL-FORTE. (Marion) Calcium 250 mg, iron 5 mg, magnesium 1.6 mg, manganese 0.3 mg, zinc 0.5 mg, vitamin A 1668 IU, D 125 IU, B_1 1.7 mg, B_2 1.7 mg, B_6 2 mg, niacinamide 15 mg, C 50 mg, E 0.83 IU/Tab. Bot. 100s.
Use: Vitamin/mineral supplement.

OS-CAL PLUS. (Marion) Calcium 250 mg, vitamins D 125 IU, A 1666 IU, C 33 mg, B_2 0.66 mg, B_1 0.5 mg, B_6 0.5 mg, niacinamide 3.33 mg, zinc 0.75 mg, manganese 0.75 mg, iron 16.6 mg/Tab. Bot. 100s.
Use: Vitamin/mineral supplement.

OSMITROL. (Travenol) Mannitol in water. **5%:** 1000 ml; **10%**: 500 ml, 1000 ml; **15%:** 150 ml, 500 ml; **20%:** 250 ml, 500 ml. Mannitol in 0.3% sodium **5%:** 1000 ml. Mannitol in 0.45% sodium **20%:** 500 ml.
Use: Osmotic diuretic.
See: Mannitol.

OSMOGLYN. (Alcon Surgical) Glycerin 50% in flavored aqueous vehicle. Plastic bot. 6 oz.
Use: Osmotic diuretic.

OSMOLITE. (Ross) Isotonic liquid food containing 1.06 calories/ml. Two quarts (2000 calories) provides 100% US RDA vitamins and minerals for adults and children. Osmolality: 300 mOsm/kg water. Ready-to-Use: Bot. Can 8 fl oz, 32 fl oz.
Use: Enteral nutritional supplement.

OSMOLITE HN. (Ross) High nitrogen isotonic liquid food containing 1.06 calories/ml; 1400 calories provides 100% US RDA vitamins and minerals for adults and children. Osmolality: 300 mOsm/kg water. Ready-to-Use: Bot. 8 fl oz. Can 8 fl oz, 32 fl oz.
Use: Enteral nutritional supplement.

OSPOLOT. Tetrahydro-2-(p-sulfa-molyphenyl)-1,2-thiazine-1,1-dioxide.
Use: Anticonvulsant drug; pending release.

OSSONATE CAPSULE. (Marcen) Cartilage mucopolysaccharide extract, chondroitin sulfate 50 mg/Cap. Bot. 100s, 500s, 1000s.

OSSONATE-PLUS, CAPS. (Marcen) Ossonate-

mucopolysaccharide extract 50 mg, acetaminophen 300 mg, salicylamide 200 mg/Cap. Bot. 100s, 500s, 1000s.
Use: Anti-arthritic agent.

OSSONATE-PLUS, INJ. (Marcen) Ossonate cartilage mucopolysaccharide extract 12.5 mg, casein hydrolysates 80 mg, sulfur 20 mg, sodium citrate 5 mg, benzyl alcohol 0.5%, phenol 0.5%/ml. Multidose 10 ml vial.
Use: Skeletal muscle relaxant, pain reliever.

OSSONATE-75. (Marcen) Chondroitin sulfate 37.5 mg, benzyl alcohol 0.5%, phenol 0.5%, sodium citrate 5 mg/ml. Vial 10 ml.
Use: Infantile and atopic eczemas, drug allergies, dermatoses associated with intestinal toxemias.

OSTEOLATE INJECTION. (Fellows) Sodium thiosalicylate 50 mg, benzyl alcohol 2%/ml. Vial 30 ml.
Use: Salicylate analgesic.

OSTEON/D. (Pasadena Research) Calcium 600 mg, phosphorus 400 mg, magnesium 240 mg, vitamin D 400 IU/6 Tab. Bot. 180s.
Use: Vitamin/mineral supplement.

OSTI-DERM LOTION. (Pedinol) Liquified phenol, glycerin, zinc oxide, magnesium carbonate, aluminum acetate solution, camphor water, in hydrated aluminum silicate gel. Tube 45 ml.
Use: Antipruritic, astringent.

OSTO-K. (Parthenon) Potassium 1 mEq (39 mg from gluconate, Cl and citrate), vitamin C 25 mg, sodium 0.52 mg/Tab. Bot. 60s.
Use: Potassium/vitamin C supplement.

OSTREOGRYCIN. B.A.N. Antimicrobial substances produced by *Streptomyces ostreogriseus.* (Specific substances are designated by a terminal letter; thus, Ostreogrycin B) Ostreocin is a mixture of Ostreogrycins B and G; Ostreogrycin B is Mikamycin B.

OSVARSAN.
See: Acetarsone.

OTIC DOMEBORO. (Miles Pharm) Acetic acid 2%, aluminum acetate solution. Plastic dropper bot 2 oz.
Use: Otic preparation.

OTIC-HC. (Hauck) Chloroxylenol 1 mg, pramoxine HCl 10 mg, hydrocortisone alcohol 10 mg, benzalkonium Cl 0.2 mg/ml. Bot. 12 ml.
Use: Anti-infective, otic.

OTIC-NEO-CORT DOME.
See: Neo-Cort Dome Otic Soln. (Miles Pharm).

OTIC-PLAIN. (Hauck) Chloroxylenol 1 mg, pramoxine HCl 10 mg, benzalkonium Cl 0.2 mg/ml. Bot. 12 ml.
Use: Anti-infective, otic.

OTIC SOLUTION NO. 1. (Foy) Hydrocortisone alcohol 10 mg, pramoxine HCl 10 mg, benzalkonium Cl 0.2 mg, acetic acid glacial 20 mg/ml w/ propylene glycol q.s.
Use: Anti-infective, otic.

OTOBIOTIC OTIC SOLUTION. (Schering) Polymixin B, hydrocortisone in propylene glycol and glycerin vehicle w/edetate disodium, sodium bisulfite, anhydrous sodium sulfite, purified water. Bot. w/dropper 15 ml.
Use: Otic preparation.

OTOCAIN. (Holloway) Benzocaine 20%, benzethonium Cl 0.1%, glycerin 1%, polyethylene glycol. Soln. Bot. 15 ml.
Use: Local anesthetic, otic.

OTOCALM-H EAR DROPS. (Parmed) Pramoxine HCl 10 mg, hydrocortisone alcohol 10%, p-Chloro-m-Xylenol 1 mg, benzalkonium Cl 0.2 mg, acetic acid glacial 20 mg, propylene glycol/ml. Bot. 10 ml.
Use: Anti-infective, otic.

OTOCORT STERILE SOLUTION. (Lemmon) Neomycin sulfate equivalent to 3.5 mg neomycin base, polymyxin B sulfate 10,000 units, hydrocortisone 10 mg/ml, propylene glycol, glycerin, potassium metabisulfite, HCl, purified water. Bot. 10 ml.
Use: Anti-infective, otic.

OTOCORT STERILE SUSPENSION. (Lemmon) Neomycin sulfate equivalent to 3.5 mg neomycin base, polymyxin B sulfate 10,000 units, hydrocortisone 10 mg/ml, cetyl alcohol, propylene glycol, polysorbate 80, thimerosal, water for injection. Bot. 10 ml.
Use: Anti-infective, otic.

OTO DROPS. (Standex) Benzocaine 0.85%, antipyrine 3.2%, glycerol q.s./0.5 oz. Bot. 0.5 oz.
Use: Local anesthetic, otic.

OTOGESIC HC SOLUTION. (Metro Med) Polymyxin B sulfate 10,000 IU, neomycin sulfate 3.5 mg, hydrocortisone 10 mg/ml, potassium metabisulfite 0.1%. Bot. 10 ml.
Use: Anti-infective, otic.

OTOGESIC HC SUSPENSION. (Metro Med) Polymyxin B sulfate 10,000 units, neomycin sulfate 3.5 mg, hydrocortisone 10 mg/ml, benzalkonium Cl 0.01%. Bot. 10 ml.
Use: Anti-infective, otic.

OTOMYCIN-HPN. (Misemer) Polymyxin B sulfate 10,000 units, neomycin sulfate 3.5 mg, hydrocortisone 10 mg/ml. Bot. w/dropper 10 ml.
Use: Anti-infective, otic.

OTOREID-HC. (Solvay) Hydrocortisone-free alcohol 10 mg (1%), polymyxin B sulfate 10,000 units, neomycin sulfate equivalent to neomycin base 3.5 mg. Dropper bot. 10 ml.
Use: Anti-infective, otic.

OTOSTAN H.C. (Standex) Pramoxine HCl 1%, hydrocortisone 1%, parachlorometaxylenol 0.1%, benzalkonium Cl 0.02%, acetic acid 2%, propylene glycol. Vial 10 ml.
Use: Otic preparation.

OTRIVIN. (Geigy) Xylometazoline HCl. **Nasal Drops:** 0.1% w/sodium Cl, phenylmercuric acetate 1:50,000. Dropper bot. 20 ml. **Nasal Spray:** 0.1% w/potassium phosphate monobasic, potassium Cl, sodium phosphate dibasic, sodium Cl, benzalkonium Cl 1:5000. Plastic

squeeze spray 15 ml. **Ped. Nasal Soln. Drops:** 0.05%. Bot. 20 ml.
Use: Nasal decongestant.

OUABAIN OCTAHYDRATE. Ouabain, U.S.P. XXII.

OUTGRO. (Whitehall) Chlorobutanol 5%, tannic acid 25%, isopropyl alcohol 83%. Bot. 13 oz.
Use: Ingrown toenail preparation.

OVARIAN EXTRACT. Aqueous extract of whole ovaries of cattle.
Use: Estrogen.

OVARIAN SUBSTANCE. (Various Mfr.) Whole ovarian substance from cattle, sheep or swine.
Use: Estrogen.

OVCON-35. (Mead Johnson Nutrition) Norethindrone 0.4 mg, ethinyl estradiol 0.035 mg/Tab. Ctn. 6×21s.
Use: Oral contraceptive.

OVCON-35, 28 day. (Mead Johnson Nutrition) Norethindrone 0.4 mg, ethinyl estradiol 0.035 mg, w/7 inert tab/Carton 6×28s.
Use: Oral contraceptive.

OVCON-50. (Mead Johnson Nutrition) Norethindrone 1 mg, ethinyl estradiol 0.05 mg/Tab. Ctn. 6×21s.
Use: Oral contraceptive.

OVCON-50, 28 day. (Mead Johnson Nutrition) Norethindrone 1 mg, ethinyl estradiol 0.05 mg, w/7 inert tab/Carton. 6×28s.
Use: Oral contraceptive.

OVIFOLLIN.
See: Estrone (Various Mfr.).

OVLIN. (Sig) **Tab.:** Ethinyl estradiol 0.02 mg, conjugated estrogens 0.2 mg/Tab. Bot. 100s, 1000s. **Inj.:** Estrone 2 mg, estradiol 0.05 mg, vitamin B_{12} 1000 mcg/ml. Vial 30 ml.
Use: Estrogen.

OVOCYLIN DIPROPIONATE. (Ciba) Estradiol dipropionate.
Use: Estrogen.

OVRAL. (Wyeth-Ayerst) Norgestrel 0.5 mg, ethinyl estradiol 0.05 mg/Tab. 6 Pilpak dispensers, 21 Tab. Tripak 63s.
Use: Oral contraceptive.

OVRAL-28. (Wyeth-Ayerst) Norgestrel 0.5 mg, ethinyl estradiol 0.05 mg/Tab. w/7 inert Tab. Pilpak dispenser 6s containing 21 Tab, 7 inert Tab.
Use: Oral contraceptive.

OVRETTE. (Wyeth-Ayerst) Norgestrel 0.075 mg/Tab. 6 Pilpak dispenser, Tab. 28s.
Use: Oral contraceptive.

O-V STATIN. (Squibb Mark) Nystatin. Oral/vaginal therapy pack containing 42 Mycostatin oral Tab. (500,000 units/Tab.), 14 Mycostatin Vaginal Tab (100,000 units/Tab.).
Use: Antifungal, vaginal.

OVULEN-21. (Searle) Ethynodiol diacetate 1 mg, mestranol 0.1 mg/Tab. Compack Disp. 21s, 6×21, 24×21. Refill 21s, 12×21.
Use: Oral contraceptive.

OVULEN-28. (Searle) Ethynodiol diacetate 1 mg, mestranol 0.1 mg/Tab. w/7 inert Tab. Compack 28s: 21 active tab., 7 placebo tab. Compack dispenser 28s. Box 6×28. Refill 28s, Box 12×28.
Use: Oral contraceptive.

OVUSTICK SELF-TEST. (Monoclonal Antibodies) Home test for ovulation. Test kit 10s.
Use: Diagnostic aid.

OXABID. (Jamieson-McKames) Magnesium oxide 140 mg or magnesium oxide heavy 400 mg/Cap. Bot. 100s.
Use: Antacid.

•**OXACILLIN, SODIUM,** U.S.P. XXII. Cap., Inj., Soln., Sterile, U.S.P. XXII. 5-Methyl-3-phenyl-4-isoxazolyl penicillin. Sodium 3,3-Dimethyl-6-(5-methyl-3-phenyl-4-isoxazole-carboxamido)-7-oxocarboxylate.
Use: Antibiotic.
See: Bactocill, Cap., Vial (Beecham Labs).
Prostaphilin, Preps. (Bristol).
Sodium oxacillin.

OXADIMEDINE HCl. N-(2-Benzoxazolyl)-N-benzyl-N′,N′-dimethylethylenediamine HCl.
Use: Antiarrhythmic.

OXAFURADENE. Name used for Nifuradene.
Use: Platelet aggregation agent.

•**OXAGRELATE.** USAN.
Use: Platelet aggregation agent.

•**OXAMARIN HYDROCHLORIDE.** USAN. 6,-7-bis[2-(Diethylamino)-ethoxy]-4-methylcoumarin dihydrochloride.
Use: Systemic hemostat.

•**OXAMISOLE HYDROCHLORIDE.** USAN.
Use: Immunoregulator.

•**OXAMNIQUINE,** U.S.P. XXII. Cap., U.S.P. XXII. 6-Hydroxymethyl-2-isopropylaminomethyl-7-nitro-1,2,3,4-tetrahydroquino-line.
Use: Treatment of schistosomiasis.
See: Vansil, Cap. (Pfizer Laboratories).

OXANAMIDE. 2-Ethyl-3-propyl glycidamide.
Use: Tranquilizer.

•**OXANDROLONE,** U.S.P. XXII. Tab., U.S.P. XX (1) Dodecahydro-3-hydroxy-6-(hydroxy-methyl)-3,3α,-6-trimethyl-1H-benz[e]indene-7-acetic acid, a-lactone. (2) 17 β-hydroxy-17-methyl-2-oxa-5α-androstan-3-one.
Use: Anabolic.
See: Anavar, Tab. (Searle).

•**OXANTEL PAMOATE.** USAN.
Use: Anthelmintic.

•**OXAPROTILINE HYDROCHLORIDE.** USAN.
Use: Antidepressant.

•**OXAPROZIN.** USAN. 3-(4,5-Diphenyloxazol-2-yl)-propionicacid.
Use: Anti-inflammatory.

•**OXARBAZOLE.** USAN.
Use: Antiasthmatic.

•**OXATOMIDE.** USAN.
Use: Anti-allergic, antiasthmatic.

•**OXAZEPAM,** U.S.P. XXII. Cap., Tab., U.S.P.

XXII. 7-Chloro-1,3-dihydro-3-hydroxy-5-phenyl-2H-1,4-benzodia-zepin-2-one. Serenid-D.
Use: Sedative.
See: Serax, Cap., Tab. (Wyeth-Ayerst).

OX BILE EXTRACT. Purified oxgall.
See: Bile Extract, Ox.

OXELADIN. B.A.N. 2-(2-Diethylaminoethoxy)-ethyl 2-eethyl-2-phenylbutyrate. Pectamol citrate.
Use: Cough suppressant.

•**OXENDOLONE.** USAN.
Use: Antiandrogen (benign prostatic hypertrophy).

•**OXETHAZAINE.** USAN. 2-Di-(N-methyl-N-phenyl-tert. butyl-carbamoyl-methyl)-aminoethanol; N,N-bis-(N-methyl-N-phenyl-t-butyl-acetamido)-beta-hydroxethyl-amino). 2,2′-[(2-Hydroxyethyl)imino]bis-[N-(α,α- dimethylphenethyl)-N-methylacetamide]. 2-Di-[(Nαα-trimethylphenethylcarbamoyl-methyl]-amino- ethanol.
Use: Local anesthetic.

•**OXETORONE FUMARATE.** USAN.
Use: Analgesic specific for migraine.

•**OXFENDAZOLE.** USAN.
Use: Anthelmintic.
See: Synanthic (Syntex).

•**OXFENICINE.** USAN.
Use: Vasodilator.

•**OXYFILCON A.** USAN.
Use: Contact lens material.

OX GALL.
See: Bile Extract, Ox.

•**OXIBENDAZOLE.** USAN.
Use: Anthelmintic.

•**OXICONAZOLE NITRATE.** USAN.
Use: Antifungal.
See: Oxistat, Crm. (Glaxo).

OXIDIZED BILE ACIDS.
See: Bile Acids, Oxidized.

•**OXIDIZED CELLULOSE,** U.S.P. XXII. Absorbable cellulose. Cellulosic acid.
Use: Local hemostatic.

•**OXIDOPAMINE.** USAN.
Use: Adrenergic.

•**OXIFUNGIN HYDROCHLORIDE.** USAN.
Use: Antifungal.

•**OXILORPHAN.** USAN.
Use: Antagonist to narcotics.

•**OXIMONAM.** USAN.
Use: Antibacterial.

OXINE.
See: Oxyquinoline sulfate (Various Mfr.).

•**OXIPEROMIDE.** USAN.
Use: Antipsychotic.

OXIPOR VHC PSORIASIS LOTION. (Whitehall) Coal tar soln. 48.5%, salicylic acid 1%, benzocaine 2%, alcohol 81%. Bot. 1.9 oz, 4 oz.
Use: Antipsoriatic.

•**OXIRAMIDE.** USAN.
Use: Cardiac depressant.

OXISTAT. (Glaxo) Oxiconazole nitrate 1%. Cream. Tube 15 Gm, 30 Gm.
Use: Anti-infective, external.

•**OXISURAN.** USAN. (Methyl-sulfinyl)-methyl-2-pyridyl ketone.
Use: Antineoplastic agent.

•**OXMETIDINE HYDROCHLORIDE.** USAN.
Use: Antagonist to histamine receptors.

•**OXMETIDINE MESYLATE.** USAN.
Use: Antagonist to histimine receptors.

•**OXOGESTONE PHENPROPIONATE.** USAN. **#1:** 20β-Hydroxy-19-norpregn-4-en-3-one hydrocinnamate. **#2:** 20β-hydroxy-19-nor-4-pregnen-3-one 20-phenylpropionate.
Use: Progestin.

OXOLAMINE. (Arcum) Crystalline hydroxycobalamin 1000 mcg/ml. Vial 10 ml.
Use: Vitamin B_{12} supplement.

OXOPHENARSINE HYDROCHLORIDE. 2-Amino-4-arsenophenol hydrochloride.

OXPENTIFYLLINE. B.A.N. 3,7-Dimethyl-1-(5-oxohexyl)xanthine. Pentoxifylline (I.N.N.).
Use: Vasodilator.
See: Trental (Hoechst).

OXPHENERIDINE. 1-(β-phenyl-β-hydroxy-ethyl)-4-carbethoxy-4-phenylpiperidine.

•**OXPRENOLOL HCl,** U.S.P. XXII, USAN. Extended release tab., U.S.P. XXII. (±) 1-[o-(Allyloxy)-phenoxy]-3-(isopropylamino)-2-propanol HCl. Trasicor. Under study.
Use: Beta-adrenergic receptor blocking agent.

OXSORALEN CAPSULES. (Elder) Methoxsalen 10 mg/Cap. Bot. 30s, 100s.
Use: Psoralen.

OXSORALEN LOTION. (Elder) Methoxsalen 1% in an inert lotion vehicle of alcohol 71%, propylene glycol, acetone, water. Bot. oz.
Use: Psoralen, topical.

OXSORALEN-ULTRA. (Elder) Methoxsalen 10 mg/Cap. Bot. 50s, 100s.
Use: Psoralen.

•**OXTRIPHYLLINE,** U.S.P. XXII. Oral Soln, ER Tab., U.S.P. XXII. Choline theophyllinate.
Use: Bronchodilator.
See: Choledyl, Tab., Elix. (Parke-Davis).
W/Guaifenesin.
See: Brondecon, Tab., Elix. (Parke-Davis).

OXY-5 ACNE-PIMPLE MEDICATION. (Norcliff Thayer) Benzoyl peroxide 5% in lotion base. Bot. fl oz.
Use: Anti-acne.

OXY-10 COVER MAXIMUM STRENGTH ACNE-PIMPLE MEDICATION. (Norcliff Thayer) Benzoyl peroxide 10%. Lot. Bot. oz.
Use: Anti-acne.

OXY-10 MAXIMUM STRENGTH ACNE-PIMPLE MEDICATION. (Norcliff Thayer) Benzoyl peroxide 10% in lotion base. Bot. fl oz.
Use: Anti-acne.

OXY-10 WASH ANTIBACTERIAL SKIN WASH. (Norcliff Thayer) Benzoyl peroxide 10%. Bot. 4 fl oz.

Use: Anti-acne.

OXYBENZONE, U.S.P. XXII. 2-Hydroxy-4-methoxybenzophenone. Methanone, (2-hydroxy-4-methoxyphenyl)phenyl-. Cyasorb UV 9 (Lederle).
Use: Ultraviolet screen.
W/Dioxybenzone, benzophenone.
See: Solbar, Lot. (Person & Covey).

OXYBENZONE WITH COMBINATIONS.
See: Coppertone, Prods. (Schering-Plough).
Noskote, Cream (Schering-Plough.
Shade, Prods. (Schering-Plough).
Sunger, Prods. (Schering-Plough).
Super Shade, Lot. (Schering-Plough).

OXYBUPROCAINE. B.A.N. 2-Diethylaminoethyl 4-amino-3-butoxybenzoate. Novesine hydrochloride.
Use: Local anesthetic.

OXYBUTYNIN CHLORIDE, U.S.P. XXII. Syr., Tab., U.S.P. XXII. 4-Diethylamino-2-butynyl-α-phenylcyclo-hexanegly-colate hydrochloride.
Use: Anticholinergic.
See: Ditropan Syr., Tab. (Marion Lab.).
Oxybutynin Cl (Mead Johnson).

OXYCEL. (Deseret) Cellulosic acid in absorbable hemostatic agent prepared from cellulose. Resembles ordinary surgical gauze or cotton. Pledget 2 × 1 × 1 in. 10s. Pad 3 × 3 in. 8 ply. 10s. Strip 5 × 0.5 in. 4 ply. 18 × 2 in. 4 ply. 10s. 36 × 0.5 in. 4 ply.
Use: Hemostatic, topical.

OXYCET. (Halsey) Oxycodone HCl 5 mg, acetaminophen 325 mg/Tab. Bot. 100s, 500s, Hospital pack 250s.
Use: Narcotic analgesic combination.

OXYCINCHOPHEN. B.A.N. 3-Hydroxy-2-phenylquinoline-4-carboxylic acid.
Use: Uricosuric.

OXY-CHINOL. (Ferndale) Potassium oxyquinoline sulfate 1 gr/Tab. Bot. 100s, 1000s.
Use: Deodorizer, bacteriostatic.

•**OXYCHLOROSENE.** USAN. Monoxychlorosene. Hydrocarbon derivative containing fourteen carbons and hypochlorous acid. The hydrocarbon chain also has a phenyl substituent which in turn holds a sulfonic acid group.
Use: Anti-infective, topical.
See: Clorpactin, Prod. (Scrip).

•**OXYCHLOROSEN SODIUM.** USAN. Sodium salt of the complex derived from hypochlorous acid and tetradecylbenzene sulfonic acid. Action of active chlorine.
Use: Anti-infective, topical.

OXY CLEAN LATHERING FACIAL. (Norcliff Thayer) Sodium tetraborate decahydrate dissolving particles in a base of surfactant cleaning agents. Soap free. Scrub 79.5 Gm.
Use: Anti-acne.

OXY CLEAN MEDICATED CLEANSER AND PADS. (Norcliff Thayer) **Cleanser and reg. strength pads:** Salicylic acid 0.5%, SD alcohol 40 B 40%, citric acid, menthol, sodium lauryl sulfate. **Max. strength pads:** Salicylic acid 2%, SD alcohol 40 B 50%, citric acid, menthol, sodium lauryl sulfate. Cleanser 120 ml Pad. 50s.
Use: Anti-acne.

OXY CLEAN SOAP. (Norcliff Thayer) Salicylic acid 3.5%, sodium borate. Bar 97.5 Gm.
Use: Anti-acne.

OXYCLOZANIDE. V.B.A.N. 3,3′,5,5′,6-Pentachloro-2′-hydroxysalicylanilide. Zanil.
Use: Anthelmintic, veterinary medicine.

•**OXYCODONE.** USAN. 7,8-Dihydro-14-hydroxy-O^3-methylmorphinone. Dihydrohydroxycodeineone Eucodal hydrochloride; Proladone pectinate.
Use: Narcotic analgesic.

OXYCODONE AND ASPIRIN. (Various Mfr.) Oxycodone HCl 4.5 mg, oxycodone terephthalate 0.38 mg, aspirin 325 mg/Tab. Bot. 100s, 500s.
Use: Narcotic analgesic combination.

•**OXYCODONE AND ACETAMINOPHEN CAPSULES,** U.S.P. XXII.
Use: Analgesic.

•**OXYCODONE AND ACETAMINOPHEN TABLETS,** U.S.P. XXII.
Use: Analgesic.

•**OXYCODONE HYDROCHLORIDE,** U.S.P. XXII, Oral Soln. **(1)**(−)-4,5α-Epoxy-14-hydroxy-3-methoxy-17-methylmorphinan-6-one, **(2)**(−)-14-Hydroxydi-hydrocodeinone.
Use: Narcotic analgesic.
See: Dihydrohydroxycodeinone HCl.
W/Acetaminophen, oxycodone terephthalate.
See: Percocet-5, Tab. (Du Pont).
Tylox, Cap. (McNeil).

OXY COVER. (Norcliff Thayer) Benzoyl peroxide 10%. Cream. 30 Gm.
Use: Anti-acne.

OXYETHYLATED TERTIARY OCTYLPHENOL-FORMALDEHYDE POLYMER.
See: Triton WR-1339 (Rohm & Haas).

OXYETHYLENE OXYPROPYLENE POLYMER.
See: Poloxalkol.
W/Danthron, B_1, carboxymethyl cellulose.
See: Evactol, Cap. (Delta).

OXYFEDRINE. B.A.N. L-3-[(β-Hydroxy-α-methylphen-ethyl-amino]-3′-methoxypropiophenone. Ildamen hydrochloride.
Use: Coronary vasodilator.

•**OXYGEN,** U.S.P. XXII.
Use: Medicinal.

•**OXYGEN 93 PERCENT,** U.S.P. XXII.
Use: Medicinal.

OXYMESTERONE. B.A.N. 4,17β-Dihydroxy-17α-methylandrost-4-en-3-one. 4-Hydroxy-17α-methyl-testosterone. Oranabol.
Use: Anabolic steroid.

OXYMETAZOLINE. B.A.N. 2-(4-t-Butyl-3-hydroxy-2,6-dimethylbenzyl)-2-imidazoline. Afrin and Hazol hydrochloride.
Use: Vasoconstrictor.

•**OXYMETAZOLINE HYDROCHLORIDE,** U.S.P. XXII. Nasal Soln., U.S.P. XXII. Phenol, 3-[(4,5-

dihydro-1H-imidazol-2-yl-)methyl]-6-(1,1-dimethyl-ethyl)-2,4-dimethyl-, monohydrochloride. 6-Tert-butyl-3-(2-imidazolin-2-ylmethyl)-2,4-dimethylphenol HCl.
Use: Decongestant, adrenergic.
See: Afrin, Nasal Spray, Soln. (Schering).
Duration Nasal Spray (Schering-Plough).
Duration Nose Drops (Schering-Plough).
Duration Nose Drops for Children (Schering-Plough).
St. Joseph Nasal Spray for Children (Schering-Plough).
St. Joseph Nose Drops for Children (Schering-Plough).

•**OXYMETHOLONE,** U.S.P. XXII. Tab., U.S.P. XXII. 17-beta-Hydroxy-2-(hydroxymethylene)-17-methyl-5α-androstan-3-one.
Use: Androgen.
See: Anadrol, Tab. (Syntex).

•**OXYMORPHONE HCl,** U.S.P. XXII. Inj., Supp., U.S.P. XXII. 14-Hydroxydihydromorphinone HCl. 4,5α-Epoxy-3,14-dihydroxy-17-methylmorphinan-6-one Hydrochloride.
Use: Analgesic, narcotic.
See: Numorphan Amp., Vial, Supp. (Du Pont).

•**OXYPERTINE.** USAN. 5,6-Dimethoxy-2-methyl-3-[2-(4-phenyl-1-piperazinyl-ethyl]indole. 1-[2-(5,6-Dimethoxy-2-methylindol-3-yl)ethyl]-4-phenylpiperazine. Integrin hydrochloride.
Use: Psychotropic.

•**OXYPHENBUTAZONE,** U.S.P. XXII. Tab., U.S.P. XXII. 1-(p-Hy-droxyphenyl)-2-phenyl-4-butyl-3,5-pyrazolidine-dione. Oxazolidin. 4-Butyl-1-(p-hydroxyphenyl)-2-phenyl 3,5-pyrazolidinedione monohydrate.
Use: Antiarthritic, anti-inflammatory analgesic, antipyretic.
See: Oxalid, Tab. (USV Labs.).

•**OXYPHENCYCLIMINE HCl,** U.S.P. XXII. Tab., U.S.P. XXII. 1-Methyl-1,4,5,6-tetrahydro-2-pyrimidylmethyl-alpha-cyclohexyl-alpha-phenylglycolate HCl. (1,4,5,6-Tetrahydro-1-methyl-2-pyrimidinyl)methyl α-phenylcyclohexane-glycolate monohydrochloride.
Use: Antispasmodic.
See: Daricon, Tab. (Beecham Labs).
W/Hydroxyzine HCl.
See: Enarax, Tab. (Beecham Labs).
W/Phenobarbital.
See: Daricon-PB, Tab. (Beecham Labs).

OXYPHENISATIN. B.A.N. 3,3-Di-(4-hydroxyphenyl)-indolin-2-one. Bydolax; Contax diacetate.
Use: Laxative.

•**OXYPHENISATIN ACETATE.** USAN. 3,3-bis(p-Hydroxyphenyl)2-indolinone diacetate. Diacetoxydiphenylisatin, Acetphenolisatin, Acetylphenylisatin, Diacetoxyphenyloxindol, Bisatin, Phenylisatin bis-(acetoxyphenyl) oxindol.
Use: Laxative.
See: Endophenolphthalein (Roche).
Isacen (No Mfr. currently lists).
Prulet, Tab. (Mission).
Prulet Liquitab. (Mission).

OXYPHENUDRINE. α-{[(p-Hydroxy-α-methylphenethyl)amino]methyl}proto-catechuyl alcohol.

•**OXYPURINOL.** USAN. 4,6-Dihydroxypyrazolo(3,4-d)pyrimidine. 1H-Pyrazolo[3,4-d]pyrimidine-4,6-diol.
Use: Xanthine oxidase inhibitor.

•**OXYQUINOLINE.** USAN.
Use: Disinfectant.

OXYQUINOLINE BENZOATE. (Merck) Pkg. lb. 8-Hydroxyquinoline benzoate.
W/Alkyl aryl sulfonate, disodium edetate, aminacrine HCl, copper sulfate, sodium sulfate.
See: Triva, Vaginal Jelly, Pow. (Boyle).
W/Benzoic acid, salicylic acid, sodium tetradecyl sulfate.
See: NP-27 Cream (Norwich).

•**OXYQUINOLINE SULFATE,** N.F. XVII. 8-Hydroxyquinoline sulfate.
Use: Disinfectant.
See: Chinosol, Tab., Pow., Vial (Vernon).

OXYQUINOLINE SULFATE W/COMBINATIONS.
See: Oxyzal Wet Dressing, Soln. (Gordon).
Rectal Medicone, Oint. (Medicone).
Rectal Medicone-HC, Oint. (Medicone).
Rectal Medicone Unguent, Oint. (Medicone).
Trapens, Tab. (Mills).
Triticoll, Tab. (Western Research).
Triva, Douche Pow. (Boyle).

OXY-SCRUB. (Norcliff Thayer) Abradant cleanser containing dissolving abradant particles of sodium tetraborate decahydrate. Tube 2.65 oz.
Use: Anti-acne.

OXYSORALEN. 8-Hydroxy-4′,5′,6,7-furocoumarin.
Use: Psoralen.
See: Methoxsalen.

OXYTETRACLOR. (Kenyon) Oxytetracycline HCl 250 mg/Cap. Bot. 100s, 1000s.
Use: Anti-infective, tetracycline.

•**OXYTETRACYCLINE,** U.S.P. XXII. Inj., Sterile, Tab., U.S.P. XXII.
Use: Antibiotic.
See: Oxytetraclor, Cap. (Kenyon).
Terramycin, Prods. (Pfizer Laboratories).

•**OXYTETRACYCLINE AND NYSTATIN CAPSULES,** U.S.P. XXII.
Use: Antibiotic, antifungal.

•**OXYTETRACYCLINE AND NYSTATIN FOR ORAL SUSPENSION,** U.S.P. XXII.
Use: Antibiotic, antifungal.

•**OXYTETRACYCLINE AND HYDROCORTISONE ACETATE OPHTHALMIC SUSPENSION,** U.S.P. XXII.
Use: Antibiotic, anti-inflammatory.

•**OXYTETRACYCLINE AND PHENAZOPYRIDINE HYDROCHLORIDES AND SULFAMETHIZOLE CAPSULES,** U.S.P. XXII.
Use: Antibiotic, urinary analgesic, antispasmodic, anti-infective.

•**OXYTETRACYCLINE CALCIUM,** U.S.P. XXII. Oral Susp., U.S.P. XXII.

Use: Antibiotic.

OXYTETRACYCLINE HYDROCHLORIDE, U.S.P. XXII. Cap., Inj., Sterile, U.S.P. XXII. 5-Hydroxytetracycline HCl. An antibiotic from *Streptomyces rimosus.*
Use: Antibiotic, antirickettsial.
See: Dalimycin, Cap. (Dalin).
Oxlopar, Cap. (Parke-Davis).
Oxy-Kesso-Tetra, Cap. (McKesson).
Terramycin HCl, Preps. (Pfizer Laboratories, Pfipharmecs).
Uri-tet, Cap. (American Urologicals).
Urobiotic (Roerig).

OXYTETRACYCLINE HYDROCHLORIDE AND HYDROCORTISONE OINTMENT, U.S.P. XXII.
Use: Antibiotic, anti-inflammatory.

OXYTETRACYCLINE HYDROCHLORIDE AND POLYMYXIN B SULFATE, U.S.P. XXII.
Use: Antibiotic.

OXYTETRACYCLINE HYDROCHLORIDE AND POLYMYXIN B SULFATE OPHTHALMIC OINTMENT, U.S.P. XXII.
Use: Antibiotic.

OXYTETRACYCLINE HYDROCHLORIDE AND POLYMYXIN B SULFATE TOPICAL POWDER, U.S.P. XXII.
Use: Antibiotic.

OXYTETRACYCLINE HYDROCHLORIDE AND POLYMYXIN B SULFATE VAGINAL TABLETS, U.S.P. XXII.
Use: Antibiotic.

OXYTETRACYCLINE-POLYMYXIN B. Mix of oxytetracycline HCl and polymyxin B sulfate.
Use: Antibiotic.
See: Terramycin HCl w/Polymyxin B.
Sulfate, Oint., Tab., Pow. (Pfizer Laboratories, Pfipharmecs).

OXYTOCICS.
See: Ergot Preps.

OXYTOCIN INJECTION, U.S.P. XXII.
Use: Oxytocic.
See: Pitocin, Amp. (Parke-Davis).
Syntocinon, Amp. (Sandoz).

OXYTOCIN NASAL SOLUTION, U.S.P. XXII.
Use: Oxytocic.

OXYTOCIN, SYNTHETIC.
See: Pitocin, Amp. (Parke-Davis).
Syntocinon, Amp. (Sandoz).
Syntocinon Nasal Spray (Sandoz).

OXY WASH. (Norcliff Thayer) Benzoyl peroxide 10%. Liq. Bot. 120 ml.
Use: Anti-acne.

OXYZAL WET DRESSING. (Gordon) Benzalkonium Cl 1:2000, oxyquinoline sulfate, distilled water. Dropper bot. 1 oz, 4 oz.
Use: Minor skin irritations.

OYSCO. (Rugby) Elemental calcium 500 mg/Tab. Bot. 60s.
Use: Calcium supplement.

OYST-CAL 500. (Goldline) Calcium carbonate 1.25 Gm (calcium 500 mg)/Tab. Bot. 60s, 120s.
Use: Calcium supplement.

OYST-CAL-D. (Goldline) Calcium 250 mg, vitamin D 125 IU/Tab. Bot. 100s, 1000s.
Use: Calcium/vitamin D supplement.

OYSTER SHELLS.
See: Os-Cal, Tab. (Marion).
W/Vitamin D-2.
See: Ostrakal, Tab. (Elder).

OYSTERCAL 500. (Nature's Bounty) Calcium carbonate 1.25 Gm (calcium 500 mg)/Tab. Bot. 100s.
Use: Calcium supplement.

OYSTERCAL-D. (Nature's Bounty) Calcium 250 mg, vitamin D 125 IU/Tab. Bot. 100s, 250s.
Use: Calcium/vitamin D supplement.

•**OZOLINONE.** USAN.
Use: Diuretic.

P

P1E1; P2E1; P3E1; P4E1; P6E1. (Alcon) Pilocarpine HCl 1%, 2%, 3%, 4% or 6% respectively, with epinephrine bitartrate 1%. Plastic dropper vial 15 ml.
Use: Agent for glaucoma.

P.A.A.M. (Kenyon) Acetylsalicylic acid 5 gr, para-aminobenzoic acid 5 gr, vitamin C 50 mg/Tab. Bot. 100s, 1000s.
Use: Salicylate analgesic, vitamin combination.

P AND S LIQUID. (Baker/Cummins) Bot. 4 oz, 8 oz.
Use: Antiseborrheic.

P AND S PLUS. (Baker/Cummins) Coal tar solution 8% (crude coal tar 1.6%, ethyl alcohol 6.4%), salicylic acid 2%. Gel 105 Gm.
Use: Tar-containing preparation, topical.

P AND S SHAMPOO. (Baker/Cummins) Salicylic acid 2%, lactic acid 0.5% Bot. 4 oz.
Use: Antiseborrheic.

PABA-"5". (Durel) P-amino benzoic acid in quick-drying moisturizing base. Bot. 4 oz.
Use: Sunscreen.

PABALAN. (Lannett) Potassium para-amino benzoate 5 gr, potassium salicylate 5 gr, ascorbic acid 50 mg/Tab. Bot. 100s, 1000s.

PABALATE. (Robins) Sodium salicylate 300 mg, sodium aminobenzoate 300 mg/EC Tab. Bot. 100s, 500s.
Use: Antirheumatic.

PABALATE-SF. (Robins) Potassium salicylate 300 mg, potassium aminobenzoate 300 mg/Tab. Bot. 100s, 500s.
Use: Antirheumatic.

PABAQUINONE CREAM. (Dermohr Pharmacal) Hydroquinone 4%, amyl dimethyl paba 3% in creamy base. Tube oz.
Use: Skin-bleaching agent.

PABA-SALICYLATE. (Various Mfr.) Sodium salicylate, p-aminobenzoate, vitamin C/Tab. Bot. 100s, 500s.
Use: Salicylate analgesic, vitamin combination.

PABA SODIUM. (Various Mfr.). Sodium p-aminobenzoate.

Use: Vitamin supplement.
PABASONE. (Pinex) Sodium salicylate 5 gr, para-aminobenzoic acid 5 gr, ascorbic acid 20 mg/Tab. Bot. 100s.
Use: Salicylate analgesic, vitamin combination.
P-A-C. Preparations of phenacetin, aspirin, caffeine.
See: A.P.C. Preparations, Empirin Preparations.
P-A-C REVISED FORMULA ANALGESIC. (Upjohn) Aspirin 400 mg, caffeine 32 mg/Tab. Bot. 100s, 1000s.
Use: Salicylate analgesic.
PACEMAKER PROPHYLAXIS PASTES WITH FLUORIDE. (Pacemaker) Silicone dioxide and diatomaceous earth, sodium fluoride 4.4%. Light abrasive, cinnamon/cherry. Medium abrasive, orange. Heavy abrasive, mint. Paste Bot. 8 oz.
Use: Dental caries preventative.
PACKER'S PINE TAR LIQUID SHAMPOO. (Rydelle) Bot. 6 fl oz.
Use: Antiseborrheic.
PACKER'S PINE TAR SOAP. (Rydelle) Bar 3.3 oz.
Use: Tar-containing preparation, topical.
PACLIN G. (Geneva) Penicillin G potassium.
Tab.: 100 M units or 200 M units: Bot. 1000s.
250 M units or 400 M units: Bot. 100s, 1000s.
Use: Antibacterial, penicillin.
PACLIN VK. (Geneva) Penicillin phenoxymethyl 125 mg or 250 mg/Tab. Bot. 100s, 1000s.
Use: Antibacterial, penicillin.
•**PADIMATE A.** USAN.
Use: Ultraviolet screen.
•**PADIMATE O.** USAN.
Use: Ultraviolet screen.
See: Coppertone Prods. (Schering-Plough).
Eclipse Prods. (Dorsey).
Escalol 506 (Van Dyk).
Noskote Prods. (Schering-Plough).
Pabafilm (Owen).
Shade Prods. (Schering-Plough).
Sunger Prods. (Schering-Plough).
Super Shade, Prods. (Schering-Plough).
Tropical Blend Sunscreen Lot. (Schering-Plough).
PAH.
See: Sodium Aminohippurate Inj. (Various Mfr.).
PAIN-A-LAY. (Glessner) Antiseptic, anesthetic soln. Bot. 4 oz w/sprayer, Bot. 4 oz, 8 oz, 1 pt.
Use: Mouth and throat product.
PAIN AND FEVER CAPSULES. (Lederle) Acetaminophen 500 mg/Cap. Bot. 50s, 100s.
Use: Analgesic.
PAIN AND FEVER LIQUID. (Lederle) Acetaminophen 160 mg/5 ml (children's strength). Unit-of-use 4 oz, Bot. 16 oz.
Use: Analgesic.
PAIN AND FEVER TABLETS. (Lederle) Acetaminophen 325 mg or 500 mg/Tab. **325 mg:** Bot. 100s, 1000s; **500 mg:** Bot. 50s, 100s.
Use: Analgesic.
PAIN-EZE. (E.J. Moore) Benzocaine, menthol, peppermint oil. Tube ⅛ oz, ¼ oz.
Use: Local anesthetic.
PAIN RELIEF, ASPIRIN FREE. (Hudson) Acetaminophen 325 mg/Tab. Bot. 100s, 200s.
Use: Analgesic.
PAIN RELIEF OINTMENT. (Walgreen) Methyl salicylate 15%, menthol 10%. Tube 1.5 oz, 3 oz.
Use: External analgesic.
PAIN RELIEVER. (Rugby) Acetaminophen 250 mg, aspirin 250 mg, caffeine 65 mg/Tab. Bot. 100s, 1000s.
Use: Analgesic combination.
PAIN RELIEVERS-TENSION HEADACHE RELIEVERS. (Weeks & Leo) Acetaminophen 325 mg, phenyltoloxamine citrate 30 mg/Tab. Bot. 40s, 100s.
Use: Analgesic combination.
PALBAR NO. 2. (Hauck) Atropine sulfate 0.012 mg, scopolamine HBr 0.005 mg, hyoscyamine HBr 0.018 mg, phenobarbital 32.4 mg/Tab. Bot. 100s.
Use: Anticholinergic/antispasmodic, sedative/hypnotic.
•**PALDIMYCIN.** USAN.
Use: Antibacterial.
PALESTROL.
See: Diethylstilbestrol (Various Mfr.).
PALGESIC. (Pan American) Isobutylallylbarbituric acid ¾ gr, phenacetin 2 gr, aspirin 3 gr, caffeine ⅔ gr/Tab. or Cap. Bot. 100s.
Use: Sedative/hypnotic, salicylate analgesic.
PALINUM.
Use: Sedative/hypnotic.
See: Cyclobarbital Calcium (Various Mfr.).
PALMIDROL. N-(2-Hydroxyethyl)palmitamide.
•**PALMOXIRATE SODIUM.** USAN.
Use: Antidiabetic.
PAMABROM. 2-Amino-2-methyl-1-propanol salt of 8-bromotheophyllinate.
W/Acetaminophen.
See: Pamprin, Tab. (Chattem Labs.).
W/Acetaminophen, pyrilamine maleate.
See: Cardui, Tab. (Chattem Labs.).
Sunril, Cap. (Emko).
W/Pyrilamine maleate, homatropine methylbromide, hyoscyamine sulfate, scopolamine HBr, methamphetamine HCl.
See: Aridol, Tabs. (MPL).
•**PAMATOLOL SULFATE.** USAN.
Use: Anti-adrenergic.
PAM.
See: Melphalan.
PAM-B12 INJ. (Pan American) Cyanocobalamin 1000 mcg/ml. Amp. 10 ml, 30 ml.
Use: Vitamin B_{12} supplement.
PAMELOR. (Sandoz) Nortriptyline HCl. Cap or Liq. **Cap.:** 10 mg, 25 mg, 50 mg or 75 mg base. **10 mg:** Bot. 100s, SandoPak 100s; **25 mg:** Bot. 100s, 500s, SandoPak 100s; **50 mg:** Bot. 100s, SandoPak 100s. **75 mg:** Bot. 100s.
Liq.: Nortriptyline HCl equivalent to 10 mg base/5 ml. Bot. pt.
Use: Antidepressant.

PAMIDRONATE DISODIUM. USAN.
Use: Bone resorption inhibitor.

PAMINE. (Upjohn) Methscopolamine bromide 2.5 mg/Tab. Bot. 100s, 500s.
Use: Anticholinergic/antispasmodic.

PAMPRIN. (Chattem) Acetaminophen 400 mg, pamabrom 25 mg, pyrilamine maleate 15 mg/ Tab. Bot. 24s, 48s.
Use: Analgesic combination.

PAMPRIN EXTRA STRENGTH MULTI-SYMPTOM RELIEF FORMULA TABLETS. (Chattem) Acetaminophen 400 mg, pamabrom 25 mg, pyrilamine maleate 15 mg/Tab. Bot. 12s, 24s, 48s.
Use: Analgesic combination.

PAMPRIN-IB TABLETS. (Chattem) Ibuprofen 200 mg/Tab. Bot. 6s, 12s, 24s.
Use: Nonsteroidal anti-inflammatory drug; analgesic.

PAMPRIN MAXIMUM CRAMP RELIEF FORMULA CAPLETS. (Chattem) Acetaminophen 500 mg, pamabrom 25 mg, pyrilamine maleate 15 mg/Tab. Bot. 8s, 16s, 32s.
Use: Analgesic combination.

PAMPRIN MAXIMUM CRAMP RELIEF FORMULA CAPSULES. (Chattem) Pamabrom 25 mg, acetaminophen 500 mg, pyrilamine maleate 15 mg/Cap. Pkg. 8s, 16s, 32s.
Use: Analgesic combination.

PANACARB. (Lannett) Bismuth subnitrate, sodium bicarbonate, magnesium carbonate, papain, diastase/Tab. Bot. 1000s.
Use: Antacid.

PANADEINE TABLETS. (Winthrop Products) Paracetamol, codeine.
Use: Narcotic analgesic combination.

PANADEINE CO. TABLETS. (Winthrop Products) Paracetamol, codeine.
Use: Narcotic analgesic combination.

PANADIPLON. USAN.
Use: Anxiolytic.

PANADO. (Winthrop Products) Paracetamol, codeine.
Use: Narcotic analgesic combination.

PANADOL. (Glenbrook) Acetaminophen 500 mg/ Tab. or Cap. **Tab:** Bot. 2s, 30s, 60s, 100s; **Cap:** Bot. 10s, 24s, 48s.
Use: Analgesic.

PANADOL CHILDREN'S. (Glenbrook) Acetaminophen. **Tab.:** 80 mg. Bot. 30s. **Liq.:** 80 mg/0.8 ml. Bot. 2 oz, 4 oz. **Drops:** 80 mg/0.5 oz. Bot. 0.5 oz.
Use: Analgesic.

PANADOL JR. (Glenbrook) Acetaminophen 160 mg/Caplet. Box. 30s.
Use: Analgesic.

PANADYL. (Misemer) Pyrilamine maleate 25 mg, phenylpropanolamine HCl 50 mg, pheniramine maleate 25 mg/Tab. Bot. 100s, 1000s.
Use: Antihistamine, decongestant.

PANAFIL. (Rystan) Papain pow. 10%, urea 10%, chlorophyllin copper complex 0.5%, hydrophilic base. Oint. Tube oz, Jar lb.
Use: Topical enzyme preparation.

PANAFIL WHITE OINTMENT. (Rystan) Papain 10,000 units enzyme activity, hydrophilic base/ Gm, urea 10%. Tube oz.
Use: Topical enzyme preparation.

PANAFORT ELIXIR. (Pan American) Lysine mono HCl 800 mg, vitamins B_{12} 30 mcg, B_1 2 mg, B_2 12 mg, B_6 12 mg, niacinamide 100 mg, panthenol 20 mg, alcohol 5%/15 ml. Bot. 8 oz.
Use: Vitamin/amino acid supplement.

PANAFORT TABLETS. (Pan American) Bot. 100s.

PANALGESIC CREAM. (Poythress) Methyl salicylate 35%, menthol 4%. Jar 4 oz.
Use: External analgesic.

PANALGESIC LIQUID. (Poythress) Methyl salicylate 55.01%, menthol 1.25%, camphor 3.1%, in alcohol 22%, emollients, color. Bot. 4 oz, pt, 0.5 gal.
Use: External analgesic.

PAN-APC. (Panray) Aspirin 3.5 gr, phenacetin 2.5 gr, caffeine 0.5 gr/Tab. Bot. 1000s.
Use: Analgesic combination.

PANAPHYLLIN. (Pan American) Theophylline 65 mg, ephedrine HCl 12 mg, guaifenesin 50 mg/5 ml. Susp. Bot. 8 oz.
Use: Bronchodilator, vasoconstrictor, expectorant.

PANASOL. (Seatrace) Prednisone 5 mg/Tab. Bot. 100s.
Use: Corticosteroid.

PANASOL-S. (Seatrace) Prednisone 1 mg/Tab. Bot. 100s, 1000s.
Use: Corticosteroid.

PANASORB DROPS. (Winthrop Products) Paracetamol, codeine.
Use: Narcotic analgesic combination.

PANASORB ELIXIR. (Winthrop Products) Paracetamol, codeine.
Use: Narcotic analgesic combination.

PANASORB SUPPOSITORIES. (Winthrop Products) Paracetamol, codeine.
Use: Narcotic analgesic combination.

PANASORB TABLETS. (Winthrop Products) Paracetamol.
Use: Analgesic.

PANC-500. (Freeda) Hesperidin 100 mg, citrus bioflavonoids 100 mg, rutin 50 mg, vitamin C 500 mg/Tab. Bot. 100s, 250s, 500s.
Use: Vitamin supplement.

PANCARD. (Pan American) Pentaerythritol tetranitrate 10 mg/Tab. Bot. 100s, 500s. Also available w/phenobarbital 20 mg/Tab. Bot. 100s.
Use: Antianginal.

PANCARD 30 TP. (Pan American) Pentaerythritol tetranitrate 30 mg/LA Panseal. Bot. 60s.
Use: Antianginal.

PANCARD 30 TPA. (Pan American) Pentaerythritol tetranitrate 30 mg, amobarbital 50 mg/LA Panseal. Bot. 60s.
Use: Antianginal, sedative/hypnotic.

PANCET. (Pan American) Propoxyphene HCl 65 mg, acetaminophen 650 mg/Tab. Bot. 100s.
Use: Narcotic analgesic combination.

PANCOF EXPECTORANT. (Pan American) Dextromethorphan HBr 15 mg, chlorpheniramine maleate 1 mg, phenylephrine HCl 5 mg/ml.
Use: Antitussive, antihistamine, decongestant.

•**PANCOPRIDE.** USAN.
Use: Antiemetic; antianxiety agent; peristaltic stimulant.

PANCREASE. (McNeil Pharm) Enteric coated pancrelipase capsules. **Regular:** Lipase 4000 units, amylase 20,000 units, protease 25,000 units/Cap. Bot. 100s, 250s; **MT4:** Lipase 4000 units, amylase 12,000 units, protease 12,000 units/Cap. Bot. 100s; **MT10:** Lipase 10,000 units, amylase 30,000 units, protease 30,000 units/Cap. Bot. 100s; **MT16:** Lipase 16,000 units, amylase 48,000 units, protease 48,000 units/Cap. Bot. 100s.
Use: Digestive enzymes.

PANCREATIC ENZYME.
W/Pepsin, ox bile.
See: Nu' Leven, Nu' Leven Plus, Tab. (Lemmon).

PANCREATIC SUBSTANCE. Substance from fresh pancreas of hog or ox, containing the enzymes amylopsin, trypsin, steapsin.
W/Bile extract, dl-methionine, choline bitartrate.
See: Licoplex, Tab. (Mills).
W/Bile salts, lipase.
See: Cotazym-B, Tab. (Organon).
W/Bile, whole (desiccated), oxidized bile acids, homatropine methylbromide.
See: Pancobile, Tab. (Solvay).
W/Lipase.
See: Cotazym, Cap., Packet (Organon).

•**PANCREATIN,** U.S.P. XXII. Cap., Tab., U.S.P. XXII. Pancreatic enzymes obtained from hog or cattle pancreatic tissue.
Use: Digestant.
See: Depancol, Tab. (Warner-Chilcott).
Elzyme, Tab. (Elder).
Panteric, Tab. (Parke-Davis).

PANCREATIN W/COMBINATIONS.
See: Entozyme, Tab. (Robins).
Nu'Leven, Tab. (Lemmon).
Pepsatal, Tab. (Kenyon).
Ro-Bile, Tab. (Solvay).
Sto-Zyme, Tab. (Jalco).
Zypan, Tab. (Standard Process).

•**PANCRELIPASE,** U.S.P. XXII. Cap., Tab., U.S.P. XXII. Formerly Lipancreatin. Preparation of hog pancreas with high content of steapsin and adequate amounts of pancreatic enzymes.
Use: Pancreatic enzymes preparation; digestive aid.
See: Accelerase, Cap. (Organon).
Cotazym, Cap., Packet (Organon).
Viokase, Pow., Tab. (Robins).
W/Mixed conjugated bile salts, cellulase.
See: Accelerase, Cap. (Organon).
Cotazym-B, Tab. (Organon).

PANCREOZYMIN. B.A.N. A hormone obtained from duodenal mucosa.
Use: Diagnostic aid.

PANCRETIDE. (Baxter) Pancreatic polypeptide in normal saline.
Use: Fibrinolytic conditions.

PANCURONIUM.
See: Pancuronium Bromide (Organon).

•**PANCURONIUM BROMIDE.** USAN. (1) 1,1′-(3α,17β-Dihydroxy-5α-androstan-2β,16β-ylene)bis-[1-methylpiperidinium]dibromide diacetate: (2) 2β,16β-dipiperidino-5α-androstane-3α, 17 β-diol diacetate dimethobromide.
Use: Skeletal muscle relaxant.
See: Pavulon, Inj. (Organon).

PANEX. (Mallard) Acetaminophen 325 mg/Tab. Bot. 1000s.
Use: Analgesic.

PANEX 500. (Mallard) Acetaminophen 500 mg/Tab. Bot. 1000s.
Use: Analgesic.

PANFIL. (Pan American) Dyphylline 200 mg/Tab. Bot. 100s.
Use: Bronchodilator.

PANFIL-G. (Pan American) **Tab.:** Dyphylline 200 mg, guaifenesin 50 mg. Bot. 100s. **Elix.:** Dyphylline 100 mg, guaifenesin 50 mg/5 ml. Bot. pt.
Use: Bronchodilator.

PANFLEX CAPSULES. (Pan American) Chlorzoxazone 250 mg, acetaminophen 300 mg/Cap.
Use: Skeletal muscle relaxant, analgesic.

PANHEMATIN. (Abbott) Hemin 313 mg/43 ml when reconstituted. Vial 100 ml.
Use: Agent for acute intermittent porphyria.

PANIDAZOLE. B.A.N. 2-Methyl-5-nitro-1-[2-(4-pyridyl)ethyl]imidazole.
Use: Amebicide.

PANITOL. (Wesley) Allylisobutyl barbituric acid 15 mg, acetaminophen 300 mg/Tab. Bot. 100s, 1000s.
Use: Sedative/hypnotic, analgesic.

PANITOL H.M.B. (Wesley) Panitol formula plus homatropine methylbromide 2.5 mg/Tab. Bot. 100s, 1000s.
Use: Sedative/hypnotic, analgesic, anticholinergic/antispasmodic.

PANMYCIN. (Upjohn) Tetracycline HCl 250 mg/Cap. Bot. 100s, 1000s.
Use: Antibacterial, tetracycline.
See: Panmycin, Cap. (Upjohn).

PAN OB FORTE TABLETS. (Pan American) Ferrous fumarate 150 mg, calcium lactate 333 mg, ergocalciferol 400 IU, vitamins C 100 mg, B_1 3 mg, B_2 3 mg, folic acid 1 mg/Tab.
Use: Vitamin/mineral supplement.

PAN OB TABLETS. (Pan American) Calcium lactate 333 mg, ferrous fumarate 150 mg, vitamins D 400 units, C 25 mg, B_1 1 mg, B_2 1 mg/Tab.
Use: Vitamin/mineral supplement.

PANOXYL ACNE GEL. (Stiefel) Benzoyl peroxide 5% or 10%, alcohol 20%, polyoxyethylene lauryl ether 6% in a hydroalcoholic gel base. Tube 2 oz, 4 oz.
Use: Anti-acne.

PANOXYL AQ ACNE GEL. (Stiefel) Benzoyl peroxide 2.5%, 5% or 10%, polyoxyethylene lauryl ether in an aqueous gel base. Tube 2 oz, 4 oz.
Use: Anti-acne.

PANOXYL BAR-5. (Stiefel) Benzoyl peroxide 5% in a rich-lathering, mild surfactant cleansing base. Bar 4 oz.
Use: Anti-acne.

PANOXYL BAR-10. (Stiefel) Benzoyl peroxide 10% in rich-lathering, mild surfactant cleansing base. Bar 4 oz.
Use: Anti-acne.

PANPARNIT HYDROCHLORIDE. Caramiphen HCl.
Use: Antiparkinson agent.

PANPAV TP PANSEALS. (Pan American) Papaverine HCl 150 mg/TR Cap.
Use: Peripheral vasodilator.

PANPRES. (Pan American) Hydralazine HCl 25 mg, hydrochlorothiazide 15 mg, resperine 0.1 mg/Tab. Bot. 100s.
Use: Antihypertensive agent.

PANRITIS. (Pan American) Salicylamide 250 mg, acetaminophen 250 mg/Tab. Bot. 100s.
Use: Analgesic combination.

PANRITIS FORTE TABLETS. (Pan American) Salicylamide 600 mg, acetaminophen 250 mg/Tab.
Use: Analgesic combination.

PANSCOL. (Baker/Cummins) Salicylic acid 3%, lactic acid 2%, phenol (less than 1%). **Oint.:** Jar 3 oz. **Lot.:** Bot. 4 oz.
Use: Emollient.

PANSHAPE M TP. (Pan American) Phentermine HCl 30 mg/Cap. Bot. 60s.
Use: Anorexiant.

PANTEMIC M. (Pan American) **Tab.:** Ferrous fumarate 300 mg. Bot. 100s. **Susp.:** 100 mg/5 ml. Bot. 8 oz.
Use: Iron supplement.

•**PANTHENOL,** U.S.P. XXII. Alcohol corresponding to pantothenic acid. Pantothenol. Pantothenylol. (±)-2,4-Dihydroxy-N-(3-hydroxypropyl)-3,3-dimethylbutyramide.
Use: Treatment of paralytic ileus and postoperative distention.
See: Ilopan, Amp., Vial (Warren-Teed).
Panadon, Cream (Gordon Labs.).
Panthoderm Cream (USV Pharm).

PANTHENOL W/COMBINATIONS.
See: Geriatrazole Prod., Vial (Kenyon).
Lifer-B, Liq. (Burgin-Arden).
Nutricol, Cap., Inj. (Nutrition Control).
Vi-Testrogen, Vial (Pharmex).

PANTHODERM CREAM. (Rorer) Dexpanthenol 2% in water-miscible cream. Tube 1 oz, Jar 2 oz, lb.
Use: Emollient.

PANTOCAINE.
See: Tetracaine HCl. (Various Mfr.).

PANTOCRIN-F. (Spanner) Plurigland, ovarian, anterior and posterior pituitary, adrenal, thyroid extracts. Vial 30 ml.

PANTOPAQUE. (Alcon Surgical) Iophendylate, ethyl iodophenylundecanoate. Amp. 3 ml 3s; 6 ml 6s; 1 ml 2s.
Use: Radiopaque agent.

PANTOPON. (Roche) Hydrochlorides of opium alkaloids, alcohol 6%, glycerin 136 mg, methyl and propyl parabens 0.2%, acetic acid and/or sodium hydroxide to adjust pH to approximately 3.3. Amp. 20 mg/ml. Box 10s.
Use: Narcotic analgesic.

PANTOTHENIC ACID. As calcium or sodium salt.
Use: Vitamin B_5 supplement.
See: Vitamin preparations.

PANTOTHENIC ACID SALTS.
See: Calcium Pantothenate.
Sodium Pantothenate.

PANTOTHENOL.
See: Panthenol, Preps. (Various Mfr.).

PANTOTHENYL ALCOHOL.
See: Panthenol, Preps. (Various Mfr.).

PANTOTHENYLOL.
See: Panthenol, Preps. (Various Mfr.).

PANVITEX GERIATRIC CAPSULES. (Forest Pharm.) Safflower oil 340 mg, vitamins A 10,000 IU, D 400 IU, B_1 5 mg, B_6 1 mg, B_2 2.5 mg, B_{12} activity 2 mcg, C 75 mg, niacinamide 40 mg, calcium pantothenate 4 mg, E 2 IU, inositol 15 mg, choline bitartrate 31.4 mg, calcium 75 mg, phosphorus 58 mg, iron 30 mg, manganese 0.5 mg, potassium 2 mg, zinc 0.5 mg, magnesium 3 mg/Cap. Bot. 100s, 1000s.
Use: Vitamin/mineral supplement.

PANVITEX GERIATRIC INJ. (Forest Pharm.) Testosterone 10 mg, vitamins B_{12} 100 mcg, B_1 50 mg, nicotinamide 50 mg, B_6 5 mg, estrone 0.5 mg, liver injection equivalent in B_{12} activity of cyanocobalamin 2 mcg, lidocaine 20 mg, panthenol 10 mg, B_2 5 mg/ml. Vial 30 ml.
Use: Vitamin/hormone supplement.

PANVITEX G.H. (Fellows) Methyltestosterone 2 mg, ethinyl estradiol 0.01 mg, vitamins A 5000 IU, D 400 IU, E 10 IU, B_1 2 mg, B_2 2 mg, B_6 0.3 mg, B_{12} 1 mcg, C 30 mg, niacinamide 20 mg, calcium pantothenate 3 mg, choline bitartrate 40 mg, inositol 20 mg, methionine 20 mg, iron sulfate 10 mg, copper 0.2 mg, molybdenum 0.5 mg, manganese 1 mg, zinc 1 mg, magnesium 5 mg, potassium 2 mg, iodine 0.15 mg/SC Tab. Bot. 100s, 1000s.
Use: Vitamin/mineral/hormone supplement.

PANVITEX PLUS MINERALS CAPSULES. (Forest Pharm.) Vitamins A 5000 IU, D 400 IU, B_1 3 mg, B_2 2.5 mg, niacinamide 20 mg, B_6 1.5 mg, calcium pantothenate 5 mg, B_{12} 2.5 mcg, C 50 mg, E 3 IU, calcium 215 mg, phosphorus 166

mg, iron 13.4 mg, magnesium 7.5 mg, manganese 1.5 mg, potassium 5 mg, zinc 1.4 mg/Cap. Bot. 100s, 1000s.
Use: Vitamin/mineral supplement.

PANVITEX PRENATAL CAPSULES. (Forest Pharm.) Ferrous fumarate 150 mg, cobalamin concentration 2 mcg, vitamins A 6000 IU, D 400 IU, B_1 1.5 mg, B_2 2.5 mg, niacinamide 15 mg, B_6 3 mg, C 100 mg, calcium 250 mg, calcium pantothenate 5 mg, folic acid 0.2 mg/Cap. Bot. 100s, 1000s.
Use: Vitamin/mineral supplement.

PANVITEX T-M. (Forest Pharm.) Vitamins A 10,000 IU, D 400 IU, B_1 10 mg, B_6 1 mg, B_2 5 mg, B_{12} 5 mcg, C 150 mg, niacinamide 100 mg, calcium 103 mg, phosphorus 80 mg, iron 10 mg, manganese 1 mg, potassium 5 mg, zinc 1.4 mg, magnesium 5.56 mg/Cap. Bot. 100s, 1000s.
Use: Vitamin/mineral supplement.

PANWARFIN. (Abbott) Warfarin sodium 2 mg, 2.5 mg, 5 mg, 7.5 mg or 10 mg/Tab. Bot. 100s, UD 100s.
Use: Anticoagulant.

PAP. (Abbott Diagnostics) Enzyme immunoassay for measurement of prostatic acid phosphatase. Test kit 100s.
Use: Diagnostic aid.

P.A.P. No. 1. (Jenkins) Phenobarbital 15 mg, acid acetylsalicylic 0.23 Gm, acetophenetidin 0.15 Gm/Tab. Bot. 1000s.
Use: Sedative/hypnotic, analgesic.

PAPA-CARIA. (Jenkins) Magnesium carbonate 100 gr, calcium carbonate 50 gr, sodium bicarbonate 120 gr, bismuth subnitrate 50 gr, cerium oxalate 25 gr, magnesium trisilicate 70 gr, powder ginger 4 gr, papain 11 gr, pancreatin 5.5 gr/oz. Pkg. 2 oz.
Use: Digestive aid.

PAPADEINE #3. (Vangard) Codeine phosphate 30 mg, acetaminophen 300 mg/Tab. Bot. 100s, 1000s.
Use: Narcotic analgesic combination.

•**PAPAIN,** U.S.P. XXII. Tab. for Topical Soln., U.S.P. XXII. A proteolytic substance derived from *Carlica papaya.*
Use: Proteolytic enzyme.
See: Papase, Tab. (Parke-Davis).
Softlens Enzymatic Contact Lens Cleaner (Allergan).

PAPAIN W/COMBINATIONS.
See: Baculin, Tab. (Amfre-Grant).
Bilate, Tab. (Central).
Cerophen, Tab. (Wendt-Bristol).
Digenzyme, Tab. (Burgin-Arden).
Kaocasil, Tab. (Jenkins).
Panacarb, Tab. (Lannett).
Panafil, Oint. (Rystan).

PAP-A-LIX. (Freeport) n-Acetyl-aminophenol 120 mg, alcohol 10%/5 ml. Bot. 4 oz, gal.
Use: Analgesic.

•**PAPAVERINE HYDROCHLORIDE,** U.S.P. XXII. Inj., Tab., U.S.P. XXII. 6,7-Dimethoxy-l-veratrylisoquinoline Hydrochloride.
Use: Smooth muscle relaxant.
See: BP-Papaverine, Cap. (Burlington).
Cerebid Cap. (Saron).
Cerespan, Cap. (Rorer).
Cirbed, Cap. (Boyd).
Delapav, Time Cap. (Dunhall).
Lapay, Graduals (Amfre-Grant).
Myobid, Cap. (Laser).
P-200, Cap. (Boots).
Pavabid, Cap. (Marion).
Pavacap, Unicells (Solvay).
Pavacaps, Cap. (Freeport).
Pavacen Cenules, Cap. (Central).
Pavaclor, Cap. (Pasadena Research).
Pavacron, Cap. (Cenci).
Pavadel, Cap. (Canright).
Pavadyl, Cap. (Bock).
Pavakey 300, Cap. (Key).
Pavakey S.A., Cap. (Key).
Pava-lyn, Cap. (Lynwood).
Pava Par, Cap. (Parmed).
Pavasule, Cap. (Jalco).
Pavatest T.D., Cap. (Fellows-Testagar).
Pavatime, Cap. (Rocky Mtn.).
Pavatym, Cap. (Everett).
Pavatran T.D. Cap. (Mayrand).
Paverolan, Lanacap (Lannett).
Pavex, Cap. (Xxtrium).
Ro-Papav, Tab. (Robinson).
Vasocap, Cap. (Keene).
Vazosan, Tab. (Sandia).
W/Codeine sulfate.
See: Copavin, Pulvule, Tab. (Lilly).
W/Codeine sulfate, aloin, sodium salicylate.
See: Copavin Compound, Elix. (Lilly).
W/Codeine sulfate, emetine HCl, ephedrine HCl.
See: Golacol, Syr. (Arcum).
W/Phenobarbital.
See: Pavadel-PB, Cap. (Canright).

PAPAVEROLINE. B.A.N. 1-(3,4-Dihydroxybenzyl)-6,7-dihydroxyisoquinoline.
Use: Vasodilator.

PARA-AMINOBENZOIC ACID. Aminobenzoic Acid, U.S.P. XXII.
See: Paba-"5", Lot. (Durel).
Pabanol, Lot. (Elder).
Presun, Lot., Gel (Westwood).
W/Acetylsalicylic acid, vitamin C.
See: P.A.A.M., Tab. (Kenyon).

PARA-AMINOSALICYLATE, SODIUM.
See: Aminosalicylate Sodium.

PARA-AMINOSALICYLIC ACID. Aminosalicylic Acid, U.S.P. XXII.

PARABAXIN. (Parmed) Methocarbamol 500 mg or 750 mg/Tab. Bot. 100s.
Use: Skeletal muscle relaxant.

PARABROM.
See: Pyrabrom.

PARABROMIDYLAMINE.

See: Brompheniramine, Dimetane, Preps. (Robins).
PARACAIN.
See: Procaine Hydrochloride (Various Mfr.).
PARACARBINOXAMINE MALEATE. Carbinoxamine.
PARACET FORTE TABS. (Major) Chlorzoxazone, acetaminophen. Bot. 100s, 1000s.
Use: Skeletal muscle relaxant.
PARACETALDEHYDE.
See: Paraldehyde, U.S.P. XXII.
PARACETAMOL. B.A.N. 4-Acetamidophenol.
Use: Analgesic; antipyretic.
PARACHLORAMINE HYDROCHLORIDE. Meclizine HCl, U.S.P. XXII.
See: Bonine, Tab. (Pfizer).
PARACHLOROMETAXYLENOL.
Use: Phenolic antiseptic.
See: D-Seb, Liq. (Cooper).
Nu-Flow, Liq. (Cooper).
W/9-aminoacridine HCl, methyl-dodecylbenzyl-trimethyl ammonium Cl, pramoxine HCl, hydrocortisone, acetic acid.
See: Drotic No. 2, Drops (Ascher).
W/Benzocaine.
See: TPO 20 (DePree).
W/Coconut oil, pine oil, castor oil, lanolin, cholesterols, lecithin.
See: Sebacide, Liq. (Paddock).
W/Hydrocortisone, pramoxine HCl, benzalkonium Cl, acetic acid.
See: Oto Drops (Solvay).
W/Hydrocortisone, pramoxine HCl, benzalkonium Cl, acetic acid, propylene glycol.
See: Otostan H.C. (Standex).
W/Lidocaine, phenol, zinc oxide.
See: Unguentine Plus, Cream (Norwich).
W/Pramoxine HCl, hydrocortisone, benzalkonium Cl, acetic acid.
See: My Cort Otic #2, Drops (Scrip).
Steramine Otic, Drops (Mayrand).
W/Resorcinol, sulfur.
See: Rezamid, Lot. (Dermik).
•**PARACHLOROPHENOL,** U.S.P. XXII. Camphorated, U.S.P XX. Phenol, 4-chloro. p-Chlorophenol.
Use: Topical antibacterial.
W/Camphor.
See: Camphorated parachlorophenol.
PARACODIN.
See: Dihydrocodeine.
PARADIONE CAPSULES. (Abbott) Paramethadione 150 mg or 300 mg/Cap. Bot. 100s.
Use: Anticonvulsant.
PARADYNE. (Spanner) Dipyrone injection 50%. Vial 10 ml.
PARAEUSAL LIQUID. (Paraeusal) Liq. Bot. 2 oz, 6 oz, 12 oz.
Use: Minor skin irritations.
PARAEUSAL SOLID. (Paraeusal) Oint. Jar 1 oz, 2 oz, 16 oz.
Use: Minor skin irritations.
•**PARAFFIN,** N. F. XVII.
Use: Stiffening agent.
PARAFLEX. (McNeil Pharm.) Chlorzoxazone 250 mg/Tab. Bot. 100s.
Use: Skeletal muscle relaxant.
PARAFON FORTE DSC. (McNeil Pharm.) Chlorzoxazone 500 mg/Capl. Bot. 100s.
Use: Skeletal muscle relaxant.
PARAFORM. Paraformaldehyde. (No Mfr. listed).
PARAFORMALDEHYDE.
Use: Essentially the same as formaldehyde.
See: Formaldehyde (Various Mfr.).
Trioxymethylene (an incorrect term for paraformaldehyde).
PARAGLYCYLARSANILIC ACID. N-Carbamylmethyl-p-aminobenzenearsonic acid, the free acid of tryparsamide.
PARAHIST A.T. SYRUP. (Pharmics) Promethazine 6.25 mg, phenylephrine HCl 5 mg, codeine phosphate 10 mg/5 ml. Syr. Bot. pt.
Use: Antihistamine, decongestant, antitussive.
PARAHIST H.D. (Pharmics) Hydrocodone bitartrate 10 mg, phenylephrine HCl 30 mg, chlorpheniramine maleate 12 mg. Sugar and alcohol free. Pt, gal.
Use: Antitussive, decongestant, antihistamine.
PARA-JEL. (Approved) Benzocaine 5%, cetyl dimethyl benzyl ammonium Cl. Tube 0.25 oz.
Use: Local anesthetic.
PARAL ORAL. (Forest) Paraldehyde 30 ml. Bot. 12s, 25s.
Use: Sedative/hypnotic.
•**PARALDEHYDE,** U.S.P. XXII. Sterile, U.S.P. XXI. 1,3,5-Trioxane, 2,4,6-trimethyl-.2,4,6-Trimethyl-s-trioxane. Paracetaldehyde. Bot. 0.25 lb, 1 lb. Amp.
Use: I.M., I.V. or orally; hypnotic and sedative.
See: Paral, Cap., Liq., Amp. (Forest).
PARAMEPHRIN.
See: Epinephrine (Various Mfr.).
•**PARAMETHADIONE,** U.S.P. XXII. Cap., Oral Soln., U.S.P. XXII. 2,4-Oxazolidinedione, 5-methyl-3,5-dimethyl-.5-Ethyl-3,5-dimethyl-2,4-oxazolidenedione.
Use: Anticonvulsant.
See: Paradione, Cap., Soln. (Abbott).
•**PARAMETHASONE ACETATE,** U.S.P. XXII. Tab., U.S.P. XXII. 16α-Methyl-6α-fluoroprednisolone-21- acetate.6α-Fluoro-11β,17,21-trihydroxy-16α-methylpregna-1,4-diene-3,20-dione 21-Acetate.
Use: Glucocorticoid.
See: Haldrone, Tab. (Lilly).
PARA-MONOCHLOROPHENOL.
See: Camphorated para-chlorophenol, Liq. (Novocol).
•**PARANYLINE HYDROCHLORIDE.** USAN.
Use: Anti-inflammatory.
•**PARAPENZOLATE BROMIDE.** USAN.
Use: Anticholinergic.
PARAPLATIN. (Bristol-Myers Oncology) Carboplatin 50 mg, 150 mg or 450 mg. Inj. Vial.

Use: Antineoplastic agent.

PARAROSANILINE EMBONATE. Pararosaniline pamoate.

•**PARAROSANILINE PAMOATE.** USAN. Bis-[tris(p-Aminophenyl)methylium (4,4′-methylene-bis[3-hydroxy-2-naphthoate])hydrate. Under study.
Use: Antischistosomal agent.

PARASYMPATHOLYTIC AGENTS. Cholinergic blocking agents.
See: Anticholinergic Agents.
Antispasmodics.
Mydriatics.
Parkinsonism.

PARASYMPATHOMIMETIC AGENTS.
See: Cholinergic Agents.

PARATHAR. (Rorer) Teriparatide acetate hPTH activity 200 units with gelatin 20 mg pow. for inj. Vial 10 ml w/10 ml vial diluent.
Use: Diagnostic aid.

PARATHYROID THERAPY. Dihydrotachysterol, U.S.P. XXII. Tachysterol.
See: Hytakerol, Soln., Cap. (Winthrop Pharm).
Parathyroid Injection (Various Mfr.).

PARATROL LIQUID. (Walgreen) Pyrethrins 0.2%, piperonyl butoxide technical 2%, deodorized kerosene 0.8%. Bot. 2 oz.
Use: Pediculicide.

PARAZONE. (Interstate) Chlorzoxazone 250 mg, acetaminophen 300 mg/Tab. Bot. 100s, 1000s.
Use: Skeletal muscle relaxant, analgesic.

•**PARBENDAZOLE.** USAN. Methyl 5-butyl-2-benzimidazolecarbamate. Helmatac. Under study.
Use: Anthelmintic.

PARBUTOXATE. β-Dimethylaminoethyl-3-amino-4-butoxybenzoate.

PARCILLIN. (Parmed) Crystalline potassium penicillin G 240 mg, 400,000 units/Tab. Bot. 100s, 1000s. Pow. for syr. 400,000 units/Tsp. 80 ml.
Use: Antibacterial, penicillin.

•**PARCONAZOLE HYDROCHLORIDE.** USAN.
Use: Antifungal.

•**PAREGORIC,** U.S.P. XXII. (Various Mfr.).
Use: Antiperistaltic.
W/Bismuth subgallate, kaolin, pectin.
See: Dysenaid Jr., Tab. (Jenkins).
W/Glycyrrhiza fluidextract, antimony potassium tartrate.
See: Brown Mixture, Liq. (Lilly).
W/Kaolin (colloidal), aluminum hydroxide, bismuth subcarbonate, pectin.
See: Kapinal, Tab. (Jenkins).
W/Kaolin, pectin.
See: Kaoparin, Susp. (McKesson).
Parepectolin, Susp. (Rorer Consumer).
W/Kaolin, pectin, bismuth subsalicylate, zinc sulfocarbonate.
W/Milk of bismuth, kaolin, pectin.
See: Mul-Sed, Liq. (Webcon).
W/Pectin, kaolin.
See: Parepectolin, Susp. (Rorer).
W/Zinc sulfocarbolate, phenyl salicylate, bismuth subsalicylate, pepsin.
See: C M with Paregoric, Liq. (Beecham Labs).
Corrective Mixture with Paregoric (Beecham Labs).

PARENABOL. Boldenone undecylenate.

PAREPECTOLIN. (Rorer Consumer) Paregoric (equivalent) 3.7 ml, pectin 162 mg, kaolin 5.5 Gm/fl oz. Susp. Bot. 4 fl oz, 8 fl oz.
Use: Antidiarrheal.

•**PAREPTIDE SULFATE.** USAN.
Use: Antiparkinsonian.

PAR ESTRO. (Parmed) Conjugated estrogens 1.25 mg/Tab. Bot. 100s.
Use: Estrogen.

PARETHOXYCAINE HCl.
W/Zirconium oxide, calamine.
See: Zotox, Spray, Cream (Commerce).

PAR-F. (Pharmics) Iron 60 mg, calcium 250 mg, vitamins C 120 mg, A 5000 IU, D 400 IU, B_1 3 mg, B_2 3.4 mg, B_{12} 12 mcg, B_6 12 mg, niacinamide 20 mg, iodine 0.15 mg, magnesium 100 mg, copper 2 mg, zinc 15 mg, E 30 IU, folic acid 1 mg/Tab. Bot. 100s.
Use: Vitamin/mineral supplement.

PARKELP. (Phillip R. Park) Pacific sea kelp. **Tab.:** Bot. 100s, 200s, 500s, 800s. **Gran.:** Bot. 2 oz, 7 oz, 1 lb, 3 lb.
Use: Iodine supplement.

PARKINSONISM. Parasympatholytic agents.
See: Akineton, Tab., Amp. (Knoll).
Artane, Elix., Tab., Sequels (Lederle).
Caramiphen HCl.
Cogentin, Tab., Amp. (Merck Sharp & Dohme).
Disipal, Tab. (Riker).
Kemadrin, Tab. (Burroughs Wellcome).
Levodopa, Cap., Tab. (Various Mfr.).
Levsin, Tab., Elix., Inj., Drops (Kremers-Urban).
Levsinex Timecaps, Cap., Syr. (Kremers-Urban).
Pagitane HCl, Tab. (Lilly).
Parsidol HCl, Tab. (Warner-Chilcott).
Phenoxene, Tab. (Merrell Dow).
Sinemet, Tab. (Merck Sharp & Dohme).
Symmetrel, Cap., Syr. (Du Pont).
Trihexyphenidyl HCl (Various Mfr.).

PARLAX SYRUP. (Robinson) Docusate sodium 20 mg/5 ml. Bot. 8 oz.
Use: Laxative.

PARLAX W/CASANTHRANOL. (Robinson) Docusate sodium 100 mg, casanthranol 50 mg/Cap. Docusate sodium 50 mg, casanthranol 25 mg/Cap. Bot. 100s, 1000s.
Use: Laxative.

PARLODEL. (Sandoz) Bromocriptine mesylate. **Tab.:** 2.5 mg. Bot. 30s. **Cap.:** 5 mg. Bot. 30s, 100s.
Use: Antiparkinson agent.

PARMETH. (Parmed) Promethazine HCl 50 mg/Cap. Bot. 100s, 1000s.

Use: Antihistamine, antiemetic/antivertigo agent.

PARMINYL. W/Salicylamide, phenacetin, caffeine, acetaminophen.
See: Dolopar, Tab. (O'Neal).

PAR-NATAL-FA. (Parmed) Vitamins A 4000 IU, D 400 IU, thiamine HCl 2 mg, riboflavin 2 mg, pyridoxine HCl 0.8 mg, ascorbic acid 50 mg, niacinamide 10 mg, iodine 0.15 mg, folic acid 0.1 mg, cobalamin concentrate 2 mcg, iron 50 mg, calcium 240 mg/Cap. Bot. 100s, 1000s.
Use: Vitamin/mineral supplement.

PARNATE. (SmithKline) Tranylcypromine sulfate 10 mg/Tab. Bot. 100s, 1000s.
Use: Antidepressant.

PARODONTAX DENTAL CREAM. (E.J. Moore) Sodium bicarbonate plus five natural herbs. Tube 60 Gm.
Use: Dental caries preventative.

PARODYNE.
See: Antipyrine (Various Mfr.).

PAROLEINE.
See: Petrolatum Liquid (Various Mfr.).

•**PAROMOMYCIN SULFATE,** U.S.P. XX. Cap., Syr., U.S.P. XXII. An antibiotic substance obtained from cultures of certain *Streptomyces* species, one of which is *Streptomyces rimosus.*
Use: Antiamebic.

PAROTHYL. (Interstate) Meprobamate 400 mg, tridihexethyl Cl 25 mg/Tab. Bot. 100s.
Use: Antianxiety agent, anticholinergic/antispasmodic.

PAROXYL.
See: Acetarsone (Various Mfr.).

PARPANIT.
See: Caramiphen HCl (Various Mfr.).

PARSIDOL HCl. (Parke-Davis) Ethopropazine HCl 10 mg or 50 mg/Tab. Bot. 100s.
Use: Antiparkinson agent.

PARSLEY CONCENTRATE.
W/Garlic concentrate.
See: Allimin, Tab. (Mosso).

PAR-Supp. (Parmed) Estrone 0.2 mg, lactose 50 mg/Vaginal Supp. Pkg. 12s.
Use: Vaginitis.

PARTEN. (Parmed) Acetaminophen 10 gr/Tab. Bot. 100s, 1000s.
Use: Analgesic.

•**PARTRICIN.** USAN. Antibiotic produced by *Streptomyces aureofaciens.*
Use: Antifungal, antiprotozoal.

PARTUSS. (Parmed) Dextromethorphan hydrobromide 60 mg, potassium guaiacolsulfonate 8 gr, chlorpheniramine maleate 6 mg, ammonium Cl 8 gr, tartar emetic 1/12 gr, chloroform 2 min/30 ml. Bot. 4 oz, pt, gal.
Use: Antitussive, expectorant, antihistamine.

PARTUSS "A". (Parmed) Acetaminophen 5 gr, salicylamide 2 gr, caffeine 0.5 gr, atropine sulfate 0.12 mg, guaifenesin 100 mg, phenylpropanolamine HCl 25 mg/Tab. Bot. 1000s.
Use: Analgesic, anticholinergic/antispasmodic, expectorant, decongestant.

PARTUSS A.C. (Parmed) Guaifenesin 100 mg, pheniramine maleate 7.5 mg, codeine phosphate 10 mg, alcohol 3.5%/5 ml. Bot 4 oz.
Use: Expectorant, antihistamine, antitussive.

PARVLEX. (Freeda) Iron 100 mg, vitamins B_1 20 mg, B_2 20 mg, B_3 20 mg, B_5 1 mg, B_6 10 mg, B_{12} 50 mcg, C 50 mg, folic acid 0.1 mg, Cu, Mn/Tab. Bot. 100s, 250s, 500s.
Use: Vitamin/mineral supplement.

P.A.S. ACID. (Kasar) Para-aminosalicylic acid 500 mg/Tab. Bot. 1000s.
Use: Antituberculous agent.

PAS-C. (Hellwig) Pascorbic. p-aminosalicylic acid 0.5 Gm with vitamin C/Tab. Bot. 1000s.
Use: Antituberculous agent.

PASDIUM. (Kasar) Sodium aminosalicylate 0.5 Gm or 1 Gm/Tab. Bot. 1000s.
Use: Antituberculous agent.

PASIJEN. (Jenkins) Passiflora 1 gr, valerian 1 gr, extract henbane 1/8 gr (total alkaloids 0.00019 gr), phenobarbital 0.25 gr/Tab. Bot. 1000s.
Use: Anticholinergic/antispasmodic, sedative/hypnotic.

PASSIFLORA. Dried flowering and fruiting tops of Passiflora incarnata.
W/Phenobarbital, extract hyoscyamus.
See: Somlyn w/Pb, Cap. (Scrip).
W/Phenobarbital, jamaica dogwood.
See: Sominol, Phenobarbital, Tab. (O'Neal).
W/Phenobarbital, valerian, hyoscyamus.
See: Aluro, Tab. (Foy).

PASTEURELLA TULARENSIS ANTIGEN. 10,000 million organisms/ml.
(Lederle)—Vial 5 ml, 20 ml.
Use: Diagnostic aid.

PATH. (Parker) Buffered neutral formalin soln. 10%. Bot. 1 gal, 5 gal. Jar 4 oz.
Use: Tissue specimen fixative.

PATHOCIL. (Wyeth-Ayerst) Sodium dicloxacillin monohydrate. Monohydrate sodium salt of 6[3-(2,6-dichlorophenyl)-5-methyl-4-isoxazolyl]penicillin. **250 mg/Cap.:** Bot. 100s. **500 mg/Cap.:** Bot. 50s. **Pow. for oral susp.:** 62.5 mg/5 ml. Bot. to make 100 ml.
Use: Antibacterial, penicillin.

•**PAULOMYCIN.** USAN.
Use: Antibacterial.

PAVABID HP. (Marion) Papaverine HCl 300 mg/Capl. Bot. 60s.
Use: Peripheral vasodilator.

PAVABID PLATEAU. (Marion) Papaverine HCl 150 mg/TR Cap. Bot. 100s, 250s, 1000s, UD 100s.
Use: Peripheral vasodilator.

PAVACAPS. (Freeport) Papaverine HCl 150 mg/TR Cap. Bot. 1000s.
Use: Peripheral vasodilator.

PAVACEN CENULES. (Central) Papaverine HCl 150 mg/TR Cap. Bot. 100s.
Use: Peripheral vasodilator.

PAVACRON CHRONCAPS. (Cenci) Papaverine HCl 150 mg/Cap. Bot. 100s, 1000s.

Use: Peripheral vasodilator.
PAVADEL. (Canright) Papaverine HCl 150 mg/Cap. Bot. 100s, 1000s.
Use: Peripheral vasodilator.
PAVADEL PB. (Canright) Papaverine HCl 150 mg, phenobarbital 45 mg/Cap. Bot. 100s.
Use: Peripheral vasodilator.
PAVADYL CAPSULES. (Bock) Papaverine HCl 150 mg/Cap. Bot. 100s.
Use: Peripheral vasodilator.
PAVAGEN. (Rugby) Papaverine 150 mg/TR Cap. Bot. 500s, 1000s, UD 100s.
Use: Peripheral vasodilator.
PAVA-LYN. (Lynwood) Papaverine HCl 150 mg/Cap. Bot. 100s.
Use: Peripheral vasodilator.
PAVASED. (Mallard) Papaverine HCl 150 mg/Cap. Bot. 100s, 500s.
Use: Peripheral vasodilator.
PAVATIME. (Rocky Mtn.) Papaverine HCl 150 mg/Cap. Bot. 100s.
Use: Peripheral vasodilator.
PAVATINE TABS. (Major) Papaverine 300 mg/Tab. Bot. 100s.
Use: Peripheral vasodilator.
PAVATINE T.D. CAPS. (Major) Papaverine 150 mg/TD Cap. Bot. 100s, 1000s.
Use: Peripheral vasodilator.
PAVATYM. (Everett) Papaverine HCl 150 mg/TR Cap. Bot. 100s, 1000s, UD 100s.
Use: Peripheral vasodilator.
PAVEROLAN. (Lannett) Papaverine 150 mg/Lanacap. Bot. 100s, 1000s.
Use: Peripheral vasodilator.
PAVRIN-T.D. (Kenyon) Papaverine HCl 150 mg/Cap. Bot. 100s, 1000s.
Use: Peripheral vasodilator.
PAVULON. (Organon) Pancuronium bromide. **1 mg/ml:** Vial 10 ml, Box 25s. **2 mg/ml:** Amp. 2 ml, 5 ml, Box 25s.
Use: Muscle relaxant, adjunct to anesthesia.
PAX-400. (Kenyon) Meprobamate 400 mg/Tab. Bot. 100s, 1000s.
Use: Antianxiety agent.
PAXAREL. (Circle) Acetylcarbromal 250 mg/Tab. Bot. 100s.
Use: Sedative/hypnotic.
PAXIPAM. (Schering) Halazepam 20 mg or 40 mg/Tab. Bot. 100s, UD 100s.
Use: Antianxiety agent.
PAZO OINTMENT. (Bristol-Myers) Benzocaine 0.8%, zinc oxide 4%, ephedrine sulfate 0.2%, camphor 2.18% in lanolin-petrolatum base. Tube 1 oz, 2 oz.
Use: Anorectal preparation.
PAZO SUPPOSITORIES. (Bristol-Myers) Benzocaine 15.44 mg, ephedrine sulfate 3.86 mg, zinc oxide 77.2 mg, camphor 42.07 mg/Supp. Box 12s, 24s.
Use: Anorectal preparation.
•**PAZOXIDE.** USAN.
Use: Antihypertensive.
PB 100. (Schlicksup) Phenobarbital 1.5 gr/Tab. Bot. 1000s.
Use: Sedative/hypnotic.
PBZ. (Geigy) Tripelennamine HCl. **Tab.:** 25 mg Bot. 100s. 50 mg Bot. 100s, 1000s. **Elix.:** Tripelennamine citrate (equivalent to HCl 25 mg)/5 ml. Bot. 473 ml.
Use: Antihistamine.
PBZ-SR. (Geigy) Tripelennamine HCl 100 mg/SR Tab. Bot. 100s.
Use: Antihistamine.
PCE DISPERTAB TABLETS. (Abbott) Erythromycin particles 333 mg/Tab. Bot. 60s, 500s.
Use: Anti-infective.
PCMX.
See: Parachlorometaxylenol.
PDP LIQUID PROTEIN. (Wesley Pharm.) Protein 15 Gm (from protein hydrolysates), cal 60/30 ml. Bot. pt, qt, gal.
Use: Protein supplement.
PEACOCK'S BROMIDES. (Natcon) **Liq.:** Potassium bromide 6 gr, sodium bromide 6 gr, ammonium bromide 3 gr/5 ml. Bot. 8 oz. **Tab.:** Potassium bromide 3 gr, sodium bromide 3 gr, ammonium bromide 1.5 gr. Bot. 100s.
Use: Sedative/hypnotic.
•**PEANUT OIL,** N.F. XVII.
Use: Pharmaceutic aid (solvent, oleaginous vehicle).
PECAZINE. B.A.N. 10-(1-Methyl-3-piperidylmethyl)-phenothiazine.
Use: Tranquilizer.
PECILOCIN. B.A.N. An antibiotic produced by Paecilomyces variotin banier (var. antibioticus). 1-(8-Hydroxy-6-methyldodeca-trans trans cis-2,4,6-tri-enoyl)-2-pyrrolidone.
See: Variotin.
PECTAMOL. (British Drug House) Diethylaminoethoxyethyl-a,a-diethylphenylacetate citrate. Bot. 4 fl oz, 16 fl oz, 80 fl oz, 160 fl oz.
Use: Antitussive.
•**PECTIN,** U.S.P. XXII. (Various Mfr.).
Use: Protectant, pharmaceutic aid (suspending agent).
PECTIN W/COMBINATIONS.
See: Diatrol, Tab. (Otis Clapp).
Donnagel Susp. (Robins).
Donnagel-PG, Susp. (Robins).
Furoxone, Liq., Tab. (Eaton).
Infantol Pink, Liq. (Scherer).
Kaopectate, Liq. (Upjohn).
Kapigam, Liq. (Solvay).
Kapinal, Tab. (Jenkins).
KBP/O, Cap. (Cole).
Parepectolin, Susp. (Rorer Consumer).
Pectocomp, Liq. (Lannett).
Pectokay, Liq. (Bowman).
PECTOCOMP. (Lannett) Pectin 4 gr, kaolin 90 gr, zinc phenolsulfonate 1⅛ gr/fl oz. Bot. pt, gal.
Use: Antidiarrheal.
PEDAMETH. (Forest) Racemethionine. **Cap.:** 200 mg. Bot. 50s, 500s. **Liq.:** 75 mg/5 ml. Bot. pt.

Use: Diaper rash product.

PEDENEX. (Approved) Caprylic acid, zinc undecylenate, sodium propionate. Tube 1.5 oz. Foot pow. spray 5 oz.
Use: Antifungal, external.

PEDIACARE 2 CHILDREN'S COLD RELIEF. (McNeil) Pseudoephedrine HCl 15 mg, chlorpheniramine maleate 1 mg/5 ml. Bot. 4 oz.
Use: Decongestant, antihistamine.

PEDIACARE 3 CHILDREN'S COLD CHEWABLE TABLETS. (McNeil) Pseudoephedrine HCl 7.5 mg, chlorpheniramine maleate 0.5 mg, dextromethorphan HBr 2.5 mg/Tab. Bot 24s.
Use: Decongestant, antihistamine, antitussive.

PEDIACARE INFANTS' COLD RELIEF. (McNeil) Pseudoephedrine HCl 7.5 mg/0.8 ml. Bot. 15 ml.
Use: Decongestant.

PEDIACOF SYRUP. (Winthrop) Codeine phosphate 5 mg, phenylephrine HCl 2.5 mg, chlorpheniramine maleate 0.75 mg, potassium iodide 75 mg/5 ml, sodium benzoate 0.2%, alcohol 5%. Bot. 16 fl oz.
Use: Antitussive, decongestant, antihistamine, expectorant.

PEDIAFLOR FLUORIDE DROPS. (Ross) Fluoride 0.5 mg/ml as sodium fluoride 1.1 mg/ml. Bot. 50 ml.
Use: Dental caries preventative.

PEDIALYTE. (Ross) Sodium 45 mEq, potassium 20 mEq, chloride 35 mEq, citrate 30 mEq, dextrose 25 Gm/Liter. 100 calories/Liter. **Plastic Bot.:** 8 fl oz. (unflavored), 32 fl oz. (unflavored, fruit). **Nursing Bot.:** Hospital use. Bot. 8 fl oz.
Use: Minerals/electrolytes, oral.

PEDIAMYCIN DROPS. (Ross) Erythromycin ethylsuccinate for oral suspension 100 mg/2.5 ml. Bot. 50 ml (Dropper enclosed).
Use: Anti-infective.

PEDIAPRED ORAL LIQUID. (Fisons) Prednisolone sodium phosphate 6.7 mg/5 ml. Bot. 4 oz.
Use: Corticosteroid.

PEDIATRIC COUGH SYRUP. (Weeks & Leo) Ammonium Cl 300 mg, sodium citrate 600 mg/oz. Bot. 4 oz.
Use: Expectorant.

PEDIATRIC MAINTENANCE SOLUTION. (Abbott) I.V. solution w/dose calculated according to age, weight, clinical condition. Bot. 250 ml.
Use: Fluids, electrolyte and nutrient replenisher.

PEDIATROL (B13). (Kenyon) Vitamins B_{12} 25 mcg, B_1 10 mg/5 ml. Bot. pt, gal.
Use: Vitamin supplement.

PEDIAZOLE SUSPENSION. (Ross) Erythromycin ethylsuccinate 200 mg, sulfisoxazole acetyl 600 mg/5 ml. Bot. Granules reconstituted to 100 ml, 150 ml, 200 ml.
Use: Anti-infective.

PEDI-BATH. (Pedinol) Colloidal sulfur, balsam peru. Bot. 6 oz.
Use: Bath dermatological, emollient.

PEDI-BOOT MIST KIT. (Pedinol) Cetyl pyridinium Cl, triacetin, chloroxylenol. Bot. 2 oz.
Use: Fungicide, sanitizer, deodorizer for shoes.

PEDI-BORO SOAK PAKS. (Pedinol) Astringent wet dressing w/aluminum sulfate, calcium acetate, coloring agent. Box 12s, 100s.
Use: Minor skin irritations.

PEDI-CORT V CREME. (Pedinol) Clioquinol 3%, hydrocortisone 1%. Tube 20 Gm.
Use: Antifungal, corticosteroid.

PEDICRAN WITH IRON. (Scherer) Vitamin B_{12} (crystallized) 25 mcg, ferric pyrophosphate, soluble (elemental iron 30 mg) 250 mg, thiamine mononitrate 10 mg, nicotinamide 10 mg, alcohol 1%/5 ml. Bot. 4 oz, pt.
Use: Vitamin/mineral supplement.

PEDICULICIDES.
See: A-200 Pyrinate (Norcliff Thayer).
Benzyl Benzoate, Preps. (Various Mfr.).
Chlorophenothane (Various Mfr.).
Cuprex, Liq. (Calgon Consumer Prods.).
DDT (Various Mfr.).
Kwell, Preps. (Reed & Carnrick).

PEDI-DRI FOOT POWDER. (Pedinol) Aluminum chlorohydroxide, zinc undecylenate, menthol, formaldehyde. Spout Cap Bot. 2 oz.
Use: Antiperspirant, deodorant, fungicidal foot powder.

PEDIOTIC. (Burroughs Wellcome) Hydrocortisone 1%, neomycin 3.5 mg (as sulfate), polymyxin B sulfate 10,000 units/ml. Susp. Bot 7.5 ml with dropper.
Use: Corticosteroid, anti-infective, otic.

PEDI-PRO FOOT POWDER. (Pedinol) Aluminum chlorhydroxide, menthol, zinc undecylenate, chloroxylenol. Bot. 2 oz.
Use: Fungicide, antiperspirant, deodorant.

PEDI-VIT A CREME. (Pedinol) Vitamin A 100,000 units/oz. Jar 2 oz, 16 oz, 5 lb.
Use: Emollient.

PEDOLATUM. (King) Salicylic acid, sodium salicylate. Oint. Pkg. 0.5 oz.
Use: External analgesic.

PEDRIC SENIOR. (Vale) Acetaminophen 320 mg.
Use: Analgesic.

PEDTE-PAK-4. (SoloPak) Zinc 1 mg, copper 0.1 mg, manganese 0.025 mg, chromium 1 mcg. Vial 3 ml.
Use: Parenteral nutritional supplement.

PEDTRACE-4. (Lyphomed) Zinc 0.5 mg, copper 0.1 mg, chromium 0.85 mcg, manganese 0.25 mg/ml. Vial 3 ml, 10 ml.
Use: Parenteral nutritional supplement.

•**PEFLOXACIN.** USAN.
Use: Antibacterial.

•**PEFLOXACIN MESYLATE.** USAN.
Use: Antibacterial.

PEGADEMASE BOVINE. Modified enzyme for use in ADA deficiency.
See: Adagen (Enzon).

PEGANONE. (Abbott) Ethotoin 250 mg/Tab. or 500 mg/Cap. Bot. 100s.
Use: Anticonvulsant.

•**PEGASPARGASE.** USAN.
Use: Antineoplastic.

PEGLICOL 5 OLEATE. USAN.
Use: Emulsifying agent.

P.E.G. OINTMENT. (Medco Lab) Polyethylene glycol. Jar 16 oz.
Use: Water soluble ointment base.

•**PEGOTERATE.** USAN.
Use: Suspending agent.

•**PEGOXOL 7 STEARATE.** USAN.
Use: Emulsifying agent.

PELAMINE. (Major) Tripelennamine HCl 50 mg/Tab. Bot. 100s, 1000s.
Use: Antihistamine.

•**PELANSERIN HYDROCHLORIDE.** USAN.
Use: Antihypertensive.

PELENTAN. Ethyl Biscoumacetate. (No Mfr. currently lists).

•**PELIOMYCIN.** USAN. An antibiotic derived from *Streptomycin luteogriseus.*
Use: Antineoplastic agent.

•**PELRINONE HYDROCHLORIDE.** USAN.
Use: Cardiotonic.

•**PEMEDOLAC.** USAN.
Use: Analgesic.

•**PEMERID NITRATE.** USAN. 4-[3-(Di-methylimino)propoxy]-1,2,2,6,6-pentamethylpiperidine dinitrate.
Use: Antitussive.

•**PEMOLINE.** USAN. 2-amino-5-phenyl-4-azolin-4-one.
Use: Childhood attention-deficit syndrome (hyperkinetic syndrome).
See: Cylert Prods. (Abbott).

PEMPIDINE. B.A.N. 1,2,2,6,6-Pentamethylpiperidine.
Use: Hypotensive.

PENAGEN-VK. (Grafton) Penicillin V. **Tab.:** 250 mg. Bot. 100s. **Pow.:** 250 mg/100 ml.
Use: Antibacterial, penicillin.

•**PENAMECILLIN.** USAN. Acetoxymethyl 6-phenyl-acetamidopenicillanate.
Use: Antibiotic.

•**PENBUTOLOL.** USAN.(−)-1-tert-Butylamino-3-(2-cyclopentylphenoxy)propan-2-ol.
Use: Beta adrenergic blocking agent.
See: Levatol (Reed and Carnrick).

PENDECAMAINE. B.A.N. NN-Dimethyl-(3-palmitamidopropyl)glycine betaine.
Use: Surface active agent.

PENECORT CREAM. (Herbert) Hydrocortisone 1% or 2.5%, benzyl alcohol, petrolatum, stearyl alcohol, propylene glycol, isopropyl myristate, polyoxyl 40 stearate, carbomer 934, sodium lauryl sulfate, edetate disodium w/sodium hydroxide to adjust pH, purified water. **1%:** Tube 30 Gm, 60 Gm. **2.5%:** Tube 30 Gm.
Use: Corticosteroid.

PENECORT TOPICAL SOLUTION 1%. (Herbert) Hydrocortisone 1%, alcohol 57%, propylene glycol, benzyl alcohol, purified water. Bot. 30 ml, 60 ml.
Use: Corticosteroid.

PENETHAMATE HI.
See: Benzylpenicillin 2-diethylaminoethyl ester HI.

PENETHAMATE HYDRIODIDE. B.A.N. 2-Diethylaminoethyl 6-phenylacetamidopenicillanate hydriodide. Benzylpenicillin 2-diethylaminoethyl ester hydriodide.
Use: Treatment of respiratory tract infections.

•**PENFLURIDOL.** USAN. 1-[4,4-bis(p-Flurophenyl)butyl]-4-(4-chloro-α,α,α-trifluoro-m-tolyl)-4-piperidi-nol. 4-(4-Chloro-3-trifluoromethylphenyl)-1-[4,4-di-(4-fluorophenyl)butyl]piperidin-4-ol.
Use: Tranquilizer.

PENFONYLIN.
See: Pentid, Prods. (Squibb).

•**PENICILLAMINE,** U.S.P. XXII. Cap., Tab., U.S.P. XXII. (Merck Sharp & Dohme) D-3-Mercaptovaline. Cuprimine.
Use: Metal complexing agent, cystinuria, rheumatoid arthritis.
See: Cuprimine, Cap. (Merck Sharp & Dohme).
Depen, Tab. (Wallace).

PENICILLIN. Unless clarified, it means an antibiotic substance or substances produced by growth of the molds *Penicillium notatum* or *P. chrysogenum.*
Use: Antibacterial.

PENICILLIN ALUMINUM. Aluminum 3,3-dimethyl-7-oxo-6-(2-phenylacetamido)-4-thia-1-azabicyclo-[3.2.0]-heptane-2-carboxylate.
Use: Antibacterial, penicillin.

PENICILLIN CALCIUM. Calcium 3,3-dimethyl-7-oxo-6-(2-phenylacetamido)-4-thia-1-azabicyclo-[3.2.0]-heptane-2-carboxylate. U.S.P. XIII.
Use: Antibacterial, penicillin.

PENICILLIN, DIMETHOXY-PHENYL. Methicillin Sodium.
Use: Antibacterial, penicillin.
See: Staphcillin, Vial (Bristol).

•**PENICILLIN G. BENZATHINE,** U.S.P. XXII. Sterile Susp., Oral Susp., Sterile, Tab. U.S.P. XXII. Benzathine penicillin G.
Use: Antibiotic.
See: Bicillin, Tab. (Wyeth-Ayerst).
Bicillin Long-Acting (Wyeth-Ayerst).
Permapen, Aqueous Susp. (Pfizer Laboratories).

•**PENICILLIN G, POTASSIUM,** U.S.P. XXII. Cap., Inj., for Oral Soln., Sterile, Tab., Tab. for Oral Soln., U.S.P. XXII. (Potassium Penicillin, Benzyl Penicillin Pot.).
Use: Antibiotic.
See: Arcocillin, Preps. (Arcum).
Biotic-T-500, Tab. (Scrip).
Cryspen 400, Tab. (Knight).
Deltapen, Syr., Tab. (Trimen).
G-Recillin-T, Tab. (Solvay).

Hyasorb, Tab. (Key Pharm.).
K-Cillin, Prods.(Mayrand).
Lanacillin, Pow. (Lannett).
Palocillin-S, Pow. (Hauck).
Palocillin-5, Tab. (Hauck).
Parcillin, Tab. (Parmed).
Pensorb, Tab. (Kenyon).
Pentids, Syr., Tab. (Squibb Mark).
Pfizerpen, Tab., Syr. (Pfizer Laboratories).
Pfizerpen, Inj. (Roerig).

PENICILLIN G POTASSIUM W/COMBINATIONS.
See: Lanacillin "200,000", "400,000" (Lannett).
Pentid, Prods. (Squibb).

•**PENICILLIN G, PROCAINE, STERILE,** U.S.P. XXII. Sterile Susp., Intramammary infusion, U.S.P. XXII. Procaine Penicillin.
Use: Antibiotic.
Parenteral, aqueous susp.}, (Procaine Penicillin, for Aqueous Inj.,) Procaine Penicillin and buffered Penicillin for aqueous, Inj.
See: Crysticillin A.S., Vial (Squibb).
Diurnal-Panicillin (Upjohn).
Duracillin A.S., Preps. (Lilly).
Pfizerpen-A.S. (Roerig).
Tu-Cillin, Inj. (Solvay).
Wycillin, Susp. (Wyeth-Ayerst).
Parenteral, in oil w/aluminum monostearate. Penicillin Procaine in Oil Inj.

PENICILLIN G PROCAINE COMBINATIONS
See: Bicillin C-R, Tubex (Wyeth-Ayerst).
Bicillin C-R 900/300 Inj. (Wyeth-Ayerst).
Duracillin F.A., Amp. (Lilly).
Duracillin Fortified, Vial (Lilly).

•**PENICILLIN G PROCAINE AND DIHYDROSTREPTOMYCIN SULFATE INTRAMAMMARY INFUSION,** U.S.P. XXII.
Use: Antibiotic.

•**PENICILLIN G PROCAINE, DIHYDROSTREPTOMYCIN SULFATE, CHLORPHENIRAMINE MALEATE, AND DEXAMETHASONE SUSPENSION, STERILE,** U.S.P. XXII.
Use: Antibiotic, antihistamine, anti-inflammatory.

•**PENICILLIN G PROCAINE, DIHYDROSTREPTOMYCIN SULFATE, AND PREDNISOLONE SUSPENSION, STERILE,** U.S.P. XXII.
Use: Antibiotic, anti-inflammatory.

•**PENICILLIN G PROCAINE AND DIHYDROSTREPTOMYCIN SULFATE SUSPENSION, STERILE,** U.S.P. XXII.
Use: Antibiotic.

•**PENICILLIN G PROCAINE, NEOMYCIN AND POLYMYXIN B SULFATES, AND HYDROCORTISONE ACETATE TOPICAL SUSPENSION,** U.S.P. XXII.
Use: Antibiotic, anti-inflammatory.

•**PENICILLIN G PROCAINE AND NOVOBIOCIN SODIUM INTRAMAMMARY INFUSION,U.S.P. XXII.**
Use: Antibiotic.

•**PENICILLIN G PROCAINE W/ALUMINUM STEARATE SUSPENSION, STERILE,** U.S.P. XXII.
Use: Antibiotic.

•**PENICILLIN G SODIUM FOR INJECTION,** U.S.P. XXII. (Various Mfr.) Sodium Benzylpenicillin.
Use: Antibiotic.

•**PENICILLIN G SODIUM, STERILE,** U.S.P. XXII.
Use: Antibiotic.

PENICILLIN HYDRABAMINE PHENOXYMETHYL. 3,3-Dimethyl-7-oxo-6-(2-phenoxyacetamido)-4-thia-1-azabicyclo[3.2.0]heptane-2-carboxylic acid compound with N,N′-bis[(1,2,3,4,-4a,9,10,10a-octahydro-7-isopropyl-1,4a-dimethyl-1-phenanthryl)methyl]ethylenediamine.
Use: Antibiotic.

PENICILLIN N. Adicillin, B.A.N.
Use: Antibiotic.

PENICILLIN O CHLOROPROCAINE. 6-[2-(Allylthio)acetamido]-3-3-dimethyl-7-oxo-4-thia-1-azabicyclo-[3.2.0]heptane-2-carboxylic acid compound with 2-(diethylamino)ethyl 4-amino-2-chlorbenzoate (1:1).
Use: Antibacterial, penicillin.

PENICILLIN O, SODIUM. Allylmercaptomethyl penicillin.
Use: Antibacterial.

PENICILLIN, PHENOXYETHYL.
Use: Antibacterial, penicillin.
See: Phenethicillin, Penicillin potassium 152.

PENICILLIN PHENOXYMETHYL BENZATHINE.
Use: Antibacterial, penicillin.
See: Penicillin V Benzathine.

PENICILLIN PHENOXYMETHYL HYDRABAMINE.
Use: Antibacterial, penicillin.
See: Penicillin V Hydrabamine.

•**PENICILLIN S BENZATHINE AND PENICILLIN G PROCAINE SUSPENSION, STERILE,** U.S.P. XXII.
Use: Antibiotic.

•**PENICILLIN V,** U.S.P. XX for Oral Susp., Tab. U.S.P. XXII. Phenoxymethyl penicillin. A biosynthetic penicillin formed by fermentation, with suitable precursors of *Penicillin notatum.*
Use: Antibiotic.
See: Biotic Pow. (Scrip).
Compocillin-V, Water, Susp. (Ross).
Ledercillin VK (Lederle).
Penagen-VK, Tab., Pow. (Gafton).
Robicillin-VK (Robins).
Uticillin VK (Upjohn).
V-Cillin, Preps. (Lilly).
V-Pen, Tab. (Century).

•**PENICILLIN V BENZATHINE,** U.S.P. XXII. Oral Susp., U.S.P. XXII.
Use: Antibiotic.
See: Pen-Vee, Prods. (Wyeth-Ayerst).

PENICILLIN V HYDRABAMINE. Hydrabamine phenoxymethyl penicillin.
Use: Antibacterial, penicillin.

See: Compocillin-V Hydrabamine, Oral Susp. (Ross).

•**PENICILLIN V POTASSIUM,** U.S.P. XXII. Oral Soln., Tab., U.S.P. XXII.
Use: Antibiotic.
See: Beepen VK, Tab., Syr. (Beecham Labs).
Betapen VK., Soln., Tab. (Bristol).
Biotic-V-Powder (Scrip).
Bopen, V-K, Tab. (Boyd).
Dowpen VK, Tab. (Merrell Dow).
Lanacillin VK, Tab., Pow. (Lannett).
Ledercillin VK, Oral Soln., Tab. (Lederle).
LV, Tab (Elder).
Pen-Vee-K, Soln., Tab. (Wyeth-Ayerst).
Pfizerpen VK, Pow., Tab. (Pfizer Laboratories).
Phenethicillin Potassium.
Repen-VK, Tab., Oral Susp. (Solvay).
Robicillin VK, Tab., Soln. (Robins).
Ro-Cillin VK, Soln., Tab. (Solvay).
Saropen-VK (Saron).
SK-Penicillin VK, Soln., Tab. (SmithKline).
Suspen, Liq. (Circle).
Uticillin VK, Tab., Soln. (Upjohn).
V-Cillin K, Tab., Oral Soln. (Lilly).
Veetids, Soln., Tab. (Squibb Mark).

PENICILLINASE. B.A.N. An enzyme that hydrolyzes penicillin, obtained from several strains of bacteria *(B.cereus).* Vial (1000 units) 20 ml.
Use: Clinical lab use only.

PENIDURAL.
Use: Antibacterial.
See: Benzathine Penicillin. B.A.N.

PEN-KERA CREME WITH KERATIN BINDING FACTOR. (Ascher) Bot. 8 oz.
Use: Emollient.

PENNATE. (Robinson) Pentaerythritol tetranitrate. **"10":** 10 mg/Tab. Bot. 100s, 1000s. **"20":** 20 mg/Tab. Bot. 100s, 1000s. **"30":** 30 mg/Timedcap. Bot. 100s, 500s, 1000s.
Use: Antianginal.

PENNPHENO. (Robinson) Phenobarbital 0.25 gr, pentaerythritol 10 mg or 20 mg/Tab. Bot. 100s, 1000s.
Use: Antianginal.

PENSORB. (Kenyon) Crystalline penicillin G potassium 250,000 units, buffered w/calcium carbonate/Tab. Bot. 100s, 1000s.
Use: Antibacterial, penicillin.

•**PENTABAMATE.** USAN. 3-Methyl-2,4-pentanediol dicarbamate.
Use: Tranquilizer.

PENTA-CAP #1. (Kenyon) Pentaerythritol tetranitrate 30 mg/Cap. Bot. 90s, 100s, 1000s.
Use: Antianginal.

PENTA-CAP PLUS. (Kenyon) Pentaerythritol tetranitrate 30 mg, amobarbital 50 mg/Cap. Bot. 100s, 1000s.
Use: Antianginal.

PENTACOSACTRIDE. D-Ser^1-Nle^4-(Val-NH$_2$)$^{25-}$ b$^{1\ 25-}$corticotrophin.
Use: Corticotrophic peptide.
See: Norleusactide (I.N.N.).

PENTACYNIUM METHYLSULPHATE. B.A.N. 4-2-[(5-Cyano-5,5-diphenylpentyl)dimethylammonio]ethyl-4-methylmorpholinium di(methylsulfate).
Use: Hypotensive.

PENTAERYTHRITOL TETRANITRATE, DILUTED, U.S.P. XXII.
Use: Vasodilator.

•**PENTAERYTHRITOL TETRANITRATE,** U.S.P. XXII. Diluted, U.S.P. XXII.
Use: Vasodilator.
See: Angijen Green, Tab. (Jenkins).
Arcotrate Nos. 1 and 2, Tab. (Arcum).
Dilac-80, Cap. (Ascher).
Duotrate-45, Cap. (Marion).
Kortrate, Cap. (Amid).
Maso-Trol, Tab. (Mason).
Metranil, Cap. (Meyer).
Nitrin, Tab. (Vale).
Penta-Cap No. 1, Cap. (Kenyon).
Penta-E, Tab. (Recsei).
Pentafin, Granucap, Tab. (Solvay).
Penta-Tal Nos. 1 and 2, Tab. (Kenyon).
Pentestan-80, Cap. (Standex).
Pentetra, Tab. (Paddock).
Pentryate, Cap., Tab. (Fellows-Testagar).
Pentryate Stronger, Cap. (Fellows-Testagar).
Pent-T-80, Cap. (Rocky Mtn.).
Pentylan, Tab. (Lannett).
Pentylan w/Phenobarbital, Tab. (Lannett).
Peritrate, Tab. (Parke-Davis).
Petro-20 mg, Tab. (Foy).
Rate, Cap., Tab. (Scrip).
Reithritol, Tab. (Bowman).
Tentrate, Tab. (Tennessee Pharm.).
Tetracap-30, Cap. (Freeport).
Tetracap-80, Cap. (Freeport).
Tetratab, Tab. (Freeport).
Tetratab No. 1, Tab. (Freeport).
Tranite, Cap., Tab. (Westerfield).
Vasolate, Cap. (Parmed).
Vasolate-80, Cap. (Parmed).

PENTAERYTHRITOL TETRANITRATE W/COMBINATIONS.
See: Angijen S.C., Tab. (Jenkins).
Angitab, Tab. (Moore Kirk).
Arcotrate No. 3, Tab. (Arcum).
Bitrate, Tab. (Arco).
Dimycor, Tab. (Standard Drug).
Penta-Cap Plus, Cap. (Kenyon).
Penta-Tal Nos. 3 and 4, Tab. (Kenyon).
Pentetra w/Phenobarbital, Tab. (Paddock).
Pentylan w/Phenobarbital, Tab. (Lannett).
Peritrate w/Nitroglycerin, Tab. (Parke-Davis).
Respet, Tab. (Westerfield).
Robam-Petn, Tab. (Robinson).

•**PENTAFILCON A.** USAN.
Use: Contact lens material.

•**PENTAGASTRIN.** USAN. N-t-Butyloxy-carbonyl-b-alanyl-L-tryptophyl-L-methionyl-L-aspartyl-L-phenylalanine amide.

Use: Gastric acid secretion stimulant.
See: Peptavlon, Amp. (Wyeth-Ayerst).

PENTALAMIDE. B.A.N. 2-Pentyloxybenzamide.
Use: Treatment of fungal infections.

•**PENTALYTE.** USAN.
Use: Electrolyte combination.

PENTAM 300. (Lyphomed) Pentamidine isethionate 300 mg/Vial.
Use: Anti-infective.

PENTAMETHONIUM BROMIDE. B.A.N. Pentamethylenedi(trimethylammonium bromide).
Use: Hypotensive.

PENTAMETHONIUM IODIDE. B.A.N. Pentamethylenedi(trimethylammonium iodide).
Use: Hypotensive.

PENTAMETHYLENETETRAZOL.
See: Pentylenetetrazol, U.S.P.

PENTAMIDINE. B.A.N. 4,4′-(Pentamethylenedioxy)-dibenzamidine.
Use: Treatment of trypanosomiasis.

PENTAMIDINE ISETHIONATE.
See: Pentam 300, Inj. (Lyphomed).

PENTAMOXANE HCl. 2-Isoamylamino-methyl-1,4-benzodioxane HCl.
Use: Tranquilizing agent.

•**PENTAMUSTINE.** USAN.
Use: Antineoplastic.

PENTAPHONATE. Dodecyltriphenylphosphonium pentachlorophenolate.
Use: Anti-infective.

PENTAPIPERIDE. B.A.N. 1-Methyl-4-(3-methyl-2-phenylvaleryloxy)piperidine.
Use: Anticholinergic.

PENTAPIPERIDE METHYLSULFATE. 4′-(1′-Methylpiperidyl)-2-phenyl-3-methyl-valerate dimethylsulfate. Valpipamate Methylsulfate.
Use: Anticholinergic.

•**PENTAPIPERIUM METHYLSULFATE.** USAN.
Use: Anticholinergic.

PENTAPYRROLIDINIUM BITARTRATE.
See: Pentolinium Tartrate.

PENTAQUINE. B.A.N. 8-(5-Isopropylaminopentylamino)-6-methoxyquinoline.
Use: Antimalarial.

PENTAQUINE PHOSPHATE. 8-[[5-(Isopropylamino)pentyl]amino]-6-methoxyquinoline phosphate.

PENTARCORT. (Dalin) Hydrocortisone alcohol 0.5%, coal tar solution 2%, clioquinol 3%, diperodone HCl 0.25%, vitamins A 850 IU, D 85 IU/Gm. Tube 15 Gm.
Use: Corticosteroid, anti-infective, topical.

PENTASODIUM COLISTINMETHANESULFONATE. Sterile Colistimethate Sodium, U.S.P. XXII.

•**PENTASTARCH.** USAN.
Use: Leukopheresis adjunct (red cell sedimenting agent).

PENTA-STRESS. (Penta) Vitamins A 10,000 IU, D 500 IU, B_1 10 mg, B_2 10 mg, B_6 1 mg, calcium pantothenate 5 mg, niacinamide 50 mg, C 100 mg, E 2 IU, B_{12} 3.3 mcg/Cap. Bot. 90s, 1000s, Jar 250s.
Use: Vitamin supplement.

PENTA-TAL. (Kenyon) Pentaerythritol tetranitrate 10 mg or 20 mg/Tab. Bot. 100s, 1000s.
Use: Antianginal.

PENTA-TAL #3, #4. (Kenyon) Pentaerythritol tetranitrate 10 mg or 20 mg, phenobarbital 15 mg/Tab. Bot. 100s, 1000s.
Use: Antianginal.

PENTAVALENT GAS GANGRENE. Antitoxin.

PENTA-VIRON. (Penta) Calcium carbonate 500 mg, ferrous fumarate 100 mg, vitamins C 50 mg, D 167 IU, A 3.333 IU, B_1 3.3 mg, B_2 3.3 mg, B_6 2 mg, calcium pantothenate 1.6 mg, niacinamide 16.7 mg, E 2 IU/Cap. Bot. 100s, 1000s, Jar 250s.
Use: Vitamin supplement.

PENTAZINE. (Century) Promethazine expectorant. Bot. 4 oz, 16 oz, gal.
Use: Antihistamine.

PENTAZINE W/CODEINE. (Century) Promethazine expectorant. Bot. 4 oz, 16 oz, gal.
Use: Antihistamine.

PENTAZINE INJ. (Century) Promethazine 50 mg/ml. Inj. Vial 10 ml.
Use: Antihistamine.

•**PENTAZOCINE,** U.S.P. XXII. 2,6-Methano-3-benzazocin-8-ol, 1,2,3,4,5,6-hexahydro-6,11-dimethyl-3-(3-methyl-2-butenyl)-1,2,3,-4,5,6-Hexahydro-cis-6,11-dimethyl-3-(3-methyl-2-butenyl)-2,6-methano-2-benzazocin-8-ol.
Use: Analgesic.

•**PENTAZOCINE HYDROCHLORIDE,** U.S.P. XXII. Tab., U.S.P. XXII.
Use: Analgesic.
W/Acetaminophen.
See: Talacen, Cap. (Winthrop Pharm).

•**PENTAZOCINE HYDROCHLORIDE AND ASPIRIN TABLETS,** U.S.P. XXII.
Use: Analgesic.
See: Talwin Compound, Tab. (Winthrop Pharm).

•**PENTAZOCINE LACTATE INJECTION,** U.S.P. XXII.
Use: Analgesic.
See: Talwin Injection, Inj. (Winthrop Pharm).

•**PENTAZOCINE AND NALOXONE HYDROCHLORIDE TABLETS.** U.S.P. XXII.
Use: Analgesic.
See: Talwin NX, Tab. (Winthrop Pharm).

PENTESTAN 10. (Standex) Pentaerythritol tetranitrate 10 mg/Tab. Bot. 100s.
Use: Antianginal.

PENTESTAN 10-P. (Standex) Pentaerythritol tetranitrate 10 mg, phenobarbital 15 mg/Tab. Bot. 100s.
Use: Antianginal.

•**PENTETATE CALCIUM TRISODIUM.** USAN.
Use: Chelating agent (plutonium).

•**PENTETATE CALCIUM TRISODIUM Yb 169.** USAN.

Use: Radioactive agent.

•**PENTETATE INDIUM DISODIUM IN 111.** USAN.
Use: Diagnostic aid, radioactive agent.

•**PENTETIC ACID.** USAN.
Use: Diagnostic aid.

PENTETRA-PARACOTE. (Paddock) Pentaerythritol tetranitrate 30 mg or 80 mg/Cap. Bot. 100s, 500s, 1000s.
Use: Antianginal.

PENTHIENATE. B.A.N. 2-Diethylaminoethyl α-cyclopentyl-α-(2-thienyl).
Use: Antispasmodic.

PENTHIENATE BROMIDE. Diethyl (2-Hydroxyethyl) methylammonium bromide α-cyclopentyl-2-thio- pheneglycolate.

PENTHRANE. (Abbott Hospital Prods.) Methoxyflurane. Bot. 15 ml, 125 ml.
Use: General anesthetic.

PENTHRICHLORAL. B.A.N. 5,5-Di(hydroxymethyl)-2-trichloromethyl-1,3-dioxan.
Use: Hypnotic; sedative.

•**PENTIAPINE MALEATE.** USAN.
Use: Antipsychotic.

PENTIDS. (Squibb Mark) Potassium Penicillin G buffered with calcium carbonate. **Tab.:** 125 mg (200,000 units). Bot. 100s. **Syr.:** 125 mg (200,000 units)/5 ml. Bot. 100 ml, 200 ml.
Use: Antibacterial, penicillin.

PENTIDS 400. (Squibb Mark) Potassium Penicillin G buffered with calcium carbonate. **Tab.:** 250 mg (400,000 units). Bot. 100s, Unimatic 100s. **Syr.:** 250 mg (400,000 units)/5 ml. Bot. 100 ml, 200 ml.
Use: Antibacterial, penicillin.

PENTIDS 800. (Squibb Mark) Potassium Penicillin G 500 mg (800,000 units)/Tab. buffered with calcium carbonate. Bot. 30s, 100s.
Use: Antibacterial, penicillin.

PENTIFYLLINE. B.A.N. 1-Hexyl-3,7-dimethyl-xanthine.
Use: Vasodilator.

PENTINA. (Freeport) Rauwolfia serpentina, 100 mg/Tab. Bot. 1000s.
Use: Antihypertensive.

•**PENTISOMICIN.** USAN.
Use: Anti-infective.

•**PENTIZIDONE SODIUM.** USAN.
Use: Antibacterial.

•**PENTOBARBITAL,** U.S.P. XXII. Elixir, U.S.P. XXI. (Various Mfr.) 5-Ethyl-5-(1-methylbutyl) barbituric acid.
Use: Sedative.
See: Nembutal, Elix., Gradumets (Abbott)
Penta, Tab. (Dunhall).

PENTOBARBITAL COMBINATIONS.
Use: Sedative/hypnotic.
See: Cafergot-PB, Supp., Tab. (Sandoz).
Nembutal, Preps. (Abbott).
Quad-Set, Tab. (Kenyon).

•**PENTOBARBITAL, SODIUM,** U.S.P. XXII. Cap. Elixir, Inj.: U.S.P. XXII. 2,4,6,(1H,3H,5H)-Pyrimidinetrione, 5-ethyl-5-(1-methyl-butyl)-, monosodium salt. Sodium 5-Ethyl-5-(1-methylbutyl) barbiturate. Embutal.
Use: Hypnotic, sedative.
See: Maso-Pent, Tab. (Mason).
Nembutal Sodium, Preps. (Abbott).
Night-Caps, Cap. (Bowman).
W/Adiphenine HCl, phamasorb, aluminum hydroxide.
See: Spasmasorb, Tab. (Hauck).
W/Atropine sulfate, hyoscine HBr, hyoscyamine sulfate.
See: Eldonal, Elix., Tab., Cap. (Canright).
W/Ephedrine.
See: Ephedrine and Nembutal-25, Cap. (Abbott).
W/Ergotamine tartrate, caffeine alkaloid, bellafoline.
See: Cafergot-P.B., Tab. (Sandoz).
W/Homatropine methylbromide, dehydrocholic acid, ox bile extract.
See: Homachol, Tab. (Lemmon).
W/Pyrilamine maleate.
See: A-N-R, Rectorette (Hauck).
W/Seco-, buta-, phenobarbital.
W/Vitamin compounds, d-methamphetamine HCl.
See: Fetamin, Tab. (Mission).

PENTOBARBITAL, SOLUBLE.
See: Pentobarbital Sodium, U.S.P.

PENTOL TABS. (Major) Pentaerythritol tetranitrate. **10 mg/Tab.:** Bot. 1000s; **20 mg/Tab.:** Bot. 100s, 1000s; **80 mg/SA Tab.:** Bot. 250s, 1000s.
Use: Antianginal.

PENTOLINIUM TARTRATE. Pentamethylene-1:5-bis (1′-methylpyrrolidinium bitartrate). N,N′-Pentamethylenedi-(1-methylpyrrolidinium hydrogen tartrate. Pentapyrrolidinium Bitartrate.
Use: Antihypertensive.

•**PENTOMONE.** USAN.
Use: Prostate growth inhibitor.

•**PENTOPRIL.** USAN.
Use: Enzyme inhibitor (angiotensin-converting).

•**PENTOSTATIN.** USAN.
Use: Potentiator.

PENTOTHAL. (Abbott Hospital Prods.) Thiopental sodium. 500 mg fliptop vial w/20 ml water diluent; 1 Gm fliptop vial w/50 ml water diluent; 250 mg, 400 mg or 500 mg syringes; 5 Gm in 250 ml and 10 Gm in 500 ml Multi-Dose container; Kits: 1 Gm/2.5%, 2.5 Gm/2.5%, 5 Gm/2.5%, 2.5 Gm/2% or 5 Gm/2%. Pentothal Rectal Susp. in AbboSert Syringe. Single-dose syringe 250 mg, 400 mg, 500 mg.
Use: Anesthetic.

•**PENTOXIFYLLINE.** USAN. Oxpentifylline. B.A.N.
Use: Oral hemorrheologic agent for peripheral vascular disease.
See: Trental (Hoechst).

PENTRAX SHAMPOO. (Rydell) Tar extract 8.75%, detergents, conditioning agents. Bot. 4 oz, 8 oz.
Use: Antiseborrheic.

•**PENTRINITROL.** USAN.
Use: Vasodilator.
PENT-T-80. (Rocky Mtn.) Pentaerythritol tetranitrate 80 mg/Time Cap. Bot. 50s.
Use: Antianginal.
PENT-T-80. (Mericon) Pentaerythritol tetranitrate 80 mg/T.D. Cap. Bot. 100s, 1000s.
Use: Antianginal.
PENNTUSS. (Pennwalt) Codeine (as polistirex) 10 mg, chlorpheniramine maleate 4 mg/5 ml. Bot. pt.
Use: Antitussive, antihistamine.
PEN-V. (Goldline) Penicillin 250 mg or 500 mg/ Tab. Bot. 100s, 1000s.
Use: Antibacterial, penicillin.
PEN-VEE K. (Wyeth-Ayerst) Potassium phenoxymethyl penicillin. 250 mg or 500 mg/Tab. Bot. 100s, 500s, Redipak 100s.
Use: Antibacterial, penicillin.
PEN-VEE K FOR ORAL SOLUTION. (Wyeth-Ayerst) Penicillin V potassium. **125 mg/5 ml:** Bot. 100 ml, 200 ml. **250 mg/5 ml:** Bot. 100 ml, 150 ml, 200 ml.
Use: Antibacterial, penicillin.
PEPCID. (Merck Sharp & Dohme) Famotidine. **Tab.:** 20 mg or 40 mg. Bot. 30s, UD 100s. **Oral Susp.:** 40 mg/5 ml. Bot. 10 doses. **I.V.:** Single dose vial 10 mg/ml or 20 mg/2 ml; Multi-dose vial 40 ml.
Use: Histamine H_2 antagonist.
•**PEPLOMYCIN SULFATE.** USAN.
Use: Antineoplastic.
•**PEPPERMINT,** N.F. XVII. Oil, Water, N.F. XVII.
Use: Pharmaceutic aid (flavor), antitussive, expectorant, nasal decongestant.
See: Vicks Prods. (Vicks).
•**PEPPERMINT OIL,** N.F. XVII.
Use: Pharmaceutic aid (flavor).
•**PEPPERMINT SPIRIT,** U.S.P. XXII.
Use: Digestive aid, flavor, perfume.
•**PEPPERMINT WATER,** N.F. XVII.
Use: Vehicle.
PEPSAMAR ESP LIQUID. (Winthrop Products) Aluminum hydroxide, glycerin.
Use: Antacid.
PEPSAMAR ESP TABLETS. (Winthrop Products) Aluminum hydroxide, magnesium hydroxide, mannitol powder.
Use: Antacid.
PEPSAMAR COMP. TABLETS. (Winthrop Products) Aluminum hydroxide, magnesium hydroxide.
Use: Antacid.
PEPSAMAR HM TABLETS. (Winthrop Products) Aluminum hydroxide, starch.
Use: Antacid.
PEPSAMAR LIQUID. (Winthrop Products) Aluminum hydroxide.
Use: Antacid.
PEPSAMAR SUSPENSION. (Winthrop Products) Aluminum hydroxide, magnesium hydroxide, sorbitol.
Use: Antacid.
PEPSAMAR TABLETS. (Winthrop Products) Aluminum hydroxide.
Use: Antacid.
PEPSATAL. (Kenyon) Pepsin 200 mg, pancreatin 200 mg, bile salts 100 mg, dehydrocholic acid 30 mg, desoxycholic acid 30 mg/Tab. Bot. 100s, 1000s.
Use: Digestive aid.
PEPSICONE GEL. (Winthrop Products) Aluminum hydroxide, magnesium hydroxide, simethicone.
Use: Antacid, antiflatulent.
PEPSICONE TABLET. (Winthrop Products) Aluminum hydroxide, magnesium hydroxide, simethicone.
Use: Antacid, antiflatulent.
PEPSIN.
Use: Digestive aid.
PEPSIN W/COMBINATIONS.
See: Biloric, Cap. (Arcum).
Donnazyme, Tab. (Robins).
Entozyme, Tab. (Robins).
Enzobile, Tab. (Mallard).
Gourmase-PB, Cap. (Solvay).
Kanulase, Tab. (Dorsey).
Leber Taurine, Liq. (Paddock).
Nu'Leven, Tab. (Lemmon).
Pepsatal, Tab. (Kenyon).
Ro-Bile, Tab. (Solvay).
Zypan, Tab. (Standard Process).
PEPSIN LACTATED, ELIXIR.
See: Peptalac, Liq. (Bowman).
•**PEPSTATIN.** USAN.
Use: Enzyme inhibitor (pepsin).
PEPTAMEN LIQUID. (Clintec Nutrition) Enzymatically hydrolyzed whey proteins, maltodextrin, starch, MCT, sunflower oil, lecithin, vitamins A, B_1, B_2, B_3, B_5, B_6, B_{12}, C, D, E, K, folic acid, biotin, choline, Ca, Cl, Cu, Fe, I, Mg, Mn, P, Zn. Can 500 ml.
Use: Enteral nutritional supplement.
PEPTAVLON. (Wyeth-Ayerst) Pentagastrin 0.25 mg, sodium Cl/ml. For evaluation of gastric acid secretion. Amp. 2 ml, Ctn. 10s.
Use: Diagnostic aid.
PEPTENZYME. (Reed & Carnrick) Alcohol 16%. Pleasantly aromatic. Bot. pt.
Use: Pharmaceutic aid.
PEPTO-BISMOL LIQUID. (Procter & Gamble) Bismuth subsalicylate 1.75%. Bot. 4 oz, 8 oz, 12 oz, 16 oz.
Use: Antidiarrheal.
PEPTO-BISMOL TABLETS. (Procter & Gamble) Bismuth subsalicylate 262.5 mg/Tab. Pkg. 24s, 42s.
Use: Antidiarrheal.
PERANDREN PHENYLACETATE. (Ciba) Testosterone phenylacetate.
Use: Androgen.
PERATIZOLE. B.A.N. 1-[-(2,4-Dimethylthiazol-5-yl)butyl]-4-(4-methylthiazol-2-yl)piperazine.

Use: Antihypertensive agent.
PERCAINE.
Use: Local anesthetic.
See: Dibucaine HCl, U.S.P.
PERCHLORACAP. (Mallinckrodt) Potassium perchlorate 200 mg/Cap. Bot. 100s.
Use: Radiographic adjunct.
PERCHLORETHYLENE.
See: Tetrachlorethylene, U.S.P. XXII.
PERCHLORPERAZINE.
See: Compazine, Preps. (SmithKline).
PERCOCET. (Du Pont) Oxycodone HCl 5 mg, acetaminophen 325 mg/Tab. Bot. 100s, 500s, UD 250s.
Use: Narcotic analgesic combination.
PERCODAN. (Du Pont) Oxycodone HCl 4.5 mg, oxycodone terephthalate 0.38 mg, aspirin 325 mg/Tab. Bot. 100s, 500s, 1000s, UD 250s.
Use: Narcotic analgesic combination.
W/Hexobarbital.
See: Percobarb, Cap. (Du Pont).
PERCODAN-DEMI. (Du Pont) Oxycodone HCl 2.25 mg, oxycodone terephthalate 0.19 mg, aspirin 325 mg/Tab. Bot. 100s.
Use: Narcotic analgesic combination.
PERIO-EZE-20. (Moyco) Oral paste.
Use: Analgesic for pain of gums and mucosa.
PERCOGESIC. (Vicks) Acetaminophen 325 mg, phenyltoloxamine citrate 30 mg/Tab. Bot. 24s, 50s, 90s.
Use: Analgesic, antihistamine.
PERCOMORPH LIVER OIL. (May be blended with 50% other fish liver oils; each Gm contains vitamins A 60,000 IU & D 8500 IU).
See: Oleum Percomorphum.
PERCY MEDICINE. (Merrick Medicine) Bismuth subnitrate 959 mg, calcium hydroxide 21.9 mg/10 ml, alcohol 5%.
Use: Antidiarrheal.
PERDIEM. (Rhone-Poulenc Rorer) Blend of psyllium 82%, senna 18% as active ingredients in granular form. Sodium content (0.08 mEq) 1.8 mg/rounded tsp. (6 Gm). Canister 100 Gm, 250 Gm, UD 6 Gm.
Use: Laxative.
PERDIEM FIBER. (Rhone-Poulenc Rorer) Psyllium 100% as active ingredient in granular form. Sodium content (0.08 mEq) 1.8 mg/rounded tsp. (6 Gm). Canister 100 Gm, 250 Gm, UD 6 Gm.
Use: Laxative.
PERE-DIOSATE. (Towne) Docusate sodium 100 mg, casanthranol 30 mg/Cap. Bot. 100s.
Use: Laxative.
PERESTAN. (Interstate) Docusate sodium 100 mg, casanthranol 30 mg/Cap. Bot. 100s, 1000s.
Use: Laxative.
•**PERFILCON A.** USAN.
Use: Contact lens material.
See: Permalens (CooperVision).
PERGALEN.
See: Sodium Apolate.
•**PERGOLIDE MESYLATE.** USAN.
Use: Dopamine agonist.
PERGONAL (MENOTROPINS). (Serono) Follicle stimulating hormone (FSH) and luteinizing hormone (LH). **75 IU:** Unit contains 1 Amp. FSH/LH and 1 Amp. sodium Cl diluent. Pkg. 10s. **150 IU:** Unit contains 1 Amp. FSH/LH and 1 Amp. sodium Cl diluent.
Use: Gonadotropin.
PERGRAVA. (Arcum) Vitamins A 2000 IU, D 300 IU, B_1 2 mg, B_2 2 mg, nicotinamide 10 mg, B_6 2 mg, B_{12} 5 mcg, C 60 mg, calcium 40 mg/Cap. Bot. 100s, 1000s.
Use: Vitamin/mineral supplement.
PERGRAVA NO. 2. (Arcum) Vitamins A 2000 IU, D 300 IU, B_1 2 mg, B_2 2 mg, nicotinamide 10 mg, B_6 2 mg, C 60 mg, calcium lactate monohydrate 200 mg, ferrous gluconate 31 mg, folic acid 0.1 mg/Cap. Bot. 100s, 1000s.
Use: Vitamin/mineral supplement.
•**PERHEXILINE.** USAN. 2-(2,2-Dicyclohexylethyl)-piperidine.
Use: Treatment of angina pectoris.
•**PERHEXILINE MALEATE.** USAN. 2-(2,2-Dicyclohexylethyl) piperidine maleate.
Use: Cardiovascular agent.
PERHYDROL.
See: Hydrogen Peroxide 30% (Various Mfr.).
PERIACTIN. (Merck Sharp & Dohme) Cyproheptadine HCl 4 mg/Tab. Bot. 100s.
Use: Antihistamine.
PERIACTIN SYRUP. (Merck Sharp & Dohme) Cyproheptadine HCl 2 mg/5 ml, alcohol 5%, sorbic acid 0.1%. Bot. 473 ml.
Use: Antihistamine.
PERI-CARE. (Sween) Vitamins A and D in petroleum ointment base. Tube 0.5 oz, 1.75 oz. Jar 2 oz, 5 oz, 8 oz.
Use: Emollient.
PERI-COLACE. (Mead Johnson) **Cap.:** Docusate sodium 100 mg, casanthranol 30 mg/Cap. Bot. 30s, 60s, 250s, 1000s, UD 100s. **Syr.:** Docusate sodium 60 mg, casanthranol 30 mg/15 ml, ethyl alcohol 10%. Bot. 8 oz, pt.
Use: Laxative.
PERI-CONATE. (Cenci) Docusate sodium 100 mg, casanthranol 30 mg/Cap. Bot. 100s, 1000s.
Use: Laxative.
PERICYAZINE. B.A.N. 2-Cyano-10-[3-(4-hydroxypiperidino)propyl]phenothiazine. Neulactil.
Use: Tranquilizer.
PERIDEX. (Procter & Gamble) Chlorhexidine gluconate 0.12%, alcohol 11.6%, glycerin, PEG-40 sorbitan diisostearate, flavor, sodium saccharin, FD&C blue No. 1, water. Bot. pt.
Use: Mouth preparation.
PERIDIN-C. (Beutlich) Hesperidin methyl chalcone 50 mg, hesperidin complex 150 mg, ascorbic acid 200 mg/Tab. Bot. 100s, 500s.
Use: Vitamin supplement.

PERI-DOS. (Goldline) Docusate sodium 100 mg, casanthranol 30 mg/Cap. Bot. 30s, 60s, 100s, 1000s.
Use: Laxative.

PERIES. (Xttrium) Medicated pads w/witch hazel, glycerin. Jar pad 40s.
Use: Hygienic wipe and local compress.

PERIMED. (Olin) Hydrogen peroxide 1.5%, povidone-iodine 6%, saccharin. Pouch 20 ml.
Use: Mouth and gum preparation.

PERI SOFCAP. (Alton) Docusate sodium with peristim. Bot. 100s, 1000s.
Use: Laxative.

PERISTOMAL COVERING.
See: Stomahesive, Wafer (Squibb).

PERITIME-80. (Kenyon; Werner) Pentaerythritol tetranitrate 80 mg/Cap. Bot. 100s.
Use: Antianginal.

PERITINIC. (Lederle) Elemental iron 100 mg, docusate sodium 100 mg, vitamins B_1 7.5 mg, B_2 7.5 mg, B_6 7.5 mg, B_{12} 50 mcg, C 200 mg, niacinamide 30 mg, folic acid 0.05 mg, pantothenic acid 15 mg/Tab. Bot. 60s.
Use: Vitamin/mineral supplement, laxative.

PERITRATE. (Parke-Davis) Pentaerythritol tetranitrate. **10 mg/Tab.:** Bot. 100s, 1000s. **20 mg/Tab.:** Bot. 100s, 1000s, UD 100s. **40 mg/Tab.:** Bot. 100s.
Use: Antianginal.

PERITRATE S.A. (Parke-Davis) Pentaerythritol tetranitrate 80 mg (20 mg in immediate release layer, 60 mg in sustained release base)/Tab. Bot. 100s, 1000s, UD 100s.
Use: Antianginal.

PERI-WASH. (Sween) Bot. 4 oz, 8 oz, 1 gal, 5 gal, 30 gal, 55 gal.
Use: Anorectal preparation.

PERI-WASH II. (Sween) Bot. 4 oz, 8 oz, 1 gal, 5 gal, 30 gal, 55 gal.
Use: Anorectal preparation.

•**PERLAPINE.** USAN. 6-(4-Methyl-1-piperazinyl) Morphanthridine.
Use: Hypnotic.

PERLATAN.
See: Estrone (Various Mfr.).

PERMANGANIC ACID, POTASSIUM SALT. Potassium Permanganate, U.S.P. XXII.

PERMAPEN. (Roerig) Benzathine penicillin G 1,200,000 units/ml. Disp. syringe 2 ml.
Use: Antibacterial, penicillin.

PERMAX. (Lilly) Pergolide mesylate.
Use: Antiparkinson agent.

PERMETHRIN. USAN. Synthetic pyrethrin.
Use: Pediculicide for treatment of head lice, ectoparasiticide.
See: Nix, Cream (Burroughs Wellcome).

PERMITIL. (Schering) Fluphenazine HCl. **2.5 mg** or **5 mg/Tab:** Bot. 100s. **10 mg/Tab.:** Bot. 1000s.
Use: Antipsychotic agent.

PERMITIL ORAL CONCENTRATE. (Schering) Fluphenazine HCl 5 mg/ml. Bot. 120 ml w/calibrated dropper. Hospital use.
Use: Antipsychotic agent.

PERNOX LOTION. (Westwood) Microfine granules of polyethylene 20%, sulfur 2%, salicylic acid 2% in a combination of soapless cleansers and wetting agents. Bot. 6 oz.
Use: Anti-acne.

PERNOX MEDICATED LATHERING SCRUB CLEANSER. (Westwood) Polyethylene granules 26%, sulfur 2%, salicylic acid 1.5% w/ soapless surface-active cleansers and wetting agents. Regular or lemon. Tube 2 oz, 4 oz.
Use: Anti-acne.

PERNOX SHAMPOO. (Westwood) Sodium laureth sulfate, water, lauramide DEA, quaternium 22, PEG-75 lanolin/hydrolyzed animal protein, fragrance, sodium Cl, lactic acid, sorbic acid, disodium EDTA, FD&C yellow No. 6 and blue No. 1. Bot. 8 oz.
Use: Cleanser and conditioner for oily hair.

PEROXIDASE. W/Glucose oxidase, potassium, iodide.
See: Diastix Reagent Strips (Ames).

PEROXIDE, DIBENZOYL. Benzoyl Peroxide, Hydrous.

PEROXIDES.
See: Hydrogen Peroxide (Various Mfr.).
Urea Peroxide.
Zinc Peroxide.

PEROXYL MOUTHRINSE. (Hoyt) Hydrogen peroxide 1.5% in mint flavored base, alcohol 6%. Bot. 8 oz.
Use: Mouth preparation.

•**PERPHENAZINE,** U.S.P. XXII. Inj., Oral Soln., Syr., Tab., U.S.P. XXII. 2-Chloro-10-[3-[4-(2-hydroxyethyl)-piperazinyl]propyl]-phenothiazine. 4-(3-(2-Chloro-phenothiazin-1-yl)propyl)-1-piperazine-ethanol.
Use: Antiemetic, tranquilizer.
See: Trilafon, Prods. (Schering).

•**PERPHENAZINE/AMITRIPTYLINE TABLETS,** U.S.P. XXII. (Various, eg, Bolar, Geneva, Goldline, Lemmon, Par, Rugby, Schein, Zenith). Perphenazine (mg): 2, 2; Amitriptyline (mg): 10, 25. Bot. 21s, 100s, 500s, 1000s; Bot. 100s, 500s, 1000s.
Use: Miscellaneous psychotherapeutic agents.
See: Etrafon, Prods. (Schering).
Triavil, Tab. (Merck Sharp & Dohme).

PERSA-GEL. (Ortho Derm) Benzoyl peroxide 5% or 10%, acetone base. Tube 1.5 oz, 3 oz.
Use: Anti-acne.

PERSA-GEL W. (Ortho Derm) Benzoyl peroxide 5% or 10% in water base. Tube 1.5 oz, 3 oz.
Use: Anti-acne.

PERSANGUE. (Arcum) Ferrous gluconate 192 mg, vitamins C 150 mg, B_1 3 mg, B_2 3 mg, B_{12} 50 mcg/Cap. Bot. 100s, 500s.
Use: Vitamin/mineral supplement.

PERSANTINE. (Boehringer Ingelheim) Dipyridamole 25 mg, 50 mg or 75 mg/Tab. **25 mg or 50 mg:** Bot. 100s, 1000s, UD 100s. **75 mg:** Bot. 100s, 500s, UD 100s.
Use: Antiplatelet agent.
PERSANTINE IV. (DuPont-Merck) Dipyridamole. Inj. For evaluation of coronary artery disease.
Use: Diagnostic aid.
•**PERSIC OIL,** N.F. XVII.
Use: Vehicle.
PERSONAL LUBRICANT. (Ortho) Glycerin, propylene glycol, sodium carboxymethylcellulose, sodium alginate, sorbic acid. Gel Tube. 60 Gm, 120 Gm.
Use: Vaginal preparation.
PERTECHNETIC ACID, SODIUM SALT. Sodium Pertechnetate Tc 99 m Solution.
PERTOFRANE. (Rorer) Desipramine HCl 25 mg or 50 mg/Cap. Bot. 100s, 1000s.
Use: Antidepressant.
PERTROPIN. (Lannett) Linolenic acid 7 min/Cap. Bot. 100s.
Use: Oral nutritional supplement.
PERTSCAN-99m. (Abbott Diagnostics) Radiodiagnostic. Inj. Tc-99m.
Use: Diagnostic aid.
PERTUSSIN AM. (Canaan Labs) Phenylpropanolamine HCl 12.5 mg, chlorpheniramine maleate 2 mg, dextromethorphan HBr 10 mg/5 ml, 9.5% alcohol. Bot. 180 ml.
Use: Decongestant, antihistamine, antitussive.
PERTUSSIN CS. (Canaan Labs) Dextromethorphan HBr 3.5 mg, guaifenesin 25 mg/5 ml, 8.5% alcohol. Bot. 90 ml.
Use: Antitussive, expectorant.
PERTUSSIN PM. (Canaan Labs) Pseudoephedrine HCl 10 mg, doxylamine succinate 1.25 mg, dextromethorphan HBr 5 mg, acetaminophen 167 mg/5 ml, alcohol 25%. Bot. 180 ml.
Use: Decongestant, antihistamine, antitussive, analgesic.
PERTUSSIN SYRUP. (Canaan Labs) Dextromethorphan HBr 15 mg/5 ml, alcohol 9.5%. Bot. 3 oz, 6 oz.
Use: Antitussive.
•**PERTUSSIS VACCINE,** U.S.P. XXII. (Various Mfr.).
Use: Active immunization against whooping cough.
•**PERTUSSIS VACCINE, ADSORBED,** U.S.P. XXII. Vial 7.5 ml.
Use: Active immunizing agent.
PERTUSSIS VACCINE AND DIPHTHERIA AND TETANUS TOXOIDS, COMBINED.
Use: Active immunizing agent.
See: Tri-Immunol, Vial (Lederle).
Triple Antigen, Vial (Wyeth-Ayerst).
Tri-Solgen, Vial, Hyporet (Lilly).
PERUVIAN BALSAM.
Use: Local protectant, rubefacient.
W/Benzocaine, zinc oxide, bismuth subgallate, boric acid.
See: Anocaine, Supp. (Mallard).
W/Benzocaine, zinc oxide, 8-hydroxyquinoline benzoate, menthol. Unit-of-Use 90s. **50 mg:** Bot. 100s, 1000s, UD 100s. **75 mg:** Bot. 100s.
See: Hemorrhoidal Oint. (Towne).
W/Ephedrine sulfate, belladonna extract, zinc oxide, boric acid, bismuth oxyiodide, subcarbonate.
See: Wyanoids, Preps. (Wyeth-Ayerst).
W/Lidocaine, bismuth subgallate, zinc oxide, aluminum subacetate.
See: Xylocaine, Supp. (Astra).
W/Oxyquinoline sulfate, pramoxine HCl, zinc oxide.
See: Zyanoid, Oint. (Elder).
PESON. Sodium Lyapolate. Polyethenesulfonate sodium.
Use: Anticoagulant.
PETERSON'S OINTMENT. (Peterson) Carbolic acid, camphor, tannic acid, zinc oxide. Tube w/ pipe 1 oz. Jar 16 oz. Can 1.4 oz, 3 oz.
Use: Anorectal preparation.
PETHADOL TABLETS. (Halsey) Meperidine HCl 50 mg or 100 mg/Tab. Bot. 100s, 1000s.
Use: Narcotic analgesic.
PETHIDINE HYDROCHLORIDE.
See: Meperidine HCl, U.S.P. XXII.
PETN.
See: Pentaerythritol tetranitrate.
PETRICHLORAL. Pentaerythritol chloral. 1,1′,1″,1‴-(Neopentanetetrayl-tetraoxy)tetrakis [2,2,2-trichloroethanol].
Use: Sedative.
PETRO-20. (Foy) Pentaerythritol tetranitrate 20 mg/Tab. Bot. 100s, 1000s.
Use: Antianginal.
•**PETROLATUM,** U.S.P. XXII.
Use: Ointment base.
See: Lipkote, Stick (Schering-Plough).
•**PETROLATUM GAUZE,** U.S.P. XXII.
Use: Surgical aid.
•**PETROLATUM, HYDROPHILIC,** U.S.P. XXII.
Use: Absorbent ointment base; topical protectant.
See: Lipkote (Schering-Plough).
PETROLATUM, LIQUID. Mineral Oil, U.S.P. XXII. Light Mineral Oil, U.S.P. XXII. Adepsine Oil, Glymol, Liquid Paraffin, Parolein, White Mineral Oil, Heavy Liquid Petrolatum.
Use: Laxative.
See: Clyserol Oil Retention Enema (Fuller Labs).
Fleet Mineral Oil Enema (Fleet).
Mineral Oil (Various Mfr.).
Nujol, Liq. (Schering-Plough).
Saxol (Various Mfr.).
PETROLATUM, LIQUID, EMULSION.
Use: Lubricant, laxative.
See: Milkinol, Liq. (Kremers-Urban).
W/Agar-Gel.
See: Agoral Plain, Liq. (Parke-Davis).
Petrogalar, Preps. (Wyeth-Ayerst).

W/Cascara.
See: Petrogalar w/Cascara, Emulsion (Wyeth-Ayerst).
W/Docusate sodium.
See: Milkinol, Liq. (Kremers-Urban).
W/Irish moss, casanthranol.
See: Neo-Kondremul (Fisons).
W/Milk of magnesia.
See: Haley's M. O., Liq. (Winthrop Consumer Products).
W/Phenolphthalein.
See: Agoral, Emulsion (Parke-Davis).
Petrogalar w/Phenolphthalein, Emulsion (Wyeth-Ayerst).
Phenolphthalein in liquid Petrolatum Emulsion.

PETROLATUM, RED VETERINARIAN. (Elder) Also known as RVP.
See: Rubrapet, Oint. (Medco).
W/Micasorb.
See: RV Plus, Oint. (Elder).
W/N-diethyl metatoluamide.
See: RV Pellent, Oint. (Elder).
W/Zinc oxide, 2-ethoxyethyl p-methoxycinnamate.
See: RV Paque, Oint. (Elder).

•**PETROLATUM, WHITE,** U.S.P. XXII.
Use: An oleaginous ointment base, topical protectant.
See: Moroline, Oint. (Schering-Plough).

PETRO-PHYLIC SOAP. (Doak) Hydrophilic Petrolatum. Cake 4 oz.
Use: Emollient, anti-infective, external.

PF4RIA. (Abbott Diagnostics) Platelet factor 4 radioimmunoassay for the quantitative measurement of total PF4 levels in plasma.
Use: Diagnostic aid.

PFEIFFER'S ALLERGY. (Pfeiffer) Chlorpheniramine maleate 4 mg/Tab. Bot. 24s.
Use: Antihistamine.

PFEIFFER'S COLD SORE. (Pfeiffer) Gum benzoin 7%, camphor, menthol, thymol, eucalyptol, alcohol 85%. Lot. Bot. 15 ml.
Use: Cold sores, fever blisters, cracked lips.

PFIZERPEN-AS. (Roerig) Procaine penicillin G 3,000,000 units in aqueous susp./Vial. Carton 5s. Multi-Vial Pack, Carton 100s.
Use: Antibacterial, penicillin.

PFIZERPEN FOR INJECTION. (Roerig) Potassium penicillin G, buffered. **Multi-Vial Pack:** 1,000,000 units or 5,000,000 units/Vial. Carton 10s, 100s; **Individual Vial:** 20,000,000 units/Vial 1s, 10s.
Use: Antibacterial, penicillin.

PFIZERPEN VK TABLETS. (Pfizer Laboratories) Penicillin V potassium 250 mg or 500 mg/Tab. **250 mg:** Bot. 1000s. **500 mg:** Bot. 100s.
Use: Antibacterial, penicillin.

PGA. *See:* Folic Acid, U.S.P. XXII.

PGE.
Use: Prostaglandin.
See: Alprostadil.

PHacid. (Baker/Cummins) Bot. 8 oz.
Use: Shampoo.

PHADIATOP RIA TEST. (Pharmacia) Determination of IgE antibodies specific to inhalant allergens in human serum. Kit 60s.
Use: Diagnostic aid.

PHANATUSS. (Pharmakon Labs) Dextromethorphan HBr 10 mg, guaifenesin 85 mg, potassium citrate 75 mg, citric acid 35 mg/5 ml, sorbitol, menthol. Syr. Bot. 118 ml.
Use: Antitussive, expectorant.

PHANQUONE. B.A.N. 4,7-Phenanthroline-5,6-quinone. Phanquinone (I.N.N.).
Use: Treatment of amebiasis.
See: Entobex.

pH ANTISEPTIC SKIN CLEANSER. (Walgreen) Alcohol 63%. Bot. 16 oz.
Use: Astringent, cleanser.

PHARAZINE. (Halsey) Bot. 4 oz, 16 oz, gal.
Use: A series of cough and cold products.

PHARMADINE. (Sherwood Pharm.) Povidone-iodine. **Oint.:** Pkt. 1 Gm, 1.5 Gm, 2 Gm, 30 Gm, 1 lb. **Perineal wash:** 240 ml. **Skin cleanser:** 240 ml. **Soln.:** 15 ml, 120 ml, 240 ml, pt, qt. **Soln., swabs:** 100s. **Soln., swabsticks:** 1 or 3/packet in 250s. **Spray:** 120 Gm. **Surgical scrub:** 30 ml, pt, qt, gal, foil-pack 15 ml. **Surgical scrub sponge/brush:** 25s. **Swabsticks, lemon glycerin:** 100s. **Whirlpool soln.:** gal.
Use: Antiseptic.

PHARMAFLUR. (Pharmics) Sodium fluoride 2.21 mg/Tab. Bot. 1000s.
Use: Dental caries preventative.

PHARMALGEN. (Pharmacia) Freeze-dried hymenopteria venom/venom protein from honey bee, yellow jacket, yellow hornet white-faced hornet, wasp, mixed vespid. Diagnostic kit: 5 × 1 ml Vial. Treatment kit: 6 × 1 ml vial or 1 × 1.1 mg multiple dose vial. Starter Kit: 6 × 1 ml, pre-diluted 0.01 mcg to 100 mcg/ml.
Use: Diagnostic aid, treatment kit.

PHARMALGEN RAST STANDARDIZED ALLERGENIC EXTRACTS-POLLENS. (Pharmacia) 100,000 allergenic units/Vial. Box 5 x 1 ml.
Use: Diagnostic aid, treatment kit.

PHAZYME. (Reed & Carnrick) Simethicone 60 mg/Core Tab. Bot. 50s, 100s, 1000s.
Use: Antiflatulent.

PHAZYME-95. (Reed & Carnrick) Simethicone 95 mg/Core Tab. Bot. 100s.
Use: Antiflatulent.

•**PHEMFILCON A.** USAN.
Use: Contact lens material.

PHENACAINE HYDROCHLORIDE, U.S.P. XXI. N,N′-Bis(p-ethoxy-phenyl)acetamidine HCl, monohydrate.
Use: Local anesthetic (ophthalmic).
W/Atropine, phenol, nut gall, zinc oxide.
See: Tanicaine, Oint., Supp. (Upjohn).
W/Cod liver oil.
See: Morusan Oint. (Beecham Labs).
W/Ephedrine. (Upjohn) Phenacaine HCl 1%, epinephrine 1:25,000. Ophth. oint. Tube 1 dr.

W/Mercarbolide. (Upjohn) Holocaine HCl 2%, mercarbolide 1:3000. Ophth. oint., Tube w/applicator tip, 1 dr.

•**PHENACEMIDE,** U.S.P. XXII. Tab., U.S.P. XXII. Phenylacetylurea.
Use: Anticonvulsant.
See: Phenurone, Tab. (Abbott).

PHENACETIN. Acetophenetidin. Ethoxyacetanilide.
Use: Antipyretic, analgesic.
NOTE: This drug has been withdrawn from the market due to liver and kidney toxicity. This drug is no longer official in the U.S.P.

PHENACETYLCARBAMIDE.
See: Phenurone, Tab. (Abbott).

PHENACETYLUREA.
See: Phenurone, Tab. (Abbott).

PHENACRIDANE. (9(p-Hexloxphenyl)-10-methylacridinium Cl).
See: Micridium (Johnson & Johnson).

PHENACTROPINIUM CHLORIDE. B.A.N. N-Phenacylhomatropinium Cl. Trophenium.
Use: Hypotensive.

PHENACYL HOMATROPHINIUM HCl. Not available.

PHENADOXONE. B.A.N. 6-Morpholino-4,4-diphenyl-heptan-3-one. Heptalgin hydrochloride.
Use: Analgesic, hypnotic.

PHENAGESIC. (Dalin) Phenylephrine HCl 10 mg, phenylpropanolamine HCl 50 mg, pyrilamine maleate 25 mg, pheniramine maleate 25 mg, acetyl-p-aminophenol 300 mg/Tab. or 5 ml. **Tab.:** Bot. 50s. **Syr.:** (without acetaminophen): Bot. 6 oz, pt.
Use: Decongestant, antihistamine, analgesic.

PHENAGLYCODOL. B.A.N. 2-p-Chlorophenyl-3-methyl-2,3-butanediol. 2-(4-Chlorophenyl)-3-methylbutane-2,3-diol.
Use: Central nervous system depressant.

PHENAHIST INJECTABLE. (T.E. Williams) Atropine sulfate 0.2 mg, phenylpropanolamine HCl 12.5 mg, chlorpheniramine maleate 5 mg/ml. Vial 10 ml.
Use: Anticholinergic/antispasmodic, decongestant, antihistamine.

PHENAHIST-TR TABLETS. (T.E. Williams) Phenylephrine HCl 25 mg, phenylpropanolamine HCl 50 mg, chlorpheniramine maleate 8 mg, hyoscyamine sulfate 0.143 mg, atropine 0.0362 mg, scopolamine HBr 0.012 mg/Tab. Bot. 100s.
Use: Decongestant, antihistamine, anticholinergic/antispasmodic.

PHENALZINE DIHYDROGEN SULFATE.
See: Nardil, Tab. (Parke-Davis).

PHENAMAZOLINE HCl. 2-(Anilinomethyl)-2-imidazoline HCl.
Use: Vasoconstrictor.

PHENAMETH TABLETS. (Major) Promethazine 25 mg/Tab. Bot. 1000s.
Use: Antihistamine, antiemetic.

PHENAMETH W/CODEINE. (Major) Promethazine HCl 6.25 mg, codeine phosphate 10 mg/5 ml, alcohol 7%. Syr. Bot. 4 oz, pt, gal.
Use: Antihistamine, antitussive.

PHENAMETH VC W/CODEINE. (Major) Phenylephrine HCl 5 mg, promethazine HCl 6.25 mg, codeine phosphate 10 mg/5 ml, alcohol 7%. Syr. Bot. pt, gal.
Use: Decongestant, antihistamine, antitussive.

PHENAMPROMIDE. B.A.N. N-(1-Methyl-2-piperidinoethyl)propionanilide.
Use: Analgesic.

PHENANTOIN. Mephenytoin. N-Methyl-5,5-phenylethylhydantoin.
See: Mesantoin, Tab. (Sandoz).

PHENAPAP. (Rugby) Pseudoephedrine HCl 30 mg, chlorpheniramine 2 mg, acetaminophen 325 mg/Tab. Bot. 30s, 100s, 1000s.
Use: Decongestant, antihistamine, analgesic.

PHENAPHEN. (Robins) Acetaminophen 325 mg/Cap. Bot. 100s, 1000s.
Use: Analgesic.

PHENAPHEN WITH CODEINE. (Robins) **No. 2:** Acetaminophen 325 mg, codeine 15 mg/Cap. **No. 3:** Acetaminophen 325 mg, codeine 30 mg/Cap. **No. 4:** Acetaminophen 325 mg, codeine 60 mg/Cap. Bot. 100s, 500s, Dis-Co packs 4 × 25s.
Use: Narcotic analgesic combination.

PHENAPHEN-650 WITH CODEINE. (Robins) Codeine phosphate 30 mg, acetaminophen 650 mg/Tab. Bot. 50s, Dis-Co packs 4 × 25s.
Use: Narcotic analgesic combination.

PHENAPHTHAZINE. Sodium dinitro phenylazonaphthol disulfonate.
See: Nitrazine Paper, Roll (Squibb).

PHENARSONE SULFOXYLATE. (5-Arsono-2-hydroxyanilino)methanesulfinic acid disodium salt.
Use: Antiamebic.

PHENASPIRIN COMPOUND. (Davis & Sly) Phenobarbital 0.25 gr, aspirin 3.5 gr/Cap. Bot. 1000s.
Use: Sedative/hypnotic, salicylate analgesic.

PHENASPIRIN COMPOUND CAPSULES. (Lannett) Aspirin 3.5 gr, phenobarbital 0.25 gr/Cap. Bot. 1000s, 5000s.
Use: Salicylate analgesic, sedative/hypnotic.

PHENATE T.D. (Hauck) Phenylpropanolamine HCl 40 mg, chlorpheniramine maleate 4 mg, acetaminophen 325 mg/CR Tab. Bot. 100s, 1000s.
Use: Decongestant, antihistamine, analgesic.

PHENATIN. (Jenkins) Acetophenetidin 0.2 Gm, acetylsalicylic acid 0.25 Gm, caffeine 30 mg, camphor monobromated 0.1 Gm/Tab. Bot. 1000s.
Use: Analgesic combination.

PHENATIN TD CAPSULE. (Jenkins) Phenylpropanolamine HCl 50 mg, chlorpheniramine maleate 1 mg, pheniramine maleate 12.5 mg, atropine sulfate 0.025 mg, scopolamine HBr 0.014

mg, belladonna alkaloids (total) 0.16 mg, hyoscyamine sulfate 0.122 mg/Cap. Bot. 1000s.
Use: Decongestant, antihistamine, anticholinergic/antispasmodic.

PHENATUSS. (Dalin) Codeine phosphate 10 mg, chlorpheniramine maleate 2 mg, phenylephrine HCl 5 mg, guaifenesin 100 mg, 1-menthol 1 mg/5 ml. Bot. 4 oz, pt, gal.
Use: Antitussive, antihistamine, decongestant, expectorant.

PHENAZINE. (Jenkins) Phendimetrazine bitartrate 50 mg/ml. Vial 10 ml.
Use: Anorexiant.

PHENAZINE. (Keene) Promethazine HCl 25 mg or 50 mg. Vial 10 ml.
Use: Antihistamine, antiemetic.

PHENAZOCINE. B.A.N. 1,2,3,4,5,6-Hexahydro-6,11-dimethyl-3-phenethyl-2,6-methano-3-benzazocin-8-ol.
Use: Analgesic; antipyretic.

PHENAZOCINE HBr. 1,2,3,4,5,6-Hexahydro-8-hydroxy-6,11-dimethyl-3-phenethyl-2,6-methano-3-benzazo-cine HBr.
Use: Analgesic.

PHENAZODINE. (Lannett) Phenazopyridine HCl 100 mg or 200 mg/Tab. Bot. 100s, 500s, 1000s.
Use: Urinary tract product.

PHENAZONE.
See: Antipyrine (Various Mfr.).

PHENAZOPYRIDINE HCl, U.S.P. XXII. Tab., U.S.P. XXII. 2,6-Diamino-3-phenylazopyridine HCl.
Use: Analgesic (urinary tract).
See: Azogesic, Tab. (Century).
Azo-Pyridon, Tab. (Solvay).
Azo-Standard, Tab. (Webcon).
Azo-Sulfizin (Solvay).
Diridone, Tab. (Premo).
Phen-Azo, Tab. (Vanguard).
Phenazodine, Tab. (Lannett).
Pyridium, Tab. (Parke-Davis).
Uri-Pak (Westerfield).
Urodine, Tab. (Saron).

PHENAZOPYRIDINE HCl W/COMBINATIONS.
See: Azo-Cyst, Tab. (Moore Kirk).
Azo Gantanol, Tab. (Roche).
Azo Gantrisin, Tab. (Roche).
Azosulfisoxazole (Various Mfr.).
Pyridium Plus, Tab.(Parke-Davis).
Rosoxol-Azo, Tab. (Robinson).
Thiosulfil-A, Tab. (Wyeth-Ayerst).
Thiosulfil-A Forte, Tab. (Wyeth-Ayerst).
Triurisul, Tab. (Sheryl).
Uridium, Tab. (Ferndale; Pharmex).
Urisan-P, Tab. (Sandia).
Uritral, Cap. (Central).
Urobiotic, Cap. (Pfizer).
Urogesic, Tab. (Edwards).
Urotrol, Tab. (Mills).

PHENBENICILLIN. B.A.N. 6-(α-Phenoxyphenylacetamido)penicillanic acid. α-Phenoxybenzylpenicillin.
Use: Antibiotic.

•**PHENBUTAZONE SODIUM GLYCERATE.** USAN. 4-Butyl-3-hydroxy-1,2-diphenyl-3-pyrazolin-5-one sodium salt compound with glycerol.
Use: Anti-inflammatory.

PHENBUTRAZATE. B.A.N. 2-(3-Methyl-2-phenylmorpholino)ethyl 2-phenylbutryate.
Use: Appetite suppressant.

PHENCAP. (Jenkins) Phenylpropanolamine HCl 50 mg, chlorpheniramine maleate 8 mg, atropine sulfate 1/180 gr/Cap. Bot. 1000s.
Use: Decongestant, antihistamine, anticholinergic/antispasmodic.

•**PHENCARBAMIDE.** USAN. S-2-Diethyl-ammoethyl diphenylthiocarbamate.
Use: Spasmolytic agent.
See: Escorpal (Farben-Fabriken).

PHENCEN-50. (Central) Promethazine HCl 50 mg, disodium edetate 0.1 mg, calcium Cl 0.04 mg, phenol 5 mg/ml. Vial 10 ml Box 12s.
Use: Antihistamine, antiemetic.

PHENCHLOR-EIGHT. (Freeport) Chlorpheniramine maleate 8 mg/TR Cap. Bot. 1000s.
Use: Antihistamine.

PHENCHLOR-TWELVE. (Freeport) Chlorpheniramine maleate 12 mg/TR Cap. Bot. 1000s.
Use: Antihistamine.

•**PHENCYCLIDINE HYDROCHLORIDE.** USAN. 1-(1-Phenylcyclohexyl)piperidine HCl.
Use: Anticholinergic.

•**PHENDIMETRAZINE TARTRATE,** U.S.P. XXII. Cap., Tab., U.S.P. XXII. d-3,4-Dimethyl-2-phenylmorpholine bitartrate.
Use: Anorexic.
See: Adipost, Cap. (Ascher).
Adphen, Tab. (Ferndale).
Anorex, Cap., Tab. (Dunhall).
Bacarate, Tab. (Solvay).
B.O.F. (Saron).
Bontril PDM, Tab. (Carnrick).
Bontril Slow Release, Cap. (Carnrick).
Delcozine, Tab. (Delco).
Di-Ap-Trol, Tab. (Foy).
Di-Metrex, Tab. (Fellows-Testagar).
Elphemet, Tab. (Canright).
Limit, Tab. (Bock).
Melfiat, Tab. (Solvay).
Melfiat 105, Cap. (Solvay).
Minus, Tab. (Amfre-Grant).
Obacin, Tab. (Kenyon).
Obalan, Tab. (Lannett).
Obepar, Tab. (Parmed).
Obe-Tite, Tab. (Scott/Cord).
Phenazine, Inj. (Jenkins).
Phen-70, Tab. (Parmed).
Phenzine, Tab. (Hauck).
Prelu-2, Cap. (Boehringer Ingelheim).
Reducto, Tab. (Arcum).
Robese "P", Tab., Vial (Rocky Mtn.).
Ropledge, Tab. (Robinson).

Slim-Tabs, Tab. (Wesley).
Statobex, Prods. (Lemmon).
Stodex, Tab., Cap. (Jalco).
Trimtabs, Tab. (Mayrand).

•**PHENELZINE SULFATE,** U.S.P. XXII. Tab., U.S.P. XXII. Phenethylhydrazine sulfate. Monoamine oxidase inhibitor, betaphenylethyl-hydrazinedihydrogen sulfate.
Use: Antidepressant.
See: Nardil, Tab. (Parke-Davis).

PHENERGAN-D. (Wyeth-Ayerst) Promethazine HCl 6.25 mg, pseudoephedrine HCl 60 mg/Tab. Bot. 100s.
Use: Antihistamine, decongestant.

PHENERGAN FORTIS. (Wyeth-Ayerst) Promethazine HCl 25 mg/5 ml, alcohol 1.5%. Bot. pt.
Use: Antihistamine.

PHENERGAN INJECTION. (Wyeth-Ayerst) Promethazine HCl 25 mg or 50 mg/ml. Inj. Amp. 1 mg Pkg. 5s, 25s, Tubex 10s.
Use: Antihistamine.

PHENERGAN PLAIN. (Wyeth-Ayerst) Promethazine HCl 6.25 mg/5 ml, alcohol 7%, saccharin. Syr. Bot. 120 ml, 180 ml, 240 ml, pt, gal.
Use: Antihistamine.

PHENERGAN SUPPOSITORIES. (Wyeth-Ayerst) Promethazine HCl 12.5 mg, 25 mg or 50 mg/ Supp. Box. 12s, Redipak.
Use: Antihistamine.

PHENERGAN SYRUP PLAIN. (Wyeth-Ayerst) Promethazine HCl 6.25 mg/5 ml. Bot. 4 oz, 6 oz, 8 oz, pt, gal.
Use: Antihistamine.

PHENERGAN TABLETS. (Wyeth-Ayerst) Promethazine HCl 12.5 mg, 25 mg or 50 mg/Tab. Bot. 100s. Redipak 100s.
Use: Antihistamine.

PHENERGAN VC. (Wyeth-Ayerst) Promethazine HCl 6.25 mg, phenylephrine HCl 5 mg/5 ml, alcohol 7%. Bot. 4 oz, 6 oz, 8 oz, pt, gal.
Use: Antihistamine, decongestant.

PHENERGAN VC WITH CODEINE. (Wyeth-Ayerst) Promethazine HCl 6.25 mg, codeine phosphate 10 mg, phenylephrine HCl 5 mg/5 ml, alcohol 7%. Bot. 4 oz, 6 oz, 8 oz, pt, gal.
Use: Antihistamine, antitussive, decongestant.

PHENERGAN WITH CODEINE. (Wyeth-Ayerst) Promethazine HCl 6.25 mg, codeine phosphate 10 mg/5 ml. Bot. 4 oz, 6 oz, 8 oz, pt, gal.
Use: Antihistamine, antitussive.

PHENERGAN WITH DEXTROMETHORPHAN. (Wyeth-Ayerst) Promethazine HCl 6.25 mg, dextromethorphan HBr 15 mg/5 ml, alcohol 7%. Bot. 4 oz, 6 oz, pt, gal.
Use: Antihistamine, antitussive.

PHENERHIST. (Rocky Mtn.) Promethazine HCl 25 mg or 50 mg/ml. Vial 10 ml.
Use: Antihistamine.

PHENERIDINE. 1-(β-Phenyl-b-ethyl)-4-carbethoxy-4-phenylpiperidine. Ethyl 1-phenethyl-4-phenyl-isonipecotate.
Use: Analgesic.

PHENETHICILLIN. B.A.N. 6-(α-Phenoxypropionamido)penicillanic acid. Broxil [potassium salt].
Use: Antibiotic.

PHENETHYL ALCOHOL. B.A.N. 2-Phenylethanol.
Use: Antiseptic.

I-PHENETHYLBIGUANIDE MONOHYDROCHLORIDE. Phenformin HCl.

PHENETRON. (Lannett) Chlorpheniramine maleate 4 mg/Tab. Bot. 1000s.
Use: Antihistamine.

PHENETRON COMPOUND TABLETS. (Lannett) Chlorpheniramine maleate 2 mg, aspirin 390 mg, caffeine 30 mg/Tab. Bot. 1000s.
Use: Antihistamine, salicylate analgesic.

PHENETRON INJECTABLE. (Lannett) Chlorpheniramine maleate. Amp. (10 mg/ml) 1 ml 25s, 100s, Vial 30 ml; (100 mg/ml) Vial 5 ml.
Use: Antihistamine.

PHENETRON SYRUP. (Lannett) Chlorpheniramine maleate 2 mg/5 ml. Bot. pt, gal.
Use: Antihistamine.

PHENETURIDE. B.A.N. (2-Phenylbutyryl)urea. Ethylphenacemide (I.N.N.) Benuride.
Use: Anticonvulsant.

PHENFORMIN HCl. Imidodicarbonimidic diamide, nN-(2-phenylethyl)-monohydrochloride. N^1-β-Phenethylbiguanide HCl.
Use: Hypoglycemic.
Note: Withdrawn from market in 1978. Available under IND exemption.

PHENGLUTARIMIDE. B.A.N. 2-(2-Diethylaminoethyl)-2-phenylglutarimide. Aturbane HCl.
Use: Treatment of the Parkinsonian syndrome.

PHENIFORM.
See: Phenformin HCl.

PHENINDAMINE TARTRATE. 2,3,4,9-Tetrahydro-2-methyl-9 phenyl-1 H-indeno-[2,1-c] pyridine bitartrate. 2,3,4,9-Tetrahydro-2-methyl-9-phenyl-IH-indeno-(2,1-c)pyridine Tartrate (1:1).
Use: Antihistamine.
See: Nolahist, Tab. (Carnrick).
Thephorin, Tab. (Roche).

W/Chlorpheniramine maleate, phenylpropanolamine HCl.
See: Nolamine, Tab. (Carnrick).

W/Phenylephrine HCl, aspirin, caffeine, aluminum hydroxide, magnesium carbonate.
See: Dristan, Tab. (Whitehall).

W/Phenylephrine HCl, caramiphen ethanedisulfonate.
See: Dondril, Tab. (Whitehall).

W/Phenylephrine HCl, chlorpheniramine maleate, drytane.
See: Comhist, Tab., Elix. (Baylor).

W/Phenylephrine HCl, chlorpheniramine maleate, belladonna alkaloids.
See: Comhist L.A., Cap. (Baylor Labs.).

W/Phenylephrine HCl, pyrilamine maleate, chlorpheniramine maleate, dextromethorphan HBr.
See: Histalet, Histalet-DM, Histalet-Forte, Syr. (Solvay).

PHENIODOL.
See: Iodoalphionic Acid (Various Mfr.).
PHENIPRAZINE. B.A.N. α-Methylphenethylhydrazine. Cavodil [hydrochloride].
Use: Monoamine oxidase inhibitor.
PHENIPRAZINE HCl. (α-Methyl-phenethyl)-hydrazine monohydrochloride.
Use: Antihypertensive.
PHENIRAMINE MALEATE. 2-[a-[2-(Dimethylamino)ethyl]benzyl]-pyridine bimaleate. Prophen- pyridamine.
Use: Antihistamine.
See: Inhiston, Tab. (Schering-Plough).
W/Combinations.
Allerstat, Cap. (Lemmon).
Chexit, Tab. (Sandoz Consumer).
Citra Forte, Cap., Syr. (Boyle).
Decobel, Cap. (Lannett).
Fitacol Stankaps (Standex).
Kenahist-S.A., Tab. (Kenyon).
Partuss AC (Parmed).
Phenagesic, Tab., Syr. (Dalin).
Poly-Histine Cap., Elix., Lipospan (Bock).
Pyma, Cap. (Fellows-Testagar).
Symptrol, Syr., Cap., Inj. (Saron).
T.A.C., Cap. (Towne).
Thor, Cap. (Towne).
Trigelamine, Oint. (E.J. Moore).
Tritussin, Syr. (Towne).
•**PHENISTIX REAGENT STRIPS.** (Ames) Urinalysis strip test for phenylketonuria. Bot. 50s, 100s, Foil wrapped 3s.
Use: Diagnostic aid.
•**PHENMETRAZINE HCl,** U.S.P. XXII. Tab., U.S.P. XXII. 3-Methyl-2-phenylmorpholine hydrochloride.
Use: Anorexic.
See: Melfiat, Tab. (Solvay).
Preludin, Tab., Endurets (Boehringer Ingelheim).
•**PHENOBARBITAL,** U.S.P. XXII. Elixir, Tab., U.S.P. XXII. 2,4,6(1H,3H,%H) Pyrimidinetrione, 5-ethyl-5-phenyl. 5-Ethyl-5-phenylbarbituric acid. Phenylethylbarbituric acid, phenylethylmalonylurea, Barbenyl, Dormiral, Duneryl, Neurobarb, Numol, Phenonyl, Somonal.
Use: Anticonvulsant, hypnotic, sedative.
See: Bar Elix. (Scrip).
Henomint, Elix. (Bowman).
Hypnette, Supp., Tab. (Fleming).
Orprine, Liq. (Pennwalt).
Pheno-Square, Tab. (Mallard).
Sedadrops, Liq. (Merrell Dow).
SK-Phenobarbital, Tab. (SmithKline).
Solu-barb, Tab. (Fellows-Testagar).
•**PHENOBARBITAL W/AMINOPHYLLINE.**
See: Aminophylline (Various Mfr.).
•**PHENOBARBITAL W/ATROPINE SULFATE.**
See: Atropine Sulfate (Various Mfr.).
P.A., Tab. (Scrip).
•**PHENOBARBITAL W/BELLADONNA.**
See: Belladonna Products and Phenobarbital Combinations.
PHENOBARBITAL WITH CENTRAL NERVOUS SYSTEM STIMULANTS.
See: Arcotrate No. 3, Tab. (Arcum).
Bronkolixir, Elix. (Winthrop Pharm).
Bronkotab, Tab. (Winthrop Pharm).
Quadrinal, Susp., Tab. (Knoll).
Sedamine, Tab. (Dunhall).
Spabelin, Elix., Tab. (Arcum).
PHENOBARBITAL COMBINATIONS.
See: Aminophylline w/Phenobarbital, Combinations.
Aspirin-Barbiturate, Combinations.
Atropine-Hyoscine-Hyoscyamine Combinations.
Atropine Sulfate w/Phenobarbital.
Belladonna Extract Combinations.
Belladonna Products and Phenobarbital Combinations.
Homatropine Methylbromide and Phenobarbital Combinations.
Hyoscyamus Products and Phenobarbital Combinations.
Mannitol Hexanitrate w/Phenobarbital Combinations.
Mephenesin and Barbiturates Combinations.
Phenobarbital w/Central Nervous System Stimulants.
Secobarbital Combinations.
Sodium Nitrite Combinations.
Theobromine w/Phenobarbital Combinations.
Theophylline w/Phenobarbital Combinations.
Veratrum Viride w/Phenobarbital Combinations.
PHENOBARBITAL W/HOMATROPINE METHYLBROMIDE.
See: Homatropine Methylbromide and Phenobarbital Combinations.
PHENOBARBITAL W/HYOSCYAMUS.
See: Hyoscyamus Products and Phenobarbital Combinations.
PHENOBARBITAL W/MANNITOL HEXANITRATE.
Use: Anticonvulsant, sedative/hypnotic.
See: Mannitol Hexanitrate w/Phenobarbital Combinations.
•**PHENOBARBITAL SODIUM,** U.S.P. XXII. Inj., Sterile, U.S.P. XXII. Tab., U.S.P. XXI. Sodium 5-ethyl-5-phenylbarbiturate. 2,4,6(1H,3H,5H)-Pyrimidinetrione, 5-ethyl-5 phenyl, monosodium salt. (Sodium Phenylethylbarbiturate, Soluble Phenobarbital). (Various Mfr.).
Use: Anticonvulsant, sedative, hypnotic.
See: Luminal Sodium, Inj. (Winthrop Pharm).
PHENOBARBITAL SODIUM IN PROPYLENE GLYCOL. Vitarine. Amp. 0.13 Gm: 1 ml, Box 25s, 100s.
Use: Anticonvulsant, hypnotic, sedative.
PHENOBARBITAL AND THEOBROMINE COMBINATIONS.

See: Theobromine w/Phenobarbital Combinations.

PHENOBARBITAL W/THEOPHYLLINE.
See: Theophylline w/Phenobarbital Combinations.

PHENOBARBITAL W/VERATRUM VIRIDE.
See: Veratrum Viride w/Phenobarbital Combinations.

PHENO-BELLA. (Ferndale) Belladonna extract 10.8 mg, phenobarbital 16.2 mg/Tab. Bot. 100s, 1000s.
Use: Anticholinergic/antispasmodic, sedative/hypnotic.

PHENOBUTIODIL. B.A.N. w-(2,4,6-Triiodophenoxy)-butyric acid. Vesipaque (Warner-Lambert).
Use: Radiopaque substance.

PHENOJECT. (Mayrand) Promethazine HCl 25 mg or 50 mg/ml. Vial 10 ml.
Use: Antihistamine, antiemetic.

•**PHENOL,** U.S.P. XXII. Liq., U.S.P. XXII. (Various Mfr.) Carbolic acid.
Use: Pharmaceutic aid (preservative), topical antipruritic.
W/Aluminum hydroxide, zinc oxide, camphor, eucalyptol, ichthammol, thyme oil.
See: Almophen, Oint. (Bowman).
W/Benzocaine, ichthammol, balsam peru, alum exsiccated, cade oil, oil eucalyptus, carbolic oil.
See: Alucaine, Oint. (Jenkins).
W/Benzocaine, triclosan,
See: Solarcaine Pump Spray (Schering-Plough).
W/Dextromethorphan.
See: Chloraseptic DM Lozenges (Eaton).
W/Resorcinol.
See: Black & White Ointment (Schering-Plough).
W/Resorcinol, boric acid, basic fuchsin, acetone.
See: Castellani's Paint, Liq. (Various Mfr.).

•**PHENOLATE SODIUM.** USAN.
Use: Disinfectant.

PHENOLAX. (Upjohn) Phenolphthalein 64.8 mg/Wafer. Bot. 100s.
Use: Laxative.

•**PHENOL, LIQUEFIED,** U.S.P. XXII.
Use: Topical antipruritic.

•**PHENOLPHTHALEIN,** U.S.P. XXII. Tab., U.S.P. XXII. (Various Mfr.) 3,3-Bis(p-hydroxyphenyl)phthalide. Pkg. 1 oz, 0.25 lb., 1 lb.
Use: Cathartic.
See: Alophen, Pill (Parke-Davis).
Espotabs, Tab. (Combe).
Evac-U-Lax, Wafer. (Mallard).
Evasof, Tab. (Lemmon).
Ex-Lax, Prods. (Sandoz Consumer).
Feen-A-Mint, Tab., Gum (Schering-Plough).
Phenolax, Wafer (Upjohn).

PHENOLPHTHALEIN W/COMBINATIONS.
See: Bilocomp, Tab. (Lannett).
Bilstan (Standex).
Correctol, Tab. (Schering-Plough).
Disolan, Cap. (Lannett).
Evac-Q-Kit, Tab., Supp. (Warren-Teed).
Dual Formula Feen-A-Mint Pills. (Schering-Plough).
Feen-A-Mint, Gum, Mint, Pill (Schering-Plough).
4-Way Cold Tab. (Bristol-Myers).
Lanothal Pills (Lannett).

PHENOLPHTHALEIN IN LIQUID PETROLATUM EMULSION. (Various Mfr.).
See: Petrolatum, Liq.

•**PHENOLPHTHALEIN YELLOW,** U.S.P. XXII.
Use: Cathartic.

PHENOLSULFONATES.
See: Sulfocarbolates.

PHENOLSULFONIC ACID. Sulfocarbolic acid.
Note: Used in Sulphodine, Tab. (Strasenburgh).

PHENOLTETRABROMOPHTHALEIN. Disulfonate Disodium.
See: Sulfobromophthalein Sodium, U.S.P. XXII.

PHENOLZINE SULFATE. β-Phenylethylhydrazine hydrogen sulfate.

PHENOMORPHAN. B.A.N. 3-Hydroxy-N-phenethylmorphinan.
Use: Narcotic analgesic.

PHENO NUX TABLETS. (Vale) Phenobarbital 16.2 mg, nux vomica extract 8.1 mg, calcium carbonate 194.4 mg/Tab. Bot. 1000s.
Use: Sedative/hypnotic, antacid.

PHENOPERIDINE. B.A.N. Ethyl 1-(3-hydroxy-3-phenylpropyl)-4-phenylpiperidine-4-carboxylate. Operidine HCl.
Use: Narcotic analgesic.

PHENOTHIATAL ELIXIR. (Fellows) Phenobarbital 0.25 gr, vitamins B_1 5 mg, hyoscine HBr 0.0065 mg, atropine sulfate 0.0194 mg, hyoscyamine 0.1037 mg/5 ml. Bot. pt, gal.
Use: Sedative/hypnotic, vitamin B, anticholinergic/antispasmodic.

PHENOTHIAZINE. Thiodiphenylamine.

PHENOTURIC. (Truett) Phenobarbital 40 mg/5 ml. Elix. Bot. pt, gal.
Use: Sedative/hypnotic.

PHENOXYBENZAMINE HCl, U.S.P. XXI. Cap., U.S.P. XXI. N-Phenoxyisopropyl-N-benzyl-beta-chlorethylamineHCl. N-(2-Chloroethyl)-N-(1-methyl-2- phenoxy-ethyl)benzylamine HCl.
Use: Antihypertensive.
See: Dibenzyline, Cap. (SmithKline).

PHENOXYMETHYL PENICILLIN.
See: Penicillin V.

PHENOXYMETHYL PENICILLIN POTASSIUM.
See: Penicillin V potassium.

PHENOXYNATE. Mixture of phenylphenols 17-18%, octyl and related alkylphenols 2-3%.
See: Surtenol, Liq. (Guardian Chem.).

PHENOXYPROPAZINE. B.A.N. (1-Methyl-2-phenoxyethyl)hydrazine. Drazine hydrogen maleate.
Use: Monoamine oxidase inhibitor.

PHENPROBAMATE. B.A.N. 3-Phenylpropyl carbamate. Gamaquil.

Use: Skeletal muscle relaxant.

•**PHENPROCOUMON,** U.S.P. XXII. Tab., U.S.P. XXII. 3-(α-Ethylbenzyl)-4-hydroxycoumarin. 4-Hydroxy-3-(1-phenylpropyl)coumarin. Marcoumar.
Use: Anticoagulant.
See: Liquamar, Tab. (Organon).

PHEN-70. (Parmed) Phendimetrazine tartrate 70 mg/Tab. Bot. 100s, 1000s.
Use: Anorexiant.

•**PHENSUXIMIDE,** U.S.P. XXII. Cap., U.S.P. XXII. N-Methyl-2-phenylsuccinimide.
Use: Anticonvulsant.
See: Milontin, Preps. (Parke-Davis).

PHENTAL. (Geneva) Belladonna alkaloids, phenobarbital 0.25 gr/Tab. Bot. 1000s.
Use: Anticholinergic/antispasmodic, sedative/hypnotic.

PHENTAMINE. (Major) Phentermine HCl 30 mg/Cap. (equivalent to 24 mg base). Bot. 100s.
Use: Anorexiant.

•**PHENTERMINE.** USAN. α,α-Dimethylphenethylamine. Phenyl-tertiarybutylamine. Duromine (an ion-exchange resin complex).
Use: Anorexiant.
See: Adipex, Tab. (Lemmon).
Adipex-8 C.T., Cap. (Lemmon).
Adipex-P, Cap. (Lemmon).
Fastin, Cap. (Beecham Labs).
Parmine, Cap. (Parmed).
Rolaphent, Tab. (Robinson).
Tora, Tab. (Solvay).
Unifast Unicelles, Cap. (Solvay).
Wilpowr, Cap. (Foy).

PHENTERMINE AS RESIN COMPLEX.
See: Ionamin, Cap. (Pennwalt).

•**PHENTERMINE HYDROCHLORIDE,** U.S.P. XXII. Cap., Nasal Jelly, Tab., U.S.P. XXII. Benzeneethanamine, α,α-dimethyl-, HCl.
Use: Anorexiant.

•**PHENTETIOTHALEIN SODIUM.** Iso-Iodeikon.
Use: Radiopaque agent.

•**PHENTOLAMINE HYDROCHLORIDE.** m-[n-(2-Imi-dazolin-2-ylmethyl)-p-toluidino]phenol HCl.
Use: Antihypertensive.
See: Regitine HCl, Tab. (Ciba).

•**PHENTOLAMINE MESYLATE,** U.S.P. XXII. For Inj., U.S.P. XXII. Phenol, 3-[[(4,5-dihydro-1H-imidazol-2-yl)methyl]-(4-methyl-phenyl)amino]-, monomethanesulfonate (salt). m-[N-(2-Imidazolin-2-ylmethyl)-p-toluidino]-phenol methanesulfonate.
Use: Anti-adrenergic.
See: Regitine Inj. (Ciba).

PHENTOLAMINE METHANESULFONATE.
Phentolamine mesylate, U.S.P. XXII.

PHENTOLOX w/APAP. (Richlyn) Phenyltoloxamine citrate 30 mg, acetaminophen 325 mg/Tab. Bot. 1000s.
Use: Antihistamine, analgesic.

PHENTOX COMPOUND. (My-K Labs) Phenylpropanolamine HCl 20 mg, phenylephrine HCl 5 mg, chlorpheniramine maleate 2.5 mg, phenyltoloxamine citrate 7.5 mg/5 ml. Bot. pt, gal.
Use: Decongestant, antihistamine.

PHENTYDRONE. 1,2,3,4-Tetrahydrofluoren-9-one.
Use: Systemic fungicide.

PHENURONE. (Abbott) Phenacemide 0.5 Gm/Tab. Bot. 100s.
Use: Anticonvulsant.

N-PHENYLACETAMIDE.
See: Acetanilid (Various Mfr.).

•**PHENYLAMINOSALICYLATE.** USAN. Phenyl 4 aminosalicylate. Fenamisal (I.N.N.) Phenypastebamin.
Use: Tuberculostatic.

PHENYLACETYLUREA.
See: Phenurone, Tab. (Abbott).

•**PHENYLALANINE,** U.S.P. XXII. $C_9H_{11}NO_2$ as L-phenylalanine.
Use: Amino acid.
See: Phenylketonuria therapy.

PHENYLALANINE MUSTARD.
See: Melphalan, U.S.P. XXII.

PHENYLAZO-DIAMINOPYRIDINE HYDROCHLORIDE.
See: Rodine, Tab. (Paddock).

PHENYLAZO SULFISOXAZOLE. (A.P.C.) Sulfisoxazole 0.5 Gm, phenylazopyridine 50 mg/Tab. Bot. 1000s.
Use: Antibacterial, sulfonamide, urinary analgesic.

PHENYLAZO TABLETS. (A.P.C.) Phenylazodiamino-pyridine HCl 1.5 gr/Tab. Bot. 1000s.
Use: Urinary analgesic.

PHENYLAZO-DIAMINO-PYRIDINE.
See: Phenazopyridine (Various Mfr.).

PHENYLAZO-DIAMINO-PYRIDINE HCl or HBr.
See: Phenazopyridine HCl or HBr (Various Mfr.).

•**PHENYLBUTAZONE,** U.S.P. XXII. Cap., Tab. U.S.P. XXII. 3,5-Pyrazolidinedione, 4-butyl-1,2-diphenyl-. 4-Butyl-1,2-diphenyl-3,5-pyrazolidinedione. 4-Butyl-1,2-diphenylpyrazolidine-3,5-dione. Benzone; Butacote; Butaphen; Butazone; Flexaz IA-But; Tetnor.
Use: Anti-inflammatory.
See: Azolid, Tab. (Rorer).
Butazolidin, Tab. (Geigy).
W/Aluminum hydroxide dried gel, magnesium trisilicate.
See: Azolid-A, Cap. (USV).
W/Aluminum hydroxide, magnesium trisilicate.
See: Butazolidin Alka, Cap. (Geigy).

PHENYLCARBINOL.
See: Benzyl Alcohol, N.F. XVII.

PHENYLCINCHONINIC ACID. Name used for cinchophen.

•**PHENYLEPHRINE HYDROCHLORIDE,** U.S.P. XXII. Inj., Nasal Soln., Ophth. Soln., U.S.P. XXII. Benzenemethanol, 3-hydroxy-α-[(methylamino)-methyl]-, hydrochloride (S)-. l-m-Hy-

droxy-a-[(me-thylamino)methyl]-benzyl alcohol hydrochloride. (Neophryn).
Use: Sympathomimetic agent, vasoconstrictor, mydriatic.
See: Alcon-Efrin, Soln. (Webcon).
Allerest Nasal Spray (Pharmacraft).
Coricidin Decongestant Nasal Mist (Schering).
Ephrine, Spray (Walgreen).
Neo-Synephrine HCl, Preps. (Winthrop Consumer Products).
Prefrin Liquifilm Ophth. Soln. (Allergan).
Pyracort-D, Spray (Lemmon).
Sinarest, Nasal Spray (Pharmacraft).
Super-Anahist Nasal Spray (Warner-Lambert).
W/Combinations.
See: Acotus, Liq. (Whorton).
Anodynos Forte, Tab. (Buffington).
Bellafedrol A-H, Tab. (Lannett).
Bur-Tuss Expectorant (Burlington).
C.D.M. Expectorant Liq. (Lannett).
Cenahist, Cap. (Century).
Cenaid, Tab. (Century).
Chlor-Trimeton Expectorant (Schering).
Chlor-Trimeton Expectorant w/Codeine (Schering).
Conar, Susp., Expectorant (Beecham Labs).
Conar-A, Tab., Susp. (Beecham Labs).
Congespirin, Tab. (Bristol-Myers).
Coricidin Demilets (Schering).
Dallergy, Syr., Cap., Tab., Inj. (Laser).
Demazin, Syr. (Schering).
Dimetane Decongestant, Tab., Elix. (Robins).
Dimetane Expectorant, Liq. (Robins).
Dimetane Expectorant-DC, Liq. (Robins).
Dimetapp, Elix., Extentabs (Robins).
Doktors, Drops, Spray (Scherer).
Drinus-M, Cap. (Amfre-Grant).
Eldatapp, Tab., Liq. (Elder).
Emagrin Forte, Tab. (Clapp).
Entex, Prods. (Norwich Eaton).
Eye-Gene, Soln. (Pearson).
4 Way Tab., Spray (Bristol-Myers).
Furacin Nasal Soln. (Eaton).
Histabid, Cap. (Meyer).
Histapp Prods. (Upsher-Smith).
Histaspan-D, Cap. (Rorer).
Histaspan-Plus, Cap. (Rorer).
Mydfrin Ophthalmic, Liq. (Alcon).
Na-Co-Al, Tab. (High).
Nasahist, Cap. (Keene).
Pediacof, Syr. (Winthrop Pharm).
Phenoptic, Soln. (Muro).
Phenylzin Drops, Ophth. Soln. (CooperVision).
Prefrin-A Ophth. Soln. (Allergan).
Prefrin-Z Ophth. Soln. (Allergan).
Pyraphed, Soln. (Lemmon).
Pyristan, Cap., Elix. (Arcum).
Queledrine, Syr. (Abbott).
Rhinall, Liq. (Scherer).
Rhinex DM, Tab. (Lemmon).
Rymed, Prods. (Edwards).
Sinex, Nasal Spray (Vicks).
Singlet, Tab. (Merrell Dow).
Spectab, Tab. (Solvay).
Spec-T Sore Throat-Decongestant Loz. (Squibb).
Sucrets Cold Decongestant Loz. (Calgon).
Tearefrin, Liq. (CooperVision).
Trind, Liq. (Mead Johnson).
Trind-DM, Liq. (Mead Johnson).
Tri-Ophtho, Soln. (Maurry).
T-Spray (Saron).
Turbilixir, Liq. (Burlington).
Turbispan Leisurecaps, Cap. (Burlington).
Tussar-DM, Liq. (Rorer).
Tympagesic, Liq. (Adria).
Vacon, Liq. (Scherer).
Valihist, Cap. (Clapp).
Vasocidin, Ophth. Soln. (CooperVision).
Vasosulf, Ophth. Soln. (CooperVision).

•**PHENYLETHYL ALCOHOL,** U.S.P. XXII. Beta-phenylethanol. Benzylcarbinol. (Various Mfr.) Phenethyl Alcohol.
Use: Antibacterial; preservative (ophthalmic).

beta-PHENYL-ETHYL-HYDRAZINE. Phenelzine dihydrogen sulfate.
See: Nardil, Tab. (Parke-Davis).

PHENYLETHYLMALONYLUREA.
See: Phenobarbital (Various Mfr.).

PHENYLGESIC TABS. (Goldline) Phenyltoloxamine citrate 30 mg, acetaminophen 325 mg/Bot. 100s, 1000s.
Use: Antihistamine, analgesic.

PHENYLIC ACID.
See: Phenol, U.S.P. XXII.

PHENYLKETONURIA THERAPY.
See: Lofenalac, Pow. (Mead Johnson).
Phenistix Reagent Strips (Ames).

•**PHENYLMERCURIC ACETATE,** N.F. XVII. (Various Mfr.) (Acetato)phenylmercury. Bot. 1 lb, 5 lb, 10 lb.
Use: Preservative (bacteriostatic).
W/9-Aminoacridine HCl, tyrothricin, urea, lactose.
See: Trinalis, Vaginal Supp. (Webcon).
W/Benzocaine, chlorothymol, resorcin.
See: Lanacane Creme (Combe).
W/Boric acid, polyoxyethylenenonylphenol or oxyquinoline benzoate.
See: Koromex, Preps. (Holland-Rantos).
W/Methylbenzethonium Cl.
See: Norforms, Aerosol, Supp. (Norwich).

PHENYLMERCURIC BORATE. (F. W. Berk) Pkg. Custom packed.
W/Benzyl alcohol, benzocaine, butyl p-aminobenzoate.
See: Dermathyn, Oint. (Davis & Sly).

PHENYLMERCURIC CHLORIDE. Chlorophenylmercury.

•**PHENYLMERCURIC NITRATE,** N.F. XVII. (Merphenyl Nitrate, Phenmerzyl Nitrate) A.P.L.—Oint. 1:1500, 1 oz, 4 oz, lb. Chicago Pharm.-Loz. w/benzocaine. Bot. 100s, 1000s. Ophth. Oint., 1:3000, Tube ⅛ oz. Soln. 1:20,000, Bot. pt, gal. Vaginal supp., 1:5000, Box 12s.

Use: Bacteriostatic.
See: Preparation H, Oint., Supp. (Whitehall).
W/Amyl, phenylphenol complex.
See: Lubraseptic Jelly (Guardian).
W/Undecylenic acid.
See: Bridex, Oint. (Briar).
PHENYLMERCURIC PICRATE.
Use: Germicide.
o-PHENYLPHENOL.
W/Amyl complex, phenylmercuric nitrate.
See: Lubraseptic Jelly. (Guardian).
PHENYLPROPANOLAMINE HYDROCHLORIDE, U.S.P. XXII. Extended-release Cap., U.S.P. XXII. (±)-Norephedrine HCl. 2-Amino-1-phenyl-1-propanol (Mydriatine).
Use: Sympathomimetic.
See: Obestat, Cap. (Lemmon).
Obestat 150, Cap. (Lemmon).
Propadrine HCl, Preps. (Merck Sharp & Dohme).
Propagest, Tab. (Carnrick).
PHENYLPROPANOLAMINE HCl W/COMBINATIONS.
See: Allerest, Prods. (Pharmacraft).
Allerstat, Cap. (Lemmon).
A.R.M., Tab. (SmithKline Prods).
Bayer Prods. (Glenbrook).
BQ Cold Tab. (Bristol-Myers).
Breacol Cough Medication, Liq. (Glenbrook).
Bur-Tuss Expectorant (Burlington).
Chexit, Tab. (Sandoz Consumer).
Comtrex, Cap., Liq., Tab. (Bristol-Myers).
Congespirin, Liq., Tab. (Bristol-Myers).
Contac, Prods. (SmithKline Prods).
Cophene No. 2, Cap. (Dunhall).
Coricidin Cough Formula (Schering).
Coricidin "D" Decongestant, Tab. (Schering).
Coricidin Sinus Headache Tab. (Schering).
Coryban-D, Cap. (Leeming).
Decobel, Cap. (Lannett).
Dex-A-Diet, Prods. (O'Connor).
Dezest, Cap. (Geneva).
Dimetane Expectorant, Liq. (Robins).
Dimetapp, Elix., Extentabs (Robins).
Drinophen, Cap. (Lannett).
Entex, Cap. (Norwich Eaton).
Entex, Liq. (Norwich Eaton).
Entex LA, Tab. (Norwich Eaton).
Halls Mentho-Lyptus Cough Formula, Liq. (Warner-Lambert).
Histabid, Cap. (Glaxo).
Histalet Forte T. D., Tab. (Solvay).
Hista-Vadrin, Syr., Tab., Cap. (Scherer).
Kleer Compound, Tab. (Scrip).
Koryza, Tab. (Fellows-Testagar).
Meditussin-X, Liq. (Hauck).
Naldecon, Drop, Syr., Tab. (Bristol).
Nasahist, Cap., Inj. (Keene).
Nolamine, Tab. (Carnrick).
Ornade, Cap. (SmithKline).
Ornex, Cap. (SmithKline).
Panadyl, Tab., Cap. (Misemer).
Partuss-A, Tab. (Parmed).
Partuss T.D., Tab. (Parmed).
Pyristan, Cap., Elix. (Arcum).
Rhinex DM, Liq. (Lemmon).
Rolanade, Cap. (Robinson).
Rymed, Prods. (Edwards).
Sanhist TD, Tab., Vial (Sandia).
Santussin, Cap., Susp. (Sandia).
Sinarest, Tab. (Pharmcraft).
Sine-Off, Tab. (SmithKline).
Sinulin, Tab. (Carnrick).
Spec-T Sore Throat-Decongestant Loz. (Squibb).
St. Joseph Cold Tablets for Children (Schering-Plough).
Sto-Caps, Cap. (Jalco).
Sucrets Cold Decongestant Loz. (Calgon).
Triaminic, Preps. (Sandoz Consumer).
Triaminicin, Chew. Tab. (Sandoz Consumer).
Triaminicol, Syr. (Sandoz Consumer).
Turbilixir, Liq. (Burlington).
Turbispan Leisurecaps, Cap. (Burlington).
Tusquelin, Syr. (Circle).
Tussagesic, Susp., Tab. (Sandoz Consumer).
U.R.I., Cap., Liq. (ICN).
•**PHENYLPROPANOLAMINE POLISTIREX.** USAN.
Use: Adrenergic (vasoconstrictor).
PHENYLPROPYLMETHYLAMINE HYDROCHLORIDE. Vonedrine HCl.
PHENYL SALICYLATE. Salol.
W/Atropine sulfate, hyoscyamine, methenamine, methylene blue, gelsemium, benzoic acid.
See: Lanased, Tab. (Lannett).
Renalgin, Tab. (Meyer).
U-Tract, Tab. (Bowman).
W/Euphorbia extract and various oils.
See: Rayderm Oint. (Velvet Pharmacal).
W/Methenamine, methylene blue, benzoic acid, hyoscyamine alkaloid, atropine sulfate.
See: Cystrea, Tab. (Moore Kirk).
Urised, Tab. (Webcon).
UTA, Tab. (ICN).
W/Methenamine, sodium biphosphate, methylene blue, hyoscyamine, alkaloid.
See: Urostat Forte, Tab. (Elder).
PHENYL-TERT-BUTYLAMINE.
See: Phentermine.
PHENYLTHILONE. 2-Ethyl-2-phenyl-3,5-thiomorpho-linedione.
Use: Anticonvulsant.
PHENYLTOLOXAMINE. B.A.N. N-2-(2-Benzylphen-oxy)ethyldimethylamine. o-Benzylphenyl-2-dimethyl-aminoethyl ether.
Use: Antihistamine.
PHENYLTOLOXAMINE CITRATE. N,N-Dimethyl-2-[(alpha-phenyl-o-tolyl)oxy]ethylamine citrate.
Use: Antihistamine.
See: Volaxin Modified, Tab. (Elder).
PHENYLTOLOXAMINE CITRATE W/COMBINATIONS.
See: Dengesic, Tab. (Scott-Alison).

Dilone, Tab. (Vicks).
Meditussin-X, Liq. (Hauck).
Myocalm, Tab. (Parmed).
Naldecon, Preps. (Bristol).
Poly-histine Prods. (Bock).
Quadrahist, Tab. (Pharmex).
S.A.C. Sinus, Tab. (Towne).
Scotgesic, Elix., Cap. (Scott/Cord).

PHENYLTOLOXAMINE RESIN W/COMBINATIONS.
See: Tussionex, Cap., Liq., Tab. (Pennwalt).

PHENYLZIN. (CooperVision) Zinc sulfate 0.25%, phenylephrine HCl 0.12%. Bot. 15 ml.
Use: Ophthalmic decongestant combination.

•**PHENYRAMIDOL HCL.** USAN. 2(β-Hydroxyphen-ethylamino)pyridine HCl. α-[2-Pyridylamino)-methyl]-benzyl alcohol hydrochloride.
Use: Analgesic.

PHENYTHILONE. 2-Ethyl-2-phenyl-3, 5-thiamorpho-linedione.

•**PHENYTOIN,** U.S.P. XXII. Oral Susp., Tab., U.S.P. XXII. 2,4-Imidazolidinedione, 5,5-diphenyl-. 5,5-Di-phenylhydantoin. Diphenylhydantoin.
Use: Anticonvulsant.
See: Dilantin Prods. (Parke-Davis).
Di-phenyl, TR Cap. (Drug. Ind.).
Ekko, Cap. (Fleming).
Toin, Unicelles (Solvay).

•**PHENYTOIN SODIUM,** U.S.P. XXII. Extended Cap., Inj., Prompt Cap., U.S.P. XXII. Sterile, U.S.P. XXI. 2,4-Imidazolidinedione, 5,5-diphenyl-, monosodium salt. 5,5-Diphenylhydantoin sodium salt. Diphenylhydantoin sodium. Alepsin, Dihydan soluble, Diphentoin, Silantin Sodium, Epanutin, Eptoin, Phenytoin soluble, Solantoin, Solantyl, Denyl Sodium, Soluble Phenytoin (5,5-diphenyl-hydantoinate Sodium).
Use: Anticonvulsant, cardiac depressant (antiarrhythmic).
See: Dilantin Sodium, Preps. (Parke-Davis).
Diphenylan Sodium, Cap. (Lannett).
Ekko Jr. and Sr., Cap. (Fleming).

PHENYTOIN SODIUM WITH PHENOBARBITAL.
Use: Anticonvulsant.
See: Dilantin with Phenobarbital Kapseals, Cap. (Parke-Davis).

PHEOCHROMOCYTOMA, AGENTS FOR.
See: Demser, Cap. (MSD).
Dibenzyline, Cap. (SKF).
Regitine, Inj. (Ciba Pharm.).

PHERAZINE DM. (Halsey) Promethazine 6.25 mg, dextromethorphan HBr 15 mg, alcohol 7%/5 ml. Bot. 4 oz, 6 oz, pt, gal.
Use: Antihistamine, antitussive.

PHERAZINE VC WITH CODEINE SYRUP. (Halsey) Phenylephrine HCl 5 mg, promethazine HCl 6.25 mg, codeine phosphate 10 mg, alcohol 7%/5 ml. Bot. pt, gal.
Use: Decongestant, antihistamine, antitussive.

PHERAZINE VC SYRUP. (Halsey) Phenylephrine HCl 5 mg, promethazine HCl 6.25 mg, alcohol 7%/5 ml. Bot. pt, gal.
Use: Decongestant, antihistamine.

PHERMINE. (Fellows) Phentermine HCl 8 mg/Tab. Bot. 100s, 1000s.
Use: Anorexiant.

PHETABAR SPACECAP. (Moore Kirk) Amobarbital 90 mg, dextroamphetamine sulfate 15 mg/timed disintegration Cap. Bot. 1000s.
Use: Sedative/hypnotic, amphetamine.

PHETHARBITAL. 5,5-Diethyl-1-phenylbarbituric acid.

PHETHENYLATE. 5-Phenyl-5-(2-thienyl)hydantoinate. Also sodium salt.

PHILJECT INJECTION. (Fellows) Procaine base 75 mg, butyl-amino-benzoate 300 mg, benzyl alcohol 250 mg/5 ml in peanut oil. Vial 5 ml.

PHILLIPS' LAXCAPS. (Glenbrook) Docusate sodium 83 mg, phenolphthalein 90 mg/Cap. Bot. 8s, 24s, 48s.
Use: Laxative.

PHILLIPS' MILK OF MAGNESIA. (Glenbrook) Magnesium hydroxide. Reg. and Mint Bot. 4 oz, 12 oz, 26 oz; Tab. Bot. 30s, 100s, 200s.
Use: Laxative, antacid.

PHILLIPS OINTMENT. (Fellows) Bismuth tribromophenate 5%. Base 1 oz, 1 lb, 5 lb.
Use: Antiseptic, topical.

PHISH OMEGA. (Pharmics) Natural salmon oil concentrate containing EPA 120 mg, DHA 100 mg/Cap. Bot. 60s.
Use: Fish oil.

PHISH OMEGA PLUS. (Pharmics) Natural fish oil concentrate containing EPA 300 mg, DHA 200 mg/Cap. Bot. 60s.
Use: Fish oil.

pHisoAc-BP. (Winthrop) Benzoyl peroxide 10% in cream base. Tube 1 oz, 1.5 oz.
Use: Anti-acne.

pHisoDerm. (Winthrop) Sodium octoxynol-2 ethane sulfonate, white petrolatum, water, mineral oil (with lanolin alcohol and oleyl alcohol), sodium benzoate, octoxynol-3 tetrasodium EDTA, methylcellulose, hydrochloric acid. **Regular:** Bot. 5 oz, 9 oz, 16 oz. **Dry type:** Bot. 5 oz, pt. Wall dispenser pt. **Oily type:** Bot. 5 oz, 16 oz. **Lightly Scented:** Bot. 5 oz, 9 oz, 16 oz. **For Baby:** Bot. 5 oz, 9 oz.
Use: Skin cleanser, conditioner.

pHisoDerm GENTLE CLEANSING BAR. (Winthrop) Sodium tallowate, sodium cocoate, petrolatum, glycerin, lanolin, sodium Cl, BHT, trisodium EDTA, titanium dioxide. Bar 99 Gm.
Use: Skin cleanser.

pHisoHex. (Winthrop) Entsufon sodium, hexachlorophene 3%, petrolatum, lanolin cholesterols, methylcellulose, polyethylene glycol, polyethylene glycol monostearate, lauryl myristyl diethanolamide, sodium benzoate, water, pH adjusted with hydrochloric acid. Emulsion, Bot. 5 oz, pt, gal. Wall dispensers pt. Unit packets

0.25 oz. Box 50s, Pedal operated dispenser 30 oz.
Use: Antiseptic, germicide skin cleanser.

•**HisoMed.** (Winthrop) Hexochlorophene.
Use: Antiseptic, germicide.

•**HisoPUFF.** (Winthrop) Nonmedicated cleansing sponge. Box sponge 1s.
Use: Skin cleanser.

•**HISO SCRUB.** (Winthrop-Breon) Hexachlorophene 3%. Disposable brush-sponge (36 × 4).
Use: Antiseptic, germicide.

•**HISTOL.** (Kenyon) Vitamins A 10,000 IU, D 1000 IU, B_1 5 mg, B_2 3 mg, B_6 1 mg, C 100 mg, calcium pantothenate 5 mg, niacinamide 25 mg/Cap. Bot. 100s, 1000s.
Use: Vitamin supplement.

•**HOLEDRINE.** B.A.N. 4-(2-Methylaminopropyl)-phenol. Veritain; Veritol.
Use: Sympathomimetic.

•**HOSCOLIC ACID.** 2,2′-Phosphinicodilacetic acid.
Use: Adjuvant.

•**HOS-FLUR ORAL RINSE SUPPLEMENT.** (Colgate-Hoyt) Acidulated phosphate sodium fluoride 0.05%, fluoride 1 ml/5 ml Bot. 250 ml, 500 ml, gal.
Use: Dental caries preventative.

•**HOSPHACAL-D.** (Lannett) Dicalcium phosphate anhydrous 330 mg, vitamin D 333 IU/Cap. Bot. 500s, 1000s.
Use: Vitamin/mineral supplement.

HOS-pHAID. (Guardian) Ammonium biphosphate 190 mg, sodium biphosphate 200 mg, sodium acid pyrophosphate 110 mg/0.5 Gm Tab. Regular or enteric coated. Bot. 90s, 500s.
Use: Urinary acidifier.

HOSPHALJEL. (Wyeth-Ayerst) Aluminum phosphate gel 700 mg/15 ml. Bot. 12 oz.
Use: Antacid.

HOSPHATE.
See: Potassium Phosphate, Inj. (Abbott).
Sodium Phosphate, Inj. (Abbott).

•**HOSPHENTASIDE.** Adenosine-5-monophosphate. Adenylic acid.
/Vitamin B_{12}, niacin.
See: Denylex Gel, Vial (Westerfield).
/Vitamin B_{12}, niacin, B_1.
See: Adenolin, Vial (Lincoln).

•**HOSPHOCOL P32.** (Mallinckrodt) Chromic phosphate P32: 10 or 15 mCi with a concentration of up to 5 mCi/ml and specific activity of up to 5 mCi/mg at time of standardization. Susp. Vial 5 ml.
Use: Radiopharmaceutical.

•**HOSPHOLINE IODIDE.** (Wyeth-Ayerst) Echothiophate Iodide for Ophthalmic Solution. Sterile echothiophate iodide powder w/potassium acetate 40 mg, diluent: chlorobutanol 0.5%, mannitol 1.2%, boric acid 0.06%, sodium phosphate exsiccated 0.026% for preparing 0.03%, 0.06%, 0.125% and 0.25% potencies/5 ml of sterile eye drops. Package: 1.5 mg for 0.03%; 3 mg for 0.06%; 6.25 mg for 0.125%; 12.5 mg for 0.25%.
Use: Agent for glaucoma.

PHOSPHOLIPIDS, SOY.
See: Granulestin Concentrate, Gran. (Associated Concentrates).

PHOSPHORATED CARBOHYDRATE SOLUTION.
See: Emetrol, Liq. (Rorer).

•**PHOSPHORIC ACID,** N.F. XVII.
Use: Solvent.

•**PHOSPHORIC ACID, DILUTED,** N.F. XVII.
Use: Pharmaceutic aid (solvent).

PHOSPHORUS.
Use: Phosphorus replacement.
See: Uro-KP-Neutral, Tab. (Star).
K-Phos Neutral, Tab. (Beach).
Neutra-Phos, Cap., Pow. (Willen).
Neutra-Phos-K, Cap., Pow. (Willen).

PHOSPHO-SODA. (Fleet) Sodium biphosphate 48 Gm, sodium phosphate 18 Gm/100 ml. Bot. 1.5 oz, 3 oz, 8 oz. Flavored, unflavored.
Use: Laxative.

PHOSPHOTEC. (Squibb) Technetium Tc 99m pyrophosphate kit. 10 vials/kit.
Use: Radiodiagnostic.

PHOTOPLEX SUNSCREEN. (Herbert) Butyl methoxydibenzoylmethane 3%, padimate O 7%. Lot. 120 ml.
Use: Sunscreen.

PHOXIN. V.B.A.N. α-Diethoxyphosphinothioyloxyimino-α-phenylacetonitrile.
Use: Insecticide; anthelmintic, veterinary medicine.

PHRENILIN FORTE CAPSULES. (Carnrick) Acetaminophen 650 mg, butalbital 50 mg/Cap. Bot. 100s.
Use: Analgesic, sedative/hypnotic.

PHRENILIN TABLETS. (Carnrick) Butalbital 50 mg, acetaminophen 325 mg/Tab. Bot. 100s.
Use: Sedative/hypnotic, analgesic.

PHRENILIN WITH CODEINE #3. (Carnrick) Acetaminophen 325 mg, butalbital 50 mg, codeine phosphate 30 mg/Cap. Bot. 100s.
Use: Narcotic analgesic combination, sedative/hypnotic.

PHRESH 3.5 FINNISH CLEANSING LIQUID. (3M Products) Water, cocamidopropyl betaine, lactic acid, polyoxyethylene distearate, polyoxyethylene monostearate, hydroxyethyl cellulose, sodium phosphate, methylparaben. Bot. 6 oz.
Use: Soapless cleansing agent.

pH-STABIL CREAM. (Hermal) Skin protection cream. Bot. 8 oz. Tube 2 oz.
Use: Skin protectant.

PHTHALAMAQUIN. (Penick) Quinetolate.
Use: Antiasthmatic.

PHTHALAZINE, I-HYDRAZINO-, MONOHYDROCHLORIDE. Hydralazine Hydrochloride, U.S.P. XXII.

•**PHTHALOFYNE.** USAN. Mono(I-ethyl-I-methyl-2-propynyl)phthalate.

Use: Anthelmintic (veterinary).
PHTHALYLSULFACETAMIDE. 4′-(Acetylsulfamoyl) phthalanilic acid. Enterosulfon.
PHYLCARDIN.
See: Aminophylline (Various Mfr.).
PHYLLINDON.
See: Aminophylline (Various Mfr.).
PHYLLOCONTIN. (Purdue Frederick) Aminophylline 225 mg/CR Tab. Bot. 100s.
Use: Bronchodilator.
PHYLLOQUINONE. 2-Methyl-3-phytyl-1,4-naphthoquinine, vitamin K.
See: Phytonadione, U.S.P., Inj., Tab. (Various Mfr.).
Vitamin K-1 (Various Mfr.).
PHYSIOLOGICAL IRRIGATING SOLUTION.
See: TIS-U-SOL, Soln. (Travenol).
Physiosol, Soln. (Abbott).
Physiolyte, Soln. (American McGaw).
PHYSIOLYTE. (American McGaw) Sodium Cl 530 mg, sodium acetate 370 mg, sodium gluconate 500 mg, potassium Cl 37 mg, magnesium Cl 30 mg/100 ml. Soln. Bot. 500 ml, 2 L, 4 L.
Use: Irrigating solution.
PHYSIOSOL IRRIGATION. (Abbott Hospital Prods) Bot. 250 ml, 500 ml, 1000 ml glass or Aqualite (semi-rigid) containers.
Use: Irrigating solution.
•**PHYSOSTIGMINE,** U.S.P. XXII. Pyrrolo [2,3-b] indol-5-ol methylcarbamate (ester), (3as-cis). 1,2,3a β,8,8aβ-Hexahydro-1,3a,8-trimethyl-pyrrolo[2,3-b]-indol-5yl-methylcarbamate. An alkaloid.
Use: Parasympathomimetic agent.
•**PHYSOSTIGMINE SALICYLATE,** U.S.P. XXII. Inj., Ophth. Soln., U.S.P. XXII. Pyrrolo[2,3-b]indol-5-ol,1,2,3,3a,8,8a-hexahydro-1,3a,8-trimethyl-, methylcarbamate (ester), (3aS-cis)-,mono(2-hydroxybenzoate). Physostigmine monosalicylate. Eserine salicylate. (Forest)—Pow., Tube 1 gr, 5 gr, 15 gr.
Use: Parasympathomimetic agent.
See: Antilirium, Amp. (Forest).
Isopto-Eserine, Ophthalmic, Soln. (Alcon).
W/Atropine sulfate.
See: Atrophysine, Inj. (Lannett).
W/l-Hyoscyamine HBr.
See: Phyatromine-H, Amp., Vial (Kremers-Urban).
W/Pilocarpine, methylcellulose.
See: Isopto P-ES, Soln. (Alcon).
•**PHYSOSTIGMINE SULFATE,** U.S.P. XXII. Ophth. Oint., U.S.P. XXII. Pyrrolo[2,3-b]indol-5-ol, 1,2,3,3a, 8,8a-hexahydro-1,3a,8-trimethyl-, methylcarbamate (ester), (3aS-cis)-,sulfate (2:1).
Use: Cholinergic (ophthalmic).
•**PHYTATE PERSODIUM.** USAN.
Use: Pharmaceutic aid.
•**PHYTATE SODIUM.** USAN. Sodium salt of inositol hexaphosphoric acid.
Use: Chelating agent (calcium).
PHYTIC ACID. Inositol hexophosphoric acid.
PHYTOMENADIONE. B.A.N. 2-Methyl-3-phytyl-1,4-naphthaquinone. Vitamin K Konakion; Mephyton.
Use: Antidote to anticoagulants.
PHYTONADIOL SODIUM DIPHOSPHATE. Disodium salt of 2-methyl-3-phytyl-1,4-naphthohydroquinone-0[1],0[4]-diphosphoric acid.
•**PHYTONADIONE,** U.S.P. XXII. Inj., Tab., U.S.P. XXII. Vitamin K 1,4-Naphthalenedione, 2-methyl-3-(3,7,11,15-tetramethyl-2-hexadecenyl)-,[R-[R*,R*-(E)]]-. Phylloquinone. 2-Methyl-3-phytyl-1,4-naphthoquinone.
Use: Prothrombogenic.
See: Aquamephyton, Inj. (Merck Sharp & Dohme).
Konakion, Amp. (Roche).
Mephyton, Tab. (Merck Sharp & Dohme).
•**PICENADOL HYDROCHLORIDE.** USAN.
Use: Analgesic.
PICLOXYDINE. B.A.N. NN′-Di-(p-Chlorophenylguanidinoformimidoyl)-piperazine. 1,4-Di-(4-chloro-phenylguanidinoformimidoyl)piperazine.
Use: Bactericide; fungicide.
•**PICOTRIN DIOLAMINE.** USAN.
Use: Keratolytic.
PICRIC ACID, TRINITROPHENOL.
See: Butesyn Picrate, Oint. (Abbott).
Silver Salts (Various Prods.).
PICROTOXIN. Cocculin.
Use: Respiratory stimulant.
P.I.D.
See: Phenindione (Various Mfr.).
PIFARNINE. USAN.
Use: Anti-ulcerative.
PIFENATE. B.A.N. Ethyl 2,2-diphenyl-3-(2-piperidyl)propionate.
Use: Analgesic.
PILE-GON. (E.J. Moore) Bismuth subgallate, balsam peru, zinc oxide, cod liver oil in petrolatum base. Tube 1.25 oz.
Use: Anorectal preparation.
PILOCAR. (Iolab) Pilocarpine HCl 0.5%, 1%, 2%, 3%, 4% or 6%. Bot. 15 ml; Twinpack 2 × 15 ml 0.5%, 1%, 2%, 3%, 4% or 6%; 1 ml Dropperettes 1%, 2%, 3% or 4%. Box 12s.
Use: Agent for glaucoma.
•**PILOCARPINE,** U.S.P. XXII. Ocular system U.S.P. XXII.
Use: Ophthalmic cholinergic, miotic.
See: Ocusert Pilo-20 and Pilo-40 (Ciba).
•**PILOCARPINE HYDROCHLORIDE,** U.S.P. XXII. Ophth. Soln., U.S.P. XXII. (Various Mfr.) Pilocarpine muriate.
Use: Cholinergic 0.5% to 8.0% soln. topically as a miotic.
See: Almocarpine (Wyeth-Ayerst).
Isopto-Carpine, Ophthalmic (Alcon).
Mi-Pilo, Soln.(Barnes-Hind).
Pilocar, Soln. (CooperVision).
Pilomiotin, Soln. (CooperVision).
Piloptic, Soln. (Muro).
W/Epinephrine HCl.

See: E-Carpine, Inj. (Alcon).
Epicar, Ophthalmic Soln. (Barnes-Hind).
W/Epinephrine bitartrate, mannitol, benzalkonium Cl.
See: E-Pilo, Soln. (CooperVision).
W/Eserine salicylate, methylcellulose.
See: Isopto P-ES, Soln. (Alcon).
•**PILOCARPINE NITRATE,** U.S.P. XXII. Ophth. Soln., U.S.P. XXII.
Use: Cholinergic (ophthalmic).
See: P.V. Carpine (Allergan).
W/Phenylephrine HCl.
Use: Parasympathomimetic agent.
See: Pilofrin Liquifilm, Ophthalmic (Allergan).
•**PILOPINE.** (International Pharm.) Pilocarpine HCl 1%, 2% or 4%. Soln. Bot. 15 ml.
Use: Agent for glaucoma.
•**PILOPINE HS GEL.** (Alcon) Pilocarpine HCl 4%. Tube 5 Gm.
Use: Agent for glaucoma.
•**PIMA SYRUP.** (Fleming) Potassium iodide 5 gr/5 ml. Bot. pt, gal.
Use: Expectorant.
•**PIMETINE HYDROCHLORIDE.** USAN. 4-Benzyl-1-(2-dimethylaminoethyl)piperidine HCl.
Use: Cardiovascular drug (anticholesteremic).
•**PIMINODINE.** B.A.N. 1-(3-Phenylaminopropyl-4-phenylpiperidine-4-carboxylic acid ethyl ester. Ethyl 4-phenyl-1-(3-phenylaminopropyl)piperidine-4-carboxylate.
Use: Narcotic analgesic.
•**PIMINODINE ESYLATE.** Ethyl 1-(30 anilinopropyl)-4-phenylisonipecotate monoethanesulfaonte.
Use: Analgesic.
•**PIMINODINE ETHANESULFONATE.** Ethyl-4-phenyl-1-[3-(phenylamino)propyl]-piperidine-4-carboxylate ethanesulfonate.
Use: Narcotic analgesic.
•**PIMOBENDAN.** USAN.
Use: Cardiotonic.
•**PIMOZIDE,** U.S.P. XXII, Tab., USAN. 1-[1-[4,4-bis(p-Fluorophenyl)butyl]-4-piperidyl]-2-benzimidazoline. Orap.
Use: Tranquilizer.
See: Orap, Tab. (McNeil Pharm).
•**PINACIDIL.** USAN.
Use: Antihypertensive.
•**PINADOLINE.** USAN.
Use: Analgesic.
•**PINDOLOL,** U.S.P. XXII. Tab., U.S.P. XXII. 1-(Indol-4-yloxy)-3-isopropyl-amino)-2-propanol.
Use: Beta-adrenergic blocking agent.
See: Visken (Sandoz).
•**PINE NEEDLE OIL,** N.F. XVII.
Use: Perfume; flavor.
•**PINE TAR,** U.S.P. XXI.
Use: Local anti-eczematic; rubefacient.
•**PINEX CONCENTRATE COUGH SYRUP.** (Last) Dextromethorphan HBr 7.5 mg/5 ml (after diluting 3 oz. concentrate to make 16 oz. solution). Bot. 3 oz.
Use: Antitussive.
PINEX COUGH SYRUP. (Last) Dextromethorphan HBr 7.5 mg/5 ml. Bot. 3 oz, 6 oz.
Use: Antitussive.
PINEX REGULAR. (Pinex) Potassium guaiacolsulfonate, oil of pine and eucalyptus, extract of grindelia, alcohol 3%/30 ml. Syr. Bot. 3 oz, 8 oz. Also cherry flavored 3 oz. Super and concentrated 3 oz.
Use: Expectorant.
•**PINOXEPIN HCl.** USAN.
Use: Tranquilizer.
PIPAMAZINE. B.A.N. 1-[3-(2-Chlorophenothiazin-10-yl)-propyl] isonipecotramide. 10-[3-(4-Carbamoylpiperidino)propyl]-2-chlorophenothiazine. Mornidine.
Use: Antiemetic.
•**PIPAMPERONE.** USAN. 1′-[3-(p-Fluorobenzoyl)propyl][1,4′-bipiperidine]-4′-carboxamide. Under study.
Use: Tranquilizer.
•**PIPAZETHATE.** USAN. 2-(2-Piperidinoethoxy)-ethyl pyrido[3,2-b][1,4]benzothiazine-10-carboxylate. Selvigon HCl.
Use: Cough suppressant.
PIPAZETHATE HYDROCHLORIDE. 2-(2-Piperidinoethoxy)ethyl-10-H-pyrido [3,2-b]-[1,4]benzothiazine-10-carboxylate HCl.
Use: Antitussive.
•**PIPECURONIUM BROMIDE.** USAN.
Use: Muscle relaxant.
PIPENZOLATE BROMIDE. B.A.N. 1-Ethyl-3-piperidyl benzilate methylbromide. 3-Benziloyloxy-1-ethyl-1-methylpiperidinium bromide.
Use: Anticholinergic.
•**PIPERACILLIN SODIUM, STERILE,** U.S.P. XXII.
Use: Antibacterial.
•**PIPERAMIDE MALEATE.** USAN. 4′-[4-[3- (Dimethylamino)propyl]-1-piperazinyl]acetanilide dimaleate.
Use: Antiparasitic.
•**PIPERAZINE,** U.S.P. XXII.
Use: Anthelmintic.
PIPERAZINE CALCIUM EDETATE. B.A.N. [Dihydrogen(ethylenedinitrilo)tetraacetato]-calcium piperazine salt. Perin.
Use: Anthelmintic.
•**PIPERAZINE CITRATE,** U.S.P. XXII. Syr., Tab., U.S.P. XXII. Piperazine, 2-hydroxy-1,2,3-propanetricarboxylate (3:2) hydrate. Piperazine citrate (3:2) hydrate. Piperazine Citrate Telra Hydrous Tripiperazine Dicitrate.
Use: Anthelmintic.
See: Bryrel, Syr. (Winthrop Products).
Pipril, Liq. (Kenyon).
Ta-Verm, Syr., Tab. (Table Rock).
Vermago, Syr. (Westerfield).
•**PIPERAZINE EDETATE CALCIUM.** USAN. Dihydrogen [(ethylenedinitrilo)tetraacetato]calciate(2-) compound with piperazine (1:1). Perin.
Use: Anthelmintic.
PIPERAZINE ESTRONE SULFATE.

See: Estropipitate.
PIPERAZINE HEXAHYDRATE. Tivazine.
PIPERAZINE PHOSPHATE.
Use: Anthelmintic.
PIPERAZINE TARTRATE.
See: Razine Tartrate, Tab. (Paddock).
PIPERIDINE PHOSPHATE.
Use: Psychiatric drug.
PIPERIDINOETHYL BENZILATE HCl. No products listed.
PIPERIDOLATE. B.A.N. 1-Ethyl-3-piperidyl diphenylacetate.
Use: Parasympatholytic.
PIPERIDOLATE HYDROCHLORIDE. 1-Ethyl-3-piperidyl diphenylacetate HCl.
Use: Anticholinergic.
PIPEROCAINE. B.A.N. 3-(2-Methylpiperidino)-propyl benzoate.
Use: Local anesthetic.
PIPERONYL BUTOXIDE. B.A.N. 5-[2-(2-Butoxyethoxy)ethoxymethyl]-6-propyl-1,3-benzodioxole.
Use: Pediculicide.
PIPEROXAN. B.A.N. 2-Piperidinomethyl-1,4-benzodioxan.
Use: Adrenergic blocking agent.
PIPEROXAN HYDROCHLORIDE. 2-(1-Piperidylmethyl)-1,4-benzodioxan HCl. Fourneau 933. Benzodioxane. Diagnosis of hypertension.
Use: Diagnostic aid.
PIPERPHENIDOL HCl. 5-Methyl-4-phenyl-1-(1-piperidyl)-3-hexanol HCl.
PIPETHANATE HCl. 2-Piperidinoethyl benzilate HCl.
Use: Tranquilizer.
•**PIPOBROMAN,** U.S.P. XXII. Tab., U.S.P. XXII. 1,4-Bis(3-bromopropionyl)piperazine. Δ2,a-thiazolidine-acetate.
Use: Antineoplastic.
See: Vercyte, Tab. (Abbott).
•**PIPOSULFAN.** USAN. 1,4-Dihydracryloylpiperazine dimethanesulfonate.
Use: Antineoplastic agent.
PIPOTHIAZINE. B.A.N. 2-Dimethylsulfamoyl-10-3-[4-(2-hydroxyethyl)piperidino]propyl phenothiazine.
Use: Neuroleptic.
•**PIPOTIAZINE PALMITATE.** USAN.
Use: Antipsychotic.
See: Piportil (Ives).
•**PIPOXOLAN HCl.** USAN. 5,5-Diphenyl-2-(2- piperidinoethyl)-1,3-dioxolan-4-one HCl. Rowapraxin.
Use: Muscle relaxant.
PIPRACIL. (Lederle) Piperacillin sodium 2 Gm, 3 Gm, 4 Gm or 40 Gm/Vial; 2 Gm, 3 Gm or 4 Gm/Infusion Bottle. Sterile.
Use: Antibacterial, penicillin.
PIPRADOL. B.A.N. α-2-Piperidylbenzhydrol.
Use: Central nervous system stimulant.
PIPRIL. (Kenyon) Piperazine citrate 0.5 Gm/5 ml. Bot. pt, gal.
Use: Anthelmintic.
PIPRINHYDRINATE. B.A.N. Diphenylpyraline salt of 8-chlorotheopylline. 4-Benzyhydryloxy-1-methylpiperidine salt of 8-chlorotheophylline. Kolton; Mepedyl.
Use: Antihistamine.
•**PIPROZOLIN.** USAN. Ethyl 3-ethyl-4-oxo-5-piperidino Δ^2, alpha-thiazolidineacetate.
Use: Choleretic.
•**PIQUINDONE HYDROCHLORIDE.** USAN.
Use: Antipsychotic.
•**PIQUIZIL HCl.** USAN. Isobutyl 4-(6,7-dimethoxy-4-quinazolinyl)-1-piperazinecarboxylate monohydrochloride.
Use: Bronchodilator.
•**PIRACETAM.** USAN. 2-Oxopyrrolidin-1-ylacetamide. Nootropyl.
Use: Cerebral stimulant.
•**PIRANDAMINE HYDROCHLORIDE.** USAN.
Use: Antidepressant.
•**PIRAZOLAC.** USAN.
Use: Antirheumatic.
PIRAZMONAM SODIUM. USAN.
Use: Antimicrobial.
•**PIRBENICILLIN SODIUM.** USAN.
Use: Antibacterial.
•**PIRBUTEROL ACETATE.** USAN. 2-tert-Butylamino-1-(5-hydroxy-6-hydroxymethyl-2-pyridyl)ethanol acetate.
Use: Bronchodilator.
•**PIRBUTEROL HYDROCHLORIDE.** USAN.
Use: Bronchodilator.
•**PIRENPERONE.** USAN.
Use: Tranquilizer.
•**PIRENZEPINE HYDROCHLORIDE.** USAN.
Use: Antiulcerative.
•**PIRETANIDE.** USAN.
Use: Diuretic.
See: Arlix, Prods. (Hoechst).
•**PIRFENIDONE.** USAN.
Use: Anti-inflammatory, antipyretic.
PIRIDAZOL.
See: Sulfapyridine, Tab. (Various Mfr.).
•**PIRIDICILLIN SODIUM.** USAN.
Use: Antibacterial.
PIRIDOCAINE HCl. Beta-(2-Piperidyl) ethyl-o-aminobenzoate.
PIRIDOXILATE. B.A.N. The reciprocal salt of (5-hydroxy-4-hydroxymethyl-6-methyl-3-pyridyl)-meth-oxyglycolic acid with [4,5-bis(hydroxymethyl)-2-methyl-3-pyridyl] oxyglycolicacid (1:1). GLYO-6.
Use: Treatment of angina.
•**PIRIDRONATE SODIUM.** USAN.
Use: Regulator (calcium).
•**PIRIPROST.** USAN.
Use: Antiasthmatic.
•**PIRIPROST POTASSIUM.** USAN.
Use: Antiasthmatic.
PIRITON.
See: Chlorpheniramine (Various Mfr.).

PIRITRAMIDE. B.A.N. 4-(4-Carbamoyl-4-piperidino-piperidino)-2,2-diphenylbutyronitrile. Dipodolor.
Use: Analgesic.

•**PIRITREXIM ISETHIONATE.** USAN.
Use: Antiproliferative agent.

•**PIRLIMYCIN HYDROCHLORIDE.** USAN.
Use: Antibacterial.

•**PIRMAGREL.** USAN.
Use: Inhibitor (thromboxane synthetase).

•**PIRMENOL HYDROCHLORIDE.** USAN.
Use: Cardiac depressant.

•**PIRNABINE.** USAN.
Use: Antiglaucoma agent.

•**PIROCTONE.** USAN.
Use: Antiseborrheic.

•**PIROCTONE OLAMINE.** USAN.
Use: Antiseborrheic.

•**PIROGLIRIDE TARTRATE.** USAN.
Use: Antidiabetic.

•**PIROLATE.** USAN.
Use: Antiasthmatic.

•**PIROLAZAMIDE.** USAN.
Use: Cardiac depressant.

•**PIROXANTRONE HYDROCHLORIDE.** USAN.
Use: Antineoplastic.

•**PIROXICAM,** U.S.P. XXII. Cap., U.S.P. XXII. N-pyridyl-methyl-hydroxy-(benzothiazine-1 idioxide)carboxamide.
Use: Anti-inflammatory.
See: Feldene, Cap. (Pfizer).

•**PIROXICAM CINNAMATE.** USAN.
Use: Anti-inflammatory.

•**PIROXICAM OLAMINE.** USAN.
Use: Anti-inflammatory, analgesic.

•**PIROXIMONE.** USAN.
Use: Cardiotonic.

•**PIRPROFEN.** USAN.
Use: Anti-inflammatory.
See: Rengasil (Geigy).

•**PIRQUINOZOL.** USAN.
Use: Anti-allergic.

PIRSEAL. (Fellows) Acetylsalicylic acid 5 gr or 10 gr/Tab. Bot. 100s, 1000s.
Use: Salicylate analgesic.

PISO's. (Pinex) Ipecac, ammonium Cl, menthol in syrup base. Bot. 3 oz, 5 oz.
Use: Expectorant.

PITAYINE.
See: Quinidine, Preps. (Various Mfr.).

PITOCIN. (Parke-Davis) Oxytocin w/chlorobutanol 0.5%, acetic acid to adjust pH. Amp. (5 units)/0.5 ml; (10 units)/1 ml. Box 10s, Steri-dose syringe; (10 units)/1 ml 10s.
Use: Oxytocic.

PITRESSIN SYNTHETIC. (Parke-Davis) Vasopressin w/chlorobutanol 0.5%, pH adjusted with acetic acid. Amp. 0.5 ml (10 pressor units), 1 ml (20 pressor units). Box 10s.
Use: Posterior pituitary hormones.

PITTS CARMINATIVE. (Commerce) Bot. 2 oz.
Use: Antiflatulent.

PITUITARY, ANTERIOR. The anterior lobe of the pituitary gland supplies protein hormones classified under following headings.
See preparation of:
Corticotropin, Preps. (Various Mfr.).
Gonadotropin, Preps. (Various Mfr.).
Growth Hormone.
Thyrotropic Principle.

PITUITARY FUNCTION TEST.
See: Metopirone, Tab. (Ciba).

PITUITARY, POSTERIOR, HORMONES.
(a) Vasopressin. Pressor principle, β-hypophamine, postlobin-V.
See: Pitressin, Amp. (Parke-Davis).
(b) Oxytocin. Oxytocic principle. α-hypophamine, postiobin-O.
See: Oxytocin, Inj.
Pitocin, Amp. (Various Mfr.).
Syntocinon, Amp. (Sandoz).

•**PITUITARY, POSTERIOR, INJECTION,** U.S.P. XXII.
Use: Hormone (antidiuretic).
See: Pituitrin, Obstetrical, Amp. (Parke-Davis).
Pituitrin, Surgical, Amp. (Parke-Davis).

•**PIVAMPICILLIN HYDROCHLORIDE.** USAN.
Use: Antibacterial.

•**PIVAMPICILLIN PAMOATE.** USAN.
Use: Antibacterial.

•**PIVAMPICILLIN PROBENATE.** USAN.
Use: Antibacterial.

PIVAZIDE. N-Benzyl-N′-pivaloylhydrazine. Tersavid.

PIVHYDRAZINE. B.A.N. 1-Benzyl-2-pivaloyl-hydrazine.
Use: Monoamine oxidase inhibitor.

PIVMECILLINAM. B.A.N. Pivaloyloxymethyl (2S,5R,6R)-6-(perhydroazepin-1-ylmethyleneamino)-penicillanate.
Use: Antibiotic.

•**PIVOPRIL.** USAN.
Use: Antihypertensive.

PIX CARBONIS.
See: Coal Tar, Preps. (Various Mfr.).

PIX JUNIPERI.
Use: Sunscreen, moisturizer.
See: Juniper Tar, Comp. (Various Mfr.).

PIZOTIFEN. B.A.N. 4-(9,10-Dihydrobenzo[4,5]-cyclohepta]1,2-b]thien-4-ylidene)-1-methyl-piperidine.
Use: Prophylaxis of migraine.

•**PIZOTYLINE.** USAN. 4-(9,10-Dihydro-4H-benzo[4,5]-cyclohepta]1,2-b]thien-4-ylidene)-1-methyl-piperidine.
Use: Anabolic, antidepressant, migraine prophylactic.

PLACEBO CAPSULES. (Cowley) No. 3 orange red; No. 4 yellow. Bot. 1000s.
Use: Placebo.

PLACEBO TABLETS. (Cowley) 1 gr white; 2 gr white; 3 gr white, red or yellow, pink, orange; 4 gr white; 5 gr white. Bot. 1000s.
Use: Placebo.

PLACENTA.
See: Gonadotropins, Chorionic, Inj. (Various Mfr.).
PLACIDYL. (Abbott) Ethchlorvynol. **200 mg/Cap.:** Bot. 100s. **500 mg/Cap.:** Bot. 100s, 500s, UD 100s. **750 mg/Cap.:** Bot. 100s.
Use: Sedative/hypnotic.
•**PLAGUE VACCINE,** U.S.P. XXII. (Cutter) 2,000 million killed *Pasteurella pestis*/ml. Vial 2 ml, 20 ml.
Use: S.C. vaccination, active immunizing agent.
PLANOCAINE.
See: Procaine HCl, Preps. (Various Mfr.).
PLANOCHROME.
See: Merbromin, Soln. (Various Mfr.).
PLANTAGO, OVATA COATING.
See: Effersyllium, Prods. (Stuart).
Konsyl, Pow. (Burton, Parsons).
L.A. Formula, Pow. (Burton, Parsons).
Metamucil, Pow. (Searle).
W/Psyllium seed, gum karaya, Brewer's yeast.
See: Plantamucin, Gran. (Elder).
W/Vitamin B_1.
See: Siblin, Gran. (Parke-Davis).
•**PLANTAGO SEED,** U.S.P. XXII. Psyllium Seed, Plantain Seed.
Use: Fecal softener.
PLANT PROTEASE CONCENTRATE.
See: Ananase, Tab. (Rorer).
PLAQUENIL SULFATE. (Winthrop-Breon) Hydroxychloroquine sulfate 200 mg/Tab. (equivalent to base 155 mg). Bot. 100s.
Use: Antimalarial, antirheumatic.
PLAQUENIL TABLET. (Winthrop Pharm.) Hydroxychloroquine sulfate.
Use: Antimalarial, antirheumatic.
PLASBUMIN-5. (Cutter) Normal serum albumin (Human) 5% U.S.P. fractionated from normal serum plasma, heat treated against hepatitis virus. Albumin 12.5 Gm/250 ml. Vial 50 ml. Bot. with IV set 250 ml, 500 ml.
Use: Plasma protein fraction.
PLASBUMIN-25. (Cutter) Normal serum albumin (Human) 25% U.S.P. fractionated from normal serum plasma, heat treated against hepatitis virus. Albumin 12.5 Gm/50 ml. Vial 20 ml. Bot. with IV set 50 ml, 100 ml.
Use: Plasma protein fraction.
PLASMA.
See: Normal Human Plasma (Various Mfr.).
PLASMA EXPANDERS OR SUBSTITUTES.
See: Dextran 6% and LMD 10% (Abbott).
Macrodex, Soln. (Pharmacia).
PLASMA-LYTE A INJECTION. (Travenol) Sodium 140 mEq, potassium 5 mEq, magnesium 3 mEq, chloride 98 mEq, acetate 27 mEq, gluconate 23 mEq/L w/pH adjusted to 7.4. Plastic bot. 500 ml, 1000 ml.
Use: Parenteral nutritional supplement.
PLASMA-LYTE 148 INJECTION. (Travenol) Sodium 140 mEq, potassium 5 mEq, magnesium 3 mEq, chloride 98 mEq, acetate 27 mEq, gluconate 23 mEq/L. Plastic bot. 500 ml, 1000 ml.
Use: Parenteral nutritional supplement.
PLASMA-LYTE M and 5% DEXTROSE INJECTION. (Travenol) Sodium 40 mEq, potassium 16 mEq, calcium 5 mEq, magnesium 3 mEq, chloride 40 mEq, acetate 12 mEq, lactate 12 mEq/L. Plastic bot. 500 ml, 1000 ml.
Use: Parenteral nutritional supplement.
PLASMA-LYTE R and 5% DEXTROSE INJECTION. (Travenol) Sodium 140 mEq, potassium 10 mEq, calcium 5 mEq, magnesium 3 mEq, chloride 103 mEq, acetate 47 mEq, lactate 8 mEq/L. Bot. 500 ml, 1000 ml.
Use: Parenteral nutritional supplement.
PLASMA-LYTE 56 and 5% DEXTROSE. (Travenol) Sodium 40 mEq, potassium 13 mEq, magnesium 3 mEq, chloride 40 mEq, acetate 16 mEq/L. Plastic bot. 500 ml, 1000 ml.
Use: Parenteral nutritional supplement.
PLASMA-LYTE 148 AND 5% DEXTROSE. (Travenol) Dextrose 50 Gm, calories 190, sodium 140 mEq, potassium 5 mEq, magnesium 3 mEq, chloride 98 mEq, acetate 27 mEq, 547 mOsm, gluconate 23 mEq/L. Soln. Bot. 500 ml, 1000 ml.
Use: Parenteral nutritional supplement.
PLASMA-LYTE 56 IN WATER. (Travenol) Sodium 40 mEq, potassium 13 mEq, magnesium 3 mEq, chloride 40 mEq, acetate 16 mEq/L. Plastic bot. 500 ml, 1000 ml.
Use: Parenteral nutritional supplement.
PLASMA-LYTE R INJECTION. (Travenol) Sodium 140 mEq, potassium 10 mEq, calcium 5 mEq, magnesium 3 mEq, chloride 103 mEq, acetate 47 mEq, lactate 8 mEq/L. Bot. 1000 ml.
Use: Parenteral nutritional supplement.
PLASMANATE. (Cutter) Plasma protein fraction (Human) 5%. U.S.P. Vial 50 ml. Bot. 250 ml, 500 ml with set.
Use: Plasma protein fraction.
•**PLASMA PROTEIN FRACTION,** U.S.P. XXII. (Hyland) For the plasma protein preparation obtained from human plasma using the Cohn fractionation technic. Bot. 250 ml.
Use: Blood-volume supporter.
See: Plasmanate, Soln. (Cutter).
Plasma-Plex, Soln. (Armour).
Plasmatein (Abbott).
PLASMATEIN. (Alpha Therapeutic) Plasma protein fraction 5%. Inj. Vial w/injection set 250 ml, 500 ml.
Use: Plasma protein fraction.
PLASMIN. B.A.N. The proteolytic enzyme derived from the activation of plasminogen. Actase is Plasmin (Human).
PLASMINOGEN. B.A.N. The specific substance derived from plasma which, when activated, has the property of lysing fibrinogen, fibrin, and some other proteins.
PLASMOCHIN NAPHTHOATE. Pamaquine naphthoate.

Use: Antimalarial.
•**PLATELET CONCENTRATE,** U.S.P. XXII.
Use: Platelet replenisher.
PLATELET FACTOR 4. (Abbott Diagnostics) Radioimmunoassay for quantitative measurement of total PF4 levels in plasma. Test kit 100s.
Use: Diagnostic aid.
PLATINOL. (Bristol-Myers/Bristol Oncology) Cisplatin 10 mg or 50 mg/Vial.
Use: Antineoplastic agent.
PLATINOL-AQ. (Bristol-Myers Oncology) Cisplatin (CDDP). 1 mg/ml. Inj. Vial. 50 ml, 100 ml.
Use: Antineoplastic agent.
•**PLAURACIN.** USAN.
Use: Growth stimulant.
PLEGINE. (Wyeth-Ayerst) Phendimetrazine tartrate 35 mg/Tab. Bot. 100s, 1000s.
Use: Anorexiant.
PLEGISOL. (Abbott Hospital Prods) Calcium Cl dihydrate 17.6 mg, magnesium Cl hexahydrate 325.3 mg, potassium Cl 119.3 mg, sodium Cl 643 mg/100 ml. Approximately 260 mOsm/L. Single Dose Container 1000 ml without sodium bicarbonate.
Use: Cardioplegic solution.
PLEWIN TABLETS. (Winthrop Products) Glycobiarsol, chloroquine phosphate.
Use: Amebicide.
PLEXOLAN CREAM. (Last) Zinc oxide, lanolin. Tube 1.25 oz, 3 oz. Jar 16 oz.
Use: Skin protectant.
PLEXON. (Sig) Testosterone 10 mg, estrone 1 mg, liver 2 mcg, pyridoxine HCl 10 mg, panthenol 10 mg, inositol 20 mg, choline Cl 20 mg, vitamin B_2 2 mg, B_{12} 100 mcg, procaine HCl 1%, niacinamide 100 mg/ml. Vial 10 ml.
Use: Hormone, vitamin/mineral supplement.
PLIAGEL. (CooperVision) Sodium Cl, potassium Cl, poloxamer 407, sorbic acid 0.25%, EDTA 0.5%. Soln. Bot. 25 ml.
Use: Soft contact lens care.
•**PLICAMYCIN,** U.S.P. XXII. Inj. U.S.P. XXII. Antibiotic derived from *Streptomyces agrillaceus* & *S. tanashiensis.*
Use: Antineoplastic.
See: Mithracin, Pow. (Miles Pharm).
PLOVA. (Washington Ethical) Psyllium mucilloid. Pow., (flavored) 12 oz. (plain) 10 0.5 oz.
Use: Laxative.
PLURAVIT DROPS. (Winthrop Products) Multivitamin.
Use: Vitamin supplement.
PMB 200. (Wyeth-Ayerst) Premarin (Conjugated Estrogens, U.S.P.) 0.45 mg, meprobamate 200 mg/Tab. Bot. 60s.
Use: Estrogen, antianxiety agent.
PMB 400. (Wyeth-Ayerst) Premarin (Conjugated Estrogens, U.S.P.) 0.45 mg, meprobamate 400 mg/Tab. Bot. 60s.
Use: Estrogen, antianxiety agent.
P.M.P. COMPOUND. (Mericon) Chlorpheniramine maleate 4 mg, phenylephrine HCl 15 mg, salicylamide 300 mg, scopolamine methylnitrate 0.8 mg/Tab. Bot. 100s, 1000s.
Use: Antihistamine, decongestant, analgesic.
PMP EXPECTORANT. (Mericon) Codeine phosphate 10 mg, phenylephrine HCl 10 mg, guaifenesin 40 mg, chlorpheniramine maleate 2 mg/5 ml. Bot. gal.
Use: Antitussive, decongestant, expectorant, antihistamine.
PNEUMOCOCCAL VACCINE, POLYVALENT. Purified capsular polysaccharides from 23 pneumococcal types.
Use: Agent for immunization.
See: Pneumovax 23, Inj. (Merck Sharp & Dohme) Pnuimune 23, Inj. (Merck Sharp & Dohme).
PNEUMOCOCCI.
W/*Haemophilus influenzae, Neisseria catarrhalis, streptococci, Klebsiella pneumoniae, staphylococci, pneumococci,* killed.
See: Mixed Vaccine No. 4 w/H. Influenzae, Inj. (Lilly).
PNEUMONIA VACCINE, KILLED DIPLOCOCCUS.
W/*Neisseria catarrhalis, Klebsiella pneumoniae, streptococci, staphylococci.*
See: Combined Vaccine No. 4 w/Catarrhalis, Inj. (Lilly).
PNEUMONIAE VACCINE, KILLED KLEBSIELLA.
W/*Neisseria catarrhalis, Diplococcus pneumoniae, streptococci, staphylococci.*
See: Combined Vaccine No. 4 w/Catarrhalis, Inj.(Lilly).
PNEUMOVAX 23. (Merck Sharp & Dohme) Pneumococcal vaccine polyvalent 0.5 ml/dose. Vial 5 dose, 1 dose X 5s.
Use: Agent for immunization.
PNS UNNA BOOT. (Pedinol) Non-sterile gauze bandage 10 yds × 3″. Box 12s.
Use: Ambulatory procedure in treatment of leg ulcers and varicosities.
PNU-IMUNE 23. (Lederle) Pneumococcal vaccine 0.5 ml dose. Vial dose 5s. Lederject disposable syringe 5 × 1 dose.
Use: Agent for immunization.
POCHLORIN. Prophyrinic and chlorophyllic compound.
Use: Anti-hypercholesteremic agent.
PODIASPRAY. (Dalin) Undecylenic acid, salicylic acid, dichlorophene. Spray-on pow. 6 oz.
Use: Fungicide, germicide.
PODIODINE. (A.V.P.) Germicidal surgical scrub and solution.
Use: Germicide.
POD-BEN-25. (C & M Pharmacal) Podophyllin 25% in benzoin tincture. Bot. 1 oz.
Use: Keratolytic.
PODOBEN. (American) Podophyllum resin extract 25%. Bot. 5 ml.
Use: Keratolytic.
•**PODOFILOX.** USAN.

Use: Cytotoxic, topical.
See: Condylox (Oclassen).

PODOFIN. (Syosset Labs) Podophyllum resin 25% in benzoin tincture. Liq. Bot. 7.5 ml.
Use: Keratolytic.

PODOPHYLLIN.
See: Podophyllum resin.

•**PODOPHYLLUM,** U.S.P. XXII.
Use: Caustic.
W/Cascara sagrada, bile salts, phenolphthalein.
See: Bilstan (Standex).
W/Oxgall, cascara sagrada, dandelion root, tincture nux vomica.
See: Oxachol, Liq. (Philips Roxane).

•**PODOPHYLLUM RESIN,** U.S.P. XXII. Topical Soln., U.S.P. XXII. (Various Mfr.) Podophyllin. Pkg. 1 oz, 0.25 lb, 1 lb.
Use: Caustic.
See: Podoben, Liq. (Maurry).
W/Salicylic acid.
See: Ver-Var, Soln. (Owen).

POINT-TWO MOUTHRINSE. (Hoyt) Sodium fluoride 0.2% in a flavored neutral liquid. Bot. 120 ml.
Use: Dental caries preventative.

POISON ANTIDOTE KIT. (Bowman) Charcoal suspension. Bot. 2 oz, 4s. Ipecac syrup, Bot. 1 oz, 1/Kit.
Use: Antidote.

POISON IVY EXTRACT. (Parke-Davis) Extract from leaves of *Rhus toxicodendron* dissolved in sterile almond oil. Vial 2 ml.
Use: Systemic poison ivy product.

•**POISON IVY EXTRACT, ALUM PRECIPITATED.** USAN. An aqueous suspension of a pyridine extract of poison ivy which is precipitated with alum and adjusted to standard concentrations.
Use: Ivy poisoning counteractant.
See: Aqua Ivy, Inj. (Miles Pharm).
Poisonivi, Extract (Cutter).
Poisonok, Extract (Cutter).

POISON IVY AND OAK PROPHYLAXIS. (Hollister-Stier) Allergenic extract for oral administration. Dropper Bot. 15 ml Pkg. 3s. Strength 1:25, 1:50, 1:100.
Use: Hyposensitization of patients allergic to poison ivy and poison oak.

POISON OAK EXTRACT. USAN.
Use: Anti-allergic.

•**POLACRILLIN.** USAN. Methacrylic acid with divinylbenzene. A synthetic ion-exchange resin, supplied in the hydrogen or free acid form. Amberlite IRP-64 (Rohm and Haas).
Use: Pharmaceutic aid.

•**POLACRILLIN POTASSIUM,** N.F. XVII. A synthetic ion-exchange resin, prepared through the polymerization of methacrylic acid and divinylbenzene, further neutralized with potassium hydroxide to form the potassium salt of methacrylic acid and divinylbenzene. Supplied as a pharmaceutical-grade ion-exchange resin in a particle size of 100- to 500-mesh.
Use: Pharmaceutic aid (tablet disintegrant).
See: Amberlite IRP-88 (Rohm and Haas).

POLADEX TABS. (Major) Dexchlorpheniramine maleate. **4 mg/Tab.:** Bot. 100s, 250s, 1000s; **6 mg/Tab.:** Bot. 100s, 1000s.
Use: Antihistamine.

POLAMETHENE RESIN CAPRYLATE. The physiochemical complex of the acid-binding ion exchange resin, polyamine-methylene resin and caprylic acid.

POLARAMINE. (Schering) Dexchlorpheniramine maleate (d-isomer of Chlor-Trimeton). **Repetab:** 4 mg/Tab. Bot. 100s; 6 mg/Tab. Bot. 100s, 1000s. **Syr.:** 2 mg/5 ml. Bot. 16 oz.
Use: Antihistamine.

POLARAMINE EXPECTORANT. (Schering) Dexchlorpheniramine maleate 2 mg, pseudoephedrine sulfate 20 mg, guaifenesin 100 mg, alcohol 7.2%/5 ml. Bot. 16 oz.
Use: Antihistamine, decongestant, expectorant.

POLARGEN T.D. TABS. (Goldline) Dexchlorpheniramine maleate 4 mg or 6 mg/Tab. Bot. 100s, 1000s.
Use: Antihistamine.

POLDEMAN AD SUSPENSION. (Winthrop Products) Kaolin.
Use: Antidiarrheal.

POLDEMAN SUSPENSION. (Winthrop Products) Kaolin.
Use: Antidiarrheal.

POLDEMICINA SUSPENSION. (Winthrop Products) Kaolin.
Use: Antidiarrheal.

•**POLICAPRAM.** USAN.
Use: Pharmaceutic aid (tablet binder).

POLIDENT DENTU-GRIP. (Block) Carboxymethylcellulose gum, ethylene oxide polymer. Pkg. 0.675 oz, 1.75 oz, 3.55 oz.
Use: Denture adhesive.

POLIDEXIDE. B.A.N. Dextran cross-linked with epichlorhydrin and 0-substituted with 2-diethylaminoethyl groups, some of them quaternized with diethylaminoethyl Cl. Secholex hydrochloride.
Use: Antihypercholesterolemic agent.

•**POLIGEENAN.** USAN. 3,6-Anhydro-4-O-β-D-galactopyranosyl-α-D-galactopyranose 2,4′-bis(potassium/sodium sulfate)-(1-3′)-polysaccharide. Polysaccharide produced by limited hydrolysis of carragheen from red algae.
Use: Enzyme inhibitor.

•**POLIGNATE SODIUM.** USAN.
Use: Enzyme inhibitor.

POLI-GRIP. (Block) Karaya gum, magnesium oxide in petrolatum mineral oil base, peppermint and spearmint flavor. Tube 0.75 oz, 1.5 oz, 2.5 oz.
Use: Denture adhesive.

POLIOMYELITIS IMMUNE GLOBULIN (HUMAN). (Various Mfr.) Preparation of gamma globulin primarily assayed for content of poliomyelitis antibodies in accordance with standard procedures licensed by National Institutes of Health.

POLIOMYELITIS VACCINE. (Squibb/Connaught) (Purified, Salk Type IPV) Amp. 5 x 1 ml. Vial 10 dose.
Use: Agent for immunization.

•**POLIOMYELITIS VACCINE INACTIVATED,** U.S.P. XXII.
Use: Active immunizing agent.

POLIOVIRUS VACCINE, INACTIVATED. (Squibb/Connaught) Amp. 1 ml. Box 5s. Vial 10 dose. Subcutaneous administration.
Use: Agent for immunization.

•**POLIOVIRUS VACCINE LIVE ORAL,** U.S.P. XXII. Poliovirus vaccine, live, oral, type I, II or III. Poliovirus vaccine, live, oral, trivalent.
Use: Active immunizing agent.
See: Orimune Trivalent I, II & III, Vial (Lederle).

POLIOVIRUS VACCINE, LIVE, ORAL, TRIVALENT. Immunization against polio strains 1, 2 & 3.
Use: Agent for immunization.
See: Orimune (Lederle).

•**POLIPROPENE 25.** USAN.
Use: Pharmaceutic aid.

POLOCAINE. (Astra) Mepivacaine 1%, 1.5% or 2%. Inj. Vial 30 ml, 50 ml.
Use: Local anesthetic.

POLOCAINE 3% INJECTION. (Astra) Mepivacaine HCl 3%. Astrapak 1.8 ml, Box 100 cartridges.
Use: Local anesthetic.

POLORIS POULTICES. (Block) Benzocaine 7.5 mg, capsicum 4.6 mg in poultice base. Pkg. 5 unit, 12 unit.
Use: Local anesthetic.

•**POLOXALENE.** USAN. Liquid nonionic surfactant polymer of polyoxypropylene polyoxyethylene type.
Use: Surfactant.

POLOXALKOL. B.A.N. A polymer of ethylene oxide, propylene oxide, and propylene glycol.
Use: Surface active agent.

POLOXALKOL. Polyoxyethylene polyoxypropylene polymer.
See: Magcyl, Cap. (Elder).
W/Casanthrol.
See: Casakol, Cap. (Upjohn).
W/Phenylephrine HCl, dextrose soln.
See: Isohalent, Soln. (Elder).

•**POLOXAMER,** N.F. XVII.
Use: Surfactant.

•**POLOXAMER 182 D.** USAN.
Use: Pharmaceutic aid (surfactant).

•**POLOXAMER 182 LF.** USAN.
Use: Food additive; pharmaceutic aid.

•**POLOXAMER 188.** USAN.
Use: Cathartic.

•**POLOXAMER 188 LF.** USAN.
Use: Pharmaceutic aid (surfactant).

•**POLOXAMER 331.** USAN.
Use: Food additive (surfactant).

POLOXAMER-IODINE.
See: Prepodyne, Soln. (West).

POLOXYL LANOLIN. B.A.N. A polyoxyethylene condensation-product of anhydrous lanolin. Aqualose.
Use: Emollient.

POLYAMINE-METHYLENE RESIN.
See: Exorbin (Various Mfr.).

POLYAMINE RESIN.
See: Polyamine-Methylene Resin (Various Mfr.).

POLYANETHOL SULFONATE, SODIUM.
See: Grobax, Vial (Roche Diagnostics).

POLYANHYDROGLUCOSE. Polyanhydroglucuronic acid.
See: Dextran, Inj., Soln. (Various Mfr.).

POLYBASE. (Paddock) Preblended polyethylene glycol suppository base for incorporation of medications where a water soluble base is indicated. Jar 1 lb, 5 lb.
Use: Suppository base.

POLYBENZARSOL. Benzarsoln.

POLY-BON DROPS. (Barrows) Vitamins A 3000 IU, D 400 IU, C 60 mg, B_1 1 mg, B_2 1.2 mg, niacinamide 8 mg/0.6 ml. Bot. 50 ml.
Use: Vitamin supplement.

•**POLYBUTESTER.** USAN.
Use: Surgical suture material.

•**POLYBUTILATE.** USAN.
Use: Surgical suture coating.

POLYCARBOPHIL. A synthetic, loosely cross-linked, hydrophilic resin of the polycarboxylic type. Sorboquel.
Use: Laxative.

POLYCILLIN. (Bristol) Ampicillin trihydrate. **250 mg/Cap.:** Bot. 100s, 500s, 1000s, UD 100s. **500 mg/Cap.:** Bot. 100s, 500s, UD 100s. **Pediatric Drops:** 100 mg/ml. Dropper bot. 20 ml.
Use: Antibacterial, penicillin.

POLYCILLIN-N. (Bristol) Sodium ampicillin 125 mg, 250 mg, 500 mg, 1 Gm or 2 Gm/Vial. Pkg. 1s, 10s. Piggyback vial 500 mg, 1 Gm, 2 Gm. Bulk vial 10 Gm.
Use: Antibacterial, penicillin.

POLYCILLIN ORAL SUSPENSION. (Bristol) Ampicillin trihydrate. **125 mg/5 ml:** Bot. 80 ml, 100 ml, 150 ml, 200 ml, UD 5 ml. **250 mg/5 ml:** Bot. 80 ml, 100 ml, 150 ml, 200 ml, UD 5 ml. **500 mg/5 ml:** Bot. 100 ml, UD 5 ml.
Use: Antibacterial, penicillin.

POLYCILLIN-PRB ORAL SUSPENSION. (Bristol) Ampicillin trihydrate 3.5 Gm, probenecid 1 Gm/Bot. Bot 9s.
Use: Antibacterial, penicillin.

POLYCITRA-K. (Willen) Potassium citrate monohydrate 1100 mg, citric acid monohydrate 334 mg, potassium ion 10 mEq/5 ml. Bot. 4 oz, pt.
Use: Systemic alkalinizer.

POLYCITRA-K CRYSTALS. (Willen) Potassium citrate monohydrate 3300 mg, citric acid 1002 mg, potassium ion 30 mEq, equivalent to 30 mEq bicarbonate/UD pkg. Box 100s.
Use: Systemic alkalinizer.

POLYCITRA-LC. (Willen) Potassium citrate monohydrate 550 mg, sodium citrate dihydrate 500 mg, citric acid monohydrate 334 mg, potassium ion 5 mEq, sodium ion 5 mEq/5 ml. Bot. 4 oz, pt.
Use: Systemic alkalinizer.

POLYCITRA SYRUP. (Willen) Potassium citrate monohydrate 550 mg, sodium citrate dihydrate 500 mg, citric acid monohydrate 334 mg, potassium ion 5 mEq, sodium ion 5 mEq/5 ml. Bot. 4 oz, pt.
Use: Systemic alkalinizer.

POLYCOSE. (Ross) **Pow.:** Glucose polymers derived from controlled hydrolysis of corn starch. Calories 380, carbohydrate 94 Gm, water 6 Gm, sodium 110 mg, potassium 10 mg, chloride 223 mg, calcium 30 mg, phosphorus 5 mg/100 Gm. Can 12.3 oz. Case 6s. **Liq.:** Calories 200, carbohydrate 50 Gm, water 70 Gm, sodium 70 mg, potassium 6 mg, chloride 140 mg, calcium 20 mg, phosphorus 3 mg/100 ml. Bot. 4 oz. Case 48s.
Use: Enteral nutritional supplement.

POLYCYCLINE INTRAVENOUS.
See: Bristacycline, Cap., Vial (Bristol).

•**POLYDEXTROSE.** USAN.
Use: Food additive.

POLYDINE OINTMENT. (Century) Povidone iodine in ointment base. Jar 1 oz, 4 oz, lb.
Use: Anti-infective, external.

POLYDINE SCRUB. (Century) Povidone iodine in scrub solution. Bot. 1 oz, 4 oz, 8 oz, pt, gal.
Use: Antiseptic.

POLYDINE SOLUTION. (Century) Povidone iodine solution. Bot. 1 oz, 4 oz, 8 oz, pt, gal.
Use: Antiseptic.

•**POLYDIOXANONE.** USAN.
Use: Surgical aid.

POLYECTIN. (Amid).
See: Am-Tuss Elixir.

POLY ENA TEST SYSTEM FOR RNP AND SM. (Wampole-Zeus) Qualitative identification of auto antibodies to extractable nuclear antigens in human serum by gel precipitation technique. Aid in the diagnosis of SLE, MCTD, PSS, SS. Box test 48s.
Use: Diagnostic aid.

POLY ENA TEST SYSTEM FOR RNP, SM, SSA AND SSB. (Wampole-Zeus) Qualitative identification of auto antibodies to extractable nuclear antigens in human serum by gel precipitation techniques. Aid in the diagnosis of SLE, MCTD, PSS, SS. Box test 96s.
Use: Diagnostic aid.

POLY ENA TEST SYSTEM FOR SSA AND SSB. (Wampole-Zeus) Qualitative identification of auto antibodies to extractable nuclear antigens in human serum by gel precipitation techniques. Aid in the diagnosis of SLE, MCTD, PSS, SS. Box test 48s.
Use: Diagnostic aid.

POLYESTRADIOL PHOSPHATE.
See: Estradurin, Amp. (Wyeth-Ayerst).

•**POLYETHADENE.** USAN. 1,2:3,4-Diepoxybutane polymer with ethylenimine. Erythritol anhydride polyethyleneimine polymer.
Use: Antacid.

•**POLYETHYLENE EXCIPIENT,** N.F. XVII.
Use: Pharmaceutic aid (stiffening agent).

•**POLYETHYLENE GLYCOL 300, 400, 600, 1500, 1540, 4000 AND 6000, N.F. XVII. Oint., N.F. XVII.**
Use: Water-soluble ointment and suppository base; tablet excipient.
See: Carbowax (Doak) 16 oz.
P.E.G. Lotion (Medco).

•**POLYETHYLENE GLYCOL 3350 AND ELECTROLYTES FOR ORAL SOLUTION,** U.S.P. XXII.
Use: Rehydration.

•**POLYETHYLENE GLYCOL MONOETHYL ETHER,** U.S.P. XXII.

•**POLYETHYLENE OXIDE,** N.F. XVII.
Use: Pharmaceutical aid.

•**POLYFEROSE.** USAN. An iron carbohydrate chelate containing approximately 45% of iron in which the metallic (Fe) ion is sequestered within a polymerized carbohydrate derived from sucrose.
Use: Hematinic.

POLY-F FLUORIDE DROPS. (Major) Fluoride 0.5 mg, vitamins A 1500 IU, D 400 IU, E 5 mg, B_1 0.5 mg, B_2 0.6 mg, B_3 8 mg, B_6 0.4 mg, B_{12} 2 mcg, C 35 mg/ml. Drops. Bot. 50 ml.
Use: Vitamin/mineral supplement.

POLYGELINE. B.A.N. A polymer of urea and polypeptides derived from denatured gelatin.
Use: Restoration of blood volume.

•**POLYGLACTIN 370 & 910.** USAN. Lactic acid polyester with glycolic acid.
Use: Synthetic absorbable suture.

•**POLYGLYCOLIC ACID.** USAN. Poly-(oxycarbonylmethylene).
Use: Surgical aid.
See: Dexon Sterile Suture (David & Geck).

•**POLYGLYCONATE.** USAN.
Use: Surgical Aid.

POLYHEXANIDE. V.B.A.N. Poly-(1-hexamethylene-biguanide hydrochloride).
Use: Antibacterial, veterinary medicine.

POLY-HISTINE CS. (Bock) Brompheniramine maleate 2 mg, phenylpropanolamine HCl 12.5 mg, codeine phosphate 10 mg/5 ml, alcohol 0.95%. Bot. pt.
Use: Antihistamine, decongestant, expectorant.

POLY-HISTINE-D CAPSULES. (Bock) Phenylpropanolamine HCl 50 mg, phenyltoloxamine citrate 16 mg, pyrilamine maleate 16 mg, pheniramine maleate 16 mg/Cap. Bot. 100s.
Use: Decongestant, antihistamine.

POLY-HISTINE-D ELIXIR. (Bock) Phenylpropanolamine HCl 12.5 mg, phenyltoloxamine citrate 4 mg, pyrilamine maleate 4 mg, pheniramine 4 mg/5 ml, alcohol 4%. Bot. pt.

Use: Antihistamine, decongestant.

POLY-HISTINE DM. (Bock) Dextromethorphan HBr 10 mg, phenylpropanolamine HCl 12.5 mg, brompheniramine maleate 2 mg/5 ml. Bot. pt.
Use: Antitussive, decongestant, antihistamine.

POLY-HISTINE-D PED CAPS. (Bock) Phenylpropanolamine HCl 25 mg, phenyltoloxamine citrate 8 mg, pheniramine maleate 8 mg, pyrilamine maleate 8 mg/Cap. Bot. 100s.
Use: Decongestant, antihistamine.

POLY-HISTINE ELIXIR. (Bock) Phenyltoloxamine citrate 4 mg, pyrilamine maleate 4 mg, pheniramine maleate 4 mg/5 ml, alcohol 4%. Elix. Bot. pt.
Use: Antihistamine.

•**POLYMACON.** USAN. Poly(2-hydroxyethyl methacrylate).
Use: Contact lens material.

•**POLYMETAPHOSPHATE P-32.** USAN.
Use: Radioactive agent.

POLYMETHINE BLUE DYE. (3,3′-Diethylhiadicarbocyanine iodide).

POLYMONINE. A formaldehyde polymer of N-methylmonoanisylamine.

POLYMOX. (Bristol) Amoxicillin trihydrate. **Cap.:** 250 mg. Bot. 100s, 500s, UD 100s; 500 mg. Bot. 50s, 100s, 500s, UD 100s. **Oral Susp.:** 125 mg or 250 mg/5 ml. Bot. 80 ml, 100 ml, 150 ml. Dosatrol 125 mg or 250 mg/Bot. 5 ml. **Ped. Drops:** 50 mg/ml. Bot. 15 ml.
Use: Antibacterial, penicillin.

POLYMYXIN. B.A.N. Generic term for antibiotics obtained from fermentations of various media by strains of *Bacillus polymyxa.*
Use: Polymyxins A, B and D active against susceptible gram-negative bacteria.

POLYMYXIN B. (Various Mfr.) (No Pharmaceutical Form Available) Antimicrobial substances produced by *Bacillus polymyxa.*
W/Bacitracin zinc, neomycin sulfate, benzalkonium Cl.
See: Biotres, Oint. (Central).

•**POLYMYXIN B SULFATE,** U.S.P. XXII. Otic Soln., Sterile, U.S.P. XXII.
Use: Antibiotic.
See: Aerosporin, Pow., Soln. (Burroughs Wellcome).

•**POLYMYXIN B SULFATE AND BACITRACIN ZINC TOPICAL AEROSOL,** U.S.P. XXII.
Use: Antibiotic.

•**POLYMYXIN B SULFATE AND BACITRACIN ZINC TOPICAL POWDER,** U.S.P. XXII.
Use: Antibiotic.

•**POLYMYXIN** B SULFATE AND HYDROCORTISONE OTIC SOLUTION, U.S.P. XXII.
Use: Antibiotic, anti-inflammatory.

POLYMYXIN B SULFATE STERILE. (Pfipharmics) Polymyxin B sulfate 500,000 units/Vial 20 ml for reconstitution.
Use: Anti-infective.

POLYMYXIN B SULFATE W/COMBINATIONS.
See: Aural Acute, Drops (Saron).
Cortisporin, Preps. (Burroughs Wellcome).
Epimycin A, Oint. (Delta).
Maxitrol, Oint., Ophthalmic Oint. (Upjohn).
Mycitracin, Oint., Ophthalmic Oint. (Upjohn).
Neomixin, Oint. (Mallard).
Neosporin, Preps. (Burroughs Wellcome).
Neosporin G.U. Irrigant, Amp. (Burroughs Wellcome).
Neotal, Oint. (Mallard).
Neo-Thrycex, Oint. (Commerce).
Otobiotic, Soln. (Schering).
Otoreid-HC, Liq. (Solvay).
P.B.N., Oint. (Jenkins).
Polysporin, Oint., Ophthalmic Oint. (Burroughs Wellcome).
Pyocidin-Otic, Soln. (Berlex).
Statrol, Liq. (Alcon).
Statrol Sterile Ophthalmic Oint. (Alcon).
Terramycin, Preps. w/Polymyxin (Pfizer).
Tigo, Oint. (Burlington).
Tribotic, Oint. (Burgin-Arden).
Trimixin, Oint. (Hance).
Triple Antibiotic Oint. (Kenyon).

POLYMYXIN E.
See: Colistin sulfate.

POLYMYXIN-NEOMYCIN-BACITRACIN OINTMENT. (Various Mfr.).
Use: Antibiotic for treatment of gram-positive and gram-negative organisms.

POLY-NEO-CORT. (Robinson) Ear drops. Bot. 12.5 ml.
Use: Anti-infective, otic.

POLYNOXYLIN. B.A.N. Poly[methylenedi(hydroxymethyl)urea]Anaflex; Ponoxylan.
Use: Antibacterial, anti-inflammatory.

POLYNOXYLIN. Poly[methylenedi(hydroxymethyl)urea]. Anaflex.

POLYOXYETHYLENE 8 STEARATE. Myrj 45. (ICI U.S.), Polyoxyl 8 Stearate.

POLYOXYETHYLENE (20) SORBITAN MONOLEATE.
See: Polysorbate 80, U.S.P. XXII. (Various Mfr.).

POLYOXYETHYLENE 20 SORBITAN TRIOLEATE. Tween 85. (ICI U.S.), Polysorbate 85.

POLYOXYETHYLENE 20 SORBITAN TRISTEAR-ATE. Tween 65. (ICI U.S.), Polysorbate 65.

POLYOXYETHYLENE 40 MONOSTEARATE. Polyoxyl 40 Stearate.
See: Myrj 52 & Myrj 52S (ICI U.S.).

•**POLYOXYETHYLENE 50 STEARATE,** N.F. XVII.
Use: Surfactant; emulsifying agent.

POLYOXYETHYLENEONYLPHENOL.
W/Alkyldimethylbenzylammonium Cl, methylrosaniline Cl, polyethylene glycol tert-dodecylthioether.
See: Hyva, Vaginal Tab. (Holland-Rantos).

POLYOXYETHYLENE SORBITAN MONOLAURATE. Polysorbate 20, N.F. XVII.
W/Ferrous gluconate.
See: Simron, Cap. (Merrell Dow).

W/Ferrous gluconate, vitamins.
See: Simron Plus, Cap. (Merrell Dow).
POLYOXYETHYLENE LAURYL ETHER.
W/Benzoyl peroxide, ethyl alcohol.
See: Benzagel, Gel (Dermik).
Desquam-X, Preps. (Westwood).
W/Hydrocortisone, sulfur.
See: Fostril HC, Lot. (Westwood).
W/Sulfur.
See: Fostril, Lot. (Westwood).
Proseca, Oint. (Westwood).
POLYOXYETHYLENE NONYL PHENOL
W/Sodium edetate, docusate sodium, 9-aminoacridine HCl.
See: Vagisec Plus, Supp. (Schmid).
•**POLYOXYL 8 STEARATE.** USAN. Polyoxyethylene 8 stearate.
Use: Surfactant.
See: Myrj 45 (Atlas).
•**POLYOXYL 10 OLEYL ETHER,** N.F. XVII.
Use: Pharmaceutic aid (surfactant).
•**POLYOXYL 20 CETOSTEARYL ETHER,** N.F. XVII.
Use: Pharmaceutic aid (surfactant).
•**POLYOXYL 35 CASTOR OIL,** N.F. XVII.
Use: Pharmaceutic aid (surfactant, emulsifying agent).
•**POLYOXYL 40 HYDROGENATED CASTOR OIL,** N.F. XVII.
Use: Pharmaceutic aid (surfactant, emulsifying agent).
•**POLYOXYL 40 STEARATE,** N.F. XVII. Macrogic Stearate 2,000 (I.N.N.) Polyoxyethylene 40 monostearate.
Use: Pharmaceutic aid (surfactant).
Use: Hydrophilic oint., surfactant; surface-active agent.
See: Myrj 52. (Atlas).
Myrj 52S. (Atlas).
W/Polyethylene glycol, chlorobutanol.
See: Blink-N-Clean (Allergan).
POLY-PRED LIQUIFILM. (Allergan) Prednisolone acetate 0.5%, neomycin sulfate equivalent to 0.35% neomycin base, polymyxin B sulfate 10,000 units/ml, polyvinyl alcohol 1.4%, thimerosal 0.001%. Dropper bot. 5 ml, 10 ml.
Use: Corticosteroid, anti-infective, ophthalmic.
•**POLYPROPYLENE GLYCOL,** N.F. XVII. An addition polymer of propylene oxide and water.
Use: Pharmaceutic aid (suspending agent).
POLYSEPT. (Dalin) Polymyxin B sulfate 5000 units, bacitracin 400 units, neomycin sulfate 5 mg, diperodon HCl 10 mg/Gm. Tube 0.5 oz.
Use: Anti-infective, external.
POLYSONIC LOTION. (Parker) Multi-purpose ultrasound lotion with high coupling efficiency. Bot. 8.5 oz, gal.
Use: For diagnostic and therapeutic medical ultrasound.
•**POLYSORBATE 20,** N.F. XVII. (Atlas) Tween 20. Polyoxyethlene 20 sorbitan monolaurate.
Use: Surface-active agent.
•**POLYSORBATE 40,** N.F. XVII. (Atlas) Tween 40. Polyoxyethylene 20 sorbitan monopalmitate.
Use: Surface-active agent.
•**POLYSORBATE 60,** N.F. XVII. (Atlas) Tween 60. Polyoxyethylene 20 sorbitan monostearate.
Use: Surface-active agent.
•**POLYSORBATE 65.** USAN. (Atlas) Tween 65. Polyoxyethylene 20 sorbitan tristearate.
Use: Surface-active agent.
•**POLYSORBATE 80,** N.F. XVII. Polyoxyethylene (20) Sorbitan Monooleate.
Use: Surfactant.
•**POLYSORBATE 85.** USAN. (Atlas) Polyoxyethylene 20 sorbitan trioleate. Tween 85.
Use: Surface-active agent.
POLYSPORIN OINTMENT. (Burroughs Wellcome) Polymyxin B sulfate 10,000 units, bacitracin zinc 500 units/Gm in special white petrolatum base. Tube 3.75 Gm.
Use: Anti-infective, external.
POLYSPORIN POWDER. (Burroughs Wellcome) Polymyxin B 10,000 units, zinc bacitracin 500 units, lactose base/Gm. Shaker vial 10 Gm.
Use: Anti-infective, external.
POLYSPORIN SPRAY. (Burroughs Wellcome) Aerosporin brand polymyxin B sulfate 200,000 units, zinc bacitracin 10,000 units, dispersed in inert propellant/Container (aerosol spray) 85 Gm. Approximate spraying time 100 seconds.
Use: Anti-infective, external.
POLYSULFIDES. Polythionate.
POLYTABS-F CHEWABLE VITAMIN. (Major) Fluoride 1 mg, vitamins A 2500 IU, D 400 IU, E 15 mg, B_1 1.05 mg, B_2 1.2 mg, B_3 13.5 mg, B_6 1.05 mg, B_{12} 4.5 mcg, C 60 mg, folic acid 0.3 mg/Tab. Bot. 100s, 1000s.
Use: Vitamin/mineral supplement.
POLYTAR BATH. (Stiefel) A 25% polytar blend of four different vegetable and mineral tars in an emulsion base. Bot. 8 fl oz.
Use: Tar-containing bath dermatological.
POLYTAR SHAMPOO. (Stiefel) A neutral soap containing 1% Polytar in a surfactant shampoo. Buffered. Plastic Bot. 6 fl oz, 12 fl oz, gal.
Use: Antiseborrheic.
POLYTAR SOAP. (Stiefel) A neutral soap containing 1% Polytar. Cake 4 oz.
Use: Tar-containing preparation.
POLYTEF. (Ethicon) Poly(tetrafluoroethylene). PTFE.
Use: Prosthetic aid.
•**POLYTHIAZIDE,** U.S.P. XXII. Tab., U.S.P. XXII. 2-Methyl-3,4-dihydro-3,(2,2,2-Trifluoroethylthiomethyl)-6- chloro-7-sulfamyl-1,2,4-benzothiadiazine, 1,1-dioxide. 6-Chloro-3,4-dihydro-2-methyl-3-[[(2,2,2,-trifluoro- ethyl)thio]-methyl]-2H-1,2,4-Benzothiadiazine-7- sulfonamide 1,1-dioxide.
Use: Diuretic; antihypertensive.
See: Renese Tab. (Pfizer Laboratories).
W/Prazosin.
See: Minizide, Cap. (Pfizer Laboratories).
W/Reserpine.

See: Renese-R, Tab. (Pfizer Laboratories).

POLYTINIC. (Pharmics) Elemental iron 100 mg, vitamin C 300 mg, folic acid 1 mg/tab. Bot. 100s.
Use: Vitamin/mineral supplement.

POLYTUSS-DM. (Rhode) Dextromethorphan HBr 15 mg, chlorpheniramine maleate 1 mg, guaifenesin 25 mg/5 ml. Bot. 4 oz, 8 oz.
Use: Antitussive, antihistamine, expectorant.

•**POLYURETHANE FOAM.** USAN.
Use: Prosthetic aid.

POLYVIDONE.
See: Polyvinylpyrrolidone.

POLY-VI-FLOR 0.5 mg CHEWABLE TABS. (Mead Johnson Nutrition) Vitamins A 2500 IU, D 400 IU, E 15 IU, C 60 mg, B_1 1.05 mg, B_2 1.2 mg, niacin 13.5 mg, B_6 1.05 mg, B_{12} 4.5 mcg, fluoride 0.5 mg, folic acid 0.3 mg/Chew. tab. Bot. 100s. **With Iron:** Above formula plus iron 12 mg, copper 1 mg, zinc 10 mg/Tab. Bot. 100s.
Use: Vitamin/mineral supplement, dental caries preventative.

POLY-VI-FLOR 1 mg CHEWABLE TABLETS. (Mead Johnson Nutrition) Vitamins A 2500 IU, D 400 IU, E 15 IU, C 60 mg, B_1 1.05 mg, B_2 1.2 mg, niacin 13.5 mg, B_6 1.05 mg, B_{12} 4.5 mcg, fluoride 1 mg, folic acid 0.3 mg/Chew. tab. Bot. 100s, 1000s. **With Iron:** Above formula plus iron 12 mg, copper 1 mg, zinc 10 mg/Tab.
Use: Vitamin/mineral supplement, dental caries preventative.

POLY-VI-FLOR 0.25 mg DROPS. (Mead Johnson Nutrition) Vitamins A 1500 IU, D 400 IU, E 5 IU, C 35 mg, B_1 0.5 mg, B_2 0.6 mg, B_6 0.4 mg, niacin 8 mg, B_{12} 2 mcg, fluoride 0.25 mg/ml. Dropper bot. 50 ml.
Use: Vitamin/mineral supplement, dental caries preventative.

POLY-VI-FLOR 0.5 mg DROPS. (Mead Johnson Nutrition) Vitamins A 1500 IU, D 400 IU, E 5 IU, C 35 mg, B_1 0.5 mg, B_2 0.6 mg, B_6 0.4 mg, niacin 8 mg, B_{12} 2 mcg, fluoride 0.5 mg/ml. Dropper bot. 30 ml, 50 ml.
Use: Vitamin/mineral supplement, dental caries preventative.

POLY-VI-FLOR 0.25 mg w/IRON DROPS. (Mead Johnson Nutrition) Vitamins A 1500 IU, D 400 IU, E 5 IU, C 35 mg, B_1 0.5 mg, B_2 0.6 mg, B_6 0.4 mg, niacin 8 mg, fluoride 0.25 mg, iron 10 mg/ml. Bot. 50 ml.
Use: Vitamin/mineral supplement, dental caries preventative.

POLY-VI-FLOR 0.5 mg W/IRON DROPS. (Mead Johnson Nutrition) Vitamins A 1500 IU, D 400 IU, E 5 IU, C 35 mg, B_1 0.5 mg, B_2 0.6 mg, B_6 0.4 mg, niacin 8 mg, fluoride 0.5 mg, iron 10 mg/ml. Dropper bot. 50 ml.
Use: Vitamin/mineral supplement, dental caries preventative.

POLYVINOX. B.A.N. Poly(butyl vinyl ether). Shostakovsky Balsam.
Use: Skin application.

•**POLYVINYL ACETATE PHTHALATE,** N.F. XVII.
Use: Pharmaceutic aid (coating agent).

•**POLYVINYL ALCOHOL,** U.S.P. XXII. Ethanol, homopolymer.
Use: Viscosity-increasing agent; pharmaceutic necessity for ophthalmic solution dosage form.
See: Liquifilm Forte (Allergan).
Liquifilm Tears (Allergan).
W/Hydroxypropyl methylcellulose.
See: Liquifilm Wetting Soln. (Allergan).

POLYVINYLPYRROLIDONE, POLYVIDONE, POVIDONE.
W/Acetrizoate Sodium
See: Salpix, Vial (Ortho).

POLYVINYLPYRROLIDONE VINYLACETATE COPOLYMERS.
See: Ivy-Rid, Spray (Mallard).
W/Benzalkonium.
See: Ivy-Chex, Aerosol (Bowman).

POLY-VI-SOL CHEWABLE TABS. (Mead Johnson Nutrition) Vitamins A 2500 IU, E 15 IU, D 400 IU, C 60 mg, B_1 1.05 mg, B_2 1.2 mg, niacin 13.5 mg, B_6 1.05 mg, B_{12} 4.5 mcg, folic acid 0.3 mg/Chew. tab. Bot. 100s. Circus Shape Tab. Bot. 100s. **With Iron:** Above formula plus iron 12 mg, zinc 8 mg/Tab. Bot. 100s. Circus shape Tab. Bot. 100s.
Use: Vitamin/mineral supplement.

POLY-VI-SOL DROPS. (Mead Johnson Nutrition) Vitamins A 1500 IU, D 400 IU, C 35 mg, B_1 0.5 mg, B_2 0.6 mg, E 5 IU, B_6 0.4 mg, niacin 8 mg, B_{12} 2 mcg/ml. Bot. 30 ml, 50 ml with calibrated "Safti-Dropper."
Use: Vitamin supplement.

POLY-VI-SOL W/IRON DROPS. (Mead Johnson Nutrition) Vitamins A 1500 IU, D 400 IU, E 5 IU, C 35 mg, B_1 0.5 mg, B_2 0.6 mg, B_6 0.4 mg, niacin 8 mg, iron 10 mg/ml. Bot. 50 ml.
Use: Vitamin/mineral supplement.

POLY-VI-SOL W/MINERALS. (Mead Johnson Nutritional) Iron 12 mg, vitamins A 2500 IU, D 400 IU, E 15 mg, B_1 1.05 mg, B_2 1.2 mg, B_3 13.5 mg, B_6 1.06 mg, B_{12} 4.5 mcg, C 60 mg, folic acid 0.3 mg, Cu, zinc 8 mg/Chew. tab. Bot. 60s, 100s.
Use: Vitamin/mineral supplement.

POLYVITAMINS.
See: Vitamin preparations.

POLY-VITAMINS W/FLUORIDE. (Various Mfr.) **Tab.:** Fluoride 0.5 mg, vitamins A 2500 IU, D 400 IU, E 15 mg, B_1 1 mg, B_2 1.2 mg, B_3 13.5 mg, B_6 1 mg, B_{12} 4.5 mcg, C 60 mg, folic acid 0.3 mg/Tab. Bot. 100s, 1000s.
Use: Vitamin/mineral supplement, dental caries preventative.

POLYVITAMIN WITH IRON. (Rugby) Iron 10 mg, vitamins A 1500 IU, D 400 IU, E 5 mg, B_1 0.5 mg, B_2 0.6 mg, B_3 8 mg, B_6 0.4 mg, C 35 mg/ml. Dropper bot. 50 ml.
Use: Vitamin/mineral supplement.

POLYVITAMIN W/IRON FLUORIDE. (Rugby) Fluoride 1 mg, vitamins A 2500 IU, D 400 IU, E 15 mg, B_1 1.05 mg, B_2 1.2 mg, B_3 13.5 mg, B_6 1.05 mg, B_{12} 4.5 mcg, C 60 mg, folic acid 0.3 mg, iron 12 mg/Tab. Bot. 100s, 1000s.
Use: Vitamin/mineral supplement, dental caries preventative.

POLYVITAMIN W/FLUORIDE. (Rugby) Fluoride 0.5 mg, vitamins A 1500 IU, D 400 IU, E 5 mg, B_1 0.5 mg, B_2 0.6 mg, B_3 8 mg, B_6 0.4 mg, B_{12} 2 mcg, C 35 mg/ml. Dropper bot. 50 ml.
Use: Vitamin/mineral supplement, dental caries preventative.

POLYVITE WITH FLOURIDE. (Geneva Generics) Flouride 0.25 mg, vitamins A 1500 IU, D 400 IU, E 5 mg, B_1 0.5 mg, B_2 0.6 mg, B_3 8 mg, B_6 0.4 mg, B_{12} 2 mcg, C 35 mg/ml. Dropper bot. 50 ml.
Use: Vitamin/mineral supplement, dental caries preventative.

•**PONALRESTAT.** USAN.
Use: Aldose reductase inhibitor.

PONARIS. (Jamol) Nasal emollient of mucosal lubricating and moisturizing botanical oils. Cajeput, eucalyptus, peppermint in iodized cottonseed oil. Bot. 1 oz w/dropper.
Use: Nasal moisturizer.

PONDIMIN. (Robins) Fenfluramine HCl 20 mg/Tab. Bot. 100s, 500s.
Use: Anorexiant.

PONSTEL KAPSEALS. (Parke-Davis) Mefenamic acid 250 mg/Cap. Bot. 100s.
Use: Nonsteroidal anti-inflammatory drug; analgesic.

PONTOCAINE 2% AQUEOUS SOLUTION. (Winthrop Pharm) Tetracaine HCl 20 mg, chlorobutanol 4 mg/ml of 2% soln. Bot. 30 ml, Box 12s. Bot. 118 ml, Box 6s.
Use: Local anesthetic.

PONTOCAINE CREAM. (Winthrop Pharm) Tetracaine HCl, equivalent to 1% tetracaine HCl base, in a bland, water-miscible cream with methylparaben and sodium metabisulfite as preservatives. Tube 1 oz. Pkg. 6s.
Use: Local anesthetic.

PONTOCAINE EYE OINTMENT. (Winthrop Pharm) Tetracaine 0.5% in a base of white petrolatum and light mineral oil. Tube 1/8 oz. Pkg. 12s.
Use: Local anesthetic.

PONTOCAINE HYDROCHLORIDE. (Winthrop Pharm) Niphanoid (instantly soluble) form consisting of a network of extremely fine, highly purified particles, resembling snow. Amp. 20 mg, Box 100s. 1% isotonic, isobaric solution: Tetracaine HCl 10 mg, sodium Cl 6.7 mg, acetone sodium bisulfite not more than 2 mg/ml. Amp. 2 ml, Box 25s.
Use: Local anesthetic.

PONTOCAINE HYDROCHLORIDE IN DEXTROSE (Hyperbaric) SOLUTIONS. (Winthrop Pharm) **0.2%:** Tetracaine HCl 2 mg/ml in a sterile solution containing dextrose 6%. Amp. 2 ml, 10s. **0.3%:** Tetracaine HCl 3 mg/ml in a sterile solution containing dextrose 6%. Amp. 5 ml, 10s.
Use: Local anesthetic.

PONTOCAINE OINTMENT. (Winthrop Pharm) Tetracaine 0.5% and menthol in an ointment consisting of white petrolatum and white wax. Tube 1 oz.
Use: Local anesthetic.

PONTOCAINE 0.5% SOLUTION FOR OPHTHALMOLOGY. (Winthrop Pharm) Tetracaine HCl 5 mg, sodium Cl 7.5 mg, chlorobutanol 4 mg/ml of 0.5% solution. Bot. 15 ml, Pkg. 12s. Bot. 59 ml, Pkg. 6s.
Use: Local anesthetic.

PO-PON-S. (Shionogi) Vitamins A 2000 IU, D 100 IU, E 5 mg, B_1 5 mg, B_2 3 mg, B_3 35 mg, B_5 15 mg, B_6 4 mg, B_{12} 6 mcg, C 100 mg, Ca, P/Tab. Bot. 60s, 240s.
Use: Vitamin/mineral supplement.

POPPY-SEED OIL, The ethyl ester of the fatty acids of the poppy w/iodine.
See: Lipiodol, Ascendant & Lafay, Amps., Vial (Savage).

PORCELANA SKIN BLEACHING AGENT. (Jeffrey Martin) **Regular:** Hydroquinone 2%. Jar 2 oz, 4 oz. **Sunscreen:** Hydroquinone 2%, octyl dimethyl PABA 2.5%. Jar 4 oz.
Use: Skin bleaching agent.

•**PORFIMER SODIUM.** USAN.
Use: Antineoplastic.

•**PORFIROMYCIN.** USAN.
Use: Antibacterial; antineoplastic.

PORK THYROID, DEFATTED.
See: Tuloidin, Tab. (Solvay).

•**POROFOCON A.** USAN.
Use: Contact lens material.

•**POROFOCON B.** USAN.
Use: Cabcurve lens (soft lenses).

PORTABIDAY. (Washington Ethical) Concentrated soln. of alkylamine lauryl sulfate, a mild detergent with pH approx. 6 for use with Portabiday Vaginal Cleansing Kit. Bot. 3 oz.
Use: Vaginal preparation.

PORTAGEN. (Mead Johnson Nutrition) A nutritionally complete dietary powder containing as a % of the calories protein 14% as caseinate, fat 41% (medium chain triglycerides 86%, corn oil 14%), carbohydrate 45% as corn syrup solids and sucrose, vitamins A 5000 IU, D 500 IU, E 20 IU, C 52 mg, B_1 1 mg, B_2 1.2 mg, B_6 1.4 mg, B_{12} 4 mcg, niacin 13 mg, folic acid 0.1 mg, choline 83 mg, biotin 0.05 mg, calcium 600 mg, phosphorus 450 mg, magnesium 133 mg, iron 12 mg, iodine 47 mcg, copper 1 mg, zinc 6 mg, manganese 0.8 mg, chloride 550 mg, sodium 300 mg, potassium 800 mg, pantothenic acid 6.7 mg, K-1 0.1 mg/Qt. 20 Kcal/fl oz. Can 1 lb.
Use: Enteral nutritional supplement.

POSITIVE AND NEGATIVE HCG URINE CONTROLS. (Wampole) Positive and negative hu-

man urine controls for Wampole urine pregnancy tests. 1 set, 1 vial each.
Use: Diagnostic aid.

POSKINE. B.A.N. O-Propionylhyoscine. Proscopine hydrobromide.
Use: Central nervous system depressant.

POSLAM PSORIASIS OINTMENT. (Last) Sulfur 5%, salicylic acid 2%. Jar 1 oz.
Use: Antipsoriatic.

POSTAFENE.
See: Bonamine, Tab. (Pfizer).

•**POSTERIOR PITUITARY INJECTION,** U.S.P. XXII.
Use: Hormone (antidiuretic).

POSTLOBIN-O.
See: Pituitary, Posterior, Hormone (b).

POSTLOBIN-V.
See: Pituitary, Posterior, Hormone (a).

POSTURE. (Wyeth-Ayerst) Calcium phosphate 300 mg or 600 mg/Tab. Bot. 60s.
Use: Calcium supplement.

POSTURE-D 300. (Wyeth-Ayerst) Calcium phosphate 300 mg, vitamin D 62.5 IU/Tab. Bot. 100s.
Use: Calcium/vitamin D supplement.

POSTURE D 600. (Wyeth-Ayerst) Calcium phosphate 600 mg, vitamin D 125 IU/Tab. Bot. 60s.
Use: Calcium/vitamin D supplement.

POTABA. (Glenwood) Potassium p-aminobenzoate. **Cap.:** 0.5 Gm. Bot. 250s, 1000s. **Pow.:** 100 Gm. 1 lb. **Tab.:** 0.5 Gm. Bot. 100s, 1000s. **Envule:** 2 Gm. Box 50s.
Use: Para-aminobenzoic acid supplement.

POTABLE-AQUA IODINE. (Wisconsin) Tab. Bot. 50s.
Use: Water purification.

POTABLE AQUA KIT. (Wisconsin) Tab. Bot. 50s with collapsible gallon container.
Use: Water purification.

POTACHLOR 10%. (My-K Labs) Potassium and chloride 20 mEq/15 ml. With alcohol 5% Bot. pt, gal. With alcohol 3.8% Bot. pt, gal, UD 15 ml and 30 ml.
Use: Potassium supplement.

POTACHLOR 20%. (My-K Labs) Potassium and chloride 40 mEq/15 ml, alcohol free. Liq. Bot. pt, gal.
Use: Potassium supplement.

POTASALAN ELIXIR. (Lannett) Potassium Cl 10%, alcohol 4%. Bot. pt, gal.
Use: Potassium supplement.

•**POTASH, SULFURATED,** U.S.P. XXII.
Use: Pharmaceutical aid (source of sulfide).

POTASSIC SALINE LACTATED INJECTION.
Use: Fluid and electrolyte replenisher.

•**POTASSIUM ACETATE,** U.S.P. XXII. Inj., U.S.P. XXII. Acetic acid, potassium salt. (Various Mfr.) **Inj.:** (Abbott) 40 mEq, 20 ml in 50 ml Vial.
Use: Electrolyte replenisher; to avoid Cl when high concentration of potassium is needed.

POTASSIUM ACID PHOSPHATE.
See: K-Phos, Tab. (Beach).
Uro-K, Tab. (Star).

POTASSIUM p-AMINOBENZOATE.
See: Potaba, Preps. (Glenwood).
W/Potassium salicylate.
See: Pabalate-SF, Tab. (Robins).
W/Pyridoxine.
See: Potaba Plus 6, Cap., Tab. (Glenwood).

POTASSIUM p-AMINOSALICYLATE.
See: Paskalium, Preps. (Glenwood).

•**POTASSIUM ASPARTATE AND MAGNESIUM ASPARTATE.** USAN.
Use: Nutrient.

•**POTASSIUM BENZOATE,** N.F. XVII.
Use: Preservative.

•**POTASSIUM BICARBONATE,** U.S.P. XXII.
Use: Electrolyte replenisher.

•**POTASSIUM BICARBONATE EFFERVESCENT TABLETS FOR ORAL SOLUTION,** U.S.P. XXII.
Use: Potassium supplement.

•**POTASSIUM BICARBONATE AND POTASSIUM CHLORIDE FOR EFFERVESCENT ORAL SOLUTION,** U.S.P. XXII.
Use: Potassium supplement.

•**POTASSIUM BICARBONATE AND POTASSIUM CHLORIDE FOR EFFERVESCENT ORAL SOLUTION,** U.S.P. XXII.
Use: Potassium supplement.

•**POTASSIUM BICARBONATE AND POTASSIUM CHLORIDE EFFERVESCENT TABLETS FOR ORAL SOLUTION,** U.S.P. XXII.
Use: Potassium supplement.

•**POTASSIUM BICARBONATE AND SODIUM BICARBONATE AND CITRIC ACID EFFERVESCENT TABLETS FOR ORAL SOLUTION,** U.S.P. XXII.
Use: Potassium supplement.

POTASSIUM BITARTRATE.
Use: Cathartic.

POTASSIUM BROMIDE.
W/Aspirin, caffeine, sodium bromide.
See: Lanabac, Tab. (Lannett).
W/Sodium bromide, strontium bromide, ammonium bromide.
See: Lanabrom, Elix. (Lannett).

•**POTASSIUM CARBONATE,** U.S.P. XXII.
Use: Potassium therapy.

•**POTASSIUM CHLORIDE,** U.S.P. XXII. Extended-Release Cap., Extended-Release Tab., In Dextrose Inj., Inj., Oral Soln., For Oral Soln., U.S.P. XXII. Elixir, U.S.P. XXI.
Use: Potassium deficiency, hypopotassemia.
Ampules:
(Abbott) **Ampules:** 20 mEq, 10 ml; 40 mEq, 20 ml. **Pintop Vials:** 10 mEq, 5 ml in 10 ml; 20 mEq, 10 ml in 20 ml; 30 mEq, 12.5 ml in 30 ml; 40 mEq, 12.5 ml in 30 ml. **Fliptop Vials:** 20 mEq, 10 ml in 20 ml; 40 mEq, 20 ml in 50 ml. **Univ. Add. Syr.:** 5 mEq/5 ml, 20 mEq/10 ml, 30 mEq/20 ml, 40 mEq/20 ml (Lilly) Amp. (40 mEq) 20 ml, 6s, 25s.
Capsules:

See: K-Norm, Cap. (Pennwalt).
Micro-K Extencaps, Cap. (Robins).
Liquid:
See: Cena-K, Liq. (Century).
Choice 10 and 20, Soln. (Whiteworth).
Kaochlor, Preps. (Adria).
Kaon-C1 20%, Liq. (Adria).
Kay Ciel, Elix. (Berlex).
Klor-Con, Liq. (Upsher-Smith).
Kloride, Elix. (Fed. Pharm.).
Klorvess, Liq. (Dorsey).
Klotrix, Tab. (Mead Johnson).
Klowess (Dorsey).
K-Lyte/C1, Tab. (Bristol).
Pan-Kloride, Liq. (U.S. Products).
Potassine, Liq. (Recsei).
Taside, Liq. (Solvay).
Powder:
See: Kaochlor-Eff, Gran. (Adria).
Kato, Pow. (Ingram).
Kay Ciel, Pow. (Berlex).
K-Lor, Pow. (Abbott).
K-Lyte/C1, Pow. (Bristol).
Potage, Pow. (Lemmon).
Tablets:
See: Kaon, Tab. (Adria).
Kaon Controlled Release Tab. (Adria).
Klorvess Effervescent Tab. (Dorsey).
K-Lyte/Cl 50, Tab. (Bristol).
K-Tab, Tab. (Abbott).
Micro-K Extencap (Robins).
Slow-K, Tab. (Ciba).
Ten-K, Cap. (Geigy).

POTASSIUM CHLORIDE. (Roxane) **Oral soln.:** Potassium Cl, sugar free. 40 mEq/30 ml. Bot. 6 oz, 500 ml, 1 L, 5 L 20%. 80 mEq/30 ml. Bot. 500 ml, 1 L, 5 L. **Pow.:** 20 mEq/4 Gm. Pkt. 30s, 100s.
Use: Potassium supplement.

•**POTASSIUM CHLORIDE IN DEXTROSE AND SODIUM CHLORIDE INJECTION,** U.S.P. XXII.

•**POTASSIUM CHLORIDE IN SODIUM CHLORIDE INJECTION,** U.S.P. XXII.

•**POTASSIUM CHLORIDE K 42.** USAN.
Use: Radioactive agent.

POTASSIUM CHLORIDE WITH POTASSIUM GLUCONATE.
See: Kolyum, Prods. (Pennwalt).

•**POTASSIUM CHLORIDE, POTASSIUM BICARBONATE, AND POTASSIUM CITRATE EFFERVESCENT TABLETS FOR ORAL SOLUTION,** U.S.P. XXII.

POTASSIUM CHLORIDE SOLUTION, (Lederle) Potassium Cl 10% or 20%. Sugar free. Bot. 16 oz, gal.
Use: Potassium supplement.

•**POTASSIUM CITRATE,** U.S.P. XXII. Tripotassium Citrate.
Use: Systemic alkalizer.
W/Sodium citrate.
See: Bicitra, Liq. (Willen).
W/Sodium citrate, citric acid.
See: Polycitra-K, Liq. (Willen).
Polycitra-LC, Liq.(Willen).

•**POTASSIUM CITRATE AND CITRIC ACID ORAL SOLUTION,** U.S.P. XXII.

POTASSIUM CLAVULANATE/AMOXICILLIN.
Use: Antibacterial, penicillin.
See: Amoxicillin and Potassium Clavulanate.

POTASSIUM CLAVULANATE/TICARCILLIN.
Use: Antibacterial, penicillin.
See: Ticarcillin and Clavulanate Potassium.

POTASSIUM ESTRONE SULFATE.
W/Estrone.
See: Dura-Keelin, Vial (Pharmex).
Estro Plus, Inj. (Rocky Mtn.).
W/Estrone, estradiol.
See: Tri-Oraphn (Standex).
W/Micro crystalline estrone.
See: Estrones Duo-Action, Vial (Med. Chem.).

•**POTASSIUM GLUCALDRATE.** USAN.
Use: Antacid.

•**POTASSIUM GLUCONATE,** U.S.P. XXII. Elixir, Tab., U.S.P. XXII. Monopotassium D-gluconate.
Use: Electrolyte replenisher.
See: Kalinate, Elix. (Bock).
Kaon, Elixir, Tab. (Warren-Teed).

•**POTASSIUM GLUCONATE AND POTASSIUM CHLORIDE ORAL SOLUTION,** U.S.P. XXII.
Use: Replacement therapy.

•**POTASSIUM GLUCONATE AND POTASSIUM CHLORIDE FOR ORAL SOLUTION,** U.S.P. XXII.
Use: Replacement therapy.

POTASSIUM GLUCONATE ELIXIR. (Mills) Elemental potassium as potassium gluconate 20 mEq, base w/sorbitol soln./Tab. Bot. 8 oz.
Use: Potassium supplement.

POTASSIUM GLUCONATE ELIXIR. (Various Mfr.) Potassium 40 mEq provided by potassium gluconate 9.36 Gm/30 ml, alcohol 5%. Bot. pt, Patient-Cup 15 ml.
Use: Potassium supplement.

•**POTASSIUM GLUCONATE, POTASSIUM CITRATE, AND AMMONIUM CHLORIDE ORAL SOLUTION,** U.S.P. XXII.
Use: Replacement therapy.

•**POTASSIUM GLUCONATE AND POTASSIUM CITRATE ORAL SOLUTION,** U.S.P. XXII.
Use: Replacement therapy.

POTASSIUM GLUTAMATE. The monopotassium salt of l-glutamic acid.

POTASSIUM G PENICILLIN.
See: Penicillin G Potassium, U.S.P. XXII.

•**POTASSIUM GUAIACOLSULFONATE,** U.S.P. XXII. Sulfoguaiacol. Potassium Hydroxymethoxybenzenesulfonate. Used in many cough preps.
Use: Expectorant.
See: Conex, Liq. (Westerfield).
Pinex Regular, Syr. (Pinex).

POTASSIUM GUAIACOLSULFONATE W/COMBINATIONS.
See: Cheralin, Syr. (Lannett).
Cherralex, Syr. (Barre).

Efricon Expectorant (Lannett).
Eucapine, Syr. (Lannett).
Formadrin, Liq. (Kenyon).
Guahist, Vial (Hickam).
Guaicohist, Vial (Pharmex).
Guaiodol-Plus, Vial (Kenyon).
Partuss, Liq. (Parmed).
Proclan, Preps. (Cenci).
Tusquelin, Syr. (Circle).

POTASSIUM HETACILLIN.
See: Versapen K, Inj., Cap. (Bristol).

•**POTASSIUM HYDROXIDE,** N.F. XVII.
Use: Pharmaceutical aid (alkalinizing agent).

•**POTASSIUM IODIDE,** U.S.P. XXII. Tab., Oral Soln., U.S.P. XXII.
Use: Expectorant; antifungal; source of iodine.
See: Pima, Syr., Expectorant (Fleming).
SSKI, Liq. (Upsher-Smith).

POTASSIUM IODIDE W/COMBINATIONS
See: Diastix, Reagent Strips (Ames).
Elixophyllin-KI, Elix. (Berlex).
Iodo-Niacin, Tab. (Cole).
KIE, Syr., Tab. (Laser).
Mudrane, Tab. (Poythress).
Mudrane-2, Tab. (Poythress).
Quadrinal, Tab., Susp. (Knoll).

POTASSIUM IODIDE AND NIACINAMIDE.
See: Iodo-Niacin, Tab. (Cole).

POTASSIUM MENAPHTHOSULPHATE. B.A.N. Dipotassium 2-methyl-1,4-disulpnatonaphthalene. Vikastab [dihydrate]
Use: Vitamin K analogue.

•**POTASSIUM METABISULFITE,** N.F. XVII.

•**POTASSIUM METAPHOSPHATE,** N.F. XVII.
Use: Buffering agent.

POTASSIUM PENICILLIN G .
Use: Antibiotic.
See: Penicillin G, Potassium U.S.P. XXII.

POTASSIUM PENICILLIN V.
Use: Antibiotic.
See: Phenoxymethyl Penicillin Potassium, U.S.P. XXII.

•**POTASSIUM PERMANGANATE,** U.S.P. XXII. Tab. for Topical Soln., U.S.P. XXI. Permanganic acid, potassium salt.
Use: Topical anti-infective.

POTASSIUM PHENETHICILLIN. Phenethicillin Potassium, U.S.P. XXII.
Use: Antibiotic.

POTASSIUM PHENOXYMETHYL PENICILLIN.
Use: Antibiotic.
See: Penicillin V Potassium, U.S.P. XXII.

•**POTASSIUM PHOSPHATE, DIBASIC,** U.S.P. XXII. Inj., U.S.P. XXII.
Use: Calcium regulator.

•**POTASSIUM PHOSPHATE, MONOBASIC,** N.F. XVII. Dipotassium hydrogen phosphate. Solution by Various Mfr. **Inj.:** (Abbott) 15 mM, 5 ml in 10 ml Vial; 45 mM, 15 ml in 20 ml Vial.
Use: Buffering agent, source of potassium.

POTASSIUM REAGENT STRIPS. (Ames) Quantitative dry reagent strip test for potassium In serum or plasma. Bot. 50s.
Use: Diagnostic aid.

POTASSIUM-REMOVING RESINS.
See: Kayexalate, Pow. (Winthrop Pharm).

POTASSIUM RHODANATE.
See: Potassium Thiocyanate.

POTASSIUM SALICYLATE.
See: Neocylate, Tab. (Central).
W/Mephenesin, colchicine alkaloid.
W/Potassium bromide, methapyrilene HCl, vitamins.
See: Alva-Tranquil, Cap., Tab., T.D. Tab. (Alva/Amco).
W/Potassium p-aminobenzoate.
See: Pabalate-SF, Tab. (Robins).

POTASSIUM SALT.
See: Potassium Sorbate, N.F. XVII.

•**POTASSIUM SODIUM TARTRATE,** U.S.P. XXII.
Use: Cathartic.

•**POTASSIUM SORBATE,** N.F. XVII. 2,4-Hexadienoic Acid, Potassium Salt.
Use: Preservative (antimicrobial).

POTASSIUM SULFOCYANATE. Potassium Rhodanate.
See: Potassium Thiocyanate (Various Mfr.).

POTASSIUM THERAPY.
See: Kaon, Elix., Tab. (Warren-Teed).
Potassium Chloride, Preps. (Various Mfr.).
Slow-K, Tab. (Ciba).
Ten-K, Cap. (Geigy).

POTASSIUM THIOCYANATE. Potassium sulfocyanate, Potassium Rhodanate.

POTASSIUM THIPHENCILLIN. Potassium 6-(phenylmercaptoacetamido)penicillanate.
Use: Anti-infective.

POTASSIUM TROCLOSENE. (Monsanto) Potassium dichloroisocyanurate. Dichloro-s-triazine-2,4,6(1H,3H,5H)trione Potassium derivative.
Use: Anti-infective.

•**POVIDONE,** U.S.P. XXII. 2-Pyrrolidinone, 1-ethyl, homopolymer.
Use: Dispersing and suspending agent.

•**POVIDONE I-125.** USAN.
Use: Radioactive agent.

•**POVIDONE I-131.** USAN.
Use: Radioactive agent.

•**POVIDONE-IODINE,** U.S.P. XXII., Topical Aerosol Soln., Oint., Cleansing Soln., Topical Soln., U.S.P. XXII. Poly(1-(2-oxo-1-pyrrolidinyl)-ethylene) Iodine Complex.
Use: Local anti-infective.
See: Betadine, Preps. (Purdue-Fredrick).
BPS, Preps. (AVP).
Efo-Dine (Fougera).
Femidine, Liq. (AVP).
Isodine, Preps. (Blair).

POVIDONE-IODINE COMPLEX.
See: Betadine, Preps. (Purdue-Frederick).
Isodine, Preps. (Blair).

POYALIVER STRONGER. (Forest Pharm.) Liver inj. (equivalent to 10 mcg B_{12}), vitamin B_{12} 100 mcg, folic acid 10 mcg, niacinamide 1%/ml. Vial 10 ml.
Use: Parenteral nutritional supplement.

POYAMIN. (Fellows) Vitamin B_{12} 1000 mcg/ml. Vial 10 ml, 30 ml.
Use: Parenteral nutritional supplement.

POYAMIN JEL INJECTION. (Forest Pharm.) Cyanocobalamin 1000 mcg/ml. Vial 10 ml.
Use: Parenteral nutritional supplement.

POYAPLEX. (Forest Pharm.) Vitamins B_1 100 mg, niacinamide 100 mg, B_6 10 mg, B_2 1 mg, panthenol 10 mg, B_{12} 5 mcg/ml. Vial 10 ml, 30 ml.
Use: Parenteral nutritional supplement.

P.P.D. TUBERCULIN.
See: Tuberculin, Purified Protein Derivative, U.S.P. (Various Mfr.).

P.P. FACTOR (PELLAGRA PREVENTIVE FACTOR).
See: Nicotinic Acid, Preps. (Various Mfr.).

•**PPG-15 STEARYL ETHER.** USAN.
Use: Pharmaceutic aid (surfactant).

•**PRACTOLOL.** USAN. 4′-[2-Hydroxy-3-(iso- propylamino)propoxy]acetanilide.
Use: Antiadrenergic (β-receptors).

PRAJMALIUM BITARTRATE. B.A.N. N-Propylajmalinium hydrogen tartrate.
Use: Treatment of heart arrhythmias.

PRALIDOXIME. B.A.N. 2-Hydroxyiminomethyl-1-methylpyridinium.
Use: Antagonist to cholinesterase inhibitors.

•**PRALIDOXIME CHLORIDE,** U.S.P. XXII. Sterile, Tabs: U.S.P. XXII. Pyridinium, 2-[(hydroxyimino)methyl]-1-methyl-,chloride. 2-Formyl-1-methylpyridinium Chloride Oxime. Pam.
Use: Cholinesterase reactivator.
See: Protopam Chloride, Tab., Vial (Wyeth-Ayerst).

•**PRALIDOXIME IODIDE.** USAN. 2-Pyridine aldoxime methiodide.
Use: Cholinesterase reactivator.
See: Protopam Iodide (Wyeth-Ayerst).

•**PRALIDOXIME MESYLATE.** USAN.
Use: Cholinesterase reactivator.

PRALIDOXIME METHIODIDE.
See: Pralidoxime Iodide (Various Mfr.).

PRAMEGEL ANTIPRURITIC GEL. (GenDerm) Pramoxine HCl 1%, menthol 0.5% in base w/ benzyl alcohol. Bot. 4 oz.
Use: Local anesthetic.

PRAMET FA. (Ross) Vitamins A 4000 IU, D-2 400 IU, C 100 mg, B_1 3 mg, B_2 2 mg, B_6 5 mg, B_{12} 3 mcg, niacinamide 10 mg, calcium pantothenate 0.92 mg, iodine 100 mcg, calcium 250 mg, copper 0.15 mg, iron 60 mg, folic acid 1 mg/Gradumet. Bot. 100s.
Use: Vitamin/mineral supplement.

PRAMILET FA. (Ross) Vitamins A 4000 IU, B_1 3 mg, B_2 2 mg, B_6 3 mg, B_{12} 3 mcg, C 60 mg, D 400 IU, calcium panthothenate 1 mg, niacinamide 10 mg, calcium 250 mg, copper 0.15 mg, iodine 0.1 mg, iron 40 mg, magnesium 10 mg, zinc 0.085 mg, folic acid 1 mg/Filmtab. Bot. 100s.
Use: Vitamin/mineral supplement.

PRAMIVERINE. B.A.N. 4,4-Diphenyl-N-isopropylcyclohexylamine.
Use: Spasmolytic.

PRAMOCAINE (I.N.N.). Pramoxine, B.A.N.
Use: Allergic dermatitis.

PRAMOSONE CREAM 0.5%. (Ferndale) Hydrocortisone acetate 0.5%, pramoxine HCl 1% in cream base. Tube 1 oz, 4 oz. Jar 4 oz, lb.
Use: Corticosteroid, local anesthetic.

PRAMOSONE CREAM 1%. (Ferndale) Hydrocortisone acetate 1%, pramoxine HCl 1% in cream base. Tube 1 oz, 4 oz. Jar 4 oz, lb.
Use: Corticosteroid, local anesthetic.

PRAMOSONE CREAM 2.5%. (Ferndale) Hydrocortisone acetate 2.5%, pramoxine HCl 1% in cream base. Tube 1 oz, 4 oz. Jar lb.
Use: Corticosteroid, local anesthetic.

PRAMOSONE LOTION 0.5%. (Ferndale) Hydrocortisone acetate 0.5%, pramoxine HCl 1% in lotion base. Bot. 1 oz, 4 oz, 8 oz.
Use: Corticosteroid, local anesthetic.

PRAMOSONE LOTION 1%. (Ferndale) Hydrocortisone acetate 1%, pramoxine HCl 1% in lotion base. Bot. 2 oz, 4 oz, 8 oz.
Use: Corticosteroid, local anesthetic.

PRAMOSONE LOTION 2.5%. (Ferndale) Hydrocortisone acetate 2.5%, pramoxine HCl 1% in lotion base. Bot 2 oz, gal.
Use: Corticosteroid, local anesthetic.

PRAMOSONE OINTMENT 1%. (Ferndale) Hydrocortisone acetate 1%, pramoxine HCl 1% in ointment base. Tube 1 oz, 4 oz. Jar 4 oz, lb.
Use: Corticosteroid, local anesthetic.

PRAMOXINE. B.A.N. 4-[3-(4-Butoxyphenoxy)-propyl]morpholine. Pramocaine (I.N.N.).
Use: Local anesthetic.

•**PRAMOXINE HYDROCHLORIDE,** U.S.P. XXII. Cream, Jelly, U.S.P. XXII. 4-[3-(p-Butoxyphenoxy)propyl]morpholine HCl.
Use: Local anesthetic.
See: Prax, Lot. (Ferndale).
Proctofoam, Aerosol (Reed & Carnrick).
Tronothane HCl, Cream, Jel (Abbott).

PRAMOXINE HCl W/COMBINATIONS
See: Anti-Itch, Lot. (Towne).
Dermarex, Cream (Hyrex).
Gentz, Jelly, Wipes (Philips Roxane).
1 + 1 Creme, 1 + 1-F Creme (Dunhall).
Otocalm-H Ear Drops (Parmed).
Perifoam, Aerosol (Rowell Labs.).
Proctofoam-HC, Aerosol (Reed-Carnrick).
Sherform-HC, Oint. (Sheryl).
Steraform Creme (Mayrand).
Steramine Otic, Drops (Mayrand).

PRAMPINE. B.A.N. O-Propionylatropine, PAMN methonitrate.
Use: Treatment of peptic ulcer.

•**PRANOLIUM CHLORIDE.** USAN.
Use: Cardiac depressant.

PRAX CREAM. (Ferndale) Pramoxine HCl 1% in cream base. Tube 1 oz. Jar 4 oz, lb.
Use: Local anesthetic.

PRAX LOTION. (Ferndale) Pramoxine HCl 1%. Bot. 15 ml, 120 ml.
Use: Local anesthetic.

•**PRAZEPAM,** U.S.P. XXII. Cap., Tab. U.S.P. XXII. 7-Chloro-1-(cyclopropylmethyl)-1,2-dihydro-5-phenyl-2H-1, 4-benzodiazepin-2-one.
Use: Muscle relaxant.
See: Centrax, Cap. (Parke-Davis).
Vestran, Cap. (Parke-Davis).

•**PRAZIQUANTEL,** U.S.P. XXII, Tab. 2-Cyclohexylcarbonyl-1,3,4,6,7,11b-hexahydro-2H-pyrazino[2,1-a]-isoquinolin-4-one.
Use: Anthelmintic.
See: Biltricide, Tab. (Miles Pharm).

PRAZITONE. B.A.N. 5-Phenyl-5-(2-piperidyl)-methylbarbituric acid.
Use: Antidepressant.

•**PRAZOSIN HYDROCHLORIDE,** U.S.P. XXII. Cap., U.S.P. XXII. 1-(4-Amino-6,7-dimethoxy-2-quinazoliny)-4-(2-furoyl)piperazine monohydrochloride.
Use: Antihypertensive.
See: Minipress, Cap. (Pfizer Laboratories).

PRE-17. (Standex) Vitamins A 4000 IU, D 400 IU, B_1 1.5 mg, B_2 2 mg, B_6 2 mg, B_{12} 2 mcg, C 50 mg, niacinamide 10 mg, calcium pantothenate 5 mg, folic acid 8 mg, iron 40 mg, calcium carbonate 240 mg/Tab. Bot. 100s.
Use: Vitamin/mineral supplement.

PRE-ATTAIN LIQUID. (Sherwood) Sodium caseinate, maltodextrin, corn oil, soy lecithin, vitamins A, B_1, B_2, B_3, B_5, B_6, B_{12}, C, D, E, K, folic acid, Ca, Cl, Cu, Fe, I, Mg, Mn, P, Zn. Can 250 ml, closed system 1000 ml.
Use: Enteral nutritional supplement.

PRECEF FOR INJECTION. (Bristol) Ceforanide 500 mg or 1 Gm/Vial or piggyback.
Use: Antibacterial, cephalosporin.

PRECISION HIGH NITROGEN DIET. (Sandoz Nutrition) Vanilla flavor: Maltodextrin, pasteurized egg white solids, sucrose, natural and artificial flavors, medium chain triglycerides, partially hydrogenated soybean oil, polysorbate 80, mono and diglycerides, vitamins, minerals. Pow. Packet 2.93 oz.
Use: Enteral nutritional supplement.

PRECISION ISOTONIC DIET. (Sandoz Nutrition) Vanilla flavor: Maltodextrin, egg white solids, sucrose, partially hydrogenated soybean oil with BHA, natural and artificial flavor, sodium caseinate, citric acid, carrageenan, mono and diglycerides, vitamins, minerals. Individual Packet 2.06 oz.
Use: Enteral nutritional supplement.

PRECISION LR DIET. (Sandoz Nutrition) Orange flavor: Maltodextrin,pasteurized egg white solids, sucrose, medium chain triglycerides, partially hydrogenated soybean oil with BHA, citric acid, natural and artificial flavors, mono and diglycerides, polysorbate 80, FD & C Yellow No. 5 and No. 6, vitamins, minerals. Pow. Packet 3 oz.
Use: Enteral nutritional supplement.

PRED-5. (Saron) Prednisone 5 mg/Tab. Bot. 100s, 1000s.
Use: Corticosteroid.

PREDAJECT. (Mayrand) Prednisolone acetate 50 mg/ml. Vial 10 ml.
Use: Corticosteroid.

PREDALONE 50. (Forest) Prednisolone acetate 50 mg/ml. Vial 10 ml.
Use: Corticosteroid.

PREDALONE T.B.A. (Forest) Prednisolone tebutate 20 mg/ml in aqueous suspension. Vial 10 ml.
Use: Corticosteroid.

PREDAMIDE OPHTHALMIC. (Maurry) Sodium sulfacetamide 10%, prednisolone acetate 0.5%, hydroxyethyl cellulose, polysorbate 80, sodium thiosulfate, benzalkonium Cl 0.025%. Bot. 5 ml, 15 ml.
Use: Anti-infective, corticosteroid, ophthalmic.

PREDCOR INJECTION. (Hauck) Prednisolone acetate 25 mg or 50 mg/ml. Vial 10 ml.
Use: Corticosteroid.

PRED-FORTE. (Allergan) Prednisolone acetate 1%, benzalkonium Cl polysorbate 80, boric acid, sodium citrate, sodium bisulfite, sodium Cl, edetate disodium, hydroxypropyl methylcellulose, purified water. Plastic dropper bot. 1 ml, 5 ml, 10 ml, 15 ml.
Use: Corticosteroid, ophthalmic.

PRED-G. (Allergan) Prednisolone acetate 1%, gentamicin sulfate 0.3%. Bot. 5 ml, 10 ml.
Use: Corticosteroid, anti-infective, ophthalmic.

PREDICORT-AP. (Dunhall) Prednisolone sodium phosphate 20 mg, prednisolone acetate 80 mg/ml. Vial 10 ml.
Use: Corticosteroid.

PREDICORT-RP. (Dunhall) Prednisolone sodium phosphate equivalent to prednisolone phosphate 20 mg, niacinamide 25 mg/ml. Vial 10 ml.
Use: Corticosteroid.

PRED MILD. (Allergan) Prednisolone acetate 0.12%, benzalkonium Cl, polysorbate 80, boric acid, sodium citrate, sodium bisulfite, sodium Cl, edetate disodium, hydroxypropyl methylcellulose, purified water. Bot. 5 ml, 10 ml.
Use: Corticosteroid, ophthalmic.

•**PREDNAZATE.** USAN.
Use: Anti-inflammatory.

•**PREDNICARBATE.** USAN.
Use: Glucocorticoid.

PREDNICEN-M. (Central) Prednisone 5 mg/Tab. Bot. 100s, 1000s.
Use: Corticosteroid.

•**PREDNIMUSTINE.** USAN.
Use: Antineoplastic.

PREDNISOLAMATE. B.A.N. Prednisolone 21-diethylaminoacetate. Deltacortril DA hydrochloride.
Use: Corticosteroid.

•**PREDNISOLONE,** U.S.P. XXII. Cream, Tab., U.S.P. XXII. Pregna-1,4-diene-3,20-dione, 11,17,21-trihy-droxy-, (11β)- 11β,17,21-Trihydroxypregna-1,4-diene-3,20 dione. Metacortandralone.
Use: Adrenocortical steroid (anti-inflammatory).
See: Cordrol, Tab. (Vita Elixir).
Delta-Cortef, Tab. (Upjohn).
Fernisolone, Tab., Inj. (Ferndale).
Orasone, Tab. (Solvay).
Orasone 50, Tab. (Solvay).
Panisolone, Tab. (Panray).
Prednis, Tab. (USV Labs.).
Ster 5, Tab. (Scrip).
Ulacort, Tab. (Fellows-Testagar).
W/Aluminum hydroxide gel, dried.
See: Predoxide, Tab. (Mallard).
W/Aspirin.
See: Sarogesic, Tab. (Saron).
W/Chloramphenicol.
See: Chloroptic-P, Ophthalmic Oint. (Allergan).
W/Hydroxyzine HCl.
W/Neomycin sulfate.
Neo-Deltef, Drops (Upjohn).
W/Sulfacetamide sodium, methylcellulose.
See: Isopto Cetapred, Susp. (Alcon).
W/Sulfacetamide sodium.
See: Cetapred Ophthalmic Oint. (Alcon).

•**PREDNISOLONE ACETATE,** U.S.P. XXII, Ophth., Sterile Susp., U.S.P. XXII. Pregna-1,4-diene-3,20-dione, 21-(acetyloxy)-11,17-dihydroxy-,(11β)-
Use: Adrenocortical steroid (anti-inflammatory).
Econopred, Susp. (Alcon).
Key-Pred, Inj. (Hyrex).
Nisolone, Vial (Ascher).
Predicort, Amp. (Dunhall).
Pred, Preps. (Allergan).
Pred-Forte, Ophthalmic Susp. (Allergan).
Savacort-50, 100, Vial (Savage).
Sigpred, Inj. (Sig).
Steraject, Vial (Mayrand).
Sterane, Inj. (Pfizer Laboratories).
Ulacort, Inj. (Fellows-Testagar).

PREDNISOLONE ACETATE W/COMBINATIONS
See: Blephamide Liquifilm, Soln. (Allergan).
Blephamide S.O.P., Ophthalmic, Oint. (Allergan).
Cetapred Opthalmic Oint. (Alcon).
Dua-Pred, Inj. (Solvay).
Metimyd, Ophthalmic Susp., Oint. (Schering).
Neo-Delta-Cortef, Preps. (Upjohn).
Panacort R-P, Vial (Ferndale).
Prednefrin, Mild, Susp. (Allergan).
Tri-Ophtho, Ophthalmic (Maurry).
Vasocidin, Preps. (CooperVision).

PREDNISOLONE ACETATE AND PREDNISOLONE SODIUM PHOSPHATE. (Various Mfr.) Prednisolone acetate 80 mg, prednisolone sodium phosphate 20 mg/ml Inj. Susp. Vial 10 ml.
Use: Corticosteroid.

•**PREDNISOLONE ACETATE OPHTHALMIC SUSPENSION.** U.S.P. XXII.
See: Prednisolone Acetate.

PREDNISOLONE BUTYLACETATE. 1,4-Pregnadiene-3,20-dione-11β,17α,21-triol-tert-butyl-acetate.
Use: Corticosteroid.
See: Hydeltra-T.B.A., Vial (Merck Sharp & Dohme).

PREDNISOLONE CYCLOPENTYLPROPIONATE. d[1],4-Pregnadiene-3,20-dione-11, 17a-diol-21-cy-clopentylpropionate(prednisolone-21-cyclopentylpropionate).
Use: Corticosteroid.

•**PREDNISOLONE HEMISUCCINATE,** U.S.P. XXII. Pregna-1,4-diene-3,20-dione, 21-(3-carboxy-1-oxopropoxy)-11, 17-dihydroxy-, (11β)−.
Use: Adrenocortical steroid (anti-inflammatory).

•**PREDNISOLONE SODIUM PHOSPHATE,** U.S.P. XXII. Inj., Ophth. Soln.: U.S.P. XXII. Pregna-1,4-diene-3,20-dione, 11,17-dihydroxy-21-(phosphonoxy)-,disodium salt, (11)-.
Use: Adrenocortical steroid (anti-inflammatory).
See: Alto-Pred Soluble, Vial (Alto).
Hydeltrasol, Inj. (Merck Sharp & Dohme).
Hydrosol, Inj. (Rocky Mtn.).
Inflamase Forte, Ophthalmic Soln. (CooperVision).
Inflamase, Ophthalmic Soln. (CooperVision).
Key-Pred SP, Inj. (Hyrex).
Liquid Pred, Inj. (Muro).
Metreton, Ophthalmic Soln. Sterile (Schering).
Pediapred, Liq. (Fisons).
P.S.P. IV (Four), Inj. (Solvay).
Savacort-S, Inj. (Savage).
Sodasone, Inj. (Fellows Testagar).
Sol-Pred, Inj. (Amfre-Grant).
W/Neomycin sulfate.
See: Neo-Hydeltrasol, Ophthalmic Soln., Ophthalmic Oint. (Merck Sharp & Dohme).
W/Niacinamide, disodium edetate, sodium bisulfite, phenol.
See: P.S.P. IV, Inj. (Solvay).
W/Prednisolone acetate.
See: Panacort R-P, Vial (Ferndale).
Solu-Pred, Vial (Kenyon).
W/Sodium Sulfacetamide.
See: Optimyd, Soln. (Schering).
Vasocidin, Liq. (CooperVision).

PREDNISOLONE TERTIARY-BUTYLACETATE.
See: Prednisolone Tebutate, U.S.P. XXII.

PREDNISOL T.B.A.. (Pasadena Research) Prednisolone tebutate 20 mg/ml. Vial 10 ml.
Use: Corticosteroid.

•**PREDNISOLONE TEBUTATE SUSPENSION, STERILE,** U.S.P. XXII. Pregna-1,4-diene-3,20-

dione, 11,17-dihydroxy-21-(3,3-dimethyl-1-oxobutyl)oxy-, (11β)−.
Use: Adrenocorticol steroid.
See: Durapred T.B.A., Inj. (Amfre-Grant).
Hydeltra-T.B.A., Vial (Merck Sharp & Dohme).
Metalone, Vial (Foy).

•**PREDNISONE,** U.S.P. XXII. Oral Soln., Syrup, Tabs., U.S.P. XXII. Pregna-1,4-diene-3,11,20-trione, 17,21-dihydroxy-. Δ1,4-Pregnadiene-17α,21-diol-3,11-20-trione. 1-Dehydro-cortisone, Metacortandracin. 17,21-Dihydroxypregna-1,4-diene-3,11,20-trione.
Use: Glucocorticoid.
See: Delta-Dome, Tab. (Miles Pharm).
Deltasone, Tab. (Upjohn).
Keysone, Tab.(Hyrex).
Lisacort, Tab. (Fellows-Testagar).
Meticorten, Tab. (Schering).
Maso-Pred, Tab. (Mason).
Orasone, Tab. (Solvay).
Pan-Sone, Tab. (Panray).
Pred-5 (Saron).
Ropred, Tab. (Robinson).
Sarogesic, Tab. (Saron).
Sterapred, Tab. (Mayrand).
W/Chlorpheniramine maleate.
See: Histone, Tab. (Blaine).
W/Phenylephrine HCl.
See: Prednefrin-S, Soln. (Allergan).

PREDNISONE INTENSOL ORAL SOLUTION. (Roxane) Prednisone concentrated oral solution 5 mg/ml. Bot. 30 ml w/calibrated dropper.
Use: Corticosteroid.

•**PREDNIVAL.** USAN. 11 beta, 17, 21-Trihydroxypregna-1,4-diene-3,20-dione 17 valerate. Under study.
Use: Topical anti-inflammatory.

PREDNYLIDENE. B.A.N. 11β,17α,21-Trihydroxy-16-methylenepregna-1,4-diene-3,20-dione. Dacortilene; Decortilen.
Use: Corticosteroid.

PREDSULFAIR. (Pharmafair) **Drops:** Prednisolone acetate 0.5%, sodium sulfacetamide 10%, hydroxypropyl methylcellulose, polysorbate 80 0.5%, sodium thiosulfate, benzalkonium Cl 0.01%. Bot. 5 ml, 15 ml. **Oint.:** Prednisolone acetate 0.5%, sodium sulfacetamide 10%, mineral oil, white petrolatum, lanolin, parabens. In 3.5 Gm.
Use: Corticosteroid, anti-infective, ophthalmic.

PREFLEX FOR SENSITIVE EYES. (Alcon Lenscare) Isotonic, aqueous solution of sorbic acid sodium phosphates, sodium Cl, tyloxapol, hydroxyethyl cellulose, polyvinyl alcohol. Bot. 1.5 oz.
Use: Soft contact lens care.

PREFRIN LIQUIFILM. (Allergan) Phenylephrine HCl 0.12%, antipyrine 0.1%, polyvinyl alcohol 1.4%, benzalkonium Cl 0.004%, edetate disodium. Bot. 0.7 fl oz.
Use: Ophthalmic decongestant.

PREFRIN-A. (Allergan) Phenylephrine 0.12%, pyrilamine maleate 0.1%, antipyrine 0.1%, benzalkonium Cl, sodium bisulfite, edetate disodium. Bot. 15 ml.
Use: Ophthalmic antihistamine, decongestant.

PREGESTIMIL. (Mead Johnson Nutrition) Protein hydrolysate formula supplies 640 calories/qt. protein 18 Gm, fat 26 Gm, carbohydrate 86 Gm, vitamins A 2000 IU, D 400 IU, E 15 IU, C 52 mg, folic acid 100 mcg, thiamine 0.5 mg, riboflavin 0.6 mg, niacin 8 mg, B_6 0.4 mg, B_{12} 2 mcg, biotin 0.05 mg, pantothenic acid 3 mg, K-1 100 mcg, choline 85 mg, inositol 30 mg, calcium 600 mg, phosphorus 400 mg, iodine 45 mcg, iron 12 mg, magnesium 70 mg, copper 0.6 mg, zinc 4 mg, manganese 0.2 mg, chloride 550 mg, potassium 700 mg, sodium 300 mg/Qt. (20 Kcal/fl oz.). Pow. Can lb.
Use: Enteral nutritional supplement.

PREGNASLIDE LATEX HCG TEST WITH FAST TRAK SLIDES. (Wampole) Latex agglutination slide test for the qualitative detection of human chorionic gonadotropin in urine. Test 24s. Test kit 96s.
Use: Diagnostic aid.

PREGNENINOLONE.
See: Ethisterone.

•**PREGNENOLONE.** F.D.A. 3-beta-Hydroxypregn-5-en-20-one. Synthetic steroid intermediate. 3-Hydroxy-20-keto-pregene-5.
Use: Treatment of rheumatoid arthritis.

•**PREGNENOLONE SUCCINATE.** USAN. 3-Hydroxy-5-pregnen-20-one, hydrogen succinate.
Use: Glucocorticoid.

PREGNOSIS SLIDE TEST. (Roche Diagnostics) Latex agglutination inhibition slide test. 50s, 200s.
Use: Diagnostic aid.

PREGNOSPIA. (Organon Technica) Monoclonal antibody-based enzyme immunoassay. 25s, 100s.
Use: Diagnostic aid.

PREGNYL. (Organon) Human chorionic gonadotropin 10,000 IU/Vial w/diluent 10 ml, mannitol, benzyl alcohol. Vial 10 ml.
Use: Chorionic gonadotropin.

PREJECT PREINJECTION TOPICAL ANESTHETIC. (Hoyt) Benzocaine 20% in polyethylene glycol base. Jar 2 oz.
Use: Local anesthetic.

PRELAN. (Lannett) Vitamins A 4000 IU, B_1 0.5 mg, B_2 2 mg, niacin 10 mg, B_6 3 mg, B_{12} 2 mcg, D 400 IU, C 50 mg, calcium 200 mg, iron 30 mg/Tab. Bot. 100s.
Use: Vitamin/mineral supplement.

PRELAN F.A. TABLETS. (Lannett) Vitamin A 4000 IU, B_1 0.5 mg, B_2 2 mg, niacin 10 mg, B_6 3 mg, B_{12} 2 mcg, D 400 IU, C 50 mg, calcium 200 mg, iron 30 mg, folic acid 1 mg/Tab. Bot. 100s.
Use: Vitamin/mineral supplement.

PRELESTRIN. (Pasadena Research) Conjugated estrogens 0.625 mg or 1.25 mg/Tab. Bot. 100s, 1000s.
Use: Estrogen.

PRELONE SYRUP. (Muro) Prednisolone 15 mg/5 ml, alcohol 5%, saccharin. Cherry flavor. 240 ml.
Use: Corticosteroid.

PRELU-2. (Boehringer Ingelheim) Phendimetrazine tartrate 105 mg/Cap. Bot. 100s.
Use: Anorexiant.

PRELUDIN TABLETS. (Boehringer Ingelheim) Phenmetrazine HCl 25 mg/Tab. or 75 mg/SA Tab. w/tartrazine. Bot. 100s.
Use: Anorexiant.

PRELUS ELIXIR. (Winthrop Products) Isoproterenol HCl.
Use: Bronchodilator.

PREMARIN. (Wyeth-Ayerst) Conjugated estrogens tablets. Water-soluble conjugated estrogens derived from natural sources. 0.3 mg, 0.625 mg, 0.9 mg, 1.25 mg or 2.5 mg/Tab.: Bot. 100s, 1000s. 0.625 mg or 1.25 mg: UD 100s. Cycle packs 21s.
Use: Estrogen.

PREMARIN INTRAVENOUS. (Wyeth-Ayerst) Conjugated Estrogens U.S.P., for Injection. Vial 25 mg/5 ml w/diluent. (Vial also contains lactose 200 mg, sodium citrate 12.5 mg, simethicone 0.2 mg). Diluent contains benzyl alcohol 2%, Water for Injection, U.S.P.
Use: Estrogen.

PREMARIN VAGINAL CREAM. (Wyeth-Ayerst) Conjugated Estrogens, U.S.P. 0.625 mg/1 Gm w/cetyl esters wax, cetyl alcohol, white wax, glyceryl monostearate, propylene glycol monostearate, methyl stearate, phenylethyl alcohol, sodium lauryl sulfate, glycerin, mineral oil. Tube w/applicator 1.5 oz. (42.5 Gm). Tube refill.
Use: Estrogen.

PREMARIN W/MEPROBAMATE.
See: PMB 200 and 400, Tab. (Wyeth-Ayerst).

PREMARIN W/METHYLTESTOSTERONE. (Wyeth-Ayerst) Premarin (Conjugated Estrogens, U.S.P.) 1.25 mg, methyltestosterone 10 mg/Yellow Tab. Premarin 0.625 mg, methyltestosterone 5 mg/Red Tab. Bot. 100s, 1000s.
Use: Estrogen, androgen combination.

W/Methyltestosterone, methamphetamine HCl, vitamins.
See: Mediatric, Cap., Liq., Tab. (Wyeth-Ayerst).

PREMATE-200. (Major) Meprobamate 200 mg, tridihexethyl Cl 25 mg/Tab. Bot. 100s.
Use: Antianxiety agent, anticholinergic.

PREMATE-400. (Major) Meprobamate 400 mg, tridihexethyl Cl 25 mg/Tab. Bot. 100s.
Use: Antianxiety agent, anticholinergic.

PREMENSTRUAL TENSION.
See: Motion Sickness.
Pamabrom (Various Mfr.).
Pyranisamine Bromotheophyllinate (Various Mfr.).

PREMSYN PMS CAPLETS. (Chattem) Acetaminophen 500 mg, pamabrom 25 mg, pyrilamine maleate 15 mg/Capl. Bot. 20s, 40s.
Use: Analgesic, diuretic, antihistamine.

PREMSYN PMS CAPSULES. (Chattem) Pamabrom 25 mg, acetaminophen 500 mg, pyrilamine maleate 15 mg/Cap. Bot. 20s, 40s.
Use: Diuretic, analgesic, antihistamine.

•**PRENALTEROL HYDROCHLORIDE.** USAN.
Use: Adrenergic.

PRENATAL. (Kenyon) Vitamins A 100 IU, D 500 IU, B_1 1 mg, C 25 mg, B_2 1 mg, niacinamide 3 mg, iron 39 mg, calcium 140 mg, phosphorus 62 mg, potassium iodide 0.065 mg, copper sulfate 1 mg, cobalt sulfate 1 mg, magnesium oxide 10 mg, manganese sulfate 14 mg, potassium sulfate 11 mg, sodium sulfate 0.4 mg, zinc oxide 0.4 mg, fluoride 1 mg/Tab. Bot. 100s, 1000s.
Use: Vitamin/mineral supplement.

PRENATAL FOLIC ACID + IRON. (Everett) Vitamins, minerals, folic acid 1 mg/Tab. Bot. 100s.
Use: Vitamin/mineral supplement.

PRENATAL NO. 2. (Kenyon) Vitamins A 4000 IU, B_1 2 mg, B_2 2 mg, B_6 0.8 mg, C 50 mg, niacinamide 10 mg, iodide 0.15 mg, folic acid 0.1 mg, B_{12} concentrate 2 mcg, iron 50 mg, calcium 240 mg/Cap. Bot. 100s, 1000s.
Use: Vitamin/mineral supplement.

PRENATAL ONE. (Major) Vitamins A 8000 IU, D 400 IU, E 30 mg, C 90 mg, folic acid 1 mg, B_1 2.5 mg, B_2 3 mg, niacin 20 mg, B_6 10 mg, B_{12} 12 mcg, calcium 200 mg, iodine, iron 65 mg, magnesium, zinc 35 mg/Tab. Bot. 100s, 500s.
Use: Vitamin/mineral supplement.

PRENATAL-S. (Goldline) Calcium 200 mg, iron 60 mg, vitamins A 8000 IU, D 400 IU, E 30 mg, B_1 1.7 mg, B_2 2 mg, B_3 20 mg, B_6 4 mg, B_{12} 8 mcg, C 60 mg, folic acid 0.8 mg, I, Mg, zinc 25 mg/Tab. Bot. 100s, 1000s.
Use: Vitamin/mineral supplement.

PRENATAL WITH FOLIC ACID. (Geneva Generics) Calcium 200 mg, iron 60 mg, vitamins A 8000 IU, D 400 IU, E 30 mg, B_1 1.7 mg, B_2 2 mg, B_3 20 mg, B_6 4 mg, B_{12} 8 mcg, C 60 mg, folic acid 0.8 mg, I, Mg/Tab. Bot. 100s.
Use: Vitamin/mineral supplement.

PRENATAL WITH FOLIC ACID. (Vitarine) Vitamins A 6000 IU, D 400 IU, E 30 IU, folic acid 1 mg, C 60 mg, B_1 1.1 mg, B_2 1.8 mg, B_6 2.5 mg, B_{12} 5 mcg, niacin 15 mg, calcium 125 mg, iron 65 mg/Tab. Bot. 100s, 1000s.
Use: Vitamin/mineral supplement.

PRENATE 90 TABLETS. (Bock) Vitamins A 8000 IU, D 400 IU, E 30 mg, C 120 mg, folic acid 1 mg, B_1 3 mg, B_2 3.4 mg, B_6 20 mg, B_{12} 12 mcg, niacinamide 20 mg, docusate sodium, calcium 250 mg, iodine, iron 90 mg, Cu, zinc 20 mg/FC Tab. Bot. 100s, 1000s.
Use: Vitamin/mineral supplement.

PRENAVITE. (Rugby) Calcium 200 mg, iron 60 mg, vitamins A 8000 IU, D 400 IU, E 30 mg, B_1

1.7 mg, B_2 2 mg, B_3 20 mg, B_6 4 mg, B_{12} 8 mcg, C 60 mg, folic acic 0.8 mg, I, Mg/Tab., sodium free. Bot. 100s, 500s.
Use: Vitamin/mineral supplement.

PRENISTAT. (Pharmex) Prednisolone sodium phosphate 20 mg, niacinamide 25 mg/ml. Vial 10 ml.
Use: Corticosteroid.

•**PRENYLAMINE.** USAN. N-(3,3-Diphenylpropyl)-a-methylphenethylamine. Segontin; Synadrin lactate.
Use: Coronary vasodilator.

PRE-PEN. (Kremers-Urban) Benzylpenicilloyl-polylysine 0.25 ml/Amp.
Use: Diagnostic aid.

PREPARATION H. (Whitehall) Phenylmercuric nitrate 1:10,000, live yeast cell derivative 2000 units skin respiratory factor, shark liver oil 3%. Supp. w/PEG 600 dilaurate. Oint. Tube 1 oz, 2 oz. Supp. 12s, 24s, 36s, 48s.
Use: Anorectal preparation.

PREPCAT. (Lafayette) Barium sulfate 1.2% w/w suspension. Bot. 480 ml, Case Bot. 24s.
Use: Radiopaque agent.

PREPCAT 2000. (Lafayette) Barium sulfate 1.2% w/w suspension. Bot. 2000 ml, Case Bot. 4s.
Use: Radiopaque agent.

PREPCORT CREAM. (Whitehall) Hydrocortisone 0.5%. Tube 0.5 oz, 1 oz.
Use: Corticosteroid.

PREPODYNE. (West) Titratable iodine. **Soln:** 1%. Bot. pt, gal. **Scrub:** 0.75%. Bot. 6 oz, gal. **Swabs:** Saturated with soln. Pkt. 1s, Box 100s. **Swabsticks:** Saturated with soln. Pkt. 1s, Box 50s. Pkt. 3s, Box 75s.
Use: Topical antiseptic.

PRESALIN. (Hauck) Aspirin 260 mg, salicylamide 120 mg, acetaminophen 120 mg, aluminum hydroxide 100 mg/Tab. Bot. 50s.
Use: Analgesic combination, antacid.

PRESSOR AGENTS.
See: Sympathomimetic agents.

PRESSOROL. (Travenol) Metaraminol bitartrate. Vial 10 ml (10 mg/ml).
Use: Vasopressor.

PRESUN 8 CREAMY. (Westwood) Padimate O 5%, oxybenzone 2%. Waterproof. Bot. 4 oz.
Use: Sunscreen.

PRESUN 8 LOTION. (Westwood) Padimate O 7.3%, oxybenzone 2.3%, SD alcohol 40 60%. Bot. 4 oz.
Use: Sunscreen.

PRESUN 15 CREAMY. (Westwood) Padimate O 8%, oxybenzone 3%, benzyl alcohol. Waterproof. Bot. 4 oz.
Use: Sunscreen.

PRESUN 15 FACIAL SUNSCREEN. (Westwood) Padimate O (Octyl dimethyl PABA) 8%, oxybenzone 3%. Bot. 2 oz.
Use: Sunscreen.

PRESUN 15 FACIAL SUNSCREEN STICK. (Westwood) Octyl dimethyl PABA 8%, oxybenzone 3%. Stick 0.42 oz.
Use: Sunscreen.

PRESUN 15 LIP PROTECTOR. (Westwood) Padimate O 8%, oxybenzone 3%. Stick 4.5 Gm.
Use: Sunscreen.

PRESUN 15 LOTION. (Westwood) Padimate O 5%, PABA 5%, oxybenzone 3%, SD alcohol 40 58%. Bot. 4 oz.
Use: Sunscreen.

PRESUN 4 CREAMY. (Westwood) Padimate O 1.4%, alcohol, titanium dioxide. Waterproof lotion. Bot. 4 oz.
Use: Sunscreen.

PRESUN 29. (Westwood) Octyl methoxycinnamate, oxybenzone, octyl salicylate. SPF 29. Waterproof. Bot. 4 oz.
Use: Sunscreen.

PRETAMAZIUM IODIDE. B.A.N. 4-(Biphenyl-4-yl)-3-ethyl-2-[4-(pyrrolidin-1-yl)styryl]thiazolium iodide.
Use: Treatment of enterobiasis.

PRETEND-U-ATE. (Vitalax) Enriched candy-appetite pacifier. Pkg. 20s.
Use: Diet aid.

PRETHCAMIDE. Mixture of crotethamide and cropropamide. Micoren (Geigy).

PRETTY FEET & HANDS. (Norcliff Thayer) Lotion 3 fl oz.
Use: Emollient.

PREVIDENT DISCLOSING DROPS. (Hoyt) Erythrosine sodium 1%. Bot. 1 oz.
Use: Disclosing dental plaque.

PREVIDENT DISCLOSING TABLET. (Hoyt) Erythrosine sodium 1%/Tab. UD strip 1000s.
Use: Disclosing dental plaque.

PREVIDENT PROPHYLAXIS PASTE. (Hoyt) Sodium fluoride containing 1.2% fluoride ion w/ pumice and alumina abrasives. Cup 2 Gm, Box 200s. Jar 9 oz.
Use: Dental caries preventative.

PREVIEW. (Lafayette) Barium sulfate 60% w/v suspension. Bot. 355 ml, Case 24 bot.
Use: Radiopaque agent.

PREVIEW 2000. Barium sulfate 60% w/v suspension. Bot. 2000 ml, Case 4 Bot.
Use: Radiopaque agent.

PREVISION. Mestranol, U.S.P. XXII.

PREXONATE TABLETS. (Tennessee Pharm.) Vitamins A acetate 5000 IU, D 500 IU, B_6 2 mg, B_1 5 mg, B_2 2 mg, C 100 mg, B_{12} 2.5 mcg, calcium pantothenate 1 mg, niacinamide 15 mg, folic acid 1 mg, iron 45 mg, calcium 500 mg, intrinsic factor 3 mg/Tab. Bot. 100s, 1000s.
Use: Vitamin/mineral supplement.

PRID SALVE. (Walker Pharmacal) Icthammol, Phenol, Lead Oleate, Rosin, Beeswax, Lard. Tin 20 Gm.
Use: Drawing salve.

•**PRIDEFINE HYDROCHLORIDE.** USAN.
Use: Antidepressant.

•**PRILOCAINE AND EPINEPHRINE INJECTION,** U.S.P. XXII.
Use: Local anesthetic.

•**PRILOCAINE HYDROCHLORIDE,** U.S.P. XXII. Inj., U.S.P. XXII. 2-(Propylamino)-o-propionotolidide HCl.
Use: Local anesthetic.
See: Citanest Hydrochloride, Vial, Amp. (Astra).

PRILOSEC. (Merck, Sharp and Dohme) Omeprazole 20 mg/Cap. Bot. 30s, UD 100s.
Use: Gastric acid suppressant.

PRIMACAINE. 2′-Diethylamino-ethyl-2-butoxy-3-aminobenzoate HCl.
Use: Local anesthetic.

PRIMADERM. (Arrow Medical) Cod liver oil concentrate (Vitamins A and D), zinc oxide in a mentholated petrolatum-lanolin base. Oint. In 30 Gm, 60 Gm.
Use: Burn preparation.

PRIMADERM-B. (Arrow Medical) Benzocaine, zinc oxide, cod liver oil in a petrolatum-lanolin base. Oint. 30 Gm, 60 Gm.
Use: Burn preparation.

•**PRIMAQUINE PHOSPHATE,** U.S.P. XXII. Tab., U.S.P. XXII. 1,4-Pentanediamine, N-(6-methoxy-8-quinolinyl)-, phosphate (1:2). (Winthrop Pharm). Tab. 26.3 mg, Bot. 100s.
Use: Prevents relapses in nearly all cases of vivax malaria.

PRIMATENE MIST SOLUTION. (Whitehall) Epinephrine 0.2 mg, alcohol 34%. Bot. 0.5 oz. Spray.
Use: Bronchodilator.

PRIMATENE MIST SUSPENSION. (Whitehall) Epinephrine bitartrate 0.3 mg. Bot. 10 ml w/ mouthpiece. Spray.
Use: Bronchodilator.

PRIMATENE M. TABLETS. (Whitehall) Theophylline 118 mg, ephedrine HCl 24 mg, pyrilamine maleate 16.6 mg/Tab. Bot. 24s, 60s.
Use: Bronchodilator, antihistamine.

PRIMATENE P TABLETS. (Whitehall) Theophylline 118 mg, ephedrine HCl 24 mg, phenobarbital 8 mg/Tab. Bot. 24s, 60s.
Use: Bronchodilator, sedative/hypnotic.

PRIMATUSS COUGH MIXTURE 4 LIQUID. (Rugby) Doxylamine succinate 3.75 mg, dextromethorphan HBr 7.5 mg/5 ml, alcohol 10% Liq. Bot. 180 ml.
Use: Antihistamine, antitussive.

PRIMATUSS COUGH MIXTURE 4D LIQUID. (Rugby) Phenylpropanolamine HCl 12.5 mg, dextromethorphan HBr 10 mg, guaifenesin 100 mg/5 ml, alcohol 10%. Liq. Bot. 180 ml.
Use: Decongestant, antitussive, expectorant.

PRIMAXIN. (Merck Sharp & Dohme) Imipenem (anhydrous equivalent), cilastatin w/sodium bicarbonate buffer. **250-250:** ADD-Vantage Vial, Tray 10s, 25s. Tray 10 infusion bottles. **500-500:** ADD-Vantage Vial, Tray 10s, 25s. Tray 10 infusion bottles.
Use: Anti-infective.

•**PRIMIDOLOL.** USAN.
Use: Anti-anginal; cardiac depressant.

•**PRIMIDONE,** U.S.P. XXII. Tab., Oral Susp., U.S.P. XXII. 4,6(1H,5H)-Pyrimidinedione, 5-ethyldihydro-5-phenyl-5-Ethyldihydro-5-phenyl-4,6(1H,5H)-pyrimidinedione. Tab. 250 mg Bot. 100s, 1000s.
Use: Anticonvulsant.

PRIMOSTRUM. A prep. of primiparous colostrum.

PRINCIPEN '125' FOR ORAL SUSPENSION. (Squibb) Ampicillin trihydrate 125 mg/5 ml, saccharin. Reconstitution to 80 ml, 100 ml, 150 ml, 200 ml, UD 5 ml 100s.
Use: Antibacterial, penicillin.

PRINCIPEN '250' CAPSULES. (Squibb) Ampicillin 250 mg/Cap. Bot. 100s, 500s, UD 100s.
Use: Antibacterial, penicillin.

PRINCIPEN '250' FOR ORAL SUSPENSION. (Squibb) Ampicillin trihydrate 250 mg/5 ml, saccharin. Reconstitution to 80 ml, 100 ml, 150 ml, 200 ml, UD 5 ml 100s.
Use: Antibacterial, penicillin.

PRINCIPEN '500' CAPSULES. (Squibb) Ampicillin trihydrate 500 mg/Cap. 100s, 500s, UD 100s.
Use: Antibacterial, penicillin.

PRINCIPEN WITH PROBENECID. (Squibb) Ampicillin (as trihydrate) 3.5 Gm, probenecid 1 Gm/ regimen. Single dose bot., 9s.
Use: Antibacterial, penicillin.

PRINIVIL. (MSD) Lisinopril. **5 mg or 40 mg/Tab.:** Bot. 100s, UD 100s. **10 mg or 20 mg/Tab.:** Bot. 30s, 100s, UD 100s.
Use: Antihypertensive.

PRINN 0.5. (Scrip) Conjugated estrogen 0.625 mg/Tab. Bot. 100s.
Use: Estrogen.

•**PRINOMIDE TROMETHAMINE.** USAN.
Use: Antirheumatic.

•**PRINOXODAN.** USAN.
Use: Cardiotonic.

PRINZIDE. (MSD) Lisinopril 20 mg, hydrochlorothiazide 12.5 mg/Tab or lisinopril 20 mg, hydrochlorothiazide 25 mg/Tab. Bot. 30s, 100s.
Use: Antihypertensive.

PRISCOLINE. (Ciba) Tolazoline HCl 25 mg/ml, tartaric acid 0.65%, chlorobutanol 0.5%. Vial 10 ml.
Use: Antihypertensive.

PRISILIDENE HYDROCHLORIDE.
See: Alphaprodine HCl (Various Mfr.).

PRISTINAMYCIN. B.A.N. An antibiotic produced by Streptomyces pristina spiralis.
Use: Anti-infective.

PRIVADORN.
See: Bromisovalum (Various Mfr.).

PRIVINE. (Ciba Consumer) Naphazoline HCl. **Nasal Soln.:** 0.05%. 20 ml w/dropper. **Nasal Spray:** 0.05%. 15 ml.
Use: Decongestant.

•**PRIZIDILOL HYDROCHLORIDE.** USAN.
Use: Antihypertensive.

PRO-50. (Dunhall) Promethazine HCl 50 mg/ml. Vial 10 ml.
Use: Antihistamine, antiemetic.

PRO-ACET DOUCHE CONCENTRATE. (Pro-Acet) Lactic, citric, and acetic acids, sodium lauryl sulfate, lactose, dextrose and sodium acetate. Pkg. polyethylene envelope 10 ml. Contents of 1 envelope to be diluted with 2 quarts of water. Douche 6 oz, 12 oz. Travel Packet, 10 ml.
Use: Vaginal preparation.

PROADIFEN HYDROCHLORIDE. USAN. 2-(Diethylamino)ethyl-2,2-diphenyl-valerate hydrochloride.
Use: Drug potentiator.

PROBALAN. (Lannett) Probenecid 0.5 Gm/Tab. Bot. 100s, 1000s.
Use: Agent for gout.

PROBAMPACIN. (Robinson) Ampicillin trihydrate 3.5 Gm, probenecid 1 Gm/UD Bottle.
Use: Antibacterial, penicillin.

PROBAMPACIN SUSPENSION. (Goldline) Bot. 60 ml.
Use: Antibacterial, penicillin.

PRO-BANTHINE. (Searle) Propantheline bromide **7.5 mg/Tab.:** Bot. 100s. **15 mg/Tab.:** Bot. 100s, 500s, UD 100s.
Use: Anticholinergic/antispasmodic.

PROBARBITAL SODIUM. 5-Ethyl-5-isopropylbarbiturate sodium.

PROBEC-T. (Stuart) Vitamins B_1 15 mg, B_2 10 mg, niacinamide 100 mg, B_6 5 mg, B_{12} 5 mcg, C 600 mg. Bot. 60s.
Use: Vitamin/mineral supplement.

PROBEN. (Richlyn) Probenecid 500 mg, colchicine 0.5 mg/Tab. Bot. 1000s.
Use: Agent for gout.

PROBEN-C. (Rugby) Probenecid 500 mg, colchicine 0.5 mg/Tab. Bot. 100s, 1000s.
Use: Agent for gout.

PROBENECID, U.S.P. XXII. Tabs., U.S.P. XXII. Benzoic acid, 4-[(dipropylamino)sulfonyl)]-p-(Dipropylsulfamoyl) benzoic acid.
Use: Uricosuric.
See: Benacen, Tab. (Cenci).
Benemid, Tab. (Merck Sharp & Dohme).
Benn, Tab. (Scrip).
Probalan, Tab. (Lannett).
Robenecid, Tab. (Robinson).
W/Ampicillin.
See: Amcill-GC, Oral Susp. (Parke-Davis).
Polycillin-PRB, Liq. (Bristol).
Principen w/Probenecid, Cap. (Squibb).
W/Ampicillin trihydrate.
See: Probampacin (Biocraft).

PROBENECID AND COLCHICINE, U.S.P. XXII.
Use: Uricosuric combination for chronic gouty arthritis.
See: Benn-C, Tab. (Scrip).
Colbenemid, Tab. (Merck Sharp & Dohme).
Robenecid w/Colchicine, Tab. (Robinson).
Robenecol, Tab. (Robinson).

PROBENZAMIDE. 0-Propoxybenzamide. (Warner-Lambert).

•**PROBICROMIL CALCIUM.** USAN.
Use: Anti-allergenic.

•**PROBUCOL,** U.S.P. XXII. (1) Acetone bis(3,5-ditertbutyl-4-hydroxyphenyl) mercaptole; (2) 4,4′-(iso-propylidenedithio)-bis[2,6-di-tert-butylphenol].
Use: Anticholesteremic.
See: Lorelco, Tab. (Merrell Dow).

•**PROCAINAMIDE HYDROCHLORIDE,** U.S.P. XXII. Cap., Inj., Tab., Ext. Rel. Tab., U.S.P. XXII. Benzamide, 4-amino-N-[2-(diethylamino)ethyl]-HCl. p-Amino-N-[2-(diethylaminoethyl]benzamide HCl.
Use: Cardiac depressant in arrhythmias.
See: Procamide SR, Tab. (Solvay).
Procan SR, Tab. (Parke-Davis).
Procapan, Cap. (Panray).
Pronestyl, Cap., Vial (Princeton).

PROCAINE BASE.
W/Benzyl alcohol, propyl-p-aminobenzoate.
Use: Local anesthetic.
See: Rectocaine, Vial (Moore-Kirk).
W/Butyl-p-aminobenzoate, benzyl alcohol, in sweet almond oil.
See: Anucaine, Amp. (Calvin).

PROCAINE BUTYRATE. p-Aminobenzoyl-di-ethylaminoethanol butyrate.

•**PROCAINE HYDROCHLORIDE,** U.S.P. XXII. Inj., Sterile, U.S.P. XXII. Benzoic acid, 4-amino-, 2-(diethylamino)-ethyl ester, HCl. 2-Diethylaminoethyl p-aminobenzoate HCl. Allocaine, Bernocaine, Chlorocaine, Ethocaine, Irocaine, Kerocaine, Syncaine. (Abbott) 1% or 2% solution. Multiple-dose Vial 30 ml.
Use: Local anesthetic.
See: Anucaine, Amp. (Calvin).
Novocain, Amp., Soln. (Winthrop Pharm).
W/Tetracaine and Nordefrin Hydrochlorides, Inj.

PROCAINE HYDROCHLORIDE AND LEVONORDEFRIN INJECTION.
Use: Local anesthetic.

•**PROCAINE PENICILLIN G SUSPENSION, STERILE,** U.S.P. XXII.
Use: Antibiotic.
See: Crysticillin, Vial (Squibb).
Penicillin G, Procaine (Various Mfr.).
Pfizerpen For Injection (Pfipharmecs).

•**PROCAINE, PENICILLIN G W/ALUMINUM STEARATE SUSPENSION, STERILE,** U.S.P. XXII.
Use: Antibiotic.
See: Penicillin G Procaine with Aluminum Stearate, Sterile, U.S.P. XXII.

•**PROCAINE HYDROCHLORIDE AND EPINEPHRINE INJECTION,** U.S.P. XXII.
Use: Local anesthetic.

•**PROCAINE AND PHENYLEPHRINE HYDROCHLORIDES INJECTION,** U.S.P. XXII.
Use: Local anesthetic (dental).

•**PROCAINE AND TETRACAINE HYDROCHLORIDES AND LEVONORDEFRIN INJECTION,** U.S.P. XXII.
Use: Local anesthetic (dental).

PROCAINE, TETRACAINE AND NORDEFRIN HYDROCHLORIDES INJECTION.
Use: Local anesthetic.

PROCAINE, TETRACAINE AND PHENYLEPHRINE HYDROCHLORIDES INJECTION.
Use: Anesthetic.

PROCALAMINE INJECTION. (Kendall McGaw) Injection of amino acid 3%, glycerin 3%, electrolytes. Bot. 1000 ml.
Use: Parenteral nutritional supplement.

PRO-CAL-SOF. (Vangard) Docusate calcium 240 mg/Cap. Bot. 100s, 1000s, UD 100s.
Use: Laxative.

PROCAN SR. (Parke-Davis) Procainamide HCl sustained release 250 mg, 500 mg, 750 mg or 1 Gm/Tab. Bot. 100s, 500s (except 1 Gm), UD 100s.
Use: Antiarrhythmic.

PRO-CAP 65. (Foy) Propoxyphene HCl 65 mg, aspirin 227 mg, phenacetin 162 mg, caffeine 32.4 mg/Cap. Bot. 500s.
Use: Narcotic analgesic combination.

PROCARBAZINE HCl, U.S.P. XXI. Cap., U.S.P. XXI. Benzamide, N-(1-methylethyl)-4-[(2-methylhy- drazino)methyl]-HCl. (Roche) Natulan.
Use: Cytostatic, Antineoplastic.
See: Matulane, Cap. (Roche).

PROCARDIA. (Pfizer) Nifedipine 10 mg or 20 mg/Cap. Bot. 100s, 300s, UD 100s.
Use: Calcium channel blocking agent.

PROCARDIA XL. (Pfizer) Nifedipine 30 mg, 60 mg or 90 mg/SR Tab. **30 mg, 60 mg:** Bot. 100s, UD 100s. **90 mg:** Bot 100s.
Use: Calcium channel blocking agent.

•**PROCATEROL HYDROCHLORIDE.** USAN.
Use: Bronchodilator.

PROCEPTION SPERM NUTRIENT DOUCHE. (Milex) Ringer type glucose douche. Bot. ample for 10 douches.
Use: Contraceptive.

•**PROCHLORPERAZINE,** U.S.P. XXII. Supp., U.S.P. XXII. 10H-Phenothiazine, 2-chloro-10-[3-(4-methyl-1-piperazinyl)propyl]-.
Use: Antiemetic.
See: Compazine, Preps. (SmithKline).
W/Isopropamide.
See: Iso-Perazine, Cap. (Lemmon).

•**PROCHLORPERAZINE EDISYLATE,** U.S.P. XXII. Inj., Oral Soln., Syr., U.S.P. XXII. 10H-Phenothiazine, 2-chloro-10-[3-(4-methyl-1-piperazinyl)propyl]-1,2-ethanedisulfonate (1:1).
Use: Tranquilizer, antiemetic.
See: Compazine, Preps. (SmithKline).

PROCHLORPERAZINE ETHANEDISULFONATE. Prochlorperazine Edisylate, U.S.P. XXII.
Use: Tranquilizing agent.

PROCHLORPERAZINE/ISOPROPAMIDE. (Various Mfr.) Isopropamide iodide 5 mg, prochlorperazine maleate 10 mg/Cap. Bot. 100s, 500s, 1000s, UD 100s.
Use: Anticholinergic/antispasmodic, antiemetic/antivertigo agent.

•**PROCHLORPERAZINE MALEATE,** U.S.P. XXII. Tab., U.S.P. XXII. 10H-Phenothiazine, 2-chloro-10-[3-(4-methyl-1-piperazinyl)-propyl]-(Z)-2-butenedio- ate (1:2).
Use: Antiemetic, tranquilizer.
See: Compazine, Preps. (SmithKline).

•**PROCINONIDE.** USAN.
Use: Adrenocortical steroid.

PROCLAN EXPECTORANT WITH CODEINE. (Cenci) Promethazine HCl, codeine phosphate, ipecac, potassium guaiacolsulfonate/5 ml. Bot.
Use: Antihistamine, antitussive, expectorant.

PROCLAN VC EXPECTORANT WITH CODEINE. (Cenci) Codeine phosphate 10 mg, promethazine HCl 5 mg, phenylephrine HCl 5 mg, fluidextract ipecac 0.17 min, potassium guaiacolsulfonate 44 mg, citric acid anhydrous 60 mg, sodium citrate 197 mg/5 ml, alcohol 7%. Bot.
Use: Antitussive, antihistamine, decongestant, expectorant.

•**PROCLONOL.** USAN. Bis(p-chlorophenyl)-cyclopropylmethanol. Under study.
Use: Acaricide, fungicide.

PRO COMFORT ATHLETE'S FOOT SPRAY. (Scholl) Tolnaftate 1%. Aerosol Can 4 oz.
Use: Antifungal, external.

PRO COMFORT JOCK ITCH SPRAY POWDER. (Scholl) Tolnaftate 1%. Aerosol can 3.5 oz.
Use: Antifungal, external.

PROCTOCORT. (Solvay) Hydrocortisone 1%. Cream 30 Gm w/rectal applicator.
Use: Corticosteroid.

PROCTOCREAM-HC. (Reed & Carnrick) Hydrocortisone acetate 1%, pramoxine HCl 1%. Cream 30 Gm.
Use: Corticosteroid, local anesthetic.

PROCTOFOAM-HC. (Reed & Carnrick) Hydrocortisone acetate 1%, pramoxine HCl 1% in hydrophilic foam base. Bot. aerosol container, Aerosol foam 10 Gm w/applicator.
Use: Corticosteroid, local anesthetic.

PROCTOFOAM N.S. (Reed & Carnrick) Pramoxine HCl 1%. Aerosol Bot. 10 Gm w/applicator.
Use: Local anesthetic.

PROCTOFORM. (Fellows) Bismuth subiodide 0.125 gr, zinc oxide 2.5 gr, bismuth subcarbonate 0.9 gr, boric acid 4 gr, isobutyl-propyl-para-aminobenzoic acid 1 gr/Supp. Box 12s.
Use: Antiseptic, analgesic.

PRO-CUTE CREAM. (Ferndale) Silicone, hexachlorophene, lanolin. 2 oz, lb.
Use: Emollient.

PRO-CUTE LOTION. (Ferndale) Hexachlorophene, silicone, lanolin. Bot. 8 oz.
Use: Emollient.

•**PROCYCLIDINE HCl,** U.S.P. XXII. Tab., U.S.P. XXII. α-Cyclohexyl-α-phenyl-1-pyrrolidinepropanol HCl.
Use: Skeletal muscle relaxant.
See: Kemadrin, Tab. (Burroughs Wellcome).

PRODERM TOPICAL DRESSING. (Hickam) Castor oil 650 mg, peruvian balsam 72.5 mg/.82 cc. Aerosol 4 oz.
Use: Prevention of decubiti.

•**PRODILIDINE HCl.** USAN. (1,2-Di- methyl-3-phenyl-3-pyrrolidyl propionate HCl.
Use: Analgesic.

•**PRODOLIC ACID.** USAN.
Use: Anti-inflammatory.

PRO-EST. (Burgin-Arden) Progesterone 25 mg, estrogenic substance 25,000 IU, sodium carboxymethylcellulose 1 mg, sodium Cl 0.9%, benzalkonium Cl 1:10,000, sodium phosphate dibasic 0.1% in water.
Use: Progestin, estrogen combination.

PRO-ESTRONE. (Pharmex) Estradiol benzoate 2.5 mg, progesterone 12.5 mg/ml. Vial 10 ml.
Use: Estrogen, progestin combination.

PROESTRONE. (Rocky Mtn.) Progesterone 25 mg, estrone 2.5 mg/ml. Vial 10 ml.
Use: Progestin, estrogen combination.

•**PROFADOL HCl.** USAN. m-(1-Methyl-3-propyl-3-pyrrolidinyl)phenol HCl.
Use: Analgesic.

PROFAMINA.
See: Amphetamine (Various Mfr.).

PROFASI HP. (Serono) Chorionic gonadotropin 5000 units or 10,000 units/Vial. With 1 vial product and 1 vial diluent (w/mannitol and benzyl alcohol).
Use: Chorionic gonadotropin.

PROFENAL. (Alcon) Suprofen 1% soln. Drop-Tainer 2.5 ml.
Use: Nonsteroidal anti-inflammatory drug, ophthalmic.

PROFESSIONAL CARE LOTION, EXTRA STRENGTH. (Walgreen) Zinc oxide 0.25% in a lotion base. Bot. 16 oz.
Use: Astringent, antiseptic, skin protectant.

PROFIBER LIQUID. (Sherwood) Sodium caseinate, dietary fiber from soy, calcium caseinate, hydrolyzed cornstarch, corn oil, soy lecithin, vitamins A, B_1, B_2, B_3, B_5, B_6, B_{12}, C, D, E, K, folic acid, biotin, choline, Ca, Cl, Cr, Cu, Fe, I, Mg, Mn, Mo, P, Se, Zn. Can 250 ml, closed system 1000 ml.
Use: Enteral nutritional supplement.

PROFILININE HEAT-TREATED. (Alpha Therapeutics) Dried plasma fraction of coagulation factors II, VII, IX and X. Heparin free. Vial, single dose with diluent.
Use: Antihemophilic.

PROFLAVINE.
Use: Topical, antiseptic.

PROFLAVINE DIHYDROCHLORIDE. 3,6-Diaminoacridine dihydrochloride.

PROFLAVINE SULFATE. 3,6-Diaminoacridine sulfate.

PROFREE/GP. (Allergan) Papain, sodium Cl, sodium borate, sodium carbonate, edetate disodium. Kit 24s.
Use: Rigid gas permeable contact lens care.

•**PROGABIDE.** USAN.
Use: Anticonvulsant, muscle relaxant.

PROGELAN. (Lannett) Progesterone 25 mg, 50 mg or 100 mg/ml in oil. Vial 10 ml.
Use: Progestin.

PROGELAN AQUEOUS. (Lannett) Progesterone 25 mg or 50 mg, aqueous susp./ml. Vial 10 ml.
Use: Progestin.

PROGENS TABS. (Major) Conjugated estrogens. **0.625 mg/Tab.:** Bot. 100s, 1000s; **1.25 mg/Tab.:** Bot. 1000s; **2.5 mg/Tab.:** Bot. 100s, 1000s.
Use: Estrogen.

PROGESTASERT. (Alza) T-shaped intrauterine device (IUD) unit containing a reservoir of progesterone 38 mg with barium sulfate dispersed in medical grade silicone fluid. In 6s w/inserter.
Use: Contraceptive, progestin.

•**PROGESTERONE,** U.S.P. XXII. Inj., Sterile Susp. U.S.P. XXII. 4-Pregnene-3,20-dione. Corpus luteum hormone. Flavolutan, Luteogan, Luteosan, Lutren.
Use: Progestin.

Aqueous. Susp.
See: Gesterol, Aqueous, Vial (Fellows-Testagar).
Progelan Aqueous, Vial (Lannett).
Prorone, Inj. (Sig).

In Oil
See: Femotrone, Inj. (Bluco).
Gesterol, Inj. (Fellows-Testagar).
Lipo-Lutin, Amp. (Parke-Davis).
Progelan, Vial (Lannett).
Progestin, Vial (Various Mfr.).
Prorone, Inj. (Sig).

Tab., Sublingual.
W/Estradiol benzoate.
See: Pro-Estrone, Vial (Pharmex).
W/Estradiol, testosterone, procaine HCl, procaine base.
See: Hormo-Triad, Vial (Bell).
W/Estrogenic substance.
See: Profoygen Aqueous (Foy).
Progex, Inj. (Pasadena Research).
W/Estrone.
See: Proestrone, Inj. (Rocky Mtn.).

PROGESTERONE INTRAUTERINE CONTRACEPTIVE SYSTEM, U.S.P. XXII.
Use: Contraceptive.

PROGESTERONE-LIKE.
See: Haloprogesterone.
Norethynodrel.

PROGESTIN. Progesterone (Various Mfr.).

PRO-GESTIVE. (Nutrition) Pepsin 200 mg, pancreatin 200 mg, bile salts 100 mg, dehydrocholic acid 30 mg/Tab. Bot. 60s.

Use: Digestive aid.

PROGESTIVE TABLETS. (NCP) Dehydrocholic acid 25 mg, bile salts 150 mg, pepsine 250 mg, pancreatin 300 mg/Tab. Bot. 60s.
Use: Digestive aid.

PROGIATRIC. (Nutrition) Calcium L-glutamate 3 Gm, l-lysine 25 mg, vitamin C 30 mg, calcium 300 mg, iron 10 mg, A 4000 IU, B_1 1 mg, B_2 1.2 mg, B_6 1 mg, B_{12} 5 mcg, folic acid 25 mcg, calcium pantothenate 1 mg, niacin 50 mg/2 Tab. Bot. 90s.
Use: Vitamin/mineral supplement.

•**PROGLUMIDE.** USAN. (±)-4-Benzamido-N,N-dipropylglutaramic acid. Nulsa (Wallace).
Use: Anticholinergic.

PROGLYCEM. (Medical Market Specialties) **Cap.:** Diazoxide 50 mg/Cap. Bot. 100s. **Oral Susp.:** Diazoxide 50 mg/ml. Bot. 30 ml w/calibrated dropper.
Use: Glucose elevating agent.

PROGUANIL HYDROCHLORIDE.
See: Chloroguanide Hydrochloride.
Paludrine, Tab. (Wyeth-Ayerst).

PROHEPTAZINE. B.A.N. Hexahydro-1,3-dimethyl-4-phenyl-1H-azepin-4-ol propionate (ester).
Use: Analgesic.

PROHIBIT. (Connaught) Purified capsular polysaccharide 25 mcg, conjugated diphtheria toxoid protein 18 mcg/0.5 ml dose. Inj. Vial 1 dose, 5 dose, 10 dose.
Use: Agent for immunization.

PRO-HYDRO. (Mills) Protein hydrolysates (45% amino acids) 50 gr, iron 46 mg, l-lysine HCl 600 mg, dl-methione 75 mg, niacinamide 30 mg, vitamins B_1 3 mg, B_2 2 mg, B_6 2 mg, B_{12} 3 mcg, C 60 mg, calcium pantothenate 12 mg/6 Tab. Bot. 168s.
W/O Iron. Same formula as above without iron.
W/Vitamin E. Same formula with vitamin E 30 IU.
Use: Vitamin/mineral supplement.

PROKINE. (Hoechst-Roussel) Sargramostim (GM-CSF).
Use: Adjunct in bone marrow transplantation.

PROLACTIN RIA. (Abbott Diagnostics) Quantitative measurement of total circulating human prolactin. Test unit 50s, 100s.
Use: Diagnostic aid.

PROLACTIN RIABEAD. (Abbott Diagnostics) Radioimmunoassay for the quantitative measurement of prolactin in human serum and plasma.
Use: Diagnostic aid.

PROLADYL. Pyrrobutamine. 1-Pyrrolidyl-3-phenyl-4-(p-chlorophenyl)-2-butene phosphate.
Use: Antihistamine.

PROLAMINE. (Thompson Medical) Phenylpropanolamine HCl 37.5 mg/Tab.
Use: Diet aid.

PROLASE. Proteolytic enzyme from *Carica papaya.*
See: Papain.
W/Mylase, cellase, calcium carbonate, magnesium glycinate.
See: Zylase, Tab. (Vitarine).

PROLASTIN. (Cutter) Alpha$_1$-proteinase inhibitor E 20 mg alpha$_1$-PI/ml when reconstituted. W/polyethylene glycol, sucrose and small amounts of other plasma proteins. Inj. Vial, single dose.
Use: Alpha$_1$-proteinase inhibitor.

PROLENE. (Ethicon) Surgical suture, nonabsorbable.

PROLENS. (Ketchum) Bot. 2 oz.
Use: Contact lens care.

•**PROLINE,** U.S.P. XXII. $C_5H_9NO_2$ as L-proline.
Use: Amino acid.

PROLINTANE. B.A.N. 1-(α-Propylphenethyl)-pyrrolidine. 1-Phenyl-2-(pyrrolidin-1-yl)pentane. Villescon.
Use: Tonic.

•**PROLINTANE HYDROCHLORIDE.** USAN.
Use: Antidepressant.

PROLIXIN. (Princeton) Fluphenazine HCl. **Tab.:** 1 mg. Bot. 50s, 500s; 2.5 mg. w/tartrazine. Bot. 50s, 500s; 5 mg. w/tartrazine. Bot. 500s, UD 100s; 10 mg. w/tartrazine. Bot. 50s, 500s. **Elixir:** 0.5 mg/ml, alcohol 14%. Dropper Bot. 60 ml. Bot. pt. **Inj.:** 2.5 mg/ml. Vial 10 ml w/methyl and propyl parabens. Unimatic syringe 1 ml, Single dose syringe 25 mg/ml. 10s.
Use: Antipsychotic agent.

PROLIXIN CONCENTRATE. (Princeton) Fluphenazine HCl 5 mg/ml, alcohol 14%. Bot. 120 ml w/dropper.
Use: Antipsychotic agent.

PROLIXIN DECANOATE. (Princeton) Fluphenazine decanoate 25 mg/ml (in sesame oil with benzyl alcohol). Unimatic syringe 1 ml. Vial 5 ml.
Use: Antipsychotic agent.

PROLIXIN ENANTHATE. (Princeton) Fluphenazine enanthate 25 mg/ml (in sesame oil with benzyl alcohol). Vial 5 ml.
Use: Antipsychotic agent.

PROLOID. (Parke-Davis) Thyroglobulin. **0.5 gr, 1 gr, 1.5 gr or 3 gr/Tab.:** Bot. 100s, 1000s. **2 gr/Tab.:** Bot. 100s.
Use: Thyroid hormone.

PROLOPRIM. (Burroughs Wellcome) Trimethoprim 100 mg/Tab. Bot. 100s, UD 100s (in sesame oil with benzyl alcohol).
Use: Urinary anti-infective.

PROMACHLOR. (Geneva) Chlorpromazine HCl 10 mg, 25 mg, 50 mg, 100 mg or 200 mg/Tab. Bot. 100s, 1000s.
Use: Antiemetic/antivertigo, antipsychotic agent.

•**PROMAZINE HCl,** U.S.P. XXII. Inj., Oral Soln., Syr., Tab., U.S.P. XXII. 10-(α-Dimethylamino-n-propyl) phenothiazine HCl. 10-[3-(Dimethylamino)propyl]- phenothiazine monohydrochloride.
Use: Ataraxic, anticholinergic.
See: Sparine, Tab., Inj. (Wyeth-Ayerst).

PROMEGA. (Parke-Davis) Omega-3 (N-3) polyunsaturated fatty acids 1000 mg, containing

EPA 350 mg, DHA 150 mg, vitamins E (3% RDA), A, B_1, B_2, B_3, Ca, Fe (> 2% RDA)/Cap., cholesterol and sodium free. Bot. 30s.
Use: Vitamin/mineral supplement.

PROMETH-50. (Seatrace) Promethazine HCl 50 mg/ml. Vial 10 ml.
Use: Antihistamine, antiemetic/antivertigo.

PROMETH EXPECTORANT. (Medwick) With or without codeine. Bot. 4 oz, pt, gal.
W/Dextromethorphan. Bot. 4 oz, pt, gal.
Use: Antihistamine, antitussive.

PROMETH EXPECTORANT VC. (Medwick) With or without codeine. Bot. 4 oz, pt, gal.
Use: Antihistamine, antitussive.

PROMETH WITH CODEINE COUGH SYRUP. (Goldline) Promethazine 6.25 mg, codeine phosphate 10 mg, alcohol 7%. Pt, gal.
Use: Antihistamine, antitussive/antivertigo.

PROMETHASTAN. (Standex) Promethazine 25 mg or 50 mg/ml. Vial 10 ml.
Use: Antihistamine, antiemetic.

PROMETHAZINE. B.A.N. 10(2-Dimethylaminopropyl)phenothiazine. Phenergan hydrochloride.
Use: Antihistamine; antiemetic, sedative.

PROMETHAZINE-50. (Kenyon) Promethazine HCl 50 mg, sodium formaldehyde sulfoxylate 0.75 mg, sodium metabisulfite 0.25 mg, disodium EDTA 0.1 mg, calcium Cl 0.04 mg, phenol 5 mg, buffered with sodium acetate/ml. Vial 10 ml.
Use: Antihistamine.

PROMETHAZINE CHLOROTHEOPHYLLINATE.
See: Promethazine Theoclate, B.A.N.

PROMETHAZINE HCl WITH CODEINE. (Various Mfr.) Promethazine HCl 6.25 mg, codeine phosphate 10 mg/5 ml, alcohol 7%. Syr. Bot. 120 ml, pt, gal.
Use: Antihistamine, antitussive.

PROMETHAZINE HYDROCHLORIDE, U.S.P. XXII. Tab., Syr., Inj., Supp., U.S.P. XXII. 10H-Phenothiazine-10- ethanamine, N,N-trimethyl-, HCl. 10-(2-Dime- thylaminopropyl)phenothiazine HCl.
Use: Antihistamine, antiemetic.
See: Fellozine, Inj. (Fellows-Testagar).
Methazine, Vial (Pharmex).
Pentazine, Expectorant, Vial (Century).
Phenergan, Preps. (Wyeth-Ayerst).
Phenerhist, Inj. (Rocky Mtn.).
Phenerject, Vial (Mayrand).
Prorex, Vial, Amp. (Hyrex).
Provigan, Inj. (Solvay).
Remsed, Tab. (Du Pont).
Rolamethazine, Prods. (Robinson).
Sigazine, Inj. (Sig).

PROMETHAZINE HCl W/COMBINATIONS.
Use: Antihistamine, antiemetic/antivertigo.
See: Mepergan, Vial, Cap. (Wyeth-Ayerst).
Phenergan-D, Tab. (Wyeth-Ayerst).
Phenergan VC Expectorant (Wyeth-Ayerst).
Rolamethazine, Prods. (Robinson).

PROMETHAZINE THEOCLATE. B.A.N. Promethazine salt of 8-chlorotheophylline. Promethazine chlorotheophyllinate. Avomine.
Use: Antihistamine; antiemetic; sedative.

PROMETHAZINE VC. (PBI) Promethazine HCl 6.25 mg, phenylephrine HCl 5 mg/5 ml, alcohol 7%. Bot. 4 oz, pt, gal.
Use: Antihistamine, decongestant.

PROMETHAZINE VC WITH CODEINE. (PBI) Promethazine HCl 6.25 mg, phenylephrine HCl 5 mg, codeine 10 mg/5 ml, alcohol 7%. Bot. 4 oz, pt, gal.
Use: Antihistamine, decongestant, antitussive.

PROMETHESTROL. B.A.N. 3,4-Di-(4-hydroxy- 3-methylphenyl)hexane. Methestrol (I.N.N.).
Use: Estrogen.

PROMETHESTROL DIPROPIONATE.
Use: Estrogen.
See: Meprane Dipropionate, Tab. (Reed & Carnrick).
W/Phenobarbital.
See: Meprane-Phenobarbital, Tab. (Reed & Carnrick).

PROMETOL. (Viobin) Concentrated wheat germ oil. **3 min/Cap.:** Bot. 100s, 250s. **10 min/Cap.:** Bot. 100s.

PROMINAL.
See: Mephobarbital.

PROMINE. (Major) Procainamide 250 mg, 375 mg or 500 mg/Cap. Bot. 100s, 250s, 1000s, UD 100s (375 mg/Cap. w/500s instead of 250s).
Use: Antiarrhythmic.

PROMINE S.R. (Major) Procainamide. **SR Tab.:** 250 mg. Bot. 100s, 250s; 500 mg. Bot. 100s, 250s, 1000s; 750 mg. Bot. 100s, 250s. **SR Cap.:** 250 mg, 375 mg or 500 mg.
Use: Antiarrhythmic.

PRO-MIN-VITE. (Drug Industries) Vitamins A 10,000 IU, D 1000 IU, E 3 IU, C 100 mg, B_1 10 mg, B_2 3 mg, B_6 2 mg, citrus bioflavonoids 25 mg, calcium pantothenate 10 mg, niacin 20 mg, B_{12} 2 mcg, biotin 0.1 mg, l-lysine 25 mg, iron 20 mg, copper 0.5 mg, manganese 2 mg, molybdenum 0.5 mg, zinc 1 mg, potassium 5 mg, magnesium 5 mg, iodine 0.1 mg/Tab. Bot. 100s, 500s.
Use: Vitamin/mineral supplement.

PROMIST HD. (Russ) Hydrocodone bitartrate 2.5 mg, pseudoephedrine HCl 30 mg, chlorpheniramine maleate 2 mg/5 ml, alcohol 5%, menthol, saccharin, sorbitol. Bot. pt.
Use: Antitussive, decongestant, antihistamine.

PROMIST LA. (Russ) Pseudoephedrine HCl 120 mg, guaifenesin 500 mg/Tab. Bot. 100s.
Use: Decongestant, expectorant.

PROMIT. (Pharmacia) Dextran 1 150 mg/ml Inj. Vial 20 ml.
Use: Dextran adjunct.

PRO-MIX R.D.P. (Navaco) Protein 15 Gm (from whey protein), fat 0.8 Gm, carbohydrate 1 Gm, sodium 46 mg, potassium 165 mg, chloride 46 mg, calcium 73.6 mg, phosphorus 64.4 mg, iron

0.3 mg, Cr, Cu, Mg, Mn, Mo, Se, Zn, 72 Cal./5 Tbsp. (20 Gm). Pow. Packet 20 Gm, can 300 Gm.
Use: Enteral nutritional supplement.

PROMOD. (Ross) Protein supplement. Nine scoops provides protein 45 Gm, 100% U.S. RDA. Pow. Can 9.7 oz.
Use: Enteral nutritional supplement.

PROMOXALAN. B.A.N. 2,2-Diisopropyl-1,3-dioxolane-4-methanol. 4-Hydroxymethyl-2,2-di-isopropyl-1,3-dioxolan.
Use: Skeletal muscle relaxant.

PROMPT. (DePree) **Spray:** Benzocaine 1.5%, parachlorometaxylenol 0.5%. Can 5 oz. **Lot.:** Benzocaine 1%, triclosan 0.2%. Bot. 4 oz. **Tab.:** Acetaminophen 5 gr, Bot. 50s, 100s, 200s.
Use: Anesthetic, analgesic.

PROMYLIN ENTERIC COATED MICROZYMES. (Shear/Kershman) Enteric coated pancrelipase. Lipase 4000 units, amylase 20,000 units, protease 25,000 units.
Use: Digestive enzymes.

PRO-NASYL. (Progonasyl Co.) o-Iodobenzoic acid 0.5%, triethanolamine 5.5% in a special neutral hydrophilic base compounded from oleic acid, mineral oil, vegetable oil. Bot. 15 ml, 60 ml.
Use: Treatment of sinusitis.

PRONESTYL. (Princeton) Procainamide. **Cap.:** 250 mg. Bot. 100s, 1000s; 375 mg. Bot. 100s; 500 mg. Bot. 100s, 1000s. **Inj.:** 100 mg/ml w/ benzyl alcohol 0.9%, sodium bisulfite 0.09%. Vial 10 ml; 500 mg/ml w/methylparaben 0.1%, sodium bisulfite 0.2%. Vial 2 ml. **Tab.:** 250 mg. Bot. 100s, 1000s, Unimatic 100s; 375 mg. Bot. 100s; 500 mg. Bot. 100s, 1000s, Unimatic 100s.
Use: Antiarrhythmic.

PRONESTYL-SR. (Princeton) Procainamide 500 mg/Tab. Bot. UD 100s.
Use: Antiarrhythmic.

PRONETHALOL. B.A.N. 2-Isopropylamino-1-(2-naphthyl)-ethanol. Alderlin hydrochloride.
Use: Adrenergic beta-receptor blocking agent.

PRONETHELOL (I.C.I.) Adrenergic beta-receptor antagonist; pending release.

PRONTO CONCENTRATE LICE KILLING SHAMPOO KIT. (Commerce) Pyrethrins 0.33%, piperonyl butoxide technical 4%. Bot. 2 oz, 4 oz.
Use: Pediculicide.

PRONTO GEL. (Commerce) Tube 2 oz.
Use: Analgesic.

PRONTO LICE KILLING SPRAY. (Commerce) 3-phenoxybenzyl d-cis and trans 2,2 dimethyl 3-(2-methylpropenyl) cyclopropanecarboxylate. Spray cans 5 oz.
Use: Pediculicide for inanimate objects.

PROPAC. (Biosearch) Protein 3 Gm (from whey protein), carbohydrate 0.2 Gm, fat 0.3 Gm, chloride 3 mg, potassium 20 mg, sodium 9 mg, calcium 24 mg, phosphorus 12 mg, 16 Cal./ Tbsp. (4 Gm). Pow. Packet 19.5 Gm, Can 350 Gm.
Use: Enteral nutritional supplement.

PROPACET 100. (Lemmon) Propoxyphene napsylate 100 mg, acetaminophen 650 mg/Tab. Bot. 100s, 500s, UD 100s.
Use: Narcotic analgesic combination.

PROPAESIN. Propyl p-Aminobenzoate. (Various Mfr.).

•**PROPAFENONE HYDROCHLORIDE.** USAN.
Use: Antiarrhythmic.
See: Rythmol, Tab. (Knoll).

PROPAGEST TABLETS. (Carnrick) Phenylpropanolamine HCl 25 mg/Tab. Bot. 100s.
Use: Decongestant.

PROPAGON-S. (Spanner) Estrone 2 mg or 5 mg/ml. Vial 10 ml.
Use: Estrogen.

PROPAIN HC. (Springbok) Acetaminophen 500 mg, hydrocodone bitartrate 5 mg/Cap. Bot. 100s, 500s.
Use: Narcotic analgesic combination.

PROPAMIDINE. B.A.N. 1,3-Di-(4-amidinophenoxy)-propane. Brolene isethionate.
Use: Bactericide; fungicide.

•**PROPANE,** N.F. XVII.
Use: Aerosol propellant.

PROPANEDIOL DIACETATE, 1,2.
See: VoSol, Liq. (Wampole).

1,2,3-PROPANETRIOL, TRINITRATE. Nitroglycerin Tab., U.S.P. XXII.

•**PROPANIDID.** USAN. [4- { (Diethylcarbamoyl)-methoxy } -3-methoxyphenyl] acetic acid propyl ester. Propyl 4-diethylcarbamoylmethoxy-3-methoxyphenylacetate. Epontol.
Use: Systemic anesthetic.

PROPANOLOL. 1-Isopropylamino-3-(l-napthyloxy)propan-2-ol. Propranolol.

•**PROPANTHELINE BROMIDE,** U.S.P. XXII. Sterile, Tabs., U.S.P. XXII. 2-Propanaminium, N-methyl-N-(1-methylethyl)-N-[2-](9H-xanthen-9-ylcarbonyl)oxy[ethyl]-, Br.
Use: Anticholinergic.
See: Pro-Banthine, Preps. (Searle).
Robantaline, Tab. (Robinson).
Spastil, Tab. (Kenyon).
W/Phenobarbital.
See: Probital, Tab. (Searle).
Robantaline with Phenobarbital (Robinson).
W/Thiopropazate dihydrochloride.
See: Pro-Banthine W/Dartal, Tab. (Searle).

PROPA PH MEDICATED ACNE CREAM WITH ALOE. (Commerce) Salicylic acid 2%. Tube 1 oz.
Use: Anti-acne.

PROPA PH MEDICATED ACNE STICK WITH ALOE. (Commerce) Salicylic acid 2%. Stick 0.05 oz.
Use: Anti-acne.

PROPA PH SKIN CLEANSER WITH ALOE. (Commerce) Salicylic acid USP 0.5%, SD alcohol 40 25%. Bot. 6 oz, 10 oz.

Use: Anti-acne.
PROPA PH MEDICATED CLEANSING PADS WITH ALOE. (Commerce) Salicylic acid 0.5%, SD alcohol 40 25%, aloe. Jar containing 45 pads.
Use: Anti-acne.
•**PROPARACAINE HCl,** U.S.P. XXII. Ophth. Soln., U.S.P. XXII. Benzoic acid, 3-amino-4-propoxy-, 2-(diethylamino)ethyl ester, HCl. Proxymetacaine, B.A.N.
Use: Anesthetic (topical, ophthalmic).
See: Alcaine Ophthalmic Soln. (Alcon).
Ophthaine HCl, Soln. (Squibb Mark).
Ophthetic, Ophthalmic Soln. (Allergan).
•**PROPATYL NITRATE.** USAN. 2-Ethyl-2-hydroxymethyl-1,3-propanedioltrinitrate. Ettriol Trinitrate. 1,1,1-Trisnitratomethylpropane. Etrynit; Gina. Investigational drug in U.S. but available in England.
Use: Coronary vasodilator.
PROPAZOLAMIDE. 2-Propionylamino-1,3,4-thiadiazole-5-sulfonamide. Ionaze (Lilly).
p-PROPENYLANISOLE. Anethole, N.F. XVII.
•**PROPENZOLATE HYDROCHLORIDE.** USAN. 1-Methyl-3-piperidyl-α-phenylcyclohexaneglycolate HCl.
Use: Anticholinergic.
PROPERIDINE. B.A.N. Isopropyl 1-methyl-4-phenyl-piperidine-4-carboxylate.
Use: Narcotic analgesic.
PROPESIN. Name used for Risocaine.
PROPHENE 65. (Halsey) Propoxyphene HCl 65 mg/Cap. Bot. 100s, 500s, 1000s.
Use: Narcotic analgesic.
PROPHENPYRIDAMINE.
See: Pheniramine (Various Mfr.).
PROPHENPYRIDAMINE MALEATE.
See: Pheniramine Maleate.
PROPHENPYRIDAMINE MALEATE W/COMBINATIONS.
See: Histjen, Cap. (Jenkins).
Hist-Span No. 2, Cap. (Kenyon).
Panadyl, Tab., Cap. (Misemer).
Polyectin, Liq. (Amid).
Trimahist Elix., Liq. (Tennessee).
Vasotus, Liq. (Sheryl).
PROPHYLLIN. (Rystan) **Pow.:** Sodium propionate 1%, water soluble chlorophyllin 0.0025%. Box packet 12s, 2.3 Gm pow./packet for preparation of 8 fl oz. Jar 4 oz., bulk powder. **Oint.:** Sodium propionate 5%, chlorophyll derivatives 0.0125%. Tube 1 oz.
Use: Anti-infective, external.
PROPICILLIN. B.A.N. 6-(α-Phenoxybutyramido)-penicillanic acid(1-Phenoxypropyl)penicillin. Brocillin & Ultrapen are the potassium salt.
Use: Antibiotic.
•**PROPIKACIN.** USAN.
Use: Antibacterial.
PROPINE STERILE OPHTHALMIC SOLUTION. (Allergan) Dipivefrin HCl 0.1%, benzalkonium Cl 0.004%, mannitol, sodium metabisulfite, edetate disodium. Bot. 5 ml, 10 ml, 15 ml.
Use: Agent for glaucoma.
PROPIODAL.
See: Entodon.
•**PROPIOLACTONE.** USAN. 2-Oxetanone; beta-propiolactone, Betaprone. Hydracrylic acid, β-lactone.
Use: Sterilization of vaccines and tissue grafts.
•**PROPIOMAZINE.** USAN. 1-[10-(2-Dimethylaminopropyl)-phenothiazine-2-yl]-1-propanone. Dorevane; Indorm.
Use: Sedative.
See: Largon, Amp. (Wyeth-Ayerst).
•**PROPIOMAZINE HYDROCHLORIDE,** U.S.P. XXII. Inj., U.S.P. XXII. 1-[10-[2-(Dimethylamino)propyl]- phenothiazin-2-yl]-1-propanone HCl.
Use: Sedative.
See: Largon, Inj. (Wyeth-Ayerst).
•**PROPIONIC ACID,** N.F. XVII.
Use: Antimicrobial.
W/Sodium propionate, docusate sodium, salicylic acid.
See: Prosal, Liq. (Gordon).
Propionate-Caprylate Mixtures.
PROPIONATE COMPOUND.
See: Propion Gel (Wyeth-Ayerst).
PROPIONATE SALTS.
See: Copper.
Potassium.
Sodium.
Zinc.
PROPIONYL ERYTHROMYCIN LAURYL SULFATE.
See: Erythromycin Propionate Lauryl Sulfate.
•**PROPIRAM FUMARATE.** USAN. N-(1-Methyl-2-pipe-ridinoethyl)-N-(2-pyridyl) propionamide fumarate. 1:1.
Use: Analgesic.
PROPISAMINE.
See: Amphetamine (Various Mfr.).
PROPITOCAINE. Prilocaine.
See: Citanest, Soln., Vial, Amp. (Astra).
PROPLEX. (Hyland) Factor IX Complex (Human), clotting Factor II (prothrombin), VII (proconvertin), IX (PTC, antihemophilic factor B) and X (Stuart-Prower factor) all dried and concentrated. Vial 30 ml w/Diluent.
Use: Antihemophilic.
PROPLEX T. (Hyland) Factor IX complex, heat treated. W/Factors II, VII, IX and X. W/heparin. Dried concentrate. Vial w/diluent.
Use: Antihemophilic.
•**PROPOFOL.** USAN.
Use: Anesthetic.
PROPONADE CAPSULES. (Blue Cross) Chlorpheniramine maleate 8 mg, phenylpropanolamine HCl 50 mg, isopropamide 2.5 mg/Cap. Bot. 100s.
Use: Antihistamine, decongestant.
PROPOQUIN. Amopyroquin HCl.
Use: Antimalarial.

PROPOXAMIDE. o-Propoxybenzamide.

•**PROPOXYCAINE HYDROCHLORIDE,** U.S.P. XXII. 2-(Diethylamino)ethyl-4-amino-2-propoxybenzoate HCl.
Use: Local anesthetic.

•**PROPOXYCAINE AND PROCAINE HYDROCHLORIDES AND LEVONORDEFRIN INJECTION,** U.S.P. XXII.
Use: Local anesthetic (dental).

PROPOXYCAINE AND PROCAINE HYDROCHLORIDES AND NOREPINEPHRINE BITARTRATE INJECTION, U.S.P. XXII.
Use: Local anesthetic (dental).
See: Ravocaine Cartridge (Cook-Waite).

PROPOXYCHLORINOL. Toloxychlorinol.

•**PROPOXYPHENE HCl,** U.S.P. XXII. Cap. U.S.P. XXII. Benzenethanol, α[2-(dimethylamino)-1-methyl-ethyl]-α-phenyl, propanoate (ester), HCl.
Use: Analgesic.
See: Darvon, Pulvules (Lilly).
Dolene, Cap. (Lederle).
Progesic, Cap. (Ulmer).
Pro-Pox 65, Cap. (Kenyon).
Ropoxy, Cap. (Robinson).
SK-65, Cap. (SmithKline).

PROPOXYPHENE HCl W/COMBINATIONS.
Use: Analgesic.
See: Darvon Compound, Pulvule (Lilly).
Darvon Compound-65, Cap. (Lilly).
Darvon With A.S.A., Cap. (Lilly).
Dolene, AP-65, Tab. (Lederle).
Dolene Compound-65, Cap. (Lederle).
Doraphen-Compound-65, Cap. (Cenci).
Ropoxy Compound-65, Cap. (Robinson).
Wygesic, Tab. (Wyeth-Ayerst).

•**PROPOXYPHENE HCl AND ACETAMINOPHEN TABLETS,** U.S.P. XXII.
Use: Analgesic.

PROPOXYPHENE HCl AND APC CAPSULES.
Use: Analgesic.

•**PROPOXYPHENE HCl, ASPIRIN AND CAFFEINE CAPSULES,** U.S.P. XXII.
Use: Analgesic.

•**PROPOXYPHENE NAPSYLATE,** U.S.P. XXII. Oral Susp., Tab., U.S.P. XXII.
Use: Analgesic.
See: Darvocet-N (Lilly).
Darvon-N, Tab. (Lilly).
W/Acetaminophen.
See: Darvocet-N, Tab. (Lilly).

•**PROPOXYPHENE NAPSYLATE AND ACETAMINOPHEN TABLETS,** U.S.P. XXII.
Use: Analgesic.

•**PROPOXYPHENE NAPSYLATE AND ASPIRIN TABLETS,** U.S.P. XXII.
Use: Analgesic.

•**PROPRANOLOL HYDROCHLORIDE,** U.S.P. XXII. Inj., Tab., U.S.P. XXII. 2-Propanol, 1-[(1-methylethyl)amino]-3-(1-naphthalenyloxy)-, HCl. Propanolol HCl. **Oral Soln.** (Roxane): 20 mg or 40 mg/5 ml. Patient cups UD 5 ml (10s). **Concentrated Oral Soln.** (Roxane): 80 mg/ml. Bot. 30 ml w/calibrated dropper.
Use: Antiarrhythmic agent.
See: Inderal, Tab., Inj. (Wyeth-Ayerst).

•**PROPRANOLOL HYDROCHLORIDE AND HYDROCHLOROTHIAZIDE TABLETS,** U.S.P. XXII.
See: Inderide, Tab. (Wyeth-Ayerst).

PROPRANOLOL HCl ITENSOL. (Roxane) Propranolol HCl 80 mg/ml concentrated oral soln. Bot. 30 ml with dropper.
Use: Beta-adrenergic blocking agent.

PROPYL p-AMINOBENZOATE. (Various Mfr.) Propaesin.
Use: Local anesthetic.
W/Procaine base, benzyl alcohol, phenol.
See: Rectocaine, Vial (Moore-Kirk).

•**PROPYL GALLATE,** N.F. XVII.
Use: Pharmaceutic aid (antioxidant).

PROPYLDOCETRIZOATE. B.A.N. Propyl 3-diacetylamino-2,4,6-tri-iodobenzoate. Pulmidol.
Use: Radio-opaque substance.

•**PROPYLENE CARBONATE,** N.F. XVII.
Use: Pharmaceutical aid (gelling agent).

•**PROPYLENE GLYCOL,** U.S.P. XXII. 1-2-Propanediol.
Use: Pharmaceutical aid (humectant, solvent).

•**PROPYLENE GLYCOL ALGINATE,** N.F. XVII.
Use: Pharmaceutical aid.

•**PROPYLENE GLYCOL DIACETATE,** N.F. XVII.
Use: Pharmaceutical aid.

PROPYLENE GLYCOL MONOSTEARATE, N.F. XVII. 1,2-Propanediol monostearate.
Use: Emulsifying agent.

•**PROPYLHEXEDRINE,** U.S.P. XXII. Inhalant, U.S.P. XXII. N,α-Dimethylcyclohexaneethylamine. Evetin HCl.
Use: Adrenergic (vasoconstrictor), appetite suppressant, antihistamine.
See: Benzedrex, Inhalant (SmithKline Prods).

•**PROPYLIODONE,** U.S.P. XXII. Sterile Oil Susp., U.S.P. XXII. 1(4H)-Pyridineacetic acid, 3,5-diiodo-4-oxo-, propyl ester. Sterile oil Susp. (peanut oil). Sterile water susp. Propyl 3,5-diiodo-4-oxopyridine-1-ylacetate. 3,5-Di-iodo-1-propoxycarbonylmethyl-4-pyridone.
Use: Radio-opaque substance.
See: Dionosil Oily (Glaxo).

iso-PROPYLNORADRENALINE.
See: Isoproterenol.

•**PROPYLPARABEN,** N.F. XVII. Propyl p-hydroxybenzoate. Propyl Chemosept (Chemo Puro).
Use: Pharmaceutic aid (antifungal preservative).

•**PROPYLPARABEN SODIUM,** N.F. XVII.
Use: Antifungal preservative.

•**PROPYLTHIOURACIL,** U.S.P. XXII. Tab., U.S.P. XXII. 4(1H)-Pyrimidinone, 2,3-dihydro-6-propyl-2-thioxopropyl. (Abbott) 50 mg/Tab. Bot. 100s, 1000s. (Lilly) 50 mg/Tab. Bot. 100s, 1000s. (Lederle) 50 mg/Tab. Bot. 100s, 1000s. 50 mg/Tab. Bot. 100s, 1000s, UD 100s.
Use: Thyroid inhibitor.

PROPYPHENAZONE. B.A.N. 4-Isopropyl-2,3-dimethyl-1-phenyl-5-pyrazolone.
Use: Analgesic.

PROQUAMEZINE. B.A.N. 10-(2,3-Bisdimethylaminopropyl)phenothiazine. Aminopromazine (I.N.N.) Myspamol.
Use: Bronchial spasmolytic.

PROQUAZONE. USAN. 1-Isopropyl-7-methyl-4-phenyl-2 (1H)-quinazolinone.
Use: Anti-inflammatory.

PROQUINOLATE. USAN.
Use: Coccidiostat.

PRORENOATE POTASSIUM. USAN.
Use: Aldosterone antagonist.

PROREX. (Hyrex) Promethazine HCl 25 mg or 50 mg/ml. Vial 10 ml.
Use: Antihistamine, antiemetic/antivertigo.

PRORONE. (Sig) Progesterone 25 mg/ml. Aqueous or oil susp. Vial 10 ml.
Use: Progestin.

PROROXAN HYDROCHLORIDE. USAN.
Use: Anti-adrenergic.

PROSCILLARIDIN. USAN. 3β, 14β-Dihydroxybufa-4,20,22-trienolide 3-rhamnoside. Talusin, Tradenal.
Use: Cardiac glycoside.

PROSOBEE. (Mead Johnson Nutrition) Milk free formula supplies 640 cal./qt, protein 19.2 Gm, fat 34 Gm, carbohydrate 64 Gm, vitamins A 2000 IU, D 400 IU, E 20 IU, C 52 mg, folic acid 100 mcg, B_1 0.5 mg, B_2 0.6 mg, niacin 8 mg, B_6 0.4 mg, B_{12} 2 mcg, biotin 50 mg, pantothenic acid 3 mg, K-1 100 mcg, choline 50 mg, inositol 30 mg, calcium 600 mg, phosphorus 475 mg, iodine 65 mcg, iron 12 mg, magnesium 70 mg, copper 0.6 mg, zinc 5 mg, manganese 1.6 mg, chloride 530 mg, potassium 780 mg, sodium 230 mg/Qt. (20 Kcal/fl oz). Concentrated liq. can 13 fl oz; Ready-to-use liq. can 8 fl oz, 32 fl oz. Pow., can 14 oz.
Use: Enteral nutritional supplement.

PROSOBEE CONCENTRATE. (Mead Johnson) P-soy protein isolate, l-methionine. CHO. corn syrup solids, soy and coconut oil, lecithin, mono and diglycerides. Protein 20.3 Gm, CHO 65.4 Gm, fat 33.6 Gm, iron 12 mg, 640 cal./serving. Concentrate 390 ml.
Use: Enteral nutritional supplement.

PRO-SOF PLUS. (Vangard) Docusate sodium 100 mg, casanthranol 30 mg/Cap. Bot. 100s, 1000s, UD 32s, 100s.
Use: Laxative.

PRO-SOF SG 100. (Vangard) Docusate sodium 100 mg/Cap. Bot. 100s, 1000s, UD 10×10s.
Use: Laxative.

PRO-SOF SG 200. (Vangard) Docusate sodium 250 mg/Cap. Bot. 100s, 500s, UD pkg. 10×10s.
Use: Laxative.

PRO-SOF SYRUP. (Vangard) Docusate sodium 20 mg/5 ml. Bot. pt.
Use: Laxative.

PRO-SOF w/CASANTHRANOL SG. (Vangard) Cansanthranol 30 mg, docusate sodium 100 mg/Cap. Bot. 100s, 1000s.
Use: Laxative.

PROSOM. (Abbott) Estazolam 1 mg or 2 mg/Tab. Bot. 100s, UD 100s.
Use: Sedative/hypnotic.

PROSTAGLANDIN E. Dinoprostone, B.A.N.
Use: Prostaglandin.

PROSTAGLANDIN F. Dinoprost, B.A.N.
Use: Prostaglandin.

•**PROSTALENE.** USAN.
Use: Prostaglandin.

PROSTAPHLIN CAPSULES. (Bristol) Sodium oxacillin 250 mg or 500 mg/Cap. Bot. 48s, 100s, Dosatrol Pack 100s.
Use: Antibacterial, penicillin.

PROSTAPHLIN FOR INJECTION. (Bristol) Crystalline oxacillin sodium 250 mg, 500 mg, 1 Gm, 2 Gm or 4 Gm/dry filled Vial. Piggyback vial 1 Gm, 2 Gm, Bulk vial 10 Gm.
Use: Antibacterial, penicillin.

PROSTAPHLIN ORAL SOLUTION. (Bristol) Sodium oxacillin reconstitute for oral soln. 250 mg/5 ml. Bot. 100 ml, Dosa-Trol Pack 25s.
Use: Antibacterial, penicillin.

PROSTIGMIN. (ICN Pharm) Injectable neostigmine methylsulfate. **1:1000**: 1 mg/ml w/phenol 0.45%. Vial 10 ml. Box 10s. **1:2000**: 0.5 mg/ml. Amp. 1 ml w/methyl and propylparabens 0.2%. Box 10s. Vial 10 ml w/phenol 0.45%. Box 10s. **1:4000**: 0.25 mg/ml Amp. 1 ml w/methyl and propylparabens 0.2%. Box 10s.
Use: Cholinergic muscle stimulant.

PROSTIGMIN BROMIDE TABLETS. (ICN Pharm) Neostigmine bromide 15 mg/Tab. Bot. 100s, 1000s.
Use: Cholinergic muscle stimulant.

PROSTIN/15 M. (Upjohn) Carboprost 250 mcg, tromethamine 83 mcg/ml. Inj. Amp. 1 ml.
Use: Abortifacient.

PROSTIN E2. Dinoprostone, B.A.N.

PROSTIN VR PEDIATRIC. (Upjohn) Alprostadil 500 mcg/ml. Amp. 1 ml. Box 5s.
Use: Agent for patent ductus arteriosus.

PROSTONIC. (Seatrace) Thiamine HCl 10 mg, alanine 130 mg, glutamic acid 130 mg, aminoacetic acid 130 mg/Cap. Bot. 100s.
Use: Palliative relief of benign prostatic hypertrophy

PROTABOLIN. (Pasadena Research) Methandriol dipropionate 50 mg/ml. Vial 10 ml.

PROTAC. (Republic) Benzocaine 10 mg, cetylpyridinium Cl 2.5 mg/Troche. In 10s.
Use: Local anesthetic, antiseptic.

•**PROTAMINE SULFATE,** U.S.P. XXII. Inj., for inj., U.S.P. XXII. (Lilly)-Amp. 1%, 5 ml; 1s, 25s; 25 ml 6s.
Use: I.V.; heparin overdosage.

•**PROTAMINE ZINC INSULIN SUSPENSION,** U.S.P. XXII.
Use: Insulin.

See: Iletin (Insulin, Lilly).
Insulin, Protamine Zinc, Susp. (Squibb).
PROTARGIN MILD.
See: Silver Protein, Mild (Various Mfr.).
PROTARGOL. (Sterwin) Strong silver protein. Pow. Bot. 25 Gm.
Use: Topical silver antiseptic.
PROTASE. (Kenyon) Standardized amount of extract of proteolytic enzymes from *Carica papaya* with 10,000 units of activity/Tab. Bot. 100s, 1000s.
Use: Digestive enzymes.
PROTEASE.
W/Pancreatin, amylase.
See: Dizymes, Cap. (Recsei).
W/Vitamins B_1, B_{12}.
See: Arcoret, Tab. (Arco).
W/Vitamins B_1, B_{12}, iron.
See: Arcoret W/Iron, Tab. (Arco).
PROTECTOL MEDICATED POWDER. (Daniels) Calcium undecyclenate 15%. Bot. 2 oz.
Use: Diaper rash product.
•**PROTEIN HYDROLYSATE INJECTION,** U.S.P. XXII.
Use: Fluid and nutrient replenisher.
See: Amigen, Inj. (Baxter Lab.).
Aminogen, Amp., Vial (Christina).
Lacotein, Vial (Christina).
Travamin, Inj. (Travenol).
Virex, Inj. (Burgin-Arden).
PROTEIN HYDROLYSATES ORAL.
Use: Enteral nutritional supplement.
See: Lofenalac, Pow. (Mead Johnson).
Nutramigen, Pow. (Mead Johnson).
Pregestimil, Pow. (Mead Johnson).
Stuart Amino Acids, Pow. (Stuart).
W/Lysine HCl, methionine, niacinamide, calcium pantothenate, vitamin B complex, C, iron.
See: Pro-Hydro, Tab. (Mills).
W/Vitamin B_{12}.
See: Stuart Amino Acids and B_{12}, Tab. (Stuart).
PROTEIN, NONSPECIFIC THERAPY.
See: Lacotein, Vial (Christina).
Mucusol, Amp., Vial (Kremers-Urban).
PROTENATE. (Hyland) Plasma protein fraction (Human) 5%. Inj. Vial 250 ml, 500 ml w/administration set.
Use: Plasma protein fraction.
PROTEOLYTIC ENZYMES.
See: Dornavac (Merck Animal Health).
Papase, Tab. (Parke-Davis).
Vardase, Prods. (Lederle).
W/Amylolytic enzyme, cellulolytic enzyme, lipolytic enzyme.
See: Arco-Lase, Tab. (Arco).
Kutrase, Cap. (Kremers-Urban).
Kuzyme, Cap. (Kremers-Urban).
Zymme, Cap. (Scrip).
W/Amylolytic enzyme, lipolytic enzyme, cellulolytic enzyme, belladonna extract.
See: Mallenzyme, Tab. (Mallard).
W/Amylolytic, cellulolytic enzymes, lipase, phenobarbital, hyoscyamine sulfate, atropine sulfate.
See: Arco-Lipase Plus, Tab. (Arco).
W/Amylolytic, cellulolytic enzymes.
See: Trienzyme, Tab. (Fellows-Testagar).
W/Amylolytic enzyme, homatropine methylbromide, d-sorbitol. (Papain).
See: Converzyme, Liq. (Ascher).
W/Calcium carbonate, glycine, amylolytic and cellulolytic enzymes.
See: Co-Gel, Tab. (Arco).
W/Neomycin palmitrate, hydrocortisone acetate, water-miscible base.
See: Biozyme, Oint. (Armour).
PROTHIONAMIDE. B.A.N. 2-Propylisonicotinthioamide.
Use: Treatment of tuberculosis.
PROTHIPENDYL. B.A.N. 10-(3-Dimethylaminopropyl)pyrido[3,2-b][1,4]benzothiazine.
Use: Tranquilizer; antiemetic.
PROTHIPENDYL HCl. [(4-Dimethyl-aminopropyl-pyrido(3,2B)Benzothiazine)] HCl-monohydrate.
Use: Sedative.
PROTICULEEN. (Spanner) Vitamin B_{12} activity 10 mcg, folic acid 10 mg, B_{12} crystalline 50 mcg, niacinamide 75 mg/ml. Multiple dose vial 10 ml. I.M. inj.
Use: Parenteral nutritional supplement.
•**PROTIRELIN.** USAN. 1-[N-(5-Oxo-L-prolyl)-L-histidyl]- -prolinamide. 5-oxo-L-histidyl-L-proline amide.
Use: Thyrotrophin releasing hormone.
See: Thypinone, Inj. (Abbott).
PROTOKYLOL. B.A.N. 1-(3,4-Dihydroxyphenyl)-2-(α-methyl-3,4-methylene-dioxyphenethylamino)-ethanol.
Use: Sympathomimetic.
PROTOPAM CHLORIDE. (Wyeth-Ayerst) **Emergency kit:** One 1 Gm/20 ml vial of pralidoxime Cl w/one 20 ml amp. diluent, disposable syringe, needle and alcohol swab. **Hospital package:** Six 20 ml vials of 1 Gm each of sterile Protopam Cl powder, without diluent or syringe.
Use: Antidote.
PROTOSAN. (Recsei) Protein 87.5%, lactose 0.5%, fat 1.3%, ash 3.5%, sodium 0.02%. Jar 1 lb, 5 lb.
Use: Nutritional supplement.
PROT-O-SEA. (Barth's) Protein 90%, containing amino acids and minerals. Bot. 100s, 500s.
Use: Nutritional supplement.
PROTOSTAT. (Ortho) Metronidazole 250 mg or 500 mg/Tab. **250 mg:** Bot. 100s. **500 mg:** Bot. 50s.
Use: Amebicide, anti-infective.
PROTOVERATRINE A.
See: Pro-Amid, Tab. (Amid).
PROTOVERATRINES A & B MALEATE.
PROTRAN PLUS. (Vangard) Meprobamate 150 mg, ethoheptazine citrate 75 mg, aspirin 250 mg/Tab. Bot. 100s. 500s.
Use: Antianxiety agent, analgesic combination.

•**PROTRIPTYLINE HYDROCHLORIDE,** U.S.P. XXII. Tab., U.S.P. XXII. N-methyl-5H-dibenzo [α,d]cycloheptene-5-propylamine HCl.
Use: Antidepressant.
See: Vivactil, Tab. (Merck Sharp & Dohme).

PROTROPIN. (Genentech) Somatrem growth hormone. Vial 5 mg w/mannitol 40 mg.
Use: Growth hormone.

PROVAL #3. (Solvay) Acetaminophen 325 mg, codeine phosphate 30 mg/Tab. Bot. 100s, 500s.
Use: Narcotic analgesic combination.

PROVATENE. (Solgar) Beta-carotene 15 mg/Soft gel perle. Bot. 60s, 180s.
Use: Vitamin A supplement.

PROVENTIL. (Schering) Albuterol sulfate 2 mg or 4 mg/Tab. Bot. 100s, 500s.
Use: Bronchodilator.

PROVENTIL INHALER. (Schering) Metered dose aerosol unit containing albuterol in propellants. Each actuation delivers 90 mcg of albuterol. Canister 17 Gm with oral adapter. Box 1s.
Use: Bronchodilator.

PROVENTIL SOLUTION. (Schering) Albuterol sulfate solution. **0.5%:** Albuterol sulfate 6 mg/ml. Bot. 20 ml. Box 1s. **0.083%:** Albuterol sulfate 0.83 mg/ml. Bot. 3 ml. Box 100s.
Use: Bronchodilator.

PROVENTIL SYRUP. (Schering) Albuterol sulfate 2 mg/5 ml. Bot. 16 oz.
Use: Bronchodilator.

PROVERA. (Upjohn) Medroxyprogesterone acetate 2.5 mg, 5 mg or 10 mg/Tab. **2.5 mg:** Bot. 25s. **5 mg:** Bot. 25s, 100s. **10 mg:** Bot. 25s, 100s, Dosepak 10s.
Use: Progestin.

PROVOCHOLINE. (Roche) Methacholine Cl for inhalation 100 mg/Vial for reconstitution. Vial 5 ml. Box 1s.
Use: Diagnostic aid.

PROX/APAP. (UAD Labs) Propoxyphene HCl 65 mg, acetaminophen 650 mg/Tab. Bot. 100s, 500s.
Use: Narcotic analgesic combination.

•**PROXAZOLE.** USAN. 5-[(2-Diethyl-amino)ethyl]-3-(α-ethyl-benzyl)-1,2,4-oxadiazole.
Use: Antispasmodic, analgesic, anti-inflammatory.

•**PROXAZOLE CITRATE.** USAN.
Use: Relaxant (smooth muscle), analgesic, anti-inflammatory.

•**PROXICROMIL.** USAN.
Use: Anti-allergic.

PROXIGEL. (Reed & Carnrick) Carbamide peroxide 11% in a water free gel base. Tube 1.2 oz.
Use: Antiseptic, cleanser.

•**PROXORPHAN TARTRATE.** USAN.
Use: Analgesic; antitussive.

PROXYMETACAINE. B.A.N. 2-Diethylaminoethyl 3-amino-4-propoxybenzoate.
Use: Local anesthetic.

PROXYPHYLLINE. B.A.N. 7-(2-Hydroxypropyl)-theophylline.
Use: Bronchodilator.

PROZAC. (Dista) Fluoxetine HCl 20 mg/Pulvule.
Use: Antidepressant.

PROZINE-50. (Hauck) Promazine HCl 50 mg/ml. Vial 10 ml.
Use: Antipsychotic agent.

PRUDENTS. (Bariatric) Acetylphenylisatin 5 mg/Tab. Bot. 30s, 100s. Chewable protein and amino acid.
Use: Laxative.

PRULET. (Mission) White phenolphthalein 60 mg/Tab. Strips 12s, 40s.
Use: Laxative.

PRUNE CONCENTRATE. W/cascarin.
See: Prucara, Tab. (ICN).

PRUNE POWDER CONCENTRATED DEHYDRATED.
See: Diacetyldihydroxyphenylisatin.
W/Cascara fluidextract aromatic and psyllium husk powder.
See: Casyllium, Pow. (Upjohn).

PRUNE PREPS.
See: Casyllium, Granules (Upjohn).

PRUN-EVAC. (Pharmex) Bot. 30s.
Use: Laxative.

PRURILO. (Whorton) Menthol 0.25%, phenol 0.25%, calamine lotion in special lubricating base. Bot. 4 oz, 8 oz.
Use: Minor skin irritations.

PSEUDO-CAR DM. (Geneva Generics) Pseudoephedrine HCl 60 mg, carbinoxamine maleate 4 mg, dextromethorphan HBr 15 mg/5 ml, alcohol $>$ 0.6%. Bot. pt, gal.
Use: Decongestant, antihistamine, antitussive.

PSEUDO-CHLOR. (Major) Pseudoephedrine HCl 120 mg, chlorpheniramine maleate 8 mg/Cap. Bot. 250s.
Use: Decongestant, antihistamine.

•**PSEUDOEPHEDRINE HYDROCHLORIDE,** U.S.P. XXII. Syrup, Tab., U.S.P. XXII. Isoephedrine HCl. α(1-Methylamino)-ethyl benzyl alcohol HCl. (+)-Pseudoephedrine HCl.
Use: Adrenergic (vasoconstrictor).
See: Cenafed, Tab., Syr. (Century).
D-Feda, Cap., Syr. (Dooner).
Novafed, Cap., Liq. (Merrell Dow).
Ro-Fedrin, Tab., Syr. (Robinson).
Sinufed, Cap. (Hauck).
Sudafed, Tab., Syr. (Burroughs Wellcome).
Sudafed S.A., Cap. (Burroughs Wellcome).
Ursinus, Inlay Tab. (Sandoz Consumer).

PSEUDOEPHEDRINE HCl W/COMBINATIONS
See: Actifed, Tab., Syr. (Burroughs Wellcome).
Ambenyl-D, Liq. (Marion).
Atridine, Tab. (Interstate).
Brexin, Cap., Liq. (Savage).
Congestac, Tab. (SmithKline Prods).
CoTylenol, Tab. (McNeil).
CoTylenol Liquid Cold Formula (McNeil).
Deconamine, Cap., Tab., Elix., Syr. (Berlex).
Dimacol, Cap., Liq. (Robins).
Dorocol, Prods. (Sandoz Consumer).

Fedrazil, Tab. (Burroughs Wellcome).
Isoclor, Preps. (American Critical Care).
Kronofed-A, Cap. (Ferndale).
Novafed A, Liq., Cap. (Merrell Dow).
Novahistine Sinus, Tab. (Merrell Dow).
Phenergan-D, Tab. (Wyeth-Ayerst).
Robitussin-DAC, Liq. (Robins).
Robitussin-PE, Liq. (Robins).
Rondec D, Drops; C, Tab.; S, Syr.; T, Filmtab (Ross).
Rondec DM, Drops, Syr. (Ross).
Sine-Off, Prods. (SmithKline Prods).
Sudafed Plus, Tab., Syr. (Burroughs Wellcome).
Triphed, Tab. (Lemmon).
Tussafed Expectorant Liq. (Cavital).
Wal-Phed, Syr., Tab. (Walgreens).

•**PSEUDOEPHEDRINE POLISTIREX.** USAN.
Use: Nasal decongestant.

•**PSEUDOEPHEDRINE SULFATE,** U.S.P. XXII.
Use: Nasal decongestant, adrenergic (bronchodilator).
See: Afrinol Repetabs (Schering).
W/Chlorpheniramine maleate.
See: Chlor-trimeton Decongestant, Tab. (Schering).
W/Dexbrompheniramine.
See: Disophrol Chronotabs, Tab. (Schering).
Drixoral S.A., Tab. (Schering).
W/Dexchlorpheniramine.
See: Polaramine Expectorant (Schering).

PSEUDOGEST. (Major) Pseudoephedrine HCl 30 mg or 60 mg/Tab. Bot. 24s, 100s.
Use: Decongestant.

PSEUDOGEST PLUS. (Major) Pseudoephedrine HCl 60 mg, chlorpheniramine maleate 4 mg/Tab. In 24s.
Use: Decongestant, antihistamine.

PSEUDO-HIST. (Holloway) Pseudoephedrine HCl 30 mg, chlorpheniramine maleate 10 mg/Cap. Bot. 100s.
Use: Decongestant, antihistamine.

PSEUDO-HIST EXPECTORANT. (Holloway) Pseudoephedrine 15 mg, hydrocodone bitartrate 2.5 mg, guaifenesin 100 mg, alcohol 5%. Bot. 480 ml.
Use: Decongestant, antitussive, expectorant.

"PSEUDO-PHEDRINE". (Whiteworth) Pseudoephedrine HCl 30 mg/Tab. Bot. 100s, 1000s.
Use: Decongestant.

PSEUDO PLUS. (Weeks & Leo) Pseudoephedrine HCl 60 mg, chlorpheniramine maleate 4 mg/Tab. Bot. 40s.
Use: Decongestant, antihistamine.

PSEUDO SYRUP. (Major) Pseudoephedrine 30 mg/5 ml. Liq. Bot. 120 ml, pt, gal.
Use: Decongestant.

PSILOCYBIN. B.A.N. (Sandoz) 3-(2-Dimethylaminoethyl)indol-4-yl dihydrogen phosphate.
Use: Psychotogenic agent.

PSORALENS.
See: Methoxsalen.
Trioxsalen.

PSORCON OINTMENT. (Dermik) Diflorasone diacetate (0.05%) 0.5 mg/Gm. Tube 15 Gm, 30 Gm, 60 Gm.
Use: Corticosteroid.

PSORIGEL. (Owen) Coal tar soln. 7.5%, alcohol 33% in hydroalcoholic gel vehicle. Tube 4 oz.
Use: Tar-containing preparation.

PSYCHOTHERAPEUTIC DRUGS.
See: Ataraxic Agents.

PSYLLIUM GRANULES.
Use: Laxative.
See: Perdiem Fiber, Gran. (Rorer Consumer).
W/Dextrose.
See: Muci-lax, Granules (Shionogi).
W/Senna.
See: Perdiem, Granules (Rorer Consumer).

•**PSYLLIUM HUSK,** U.S.P. XXII.
Use: Cathartic.
W/Cascara fluidextract aromatic, prune powder.
Use: Cathartic.
See: Casyllium, Pow. (Upjohn).

PSYLLIUM HYDROCOLLOID.
Use: Laxative.
See: Effersyllium, Pow. (Stuart).

•**PSYLLIUM HYDROPHILIC MUCILLOID FOR ORAL SUSPENSION,** U.S.P. XXII.
Use: Bulk producing laxative.
See: Aquamucil, Liq. (Cenci).
Konsyl, Pow. (Lafayette).
Modane Versabran, Pow. (Adria).
Mucillium, Pow. (Whiteworth).
W/Dextrose.
See: Hydrocil Plain (Solvay).
Konsyl-D Pow. (Lafayette).
V-lax, Pow. (Century).
W/Dextrose, casanthranol.
See: Hydrocil Fortified (Solvay).
W/Oxyphenisatin acetate.
See: Plova, Pow. (WEL).
W/Standardized senna concentrate.
See: Senokot w/Psyllium, Pow. (Purdue Frederick).

PSYLLIUM SEED GEL.
Use: Laxative.
W/Planta Ovata, gum Karaya, Brewer's yeast.
See: Plantamucin, Granules (Elder).

P.T.E.-4. (Lyphomed) Zinc 1 mg, copper 0.1 mg, chromium 1 mcg, manganese 25 mcg/ml. Vial 3 ml.
Use: Mineral supplement.

P.T.E.-5. (Lyphomed) Zinc 1 mg, copper 0.1 mg, chromium 1 mcg, manganese 25 mcg, selenium 15 mcg/ml. Vial 3 ml, 10 ml.
Use: Mineral supplement.

PTEROIC ACID. The compound formed by the linkage of carbon 6 of 2-amine-4-hydroxypteridine by means of a methylene group with the nitrogen of p-aminobenzoic acid.

PTEROYLGLUTAMIC ACID.
See: Folic Acid, Preps. (Various Mfr.).

PTEROYLMONOGLUTAMIC ACID. Pteroylglutamic acid.
See: Folic Acid, Preps. (Various Mfr.).

PTFE. (Ethicon) Polytef.

PTU.
See: Propylthiouracil.

PULMOCARE. (Ross) High fat, low-carbohydrate liquid diet for pulmonary patients containing 1500 calories/Liter; 1420 calories provides 100% U.S. RDA vitamins and minerals. Calorie:Nitrogen ratio is 150:1. Osmolarity: 490 mosm/Kg water. Can 8 fl oz.
Use: Enteral nutritional supplement.

PULMOSIN. (Spanner) Guaiacol 0.1 Gm, eucalyptol 0.08 Gm, camphor 0.05 Gm, iodoform 0.02 Gm/2 ml. Multiple dose vial 30 ml. Inj. I.M.

PUMICE, U.S.P. XXII.
Use: Abrasive (dental).

PURA. (D'Franssia) High potency vitamin E cream.
Use: Emollient.

PUREBROM COMPOUND ELIXIR. (Purepac) Brompheniramine maleate 4 mg/5 ml, phenylephrine HCl, phenylpropanolamine HCl, alcohol. Bot. pt, gal.
Use: Antihistamine, decongestant.

PURGE EVACUANT. (Fleming) Castor oil 95%. Bot. 1 oz, 2 oz.
Use: Laxative.

PURI-CLENS. (Sween) UD 2 oz. Bot. 8 oz.
Use: Wound deodorizer, cleanser.

PURIFIED OXGALL.
See: Bile Extract, Ox (Various Mfr.).

PURIFIED PROTEIN DERIVATIVE OF TUBERCULIN.
Use: Mantoux TB test.
See: Tuberculin, Old, Vial (Parke-Davis).

PURINETHOL. (Burroughs Wellcome) Mercaptopurine 50 mg/Tab. Bot. 25s, 250s.
Use: Antineoplastic agent.

PUROMYCIN. USAN. 3′-(L-α-Amino-p-methoxhydrocinnamamido)-3′-deoxy-N,N-dimethyladenosine.
Use: Antibiotic.

PUROMYCIN HYDROCHLORIDE. USAN.
Use: Antineoplastic; antiprotozoal.

PURPLE FOXGLOVE.
See: Digitalis, Preps. (Various Mfr.).

PURPOSE DRY SKIN CREAM. (Ortho Derm) Water, white petrolatum, propylene glycol, glyceryl stearate, almond oil, sodium lactate, steareth-20, cetyl alcohol, mineral oil, ethyl esters wax, xanthan gum, steareth-2, sorbic acid, lactic acid, fragrance. Tube 3 oz.
Use: Emollient.

PURPOSE SHAMPOO. (Ortho Derm) Water, amphoteric-19, PEG-44 sorbitan laurate, PEG-150 distearate, sorbitan laurate, boric acid, fragrance, benzyl alcohol. Bot. 8 oz.
Use: Shampoo.

PURPOSE SOAP. (Ortho) Sodium and potassium salts of fatty acids, glycerin, fragrance. Bar 3.6 oz, 6 oz.
Use: Therapeutic skin cleanser.

PURSETTES PREMENSTRUAL TABLETS. (Jeffrey Martin) Acetaminophen 500 mg, pamabrom 25 mg, pyrilamine maleate 15 mg/Tab. Bot. 24s.
Use: Analgesic, diuretic, antihistamine.

P.V. CARPINE LIQUIFILM. (Allergan) Pilocarpine nitrate 1%, 2% or 4%, polyvinyl alcohol 1.4%, sodium acetate, sodium Cl, citric acid, menthol, camphor, phenol, eucalyptol, chlorobutanol 0.5%, purified water. Dropper bot. 15 ml.
Use: Agent for glaucoma.

PVP-I OINTMENT. (Day-Baldwin) Povidone-iodine. Tube 1 oz, Jar lb, Foilpac 1.5 Gm.
Use: Antiseborrheic, antiseptic.

P-V-TUSSIN. (Solvay) Hydrocodone bitartrate 2.5 mg, phenylephrine HCl 5 mg, ammonium Cl 50 mg, pyrilamine maleate 6 mg, chlorpheniramine maleate 2 mg, phenindamine tartrate 5 mg/5 ml, alcohol 5%. Bot. pt, gal.
Use: Antitussive, decongestant, expectorant, antihistamine.

P-V TUSSIN TABLETS. (Solvay) Hydrocodone bitartrate 5 mg, phenindamine tartrate 25 mg, guaifenesin 200 mg/Tab. Bot. 100s.
Use: Antitussive, antihistamine, expectorant.

PY-CO-PAY TOOTH POWDER. (Block) Sodium Cl, sodium bicarbonate, calcium carbonate, magnesium carbonate, tricalcium phosphate, eugenol, methyl salicylate. Can 7 oz.
Use: Dentifrice.

PYLODATE. (Kenyon) Phenylazodiaminopyridine HCl 100 mg, methenamine mandelate 500 mg/Tab. Bot. 100s, 1000s.
Use: Urinary antiseptic.

PYMA. (Forest Pharm.) **TR Cap.:** Pyrilamine maleate 50 mg, chlorpheniramine maleate 6 mg, pheniramine maleate 20 mg, phenylephrine HCl 15 mg. Bot. 30s, 100s, 1000s. **Inj.:** Chlorpheniramine maleate 5 mg, phenylpropanolamine HCl 12.5 mg, atropine sulfate 0.2 mg/ml. Vial 10 ml.
Use: Antihistamine, decongestant, anticholinergic/antispasmodic.

PYOCIDIN-OTIC SOLUTION. (Forest) Hydrocortisone 5 mg, polymyxin B sulfate 10,000 USP units/ml in a vehicle containing water and propylene glycol. Bot. 10 ml w/sterile dropper.
Use: Corticosteroid, anti-infective otic.

•**PYRABROM.** USAN. Pyrilamine 8-bromotheophyllinate. Glybrom.
Use: Antihistamine.

PYRACOL. (Davis & Sly) Pyrathyn HCl 0.08 Gm, ammonium Cl 0.778 Gm, citric acid 0.52 Gm, menthol 0.006 Gm/fl oz. Bot. pt.

PYRADIN. (Jenkins) Acetophenetidin 4 gr, antipyrine 1 gr, caffeine 1/8 gr, tincture hyoscyamus 8 min. (total alkaloids 0.00032 gr), tincture gelsemium 4 min./Tab. Bot. 1000s.
Use: Analgesic, anticholinergic/antispasmodic.
PYRADONE.
See: Aminopyrine (Various Mfr.).
PYRAMINYL.
See: Pyrilamine Maleate (Various Mfr.).
PYRANEURIN INJ. (Nutrition) Vitamins B_1 100 mg, B_6 100 mg/ml, benzyl alcohol 1.5%. Vial. 10 ml.
Use: Vitamin B supplement.
PYRANILAMINE MALEATE.
See: Pyrilamine Maleate, Preps. (Various Mfr.).
PYRANISAMINE BROMOTHEOPHYLLINATE.
See: Pyrabrom (Various Mfr.).
PYRANISAMINE MALEATE.
See: Pyrilamine Maleate, Preps. (Various Mfr.).
PYRANISTAN. (Standex) Chlorprophenpyridamine 60 mg/10 ml.
Use: Antihistamine.
PYRANISTAN COMPOUND. (Standex) Chlorpheniramine maleate 2 mg, salicylamide 3.5 gr, phenacetin 2.5 gr, caffeine 0.5 gr/Tab. Bot. 100s.
Use: Antihistamine, analgesic.
PYRANISTAN CREME. (Standex) Coal tar extract 5%, pyrilamine maleate 1%, benzocaine 2.5%, benzalkonium Cl 1%. Jar 1 oz.
Use: Tar-containing preparation, antihistamine, analgesic.
PYRANISTAN STANKAPS. (Standex) Chlorpheniramine maleate 12 mg/Cap. Bot. 100s.
Use: Antihistamine.
PYRANISTAN SYRUP. (Standex) d-Methorphan HBr 30 mg, guaifenesin 75 mg, sodium citrate 150 mg, chlorpheniramine maleate 3 mg/fl oz. Bot. pt.
Use: Antitussive, expectorant, antihistamine.
PYRANISTAN TAB. (Standex) Chlorpheniramine maleate 4 mg/Tab. Bot. 100s.
Use: Antihistamine.
•**PYRANTEL PAMOATE,** U.S.P. XXII. Oral Susp., U.S.P. XXII.
Use: Anthelmintic.
See: Antiminth, Oral Susp. (Pfizer Laboratories).
•**PYRANTEL TARTRATE.** USAN. 1,4,5,6-Tetrahydro-1-methyl-2-[trans-2-(2-thienyl)vinyl]-pyrimidine Tartrate.
Use: Anthelmintic.
PYRATHIAZINE HYDROCHLORIDE. (N-(2-Pyrrolidinoethyl)-phenothiazine.
•**PYRAZINAMIDE,** U.S.P. XXII. Tab., U.S.P. XXII. Pyrazinecarboxamide. 2-Carbamyl pyrazine. Pyrazinecarboxamide. Aldinamide, Zinamide. Pyrazinoic acid 0.5 Gm/Tab. Bot. 500s. Lederle-500 mg/Tab. Bot. 500s.
Use: Antibacterial (tuberculostatic).
PYRAZINECARBOXAMIDE. Pyrazinamide, U.S.P. XXII.
PYRAZODINE. (Cenci) Phenazopyridine HCl 100 mg/Cap. Bot. 100s, 1000s.
Use: Urinary tract analgesic.
•**PYRAZOFURIN.** USAN.
Use: Antineoplastic.
PYRAZOLE. Under study.
Use: Antitumor.
PYRAZOLINE.
See: Antipyrine (Various Mfr.).
PYRBENZINDOLE.
See: Benzindopyrine Hydrochloride (Various Mfr.).
PYRIBENZAMINE.
See: PBZ, Prods. (Geigy).
PYRICAIN. (Jenkins) Cetylpyridium Cl 4 mg, sodium propionate 10 mg, benzocaine 5 mg/Tab. Bot. 1000s.
PYRICARDYL.
See: Nikethamide, Inj. (Various Mfr.).
PYRIDAMOLE TABS. (Major) Dipyridamole 25 mg, 50 mg or 75 mg/Tab. **25 mg:** Bot. 1000s, 2500s; **50 mg or 75 mg:** 100s, 1000s.
Use: Antianginal, antiplatelet.
PYRIDATE TABS. (Major) Phenazopyridine 100 mg or 200 mg/Tab. Bot. 1000s.
Use: Urinary analgesic, anti-infective.
PYRIDENE. (Approved) Phenylazo-diaminopyridine HCl 100 mg/Tab. Bot. 24s, 100s, 1000s.
Use: Urinary tract analgesic.
PYRIDINE-BETA-CARBOXYLIC ACID DIETHYL AMIDE.
See: Nikethamide, Inj. (Various Mfr.).
PYRIDIUM. (Parke-Davis) Phenazopyridine HCl 100 mg or 200 mg/Tab. Bot. 100s, 1000s, UD 100s.
Use: Urinary analgesic, anti-infective.
W/Hyoscyamine HBr, butabarbital.
See: Pyridium Plus, Tab. (Parke-Davis).
PYRIDIUM PLUS. (Parke-Davis) Formerly Dolonil. Phenazopyridine HCl 150 mg, hyoscyamine HBr 0.3 mg, butabarbital 15 mg/Tab. Bot. 100s.
Use: Urinary analgesic, anticholinergic/antispasmodic, sedative/hypnotic.
•**PYRIDOSTIGMINE BROMIDE,** U.S.P. XXII. Syr., Tab., U.S.P. XXII. Pyridinium 3-[[(dimethylamino)-carbonyl]oxy]-1-methyl-, bromide. Dimethyl carbamic ester of 3-hydroxy-1-methylpyridinium bromide.
Use: Cholinergic.
See: Mestinon, Tab., Syr., Amp. (Roche).
Regonal (Organon).
PYRIDOX. (Oxford) **No. 1:** Pyridoxine HCl 100 mg/Tab. **No. 2:** Pyridoxine HCl 200 mg/Tab. Bot. 100s.
Use: Vitamin B_6 supplement.
PYRIDOXAL. Vitamin B_6. 3-Hydroxy-4-formyl-5-hydroxy-methyl-2-methylpyridine.
Use: Vitamin B_6 supplement.
PYRIDOXAMINE. Vitamin B_6. 3-Hydroxy-4-aminomethyl-5-hydroxymethyl-2-methylpyridine.
Use: Vitamin B_6 supplement.

•**PYRIDOXINE HYDROCHLORIDE,** U.S.P. XXII. Inj., Tab., U.S.P. XXII. Vitamin B_6. 3,4-Pyridinedimethanol, 5-hydroxy-6-methyl-, hydrochloride. Pyridoxol hydrochloride.
Use: Enzyme co-factor vitamin.
See: Beesix, Vial (Fellows-Testagar).
Hexa Betalin, Amp., Tab., Vial (Lilly).
Hexavibex, Vial (Parke-Davis).
Pan B_6, Tab. (Panray).

PYRIDOXOL. 3-Hydroxy-4,5-hydroxymethyl-2-methylpyridine.
See: Pyridoxine, Vitamin B_6.

PYRIDYL CARBINOL.
See: Roniacol, Elix., Tab. (Roche).

PYRILAMINE BROMOTHEOPHYLLINATE.
See: Pyrabrom.
W/2-amino-2-methyl-1-propanol.
See: Bromaleate.

•**PYRILAMINE MALEATE,** U.S.P. XXII. Tab., U.S.P. XXII. 2-[[2-(Dimethylamino)ethyl](p-methoxy-benzyl)-amino]-pyridine maleate (1:1). Pyranisamine, Pyranilamine, Pyraminyl, Anisopyradamine. Available: Cap. sustained action, Cream, Ophthalmic Soln., Syr., Tab.
Use: Antihistamine.
See: Pyma, Cap., Vial (Fellows-Testagar).
Pyristan, Cap., Elix. (Arcum).
W/Combinations.
See: Antihistamine Cream (Towne).
Anti-Itch Cream (Towne).
Cardui, Tab. (Chattem Labs.).
Corizahist, Tab. (Mason).
Coton, Syr., Tab. (Solvay).
Femicin, Tab. (Norcliff Thayer).
Histjen, Cap. (Jenkins).
Hist-Span No. 2, Cap. (Kenyon).
Kenahist S.A., Tab.(Kenyon).
Miles Nervine, Tab. (Miles).
Nasal Spray (Penta).
Prefrin-A Ophth. Soln. (Allergan).
Triaminic Prods. (Sandoz Consumer).

•**PYRIMETHAMINE,** U.S.P. XXII. Tab., U.S.P. XXII. 2,4-Pyrimidinediamine, 5-(4-chlorophenyl) 6-ethyl-.2,4-Diamino-5-(p-chlorophenyl)-6-ethylpyrimidine. Daraprim.
Use: Antimalarial.
See: Daraprim, Tab. (Burroughs Wellcome).
W/Sulfadoxine.
See: Fansidar, Tab. (Roche).

PYRIMITHATE. V.B.A.N. 0-2-Dimethylamino-6-methylpyrimidin-4-y100-diethyl phosphorothioate.
Use: Insecticide, veterinary medicine.

•**PYRINOLINE.** USAN.
Use: Cardiac depressant.

PYRINYL. (Various Mfr.) Pyrethrins 0.2%, piperonyl butoxide technical 2%, deodorized kerosene 0.8%. Liq. Bot. 60, 120 ml.
Use: Pediculicide.

PYRISTAN. (Arcum) Phenylephrine HCl 8 mg, phenylpropanolamine HCl 15 mg, chlorpheniramine maleate 3 mg, pyrilamine maleate 10 mg/Cap. Bot. 50s, 500s. Elix. Bot. 4 oz, pt, gal.
Use: Decongestant, antihistamine.

PYRISUL. (Kenyon) Sulfamethylthiadiazole 250 mg, phenylazodiamine pyridine 50 mg/Tab. Bot. 100s, 1000s.
Use: Anti-infective.

PYRISUL-FORTE. (Kenyon) Sulfamethylthiadiazole 500 mg, phenylazodiamine pyridine 50 mg/Tab. Bot. 100s, 1000s.
Use: Anti-infective.

PYRISUL PLUS. (Kenyon) Sulfamethylthiadiazole 250 mg, methenamine mandelate 250 mg, phenylazodiamine pyridine 50 mg/Tab. Bot. 100s, 1000s.
Use: Anti-infective.

PYRITHEN.
See: Chlorothen Citrate (Various Mfr.).

PYRITHIDIUM BROMIDE. V.B.A.N. 3-Amino-8-(2-amino-1,6-dimethylpyrimidinium-4-ylamino)-6-(4-aminophenyl)-5-methylphenanthridinium dibromide.
Use: Antiprotozoan, veterinary medicine.

•**PYRITHIONE SODIUM.** USAN.
Use: Antibacterial, topical; antifungal, topical.

•**PYRITHIONE ZINC.** USAN. Bis [1-hydroxy-2-(1H)-pyridinethionato]zinc. Zinc bis(pyridine-2-thiol 1-oxide. Zinc Omadine.
Use: Treatment of seborrhea.
See: Danex Shampoo (Herbert).
Zincon Shampoo (Lederle).

PYRITINOL. B.A.N. Di(5-hydroxy-4-hydroxymethyl-6-methyl-3-pyridylmethyl) disulfide.
Use: Cerebral neuroactivator which increases vigilance and increases or normalizes cerebral metabolism and blood flow.

PYRODYN. (Fellows) Dipyrone 0.5 Gm/ml. Vial 30 ml.
Use: Analgesic.

PYROGALLIC ACID OINTMENT. (Gordon) Pyrogallic acid 25%, chlorobutanol. Jar 1 oz, 1 lb.
Use: Verruca therapy.

PYROGALLOL. Pyrogallic acid.

PYROHEP TABS. (Major) Cyproheptadine HCl 4 mg/Tab. Bot. 250s, 500s.
Use: Antihistamine.

PYROPHENINDANE. 1-(1-Methyl-3-pyrroli-dylmethyl)-3-phenylindane. (Mead Johnson).

•**PYROVALERONE HCl.** USAN. 4′-Methyl-2-(1-pyrrolidinyl)valerophenone HCl.
Use: Central stimulant.

•**PYROXAMINE MALEATE.** USAN.
Use: Antihistamine.

PYROXYLIN, U.S.P. XXI. Soluble guncotton. Cellulose nitrate.
Use: Pharmaceutic necessity for Collodion.

PYRRALAN COMPOUND CAPSULES. (Lannett) Thenylpyramine fumarate 25 mg, acetylsalicylic acid 3.25 gr, phenacetin 2.5 gr, caffeine 0.25 gr/Cap. Bot. 100s, 500s, 1000s.
Use: Antihistamine, analgesic.

PYRRALAN EXPECTORANT. (Lannett) Thenylpyramine fumarate 80 mg, ephedrine HCl 30 mg, ammonium Cl 500 mg/fl oz. Bot. pt, gal.
Use: Antihistamine, bronchodilator, expectorant.

PYRRALAN EXPECTORANT "DM." (Lannett) Same formula as Pyrralan Expectorant w/d-methorphan HBr 10 mg/5 ml. Bot. pt, gal.
Use: Antitussive, antihistamine, bronchodilator, expectorant.

PYRROBUTAMINE PHOSPHATE, U.S.P. XXI. 1-[4-(p-Chlorphenyl)-3-phenyl-2-butenyl]pyrrolidine diphosphate. 1-[α-(p-Chlorobenzyl)cinnamyl]pyrrolidine phosphate (1:2).
Use: Antihistamine.
W/Clopane HCl, Histadyl.
See: Co-Pyronil, Preps. (Lilly).

•**PYRROCAINE.** USAN. 1-Pyrrolidine-aceto-2′,6′-xylidide. Endocaine.
Use: Local anesthetic.

PYRROCAINE HYDROCHLORIDE. 1-Pyr- rolidineaceto-2′,6′-xylidide HCl.
Use: Local anesthetic (dental).

PYRROCAINE HYDROCHLORIDE AND EPINEPHRINE INJ.
Use: Local anesthetic (dental).

•**PYRROLIPHENE HYDROCHLORIDE.** USAN. d-a-Benzyl-β-methyl-α-phenyl-1-pyrrolidine-propanol acetate HCl. α-d-2-Acetoxy-1,2-dephenyl-3-methyl-4-pyrrolidinobutane HCl.
Use: Analgesic.

•**PYRROLNITRIN.** USAN. 3-Chloro-4-(3-chloro-2-nitrophenyl)pyrrole. Under study.
Use: Antifungal.

PYRROXATE. (Upjohn) Chlorpheniramine maleate 4 mg, phenylpropanolamine HCl 25 mg, acetaminophen 500 mg/Cap. Blister pkg. 24s. Bot. 500s.
Use: Antihistamine, decongestant, analgesic.

•**PYRVINIUM PAMOATE,** U.S.P. XXII. Tab., Oral Susp., U.S.P. XXII. Quinolinium, 6-(dimethylamino-2-[2-(2,5-dimethyl-1-phenyl-1H-pyrrol-3-yl)ethenyl]-1-methyl-, salt with 4,4′-methyl-enebis[3-hydroxy-2-naphthalenecarboxylic]
Use: Anthelmintic.

Q

QB LIQUID. (Major) Theophylline 150 mg, guaifenesin 90 mg. Bot. pt, gal.
Use: Bronchodilator, expectorant.

QT QUICK TANNING LOTION. (Schering-Plough) Padimate O, dihydroxyacetone (SPF 2). Bot. 4 oz.
Use: Sunscreen, artificial tanner.

QUA-BID. (Quaker City Pharmacal) Papaverine HCl 150 mg/TR Cap. Bot. 100s, 1000s.
Use: Peripheral vasodilator.

•**QUADAZOCINE MESYLATE.** USAN.
Use: Antagonist (opioid).

QUADRABARB. (Harvey) Secobarbital sodium 3/8 gr, pentobarbital sodium 3/8 gr, butabarbital sodium 3/8 gr, phenobarbital 3/8 gr/Tab. Bot. 1000s.
Use: Sedative/hypnotic.

QUADRIHIST. (Pharmex) Pyrilamine maleate, phenyltoloxamine dihydrogen citrate, prophenpyridamine maleate/Tab. Bot. 36s, 1000s.
Use: Antihistamine.

QUADRINAL. (Knoll) Ephedrine HCl 24 mg, phenobarbital 24 mg, theophylline calcium salicylate 130 mg, potassium iodide 320 mg/Tab. Bot. 100s, 1000s.
Use: Bronchodilator, sedative/hypnotic, expectorant.

QUADRODIDE.
See: Quadrinal, Susp., Tab. (Knoll).

QUADRUPLE SULFONAMIDES.
See: Sulfonamides.

QUAD-SET. (Kenyon) Secobarbital 25 mg, pentobarbital 25 mg, butabarbital 25 mg, phenobarbital 25 mg/Tab. Bot. 100s, 1000s.
Use: Sedative/hypnotic.

QUARZAN. (Roche) Clidinium bromide 2.5 mg or 5 mg/Cap. Bot. 100s.
Use: Anticholinergic/antispasmodic.

•**QUAZEPAM.** USAN.
Use: Sedative; hypnotic.
See: Doral (Baker Cummins).

•**QUAZINONE.** USAN.
Use: Cardiotonic.

•**QUAZODINE.** USAN.
Use: Cardiotonic; bronchodilator.

•**QUAZOLAST.** USAN.
Use: Anti-asthmatic.

QUELICIN. (Abbott Hospital Prods) Succinylcholine Cl. **20 mg/ml:** Fliptop vial 10 ml, Abboject Syringe 5 ml; **50 mg/ml:** Amp. 10 ml; **100 mg/ml:** Amp. 10 ml; **Quelicin-500:** 5 ml in Pintop vial 10 ml; **Quelicin-1000:** 10 ml in Pintop vial 20 ml.
Use: Muscle relaxant.

QUELIDRINE SYRUP. (Abbott) Dextromethorphan HBr 10 mg, chlorpheniramine maleate 2 mg, ephedrine HCl 5 mg, phenylephrine HCl 5 mg, ammonium Cl 40 mg, ipecac fluidextract 0.005 ml, ethyl alcohol 2%/5 ml. Bot. 4 oz.
Use: Antitussive, antihistamine, bronchodilator, decongestant, expectorant.

QUELTUSS. (Forest) Dextromethorphan HBr 15 mg, guaifenesin 100 mg/Tab. or 5 ml. **Tab.:** Bot. 100s, 1000s. **Syr.:** Bot. 4 oz, pt.
Use: Antitussive, expectorant.

QUERCETIN. Active constituent of rutin. Quertine.

QUERTINE. Quercetin. 3,3′,4′,5,7-Pentahydroxyflavone.
Use: Bioflavonoid supplement.

QUESTRAN. (Bristol) Cholestyramine resin 4 Gm active ingredient/9 Gm Powder Packet. Box packet 50s. Can 378 Gm (42 dose).
Use: Antihyperlipidemic, antipruritic.

QUESTRAN LIGHT. (Bristol Labs) Anhydrous cholestyramine 4 Gm/Packet or scoopful. Pow. for Oral Susp. Can 210 Gm (42 doses), carton packet 5 Gm (60s).
Use: Antihyperlipidemic.

QUIAGEL. (Rugby) Kaolin 6 Gm, pectin 142.8 mg, hyoscyamine sulfate 0.1037 mg, atropine sulfate 0.0194 mg, scopolamine HBr 0.0065 mg/30 ml. Susp. Bot. pt, gal.
Use: Antidiarrheal.

QUIAGEL PG. (Rugby) Powdered opium 24 mg, kaolin 6 Gm, pectin 142.8 mg, hyoscyamine sulfate 0.1037 mg, atropine sulfate 0.0194 mg, scopolamine HBr 0.0065 mg/30 ml, alcohol 5%. Susp. Bot. 180 ml, pt, gal.
Use: Antidiarrheal.

QUIBRON. (Bristol) Theophylline (anhydrous) 150 mg, guaifenesin 90 mg/Cap. or 15 ml. **Cap.:** Bot. 100s, 1000s, Box 100s individually wrapped. **Liq.:** Bot. pt, gal.
Use: Antiasthmatic combination.

QUIBRON-300. (Bristol) Theophylline (anhydrous) 300 mg, guaifenesin 180 mg/Cap. Bot. 100s.
Use: Antiasthmatic combination.

QUIBRON PLUS. (Bristol) Ephedrine HCl 25 mg, theophylline (anhydrous) 150 mg, butabarbital 20 mg, guaifenesin 100 mg/Cap. Bot. 100s.
Use: Antiasthmatic combination.

QUIBRON-T DIVIDOSE TABLETS. (Bristol) Theophylline anhydrous 300 mg/Tab. Dividose design breakable into 100, 150 or 200 mg portions. Immediate release. Bot. 100s.
Use: Antiasthmatic combination.

QUIBRON-T/SR DIVIDOSE TABLETS. (Bristol) Theophylline anhydrous 300 mg/Tab. Dividose design breakable into 100 mg, 150 mg or 200 mg portions. Sustained release. Bot. 100s.
Use: Antiasthmatic combination.

QUICK PEP. (Thompson) Caffeine 150 mg, dextrose 300 mg/Tab. Bot. 32s.
Use: Analeptic.

QUICK-K. (Western Research) Potassium bicarbonate 650 mg (6.5 mEq) potassium/Tab. Bot. 30s, 100s.
Use: Potassium supplement.

QUICK-SEPT. (Bausch & Lomb) **Sensitive eyes saline soln:** Isotonic sodium Cl, borate buffer, sorbic acid 0.1%, EDTA. **Sensitive eyes saline/cleaning soln.:** Isotonic solution of sodium Cl, borate buffer, surfactant, sorbic acid, EDTA.
Use: Soft contact lens care.

QUIEBAR. (Nevin) Butabarbital sodium. **Spantab:** 1.5 gr/TR Spantab. Bot. 50s, 500s. **Elix.:** 30 mg/5 ml. Bot. pt, gal. **Tab.:** 15 mg. Bot. 100s, 1000s; 30 mg. Bot. 1000s. **A.C. Cap.:** Bot. 100s, 500s.
Use: Sedative/hypnotic.

QUIEBEL. (Nevin) Butabarbital sodium 15 mg, belladonna extract 15 mg/Cap. Bot. 100s, 1000s. Elix. pt, gal.
Use: Sedative/hypnotic, anticholinergic/antispasmodic.

QUIECOF. (Nevin) Dextromethorphan HBr 7.5 mg, chlorpheniramine maleate 0.75 mg, guaiacol glyceryl ether 25 mg. Bot. 4 oz, pt, gal.
Use: Antitussive, antihistamine, expectorant.

QUIESS. (Forest) Hydroxyzine HCl 25 mg/ml. Vial 10 ml.
Use: Antianxiety agent, antihistamine.

QUIET NIGHT. (PBI) Pseudoephedrine HCl 10 mg, doxylamine succinate 1.25 mg, dextromethorphan HBr 5 mg, acetaminophen 167 mg/5 ml. Liq. Bot. 180 ml, 300 ml.
Use: Decongestant, antihistamine, antitussive, analgesic.

QUIET TIME. (Whiteworth) Acetaminophen 600 mg, ephedrine sulfate 8 mg, dextromethorphan HBr 15 mg, doxylamine succinate 7.5 mg, alcohol 25 mg/30 ml. Bot. 180 ml.
Use: Analgesic, decongestant, antitussive, antihistamine.

QUIET WORLD. (Whitehall) Acetaminophen 2.5 gr, aspirin 3.5 gr, pyrilamine maleate 25 mg/Tab. Bot. 12s, 30s.
Use: Salicylate analgesic combination, antihistamine.

QUIK-CEPT. (Laboratory Diagnostics) Slide test for pregnancy, rapid latex inhibition test. Kit 25s, 50s, 100s.
Use: Diagnostic aid.

QUIK-CULT. (Laboratory Diagnostics) Slide test for fecal occult blood. Kit 150s, 200s, 300s and tape test.
Use: Diagnostic aid.

QUINACILLIN. B.A.N. 6-(3)Carboxyquinoxaline-2-carboxamideo) penicillanic acid.
Use: Antibiotic.

•**QUINACRINE HYDROCHLORIDE,** U.S.P. XXII. Tab., U.S.P. XXII. 1,4-Pentanediamine,N[4]-(6-chloro-2-methoxy-9-acridinyl)-N[1],N[1]-diethyl-, dihydrochloride, dihydrate. 6-Chloro-9- [4-(diethylamino)-1-methyl-butyl]amino -2-methoxyacridine dihydrochloride. 3-Chloro-7-methoxy-9-(1-methyl-4-diethylamino-butylamino)-acridine di-HCl dihydrate.
Use: Anthelmintic, antimalarial.
See: Atabrine HCl, Tab. (Winthrop Pharm).

QUINAGLUTE DURA-TABS. (Berlex) Quinidine gluconate 324 mg/Tab. Bot. 100s, 250s, 500s, UD 100s. Unit-of-use 90s, 120s.
Use: Antiarrhythmic.

QUINALAN GLUCONATE SR TABS. (Lannett) Quinidine gluconate 324 mg/Tab. Bot. 100s, 250s, 500s.
Use: Antiarrhythmic.

QUINALBARBITONE SODIUM. B.A.N. Monosodium derivative of 5-allyl-5-(1-methylbutyl)-barbituric acid.
Use: Hypnotic; sedative.

•**QUINALDINE BLUE.** USAN. 1-Ethyl-2-[3-(1-ethyl-2(1H) quinolylidene) propenyl]-quinolinium Cl. Vernitest reagent. (Fuller)
Use: Diagnostic agent (obstetrics).

QUINAMINOPH TABS. (Goldline) Quinine sulfate 260 mg/Tab. Bot. 100s, 500s.
Use: Antimalarial, nocturnal leg cramps.

QUINAMM. (Merrell Dow) Quinine sulfate 260 mg/Tab. Bot. 100s.
Use: Antimalarial, nocturnal leg cramps.

•**QUINAPRIL HYDROCHLORIDE.** USAN.
Use: Enzyme inhibitor (angiotensin-converting).

•**QUINAZOSIN HYDROCHLORIDE.** USAN. 2-(4-Allyl-1 piperazinyl)-4-amino-6,7-dimethoxy-quinazoline dihydrochloride.
Use: Hypotensive.

•**QUINBOLONE.** USAN. 17-beta-(1-Cyclo-penten-1-yloxy)-androsta-1,4-dien-3-one.
Use: Anabolic agent.

•**QUINDECAMINE ACETATE.** USAN. 4,4′-(Decamethylenediimino) diquinaldine diacetate dihydrate.
Use: Topical anti-infective.

•**QUINDONIUM BROMIDE.** USAN. 2,3-3α,5,6,11,12,12α-Octahydro-8-hydroxy-1H-benzo-[α]-cyclopenta[f]-quinolizinium bromide.
Use: Cardiovascular agent.

•**QUINELORANE HYDROCHLORIDE.** USAN.
Use: Dopaminergic agonist; antidyskinetic; antihyperprolactinemic; antihypertensive.

QUINESTRADOL. B.A.N. 3-Cyclopentyloxyestra-1,3,5(10)-triene-16α,17β-diol.
Use: Estrogen.

•**QUINESTROL,** U.S.P. XXII. Tab., U.S.P. XXII. 3-(Cyclopentyloxy)-19-nor-17-α-pregna-1,3,5(10)-triene-20-yn-17-ol.
Use: Estrogen.
See: Estrovis, Tab. (Parke-Davis).

•**QUINETHAZONE,** U.S.P. XXII. Tab., U.S.P. XXII. 7-Chloro-2-ethyl-6-sulfamyl-1,2,3,4-tetra-hydro-4-quinazolinone. 7-Chloro-2-ethyl-1,2,3,4-tetrahydro-4-oxo-6-quinazolinesulfonamide.
Use: Diuretic.
See: Hydromox, Tab. (Lederle).
W/Reserpine.
See: Hydromox R, Tab. (Lederle).

•**QUINETOLATE.** USAN. 6-(Diethylcarbamoyl)-3-cyclohexene-1-carboxylic acid comp. with 4- ((2-(dime-thylamino) ethyl)amino)6-methoxy- quinoline(2:1) Phthalamaquin (Penick).
Use: Anti-asthmatic.

•**QUINFAMIDE.** USAN.
Use: Anti-amoebic.

•**QUINGESTANOL ACETATE.** USAN. 3-(Cyclopentyloxy)-19-nor-17α-pregna-3,5-dien-20-yn-17-ol acetate. Under study.
Use: Progesterone.

•**QUINGESTRONE.** USAN. 3-(Cyclopentyloxy)pregna-3,5-dien-20-one.
Use: Progesterone.

QUINIDEX EXTENTABS. (Robins) Quinidine sulfate 300 mg/Tab. Bot. 100s, 250s. Dis-co pack 100s.
Use: Antiarrhythmic.

QUINIDEX L-A.
See: Quinidex Extentabs (Robins).

•**QUINIDINE GLUCONATE,** U.S.P. XXII., Inj., U.S.P. XXII. Cinchonan-9-ol, 6′-methoxy-,(9s)-, mono-D-gluconate (salt). (Lilly) Amp. (80 mg/ml) 10 ml.
Use: Quinidine therapy; cardiac depressant.
See: Duraquin, Tab. (Parke-Davis).
Quinaglute, Dura-Tab. (Berlex).
Quinalan, Tab. (Lannett).

QUINIDINE POLYGALACTURONATE.
See: Cardioquin Tab. (Purdue Frederick).

•**QUINIDINE SULFATE,** U.S.P. XXII. Cap., Extended-release Tab., U.S.P. XXII. Cinchonan-9-ol, 6′-methoxy-,(9s)-, sulfate (2:1) (salt), dihydrate.
Use: Cardiac depressant.
See: Cin-Quin (Solvay).
Quinidex Extentabs (Robins).
Quinora, Tab. (Key).

QUININE ASCORBATE. USAN.
Use: As a deterrent to smoking.

QUININE BISULFATE.
Use: Analgesic, antipyretic, antimalarial.

QUININE DIHYDROCHLORIDE.
Use: Antimalarial.

QUININE ETHYLCARBONATE.
See: Euquinine (Various Mfr.).

QUININE GLYCEROPHOSPHATE. Quinine compound with glycerol phosphate.

•**QUININE SULFATE,** U.S.P. XXII. Cap., Tab., U.S.P. XXII. Cinchonan-9-ol,6′-methoxy-(8α,9R)-sulfate (2:1) (salt) dihydrate.
Use: Antimalarial.
See: Quinamm, Tab. (Merrell Dow).
Quine, Cap. (Solvay).
W/Aminophylline.
See: Strema, Cap. (Foy).
W/Atropine sulfate, emetine HCl, aconitine, camphor monobromate.
See: Coryza, Tab. (Bowman).
W/Niacin, vitamin E.
See: Myodyne, Tab. (Paddock).

QUININE AND UREA HYDROCHLORIDE.
Use: Sclerosing agent.

QUINISOCAINE (I.N.N.). Dimethisoquin, B.A.N.

QUINNONE CREAM. (Dermohr Pharmacal) Hydroquinone 4% in creamy base. Tube 1 oz.
Use: Skin bleaching agent.

QUINOPHAN.
See: Cinchophen (Various Mfr.).

QUINORA. (Key) Quinidine sulfate 300 mg/Tab. Bot. 100s, 1000s, UD 100s.
Use: Antiarrhythmic.

QUINOXYL.
See: Chiniofon

•**QUINPIROLE HYDROCHLORIDE.** USAN.
Use: Antihypertensive.

QUINPRENALINE. Quinterenol Sulfate.

QUIN-260 TABS. (Major) Quinine sulfate 260 mg/Tab. Bot. 250s.
Use: Antimalarial, nocturnal leg cramps.

QUIN-RELEASE. (Major) Quinidine gluconate 324 mg/SR Tab. Bot. 100s, 250s, 500s, UD 100s.
Use: Antiarrhythmic.

QUINSANA PLUS. (Mennen) Undecylenic acid 2%, zinc undecylenate 20%. Pow. 81 Gm, 165 Gm.
Use: Antifungal, external.

QUINTABS. (Freeda) Vitamins A 10,000 IU, D 400 IU, E 25 mg, B_1 25 mg, B_2 25 mg, B_3 100 mg, B_5 25 mg, B_6 25 mg, B_{12} 25 mcg, C 300 mg, folic acid 0.1 mg, inositol 50 mg, PABA 30 mg/Tab. Bot. 100s, 250s, 500s.
Use: Vitamin supplement.

QUINTABS-M. (Freeda) Iron 15 mg, Vitamins A 10,000 IU, D 400 IU, E 41.3 mg, B_1 30 mg, B_2 30 mg, B_3 150 mg, B_5 30 mg, B_6 30 mg, B_{12} 30 mcg, C 300 mg, folic acid 0.4 mg, Ca, Cu, K, Mg, Mn, Se, Zn, PABA/Tab. Sodium free. Bot. 100s, 250s, 500s.
Use: Vitamin/mineral supplement.

QUINTERENOL SULFATE. USAN. 8-Hydroxy-alpha-[(isopropylamino)methyl]-5-quinoline-methanol [sulfate (2:1).
Use: Bronchodilator.

QUINUCLIUM BROMIDE. USAN.
Use: Antihypertensive.

QUIPAZINE MALEATE. USAN. 2-(1-Piperazinyl) quinoline maleate.
Use: Oxytocic.

QUIPENYL NAPHTHOATE.
See: Pamaquine naphthoate.
Plasmochin naphthoate.

QUIPHILE. (Geneva Generics) Quinine sulfate 260 mg/Tab. Bot. 100s.
Use: Antimalarial.

QUIAGEN SOFT GELATIN CAPS. (Goldline) Theophylline, glyceryl guaiacolate. Bot. 100s, 500s.
Use: Bronchodilator.

Q-VEL SOFTGELS. (Ciba Consumer) Quinine sulfate 64.8 mg, vitamin E 400 IU (as dl-alpha tocopheryl acetate), lecithin/Cap. Bot. 30s.
Use: Antimalarial, nocturnal leg cramps.

R

R-3 SCREEN TEST. (Wampole) A three-minute latex-eosin slide test for the qualitative detection of rheumatoid factor activity in serum. Kit 100s.
Use: Diagnostic aid.

RABIES IMMUNE GLOBULIN, U.S.P. XXII.
Use: Immunizing agent (passive).

RABIES VACCINE, U.S.P. XXII. (Lilly) 1 dose Vial of 1.1 ml. The suspending fluid consists of cysteine HCl 0.1%, lactose 5%, gelatin 0.2%, dibasic potassium phosphate 0.25%. Vaccine preserved w/thimerosal 1:10,000. (Lederle) 1000 units/Vial. Antirabies Serum.
Use: Immunizing agent, active.

RACEMETHIONINE, U.S.P. XXI. Cap., Tab., U.S.P. XXI. Dl-2-Amino-4-(methylthio)butyric acid. Methionine.
Use: Acidifier (urinary).
See: Amurex, Cap. (Solvay).
Odonil, Cap. (Kenyon).
Odor-Scrip, Cap. (Scrip).
Oradash, Cap. (Lambda).
Pedameth. Cap., Liq. (Forest).

RACEMETHIONINE W/COMBINATIONS.
See: Aminomin, Vial (Pharmex).
Aminovit, Vial (Hickam).
Ardiatric, Tab. (Burgin-Arden).
Cho-Meth, Vial (Kenyon).
Geriatrazole, Vial (Kenyon).
Geriatro-B, Vial (Kenyon).
Hi-Pro Wafers, Tab. (Mills).
Licoplex, Tab. (Mills).
Limvic, Tab. (Briar).
Lipo-K, Cap. (Marcen).
Lychol-B, Inj. (Burgin-Arden).
Minoplex, Vial (Savage).
Pro-Hydro, Tab. (Mills).
Vio-Geric, Tab. (Solvay).
Vio-Geric-H, Tab. (Solvay).
Vi-Testrogen, Vial (Pharmex).

RACEMETHORPHAN. B.A.N. (±)-3-Methoxy-N-methylmorphinan
Use: Narcotic analgesic.

RACEMIC CALCIUM PANTOTHENATE.
See: Calcium Pantothenate, Racemic.

RACEMIC DESOXY-NOR-EPHEDRINE.
See: Amphetamine (Various Mfr.).

RACEMIC EPHEDRINE HCl. Racephedrine HCl.

RACEMIC PANTOTHENIC ACID.
See: Vitamin, Preps.

RACEMORAMIDE. B.A.N. (±)-1-(3-Methyl-4-morpholino-2,2-diphenylbutyryl)pyrrolidine.
Use: Narcotic analgesic.

RACEMORPHAN HBr. B.A.N. (±)-3-Hydroxy-N-methylmorphinan.
Use: Narcotic analgesic.

RACEPHEDRINE HYDROCHLORIDE. (Upjohn) dl-a-[1-(Methylamino)ethyl]benzyl alcohol HCl. **Cap.:** ⅜ gr. Bot. 40s, 250s, 1000s. **Soln.:** 1%. Bot. 1 fl oz, pt, gal.
Use: Vasoconstrictor, nasal decongestant.
See: Ephedrine Combinations
W/Aminophylline, phenobarbital.
See: Amodrine, Tab. (Searle).
W/Theophylline sodium glycinate, phenobarbital.
See: Synophedal, Tab. (Central).

•**RACEPHENICOL.** USAN.
Use: Antibacterial.

•**RACEPINEPHRINE,** U.S.P. XXII.
Use: Bronchodilator.

•**RACEPINEPHRINE HYDROCHLORIDE,** U.S.P. XXII. Inhalation Soln., U.S.P. XXII.
Use: Bronchodilator.

•**RACTOPAMINE HYDROCHLORIDE.** USAN.
Use: Veterinary growth stimulant.

RADIOACTIVE ISOTOPES.

See: Medotope, Prods. (Squibb).
Radio-Gold, Soln.
Radio-Iodinated Serum Albumin (Human).
Sodium Radio-Chromate, Inj.
Sodium Radio-Iodide, Soln.
Sodium Radio Phosphate, Soln.

RADIOACTIVE ISOTOPES.
See: Aggregated Radioiodinated Albumin, Human I-131.
Chlormerodrin Hg-197, Inj.
Chlormerodrin Hg-203, Inj.
Cyanocobalamin Co-57, Cap.
Cyanocobalamin Co-60, Cap.
Gold Au-198, Inj.
Radiodinated Serum Albumin, Human I-125.
Radiodinated Serum Albuminia, Human I-131.
Selenomethionine Se-75, Inj.
Sodium Chromate Cr-51, Inj.
Sodium Iodide I-125, Soln., Cap.
Sodium Iodide I-131, Soln., Cap.
Sodium Phosphate P-32, Cap., Inj.
Sodium Rose Bengal I-131, Inj.
Strontium Nitrate Sr-85, Inj.
Technetium Tc-99m, Kit, Inj.
Triolein I-131, Cap., Soln.
Xenon Xe-133, Inj.

RADIOGOLD (^{198}Au), SOLUTION. Gold Au-198 Injection, U.S.P. XXII.
Use: Irradiation therapy.
See: Auretope, Vial (Squibb).

RADIO-IODIDE (^{131}I), SODIUM.
Use: Radioactive isotopes.
See: Iodotope (Squibb).
Radiocaps (Abbott).

RADIO-IODINATED (^{131}I) SERUM ALBUMIN. (Human), Iodinated I-131 Albumin Injection, U.S.P. XXII.

RADIO-IODINATED SERUM ALBUMIN (Human),(^{125}I).
See: Albumotope (^{125}I) (Squibb).

RADIO-PHOSPHATE (^{32}P), SODIUM.
Use: Radioactive isotopes.

RADIOSELENOMETHIONINE 75 Se. Selenomethionine Se 75.

RADIOTOLPOVIDONE I-131. Tolpovidone I-131.
See: Raovin (Abbott).

•**RAFOXANIDE.** USAN.
Use: Anthelmintic.

RAGUS. (Miller) Magnesium 27 mg, vitamins C 100 mg, calcium 580 mg, phosphorus 450 mg, l-lysine 25 mg, dl-methionine 50 mg, A 5000 IU, D 400 IU, E 10 mg, B_1 20 mg, B_2 3 mg, B_6 5 mg, B_{12} 9 mcg, niacinamide 80 mg, pantothenic acid 5 mg, iron 20 mg, copper 1 mg, manganese 2 mg, potassium 10 mg, zinc 2 mg, iodine 0.1 mg/3 Tab. Bot. 100s.
Use: Vitamin/mineral supplement.

R A LOTION. (Medco Lab) Resorcinol 3%, calamine, starch, sodium borate, bentonite, alcohol 43%. Plastic bot. 4 oz, 8 oz, 16 oz.
Use: Anti-acne.

•**RAMIPRIL.** USAN.
Use: Antihypertensive, enzyme inhibitor (angiotensin-converting).
See: Altace (Hoechst-Roussel).

RAMSES BENDEX. (Schmid) Flexible cushioned diaphragm; arcing spring. 65-90 mm. Pkg. w/ Ramses Vaginal Jelly Tube 1 oz, 3 oz.
Use: Contraceptive.

RAMSES DIAPHRAGM. (Schmid) Flexible cushioned diaphragm 50-95 mm. Pkg. diaphragm, tube of Ramses Vaginal Jelly. Pkg. diaphragm alone.
Use: Contraceptive.

RAMSES EXTRA. (Schmid) Condom with nonoxynol 9 5.6%. In 12s.
Use: Contraceptive.

RAMSES JELLY. (Schmid) Nonoxynol 9. Tube w/applicator 5 oz.
Use: Contraceptive.

RANDOLECTIL. (Farbenfabriken Bayer) Butaperazine.
Use: Psychotropic agent.

R & C SHAMPOO. (Reed & Carnrick) Pyrethrin shampoo. Bot. 2 oz, 4 oz.
Use: Pediculicide.

R & C SPRAY III. (Reed & Carnrick) Spray containing pyrethroid (sumethrin) 0.382%, other isomers 0.018%, petroleum distillate 4.255%. Aerosol Container 5 oz.
Use: Pediculicide.

RANESTOL. Triclofenol piperazine.
Use: Anthelmintic.

•**RANIMYCIN.** USAN.
Use: Antibacterial.

RANITIDINE.
Use: Histamine H_2 antagonist.
See: Zantac, Tab., Inj., Syr. (Glaxo).

•**RANITIDINE HYDROCHLORIDE IN SODIUM CHLORIDE INJECTION.** U.S.P. XXII
Use: Histamine H_2 anatagonist.
See: Zantac Inj. Premixed (Glaxo).

•**RANOLAZINE HYDROCHLORIDE.** USAN.
Use: Antianginal.

RAPID TEST STREP. (SmithKline Diagnostics) Latex slide agglutination test for identification of group A Streptococci. In 25s, 100s.
Use: Diagnostic aid.

RASTINON. Tolbutamide, U.S.P. XXII.

RATTLESNAKE BITE THERAPY.
See: Antivenin, Snake Polyvalent (Wyeth-Ayerst).

RAUDILAN PB TABLETS. (Lannett) Rauwolfia serpentina root 50 mg, phenobarbital 15 mg/ Tab. Bot. 100s, 500s, 1000s.
Use: Antihypertensive.

RAUDIXIN. (Princeton) Rauwolfia whole root w/ tartrazine. 50 mg or 100 mg/Tab. Bot. 100s, 1000s.
Use: Antihypertensive.

RAUDOLFIN. (Premo) Rauwolfia serpentina 50 mg or 100 mg/Tab. Bot. 1000s.
Use: Antihypertensive.

RAUNEED. (Hanlon) Rauwolfia 50 mg or 100 mg/Tab. Bot. 100s.
Use: Antihypertensive.
RAUNESCINE. (Penick) An alkaloid of Rauwolfia serpentina. Under study.
Use: Antihypertensive.
RAUNORMINE. (Penick) 11-Desmethoxy reserpine.
RAURINE. (Westerfield) Reserpine. **Tab.:** 0.1 mg. Bot. 100s. **Delayed Action Cap.:** 0.5 mg. Bot. 100s.
Use: Antihypertensive.
RAUSERFIA. (New Eng. Phr. Co.) Rauwolfia serpentina 50 mg or 100 mg/Tab. Bot. 100s.
Use: Antihypertensive.
RAUTINA. (Fellows) Rauwolfia serpentina whole root 50 mg or 100 mg/Tab. Bot. 1000s.
Use: Antihypertensive.
RAUVAL. (Vale) Rauwolfia whole root 50 mg or 100 mg/Tab. Bot. 100s, 500s, 1000s.
Use: Antihypertensive.
RAUVERAT. (Kenyon) Rauwolfia serpentina whole root pow. 50 mg, veratrum viride extract equivalent to total alkaloids 1.1 mg/Tab. Bot. 100s, 1000s.
Use: Antihypertensive.
RAUVERID. (Forest) Rauwolfia serpentina pow. whole root 50 mg/Tab. Bot. 100s.
Use: Antihypertensive.
RAU-VER-TIN. (Kenyon) Rauwolfia serpentina 40 mg, veratrum viride 25 mg, rutin 20 mg, mannitol hexanitrate 30 mg/Tab. Bot. 100s, 1000s.
Use: Antihypertensive.
RAUWOLFIA CANESCENS ALKALOID.
See: Harmonyl, Tab. (Abbott).
RAUWOLFIA SERPENTINA ACTIVE PRINCIPLES (ALKALOIDS). Deserpidine, Rescinnamine.
See: Reserpine, Inj. (Various Mfr.).
RAUWOLFIA SERPENTINA ALKALOIDAL EXTRACT.
See: Alseroxylon (Various Mfr.).
•**RAUWOLFIA SERPENTINA,** U.S.P. XXII. Powder, Tab., U.S.P. XXII.
Use: Antihypertensive.
See: Rau, Tab. (Scrip).
Raudixin, Tab. (Princeton).
Rauja, Tab. (Table Rock).
Raumason, Tab. (Mason).
Rauneed, Tab. (Hanlon).
Rautina, Tab. (Fellows-Testagar).
Rauval, Tab. (Vale).
Rawfola, Tab. (Foy).
Serfia, Tab. (Westerfield).
Serfolia, Tab. (Mallard).
T-Rau, Tab. (Tennessee Pharm.).
Wolfina, Tab. (Westerfield).
W/Bendroflumethiazide.
See: Rautrax-N, Tab. (Princeton).
Rauzide, Tab. (Princeton).
W/Bendroflumethiazide, potassium Cl (400).
See: Rautrax, Tab. (Princeton).
W/Mannitol hexanitrate, rutin.
See: Maxitate W/Rauwolfia, Tab. (Pennwalt).
W/Phenobarbital.
See: Raudilan PB, Tab. (Lannett).
RAUWOLSCINE. An alkaloid of *Rauwolfia canescens.* Under study.
Use: Antihypertensive.
RAUZIDE. (Princeton) Rauwolfia serpentina pow. 50 mg, bendroflumethiazide 4 mg, tartrazine/Tab. Bot. 100s.
Use: Antihypertensive.
RAVOCAINE. (Cook-Waite) Propoxycaine HCl 4 mg, procaine 20 mg, norepinephrine bitartrate equivalent to 0.033 mg levophed base, sodium Cl 3 mg, acetone sodium bisulfite not more than 2 mg. Cartridge 1.8 ml.
Use: Local anesthetic.
RAVOCAINE AND NOVOCAIN WITH LEVOPHED. (Cook-Waite) Propoxycaine HCl 7.2 mg, procaine 36 mg, norepinephrine 0.12 mg, acetone sodium bisulfite 1.8 ml. Inj. Dental Cartridge.
Use: Local anesthetic.
RAVOCAINE AND NOVOCAIN WITH NEO-COBEFRIN. (Cook-Waite) Propoxycaine HCl 7.2 mg, procaine 36 mg, levonordefrin 0.09 mg, acetone sodium bisulfite 1.8 ml. Inj. Dental cartridge.
Use: Local anesthetic.
RAWFOLA. (Foy) Rauwolfia serpentina 50 mg/Tab. Bot. 1000s.
Use: Antihypertensive.
RAWL VITE. (Rawl) Vitamins A 10,000 IU, D 500 IU, B_1 10 mg, B_2 5 mg, B_6 1 mg, calcium pantothenate 5 mg, nicotinamide 50 mg, C 125 mg, E 2.5 IU/Tab. Bot. 100s.
Use: Vitamin supplement.
RAWL WHOLE LIVER VITAMIN B COMPLEX. (Rawl) Whole liver 500 mg, amino acids found in the whole liver, vitamins B_1 1 mg, B_2 2 mg, niacinamide 5 mg, choline Cl 12 mg, B_6 0.2 mg, calcium pantothenate 0.2 mg, inositol 5 mg, biotin 0.6 mcg, B_{12} 0.3 mcg/Cap. Bot. 100s, 500s.
Use: Vitamin/mineral supplement.
RAY BLOCK. (Del-Ray) Padimate O 5%, benzophenone-3 3%, SD alcohol. Bot. 4 oz.
Use: Sunscreen.
RAY-D. (Nion) Vitamin D 400 IU, thiamine mononitrate 1 mg, riboflavin 2 mg, niacin 10 mg, iodine 0.1 mg, calcium 375 mg, phosphorus 300 mg/6 Tab. In base of brewer's yeast. Bot. 100s, 500s.
Use: Vitamin/mineral supplement.
RAYDERM OINTMENT. (Velvet Pharmacal) Euphorbia extract, phenyl salicylate, neatsfoot oil, olive oil, lanolin in emulsion base preserved with methyl and propylparabens. Tube 1.5 oz, Jar lb.
Use: Burn preparation.
RAY-NOX. (Torch) PABA and para-aminobenzoic sodium. Jar 2 oz, 1 lb.
Use: Sunscreen.

•**RAYON, PURIFIED,** U.S.P. XXII.
Use: Surgical aid.

RAYTHESIN. (Raymer).
See: Propyl p-Aminobenzoate.

RAZEPAM. (Major) Temazepam 15 mg or 30 mg/Cap. Bot. 100s.
Use: Sedative/hypnotic.

RAZOXANE. B.A.N. 1,2-Bis(3,5-dioxopiperazin-1-yl)propane.
Use: Antineoplastic.

RCF. (Ross) Carbohydrate free low iron soy protein formula base. Carbohydrate and water must be added. For infants unable to tolerate the amount or type of carbohydrate in conventional formulas. Can 14 fl oz. (Concentrated liq.).
Use: Enteral nutritional supplement.

REA-LO. (Whorton) Urea in water soluble moisturizing oil base. **Lot.:** 15%. Bot. 4 oz, pt. **Cream:** 30%. Jar 2 oz, 16 oz.
Use: Emollient.

REALPHENE.
See: Acetarsone, Tab. (City Chem.).

•**RECAINAM HYDROCHLORIDE.** USAN.
Use: Antiarrhythmic.

•**RECAINAM TOSYLATE.** USAN.
Use: Antiarrhythmic.

RECINDAL. (Winthrop Products) Dextromethorphan HBr.
Use: Antitussive, decongestant.

•**RECLAZEPAM.** USAN.
Use: Sedative.

RECLOMIDE. (Major) Metoclopramide HCl 10 mg/Tab. Bot. 100s, 500s, 1000s, UD 100s.
Use: GI stimulant.

RECOMBIVAX-HB. (Merck, Sharp & Dohme) Hepatitis B vaccine recombinant. **Pediatric:** 5 mcg/0.5 ml. Single dose vial 0.5 ml; **Adult:** 10 mcg/ml. Vial 3 ml.
Use: Agent for immunization.

RECORTEX 10X IN OIL. (Forest Pharm.) 1000 mcg/ml. Vial 10 ml.

RECOVER. (Commerce) Bot. 2.25 oz.
Use: Skin discoloration cover-up cream.

RECTACORT. (Century) Hydrocortisone acetate 10 mg, zinc oxide 11%, bismuth subgallate 2.25%, balsam peru 1.8%, bismuth resorcin compound 1.75%, benzyl benzoate 1.2%. Supp. Pkg. 12s.
Use: Anorectal preparation.

RECTAGENE MEDICATED RECTAL BALM. (Pfeiffer) Benzocaine 3%, phenylephrine HCl 0.2%, bismuth subgallate 1%, zinc oxide 1.5%, pyrilamine maleate, cetalkonium Cl in a polyethylene glycol base. Oint. 30 Gm.
Use: Anorectal preparation.

RECTAL MEDICONE. (Medicone) Benzocaine 2 gr, balsam peru 1 gr, hydroxyquinoline sulfate 0.25 gr, menthol 1/7 gr, zinc oxide 3 gr/Supp. Box 12s, 24s.
Use: Antiseptic, local anesthetic.

RECTAL MEDICONE UNGUENT. (Medicone) Benzocaine 20 mg, oxyquinoline sulfate 5 mg, menthol 4 mg, zinc oxide 100 mg, balsam peru 12.5 mg, petrolatum 625 mg, lanolin 210 mg/Gm. Tube 1.5 oz.
Use: Anorectal preparation.

RECTOCAINE. (Moore Kirk) Phenol 1%, propyl-p-aminobenzoate 7%, benzyl alcohol 7%, procaine 0.5%. Amp. 5 ml.
Use: Local anesthetic, rectal.

RECTULES. (Forest Pharm.) Chloral hydrate 10 or 20 gr in water-soluble base. Supp. Pkg. 12s.
Use: Sedative/hypnotic.

•**RED BLOOD CELLS,** U.S.P. XXII. Human red blood cells given by IV infusion.
Use: Blood replenisher.

RED CELL TAGGING SOLUTION.
See: A-C-D Solution (Squibb).

RED CROSS TOOTHACHE KIT. (Mentholatum) Complete kit containing toothache drops w/cotton pellets and tweezers.
Use: Local anesthetic.

•**RED FERRIC OXIDE,** N.F. XVII.
Use: Pharmaceutic aid (color).

RED MERCURIC IODIDE.
See: Auralcaine, Liq. (Truett).

REDITEMP-C. (Wyeth-Ayerst) Ammonium nitrate, water and special additives. Pkg. large and small sizes. 4 × 10s.
Use: For short-term topical cold application.

REDUCTO, IMPROVED. (Arcum) Phendimetrazine bitartrate 35 mg/Tab. Bot. 100s, 1000s.
Use: Anorexiant.

REESE'S PINWORM. (Reese) Pyrantel pamoate 144 mg. Liq. 30 ml.
Use: Anthelmintic.

REFRESH. (Allergan) Polyvinyl alcohol 1.4%, povidone 0.6%, sodium Cl 0.3 ml. UD 30s (single dose container).
Use: Artificial tear solution.

REFRESH PM. (Allergan) White petrolatum 55%, mineral oil 41.5%, petrolatum, lanolin alcohol 2%, sodium Cl. Tube 0.12 oz.
Use: Ocular lubricant.

REGITINE. (Ciba) Phentolamine mesylate 5 mg/Vial (w/mannitol 25 mg in lyophilized form). Pkg. 2s, 6s.
Use: Diagnostic aid.

REGLAN. (Robins) Metoclopramide HCl. **Inj.: 10 mg/2 ml:** Amp. 2 ml, 10 ml; **5 mg/ml:** Vial 2 ml, 10 ml, 30 ml. **Syr.:** 5 mg (as monohydrochloride monohydrate)/5 ml. Bot. pt, Dis-Co Pack 10×10s. **Tab.: 5 mg:** Bot. 100s. **10 mg:** Bot. 100s, 500s, Dis-co Pak 100s.
Use: Antiemetic, GI stimulant.

REGONOL. (Organon) Pyridostigmine bromide 5 mg/ml. Amp 2 ml, Vial 5 ml.
Use: Cholinergic muscle stimulant.

•**REGRAMOSTIM.** USAN.
Use: Biological response modifier; antineoplastic adjunct.

•**REGROTON.** (Rorer) Chlorthalidone 50 mg, reserpine 0.25 mg/Tab. Bot. 100s, 1000s.
Use: Antihypertensive.

REGROTON DEMI. (Rorer) Chlorthalidone 25 mg, reserpine 0.125 mg/Tab. Bot. 100s, 1000s.
Use: Antihypertensive.

REGULACE CAPSULES. (Republic) Docusate sodium 100 mg, casanthranol 30 mg/Cap. Bot. 60s, 100s, 1000s.
Use: Laxative.

REGULAX SS. (Republic) Docusate sodium. **100 mg/Cap.:** Bot. 60s, 100s, 1000s; **250 mg/Cap.:** Bot. 100s.
Use: Laxative.

REGULOID, Orange. (Rugby) Psyllium mucilloid 3.4 Gm, sucrose 70%/rounded tsp. Pow. 420 Gm, 630 Gm.
Use: Laxative.

REGUTOL. (Schering-Plough) Docusate sodium 100 mg/Tab. Box 30s, 60s, 90s.
Use: Laxative.

REHYDRALYTE. (Ross) Sodium 75 mEq, potassium 20 mEq, chloride 65 mEq, citrate 30 mEq, dextrose 25 Gm/L, 100 calories/L. Ready-to-use Bot. 8 oz.
Use: Fluid/electrolyte replacement.

RELA. (Schering) Carisoprodol 350 mg w/tartrazine/Tab. Bot. 100s.
Use: Muscle relaxant.

RELAXADON. (Geneva Generics) Atropine sulfate 0.0194 mg, scopolamine 0.0065 mg, hyoscyamine HBr or SO_4 0.1037 mg, phenobarbital 16.2 mg/Tab. Bot. 1000s.
Use: Anticholinergic/antispasmodic, sedative/hypnotic.

RELAXIN. A purified ovarian hormone of pregnancy (obtained from sows) responsible for pubic relaxation or separation of the symphysis pubis in mammals.
See: Lutrexin, Tab. (Hynson, Westcott & Dunning).

RELEFACT TRH. (Hoechst) Protirelin 0.5 mg/ml. Amp. 1 ml Box 5s.
Use: Diagnostic aid.

RELIEF EYE DROPS. (Allergan) Phenylephrine HCl 0.12%, antipyrine 0.1%, polyvinyl alcohol 1.4%, edetate disodium. Bot. 0.3 ml, 1 ml.
Use: Ophthalmic decongestant.

•**RELOMYCIN.** USAN. A macrolide antibiotic produced by a variant strain of *Streptomyces hygroscopicus.*
Use: Antibiotic.

REMCOL COLD CAPSULES. (Shionogi) Phenylpropanolamine HCl 25 mg, chlorpheniramine maleate 2 mg, acetaminophen 300 mg/Cap. In 24s.
Use: Decongestant, antihistamine, analgesic.

REMCOL-C. (Shionogi) Chlorpheniramine maleate 2 mg, dextromethorphan HBr 15 mg, acetaminophen 300 mg/Cap. In 24s.
Use: Antihistamine, antitussive, analgesic.

REM COUGH MEDICINE. (Last) Dextromethorphan HBr 5 mg/5 ml. Bot. 3 oz, 6 oz.
Use: Antitussive.

REMEGEL SOFT CHEWABLE ANTACID TABLETS. (Warner-Lambert) Aluminum hydroxide-magnesium carbonate 476.4 mg/Chew. Tab. Pkg. 8s, 24s.
Use: Antacid.

REMIVOX. (Janssen) Lorcainide HCl.
Use: Antiarrhythmic.

REMOVING CREAM. (O'Leary) Specially formulated to remove Covermark. Jar 4 oz.

•**REMOXIPRIDE.** USAN.
Use: Antipsychotic.

RENACIDIN. (Guardian) The composition of this powder, as manufactured, is in terms of 156 to 171 Gm citric acid (anhydrous) and 21 to 30 Gm d-gluconic acid (as the lactone) w/purified magnesium hydroxycarbonate 75 to 87 Gm, magnesium acid citrate 9 to 15 Gm, calcium (as carbonate) 2 to 6 Gm, water 17 to 21 Gm per 300 Gm. Bot. 25 Gm 6s; 150 Gm, 300 Gm.
Use: Genitourinary irrigant.

RENALTABS-S.C. (Forest Pharm.) Methenamine 40.8 mg, benzoic acid 4.5 mg, phenyl salicylate 18.1 mg, hyoscyamine sulfate 1/2000 gr, atropine sulfate 0.03 mg, methylene blue 5.4 mg, gelsemium 6.1 mg/Tab. Bot. 1000s.
Use: Urinary anti-infective.

RENAMIN. (Clintec) Sterile hypertonic soln. of essential and non-essential amino acids. Bot. 250 ml, 500 ml.
Use: Parenteral nutritional supplement.

RENANOLONE. 3α-Hydroxypregnane-11,20-dione.
Use: Steroid anesthetic.

RENBU. (Wren) Butabarbital sodium 32.4 mg/Tab. Bot. 100s, 1000s.
Use: Sedative/hypnotic.

RENESE. (Pfizer Laboratories) Polythiazide 1 mg, 2 mg or 4 mg/Tab. Bot. 100s, 1000s.
Use: Diuretic, antihypertensive.

RENESE-R TABLETS. (Pfizer Laboratories) Polythiazide 2 mg, reserpine 0.25 mg/Tab. Bot. 100s, 1000s.
Use: Antihypertensive.

RENGASIL. (Geigy) Pirprofen. Investigational drug.
Use: Anti-inflammatory agent.

RENOFORM.
See: Epinephrine, Preps. (Various Mfr.).

RENOGRAFIN-60,-76. (Squibb Diagnostics) **-60:** Diatrizoate meglumine 52%, sodium diatrizoate 8%, iodine 29.2%. Vial 10 ml, 100 ml, 10s; 30 ml, 50 ml, 25s. **-76:** Diatrizoate meglumine 66%, sodium diatrizoate 10%, iodine 37%. Vial 20 ml, 50 ml, 25s; 100 ml, 200 ml, 10s.
Use: Radiopaque agent.

RENO-M-DIP. (Squibb Diagnostics) Diatrizoate meglumine, iodine 14.1%. 30% for drip infusion pyelography. Inj. Bot. 300 ml. Also w/soln. admin. sets. (Formerly Renografin-Dip).

Use: Radiopaque agent.

RENO-M-30. (Squibb Diagnostics) Diatrizoate meglumine 30%, iodine 14.1%. Vial 50 ml, 100 ml, Box 25s.
Use: Radiopaque agent.

RENO-M-60. (Squibb Diagnostics) Diatrizoate meglumine 60%, iodine 28%. Vial 10 ml, 30 ml, 50 ml, 100 ml.
Use: Radiopaque agent.

RENO-SED. (Vita Elixir) Methenamine 2 gr, salol 0.5 gr, methylene blue 1/10 gr, benzoic acid 1/8 gr, atropine sulfate 1/1000 gr, hyoscyamine sulfate 1/2000 gr/Tab.
Use: Urinary anti-infective.

RENOVIST INJ. (Squibb Diagnostics) Diatrizoate methylglucamine 34.3%, diatrizoate sodium 35%, iodine 37%. Vial 50 ml, Box 25s.
Use: Radiopaque agent.

RENOVIST II. (Squibb Diagnostics) Diatrizoate sodium 29.1%, meglumine diatrizoate 28.5%, iodine 31%. Inj. Vial 30 ml, 60 ml, Box 25s.
Use: Radiopaque agent.

RENOVUE-65. (Squibb Diagnostics) Iodamide meglumide 65%, organically bound iodine 30%, edetate disodium. Vial 50 ml.
Use: Radiopaque agent.

RENOVUE-DIP. (Squibb Diagnostics) Iodamide meglumide 24%, iodine 11.1%. Infusion Bot. 300 ml.
Use: Radiopaque agent.

RENPAP. (Wren) Acetaminophen 4 gr, salicylamide 3 gr, caffeine 2/3 gr, allylisobutylbarbituric acid 3/4 gr/Tab. Bot. 100s, 1000s.
Use: Salicylate analgesic.

RENTUSS. (Wren) **Tab.:** Dextromethorphan HBr 10 mg, guaifenesin 100 mg, phenylephrine HCl 5 mg, phenylpropanolamine HCl 25 mg, chlorpheniramine maleate 2 mg, acetaminophen 300 mg. Bot. 100s, 500s, 1000s. **Syr.:** Same except guaifenesin 50 mg, acetaminophen 120 mg/5 ml. Pt, gal.
Use: Antitussive, expectorant, decongestant, antihistamine, analgesic.

RENU EFFERVESCENT ENZYMATIC CLEANER. (Bausch & Lomb) Subtilisin, polyethylene glycol, sodium carbonate, sodium Cl, tartaric acid. Tab. In 10s, 20s.
Use: Soft contact lens care.

RENU LIQUID. (Biosearch) P-Ca and Na caseinates, CHO-maltodextrin sucrose, F-partially hydrogenated soy oil, mono and diglycerides, soy lecithin, protein 35 Gm, CHO 125 Gm, fat 40 Gm, sodium 500 mg, potassium 1250 mg/L, 1 Cal/ml, 300 mOsm/kg, H_2O. In 250 ml ready to use.
Use: Enteral nutritional supplement.

RENU MULTI-ACTION. (Bausch & Lomb) Isotonic soln. w/sodium Cl, sodium borate, boric acid, poloxamine, polyaminopropyl biguanide 0.00005%, EDTA. Soln. Bot. 240 ml, 360 ml.
Use: Soft contact lens care.

RENU SALINE. (Bausch & Lomb) Isotonic buffered soln. of sodium Cl, boric acid, polyaminopropyl biguanide 0.00003%, EDTA. Soln. Bot. 240 ml, 360 ml.
Use: Soft contact lens care.

RENU THERMAL ENZYMATIC CLEANER. (Bausch & Lomb) Subtilisin, sodium carbonate, sodium Cl, boric acid. Tab. 8s, 16s.
Use: Soft contact lens care.

REPAN. (Everett) Butalbital 50 mg, caffeine 40 mg, acetaminophen 325 mg/Tab. Bot. 100s.
Use: Analgesic combination.

•**REPIRINAST.** USAN.
Use: Antiallergic; antiasthmatic.

REPLETE LIQUID. (Clintec Nutrition) K caseinate, Ca caseinate, maltodextrin, sucrose, corn oil, lecithin, vitamins A, B_1, B_2, B_3, B_5, B_6, B_{12}, C, D, E, K, folic acid, biotin, choline, Ca, Cl, Cu, Fe, I, Mg, Mn, P, Zn. In 250 ml.
Use: Enteral nutritional supplement.

REPOSANS-10. (Wesley) Chlordiazepoxide HCl 10 mg/Cap. Bot. 1000s.
Use: Antianxiety agent.

REP-PRED 40. (Central) Methylprednisolone acetate 40 mg/ml, polyethylene glycol, myristal-gamma-picolinium-chloride. Vial 5 ml.
Use: Corticosteroid.

REP-PRED 80. (Central) Methylprednisolone acetate 80 mg/ml, polyethylene glycol, myristyl-gamma-picolinium-chloride. Vial 5 ml.
Use: Corticosteroid.

REPRIEVE. (Mayer) Caffeine 32 mg, salicylamide 225 mg, vitamin B_1 50 mg, homatropine methylbromide 0.5 mg/Tab. Bot. 8s, 16s.
Use: Analgesic combination.

•**REPROMICIN.** USAN.
Use: Antibacterial.

•**REPROTEROL HYDROCHLORIDE.** USAN.
Use: Bronchodilator.

REPTILASE-R. (Abbott Diagnostics) Diagnostic for the investigation of fibrin formation and disturbances in fibrin formation due to causes other than thrombin inhibition.
Use: Diagnostic aid.

REQUA'S CHARCOAL TABLETS. (Requa) Wood charcoal 10 gr/Tab. Pkg. 50s. Can 125s.
Use: Antiflatulent.

RESA. (Vita Elixir) Reserpine 0.25 mg/Tab.
Use: Antihypertensive.

RESAID S.R. (Geneva Generics) Phenylpropanolamine HCl 75 mg, chlorpheniramine maleate 12 mg/SR Cap. Bot. 100s, 1000s.
Use: Decongestant, antihistamine.

RESCINNAMINE. Methyl 18β-Hydroxy-11,17 α-dimethoxy-3β20α-yohimban-16β-carboxylate 3,4,5- Trimeth-oxycinnamate (Ester). Methyl 0-(3,4,5-trimethoxy-cinnamoyl)reserpate.
Use: Antihypertensive.
See: Anaprel.
Moderil, Tab. (Pfizer Laboratories).

•**RESCON CAPSULES.** (Ion) Pseudoephedrine 120 mg, chlorpheniramine maleate 12 mg/TR Cap. Bot. 100s.
Use: Decongestant, antihistamine.

RESCON-GG CAPSULES. (Ion) Pseudoephedrine HCl 120 mg, chlorphoniramine maleate 8 mg/Cap. Bot. 100s.
Use: Decongestant, antihistamine.

RESCON-GG LIQUID. (Ion) Phenylephrine HCl 5 mg, guaifenesin 100 mg/5 ml Bot. 4 oz.
Use: Decongestant, expectorant.

RESCON JR. (Ion) Pseudoephedrine HCl 60 mg, chlorpheniramine maleate 4 mg/Cap. Bot. 100s.
Use: Decongestant, antihistamine.

RESCON LIQUID. (Ion) Phenylpropanolamine HCl 12.5 mg, chlorpheniramine maleate 2 mg/5 ml. Bot. 4 oz.
Use: Decongestant, antihistamine.

RESECTISOL. (Kendall McGaw) Mannitol soln. 5 Gm/1000 ml in distilled water (275 mOsm/L.). In 2000 ml.
Use: Genitourinary irrigant.

RESERPANEED. (Hanlon) Reserpine 0.25 mg/Tab. Bot. 100s, 1000s.
Use: Antihypertensive.

•**RESERPINE,** U.S.P. XXII. Elix., Inj., Tab., U.S.P. XXII. Yohimban-16-carboxylic acid, 11,17-dimethoxy-18-[(3,4,5-trimethoxybenzyol)oxy]-, methyl ester. Pure alkaloid from Rauwolfia serpentina.
Use: Antihypertensive.
See: Arcum R-S, Tab. (Arcum).
Broserpine, Tab. (Brothers).
De Serpa, Tab. (De Leon).
Elserpine, Tab. (Canright).
Maso-Serpine, Tab. (Mason).
Rauloydin, Tab. (Solvay).
Raurine, Tab. (Westerfield).
Reserjen, Tab. (Jenkins).
Reserpaneed, Tab. (Hanlon).
Serpalan, Tab. (Lannett).
Serpanray, Tab., Amp. (Panray).
Serpasil Preps. (Ciba).
Sertabs, Tab. (Table Rock).
Sertina, Tab. (Fellows-Testagar).
SK-Reserpine, Tab. (SmithKline).
Tensin (Standex).
T-Serp, Tab. (Tennessee).
Vio-Serpine, Tab. (Solvay).
Zepine, Tab. (Foy).

RESERPINE W/COMBINATIONS
See: Demi-Regroton, Tab. (Rorer).
Diupres, Tab. (Merck Sharp & Dohme).
Harbolin, Tab. (Arcum).
Hydromox R, Tab. (Lederle).
Hydropres-25 or -50, Tab. (Merck Sharp & Dohme).
Hydroserp, Tab. (Zenith).
Hydroserpine, Tab. (Geneva).
Hydrotensin-50, Tab. (Mayrand).
Mallopress, Tab. (Mallard).
Metatensin, Tab. (Merrell Dow).
Naquival, Tab. (Schering).
Regroton, Tab. (Rorer).
Renese-R, Tab. (Pfizer Laboratories).
Salutensin, Tab. (Bristol).
Ser-Ap-Es, Tab. (Ciba).
Serapine, Tab. (Cenci).
Serpasil-Apresoline, Tab. (Ciba).
Serpasil-Esidrix, Tab. (Ciba).
Thia-Serp-25, Tab. (Robinson).
Thia-Serp-50, Tab. (Robinson).
Thia-Serpa-Zine, Tab. (Robinson).
Unipres, Tab. (Solvay).

•**RESERPINE AND CHLOROTHIAZIDE TABLETS,** U.S.P. XXII.
Use: Antihypertensive.

•**RESERPINE AND HYDROCHLOROTHIAZIDE TABLETS.** U.S.P. XXII.
Use: Antihypertensive.

•**RESERPINE, HYDRALAZINE HCl and HYDROCHLOROTHIAZIDE,** U.S.P. XXII.
Use: Antihypertensive.

RESINOL MEDICINAL OINTMENT. (Mentholatum) Zinc oxide 12%, calamine 6%, resorcinol 2% in a lanolin and petrolatum base. Jar 3.5 oz, 1.25 oz.
Use: Skin protectant.

RESIN UPTAKE KIT WITH LIOTHYRONINE I-125 BUFFER SOLUTION.
See: Thyrostat-3 (Squibb).

RESINS, ANTACID.
See: Polyamine methylene Resins.

RESOL. (Wyeth-Ayerst) Sodium 50 mEq, potassium 20 mEq, Cl 50 mEq, citrate 34 mEq, calcium 4 mEq, magnesium 4 mEq, phosphate 5 mEq, glucose 20 Gm/L. Contains 80 calories/L. Ctn. 32 fl oz.
Use: Fluid/electrolyte replacement.

RESONIUM-A. (Winthrop Products) Sodium polystyrene sulfonate.
Use: Potassium removing resin.

RESORCIN.
See: Resorcinol (Various Mfr.).

•**RESORCINOL,** U.S.P. XXII. Compound Oint., U.S.P. XXII. 1,3-Benzenediol.
Use: Topical antifungal.

•**RESORCINOL AND SULFUR LOTION.** U.S.P. XXII.
Use: Scabicide, parasiticide, antifungal.

RESORCINOL W/COMBINATIONS
See: Acnomel, Cake, Cream. (SmithKline Prods).
Bicozene, Cream (Ex-Lax).
Biscolan, Supp. (Lannett).
Black and White Ointment, (Schering-Plough).
Castaderm, Preps. (Lannett).
Clearasil, Stick (Vicks).
Lanacane Creme (Combe).
Mazon, Oint. (Thayer).
RA Lot. (Medco).
Rezamid Lot. (Dermick).

•**RESORCINOL MONOACETATE,** U.S.P. XXII. (Various Mfr.) Resorcin acetate.

Use: Antiseborrheic, keratolytic.
See: Euresol, Liq. (Knoll).
W/Salicylic acid, ethyl alcohol, castor oil.
See: Resorcitate w/oil, Lot. (Almay).
W/Salicylic acid, LCD, betanaphthol, castor oil, isopropyl alcohol.
See: Neomark, Liq. (C&M Pharm.).

RESORCINOLPHTHALEIN SODIUM.
See: Fluorescein Sodium, U.S.P. XXII. (Various Mfr.).
W/Oil. Resorcinol monoacetate 1.5%, salicylic acid 1.5%, castor oil 1.5%, ethyl alcohol 81%. Bot. 8 fl oz.
Use: Topical antiseborrheic.

RESOURCE INSTANT CRYSTALS. (Sandoz Nutrition) Vanilla flavor: maltodextrin, sucrose, hydrogenated soy oil, sodium caseinate, calcium caseinate, soy protein isolate, potassium citrate, polyglycerol esters of fatty acids, artificial flavors, vitamins and minerals. Instant Crystals 1.5 oz. or 2 oz. packets.
Use: Enteral nutritional supplement.

RESPAIRE-60 SR. (Laser) Pseudoephedrine HCl 60 mg, guaifenesin 200 mg/S.R. Cap. Bot. 100s, 1000s.
Use: Decongestant, expectorant.

RESPAIRE-120 SR. (Laser) Pseudoephedrine HCl 120 mg, guaifenesin 250 mg/SR Cap. Bot. 100s, 1000s.
Use: Decongestant, expectorant.

RESPBID. (Boehringer Ingelheim) Theophylline 250 mg or 500 mg/Tab. Bot. 100s.
Use: Bronchodilator.

RESPIHALER DECADRON PHOSPHATE. (Merck Sharp & Dohme).
See: Decadron phosphate, respihaler (Merck Sharp & Dohme).

RESPINOL-G TABLETS. (Misemer) Pseudoephedrine HCl 60 mg, guaifenesin 400 mg/Tab. Bot 100s.
Use: Decongestant, expectorant.

RESPIRACULT. (Medical Tech. Corp.) Culture test for group A beta-hemolytic streptococci. In 10s.
Use: Diagnostic aid.

RESPIRALEX. (Medical Tech. Corp.) Latex agglutination test to detect group A streptococci in throat and nasopharynx. Kit 1s.
Use: Diagnostic aid.

RESPORAL TR TABLETS. (Pioneer Pharm) Pseudoephedrine sulfate 120 mg, dexbrompheniramine maleate 6 mg. In 10s, 20s, 30s, 50s, 100s, 1000s.
Use: Decongestant, antihistamine.

RES-Q. (Boyle) Activated charcoal 50%, magnesium hydroxide 25%, tannic acid (Universal antidote). Pkg. 0.5 oz.
Use: Antidote.

REST EASY. (Walgreen) Acetaminophen 1000 mg, pseudoephedrine HCl 60 mg, dextromethorphan HBr 30 mg, doxylamine succinate 7.5 mg/30 ml. Bot. 6 oz, 16 oz.
Use: Analgesic, decongestant, antitussive, antihistamine.

RESTORIL. (Sandoz) Temazepam 15 mg or 30 mg/Cap. Bot. 100s, 500s, UD 25s and 100s.
Use: Sedative/hypnotic.

RETADIAMONE. (Rocky Mtn.) Testosterone enanthate 90 mg, estradiol valerate 4 mg/ml. Vial 10 ml. In sesame oil. Also available in double strength. Vial 5 ml.
Use: Androgen, estrogen.

RETANDROS. (Rocky Mtn.) Testosterone enanthate 200 mg/ml in sesame oil. Vial 10 ml.
Use: Androgen.

RETESTRIN. (Rocky Mtn.) Estradiol-17 valerate in sesame oil 10 mg or 40 mg/ml. Vial 10 ml.
Use: Estrogen.

RETIN-A CREAM. (Ortho) Tretinoin 0.1%, 0.05% or 0.025%. Tube 20 Gm, 45 Gm.
Use: Anti-acne.

RETIN-A GEL. (Ortho) Tretinoin 0.01% or 0.025%, alcohol 90%. Tube 15 Gm, 45 Gm.
Use: Anti-acne.

RETIN-A LIQUID. (Ortho) Tretinoin (retinoic acid, Vitamin A acid) 0.05%, polyethylene glycol 400, butylated hydroxytoluene and alcohol 55%. Bot. 28 ml.
Use: Anti-acne.

RETINOIC ACID. Tretinoin, U.S.P. XXII.
Use: Keratolytic.
See: Retin A Prods. (Ortho).

ALL TRANS-RETINOIC ACID. Tretinoin, U.S.P. XXII.

RETINOL. B.A.N. 3,7-Dimethyl-9-(2,6,6-trimethylcyclohex-1-enyl)nona-2,4,6,8-all-trans-tetraen-1-ol.
See: Vitamin A alcohol.

RETROVIR. (Burroughs Wellcome) Zidovudine 100 mg/Cap. Bot. 100s.
Use: Antiviral agent.

REVS CAFFEINE T.D. CAPSULES. (Vitarine) Caffeine 250 mg/Cap. Bot. 100s, 1000s.
Use: CNS stimulant.

REXAHISTINE. (Econo-Rx) Phenylephrine HCl 5 mg, chlorpheniramine maleate 1 mg, menthol 1 mg, sodium bisulfite 0.1%, alcohol 5%/5 ml. Bot. Gal.
Use: Decongestant, antihistamine.

REXAHISTINE DH. (Econo-Rx) Codeine phosphate 10 mg, phenylephrine HCl 10 mg, chlorpheniramine maleate 2 mg, menthol 1 mg, alcohol 5%/5 ml. Bot. gal.
Use: Antitussive, decongestant, antihistamine.

REXAHISTINE EXPECTORANT. (Econo-Rx) Codeine phosphate 10 mg, phenylephrine HCl 10 mg, chlorpheniramine maleate 2 mg, guaifenesin 100 mg, menthol 1 mg, alcohol 5%/5 ml. Bot. Gal.
Use: Antitussive, decongestant, antihistamine, expectorant.

REXIGEN. (Ion) Phendimetrazine tartrate 35 mg/Tab. Bot. 100s.
Use: Anorexiant.

REXIGEN FORTE CAPSULES. (Ion) Phendimetrazine tartrate 105 mg/SR Cap. Bot. 100s.
Use: Anorexiant.

REZAMID LOTION. (Dermik) Sulfur 5%, resorcinol 2%, alcohol 28.5% in flesh-tinted base. Bot. 2 oz.
Use: Antitreatment.

RF LATEX TEST. (Laboratory Diagnostics) Rapid latex agglutination test for the qualitative screening and semi-quantitative determination of rheumatoid factor. Kit 100s.
Use: Diagnostic aid.

R-GEN. (Owen) Purified water, amphoteric 2, hydrolyzed animal protein, lauramine oxide, methylparaben, benzalkonium Cl, tetrasodium, EDTA, propylparaben, fragrance. Bot. 8 oz.
Use: Protein hair repair shampoo.

R-GEN ELIXIR. (Goldline) Iodinated glycerol 60 mg/5 ml. Bot. pt.
Use: Expectorant.

R-GENE 10. (KabiVitrum) Arginine HCl 10% (950 mOsm/L) with Cl ion 47.5 mEq/100 ml. Inj. 500 ml.
Use: Pituitary (growth hormone) function test.

R-HCTZ-H. (Lederle) Reserpine 0.1 mg, hydrochlorothiazide 15 mg, hydralazine HCl 25 mg/Tab. Bot. 100s, 500s.
Use: Antihypertensive.

RHEABAN. (Leeming) Colloidal activated attapulgite 750 mg/Tab. In 12s.
Use: Antidiarrheal.

RHEOMACRODEX. (Pharmacia) Dextran 40 10% in sodium Cl 0.9% or in dextrose 5%. Soln. Bot. 500 ml.
Use: Plasma expander.

RHEUMASAL. (Jenkins) Sodium salicylate 5 gr, potassium iodide 1 gr, gelsemium extract 0.25 gr, cimicifuga extract ⅛ gr/Tab. Bot. 1000s.
Use: Salicylate analgesic.

RHEUMATEX. (Wampole) Latex agglutination test for the qualitative detection and quantitative determination of rheumatoid factor in serum. Kit 100s.
Use: Diagnostic aid.

RHEUMATON. (Wampole) Two-minute hemagglutination slide test for the qualitative and quantitative determination of rheumatoid factor in serum or synovial fluid. Test kit 20s, 50s, 150s.
Use: Diagnostic aid.

RHEUMATREX DOSE PACK. (Lederle) Methotrexate 2.5 mg. Tab.: 4 cards, each w/three tablets.
Use: Antirheumatic agent.

RHINALL DROPS. (Scherer) Phenylephrine HCl 0.25%, sodium bisulfite. Bot. oz.
Use: Decongestant.

RHINALL SPRAY. (Scherer) Phenylephrine HCl 0.25%. Bot. oz.
Use: Decongestant.

RHINALL 10. (Scherer) Phenylephrine HCl 0.2%. Drop. Bot. oz.
Use: Decongestant.

RHINDECON. (McGregor) Phenylpropanolamine HCl 75 mg/SR Cap. Dye Free. Bot 60s.
Use: Decongestant.

RHINOCAPS. (Ferndale) Aspirin 162 mg, acetaminophen 162 mg, phenylpropanolamine HCl 20 mg/Cap. Bot. 100s.
Use: Analgesic, decongestant.

RHINOGESIC. (Vale) Phenylephrine HCl 5 mg, chlorpheniramine maleate 2 mg, salicylamide 250 mg, acetaminophen 150 mg/Tab. Bot. 100s, 1000s.
Use: Decongestant, antihistamine, analgesic.

RHINOGESIC-GG. (Vale) Phenylephrine HCl 5 mg, chlorpheniramine maleate 2 mg, salicylamide 250 mg, acetaminophen 150 mg, guaifenesin 100 mg/Tab. Bot. 100s, 1000s.
Use: Decongestant, antihistamine, analgesic, expectorant.

RHINOLAR. (McGregor) Phenylpropanolamine HCl 75 mg, chlorpheniramine maleate 8 mg, methscopolamine nitrate 2.5 mg/SR Cap. Dye Free. Bot. 60s.
Use: Decongestant, antihistamine, anticholinergic.

RHINOLAR-EX. (McGregor) Phenylpropanolamine HCl 75 mg, chlorpheniramine maleate 8 mg/SR Cap. Dye free. Bot. 60s.
Use: Decongestant, antihistamine.

RHINOLAR-EX 12. (McGregor) Phenylpropanolamine HCl 75 mg, chlorpheniramine maleate 12 mg/SR Cap. Dye free. Bot. 60s.
Use: Decongestant, antihistamine.

RHODANATE.
See: Potassium Thiocyanate.

RHODANIDE. More commonly Rhodanate, same as thiocyanate.
See: Potassium thiocyanate.

•**RHO (D) IMMUNE GLOBULIN,** U.S.P. XXII.
See: Gamulin Rh, Vial (Parke-Davis).

RhoGAM. (Ortho Diagnostic) Rh_o (D) immune globulin (human). Single-dose vial Pkg. 5s; Prefilled syringe Pkg. 5s, 25s.
Use: Agent for immunization.

RHULICREAM. (Rydelle) Zirconium oxide 1%, benzocaine 1%, menthol 0.7%, camphor 0.3%, isopropyl alcohol 8.8%, parabens. Cream 60 Gm.
Use: Topical poison ivy product.

RHULIGEL. (Rydelle) Phenylcarbinol 2%, menthol 0.3%, camphor 0.3%, SD alcohol 23A 31%. Gel 60 Gm.
Use: Topical poison ivy product.

RHULISPRAY. (Rydelle) Phenylcarbinol 0.67%, calamine 4.7%, menthol 0.025%, camphor 0.25%, benzocaine 1.15%, alcohol 28.8%. Aerosol 120 Gm.
Use: Topical poison ivy product.

RHYTHMIN. (Sidmak) Procainamide 250 mg or 500 mg/SR Tab. Bot. 100s, 500s, 1000s.
Use: Antiarrhythmic.

RHYTHMOL. (Knoll) Propafenone HCl 150 mg or 300 mg/Tab. Bot. 100s, UD 100s.
Use: Antiarrhythmic.

•**RIBAMINOL.** USAN. Ribonucleic acid compound, 2-(diethylamino)-ethanole. Under study.
Use: Learning and memory enhancer.

•**RIBAVIRIN,** U.S.P. XXII. Soln. for inhalation.
Use: Antiviral.
See: Virazole, Inj. (ICN).

•**RIBOFLAVIN,** U.S.P. XXII. Inj., Tab., U.S.P. XXII. Vitamins B_2, G, yellow enzyme, lactoflavin.
Use: Vitamin (enzyme orco-factor).
W/Nicotinamide. (Lilly) Riboflavin 5 mg, nicotinamide 200 mg/ml Amp. 1 ml, Box 100s.
Use: I.M., I.V.; Vitamin B therapy.
W/Vitamins.
See: Vitamin Preparations.

RIBOFLAVIN, METHYLOL.

•**RIBOPRINE.** USAN. N-(3-Methyl-2-butenyl) adrenosin.
Use: Antineoplastic agent.

RIBOZYME INJECTION. (Fellows) Riboflavin-5-Phosphate Sodium 50 mg/ml Vial 10 ml.

RICINOLEATE SODIUM.
See: Preceptin, Gel (Ortho).

RICOLON SOLUTION. (Winthrop Products) Ricolon concentrate.
Use: Leucocytotic preparation.

RID. (Leeming) Piperonyl butoxide 3%, pyrethrins 0.3%, petroleum distillate 1.2%, benzyl alcohol 2.4%. Bot. 2 oz, 4 oz.
Use: Pediculicide.

RID-A-PAIN DROPS. (Pfeiffer) Benzocaine 2.5%, cetalkonium Cl 0.02%, alcohol 20%, hamamelis water, propylene glycol, sodium benzoate, urea, menthol, camphor. Soln. Bot. 15 ml.
Use: Local anesthetic.

RID-A-PAIN OINTMENT. (Pfeiffer) Methyl salicylate 10%, methyl nicotinate 0.5%, menthol, camphor. Oint. 120 ml.
Use: External analgesic.

RID-A-PAIN WITH CODEINE. (Pfeiffer) Codeine phosphate 1 mg, acetaminophen 97.2 mg, aspirin 226.8 mg, caffeine 32.4 mg, salicylamide 32.4 mg/Tab. In 24s, 48s.
Use: Narcotic analgesic combination.

RID LICE CONTROL SPRAY. (Leeming) Synthetic pyrethroids 0.5%, related compounds 0.065%, aromatic petroleum hydrocarbons 0.664%. Can 5 oz.
Use: Pediculicide.

RID LICE ELIMINATION SYSTEM. (Leeming) Rid lice killing shampoo, nit removal comb, Rid lice control spray and instruction booklet/unit.
Use: Pediculicide.

RID LICE SHAMPOO-KIT. (Leeming) Pyrethrins 0.3%, piperonyl butoxide 3%. Bot. 2 oz, 4 oz.
Use: Pediculicide.

RIDAURA CAPSULES. (Smith Kline & French) Auranofin 3 mg/Cap. Bot. 60s.
Use: Antirheumatic.

RIFADIN. (Merrell Dow) Rifampin. **150 mg/Cap.:** Bot. 30s. **300 mg/Cap.:** Bot. 30s, 60s, 100s.
Use: Antituberculous agent.

RIFAMATE. (Merrell Dow) Rifampin 300 mg, isoniazid 150 mg/Cap. Bot. 60s.
Use: Antituberculous agent.

•**RIFAMETANE.** USAN.
Use: Antibacterial.

•**RIFAMIDE.** USAN.
Use: Antibacterial.

RIFAMPICIN. B.A.N. 3-(4-Methylpiperazin-1-ylimino-methyl)rifamycin SV.
Use: Antibiotic.
See: Rifadin, Cap. (Merrell Dow).
Rimactane, Cap. (Ciba).

•**RIFAMPIN,** U.S.P. XXII. Cap., U.S.P. XXII. Hydrazone 3-(4-Methyl-piperazinylimino-methyl rifamycin SV.
Use: Antibacterial (tuberculostatic).
See: Rifadin, Cap. (Merrell Dow).
Rifomycin (Various Mfr.).
Rimactane, Cap. (Ciba).

•**RIFAMPIN AND ISONIAZID CAPSULES,** U.S.P. XXII.
Use: Antibacterial (tuberculostatic).

RIFAMYCIN. B.A.N. Rifamycin SV, an antibiotic produced by certain strains of *Streptomyces mediterranei.* 3-[[(4-Methyl-1-piperazinyl)imino]-methyl]-.
Use: Antibacterial (tuberculostatic).
See: Rifampin, U.S.P. XXII.

•**RIFAPENTINE.** USAN.
Use: Antibacterial.

RIMACTANE. (Ciba) Rifampin 300 mg/Cap. Bot. 30s, 60s, 100s.
Use: Antituberculous agent.

RIMACTANE/INH. (Ciba) Dual pack: 60 Rimactane 300 mg/Cap., 30 Isoniazid 300 mg/Tab.
Use: Antituberculous agent.

•**RIMANTADINE HCl.** USAN. Alpha-methyl-1-adamantanemethylamine HCl.
Use: Antiviral.

•**RIMCAZOLE HYDROCHLORIDE.** USAN.
Use: Antipsychotic.

•**RIMEXOLONE.** USAN.
Use: Anti-inflammatory.

RIMITEROL. B.A.N. erythro-3,4-Dihydroxy-α-(2-piperidyl)benzyl alcohol.
Use: Bronchodilator.

•**RIMITEROL HYDROBROMIDE.** USAN. α-(3,4-Dihydroxy-phenyl)-2-piperidinemethanol HBr.
Use: Bronchodilator.

RIMSO-50. (Research Industries) Dimethyl sulfoxide in a 50% aqueous soln. Bot. 50 ml.
Use: Interstitial cystitis, intravesical instillation.

RINADE. (Econo Med) Chlorpheniramine maleate 8 mg, phenylephrine HCl 20 mg, methscopolamine nitrate 2.5 mg/Cap. Bot. 120s.
Use: Antihistamine, decongestant, anticholinergic.

RINADE-BID. (Econo Med) Chlorpheniramine maleate 8 mg, pseudoephedrine HCl 120 mg/SR Cap. Dye free. Bot. 100s.
Use: Antihistamine, decongestant.

•**RINGER'S INJECTION,** U.S.P. XXII. Lactated, U.S.P. XXII. (Abbott) 250 ml, 500 ml, 1000 ml; (Invenex) 250 ml, 500 ml, 1000 ml; Abbo-Vac glass or flexible containers, Vial 50 ml Pkg. 25s. (Lilly) Amp. 20 ml, Pkg. 6s. (Cutter) Bot. 500 ml, 1000 ml.
Use: Fluid and electrolyte replenisher, irrigating soln.
W/Dextrose. (Cutter) 5% soln. Bot. 1000 ml.

•**RINGER'S INJECTION, LACTATED,** U.S.P. XXII.
Use: Fluid and electrolyte replenisher.

•**RINGER'S IRRIGATION,** U.S.P. XXII. (Abbott) 500 ml, 1000 ml.
Use: Irrigation soln.

RINOCIDIN CAPSULES. (Cenci) Phenylephrine HCl 10 mg, chlorpheniramine maleate 1 mg, pyrilamine maleate 1.5 mg, vitamin C 50 mg, caffeine 30 mg, acetophenetidin 130 mg, salicylamide 200 mg/Cap. Bot. 48s.
Use: Decongestant, antihistamine, analgesic.

RINOCIDIN EXPECTORANT. (Cenci) Codeine phosphate 10.08 mg, phenylephrine HCl 10 mg, chlorpheniramine maleate 2 mg, pyrilamine maleate 6.25 mg, ammonium Cl 60 mg, sodium citrate 85 mg/5 ml. Bot. pt, gal. Also availalable without codeine. Bot. pt, gal.
Use: Antitussive, decongestant, antihistamine, expectorant.

RIOPAN. (Whitehall) Magaldrate. **Tab.:** Magaldrate 480 mg, sodium > 0.1 mg/Tab. (Chew or Swallow). In 60s, 100s. **Susp.:** Magaldrate 540 mg, sodium > 0.1 mg/5 ml. Bot. 6 oz, 12 oz. Individual Cup 30 ml each.
Use: Antacid.

RIOPAN EXTRA STRENGTH. (Whitehall) Magaldrate 1080 mg, sodium ≤ 0.3 mg/5 ml. Liq. Bot. 176 ml, 355 ml, UD 30 ml (10s).
Use: Antacid.

RIOPAN PLUS. (Whitehall) **Chew. Tab.:** Magaldrate 480 mg, simethicone 20 mg, sodium > 0.1 mg/Chew Tab. Bot. 20s, 24s, 60s, 100s. **Susp.:** Magaldrate 540 mg, simethicone 20 mg, sodium > 0.1 mg/5 ml. Bot. 6 oz, 12 oz. Individual Cup 30 ml each. 10 cup/Tray.
Use: Antacid, antiflatulent.

RIOPAN PLUS 2 CHEW TABLETS. (Wyeth-Ayerst) Magaldrate 1880 mg, simethicone 20 mg/Chew. Tab. Bot. 60s.
Use: Antacid, antiflatulent.

RIOPAN PLUS 2 SUSPENSION. (Wyeth-Ayerst) Magaldrate 1080 mg, simethicone 30 mg, sodium 0.3 mg/5 ml. Bot. 6 oz, 12 oz. Cup 30 ml Packer 10 × 10s.
Use: Antacid, antiflatulent.

•**RIOPROSTIL.** USAN.
Use: Gastric antisecretory.

•**RIPAZEPAM.** USAN.
Use: Tranquilizer (minor).

•**RISEDRONATE SODIUM.** USAN.
Use: Regulator (calcium).

•**RISOCAINE.** USAN.
Use: Anesthetic (local).

•**RISOTILIDE HYDROCHLORIDE.** USAN.
Use: Antiarrhythmic.

•**RISTIANOL PHOSPHATE.** USAN.
Use: Immunoregulator.

RISTOCETIN. B.A.N. An antibiotic from species of *Actinomycetes Norcardia lurida.*
Use: Antibiotic.

RITALIN HYDROCHLORIDE. (Ciba) Methylphenidate HCl. **5 mg or 10 mg/Tab.:** Bot. 100s, 500s, 1000s. **20 mg/Tab.:** Bot. 100s, 1000s, 10 mg Accu-Pak 100s.
Use: CNS stimulant.

RITALIN-SR. (Ciba) Methylphenidate HCl 20 mg/SR Tab. Bot. 100s.
Use: CNS stimulant.

•**RITANSERIN.** USAN.
Use: Serotonin antagonist.

RITE-DIET. (E.J. Moore) Methylcellulose, benzocaine, vitamins A, D, B_1, B_2, C plus iron, calcium, potassium, niacinamide/Cap. Bot. 42s.
Use: Diet aid with vitamins.

•**RITODRINE.** USAN. Erythro-p-Hydroxy-α-[1-[(p-hydroxyphenethyl)amino]ethyl] benzyl alcohol
Use: Smooth muscle relaxant.
See: Prempar HCl.
Yutopar, Tab., Inj. (Astra).

•**RITODRINE HYDROCHLORIDE,** U.S.P. XXII. Inj., Tab., U.S.P. XXII.
Use: Relaxant (smooth muscle).

•**RITOLUKAST.** USAN.
Use: Antiasthmatic.

RMS SUPPOSITORIES. (Upsher-Smith) Morphine sulfate 5 mg, 10 mg, 20 mg or 30 mg/Supp. Box 12s.
Use: Narcotic analgesic.

ROAMPICILLIN. (Robinson) Ampicillin 250 mg/Tab. Bot. 100s.
Use: Antibacterial, penicillin.

ROAMPICILLIN POWDER. (Robinson) Ampicillin 125 mg or 250 mg/5 ml. Pow. Vial 80 ml, 100 ml, 150 ml, 200 ml.
Use: Antibacterial, penicillin.

ROBAFEN. (Major) Guaifenesin 100 mg/5 ml, alcohol 3.5%. Syr. Bot. 118 ml, 240 ml, pt, gal.
Use: Expectorant.

ROBAMATE. (Robinson) Meprobamate. Tab. **200 mg:** Bot. 100s. **400 mg:** Bot. 1000s.
Use: Antianxiety agent.

ROBAMOL. (Cenci) Methocarbamol 750 mg/Tab. Bot. 100s, 1000s.
Use: Skeletal muscle relaxant.

ROBANTALINE. (Robinson) Propantheline bromide 15 mg/Tab. Bot. 100s, 500s, 1000s.
Use: Anticholinergic.

ROBANTALINE WITH PHENOBARBITAL. (Robinson) Propantheline bromide, phenobarbital/Tab. Bot. 100s, 500s, 1000s.

Use: Anticholinergic.
ROBANUL.
See: Robinul, Preps. (Robins).
ROBARB. (Robinson) Amobarbital 0.25 gr, 0.5 gr or 1 gr/Cap. Bot. 100s.
Use: Sedative/hypnotic.
ROBATEN DAC. (Major) Pseudoephedrine 30 mg, codeine phosphate 10 mg, guaifenesin 100 mg, alcohol 1.4%. Bot. Pt.
Use: Decongestant, antitussive, expectorant.
ROBATHOL BATH OIL. (Pharmaceutical Specialties) Cottonseed oil, alkyl aryl polyether alcohol. Lanolin free. Bot. 240 ml, 480 ml, gal.
Use: Bath dermatological.
ROBAXIN. (Robins) Methocarbamol. **Tab.:** 500 mg, Bot. 100s, 500s, UD 100s. **Inj.:** 1 Gm/10 ml of a 50% aqueous soln. of polyethylene glycol 300. Vial 10 ml.
Use: Skeletal muscle relaxant.
ROBAXIN-750. (Robins) Methocarbamol 750 mg/Tab. Bot. 100s, 500s, Dis-Co Pak 100s.
Use: Skeletal muscle relaxant.
ROBAXISAL. (Robins) Methocarbamol (Robaxin) 400 mg, aspirin 325 mg/Tab. Bot. 100s, 500s, Dis-Co pack 100s.
Use: Muscle relaxant, analgesic.
ROBENECID. (Robinson) Probenecid 0.5 Gm/Tab. Bot. 100s, 1000s.
Use: Agent for gout.
ROBENECID WITH COLCHICINE. (Robinson) Colchicine 0.5 mg, probenecid 500 mg/Tab. Bot. 100s.
Use: Agent for gout.
ROBENECOL. (Robinson) Probenecid with colchicine/Tab. Bot. 100s, 1000s.
Use: Agent for gout.
•**ROBENIDINE HYDROCHLORIDE.** USAN.
Use: Coccidiostat.
ROBESE. (Rocky Mtn.) Dextroamphetamine sulfate 5 mg/Tab. Bot. 100s, 1000s.
Use: CNS stimulant.
ROBESE C. CAP NON-AMPHETAMINE W.C. (Rocky Mtn.) Carboxymethylcellulose 500 mg, benzocaine 9 mg, vitamins A 5000 IU, D 400 IU, B_1 2 mg, B_2 2.5 mg, niacinamide 20 mg, ascorbic acid 50 mg, B_6 1 mg, calcium pantothenate 1 mg, iron 15 mg/3 Cap. Bot. 48s, 96s.
Use: Diet aid.
ROBESE C. INJ. NON-AMPHETAMINE W.C. (Rocky Mtn.) Caffeine 250 mg, sodium benzoate 250 mg/2 ml. Vial 30 ml.
Use: Diet aid.
ROBESE "P" INJ. (Rocky Mtn.) Phenylpropanolamine HCl 75 mg, protein hydrolysate containing amino acid 100 ml, leucine 0.415 Gm, valine 0.30 Gm, lysine 0.35 Gm, isoleucine 0.24 Gm, phenylalanine 0.28 Gm, arginine 0.15 Gm, threonine 0.18 Gm, methionine 0.22 Gm, histidine 0.12 Gm, tryptophan 0.05 Gm/ml. Vial 10 ml.
ROBESE "P" TABLETS. (Rocky Mtn.) Phendimetrazine tartrate 35 mg/Tab. Bot. 100s, 1000s.
Use: Anorexiant.
ROBICILLIN VK. (Robins) Penicillin V Potassium. **250 mg.:** (400,000 units)/Tab. Bot. 100s, 1000s. **500 mg:** (800,000 units)/Tab. Bot. 100s, 500s.
Use: Antibacterial, penicillin.
ROBIMYCIN. (Robins) Erythromycin 250 mg/Tab. Bot. 100s, 500s.
Use: Antibacterial, erythromycin.
ROBINUL. (Robins) Glycopyrrolate 1 mg/Tab. Bot. 100s, 500s.
Use: Anticholinergic.
ROBINUL FORTE TABLETS. (Robins) Glycopyrrolate 2 mg/Tab. Bot. 100s.
Use: Anticholinergic.
ROBINUL INJECTABLE. (Robins) Glycopyrrolate 0.2 mg/ml, benzyl alcohol 0.9%. Vial 1 ml, 2 ml, 5 ml, 20 ml.
Use: Anticholinergic.
ROBITET. (Robins) Tetracycline HCl. Cap. **250 mg:** Bot. 100s, 1000s; **500 mg:** Bot. 100s, 500s.
Use: Antibacterial.
ROBITUSSIN. (Robins) Guaifenesin 100 mg/5 ml, alcohol 3.5%. Bot 1 oz, 4 oz, 8 oz, 1 pt, gal. UD 5 ml, 10 ml, 15 ml.
Use: Expectorant.
ROBITUSSIN A-C. (Robins) Guaifenesin 100 mg, codeine phosphate 10 mg/5 ml, alcohol 3.5%, saccharin, sorbitol. Bot. 2 oz, 4 oz, pt, gal.
Use: Expectorant, antitussive.
ROBITUSSIN-CF. (Robins) Guaifenesin 100 mg, phenylpropanolamine HCl 12.5 mg, dextromethorphan HBr 10 mg/5 ml, alcohol 4.75%, saccharin, sorbitol. Syr. Bot. 4 oz, 8 oz, pt.
Use: Expectorant, decongestant, antitussive.
ROBITUSSIN-DAC. (Robins) Guaifenesin 100 mg, pseudoephedrine HCl 30 mg, codeine phosphate 10 mg/5 ml, alcohol 1.9%, saccharin, sorbitol. Syr. Bot. 4 oz, pt.
Use: Expectorant, decongestant, antitussive.
ROBITUSSIN DIS-CO. (Robins) Guaifenesin 100 mg, alcohol 3.5%/5 ml. Syr. UD pack 5 ml, 10 ml, 15 ml; (10 x 10s).
Use: Expectorant.
ROBITUSSIN-DM. (Robins) Guaifenesin 100 mg, dextromethorphan HBr 15 mg/5 ml, alcohol 1.4%, saccharin. Syr. Bot. 4 oz, 8 oz, pt, gal, UD 5 ml, 10 ml (100s).
Use: Expectorant, antitussive.
ROBITUSSIN NIGHT RELIEF. (Robins) Acetaminophen 1000 mg, phenylephrine HCl 10 mg, pyrilamine maleate 50 mg, dextromethorphan HBr 30 mg/oz, alcohol 25%, saccharin, sorbital. Bot. 4 oz, 8 oz.
Use: Analgesic, decongestant, antihistamine, antitussive.
ROBITUSSIN-PE. (Robins) Guaifenesin 100 mg, pseudoephedrine HCl 30 mg/5 ml, alcohol 1.4%, saccharin. Syr. Bot. 4 oz, 8 oz, pt.
Use: Expectorant, decongestant.

ROBOLIC. (Rocky Mtn.) Methandriol dipropionate 50 mg/ml. Vial 10 ml.

ROBOMOL-500. (Major) Methocarbamol 500 mg/Tab. Bot. 100s, 500s.
Use: Skeletal muscle relaxant.

ROBOMOL-750. (Major) Methocarbamol 750 mg/Tab. Bot. 500s, UD 100s.
Use: Skeletal muscle relaxant.

ROBOMOL/ASA TABS. (Major) Methocarbamol w/ASA. Bot. 100s, 500s.
Use: Skeletal muscle relaxant, analgesic.

ROCAINE. (Rocky Mtn.) Lidocaine HCl 1% or 2%. Vial 50 ml.
Use: Local anesthetic.

ROCALOSAN. (Rocky Mtn.) Calcium glycerophosphate 1%, calcium levulinate 1.5%. Vial 30 ml.

ROCALTROL. (Roche) Calcitriol 0.25 mcg or 0.5 mcg/Cap. **0.25 mcg:** Bot. 30s, 100s. **0.5 mcg:** Bot. 100s.
Use: Management of hypocalcemia in patients undergoing chronic renal dialysis.

•**ROCASTINE HYDROCHLORIDE.** USAN.
Use: Antihistamine.

ROCEPHIN. (Roche) Ceftriaxone sodium 250 mg, 500 mg, 1 Gm, or 2 Gm/Vial to be reconstituted for IV or IM administration. Box 10s. Piggyback Bot. 1 Gm or 2 Gm Box 10s. Bulk Pharmacy Container 10 Gm Box 1s. ADD-Vantage Vial 1 Gm or 2 Gm Box 10s. Frozen Premix 1 Gm or 2 Gm Iso-osmotic in 50 ml plastic container, not to be stored above -20 degrees C.
Use: Antibacterial, cephalosporin.

ROCHLOMETHIAZIDE. (Robinson) Trichlormethiazide 4 mg/Tab. Bot. 100s, 500s.
Use: Diuretic, antihypertensive.

ROCHORIC. (Rocky Mtn.) Chorionic gonadotropin 10,000 IU/10 ml. Univial 10 ml.
Use: Chorionic gonadotropin.

RO-CHLOROZIDE. (Robinson) Chlorothiazide 250 mg or 500 mg/Tab. Bot. 100s, 1000s.
Use: Diuretic.

ROCORT LOTION. (Rocky Mtn.) Hydrocortisone 0.5%. Bot. 4 oz.
Use: Corticosteroid, topical.

ROCYCLO INJECTION. (Robinson) Dicyclomine HCl 10 mg/ml. Vial 10 ml.
Use: Anticholinergic.

ROCYCLO-PHEN. (Robinson) Dicyclomine HCl, phenobarbital. Tab. Bot. 100s, 500s.
Use: Anticholinergic, sedative/hypnotic.

ROCYCLO-10. (Robinson) Dicyclomine HCl 10 mg/Cap. Bot. 100s, 500s.
Use: Anticholinergic.

ROCYCLO-20. (Robinson) Dicyclomine HCl 20 mg/Tab. Bot. 100s, 500s.
Use: Anticholinergic.

RODELTA T.B.A. (Rocky Mtn.) Prednisolone tertiary butylacetate 20 mg/10 ml. Vial 10 ml.
Use: Corticosteroid.

RODESINE. (Rocky Mtn.) Adenosine 5 monophosphoric acid 25 mg, sodium nicotinate 20 mg, vitamin B_{12} crystalline 75 mcg, benzyl alcohol 1.5%/ml. Vial 10 ml.
Use: Anti-inflammatory agent.

RO-DIET. (Robinson) Diethylpropion HCl 25 mg/Tab. Bot. 100s, 1000s.
Use: Anorexiant.

RO-DIET TIMED. (Robinson) Diethylpropion HCl 75 mg/TD Tab. Bot. 100s, 1000s.
Use: Anorexiant.

•**RODOCAINE.** USAN.
Use: Local anesthetic.

RODOX. (Rocky Mtn.) Docusate sodium 100 mg or 250 mg/Cap. Bot. 100s.
Use: Laxative.

RODOX/W. (Rocky Mtn.) Docusate sodium 100 mg, casanthranol 75 mg/Cap. Bot. 100s, 1000s.
Use: Laxative.

RODRYL. (Rocky Mtn.) Diphenhydramine HCl 10 mg/ml. Vial 30 ml.
Use: Antihistamine.

RODRYL-50. (Rocky Mtn.) Diphenhydramine HCl 50 mg/ml. Vial 10 ml.
Use: Antihistamine.

ROENTGENOGRAPHY.
See: Iodine Products, Diagnostic.

RO-FEDRIN. (Robinson) Pseudoephedrine HCl 60 mg/Tab. Bot. 100s, 1000s.
Use: Decongestant.

RO-FEDRINE SYRUP. (Robinson) Pseudoephedrine HCl 30 mg/5 ml. Bot. pt.
Use: Decongestant.

ROFERON-A. (Roche) Interferon alfa-2a, recombinant as 3 million or 18 million IU/Vial in injectable soln. Available as sterile pow. in 18 million IU w/diluent. Subcutaneous or intramuscular inj. 3 million IU/ml Box 10s. 18 million IU/0.5 ml Box 1s.
Use: Antineoplastic agent.

•**ROFLURANE.** USAN. 2-Bromo-1, 1,2-trifluoroethyl methyl ether.
Use: General anesthetic.

ROGAINE. (Upjohn) Minoxidil 20 mg/ml Topical Soln. Bot. 60 ml w/applicator.
Use: Male pattern baldness.

ROGENIC. (Forest) **SC Tab.:** Iron 60 mg, vitamin C 100 mg, B_6 6 mg, B_{12} 25 mcg, desiccated liver. Bot. 100s, 1000s. **Inj.:** Vitamin B_{12} 500 mcg, peptonized iron 20 mg, liver 10 mcg/ml. Vial 10 ml.
Use: Vitamin/mineral supplement.

RO-HIST. (Robinson) Tripelennamine HCl 50 mg/Tab. Bot. 100s, 1000s.
Use: Antihistamine.

ROHIST. (Rocky Mtn.) Chlorpheniramine 12 mg/TD Tab. Bot. 100s.
Use: Antihistamine.

ROHIST C. (Rocky Mtn.) Chlorpheniramine 100 mg/ml. Vial 10 ml.
Use: Antihistamine.

ROHIST-D. (Rocky Mtn.) Chlorpheniramine 5 mg, phenylpropanolamine HCl 12.5 mg, atropine

sulfate 0.2 mg, vitamin C 100 mg/Cap. Bot. 100s. Vial 10 ml.
Use: Antihistamine, decongestant, anticholinergic/antispasmodic.

ROHIST PLUS. (Rocky Mtn.) Chlorpheniramine 12 mg, d-desoxyephedrine HCl 8 mg/TR Tab. Bot. 100s.
Use: Antihistamine, decongestant.

RO HONEY PROTEIN. (Rocky Mtn.) Protein 70%. Bot. 250s.
Use: Protein supplement.

ROHYDRA. (Robinson) **Cap.:** Diphenhydramine HCl 25 mg or 50 mg. Bot. 100s, 1000s. **Elix.:** Diphenhydramine HCl 80 mg, ammonium Cl 12 gr, sodium citrate 5 gr, menthol 0.1 gr/fl oz. Bot. pt, gal.
Use: Antihistamine, expectorant.

RO-HYDRAZIDE. (Robinson) Hydrochlorothiazide 100 mg/Tab. Bot. 100s, 1000s.
Use: Diuretic.

ROLA-BEE. (Robinson) Vitamins B_1 15 mg, B_2 10 mg, niacinamide 50 mg, calcium pantothenate 10 mg, B_6 5 mg, C 250 mg/Cap. Bot. 100s, 1000s.
Use: Vitamin supplement.

ROLABROMOPHEN. (Robinson) Brompheniramine maleate 4 mg/Tab. Bot. 100s, 5000s.
Use: Antihistamine.

ROLABROMOPHEN DECONGESTANT ELIXIR. (Robinson) Brompheniramine maleate 4 mg, phenylephrine HCl 5 mg, phenylpropanolamine HCl 5 mg, alcohol 2.3%/5 ml. Bot. pt, gal.
Use: Antihistamine, decongestant.

ROLABROMOPHEN ELIXIR. (Robinson) Brompheniramine maleate 2 mg, alcohol 3%/5 ml. Bot. pt, gal.
Use: Antihistamine.

ROLABROMOPHEN EXPECTORANT. (Robinson) Brompheniramine maleate 2 mg, phenylephrine HCl 5 mg, phenylpropanolamine HCl 5 mg, guaifenesin 100 mg, alcohol 3.5%/5 ml. Bot. pt, gal.
Use: Antihistamine, decongestant, expectorant.

ROLABROMOPHEN FORTE. (Robinson) Brompheniramine maleate-forte extended. Bot. 100s, 500s, 1000s.
Use: Antihistamine.

ROLABROMOPHEN INJECTION. (Robinson) Brompheniramine maleate. Inj. **10 mg/ml:** Vial 30 ml; **100 mg/ml:** Vial 10 ml.
Use: Antihistamine.

ROLABROMOPHEN TIMED. (Robinson) Brompheniramine maleate 8 mg or 12 mg/TD Tab. Bot. 100s, 1000s.
Use: Antihistamine.

ROLAIDS ANTACID TABLETS. (Warner-Lambert) Dihydroxyaluminum sodium carbonate 334 mg/Tab. Roll 12s.
Use: Antacid.

ROLAIDS CALCIUM RICH. (Warner-Lambert) Calcium Carbonate 550 mg. Chew. Tab. Roll 12s, Bot. 75s, 150s.
Use: Antacid.

ROLAIDS SODIUM FREE TABLETS. (Warner-Lambert) Magnesium hydroxide 64 mg, calcium carbonate 317 mg. Roll 12s, Bot. 75s, 150s.
Use: Antacid.

ROLA-METHAZINE. (Robinson) Promethazine HCl 12.5 mg, 25 mg or 50 mg/Tab. Bot. 100s, 500s, 1000s.
Use: Antihistamine, antiemetic, sedative.

ROLA-METHAZINE EXPECTORANT PLAIN. (Robinson) Promethazine with expectorant. Bot. pt, gal.
Use: Antihistamine, expectorant.

ROLA-METHAZINE INJECTION. (Robinson) Promethazine HCl 25 mg/ml. Inj. Vial 10 ml.
Use: Antiemetic, antihistamine.

ROLA-METHAZINE PEDIATRIC LIQUID. (Robinson) Promethazine pediatric liq. Bot. pt, gal.
Use: Antihistamine.

ROLA-METHAZINE VC EXPECTORANT. (Robinson) Promethazine VC. Bot. pt, gal.
Use: Antihistamine, expectorant.

ROLA-METHAZINE VC EXPECTORANT WITH CODEINE. (Robinson) Promethazine VC expectorant, codeine. Bot. pt, gal.
Use: Antihistamine, expectorant, antitussive.

ROLA-METHAZINE WITH CODEINE. (Robinson) Promethazine expectorant, codeine. Bot. pt, gal.
Use: Antihistamine, expectorant, antitussive.

ROLANADE. (Robinson) Chlorpheniramine maleate 8 mg, phenylpropanolamine HCl 50 mg, atropine sulfate 1/180 gr/Cap. Bot. 100s, 500s, 1000s.
Use: Antihistamine, decongestant, anticholinergic/antispasmodic.

ROLAPHENT. (Robinson) Phentermine 8 mg/Tab. Bot. 100s.
Use: Anorexiant.

ROLATHIMIDE. (Robinson) Glutethimide 0.5 Gm/Tab. Bot. 100s, 500s.
Use: Hypnotic.

ROLAZID. (Robinson) Isonicotinic acid hydrazide 100 mg or 300 mg/Tab. Bot. 100s, 1000s.
Use: Antituberculous agent.

ROLAZINE. (Robinson) Hydralazine HCl 25 mg or 50 mg/Tab. Bot. 100s, 500s, 1000s.
Use: Antihypertensive.

ROLCEDIN. (Robinson) Chlorpheniramine maleate 2 mg, salicylamide 3.5 gr, acetophenetidin 2.5 gr, caffeine 0.5 gr/Tab. Bot. 100s, 1000s.
Use: Antihistamine, analgesic.

ROLECITHIN. (Robinson) **Cap.:** Soya lecithin 259.2 mg, soy bean oil 170.2 mg, vitamin D 150 units/Cap. **Tab.:** Soya lecithin 7 gr/Tab. Bot. 100s, 250s, 1000s.
Use: Nutritional supplement.

•**ROLETAMIDE.** USAN. 3′,4′,5′-Trimethoxy-3-(3-pyrrolin-1-yl)acrylophenone.
Use: Hypnotic.

•**ROLGAMIDINE.** USAN.
Use: Antidiarrheal.

ROLICAP. (Arcum) Vitamins A acetate 5000 IU, D_2 400 IU, B_1 3 mg, B_2 2.5 mg, B_6 10 mg, C 50 mg, niacinamide 20 mg, B_{12} 1 mcg/Chew. Tab. Bot. 100s, 1000s.
Use: Vitamin supplement.

ROLICYPRAM. B.A.N. (+)-5-Oxo-N-(trans-2-phenylcyclopropyl) L pyrrolidine 2 carboxamide.
Use: Antidepressant.

•**ROLICYPRINE.** USAN. (+)-5-Oxo-N-(trans-2-phenylcyclopropyl)-L-2-pyrrolidinecarboxamide.
Use: Antidepressant.

ROLIDIOL. (Robinson) Ethinyl estradiol 0.02 mg or 0.05 mg/Tab. Bot. 100s, 1000s.
Use: Estrogen.

ROLIDRIN-6. (Robinson) Nylidrin HCl 6 mg/Tab. Bot. 100s, 1000s.
Use: Vasodilator.

ROLIDRIN-12. (Robinson) Nylidrin HCl 12 mg/Tab. Bot. 100s, 1000s.
Use: Vasodilator.

RO-LINOIL. (Robinson) Linolenic acid 51%, linoleic acid 17%, oleic acid 23%, stearic acid 2%, palmitic acid 7%. Cap. 200 min. Bot. 100s, 500s.
Use: Unsaturated free fatty acid supplement.

•**ROLIPRAM.** USAN.
Use: Tranquilizer.

ROLISOX-10. (Robinson) Isoxsuprine HCl 10 mg/Tab. Bot. 100s.
Use: Vasodilator.

ROLISOX-20. (Robinson) Isoxsuprine HCl 20 mg/Tab. Bot. 100s.
Use: Vasodilator.

ROLITETRACYCLINE, STERILE, U.S.P. XXII. Inj., U.S.P. XXII. N-(Pyrrolidinomethyl) tetracycline. 4-(Dimethylamino)-1,4,4a,5,5a,6,11,12a-octahydro-3,6,10,12,12a-pentahydroxy-6-methyl-1,11-dioxo-N-(1-pyrrolidinylmethyl)-2-naphthacenecarboxamide. Tetrex PMT nitrate Inj. Syntetrin Inj. (Bristol) Velacycline (Squibb).
Use: Antibacterial.

ROLITETRACYCLINE NITRATE. USAN. Tetrim.
Use: Antibacterial.

ROLODINE. USAN. 4-(Benzylamino)-2-methyl-7H-pyrrolo-[2,3-d]-pyrimidine.
Use: Muscle relaxant.

ROLSERP. (Robinson) Reserpine. **Tab.:** 0.1 mg, 0.25 mg or 0.5 mg. Bot. 100s, 1000s. **Inj.:** 5 mg/ml Vial 10 ml. **Timed cap:** 0.25 mg, 0.5 mg or 0.75 mg. Bot. 100s, 500s, 1000s, Bulk Pack 5000s. **Elix.:** 0.25 mg/5 ml. Bot. 16 oz.
Use: Antihypertensive.

ROLUTIN. (Rocky Mtn.) Hydroxyprogesterone caproate in oil 125 mg/10 ml Vial 10 ml.
Use: Progestin.

ROLUTIN 2X. (Rocky Mtn.) Hydroxyprogesterone caproate in oil 125 mg/5 ml Vial 5 ml.
Use: Progestin.

ROLZYME. (Robinson) Pepsin 250 mg, pancreatin 200 mg, bile salts 150 mg, dehydrocholic acid 25 mg/Tab. Bot. 100s, 1000s.
Use: Enzyme supplement.

ROMACH ANTACID TABLETS. (Last) Magnesium carbonate 400 mg, sodium bicarbonate 250 mg/Tab. Strip pack 60s, 500s.
Use: Antacid.

ROMAPHED. (Robinson) Aminophylline, ephedrine, amobarbital. Tab. Bot. 100s, 500s, 1000s.
Use: Antiasthmatic combination.

•**ROMAZARIT.** USAN.
Use: Anti-inflammatory; antirheumatic.

ROMETHOCARB. (Robinson) Methocarbamol 500 mg or 750 mg/Tab. Bot. 100s, 500s.
Use: Skeletal muscle relaxant.

ROMEX COUGH & COLD CAPSULES. (APC) Guaifenesin 65 mg, dextromethorphan HBr 10 mg, chlorpheniramine maleate 1.5 mg, pyrilamine maleate 12.5 mg, phenylephrine HCl 5 mg, acetaminophen 160 mg/Cap. Bot. 21s.
Use: Expectorant, antitussive, antihistamine, decongestant.

ROMEX COUGH & COLD TABLETS. (APC) Dextromethorphan HBr 7.5 mg, phenylephrine HCl 2.5 mg, ascorbic acid 30 mg. Box 15s.
Use: Antitussive, decongestant.

ROMEX TROCHES & LIQUID. (APC) **Troche:** Polymyxin B sulfate 1000 units, benzocaine 5 mg, cetalkonium Cl 2.5 mg, gramicidin 100 mcg, chlorpheniramine maleate 0.5 mg, tyrothricin 2 mg. Pkg. 10s. **Liq.**: Guaifenesin 200 mg, dextromethorphan HBr 60 mg, chlorpheniramine maleate 12 mg, phenylephrine HCl 30 mg/fl oz. Bot. 4 oz.
Use: Antibacterial, antihistamine, expectorant, antitussive, decongestant.

ROMINAL W/C. (Robinson) Vitamins B_1 25 mg, B_2 12.5 mg, nicotinamide 75 mg, B_6 3 mg, calcium pantothenate 10 mg, C 250 mg, B_{12} 3 mcg/Cap. Bot. 100s.
Use: Vitamin supplement.

ROMINE. (Rocky Mtn.) Dimenhydrinate 50 mg, propylene glycol/ml. Vial 10 ml.
Use: Antiemetic/antivertigo.

RONDEC ORAL DROPS. (Ross) Carbinoxamine maleate 2 mg, pseudoephedrine HCl 25 mg/ml. Bot. 30 ml w/dropper.
Use: Antihistamine, decongestant (pediatric).

RONDEC SYRUP. (Ross) Carbinoxamine maleate 4 mg, pseudoephedrine HCl 60 mg/5 ml. Syr. Bot. 4 oz, pt.
Use: Antihistamine, decongestant (pediatric).

RONDEC-DM ORAL DROPS. (Ross) Carbinoxamine maleate 2 mg, pseudoephedrine HCl 25 mg, dextromethorphan HBr 4 mg/ml, alcohol 6%. Bot. 30 ml w/dropper.
Use: Antihistamine, decongestant, antitussive.

RONDEC-DM SYRUP. (Ross) Carbinoxamine maleate 4 mg, pseudoephedrine HCl 60 mg, dextromethorphan HBr 15 mg/5 ml, alcohol 6%. Bot. 4 oz, pt.
Use: Antihistamine, decongestant, antitussive.

RONDEC-TR. (Ross) Carbinoxamine 8 mg, pseudoephedrine HCl 120 mg/SR Tab. Bot. 100s.
Use: Antihistamine, decongestant.

RONDOMYCIN. (Wallace) Methacycline HCl. 150 mg or 300 mg/Cap. **150 mg**: Bot. 100s. **300 mg**: Bot. 50s.
Use: Antibacterial, tetracycline.

RONICOTIN. (Rocky Mtn.) Nicotinic acid 500 mg/Tab. Bot. 100s, 1000s.
Use: Vasodilator.

•**RONIDAZOLE.** USAN.
Use: Antiprotozoal.

RONIL. (Rocky Mtn.) Milk sugar 3 gr/TD Tab. Bot. 100s.
Use: Placebo.

•**RONNEL.** USAN. Fenchlorphos.
Use: Insecticide (systemic).
See: Korlan (Dow).
Trolene (Dow).

RONVET. (Geneva) Erythromycin stearate 250 mg/Tab. Bot. 100s.
Use: Antibacterial.

RO OPTHO. (Rocky Mtn.) Sodium sulfacetamide 100 mg, prednisolone 5 mg, phenylephrine HCl 0.12%/ml. Bot. 5 ml.
Use: Anti-infective, ophthalmic; corticosteroid.

RO-PAPAV. (Robinson) Papaverine HCl. 150 mg/TD Tab. Bot. 100s, 250s, 1000s.
Use: Smooth muscle relaxant.

RO-PHYLLINE. (Robinson) Theophylline 80 mg/15 ml, alcohol 20%, fruit-flavored, sugar-free. Soln. Bot. pt, gal.
Use: Antiasthmatic.

•**ROPITOIN HYDROCHLORIDE.** USAN.
Use: Cardiac depressant.

•**ROPIZINE.** USAN.
Use: Anticonvulsant.

ROPLEDGE. (Robinson) Phendimetrazine tartrate 35 mg/Tab. Bot. 100s, 1000s.
Use: Anorexiant.

ROPOXY. (Robinson) Propoxyphene HCl 65 mg/Cap. Bot. 100s, 500s, 1000s.
Use: Analgesic.

ROPOXY COMPOUND-65. (Robinson) Propoxyphene compound. Cap. Bot. 100s, 500s.
Use: Analgesic.

ROPRED. (Robinson) Prednisone 1 mg, 2.5 mg, 5 mg or 20 mg/Tab. Bot. 100s, 500s, 1000s.
Use: Corticosteroid.

RO-PRENATE. (Robinson) Prenatal vitamins and minerals. Tab. Bot. 100s, 1000s.
Use: Vitamin/mineral supplement.

ROPREDLONE. (Robinson) Prednisolone. **Tab.:** 1 mg or 5 mg. Bot. 100s, 500s, 1000s. Inj. **Vial:** 25 mg, 50 mg, 100 mg/ml Vial 10 ml.
Use: Corticosteroid.

ROQUINE. (Robinson) Chloroquine phosphate 0.25 Gm/Tab. Bot. 100s, 500s, 1000s.
Use: Antimalarial, amebicide.

ROSA GALLICAL.
See: Estivin, Soln. (Alcon).

ROSANILINE DYES.
See: Fuchsin, Basic (Various Mfr.).
Methylrosaniline Cl, Soln., Inj. (Various Mfr.).

•**ROSARAMICIN.** USAN.
Use: Antibacterial.

•**ROSARAMICIN BUTYRATE.** USAN.
Use: Antibacterial.

•**ROSARAMICIN PROPIONATE.** USAN.
Use: Antibacterial.

•**ROSARAMICIN SODIUM PHOSPHATE.** USAN.
Use: Antibacterial.

•**ROSARAMICIN STEARATE.** USAN.
Use: Antibacterial.

ROSCORB 5. (Rocky Mtn.) Vitamin C 500 mg/Tab. Bot. 100s, 1000s.
Use: Vitamin supplement.

ROSE BENGAL. (Americal) Rose bengal 1%. Bot. 5 ml.
Use: Diagnostic for staining dead ocular tissue.

•**ROSE BENGAL SODIUM I-125.** USAN.
Use: Radioactive agent.

•**ROSE BENGAL SODIUM I-131 INJECTION,** U.S.P. XXII. Sodium 4,5,6,7-Tetrachloro-2′,-4′,5′,7′-tetraiodofluorescein.
Use: Diagnostic aid (hepatic function).

ROSE BENGAL STRIPS. (Barnes-Hind) Rose bengal 1.3 mg. For disclosing corneal injury and pathology. Strip box 100s.
Use: Diagnostic aid.

ROSE-C LIQUID. (Barth's) Vitamin C 300 mg, rose hip extract/Tsp. Dropper Bot. 2 oz, 8 oz.
Use: Vitamin C supplement.

ROSE HIPS. (Burgin-Arden) Vitamin C 300 mg, in base of sorbitol. Bot. 4 oz, 8 oz.
Use: Vitamin C supplement.

ROSE HIPS VITAMIN C. (Kirkman) Vitamin C. **100 mg/Tab:** Bot. 100s, 250s. **250 mg or 500 mg/Tab:** Bot. 100s, 250s, 500s.
Use: Vitamin C supplement.

•**ROSE OIL,** N.F. XVII.
Use: Perfume.

•**ROSE WATER, STRONGER,** N.F. XVII.
Use: Perfume.

•**ROSE WATER OINTMENT,** U.S.P. XXII.
Use: Emollient, ointment base.

ROSIN, U.S.P. XXI.
Use: Stiffening agent, pharmaceutical necessity

•**ROSOXACIN.** USAN.
Use: Antibacterial, antigonococcal.
See: Rosoxacin, Pow. (Winthrop Products).

ROSOXOL TABLETS. (Robinson) Sulfisoxazole 500 mg/Tab. Bot. 100s, 1000s.
Use: Antibacterial, sulfonamide.

ROSOXOL-AZO. (Robinson) Sulfisoxazole, phenazopyridine HCl/Tab. Bot. 100s, 1000s.
Use: Antibacterial, sulfonamide, urinary analgesic.

ROSS SLD. (Ross) Low-residue nutritional supplement for patients restricted to a clear liquid feeding or with fat malabsorption disorders. Packet 1.35 oz. Ctn. 6s. Case 4 ctn. Can 13.5 oz. Case 6s.
Use: Nutritional supplement.

RO-SULFIRAM-500. (Robinson) Disulfiram 500 mg/Tab. Bot. 50s, 500s.
Use: Antialcoholic agent.

RO-SUPER-B TABLETS. (Robinson) Vitamins B_1 50 mg, B_2 20 mg, B_6 5 mg, B_{12} 15 mcg, C 300 mg, desiccated liver 100 mg, dried yeast 100 mg, niacinamide 25 mg, calcium pantothenate 5 mg, iron 10 mg/Tab. Bot. 100s, 250s, 1000s.
Use: Vitamin/mineral supplement.

ROTALEX TEST. (Medical Tech. Corp.) Latex slide agglutination test for detection of rotavirus in feces. Kit 1s.
Use: Diagnostic aid.

ROTAZYME II. (Abbott Diagnostics) Enzyme immunoassay for detection of rotavirus antigen in feces. Test kit 50s.
Use: Diagnostic aid.

ROTENSE. (Robinson) Aspirin, phenacetin, caffeine, allybarbituric acid/Tab. Bot. 100s, 1000s.
Use: Analgesic, sedative/hypnotic.

ROTHERAMIN. (Robinson) Vitamins A 25,000 IU, D 1000 IU, B_1 10 mg, B_2 5 mg, niacinamide 100 mg, B_6 1 mg, B_{12} 5 mcg, C 150 mg, calcium 103.6 mg, phosphorus 80.2 mg, iron 10 mg, magnesium 5.5 mg, manganese 1 mg, potassium 5 mg, zinc 1.4 mg/Cap. or Tab. Bot. 100s, 250s, 1000s.
Use: Vitamin/mineral supplement.

RO-THYRONINE. (Robinson) Liothyronine sodium 25 mcg or 50 mcg/Tab. Bot. 100s, 500s, 1000s.
Use: Thyroid hormone.

RO-THYROXINE. (Robinson) L-thyroxine sodium 0.1 mg or 0.2 mg/Tab. Bot. 100s, 500s, 1000s.
Use: Thyroid hormone.

•**ROTOXAMINE TARTRATE.** USAN. (−)-2-[p-Chloro-α-[2-(dimethylamino)ethoxy]-benzyl pyridine tartrate (1:1).
Use: Antihistamine.

RO-TRAN. (Robinson) Salicylamide 250 mg, powdered extract of valerian 15 mg, powdered extract of passiflora 15 mg/Tab. Bot. 100s.
Use: Antianxiety agent.

ROTRILATE. (Robinson) Trimethylcyclohexyl mandelate 200 mg/Tab. Bot. 100s, 1000s.

RO TRIM. (Rocky Mtn.) d-Amphetamine sulfate 15 mg, atropine sulfate 1/180 gr, aloin 0.25 gr, phenobarbital 0.25 gr/Cap. Bot. 100s.
Use: Anorexiant.

ROTRIM T. (Rocky Mtn.) Thyroid 3 gr/T.R. Tab. Bot. 100s.
Use: Thyroid hormone.

ROTYL HCl. (Rocky Mtn.) Dicylomine HCl 10 mg/ml. Vial 10 ml.
Use: Smooth muscle relaxant, antispasmodic.

ROVAMYCINE. Spiramycin (Orphan drug).
Use: Chronic cryptosporidiosis in immunodeficient patients.
Sponsor: Rhone-Poulenc.

ROVIMINS T.F. (Rocky Mtn.) Zinc sulfate 50 mg, magnesium sulfate 50 mg, vitamins A 25,000 IU, D 400 IU, B_1 20 mg, B_2 30 mg, B_6 3 mg, B_{12} 25 mcg, calcium pantothenate 30 mg, niacinamide 100 mg, C 400 mg, E 2 IU, manganese 3 mg, potassium sulfate 5 mg, copper oxide 1 mg, iodine 0.15 mg/Pill. Bot. 100s, 1000s.
Use: Vitamin/mineral supplement.

ROWASA. (Solvay) Mesalamine 4 Gm/60 ml. Rectal Susp. Bot. Units of 7 disposable bot.
Use: Ulcerative colitis, proctosigmoiditis, proctitis.

ROWASA SUPPOSITORIES. (Solvay) Mesalamine 500 mg/Supp. Individually wrapped in foil. Box 12s, 24s.
Use: Ulcerative proctitis.

•**ROXADIMATE.** USAN.
Use: Sunscreen.

ROXANOL ORAL SOLUTION. (Roxane) Morphine sulfate concentrated oral soln, sugar-free and alcohol free. **20 mg/ml:** Bot. 30 ml or 120 ml w/calibrated dropper. **100 mg/5 ml:** Bot. 240 ml w/calibrated spoon.
Use: Narcotic analgesic.

ROXANOL SR TABLETS. (Roxane) Morphine sulfate 30 mg/SR Tab. Bot. 50s, 250s, UD 100s.
Use: Narcotic analgesic.

•**ROXARSONE.** USAN. 3-Nitro-4-hydroxy-phenylarsonic acid.
Use: Coccidiostat and antibacterial.

ROXATIDINE ACETATE HYDROCHLORIDE. USAN.
Use: Antiulcer agent.

ROXICET ORAL SOLUTION. (Roxane) Oxycodone HCl 5 mg, acetaminophen 325 mg/5 ml. Bot. 5 ml, 500 ml.
Use: Narcotic analgesic.

ROXICET TABLETS. (Roxane) Oxycodone HCl 5 mg, acetaminophen 325 mg, 0.4% alcohol/Tab. Bot. 100s, UD 4 X 25s.
Use: Narcotic analgesic.

ROXICODONE. (Roxane) **Liq.:** Oxycodone HCl 5 mg/5 ml. Bot. 500 ml. **Tab.:** Oxycodone HCl 5 mg. Bot. 100s, UD 4 X 25s.
Use: Narcotic analgesic.

ROXIPRIN TABLETS. (Roxane) Oxycodone HCl 4.5 mg, oxycodone terephthalate 0.38 mg, aspirin 325 mg/Tab. Bot. 100s, 1000s, UD 4 X 25s.
Use: Narcotic analgesic.

•**ROXITHROMYCIN.** USAN.
Use: Antibacterial.

ROXYN. (Rocky Mtn.) d-Desoxyephedrine HCl 15 mg/Tab. Bot. 100s.
Use: Anorexiant.

ROZINC. (Rocky Mtn.) Zinc sulfate 220 mg/Cap. Bot. 100s, 1000s.
Use: Zinc supplement.

R-S LOTION. (Hill) No. 2: Sulfur 8%, resorcinol monoacetate 4%. Bot. 2 oz.
Use: Topical drying medication.

R-TANNATE TABLETS. (Various Mfr.) Phenylephrine tannate 25 mg, chlorpheniramine tannate 8 mg, pyrilamine tannate 25 mg. In 100s.
Use: Decongestant, antihistamine.

R-TANNATE PEDIATRIC SUSPENSION. (Various Mfr.) Phenylephrine tannate 5 mg, chlor-

phenramine tannate 2 mg, pyrilamine tannate 12.5 mg, saccharin. In 480 ml.
Use: Decongestant, antihistamine.

RUBACELL. (Abbott Diagnostics) Passive hemagglutination (PHA) test for the detection of antibody to rubella virus in serum or recalcified plasma.
Use: Diagnostic aid.

RUBACELL II. (Abbott) Passive hemagglutination (PHA) test to detect antibody to rubella in serum or recalcified plasma. In 100s, 1000s.
Use: Diagnostic aid.

RUBAQUICK DIAGNOSTIC KIT. (Abbott Diagnostics) Rapid passive hemagglutination (PHA) for the detection of antibodies to rubella virus in serum specimens.
Use: Diagnostic aid.

RUBA-TECT. (Abbott Diagnostics) Hemagglutination inhibition test for the detection and quantitation of rubella antibody in serum. In 100s.
Use: Diagnostic aid.

RUBAZYME. (Abbott Diagnostics) Enzyme immunoassay for 1 gG antibody to rubella virus. Test kit 100s, 1000s.
Use: Diagnostic aid.

RUBAZYME-M. (Abbott Diagnostics) Enzyme immunoassay for IgM antibody to rubella virus in serum. Test kit 50s.
Use: Diagnostic aid.

•**RUBELLA & MUMPS VIRUS VACCINE, LIVE,** U.S.P. XXII.
Use: Active immunizing agent.
See: Biavax II, Inj. (Merck Sharp & Dohme).

•**RUBELLA VIRUS VACCINE, LIVE,** U.S.P. XXII.
Use: Active immunizing agent.
See: Cendevax, Inj. (SmithKline).
Meruvax, Inj. (Merck Sharp & Dohme).
W/Measles vaccine.
See: M-R-Vax, Inj. (Merck Sharp & Dohme).
W/Measles vaccine, mumps vaccine.
See: M-M-R, Inj. (Merck Sharp & Dohme).

RUBELLA VIRUS VACCINE, LIVE ATTENUATED. Live attenuated strain of rubella virus HPV-77.
Use: Agent for immunization.
W/Measles vaccine.
See: Lirubel, Vial (Merrell Dow).
W/Measles vaccine, mumps vaccine.
See: Lirutrin, Vial (Merrell Dow).

RUBESOL-1000. (Central) Cyanocobalamin. U.S.P. 1000 mcg/ml. Vial 10 ml, 30 ml Box 12s.
Use: Vitamin supplement.

•**RUBIDIUM CHLORIDE Rb 86.** USAN.
Use: Radioactive agent.

RUBRAMIN PC. (Squibb Marsam) Vitamin B_{12} U.S.P. (cyanocobalamin), benzyl alcohol 1%, sodium Cl, sodium hydroxide or HCl acid. (100 mcg/ml; cobalt content 4 mcg/ml) Vial 10 ml. (1000 mcg/ml; cobalt content 40 mcg/ml) Vial 1, 10 ml Unimatic: 100 mcg/ml 1 dose syringe 1s, 10s. 1,000 mcg/ml 1 dose syringe 1s, 10s.
Use: Vitamin supplement.

RUBRAPLEX. (Lannett) Vitamins B_1 2.5 mg, B_2 2 mg, B_6 0.5 mg, B_{12} 5 mcg, calcium pantothenate 1 mg, niacinamide 20 mg/Cap. Bot. 100s, 1000s.
Use: Vitamin supplement.

RUBRATOPE-57. (Squibb) Cyanocobalamin Co 57 Capsules; Soln U.S.P.
Use: Vitamin supplement.

RUBRAVITE LIQUID. (Lannett) Vitamins B_1 10 mg, B_{12} 25 mcg/5 ml. Bot. pt.
Use: Vitamin supplement.

RUFEN. (Boots) Ibuprofen 400 mg, 600 mg or 800 mg/Tab. Bot. 100s, 500s, UD 100s.
Use: Nonsteroidal anti-inflammatory drug; analgesic.

RUFOCROMOMYCIN. B.A.N. An antibiotic produced by *Streptomyces rufochromogenus.*
Use: Antibacterial.

RUFOLEX. (Lannett) Vitamins B_1 1.5 mg, B_2 1.5 mg, B_6 1 mg, B_{12} 5 mcg, C 50 mg, niacinamide 10 mg, ferrous fumarate 200 mg, d-sorbitol 200 mg, folic acid 0.25 mg/Cap. Bot. 100s.
Use: Vitamin/mineral supplement.

RU-LETS M 500. (Rugby) Vitamin C 500 mg, niacinamide 100 mg, calcium pantothenate 20 mg, B_1 15 mg, B_2 10 mg, B_6 5 mg, A 10,000 IU, B_{12} 12 mcg, D 400 IU, E 30 mg, magnesium 80 mg, iron 20 mg, copper 2 mg, zinc 1.5 mg, manganese 1 mg, iodine 0.15 mg/Tab. Bot. 100s.
Use: Vitamin/mineral supplement.

RULOX. (Rugby) **#1 Tab.:** Aluminum hydroxide 200 mg, magnesium hydroxide 200 mg. **#2 Tab.:** Aluminum hydroxide 400 mg, magnesium hydroxide 400 mg. Bot. 100s, 1000s.
Use: Antacid.

RULOX SUSPENSION. (Rugby) Aluminum hydroxide 225 mg, magnesium hydroxide 200 mg/5 ml, sodium 0.82 mg. Susp. Bot. 360 ml, 780 ml, gal.
Use: Antacid.

RUM-K. (Fleming) Potassium Cl 10 mEq/5 ml in butter/rum flavored base. Bot. pt, gal.
Use: Potassium supplement.

RUSCORB. (Robinson) **20/100:** Rutin 20 mg, C 100 mg/Tab. **50/300:** Rutin 50 mg, C 300 mg/Tab. Bot. 100s, 1000s.
Use: Vitamin supplement.

RUST INHIBITOR.
See: Anti-Rust, Tab. (Winthrop Pharm).
Sodium Nitrite, Tab. (Various Mfr.).

•**RUTAMYCIN.** USAN. From strain of *Streptomyces rutgersensis.* Under study.
Use: Antifungal antibiotic.

RUTGERS 612.
See: Ethohexadiol. (Various Mfr.).

RUTIN. (Various Mfr.) 3-Rhamnoglucoside of 5,7,3′,4′-tetrahydroxyflavonol. Eldrin, globulariacitrin, myrticalorin, oxyritin, phytomelin, rutoside, sophorin. Tab. 20 mg, 50 mg, 60 mg, 100 mg.
Use: Vascular disorders.

RUTIN COMBINATIONS

See: Hexarutan, Tab. (Westerfield).
Hyrunal, Tab. (Kenyon).
Vio-Geric-H, Tab. (Solvay).

RUTOSIDE.
See: Rutin, Tab. (Various Mfr.).

RU-TUSS II. (Boots) Phenylpropanolamine HCl 75 mg, chlorpheniramine maleate 12 mg/Cap. Bot. 100s.
Use: Decongestant, antihistamine.

RU-TUSS EXPECTORANT. (Boots) Pseudoephedrine HCl 30 mg, dextromethorphan HBr 10 mg, guaifenesin 100 mg/5 ml, alcohol 10%. Bot. pt.
Use: Decongestant, antitussive, expectorant.

RU-TUSS LIQUID. (Boots) Phenylephrine HCl 30 mg, chlorpheniramine maleate 2 mg/30 ml, alcohol 5%. Bot. pt.
Use: Decongestant, antihistamine.

RU-TUSS TABLETS. (Boots) Phenylephrine HCl 25 mg, phenylpropanolamine HCl 50 mg, chlorpheniramine maleate 8 mg, hyoscyamine sulfate 0.19 mg, atropine sulfate 0.04 mg, scopolamine hydrobromide 0.01 mg/Tab. Bot. 100s, 500s.
Use: Decongestant, antihistamine, anticholinergic/antispasmodic.

RU-TUSS w/HYDROCODONE. (Boots) Hydrocodone bitartrate 1.67 mg, phenylephrine HCl 5 mg, phenylpropanolamine HCl 3.3 mg, pheniramine maleate 3.3 mg, pyrilamine maleate 3.3 mg/5 ml, alcohol 5%. Bot. 473 ml.
Use: Antitussive, decongestant, antihistamine.

RU-VERT M. (Solvay) Meclizine HCl 25 mg/Tab. Bot. 100s.
Use: Antiemetic, antivertigo.

RVPaba. (Elder) p-Aminobenzoic acid 5% in neutral red petrolatum-wax base/Lipstick. Stick 3.75 Gm.
Use: Sunscreen.

RVPAQUE. (Elder) Red petrolatum, zinc oxide, cinoxate, in water-resistant base. Tube 0.5 oz, 1.25 oz.
Use: Sunscreen.

RYMED. (Edwards) Pseudoephedrine HCl 30 mg, guaifenesin 250 mg/Cap. Bot. 100s.
Use: Decongestant, expectorant.

RYMED LIQUID. (Edwards) Pseudoephedrine HC1 30 mg, guaifenesin 100 mg/5 ml, alcohol 1.4%. Bot. pt.
Use: Decongestant, expectorant.

RYMED-TR. (Edwards) Phenylpropanolamine HCl 75 mg, guaifenesin 400 mg/Tab. Bot. 100s.
Use: Decongestant, expectorant.

RYNA. (Wallace) Chlorpheniramine 2 mg, pseudoephedrine HCl 30 mg/5 ml. Bot. 4 oz, pt.
Use: Antihistamine, decongestant.

RYNA-C. (Wallace) Codeine phosphate 10 mg, pseudoephedrine HCl 30 mg, chlorpheniramine maleate 2 mg, saccharin, sorbitol/5 ml. Bot. 4 oz, pt.
Use: Antitussive, decongestant, antihistamine.

RYNA-CX. (Wallace) Guaifenesin 100 mg, pseudoephedrine HCl 30 mg, codeine phosphate 10 mg, alcohol 7.5%, saccharin, sorbitol/5 ml. Bot. 4 oz, pt.
Use: Expectorant, decongestant, antitussive.

RYNATAN. (Wallace) **Tab.:** Phenylephrine tannate 25 mg, chlorpheniramine tannate 8 mg, pyrilamine tannate 25 mg. Bot. 100s, 500s. **Pediatric Susp.:** Phenylephrine tannate 5 mg, chlorpheniramine tannate 2 mg, pyrilamine tannate 12.5 mg/5 ml. Bot. pt.
Use: Decongestant, antihistamine.

RYNATUSS. (Wallace) Carbetapentane tannate 60 mg, chlorpheniramine tannate 5 mg, ephedrine tannate 10 mg, phenylephrine tannate 10 mg/Tab. Bot. 100s, 500s.
Use: Decongestant, antihistamine.

RYNATUSS PEDIATRIC SUSPENSION. (Wallace) Carbetapentane tannate 30 mg, chlorpheniramine tannate 4 mg, ephedrine tannate 5 mg, phenylephrine tannate 5 mg, saccharin, tartrazine/5 ml. Susp. Bot. 8 oz, pt.
Use: Decongestant, antihistamine.

RYTHMOL. (Knoll) Propafenone HCl 150 mg or 300 mg/Tab. Bot. 100s, 500s.
Use: Antiarrhythmic.

S

S-2 INHALANT & NEBULIZERS. (Nephron) Racemic epinephrine HCl 1.25%. Bot. 0.25 oz, 0.5 oz, 1 oz.
Use: Bronchodilator.

SAC-500. (Western Research) Vitamin C 500 mg/TR Cap. Bot. 1000s.
Use: Vitamin supplement.

•**SACCHARIN,** N.F. XVII. 1,2-Benzisothiazolin-3-one-1,1-dioxide.
(Merck)—Pkg. 1 oz, 0.25 lb, 1 lb.
(Squibb) Tabs. 0.25, 0.5 gr. Bot. 500s, 1000s; 1 gr. Bot. 1000s.
Use: Sweetening agent when sugar is contraindicated.
See: Necta Sweet, Tab. (Norwich Eaton).

•**SACCHARIN CALCIUM,** U.S.P. XXII. 1,2-Benzisothiazolin-3-one 1, 1-dioxide calcium salt hydrate (2:7).
Use: Non-nutritive sweetener.

•**SACCHARIN SODIUM,** U.S.P. XXII. Oral Soln., Tab., U.S.P. XXII. (Benzosulfimide Sodium, Soluble Gluside, Soluble Saccharine) Pow., Bot. 1 oz, 0.25 lb, 1 lb. Tab. usual sizes. (Various Mfr.).
Use: Sweetening agent and test for circulation time of blood.
See: Crystallose, Crystals, Liq. (Jamieson).
Ril Sweet, Liq. (Schering-Plough).
Sweeta (Squibb Mark).

SACCHARIN SOLUBLE.
See: Saccharin Sodium, Tab., Pow. (Various Mfr.).

SAFESKIN. (C & M Pharmacal) A dermatologically acceptable detergent for patients who are sensitive to ordinary detergents. No whiteners, brighteners or other irritants. Bot. qt.
Use: Laundry detergent for sensitive skin.

SAFE SUDS. (Ar-Ex) Hypoallergenic, all-purpose detergent for patients whose hands or respiratory membranes are irritated by soaps or detergents. pH 6.8. No enzymes, phosphates, lanolin, fillers, bleaches. Bot. 22 oz.
Use: Laundry detergent for sensitive skin.

SAFETY-COATED ARTHRITIS PAIN FORMULA. (Whitehall) Enteric coated aspirin 500 mg/Tab. Bot. 24s, 60s.
Use: Salicylate analgesic.

•**SAFFLOWER OIL,** U.S.P. XXII.
See: Safflower Oil Cap. (Various Mfr.).
W/Choline bitartrate, soybean lecithin, inositol, natural tocopherols, B_6, B_{12}, and panthenol.
See: Nutricol, Cap., Vial (Nutrition).

SAFROLE. 4-Allyl-1,2-(methylenedioxy) benzene.

SALAC CLEANSER. (Gen Derm) Salicylic acid 2% in a surfactant blend. Liq. Bot. 177 ml.
Use: Anti-acne.

SALACETIN.
See: Acetylsalicylic Acid (Various Mfr.).

SALACID 25%. (Gordon) Salicylic acid 25% in ointment base. Jar 2 oz, lb.
Use: Keratolytic.

SALACID 60%. (Gordon) Salicylic acid 60% in ointment base. Jar 2 oz.
Use: Keratolytic.

SALACTIC FILM. (Pedinol) Salicylic acid 16.7%, lactic acid 16.7% in flexible collodion w/color. Applicator bot. 0.5 oz.
Use: Keratolytic.

•**SALANTEL.** USAN.
Use: Anthelmintic.

SALATAR CREAM. (Lannett) Coal tar soln 5%, salicylic acid 3%. Jar 4 oz, lb.
Use: Antiseborrheic, keratolytic.

SALAZIDE-DEMI TABLETS. (Major) Hydroflumethiazide 25 mg, reserpine 0.125 mg. 100s.
Use: Antihypertensive combination.

SALAZIDE TABS. (Major) Hydroflumethiazide 50 mg, reserpine 0.125 mg. Bot. 100s, 500s, 1000s.
Use: Antihypertensive combination.

SALAZOSULFAPYRIDINE (I.N.N.). Sulphasalazine. B.A.N.

SALAZOSULPHADIMIDINE. B.A.N. 4′-(4,6-Dimethylpyrimidin-2-ylsulphamoyl)-4-hydroxyazobenzene-3-carboxylic acid.
Use: Sulfonamide.

SALBUTAMOL. B.A.N. 1-(4-Hydroxy-3-hydroxymethylphenyl)-2-(t-butylamino)ethanol.
Use: Bronchodilator.

SALCATONIN. B.A.N. A component of natural salmon calcitonin.
Use: Treatment of hypercalcemia and Paget's disease.

SALCEGEL. (Apco) Sodium salicylate 5 gr, calcium ascorbate 25 mg, calcium carbonate 1 gr, dried aluminum hydroxide gel 2 gr/Tab. Bot. 100s.
Use: Analgesic.

•**SALCOLEX.** USAN.
Use: Analgesic, anti-inflammatory.

•**SALETHAMIDE MALEATE.** USAN. N-[2-Diethyl(amino)ethyl]-salicylamide maleate. Under study.
Use: Analgesic.

SALETIN.
See: Acetylsalicylic Acid (Various Mfr.).

SALETO. (Hauck) Aspirin 210 mg, acetaminophen 115 mg, salicylamide 65 mg, caffeine anhydrous 16 mg/Tab. Bot. 50s, 100s, 1000s.
Use: Analgesic combination.

SALETO D. (Hauck) Acetaminophen 240 mg, salicylamide 120 mg, caffeine 16 mg, phenylpropanolamine HCl 18 mg/Cap. Bot. 20s, 50s.
Use: Analgesic, decongestant.

SALFLEX. (Carnrick Labs) Salsalate 500 mg or 750 mg/Tab. Bot. 100s.
Use: Salicylate analgesic.

•**SALICYL ALCOHOL.** USAN.
Use: Local anesthetic.

•**SALICYLAMIDE,** U.S.P. XXII.
Use: Analgesic.

SALICYLAMIDE. B.A.N. (Bryant) o-Hydroxybenzamide. Salimed.
Use: Analgesic; antipyretic.

SALICYLAMIDE W/COMBINATIONS
See: Akes-N-Pain, Cap. (E.J. Moore).
Anodynos, Tab. (Buffington).
Anodynos Forte, Tab. (Buffington).
Arthol, Tab. (Towne).
Cenaid, Tab. (Century).
Centuss, MLT Tab. (Century).
Codalan, 1,2,3, Tab. (Lannett).
Dapco, Tab. (Mericon).
Decohist, Cap. (Towne).
Dengesic, Tab. (Scott-Alison).
Duoprin, Tab. (Dunhall).
Emagrin, Tab. (Otis Clapp).
Emersal, Liq. (Medco).
F.C.A.H., Cap. (Scherer).
Myocalm, Tab. (Parmed).
Neo-Pyranistan (Standex).
Nokane, Tab. (Wren).
Panritis, Tab. (Pan Amer.).
Partuss-A, Tab. (Parmed).
Partuss T.D., Tab. (Parmed).
P.M.P. Compound, Tab. (Mericon).
Presalin, Tab. (Mallard).
Pyranistan Compound (Standex).
Renpap, Tab. (Wren).
Rhinex, Tab. (Lemmon).
Rinocidin, Cap. (Cenci).
S-A-C, Tab. (Lannett).
S.A.C., Preps. (Towne).
Saleto, Preps. (Mallard).
Salipap, Tab. (Freeport).

Salocol, Tab. (Mallard).
Salphenyl, Liq., Cap. (Mallard).
Sanger Special, Tab. (E.J. Moore).
Scotgesic, Cap., Elix. (Scott/Cord).
Sedacane, Cap. (E.J. Moore).
Sedalgesic, Tab. (Table Rock).
Sedragesic, Tab. (Lannett).
Sinulin, Tab. (Reed & Carnrick).
Sleep, Tab. (Towne).
Triaprin-DC, Cap. (Dunhall).

SALICYLANILIDE. N-Phenyl salicylamide.
Use: Antifungal agent.

SALICYLATED BILE EXTRACT. Chologestin.

•**SALICYLATE MEGLUMINE.** USAN.
Use: Antirheumatic, analgesic.

SALICYLAZOSULFAPYRIDINE.
See: Sulfasalazine, U.S.P. XXII.

•**SALICYLIC ACID,** U.S.P. XXII. Collodion, Plaster, Gel, U.S.P. XXII. Benzoic acid, 2-hydroxy. Orthohydroxybenzoic acid. Cryst. Pkg. 1 oz, 0.25 lb, 1 lb; Pow. Pkg. 0.25 lb, 1 lb.
Use: Keratolytic.
See: Calicylic, Creme (Gordon).
Listrex Scrub, Liq. (Warner-Lambert).
Salonil, Cream (Torch).
Sebulex, Cream (Westwood).
Wart-Off, Liq. (Leeming).

SALICYLIC ACID COMBINATIONS
See: Acnaveen, Bar (Cooper).
Acno (Cummins).
Akne Drying Lot., Liq. (Alto).
Cuticura (Purex).
Derma-Cover, Liq. (Scrip).
Duofilm, Liq. (Stiefel).
Duo-WR, Soln. (Whorton).
Fostex, Cream, Liq. (Westwood).
Foursalco, Tab. (Jenkins).
Ionax, Liq. (Owen).
Ionil, Liq. (Owen).
Ionil T, Liq. (Owen).
Keralyt, Gel (Westwood).
Komed, Lot. (Barnes-Hind).
Pernox, Lot. (Westwood).
Podiaspray, Aerosol Pow. (Dalin).
Pragmatar, Oint. (Menley & James).
Salatar, Cream (Lannett).
Sal-Dex, Liq. (Scrip).
Salicylic Acid Soap (Stiefel).
Saligel, Gel (Stiefel).
Salsprin, Tab. (Seatrace).
Sebaveen, Shampoo (Cooper).
Sebucare, Liq. (Westwood).
Sebulex Shampoo, Liq. (Westwood).
Therac, Lot. (C&M Pharm.).
Tinver, Lot. (Barnes-Hind).
Vanseb, Dandruff Shampoo (Herbert).
Vanseb-T Tar Shampoo (Herbert).
Vericin, Oint. (Gordon).
Ver-Var, Soln. (Owen).
Zemacol, Lotion (Norwich).

SALICYLIC ACID CREAM. (Durel) Salicylic acid 5%, in Duromantel cream.
Use: Antiseborrheic, keratolytic.

SALICYLIC ACID SOAP. (Stiefel) Neutral soap containing salicylic acid 3.5%. Cake 4 oz.
Use: Antiseborrheic, keratolytic.

SALICYLIC ACID & SULFUR SOAP. (Stiefel) Salicylic acid 3%, sulfur 10% in neutral soap bar. Cake 4.1 oz.
Use: Antiseborrheic, keratolytic.

•**SALICYLIC ACID TOPICAL FOAM,** U.S.P. XXII.
Use: Keratolytic.

SALICYLSALICYLIC ACID. Salsalate. USAN.
Use: Analgesic.
See: Arcylate, Tab. (Hauck)
Disalcid, Tab. (Riker).
W/Aspirin.
See: Causalin, Tab. (Amfre-Grant).
Duragesic, Tab. (Meyer).
Persistin, Tab. (Fisons).

SALICYLSULPHONIC ACID. Sulfosalicylic acid. Dextrotest (Ames).

SALIGEL. (Stiefel) Salicylic acid 5% in a special hydroalcoholic gel base. Tube 2 oz.
Use: Anti-acne.

SALIGENIN. (City Chem.) Salicyl alcohol. Bot. 25 Gm, 100 Gm.
W/Merodicein.
See: Thantis, Loz. (Hyson, Westcott & Dunning).

SALINAZID. B.A.N. 2′-Salicylideneisonicotinohydrazide.
Use: Treatment of tuberculosis.

SALINE SOLUTION. (Akorn) Saline solution, isotonic, preserved. Bot. 12 oz.
Use: Contact lens soaking agent.

SALINE SPRAY. (Akorn) Isotonic nonpreserved saline aerosol soln. Bot. 2 oz, 8 oz, 12 oz.
Use: Soft contact lens care.

SALINEX NASAL DROPS. (Muro) Buffered nasal isotonic saline drops. Bot. 15 ml w/dropper.
Use: Nasal moisturizer.

SALINEX NASAL MIST. (Muro) Sodium Cl 0.4%. Drops 15 ml, spray 50 ml.
Use: Nasal moisturizer.

SALIPAP. (Freeport) Salicylamide 5 gr, acetaminophen 5 gr/Tab. Bot. 1000s.
Use: Analgesic.

SALIPRAL. (Kenyon) Allylisobutyl-barbituric acid ¾ gr, aspirin 3 gr, phenacetin 2 gr, caffeine ⅔ gr/Tab. Bot. 1000s.
Use: Sedative, analgesic.

SALIPRAL-C. (Kenyon) Same formula as above w/vitamin C/Cap. Bot. 100s, 1000s.
Use: Sedative, analgesic, vitamin C supplement.

SALITHOL LIQUID. (Madland) Methyl salicylate, menthol, camphor. Bot. pt, gal. Oint. Jar 1 lb, 5 lb.
Use: External analgesic.

SALIVART. (Westport Pharm.) Sodium carboxymethylcellulose 1 gr, sorbitol 3 gr, sodium, potassium, calcium Cl 0.015 gr, magnesium Cl

0.005 gr, dibasic potassium phosphate, nitrogen (as propellant). Spray can 75 ml.
Use: Mouth preparation.

SALIVA SUBSTITUTE. (Roxane) Sorbitol, sodium carboxymethylcellulose, methylparaben. Dye free. Soln. bot. 120 ml.
Use: Mouth preparation.

SALMEFAMOL. B.A.N. 1-(4-Hydroxy-3-hydroxymethylphenyl)-2-(4-methoxy-α-methylphenethylamino)ethanol.
Use: Bronchodilator.

•**SALMETEROL XINAFOATE.** USAN.
Use: Bronchodilator.

SALOCOL. (Hauck) Acetaminophen 115 mg, aspirin 210 mg, salicylamide 65 mg, caffeine 16 mg/Tab. Bot. 1000s.
Use: Analgesic combination.

SAL-OIL-T. (Syosset) Coal tar 10%, salicylic acid 6%, allantoin vegetable oils. Soln. Bot. 60 ml.
Use: Antiseborrheic, keratolytic.

SALONIL. (Torch) Salicylic acid 40% in lanolin. Jar. lb.
Use: Antiseborrheic, keratolytic.

SALPABA W/COLCHICINE. (Madland) Sodium salicylate 0.25 Gm, para-aminobenzoic acid 0.25 Gm, vitamin C 20 mg, colchicine 0.25 mg/Tab. Bot. 100s, 1000s.
Use: Agent for gout.

SALPHENYL CAPSULES. (Hauck) Salicylamide 200 mg, acetaminophen 130 mg, chlorpheniramine maleate 2 mg, phenylephrine HCl 10 mg/Cap. Bot. 100s.
Use: Analgesic, antihistamine, decongestant.

•**SALSALATE.** USAN.
Use: Analgesic, antipyretic, anti-inflammatory.
See: Disalcid, Tab. (Riker).
Salsitab, Tab. (Upsher-Smith).

SALSITAB. (Upsher-Smith) Salsalate 500 mg or 750 mg/Tab. Bot. 100s, 500s, UD 100s.
Use: Analgesic.

SALTEN. (Wren) Salicylamide 10 gr/Tab. Bot. 100s, 1000s.
Use: Salicylate analgesic.

SALT SUBSTITUTES.
Use: Sodium-free seasoning agent.
See: Adolph's Salt Substitute (Adolph's).
Adolph's Seasoned Salt Substitute (Adolph's).
Diasal Salt (Savage).
Morton Salt Substitute (Morton Salt).
NoSalt (Norcliff Thayer).
NoSalt Seasoned (Norcliff Thayer).
Nu-Salt (Cumberland Pkg.).

SALT TABLETS. (Cross) Sodium Cl 650 mg/Tab. Dispenser 500s.
Use: Salt replenisher.

SALURON. (Bristol Labs.) Hydroflumethiazide 50 mg/Tab. Bot. 100s.
Use: Diuretic.

SALUTENSIN. (Bristol Labs.) Hydroflumethiazide 50 mg, reserpine 0.125 mg/Tab. Bot. 100s, 1000s.
Use: Antihypertensive combination.

SALUTENSIN-DEMI. (Bristol Labs.) Hydroflumethiazide 25 mg, reserpine 0.125 mg/Tab. Bot. 100s.
Use: Antihypertensive combination.

SALVARSAN.
Use: Antisyphilitic.
See: Arsphenamine (Various Mfr.).

SALVITE-B. (Faraday) Sodium Cl 7 gr, dextrose 3 gr, B_1 1 mg/Tab. Bot. 100s, 1000s.

SANAMYCIN. B.A.N. Actinomycin.
Use: Antineoplastic agent.

SANCHIA SILICONE PROTECTIVE CREAM. (Otis Clapp) Silicone and lanolin in greaseless cream base. Tube 3 oz, Jar 16 oz.
Use: Protective agent.

SANCURA. (Thompson) Benzocaine, chlorobutanol, chlorothymol, benzoic acid, salicylic acid, benzyl alcohol, cod liver oil, lanolin in a washable petrolatum base. Oint. 30 Gm, 90 Gm.
Use: Local anesthetic.

•**SANCYCLINE.** USAN. 6-Demethyl-6-deoxytetracycline. Formerly Norcycline.
Use: Antibiotic.

SANDIMMUNE. (Sandoz) Cyclosporine. **Oral soln.:** 100 mg/ml. Bot. 50 ml with graduated pipette. **Inj.:** 50 mg/ml Amp. 5 ml.
Use: Immunosuppressive agent.

SANDOGLOBULIN. (Sandoz) Immune globulin: Reconstitution fluid 1 Gm/33 ml; 3 Gm/100 ml; 6 Gm/200 ml.
Use: Immune serum.

SANDOPTAL. Isobutyl allylbarbituric acid.
See: Butalbital.
W/Caffeine, aspirin, phenacetin.
See: Fiorinal, Tab., Cap. (Sandoz).
W/Caffeine, aspirin, phenacetin, codeine phosphate.
See: Fiorinal w/Codeine, Cap. (Sandoz).

SANDOPTAL SODIUM.
W/Sodium diethylbarbiturate, sodium phenylethylbarbiturate, scopolamine HBr, dihydroergotamine methanesulfonate.
See: Plexonal (Sandoz).

SANDOSTATIN. (Sandoz) Octreotide acetate 0.05 mg, 0.1 mg or 0.5 mg. Inj. Amp. 1 ml.
Use: Adjunctive treatment of certain tumors.

SANESTRO. (Sandia) Estrone 0.7 mg, estradiol 0.35 mg, estriol 0.14 mg/Tab. Bot. 100s, 1000s.
Use: Estrogen combination.

SANGER HER CAPS. (E. J. Moore) Acetaminophen 227 mg, aspirin 227 mg, caffeine anhydrous 32.4 mg/Cap. Bot. 18s.
Use: Analgesic.

SANGER SPECIAL C-12. (E.J. Moore) Salicylamide, co. colocynth extract, dried ferrous sulfate, blue cohosh/Tab. Bot. 24s.

SANGER VAGINAL ITCH CREAM. (E.J. Moore) Benzocaine, dibucaine, tetracaine. Tube 1.25 oz.
Use: Local anesthetic combination.

SANGUIS. (Sig) Liver 10 mcg, vitamin B_{12} 100 mcg, folic acid 1 mcg/ml. Vial 10 ml.

Use: Nutritional supplement.

SANHIST T.D. 5. (Sandia) Phenylpropanolamine HCl 50 mg, chlorpheniramine maleate 5 mg, ascorbic acid 100 mg/Tab. Bot. 100s, 1000s.
Use: Decongestant, antihistamine.

SANHIST T.D. 12. (Sandia) Phenylpropanolamine HCl 50 mg, chlorpheniramine maleate 12 mg, ascorbic acid 100 mg, methscopolamine nitrate 4 mg/Tab. Bot. 100s, 1000s.
Use: Decongestant, antihistamine combination.

SANILENS. (Ketchum) Bot. 4 oz.
Use: Contact lens care.

SANI-SUPP. (G & W Labs) Glycerin, sodium stearate. Supp. 10s, 12s, 24s, 25s, 48s, 50s, 100s, 1000s.
Use: Laxative.

SANITUBE. (Sanitube Co.) Calomel 30%, oxyquinoline benzoate, triethanolamine soap in a non-irritating excipient base. Oint. 5 Gm.
Use: Topical agent for prophylaxis of syphilis and gonorrhea.

SANI-VESS. (Forest Pharm.) Papain, sodium bicarbonate, citric acid, tartaric acid, lactose, thymol, aromatics. Pkg. 6 oz.

SANLUOL.
See: Arsphenamine (Various Mfr.).

SANOREX. (Sandoz) Mazindol 1 mg or 2 mg/Tab. Bot. 100s.
Use: Anorexiant.

SANSERT. (Sandoz) Methysergide maleate 2 mg/Tab. Bot. 100s.
Use: Agent for migraine.

SANSTRESS. (Sandia) Vitamins A 25,000 IU, D 400 IU, B_1 10 mg, B_2 5 mg, niacinamide 100 mg, B_6 1 mg, B_{12} 5 mcg, C 150 mg, calcium 103 mg, phosphorus 80 mg, iron 10 mg, copper 1 mg, iodine 0.1 mg, magnesium 5.5 mg, manganese 1 mg, potassium 5 mg, zinc 1.4 mg/Cap. Bot. 100s, 1000s.
Use: Vitamin/mineral supplement.

SANTISEPTIC LOTION. (Santiseptic) Menthol, phenol, benzocaine, zinc oxide, calamine. Bot. 4 oz.
Use: Minor skin irritations.

SANTUSSIN ADULT SUSPENSION. (Sandia) Noscapine 10 mg, phenylpropanolamine HCl 12.5 mg, chlorpheniramine maleate 1.5 mg, acetaminophen 60 mg, guiachlor compound (alcohol 12% by volume) 75 mg, guaifenesin 5 mg, ammonium Cl 70 mg/5 ml. Bot. 16 oz, gal.
Use: Decongestant, antihistamine, analgesic, expectorant.

SANTUSSIN CAPSULES. (Sandia) Noscapine 10 mg, phenylpropanolamine HCl 12.5 mg, chlorpheniramine maleate 1.5 mg, acetaminophen 120 mg, guaifenesin 100 mg/Cap. Bot. 100s, 1000s.
Use: Decongestant, antihistamine, analgesic, expectorant.

SANTUSSIN PEDIATRIC SUSPENSION. (Sandia) Noscapine 5 mg, phenylpropanolamine HCl 6.25 mg, chlorpheniramine maleate 0.75 mg, acetaminophen 30 mg, guiachlor compound (alcohol 12% by volume) 37.5 mg/5 ml. Bot. 16 oz, gal.
Use: Decongestant, antihistamine, analgesic, expectorant.

SANTYL. (Knoll) Proteolytic enzyme derived from *Clostridium histolyticum.* 250 units/Gm. Oint. Tube 15 Gm, 30 Gm.
Use: Topical enzyme preparation.

SAPONATED CRESOL SOLUTION.
See: Cresol (Various Mfr.).

SAPONINS, WATER SOLUBLE.

•**SARAFLOXACIN HYDROCHLORIDE.** USAN.
Use: Anti-infective.

SARAPIN. (High) An aqueous distillate of *Sarracenia purpurea,* pitcher plant, prepared for parenteral administration. Amp. 10 ml, 12s. Multidose vials 50 ml.
Use: Relief of neuromuscular or neuralgic pain.

SARATOGA. (Blair) Boric acid, zinc oxide, eucalyptol, white petrolatum. Oint. Tube 1 oz, 2 oz.
Use: Minor skin irritations.

L-SARCOLYSIN. Melphalan, U.S.P. XXII.

SARDO BATH OIL CONCENTRATE. (Schering-Plough) Mineral oil, isopropyl palmitate. Bot. 3.75 oz, 7.75 oz.
Use: Emollient.

SARDOETTES MOISTURIZING TOWELETTES. (Schering-Plough) Mineral oil, isopropyl palmitate, impregnated towelling material. Packet. Box 25s.
Use: Emollient.

SARGRAMOSTIM (GM-CSF).
Use: Adjunct in bone marrow transplantation.
See: Leukine (Immune).
Prokine (Hoechst-Roussel).

SARISOL NO. 2. (Halsey) Butabarbital sodium 30 mg/Tab. Bot. 100s, 1000s.
Use: Sedative/hypnotic.

•**SARMOXICILLIN.** USAN.
Use: Antibacterial.

SARNA. (Stiefel) Camphor 0.5%, menthol 0.5%, phenol 0.5% in a soothing emollient base. Bot. 7.4 oz.
Use: Emollient.

SAROCYCLINE CAPSULES. (Saron) Tetracycline HCl 250 mg/Cap. Bot. 100s.
Use: Anti-infective, tetracycline.

SARODANT. (Saron) Nitrofurantoin 50 mg/Tab. Bot. 100s, 1000s.
Use: Urinary anti-infective.

SAROFLEX. (Saron) Chlorzoxazone 250 mg, acetaminophen 300 mg/Cap.
Use: Muscle relaxant, analgesic.

SAROLAX. (Saron) Docusate sodium 200 mg, yellow phenolphthalein 15 mg, dehydrocholic acid 20 mg/Cap. Bot. 100s.
Use: Laxative.

•**SARPICILLIN.** USAN.
Use: Antibacterial.

SASTID (AL). (Stiefel) Sulfur 1.6%, salicylic acid 1.6%, 20% aluminum oxide scrub particles. Tube 2.9 oz.
Use: Anti-acne.

SASTID PLAIN THERAPEUTIC SHAMPOO AND ACNE WASH. (Stiefel) Sulfur 1.6%, salicylic acid 1.6% in a surfactant base. Tube 2.5 oz.
Use: Anti-acne.

SASTID SOAP. (Stiefel) Precipitated sulfur 10%, salicylic acid 3%. Bar 4.3 oz.
Use: Anti-acne.

SAUREX. (Enzyme Process) Phosphorous 30 mg, pepsin 1:10,000 equal to 100 mg pepsin 1:3000, betaine HCl 125 mg/Tab. Bot. 100s, 250s.
Use: Digestive aid.

SAXOL.
See: Petrolatum Liquid (Various Mfr.).

SCABENE LOTION. (Stiefel) Lindane 1% in lotion base. Bot. 2 oz, 16 oz.
Use: Pediculicide.

SCABENE SHAMPOO. (Stiefel) Lindane 1% in shampoo base. Bot. 2 oz, 16 oz.
Use: Pediculicide.

SCABICIDES.
See: Benzyl Benzoate (Various Mfr.).
Cuprex, Liq. (Calgon).
Eurax, Cream, Lot. (Geigy).
Kwell, Lot., Cream, Shampoo (Reed & Carnrick).

SCADAN SCALP LOTION. (Miles Pharm) Cetyl trimethyl ammonium bromide (cetab) 1%, stearyl dimethyl benzyl ammonium Cl 0.1%. Bot. 4 oz.
Use: Antiseborrheic.

SCAN. (Parker) Water soluble gel for ultrasound B scan procedures. Bot. 8 oz, gal.
Use: Ultrasound B scan procedures.

SCARLET RED. (Lilly) Oint. 5%. Tube 1 oz.
Use: Wound-healing agent.

SCHAMBERG'S. (C & M Pharmacal) Menthol 0.15%, phenol 1%, zinc oxide, peanut oil, lime water. Bot. pt, gal.
Use: Antipruritic, counterirritant.

•**SCHICK TEST CONTROL,** U.S.P. XXII.
Use: Diagnostic aid (dermal reactivity indicator).
See: Diphtheria Toxin, Diagnostic, Inactivated, (Various Mfr.).

SCHLESINGER'S SOLUTION.
See: Morphine HCl (Various Mfr.).

SCLAVO BIOLOGICALS. (Sclavo) A wide variety of generic forms of biological products.

SCLAVOTEST-PPD. (Sclavo) Tuberculin purified protein derivative (PPD) multiple puncture device. Test package. 25s, 100s.
Use: Diagnostic aid.

SCLEREX. (Miller) Inositol 2 Gm, magnesium complex 34 mg, vitamins C 100 mg, calcium succinate 25 mg, A 2500 IU, D 200 IU, E 100 IU, B_1 5 mg, B_2 5 mg, B_6 5 mg, B_{12} 5 mcg, niacin 10 mg, niacinamide 30 mg, pantothenic acid 7.5 mg, folic acid 0.1 mg, iron 10 mg, copper 1 mg, manganese 2 mg, zinc 9 mg, iodine 0.1 mg/3 Tab. Bot. 60s.
Use: Vitamin/mineral supplement.

SCLEROSING AGENTS.
See: Glucose, Liq. (Various Mfr.).
Invert Sugar (Various Mfr.).
Quinine & Urea HCl.
Sodium Morrhuate, Inj. (Various Mfr.).
Sotradecol Sodium, Vial (Elkins-Sinn).

SCOOBY-DOO CHILDREN'S CHEWABLE TABLETS. (Vita-Fresh) Vitamins A 5000 IU, D 400 IU, E 30 mg, B_1 1.5 mg, B_2 1.7 mg, B_3 20 mg, B_5 10 mg, B_6 2 mg, B_{12} 6 mcg, C 60 mg, folic acid 0.4 mg, biotin 45 mcg/Chew. Tab. w/aspartame. Bot. 60s.
Use: Vitamin/mineral supplement.

SCOOBY-DOO CHILDREN'S COMPLETE FORMULA TABLETS. (Vita-Fresh) Calcium 25 mg, iron 18 mg, vitamins A 5000 IU, D 400 IU, E 30 mg, B_1 1.5 mg, B_2 1.7 mg, B_3 20 mg, B_5 10 mg, B_6 2 mg, B_{12} 6 mcg, C 60 mg, folic acid 0.4 mg, Cu, I, Mg, P, zinc 15 mg, biotin 45 mcg/Tab., aspartame. Bot. 60s.
Use: Vitamin/mineral supplement.

SCOOBY-DOO PLUS EXTRA C. (Vita-Fresh) Vitamins A 5000 IU, D 400 IU, E 30 mg, B_1 1.5 mg, B_2 1.7 mg, B_3 20 mg, B_5 10 mg, B_6 2 mg, B_{12} 6 mcg, C 300 mg, folic acid 0.4 mg, biotin 45 mcg/Tab w/aspartame. Bot. 60s.
Use: Vitamin/mineral supplement.

SCOOBY-DOO CHILDREN'S CHEWABLE PLUS IRON TABLETS. (Vita-Fresh) Iron 18 mg, Vitamins A 5000 IU, D 400 IU, E 30 mg, B_1 1.5 mg, B_2 1.7 mg, B_3 20 mg, B_5 10 mg, B_6 2 mg, B_{12} 6 mcg, C 60 mg, folic acid 0.4 mg, biotin 45 mcg/Chew. Tab. w/aspartame. Bot. 60s.
Use: Vitamin/mineral supplement.

•**SCOPAFUNGIN.** USAN.
Use: Antifungal, antibacterial.

SCOPE. (Procter & Gamble) Cetylpyridinium Cl 0.45%, domiphen bromide 0.005%, SD alcohol 38F 18.5%. Liq. Bot. 180 ml, 360 ml, 540 ml, 720 ml, 960 ml, 1200 ml.
Use: Mouthwash.

SCOPINE CHRONCAP. (Cenci) Scopolamine HBr 0.0195 mg, atropine sulfate 0.0582 mg, hyoscyamine sulfate 0.311 mg, phenobarbital 50 mg/Cap. Bot. 100s.
Use: Anticholinergic/antispasmodic, sedative/hypnotic.

SCOPOLAMINE. Hyoscine, l-Scopolamine, Epoxytropine tropate.
See: Hyoscine Preps. (Various Mfr.).

SCOPOLAMINE HBR. (Invenex) Scopolamine HBr 0.3 mg/ml. Inj. Vial 1 ml.
Use: Preanesthetic sedation, obstetric amnesia, calming agent.

SCOPOLAMINE HBR. (Burroughs Wellcome) Scopolamine HBr 0.86 mg/ml Inj. Amp. 0.5 ml.
Use: Preanesthetic sedation, obstetric amnesia, calming agent.

SCOPOLAMINE HBR. (Various Mfr.) Scopolamine HBr 0.4 mg and 1 mg/ml Inj. Amp., Vial 1 ml.
Use: Preanesthetic sedation, obstetric amnesia, calming agent.

SCOPOLAMINE AMINOXIDE HBr.
W/Acetylcarbromal and bromisovalum.
See: Tranquinal, Tab. (Barnes-Hind).

SCOPOLAMINE HYDROBROMIDE, U.S.P. XXII. Inj., Ophth. Oint., Ophth. Soln., Tab., U.S.P. XXII. Benzeneacetic acid, α-(hydroxymethyl)-, 9-methyl-3-oxa-9-azatricyclo [3.3.1.02,4]non-7-yl ester, hydrobromide, trihydrate. 6β, 7β-Epoxy-lαH,5αH-tropan-3α-ol(−)-tropate(ester)hydrobromide trihydrate. Hyoscine HBr.
Use: Sedative/hypnotic, anticholinergic, mydriatic, cyclopegic.
W/Atropine and hyoscyamine.
See: Atropine sulfate tab.
Belladonna alkaloids.
W/Butabarbital, chlorpheniramine maleate.
See: Pedo-Sol, Elix., Tab. (Warren).
W/Homatropine methylbromide, atropine sulfate, butabarbital, hyoscyamine sulfate.
See: Butabell HMB, Elix., Tab. (Saron).
W/Hydroxypropyl methylcellulose.
See: Isopto HBr, Soln. (Alcon).
W/Hyoscyamine sulfate, atropine sulfate, phenobarbital.
See: DeTal, Elix., Tab. (DeLeon).
Donnacin, Elix., Tab. (Pharmex).
Fenatron, Preps. (Panray).
Hyonal C.T., Tab. (Paddock).
Hytrona, Tab. (Webcon).
Nilspasm, Tab. (Parmed).
Peece Kaps (Scrip).
Peece TC, Cap. (Scrip).
Scopine, Cap. (Cenci).
Sedamine, Tab. (Dunhall).
Sedapar, Tab. (Parmed).
Setamine, Tab. (Solvay).
Spasaid, Cap. (Century).
Stannitol (Standex).
W/Pamabrom, pyrilamine maleate, homatropine methylbromide, hyoscyamine sulfate, methamphetamine HCl.
See: Aridol, Tab. (MPL).
W/Phenylephrine, phenylpropanolamine, atropine sulfate, chlorpheniramine maleate, acetaminophen, hyoscyamine HBr.
See: Koryza Tab. (Fellows-Testagar).

SCOPOLAMINE HYDROBROMIDE COMBINATIONS.
See: Belladonna Products.
Hyoscine HBr. (Various Mfr.).

SCOPOLAMINE METHOBROMIDE.
See: Methscopolamine Bromide, Preps. (Various Mfr.).

SCOPOLAMINE METHYLBROMIDE.
See: Methscopolamine Bromide, Preps. (Various Mfr.).

SCOPOLAMINE METHYL NITRATE.
See: Methscopolamine Nitrate, Preps. (Various Mfr.).

SCOPOLAMINE SALTS.
See: Belladonna Products.
Hyoscine salts.

SCORBEX/12. (Pasadena) Vitamins B_1 20 mg, B_2 3 mg, B_3 75 mg, B_5 5 mg, B_6 5 mg, B_{12} 1000 mcg, C 100 mg/ml. Vial dual compartment 10 ml.
Use: Vitamin supplement.

SCOTAVITE. (Scott/Cord) Vitamins A 25,000 IU, D 400 IU, B_1 10 mg, B_2 10 mg, B_6 5 mg, B_{12} 5 mcg, niacinamide 100 mg, calcium pantothenate 20 mg, C 200 mg, d-alpha tocopheryl 15 IU, acid succinate iodine 0.15 mg/Tab. Bot. 100s, 500s.
Use: Vitamin/mineral supplement.

SCOTCIL. (Scott/Cord) Potassium penicillin 400,000 units, calcium carbonate. **Tab.:** Bot. 100s, 500s. **Pow.** 80 ml, 150 ml.
Use: Antibacterial, penicillin.

SCOTCOF. (Scott/Cord) Dextromethorphan HBr 6.85 mg, chlorpheniramine maleate 1.8 mg, phenylephrine HCl 4.4 mg, guaifenesin 66 mg, ammonium Cl 30 mg, chloroform 0.125 mg, alcohol 4.1%/5 ml. Bot. 4 oz, pt, gal.
Use: Antitussive, antihistamine, decongestant, expectorant.

SCOTGESIC. (Scott/Cord) **Cap.:** Acetaminophen 240 mg, salicylamide 100 mg, phenyltoloxamine dihydrogen citrate 30 mg, butabarbital ⅛ gr. Bot. 100s, 500s, 1000s. **Liq.:** Butabarbital 12.15 mg, acetaminophen 300 mg, salicylamide 60 mg, phenyltoloxamine citrate 30 mg/15 ml. Bot. 4 oz, pt.
Use: Analgesic, sedative/hypnotic.

SCOTNORD. (Scott/Cord) Chlorpheniramine maleate 8 mg, phenylephrine HCl 20 mg, methscopolamine nitrate 2.5 mg/Cap. Bot. 100s, 500s.
Use: Antihistamine, decongestant combination.

SCOTONIC. (Scott/Cord) Vitamins B_1 10 mg, B_2 5 mg, B_6 1 mg, niacinamide 50 mg, choline Cl 100 mg, inositol 100 mg, B_{12} 25 mcg, calcium 19 mg, iron 50 mg, folic acid 0.15 mg, alcohol 15%, sodium benzoate 0.1%/45 ml. Bot. pt, gal.
Use: Vitamin/mineral supplement.

SCOTRATE. (Robinson) Scopolamine methyl nitrate 0.5 mg/ml Multiple dose vial 30 ml.

SCOTREX. (Scott/Cord) Tetracycline. **Cap.:** 250 mg. Bot. 16s, 100s, 500s; **Syr.:** 250 mg/5 ml Bot. 2 oz, pt.
Use: Anti-infective.

SCOTT'S EMULSION. (Beecham Products) Vitamins A 1250 IU, D 1400 IU/4 tsp. Bot. 6.25 oz, 12.5 oz.
Use: Vitamin A and D supplement.

SCOT-TUSSIN SUGAR-FREE. (Scot-Tussin) Dextromethorphan HBr 15 mg, chlorpheniramine maleate 2 mg/5 ml. Bot. 4 oz, 8 oz, 16 oz, gal.
Use: Antitussive, antihistamine.

SCOT-TUSSIN SUGAR-FREE 5-ACTION. (Scot-Tussin) Phenylephrine HCl 4.17 mg, pheniramine maleate 13.33 mg, sodium citrate 83.33 mg, sodium salicylate 83.33 mg, caffeine citrate 25 mg/5 ml Nonnarcotic, non-alcoholic. Bot. 4 oz, 8 oz, 16 oz, gal.
Use: Decongestant, antihistamine, analgesic combination.

SCOT-TUSSIN DM LIQUID. (Scot-Tussin) Dextromethorphan HBr 15 mg, chlorpheniramine maleate 2 mg/5 ml, alcohol 10%. Bot. 4 oz, 8 oz. Sugar free.
Use: Antitussive, antihistamine.

SCOT-TUSSIN DM2 SYRUP. (Scot-Tussin) Dextromethorphan HBr 15 mg, guaifenesin 100 mg, 1.4% alcohol. 120 ml, 240 ml.
Use: Antitussive, expectorant.

SCOTT-TUSSIN SUGAR FREE EXPECTORANT. (Scot-Tussin) Guaifenesin 100 mg/5 ml, alcohol 3.5%. Dye free, sodium free, sugar free.
Use: Expectorant.

SCOT-TUSSIN WITH SUGAR. (Scot-Tussin) Phenylephrine HCl 4.17 mg, pheniramine maleate 13.3 mg, sodium citrate 83.33 mg, sodium salicylate 83.33 mg, caffeine citrate 25 mg/5 ml. Bot. 4 oz, 8 oz, 16 oz. gal.
Use: Decongestant, antihistamine, analgesic combination.

SCOTUSS. (Scott/Cord) Dextromethorphan 15 mg, chlorpheniramine maleate 1 mg, phenylephrine HCl 5 mg, phenylpropanolamine HCl 5 mg, N-acetyl-P-aminophenol 120 mg, guaifenesin 100 mg, alcohol 8.2%/5 ml. Bot. 4 oz, pt, gal.
Use: Antitussive, antihistamine, decongestant, expectorant.

SCOTUSS PEDIATRIC COUGH SYRUP. (Scott/Cord) Dextromethorphan HBr 7.5 mg, guaifenesin 50 mg, chlorpheniramine maleate 0.5 mg, phenylephrine HCl 2.5 mg, acetaminophen 60 mg, phenylpropanolamine HCl 2.5 mg, methylparaben 0.15%, propylparaben 0.05%/5 ml. Bot. 4 oz, pt.
Use: Antitussive, expectorant, antihistamine, decongestant, analgesic.

SCRIP-DRI. (Scrip) Formalin soln., formaldehyde in perfumed aqueous base. Bot. 2 oz.

SCRIP SUPER DRI. (Scrip) Formalin soln. in perfumed aqueous base. Bot. 2 oz.

SCURENALINE.
See: Epinephrine, Preps. (Various Mfr.).

SCUROFORME.
See: Butyl Aminobenzoate (Various Mfr.).

S.D.M. #5. (ICI Americas) Mannitol hexanitrate 7% in lactose.
Use: Vasodilator.

S.D.M. #17. (ICI Americas) Nitroglycerin 10% in lactose.
Use: Vasodilator.

S.D.M. #23. (ICI Americas) Pentaerythritol tetranitrate 20% in lactose.
Use: Vasodilator.

S.D.M. #27. (ICI Americas) Nitroglycerin 10% in propylene glycol.
Use: Vasodilator.

S.D.M. #35. (ICI Americas) Pentaerythritol tetranitrate 35% in mannitol.
Use: Vasodilator.

S.D.M. #37. (ICI Americas) Nitroglycerin 10% in ethanol.
Use: Vasodilator.

S.D.M. #40. (ICI Americas) Isorsorbide dinitrate 25% in lactose.
Use: Vasodilator.

S.D.M. #50. (ICI Americas) Isosorbide dinitrate 50% in lactose.
Use: Vasodilator.

SEA GREENS. (Modern) Iodine 0.25 mg/Tab. Bot. 220s, 460s.

SEALE'S LOTION-MODIFIED. (C & M Pharm.) Sulfur 6.4%, zinc oxide, bentonite, sodium borate, acetone. Bot. pt.
Use: Anti-acne.

SEA MASTER. (Barth's) Vitamins A 10,000 units D 400 units/Cap Bot. 100s, 500s.
Use: Vitamin A and D supplement.

SEA-OMEGA 30. (Rugby) N-3 fat content (mg) EPA 180, DHA 140. In 100s.
Use: Nutritional supplement.

SEA-OMEGA 50. (Rugby) Omega-3 polyunsaturated fatty acid 1000 mg/Cap. containing EPA 300 mg, DHA 200 mg, vitamin E 1 IU. Bot. 30s 50s.
Use: Nutritional supplement.

SEA & SKI BABY LOTION FORMULA. (Carter Products) Octyl-dimethyl PABA. SPF 2. Lot. Bot. 120 ml.
Use: Sunscreen.

SEA & SKI GOLDEN TAN. (Carter Products) Padimate O. SPF 4. Lot. Bot. 120 ml.
Use: Sunscreen.

SEBACIDE CLEANSER. (Paddock) Coconut oil, pine oil, castor oil, lecithin, alrosol, tri-potassium EDTA, DSS, alromine RA, sodium lauryl sarcosinate, tetrasodium pyrophosphate, potassium carbonate 0.35%, parachlorometaxylenol. Bot. oz, pt, gal.
Use: Skin cleanser.

SEBA-LO. (Whorton) Acetone-alcohol cleanser. Bot. 4 oz.
Use: Skin cleanser.

SEBANA SHAMPOO. (Myers) Salicylic acid 2% Bot. 4 oz, 8 oz, pt, qt, 0.5 gal.
Use: Antiseborrheic.

SEBANATAR SHAMPOO. (Myers) Salicylic acid 2%, liquor carbonis detergens 3%. Bot. 4 oz, 8 oz, pt, qt, 0.5 gal, gal.
Use: Antiseborrheic.

SEBA-NIL CLEANSING MASK. (Owen Galderma) Astringent face mask containing bentonite, polyethylene, SD alcohol-40, sulfated castor oil, titanium dioxide, kaolin, chromium oxide, methylparaben. Tube 3.7 oz.
Use: Anti-acne.

SEBAQUIN SHAMPOO. (Summers) Iodoquinol 3% in a neutral, soapless detergent, lathering base. Bot. 4 oz.
Use: Antiseborrheic.
SEBASORB LOTION FOR ACNE. (Summers) Activated attapulgite 10%, polysorbate 80, colloidal sulfur 2%, salicylic acid 2%. Bot. 2 oz. w/ dispenser top.
Use: Anti-acne.
SEBEX. (Rugby) Pyrithione zinc 2%. Shampoo. Bot. 120 ml.
Use: Antiseborrheic.
SEBEX-T. (Rugby) Coal tar soln 5%, colloidal sulfur 2%, salicylic acid 2%. Shampoo. Bot. 120 ml.
Use: Antiseborrheic.
SEBIZON LOTION. (Schering) Sulfacetamide sodium 100 mg, methylparaben 1 mg, trisodium edetate, sodium thiosulfate, propylene glycol, isopropyl myristate, propylene glycol monostearate, polyethylene glycol 400 monostearate, water. Tube 3 oz.
Use: Antiseborrheic.
SEBUCARE SCALP LOTION. (Westwood) Laureth-4, salicylic acid 1.5%, alcohol 61%, water, PPG 40 butyl ether, dihydroabietyl alcohol, fragrance. Bot. 4 oz.
Use: Antiseborrheic.
SEBULEX CREAM SHAMPOO. (Westwood) Same formula as Sebulex in a cream shampoo. Tube 4 oz.
Use: Antiseborrheic.
SEBULEX SHAMPOO. (Westwood) Sulfur 2%, salicylic acid 2%. Cream 4.2 oz, Liq. 4 oz.
Use: Antiseborrheic.
SEBULEX WITH CONDITIONERS. (Westwood) Sulfur 2%, salicylic acid 2%. Bot. 4 oz, 8 oz.
Use: Antiseborrheic.
SEBULON. (Westwood) Pyrithione zinc 2%. Shampoo. Bot. 120 ml, 240 ml.
Use: Antiseborrheic.
SEBUTONE CREAM SHAMPOO. (Westwood) Tar equivalent to coal tar, U.S.P. 5%, sulfur 2%, salicylic acid 2%, in sebulytic-type surface-active soapless cleansers, wetting agents. Tube 4 oz.
Use: Antiseborrheic, antipsoriatic.
SEBUTONE THERAPEUTIC TAR SHAMPOO. (Westwood) Tar equivalent to coal tar, U.S.P. 0.5%, sulfur 2%, salicylic acid 2%, in sebulytic-type surface-active soapless cleansers, wetting agents. Bot. 4 oz, 8 oz.
Use: Antiseborrheic, antipsoriatic.
•**SECALCIFEROL.** USAN.
Use: Antihypocalcemic.
SECBUTOBARBITONE. B.A.N. 5-sec-Butyl-5-ethylbarbituric acid. Butabarbitone.
Use: Sedative/hypnotic.
•**SECOBARBITAL,** U.S.P. XXII. Elix, U.S.P. XXII. 5-Allyl-5-(methylbutyl)-barbituric acid. Pow., Bot. ⅛ oz, 1 oz.
Use: Hypnotic.
See: Seco-8, Cap. (Fleming).
SECOBARBITAL COMBINATIONS.
See: Amoseco, Cap. (Robinson).
Efed, Syr., Tab. (Alto).
Monosyl, Tab. (Arcum).
Quad-Set, Tab. (Kenyon).
SECOBARBITAL ELIXIR.
See: Seconal Elix. (Lilly).
•**SECOBARBITAL SODIUM,** U.S.P. XXII. Cap., Inj., Sterile, U.S.P. XXII. Sodium 5-allyl-5-(1-methyl-butyl)-barbiturate. Quinalbarbitone Sodium. B.A.N.
Use: Sedative/hypnotic.
Generic Products:
(Bowman) Secobarbital sodium 1.5 gr/Tab.
(Hance)—Cap. 1.5 gr, Bot. 100s, 1000s.
(Lannett)—Cap. ¾ gr, 1.5 gr, Bot. 100s, 500s.
(Parke-Davis)—Cap. 1.5 gr, Bot. UD 100s.
(Robinson) Cap. ¾ gr, 1.5 gr, Pow. oz.
See: Seco-8, Cap. (Fleming).
Seconal Sodium, Preps. (Lilly).
•**SECOBARBITAL SODIUM AND AMOBARBITAL SODIUM CAPSULES,** U.S.P. XXII.
Use: Sedative/hypnotic.
See: Tuinal, Cap. (Lilly).
SECRAN LIQUID. (Scherer) Vitamins B_1 10 mg, B_3 10 mg, B_{12} 25 mcg, alcohol 17%. Bot. pt.
Use: Vitamin B supplement.
SECRAN PRENATAL TABS. (Scherer) Vitamins A acetate 8000 units, D 400 IU, E 30 IU, C 60 mg, niacinamide 20 mg, B_2 2 mg, B_1 1.7 mg, B_6 2.5 mg, B_{12} 8 mcg, folic acid 1 mg, calcium 250 mg, magnesium, elemental zinc 20 mg, iron 60 mg/Tab. Bot. 100s, 240s.
Use: Vitamin/mineral supplement.
SECRETIN. B.A.N. A hormone obtained from duodenal mucosa.
Use: Diagnostic for pancreatic dysfunction.
SECRETIN FERRING POWDER. (Ferring) Secretin 75 cu/10 ml Vial. 10 cu/ml when reconstituted with 7.5 ml.
Use: Diagnostic aid.
SECTRAL. (Wyeth-Ayerst) Acebutolol HCl 200 or 400 mg/Cap. Bot. 100s, UD 100s.
Use: Antihypertensive.
SEDACANE. (E.J. Moore) Acetaminophen 120 mg, salicylamide 210 mg, caffeine 30 mg, calcium gluconate 60 mg/Cap. Bot. 12s.
Use: Analgesic combination.
SEDAFORM.
See: Chlorobutanol (Various Mfr.).
SEDAJEN. (Jenkins) Phenobarbital 5⁄16 gr, passiflora 1.5 gr, hyoscyamus ¾ gr (total alkaloids 0.0003 gr)/Tab. Bot. 1000s.
Use: Sedative/hypnotic.
SEDALGESIC INSERTS. (Table Rock) Aspirin 195 mg, secobarbital 30 mg/Insert. Box 12s.
Use: Analgesic, sedative/hypnotic.
SEDALGESIC TABLETS. (Table Rock) Bromisovalum 150 mg, acetaminophen 100 mg, salicylamide 100 mg/Tab. Bot. 100s, 500s.

Use: Sedative, analgesic.
SEDAMINE. (Approved) Phosphorated carbohydrate. Soln. Bot. 4 oz.
Use: Antiemetic.
SEDAMINE. (Dunhall) Hyoscyamine sulfate 0.1037 mg, atropine sulfate 0.0194 mg, hyoscine HBr 0.0065 mg, phenobarbital 16.2 mg/Tab. Bot. 100s, 1000s.
Use: Anticholinergic/antispasmodic, sedative/hypnotic.
SEDAPAP #3 CAPSULES. (Mayrand) Acetaminophen 500 mg, butalbital 50 mg, codeine phosphate 30 mg/Cap. Bot. 100s.
Use: Narcotic analgesic combination.
SEDAPAP-10 TABLETS. (Mayrand) Acetaminophen 10 gr, butabarbital 50 mg/Tab. Bot. 100s.
Use: Analgesic, sedative/hypnotic.
SEDAPAR. (Parmed) Atropine sulfate 0.0195 mg, hyoscine HBr 0.0065 mg, hyoscyamine sulfate 0.1040 mg, phenobarbital 0.25 gr/Tab. Bot. 1000s.
Use: Anticholinergic/antispasmodic, sedative/hypnotic.
SEDATANS TABLETS. (Lannett) Tab. Bot. 100s, 1000s.
SEDATIVE/HYPNOTIC AGENTS.
See: Bromides (Various Mfr.).
Barbiturates (Various Mfr.).
Butisol Sodium (McNeil).
Carbamide (Urea) Compounds (Various Mfr.).
Chloral Hydrate Preps (Various Mfr.).
Chlorobutanol (Various Mfr.).
Dalmane, Cap. (Roche).
Doral (Baker Cummins).
Flurazepam (Various Mfr.).
Halcion (Upjohn).
Intasedol, Elix. (Elder).
Largon, Inj. (Wyeth-Ayerst).
Lotusate, Cap. (Winthrop).
Noludar, Tab., Cap. (Roche).
Paraldehyde, Preps. (Various Mfr.).
Phenergan HCl, Preps. (Wyeth-Ayerst).
Placidyl, Cap. (Abbott).
Plexonal, Tab. (Sandoz).
ProSom (Abbott).
Restoril, Cap. (Sandoz).
Temazepam (Various Mfr.).
Valmid, Tab. (Lilly).
Vingesic, Cap. (Amid).
•**SEDECAMYCIN.** USAN.
Use: Antibacterial (veterinary).
SEDEVAL.
See: Barbital (Various Mfr.).
SEDRAGESIC TABLETS. (Lannett) Acetaminophen 0.325 Gm, salicylamide 0.195 Gm, d-amphetamine sulfate 2.5 mg, hexobarbital 8 mg, secobarbital sodium 2.7 mg, butabarbital sodium 2.7 mg, phenobarbital 2.7 mg/Tab. Bot. 100s, 1000s.
Use: Analgesic, sedative/hypnotic.
SEDRAL. (Vita Elixir) Phenobarbital ⅛ gr, theophylline 2 gr, ephedrine ⅜ gr/Tab.
Use: Sedative/hypnotic, bronchodilator.
•**SEELAZONE.** USAN.
Use: Anti-inflammatory, uricosuric.
•**SEGLITIDE ACETATE.** USAN.
Use: Antidiabetic.
SELDANE. (Merrell Dow) Terfenadine 60 mg/Tab. Bot. 100s.
Use: Antihistamine.
SELEGILINE HCl.
Use: Antiparkinson agent.
See: Eldepryl (Somerset).
SELENICEL. (Pasadena Research) Selenium yeast complex 200 mcg, vitamins C 100 mg, E 100 mg/Cap. Bot. 90s.
Use: Vitamin supplement.
•**SELENIOUS ACID,** U.S.P. XXII, Inj., U.S.P. XXII.
SELENIUM. (Nion) Selenium 50 mcg/Tab. Bot. 100s.
Use: Parenteral nutritional supplement.
SELENIUM DISULFIDE.
See: Selenium Sulfide, Detergent, Susp. (Various Mfr.).
•**SELENIUM SULFIDE,** U.S.P. XXII., Lot., U.S.P. XXII.
Use: Treatment of dandruff, antifungal, antiseborrheic.
See: Exsel Lotion (Herbert).
Iosel 250, Liq. (Owen).
Selsun, Susp. (Abbott).
•**SELENOMETHIONINESe 75 INJECTION,** U.S.P. XXII. 2-Amino-4-(methylselenyl) butyric acid (^{75}Se).
Use: Diagnostic aid (pancreas function determination).
See: Sethotope, Inj. (Squibb).
SELE-PAK. (SoloPak) Selenium 40 mcg/ml. Inj. Vial 10 ml, 30 ml.
Use: Parenteral nutritional supplement.
SELESTOJECT. (Mayrand) Betamethasone sodium phosphate 4 mg/ml (equivalent to 3 mg betamethasone alcohol). Soln. Vial 5 ml.
Use: Corticosteroid.
SELORA POWDER. (Winthrop) Potassium Cl.
Use: Salt substitute.
SELEPEN. (Lyphomed) Selenium 40 mcg/ml. Vial 3 ml, 10 ml.
Use: Parenteral nutritional supplement.
SELSUN BLUE. (Ross) Selenium sulfide 1% in lotion base. Bot. 4 oz, 7 oz, 11 oz. Dry, oily, normal extra conditioning, and extra medicated (contains 0.5% menthol) formulas.
Use: Antiseborrheic.
SELSUN SUSPENSION. (Abbott) Selenium sulfide 2.5%. Bot. 4 fl oz.
Use: Antiseborrheic.
•**SEMATILIDE HYDROCHLORIDE.** USAN.
Use: Antiarrhythmic.
•**SEMDURAMICIN.** USAN.
Use: Coccidiostat.
•**SEMDURAMICIN SODIUM.** USAN.
Use: Coccidiostat.

SEMICID. (Whitehall) Nonoxynol-9 100 mg/Vag. Supp. Box 10s, 20s.
Use: Contraceptive.

SEMILENTE ILETIN I. (Lilly) Insulin zinc suspension from beef and pork 40 or 100 units/ml. Vial 10 ml.
Use: Antidiabetic agent.

SEMILENTE INSULIN.
See: Iletin, Vial (Lilly).

•**SEMUSTINE.** USAN.
Use: Antineoplastic.

SENILAVITE. (Defco) Vitamins A 5000 IU, C 100 mg, B_1 2.5 mg, B_2 2 mg, nicotinamide 10 mg, B_6 1 mg, calcium pantothenate 5 mg, B_{12} w/intrinsic factor concentrate 0.133 IU, ferrous fumarate 150 mg, glutamic acid HCl 150 mg, docusate sodium 50 mg/Cap. Bot. 100s.
Use: Vitamin/mineral supplement.

SENILEZOL ELIXIR. (Edwards) Vitamins B_1 0.42 mg, B_2 0.42 mg, B_3 1.67 mg, B_5 0.83 mg, B_6 0.17 mg, B_{12} 0.83 mcg, ferric pyrophosphate 3.3 mg, alcohol 15%. Bot. pt.
Use: Vitamin/mineral supplement.

SENIOR FORMULA CAPSULES. (Life's Finest) Calcium 125 mg, iron 5 mg, vitamins A 2500 IU, D 200 IU, E 15.1 mg, B_1 1.1 mg, B_2 1.2 mg, B_3 15 mg, B_5 7.5 mg, B_6 1.5 mg, B_{12} 4.5 mcg, C 45 mg, folic acid 0.2 mg, Cr, Cu, Mg, Mn, P, Se, zinc 3.75 mg/Cap. Bot. 60s, 90s, 180s.
Use: Vitamin/mineral supplement.

•**SENNA,** U.S.P. XXII. Fluidextract, Syr., U.S.P. XXII. Alexandrian.
Use: Cathartic.
See: Casafru, Liq. (Key).

SENNA CONCENTRATE, STANDARDIZED.
Use: Cathartic.
See: Senokot, Gran., Tab., Supp. (Purdue Frederick).
X-Prep, Pow. (Gray).
W/Docusate sodium.
See: Gentlax S. Tab. (Blair).
Senokap-DSS, Cap. (Purdue Frederick).
Senokot S. Tab. (Purdue Frederick).
W/Guar gum.
See: Gentlax B Tab., Granules (Blair).
W/Psyllium.
See: Perdiem, Granules. (Rorer Consumer).
Senokot w/Psyllium Pow. (Purdue Frederick).

SENNA FRUIT EXTRACT, STANDARIZED.
Use: Cathartic.
See: Senokot Syr. (Purdue Frederick).
X-Prep, Liq. (Gray).

SENNA-GEN TABS. (Goldline) Bot. 100s, 1000s.
Use: Laxative.

SENNA POWDER COMPOUND. (Penick) Licorice compound. Pow. Bot. 0.25 lb, 1 lb.
Use: Laxative.

SENNOSIDES, U.S.P. XXII. Tab., U.S.P. XXII.
Use: Laxative, stool softener.
See: Gentle Nature (Sandoz Consumer).

SENOKOT TABLETS and GRANULES. (Purdue Frederick) **Granules:** Standardized senna concentrate. Can 2 oz, 6 oz, 12 oz. **Tab.:** Bot. 50s, 100s, 1000s, Unit strip pack 100s, Box 20s.
Use: Laxative.

SENOKOT S TABLETS. (Purdue Frederick) Standardized senna concentrate, docusate sodium. Tab. Bot. 30s, 60s, 1000s.
Use: Laxative.

SENOKOT SUPPOSITORIES. (Purdue Frederick) Standardized senna concentrate. Pkg. 6s.
Use: Laxative.

SENOKOT SYRUP. (Purdue Frederick) Standardized extract of senna fruit. Bot. 2 oz, 8 oz.
Use: Laxative.

SENOLAX. (Schein) Senna concentrate 217 mg/Tab. Bot. 100s, 1000s.
Use: Laxative.

SENSITIVE EYES DAILY CLEANER. (Bausch & Lomb) Isotonic solution, borate buffer, surfactant cleaner, sodium Cl, hydroxypropyl methylcellulose, sorbic acid 0.25%, EDTA 0.5%. Thimerosal free. Soln. Bot. 30 ml.
Use: Soft contact lens care.

SENSITIVE EYES DROPS. (Bausch & Lomb) Isotonic solution with a borate buffer system, sorbic acid 0.1%, EDTA. Soln. Bot. 30 ml, 60 ml.
Use: Soft contact lens care.

SENSITIVE EYES SALINE. (Bausch & Lomb) Sodium Cl, borate buffer, sorbic acid 0.1%, EDTA. Soln. Bot. 118 ml, 237 ml, 355 ml.
Use: Soft contact lens care.

SENSODYNE TOOTHPASTE. (Block) Glycerin, sorbitol, sodium methyl cocoyltaurate, PEG-40 stearate, strontium Cl hexahydrate 10%, methyl and propylparabens, tint. Tube 2.1 oz, 4 oz.
Use: Preparation for sensitive teeth.

SENSORCAINE. (Astra) Bupivacaine HCl 0.25%, 0.50% or 0.75%. Amp. 30 ml. Vial 10 ml, 30 ml, 50 ml.
Use: Local anesthetic.

•**SEPAZONIUM CHLORIDE.** USAN.
Use: Anti-infective, topical.

•**SEPERIDOL HCl.** USAN. 4-[4-(4-Chloro-α,α,α-trifluoro-m-tolyl)-4-hydroxypiperidino]-4′-fluorobutyrophenone HCl. Under study.
Use: Neuroleptic, antipsychotic.

SEPO. (Otis Clapp) Benzocaine. Loz. Bot. 80s, Safety pack 500s.
Use: Local anesthetic.

SEPTA. (Circle) Bacitracin 400 units, neomycin sulfate 5 mg, polymyxin B sulfate 5000 units/Gm. Ointment base. Tube oz.
Use: Anti-infective, external.

SEPTI-CHEK. (Roche Diagnostics) Blood culture and simultaneous sub-culture system with three media to support clinically significant pathogens. Quick and easy assembly forms a closed system to protect sub-cultures from contamination.
Use: Diagnostic aid.

SEPTIPHENE. 4-Chloro-α-phenyl-o-cresoln. Santophen 1. (Monsanto).
Use: Disinfectant.

SEPTI-SOFT. (Vestal) Hexachlorophene 0.25%. Liq. Bot. 240 ml, pt, gal.
Use: Antiseptic, germicide.

SEPTISOL. (Vestal) **Soln.:** Hexachlorophene 0.25%. Bot. 240 ml, qt, gal. **Foam:** Hexachlorophene 0.23%, alcohol 46%. In 180 ml, 600 ml.
Use: Antiseptic, germicide.

SEPTO. (Vita Elixir) Methylbenzethonium Cl, ethanol 2%, menthol.
Use: Antiseptic, germicide.

SEPTRA. (Burroughs Wellcome) Sulfamethoxazole 400 mg, trimethoprim 80 mg/Tab. Bot. 100s, 500s, UD 100s.
Use: Anti-infective.

SEPTRA DS. (Burroughs Wellcome) Trimethoprim 160 mg, sulfamethoxazole 800 mg/Tab. Bot. 100s, 250s, UD 100s.
Use: Anti-infective.

SEPTRA GRAPE SUSPENSION. (Burroughs Wellcome) Trimethoprim 40 mg, sulfamethoxazole 200 mg/5 ml. Bot. 473 ml.
Use: Anti-infective.

SEPTRA I.V. (Burroughs Wellcome) Trimethoprim 80 mg, sulfamethoxazole 400 mg/5 ml. Amp. 5 ml, Vial 10 ml, 20 ml, *Add-Vantage* Vial 5 ml, 10 ml.
Use: Anti-infective.

SEPTRA IV ADD-VANTAGE. (Burroughs Wellcome) Trimethoprim 80 mg, sulfamethoxazole 400 mg/5 ml vial or trimethoprim 160 mg, sulfamethoxazole 800 mg/10 ml vial. Box 10s.
Use: Anti-infective.

SEPTRA SUSPENSION. (Burroughs Wellcome) Trimethoprim 40 mg, sulfamethoxazole 200 mg/5 ml. Bot. 100 ml, 473 ml.
Use: Anti-infective.

•**SERACTIDE ACETATE.** USAN. Ala^{26}-Gly^{27}-$SER^{31\alpha1\text{-}39}$ corticotrophin acetate.
Use: Corticotrophic peptide, hormone (adrenocorticotropic).
See: Acthar Gel (Armour).

SER-A-GEN. (Goldline) Hydrochlorothiazide 15 mg, reserpine 0.1 mg, hydralazine HCl 25 mg/Tab. Bot. 100s, 1000s.
Use: Antihypertensive combination.

SERALAZIDE. (Lannett) Hydrochlorothiazide 15 mg, reserpine 0.1 mg, hydralazine HCl 25 mg/Tab. Bot. 100s, 1000s.
Use: Antihypertensive combination.

SERALYZER. (Ames) A system for the measurement of enzymes, potassium levels, blood chemistries and therapeutic drug assays consisting of a reflectance photometer and a series of solid-phase reagent strips.
Use: Diagnostic aid.

SER-AP-ES. (Ciba) Reserpine 0.1 mg, hydralazine HCl 25 mg, hydrochlorothiazide 15 mg/Tab. Bot. 100s, 1000s, Accu-Pak 100s.
Use: Antihypertensive combination.

SERAPINE TABLETS. (Cenci) Hydralazine HCl 25 mg, hydrochlorothiazide 15 mg, reserpine 0.1 mg/Tab. Bot. 100s, 1000s.
Use: Antihypertensive combination.

SERAX. (Wyeth-Ayerst) Oxazepam. **Cap.**: 10 mg, 15 mg or 30 mg. Bot. 100s, 500s, Redipak 25s, 100s. **Tab.**: 15 mg. Bot. 100s.
Use: Antianxiety agent.

•**SERAZAPINE HYDROCHLORIDE.** USAN.
Use: Anxiolytic.

SEREEN. (Foy) Chlordiazepoxide HCl 10 mg/Cap. Bot. 500s, 1000s.
Use: Antianxiety agent.

SERENE. (Approved) Salicylamide 2 gr, scopolamine aminoxide HBr 0.2 mg/Cap. Bot. 24s, 60s.
Use: Analgesic, sedative.

SERENTIL. (Boehringer Ingelheim) Mesoridazine besylate. **Inj.**: 25 mg/ml Amp. 1 ml. **Tab.**: 10 mg, 25 mg, 50 mg or 100 mg. Bot. 100s. **Oral Conc.:** 25 mg/ml w/dropper.
Use: Antipsychotic.

SERICINASE. A proteolytic enzyme.

•**SERINE,** U.S.P. XXII. $C_3H_7NO_3$ as L-serine.
Use: Amino acid.

•**SERMETACIN.** USAN.
Use: Anti-inflammatory.

•**SERMORELIN ACETATE.** USAN.
Use: Growth hormone-releasing factor (human); diagnostic aid (growth failure).

SERNYLAN. Phencyclidine. B.A.N. 1-(1-Phenycyclohexyl)-piperidine HCl.
Use: Anesthetic.

SEROMYCIN. (Lilly) Cycloserine 250 mg/Pulvule. Bot. 40s.
Use: Antituberculous agent.

SEROPHENE. (Serono) Clomiphene citrate 50 mg/Tab. Bot. 10s, 30s.
Use: Ovulation stimulant.

SERPALAN TABLETS. (Lannett) Reserpine alkaloid 0.1 mg or 0.25 mg/Tab. Bot. 100s, 500s, 1000s.
Use: Antihypertensive.

SERPASIL. (Ciba) Reserpine. **0.25 mg/Tab.:** Bot. 100s, 500s, 1000s, UD 100s; **0.1 mg/Tab.:** Bot. 100s, 1000s.
Use: Antihypertensive.

SERPASIL-APRESOLINE. (Ciba) **#1:** Reserpine 0.1 mg, hydralazine HCl 25 mg/Tab. Bot. 100s. **#2:** Reserpine 0.2 mg, hydralazine HCl 50 mg/Tab. Bot. 100s.
Use: Antihypertensive combination.

SERPASIL-ESIDRIX. (Ciba) **#1:** Reserpine 0.1 mg, hydrochlorothiazide 25 mg/Tab. **#2:** Reserpine 0.1 mg, hydrochlorothiazide 50 mg/Tab. Bot. 100s, 1000s.
Use: Antihypertensive combination.

SERPAZIDE TABLETS. (Major) Reserpine 0.1 mg, hydralazine HCl 25 mg, hydrochlorothiazide 15 mg/Tab. Bot. 100s, 1000s.
Use: Antihypertensive combination.

SERTABS. (Table Rock) Reserpine 0.25 mg or 0.5 mg/Tab. Bot. 100s, 500s.
Use: Antihypertensive.

SERTINA. (Fellows) Reserpine 0.25 mg/Tab. Bot. 1000s, 5000s.
Use: Antihypertensive.

•**SERTRALINE HYDROCHLORIDE.** USAN.
Use: Antidepressant

SERUM, ALBUMIN, NORMAL HUMAN.
See: Albumin Human, U.S.P. XXII. (Various Mfr.).

SERUM, ALBUMIN, HUMAN, RADIOIODINATED.
See: Iodinated I-125.
Albumin Injection, U.S.P. XXII.

SERUM, ANTIHEMOPHILUS INFLUENZAE TYPE B (RABBIT). Antihaemophilus (influenzae Type B Serum, Rabbit). (Squibb).

SERUM, GLOBULIN (HUMAN), IMMUNE.
See: Globulin Immune Serum (Human), (Various Mfr.).

SERUM, MEASLES IMMUNE, HUMAN.
See: Measles Virus Vaccine Live, U.S.P. XXII.

SERUM PERTUSSIS IMMUNE, HUMAN.
See: Pertussis Vaccine Adsorbed, U.S.P. XXII.

SERUTAN. (Beecham Products) Psyllium. **Granules:** Pkg. 6 oz, 18 oz. **Pow.:** 7 oz, 14 oz, 21 oz. (Fruit flavored): 6 oz, 12 oz, 18 oz.
Use: Laxative.

•**SESAME OIL,** N.F. XVII.
Use: Pharmaceutic aid (solvent).

SESTRON. N-Ethyl-3,3′-diphenyl-dipropylamine. Profenil. (Smith, Miller & Patch).

SETHOTOPE. (Squibb) Selenomethionine selenium 75; available as 0.25 or 1 mCi.

•**SETOPERONE.** USAN.
Use: Antipsychotic.

•**SEVOFLURANE.** USAN. Fluoromethyl 2,2,2-trifluoro-1-(trifluoromethyl)ethyl ether.
Use: Anesthetic (inhalation).

SHADE. (Schering-Plough) SPF 15. Contains one or more of the following ingredients: Padimate O, oxybenzone, ethylhexyl-p-methoxycinnamate. Bot. 118 ml, 120 ml, 240 ml.
Use: Sunscreen.

SHADE CREAM. (O'Leary) Jar 0.25 oz.
Use: Contouring cream.

SHEIK ELITE. (Schmid) Condom with nonoxynol 9 5.6%. In 12s.
Use: Contraceptive.

•**SHELLAC,** N.F. XVII.
Use: Pharmaceutic aid (tablet coating agent).

SHEPARD'S CREAM LOTION. (Dermik) Creamy lotion with no lanolin or mineral oil, for entire body. Scented or unscented. Bot. 8 oz, 16 oz.
Use: Emollient.

SHEPARD'S MOISTURIZING SOAP. (Dermik) Mildly scented, superfatted with lanolin. Bar 4 oz.
Use: Emollient.

SHEPARD'S SKIN CREAM. (Dermik) Scented or unscented, w/no lanolin or mineral oil. Jar 4 oz.
Use: Emollient.

SHERFORM-HC CREME. (Sheryl) Hydrocortisone 1%, pramoxine HCl 0.5%, clioquinol 3%. Oint. Tube 0.5 oz.
Use: Corticosteroid, local anesthetic, antifungal.

SHERHIST. (Sheryl) Phenylephrine HCl, pyrilamine maleate/Tab. Bot. 100s. Liq. Bot. pt.
Use: Decongestant, antihistamine.

SHERNATAL TABLETS. (Sheryl) Phosphorus-free calcium, non-irritating iron, trace minerals and essential vitamins. Tab. Bot. 100s.
Use: Vitamin/mineral supplement.

SHERRY-JEN TONIC. (Jenkins) Vitamins B_1 8 mg, B_2 4 mg, cyanocobalamin 4 mcg, nicotinamide 20 mg, calcium pantothenate 5 mg, B_6 1 mg, inositol 30 mg, choline bitartrate 60 mg, ferric ammonium citrate 60 mg, alcohol 9%/fl oz. Bot. 4 oz, 8 oz, gal.
Use: Vitamin/mineral supplement.

SHERTUS LIQUID. (Sheryl) Dextromethorphan HBr, chlorpheniramine maleate, phenylephrine HCl, ammonium Cl. Liq. Bot. pt.
Use: Antitussive, antihistamine, decongestant, expectorant.

SHOHL'S SOLUTION. Sodium Citrate and Citric Acid Oral Soln, U.S.P. XXII.
Use: Systemic alkalizer.

SHOSTAKOVSKY BALSAM. Polyvinox. B.A.N.

SHUR SEAL GEL. (Milex) Nonoxynol-9 6 Gm/5 oz pre-measured pak. Box 24s.
Use: Contraceptive.

SIALCO. (Foy) Chlorpheniramine maleate 4 mg, salicylamide 150 mg, acetaminophen 125 mg, phenylephrine HCl 5 mg/Tab. Bot. 100s, 500s, 1000s.
Use: Antihistamine, analgesic, decongestant.

SIBELIUM. (Janssen) Flunarizine HCl.
Use: Vasodilator.

SIBLIN. (Warner-Lambert Consumer) Water-absorbent material from plantago/Tsp. Box lb.
Use: Laxative.

•**SIBUTRAMINE HYDROCHLORIDE.** USAN.
Use: Antidepressant; appetite suppressant.

SIDEROL. (Doral) Chelated iron ammonium citrate 720 mg, folic acid 400 mcg, vitamins B_{12} 25 mcg, B_1 50 mg, B_6 1 mg, niacin 60 mg, panthenol 10 mg, PABA 6 mg, l-lysine HCl 100 mg, inositol 10 mg, choline citrate 50 mg, methionine 6.25 mg, Cu, Zn, Mn, K, Mg, in base with sorbitol, liver fraction no. 1, beef peptone/ml. Bot. 6 oz.
Use: Nutritional supplement.

SIGAMINE. (Sig) Cyanocobalamin injection 1000 mcg/ml. Vial 10 ml, 30 ml. Also Sigamine L.A. Vial 10 ml.
Use: Vitamin B_{12} supplement.

SIGAZINE. (Sig) Promethazine HCl 50 mg/ml. Vial 10 ml.
Use: Antihistamine.

SIGESIC. (Rand) Cap. Bot. 100s, 1000s.
Use: Analgesic, sedative.

SIGNA CREME. (Parker) Conductive cosmetic quality electrolyte cream. Bot. 5 oz, 2 L, 4 L.

Use: High conductive electrode cream for diagnostic electrocardiograms.

SIGNA GEL. (Parker) Conductive saline electrode gel. Tube 250 Gm.
Use: Defibrillation, ECG, EMG, electrosurgery.

SIGNA PAD. (Parker) Pre-moistened electrode pads.
Use: ECG procedures.

SIGNATAL C. (Sig) Calcium 230 mg, iron 49.3 mg, vitamins A 4000 IU, D 400 IU, B_1 2 mg, B_2 2 mg, B_6 1 mg, B_{12} 2 mcg, folic acid 0.1 mg, niacinamide 10 mg, C 50 mg, iodine 0.15 mg/SC Tab. Bot. 100s, 1000s.
Use: Vitamin/mineral supplement.

SIGNATE. (Sig) Dimenhydrinate 50 mg, propylene glycol 50%, benzyl alcohol 5%/ml. Vial 10 ml.
Use: Antiemetic/antivertigo.

SIGNEF "SUPPS". (Fellows) Hydrocortisone 15 mg/Supp. 12s w or w/out appl.
Use: Corticosteroid, vaginal.

SIGPRED. (Sig) Prednisolone acetate. Vial 10 ml.
Use: Corticosteroid.

SIGTAB. (Upjohn) Vitamins A 5000 IU, D 400 IU, B_1 10.3 mg, B_2 10 mg, C 333 mg, niacin 100 mg, B_6 6 mg, pantothenic acid 20 mg, folic acid 0.4 mg, B_{12} 18 mcg, E 16.5 mg/Tab. Bot. 30s, 90s, 500s.
Use: Vitamin supplement.

SILACLEAN. (Professional Supplies) Benzalkonium Cl, EDTA. Soln. Bot. 60 ml.
Use: Hard contact lens care.

•**SILAFILCON A.** USAN.
Use: Contact lens material.

•**SILANDRONE.** USAN. 17 β-(Trimethylsioloxy)-androst-4-en-3-one.
Use: Androgen.

SILEXIN LOZENGES. (Otis Clapp) Dextromethorphan HBr 5 mg, benzocaine 7.9 mg/Loz. In 400s.
Use: Antitussive, local anesthetic.

SILEXIN SYRUP. (Otis Clapp) Dextromethorphan HBr, guaifenesin in sugar, salt and alcohol free vehicle. Bot. 1 oz, 4 oz, 16 oz.
Use: Antitussive, expectorant.

SILEXIN TABS. (Otis Clapp) Dextromethorphan HBr, benzocaine/Tab. 400s.
Use: Antitussive, local anesthetic.

•**SILICON DIOXIDE,** N.F. XVII.
Use: Pharmaceutic aid (suspending agent, anticaking agent, disintegrating agent).

•**SILICEOUS EARTH, PURIFIED,** N.F. XVII.
Use: Filtering medium.

SILICONE. (Dow Chemicals) Dimethicone. Liq., Bot. oz. Bulk Pkg. Oint.
See also:
W/Lanolin.
See: Sanchia Silicone Protective Cream (Otis Clapp).
W/Nitro-Cellulose, castor oil.
See: Covicone, Cream (Abbott).
W/Triethylene glycol, mineral oil.
See: Allergex, Liq., Spray (Hollister-Stier).

•**SILICONE DIOXIDE, COLLOIDAL,** N.F. XVII.
Use: Tablet diluent, suspending & thickening agent.

SILICONE OINTMENT. Dimethicone Dimethyl polysiloxane.
See: Covicone Cream (Abbott).

SILICONE OINTMENT NO. 2. (C & M Pharmacal) High viscosity silicone 10% in a blend of petrolatum and hydrophobic starch. Jar 2 oz, lb.
Use: Protective agent.

SILICONE POWDER. (Gordon) Talc with silicone. Pkg. 4 oz, 1 lb, 5 lb.
Use: Dusting powder to prevent tape from adhering to clothing.

SILMAGEL. (Lannett) Aluminum hydroxide 2.5 gr, magnesium trisilicate 3.85 gr/Tab. Bot. 1000s, 5000s.
Use: Antacid.

•**SILODRATE.** USAN. Magnesium aluminosilicate hydrate.
Use: Antacid.

SILTEX. (E.J. Moore) Camphor, menthol, allantoin, tincture of benzoin in lanolin-petrolatum base. Tube 0.25 oz.
Use: Chapped lips, cold sores, fever blisters.

SILVADENE. (Marion) Silver sulfadiazine (10 mg/Gm) 1%, base w/white petrolatum, stearyl alcohol, isopropyl myristate, sorbitan mono-oleate, polyoxyl 40 stearate, propylene glycol, water, methylparaben. Cream Jar 50 Gm, 400 Gm, 1000 Gm, Tube 20 Gm.
Use: Antimicrobial, topical.

SILVER COMPOUNDS.
See: Silver Iodide, Colloidal.
Silver Nitrate, Preps. (Various Mfr.).
Silver Picrate (City Chem.).
Silver Protein, Mild (Various Mfr.).
Silver Protein, Strong (Various Mfr.).

•**SILVER NITRATE,** U.S.P. XXII. Ophth. Soln., Toughened, U.S.P. XXII. Nitric acid silver.
Use: Astringent, caustic, antiseptic.

SILVER NITRATE OINTMENT. (Gordon) Silver nitrate 1% in ointment base. Jar oz.
Use: Astringent, epithelial stimulant.

•**SILVER NITRATE OPHTHALMIC SOLUTION,** U.S.P. XXII. (Wax Amp.).
Use: Astringent, anti-infective.
Generic Products:
(Gordon)-Soln. 10%, 25% or 50%. Bot. 1 oz.
(Lilly)—Amp. 1%, 100s.
(Parke-Davis)—Cap. 1%, 100s.

•**SILVER NITRATE, TOUGHENED,** U.S.P. XXII. Silver nitrate plus silver Cl 4%.
Use: Caustic.

SILVER PICRATE. (City Chem.) 1 oz.
Use: Antiseptic.

SILVER PROTEIN, MILD. Argentum Vitellinum, Cargentos, Mucleinate Mild, Protargin Mild.
See: Argyrol Prods. (CooperVision).

SILVER PROTEIN, STRONG.
See: Protargol, Pow. (Sterling).

•**SILVER SULFADIAZINE.** USAN.
Use: Anti-infective, topical.
See: Silvadene, Oint. (Marion).

SIMAAL GEL. (Schein) Aluminum hydroxide 200 mg, magnesium hydroxide 200 mg, simethicone 20 mg/5 ml. Bot. 360 ml, gal.
Use: Antacid, antiflatulant.

SIMAAL 2 GEL. (Schein) Aluminum hydroxide 400 mg, magnesium hydroxide 400 mg, simethicone 30 mg/5 ml. Bot. 360 ml.
Use: Antacid, antiflatulant.

•**SIMETHICONE,** U.S.P. XX, Emulsion, Oral Susp., Tab., U.S.P. XXII. Mixture of liquid dimethyl polysiloxanes with silica aerogel.
Use: Antiflatulent, pharmaceutic aid (release agent).
See: Mylicon, Tab., Liq. (Stuart).
Mylicon-80, Tab. (Stuart).
Silain, Tab. (Robins).
Ingredients of:
Mylanta, Tab., Liq. (Stuart).
Phazyme, Tab. (Reed & Carnick).
W/Aluminum hydroxide, magnesium hydroxide.
See: Di-Gel, Liq., Tab. (Schering-Plough).
Mylanta, Mylanta II, Tab., Liq. (Stuart).
Silain-Gel, Liq. (Robins).
Simeco, Liq. (Wyeth-Ayerst).
Simethox, Liq. (Quality Generics).
W/Enzymes.
See: Phazyme, Tab. (Reed & Carnrick).
W/Hyoscyamine sulfate, atropine sulfate, hyoscine HBr, butabarbital sodium
See: Sidonna, Tab. (Reed & Carnrick).
W/Hyoscyamine sulfate, atropine sulfate, scopolamine HBr, phenobarbital.
See: Kinesed, Chew. Tab. (Stuart).
W/Magnesium aluminum hydroxide.
See: Maalox Plus, Susp. (Rorer).
W/Magnesium carbonate.
See: Di-Gel, Tab., Liq. (Schering-Plough).
W/Magnesium hydroxide.
See: Laxsil, Liq. (Reed & Carnrick).
W/Magnesium hydroxide, dried aluminum hydroxide gel.
See: Maalox Plus, Tab. (Rorer).
W/Pancreatin.
See: Phazyme, Tab. (Reed & Carnrick).
Phazyme-95, Tab. (Reed & Carnrick).
W/Pancreatin, phenobarbital.
See: Phazyme-PB, Tab. (Reed & Carnrick).

SIMILAC 13/SIMILAC 13 WITH IRON. (Ross) Milk-based infant formula ready-to-feed containing 13 calories/fl oz, 1.8 mg iron/100 calories. Bot. 4 fl oz.
Use: Enteral nutritional supplement.

SIMILAC 24 LBW. (Ross) Low-iron infant formula, ready-to-feed, 24 cal/fl oz. Bot. 4 fl oz.
Use: Enteral nutritional supplement.

SIMILAC 24/SIMILAC 24 WITH IRON. (Ross) Milk-based infant formula ready-to-feed (24 cal/fl oz), iron 1.8 mg/100 calories. Bot. 4 fl oz.
Use: Enteral nutritional supplement.

SIMILAC 27. (Ross) Milk-based ready-to-feed infant formula (27 cal/fl oz). Bot. 4 fl oz.
Use: Enteral nutritional supplement.

SIMILAC NATURAL CARE HUMAN MILK FORTIFIER. (Ross) Liquid fortifier designed to be mixed with human milk or fed alternately with human milk to low-birth-weight infants. Supplied as 24 cal/fl oz. Bot. 4 fl oz.
Use: Enteral nutritional supplement.

SIMILAC PM 60/40. (Ross) Milk-based formula ready-to-feed or powder with 60:40 whey to casein ratio (20 cal/fl oz). **Bot.:** Hospital use. 4 fl oz. ready-to-feed. **Pow.:** Can lb.
Use: Enteral nutritional supplement.

SIMILAC 20/SIMILAC WITH IRON 20. (Ross) Milk-based infant formula. Standard dilution (20 cal/fl oz). Similac with iron: Iron 1.8 mg/100 cal. **Pow.:** Can lb. **Concentrated Liq.:** Can 13 fl oz. **Ready-to-feed:** Can 8 fl oz, 32 fl oz. Bot. 4 fl oz, 8 fl oz.
Use: Enteral nutritional supplement.

SIMILAC SPECIAL CARE 20. (Ross) Infant formula ready-to-feed (20 cal/fl oz). Bot. 4 fl oz.
Use: Enteral nutritional supplement.

SIMILAC SPECIAL CARE 24. (Ross) Infant formula ready-to-feed (24 cal/fl oz). Bot. 4 fl oz.
Use: Enteral nutritional supplement.

SIMRON. (Merrell Dow) Iron (supplied as ferrous gluconate) 10 mg/Cap. Bot. 100s.
Use: Iron supplement.

SIMRON PLUS. (Merrell Dow) Iron 10 mg (supplied as ferrous gluconate), vitamins B_{12} 3.33 mcg, ascorbic acid 50 mg, B_6 1 mg, folic acid 0.1 mg/Cap. Bot. 100s.
Use: Vitamin/iron supplement.

•**SIMTRAZENE.** USAN. 1,4-Dimethyl-1,4-diphenyl-2-tetrazene.
Use: Antineoplastic agent.

SINAC. (Marin) Phenacetin 150 mg, acetaminophen 150 mg, phenylpropanolamine HCl 25 mg, phenyltoloxamine citrate 22 mg/Tab. Bot. 30s, 100s.
Use: Analgesic, decongestant, antihistamine.

SINAPILS. (Pfeiffer) Phenylpropanolamine HCl 12.5 mg, chlorpheniramine maleate 1 mg, acetaminophen 324 mg, caffeine 32.5 mg/Tab. Bot. 36s.
Use: Decongestant, antihistamine, analgesic.

SINAREST. (Pharmacraft) Acetaminophen 325 mg, chlorpheniramine maleate 2 mg, phenylpropanolamine HCl 18.7 mg/Tab. Bot. 20s, 40s, 80s.
Use: Analgesic, antihistamine, decongestant.

SINAREST 12 HOUR. (Pharmacraft) Oxymetazoline HCl 0.05%. Spray Bot. 15 ml.
Use: Nasal decongestant.

SINAREST DECONGESTANT NASAL SPRAY. (Pharmacraft) Oxymetazoline HCl 0.05%. Bot. 0.5 oz.
Use: Nasal decongestant.

SINAREST, EXTRA-STRENGTH. (Pharmacraft) Acetaminophen 500 mg, chlorpheniramine ma-

leate 2 mg, phenylpropanolamine HCl 18.7 mg/Tab. 24s.
Use: Analgesic, antihistamine, decongestant.

SINAREST, NO DROWSINESS. (Pharmacraft) Pseudoephedrine HCl 30 mg, acetaminophen 500 mg/Tab. Pkg. 20s.
Use: Decongestant, analgesic.

•**SINCALIDE.** USAN.
Use: Choleretic.

SINE-AID SINUS HEADACHE CAPLETS, EXTRA STRENGTH. (McNeil Prods) Acetaminophen 500 mg, pseudoephedrine HCl 30 mg/Capl. Bot. 24s, 50s.
Use: Analgesic, decongestant.

SINE-AID SINUS HEADACHE TABLETS. (McNeil Prods) Acetaminophen 325 mg, pseudoephedrine HCl 30 mg/Tab. Bot. 24s, 50s, 100s.
Use: Analgesic, decongestant.

•**SINEFUNGIN.** USAN.
Use: Antifungal.

SINEMET 10/100. (Merck Sharp & Dohme) Carbidopa 10 mg, levodopa 100 mg/Tab. Bot. 100s, UD 100s.
Use: Antiparkinson agent.

SINEMET 25/100. (Merck Sharp & Dohme) Carbidopa 25 mg, levodopa 100 mg/Tab. Bot. 100s, UD 100s.
Use: Antiparkinson agent.

SINEMET 25/250. (Merck Sharp & Dohme) Carbidopa 25 mg, levodopa 250 mg/Tab. Bot. 100s, UD 100s.
Use: Antiparkinson agent.

SINE-OFF MAXIMUM STRENGTH ALLERGY-SINUS FORMULA CAPLETS. (SmithKline Prods) Chlorpheniramine maleate 2 mg, pseudoephedrine HCl 30 mg, acetaminophen 500 mg/Cap. Pkg. 20s.
Use: Antihistamine, decongestant, analgesic.

SINE-OFF MAXIMUM STRENGTH NO DROWSINESS FORMULA CAPLETS. (SmithKline Prods) Pseudoephedrine HCl 30 mg, acetaminophen 500 mg/Cap. Pkg. 20s.
Use: Decongestant, analgesic.

SINE-OFF TABLETS. (SmithKline Prods) Chlorpheniramine maleate 2 mg, phenylpropanolamine HCl 12.5 mg, aspirin 325 mg/Tab. Pkg. 24s, 48s, 100s.
Use: Antihistamine, decongestant, analgesic.

SINEQUAN. (Roerig) Doxepin HCl. **Cap.:** 10 mg Bot. 100s, 1000s, UD 100s; 25 mg or 50 mg Bot. 90s, 100s, 1000s, UD 100s; 75 mg Bot. 100s, 1000s, UD 100s; 100 mg Bot. 100s, 1000s, UD 100s; 150 mg Bot. 50s, 500s, UD 100s. **Oral Concentrate:** 10 mg/ml Bot. 120 ml.
Use: Antidepressant.

SINEX. (Vicks) Phenylephrine HCl 0.5%, cetylpyridinium Cl 0.04%, thimerosal 0.001% preservative. Nasal Spray. Bot. 0.5 oz, 1 oz.
Use: Nasal decongestant.

SINEX LONG ACTING. (Vicks) Oxymetazoline HCl 0.05% in aqueous soln., thimerosal 0.001%. Nasal spray. Bot. 0.5 oz, 1 oz.
Use: Nasal decongestant.

SINGLET. (Lakeside) Pseudoephedrine HCl 60 mg, chlorpheniramine maleate 4 mg, acetaminophen 650 mg/Tab. Bot. 100s.
Use: Decongestant, antihistamine, analgesic.

SINOCON TR. (Vangard) Phenylpropanolamine HCl 20 mg, phenylephrine HCl 5 mg, phenyltoloxamine citrate 7.5 mg, chlorpheniramine maleate 2.5 mg/Tab. Bot. 100s, 1000s.
Use: Decongestant, antihistamine.

SINO-EZE MLT. (Richlyn) Salicylamide 3.5 gr, acetaminophen 100 mg, phenylephrine HCl 5 mg, chlorpheniramine maleate 2 mg/Tab. Bot. 1000s.
Use: Analgesic, decongestant, antihistamine.

SINOGRAFIN. (Squibb) Meglumine diatrizoate 52.7%, meglumine iodipamide 26.8%. Vial 10 ml.
Use: Diagnostic aid.

SINO-TUSSIN MLT. (Richlyn) Dextromethorphan HBr 10 mg, salicylamide 3.5 gr, acetaminophen 100 mg, phenylephrine HCl 5 mg, chlorpheniramine maleate 2 mg/Tab. Bot. 1000s.
Use: Antitussive, analgesic, decongestant, antihistamine.

SINOVAN TIMED. (Drug Industries) Chlorpheniramine maleate 8 mg, phenylephrine HCl 20 mg, methscopolamine nitrate 2.5 mg/Cap. Bot. 100s, 1000s.
Use: Antihistamine, decongestant, anticholinergic.

SINUBID. (Parke-Davis) Acetaminophen 600 mg, phenylpropanolamine HCl 100 mg, phenyltoloxamine 66 mg/Tab. Bot. 100s.
Use: Analgesic, decongestant, antihistamine.

SINUCOL. (Tennessee Pharm.) Chlorpheniramine maleate 8 mg, phenylephrine HCl 20 mg, methscopolamine nitrate 2.5 mg/Cap. Bot. 100s, 500s. Inj. Vial 10 ml.
Use: Antihistamine, decongestant, anticholinergic.

SINUESE. (Jenkins) Potassium guaiacolsulfonate 40 mg, sodium iodide 50 mg, menthol, camphor, guaiacol, eucalyptol/ml. Vial 30 ml, 12s.
Use: Expectorant combination.

SINUFED TIMECELLE. (Hauck) Pseudoephedrine HCl 60 mg, guaifenesin 300 mg/Cap. Bot. 100s.
Use: Decongestant, expectorant.

SINULIN TABLETS. (Carnrick) Phenylpropanolamine HCl 25 mg, chlorpheniramine maleate 4 mg, acetaminophen 650 mg/Tab. Bot. 20s, 100s. Blister 24s.
Use: Decongestant, antihistamine, analgesic.

SINUPAN. (Ion) Phenylephrine HCl 40 mg, guaifenesin 200 mg/SR Cap. Bot. 100s.
Use: Decongestant, expectorant.

SINUSEZE. (Amlab) Acetaminophen 325 mg, phenylpropanolamine HCl 25 mg, phenyltoloxamine citrate 22 mg/Tab. Bot. 36s.
Use: Analgesic, decongestant, antihistamine.

SINUS TABLETS. (Kenyon) Phenacetin 150 mg, acetaminophen 150 mg, phenyltoloxamine dihydrogen citrate 22 mg/Tab. Bot. 100s, 1000s.
Use: Analgesic, antihistamine.

SINUS TABLETS. (Walgreen) Acetaminophen 325 mg, chlorpheniramine maleate 2 mg, pseudoephedrine HCl mg/Tab. Bot. 30s.
Use: Analgesic, antihistamine, decongestant.

SINUTAB MAXIMUM STRENGTH. (Parke-Davis Prods) Acetaminophen 500 mg, pseudoephedrine HCl 30 mg, chlorpheniramine maleate 2 mg/Tab. or Cap. Blister pack 24s.
Use: Analgesic, decongestant, antihistamine.

SINUTAB MAXIMUM STRENGTH NIGHTTIME SINUS FORMULA. (Parke-Davis Prods) Acetaminophen 1000 mg, diphenhydramine HCl 50 mg, pseudoephedrine 60 mg/oz. Bot. 4 oz.
Use: Analgesic, antihistamine, decongestant.

SINUTAB II MAXIMUM STRENGTH NO DROWSINESS FORMULA. (Parke-Davis Prods) Acetaminophen 500 mg, pseudoephedrine HCl 30 mg/Tab. or Cap. Pack 24s.
Use: Analgesic, decongestant.

SINUTROL. (Weeks & Leo) Phenylpropanolamine HCl 25 mg, phenyltoloxamine citrate 22 mg, acetaminophen 325 mg/Tab. Bot. 40s, 90s.
Use: Decongestant, antihistamine, analgesic.

SIROIL. (Siroil) Mercuric oleate, cresol, vegetable and mineral oil. Emulsion. Bot. 8 oz.
Use: Antiseptic.

SIR-O-LENE. (Siroil) Tube 4 oz.
Use: Emollient.

SISOMICIN. USAN.
Use: Antibacterial.

SISOMICIN SULFATE, U.S.P. XXII. Inj., U.S.P. XXII.
Use: Antibacterial.

SITABS. (Canright) Lobeline sulfate 1.5 mg, benzocaine 2 mg, aluminum hydroxide—magnesium carbonate co-dried gel 150 mg/Loz. Bot. 100s.
Use: Smoking deterrent.

SITOGLUSIDE. USAN.
Use: Antiprostatic hypertrophy.

SIXAMEEN. (Spanner) Vitamins B_1 100 mg, B_6 100 mg/ml. Vial 10 ml.
Use: Vitamin B supplement.

SKEETER STIK. (Outdoor Recreation) Lidocaine 4%, phenol 2%, isopropyl alcohol 45.5% in a propylene glycol base. Stick 1s.
Use: Local anesthetic.

SKELAXIN. (Carnrick) Metaxalone 400 mg/Tab. Bot. 100s.
Use: Skeletal muscle relaxant.

SKELETAL MUSCLE RELAXANTS.
See: Anectine, Soln., Pow. (Burroughs Wellcome).
Flexeril, Tab. (Merck Sharp & Dohme).
Mephenesin (Various Mfr.).
Metubine Iodide, Vial (Lilly).
Neostig, Tab. (Freeport).
Paraflex, Tab. (McNeil).
Parafon Forte, Tab. (McNeil).
Quelicin, Fliptop and pintop Vials, Syringe w/ lancet, Amp. (Abbott).
Rela, Tab. (Schering).
Robaxin, Tab., Inj. (Robins).
Skelaxin, Tab. (Carnrick).
Soma, Preps. (Wallace).
Sucostrin, Vial, Amp. (Squibb).
Syncurine, Vial (Burroughs Wellcome).
Trancopal, Cap. (Winthrop).
d-Tubocurarine Chloride (Various Mfr.).

SKIN DEGREASER. (Health & Medical Techniques) Freon 100%. Bot. 2 oz, 4 oz.
Use: Presurgical skin degreaser.

SKIN SHIELD LIQUID BANDAGE. (Commerce) Dyclonine HCl, benzethonium Cl. Bot. 0.45 oz.
Use: Local anesthetic.

SLEEP II. (Walgreen) Diphenhydramine HCl 25 mg/Tab. Bot. 16s, 32s, 72s.
Use: Sleep aid.

SLEEP CAP. (Weeks & Leo) Diphenhydramine HCl 50 mg/Cap. Bot. 25s, 50s.
Use: Sleep aid.

SLEEP-EZE TABLETS. (Whitehall) Diphenhydramine HCl 25 mg/Tab. Pkg. 12s, 26s, 52s.
Use: Sleep aid.

SLEEP-EZE 3. (Whitehall) Diphenhydramine HCl 25 mg/Tab. Pkg. 12s, 26s, 52s.
Use: Sleep aid.

SLEEP TABS. (Towne) Scopolamine aminoxide HBr 0.2 mg, salicylamide 250 mg/Tab. Bot. 36s, 90s.
Use: Sleep aid.

SLENDER. (Carnation) Skim milk, vegetable oils, caseinates, vitamins, minerals. **Liq.:** 220 cal/10 oz can. **Pow.:** 173 or 200 cal mixed w/6 oz. skim or lowfat milk. Pkg oz.
Use: Diet aid.

SLENDER-X. (Progressive Drugs) Phenylpropanolamine, methylcellulose, caffeine, vitamins/ Tab. Pkg. 21s, 42s, 84s. Gum 20s, 60s.
Use: Diet aid.

SLIMETTES. (Blue Cross) Phenylpropanolamine HCl 35 mg, caffeine 140 mg/Cap. Box 20s.
Use: Diet aid.

SLIM-FAST. (Thompson Medical) Meal replacement powder mixed with milk to replace 1, 2 or 3 meals a day.
Use: Diet aid.

SLIM-LINE. (Thompson Medical) Benzocaine, dextrose/Chewing gum. Box 24s.
Use: Diet aid.

SLIM PLAN PLUS WITHOUT CAFFEINE. (Whiteworth) Phenylpropanolamine HCl 75 mg/ Tab. Box 40s.
Use: Diet aid.

SLIM-TABS. (Wesley) Phendimetrazine tartrate 35 mg/Tab. Bot. 1000s.

Use: Anorexiant.

SLOAN'S LINIMENT. (Warner-Lambert Prods) Capsicum oleoresin 0.62%, methyl salicylate 2.66%, camphor oil 3.35%, turpentine oil 46.76%, pine oil 6.74%. Bot. 2 oz, 7 oz.
Use: External analgesic.

SLO-BID GYROCAPS. (Rorer) Theophylline anhydrous 50 mg, 100 mg, 200 mg or 300 mg/TR Cap. Bot. 100s, 1000s, UD.
Use: Bronchodilator.

SLO-PHYLLIN 80 SYRUP. (Rorer) Theophylline anhydrous 80 mg/15 ml. Nonalcoholic. Bot. 4 oz, pt, gal, UD 15 ml.
Use: Bronchodilator.

SLO-PHYLLIN GG. (Rorer) Theophylline anhydrous 150 mg, guaifenesin 90 mg/Cap. or 15 ml Syr. **Cap.:** Bot. 100s. **Syr.:** Bot. pt.
Use: Bronchodilator, expectorant.

SLO-PHYLLIN GYROCAPS. (Rorer) Theophylline anhydrous 60 mg, 125 mg or 250 mg/TR Cap. Bot. 100s, 1000s, UD 100s.
Use: Bronchodilator.

SLO-PHYLLIN TABLETS. (Rorer) Theophylline anhydrous 100 mg or 200 mg/Tab. Bot. 100s, 1000s, UD.
Use: Bronchodilator.

SLO-SALT. (Mission) Sodium Cl 600 mg/SR Tab. Bot. 100s.
Use: Salt replacement.

SLO-SALT-K. (Mission) Potassium Cl 150 mg, sodium Cl 410 mg/Tab. Bot. 1000s, Strip 100s.
Use: Potassium/sodium supplement.

SLOW-K. (Ciba) Potassium Cl Bot. 100s, 1000s, Accu-Pak units 100s, Consumer Pack 100s.
Use: Potassium supplement.

•**SLOW FE.** (Ciba) Dried ferrous sulfate 160 mg/Tab. Bot. 30s, 100s.
Use: Iron supplement.

SLOW-MAG. (Searle) Magnesium 64 mg/Delayed-release Tab. 60s.
Use: Magnesium supplement.

SLT. (Western Research) Sodium levothyroxine 0.1 mg, 0.2 mg or 0.3 mg/Tab. Bot. 1000s.
Use: Hypothyroidism treatment.

•**SLT LOTION.** (C & M Pharmacal) Salicylic acid 3%, lactic acid 5%, coal tar soln. 2%. Bot. 4.3 oz.
Use: Antiseborrheic.

SLYN-LL. (Edwards) Phendimetrazine tartrate 105 mg/TR Cap. Bot. 100s.
Use: Anorexiant.

S-M-A FORMULA. (Wyeth-Ayerst) A series of liquid feeding formulas:
Iron Fortified, Infant Formula-Powder.
Iron Fortified, Infant Formula-Ready to Feed.
Iron Fortified, Infant Formula-Liquid.
Lo-Iron, Infant Formula-Liquid.
Lo-Iron, Infant Formula-Powder.
Lo-Iron, Infant Formula-Ready to Feed.
Use: Enteral nutritional supplement.

SMALL FRY CHEWABLE TABS. (Approved) Vitamins A 5000 IU, D 1000 IU, B_{12} 5 mcg, B_1 3 mg, B_2 2.5 mg, B_6 1 mg, C 50 mg, niacinamide 20 mg, calcium pantothenate 1 mg, E 1 IU, l-lysine 15 mg, biotin 10 mg/Tab. Bot. 100s, 250s, 365s.
Use: Vitamin/mineral supplement.

•**SMALLPOX VACCINE,** U.S.P. XXII. (Lederle)—Tube 1s, 5s, 10s, vaccinations. 1 vaccination and needle in glass capillary tube. (Wyeth-Ayerst)—Tube 1s, 5s, 10s, vaccinations.
Use: Active immunizing agent.

SN-13, 272.
See: Primaquine Phosphate, U.S.P. XXII. (Various Mfr.).

SNAKE VENOM.
Use: S.C., I.M., orally; trypanosomiasis.
See: Antivenin (Wyeth-Ayerst).

SNOOTIE BY SEA & SKI. (Carter Products) Padimate O. SPF 10. Lot. Bot. 30 ml.
Use: Sunscreen.

SOACLENS. (Alcon Lenscare) Thimerosal 0.004%, EDTA 0.1%. Bot. 4 oz.
Use: Contact lens care.

SOAKARE. (Allergan) Benzalkonium Cl 0.01%, edetate disodium, sodium hydroxide, purified water. Bot. 4 fl oz.
Use: Hard contact lens care.

SOAPS, GERMICIDAL.
See: Dial, Preps. (Armour).
Fostex, Cake, Cream, Liq. (Westwood).
pHisoHex, Liq. (Winthrop).
Thylox, Shampoo, Soap (Dent).

SOAP SUBSTITUTES.
See: Acne-Dome, Cleanser (Miles Pharm).
Domerine, Shampoo (Miles Pharm).
Lowila, Cleanser (Westwood).
pHisoDerm, Preps. (Winthrop).

•**SODA LIME,** N.F. XVII.
Use: Carbon dioxide absorbant.

SODA MINT. (Bowman) Sodium bicarbonate 5 gr, peppermint oil q.s./Tab. Bot. 100s, 1000s.
Use: Antacid.

SODA MINT. (Lilly) Sodium bicarbonate 5 gr, peppermint oil q.s./Tab. Bot. 100s.
Use: Antacid.

SODASONE. (Fellows) Prednisolone sodium phosphate 20 mg, niacinamide 25 mg/ml. Vial 10 ml.
Use: Corticosteroid.

•**SODIUM ACETATE,** U.S.P. XXII. Inj., Soln., U.S.P. XXII. Acetic acid, sodium salt, trihydrate. (Abbott) 40 mEq, 20 ml in 50 ml Fliptop Vial.
Use: Alkalinizer; pharmaceutic aid.

SODIUM ACETATE & THEOPHYLLINE.

•**SODIUM ACETAZOLAMIDE.** Acetazolamide sodium, U.S.P. XXII.
Use: Carbonic anhydrase inhibitor.

SODIUM ACETOSULFONE. Sodium 2-N-acetylsulfamyl-4,4′-diaminodiphenylsulfone.
Use: Leprostatic agent.
See: Promacetin, Tab. (Parke-Davis).

SODIUM ACETRIZOATE INJECTION. B.A.N. Sodium 3-acetamino-2,4,6-triiodobenzoate, Diaginol.
Use: Radiopaque substance.

SODIUM ACID PHOSPHATE.
See: Sodium Biphosphate (Various Mfr.).

SODIUM ACTINOQUINOL. 8-Ethoxy-5-quinoline sulfonic acid sodium salt.
Use: Treatment of flash burns (ophthalmic).
See: Uviban.

SODIUM ALGINATE, N.F. XVII.
Use: Suspending agent.
See: Algin.
Kelgin (Kelco).

SODIUM AMINOBENZOATE. Sodium p-aminobenzoate.
Use: Dermatomyositis and scleroderma.

SODIUM AMINOPTERIN. Aminopterin Sodium.

SODIUM AMINOSALICYLATE.
See: Aminosalicylate Sodium, U.S.P. XXII.

SODIUM AMOBARBITAL. Amobarbital Sodium, U.S.P. XXII.

•**SODIUM AMYLOSULFATE.** USAN. Sodium salt of potato amylopectin. Depepsin.
Use: Peptic ulcer.

SODIUM ANAZOLENE. 4-[(4-Anilino-5-sulfo-1-naphthyl)azo]-5-hydroxy-2,7-naphthalene disulfonic acid trisodium salt.
Use: Diagnostic aid.

SODIUM ANOXYNAPHTHONATE. B.A.N. Sodium 4′-anilino-8-hydroxy-1,1′-azonaphthalene-3,-5′,6-tri-sulfonate.
Use: Investigation of cardiac disease.
See: Anazolene Sodium (I.N.N.).

SODIUM ANTIMONYLGLUCONATE. B.A.N. Sodium salt of a trivalent antimony derivative of gluconic acid.
Use: Treatment of schistosomiasis.

SODIUM APOLATE. B.A.N. Sodium ethenesulfonate polymer.
Use: Anticoagulant.

•**SODIUM ARSENATE AS 74.** USAN.
Use: Radioactive agent.

•**SODIUM ASCORBATE,** U.S.P. XXII. Monosodium L-ascorbate.
Use: Pharmaceutic necessity for ascorbic acid injection.
See: Cenolate, Inj. (Abbott).
Liqui-Cee, Bot. (Arnar-Stone).
Sodascorbate, Tab. (Mosso).
Vitac Injection, Vial (Hickman).

SODIUM AUROTHIOMALATE.
See: Gold Sodium Thiosulfate, U.S.P. XXII.

•**SODIUM BENZOATE,** N.F. XVII.
Use: Pharmaceutic aid (antifungal agent, preservative).

SODIUM BENZOATE AND SODIUM PHENYLACETATE.
Use: For urea cycle enzymopathies.
See: Ucephan (Kendall-McGaw).

SODIUM BENZYLPENICILLIN. Penicillin G Sodium, U.S.P. XXII. Sodium Penicillin G.
Use: Antibiotic.

•**SODIUM BICARBONATE,** U.S.P. XXII. Inj., Oral Pow., Tab., U.S.P. XXII. (Abbott) Inj. **4.2%:** (5 mEq) Infant 10 ml Syringe (21 G × 1.5 in. needle). **7.5%:** (44.6 mEq) 50 ml Syringe (18 G × 1.5 in. needle) or 50 ml Amp. **8.4%:** (10 mEq) Pediatric 10 ml Syringe (21 G × 1.5 in. needle) or (50 mEq) 50 ml Syringe (18 G × 1.5 in. needle) or 50 ml Vial.
Use: Antacid, electrolyte replenisher, systemical alkalizer.
W/Bismuth subcarbonate and Magnesia.
See: Anachloric A, Tab. (Upjohn).
W/Sodium Bitartrate.
See: Ceo-Two, Supp. (Beutlich).
Col-Evac, Supp. (Fellows).
W/Sodium carboxymethylcellulose, alginic acid.
See: Pretts, Tab. (Marion).

SODIUM BIPHOSPHATE.
Use: Cathartic.
See: Sodium Phosphate Monobasic, U.S.P. XXII.

SODIUM BISMUTH TARTRATE.
See: Bismuth Sodium Tartrate, Preps.

SODIUM BISULFITE. Sulfurous acid, monosodium salt. Monosodium sulfite.
Use: Antioxidant.

•**SODIUM BORATE,** N.F. XVII.
Use: Pharmaceutic aid (alkalinizing agent).

SODIUM BUTABARBITAL.
See: Butabarbital Sodium, U.S.P. XXII.

SODIUM CALCIUM EDETATE. B.A.N. Calcium chelate of thedisodium salt of ethylenediamine-NNN′-N′-tetra-acetic acid.
Use: Treatment of lead poisoning.
See: Calcium Disodium Versenate.

SODIUM CALCIUM EDETATE.
See: Calcium Disodium Versenate, Amp., Tab. (Riker).

•**SODIUM CARBONATE,** N.F. XVII.
Use: Pharmaceutic aid (alkalinizing agent).

SODIUM CARBOXYMETHYLCELLULOSE. Carboxymethylcellulose Sodium, U.S.P. XXII. CMC. Cellulose Gum.

SODIUM CELLULOSE GLYCOLATE.
See: Carboxymethylcellulose, Sodium (Various Mfr.).

SODIUM CEPHALOTHIN. Cephalothin Sodium, U.S.P. XXII.
Use: Antibiotic.

•**SODIUM CHLORIDE,** U.S.P. XXII. Inhalation Soln., Inj., Bacteriostatic for Inj., Irrigation, Ophth. Oint., Ophth. Soln., Tab., Tab. for Soln., U.S.P. XXII.
Use: Fluid and irrigation, electrolyte replenisher, isotonic vehicle.

•**SODIUM CHLORIDE AND DEXTROSE TABLETS,** U.S.P. XXII.
Use: Electrolyte and nutrient replenisher.

•**SODIUM CHLORIDE INJECTION,** U.S.P. XXII. (Abbott) Normal saline 0.9% in 150 ml, 250 ml, 500 ml, 1000 ml cont.; **Partial-fill:** 50 ml in 200

ml, 50 ml in 300 ml, 100 ml in 300 ml; **Fliptop vial:** 10 ml, 20 ml, 50 ml, 100 ml; **Bacteriostatic vial:** 10 ml, 20 ml, 30 ml; 50 mEq, 20 ml in 50 ml fliptop or pintop vial; 100 mEq, 40 ml in 50 ml fliptop vial; 50 mEq, 20 ml univ. add. syr.; sodium Cl 0.45%, 500 ml, 1000 ml; sodium Cl 5%, 500 ml; sodium Cl irrigating soln., 250 ml, 500 ml, 1000 ml, 3000 ml; (Upjohn) Sodium Cl 9 mg/ml w/benzyl alcohol 9.45 mg. Vial 20 ml (Winthrop) **Carpuject:** 2 ml fill cartridge, 22 gauge 1 1/4 inch needle or 25 gauge 5/8 inch needle.
Use: Fluid and irrigation, electrolyte replenisher, isotonic vehicle.

•**SODIUM CHLORIDE Na 22.** USAN.
Use: Radioactive agent.

SODIUM CHLORIDE SUBSTITUTES.
See: Salt substitutes.

SODIUM CHLORIDE TABLETS, U.S.P. XXII. Sodium Cl 15 1/2 gr/Tab. Bot. 1000s.
Use: Preparation of normal saline solution.

SODIUM CHLORIDE THERAPY.
See: Thermolene, Tab. (Lannett).
Thermotabs., Tab. (Calgon).

SODIUM CHLOROTHIAZIDE FOR INJECTION. Chlorothiazide Sodium for Injection, U.S.P. XXII.
Use: Diuretic.

SODIUM CHOLATE. (City Chem.) Sodium cholate Bot. 100 Gm.

•**SODIUM CHROMATE Cr 51 INJ.,** U.S.P. XXII.
Use: Diagnostic aid (blood volume determination).
See: Radio Chromate Cr 51 Sodium.

•**SODIUM CITRATE,** U.S.P. XXII. 1,2,3-Propanetricarboxylic acid, 2-hy-droxy-, trisodium salt. Trisodium citrate. Trisodium citrate dihydrate.
Use: Anticoagulant.
See: Anticoagulant Citrate Dextrose Solution, U.S.P. XXII.
Anticoagulant Citrate Phosphate Dextrose Solution, U.S.P. XXII.

•**SODIUM CITRATE AND CITRIC ACID ORAL SOLUTION,** U.S.P. XXII. Shohl's Solution.
Use: Systemic alkalinizer.

SODIUM CLOXACILLIN.
See: Cloxacillin Sodium, U.S.P. XXII.

SODIUM COLISTIMETHATE. Colistimethane Sodium, Sterile, U.S.P. XXII. Antibiotic produced by *Aerobacillus colistinus*.

SODIUM COLISTIN METHANESULFONATE. Colistimethane Sodium, U.S.P. XXII. The sodium methanesulfonate salt of an antibiotic substance elaborated by *Aerobacillus colistinus.*
Use: Antibiotic.

•**SODIUM DEHYDROACETATE,** N.F. XVII.
Use: Pharmaceutic aid (antimicrobial preservative).

SODIUM DEXTROTHYROXINE. Sodium D-3,3′,5,5′-tetraiodothyronine. Sodium D-3-(4-(4-Hydroxy-3,5-diiodophenoxy)-3,5-diiodophenyl)-alanine.
Use: Anticholesteremic.

SODIUM DIATRIZOATE. Diatrizoate Sodium, U.S.P. XXII.
Use: Radiopaque medium.

SODIUM DIBUNATE. B.A.N. Sodium 2,7-di-t-butylnaphthalene-1-sulfonate.
Use: Cough suppressant.

SODIUM DICLOXACILLIN. Dicloxacillin Sodium, U.S.P. XXII.
Use: Antibiotic.

SODIUM DICLOXACILLIN MONOHYDRATE.
Use: Antibiotic.
See: Pathocil, Preps. (Wyeth-Ayerst).

SODIUM DIHYDROGEN PHOSPHATE. Sodium Biphosphate, U.S.P. XXII.

SODIUM DIMETHOXYPHENYL PENICILLIN.
See: Methicillin Sodium (Various Mfr.).

SODIUM DIOCTYL SULFOSUCCINATE.
See: Docusate Sodium, U.S.P. XXII.

SODIUM DIPHENYLHYDANTOIN. Phenytoin Sodium, U.S.P. XXII. Diphenylhydantoin Sodium.
Use: Anticonvulsant.

SODIUM DIPROTRIZOATE, B.A.N. Sodium 3,5-dipropionamide-2,4,6-triiodobenzoate.

SODIUM EDETATE, Edetate Disodium, U.S.P. XXII. Tetrasodium ethylenediaminetetraacetate.
Use: Chelating agent.
See: Vagisec products (Julius Schmid).

SODIUM ETHACRYNATE For Inj. Ethacrynate Sodium for Injection, U.S.P. XXII.
Use: Diuretic.

•**SODIUM ETHASULFATE.** USAN.
Use: Detergent.

SODIUM ETHYL-MERCURI-THIO-SALICYLATE.
See: Thimerosal, (Various Mfr.).
Merthiolate, Preps. (Lilly).

SODIUM FEREDETATE (I.N.N.). Sodium iron edetate. B.A.N.

SODIUM FLUORESCEIN, Fluorescein Sodium U.S.P. XXII. Resorcinolphthalein sodium.
Use: Diagnostic aid (corneal trauma indicator).

•**SODIUM FLUORIDE,** U.S.P. XXII. Oral Soln., Tab, U.S.P. XXII.
Use: Dental caries prophylactic.
See: Dentafluor, Tab., Drops (Saron).
Flura Drops, Drops (Kirkman).
Flura-Loz, Loz. (Kirkman).
Karidium, Liq., Tab. (Lorvic).
Kari-Rinse, Liq. (Lorvic).
Luride, Tab. (Hoyt).
NaFeen, Tab., Liq. (Pacemaker).
Pediaflor, Drops (Ross).
Solu-Flur, Tab. (Robinson).
T-Fluoride, Tab. (Tennessee Pharm.).
W/Vitamins.
See: Fluorac, Tab. (Rorer).
Mulvidren-F, Tab. (Stuart).
So-Flo, Tab., Drop (Professional Pharm.).
W/Vitamins A, D, C.
See: Cari-Tab, Softab. (Stuart).
Tri-Vi-Flor, Drops, Tab. (Mead Johnson).

•**SODIUM FLUORIDE AND PHOSPHORIC ACID GEL,** U.S.P. XXII.

Use: Dental caries prophylactic.
•**SODIUM FLUORIDE AND PHOSPHORIC ACID TOPICAL SOLUTION,** U.S.P. XXII.
Use: Dental caries prophylactic.
SODIUM FOLATE. Monosodium folate.
Use: Water-soluble, hematopoietic vitamin.
SODIUM FORMALDEHYDE SULFOXYLATE, N.F. XVII. (Various Mfr.) $H_2C(OH)SO_2Na$.
Use: Reducing agent, preservative.
SODIUM-FREE SALT.
See: Co-Salt, Bot. (Rorer).
Diasal, Prep. (Savage).
SODIUM GAMMA-HYDROXYBUTYRIC ACID. Under study.
Use: Anesthetic adjuvant.
SODIUM GENTISATE.
See: Gentisate, Sodium.
SODIUM GLUCALDRATE. B.A.N. Sodium gluconatodihydroxyaluminate.
Use: Treatment of gastric hyperacidity.
SODIUM GLUCASPALDRATE, B.A.N. Octasodium tetrakis (gluconato)-bis (salicylato), μ-diacetatodialuminate(III) dihydrate.
Use: Analgesic.
•**SODIUM GLUCONATE,** U.S.P. XXII.
SODIUM GLUCOSULFONE INJ. Disodium 1,1′-[Sulfonylbis(p-phenyleneimino)]bis-[D-gluco-2,3,4,5,6-pentahydroxy-1-hexanesulfonate].
Use: Leprostatic.
SODIUM GLUTAMATE.
See: Glutamate.
SODIUM GLYCEROPHOSPHATE. Glycerol phosphate sodium salt.
Use: Pharmaceutic necessity.
SODIUM GLYCOCHOLATE, A BILE SALT.
See: Bile Salts.
W/Phenolphthalein, cascara sagrada extract, sodium taurocholate, aloin.
See: Oxiphen, Tab. (Webcon).
W/Sodium nitrite, blue flag.
See: So-Nitri-Nacea, Cap. (Scrip).
W/Sodium, taurocholate, sodium salicylate, phenolphthalein, bile extract, cascara sagrada extract.
See: Glycols, Tab. (Bowman).
SODIUM HEPARIN. Heparin Sodium, U.S.P. XXII.
Use: Anticoagulant.
SODIUM HEXACYCLONATE. Sodium 1-hydroxy-methylcyclohexaneacetate.
SODIUM HEXOBARBITAL. Sodium 5-(1-cyclohexen-1-yl)-1,5-dimethylbarbiturate.
Use: Intravenous general anesthetic.
SODIUM HYDROGEN CITRATE. (Various Mfr.).
•**SODIUM HYDROXIDE,** N.F. XVII. Caustic Soda.
Use: Pharmaceutic aid (alkalizing agent).
SODIUM HYDROXYDIONE SUCCINATE. Sodium 21-hydroxypregnane-3,20-dione succinate.
•**SODIUM HYPOCHLORITE SOLUTION,** U.S.P. XXII.
Use: Local anti-infective, disinfectant.
See: Antiformin.
Dakin's Soln.
Hyclorite.
SODIUM HYPOPHOSPHITE. Sodium phosphinate.
Use: Pharmaceutic necessity.
SODIUM HYPOSULFITE.
See: Sodium Thiosulfate (Various Mfr.).
W/Potassium guaiacolsufonate.
See: Guaiadol Aqueous, Vial (Medical Chem.).
W/Potassium guaiacolsulfonate, chlorpheniramine maleate, sodium bisulfite.
See: Gomahist, Inj. (Burgin-Arden).
W/Sulfur, sodium citrate, phenol, benzyl alcohol.
See: Sulfo-Iodide, Inj. (Marcen).
SODIUM IODIPAMIDE. Disodium 3,3′-(Adipoyldiimino) bis-[2,4,6-triiodobenzoate].
Use: Radiopaque medium.
SODIUM ortho-IODOHIPPURATE. Iodohippurate Sodium, I-131 Injection, U.S.P. XXII.
See: Hipputope (Squibb).
SODIUM IODOMETHAMATE. Disodium 1,4-dihydro-3,5-diiodo-1-methyl-4-oxo-2,6-pyridine dicarboxylate. (Iodoxyl, Pyelecton, Uropac).
SODIUM IODOMETHANE SULFONATE. Methiodal Sodium, U.S.P. XXII.
SODIUM IOTHALAMATE. Iothalmate Sodium Inj. U.S.P. XXII.
Use: Radiopaque medium.
SODIUM IOTHIOURACIL. Sodium 5-iodo-2-thiouracil.
SODIUM IPODATE. Ipodate Sodium, U.S.P. XXII.
Use: Radiopaque.
See: Biloptin.
Oragrafin Sodium, Cap. (Squibb).
SODIUM IRONEDETATE. B.A.N. Iron chelate of the monosodium salt of ethylenediamine-NNN′N′-tetra-acetic acid.
Use: Treatment of iron-deficiency anemia.
See: Sodium Feredetate (I.N.N.).
SODIUM ISOAMYLETHYLBARBITURATE.
See: Amytal Sodium, Preps. (Lilly).
•**SODIUM LACTATE INJECTION,** U.S.P. XXII. Propanoic acid, 2-hydroxy-, monosodium salt. Monosodium lactate. (Abbott) 1/6 Molar, 250 ml, 500 ml or 1000 ml; 50 mEq, 10 ml in 20 ml fliptop vial.
Use: Fluid and electrolyte replenisher.
•**SODIUM LACTATE SOLUTION,** U.S.P. XXII.
Use: Replenisher (electrolyte).
•**SODIUM LAURYL SULFATE,** N.F. XVII. Sulfuric acid monododecyl ester sodium salt. Sodium monododecyl sulfate.
Use: Pharmaceutic aid (Surfactant).
See: Duponol.
W/Aluminum ammonium sulfate, boracic acid, citric acid, menthol.
See: Femid Green Label, Pow. (Cenci).
W/Hydrocortisone.
See: Nutracort, Cream, Lot. (Owen).
W/Iodoquinol, phenylmercuric acetate, lactose, potassium alum., papain.

See: Baculin, Tab. (Amfre-Grant).
SODIUM LEVOTHYROXINE. Levothyroxine Sodium, U.S.P. XXII.
SODIUM LIOTHYRONINE. Liothyronine Sodium, U.S.P. XXII.
Use: Thyroid hormone.
SODIUM LYAPOLATE. Polyethylene sulfonate sodium. Peson (Hoechst). Sodium Apolate, B.A.N.
Use: Anticoagulant.
SODIUM MALONYLUREA.
See: Barbital Sodium (Various Mfr.).
SODIUM MERCAPTOMERIN. Mercaptomerin Sodium, U.S.P. XXII.
Use: Diuretic.
•**SODIUM METABISULFITE,** N.F. XVII.
SODIUM METHIODAL. Methiodal Sodium, U.S.P. XXII. Sodium monoiodomethanesulfonate. Sodium Iodomethanesulfonate, Inj.
Use: Radiopaque medium.
SODIUM METHOHEXITAL FOR INJECTION. Methohexital Sodium for Injection, U.S.P. XXII.
Use: General anesthetic.
See: Brevital Sodium, Pow. (Lilly).
SODIUM METHOXYCELLULOSE. Mixture of methylcellulose and sodium CMC.
SODIUM METRIZOATE, B.A.N. Sodium 3-acetamido-2,4,6-triiodo-5-(N-methyl-acetamido) benzoate.
Use: Contrast medium.
•**SODIUM MONOFLUOROPHOSPHATE,** U.S.P. XXII.
SODIUM MORRHUATE, INJ. Morrhuate Sodium Inj., U.S.P. XXII.
Use: Sclerosing agent.
SODIUM NAFCILLIN. Nafcillin Sodium, U.S.P. XXII.
Use: Antibacterial.
SODIUM NICOTINATE. Sodium pyridine-3-carboxylate (Various Mfr.).
W/Adenosine 5 monophosphoric acid.
Use: I.V., nicotinic acid therapy.
See: Rodesine, Inj. (Rocky Mtn.).
SODIUM NITRATE. (Various Mfr.) Granules, Pkg. lb.
•**SODIUM NITRITE,** U.S.P. XXII. Inj., U.S.P. XXII. (Various Mfr.) Granules, Bot. 0.25 lb, 1 lb.
Use: Antidote to cyanide poisoning, antioxidant.
W/Sodium Thiosulfate, amyl nitrite.
Use: Vasodilator and antidote to cyanide poisoning.
See: Cyanide Antidote Pkg. (Lilly).
SODIUM NITRATE COMBINATIONS.
See: Hyperlon, Tab. (Kenyon).
Veraphen, Tab. (Davis and Sly).
•**SODIUM NITROPRUSSIDE,** U.S.P. XXII. Sterile, U.S.P. XXII.
Use: Hypotensive agent.
See: Keto-Diastix (Ames).
Nipride, Vial (Roche).
Nitropress, Vial (Abbott).
SODIUM NORAMIDOPYRINE METHANESULFONATE. Dipyrone. B.A.N.
SODIUM NOVOBIOCIN. Sodium salt of antibacterial substance produced by *Streptomyces niveus.* Novobiocin monosodium salt.
Use: Antibiotic.
See: Albamycin, Cap., Syr., Vial (Upjohn).
•**SODIUM OXYBATE.** USAN. Sodium 4-hydroxybutyrate.
Use: Adjunct to anesthesia.
SODIUM PANTOTHENATE.
Use: Orally, dietary supplement.
SODIUM PARA-AMINOBENZOATE.
See: p-Aminobenzoate, Sodium (Various Mfr.).
SODIUM PARA-AMINOHIPPURATE INJECTION.
Use: I.V., to determine kidney tubular excretion function.
SODIUM PARA-AMINOSALICYLATE.
See: p-Aminosalicylate, Sodium (Various Mfr.).
SODIUM PENICILLIN G. Penicillin G Sodium, Sterile, U.S.P. XXII. Sodium benzylpenicillin.
SODIUM PENICILLIN O. Sodium-6-[2-(allylthio)-acetamido]-3,3-dimethyl-7-oxo-4-thia-1-azabicyclo-[3.2.0]heptane-2-carboxylate.
SODIUM PENTOBARBITAL. Pentobarbital Sodium, U.S.P. XXII.
Use: Hypnotic.
SODIUM PERBORATE. Sodium Peroxyborate. Sodium peroxyhydrate.
SODIUM PEROXYBORATE.
See: Sodium Perborate. (Various Mfr.).
SODIUM PEROXYHYDRATE.
See: Sodium Perborate (Various Mfr.).
•**SODIUM PERTECHNETATE Tc 99 m INJECTION,** U.S.P. XXII. Pertechnetic acid, sodium salt.
Use: Diagnostic aid (brain scanning; thyroid scanning).
See: Minitec (Squibb).
SODIUM PHENOBARBITAL. Phenobarbital Sodium, U.S.P. XXII.
Use: Anticonvulsant, hypnotic.
SODIUM PHENYLETHYLBARBITURATE. Phenobarbital Sodium, U.S.P. XXII.
•**SODIUM PHOSPHATE,** U.S.P. XXII. Dried, Inj., U.S.P. XXII. Effervescent, U.S.P. XXI. Disodium hydrogen phosphate. (Abbott) 3 mM P and 4 mEq sodium. 15 ml in 30 ml fliptop vial.
Use: Cathartic, buffering agent, source of phosphate.
W/Gentamicin sulfate, monosodium phosphate, sodium Cl, benzalkonium Cl.
See: Garamycin Ophthalmic Soln. (Schering).
W/Sodium biphosphate.
See: Enemeez, Enema (Armour).
Fleet Enema (Fleet).
Phospho-Soda, Liq. (Fleet).
Saf-tip, Enemas (Fuller).
•**SODIUM PHOSPHATE, DIBASIC,** U.S.P. XXII.
Use: Laxative.
•**SODIUM PHOSPHATE, DRIED,** U.S.P. XXII.

Use: Cathartic.

•**SODIUM PHOSPHATE, MONOBASIC,** U.S.P. XXII. Monosodium Phosphate Sodium Acid Phosphate, Sodium Dihydrogen Phosphate, Sodium Biphosphate.
Use: Cathartic.
See: Travad, Enema (Flint).
W/Gentamicin sulfate, disodium phosphate, sodium Cl, benzalkonium Cl.
See: Garamycin Ophthalmic Soln. (Schering).
W/Methenamine.
See: Uro-Phosphate, Tab. (Poythress).
W/Methenamine mandelate, levo-hyoscyamine sulfate.
See: Levo-Uroquid, Tab. (Beach).
W/Methenamine, phenyl salicylate, methylene blue, hyoscyamine, alkaloid.
See: Urostat Forte, Tab. (Elder).
W/Sodium acid pyrophos, sodium bicarbonate.
See: Vacuetts, Supp. (Dorsey).
W/Sodium phosphate.
See: Enemeez Enema (Armour).
Fleet Enema (Fleet).
Phospho-Soda, Liq. (Fleet).
Saf-tip Enemas (Fuller).

•**SODIUM PHOSPHATES ENEMA,** U.S.P. XXII.
Use: Cathartic.

•**SODIUM PHOSPHATES ORAL SOLUTION,** U.S.P. XXII.
Use: Cathartic.

•**SODIUM PHOSPHATE P32 SOLUTION,** U.S.P. XXII. Phosphoric -32P acid, disodium salt. Disodium phosphate -32P.
Use: Antineoplastic, antipolycythemic. Diagnostic. aid (ocular tumor localization.).

SODIUM PHYTATE. Nonasodium phytate: Sodium cyclohexanehexyl (hexaphosphate).
Use: Chelating agent.

SODIUM PICOSULPHATE. B.A.N. Disodium 4,4′-(2-pyridyl)methylenedi(phenyl sulfate).
Use: Laxative.

•**SODIUM POLYPHOSPHATE.** USAN.
Use: Pharmaceutic aid.

•**SODIUM POLYSTYRENE SULFONATE,** U.S.P. XXII, Susp., U.S.P. XXII. Benzene, ethenyl-, homopolymer, sulfonated, sodium salt. Styrene polymer, sulfonated, sodium salt.
Use: Ion exchange resin (potassium).
See: Kayexalate, Pow. (Winthrop).

•**SODIUM PROPIONATE,** N.F. XVII. 5% Soln. Eye drops (Crookes-Barnes) Lacrivial 15 ml.
Use: Preservative.
W/Chlorophyll "a'
See: Prophyllin, Pow., Oint. (Rystan).
W/Neomycin sulfate.
See: Otobiotic, Ear Drops (Schering).
W/Propionic acid, docusate sodium, salicylic acid.
See: Prosal, Liq. (Gordon).

SODIUM PSYLLIATE.
Use: Sclerosing agent.

•**SODIUM PYROPHOSPHATE.** USAN.
Use: Pharmaceutic aid.

SODIUM RADIO CHROMATE INJ. Sodium Chromate Cr 51 Inj., U.S.P. XXII.

SODIUM RADIO IODIDE SOLUTION. Sodium Iodide I-131 Solution, U.S.P. XXII.
Use: Thyroid tumors, hyperthyroidism, cardiac dysfunction.

SODIUM RADIO-PHOSPHATE, P-32 Soln. Radio-Phosphate P32 Solution. Sodium phosphate P-32 Solution, U.S.P. XXII.

SODIUM REMOVING RESINS.
See: Resins.

SODIUM RHODANATE.
See: Sodium Thiocyanate.

SODIUM RHODANIDE.
See: Sodium Thiocyanate.

SODIUM SACCHARIN. Saccharin Sodium, U.S.P. XXII.
Use: Noncaloric sweetener.

•**SODIUM SALICYLATE,** U.S.P. XXII. Tab., U.S.P. XXII.
Use: Analgesic.
W/Iodide. (Various Mfr.).
Use: Intravenous injection.
W/Iodide, cholchicine. (Various Mfr.).
Use: I.V., gout.

SODIUM SALICYLATE, NATURAL.
Use: Analgesic.
See: Alysine, Elix. (Merrell Dow).

SODIUM SALICYLATE COMBINATIONS.
See: Apcogesic, Tab. (Apco).
Bisalate, Tab. (Allison).
Bufosal, Gran. (Table Rock).
Corilin, Liq. (Schering).
Nucorsal, Tab. (Westerfield).
Pabalate, Tab. (Robins).
pHisoDan, Liq. (Winthrop).

SODIUM SECOBARBITAL. Secobarbital Sodium, U.S.P. XXII.
Use: Hypnotic.

SODIUM SECOBARBITAL AND SODIUM AMOBARBITAL CAPSULES.
Use: Sedative.
See: Tuinal, Cap. (Lilly).

•**SODIUM STARCH GLYCOLATE,** N.F. XVII.
Use: Pharmaceutic aid (tablet excipient).

•**SODIUM STEARATE,** N.F. XVII. Octadecanoic acid, sodium salt.
Use: Emulsifying and stiffening agent.

•**SODIUM STEARYL FUMARATE,** N.F. XVII.
Use: Pharmaceutic aid (tablet lubricant).

SODIUM STIBOGLUCONATE. B.A.N. Sodium salt of a pentavalent antimony derivative of gluconic acid.
Use: Treatment of leishmaniasis.

SODIUM SUCCINATE.
Use: Alkalinize urine and awaken patients following barbiturate anesthesia.

SODIUM SULAMYD Ophthalmic Oint. 10% Sterile. (Schering) Sulfacetamide sodium 10%. W/methylparaben, propylparaben, benzalkonium Cl, sorbitan monolaurate, water. Tube 0.125 oz.
Use: Anti-infective, ophthalmic.

SODIUM SULAMYD Ophthalmic Soln. 10% Sterile. (Schering) Sulfacetamide sodium 10% W/methylcellulose 0.5%, sodium thiosulfate 0.31%, methylparaben, propylparaben. Bot. 5 ml. Box 25s; 15 ml Box 1s.
Use: Anti-infective, ophthalmic.

SODIUM SULAMYD Ophthalmic Soln 30% Sterile. (Schering) Sulfacetamide sodium 30% w/sodium thiosulfate 0.15%, methylparaben, propylparaben as preservative. Bot. 15 ml. Box 1s.
Use: Anti-infective, ophthalmic.

SODIUM SULFABROMOMETHAZINE. Sodium N^1-(5-Bromo-4,6-dimethyl-2-pyrimidinyl) sulfanilamide.
Use: Antibacterial.

SODIUM SULFACETAMIDE.
See: Sulfacetamide Sodium Preps. (Various Mfr.).

SODIUM SULFADIAZINE.
See: Sulfadiazine Sodium Preps. (Various Mfr.).

SODIUM SULFAMERAZINE.
See: Sulfamerazine Sodium Preps. (Various Mfr.).

SODIUM SULFAPYRIDINE.
See: Sulfapyridine Sodium Pow. (Pfaltz & Bauer).

•**SODIUM SULFATE,** U.S.P. XXII. Inj., U.S.P. XXII.
Use: Cathartic.

•**SODIUM SULFATE S 35.** USAN.
Use: Radioactive agent.

SODIUM SULFATHIAZOLE.
Use: Antibacterial.
See: Sulfathiazole Sodium, Inj. (Various Mfr.).

SODIUM SULFOACETATE. W/Sodium alkyl aryl polyether sulfonate, docusate sodium, kerohydric, sulfur, salicylic acid, hexachlorophene.
See: Sebulex, Liq., Cream (Westwood).

SODIUM SULFOBROMOPHTHALEIN. Sulfobromophthalein Sodium, U.S.P. XXII.
Use: Diagnostic aid (hepatic function determination).

SODIUM SULFOCYANATE.
See: Sodium Thiocyanate. (Various Mfr.).

SODIUM SULFOXONE. Sulfoxone Sodium, U.S.P. XXII. Disodium sulfonyl-bis(p-phenyleneimino)dimethanesulfonate.
See: Diasone Sodium, Tab. (Abbott).

SODIUM SURAMIN.
See: Suramin Sodium.

SODIUM TAUROCHOLATE, A BILE SALT.
See: Bile Salts.
W/Phenolphthalein, cascara sagrada extract, sodium glycocholate, aloin.
See: Oxiphen, Tab. (Webcon).

SODIUM TETRADECYL SULFATE.
See: Sotradecol, Inj. (Elkins-Sinn).

SODIUM TETRAIODOPHENOLPHTHALEIN.
See: Iodophthalein Sodium (Various Mfr.).

SODIUM THIACETPHENARSAMIDE. The trivalent organic arsenical p-[bis-(carboxymethylmercapto)-arsino] benzamide. Ceparsolate Sodium (Abbott).

SODIUM THIAMYLAL FOR INJECTION. Thiamylal Sodium For Injection, U.S.P. XXII.
Use: General anesthetic.
See: Surital, Inj. (Parke-Davis).

SODIUM THIOCYANATE. Sodium Sulfocyanate. Sodium Rhodanide.

SODIUM THIOPENTAL.
See: Thiopental Sodium, U.S.P. XXII.

SODIUM THIOSALICYLATE.
See: Osteolate, Vial (Fellows-Testagar).
Rexolate, Vial (Hyrex).
Thiolate (Hickam; Pharmex).
Th-Sal, Vial (Foy).

•**SODIUM THIOSULFATE,** U.S.P. XXII. Inj., U.S.P. XXII. Sodium hyposulfite. "Hypo." Thiosulfuric acid, disodium salt, pentahydrate. Disodium thiosulfate pentahydrate.
Use: For argyria, cyanide, iodine poisoning, arsphenamine reactions; prevention of spread of ringworm of feet.
W/Salicylic acid, hydrocortisone acetate, alcohol.
See: Komed HC, Lot. (Barnes-Hind).
W/Salicylic acid, isopropyl alcohol.
See: Tinver, Lot (Barnes-Hind).
W/Salicylic acid, resorcinol, alcohol.
See: Mild Komed, Lot. (Barnes-Hind).
Komed, Lot. (Barnes-Hind).
W/Sodium nitrite, amyl nitrite.
See: Cyanide Antidote Pkg. (Lilly).

SODIUM L-THYROXINE.
See: Letter, Tab. (Armour).
Levoid, Inj., Tab. (Nutrition Control).
Roxstan, Tab. (Solvay).
Synthroid, Tab., Inj. (Flint).

SODIUM TOLBUTAMIDE. Tolbutamide Sodium, U.S.P. XXII.
Use: Diagnostic aid (diabetes).

SODIUM TRICLOFOS. Sodium trichloroethylphosphate.
Use: Sedative, hypnotic.

•**SODIUM TRIMETAPHOSPHATE.** USAN.
Use: Pharmaceutic aid.

SODIUM TYROPANOATE. B.A.N. Sodium 3-butyramido-α-ethyl-2,4,6-triiodohydrocinnamate. Radiopaque.
Use: Cholecystographic agent.

SODIUM VINBARBITAL INJECTION.
Use: Sedative.

SODIUM WARFARIN. Warfarin Sodium, U.S.P. XXII.
Use: Anticoagulant.

SOD-LATE 10. (Schlicksup) Sodium salicylate 10 gr/Tab. Bot. 1000s.
Use: Analgesic.

SODOL COMPOUND. (Major) Carisoprodol 200 mg, aspirin 325 mg/Tab. Bot. 100s, 500s.
Use: Skeletal muscle relaxant.

SODOL TABS. (Major) Carisoprodol 350 mg/Tab. Bot. 100s, 250s, 500s and 1000s.
Use: Skeletal muscle relaxant.

SOFARIN. (Lemmon) Warfarin sodium. **Tab.: 2 mg or 2.5 mg** Bot 100s; **5 mg** Bot. 100s, 1000s.
Use: Anticoagulant.

SOFCAPS. (Alton) Docusate sodium 100 mg or 250 mg/Cap. Bot. 100s, 1000s.
Use: Laxative.

SOFENOL 5. (C & M Pharmacal) Moisturizing lotion formulation. Bot. 8 oz.
Use: Emollient.

SOFLENS ENZYMATIC CONTACT LENS CLEANER. (Allergan) Papain, sodium Cl, sodium carbonate, sodium borate, edetate disodium/Tab. Vial 12s, 24s, 48s, Refill 24s, 36s.
Use: Soft contact lens care.

SOF/PRO CLEAN. (Sherman) Buffered hypertonic salt solution, non-ionic detergents, thimerosal 0.004%, EDTA 0.1%. Soln. Bot. 30 ml.
Use: Soft contact lens care.

SOFT MATE COMFORT DROPS. (Barnes-Hind) Sterile, aqueous, isotonic, buffered, lubricating and rewetting solution w/edetate disodium 0.1%, thimerosal 0.004%.
Use: Soft contact lens care.

SOFT MATE DAILY CLEANING SOLUTION. (Barnes-Hind) Sterile aqueous isotonic solution w/sodium Cl, octylphenoxy (oxyethylene) ethanol, hydroxyethylcellulose, thimerosal 0.004%, edetate disodium 0.2%. Bot. 30 ml.
Use: Soft contact lens care.

SOFT MATE DAILY CLEANING SOLUTION II. (Barnes-Hind) Sterile aqueous isotonic solution w/sodium Cl, octylphenoxyl (oxyethylene) ethanol, hydoxyethylcellulose, potassium sorbate 0.13%, edetate disodium 0.2%. Bot. 0.5 oz, 8 oz.
Use: Soft contact lens care.

SOFT MATE DISINFECTING SOLUTION. (Barnes-Hind) Sterile, aqueous, isotonic solution w/sodium Cl, povidone, octylphenoxy (oxyethylene) ethanol, chlorhexidine gluconate 0.005%, edetate disodium 0.1%. Thimerosal free. Bot. 4 oz, 8 oz.
Use: Soft contact lens care.

SOFT MATE DISINFECTION AND STORAGE SOLUTION. (Barnes-Hind) Sterile aqueous isotonic solution w/sodium Cl, povidone, octylphenoxl (oxyethylene) ethanol with a borate buffer, thimerosal 0.001%, edetate disodium 0.1%, chlorhexidine gluconate 0.005%. Bot. 8 oz.
Use: Soft contact lens care.

SOFT MATE LENS DROPS. (Barnes-Hind) Sterile aqueous isotonic solution w/sodium Cl, potassium sorbate 0.13%, edetate disodium 0.025%. Thimerosal free. Bot. 2 oz.
Use: Soft contact lens care.

SOFT MATE PRESERVATIVE-FREE SALINE SOLUTION. (Barnes-Hind) Sterile aqueous isotonic solution w/sodium Cl, borate buffer. Contains no preservatives. Bot. 0.5 oz, 30 single use.
Use: Soft contact lens care.

SOFT MATE PROTEIN REMOVER SOLUTION. (Barnes-Hind) Sterile aqueous solution buffered with borates. Preservative free. 8 single use vials, 8 ml each.
Use: Soft contact lens care.

SOFT MATE PS COMFORT DROPS. (Barnes-Hind) Sterile aqueous isotonic solution w/potassium sorbate 0.13%, edetate disodium 0.1%. Bot. 15 ml.
Use: Contact lens care.

SOFT MATE PS DAILY CLEANING SOLUTION. (Barnes-Hind) Sterile aqueous isotonic solution w/sodium Cl, octylphenoxy (oxyethylene) ethanol, hydroxyethylcellulose, potassium sorbate 0.13%, edetate disodium 0.2%. Bot. 30 ml.
Use: Soft contact lens care.

SOFT MATE PS SALINE SOLUTION. (Barnes-Hind) Sterile aqueous isotonic solution w/sodium Cl, potassium sorbate 0.13%, edetate disodium 0.025%. Bot. 8 oz, 12 oz.
Use: Soft contact lens care.

SOFT MATE RINSING SOLUTION. (Barnes-Hind) Sterile aqueous isotonic solution w/sodium Cl, thimerosal 0.001%, edetate disodium 0.1%, chlorhexidine gluconate 0.005%. Bot. 8 oz.
Use: Soft contact lens care.

SOFT MATE SALINE SOLUTION. (Barnes-Hind) Sterile aqueous isotonic solution of sodium Cl. Preservative free. Bot. 8 oz, 12 oz.
Use: Soft contact lens care.

SOFT MATE SOFT LENS CLEANERS. (Barnes-Hind) Kit containing: Soft Mate daily cleaning solution II (4 oz.); soft mate weekly cleaning solution (1.2 oz.); Hydra-Mat II cleaning and storage unit.
Use: Soft contact lens care.

SOFT'N SOOTHE. (Ascher) Benzocaine, menthol, moisturizers. Tube 50 Gm.
Use: Local anesthetic, emollient.

SOFT RINSE 135. (Professional Supplies) Salt tablets for normal saline solution 135 mg/Tab. In 365s with 15 ml. Bot.
Use: Soft contact lens care.

SOFT RINSE 250. (Professional Supplies) Salt tablets for normal saline solution 250 mg/Tab. In 200s, with 27.7 ml. Bot.
Use: Soft contact lens care.

SOFT-STRESS CAPSULES. (Marlyn) Calcium 50 mg, iron 4.5 mg, vitamins A 6250 IU, D 100 IU, E 50 mg, B_1 6.25 mg, B_2 6.25 mg, B_3 6.25 mg, B_5 6.25 mg, B_6 6.25 mg, B_{12} 6.25 mcg, C 125 mg, folic acid 0.05 mg, choline, Cr, Cu, K, Mg, P, PABA, Se, biotin 6.25 mcg, inositol, lecithin, zinc 3.75 mg/Cap. In 30 packs of 4.
Use: Vitamin/mineral supplement.

SOLAGEST. (Canright) Pancreatin 10.5 gr, hyoscyamine sulfate 0.072 mg, atropine sulfate 0.013 mg, hyoscine HBr 0.0047 mg, pentobarbital sodium 10.8 mg/Tab. Bot. 100s, 1000s.
Use: Anticholinergic/antispasmodic, digestive aid.

SOLANEED. (Hanlon) Vitamin A 25,000 units/ Cap. Bot. 100s.
Use: Vitamin A supplement.

SOLAPSONE. B.A.N. Tetrasodium salt of bis-[4-(3-phenyl-1,3-disulfopropylamino)phenyl]sulfone.
Use: Antileprotic.
See: Solasulfone (I.N.N.).

SOLAQUIN. (Elder) Hydroquinone 2%, ethyl dihydroxypropyl PABA 5%, dioxybenzone 3%, oxybenzone 2%. Tube oz.
Use: Skin bleaching agent with sunscreen.

SOLAQUIN FORTE CREAM. (Elder) Hydroquinone 4%, ethyl dihydroxypropyl PABA 5%, dioxybenzone 3%, oxybenzone 2% in a vanishing cream base. Tube 0.5 oz, 1 oz.
Use: Skin bleaching agent with sunscreen.

SOLAQUIN FORTE GEL. (Elder) Hydroquinone 4%, ethyl dihydroxypropyl PABA 5%, dioxybenzone 3%, oxybenzone 2%. Tube 0.5 oz, 1 oz.
Use: Skin bleaching agent with sunscreen.

SOLARCAINE. (Schering-Plough) **Cream:** Benzocaine 1%, triclosan. Tube oz. **Lot.:** Benzocaine 0.5%, triclosan. Bot. 3 oz, 6 oz. **Spray (aerosol):** Benzocaine 20%, triclosan 0.13%, isopropyl alcohol 35%. Can 3 oz, 5 oz.
Use: Local anesthetic.

SOLAR CREAM. (Doak) PABA, titanium dioxide, magnesium stearate in a flesh-colored, water-repellent base. Tube oz.
Use: Sunscreen.

SOLARGENTUM.
See: Mild silver protein (Various Mfr.).

SOLATENE. (Roche) Beta-carotene 30 mg/Cap. Bot. 100s.
Use: Reduce photosensitivity in patients with erythropoietic protoporphyria (EPP).

SOLBAR PF 15 CREAM. (Person & Covey) Octyl methoxycinnamate 7.5%, oxybenzone 5%. Bot. 1 oz, 4 oz.
Use: Sunscreen.

SOLBAR PF PABA FREE 15. (Person & Covey) Oxybenzone 5%, octyl methoxycinnamate 7.5%. Sunscreen SPF 15. Tube 2.5 oz.
Use: Sunscreen.

SOLBAR PLUS 15. (Person & Covey) Padimate 6%, oxybenzone 4%, dioxybenzone 2%. Tube 1 oz, 4 oz.
Use: Sunscreen.

SOLFOTON. (Poythress) Phenobarbital 16 mg/ Tab. or Cap. Bot. 100s, 500s.
Use: Sedative/hypnotic.

SOLFOTON S/C TABS. (Poythress) Phenobarbital 16 mg/SC Tab. Bot. 100s.
Use: Sedative/hypnotic.

SOLGANAL. (Schering) Aurothioglucose 50 mg/ ml in sesame oil. Vial 10 ml; Box 1s.
Use: I.M., gold therapy, antiarthritic.

SOLIWAX. Docusate Sodium, U.S.P. XXII. Docusate Sodium, Solasulfone (I.N.N.).

SOLPADEINE TABLETS. (Winthrop) Paracetamol.
Use: Analgesic.

SOLTICE QUICK-RUB. (Chattem) Methyl salicylate, camphor, menthol, eucalyptol. Cream Bot. 1.33 oz, 3.75 oz.
Use: External analgesic.

SOLU-BARB 0.25 TABLETS. (Forest Pharm.) Phenobarbital 0.25 gr/Tab. Bot. 24s.
Use: Sedative/hypnotic.

SOLUCAP C. (Jamieson-McKames) Vitamin C 1000 mg/Capsulet. Bot. 100s.
Use: Vitamin C supplement.

SOLUCAP E. (Jamieson-McKames) Vitamin E 100 IU 400 IU or 1000 IU/Cap. Bot. 100s.
Use: Vitamin E supplement.

SOLU-CORTEF. (Upjohn) **100 mg:** Hydrocortisone sodium succinate, benzyl alcohol. Plain vial, 2 ml Act-O-Vial. **250 mg:** Hydrocortisone sodium succinate, benzyl alcohol. 2 ml Act-O-Vial. **500 mg:** Hydrocortisone sodium succinate, benzyl alcohol. 4 ml Act-O-Vial. **1000 mg:** Hydrocortisone sodium succinate, benzyl alcohol. 8 ml Act-O-Vial.
Use: Corticosteroid.

SOLU-EZE. (Forest) Hydroxyquinoline 0.12%, carbitol acetate 12.1%. Bot. 3 oz.

SOLU-FLUR. (Robinson) Sodium fluoride 2.21 mg/Tab. Bot. 100s, 1000s.
Use: Dental caries preventative.

SOLU-MEDROL. (Upjohn) **40 mg:** Methylprednisolone sodium succinate/vial, benzyl alcohol. Unitvial 1 ml. **125 mg:** Methylprednisolone sodium succinate/vial, benzyl alcohol. Act-O-Vial 2 ml, 5s, 25s. 25-Pack, 25s, 50s. **500 mg:** Methylprednisolone sodium succinate/vial, benzyl alcohol. Vial 8 ml, Vial 8 ml w/diluent. **1000 mg:** Methylprednisolone sodium succinate/vial, benzyl alcohol. Vial 16 ml, vial 16 ml w/diluent. **2000 mg:** Methylprednisolone sodium succinate powder for injection, benzyl alcohol. Vial 30.6 ml, vial 30.6 ml w/diluent.
Use: Corticosteroid.

SOLUMOL. (C & M Pharmacal) Petrolatum, mineral oil, cetyl-stearyl alcohol, sodium lauryl sulfate, glycerin, propylene glycol, sorbic acid, purified water. Jar lb.
Use: Ointment base.

SOLU-PRED. (Kenyon) Prednisolone sodium phosphate equivalent to prednisolone phosphate 20 mg, niacinamide 25 mg, disodium edetate 0.5 mg, sodium bisulfite 1 mg, phenol 5 mg/ml. Vial 10 ml.
Use: Corticosteroid.

SOLUREX. (Hyrex) Dexamethasone sodium phosphate 4 mg/ml. W/methyl and propyl parabens, sodium bisulfite. Vial 5 ml, 10 ml, 30 ml.
Use: Corticosteroid.

SOLUREX L.A. (Hyrex) Dexamethasone acetate 8 mg/ml, polysorbate 80, carboxymethylcellulose, sodium bisulfite, EDTA, benzyl alcohol. Susp. Vial 5 ml.
Use: Corticosteroid.

SOLUVITE CT W/FLUORIDE. (Pharmics) Vitamins A 2500 IU, D 400 IU, B_1 1.05 mg, B_2 1.2 mg, B_6 1.05 mg, B_{12} 4.5 mcg, C 60 mg, niacin 13.5 mg, E 15 IU, fluoride 1 mg, folic acid 0.3 mg/Tab. Bot. 100s, 1000s.
Use: Vitamin/mineral supplement.

SOLUVITE-F DROPS. (Pharmics) Vitamins A 1500 IU, D 400 IU, C 35 mg, fluoride 0.25 mg/0.6 ml. Bot. 57 ml.
Use: Vitamin/mineral supplement.

SOLVENT-G. (Syossett) Alcohol 47.5%, laureth-4, isopropyl alcohol 4%, propylene glycol. Lot. Bot. 50 ml.
Use: Lotion base.

SOLVISYN-A. (Towne) Water soluble vitamin A. **Cap.:** 10,000 units, 25,000 units or 50,000 units. Bot. 100s, 1000s.
Use: Vitamin A supplement.

•**SOLYPERTINE TARTRATE.** USAN. 7- 2-[4-(o-Methoxy-phenyl)-1-piperazinyl]ethyl 5H-1,3-dioxolo[4,5-f]in-dole tartrate.
Use: Antiadrenergic.

SOMA. (Wallace) Carisoprodol 350 mg/Tab. Bot. 100s, 500s, UD 100s.
Use: Skeletal muscle relaxant.

SOMA COMPOUND TABS. (Wallace) Carisoprodol 200 mg, aspirin 325 mg/Tab. Bot. 100s, 500s. UD 500s.
Use: Skeletal muscle relaxant, salicylate analgesic.

SOMA COMPOUND W/CODEINE. (Wallace) Carisoprodol 200 mg, aspirin 325 mg, codeine phosphate 16 mg/Tab. Bot. 100s.
Use: Skeletal muscle relaxant, analgesic combination.

•**SOMAGREBOVE.** USAN.
Use: Galactopoietic agent (veterinary).

•**SOMALAPOR.** USAN.
Use: Growth hormone (veterinary).

•**SOMANTADINE HYDROCHORIDE.** USAN.
Use: Antiviral.

•**SOMATREM.** USAN.
Use: Growth hormone.
See: Protropin, Inj. (Genentech).

•**SOMATROPIN.** USAN. Growth hormone derived from the anterior pituitary gland.
Use: Growth stimulant.
See: Humatrope, Inj. (Lilly).

•**SOMAVUBOVE.** USAN.
Use: Galactopoietic agent (veterinary).

•**SOMENOPOR.** USAN.
Use: Growth hormone (veterinary).

SOMINEX 2. (Beecham Products) Diphenhydramine HCl 25 mg/Tab. Blister pack 16s, 32s, 72s.
Use: Sleep aid.

SOMINEX 2 PAIN RELIEF FORMULA. (Beecham Products) Diphenhydramine HCl 25 mg, acetaminophen 500 mg/Tab. Blister pack 16s. Bot. 32s, 72s.
Use: Sleep aid, analgesic.

SOMNATABS. (Thurston) Powdered extract of Passiflora incarnata 3 gr, powdered extract of Piscidia erythrina 2 gr, powdered extract of Viburnum opulus 1 gr, powdered extract of hyoscyamus ⅛ gr/Tab. Bot. 50s, 100s, 500s.

SONACIDE. (Wyeth-Ayerst) Potentiated acid glutaraldehyde. Bot. 1 gal, 5 gal.
Use: Sterilizing and disinfecting.

SONDRATE ELIXIR. (Kenyon) Chloral hydrate 1.6 Gm/fl oz. Bot. 4 oz, pt, gal.
Use: Sedative/hypnotic.

SONERYL.
See: Butethal (Various Mfr.).

SOOTHADERM. (Pharmakon Labs) Pyrilamine maleate 2.07 mg, benzocaine 2.08 mg, zinc oxide 41.35 mg/ml, camphor, menthol. Lot. Bot. 118 ml.
Use: Antihistamine, local anesthetic.

SOOTHE. (Alcon) Tetrahydrozoline 0.05%, benzalkonium Cl 0.004%, adsorbobase. Bot. 15 ml.
Use: Decongestant, ophthalmic.

SOOTHE. (Walgreen) Bismuth subsalicylate 100 mg/Tsp. Bot. 9 oz.
Use: Antidiarrheal.

SOPRODOL. (Schein) Carisoprodol 350 mg/Tab. Bot. 100s, 500s.
Use: Skeletal muscle relaxant.

SOQUETTE. (Barnes-Hind) Polyvinyl alcohol, benzalkonium Cl 0.01%, EDTA 0.2%. Bot. 4 fl oz.
Use: Hard contact lens care.

SORBASE COUGH SYRUP. (Fort David) Dextromethorphan HBr 10 mg, guaifenesin 100 mg/5 ml in sorbitol base. Bot. 4 oz, pt, gal.
Use: Antitussive, expectorant.

•**SORBIC ACID,** N.F. XVII.
Use: Preservative (antimicrobial).

SORBIDE T.D. (Mayrand) Isosorbide dinitrate 40 mg/TR Cap. Bot. 100s.
Use: Antianginal.

SORBIDE NITRATE. B.A.N. 1,4:3,6-Dianhydrosorbitol 2,5-dinitrate. Isosorbide Dinitrate (I.N.N.).
Use: Coronary vasodilator.

SORBIDON HYDRATE. (Gordon) Water-in-oil ointment. Jar 2 oz, 0.5 oz, 1 lb, 5 lb.
Use: Emollient.

SORBIMACROGOL OLEATE 300.
See Polysorbate 80.

•**SORBINIL.** USAN.
Use: Enzyme inhibitor.

•**SORBITAN MONOLAURATE,** N.F. XVII. Mixture of laurate esters of sorbitol and its anhydrides.
Use: Surface-active agent, emulsifying agent.
See: Span 20 (ICI U.S.).

•**SORBITAN MONOOLEATE,** N.F. XVII. Mixture of oleate esters of sorbitol and its anhydrides.
Use: Surface-active agent.
See: Span 80 (ICI U.S.).

SORBITAN MONOOLEATE POLYOXYETHYLENE DERIVATIVES.
See: Polysorbate 80, N.F. XVII.

•**SORBITAN MONOPALMITATE,** N.F. XVII. Mixture of palmitate esters of sorbitol and its anhydrides.
Use: Surface-active agent.
See: Span 40 (ICI U.S.).

•**SORBITAN MONOSTEARATE,** N.F. XVII. Mixture of stearate esters of sorbitol and its anhydrides.
Use: Surface-active agent.
See: Span 60 (ICI U.S.).

•**SORBITAN SESQUIOLEATE.** USAN. Sorbitan mono-oleate and sorbitan dioleate.
Use: Surfactant.
See: Arlacel C (ICI U.S.).

•**SORBITAN TRIOLEATE.** USAN.
Use: Surfactant.
See: Span 85 (ICI U.S.).

•**SORBITAN TRISTEARATE.** USAN.
Use: Pharmaceutic aid (surfactant).
See: Span 65 (ICI U.S.).

SORBITANS.
See: Polysorbate 80, U.S.P.

•**SORBITOL,** N.F. XVII. Solution, U.S.P. XXII.
Use: Diuretic, dehydrating agent, humectant, pharmaceutic aid (sweetening agent, tablet excipient).
See: Sorbo (ICI U.S.).
W/Homatropine methylbromide.
See: Probilagol Liq. (Purdue Frederick).
W/Mannitol.
See: Sorbitol-mannitol Irrigation (Abbott).

SORBITON. (Kenyon) Vitamin B_{12} 5 mcg, folic acid 0.1 mg, ferrous fumarate 100 mg, D-sorbitol 500 mg/Tab. Bot. 100s, 1000s.
Use: Vitamin/mineral supplement.

SORBITRATE. (ICI Pharma) Isosorbide dinitrate. **Tab.:** 5 mg Bot. 100s, 500s, UD 100s; 10 mg Bot. 500s, UD 100s; 20 mg, 30 mg, 40 mg Bot. 100s, UD 100s. **Sustained action tab.** 40 mg Bot. 100s, UD 100s; **Sublingual tab.** 2.5 mg, 5 mg, 10 mg Bot. 100s, UD 100s. **Chew. tab.** 5 mg Bot. 100s, 500s, UD 100s; 10 mg Bot. 100s, 500s, UD 100s.
Use: Antianginal.

SORBO. (ICI Americas) Sorbitol Solution, U.S.P. XXII.

SORBUTUSS. (Dalin) Dextromethorphan HBr 10 mg, guaifenesin 100 mg, ipecac fluidextract 0.05 min., potassium citrate 85 mg, citric acid 35 mg/5 ml. Bot. 3 oz, pt.
Use: Antitussive, expectorant combination.

SORDINOL. Clopenthixol, B.A.N.
Use: Tranquilizer.

SORETHYTAN (20) MONO-OLEATE.
See: Polysorbate 80, (Various Mfr.).

SORETTS LOZENGES. (Lannett) Benzocaine 32 mg, extract licorice 8 mg, menthol 0.5 mg/Loz. Bot. 500s, 1000s.
Use: Local anesthetic.

SOSEGON SOLUTION. (Winthrop) Pentazocine.
Use: Analgesic.

SOSEGON SUSPENSION. (Winthrop) Pentazocine.
Use: Analgesic.

SOSEGON TABLETS. (Winthrop) Pentazocine.
Use: Analgesic.

SOTALOL. B.A.N. (±)-4′-(1-Hydroxy-2-isopropylaminoethyl)methanesulf-onanilide.
Use: Beta adrenergic blocking agent.

•**SOTALOL HYDROCHLORIDE.** USAN. 4′-[1-Hydroxy-2-(isopropylamino)-ethyl]methanesulfonanilide hydrochloride. Under study.
Use: Adrenergic β-receptor antagonist.

•**SOTERENOL HYDROCHLORIDE.** USAN.
Use: Adrenergic (bronchodilator).

SOTRADECOL. (Elkins-Sinn) Sodium tetradecyl sulfate 1% or 3%. Inj. Dosette amp. 2 ml.
Use: Sclerosing agent.

SOXA-FORTE. (Vita Elixir) Sulfisoxazole 0.5 Gm, phenazopyridine 50 mg/Tab.
Use: Anti-infective.

SOXA TABLETS. (Vita Elixir) Sulfisoxazole 0.5 Gm/Tab. Bot. 100s, 1000s.
Use: Anti-infective.

SOYACAL. (Alpha Therapeutic) Intravenous fat emulsion 10% or 20%. Vial 250 ml, 500 ml.
Use: Parenteral nutritional supplement.

SOYALAC. (Loma Linda) Infant formula based on an extract from whole soybeans containing all essential nutrients. **Ready to Serve Liq:** Can 32 fl oz. **Double Strength Conc.:** Can 13 fl oz. **Pow.:** Can 14 oz.
Use: Nutritional supplement.

SOYALAC-i. (Loma Linda) Soy protein isolate infant formula containing no corn derivatives and a negligible amount of soy carbohydrates. Contains all essential nutrients in various forms. **Ready to Serve Liq:** Can 32 fl oz. **Double Strength Conc.:** Can 13 fl oz.
Use: Nutritional supplement.

SOYA LECITHIN. Soybean extract. 100s.
Use: Phosphorus therapy.
See: Neo-Vadrin (Scherer).

SOYBEAN LECITHIN.
W/Safflower oil, choline bitartrate, whole liver, inositol, methionine, natural tocopherols, vitamins B_6, B_{12}, panthenol.
See: Nutricol, Cap., Vial (Nutrition Control).

•**SOYBEAN OIL,** U.S.P. XXII.
Use: Pharmaceutic necessity.

SPABELIN No. 1. (Arcum) Phenobarbital 15 mg, belladonna powdered extract ⅛ gr/Tab. Bot. 100s, 1000s.
Use: Sedative/hypnotic.

SPABELIN NO. 2. (Arcum) Phenobarbital 30 mg, belladonna powdered extract ⅛ gr/Tab. Bot. 100s, 1000s.
Use: Sedative/hypnotic.

SPABELIN ELIXIR. (Arcum) Hyoscyamine sulfate 81 mcg, atropine sulfate 15 mcg, scopolamine HBr 5 mcg, phenobarbital 16.2 mg/5 ml. Bot. 16 oz, gal.

SPAN 20. (ICI Americas) Sorbitan Monolaurate, N.F. XVII.
SPAN 40. (ICI Americas) Sorbitan Monopalmitate, N.F. XVII.
SPAN 60. (ICI Americas) Sorbitan Monostearate, N.F. XVII.
SPAN 65. (ICI Americas) Sorbitan tristearate. Mixture of stearate esters of sorbitol and its anhydrides.
Use: Surface-active agent.
SPAN 80. (ICI Americas) Sorbitan Mono-oleate, N.F. XVII.
SPAN 85. (ICI Americas) Sorbitan trioleate. Mixture of oleate esters of sorbitol and its anhydrides.
Use: Surface-active agent.
SPAN C. (Freeda) Citrus bioflavonoids 300 mg, rutin 50 mg, vitamin C 200 mg/Tab. Bot. 100s, 250s, 500s.
Use: Vitamin supplement.
SPAN FF. (Metro Med) Ferrous fumarate 325 mg/Cap. Bot. 60s, 500s.
Use: Iron supplement.
SPAN PD. (Metro Med) Phentermine HCl 37.5 mg/Cap. Bot. 100s.
Use: Anorexiant.
SPAN-RD. (Metro Med) d-Methamphetamine HCl 12 mg, dl-methamphetamine HCl 6 mg, butabarbital 30 mg/Tab. Bot. 100s, 1000s.
Use: Amphetamine, sedative/hypnotic.
SPANTUSS LIQUID. (Arco) Dextromethorphan HBr 15 mg, chlorpheniramine maleate 4 mg, phenylephrine HCl 5 mg, acetaminophen 120 mg/5 ml. Bot. 4 oz, pt.
Use: Antitussive, antihistamine, decongestant, analgesic.
•**SPARFOSATE SODIUM.** USAN.
Use: Antineoplastic.
SPARINE. (Wyeth-Ayerst) Promazine HCl. 25 mg, 50 mg or 100 mg/Tab. Bot. 50s.
Use: Antipsychotic.
SPARKLES GRANULES. (Lafayette) Effervescent gran 6 Gm/Packet. Each 6 Gm produces 500 ml of carbon dioxide gas. Ctn. 25 packets. Pkg. 2 Ctn.
Use: Carbon dioxide production as an aid during air contrast stomach examinations.
SPARKLES TABLETS. (Lafayette) Effervescent tablets. Each 4.3 Gm of tablets produces 250 ml of carbon dioxide gas. Bot. 43 Gm tab. (10 doses).
Use: Carbon dioxide production as an aid during air contrast stomach examination.
SPARSOMYCIN. USAN.
Use: Antineoplastic.
SPARTEINE SULFATE. USAN.
Use: Oxytocic.
W/Sodium Cl.
SPASLOIDS. (Harvey) Hyoscyamine sulfate 0.1040 mg, atropine sulfate 0.0195 mg, hyoscine HBr 0.0065 mg, phenobarbital 0.25 gr/Tab. Bot. 1000s.
Use: Anticholinergic/antispasmodic, sedative/hypnotic.
SPASMATOL. (Pharmed) Homatropine MBr 3 mg, pentobarbital 12 mg, mephobarbital 8 mg/Tab. Bot. 100s, 1000s.
Use: Anticholinergic/antispasmodic, sedative/hypnotic.
SPASMED. (Jenkins) Hyoscyamine HBr 0.1037 mg, atropine sulfate 0.0194 mg, hyoscine HBr 0.0065 mg, tri-bar (1/3 each sodium butabarbital, sodium pentobarbital, sodium phenobarbital) 16.2 mg/Tab. or 5 ml. **Tab.:** Bot. 1000s. **Elix:** Bot. 4 oz, pt, gal. Alcohol 15%.
Use: Sedative/hypnotic, anticholinergic/antispasmodic.
SPASMED JR. (Jenkins) Homatropine methylbromide 1/96 gr, phenobarbital sodium 1/8 gr, lactose, special mint flavor/Tab. Bot. 1000s.
Use: Sedative/hypnotic.
SPASMID. (Dalin) Methscopolamine nitrate 2.5 mg, phenobarbital 8 mg/Tab. or 5 ml. **Elix.:** Bot. 4 oz, pt. **Tab.:** Bot. 50s, 100s.
Use: Anticholinergic/antispasmodic, sedative/hypnotic.
SPASMODINE. (Noyes) Alcohol 4%, emulsion of infused oils lobelia, stillingia, cajeput, lavender, cassia, eucalyptol. Mixture 3 oz, pt, gal.
Use: Expectorant.
SPASMOJECT. (Mayrand) Dicyclomine HCl 10 mg/ml. Vial 10 ml.
Use: Anticholinergic/antispasmodic.
SPASMOLIN. (Richlyn) Phenobarbital 16.2 mg, hyoscyamine sulfate 0.1037 mg, atropine sulfate 0.0194 mg, hyoscine HBr 0.0065 mg/Tab. Bot. 1000s.
Use: Sedative/hypnotic, anticholinergic/antispasmodic.
SPASMOLYN. (Heun) Mephenesin 0.5 Gm./Tab. Bot. 100s.
Use: Anticholinergic/antispasmodic.
SPASMOLYTIC AGENTS.
See: Antispasmodics.
SPASMOPHEN. (Lannett) Phenobarbital 15 mg, hyoscyamine sulfate 0.1037 mg, atropine sulfate 0.0194 mg, hyoscine HBr 0.1037 mg/Tab. or 5 ml. **Tab.** Bot. 1000s. **Liq.** Bot. pt, gal.
Use: Sedative/hypnotic, anticholinergic, antispasmodic.
SPASNO-LIX. (Freeport) Phenobarbital 16.2 mg, hyoscyamine sulfate 0.1037 mg, atropine sulfate 0.0194 mg, hyoscine HBr 0.0065 mg, alcohol 21-23 %/5 ml. Bot. 4 oz.
Use: Sedative/hypnotic, anticholinergic/antispasmodic.
SPASODIL. (Rand) Ethaverine HCl 50 mg or 100 mg/Tab. Bot. 100s, 1000s.
Use: Peripheral vasodilator.
SPASQUID. (Geneva Generics) Atropine sulfate 0.0194 mg, scopolamine HBr 0.0065 mg, hyoscyamine HBr 0.1037 mg, phenobarbital 16.2 mg/5 ml, alcohol 23%. Elix. Bot. pt, gal.

Use: Anticholinergic/antispasmodic, sedative/hypnotic.

SPASTIL. (Kenyon) Propantheline Br 15 mg/Tab. Bot. 100s, 1000s.
Use: Anticholinergic/antispasmodic.

SPASTYL. (Pharmex) Dicyclomine HCl 10 mg/ml. Vial 10 ml.
Use: Anticholinergic/antispasmodic.

S.P.B. TABLET. (Sheryl) Therapeutic B complex formula with ascorbic acid 300 mg. Tab. 100s.
Use: Vitamin supplement.

SPD. (A.P.C.) Methyl salicylate, methyl nicotinate, dipropylene glycol salicylate, oleoresin capsicum, camphor, menthol. Cream Bot. 4 oz, Tube 1.5 oz.
Use: External analgesic.

•**SPEARMINT,** N.F. XVII.
Use: Flavor.

•**SPEARMINT OIL,** N.F. XVII.
Use: Flavor.

SPECIAL FORMULA OINTMENT "RF". (Lannett) Zinc oxide 10%, boric acid 4%, starch 10%, camphor 1%, menthol 0.5% in a petrolatum-aquaphor base. Jar lb.
Use: Dermatological.

SPECIAL SHAMPOO. (Del-Ray) Non medicated shampoo.
Use: Cleansing shampoo.

SPECTAZOLE. (Ortho) Econazole nitrate 1% in a water miscible base. Tube 15 Gm, 30 Gm, 85 Gm.
Use: Antifungal, topical.

SPECTINOMYCIN. Formerly Actinospectocin. An antibiotic isolated from broth cultures of *Streptomyces spectabilis.*
Use: Antibacterial.
See: Trobicin, Vial, Amp. (Upjohn).

•**SPECTINOMYCIN HYDROCHLORIDE, STERILE,** U.S.P. XXII. For Susp., U.S.P. XXII. An antibiotic produced by *Streptomyces spectabilis.*
Use: Antibacterial.

SPECTRA 360. (Parker) Salt-free electrode gel. Tube 8 oz.
Use: T.E.N.S. application, ECG pediatric, long-term procedures.

SPECTROBID POWDER FOR ORAL SUSPENSION. (Roerig) Bacampicillin pow. 125 mg/5 ml. In 70 ml, 100 ml, 140 ml, 200 ml.
Use: Antibacterial, penicillin.

SPECTROBID TABLETS. (Roerig) Bacampicillin HCl 400 mg/Tab. Bot. 100s.
Use: Antibacterial, penicillin.

SPECTRO-BIOTIC. (A.P.C.) Bacitracin 400 units, neomycin sulfate 5 mg, polymyxin B sulfate 5000 units/Gm. Oint. 0.5 oz, 1 oz.
Use: Anti-infective, topical.

SPECTRO-JEL. (Recsei) Soap free. Methylcellulose, carboxypolymethylene, cetyl alcohol, sorbitan mono-oleate, fumed silica, triethanolamine stearate, glycol polysiloxane, propylene glycol, glycerin, isopropyl alcohol 5%. Bot. 4 oz, pt, gal.
Use: Skin cleanser.

SPEC-T SORE THROAT ANESTHETIC LOZENGES. (Squibb Mark) Benzocaine 10 mg/Loz. Box 10s.
Use: Local anesthetic.

SPEC-T SORE THROAT/COUGH SUPPRESSANT LOZENGES. (Squibb) Benzocaine 10 mg, dextromethorphan HBr 10 mg, tartrazine.
Use: Local anesthetic, antitussive.

SPEC-T SORE THROAT/DECONGESTANT LOZENGES. (Squibb) Benzocaine 10 mg, phenylephrine HCl 5 mg, phenylpropanolamine HCl 10.5 mg w/tartrazine. Loz. Pkg. 10s.
Use: Local anesthetic, decongestant.

SPERMACETI.
Use: Stiffening agent; pharmaceutic necessity for cold cream.

SPERMINE. Diaminopropyltetramethylene.

SPERTI OINTMENT. (Whitehall) Live yeast cell derivative supplying 2000 units skin respiratory factor/Gm, shark liver oil 3%, phenylmercuric nitrate 1:10,000. Tube oz.
Use: Healing ointment.

SPHERULIN. (Berkeley Biologicals) Coccidioidin: 1:100 equivalent, vial 1 ml, 5 ml, 1:10 equivalent, Vial 0.5 ml.
Use: Skin test.

SPIDER-BITE ANTIVENIN.
See: Antivenin Crotalidae and Micrurus, U.S.P. XXII.

SPIDER-MAN CHILDREN'S CHEWABLE VITAMIN. (Nature's Bounty) Vitamins A 2500 IU, D 400 IU, E 15 mg, B_1 1.05 mg, B_2 1.2 mg, B_3 13.5 mg, B_6 1.05 mg, B_{12} 4.5 mcg, C 60 mg, folic acid 0.3 mg/Tab., xylitol, sorbitol. Bot. 75s, 130s.
Use: Vitamin supplement.

•**SPIPERONE.** USAN. 8-[3-(p-Fluorobenzoyl)-propyl]-1-phenyl-1,3,8-triazaspiro-[4.5]decan-4-one.
Use: Tranquilizer.

•**SPIRAMYCIN.** USAN. Antibiotic substance from cultures of *Streptomyces ambofaciens.*
Use: Antibiotic.

•**SPIRAPRIL HYDROCHLORIDE.** USAN.
Use: ACE inhibitor.

SPIRILENE. B.A.N. 8-[4-(4-Fluorophenyl)pent-3-enyl]-1-phenyl-1,3,8-triazaspiro[4,5]decan-4-one.
Use: Tranquilizer.

SPIROBARBITAL SODIUM. 1-Ethyl-2,4-dimethyl-8-thio-7,9-diazaspiro[4.5]decane-6,8,10-trione sodium salt.

•**SPIROGERMANIUM HYDROCHLORIDE.** USAN.
Use: Antineoplastic.

•**SPIROMUSTINE.** USAN. Formerly spirohydantoin mustard.
Use: Antineoplastic.

•**SPIRONOLACTONE,** U.S.P. XXII. Tab., U.S.P. XXII. 17-Hydroxy-7α-mercapto-3-oxo-17α-pregn-4-ene-21-carboxylic acid -lactone 7-acetate: 3-(3-oxo-7 α-acetylthio-17β-hydroxy-4-androsten-17 α-yl) propionic acid -lactone.
Use: Diuretic.
See: Aldactone, Tab. (Searle).

W/Hydrochlorothiazide.
See: Aldactazide, Tab. (Searle).

SPIRONAZIDE. (Schein) Spironolactone 25 mg, hydrochlorothiazide 25 mg/Tab. Bot. 100s, 500s, 1000s, UD 100s.
Use: Diuretic combination.

SPIROPITAN. (Janssen) Spiperone.
Use: Antipsychotic.

SPIROPLATIN. USAN.
Use: Antineoplastic.

SPIROTRIAZINE HCl. 2,4-Diamino-5(p-chlorophenyl)-9-methyl-1,3,5-triazaspiro [5.5]undeca-1,3-diene HCl.
Use: Anthelmintic.

SPIROXASONE. USAN.
Use: Diuretic.

SPIROZIDE. (Rugby) Spironolactone 25 mg, hydrochlorothiazide 25 mg/Tab. Bot. 100s, 500s, 1000s.
Use: Diuretic combination.

SPL-SEROLOGIC TYPES I AND III. (Delmont Labs) Staphylococcus aureus 120 to 180 million units, staphylococcus bacteriophage plaque forming units 100 to 1000 million/ml. Inj. Amp. 1 ml, Vial 10 ml.
Use: Anti-infective.

SPONGE, ABSORBABLE GELATIN, U.S.P. XXII.
Use: Local hemostatic.

SPORTSCREME. (Thompson) Triethanolamine salicylate 10% in a nongreasy base. Cream 37.5 Gm, 90 Gm.
Use: External analgesic.

SPRAY SKIN PROTECTANT. (Morton) Isopropyl alcohol, polyvinylpyrolidone, vinyl alcohol, plasticizer, propellant. Aerosol can 6 oz.
Use: Protective skin coating.

SPREADING FACTOR.
See: Hyaluronidase (Various Mfr.).

SPRX-105. (Reid-Provident) Phendimetrazine tartrate 105 mg/SR Cap. Bot. 28s, 500s.
Use: Anorexiant.

SPS. (Carolina Medical Prod. Co.) Sodium polystyrene sulfonate 15 Gm, sorbitol solution 21.5 ml, alcohol 0.18 ml/60 ml Susp. Bot. 60 ml, 120 ml.
Use: Potassium removing resin.

S-P-T. (Fleming) Pork thyroid, desiccated. 1 gr, 2 gr, 3 gr, 5 gr/Cap. Bot. 100s, 1000s.
Use: Thyroid hormone.

SRC EXPECTORANT. (Edwards) Hydrocodone bitartrate 5 mg, pseudoephedrine HCl 60 mg, guaifenesin 200 mg, alcohol 12.5%. Bot. pt.
Use: Antitussive, decongestant, expectorant.

SSKI. (Upsher-Smith) Potassium iodide. 300 mg/0.3 ml Soln. Dropper Bot. 1 oz, 8 oz.
Use: Expectorant.

S-SPAS. (Southern States) Pentobarbital 16.2 mg, atropine sulfate 0.0194 mg, hyoscyamine sulfate 0.1037 mg, hyoscine HBr 0.0065 mg/Tab. or 5 ml **Liq.** Bot. pt. **Tab.** Bot. 100s, 1000s.
Use: Sedative/hypnotic, anticholinergic/antispasmodic.

S.T. 37. (Beecham Products) Hexylresorcinol 0.1% in glycerin aqueous soln. Bot. 5.5 oz, 12 oz.
Use: Antiseptic, topical.

STADOL. (Bristol) Butorphanol tartrate. **1 mg/ml:** Vial 1 ml. **2 mg/ml:** Vial 1 ml, 2 ml, 10 ml.
Use: Analgesic.

STAFTABS. (Modern) Fine bone flour containing Ca, P, Fe, I, vitamin D, Mg/Tab. Bot. 85s, 160s.
Use: Vitamin/mineral supplement.

STAINLESS IODIZED OINTMENT. (Day-Baldwin) Jar lb.

STAINLESS IODIZED OINTMENT WITH METHYL SALICYLATE 5%. (Day-Baldwin) Jar lb.

STALL. (Cenci) o-Hydroxybenzoic acid 0.5%, thymol 0.5%, ethyl alcohol S.D. 70%. Bot. 0.5 oz, 2 oz. w/dropper.
Use: Otic preparation.

•**STALLIMYCIN HYDROCHLORIDE.** USAN.
Use: Antibacterial.

STAMYL TABLETS. (Winthrop) Pancreatin.
Use: Digestive aid.

STANACAINE. (Standex) Lidocaine HCl 2% Bot. 50 ml.
Use: Local anesthetic.

STANACILLIN. (Standex) Buffered penicillin 250,000 units/Tab. or 500,000 units/Tab. Bot. 100s.
Use: Antibacterial.

STANACILLIN PO. (Standex) Buffered penicillin Pow. 250,000 units Bot. 60 ml; 500,000 units Bot. 80 ml.
Use: Antibacterial.

STAN A SYN. (Standex) Vitamin A palmitate 50,000 IU/Cap. Bot. 100s.
Use: Vitamin A supplement.

STAN A SYN CREME. (Standex) Vitamins A and D. 1 oz.
Use: Vitamin supplement.

STAN A SYN FORTE. (Standex) Vitamin A palmitate 10,000 IU/Cap. Bot. 100s.
Use: Vitamin A supplement.

STAN A SYN FORTE S. (Standex) Vitamin A soluble 10,000 IU/Cap. Bot. 100s.
Use: Vitamin A supplement.

STAN A SYN JR. (Standex) Vitamin A palmitate 25,000 IU/Cap. Bot. 100s.
Use: Vitamin A supplement.

STAN A SYN S. (Standex) Vitamin A soluble 50,000 IU/Cap. Bot. 100s.
Use: Vitamin A supplement.

STANBACK PAIN RELIEF POWDERS. (Stanback) Aspirin 650 mg/Pow. Pkg. 2s, 6s, 24s, 50s.
Use: Salicylate analgesic.

STANBACK MAX-EXTRA STRENGTH. (Stanback) Aspirin 850 mg/Pow. Pkg. 4s, 36s.
Use: Salicylate analgesic.

STANDEX. (Standex) Vitamins A 1333 IU, D 133 IU, B_1 0.33 mg, B_2 0.4 mg, C 10 mg, niacinamide 3.3 mg, iron 3.3 mg, calcium 15 mg, phosphorous 29 mg, sodium carboxymethylcellulose 100 mg/Cap. Bot. 100s.
Use: Vitamin/mineral supplement.

STANNITOL ELIXIR. (Standex) Phenobarbital 0.25 gr, hyoscyamine sulfate 0.1037 mg, atropine sulfate 0.0194 mg, scopolamine HBr 0.0065 mg, alcohol 23%/5 ml. Bot. pt.
Use: Sedative/hypnotic, anticholinergic/antispasmodic.

STANNITOL INJ. (Standex) Dicyclomine HCl 10 mg/ml. Vial 10 ml.
Use: Anticholinergic/antispasmodic.

STANNITOL TAB. (Standex) Phenobarbital 0.25 gr, atropine sulfate 0.0195 mg, hyoscine HBr 0.0065 mg, hyoscyamine sulfate 0.1040 mg/Tab. Bot. 100s.
Use: Sedative/hypnotic, anticholinergic/antispasmodic.

•**STANNOUS CHLORIDE.** USAN.
Use: Pharmaceutic aid.

•**STANNOUS FLUORIDE,** U.S.P. XXII. Gel, U.S.P. XXII. Tin fluoride.
Use: Dental caries prophylactic.

STANNOUS FLUORIDE. (City Chem.) Stannous fluoride. Bot. 4 oz, lb.
Use: Dental caries preventative.

•**STANNOUS PYROPHOSPHATE.** USAN.
Use: Diagnostic aid (bone imaging).

•**STANNOUS SULFUR COLLOID.** USAN.
Use: Diagnostic aid (bone, liver, and spleen imaging).

STANOLONE. B.A.N. Androstanolone, dihydrotestosterone, androstane-17(β)-ol-3-one. 17 β-Hydroxy-5 α-androstan-3-one.
See: Anabolic steroid.

•**STANOZOLOL,** U.S.P. XXII. Tab., U.S.P. XXII. 17 β-Hydroxy-17 α-methylandrostano[3,2-c] pyrazole. 17-Methyl-2′H-5 α-androst-2-eno(3,2-c)pyrazol-17 β-ol. Formerly Androstanazole.
Use: Anabolic agent (androgen).
See: Stromba.
Winstrol Tab. (Winthrop).

STANPRO-75. (Standex) Phenylpropanolamine 75 mg/ml. Vial 30 ml.
Use: Decongestant.

STANTEEN CAP. (Standex) Vitamins A 5000 IU, D 400 IU, B_1 3 mg, B_2 2.5 mg, C 50 mg, niacinamide 20 mg, calcium 46 mg, phosphorous 35 mg, iron 1.34 mg, B_6 1 mg, calcium pantothenate 2 mg, B_{12} 2 mcg, magnesium 1 mg, manganese 1.5 mg, potassium 5 mg, zinc 1.4 mg/Cap. Bot. 100s.
Use: Vitamin/mineral supplement.

STAPHAGE LYSATE (SPL). (Delmont) Phage-lysed staphylococci 120-180 million/ml Amp. 1 ml, package 10s for inj.; multidose Vial 10 ml for other methods of administration.
Use: Anti-infective.

STAPHCILLIN. (Bristol) Methicillin sodium w/3 mEq sodium/Gm, 1 Gm/Vial. Vial 1 Gm, 4 Gm, 6 Gm; Piggyback Vial 1 Gm, 4 Gm.
Use: Antibacterial; penicillin.

•**STARCH,** N.F. XVII.
Use: Dusting powder; tablet disintegrant.
See: Mexsana, Pow. (Schering-Plough).

STARCH GLYCERITE.
Use: Emollient.

•**STARCH, PREGELATINIZED,** N.F. XVII.
Use: Pharmaceutic aid (tablet excipient).

•**STARCH, TOPICAL,** U.S.P. XXII.
Use: Dusting powder.

STAR-OTIC. (Star) Burrows soln. 10%, acetic acid 1%, boric acid 1%. Dropper bot. 15 ml.
Use: Otic preparation.

STATICIN 1.5%. (Westwood) Erythromycin 15 mg/ml, alcohol 55%, propylene glycol, laureth-4 fragrance. Soln. Bot. 60 ml.
Use: Anti-acne.

•**STATOLON.** USAN. Antiviral agent derived from *Penicillium stoloniferum.*
Use: Antiviral agent.

STATOMIN MALEATE II. (Bowman) Chlorpheniramine maleate 2 mg, acetaminophen 324 mg, caffeine 32 mg/Tab. Bot. 1000s.
Use: Antihistamine, analgesic.

STATROL. (Alcon) Polymyxin B sulfate 16 units/ml or 250 units/ml, neomycin 3.5 mg/ml, hydroxypropyl methylcellulose 0.5%. Droptainer 5 ml.
Use: Anti-infective, ophthalmic.

STATROL STERILE OPHTHALMIC OINTMENT (Alcon) Polymyxin B sulfate 10,000 units, neomycin 3.5 mg/Gm. Tube 3.5 Gm.
Use: Anti-infective, ophthalmic.

STA-WAKE DEXTABS. (Approved) Caffeine 1.5 gr, dextrose 3 gr/Tab. Bot. 36s, 1000s.
Use: CNS stimulant.

STAY-ALERT. (E.J. Moore) Caffeine 250 mg/Cap. Bot. 12s, 18s.
Use: CNS stimulant.

STAY AWAKE CAPSULES. (Whiteworth) Caffeine 250 mg/Cap. Bot. 30s.
Use: CNS Stimulant.

STAY-BRITE. (Sherman) EDTA 0.25%, benzalkonium Cl 0.01%. Spray 30 ml.
Use: Hard contact lens care.

STAYMINS. (Stayner) Vitamins A 5000 IU, D 500 IU, B_1 1.5 mg, B_2 1.5 mg, niacinamide 10 mg, B_6 0.5 mg, C 50 mg, B_{12} 2 mcg/5 ml. Bot. 16 oz.
Use: Vitamin supplement.

STAYMINS TABLETS. (Stayner) Vitamins A 5000 IU, D 500 IU, E 1 IU, B_1 2.5 mg, B_2 2.5 mg, B_6 0.5 mg, B_{12} 2 mcg, C 50 mg, calcium pantothenate 5 mg, niacinamide 20 mg, inositol 10 mg, choline bitartrate 10 mg/Tab. Bot. 100s, 1000s.
Use: Vitamin/mineral supplement.

STAYNERAL TABLETS. (Stayner) Vitamins A 5000 IU, D 500 IU, E 5 IU, B_1 5 mg, B_2 5 mg,

B_6 1 mg, C 100 mg, B_{12} 2 mcg, niacinamide 25 mg, calcium pantothenate 5 mg, calcium 50 mg, phosphorous 40 mg, iron 10 mg, manganese 0.5 mg, zinc 0.1 mg, magnesium 0.5 mg, iodine 0.2 mg, copper 0.1 mg/Tab. Bot. 100s, 1000s.
Use: Vitamin/mineral supplement.

STAY TRIM. (Schering-Plough) Phenylpropanolamine. **Gum:** 8.33 mg. In 20s. **Mints:** 12.5 mg. Tab. Roll 36s.
Use: Diet aid.

STAY-UPS. (Faraday) Tab. Bot. 30s.
Use: To combat fatigue.

STAY-WET. (Sherman) Polyvinyl alcohol, hydroxyethylcellulose, povidone, sodium Cl, potassium Cl, sodium carbonate, benzalkonium Cl 0.01%, EDTA 0.025%. Soln. Bot. 30 ml.
Use: Hard contact lens care.

STAZE. (Commerce) Karaya gum. Tube 1.75 oz, 3.5 oz.
Use: Denture adhesive.

STEAPSIN.
W/Oxidized bile acids, ox bile, homatropine methylbromide.
See: Oxacholin, Tab. (Philips Roxane).

•**STEARIC ACID,** N.F. XVII. Purified, N.F. XVII. Octadecanoic acid.
Use: Pharmaceutic aid (emulsion adjunct, tablet lubricant).

•**STEARYL ALCOHOL,** N.F. XVII.
Use: Pharmaceutic aid (emulsion adjunct).

•**STEFFIMYCIN.** USAN.
Use: Antibacterial, antiviral.

STELAZINE. (SmithKline) Trifluoperazine HCl. **Tab.** 1 mg, 2 mg, 5 mg or 10 mg. Bot. 100s, 1000s, UD 100s. **Inj.** 2 mg/ml, Vial 10 ml Box 1s, 20s. **Oral Conc.:** 10 mg/ml Bot. 2 fl oz, Ctn. 12s.
Use: Antipsychotic.

•**STENOBOLONE ACETATE.** USAN. 17-beta-Hydroxy-2-methyl-5-alpha-androst-1-en-3-one acetate.
Use: Inj. anabolic.

STERAJECT. (Mayrand) Prednisolone acetate 25 mg/ml or 50 mg/ml. Vial 10 ml.
Use: Corticosteroid.

STERAPRED DS. (Mayrand) Prednisone 10 mg/Tab. Uni-pak 21s.
Use: Corticosteroid.

STERAPRED-UNIPAK. (Mayrand) Prednisone 5 mg/Tab. Dosepak tab 21s.
Use: Corticosteroid.

STERCULIA GUM.
See: Karaya Gum (Various Mfr.).
W/Vitamin B_1.
See: Imbicoll w/Vitamin B_1 (Upjohn).

STERICOL. (Alton) Isopropyl alcohol 91%. Bot. 16 oz, 32 oz, gal.
Use: Antibacterial, external.

•**STERILE AUROTHIOGLUCOSE SUSPENSION,** U.S.P. XXII. Authothioglucose Injection. Gold thioglucose. Gold, (l-thio-D-glucopyranosato)-. (l-Thio-D glucopyranosato) gold.
Use: Antirheumatic.
See: Solganal, Vial (Schering).

•**STERILE ERYTHROMYCIN GLUCEPTATE,** U.S.P. XXII. Erythromycin monoglucoheptonate (salt). Erythromycin glucoheptonate (1:1) (salt).
Use: Antibacterial.

STERILE THIOPENTAL SODIUM. Thiopental sodium, U.S.P. XXII.
See: Pentothal Sodium, Amp. (Abbott).

STERI-UNNA BOOT. (Pedinol) Glycerin, acacia gum, zinc oxide, white petrolatum, amylum in oil base. 10 Yds. × 3.5 in. sterilized bandage.
Use: Treatment of leg ulcers, varicosities, sprains, strains and to reduce swelling after surgery.

STEROLOX. (Kenyon) Benzethonium Cl, benzoic acid, salicylic acid, thymol, menthol, isopropyl alcohol 50%. Bot. 2 oz, pt, gal.

S-T FORTE SUGAR FREE LIQUID. (Scot-Tussin) Hydrocodone bitartrate 2.5 mg, phenylephrine HCl 5 mg, phenylpropanolamine HCl 5 mg, pheniramine maleate 13.33 mg, guaifenesin 80 mg/5 ml, alcohol 5%. Bot. 4 oz, 8 oz, pt, gal.
Use: Antitussive, decongestant, antihistamine, expectorant.

S-T FORTE SYRUP. (Scot-Tussin) Hydrocodone bitartrate 2.5 mg, phenylephrine HCl 5 mg, phenylpropanolamine HCl 5 mg, pheniramine maleate 13.33 mg, guaifenesin 80 mg/5 ml, alcohol 5%. Bot. 8 oz, pt, gal.
Use: Antitussive, decongestant, antihistamine, expectorant.

STIBAMINE GLUCOSIDE. B.A.N. Sodium 4- glucosylaminophenylstibonate.
Use: Treatment of leishmaniasis.

STIBOCAPTATE. B.A.N. Antimony(III) sodium meso-2, 3-dimercaptosuccinate.
Use: Treatment of schistosomiasis.

STILBAMIDINE. B.A.N. 4, 4′-Diamidinostilbene.
Use: Treatment of trypanosomiasis.

STILBAMIDINE ISETHIONATE. 2-Hydroxyethane-sulfonic acid compound with 4, 4′-stilbenedicarboxamidine.
Use: Antiprotozoal.

•**STILBAZIUM IODIDE.** USAN. 1-Ethyl-2, 6-bis(p-1-pyrrolidinyl-styryl)-pyridinium iodide.
Use: Anthelmintic.
See: Monopar.

STILBESTROL.
See: Diethylstilbestrol, U.S.P. XXII. (Various Mfr.).

STILBESTRONATE.
See: Diethylstilbestrol Dipropionate (Various Mfr.).

STILBOESTROL.
See: Diethylstilbestrol (Various Mfr.).

STILBOESTROL DP.
See: Diethylstilbestrol Dipropionate (Various Mfr.).

STILLMAN'S. (Stillman) Cream. Jar 7/8 oz, Cream Bella Aurora: 7/8 oz.

•**STILONIUM IODIDE.** USAN.
Use: Antispasmodic.

STILPHOSTROL. (Miles Pharm) Diethylstilbestrol diphosphate. Amp. (250 mg/5 ml as sodium salt) 5 ml. Box 20s. Tab. 50 mg. Bot. 50s.
Use: Antineoplastic agent.

STILRONATE.
See: Diethylstilbestrol Dipropionate (Various Mfr.).

STIMATE. (Armour) Desmopressin acetate 4 mcg/ml. Vial 10 ml.
Use: Posterior pituitary hormone.

STIMURUB. (Otis Clapp) Menthol, methyl salicylate, oleo resin of capsicum, in greaseless base. Tube 36 × 0.25 oz, 1 oz, Jar. 16 oz.
Use: External analgesic.

STING-EZE. (Wisconsin) Bot. 0.5 oz.
Use: Antihistamine, topical.

STING-KILL. (MiLance) Benzocaine 18.9%, menthol 0.9%. Swab 14 ml, 0.5 ml (5s).
Use: Local anesthetic.

STIRIMAZOLE. B.A.N. 2-(4-Carboxystyryl)-5-nitro-1-vinylimidazole.
Use: Treatment of amebiasis, trichomoniasis, trypanosomiasis.

•**STIRIPENTOL.** USAN.
Use: Anticonvulsant.

•**STIROFOS.** USAN.
Use: Insecticide (veterinary).

ST. JOSEPH ASPIRIN FOR ADULTS. (Schering-Plough) Aspirin 5 gr/Tab. Bot. 36s, 100s, 200s.
Use: Salicylate analgesic.

ST. JOSEPH ASPIRIN-FREE ELIXIR FOR CHILDREN. (Schering-Plough) Acetaminophen 160 mg/5 ml. Alcohol Free. Bot. 2 oz, 4oz.
Use: Analgesic.

ST. JOSEPH ASPIRIN-FREE INFANT DROPS. (Schering-Plough) Acetaminophen 100 mg/ml/ 0.8 ml dropper. Aspirin and sugar free. Bot. 0.5 oz.
Use: Analgesic.

ST. JOSEPH ASPIRIN-FREE TABLETS FOR CHILDREN. (Schering-Plough) Acetaminophen 80 mg/Tab. Bot. 30s.
Use: Analgesic.

ST. JOSEPH COLD TABLETS FOR CHILDREN. (Schering-Plough) Aspirin 81 mg, phenylpropanolamine HCl 3.125 mg/Tab. Bot. 30s.
Use: Analgesic, decongestant.

ST. JOSEPH COUGH SYRUP FOR CHILDREN. (Schering-Plough) Dextromethorphan HBr 7.5 mg/5 ml. Bot. 2 oz, 4 oz.
Use: Antitussive.

STOMACH SUBSTANCE DESICCATED.
W/Vitamin B_{12}, cobalt gluconate, ferrous gluconate.

STOMAL. (Foy) Phenobarbital 16.2 mg, hyoscyamine sulfate 0.1037 mg, atropine sulfate 0.0194 mg, scopolamine HBr 0.0065 mg/Tab. Bot. 1000s.
Use: Sedative/hypnotic, anticholinergic/antispasmodic.

STOOL SOFTENER. (Amlab) Docusate sodium 100 mg or 250 mg/Cap. Bot. 100s.
Use: Laxative.

STOOL SOFTENER. (Weeks & Leo) Docusate sodium 100 mg or 250 mg/Cap. Bot. 30s, 100s. Calcium docusate 240 mg/Cap. Bot. 100s.
Use: Laxative.

STOP. (Oral-B) Stannous fluoride 0.4%. Tube 2 oz.
Use: Dental caries preventative.

STOPAYNE CAPSULES. (Springbok) Codeine phosphate 30 mg, acetaminophen 357 mg/Cap. Bot. 100s, 500s, UD 100s.
Use: Antitussive, analgesic.

STOPAYNE SYRUP. (Springbok) Acetaminophen 120 mg, codeine phosphate 12 mg/5 ml. Bot. 4 oz, 16 oz.
Use: Analgesic, antitussive.

STOP-ZIT. (Purepac) Denatonium benzoate in a clear nail polish base. Bot. 0.75 oz.
Use: Thumbsucking/nail-biting deterrent.

•**STORAX,** U.S.P. XXII.
Use: Pharmaceutic necessity for Compound Benzoin Tincture.

STOVARSOL.
Use: Amebicide.
See: Acetarsone, Tab.

STOXIL. (SKF) Idoxuridine. **Ophthalmic Soln.:** 0.1%, thimerosal 1:50,000. Bot. 15 ml with dropper. **Ophthalmic oint.:** 0.5%, petrolatum base (5 mg/Gm.) Tube 4 Gm.
Use: Antiviral.

STREMA. (Foy) Quinine sulfate 260 mg/Cap. Bot. 100s, 500s, 1000s.
Use: Antimalarial.

STREN-TAB. (Barth's) Vitamins C 300 mg, B_1 10 mg, B_2 10 mg, niacin 33 mg, B_6 2 mg, pantothenic acid 20 mg, B_{12} 4 mcg/Tab. Bot. 100s, 300s, 500s.
Use: Vitamin supplement.

STREPTASE (Hoechst-Roussel) Streptokinase I.V. infusion. 250,000 IU/Vial 6.5 ml; 750,000 IU/Vial 6.5 ml Vial ctn. 10s.
Use: Thrombolytic enzyme.

STREPTOCOCCI.
W/*Haemophilus influenzae, Neisseria catarrhalis, Klebsiella pneumoniae, staphylocci, pneumococci,* killed.
See: Mixed Vaccine No. 4 W-H. Influenzae (Lilly).

STREPTOCOCCI VACCINE, KILLED.
W/*Neisseria catarrhalis, Klebsiella pneumoniae, Diplococcus pneumoniae, staphylococci.*
See: Combined Vaccine No. 4 w/Catarrhalis (Lilly).

STREPTODORNASE. B.A.N. An enzyme obtained from cultures of various strains of *Streptococcus hemolyticus.*

See: Streptokinase.

STREPTODUOCIN. B.A.N. A mixture of equal parts of streptomycin and dihydrostreptomycin sulfates.
Use: Antibiotic.

STREPTOHYDRAZID. Streptomyclideneisonicotinyl hydrazine sulfate. Streptonicozid. B.A.N. Streptomycin isoniazid.
Use: Antituberculous agent.

STREPTOKINASE. B.A.N. An enzyme obtained from cultures of various strains of *Streptococcus hemolyticus.*
See: Kabikinase.
Streptase, Inj. (Hoechst).

STREPTOLYSIN O TEST. (Laboratory Diagnostics) Diagnosis of "Group A" streptococcal infections. Reagent 6 × 10 ml, buffer 6 × 40 ml, Control Serum, 6 × 10 ml or Kit.
Use: Diagnostic aid.

STREPTOMYCIN CALCIUM CHLORIDE. Streptomycin Calcium Chloride Complex.

STREPTOMYCIN ISONIAZID.
See: Streptohydrazid.

•**STREPTOMYCIN SULFATE INJECTION,** U.S.P. XXII. Sterile, U.S.P. XXII. (Various Mfr.).
Use: Antibacterial (tuberculostatic).
W/Dihydrostreptomycin sulfate.
See: Streptoduocin, Inj. (Various Mfr.).

STREPTOMYCYLIDENE ISONICOTINYL HYDRAZINE SULFATE.
See: Streptohydrazid.

•**STREPTONICOZID.** USAN. Streptomycylidene isonicotinyl hydrazine sulfate.
Use: Antibiotic.
See: Streptohydrazid.

STREPTONIGRIN. USAN. Antibiotic isolated from both filtrates of *Streptomyces flocculus.* 5-Amino-6-(7-amino-5, 8-dihydro-6-methoxy-5, 8-dioxo-2-quinolyl)-4-(2-hydroxy-3, 4-dimethoxyphenyl)-3-methylpicolinic acid.
Use: Antineoplastic agent.
See: Nigrin (Pfizer).

STREPTOVARICIN. An antibiotic composed of several related components derived from cultures of *Streptomyces variabilis.*
See: Dalacin (Upjohn).

STREPTOZOCIN. USAN.
Use: Antineoplastic.
See: Zanosar, Pow. (Upjohn).

STREPTOZYME. (Wampole) Rapid hemagglutination slide test for the qualitative detection and quantitative determination of streptococcal extracellular antigens in serum, plasma and peripheral blood. Kit 15s, 50s, 150s.
Use: Diagnostic aid.

STRESS-BEE CAPSULES. (Rugby) Vitamins B_1 10 mg, B_2 10 mg, B_3 100 mg, B_5 20 mg, B_6 2 mg, B_{12} 6 mcg, C 300 mg/Cap. Bot. 100s.
Use: Vitamin supplement.

STRESSCAPS. (Lederle) Vitamins B_1 10 mg, B_2 10 mg, niacinamide 100 mg, C 300 mg, B_6 2 mg, B_{12} 6 mcg, calcium pantothenate 20 mg/Cap. Bot. 100s.
Use: Vitamin supplement.

STRESS FORMULA. (Various Mfr.) Vitamins E 30 mg, B_1 15 mg, B_2 15 mg, B_3 100 mg, B_5 20 mg, B_6 5 mg, B_{12} 12 mcg, C 600 mg, folic acid 0.4 mg, biotin 45 mcg/Cap. or Tab. **Cap.:** Bot. 60s, 100s, 1000s. **Tab.:** Bot. 30s, 60s, 100s, 250s, 300s, 400s, 1000s, UD 100s.
Use: Vitamin supplement.

STRESS FORMULA 600. (Halsey)
Use: Vitamin supplement.

STRESS FORMULA 600 W/IRON. (Halsey)
Use: Vitamin supplement.

STRESS FORMULA 600 PLUS IRON. (Schein) Iron 27 mg, vitamins E 30 IU, B_1 15 mg, B_2 15 mg, B_3 100 mg, B_5 20 mg, B_6 5 mg, B_{12} 12 mcg, C 600 mg, folic acid 0.4 mg, biotin 45 mcg/Tab. Bot. 60s, 250s.
Use: Vitamin/mineral supplement.

STRESS FORMULA 600 W/ZINC. (Halsey)
Use: Vitamin/mineral supplement.

STRESS FORMULA WITH ZINC. (Towne) Vitamins E 45 IU, C 600 mg, folic acid 400 mcg, B_1 20 mg, B_2 10 mg, niacinamide 100 mg, B_6 10 mg, B_{12} 25 mcg, biotin 40 mcg, pantothenic acid 25 mg, copper 3 mg, zinc 23.9 mg/Tab. Bot. 60s.
Use: Vitamin/mineral supplement.

STRESSTABS 600. (Lederle) Vitamins B_1 15 mg, B_2 10 mg, B_6 5 mg, B_{12} 12 mcg, C 600 mg, niacinamide 100 mg, E 30 IU, biotin 45 mcg, folic acid 400 mcg, calcium pantothenate 20 mg/Tab. Bot. 30s, 60s, UD 10 × 10s.
Use: Vitamin/mineral supplement.

STRESSTABS 600 ADVANCED FORMULA. (Lederle) Vitamins E 30 mg, B_1 15 mg, B_2 10 mg, B_3 100 mg, B_5 20 mg, B_6 5 mg, B_{12} 12 mcg, C 600 mg, folic acid 0.4 mg, biotin 45 mcg. Bot. 30s, 60s, UD 100s.
Use: Vitamin supplement.

STRESSTABS 600 WITH IRON TABLETS. (Lederle) Ferrous fumerate 27 mg, E 30 IU, B_1 15 mg, B_2 15 mg, B_3 100 mg, B_5 20 mg, B_6 5 mg, B_{12} 12 mcg, C 600 mg, folic acid 0.4 mg, biotin 45 mcg/Tab. Bot. 30s, 60s.
Use: Vitamin/mineral supplement.

STRESSTABS 600 WITH ZINC. (Lederle) Vitamins B_1 15 mg, B_2 10 mg, B_3 100 mg, B_5 20 mg, B_6 5 mg, B_{12} 12 mcg, C 600 mg, E 30 IU, folic acid 0.4 mg, biotin 45 mcg, Cu, zinc 23.9 mg/Tab. Bot. 30s, 60s.
Use: Vitamin/mineral supplement.

STRESSTEIN. (Sandoz Nutrition) Maltodextrin, medium chain triglycerides, L-leucine, soybean oil, L-isoleucine, L-valine, L-glutamic acid, L-arginine, L-lysine acetate, L-alanine, L-threonine, L-phenylalamine, L-asparticacid, L-histidine, L-methionine, glycine, polyglycerol esters of fatty acids, L-serine, L-proline, sodium Cl, L-tryptophan, L-cysteine, sodium citrate, vitamins, minerals. Pow. 3.4 oz. packets.

Use: Enteral nutritional supplement.

STRI-DEX B.P. (Glenbrook) Benzoyl peroxide 10% in greaseless, vanishing cream base.
Use: Anti-acne.

STRI-DEX LOTION. (Glenbrook) Salicylic acid 0.5%, alcohol 28%, sulfonated alkyl benzenes, citric acid, sodium carbonate, simethicone, water. Bot. 4 oz.
Use: Anti-acne.

STRI-DEX MAXIMUM STRENGTH PADS. (Glenbrook) Salicylic acid 2%, SD alcohol 44%, citric acid.
Use: Anti-acne.

STRI-DEX REGULAR STRENGTH PADS. (Glenbrook) Salicylic acid 0.5%, SD alcohol 28%, citric acid. In 42s, 75s.
Use: Anti-acne.

STROMBA AMPULES. (Winthrop) Stanozolol.
Use: Anabolic steroid.

STRONTIUM BROMIDE. Crystals or Granules, Bot. 0.25 lb, lb. Amp. 1 Gm/10 ml.
Use: Sedative, antiepileptic.

W/Bromides of sodium, potassium, ammonium.
See: Lanabrom, Elix. (Lannett).

•**STRONTIUM CHLORIDE Sr 85.** USAN.
Use: Radioactive agent.

STRONTIUM LACTATE TRIHYDRATE.

•**STRONTIUM NITRATE Sr 85.** USAN.
Use: Radioactive agent.

STRONTIUM SR 85 INJECTION.
Use: Diagnostic aid (bone scanning).

STROPHANTHIN. K-strophanthin.

STROPHEN. (Kenyon) Prednisone 0.75 mg, salicylamide 5 gr, aluminum hydroxide gel 75 mg, vitamin C 20 mg/Tab. Bot. 100s, 1000s.
Use: Arthritis.

STROVITE PLUS TABLETS. (Everett) Vitamins A 5000 IU, E 30 mg, B_1 20 mg, B_2 20 mg, B_3 100 mg, B_5 25 mg, B_6 25 mg, B_{12} 50 mcg, C 500 mg, iron 27 mg, zinc 22.5 mg, biotin 150 mcg, Cr, Cu, Mg, Mn. Bot. 100s.
Use: Vitamin/mineral supplement.

STROVITE TABLETS. (Everett) Vitamins B_1 15 mg, B_2 15 mg, B_3 100 mg, B_5 18 mg, B_6 4 mg, B_{12} 5 mcg, C 500 mg, folic acid 0.5 mg Bot. 100s.
Use: Vitamin supplement.

STYPT-AID. (Pharmakon Labs) Benzocaine 28.71 mg, methylbenzethonium HCl 9.95 mg, aluminum Cl hexahydrate 55.43 mg, ethyl alcohol 70.97%/ml in a glycerine, menthol base. Spray. 60 ml.
Use: Local anesthetic.

STUART FORMULA. (Stuart) Vitamins A 5000 IU, B_1 1.5 mg, B_2 1.7 mg niacin 20 mg, B_6 2 mg, B_{12} 6 mcg, C 60 mg, D 400 IU, E 15 IU, iron 18 mg, phosphate 125 mg, folic acid 0.4 mg, Ca, I, Mg, P/Tab. Bot. 100s, 250s.
Use: Vitamin/mineral supplement.

STUARTINIC. (Stuart) Vitamins B_{12} 25 mcg, B_1 6 mg, B_2 6 mg, niacinamide 20 mg, B_5 10 mg, calcium pantothenate 10 mg, B_6 1 mg, C 525 mg, iron 100 mg/Tab. Bot. 60s.
Use: Vitamin/mineral supplement.

STUARTNATAL 1 + 1. (Stuart) Vitamins A 4000 IU, B_1 1.5 mg, B_2 3 mg, niacin 20 mg, B_6 10 mg, B_{12} 12 mcg, C 120 mg, D 400 IU, E 11 mg, folic acid 1 mg, calcium 200 mg, iron 65 mg, zinc 25 mg, copper 2 mg/Tab. Bot. 100s, 500s.
Use: Vitamin/mineral supplement.

STUART PRENATAL. (Stuart) Vitamins A 4000 IU, B_1 1.5 mg, B_2 1.7 mg, B_6 2.6 mg, B_{12} 4 mcg, C 100 mg, D 400 IU, E 11 mg, niacin 18 mg, iron 60 mg, calcium 200 mg, copper 2 mg, zinc 25 mg, folic acid 0.8 mg/Tab. Bot. 100s.
Use: Vitamin/mineral supplement.

STULEX. (Bowman) Docusate sodium 250 mg/Tab. Bot. 100s, 1000s.
Use: Laxative.

STYE. (Commerce) Yellow mercuric oxide 1%, boric acid, zinc sulfate, light mineral oil, white petrolatum, cod liver oil, anhydrous lanolin. Tube 0.125 oz.
Use: Ophthalmic preparation.

STYPTIRENAL.
See: Epinephrine (Various Mfr.).

STYPTO-CAINE SOLUTION. (Pedinol) Hydroxyquinoline sulfate, tetracaine HCl, aluminum Cl, aqueous glycol base. Bot. 2 oz.
Use: Hemostatic.

STYRAMATE. B.A.N. 1-Phenyl-1,2-ethanediol 2-carbamate. β-Hydroxyphenethyl carbamate. 2-Hydroxy-2-phenylethyl carbamate.
Use: Skeletal muscle relaxant.

STYRENE POLYMER, SULFONATED, SODIUM SALT. Sodium Polystyrene Sulfonate, U.S.P. XXII.

STYRONATE RESINS. Ammonium and potassium salts of sulfonated styrene polymers.
Use: Conditions requiring sodium restriction.

SUBLIMAZE. (Janssen) Fentanyl 0.05 mg as citrate/ml. Amp. 10 ml, 20 ml. Pkg. 2s, 5s.
Use: Narcotic analgesic.

•**SUCCIMER.** USAN.
Use: Diagnostic aid.

SUCCINATES.
See: Calcium succinate.
Sodium succinate.
Succinic acid.

SUCCINCHLORIMIDE. N-Chlorosuccinimide.

SUCCINIC ACID.

W/9-Aminoacridine HCl, phenyl mercuric acetate, sodium lauryl acetate.

W/9-Aminoacridine undecylenate, N-myristyl-3-hydroxybutylamine HCl, methylbenzethonium Cl.
See: Cenasert, Tab. (Central).

•**SUCCINYLCHOLINE CHLORIDE,** U.S.P. XXII. Inj., Sterile, U.S.P. XXII. Ethanaminium, 2,2′-[(1,4-dioxo-1,4-butanediyl)bis(oxy)]bis-N,NN-trimethyl-, dichlo- ride. Choline Cl succinate (2:1).
Use: Skeletal muscle relaxant.
See: Anectine Cl, Amp. (Burroughs Wellcome).

Quelicin, Amp., Additive Syringe, Fliptop and Pintop Vial (Abbott).
Sucostrin, Amp., Vial (Squibb Marsam).

SUCCINYLSULFATHIAZOLE. 4′-(2-Thiazolysulfamoyl).
Use: Intestinal antibacterial.

SUCOSTRIN. (Squibb-Marsam) Succinylcholine Cl 20 mg/ml Inj. Vial 10 ml.
Use: Muscle relaxant.

SUCOSTRIN CHLORIDE. (Squibb-Marsam) Succinylcholine Cl 20 mg/ml, methylparaben 0.1%, propylparaben 0.01%. Vial 10 ml; High potency 100 mg/ml. Vial 10 ml.
Use: Muscle relaxant.

•**SUCRALFATE.** USAN. Beta-D-fructofuranosyl-alpha-D-glucopyranoside octakis (hydrogen sulfate) aluminum hydroxide complex.
Use: Duodenal ulcer therapy.
See: Carafate, Tab. (Marion).

SUCRALOX. B.A.N. A polymerized complex of sucrose and aluminum hydroxide.
Use: Treatment of gastric hyperacidity.

SUCRETS CHILDREN'S SORE THROAT LOZENGES. (Beecham) Dyclonine HCl 1.2 mg/Loz. Cherry flavor. Tin 24s.
Use: Local anesthetic.

SUCRETS COLD DECONGESTANT LOZENGE. (Beecham) Phenylpropanolamine HCl 25 mg/Loz. Box 24s.
Use: Decongestant.

SUCRETS COUGH CONTROL LOZENGE. (Beecham) Dextromethorphan HBr 5 mg/Loz. Tin 24s.
Use: Antitussive.

SUCRETS MAXIMUM STRENGTH SORE THROAT LOZENGES. (Beecham) Dyclonine HCl 3 mg/Loz. Tin 24s, 48s, 55s.
Use: Local anesthetic.

SUCRETS MAXIMUM STRENGTH SORE THROAT SPRAY & GARGLE. (Beecham) Dyclonine HCl 0.1%, alcohol 10%, sorbitol. Spray Bot. 6 oz, 12 oz. Gargle Bot. 12 oz.
Use: Local anesthetic.

SUCRETS SORE THROAT LOZENGE. (Beecham) Hexylresorcinol 2.4 mg/Loz. **Regular:** Tin 24s, 48s. **Mentholated:** Tin 24s.
Use: Antiseptic.

•**SUCROSE,** N.F. XVII. Compressible, Confectioners, N.F. XVII. Saccharose. Sugar. α-D-Glucopyranoside, β-D-fructo-furanosyl-.
Use: I.V.; diuretic and dehydrating agent; pharmaceutic aid (sweetening agent).

•**SUCROSE OCTAACETATE,** N.F. XVII.
Use: Alcohol denaturant.

SUDAFED CHILDREN'S LIQUID. (Burroughs Wellcome) Pseudoephedrine HCl 30 mg/5 ml. Bot. 4 oz, pt.
Use: Decongestant.

SUDAFED 12 HOUR CAPSULES. (Burroughs Wellcome) Pseudoephedrine HCl 120 mg/SA Cap. Box 10s, 20s, 40s.
Use: Decongestant.

SUDAFED COUGH SYRUP. (Burroughs Wellcome) Pseudoephedrine HCl 15 mg, dextromethorphan HBr 5 mg, guaifenesin 100 mg, alcohol 2.4%. Bot. 4 oz.
Use: Decongestant, antitussive, expectorant.

SUDAFED PLUS. (Burroughs Wellcome) **Tab.:** Pseudoephedrine HCl 60 mg, chlorpheniramine maleate 4 mg/Tab. Box 24s, 48s. **Syr.:** Pseudoephedrine HCl 30 mg, chlorpheniramine maleate 2 mg. Bot. 4 oz.
Use: Decongestant, antihistamine.

SUDAFED SINUS MAXIMUM STRENGTH. (Burroughs Wellcome) Pseudoephedrine 30 mg, acetaminophen 500 mg. Capl. 24s.
Use: Decongestant, analgesic.

SUDAFED TABLETS. (Burroughs Wellcome) Pseudoephedrine HCl 30 mg or 60 mg/Tab. **30 mg:** Box 24s, 48s. Bot. 100s, 1000s. **60 mg:** Bot. 100s, 1000s.
Use: Decongestant.

SUDANYL. (Dover) Pseudoephedrine HCl. Sugar, lactose and salt free. Tab. UD Box 500s.
Use: Decongestant.

SUDDEN TAN LOTION. (Schering-Plough) Padimate O, dihydroxyacetone. Bot. 4 oz.
Use: Artificial tanning agent, sunscreen.

•**SUDOXICAM.** USAN. 4-Hydroxy-2-methyl-N-thiazol-2-yl-2H-1,2-benzothiazine-3-carboxamide 1,1-dioxide.
Use: Anti-inflammatory.

SUDRIN. (Bowman) Pseudoephedrine HCl 30 mg or 60 mg/Tab. Bot. 100s, 1000s.
Use: Decongestant.

SUFENTA. (Janssen) Sufentanil citrate 50 mcg/ml. Amp. 1 ml, 2 ml, 5 ml.
Use: Narcotic analgesic.

•**SUFENTANIL.** USAN.
Use: Analgesic.

•**SUFENTANIL CITRATE.** USAN.
Use: Narcotic analgesic.

•**SUFOTIDINE.** USAN.
Use: Antagonist (to histamine H_2 receptors).

SUFREX. (Janssen) Ketanserin tartrate.
Use: Serotonin antagonist.

•**SUGAR, COMPRESSIBLE,** U.S.P. XXII.
Use: Pharmaceutic aid (sweetening agent, tablet excipient).

•**SUGAR, CONFECTIONER'S,** N.F. XII.
Use: Pharmaceutic aid (sweetening agent, tablet excipient).

•**SUGAR SPHERES,** N.F. XVII.
Use: Pharmaceutic aid (sweetening agent).

SULAMYD SODIUM.
Use: Ophthalmic sulfonamide.
See: Sodium Sulamyd, Ophth. Soln. (Schering).

•**SULAZEPAM.** USAN. 7-Chloro-1,3-dihydro-1-methyl-5-phenyl-2H-1,4-benzodiazepine-2-thione.
Use: Tranquilizer (minor).

SULAZO. (Freeport) Sulfisoxazole 500 mg, phenylazodiaminopyridine HCl 50 mg/Tab. Bot. 1000s.

Use: Urinary anti-infective.
•**SULBACTAM BENZATHINE.** USAN.
Use: Synergistic (penicillin/cephalosporin).
•**SULBACTAM PIVOXIL.** USAN.
Use: Inhibitor, synergist (penicillin/cephalosporin).
•**SULBACTAM SODIUM.** USAN.
Use: Inhibitor (beta-lactamase), synergist (penicillin/cephalosporin).
•**SULBENOX.** USAN.
Use: Growth stimulant (veterinary).
•**SULCONAZOLE NITRATE.** USAN.
Use: Antifungal.
See: Exelderm (Westwood).
SULF-10. (Iolab Pharm.) Sodium sulfacetamide 10%. Bot. 15 ml, Dropperette 1 ml. Box 12s.
Use: Anti-infective, ophthalmic.
SULFA-10 OPHTHALMIC. (Maurry) Sodium sulfacetamide 10%, hydroxyethylcellulose, sodium borate, boric acid, disodium edetate, sodium metabisulfite, sodium thiosulfate 0.2%, chlorobutanol 0.2%, methylparaben 0.015%. Bot. 15 ml.
Use: Anti-infective, ophthalmic.
•**SULFABENZ.** USAN.
Use: Antibacterial, coccidiostat.
•**SULFABENZAMIDE,** U.S.P. XXII. Benzamide, N-(4-aminophenyl) sulfunyl)-N-Sulfanilylbenzamide. Sulfanilylbenzamide, N′ benzoylsulfanilamide.
See: Sultrin, Vag. Tab., Cream (Ortho).
SULFABROMETHAZINE SODIUM.
Use: Antibacterial.
SULFACARBAMIDE (I.N.N.). Sulphaurea. B.A.N.
SULFACET. (Dermik).
See: Sulfacetamide.
•**SULFACETAMIDE,** U.S.P. XXII. Acetamide, N-(4-aminophenyl) sulfonyl)-N-Sulfanilylacetamine. N-acetylsulfanilamide.
Use: Antibacterial.
See: Isopto-Cetamide, Ophth. Soln. (Alcon).
SULFACETAMIDE W/COMBINATIONS.
See: Acet-Dia-Mer Sulfonamides.
Cetapred, Oint. (Alcon).
Chero-Trisulfa (V), Susp. (Vita Elixir).
Sulf-10, Ophth. Soln. (CooperVision).
Sultrin, Tab., Cream (Ortho).
Triurisul, Tab. (Sheryl).
Uridium, Tab. (Pharmex).
Urotrol, Tab. (Mills).
•**SULFACETAMIDE SODIUM,** U.S.P. XXII. Ophth. Oint., Ophth. Soln., U.S.P. XXII. Acetamide, N-[(4-aminophenyl)sulfonyl]-,monosodium salt, monohydrate. N-Sulfanilylacetamide monosodium salt monohydrate.
Use: Antibacterial, ophthalmic.
See: Bleph 10, Liquifilm (Allergan).
Centamide, Ophth. Oint. (Alcon).
Sebizon Lot. (Schering).
Sodium Sulamyd Ophth. Oint. 30% (Schering).
Sulf-10, Drops (Maurry).
Sulf-10, Soln., Drops (Smith, Miller & Patch).
W/Methylcellulose.
See: Sodium Sulamyd Ophth. Soln. 10% (Schering).
W/Phenylephrine HCl, methylparaben, propylparaben.
See: Vasosulf, Liq. (CooperVision).
W/Prednisolone.
See: Cetapred Ophth. Oint. (Alcon).
Vasocidin, Soln. (CooperVision).
W/Prednisolone acetate.
See: Blephamide S.O.P., Ophth. Oint. (Allergan).
Metimyd, Ophth. Oint., Susp. (Schering).
W/Prednisolone, methylcellulose.
See: Isopto Cetapred, Susp. (Alcon).
W/Prednisolone acetate, phenylephrine.
See: Blephamide Liquifilm, Ophth. Susp. (Allergan).
Tri-Ophtho, Ophth. Drops (Maurry).
W/Prednisolone phosphate.
See: Optimyd Soln., Sterile (Schering).
W/Prednisolone sodium phosphate, phenylephrine, sulfacetamide sodium.
Vasocidia, Ophth. Soln. (CooperVision).
W/Sulfur.
See: Sulfacet-R, Lot. (Dermik).
•**SULFACETAMIDE SODIUM AND PREDNISOLONE ACETATE OPHTHALMIC OINTMENT,** U.S.P. XXII.
Use: Antibiotic, anti-inflammatory.
See: AK-Cide (Akorn).
Blephamide S.O.P. (Allergan).
Cetapred (Alcon).
Metimyd (Schering).
Predsulfair (Pharmafair).
Vasocidin (Iolab Pharm).
SULFACETAMIDE, SULFADIAZINE, & SULFAMERAZINE ORAL SUSPENSION.
See: Acet-Dia-Mer-Sulfonamides.
SULFACET-R LOTION. (Dermik) Sodium sulfacetamide 10%, sulfur 5%, in flesh-tinted base. Bot. 25 Gm.
Use: Anti-acne, antiseborrheic.
SULFACHLORPYRIDAZINE. B.A.N. N^1-(6-chloro-3-pyridazinyl) sulfanilamide.
SULFADIASULFONE SODIUM. Acetosulfone sodium.
•**SULFADIAZINE,** U.S.P. XXII.; Tab., U.S.P. XXII. 2-Sulfanilamidopyridine, N′-2-pyrimidinylsulfanilamide. Benzenesulfonamide, 4-amino-N-2-pyrimidi-nyl-.
Use: Antibacterial.
See: Microsulfon, Tab. (Consolid. Mid.).
SULFADIAZINE COMBINATIONS.
See: Acet-Dia-Mer-Sulfonamides. (Various Mfr.).
Chemozine, Tab., Susp. (Tennessee Pharm.).
Cherasulfa, Liq, Tab. (Cenci).
Chero-Trisulfa, Susp. (Vita Elixir).
Dia-Mer-Sulfonamides (Various Mfr.).
Dia-Mer-Thia-Sulfonamide (Various Mfr.).
Lantrisul, Tab., Susp. (Lannett).
Meth-Dia-Mer-Sulfonamides (Various Mfr.).

Silvadene (Marion).
Sulfajen, Cream (Jenkins).
Terfonyl, Liq., Tab. (Squibb).
Triosulf, Tab. (Jenkins).
Triple Sulfa, Tab. (Various Mfr.).

SULFADIAZINE AND SULFAMERAZINE. Citrasulfas.
See: Dia-Mer-Sulfonamides.

SULFADIAZINE SODIUM, U.S.P. XXII. Sterile Inj., U.S.P. XXII. Benzenesulfonamide, 4-amino-N-2- pyrimidinyl-, monosodium salt. N^1-2-Pyrimidinylsulfanilamide monosodium salt.
Use: Antibacterial.
W/Sodium bicarbonate.
(Pitman-Moore)—Tab. 2.5 gr Bot. 100s, 500s, 1000s; 5 gr Bot. 1000s.

SULFADIAZINE, SULFAMERAZINE & SULFACETAMIDE SUSPENSION.
See: Acet-Dia-Mer-Sulfonamides.
Coco Diazine (Lilly).

SULFADIMETHOXINE. Sulphadi-methoxine. B.A.N. N′-(2,6-Dimethoxy-4-pyrimidinyl) sulfanilamide.
Use: Antibacterial.

SULFADIMETINE. N^1-(2-6-Dimethyl-4-pyrimidyl) sulfanilamide. Sulfisomidine.
See: Elkosin (Ciba).

SULFADIMIDINE.
See: Sulfamethazine.

SULFADINE.
See: Sulfadimidine.
Sulfamethazine.
Sulfapyridine, Tab. (Various Mfr.).

SULFADOXINE, U.S.P. XXII. N^1-(5,6-dimethoxy-4-pyrimidinyl) sulfanilamide. 4-(4-Aminobenzene-sulfonamido)-5,6-dimethoxypyrimidine. Fanasil Fanzil (Roche).
Use: Antibacterial.
W/Pyrimethamine.
See: Fansidar, Tab. (Roche).

SULFADOXINE AND PYRIMETHAMINE TABLETS, U.S.P. XXII.
Use: Antibacterial, antimalarial.

SULFAETHIDOLE. Sulphaethicole. B.A.N. Sulfaethylthiadiazole. N^1-(5-ethyl-1,3,4-thiadiazole-2-yl) sulfanilamide. Sulfaethylthiadiazole. Sethadil.
Use: Antibacterial.

SULFAETHYLTHIADIAZOLE.
See: Sulfaethidole.

SULFAFURAZOLE. B.A.N. 5-(4-Aminobenzene-sul-phonamido)-3,4-dimethylisoxazole. Gantrisin. Sulphafurazole. Sulfisoxazole.

SULFAGUANIDINE. (N-Guanylsulfanilamide; Abiguanil; Ganidan; Guamide).
Use: G.I. tract infections.
W/Sulfamethazine, sulfamerazine, sulfadiazine.
See: Quadetts, Tab. (Elder).
Quad-Ramoid, Susp. (Elder).

SULFA-GYN. (Mayrand) Sulfathiazole 3.42%, sulfacetamide 2.86%, sulfabenzamide 3.7%, urea 0.64%. Tube 85 Gm.
Use: Anti-infective, vaginal.

SULFAIR 15. (Pharmafair) Sodium sulfacetamide 15%. Soln. Bot. 15 ml.
Use: Anti-infective, sulfonamide (ophthalmic).

SULFAJEN CREAM. (Jenkins) Sulfamerazine 0.167 Gm, sulfadiazine 0.167 Gm, sulfamethazine 0.167 Gm/5 ml. Bot. 3 oz, 4 oz, gal.
Use: Anti-infective, sulfonamide.

•**SULFALENE.** USAN. N′-(3-Methoxypyrazinyl) sulfanilamide. Sulfametopyrazine. B.A.N.
Use: Antibacterial.

•**SULFAMERAZINE,** U.S.P. XXII. Tab., U.S.P. XXII. Benzenesulfonamide, 4-amino-N-(4-methyl-2- pyrimidinyl)-. N^1-(4-Methyl-2-pyrimidinyl)-sulfanilamide. (Sumedine).
Use: Infections caused by susceptible bacteria.

SULFAMERAZINE COMBINATIONS.
Use: Antibacterial.
See: Chemozine Tab., Susp. (Tennessee Pharm.).
Cherasulfa, Liq, Tab. (Cenci).
Chero-Trisulfa-V, Susp. (Vita Elixir).
Terfonyl, Liq., Tab. (Squibb).
Triple Sulfa, Tab. (Various Mfr.).

SULFAMERAZINE SODIUM.
Use: Antibacterial.

SULFAMERAZINE & SULFADIAZINE.
See: Dia-Mer-Sulfonamides.

SULFAMERAZINE, SULFADIAZINE & SULFAMETHAZINE.
Use: Antibacterial.
See: Meth-Dia-Mer-Sulfonamides.

SULFAMERAZINE, SULFADIAZINE & SULFATHIAZOLE.
Use: Antibacterial.
See: Dia-Mer-Thia-Sulfonamides.

•**SULFAMETHAZINE,** U.S.P. XXII. Benzenesulfonamide, 4-amino-N-(4,6-dimethyl-2- pyrimidinyl)-. 4,6-Dimethyl-2-sulfanilamidopyrimidine. NI-(4,6-Dimethyl-2-pyrimidinyl)sulfanilamide.
Use: Antibacterial.
See: Neotrizine, Susp., Tab. (Lilly).
W/Sulfacetamide, sulfadiazine, sulfamerazine.
See: Sulfa-Plex, Vag. Cream (Solvay).
W/Sulfadiazine, sulfamerazine.
See: Lantrisul, Tab., Susp. (Lannett).
Sulfaloid, Susp. (Westerfield).
Terfonyl, Liq., Tab. (Squibb).
Triple Sulfa, Tab. (Various Mfr.).
W/Sulfadiazine, sulfamerazine, sodium citrate.
See: Cherasulfa, Liq., Tab. (Cenci).
Triple Sulfa, Susp. (Standex).

•**SULFAMETHIZOLE,** U.S.P. XXII. Oral Susp., Tab., U.S.P. XXII. N′-(5/Methyl-1,3,4-thiadiazole-2-yl)-sulfanilamide. Methisul, Mizol, Uolueosil. Sulphamethizole.
Use: Antibacterial.
See: Bursul, Tab. (Burlington).
Microsul, Tab. (Star).
Proklar-M, Liq., Tab. (Westerfield).
Sulfasol, Tab. (Hyrex-Key).
Sulfstat, Forte, Tab. (Saron).

Sulfurine, Tab. (TableRock).
Thiosulfil, Forte, Tab. (Wyeth-Ayerst).
Urifon, Tab. (Amid).

SULFAMETHIZOLE W/COMBINATIONS.
Use: Antibacterial.
See: Microsul-A, Tab. (Star).
Thiosulfil-A, Tab. (Wyeth-Ayerst).
Thiosulfil-A Forte, Tab. (Wyeth-Ayerst).
Triurisul, Tab. (Sheryl).
Urobiotic, Cap. (Pfizer).
Urotrol, Tab. (Mills).

SULFAMETHOPRIM. (Par Pharm) Sulfamethoxazole 400 mg, trimethoprim 80 mg/Tab. Bot. 100s, 500s.
Use: Anti-infective.

•**SULFAMETHOXAZOLE,** U.S.P. XXII. Oral Susp., Tab., U.S.P. XXII. Sulphamethoxazole, Methyl sulfanilamidoisoxazole. 5-Methyl-3-sulfanilamido-isoxazole. N'-(5-methyl-3-isoxazolyl) sulfanilamide.
Use: Antibacterial.
See: Gantanol, Preps. (Roche).
W/Trimethoprim.
See: Bactrim, Prods. (Roche).
Septra, Tab. (Burroughs Wellcome).
Septra DS, Tab. (Burroughs Wellcome).

SULFAMETHOXAZOLE AND PHENAZOPYRIDINE HCl.
Use: Urinary anti-infective.
See: Azo-Gantanol, Tab. (Roche).

•**SULFAMETHOXAZOLE AND TRIMETHOPRIM CONCENTRATE FOR INJECTION,** U.S.P. XXII.
Use: Urinary antibacterial.

•**SULFAMETHOXAZOLE AND TRIMETHOPRIM ORAL SUSPENSION,** U.S.P. XXII.
Use: Urinary antibacterial.

•**SULFAMETHOXAZOLE AND TRIMETHOPRIM TABLETS,** U.S.P. XXII.
Use: Urinary antibacterial.

SULFAMETHOXYDIAZINE. Sulfameter.
Use: Antibacterial.
See: Sulla, Tab. (Robins).

SULFAMETHOXYPYRIDAZINE. B.A.N. N^1-(6-Methoxy-3-pyridazinyl) sulfanilamide. 3-(4-Aminobenzenesulfonamido)-6-methoxypyridazine.
Use: Antibacterial.

SULFAMETHOXYPYRIDAZINE ACETYL.
Use: Antibacterial.

SULFAMETHYLTHIADIAZOLE.
Use: Antibacterial.
See: Sulfamethizole Preps.

SULFAMETIN. N^1-(5-Methoxy-2-pyrimidinyl)sulfanilamide. (Formerly sulfamethoxydiazine).
Use: Antibacterial.
See: Sulla, Tab. (Robins).

SULFAMETOPYRAZINE. B.A.N. 2-(4-Aminobenzenesulfonamido)-3-methoxypyrazine.
Use: Antibacterial.
See: Sulfalene (I.N.N.).

SULFAMEZANTHENE.
Use: Antibacterial.
See: Sulfamethazine.

SULFAMIDE SUSPENSION. (Rugby) Prednisolone acetate 0.5%, sodium sulfacetamide, hydroxypropyl methylcellulose, polysorbate 80, sodium thiosulfate, benzalkonium Cl 0.01%. Susp. Bot. 5 ml, 15 ml.
Use: Steroid/sulfonamide combination, ophthalmic.

•**SULFAMONOMETHOXINE.** USAN. N^1-(6-methoxy-4-pyrimidinyl) sulfanilamide.
Use: Antibacterial.

•**SULFAMOXOLE.** USAN. N'-(4,5-dimethyl-2-oxazolyl) sulfanilamide.
Use: Antibacterial.

p-SULFAMOYLBENZYLAMINE HCl. Sulfbenzamide.

SULFAMYLON CREAM. (Winthrop) Mafenide acetate equivalent to 85 mg of base/Gm, cetyl alcohol, stearyl alcohol, cetyl esters wax, polyoxyl 40 stearate, polyoxyl 8 stearate, glycerin, water, methylparaben and propylparaben, sodium metabisulfite, edetate disodium. Tube 2 oz, 4 oz, Can 14.5 oz.
Use: Burn preparation.

SULFANILAMIDE. p-Aminobenzene sulfonamide.
Use: Antibacterial.

SULFANILAMIDE COMBINATIONS.
Use: Antibacterial.
See: AVC/Dienestrol Cream, Supp. (Merrell Dow).
AVC, Cream, Supp. (Merrell Dow).
D.I.T.I. Cream (Kenyon).
K.D.C. Vag. Cream (Kenyon).
Par Cream (Parmed).
Vagacreme, Cream (Delta).
Vagisan Creme (Sandia).
Vagisul, Creme (Sheryl).
Vagitrol, Cream, Supp. (Lemmon).

2-SULFANILAMIDOPYRIDINE. Sulfadiazine, U.S.P. XXII.
Use: Antibacterial.

•**SULFANILATE ZINC.** USAN.
Use: Antibacterial.

N-SULFANILYLACETAMIDE.
Use: Antibacterial.
See: Sulfacetamide, Tab. (Various Mfr.).

SULFANILYLBENZAMIDE.
Use: Antibacterial.
See: Sulfabenzamide.

•**SULFANITRAN.** USAN. 4'-[(p-Nitrophenyl) sulfamoyl]- acetanilide.
Use: Antibacterial.

SULFAPHENAZOLE. Sulphaphenzaole. B.A.N. N'-(1-phenyl-5-pyrazolyl) sulfanilamide. 5-(4-Aminobenzenesulphonamido)-1-phenylpyrazole.
See: Orisulf (Ciba).

SULFAPYRAZOLE. V.B.A.N. N^1-(3-Methyl-1-phenylpyrazol-5-yl)sulfanilamide.
Use: Sulphonamide, (veterinary).

•**SULFAPYRIDINE,** U.S.P. XXII. Tab., U.S.P. XXII. Benzenesulfonamide, 4-amino-N-2-pyridinyl-. 2-

Sulfanilamidopyridine. N′-2-Pyridylsulfanilamide. (Pfaltz & Bauer) Pow. Bot. lb.
Use: Dermatitic herpetiformis suppressant.

SULFARSPHENAMINE. Disodium-[arsenobis[6-hydroxy-m-phenylene)imino]]-dimethanesulfonate.

•**SULFASALAZINE,** U.S.P. XXII. Tab., U.S.P. XXII. 5-[[p-(2-Pyridylsulfamoyl)-phenyl]azo]salicylic acid. 4-Hydroxy-4′-(2-pyridylsulfamoyl)azobenzene-3-car- boxylic acid. Sulphasalazine. B.A.N. (Lederle) Tab. 0.5 Gm. Bot. 500s.
Use: Antibacterial.
See: Azulfidine, Tab., Susp. (Pharmacia).
Salazopyrin.
Salicylazosulfapyridine.
Salazopyrin.
S.A.S.-50, Tab. (Solvay).
S.A.S.P., Tab. (Zenith).
Sulcolon, Tab. (Lederle).
Sulfapyridine (I.N.N.).

SULFASOMIZOLE. USAN. 5-(4-Aminobenzenesulfonamido)-3-methylisothiazole. N′-(3-methyl-iso-thiazolyl)sulfanilamide.
Use: Antibacterial, sulfonamide.
See: Bidizole.

SULFASYMASINE. N′-(4,6-Diethyl-S-triazin-2-yl) sulfanilamide.
Use: Antibacterial, sulfonamide.

SULFA-TER-TABLETS. (A.P.C.) Trisulfapyrimidines, U.S.P. Bot. 1000s.

SULFATHIAZOLE, U.S.P. XXII. Benzenesulfonamide, 4-amino-N-2-thiazolyl-N<csq>-2-Thiazolylsulfanilamide. 2-Sulfanilamidothiazole.
Use: Antibacterial.
W/Chlorophyllin.
See: Thiaphyll Cream (Lannett).

SULFATHIAZOLE COMBINATIONS.
See: Sultrin, Tab., Cream (Ortho).

SULFATHIAZOLE CARBAMIDE.
See: Otosmosan, Liq. (Wyeth-Ayerst).

SULFATHIAZOLE, SULFACETAMIDE, AND SULFABENZAMIDE VAGINAL CREAM.
See: Triple Sulfa Vaginal Cream.

SULFATHIAZOLE, SULFACETAMIDE, AND SULFABENZAMIDE VAGINAL TABLETS.
See: Triple Sulfa Vaginal Tablets.

SULFATRIM. (Various Mfr.) **Susp.:** Trimethoprim 40 mg, sulfamethoxazole 200 mg/5 ml. Susp. Bot. 480 ml. **Tab.:** Trimethoprim 80 mg, sulfamethoxazole 400 mg/Tab. Bot. 100s, 500s.
Use: Anti-infective.

SULFATRIM DS TABS. (Goldline) Trimethoprim 800 mg, sulfamethoxazole 160 mg/Tab. Bot. 100s, 500s.
Use: Anti-infective.

SULFATRIM SS TABS. (Goldline) Trimethoprim 400 mg, sulfamethoxazole 80 mg/Tab. Bot. 100s.
Use: Anti-infective.

SULFA-TRIP. (Major) Sulfathiazole 3.42%, sulfacetamide 2.86%, sulfabenzamide 3.7%, urea 0.64%. Cream 82.5 Gm.
Use: Anti-infective, vaginal.

SULFA TRIPLE NO. 2. (Richlyn) Sulfadiazine 162 mg, sulfamerizine 162 mg, sulfamethazine 162 mg/Tab. Bot. 1000s.
Use: Anti-infective.

•**SULFAZAMET.** USAN. N′-(3-Methyl-1-phenylpyrazol-5-yl) sulfanilamide.
Use: Antibacterial.
See: Vesulong (Ciba).

SULFHYDRYL ION.
See: Hydrosulphosol (Lientz).

•**SULFINALOL HYDROCHLORIDE.** USAN.
Use: Antihypertensive.

•**SULFINPYRAZONE,** U.S.P. XXII. Cap., Tab., U.S.P. XXII. 1,2-Diphenyl-4-(2-phenylsulphinylethyl)pyrazolidine-3,5-dione. 1,2-Diphenyl-4-(2-phenylsulfinyl- ethyl-3,5-pyrazolidine-dione. Sulphinpyrazone. B.A.N.
Use: Uricosuric.
See: Anturane, Tab., Cap. (Ciba).

SULFISOMIDINE. Sulfadimetine. Sulphasomidine. B.A.N.

•**SULFISOXAZOLE,** U.S.P. XXII. Tab., U.S.P. XXII. N′-(3,4-Dimethyl-5-isoxazolyl)sulfaniamide.
Use: Anti-infective sulfa, treatment of urinary infections.
See: Gantrisin Preps. (Roche).
G-Sox, Tab. (Scrip).
Rosoxol, Tab. (Robinson).
SK-Soxazole, Cap. (SmithKline).
Soxa, Tab. (Vita Elixir).
Sulfisoxazole, Tab. (Purepac).
Sulfium, Ophthalmic, Soln., Oint. (Alcon).
Sulfizin, Tab. (Solvay).
Velmatrol, Tab. (Kenyon).
W/Aminoacridine HCl, allantoin.
See: Vagilia, Cream (Lemmon).
W/Phenazopyridine.
See: Azo-Gantrisin, Tab. (Roche).
Azo-Soxazole, Tab. (Quality Generics).
Azo-Sulfisoxazole, Tab. (Richlyn; Century).
Azo-Urizole, Tab. (Jenkins).
Rosoxol-Azo, Tab. (Robinson).
W/Phenylazodiaminopyridine HCl.
See: Azo-Sulfizin (Solvay).
Velmatrol-A Tab. (Kenyon).

•**SULFISOXAZOLE, ACETYL,** U.S.P. XXII. Oral Susp., U.S.P. XXII. Acetamide, N-(4-amino-phenyl)sulfonyl-N-(3,4-dimethyl-5-isoxazolyl)-. N-(3,4-Dimethyl-5-isoxazolyl)-N-sulfanilylacetamide.
Use: Antibacterial.
W/Erythromycin Ethylsuccinate.
See: Pediazol, Susp. (Ross).

SULFISOXAZOLE DIETHANOLAMINE. Sulfisoxazole Diolamine.

•**SULFISOXAZOLE DIOLAMINE.** U.S.P. XXII. Inj., Ophth. Oint, Ophth. Soln., U.S.P. XXII. 2,2′-Iminodiethanol salt of N^1-(3,4-Dimethyl-5-isoxazolyl)sulfanilamide compound with 2,2′-iminodiethanol(1:1). Gantrisin diolamine.
Use: Antibacterial.
See: Gantrisin, Ophth. Soln., Oint. (Roche).

SULFOAM MEDICATED ANTIDANDRUFF SHAMPOO. (Bradley) Sulfur 2% with cleansers, conditioners. Bot. 4 oz, 8 oz, 15.5 oz.
Use: Antiseborrheic.

•**SULFOBROMOPHTHALEIN SODIUM,** U.S.P. XXII. Inj., U.S.P. XXII.
Use: Liver function test.

SULFOCARBOLATES. Salts of phenolsulfonic acid, Usually Ca, Na, K, Cu, Zn.

SULFOCYANATE.
See: Potassium Thiocyanate.

SULFO-GANIC. (Marcen) Thioglycerol 20 mg, sodium citrate 5 mg, phenol 0.5%, benzyl alcohol 0.5%/ml. Vial 10 ml, 30 ml.
Use: I.M., adjunctive treatment in arthritides due to sulfur metabolism disorders or deficiencies.

SULFOGUAIACOL.
See: Potassium Guaiacolsulfonate.

SULFOIL. (C & M Pharmacal) Sulfonated castor oil, water. Bot. pt, gal.
Use: Skin and hair cleanser.

SULFOLAX CALCIUM. (Major) Docusate calcium 240 mg/Cap. Bot. 100s.
Use: Laxative.

SULFO-LO. (Whorton) Sublimed sulfur, freshly precipitated polysulfides of zinc, potassium, sulfate, calamine in aqueous-alcoholic suspension. **Lot.:** Bot. 4 oz, 8 oz. **Soap:** 3 oz.
Use: Anti-acne.

•**SULFOMYXIN.** USAN.
Use: Antibacterial.

SULFONAMIDE, DOUBLES.
See: Dia-Mer-Sulfonamides.

SULFONAMIDE PREPS.
See: Acet-Dia-Mer (Various Mfr.).
Dia-Mer Sulfonamides (Various Mfr.).
Dia-Mer-Thia (Various Mfr.).
Meth-Dia-Mer, Preps. (Various Mfr.).

SULFONAMIDES, VETERINARY USE.
See: S.Q. (Merck Animal Health).
Sulfabrom (Merck Animal Health).
Sulfastrep w/streptomycin (Merck Animal Health).
Sulfathalidine (Merck Animal Health).
Sul-Thi-Zol (Merck Animal Health).

SULFONAMIDES, QUADRUPLE.
See: Quadetts, Tab. (Elder).
Quad-Ramoid, Susp. (Elder).

SULFONAMIDES, TRIPLE.
See: Acet-Dia-Mer Sulfonamides.
Dia-Mer-Thia Sulfonamides.
Meth-Dia-Mer Sulfonamides.

SULFONES.
See: Avlosulfon, Tab. (Wyeth-Ayerst).
Dapsone.
Diasone, Enterabs (Abbott).
Glucosulfone Sodium.
Promacetin, Tab. (Parke-Davis).

SULFONETHYLMETHANE. 2,2-Bis-(ethylsulfonyl)butane.

SULFONITHOCHOLYLGLYCINE.
See: S.L.C.G., Kit (Abbott).

SULFONMETHANE. 2,2-Bis(ethylsulfonyl)propane.

SULFONPHTHAL.
See: Phenolsulfonphthalein, Preps. (Various Mfr.).

•**SULFONTEROL HYDROCHLORIDE.** USAN.
Use: Bronchodilator.

SULFONYLUREAS.
See: Diabinese, Tab. (Pfizer).
Dymelor, Tab. (Lilly).
Orinase, Tab., Vial (Upjohn).
Tolinase, Tab. (Upjohn).

SULFORCIN LOTION. (Owen) Sulfur 5%, resorcinol 2%, alcohol 11.65%, methylparaben. Bot. 4 oz.
Use: Anti-acne, antiseborrheic.

SULFORMETHOXINE. Name used for Sulfadoxine.

SULFORTHOMIDINE. Name used for Sulfadoxine.

SULFOSALICYLATE W/METHENAMINE
See: Hexalet, Tab. (Webcon).

SULFOSALYCYLIC ACID. Salicylsulphonic acid.

•**SULFOXONE SODIUM,** U.S.P. XXII. Tab., U.S.P. XXII.

SULFOXYL REGULAR. (Stiefel) Benzoyl peroxide 5%, sulfur 2%. Bot. 2 oz.
Use: Anti-acne.

SULFOXYL STRONG. (Stiefel) Benzoyl peroxide 10%, sulfur 5%. Bot. 2 oz.
Use: Anti-acne.

SULFUR-8 HAIR & SCALP CONDITIONER. (Schering-Plough) Sulfur 2%, menthol 1%, triclosan 0.1%. Jar 2 oz, 4 oz, 8 oz.
Use: Antiseborrheic.

SULFUR-8 LIGHT FORMULA HAIR & SCALP CONDITIONER. (Schering-Plough) Sulfur, triclosan, menthol. Jar 2 oz, 4 oz.
Use: Antiseborrheic.

SULFUR-8 SHAMPOO. (Schering-Plough) Triclosan 0.2%. Bot. 6.85 oz, 10.85 oz.
Use: Antiseborrheic.

SULFUR, ANTIARTHRITIC.
See: Thiocyl, Amp. (Torigian).

•**SULFURATED LIME TOPICAL SOLUTION,** U.S.P. XXII. Vleminckx Lotion.
Use: Scabicide, parasiticide.

SULFUR COMBINATIONS.
See: Acnaveen, Bar (Cooper).
Acne-Aid, Cream, Lot. (Stiefel).
Acnederm, Liq. (Lannett).
Akne Oral Kapsulets, Cap. (Alto).
Acnomel, Cake, Cream (SmithKline Prods).
Acno, Soln., Lot. (Cummins).
Acnotex, Liq. (C&M Pharm.).

Akne, Drying Lot. (Alto).
Antrocol, Tab., Cap. (Poythress).
Aracain Rectal Oint. (Commerce).
Clearasil, Stick (Vicks).
Derma Cover-HC, Liq. (Scrip).
Epi-clear, Lot. (Squibb).
Exzit, Preps. (Miles Pharm).
Fomac, Cream (Dermik).
Fostex, Liq. Cream, Bar (Westwood).
Fostex, Cream, Liq. (Westwood).
Fostex CM, Cream (Westwood).
Fostril, Cream (Westwood).
Furol Cream (Torch).
Hydro Surco, Lot. (Almo).
Klaron, Lot. (Dermik).
Liquimat, Liq. (Owen).
Lotio-P (Alto).
Neutrogena Disposables (Neutrogena).
Pernox, Lot. (Westwood).
pHisoDan, Liq. (Winthrop).
Postacne, Lot. (Dermik).
Pragmatar, Oint. (Menley & James).
Proseca, Liq. (Westwood).
Rezamid, Lot. (Dermik).
Sastid Soap (Stiefel).
Sebaveen, Shampoo (Cooper).
Sebulex Shampoo, Liq. (Westwood).
Sulfacet-R, Lot. (Dermik).
Sulfo-lo, Lot. (Wharton).
Sulforcin, Pow., Lot. (Owen).
Sulfur-8, Prods. (Schering-Plough).
Teenac, Cream (Elder).
Vanseb, Cream (Herbert).
Vanseb-T Tar Shampoo (Herbert).
Xerac, Oint. (Person & Covey).

•**SULFUR DIOXIDE,** N.F. XVII.
Use: Antixodant, pharmaceutic aid.

•**SULFUR OINTMENT,** U.S.P. XXII.
Use: Scabicide, parasiticide.

•**SULFUR, PRECIPITATED,** U.S.P. XXII.
Use: Scabicide, parasiticide.
See: Bensulfoid, Pow., Lot. (Poythress).
Epi-Clear, Lot. (Squibb).
Ramsdell's Sulfur Cream (Fougera).
Sulfur Soap (Steifel Labs).

SULFUR, SALICYL DIASPORAL.
See: Diasporal, Cream (Doak).

SULFUR SOAP. (Stiefel) Precipitated sulfur 10%. Cake 4.1 oz.
Use: Anti-acne.

SULFUR, SUBLIMED, U.S.P. XXII. Flowers of Sulfur.
Use: Parasiticide, scabicide.

SULFUR, TOPICAL.
See: Thylox, Liq., Soap (Dent).

SULFURIC ACID, N.F. XVII.
Use: Pharmaceutic aid (acidifying agent).

SULFURINE. (Table Rock) Sulfamethizole 0.5 Gm/Tab. Bot. 100s, 500s.
Use: Urinary anti-infective.

SULGLYCOTIDE. B.A.N. The sulfuric polyester of a glycopeptide isolated from pig duodenum.
Use: Treatment of peptic ulcer.

•**SULINDAC,** U.S.P. XXII. Tab., U.S.P. XXII.
Use: Anti-inflammatory.
See: Clinoril, Tab. (Merck Sharp & Dohme).

•**SULISOBENZONE.** USAN. 5-Benzoyl-4-hydroxy-2-methoxybenzenesulfonic acid.
Use: Sunscreen agent.
See: Uval, Lot. (Dorsey).
Uvinul MS-40 (General Aniline & Film).

•**SULMARIN.** USAN.
Use: Hemostatic.

SULNAC. (NMC Labs) Sulfathiazol 3.42%, sulfacetamide 2.86%, sulfabenzamide 3.7%, urea 0.64% in cream base. Tube 2.75 oz.
Use: Anti-infective.

•**SULNIDAZOLE.** USAN.
Use: Antiprotozoal.

SULOCARBILATE. 2-Hydroxyethyl-p-sulfamylcarbanilate.

•**SULOCTIDIL.** USAN.
Use: Vasodilator.

•**SULOFENUR.** USAN.
Use: Antineoplastic.

•**SULOXIFEN OXALATE.** USAN.
Use: Bronchodilator.

SULOXYBENZONE. 4-p-Anisoyl-3-hydroxybenzene sulfonic acid. 2-Hydroxy-4′-methoxy-5-sulfoben-zophenone. Cyasorb UV 284 (Lederle).

SULPHABENZIDE.
See: Sulfabenzamide.

SULPHALOXIC ACID. B.A.N. 4′-[(Hydroxymethylcarbamoyl)-sulfamoyl]phthalanilic acid.
See: Enteromide calcium salt.

SULPHAMETHOXYDIAZINE. B.A.N. 2-p-Aminobenzenesulphonamido-5-methoxypyrimidine, 5-Methoxy-2-sulphanilamidopyrimidine Durenate.

SULPHAMOPRINE. B.A.N. 2-(4-Aminobenzenesul-fonamido)-4,6-dimethoxypyrimidine.

SULPHAMOXOLE. B.A.N. 2-(4-Aminobenzenesul-fonamido)-4,5-dimethyloxazole.

SULPHAN BLUE. B.A.N. Sodium 4-(4-diethylaminobenzylidene)cyclohexa-2,5-dienylidenediethylammonium-α-benzene-2,4-disulfonate.
Use: Investigation of the cardiovascular system.
See: Blue VRS.
Disulphine Blue VNS.

SULPHAPROXYLINE. B.A.N. N^1-(4-Isopropoxyben-zoyl)-4-aminobenzenesulfonamide.

SULPHASOMIDINE. B.A.N. 4-(4-Aminobenzenesul-fonamido)-2,6-dimethylpyrimidine.
See: Sulfisomidine (I.N.N.).
Elkosin.

SULPHATHIOUREA. B.A.N. 4-Aminobenzenesulfonylthiourea.

SULPHATOLAMIDE. B.A.N. 4-Aminobenzenesulphonylthiourea salt of α-amino-p-toluenesulfonamide.

SULPHAUREA. B.A.N. 4-Aminobenzesulfonylurea.
See: Sulfacarbamide (I.N.N.).

SULPHO-LAC ACNE MEDICATION. (Bradley) Sulfur 5%, zinc sulfate 27%, Vleminckx's Soln. 53%. Tube 1 oz, Jar 1.75 oz.
Use: Anti-acne.

SULPHO-LAC SOAP. (Bradley) Sulfur 5%, trisodium HEDTA, casamine OTB in soap base. Bar 3 oz.
Use: Anti-acne.

SULPHOMYXIN. Penta-(N-sulphomethyl) polymyxin B.

SULPHOMYXIN SODIUM. B.A.N. A mixture of sulfomethylated polymyxin B and sodium bisulfite.
Use: Antibiotic.

SULPHRIN SUSPENSION. (Bausch & Lomb) Sodium sulfacetamide 100 mg, prednisolone acetate 5 mg. Bot. 5 ml.
Use: Steroid/sulfonamide combination.

SULPIK. (Durel) Sulfur 5%, salicylic acid 3%, in Duromantel cream.
Use: Antiseborrheic.

SULPIK T. (Durel) Sulfur 5%, salicylic acid 3%, LCD (coal tar solution) 3%. In Duromantel Cream.
Use: Antiseborrheic.

•**SULPIRIDE.** USAN. (1) N-[(1-ethyl-2-pyrrolidinyl)methyl]-5-sulfamoyl-o-anisamide; (2) N-[(Ethyl-1-pyrrolidinyl-2)-methyl]methoxy-2-sulfamoyl-5-benza-mide. Dogmatyl (Laboratories Delagrange, France).
Use: Antidepressant.

•**SULPROSTONE.** USAN.
Use: Prostaglandin.

SUL-RAY ACNE CREAM. (Last) Sulfur 2% in cream base. Jar 1.75 oz, 6.75 oz, 20 oz.
Use: Anti-acne.

SUL-RAY ALOE VERA ANALGESIC RUB. (Last) Camphor 3.1 %, menthol 1.25%. Bot. 4 oz, 8 oz.
Use: External analgesic.

SUL-RAY ALOE VERA SKIN PROTECTANT CREAM. (Last) Zinc oxide 1%, allantoin 0.5%. Jar oz.
Use: Skin protectant.

SUL-RAY SHAMPOO. (Last) Sulfur shampoo 2%. Bot. 8 oz.
Use: Antiseborrheic.

SUL-RAY SOAP. (Last) Sulfur soap. Bar 3 oz.
Use: Anti-acne.

•**SULTAMICILLIN.** USAN.
Use: Antibacterial.

SULTEN-10. (Bausch & Lomb) Sodium sulfacetamide 10%. Bot 15 ml.
Use: Sulfonamide, ophthalmic.

•**SULTHIAME.** USAN. Formerly Sulphenytame. p-(Tetrahydro-2H-1,2-thiazin-2-yl)-benzenesulfonamide-S,S-dioxide.
Use: Anticonvulsant.

SULTRIN Triple Sulfa Vaginal Tablets. (Ortho) Sulfathiazole 172.5 mg, sulfacetamide 143.75 mg, sulfabenzamide 184 mg/Tab. Pkg. 20s w/ applicator.
Use: Anti-infective, vaginal.

SULTRIN Triple Sulfa Cream. (Ortho) Sulfathiazole 3.42%, sulfacetamide 2.86%, sulfabenzamide 3.7%, urea 0.64%. Tube 78 Gm with measured dose applicator.
Use: Anti-infective, vaginal.

•**SULUKAST.** USAN.
Use: Antiasthmatic.

SULVESOR LOTION. (Durel) Sulfur 2%, resorcinol 1%, neocalamine, talc, titanium dioxide, alcohol 34%. 2 oz, 4 oz, gal.
Use: Antifungal, keratolytic, antiseborrheic.

SUMACAL POWDER. (Biosearch) CHO 95 Gm, Cal 380, sodium 100 mg, Cl 210 mg, potassium > 39 mg, calcium > 20 mg/100 Gm. Pow. 400 Gm.
Use: Enteral nutritional supplement.

•**SUMAROTENE.** USAN.
Use: Keratolytic.

•**SUMATRIPTAN SODIUM.** USAN.
Use: Antimigraine.

•**SUMATRIPTAN SUCCINATE.** USAN.
Use: Antimigraine.

SUMMER'S EVE DISPOSABLE DOUCHE. (Fleet) Single or twin 4.5 oz. disposable units. Regular, herbal, vinegar and water, white flowers, hint of musk, post-menstrual.
Use: Vaginal preparation.

SUMMER'S EVE MEDICATED DISPOSABLE DOUCHE. (Fleet) Povidone-iodide. Single or twin 4.5 oz. disposable units.
Use: Vaginal preparation.

SUMYCIN. (Squibb Mark) Tetracycline HCl. **Cap.:** 250 mg. Bot. 100s, 1000s, Unimatic 100s; 500 mg. Bot. 100s, 500s, Unimatic 100s. **Tab.:** 250 mg. Bot. 100s, 1000s; 500 mg. Bot. 100s, 500s.
Use: Anti-infective.

SUNBURN REMEDY.
See: Solarcaine, Prods. (Schering-Plough).

•**SUNCILLIN SODIUM.** USAN. 3,3-Dimethyl-7-oxo-6-[2-phenyl-D-2-(sulfoamino)acetamido]-4-thia-1-azabicyclo[3.2.0]heptane-2-carboxylic acid disodium salt.
Use: Antibacterial.

SUNDOWN. (Johnson & Johnson) A series of products marketed under the Sundown name including: **Moderate** (SPF 4): Padimate O, oxybenzone. **Extra** (SPF 6): Oxybenzone, padimate O. **Maximal** (SPF 8): Oxybenzone, padimate O. **Ultra** (SPF 15): Oxybenzone, padimate O, octyl methoxycinnamate.
Use: Sunscreen.

SUNDOWN SUNBLOCK CREAM ULTRA SPF 24. (Johnson & Johnson) Padimate O, oxybenzone.
Use: Sunscreen.

SUNDOWN SUNBLOCK STICK SPF 15. (Johnson & Johnson) Octyl dimethyl PABA, oxybenzone. Stick 0.35 oz.
Use: Sunscreen.

SUNDOWN SUNBLOCK STICK SPF 20. (Johnson & Johnson) Octyl dimethyl PABA, octyl methoxycinnamate, oxybenzone, titanium dioxide.
Use: Sunscreen.
SUNDOWN SUNBLOCK ULTRA SPF 20. (Johnson & Johnson) Octyl dimethyl PABA, octyl methoxycinnamate, oxybenzone, titanium dioxide.
Use: Sunscreen.
SUNDOWN SUNSCREEN STICK SPF 8. (Johnson & Johnson) Octyl dimethyl PABA, oxybenzone. Stick 0.35 oz.
Use: Sunscreen.
SUNICE. (Citroleum) Allantoin 0.25%, menthol 0.25%, methyl salicylate 10%/Cream 3 oz.
Use: Burn preparation.
SUNSTICK. (Rydelle) Digalloyl trioleate 2.5% in emollient base. Cont. 0.14 oz.
Use: Sunscreen for lips.
SUPAC. (Mission) Acetaminophen 160 mg, aspirin 230 mg, caffeine 33 mg, calcium gluconate 60 mg/Tab. Filmstrip 24s, Bot. 100s, 1000s.
Use: Analgesic combination.
SUPER AFKO-HIST. (APC) Chlorpheniramine maleate 2 mg, aspirin 230 mg, phenacetin 160 mg, caffeine 32 mg/Tab. Bot. 1000s.
Use: Antihistamine, analgesic.
SUPER AYTINAL TABLETS. (Walgreen) Vitamins A 7000 IU, B_1 5 mg, B_2 5 mg, B_5 10 mg, B_6 3 mg, B_{12} 9 mcg, C 90 mg, pantothenic acid 10 mg, D 400 IU, E 30 IU, niacin 30 mg, biotin 55 mcg, folic acid 0.4 mg, iron 30 mg, calcium 162 mg, phosphorous 125 mg, iodine 150 mcg, copper 3 mg, manganese 7.5 mg, magnesium 100 mg, potassium 7.7 mg, zinc 24 mg, chloride 7 mg, cromium 15 mcg, selenium 15 mcg, molybdenum 15 mcg, choline bitartrate 1000 mcg, inositol 1000 mcg, PABA 1000 mcg, rutin 1000 mcg, yeast 12 mg. Bot. 50s, 100s, 365s.
Use: Vitamin/mineral supplement.
SUPER-B. (Towne) Vitamins B_1 50 mg, B_2 20 mg, B_6 5 mg, B_{12} 15 mcg, C 300 mg, desiccated liver 100 mg, dried yeast 100 mg, niacinamide 25 mg, calcium pantothenate 5 mg, iron 10 mg/Captab. Bot. 50s, 100s, 150s, 250s.
Use: Vitamin/mineral supplement.
SUPER B KAPSULES. (Pharmex) High potency vitamin B. Cap. Bot. 50s, 100s.
Use: Vitamin B supplement.
SUPER C-1000. (Pharmex) Vitamin C 1000 mg/Tab. Bot. 100s.
Use: Vitamin C supplement.
SUPER CALICAPS M-Z. (Nion) Calcium 1200 mg, magnesium 400 mg, zinc 15 mg, vitamin A 5000 IU, D 400 IU, selenium 15 mcg/3 Tab. Bot. 90s.
Use: Vitamin/mineral supplement.
SUPER CALCIUM 1200. (Schiff) Calcium carbonate 1512 mg (600 mg calcium)/Cap. Bot. 60s, 120s.
Use: Calcium supplement.
SUPER D. (Upjohn) Vitamin A 10,000 IU, D 400 IU/Perle. Bot. 100s.
Use: Vitamin A and D supplement.
SUPER D PERLES. (Upjohn) Vitamin A 10,000 IU, D 400 IU/Cap. Bot. 100s.
Use: Vitamin A and D supplement.
SUPER EPA. (Advanced Nutritional Tech.) Omega-3 polyunsaturated fatty acids 1200 mg/Cap. containing EPA 360 mg, DHA 240 mg. Bot. 60s, 90s.
Use: Nutritional supplement.
SUPERE-PECT. (Barth's) Alpha tocopherol 400 IU, apple pectin 100 mg/Cap. Bot. 50s, 100s, 250s.
Use: Vitamin E supplement.
SUPER HYDRAMIN PROTEIN POWDER. (Nion) Protein 41%, carbohydrate 21.8%, fat 1% in powder form. Can lb.
Use: Nutritional supplement.
SUPERINONE. Tyloxapol.
See: Triton WR-1339 (Rohm & Haas).
SUPER NUTRI-VITES. (Faraday) Vitamins A 36,000 IU, D 400 IU, B_1 25 mg, B_2 25 mg, B_6 50 mg, B_{12} 50 mcg, niacinamide 50 mg, calcium pantothenate 12.5 mg, choline bitartrate 150 mg, inositol 150 mg, betaine HCl 25 mg, PABA 15 mg, glutamic acid 25 mg, desiccated liver 50 mg, C 150 mg, E 12.5 IU, manganese gluconate 6.15 mg, bone meal 162 mg, iron gluconate 50 mg, copper gluconate 0.25 mg, zinc gluconate 2.2 mg, potassium iodide 0.1 mg, calcium 53.3 mg, phosphorous 24.3 mg, magnesium gluconate 7.2 mg/Protein coated tab. Bot. 60s, 100s.
Use: Vitamin/mineral/nutritional supplement.
SUPER PLENAMINS MULTIPLE VITAMINS AND MINERALS. (Rexall) Vitamins A 8000 IU, D_2 400 IU, Vit. B_1 2.5 mg, B_2 2.5 mg, C 75 mg, niacinamide 20 mg, B_6 1 mg, B_{12} 3 mcg, biotin 20 mcg, E 10 IU, pantothenic acid 3 mg, liver concentrate 100 mg, iron 30 mg, calcium 75 mg, phosphorous 58 mg, iodine 0.15 mg, copper 0.75 mg, manganese 1.25 mg, magnesium 10 mg, zinc 1 mg/Tab. Bot. 36s, 72s, 144s, 288s, 365s.
Use: Vitamin/mineral supplement.
SUPER POLI-GRIP/WERNET'S CREAM (Block) Carboxymethylcellulose gum, ethylene oxide polymer, petrolatum-mineral oil base. Cream Tube 0.7 oz, 1.4 oz, 2.4 oz.
Use: Denture adhesive.
SUPER SHADE SPF-25. (Schering-Plough) Ethylhexyl p-methoxycinnamate, padimate 0 oxybenzone, SPF-25. Bot. 4 fl oz.
Use: Sunscreen.
SUPER SHADE SUNBLOCK STICK SPF-25. (Schering-Plough) Ethylhexyl p-methoxycinnamate, oxybenzone, padimate 0. Stick. SPF-25. Tube 0.43 oz.
Use: Sunscreen.
SUPER STRESS. (Towne) Vitamins C 600 mg, E 30 IU, B_1 15 mg, B_2 15 mg, niacin 100 mg, B_6 5 mg, B_{12} 12 mcg, pantothenic acid 20 mg/Tab. Bot. 60s.

Use: Vitamin supplement.

SUPER STRESS PLUS IRON. (Towne) Vitamins C 600 mg, E 30 IU, B_1 15 mg, niacin 100 mg, B_6 5 mg, B_{12} 12 mcg, pantothenic acid 20 mg, folic acid 0.4 mg, iron 27 mg/Tab. Bot. 60s.
Use: Vitamin/mineral supplement.

SUPER-T. (Towne) Vitamins A palmitate 10,000 IU, D 400 IU, B_1 10 mg, B_2 10 mg, B_6 1 mg, B_{12} 6 mcg, C 200 mg, niacinamide 100 mg, E 15 IU, calcium 103 mg, phosphorous 80 mg, iron 10 mg, iodine 0.1 mg, copper 1 mg, potassium 5 mg, magnesium 5.5 mg, manganese 1 mg, zinc 1.4 mg/Captab. Bot. 100s, 130s.
Use: Vitamin/mineral supplement.

SUPER THERA 46. (Faraday) Vitamin A 36,000 IU, essential vitamins, minerals, amino acids w/ nutrient factors, digestive enzymes, B_{12} 25 mcg/ Tab. Bot. 100s.
Use: Nutritional supplement.

SUPER TROCHE. (Weeks & Leo) Benzocaine 5 mg, cetalkonium Cl 1 mg/Loz. Bot. 15s, 30s.
Use: Local anesthetic.

SUPER TROCHE PLUS. (Weeks & Leo) Benzocaine 10 mg, cetalkonium Cl 2 mg/Loz. Bot. 12s.
Use: Local anesthetic.

SUPER-T WITH ZINC. (Towne) Vitamins A 10,000 IU, D 400 IU, E 15 IU, C 200 mg, B_1 10 mg, B_2 10 mg, B_6 5 mg, B_{12} 6 mcg, niacinamide 50 mg, iron 18 mg, iodine 0.1 mg, copper 2 mg, manganese 1 mg, zinc 15 mg/Cap. Bot. 130s.
Use: Vitamin/mineral supplement.

SUPERVIM TABLETS. (U.S. Ethicals) Vitamins, minerals. Bot. 100s.
Use: Vitamin/mineral supplement.

SUPER WERNET'S POWDER. (Block) Carboxymethylcellulose gum, ethylene oxide polymer. Bot. 0.63 oz, 1.75 oz, 3.55 oz.
Use: Denture adhesive.

SUPER WESVITE. (Western Research) Vitamins A 10,000 IU, B_1 15 mg, B_2 15 mg, B_6 25 mg, B_{12} 25 mcg, C 100 mg, D 400 IU, E 30 IU, biotin 500 mcg, calcium 100 mg, calcium pantothenate 25 Gm, choline bitartrate 10 mg, lemon bioflavonoids 10 mg, copper 2 mg, pantothenic acid 25 mg, inositol 20 mg, iron 20 mg, magnesium 50 mg, folic acid 400 mcg, hesperidin complex 10 mg, rutin 20 mg, potassium 25 mg, molybdenum 100 mcg, manganese 6 mg, niacin 40 mg, para-aminobenzoic acid 8 mg, phosphorus 52 mg, potassium iodide 0.1 mg, zinc 5 mg, iodine 100 mcg/Tab. Bot. 1008s.
Use: Vitamin/mineral/amino acid supplement.

SUPLEX. (Rocky Mtn.) Vitamins B_1 100 mg, B_2 2 mg, B_6 4 mg, niacinamide 100 mg, panthenol 12 mg/ml. Vial 30 ml.
Use: Vitamin supplement.

SUPLICAL. (Parke-Davis Prods) Calcium 600 mg/Square. Bot. 30s, 60s.
Use: Calcium supplement.

SUPPAP-120. (Raway) Acetaminophen 120 mg/ Supp. 12s, 50s, 100s, 500s, 1000s.
Use: Analgesic.

SUPPAP-325. (Raway) Acetaminophen 325 mg/ Supp. 100s.
Use: Analgesic.

SUPPAP-650. (Raway) Acetaminophen 650 mg/ Supp. 50s, 100s, 500s, 1000s.
Use: Analgesic.

SUPPORT-500. (Doral) Vitamins A 12,500 IU, D 50 IU, B_1 10 mg, B_2 5 mg, niacinamide 25 mg, B_6 2 mg, calcium pantothenate 10 mg, C 500 mg, E 50 IU, magnesium sulfate 70 mg, manganese sulfate 4 mg, zinc 80 mg/Cap.
Use: Vitamin/mineral supplement.

SUPRA MIN. (Towne) Vitamins A 10,000 IU, D 400 IU, E 30 IU, C 250 mg, folic acid 0.4 mg, B_1 10 mg, B_2 10 mg, niacin 100 mg, B_6 5 mg, B_{12} 6 mcg, pantothenic acid 20 mg, iodine 150 mcg, iron 100 mg, magnesium 2 mg, copper 20 mg, manganese 1.25 mg/Tab. Bot. 130s.
Use: Vitamin/mineral supplement.

SUPRARENAL. Dried, partially defatted and powdered adrenal gland of cattle, sheep or swine.

SUPRAZINE TABS. (Major) Trifluoperazine 1 mg/ Tab. Bot 100s, 250s, 1000s; 2 mg/Tab. Bot. 100s, 250s, 1000s, UD 100s; 5 mg/Tab. Bot. 100s, 250s, 1000s; 10 mg/Tab. Bot. 100s, 250s, 1000s.
Use: Antipsychotic.

SUPRINS. (Towne) Vitamins A palmitate 10,000 IU, D 400 IU, B_1 10 mg, B_2 10 mg, B_6 5 mg, B_{12} 6 mcg, C 250 mg, calcium pantothenate 20 mg, niacinamide 100 mg, biotin 25 mcg, E 15 IU, calcium 103 mg, phosphorous 80 mg, iron 10 mg, iodine 0.1 mg, copper 1 mg, zinc 20 mg, manganese 1.25 mg/Captab. Bot. 100s.
Use: Vitamin/mineral supplement.

SUPROCLONE. USAN.
Use: Sedative.

SURAMIN SODIUM. Hexa-Sodium bis-(m-aminobenzoyl-m-amino-p-methylbenzoyl-1-naph-thylamino-4,6,8-trisulfonate) carbamide. (Bayer 205; Germanin).

SURBEX FILMTAB. (Abbott) Thiamine mononitrate 6 mg, vitamins B_2 6 mg, nicotinamide 30 mg, B_6 2.5 mg, calcium pantothenate 10 mg, B_{12} 5 mcg. Filmtab. Bot. 100s.
Use: Vitamin B supplement.

W/Vitamin C. (Abbott) Same as Surbex Filmtab, except vitamin C 250 mg/Filmtab. Bot. 100s, 500s.

SURBEX-T FILMTAB. (Abbott) Vitamins B_1 15 mg, B_2 10 mg, niacinamide 100 mg, B_6 5 mg, B_{12} 10 mcg, calcium pantothenate 20 mg, C 500 mg/Filmtab. Bot. 100s, UD 100s.
Use: Vitamin/mineral supplement.

SURBEX-750 WITH IRON. (Abbott) Vitamins B_1 15 mg, B_2 15 mg, B_6 25 mg, B_{12} 12 mcg, C 750 mg, calcium pantothenate 20 mg, E 30 IU, niacinamide 100 mg, iron 27 mg, folic acid 0.4 mg/Tab. Bot. 50s.

Use: Vitamin/mineral supplement.

SURBEX-750 WITH ZINC. (Abbott) Vitamins B_1 15 mg, B_2 15 mg, B_6 20 mg, B_{12} 12 mcg, C 750 mg, E 30 IU, pantothenic acid 20 mg, niacin 100 mg, folic acid 0.4 mg, zinc 22.5 mg/Tab. Bot. 50s.
Use: Vitamin/mineral supplement.

SURBU-GEN-T. (Goldline) Vitamins B_1 15 mg, B_2 10 mg, B_3 100 mg, B_5 20 mg, B_6 5 mg, B_{12} 10 mcg, C 500 mg/Tab. Bot. 100s.
Use: Vitamin supplement.

SURFACE-ACTIVE AGENTS.
See: Antiseptics, surface-active.

SURFAK. (Hoechst) Docusate calcium 50 mg or 240 mg/Cap. **50 mg:** Bot. 30s, 100s; **240 mg:** Bot. 30s, 100s, 500s, UD Pack 100s.
Use: Laxative.

•**SURFILCON A.** USAN.
Use: Hydrophilic contact lens material.

SURFOL POST IMMERSION BATH OIL. (Stiefel) Mineral oil, isopropyl myristate, isostearic acid, PEG-40, sorbitan peroleate. Bot. 8 oz.
Use: Emollient.

•**SURFOMER.** USAN.
Use: Hypolipidemic.

SURGASOAP. (Wade) Castile vegetable oils. Bot. qt, gal.
Use: Surgical soap.

SURGEL LIQUID. (Ulmer) Patient lubricant fluid. Bot. 4 oz, 8 oz, gal.

•**SURGIBONE.** USAN. Bone and cartilage obtained from bovine embryos and young calves.
Use: Prosthetic aid (internal bone splint).
See: Unilab Surgibone (Unilab).

SURGICAL SIMPLEX P. (Howmedica) Methyl methacrylate 20 ml poly 6.7 Gm, methyl methacrylate-styrene copolymer 33.3 Gm. **Pow.** 40 Gm. **Liq.** 20 ml.
Use: Bone cement.

SURGICAL SIMPLEX P RADIOPAQUE. (Howmedica) Methyl methacrylate 20 ml, poly 6 Gm, methyl methacrylate-styrene copolymer 30 Gm. **Pow.** 40 Gm. **Liq.** 20 ml.
Use: Bone cement.

•**SURGICAL SUTURE, ABSORBABLE,** U.S.P. XXII.
Use: Surgical aid.

•**SURGICAL SUTURE, NONABSORBABLE,** U.S.P. XXII.
Use: Surgical aid.

SURGICEL. (Johnson & Johnson) Sterile absorbable knitted fabric prepared by controlled oxidation of regenerated cellulose. Sterile strip 2″×14″, 4″×8″, 2″×3″, 0.5″×2″.
Use: Absorbable hemostat.

SURGIDINE. (Continental) Iodine 0.8% in iodine complex. Bot. 8 oz, gal. Foot operated dispenser 8 oz, gal.
Use: Antiseptic, germicide.

SURGI-KLEEN. (Sween) Bot. 2 oz, 8 oz, 16 oz, 21 oz, gal, 5 gal, 30 gal, 55 gal.
Use: Skin cleanser, shampoo.

SURGILUBE. (Day-Baldwin) Sterile bacteriostatic. **Foilpac:** 3 Gm, 5 Gm; **Tube:** 5 Gm, 2 oz, 4.5 oz.
Use: Surgical lubricant.

•**SURICAINIDE MALEATE.** USAN.
Use: Cardiac depressant (antiarrhythmic).

SURIN OINTMENT. (McKesson) Tube 1.25 oz.

SURITAL SODIUM. (Parke-Davis) Thiamylal sodium. Steri-Vial 1 Gm 25s; 5 Gm 10s; 10 Gm 10s.
Use: General anesthetic.

SURMONTIL. (Wyeth-Ayerst) Trimipramine maleate 25 mg, 50 mg or 100 mg/Cap. Bot. 100s, Redipak.
Use: Antidepressant.

SUROFENE. Hexachlorophene.

•**SURONACRINE MALEATE.** USAN.
Use: Cholinergic, cholinesterase inhibitor.

SURVANTA. (Ross) Beractant.
Use: Lung surfactant.

SUSANO. (Blue Cross) Phenobarbital 0.25 gr, hyoscyamine sulfate 0.1037 mg, atropine sulfate 0.0194 mg, scopolamine HBr 0.0065 mg/Tab. Bot. 1000s.
Use: Sedative/hypnotic, anticholinergic/antispasmodic.

SUSANO ELIXIR. (Blue Cross) Phenobarbital 0.25 gr, hyoscyamine sulfate 0.1037 mg, atropine sulfate 0.0194 mg, scopolamine HBr 0.0065 mg/5 ml. Bot. 16 oz, gal.
Use: Sedative/hypnotic, anticholinergic/antispasmodic.

SUSPEN. (Circle) Penicillin V potassium 250 mg/5 ml. Bot. 100 ml.
Use: Antibacterial, penicillin.

SUS-PHRINE INJECTION. (Forest) Epinephrine 1:200 Amp. 0.3 ml, 12s, 25s. Multiple Dose Vial 5 ml, 1s.
Use: Bronchodilator.

SUS SCROFA LINNE var DOMESTICUS.
W/Proteolytic enzyme, autolyzed.
See: Saromide Inj., Vial (Saron).

SUSTACAL HC. (Mead Johnson Nutrition) High calorie nutritionally complete food. Protein 16%, fat 34%, carbohydrate 50%. Can 8 oz. Vanilla, chocolate or eggnog.
Use: Enteral nutritional supplement.

SUSTACAL LIQUID. (Mead Johnson Nutrition) Protein 24%, fat 21%, carbohydrate 55% with appropriate vitamin and mineral levels to meet 100% of the US RDAs. Vanilla, eggnog or chocolate flavor. Can 8 fl oz, 12 fl oz, 32 fl oz.
Use: Enteral nutritional supplement.

SUSTACAL POWDER. (Mead Johnson Nutrition) Caloric distribution and nutritional value when added to milk are similar to that of Sustacal liquid except lactose. Pow. Vanilla: 1.9 oz, packet 4s, can lb; Chocolate: 1.9 oz. packet 4s.
Use: Enteral nutritional supplement.

SUSTACAL PUDDING. (Mead Johnson Nutrition) Ready-to-eat fortified pudding containing at least 15% of the US RDAs for protein, vitamins

and minerals, in a 240 calorie serving. Protein 11%, fat 36%, carbohydrate 53%. Chocolate, vanilla and butterscotch flavor. Tin 5 oz, 110 oz.
Use: Enteral nutritional supplement.

SUSTAGEN. (Mead Johnson Nutrition) High-calorie, high-protein supplement. Protein 24%, fat 8%, carbohydrate 68%, essential vitamins and minerals. Prepared from nonfat milk, corn syrup solids, powdered whole milk, calcium caseinate, dextrose. Vanilla: Can 1 lb, 5 lb. Chocolate: Can 1 lb.
Use: Enteral nutritional supplement.

SUSTAIRE. (Pfizer Laboratories) Theophylline 100 mg or 300 mg/SR Tab. Bot. 100s.
Use: Bronchodilator.

•**SUTILAINS,** U.S.P. XXII. Oint., U.S.P. XXII. Proteolytic enzyme.
Use: Debriding agent.
See: Travase, Oint. (Flint).

SUVAPLEX TABLET. (Tennessee Pharm.) Vitamins A 5000 IU, D 500 IU, B_1 2.5 mg, B_2 2.5 mg, B_6 0.5 mg, B_{12} 1 mcg, C 37.5 mg, calcium pantothenate 5 mg, niacinamide 20 mg, folic acid 0.1 mg/Tab. Bot. 100s.
Use: Vitamin/mineral supplement.

SUXAMETHONIUM BROMIDE. B.A.N. Bis-2-dimethylaminoethyl succinate bismethobromide 00′-Succinyldi-(2-oxyethyltrimethylammonium bromide).
Use: Neuromuscular blocking agent.

SUXAMETHONIUM CHLORIDE. B.A.N.
See: Succinylcholine Cl.

•**SUXEMERID SULFATE.** USAN. Bis-(1,2,2,6,6-pentamethyl-4-piperidyl)succinate sulfate.
Use: Antitussive.

SUXETHONIUM BROMIDE. B.A.N. 00′-Succinyldi-[(2-oxyethyl) ethyldimethylammonium bromide].
Use: Neuromuscular blocking agent.

SWAMP ROOT. Compound of various organic roots in an alcohol base.
Use: Diuretic to the kidney.

SWEEN-A-PEEL. (Sween) Wafer 4×4. Box 5s, 20s; Sheet 12×12s. Box 2s, 12s.
Use: Skin protectant.

SWEEN CREAM. (Sween) Vitamin A and D cream. Tube 0.5 oz, 2 oz, 5 oz. Jar 2 oz, 9 oz.
Use: Skin treatment.

SWEEN KIND LOTION. (Sween) Bot. 21 oz, gal.
Use: Skin cleasner.

SWEEN PREP. (Sween) Box wipes 54s. Dab-o-matic 2 oz. Spray top 4 oz.
Use: Medicated skin barrier.

SWEEN SOFT TOUCH. (Sween) Bot. 2 oz, 16 oz, 21 oz, 32 oz, 1 gal, 5 gal.
Use: Medicated, antimicrobial lotion skin cleanser.

SWEETA. (Squibb Mark) Saccharin sodium, sorbitol. Bot. 24 ml, 2 oz, 4 oz.
Use: Sweetening agent.

SWEETASTE. (Purepac) Saccharin, sodium bicarbonate. 0.25 gr, 0.5 gr or 1 gr/Tab. Bot. 1000s.
Use: Sweetening agent.

SWEETENING AGENTS.
See: Ril-Sweet (Schering-Plough).
Saccharin, Preps. (Various Mfr.).
Sucaryl, Preps. (Abbott).
Sweetaste, Tab. (Purepac).

SWIM EAR. (Fougera) Boric acid 2.75% in isopropyl alcohol. Bot. oz.
Use: Otic preparation.

SWISS KRISS. (Modern) Senna leaves, herbs. Can 1.5 oz, 3.25 oz. Tab. 24s, 120s, 250s.
Use: Laxative.

SYLLACT. (Wallace) Psyllium seed husks 3.3 Gm/tsp, saccharin. Pow. Bot. 11 oz.
Use: Laxative.

SYMADINE. (Solvay) Amantadine HCl 100 mg/Cap. In 100s.
Use: Antiviral, antiparkinson agent.

•**SYMCLOSENE.** USAN. Trichloroisocyanuric acid.
Use: Local anti-infective.

•**SYMETINE HCl.** USAN. 4,4′-(Ethylenedioxy)-bis-[N-hexyl-N-methylbenzylamine dihydrochloride].
Use: Antiamebic.

SYMMETREL. (DuPont) Amantadine HCl. **Cap.:** 100 mg. Bot. 100s, 500s, UD 100s. **Syr.:** 50 mg/5 ml. Bot. pt.
Use: Antiviral, antiparkinson agent.

SYMPATHOLYTIC AGENTS.
See: Adrenergic blocking agents.
D.H.E. 45, Amp. (Sandoz).
Dibenzyline, Cap. (SmithKline).
Dihydroergotamine.
Ergotamine Tartrate.
Gynergen, Amp., Tab. (Sandoz).

SYMPATHOMIMETIC AGENTS.
See: Adrenalin (Parke-Davis).
Adrenergic agents.
Aerolate Jr. and Sr., Cap. (Fleming).
Aerolone Compound (Lilly).
Afrin, Preps. (Schering).
Amesec, Enseal, Pulvules (Lilly).
Aramine, Amp., Vial (Merck Sharp & Dohme).
Arlidin HCl, Tab. (Rorer).
Benzedrine Sulfate, Spansule, Tab. (SmithKline).
Brethine, Amp., Tab (Geigy).
Bronkephrine, Amp., (Winthrop).
Bronkometer (Winthrop).
Bronkosol Soln. (Winthrop).
Delcobese, Tab. (Delco).
Demazin, Tab., Syr. (Schering).
Desoxyn, Gradumet, Tab. (Abbott).
Dexamyl Tab. (SmithKline).
Dexedrine, Elix., Spansule, Tab. (SmithKline).
D-Feda, Cap., Liq. (Dooner).
Didrex, Liq., Tab. (Upjohn).
Dimetapp, Elix., Tab. (Robins).
Drinus Graduals (Amfre-Grant).
Duovent, Tab. (Riker).

Ectasule Minus Jr. and Sr., Cap. (Fleming).
Ectasule III, Cap. (Fleming).
Ephedrine, Preps.
Epinephrine salts.
Extendryl, Cap., Syr., Tab. (Fleming).
Fedrazil, Tab. (Burroughs Wellcome).
Fiogesic, Tab. (Sandoz).
Isoephedrine HCl.
Isuprel HCl, Preps. (Winthrop).
Levophed Bitartrate, Amp. (Winthrop).
Metaproterenol Sulfate (Various Mfr.).
Napril, Cap. (Marion).
Neo-Synephrine HCl, Preps. (Winthrop).
Nolamine, Tab. (Carnrick).
Norisodrine Sulfate, Soln. (Abbott).
Obedrin-LA, Tab. (Beecham Labs).
Obetrol, Tab. (Obetrol).
Orthoxine, Orthoxine and Aminophylline (Upjohn).
Orthoxine HCl, Tab., Syr. (Upjohn).
Otrivin, Soln., Spray (Geigy).
Phenylephrine HCl, Preps.
Phenylpropanolamine HCl.
Pseudoephedrine HCl, Syr., Tab.
Rondec DSC & T (Ross).
Slo-Fedrin, Slo-Fedrin A (Dooner).
Sudafed, Tab., Syr. (Burroughs Wellcome).
Triaminic, Preps. (Dorsey).
Triaminicol, Syr. (Dorsey).
Tussagesic, Susp., Tab. (Dorsey).
Tussaminic, Tab. (Dorsey).
Ursinus, Tab. (Dorsey).
Vasoxyl HCl, Amp., Vial (Burroughs Wellcome).
Wyamine Sulfate, Amp., Vial (Wyeth-Ayerst).

SYMPTROL. (Saron) Phenylpropanolamine HCl 50 mg, chlorpheniramine maleate 8 mg/SR Cap. Bot. 50s.
Use: Decongestant, antihistamine.

SYNA-CLEAR. (Pruvo) Decongestant, vitamin C. 25 mg/Tab. Bot. 12s, 30s.
Use: Decongestant, vitamin supplement.

SYNACORT. (Syntex) Hydrocortisone. Cream. **1%:** Tube 15 Gm, 30 Gm, 60 Gm. **2.5%:** Tube 30 Gm.
Use: Corticosteroid.

SYNALAR. (Syntex) Fluocinolone acetonide. **Cream 0.01%:** Tube 15 Gm, 30 Gm, 45 Gm, 60 Gm, 120 Gm, Jar 425 Gm. **0.025%:** Tube 15 Gm, 30 Gm, 60 Gm, 120 Gm, Jar 425 Gm. **Oint. 0.025%:** Tube 15 Gm, 30 Gm, 60 Gm, 120 Gm, Jar 425 Gm. **Soln. 0.01%:** Bot. 20 ml, 60 ml.
Use: Corticosteroid.

SYNALAR-HP CREAM. (Syntex) Fluocinolone acetonide 0.2% in water-washable aqueous base. Tube 12 Gm.
Use: Corticosteroid, topical.

SYNALGOS-DC CAPSULES. (Wyeth-Ayerst) Dihydrocodeine bitartrate 16 mg, aspirin 356.4 mg, caffeine 30 mg/Cap. Bot. 100s, 500s.
Use: Analgesic combination.

SYNAPP-R. (Blue Cross) Acetaminophen 325 mg, phenylpropanolamine HCl 25 mg, phenyltoloxamine citrate 22 mg/Tab. Bot. 40s.
Use: Analgesic, decongestant, antihistamine.

SYNAREL. (Syntex) Nafarelin acetate 2 mg/ml (as nafarelin base). Soln. Bot. 10 ml with metered pump spray.
Use: Gonadotropin-releasing hormone.

SYNATUSS-ONE. (Freeport) Guaifenesin 100 mg, dextromethorphan HBr 15 mg, alcohol 1.4%/5 ml. Bot. 4 oz.
Use: Expectorant, antitussive.

SYNCAINE.
See: Procaine HCl, Inj., Tab. (Various Mfr.).

SYNCORT.
See: Desoxycorticosterone Acetate, Inj., Pellets (Various Mfr.).

SYNCORTYL.
See: Desoxycorticosterone Acetate, Inj., Pellets (Various Mfr.).

SYNDOLOR CAPSULES. (Knight) Bot. 100s, 1000s.
Use: Analgesic.

SYNEMOL. (Syntex) Fluocinolone acetonide 0.025% in water-washable aqueous emollient base. Tube 15 Gm, 30 Gm, 60 Gm, 120 Gm.
Use: Corticosteroid, topical.

SYNEPHRICOL. (Winthrop) Paracetamol.
Use: Cold treatment.

SYNKAYVITE. (Roche) Menadiol sodium disphosphate. **Amp.:** 5 mg or 10 mg/ml, sodium metabisulfite 2.5 mg, phenol 0.45%. Amp. 1 ml Box 10s; 37.5 mg/ml. Amp. 2 ml Box 10s. **Tab.:** 5 mg Bot. 100s.
Use: Agent for hypoprothrombinemia, anticoagulant.

SYNKONIN.
See: Hydrocodone (Various Mfr.).

SYNOPHYLATE. (Central) Theophylline sodium glycinate. **Elix.:** Theophylline 165 mg/15 ml, alcohol 20%. Bot. pt, gal. **Tab.:** Theophylline 165 mg/Tab. Bot. 100s, 1000s.
Use: Bronchodilator.

SYNOPHYLATE-GG. (Central) Theophylline sodium glycinate 300 mg, guaifenesin 100 mg, alcohol 10% Syr. pt, gal.
Use: Bronchodilator, expectorant.

SYNTHALOIDS. (Buffington) Benzocaine, calcium-iodine complex/Loz. Salt free. Bot. 100s, 1000s, Unit box 8s, 16s, Box 24s, Dispens-A-Kit 500s, Aidpak 100s, Medipak 200s.
Use: Local anesthetic.

SYNTHOESTRIN.
See: Diethylstilbestrol, Preps. (Various Mfr.).

SYNTHROID. (Flint) Sodium levothyroxine 25 mcg, 50 mcg, 75 mcg, 100 mcg, 125 mcg, 150 mcg, 200 mcg or 300 mcg/Tab. Bot. 100s, 1000s.
Use: Thyroid hormone.

SYNTHROID INJECTION. (Flint) Lyophilized sodium levothyroxine 500 mcg/vial. (100 mcg/ml when reconstituted.) Vial 10 ml.
Use: Thyroid hormone.

SYNTOCINON AMPULS. (Sandoz) Synthetic oxytocin, chlorobutanol 0.5%, alcohol 0.61%. Amp. (10 IU/ml) 1 ml.
Use: Oxytocic.

SYNTOCINON NASAL SPRAY. (Sandoz) Synthetic oxytocin 40 IU/ml, exsiccated sodium phosphate, citric acid, sodium Cl, glycerin, sorbitol, methyl and propylparaben, chlorobutanol 0.05%, purified water, U.S.P. q.s. Squeeze bot. 2 ml, 5 ml.
Use: Oxytocic.

SYPHILIS (FTA-ABS) FLUORO KIT. (Clinical Sciences) Test for syphilis.
Use: Diagnostic aid.

SYRACOL. (Hauck) Phenylpropanolamine HCl 12.5 mg, dextromethorphan 7.5 mg. Liq. 60 ml, 120 ml.
Use: Decongestant, antitussive.

SYRAJEN. (Jenkins) Codeine phosphate 10.9 mg, chlorpheniramine maleate 2 mg, potassium guaiacolsulfonate 44 mg, citric acid 60 mg, sodium citrate 197 mg/5 ml. Bot. 4 oz, gal.
Use: Antitussive, antihistamine, expectorant.

SYROSINGOPINE. B.A.N. 4-Ethoxy-carbonyl-3,5-dimethoxybenzoic acid ester of methyl reserpate. Methyl 18β-Hydroxy-11-17α-dimethoxy-3β, 20α- yohimban-16β-carboxylate-4-Hydroxy-3,5-dimethoxybenzoate Ethyl Carbonate (Ester). Methyl O-(4-ethoxycarbonyloxy-3,5-dimethoxybenzoyl)reserpate.
Use: Antihypertensive.

SYROXINE TABS. (Major) Sodium levothyroxine 0.1 mg, 0.2 mg or 0.3 mg/Tab. Bot. 100s, 250s, 1000s, UD 100s. (3 mg 1000s.).
Use: Thyroid hormone.

SYRPALTA. (Emerson) Syrup containing combination of fruit flavors. Bot. pt, gal.
Use: Vehicle for masking drug taste.

•**SYRUP,** N.F. XVII.
Use: Flavored vehicle.

SYRVITE. (Various Mfr.) Vitamins A 2500 IU, D 400 IU, E 15 mg, B_1 1.05 mg, B_2 1.2 mg, B_3 13.5 mg, B_6 1.05 mg, B_{12} 4.5 mcg, C 60 mg/5 ml. Liq. Bot. pt, gal.
Use: Vitamin supplement.

T

T-3 RIABEAD. (Abbott Diagnostics) Radioimmunoassay for qualitative measurement of total circulating serum liothyronine. Test kit 50s, 100s.
Use: Diagnostic aid.

T-4 RIA (PEG). (Abbott Diagnostics) For quantitative measurement of total circulating serum thyroxine. Diagnostic kit 50s, 100s, 500s.
Use: Diagnostic aid.

TA. (Wampole-Zeus) Anti-thyroid antibodies by IFA. To identify two thyroid autoantibodies in a single test. Test 48s.
Use: Diagnostic aid.

TABASYN. (Freeport) Chlorpheniramine maleate 2 mg, phenylephrine HCl 10 mg, acetaminophen 5 gr, salicylamide 5 gr/Tab. Bot. 1000s.
Use: Antihistamine, decongestant, analgesic.

TABAZONE TABS. (Major) Oxyphenbutazone 100 mg/Tab. Bot. 100s.
Use: Antirheumatic agent.

TABRON FILMSEAL TABLETS. (Parke-Davis) Ferrous fumarate 304.2 mg (representing elemental iron 100 mg), docusate sodium 50 mg, vitamins E 30 IU, B_1 6 mg, B_2 6 mg, niacinamide 30 mg, B_5 10 mg, B_6 5 mg, C 500 mg, folic acid 1 mg, B_{12} 25 mcg/Filmseal Tab. Bot. 100s, UD pkg. 100s.
Use: Vitamin/mineral supplement.

TAC-3. (Herbert) Triamcinolone acetonide 3 mg/ml. Susp.: Vial 5 ml.
Use: Corticosteroid.

TAC-40. (Parnell) Triamcinolone acetonide 40 mg/ml. Inj. Susp. Vial 5 ml.
Use: Corticosteroid.

TACARYL. (Westwood) Methdilazine HCl. **Tab.:** 8 mg. Bot. 100s. **Syr.**: 4 mg/5 ml. Bot. 16 oz.
Use: Antipruritic.

TACARYL CHEWABLE TAB. (Westwood) Methdilazine 3.6 mg/Tab. Bot. 100s.
Use: Antipruritic.

TACE. (Merrell Dow) Chlorotrianisene 12 mg, 25 mg or 72 mg/Cap. **12 mg:** Bot. 28s, 100s, 500s; **25 mg:** Bot. 60s. **72 mg:** Pkg. 48s.
Use: Estrogen.

TACHYSTEROL.
See: Dihydrotachysterol, Tab. (Philips Roxane).

TACITIN. (Ciba) Under study. Benzoctamine, B.A.N.

•**TACLAMINE HYDROCHLORIDE.** USAN.
Use: Tranquilizer (minor).

TA CREAM. (C & M Pharmacal) Triamcinolone acetonide 0.025% or 0.05%. Jar 2 oz, 8 oz, lb.
Use: Corticosteroid, topical.

TACRINE. B.A.N. 9-Amino-1,2,3,4-tetrahydroacridine.
Use: CNS stimulant.

TAGAMET. (SKF) Cimetidine. **FC Tab.: 200 mg** Bot. 100s. **300 mg** Bot. 100s, UD 100s. **400 mg** Bot. 60s, UD 100s. **800 mg** Bot. 30s. **Liq.**: 300 mg (as HCl)/5 ml, alcohol 2.8%. Bot. 240 ml, UD 5 ml (10s). **Inj.: 300 mg** (as HCl)/2 ml with phenol 10 mg in an aqueous soln/Vial. Disp. syringe 2 ml, 8 ml. **300 mg** (as HCl)/2 ml in 50 ml sodium Cl 0.9%. SD Viaflex Plus container.
Use: Anti-ulcer agent.

TALACEN. (Winthrop Pharm) Pentazocine HCl 25 mg, acetaminophen 650 mg/Capl. Bot. 100s, UD 250s, (10 × 25s).
Use: Analgesic combination.

•**TALAMPICILLIN HYDROCHLORIDE.** USAN.

Use: Antibacterial.
•**TALBUTAL,** U.S.P. XXII. Tab., U.S.P. XXII. 5-Allyl-5-sec-butylbarbituric acid.
Use: Hypnotic.
See: Lotusate, Cap. (Winthrop Pharm).
•**TALC,** U.S.P. XXII. A native hydrous magnesium silicate.
Use: Dusting powder, pharmaceutical aid.
•**TALERANOL.** USAN.
Use: Enzyme inhibitor.
•**TALISOMYCIN.** USAN.
Use: Antineoplastic.
•**TALMETACIN.** USAN.
Use: Analgesic, antipyretic, anti-inflammatory.
•**TALNIFLUMATE.** USAN.
Use: Anti-inflammatory, analgesic.
TALOIN. (Adria) Methylbenzethonium Cl, zinc oxide, calamine, eucalyptol in a water-repellent base. Oint. Tube 2 oz.
Use: Skin protectant, antiseptic.
•**TALOPRAM HYDROCHLORIDE.** USAN.
Use: Potentiator (catecholamine).
•**TALOSALATE.** USAN.
Use: Analgesic, anti-inflammatory.
TALOXIMINE. B.A.N. 4-(2-Dimethylaminoethoxy)-1,2-dihydro-1-hydroxyiminophthalazine.
Use: Respiratory stimulant.
•**TALUDIPINE HYDROCHLORIDE.** USAN.
Use: Antihypertensive.
TALWIN COMPOUND. (Winthrop Pharm) Pentazocine HCl 12.5 mg, aspirin 325 mg/Tab. Bot. 100s.
Use: Narcotic analgesic.
TALWIN INJECTION. (Winthrop Pharm) Pentazocine lactate 30 mg/ml. Inj. Vial 10 ml. Uni-Amp 1 ml, 1.5 ml, 2 ml. Uni-Nest amp 1 ml, 2 ml. Carpuject 1 ml, 1.5 ml, 2 ml.
Use: Narcotic analgesic.
TALWIN NX. (Winthrop Pharm) Pentazocine HCl 50 mg, naloxone 0.5 mg/Tab. Bot. 100s, UD 250s.
Use: Narcotic analgesic.
TAMBOCOR. (Riker) Flecainide acetate 100 mg/Tab. Bot. 100s.
Use: Antiarrhythmic.
•**TAMERIDONE.** USAN.
Use: Sedative (veterinary).
•**TAMETRALINE HYDROCHLORIDE.** USAN.
Use: Antidepressant.
TAMINE S.R. (Geneva Generics) Phenylpropanolamine HCl 15 mg, phenylephrine HCl 15 mg, brompheniramine maleate 12 mg/SC Tab. Bot. 100s, 1000s.
Use: Decongestant, antihistamine.
•**TAMOXIFEN CITRATE,** U.S.P. XXII. Tab., U.S.P. XXII. (Z)-(4-(1,2-diphenyl-1-butenyl) phenoxy)-N,N-dime-thylethanamine 2-hydroxy-1,2,3-propanetricarboxylate (1:1).
Use: Treatment of mammary carcinoma, anti-estrogen.
See: Nolvadex, Tab. (Stuart).
•**TAMPRAMINE FUMARATE.** USAN.
Use: Antidepressant.
TAMP-R-TEL. (Wyeth-Ayerst) A tamper-resistant package for narcotic drugs which includes the following:
Codeine phosphate 30 mg/ml, 60 mg/ml.
Hydromorphone HCl 1 mg, 2 mg, 3 mg, 4 mg/Tubex.
Meperidine HCl 25 mg/ml and **Promethazine HCl** 25 mg/ml 2 ml.
Meperidine HCl 25 mg/ml, 50 mg/ml, 75 mg/ml, 100 mg/ml.
Morphine Sulfate 2 mg/ml, 4 mg/ml, 8 mg/ml, 10 mg/ml, 15 mg/ml.
Pentobarbital, Sodium 100 mg/2 ml.
Phenobarbital, Sodium 30 mg/ml, 60 mg/ml, 130 mg/ml.
Secobarbital, Sodium 100 mg/2 ml.
TANAC LIQUID. (Commerce) Benzalkonium Cl 0.12%, benzocaine 10%, tannic acid 6%. Saccharin. Bot. 0.3 oz, 0.5 oz.
Use: Mouth sores, cold sores, fever blisters.
TANAC ROLL-ON. (Commerce) Tannic acid 6%, benzalkonium Cl 0.12%, benzocaine 5%. Bot. 0.3 oz.
Use: Cold sores, fever blister, cracked lips.
TANAC STICK. (Commerce) Benzocaine 7.5%, tannic acid 6%, octyl dimethyl PABA 0.75%, allantoin 0.2%, benzalkonium Cl 7.5%, saccharin. Stick 0.1 oz.
Use: Cold sores, fever blisters, dry lips.
TANADEX. (Commerce) Tannic acid 2.86%, phenol 1.05%, benzocaine 0.47%. Bot. 3 oz.
Use: Throat gargle.
TAN-A-DYNE. (Archer-Taylor) Tannic acid compound, iodine. Bot. 4 oz, pt, gal.
Use: Swab and gargle concentrate.
TANBISMUTH.
See: Bismuth Tannate.
•**TANDAMINE HYDROCHLORIDE.** USAN.
Use: Antidepressant.
•**TANDOSPIRONE CITRATE.** USAN.
Use: Antianxiety agent.
•**TANNIC ACID.** U.S.P. XXII. Gallotannic acid. Glycerite. Tannin.
Use: 1% to 20% solution as an astringent.
See: Amertan, Oint. (Lilly).
W/Benzocaine, benzyl alcohol, diisobutylphenoxyethoxyethyl dimethyl benzyl ammonium Cl.
See: Kankex, Liq. (E. J. Moore).
W/Benzocaine, phenol, thymol iodide, ephedrine HCl, zinc oxide, balsam peru.
See: Hemocaine, Oint. (Mallard).
W/Bisacodyl.
See: Clysodrast, Packet (Barnes-Hind).
W/Boric acid, salicylic acid, isopropyl alcohol.
See: Sal Dex Boro, Liq. (Scrip).
W/Chlorobutanol, isopropyl alcohol.
See: Outgro, Soln. (Whitehall).
W/Cyanocobalamin, zinc acetate, glutathione, phenol.
See: Depinar, Amp. (Armour).
W/Merthiolate.

See: Amertan, Oint. (Lilly).
W/Salicylic acid, boric acid.
See: Tan-Bor-Sal, Liq. (Gordon).

TANNIC SPRAY. (Gebauer) Tannic acid 4.5%, chlorobutanol 1.3%, menthol > 1%, benzocaine > 1%, propylene glycol 33%, ethanol 60%. Bot. 2 oz, 4 oz.
Use: Relief of minor burns.

TANPHETAMIN.
See: Dextroamphetamine tannate.

TAO. (Roerig) Troleandomycin equivalent to 250 mg oleandomycin/Cap. Bot. 100s.
Use: Anti-infective.

TAPAL AMPULS. (Winthrop Products) Dipyrone.
Use: Analgesic, antipyretic, anti-inflammatory.

TAPAL TABLETS. (Winthrop Products) Dipyrone.
Use: Analgesic, antipyretic, anti-inflammatory.

TAPAR TABLETS. (Warner-Chilcott) Acetaminophen 325 mg/Tab. Bot. 100s.
Use: Analgesic.

TAPAZOLE. (Lilly) Methimazole. 1-methyl-2-mercaptoimidazole.
5 mg or 10 mg/Tab. Bot. 100s.
Use: Antithyroid agent.

•**TAPE, ADHESIVE,** U.S.P. XXII.
Use: Surgical aid.

TA-POFF. (Ulmer) Adhesive tape remover. Bot. pt. Aerosoln. Can 6 oz.

TAPULINE. (Wesley) Activated attapulgite 600 mg, pectin 60 mg, homatropine methylbromide 0.5 mg/Chew. Tab. Bot. 100s, 1000s.
Use: Antidiarrheal.

TAR.
See: Coal Tar, Preps.

TARACTAN. (Roche) Chlorprothixene. **Tab.:** 10 mg, 25 mg, 50 mg or 100 mg. Bot. 100s, 500s. **Concentrate:** 100 mg/5 ml. Bot. pt. **Amp.:** 25 mg/2 ml. Box 10s.
Use: Antipsychotic agent.

TAR DISTILLATE. (Doak) Decolorized fractional distillate of crude coal tar. Each ml equivalent to 1 Gm whole crude coal tar. Bot. 2 oz, 16 oz.
Use: Active ingredient for dermatologic preparations.

TARLENE LOTION. (Medco Lab) Refined crude coal tar, salicylic acid, propylene glycol. Plastic applicator bot. 2 oz.
Use: Antiseborrheic.

TARNPHILIC. (Medco Lab) Coal tar 1%, polysorbate 0.5% in aquaphilic base. Jar 16 oz.
Use: Antipsoriatic.

TARPASTE. (Doak) Coal tar 5% distilled in zinc paste. Tube 1 oz, Jar 4 oz, (w/hydrocortisone 0.5%. Tube oz).
Use: Antiseborrheic.

TAR-QUIN-HC. (Jenkins) Hydrocortisone 0.5%, liquor carbonis detergens 3%, clioquinol 1%. Oint. Tube 0.5 oz.
Use: Corticosteroid combination.

TARSUM SHAMPOO/GEL. (Summers) Coal tar 10%, salicylic acid 5% in shampoo base. Bot. 4 oz.
Use: Antipruritic, antipsoriatic.

TARTAR EMETIC.
See: Antimony Potassium Tartrate, U.S.P.

•**TARTARIC ACID,** N.F. XVII.
Use: Buffer.

TASHAN, Skin Cream. (Block) Vitamin A palmitate, D_2, D-panthenol, Vitamin E. Tube oz.
Use: Emollient.

TAUROCHOLIC ACID.
W/Pancreatin, pepsin.
See: Enzymet, Tab. (Westerfield).

TAUROLIN. B.A.N. 4,4′-Methylenedi(tetrahydro-1,2,4-thiadiazine-1-dioxide).
Use: Antibacterial.

TAUROPHYLLIN. (Vale) Ox bile extract 32.4 mg, phenolphthalein 32.4 mg, cascara sagrada extract 32.4 mg/Tab. Bot. 100s, 1000s, 5000s.
Use: Laxative.

TAURULTAM. B.A.N. Tetrahydro-1,2,4-thiadiazine 1,1-dioxide.
Use: Antibacterial, antifungal.

TA-VERM. (Table Rock) Piperazine citrate 100 mg/ml. **Syr.:** Bot. pt, gal. **Tab.:** 500 mg. Bot. 100s, 500s.
Use: Anthelmintic.

TAVILEN PLUS. (Table Rock) Liver soln. 1 Gm, ferric pyrophosphate soluble 500 mg, vitamins B_{12} 24 mcg, B_1 6 mg, B_2 7.2 mg, B_6 3 mg, panthenol 3 mg, niacinamide 60 mg, l-lysine HCl 300 mg, alcohol 5%/ml. Bot. pt, gal.
Use: Vitamin/mineral supplement.

TAVIST. (Sandoz) Clemastine fumarate 2.68 mg/Tab. Bot. 100s.
Use: Antihistamine.

TAVIST SYRUP. (Sandoz) Clemastine fumarate 0.67 mg/5 ml. Bot. 4 oz.
Use: Antihistamine.

TAVIST-1 TABLETS. (Sandoz) Clemastine fumarate 1.34 mg/Tab. Bot. 100s.
Use: Antihistamine.

TAVIST-D. (Sandoz) Clemastine fumarate 1.34 mg, phenylpropanolamine HCl 75 mg/Tab. Bot. 100s.
Use: Antihistamine, decongestant.

•**TAZADOLENE SUCCINATE.** USAN.
Use: Analgesic.

TAZICEF INJECTION. (SmithKline) Ceftazidime. Inj. **Vial:** 1 Gm/20 ml, 2 Gm/60 ml or 6 Gm/100 ml. **Piggyback:** 1 Gm/100 ml or 2 Gm/100 ml. **Pharmacy Bulk:** 6 Gm/100 ml.
Use: Antibacterial, cephalosporin.

TAZIDIME. (Lilly) Ceftazidime. Pow. 500 mg/10 ml Traypak 25s; 1 Gm/10 ml Traypak 10s; 2 Gm/20 ml Traypak 10s; 2 Gm/100 ml Traypak 10s; 6 Gm/100 ml Traypak 6s. ADD-Vantage Vial 1 Gm, 2 Gm. Traypak 10s.
Use: Antibacterial, cephalosporin.

•**TAZIFYLLINE HYDROCHLORIDE.** USAN.
Use: Antihistamine.

•**TAZOBACTAM SODIUM.** USAN.
Use: Antibacterial, beta-laxtamase inhibitor.

•**TAZOLOL HYDROCHLORIDE.** USAN.

Use: Cardiotonic.

TBA-PRED. (Keene) Prednisolone tebutate 10 mg/ml Susp. Vial 10 ml.
Use: Corticosteroid.

TC SUSPENSION. (Rorer) Aluminum hydroxide 600 mg, magnesium hydroxide 300 mg/5 ml, sorbitol, sodium 0.8 mg. Liq. UD 15 ml, 30 ml (100s).
Use: Antacid.

T-CORT. (Torch) Triamcinolone acetonide micronized. Pow. Bot. 1 Gm, 10 Gm.
Use: Extemporaneous prescription compounding.

T/DERM TAR EMOLLIENT. (Neutrogena) Neutar solubized coal tar extract 5% in oil base. Bot. 4 oz.
Use: Antipsoriatic, antipruritic.

T-DRY. (Jones Medical) Pseudoephedrine HCl 120 mg, chlorpheniramine maleate 12 mg/SR Cap. Bot. 100s.
Use: Decongestant, antihistamine.

T-DRY JR. (Jones Medical) Pseudoephedrine HCl 60 mg, chlorpheniramine maleate 4 mg/SR Cap. Bot. 100s.
Use: Decongestant, antihistamine.

TDx CORTISOL. (Abbott Diagnostics) Fluorescence polarization immunoassay for the quantitative determination of cortisol in serum, plasma or urine.
Use: Diagnostic aid.

TDx THYROXINE. (Abbott Diagnostics) Automated assay for quantitation of unsaturated thyroxine binding sites in serum or plasma.
Use: Diagnostic aid.

TDx TOTAL ESTRIOL. (Abbott Diagnostics) Fluorescence polarization immunoassay for the quantitative determination of total estriol in serum, plasma or urine.
Use: Diagnostic aid.

TDx TOTAL T3. (Abbott Diagnostics) Automated assay for quantitation of total circulating triiodothyronine (T3) in serum or plasma.
Use: Diagnostic aid.

TDx T-UPTAKE. (Abbott Diagnostics) Automated assay for the determination of thyroxine binding capacity in serum or plasma.
Use: Diagnostic aid.

TEAR AID. (Ketchum) Vial 15 ml.
Use: Decongestant.

TEARGEN. (Goldline) Bot. 15 ml.
Use: Artificial tear solution.

TEARGEN II. (Goldline) Hydroxypropyl methylcellulose 0.3%, dextran 70 0.1%, benzalkonium Cl 0.01%, EDTA 0.05%. Bot. 15 ml.
Use: Artificial tear solution.

TEARISOL. (CooperVision) An isotonic buffered aqueous soln. of hydroxypropyl methylcellulose 0.5%, edetate disodium 0.01%, benzalkonium Cl 0.01%, boric acid, sodium carbonate, potassium Cl. Bot. 15 ml.
Use: Artificial tear solution.

TEARS NATURALE. (Alcon) Duasorb water soluble polymeric system, benzalkonium Cl 0.01%, disodium edetate 0.05%. Droptainer 15 ml, 30 ml.
Use: Artificial tear solution, ocular lubricant.

TEARS NATURALE II. (Alcon) Sterile isotonic solution of Duosorb water soluble polymeric system, edetate disodium 0.1%, Polyquad 0.001% as preservative. Droptainer 15 ml.
Use: Artificial tear solution, ocular lubricant.

TEARS PLUS. (Allergan) Polyvinyl alcohol, povidone. Bot. 0.5 oz, 1 oz.
Use: Artificial tear solution.

TEARS RENEWED. (Akorn) Dextran 70, sodium Cl, hydroxypropyl methylcellulose, benzalkonium Cl 0.01%, EDTA 0.05%. Soln. Bot. 15 ml.
Use: Artificial tear solution.

TEA TREE OIL. (Metabolic Prod.) Australian oil of Melaleuca alternifolia 100% pure. Bot. 1 oz, 4 oz, 8 oz, 16 oz. **Cream** Bot. 8 oz. **Oint.** Tube 1 oz, 3 oz.
Use: Antiseptic, antifungal.

TEBAMIDE. (G & W) Trimethobenzamide HCl 100 mg/Supp. In 10s.
Use: Antiemetic/antivertigo.

•**TEBUFELONE.** USAN.
Use: Analgesic; anti-inflammatory.

•**TEBUQUINE.** USAN.
Use: Antimalarial.

T.E.C. (Invenex) Zinc 1 mg, copper 0.4 mg, cromium 4.0 mcg, manganese 0.1 mg. Vial 10 ml.
Use: Mineral supplement.

•**TECELEUKIN.** USAN.
Use: Immunostimulant.

TECHENESCAN MAA. Preparation of Tc 99m Aggregated Albumin (Human).
Use: Plasma protein fraction.

TECHNEPLEX. (Squibb) Technetium Tc 99m penetate. Kit vial 10s.
Use: Radiopaque agent.

TECHNETIUM 99m-IRON-ASCORBATE-DTPA.
See: Renotec (Squibb).

•**TECHNETIUM Tc-99m ALBUMIN AGGREGATED INJECTION,** U.S.P. XXII.
Use: Diagnostic aid (lung imaging).

TECHNETIUM Tc-99m ALBUMIN COLLOID INJECTION, U.S.P. XXII.
Use: Diagnostic aid (lung imaging).

TECHNETIUM Tc-99m ALBUMIN INJECTION, U.S.P. XXII.
Use: Radioactive agent.

•**TECHNETIUM Tc-99m** BICISATE. USAN.
Use: Diagnostic aid, radioactive, brain disorders.

•**TECHNETIUM Tc 99m DISOFENIN INJECTION,** U.S.P. XXII.
Use: Radioactive agent; diagnostic aid (hepatobiliary function determination).

•**TECHNETIUM Tc-99m ETIDRONATE INJECTION,** U.S.P. XXII.
Use: Radioactive agent.

TECHNETIUM Tc-99m GENERATOR SOLUTION. (New England Nuclear) Pertechnetate sodium Tc 99 m.
Use: Radiodiagnostic.

•**TECHNETIUM Tc-99m FERPENTETATE INJECTION,** U.S.P. XXII.
Use: Radioactive agent.

•**TECHNETIUM Tc-99m GLUCEPATE INJECTION.** USAN.
Use: Radioactive agent.

•**TECHNETIUM Tc-99m LIDOFENIN INJECTION.** U.S.P. XXII.
Use: Radioactive agent.

•**TECHNETIUM Tc-99m MEDRONATE INJECTION,** U.S.P. XXII.
Use: Diagnostic aid (skeletal imaging), radioactive agent.
See: Macrotec, Inj. (Squibb).

•**TECHNETIUM Tc 99m MERTIATIDE.** USAN.
Use: Diagnostic aid, renal function.

•**TECHNETIUM Tc-99m OXIDRONATE INJECTION,** U.S.P. XXII.
Use: Diagnostic aid (skeletal imaging), radioactive agent.

•**TECHNETIUM Tc-99m PENTETATE INJECTION,** U.S.P. XXII.
Use: Radioactive agent.

•**TECHNETIUM Tc-99m PYROPHOSPHATE INJECTION,** U.S.P. XXII.
Use: Radioactive agent.

•**TECHNETIUM Tc-99m (Pyro- and trimetra-) PHOSPHATES INJECTION,** U.S.P. XXII.
Use: Radioactive agent.

•**TECHNETIUM Tc-99m SESTAMIBI.** USAN.
Use: Diagnostic aid, cardiac disease.

•**TECHNETIUM Tc-99m SIBOROXIME.** USAN.
Use: Diagnostic aid; radioactive agent.

•**TECHNETIUM Tc-99m SODIUM INJECTION,** U.S.P. XXII.
Use: Radioactive agent.

•**TECHNETIUM Tc-99m SUCCIMER INJECTION,** U.S.P. XXII.
Use: Radioactive agent.

TECHNETIUM Tc-99m SULFUR COLLOID KIT.
Use: Radioactive agent.
See: Tesuloid (Squibb).

•**TECHNETIUM Tc-99m SULFUR COLLOID INJECTION,** U.S.P. XXII.
Use: Diagnostic aid (liver scanning).

•**TECHNETIUM Tc-99m TEBOROXIME.** USAN.
Use: Diagnostic aid, cardiac disease.

TECLOSINE. Under study.
Use: Amebicide.

TECLOTHIAZIDE. B.A.N. 6-Chloro-3,4-dihydro-3-trichloromethyl-1,2,4-benzothiadiazine-7-sulfonamide 1,1-dioxide.
Use: Diuretic.

•**TECLOZAN.** USAN. N,N′-(p-Phenylenedimethylene)-bis]2,2-dichloro-N-(2-ethoxy-ethyl)-acetamide].
Use: Amebicide.
See: Falmonox (Winthrop Products).

TEDRAL. (Parke-Davis) **Tab.:** Theophylline 118 mg, ephedrine HCl 24 mg, phenobarbital 8 mg/Tab. Bot. 24s, 100s, 1000s, UD 100s. **Susp. (Pediatric):** Theophylline 65 mg, ephedrine HCl 12 mg, phenobarbital 4 mg/5 ml. Bot. 8 oz.
Use: Antiasthmatic combination.

TEDRAL ELIXIR. (Parke-Davis) Theophylline 32.5 mg, ephedrine HCl 6 mg, phenobarbital 2 mg/5 ml, alcohol 15%. (Pediatric). Bot. pt.
Use: Antiasthmatic combination.

TEDRAL-SA. (Parke-Davis) Theophylline 180 mg, ephedrine HCl 48 mg, phenobarbital 25 mg/SA Tab. Bot. 100s, 1000s.
Use: Antiasthmatic combination.

TEDRIGEN. (Goldline) Theophylline 130 mg, ephedrine HCl 24 mg, phenobarbital 8 mg/Tab. Bot. 100s, 1000s.
Use: Antiasthmatic combination.

TEEBAZONE. Tibione. 4-Acetylamino-benzaldehyde thiosemicarbazone. Under study.
Use: Antituberculous agent.

TEEPHEN. (Robinson) **Cap.** or **Tab.:** Theophylline 2 gr, ephedrine ⅜ gr, phenobarbital ⅛ gr/Bot. 100s, 1000s, Bulk Pack 5000s. **Supp.:** Same formula as Cap. and Tab. Box 12s. **Susp.:** Theophylline 1 gr, ephedrine HCl ⅕ gr, phenobarbital 1/15 gr/5 ml. Bot. 8 oz.
Use: Antiasthmatic combination.

TEEV. (Keene) Estradiol valerate 4 mg, testosterone enanthate 90 mg/ml Inj. Vial 10 ml.
Use: Estrogen/androgen combination.

•**TEFLURANE.** USAN. 2-Bromo-1,1,1,2-tetrafluoroethane.
Use: General inhalation anesthetic.

TEGACID.
See: Glyceryl monostearate.

•**TEGAFUR.** USAN. (Mead Johnson).
Use: Antineoplastic.

TEGAMIDE. (G&W) Trimethobenzamide HCl 100 mg or 200 mg/Supp. Box 10s, 50s.
Use: Anticholinergic.

TEGISON. (Roche) Etretinate 10 mg or 25 mg/Cap. Prescription Pak 30s.
Use: Antipsoriatic.

TEGOPEN. (Bristol) Cloxacillin sodium. **Cap.:** 250 mg or 500 mg. Bot. 100s. **Granules for Soln.:** 125 mg/5 ml. Bot. 100 ml, 200 ml.
Use: Antibacterial, penicillin.

TEGRETOL. (Geigy) Carbamazepine. **Tab.:** 200 mg. Bot. 100s, 1000s, UD 100s. **Chew Tab.:** 100 mg. Bot. 100s. UD 100s.
Use: Anticonvulsant.

TEGRIN CREAM. (Block) Allantoin 2%, coal tar extract 5% in cream base. Tube 2 oz, 4.4 oz.
Use: Antipsoriatic.

TEGRIN MEDICATED. (Block) **Lot.:** Crude coal tar 5%, allantoin 1.7%. Lot. 180 ml. **Shampoo:** Crude coal tar 7%, sodium lauryl sulfate, ammonium lauryl sulfate, alcohol 6.4%. Cream 110 ml.
Use: Antiseborrheic.

T.E.H. COMPOUND. (Various Mfr.) Theophylline 130 mg, ephedrine sulfate 25 mg, hydroxyzine HCl 10 mg/Tab. Bot. 100s, 500s.
Use: Antiasthmatic combination.

•**TEICOPLANIN.** USAN.
Use: Antibacterial.

TELACHLOR. (Major) Chlorpheniramine maleate 8 mg/SR Cap. Bot. 100s, 250s, 1000s.
Use: Antihistamine.

TELACHLOR TD CAPS. (Major) Chlorpheniramine maleate 8 mg or 12 mg/TD Tab. Bot. 1000s.
Use: Antihistamine.

TELDRIN MAXIMUM STRENGTH CAPSULES. (SmithKline Prods) Chlorpheniramine maleate 12 mg/Spansule. Pkg. 12s, 24s, 48s.
Use: Antihistamine.

TELDRIN TABLETS. (SmithKline Prods) Chlorpheniramine maleate 4 mg/Tab.
Use: Antihistamine.

TELEFON. (Kenyon) Ferrous sulfate 150 mg/Cap. Bot. 100s, 1000s.
Use: Iron supplement.

TELEPAQUE. (Winthrop Pharm) Iopanoic acid 0.5 Gm/Tab. Bot. 30s, 150s.
Use: Radiopaque agent.

TELODRON. (Norden) Chlorpheniramine maleate.
Use: Antihistamine.

TEM. Tretamine, B.A.N.
See: Triethylenemelamine, Tab. (Lederle).

•**TEMAFLOXCIN HYDROCHLORIDE.** USAN.
Use: Antibacterial (microbial DNA topoisomerase inhibitor).

TEMARIL. (Herbert) Trimeprazine tartrate. **Tab.:** 2.5 mg. Bot. 100s, 1000s, Single Unit Pak 100s. **Syr.:** 2.5 mg/5 ml, alcohol 5.7%. Bot. 4 oz. **Spansule:** 5 mg. Bot. 50s, Single Unit Pak 100s.
Use: Antipruritic.

TEMARIL SUSTAINED RELEASE SPANSULES. (Herbert) Trimeprazine tartrate 5 mg/SR Cap. Bot. 50s, UD 100s.
Use: Antipruritic.

TEMARIL SYRUP. (Herbert) Trimeprazine tartrate 2.5 mg/5 ml. Syr. Bot. 4 oz.
Use: Antipruritic.

TEMARIL TABLETS. (Herbert) Trimeprazine tartrate 2.5 mg/Tab. Bot. 100s, 1000s, UD 100s.
Use: Antipruritic.

•**TEMATROPIUM METHYLSULFATE.** USAN.
Use: Anticholinergic.

•**TEMAZEPAM.** USAN. 7-Chloro-1,3-dihydro-3-hydroxy-1-methyl-5-phenyl-2H-1,4-benzodiazepin-2-one.
Use: Minor tranquilizer.
See: Restoril, Cap. (Sandoz).

•**TEMEFOS.** USAN.
Use: Ectoparasiticide.

•**TEMELASTINE.** USAN.
Use: Antihistamine.

TEMETAN. (Nevin) Acetaminophen. **Tab.:** 324 mg. Bot. 100s, 500s. **Elix.:** 324 mg/5 ml. Bot. pt.
Use: Analgesic.

•**TEMOCILLIN.** USAN.
Use: Antibacterial.

•**TEMODOX.** USAN.
Use: Growth stimulant.

TEMOVATE CREAM. (Glaxo) Clobetasol propionate 0.05%. Tube 15 Gm, 30 Gm, 45 Gm.
Use: Corticosteroid, topical.

TEMOVATE OINTMENT. (Glaxo) Clobetasol propionate 0.05%. Tube 15 Gm, 30 Gm, 45 Gm.
Use: Corticosteroid, topical.

TEMPO. (Thompson Medical) Calcium carbonate 414 mg, aluminum hydroxide 133 mg, magnesium hydroxide 81 mg, simethicone 20 mg/Tab. Bot. 10s, 30s, 60s.
Use: Antacid, antiflatulent.

TEMPRA. (Mead Johnson Nutrition) Acetaminophen. **Drops:** 100 mg/ml. Grape flavor. Bot. w/ dropper 15 ml. **Syr.:** 160 mg/5 ml. Cherry flavor. Bot. 4 oz, pt. **Chew. Tab.:** 80 mg or 160 mg. Bot. 30s.
Use: Analgesic.

TENEX. (Robins) Guanfacine HCl 1 mg/Tab. Bot. 100s, 500s, UD 100s.
Use: Antihypertensive.

•**TENIDAP.** USAN.
Use: Anti-inflammatory.

•**TENIPOSIDE.** USAN.
Use: Antineoplastic agent.

TEN-K. (Geigy) Potassium Cl 750 mg (10 mEq)/CR Cap. Bot. 100s, 500s, UD, blister pak 100s.
Use: Potassium supplement.

TENORETIC TABLETS. (ICI Pharma) **50 mg:** Atenolol 50 mg, chlorthalidone 25 mg/Tab. Bot. 100s. **100 mg:** Atenolol 100 mg, chlorthalidone 25 mg/Tab Bot. 100s.
Use: Antihypertensive.

TENORMIN. (ICI Pharma) **Oral:** Atenolol 50 mg or 100 mg/Tab. Bot. 100s, UD 100s. **Parenteral:** 5 mg/10 ml. Amp. 10 ml.
Use: Antihypertensive.

•**TENOXICAM.** USAN.
Use: Anti-inflammatory.

TENSEZE. (A.P.C.) Phenyltoloxamine citrate 88 mg, salicylamide 130 mg/Cap. Bot. 10s.
Use: Antianxiety agent.

TENSILON. (ICN Pharm.) Edrophonium Cl. **Vial:** 10 mg/ml, phenol 0.45%, sodium sulfite 0.2%. **Amp.** 10 mg/ml, sodium sulfite 0.2%.
Use: Cholinergic muscle stimulant.

TENSIN. (Standex) Reserpine 0.25 mg/Tab. Bot. 100s.
Use: Antihypertensive.

TENSIVE CONDUCTIVE ADHESIVE GEL. (Parker) Non-flammable conductive adhesive electrode gel, eliminates tape and tape irritation. Tube 60 Gm.
Use: For TENS, EMS, EMG, EEG and other electromedical procedures.

TENSOCAINE TABLETS. (Winthrop Products) Acetaminophen.
Use: Analgesic.

TENSOLAX TABLETS. (Winthrop Products) Chlormezanone.
Use: Analgesic, muscle relaxant.

TENSOLATE. (Apco) Phenobarbital 0.25 gr, hyoscyamine sulfate 0.1037 mg, atropine sulfate 0.0194 mg, hyoscine HBr 0.0065 mg/Tab. Bot. 100s.
Use: Sedative/hypnotic, anticholinergic/antispasmodic.

TENSOPIN. (Apco) Phenobarbital 0.25 gr, homatropine methylbromide 2.5 mg/Tab. Bot. 100s.
Use: Sedative/hypnotic, anticholinergic/antispasmodic.

TENSTAN. (Standex) Isobutylallylbarbituric acid ¾ gr, caffeine ⅔ gr, aspirin 3 gr, phenacetin 2 gr/Tab. Bot. 100s.
Use: Analgesic.

TENTRATE. (Tennessee Pharm.) Pentaerythritol tetranitrate 20 mg/Tab. Bot. 100s, 1000s.
Use: Antianginal.

TENUATE. (Lakeside) Diethylpropion HCl 25 mg/Tab. Bot. 100s.
Use: Anorexiant.

TENUATE DOSPAN. (Lakeside) Diethylpropion HCl 75 mg/CR Tab. Bot. 100s, 250s.
Use: Anorexiant.

TEPANIL. (Riker) Diethylpropion HCl 25 mg/Tab. Bot. 100s.
Use: Anorexiant.

TEPANIL TEN-TAB. (Riker) Diethylpropion 75 mg/Tab. Bot. 30s, 100s, 250s.
Use: Anorexiant.

•**TEPOXALIN.** USAN.
Use: Antipsoriatic.

•**TEPROTIDE.** USAN.
Use: Enzyme-inhibitor (angiotensin-converting).

TEQUINOL SODIUM. Name used for Actinoquinol Sodium.

TERALASE. W/Pancreatin, polysorbate-80.
See: Digolase, Cap. (Boyle).

TERAZOL 3. (Ortho) Terconazole 80 mg/Vaginal Supp. In 3s.
Use: Antifungal, vaginal.

TERAZOL 7. (Ortho) Terconazole 0.4% Cream. In 45 Gm.
Use: Antifungal, vaginal.

•**TERAZOSIN HYDROCHLORIDE.** USAN. (1) Piperazine, 1-(4-amino-6,7-dimethoxy-2-quinazolinyl)-4-[(tetrahydro-2-furanyl)carbonyl]-, monohydrochloride, dihydrate; (2) 1-(4-Amino-6,7-dimethoxy-2-quinazolinyl)-4-(tetrahydro-2-furoyl)piperazine monohydrochloride dihydrate.
Use: Antihypertensive.
See: Hytrin, Tab. (Abbott and Burroughs Wellcome).

•**TERBINAFINE.** USAN.
Use: Antifungal.

•**TERBUTALINE SULFATE,** U.S.P. XXII. Inj., Tab., U.S.P. XXII. a-[(tert-Butylamino)methyl]-3,5-dihydroxybenzyl alcohol sulfate.
Use: Bronchodilator.
See: Brethine, Amp., Tab. (Geigy).

TERCODRYL. (Approved) Codeine phosphate ¾ gr, pyrilamine maleate 25 mg/fl oz. Bot. 4 oz.
Use: Antitussive, antihistamine.

•**TERCONAZOLE.** USAN. Triaconazole.
Use: Antifungal.
See: Terazol 3, Vaginal Supp. (Ortho).
Terazol 7, Vaginal Cream (Ortho).

•**TERFENADINE.** USAN. U.S.P. XXII.
Use: Antihistamine.
See: Seldane, Tab. (Merrell Dow).

TERG-A-ZYME. (Alconox) Alconox with enzyme action. Box 4 lb. Ctn. 9×4 lb, 25 lb, 50 lb, 100 lb, 300 lb.
Use: Biodegradeable detergent and wetting agent.

TERIDOL JR. (Approved) Terpin hydrate, cocillana, potassium guaiacolsulfonate, ammonium Cl. Bot. 3 oz.
Use: Expectorant.

•**TERIPARATIDE ACETATE.** USAN.
Use: Diagnostic aid (hypocalcemia).

•**TERODILINE HYDROCHLORIDE.** USAN.
Use: Vasodilator (coronary).

•**TEROXALENE HYDROCHLORIDE.** USAN 1-(3-Chloro-p-tolyl)-4-[6-(p-tert-pentylphenoxy)-hexyl] piperazine hydrochloride.
Use: Antischistosomal.

•**TEROXIRONE.** USAN.
Use: Antineoplastic.

TERPACOF. (Jenkins) Codeine phosphate 10 mg, terpin hydrate 88 mg/5 ml. Bot. 3 oz, gal.
Use: Antitussive, expectorant.

TERPATE. (Geneva) Pentaerythritol tetranitrate 10 mg or 20 mg/Tab. Bot. 100s.
Use: Antianginal.

TERPEX JR. (Approved) d-Methorphan 25 mg, terpin hydrate, potassium guaiacolsulfonate, cocillana, ammonium Cl. Bot. 4 oz.
Use: Antitussive, expectorant.

TERPHAN ELIXIR. (Vale) Terpin hydrate 85 mg, dextromethorphan hydrobromide 10 mg/5 ml, alcohol 40% Bot. Gal.
Use: Expectorant, antitussive.

TERPIN-DEX. (Halsey) Dextromethorphan HBr 10 mg, terpin hydrate 85 mg/5 ml, alcohol 41.5%. Elix. Bot. 120 ml.
Use: Antitussive, expectorant.

•**TERPIN HYDRATE,** U.S.P. XXII. Elixir, with Codeine Elixir, U.S.P. XXII. cis-p-Menthane-1,8-diol hydrate.
Cryst., Pow., Pkg. 0.25 lb, 4 oz, 1 lb.
Use: Expectorant for chronic cough.
See: Creoterp (Jenkins).
Terp, Liq. (Scrip).

TERPIN HYDRATE W/COMBINATIONS
See: Histogesic, Tab. (Century).
Ipaterp C.T., Tab. (Fellows).
Prunicodeine, Liq. (Lilly).

Toclonol Expectorant, Liq. (Cenci).
Toclonol W/Codeine, Liq. (Cenci).
W/Dextromethorphan, phenylpropanolamine HCl, pheniramine maleate, pyrilamine maleate.
See: Tussaminic, Tab. (Dorsey).
W/Dextromethorphan, phenylpropanolamine HCl, pheniramine maleate, pyrilamine maleate, acetaminophen.
See: Chexit, Tab. (Dorsey).
Tussagesic, Tab., Liq. (Dorsey).

•**TERPIN HYDRATE AND DEXTROMETHORPHAN HYDROBROMIDE ELIXIR,** U.S.P. XXII.
Use: Expectorant, antitussive.
See: Dicodethal, Elix. (Lannett).

TERRA-CORTRIL. (Pfizer) Hydrocortisone 15 mg, terramycin HCl 5 mg/ml. Ophth. Susp. Bot. w/dropper 5 ml.
Use: Corticosteroid, anti-infective, ophthalmic.

TERRAMYCIN. (Pfizer Laboratories) Oxytetracycline **Cap.:** HCl salt 250 mg. Bot. 16s, 100s, 500s, UD 100s. **Oint., Ophth.:** Oxytetracycline HCl 5 mg, polymyxin B sulfate 1 mg/Gm. Tube 3.75 Gm. **Oint., Topical:** Oxytetracycline HCl 100 mg, polymyxin B sulfate 10,000 units/Gm. Tube 0.5 oz, 1 oz. **Pow. Topical:** Oxytetracycline HCl 30 mg, polymyxin B sulfate 10,000 units/Gm. Bot. 28.4 Gm. **Tab., Oral:** Oxytetracycline HCl 250 mg/Tab. Bot. 100s. **Tab., Vaginal:** Oxytetracycline HCl 100 mg, polymyxin B sulfate 100,000 units/Tab. Box 10s.
Use: Anti-infective.

TERRAMYCIN CAPSULES. (Pfizer Laboratories) Oxytetracycline HCl 250 mg/Cap. Bot. 100s, 500s.
Use: Antibacterial, tetracycline.

TERRAMYCIN TOPICAL OINTMENT. (Leeming) Oxytetracycline HCl 30 mg, polymyxin B sulfate 10,000 units/Gm. Tube 0.5 oz, 1 oz. Ctn. 12s.
Use: Anti-infective, external.

TERRAMYCIN TOPICAL POWDER WITH POLYMYXIN B SULFATE. (Leeming) Oxytetracycline HCl 30 mg, polymyxin B sulfate 10,000 units/Gm. Bot. oz.
Use: Anti-infective, external.

TERSAVID. N^1-pivaloyl-N^2-benzyl-hydrazine.
Use: Monoamine oxidase inhibitor.

TERTIARY AMYL ALCOHOL.
See: Amylene Hydrate (Various Mfr.).

TESAMONE. (Dunhall) Testosterone aqueous suspension.
'25' (25 mg/ml), '50' (50 mg/ml) or '100' (100 mg/ml) Amp. 10 ml.
Use: Androgen.

•**TESICAM.** USAN. 4'-Chloro-1,2,3,4-tetrahydro-1,3-dioxo-4-isoquinolinecarboxanilide.
Use: Anti-inflammatory.

•**TESIMIDE.** USAN.
Use: Anti-inflammatory.

TESIONATE 100. (Seatrace) Testosterone cypionate 100 mg/ml. Vial 10 ml.
Use: Androgen.

TESIONATE 200. (Seatrace) Testosterone 200 mg/ml. Vial 10 ml.
Use: Androgen.

TESLAC. (Squibb Mark) Testolactone 50 mg/Tab. Bot. 100s.
Use: Antineoplastic agent.

TESOGEN. (Sig) Testosterone 25 mg, estrone 2 mg/ml. Vial 10 ml.
Use: Androgen.

TESOGEN L.A. (Sig) Testosterone enanthate 50 mg, estradiol valerate 2 mg/ml; testosterone enanthate 90 mg, estradiol valerate 4 mg/ml; or testosterone enanthate 180 mg, estradiol valerate 8 mg/ml. Vial 10 ml.
Use: Androgen, estrogen combination.

TESONE. (Sig) Testosterone 25 mg, 50 mg or 100 mg/ml. Vial 10 ml.
Use: Androgen.

TESONE L.A. (Sig) Testosterone enanthate 200 mg/ml. Vial 10 ml.
Use: Androgen.

TESSALON PERLES. (Forest Pharm.) Benzonatate 100 mg/Cap. Bot. 100s.
Use: Antitussive.

TESTAMONE 100. (Dunhall) Testosterone 100 mg/ml. Inj. Vial 10 ml.
Use: Androgen.

TESTANATE No. 1. (Kenyon) Testosterone enanthate 100 mg, lipophilic soln. 200 mg/ml. Vial 10 ml.
Use: Androgen.

TESTANATE No. 2. (Kenyon) Testosterone enanthate 90 mg, estradiol valerate 4 mg/ml. Vial 10 ml.
Use: Androgen, estrogen combination.

TESTANATE No. 3. (Kenyon) Testosterone enanthate 180 mg, estradiol valerate 8 mg/ml. Vial 10 ml.
Use: Androgen, estrogen combination.

TES-TAPE. (Lilly) Diagnostic test for glucose in urine. Glucose oxidase, glucose peroxidase, orthotolidine. Single Pkg. test 100s.
Use: Diagnostic aid.

TESTARR GRANULES, FLAKES, PLAIN & FORTIFIED. (Fellows) Plantago seed mucilage. Also available w/thiamine. Pkg. 180 Gm, 390 Gm.
Use: Laxative.

TESTAVOL-S. (Fellows) Vitamin A palmitate 50,000 units/Cap. Bot. 100s, 1000s.
Use: Vitamin A supplement.

TEST-ESTRO CYPIONATES. (Rugby) Estradiol cypionate 2 mg, testosterone cypionate 50 mg/ml. Inj. Vial 10 ml.
Use: Estrogen, androgen combination.

TESTEX. (Pasadena Research) Testosterone propionate in sesame oil 50 mg or 100 mg/ml. Vial 10 ml.
Use: Androgen.

TESTOJECT. (Mayrand) Testosterone cypionate 100 mg/ml. Vial 10 ml.
Use: Androgen.

TESTOJECT-50. (Mayrand) Testosterone 50 mg/ml. Vial 10 ml.
Use: Androgen.

TESTOJECT-LA. (Mayrand) Testosterone cypionate 200 mg/ml in oil. Vial 10 ml.
Use: Androgen.

•**TESTOLACTONE,** U.S.P. XXII. Sterile Suspension, Tab., U.S.P. XXII. 13-Hydroxy-3-oxo-13, 17-secoandrosta-1,4-dien-17oic acid-8-lactone.
Use: Antineoplastic agent.
See: Teslac, Vial, Tab. (Squibb Mark).

TESTOLIN. (Pasadena Research) Testosterone suspension **25 mg/ml:** Vial 10 ml, 30 ml. **50 mg or 100 mg/ml:** Vial 10 ml.
Use: Androgen.

•**TESTOSTERONE,** U.S.P. XXII. Pellets, Sterile Susp., U.S.P. XXII. 17 β-Hydroxyandrost-4-en-3-one.
Use: Androgen.
See: Android-T, Vial (Brown).
Androlan, Vial (Lannett).
Andronaq, Aqueous Susp., Vial (Central).
Depotest, Vial (Hyrex).
Dura-Testrone, Vial (Pharmex).
Homogene-S, Inj., Vial (Spanner).
Malotrone Aqueous Inj. (Bluco).
Neo-Hombreol-F, Aq. Susp., Vial (Organon).
Tesone, Inj. (Sig).
Testolin, Vial (Pasadena Research).
Testrone, Vial (Pharmex).

TESTOSTERONE W/COMBINATIONS
See: Andesterone, Vial (Lincoln).
Androne, Vial (Rocky Mtn.).
Angen, Vial (Davis & Sly).
Depo-Testadiol, Vial (Upjohn).
Glutest, Vial (Brown).
Mal-O-Fem, Aqueous Susp., Vial (Fellows).
Terogen, Vial (Pasadena Research).
Tesogen, Inj. (Sig).
Testrone, Vial (Pharmex).
Vi-Testrogen, Vial (Pharmex).

TESTOSTERONE CYCLOPENTANE PROPIONATE. Testosterone Cypionate, U.S.P. XXII.

•**TESTOSTERONE CYPIONATE,** U.S.P. XXII. Inj., U.S.P. XXII. 17-β-Hydroxyandrost-4-en-3-one cy- clopentanepropionate. Androst-4-en-3-one, 17-(3-cyclopentyl-1-oxopropoxy)-, (17β-Testosterone cyclopentanepropionate).
Use: Androgen.
See: Andro-Cyp 100, Inj. (Keene).
Andro-Cyp 200, Inj. (Keene).
Depo-Testosterone, Inj. (Upjohn).
Dep-Test, Inj. (Sig).
Depotest, Vial (Hyrex).
D-Test 100, 200, Inj. (Burgin-Arden).
Durandro, Inj. (Ascher).
Testoject, Vial (Mayrand).
W/Combinations.
See: D-Diol, Inj. (Burgin-Arden).
Depotestogen, Vial (Hyrex).
Depo-Testadiol, Soln. (Upjohn).
Dep-Testradiol, Inj. (Rocky Mtn.).
Duo-Cyp (Keene).
Duracrine, Inj. (Ascher).
Span F. M., Inj. (Scrip).
T.E. Ionate P.A., Inj. (Solvay).

•**TESTOSTERONE ENANTHATE,** U.S.P. XXII. Inj., U.S.P. XXII. Androst-4-en-3-one, 17-(1-oxoheptyl)- oxy-(17β)-. Testosterone heptanoate. 17β-Hydroxyandrost-4-en-3-one heptanoate.
Use: Androgen.
See: Andryl, Inj. (Keene).
Arderone 100, 200, Inj. (Burgin-Arden).
Delatest, Inj. (Dunhall).
Delatestryl, Inj., Vial (Squibb).
Dura-Testosterone, Vial (Pharmex).
Everone 200 mg, Vial (Hyrex).
Retandros-200, Inj. (Rocky Mtn.).
Span-Test 100 and 200. (Scrip).
Tesone L. A., Inj. (Sig).
Testate, Inj. (Savage).
Testrin-P.A., Inj. (Pasadena Research).
W/Estradiol valerate.
See: Ardiol 90/4, 180/8, Inj. (Burgin-Arden).
Deladumone, Vial (Squibb Mark).
Delatestadiol, Vial (Dunhall).
Ditate, Ditate DS, Vial (Savage).
Duoval-P.A., Inj. (Solvay).
Repose-TE. (Paddock).
Retadiamone, Vial (Rocky Mtn.).
Span-Est-Test 4, Inj. (Scrip).
Teev, Preps. (Keene).
Testanate No. 2 and 3, Vial (Kenyon).
Valertest, Amp., Vial (Hyrex).

TESTOSTERONE HEPTANOATE.
Use: Androgen.
See: Testosterone enanthate.

•**TESTOSTERONE KETOLAURATE.** USAN. Testosterone 3-oxododecanoate.
Use: Androgen.

•**TESTOSTERONE PHENYLACETATE.** USAN. Perandren phenylacetate.
Use: Androgen.

TESTRAMONE. (Harvey) Testosterone 12.5 mg, vitamins B_1 10 mg, B_2 2 mg, B_6 5 mg, niacinamide 40 mg, inositol 50 mg, choline Cl 10 mg, methionine 10 mg/ml. Vial 10 ml.
Use: Androgen, vitamin supplement.

TESTRED. (ICN) Methyltestosterone 10 mg/Cap. Bot. 100s.
Use: Androgen.

TESTRED CYPIONATE 200. (ICN) Testosterone cypionate 200 mg/ml. Vial 10 ml.
Use: Androgen.

TESTRIN-P.A. (Pasadena Research) Testosterone enanthate 200 mg, in sesame oil with chlorobutanol/ml. Vial 10 ml.
Use: Androgen.

TESTRONE. (Pharmex) Testosterone 25 mg, estrone 2 mg/ml. Vial 10 ml.
Use: Androgen.

TESTURIA. (Wyeth-Ayerst) Combination kit containing 5 × 20 sterile dip strips and 5 × 20 culture trays of trypticase soy agar.

Use: Diagnostic aid.

TESULOID. (Squibb) Technetium Tc 99m sulfur colloid. 5 vials/kit.
Use: Radiopaque agent.

•**TETANUS ANTITOXIN,** U.S.P. XXII.
Use: Passive immunizing agent.
See: Homo-Tet, Vial, Syringe (Savage).

TETANUS AND DIPHTHERIA TOXOIDS ADSORBED FOR ADULT USE, U.S.P. XXII.
Use: Active immunizing agent for persons over 7 yrs. old.
Generic Products:
(Squibb/Connaught) Vial 5 ml for I.M. use.
(Lederle) Vial 5 ml.

TETANUS-DIPHTHERIA TOXOIDS ADSORBED, ALUMINUM PHOSPHATE ADSORBED. (Wyeth-Ayerst) Vial 5 ml, Tubex 0.5 ml.
Use: Agent for immunization.

TETANUS AND DIPHTHERIA TOXOIDS ADSORBED PUROGENATED. (Lederle) Adult Lederject disposable syringe 10 × 0.5 ml. Vial 5 ml New package.
Use: Agent for immunization.

•**TETANUS IMMUNE GLOBULIN,** U.S.P. XXII. (Hyland) Gamma globulin fraction of the plasma of persons who have been hyperimmunized with tetanus toxoid, 16.5%. Vial 250 units.
Use: Prophylaxis of injured, against tetanus (passive immunizing agent).
See: Gamulin-T, Vial (Merrell Dow).
Homo-Tet Vial, 1 ml (Savage).
Hu-Tet, Vial (Hyland).
Hyper-Tet Injection Vial, 250 units (Cutter).
Immu-Tetanus, Vial, Disp. Syr. (Parke-Davis).
T-I-Gammagee, Disp. Syr. (Merck Sharp & Dohme).

TETANUS IMMUNE GLOBULIN, HUMAN, (Wyeth-Ayerst) 250 units/Tubex, 1 ml Dissolved in glycine 0.3 M; contains thimerosal 0.01%.
See: Ar-Tet, Syringe, Vial (Armour).

•**TETANUS TOXOID,** U.S.P. XXII.
(Squibb/Connaught)—Vial 7.5 ml for I.M. or S.C. use.
(Lederle)—Vial 0.5 ml, 5 ml.
(Wyeth-Ayerst)—Vial 7.5 ml Tubex 0.5 ml.
Use: Agent for immunization.

•**TETANUS TOXOID, ADSORBED,** U.S.P. XXII. (Serums and Vaccines of America) 20 Lf purified tetanus toxoid, 0.01% thimerosal as preservative/ml. Box 2 ampuls of 0.5 ml. Vial 5 ml, 7.5 ml, 0.5 ml. Amp. for booster injection.
(Squibb/Connaught) Vial 5 ml for I.M. use.
(Lederle)—Vial 5 ml Steri-Dose syringe 0.5 ml 10s.
(Wyeth-Ayerst)—Vial 5 ml Tubex 0.5 ml.
Use: Active immunizing agent against tetanus.

TETANUS TOXOID ADSORBED PUROGENATED. (Lederle) Vial 5 ml. Lederject disposable syringe 0.5 ml. Box 10s, 100s.
Use: Agent for immunization.

TETANUS TOXOID, ALUM PRECIPITATED.
Use: Agent for immunization.
See: (Cutter)—Vial 5 ml.
(Lilly)—Vial 1 ml, 5 ml. Hyporets 0.5 ml, 10s, 100s.
(Merck Sharp & Dohme)—Vial 5 ml.

•**TETANUS TOXOID, ALUMINUM PHOSPHATE ADSORBED,** U.S.P. XXII.
Use: Active immunizing agent.
See: (Lederle) Vial 5 ml, 10s. Lederject Disp. Syringe 10 × 0.5 ml.
(Wyeth-Ayerst) Vial 5 ml, Tubex 0.5 ml.

TETANUS TOXOID, FLUID PUROGENATED.
(Lederle)—Vial 7.5 ml Lederject disposable syringe.
0.5 ml. Box 10s, 100s.
Use: Agent for immunization.

TETANUS TOXOID PURIFIED, FLUID.
(Wyeth-Ayerst)—Vial 7.5 ml, Tubex 0.5 ml.
Use: Agent for immunization.

TETIOTHALEIN SODIUM.
See: Iodophthalein Sodium. (Various Mfr.).

TETRABEAD. (Abbott Diagnostics) Solid phase radioimmunoassay for the quantitative measurement of total circulating serum thyroxine.
Use: Radiopaque agent.

TETRABEAD-125. (Abbott Diagnostics) T-3 uptake radioassay for the measurement of thyroid function by indirectly determining the degree of saturation of serum thyroxine binding globulin (TBG).
Use: Radiopaque agent.

TETRABENAZINE. B.A.N. 1,3,4,6,7,11b-Hexahydro-3-isobutyl-9, 10-dimethoxybenzo[a] quinolizin-2-one.
Use: Tranquilizer.

•**TETRACAINE,** U.S.P. XXII. Oint., Ophth. Oint., Inj., U.S.P. XXII. 2-Dimethylaminoethyl p-butylaminobenzoate.
Use: Local anesthetic.

•**TETRACAINE AND MENTHOL OINTMENT,** U.S.P. XXII.
Use: Local anesthetic.

•**TETRACAINE HYDROCHLORIDE,** U.S.P. XXII. Cream, Inj., Ophth. Soln., Topical Soln., Sterile, U.S.P. XXII. 2-(Dimethyl-amino)-ethyl p-(butylamino)-benzoate HCl. Benzoic acid, 4-(butylamino)-, 2-(dimethylamino)ethyl ester, monohydrochloride.
Use: Local anesthetic, topical anesthetic, spinal anesthetic.
See: Bristacycline, Cap. (Bristol).
Pontocaine Hydrochloride Prods. (Winthrop Pharm).
W/Benzocaine, butyl aminobenzoate.
See: Cetacaine, Liq., Oint., Spray (Cetylite).
W/Hexachlorophene, dimethyl polysiloxane, methyl salicylate, pyrilamine maleate, zinc oxide.
W/Isocaine, benzalkonium Cl.
See: Isotraine Oint. (Philips Roxane).

TETRACAINE HYDROCHLORIDE 0.5%.

(Alcon) 0.5%/1 ml Drop-Tainer, Ophth. 15 ml Steri-Unit, 2 ml (Cooper Vision) Dropperettes 1 ml in 10s.
Use: Local anesthetic, ophthalmic.

TETRACAP. (Circle) Tetracycline HCl 250 mg/Cap. Bot. 100s.
Use: Antibacterial, tetracycline.

TETRACHLORETHYLENE, U.S.P. XXI. Cap., U.S.P. XXI. Perchlorethylene, tetrachlorethylene.
Use: Anthelmintic (hookworms and some trematodes).

TETRACLOR. (Kenyon) Tetracycline HCl 250 mg/Cap. Bot. 100s, 1000s.
Use: Antibacterial, tetracycline.

TETRACLOR-L. (Kenyon) Tetracycline HCl 125 mg/5 ml. Bot. pt.
Use: Antibacterial, tetracycline.

TETRACON. (Professional Pharmacal) Tetrahydrozoline HCl 0.5 mg, disodium edetate 1 mg, boric acid 12 mg, benzalkonium Cl 0.1 mg, sodium Cl 2.2 mg, sodium borate 0.5 mg/ml, water. Bot. 15 ml.
Use: Ocular decongestant.

TETRACOSACTIDE. (I.N.N.) Tetracosactrin, B.A.N.

TETRACOSACTRIN. B.A.N. β^{1-24}-Corticotrophin.
Use: Corticotrophic peptide.
See: Cortrosyn.
Cosyntropin.
Synacthen.
Tetracosactide (I.N.N.).

•**TETRACYCLINE,** U.S.P. XXII. Boluses, Oral Susp., U.S.P. XXII. 4-(Dimethylamino)-1,4,4a,5,5a,6,11,12a-octahydro-3,-6,10,12,12a-penta hy- droxy-6-methyl-1,11-dioxo-2-naphthacenecarboxamide.
Use: Antibiotic.
See: Robitet, Syr. (Robins).
Sumycin, Syrup (Squibb).
W/N-acetyl-para-amino-phenol, phenyltoloxamine citrate.
Use: Antibacterial; anti-amebic; antirickettsial.
See: Paltet, Cap. (Hauck).
Tetrex, Bid Cap., Cap., Vial (Bristol).

TETRACYCLINE AND AMPHOTERICIN B, U.S.P. XXI. Cap., Oral Susp., U.S.P. XXI.

•**TETRACYCLINE HYDROCHLORIDE,** U.S.P. XXII. Cap., Inj., Oint., Ophth Oint., Soluble Powder, Topical Soln., Ophth. Susp., Sterile, Tab., U.S.P. XXII.
Use: Antibiotic.
See: Achromycin, Preps. (Lederle).
Amer-Tet, Tab. (Robinson).
Amer-Tet, Susp. (Robinson).
Bicycline, Cap. (Knight).
Centet 250, Tab. (Central).
Cyclopar, Cap. (Parke-Davis).
Fed-Mycin, Cap. (Amfre-Grant).
G-Mycin, Cap., Syr. (Coast).
Maso-Cycline, Cap. (Mason).
Panmycin, Cap. (Upjohn).
Robitet, Cap. (Robins).
Sarocycline, Cap., Inj., Syr. (Saron).
Scotrex, Cap. (Scott/Cord).
Sumycin, Cap., Tab., Syr. (Squibb Mark).
Tet-Cy, Cap. (Metro).
Tetra-C, Cap. (Century).
Tetracap 250, Cap. (Circle).
Tetrachor, Tetrachor-L, Cap., Liq. (Kenyon).
Tetracyn, Cap. (Pfizer Laboratories).
Tetralan "250", "500", Cap. (Lannett).
Tetram and Tetram-S, Cap., Syr. (Dunhall).
Tetramax, Cap. (Rand).
Topicycline, Liq. (Proctor & Gamble).
Trexin, Cap. (A.V.P. Pharm.).
W/Citric Acid.
See: Achromycin V, Cap., Drop, Susp., Syr. (Lederle).
W/Nystatin.
See: Comycin, Cap. (Upjohn).

•**TETRACYCLINE HYDROCHLORIDE AND NYSTATIN CAPSULES,** U.S.P. XXII.
Use: Antibiotic, antifungal.
See: Comycin, Cap. (Upjohn)

•**TETRACYCLINE ORAL SUSPENSION,** U.S.P. XXII.
Use: Antibiotic.
See: Brand names under Tetracycline.

TETRACYN. (Pfizer Laboratories) Tetracycline HCl 250 mg or 500 mg/Cap. **250 mg:** Bot. 1000s. **500 mg:** Bot. 100s.
Use: Antibacterial, tetracycline.

TETRAETHYLAMMONIUM BROMIDE (TEAB). Diagnostic and therapeutic agent in peripheral vascular disorders. Diagnostic in hypertension.
Use: Diagnostic aid.

TETRAETHYLAMMONIUM CHLORIDE.
Use: Ganglionic blocking agent.

TETRAETHYLTHIURAM DISULFIDE.
See: Disulfiram.

•**TETRAFILCON A.** USAN.
Use: Contact lens material.

TETRAHYDROPHENOBARBITAL CALCIUM.
See: Cyclobarbital Calcium, Preps.

TETRAHYDROXYQUINONE. Name used for Tetroquinone.

TETRAHYDROZOLINE. B.A.N. 2-(1,2,3,4-Tetrahydro-1-naphthyl)-2-imidazoline.
Use: Vasoconstrictor.

•**TETRAHYDROZOLINE HYDROCHLORIDE,** U.S.P. XXII. Nasal Soln., Ophth. Soln. U.S.P. XXII. 2-(1,2,3,4-Tetrahydro-1-naphthyl)-2-imidazoline HCl.
Use: Adrenergic (vasoconstrictor).
See: Murine Plus (Abbott).
Tyzine, Soln. (Key).
Visine, Soln. (Leeming).

TETRAIODOPHENOLPHTHALEIN SODIUM.
See: Iodophthalein Sodium.

TETRAIODOPHTHALEIN SODIUM.
See: Iodophthalein Sodium.

TETRALAN "250." (Lannett) Tetracycline HCl 250 mg/Cap. Bot. 100s, 1000s.
Use: Antibacterial, tetracycline.

TETRALAN "500." (Lannett) Tetracycline HCl 500 mg/Cap. Bot. 100s, 1000s.
Use: Antibacterial, tetracycline.

TETRAM. (Dunhall) Tetracycline 250 mg/Cap. Bot. 100s.
Use: Antibacterial, tetracycline.

TETRAMAX. (Rand) Tetracycline HCl 250 mg/Cap. Bot. 100s, 1000s.
Use: Antibacterial, tetracycline.

TETRAMETHYLENE DIMETHANESULFONATE.
See: Busulfan, U.S.P. XXII.

TETRAMETHYLTHIURAM DISULFIDE. Thiram.
Use: Anti-infective, antifungal.
See: Rezifilm, Aerosol (Squibb).

TETRAMISOLE. V.B.A.N. (±)-2,3,5,6-Tetrahydro-6- phenylimidazo[2,1-b]thiazole.
Use: Anthelmintic, Veterinary medicine.

•**TETRAMISOLE HYDROCHLORIDE.** USAN. ±2,3,5,6-Tetrahydro-6-phenylimidazo [2,1-b]-thiazole HCl.
Use: Anthelmintic.
See: Ripercol (American Cyanamid).

TETRANEED. (Hanlon) Pentaerythritol tetranitrate 80 mg/Time Cap. Bot. 100s.
Use: Antianginal.

TETRANTOIN. 7,8-Benzo-1,3-diazaspiro(4,5)-decane-2,4-dione. 3′,4′-Dihydrospiro-[imidazolidine-4,2′(1′H)-naphthalene]-2,5-dione.
Use: Anticonvulsant.

TETRATAB. (Freeport) Pentaerythritol tetranitrate 10 mg/Tab. Bot. 1000s.
Use: Antianginal.

TETRATAB NO. 1. (Freeport) Pentaerythritol tetranitrate 20 mg/Tab. Bot. 1000s.
Use: Antianginal.

TETRAZYME. (Abbott Diagnostics) Enzyme immunoassay for quantitative measurement of total circulating serum thyroxine (free and protein bound). Test kit 100s, 500s.
Use: Diagnostic aid.

TETROQUINONE. USAN. Tetrahydroxy-p-benzoquinone.
Use: Treat keloids, keratolytic (systemic).
See: Kelox (Elder).

TETROXOPRIM. USAN.
Use: Antibacterial.

TETRYDAMINE. USAN. 4,5,6,7-Tetrahydro-2-methyl-3-(methylamino)-tetrahydroindazole.
Use: Analgesic, anti-inflammatory.

TETRYZOLINE (I.N.N.). Tetrahydrozoline, B.A.N.

TETTERINE. (Shuptrine) **Oint.:** Antifungal agents in green petrolatum base. Tin oz; Antifungal agents in white petroleum base. Tube oz. **Pow.:** Fungicide, germicide formula powder for heat and diaper rash. Can 2.25 oz. **Soap:** Bar 3.25 oz.
Use: Antifungal.

TEXACORT SCALP LOTION. (GenDerm Co.) Hydrocortisone 1%, alcohol 33%. Lipid free. Dropper Bot. 1 fl oz.
Use: Corticosteroid.

T-FLUORIDE. (Tennessee) Sodium fluoride 2.21 mg/Tab. Bot. 100s, 1000s.
Use: Dental caries preventative.

T/GEL SCALP SOLUTION. (Neutrogena) Neutar coal tar extract 2%, salicyclic acid 2%. Bot. 2 oz.
Use: Antipsoriatic, antiseborrheic.

T/GEL THERAPEUTIC SHAMPOO. (Neutrogena) Neutar coal tar extract 2% in mild shampoo base. Bot. 4.4 oz, 8.5 oz.
Use: Antipsoriatic, antiseborrheic.

T/GEL THERAPEUTIC CONDITIONER. (Neutrogena) Neutar coal tar extract 1.5% in oil free conditioner base. Bot. 1.4 oz.
Use: Antipsoriatic, antiseborrheic.

T-GEN SUPPOSITORIES. (Goldline) Trimethobenzamide HCl 100 mg/Pediatric Supp. or 200 mg/Adult Supp. Box 10s, 50s.
Use: Anticholinergic.

T-GESIC CAPSULE. (T.E. Williams) Hydrocodone bitartrate 5 mg, acetaminophen 325 mg, caffeine 40 mg, butalbital 30 mg/Cap. Bot. 100s.
Use: Narcotic analgesic combination, sedative/hypnotic.

•**THALIDOMIDE.** USAN. a-(N-Phthalimido)glutarimide. 2-Phthalimidoglutarimide.
Use: Hypnotic, sedative.

THALITONE. (Boehringer Ingelheim) Chlorthalidone 25 mg/Tab. Bot. 100s.
Use: Diuretic.

•**THALLOUS CHLORIDE TL-201 INJECTION,** U.S.P. XXII.
Use: Diagnostic aid (radioactive agent).

THAM SOLUTION. (Abbott) Tromethamine 18 Gm, acetic acid 2.5 Gm. Single-dose container.
Use: Parenteral nutritional supplement.

THAM-E. (Abbott) Tromethamine 36 Gm, sodium Cl 30 mEq/L, potassium Cl 5 mEq/L, chloride 35 mEq/L. Total osmolarity 367 mOsm/L. Single dose container 150 ml.
Use: Parenteral nutritional supplement.

THEAMIN. Monoethanolamine salt of theophylline.
See: Monotheamin, Supp. (Lilly).
W/Amobarbital.
See: Monotheamin and Amytal, Pulvule (Lilly).

THEBACON. B.A.N. O^6-Acetyl-O^3-methyl-Δ^6-morphine.
Use: Narcotic analgesic; cough suppressant.

THEDRAZOL. (Kenyon) Pentylenetetrazol 100 mg, nicotinic acid 50 mg/Tab. Bot. 100s, 1000s.
Use: Antihypertensive.

THEDRAZOL-L. (Kenyon) Pentylenetetrazol 100 mg, niacin 50 mg/5 ml. Bot. 4 oz, pt, gal.
Use: Antihypertensive.

THEELIN AQUEOUS SUSPENSION. (Parke-Davis) A suspension of estrone in isotonic sodium

Cl solution for I.M. administration. Steri-Vial 2 mg (20,000 IU)/ml, Vial 10 ml.
Use: Estrogen.

THEELIN INJECTION. (Morton) Estrone suspension 2 mg or 5 mg/ml. Vial 10 ml. For I.M. administration.
Use: Estrogen.

THENALIDINE. B.A.N. 1-Methyl-4-N-(2-thenyl)-anilinopiperidine.
Use: Antihistamine.

THENALIDINE TARTRATE. 1-Methyl-4-(N-2-thenylanilino) piperidine tartrate.
Use: Antihistamine, antipruritic.

•**THENIUM CLOSYLATE.** USAN. N,N-Dimethyl, N2-phenoxy-ethyl-N-2-thenylammonium p-chlorobenzenesulfonate.
Use: Canine hookworm.
See: Bancari (Burroughs Wellcome).

THENYLDIAMINE. B.A.N. 2-(N-2-Pyridyl-N-2-thenyl-amino)ethyldimethylamine.
Use: Antihistamine.

THENYLDIAMINE HYDROCHLORIDE. 2-[(2-Dimethylaminoethyl)-3-thenyl-amino] pyridine HCl, thenyldramine Cl. Dethylandiomine.
Use: Antihistamine.

THENYLPYRAMINE.
See: Methapyrilene Hydrochloride, Preps.

THEO-24. (Searle) Theophylline anhydrous 100 mg, 200 mg or 300 mg/CR Cap. **100 mg:** Bot. 100s, UD 100s; **200 mg** or **300 mg:** Bot. 100s, 500s, UD 100s.
Use: Bronchodilator.

THEOBID DURACAP. (Russ) Theophylline anhydrous 260 mg/TR Cap. Bot. 60s, 500s.
Use: Bronchodilator.

THEOBID JR DURACAP. (Russ) Theophylline anhydrous 130 mg/TR Cap. Bot 60s.
Use: Bronchodilator.

THEOBROMA OIL. Cocoa Butter, N.F. XVII.
Use: Suppository base.

THEOBROMINE WITH PHENOBARBITAL COMBINATIONS.
See: Harbolin, Tab. (Arcum).
Theocardone, Tab. (Lemmon).
T.P. KI, Tab. (Wendt-Bristol).

THEOBROMINE CALCIUM GLUCONATE.
(Bates)—Tab., Bot. 100s, 1000s. Also available w/phenobarbital.
(Grant)—Tab., Bot. 100s, 500s, 1000s.
Use: Diuretic, smooth muscle relaxant.

THEOBROMINE SODIUM ACETATE. Theobromine calcium salt mixture with calcium salicylate.
Use: Diuretic, smooth muscle relaxant.

THEOBROMINE SODIUM SALICYLATE.
See: Doan's Pills (Purex).
W/Calcium lactate, phenobarbital.
See: Theolaphen, Tab. (Elder).

THEOCHRON. (Forest Labs) Theophylline 200 mg or 300 mg/TR Tab. **200 mg:** Bot. 100s, 500s, 1000s. **300 mg:** Bot. 100s, 500s.
Use: Bronchodilator.

THEOCLEAR 80 SYRUP. (Central) Theophylline 80 mg/15 ml. Bot. pt, gal.
Use: Bronchodilator.

THEOCLEAR L.A.-130 (Central) Theophylline 130 mg/Cenule. Bot. 100s.
Use: Bronchodilator.

THEOCLEAR L.A.-260 (Central) Theophylline 260 mg/Cenule. Bot. 100s, 1000s.
Use: Bronchodilator.

THEOCOLATE. (PBI) Theophylline 150 mg, guaifenesin 90 mg/15 ml Liq. Bot. pt, gal.
Use: Antiasthmatic combination.

THEODRENALINE. B.A.N. 7-[2-(3,4,β-Trihydroxyphenethylamino)ethyl]theophylline.
Use: Analeptic.

THEODRINE. (Rugby) Theophylline 130 mg, ephedrine HCl 24 mg, phenobarbital 8 mg/Tab. Bot. 100s, 1000s.
Use: Antiasthmatic combination.

THEO-DUR. (Schering) Theophylline 450 mg/SR Tab. Bot. 100s, UD 100s.
Use: Bronchodilator.

THEO-DUR SPRINKLE. (Key) Theophylline 50 mg, 75 mg, 125 mg or 200 mg/SA Cap. Bot. 100s.
Use: Bronchodilator.

THEO-DUR TABLETS. (Key) Theophylline 100 mg, 200 mg or 300 mg/SA Tab. Bot. 100s, 500s, 1000s, 5000s, UD 100s.
Use: Bronchodilator.

•**THEOFIBRATE.** USAN.
Use: Antihyperlipoproteinemic.

THEOGEN. (Sig) Conjugated estrogens 2 mg/ml. Vial 10 ml, 30 ml.
Use: Estrogen.

THEOGEN I.P. (Sig) Estrone 2 mg, potassium estrone sulfate 1 mg/ml. Vial 10 ml.
Use: Estrogen.

THEOLAIR. (Riker) Theophylline 125 mg or 250 mg/Tab. Box 100s, 250s as foil strip 10s. Bot. 100s.
Use: Bronchodilator.

THEOLAIR LIQUID. (Riker) Theophylline 80 mg/15 ml. Bot. pt.
Use: Bronchodilator.

THEOLAIR-SR 200. (Riker) Theophylline 200 mg/SR Tab. Bot. 100s, Box 100s as foil strip 10s.
Use: Bronchodilator.

THEOLAIR-SR 250. (Riker) Theophylline 250 mg/SR Tab. Bot. 100s, 250s.
Use: Bronchodilator.

THEOLAIR-SR 300. (Riker) Theophylline 300 mg/SR Tab. Bot. 100s. Box 100s as foil strip 10s.
Use: Bronchodilator.

THEOLAIR-SR 500. (Riker) Theophylline 500 mg/SR Tab. Bot. 100s, 250s.
Use: Bronchodilator.

THEOLATE LIQUID. (Goldline) Theophylline, glyceryl guaiacolate. Bot. pt, gal.
Use: Antiasthmatic combination.

THEOMAX DF SYRUP. (Goldline) Theophylline 32.5 mg, ephedrine sulfate 6.25 mg, hydroxyzine HCl 2.5 mg/5 ml. Bot. pt, gal.
Use: Antiasthmatic combination.

THEO-ORGANIDIN. (Wallace) Theophylline anhydrous 120 mg, iodinated glycerol 30 mg/15 ml, alcohol 15%, saccharin. Bot. pt, gal.
Use: Antiasthmatic combination.

THEOPHENYLLIN. (H.L. Moore) Theophylline 130 mg, ephedrine HCl 24 mg, phenobarbital 8 mg/Tab. Bot. 1000s.
Use: Antiasthmatic combination.

THEOPHYL-SR. (McNeil Pharm) Theophylline 125 mg. Bot. 100s.
Use: Bronchodilator.

•**THEOPHYLLINE,** Cap., U.S.P. XXII. Tab., U.S.P. XXII. Extended release cap., U.S.P. XXII. 1,3-Dimethylxanthine. 1H-Purine-2,6-dione,3,-7-dihydro-1,3-dimethyl-, monohydrate.
Use: Coronary vasodilator and diuretic; pharmaceutic necessity for Aminophylline Injection.
See: Accurbron, Liq. (Merrell Dow).
Aerolate, Cap., Elix. (Fleming).
Aquaphyllin, Syr. (Ferndale).
Bronkodyl, Cap. (Winthrop Pharm).
Duraphyl, Tab. (McNeil Pharm).
Elixicon, Susp. (Berlex).
Elixophyllin, Elix., Cap. (Berlex).
Elixophyllin SR, Cap. (Berlex).
Lanophyllin, Elix. (Lannett).
Lodrane, Cap. (Poythress).
Optiphyllin, Elix. (Fougera).
Oralphyllin, Liq. (Consoln. Midland).
Quibron-T Dividose, Tab. (Bristol).
Quibron-T/SR Dividose, Tab. (Bristol).
Slo-bid, Cap. (Rhone-Poulenc Rorer).
Slo-Phyllin, Cap., Syr., Tab. (Rhone-Poulenc Rorer).
Somophyllin, Cap. (Fisons).
Sustaire, Tab. (Pfizer Laboratories)
Theo-II, Elix. (Fleming).
Theobid, Cap. (Russ)
Theobid Jr, Cap. (Russ)
Theoclear 80, Liq. (Central).
Theoclear L.A., Cenule (Central).
Theo-Dur, Tab. (Key).
Theolair, Tab., Liq. (Riker).
Theolair SR, Tab. (Riker).
Theospan, Cap. (Laser).
Theostat, Prods. (Laser).
Theovent Long-Acting, Cap. (Schering).

THEOPHYLLINE W/COMBINATIONS.
See: Asma-lief, Tab., Susp. (Quality Generics).
B.A. Prods. (Federal).
Bronkaid, Tab. (Brew).
Co-Xan, Liq. (Central).
Elixophyllin-KI, Elix. (Berlex).
Eponal, Tab. (Cenci).
Lardet, Tab. (Standex).
Lardet Expectorant, Tab. (Standex).
Liquophylline, Liq. (Paddock).
Marax DF, Syr. (Roerig).
Marax, Tab. (Roerig) Mersaline, Inj. (Standex).
Mersaphyllin, Vial (Pharmex).
Quibron, Cap., Liq.(Bristol).
Quibron-300, Cap. (Bristol).
Quibron Plus, Cap. (Bristol).
Slo-Phyllin GG, Cap., Syr. (Rhone-Poulenc Rorer).
Synophylate, Liq. (Central).
Tedral SA, Tab. (Parke-Davis).
Theocol, Cap., Liq. (Quality Generics).
Theofenal, Tab. (Cumberland).
Theolair Plus, Tab., Liq. (Riker).
Theo-Organidin, Elix. (Wampole).

THEOPHYLLINE WITH PHENOBARBITAL COMBINATIONS.
See: Asma-Lief, Tab., Susp. (Quality Generics).
Bronkolixir, Elix. (Winthrop Pharm).
Bronkotab, Tab. (Winthrop Pharm).
Ceepa, Tab. (Geneva).

THEOPHYLLINE AMINOISOBUTANOL. Theophylline w/2-amino-2-methyl-1-propanol.
See: Butaphyllamine (Various Mfr.).

THEOPHYLLINE-CALCIUM SALICYLATE.
W/Ephedrine HCl, phenobarbital, potassium iodide.
See: Quadrinal, Tab., Susp. (Knoll).
W/Phenobarbital, ephedrine HCl, guaifenesin.
See: Verequad, Tab., Susp. (Knoll).
W/Potassium iodide.
See: Theokin, Tab., Elix. (Knoll).

THEOPHYLLINE, 8-CHLORO, DIPHENHYDRAMINE. Dimenhydrinate, U.S.P. XXII.
See: Dramamine, Preps. (Searle).

THEOPHYLLINE CHOLINE SALT.
See: Choledyl, Tab., Elix. (Parke-Davis).

•**THEOPHYLLINE, EPHEDRINE HYDROCHLORIDE, AND PHENOBARBITAL TABLETS,** U.S.P. XXII.
Use: Bronchodilator, sedative.

THEOPHYLLINE ETHYLENEDIAMINE.
See: Aminophylline, Preps. (Various Mfr.).

THEOPHYLLINE EXTENDED-RELEASE CAPSULES, U.S.P. XXII.
Use: Bronchodilator.

•**THEOPHYLLINE AND GUAIFENESIN CAPSULES,** U.S.P. XXII.
Use: Smooth muscle relaxant, expectorant.

THEOPHYLLINE AND GUAIFENESIN ORAL SOLUTION, U.S.P. XXII.
Use: Smooth muscle relaxant, expectorant.

THEOPHYLLINE OLAMINE. Theophylline compound with 2-amino-ethanol (1:1).
Use: Smooth muscle relaxant.

THEOPHYLLINE REAGENT STRIPS. (Ames) Seralyzer reagent strip. Bot. 25s. A quantitative strip test for theophylline in serum or plasma.
Use: Diagnostic aid.

•**THEOPHYLLINE SODIUM GLYCINATE,** U.S.P. XXII. Elixir, Tab., U.S.P. XXII.
Use: Smooth muscle relaxant.
See: Synophylate, Elix., Tab. (Central).

Theofort, Elix. (Federal Pharm.).
W/Guaifenesin.
See: Asbron G, Tab., Elix. (Dorsey).
Synophylate-GG, Tab., Syr. (Central).
W/Phenobarbital.
See: Synophylate w/Phenobarbital, Tab. (Central).
W/Potassium iodide.
See: TSG-KI, Elix. (Elder).
W/Potassium iodide, ephedrine HCl, codeine phosphate.
See: TSG Croup Liquid. (Elder).
W/Racephedrine, phenobarbital.
See: Synophedal, Tab. (Central).

THEO-R-GEN. (Goldline) Theophylline 120 mg, iodinated glycerol 30 mg/15 ml, alcohol 15%. Elix. Bot. 480 ml.
Use: Antiasthmatic combination.

THEOSPAN-SR 130. (Laser) Theophylline anhydrous 130 mg/Cap. Bot. 100s, 1000s.
Use: Bronchodilator.

THEOSPAN-SR 260. (Laser) Theophylline anhydrous 260 mg/Cap. Bot. 100s, 1000s.
Use: Bronchodilator.

THEOSTAT 80 SYRUP. (Laser) Theophylline anhydrous 80 mg/15 ml. Bot. pt, gal.
Use: Bronchodilator.

THEO-TIME. (Major) Theophylline 100 mg, 200 mg or 300 mg/TR Tab. Bot. 100s, 500s.
Use: Bronchodilator.

THEO-TIME SR TABS. (Major) Theophylline 100 mg, 200 mg or 300 mg/SR Tab. Bot. 100s, 500s.
Use: Bronchodilator.

THEOVENT LONG-ACTING. (Schering) Theophylline anhydrous 125 mg or 250 mg/Cap. Bot. 100s.
Use: Bronchodilator.

THERA BATH. (Walgreen) Mineral oil 90%. Bot. 16 oz.
Use: Emollient.

THERA BATH WITH VITAMIN E. (Walgreen) Mineral oil 91%, vitamin E 2000 IU/16 oz.
Use: Emollient.

THERABID. (Mission) Vitamins C 500 mg, B_1 15 mg, B_2 10 mg, niacinamide 100 mg, calcium pantothenate 20 mg, B_6 10 mg, B_{12} 5 mcg, A 5000 IU, D 200 IU, E 30 mg/Tab. Bot. 100s.
Use: Vitamin supplement.

THERABLOAT. (Norden) Poloxalene.

THERABRAND. (Approved) Vitamins A 25,000 IU, D 1000 IU, B_1 10 mg, B_2 10 mg, niacinamide 100 mg, C 200 mg, B_6 5 mg, calcium pantothenate 20 mg, B_{12} 5 mcg/Cap. Bot. 100s, 1000s.
Use: Vitamin supplement.

THERABRAND-M. (Approved) Vitamins A 25,000 IU, D 1000 IU, C 200 mg, B_1 10 mg, B_2 10 mg, B_6 5 mg, niacinamide 100 mg, calcium pantothenate 20 mg, E 5 IU, B_{12} 5 mcg, iodine 0.15 mg, iron 15 mg, copper 1 mg, calcium 125 mg, manganese 1 mg, magnesium 6 mg, zinc 1.5 mg/Cap. Bot. 100s, 1000s.
Use: Vitamin/mineral supplement.

THERAC. (C & M Pharmacal) Colloidal sulfur 4%, salicylic acid 2.35% in lotion base. Bot. 2 oz.
Use: Anti-acne.

THERACAP. (Arcum) Vitamin A 10,000 IU, D 400 IU, B_1 10 mg, B_2 5 mg, niacinamide 150 mg, C 150 mg/Cap. Bot. 100s, 1000s.
Use: Vitamin supplement.

THERACAPS. (Alton) Bot. 100s, 1000s.
Use: Vitamin supplement.

THERACAPS M. (Alton) Bot. 100s, 1000s.
Use: Vitamin/mineral supplement.

THERA-COMBEX H-P. (Parke-Davis Prods) Vitamins C 500 mg, B_1 25 mg, B_2 15 mg, B_{12} 5 mcg, niacinamide 100 mg, panthenol 20 mg/Cap. Bot. 100s.
Use: Vitamin supplement.

THERACYS. (Connaught) BCG Live 27 mg (3.4 x 10 CFU)/vial. Freeze-dried suspension for reconstitution. Vial with diluent (1 ml/vial).
Use: Antineoplastic agent.

THERA-FLUR. (Colgate-Hoyt) Fluoride 0.5% (from sodium fluoride 1.1%). pH 4.5. Gel-Drops. Bot. 24 ml, 60 ml.
Use: Dental caries preventative.

THERA-FLUR-N. (Colgate-Hoyt) Neutral sodium fluoride 1.1%. Bot. 24 ml, 60 ml.
Use: Dental caries preventative.

THERAFORTIS. (General Vitamin) Vitamins A 12,500 IU, D 1000 IU, B_1 5 mg, B_2 5 mg, B_6 1 mg, B_{12} 3 mcg, niacinamide 50 mg, pantothenic acid salt 10 mg, C 150 mg, folic acid 0.5 mg/Cap. Bot. 100s, 1000s.
Use: Vitamin supplement.

THERAGENERIX-H. (Goldline) Iron 66.7 mg, vitamins A 8333 IU, D 133 IU, E 5 IU, B_1 3.3 mg, B_2 3.3 mg, B_3 33.3 mg, B_5 11.7 mg, B_6 3.3 mg, B_{12} 50 mcg, C 100 mg, folic acid 0.33 mg, Cu, Mg/Tab. Bot. 100s, 1000s.
Use: Vitamin/mineral supplement.

THERA-GESIC. (Mission) Methylsalicylate, menthol. Balm. In 90 Gm, 150 Gm.
Use: External analgesic.

THERAGRAN. (Squibb) Vitamins A 5500 IU, C 120 mg, B_1 3 mg, B_2 3.4 mg, niacin 30 mg, B_6 3 mg, B_{12} 9 mcg, D 400 IU, pantothenic acid 10 mg, folic acid 0.4 mg, biotin 15.5 mcg/Tab. Bot. 30s, 60s, 100s, 180s, 1000s, Unimatic 100s.
Use: Vitamin supplement.

THERAGRAN JR. (Squibb) Vitamins A 5000 IU, D 400 IU, E 30 mg, B_1 1.5 mg, B_2 1.7 mg, B_3 20 mg, B_6 2 mg, B_{12} 6 mcg, C 60 mg, folic acid 0.4 mg/Tab. Bot. 75s.
Use: Vitamin supplement.

THERAGRAN JR. WITH EXTRA VITAMIN C. (Squibb) Vitamins A 5000 IU, D 400 IU, E 30 mg, B_1 1.5 mg, B_2 1.7 mg, B_3 20 mg, B_6 2 mg, B_{12} 6 mcg, C 250 mg, folic acid 0.4 mg/Tab. Bot. 75s.

Use: Vitamin supplement.

THERAGRAN JR. WITH IRON. (Squibb) Iron 18 mg, vitamins A 5000 IU, D 400 IU, E 30 mg, B_1 1.5 mg, B_2 1.7 mg, B_3 20 mg, B_6 2 mg, B_{12} 6 mcg, C 60 mg, folic acid 0.4 mg, tartrazine/Tab. Bot. 75s.
Use: Vitamin/mineral supplement.

THERAGRAN HEMATINIC. (Squibb) Iron 66.7 IU, vitamins A 8333 IU, D 133 IU, E 5 IU, B_1 3.3 mg, B_2 3.3 mg, B_3 33.3 mg, B_5 11.7 mg, B_6 3.3 mg, B_{12} 50 mcg, C 100 mg, folic acid 0.33 mg, Cu, Mg, tartrazine, sodium bisulfite/Tab. Bot. 90s.
Use: Vitamin/mineral supplement.

THERAGRAN-M. (Squibb) Vitamins A 5500 IU, D 400 IU, C 120 mg, B_1 3 mg, B_2 3.4 mg, niacinamide 30 mg, calcium pantothenate 10 mg, B_6 3 mg, E 30 IU, B_{12} 9 mcg, Ca, iodine 150 mcg, iron 27 mg, magnesium 100 mg, copper 2 mg, zinc 22.5 mg, magnanese 7.5 mg, folic acid 0.4 mg, biotin 15 mcg, cromium 15 mcg, selenium 10 mcg, molybdenum 15 mcg, potassium 7.5 mg/Tab. Bot. 30s, 60s, 100s, 180s, 1000s, Unimatic 100s.
Use: Vitamin/mineral supplement.

THERAGRAN STRESS FORMULA. (Squibb) Iron 27 mg, vitamins E 30 IU, B_1 15 mg, B_2 15 mg, B_3 100 mg, B_5 20 mg, B_6 5 mg, B_{12} 12 mcg, C 600 mg, folic acid 0.4 mg, biotin 45 mcg/Tab. Bot. 75s.
Use: Vitamin/mineral supplement.

THERA H TABS. (Major) Bot. 100s, 250s.
Use: Vitamin/mineral supplement.

THERA-M. (Various Mfr.) Iron 12 mg, vitamins A 10,000 IU, D 400 IU, E 15 mg, B_1 10 mg, B_2 10 mg, B_3 100 mg, B_5 20 mg, B_6 5 mg, B_{12} 5 mcg, C 200 mg, Co, I, Mg, Mn, zinc 1.5 mg/Tab. Bot. 100s, 250s, 1000s, UD 100s.
Use: Vitamin/mineral supplement.

THERAMIN. (Arcum) Vitamins A 10,000 IU, D 400 IU, B_1 10 mg, B_2 5 mg, niacinamide 100 mg, B_6 5 mg, B_{12} 10 mcg, C 150 mg, calcium pantothenate 15 mg, calcium 103.6 mg, iodine 0.1 mg, iron 15 mg, phosphorus 80 mg, magnesium 6 mg/Tab. Bot. 30s, 100s, 1000s.
Use: Vitamin/mineral supplement.

THERANEED. (Hanlon) Vitamins A 16,000 IU, B_1 10 mg, B_2 10 mg, B_6 2 mg, C 300 mg, calcium pantothenate 10 mg, niacinamide 10 mg, B_{12} 10 mcg/Cap. Bot. 100s.
Use: Vitamin supplement.

THERAPALS. (Faraday) Vitamins A 25,000 IU, D 400 IU, B_1 10 mg, B_2 5 mg, niacinamide 150 mg, B_6 0.5 mg, E 5 IU, C 150 mg, B_{12} 10 mcg, calcium 103 mg, cobalt 0.1 mg, copper 1 mg, K 0.15 mg, magnesium 6 mg, manganese 1 mg, molybdenum 0.2 mg, phosphorus 80 mg, potassium 5 mg, zinc 1.2 mg/Tab. Bot. 100s, 250s, 1000s.
Use: Vitamin/mineral supplement.

THERAPEUTIC V & M. (Whiteworth) Vitamins A 10,000 IU, D 400 IU, B_1 10 mg, B_2 10 mg, B_6 5 mg, B_{12} 5 mcg, niacinamide 100 mg, calcium pantothenate 20 mg, C 200 mg, E 15 IU, iodine 0.15 mg, iron 12 mg, copper 2 mg, manganese 1 mg, magnesium 60 mg, zinc 1.5 mg/Tab.
Use: Vitamin/mineral supplement.

THERAPEUTIC VITAMIN CAPSULES. (Lannett) Vitamins A 25,000 IU, D 1000 IU, B_1 10 mg, B_2 5 mg, niacinamide 150 mg, C 150 mg/Cap. or Tab. **Cap.:** Bot. 100s, 500s, 1000s. **Tab.:** Bot. 1000s.
Use: Vitamin supplement.

THERAPEUTIC VITAMIN CAPSULES AND TABLETS—IMPROVED FORMULA. (Lannett) Vitamins A 25,000 IU, D 1000 IU, thiamine mononitrate 12.5 mg, B_2 12.5 mg, niacinamide 100 mg, B_6 5 mg, B_{12} 5 mcg, calcium pantothenate 25 mg, C 200 mg/Cap. or Tab. **Cap.:** Bot. 100s, 500s, 1000s. **Tab.:** Bot. 1000s.
Use: Vitamin supplement.

THERAPEUTIC VITAMIN FORMULA W/MINERALS. (Towne) Vitamins A palmitate 10,000 IU, D 400 IU, B_1 15 mg, B_2 10 mg, B_6 5 mg, B_{12} 12 mcg, C 200 mg, niacinamide 100 mg, calcium pantothenate 20 mg, E 15 IU, calcium 103 mg, iron 10 mg, manganese 1 mg, potassium 5 mg, zinc 1.5 mg, magnesium 6 mg/Cap. Bot. 30s, 60s, 100s, 250s.
Use: Vitamin/mineral supplement.

THERAPEUTIC VITAMIN FORMULA W/MINERALS. (Towne) Vitamins A palmitate 25,000 IU, D 1000 IU, B_1 10 mg, B_2 5 mg, B_6 1 mg, B_{12} 5 mcg, C 150 mg, niacinamide 100 mg, calcium 103 mg, phosphorus 80 mg, iron 10 mg, iodine 0.1 mg, manganese 1 mg, potassium 5 mg, copper 1 mg, zinc 1.4 mg, magnesium 5.5 mg/Cap. Bot. 100s, 1000s.
Use: Vitamin/mineral supplement.

THERAPHON. (Approved) Vitamins A 25,000 IU, D 1000 IU, B_1 10 mg, B_2 5 mg, C 150 mg, niacinamide 150 mg/Cap. Bot. 100s, 1000s.
Use: Vitamin supplement.

THERAPLEX. (Kenyon) Vitamins A 25,000 IU, D 1000 IU, B_1 10 mg, B_2 10 mg, niacinamide 150 mg, B_{12} 5 mcg/Tab. Bot. 100s, 1000s.
Use: Vitamin supplement.

THERAPLEX-PLUS. (Kenyon) Vitamins A palmitate 25,000 IU, D 1000 IU, B_1 10 mg, B_2 5 mg, B_6 1 mg, B_{12} 5 mcg, C 150 mg, niacinamide 100 mg, dicalcium phosphate 360 mg, calcium 106 mg, phosphorus 82 mg, ferrous sulfate 34 mg, manganese sulfate 3 mg, potassium sulfate 11 mg, zinc sulfate 3.9 mg, magnesium sulfate 40 mg/Cap. Bot. 100s, 1000s.
Use: Vitamin/mineral supplement.

THERA-STAY. (Stayner) Vitamins A 25,000 IU, D 1000 IU, B_1 12.5 mg, B_2 12.5 mg, niacinamide 100 mg, B_6 5 mg, calcium pantothenate 25 mg, B_{12} 5 mcg, C 200 mg/Cap. Bot. 100s.
Use: Vitamin supplement.

THERA-STAY "M". (Stayner) Vitamins A 25,000 IU, D 1000 IU, B_1 10 mg, B_2 5 mg, B_6 1 mg, B_{12} 5 mcg, C 150 mg, niacinamide 100 mg, cal-

cium 104 mg, phosphorus 80 mg, iron 10 mg, iodine 0.1 mg, manganese 1 mg, potassium 5 mg, copper 1 mg, zinc 1.4 mg, magnesium 5.5 mg, E 2 IU/Cap. Bot. 100s, 500s.
Use: Vitamin/mineral supplement.

THERATINIC. (Jamieson-McKames) Vitamin B_{12} 5 mcg, fortified iron 59 mg, niacin 50 mg, pyridoxine 0.3 mg, cyancobalamin 2 mcg, folic acid 2 mg/2 ml, sodium citrate 1%, phenol 0.5%, procaine HCl 1%.
Use: Vitamin/mineral supplement.

THERAVEE HEMATINIC VITAMIN. (Vangard) Vitamins A 2.5 mg, D 3.3 mcg, thiamine 3.3 mg, riboflavin 3.3 mg, pyridoxine HCl 3.3 mg, niacinamide 33.3 mg, calcium pantothenate 11.7 mg, E 5 mg, copper 0.67 mg, magnesium 41.7 mg, iron 66.7 mg, B_{12} 50 mcg, folic acid 0.33 mcg, C 100 mg/Tab. Bot. 100s, UD 10×10s.
Use: Vitamin/mineral supplement.

THERAVEE M VITAMIN. (Vangard) Vitamins A 3 mg, D 10 mcg, E 15 mg, C 200 mg, thiamine 10.3 mg, riboflavin 10 mg, niacin 100 mg, B_6 4.1 mg, B_{12} 5 mcg, pantothenic acid 18.4 mg, iodine 150 mcg, iron 12 mg, magnesium 65 mg, copper 2 mg, zinc 1.5 mg, manganese 1 mg/Tab. Bot. 100s, 1000s, UD 10×10s.
Use: Vitamin/mineral supplement.

THERAVEE VITAMIN. (Vangard) Vitamins A 10,000 IU, D 400 IU, E 14 IU, C 200 mg, thiamine 10.3 mg, riboflavin 10 mg, niacin 100 mg, B_6 4 .1 mg, B_{12} 5 mcg, pantothenic acid 18.4 mg/Tab. Bot. 100s, UD Pkg. 250s.
Use: Vitamin supplement.

THERAVILAN CAPSULES. (Lannett) Vitamins A 25,000 IU, D 1000 IU, B_1 10 mg, B_2 5 mg, B_6 1 mg, C 150 mg, B_{12} 5 mcg, niacinamide 100 mg, dicalcium phosphate anhydrous 360 mg, ferrous sulfate dried 34 mg, potassium iodide 0.133 mg, manganese sulfate dried 3 mg, cobalt sulfate 0.49 mg, potassium sulfate 11 mg, sodium molybdate 0.45 mg, copper sulfate monohydrate 2.8 mg, zinc sulfate dried 3.9 mg, magnesium sulfate dried 40 mg/Cap. or Tab. **Cap.:** Bot. 100s, 500s, 1000s. **Tab.:** Bot. 100s, 1000s.
Use: Vitamin/mineral supplement.

THERAVIM CAPSULES. (Robinson) Vitamins A 25,000 IU, D 400 IU, B_1 10 mg, B_2 5 mg, C 150 mg, niacinamide 150 mg/Cap. Bot. 50s, 100s, 500s, 1000s, Bulk Pack 5000s. W/Vitamin B_{12} 5 mcg/Cap. Bot. 100s, 250s, 1000s.
Use: Vitamin supplement.

THERAVIM HI-PO. (Robinson) Vitamins A 25,000 IU, D 400 IU, B_1 10 mg, B_2 10 mg, B_6 5 mg, B_{12} 5 mcg, C 200 mg, E 15 IU, niacinamide 100 mg, calcium pantothenate 20 mg/Cap. or Tab. Bot. 100s, 1000s.
Use: Vitamin supplement.

THERAVIM M. (Geneva Generics) Iron 27 mg, vitamins A 5500 IU, D 400 IU, E 30 mg, B_1 3 mg, B_2 3.4 mg, B_3 30 mg, B_5 10 mg, B_6 3 mg, B_{12} 9 mcg, C 120 mg, folic acid 0.4 mg, Cl, Cr, Cu, I, K, Mg, Mn, Mo, Se, zinc 15 mg, biotin 15 mcg/Tab. Bot. 100s, 1000s.
Use: Vitamin/mineral supplement.

THEREMS. (Rugby) Vitamins A 5500 IU, D 400 IU, E 30 mg, B_1 3 mg, B_2 3.4 mg, B_3 30 mg, B_5 10 mg, B_6 3 mg, B_{12} 9 mcg, C 120 mg, folic acid 0.4 mg, biotin 15 mcg/Tab. Bot. 130s, 1000s.
Use: Vitamin supplement.

THEREMS-M. (Rugby) Iron 27 mg, vitamins A 5500 IU, D 400 IU, E 30 mg, B_1 3 mg, B_2 3.4 mg, B_3 30 mg, B_5 10 mg, B_6 3 mg, B_{12} 9 mcg, C 120 mg, folic acid 0.4 mg, Cl, Cr, Cu, I, K, Mg, Mn, Mo, Se, zinc 15 mg, biotin 15 mcg/Tab. Bot. 90s, 100s, 1000s.
Use: Vitamin/mineral supplement.

THEREVAC. (Bowman) Docusate potassium 283 mg, benzocaine 20 mg/Tube capsule w/soft soap in PEG 400 and glycerin base. Unit 4 ml, packages 4s, 12s, 50s. Disposable enema.
Use: Laxative.

THEREVAC PLUS. (Jones Medical) Docusate sodium 283 mg, benzocaine 20 mg in a base of soft soap, PEG 400, glycerin/Cap. 3.9 Gm Jar 30s. Disposable enema.
Use: Laxative.

THEREVAC-SB. (Jones Medical) Docusate sodium 283 mg in a base of soft soap, PEG 400, glycerin/Cap. 3.9 Gm Bot. 30s. Disposable enema.
Use: Laxative.

THEREX NO. 1. (Blue Cross) Vitamins A 10,000 IU, D 400 IU, E 15 IU, C 200 mg, B_1 10 mg, B_2 10 mg, niacinamide 100 mg, B_6 5 mg, B_{12} 5 mcg, calcium pantothenate 20 mg/Tab. Bot. 100s.
Use: Vitamin supplement.

THEREX AND ZINC. (Blue Cross).
Use: Dietary supplement.

THEREX-M. (Blue Cross) Vitamins A 10,000 IU, D 400 IU, E 15 IU, C 200 mg, B_1 10 mg, B_2 10 mg, niacinamide 100 mg, B_6 5 mg, B_{12} 5 mcg, calcium pantothenate 20 mg, iodine 150 mcg, iron 12 mg, magnesium 65 mg, copper 2 mg, zinc 1.5 mg, manganese 1 mg/Tab. Bot. 100s.
Use: Vitamin/mineral supplement.

THEREX-Z. (Blue Cross) Vitamins A 10,000 IU, D 400 IU, E 15 IU, C 200 mg, B_1 10 mg, B_2 10 mg, niacinamide 100 mg, B_{12} 5 mcg, B_6 5 mg, calcium pantothenate 20 mg, iodine 150 mcg, copper 2 mg, iron 12 mg, zinc 22.5 mg/Tab. Bot. 100s.
Use: Vitamin/mineral supplement.

THERMA-KOOL. (Nortech) Compresses in following sizes: 3″ × 5″, 4″ × 9″, 8.5″ × 10.5″.
Use: Cold or hot compress.

THERMAZENE. (Sherwood) Silver sulfadiazine 1% in white petroleum cream. 50 Gm, 400 Gm, 1000 Gm.
Use: Burn preparation.

THERMODENT. (Mentholatum) Strontium Cl 10%. Tube.

Use: Toothpaste for sensitive teeth.

THERMOLENE. (Lannett) Sodium Cl 7 gr, dextrose 3 gr, vitamin B_1 1 mg/Tab. Bot. 1000s.
Use: Fluid/electrolyte replacement.

THERMOLOID. (Mills) Thyroid 1 gr, 2 gr, 3 gr, 4 gr or 5 gr/Tab. Bot. 100s.
Use: Thyroid hormone.

THEROAL. (Vangard) Theophylline 24 mg, ephedrine HCl 24 mg, phenobarbital 8 mg/Tab. Bot. 100s, 1000s.
Use: Antiasthmatic combination.

THIA. (Sig) Thiamine HCl 100 mg/ml. Vial 30 ml.
Use: Thiamine supplement.

•**THIABENDAZOLE,** U.S.P. XXII. Oral Susp., Tab. U.S.P. XXII. 1H-Benzimidazole,2-(4-thiazolyl)-2-(4-Thiazolyl)-benzimidazole.
Use: Anthelmintic.
See: Mintezol, Tab., Susp. (Merck Sharp & Dohme).

THIABENDAZOLE, VETERINARY USE. 2-(4-Thiazolyl)-1H-benzimidazole.

THIACETARSAMIDE SODIUM. Sodium mercaptoacetate S,S-diester with p-carbamoyldithiobenzenearsonous acid.
Use: Antitrichomonal.

THIACETAZONE, B.A.N. p-Acetylaminobenzaldehyde thiosemicarbamazone.
Use: Treatment of tuberculosis and leprosy.

THIACIDE. (Beach) Methenamine mandelate 500 mg, potassium acid phosphate 250 mg/Tab. Bot. 100s.
Use: Urinary anti-infective.

THIA-DIA-MER-SULFONAMIDES. Sulfadiazine, sulfamerazine, sulfathiazole.
See: Trionamide, Tab. (O'Neal).

THIAHEP INJECTION. (Lannett) Liver extract (derived from 10 U.S.P. units injectable) 100 mg, liver extract (derived from 10 U.S.P. units crude liver) 100 mg, iron peptonate 20 mg, niacinamide 50 mg, pyridoxine HCl 0.3 mg, riboflavin 3 mg/2 ml multiple dose Vial 300 ml.
Use: Nutritional supplement.

THIALBARBITAL.
See: Kemithal.

THIALBARBITONE. B.A.N. 5-Allyl-5-(cyclohex-2-enyl)-2-thiobarbituric acid.
Use: Anesthetic.

THIAMAZOLE (I.N.N.). Methimazole, B.A.N.

THIAMBUTOSINE. B.A.N. 1-(4-Butoxyphenyl)-3-(4-dimethylaminophenyl)thiourea.
Use: Treatment of leprosy.

THIAMINE HYDROCHLORIDE, U.S.P. XXII. Elixir, Inj., Tab., U.S.P. XXII. 3-[(4-amino-2-methyl-5-pyrimidinyl)-methyl]-5-(2-hydroxyethyl)-4-methyl-, Cl, monohydrochloride. Aneurine HCl, thiamine Cl, vitamin B_1 HCl. Thiazolium,
Use: Enzyme co-factor vitamin.
See: Apatate (Kenwood).
Betalin S, Amp., Elixir, Tab. (Lilly).
Thia, Vial (Sig).

THIAMINE MONONITRATE, U.S.P. XXII. Elixir, U.S.P. XXII. Thiazolium, 3-[(4-amino-2-methyl-5-pyrimidinyl)-methyl]-5-(2-hydroxyethyl)-4-methyl-, nitrate (salt). (Various Mfr.) Thiamine nitrate.
Use: Enzyme co-factor vitamin.
W/Sodium salicylate, colchicine.
See: Sodsylate, Tab. (Durst).

•**THIAMIPRINE.** USAN. 2-Amino-6-[(1-methyl-4-nitroimidazol-5-yl)thio] purine.
Use: Antileukemic.

•**THIAMPHENICOL.** USAN.
Use: Antibacterial.

•**THIAMYLAL SODIUM, FOR INJECTION,** U.S.P. XXII. Sodium 5-allyl-5-(1-methylbutyl)-2-thiobarbiturate.
Use: Anesthetic (systemic).
See: Surital Sodium, Prep. (Parke-Davis).

THIAPHYLL CREAM. (Lannett) Sulfathiazole 5%, chlorophyllin 1%. Jar 4 oz, lb.
Use: Wound healing agent.

THIA-SERP-25. (Robinson) Hydrochlorothiazide 25 mg, reserpine alkaloid 0.125 mg/Tab. Bot. 100s, 1000s.
Use: Antihypertensive.

THIA-SERP-50. (Robinson) Hydrochlorothiazide 50 mg, reserpine alkaloid 0.125 mg/Tab. Bot. 100s, 1000s.
Use: Antihypertensive.

THIA-SERPA-ZINE. (Robinson) Reserpine alkaloid, hydrochlorothiazide, hydralazine HCl. Tab. Bot. 100s, 1000s.
Use: Antihypertensive.

THIA-TWELVE. (Rocky Mtn.) Vitamins B_{12} crystallized 1000 mcg, B_1 100 mg/ml. Vial 10 ml.
Use: Vitamin supplement.

•**THIAZESIM.** USAN. 5-(2-Dimethylaminoethyl) 2,3-dihydro-2-phenyl-1,5-benzothiazepin-4-one.
Use: Antidepressant.

THIAZESIM HCl. 5-[2-(Dimethylamino)-ethyl]-2,3-dihydro-2-phenylbenzo-1,5-thiazepin-4-(5H)-one hydrochloride.
Use: Antidepressant.

•**THIAZINAMINIUM CHLORIDE.** USAN.
Use: Anti-allergic.

THIETHANOMELAMINE.
See: Tretamine, B.A.N.

THIETHYLENE THIOPHOSPHORAMIDE.
See: Thiotepa, B.A.N.

•**THIETHYLPERAZINE.** USAN. 2-Ethylthio-10-[3-(4-methylpiperazin-1-yl)propyl]phenothiazine.
Use: Central nervous system depressant.
See: Torecan.

THIETHYLPERAZINE MALEATE, U.S.P. XXI. Inj., Supp., Tab., U.S.P. XXI. Torecan, 2-Ethylmercapto-10-[3′-(1″-methyl-piperazinyl-4″)propyl-1″]phenothiazine maleate. 2-(Ethylthio)-10-[3-(4-methyl-1-piperazinyl)propyl]phenothiazine maleate (1:2).
Use: Antiemetic.
See: Torecan, Amp., Supp., Tab. (Boehringer Ingelheim).

THIHEXINOL METHYLBROMIDE. alpha-Dithienyl-(4-dimethylamino-cyclohexyl)-carbinolmeth-

bromide. [4-(Hydroxydi-2-thienylmethyl)cyclohexyl] trime- thylammonium Bromide.
Use: Anticholinergic.

•**THIMERFONATE SODIUM.** USAN. Ethyl(hydrogen p-mercaptobenzenesulfonato)mercury sodium salt; Sodium p-[(ethylmercuri)-thio] benzenesulfonate. Sulfo-Merthiolate (Lilly).
Use: Topical anti-infective.

•**THIMEROSAL,** U.S.P. XXII. Topical Aerosol, Topical Soln., Tr., U.S.P. XXII. Sodium Ethylmercurithiosalicylate. Sodium Ethyl (Sodium o-mercaptobenzoate)mercury.
Use: Local anti-infective; pharmaceutical aid (preservative).
See: Aeroaid, Aerosol (Aeroceuticals).
Merphol Tincture 1:1000, Liq.(Bowman).
Mersol, Liq. (Century).
Merthiolate, Prep. (Lilly).

THIOCARBANIDIN. Under study.
Use: Antituberculous agent.

THIOCARLIDE. B.A.N. 1,3-Di-(4-isopentyloxyphenyl)thiourea.
Use: Treatment of tuberculosis.

THIOCYANATE SODIUM. Sodium thiocyanate.
Use: Antihypertensive.

THIOCYL. (Torigian) Sodium thiosalicylate 100 mg/2 ml. Amp. 2 ml, Box 25s, 100s.
Use: Salicylate analgesic.

THIODINONE. Name used for Nifuratel.

THIODIPHENYLAMINE.
See: Phenothiazine.

THIOFURADENE. 1[(5-Nitrofurfurylidene)-amino]-2-imidazolidinethione.

THIOGLYCEROL.
W/Sodium citrate, phenol, benzyl alcohol.
See: Sulfo-ganic, Vial (Marcen).

•**THIOGUANINE,** U.S.P. XXII. Tab. U.S.P. XXII. 6H-Purine-6-thione,2-amino-1,7-dihydro-.2-Amino-purine-6-thiol, hemihydrate. Tabloid (Burroughs Wellcome) 40 mg, Bot. 25s.
Use: Antineoplastic agent.

THIOHEXAMIDE. N-(p-Methyl-mercaptophenylsulfonyl)-N′-cyclohexylurea.
Use: Blood sugar lowering compound.

THIOISONICOTINAMIDE. Under study.
Use: Antituberculosis drug.

THIOLA. (Mission) Tiopronin 100 mg/Tab. Bot. 100s.
Use: Kidney stone preventative.

THIOMERSAL. B.A.N. Sodium salt of(2-carboxyphenylthio)ethylmercury.
Sodium ethylmercurithiosalicylate. Thimerosal. Thiomersalate.
Use: Antiseptic; preservative.
See: Merthiolate.

THIOMESTERONE. B.A.N. $1\alpha,7\alpha$-Bis-(acetylthio)-17β-hydroxy-17α-methylandrost-4-en-3-one.
Use: Anabolic steroid.

•**THIOPENTAL SODIUM,** U.S.P. XXII. Inj., U.S.P. XXII. Sodium5-ethyl-5-(1-methylbutyl)-2-thiobarbiturate. Thiopentone sodium.
Use: Anesthetic (intravenous), anticonvulsant.
See: Pentothal Sodium, Amp. (Abbott).

THIOPHOSPHORAMIDE.
See: ThioTepa, Vial (Lederle).

THIOPROPAZATE. B.A.N. 10-[3-[4-(2-Acetoxyethyl)piperazin-1-yl]propyl]-2-chlorophenothiazine.
Use: Tranquilizer.

THIOPROPAZATE HYDROCHLORIDE. 2-Chloro-10-[3-[(2-acetoxyethyl)-4-piperazinyl]-propyl]phenothiazine dihydrochloride.4-[3-(2-Chlorophenothiazine-10-yl)propyl]-1-piperazine ethanol Acetate Dihydrochloride.
Use: Tranquilizer.

THIOPROPERAZINE. B.A.N. 2-Dimethylsulfamoyl-10-[3-(4-methylpiperazin-1-yl)propyl]phenothiazine.
Use: Tranquilizer; antiemetic.

THIOPROPERAZINE MESYLATE. N,N-Dimethyl-10-[3-(4-methyl-1-piperazinyl)propyl] phenothiazine-2-sulfonamide dimethanesulfonate.
Use: Central depressant; antiemetic.

•**THIORIDAZINE,** U.S.P. XXII. Oral Susp., U.S.P. XXII. 10-[2-(1-Methyl-2-piperidyl)ethyl]-2-methylthiopheno- thiazine.
Use: Tranquilizer, sedative.
See: Mellaril, Susp. (Sandoz).

•**THIORIDAZINE HCl,** U.S.P. XXII. Oral Soln., Tab., U.S.P. XXII. 10-[-2-(1-Methyl-2-piperidyl)-ethyl]-2- (methylthio) phenothiazine hydrochloride. 10H-Phenothiazine, 10-[2-(1-methyl-2-piperidinyl)-ethyl]-2-(methylthio)-, monohydrochloride.
Use: Tranquilizer.
See: Mellaril, Tab., Soln. (Sandoz).

THIORIDAZINE HYDROCHLORIDE INTENSOL ORAL SOLUTION. (Roxane) Thioridazine HCl oral concentrated soln. 30 mg or 100 mg/ml. Bot. 120 ml w/calibrated dropper.
Use: Antipsychotic agent.

•**THIOSALAN.** USAN. 3,4′,5-Tribromo-2-mercaptobenzanilide. Under study.
Use: Germicide, disinfectant.

THIOSALICYLIC ACID SALT.

THIOSTAN. (Standex) Sodium thiosalicylate 50 mg/30 ml. Bot. oz.
Use: Salicylate analgesic.

THIOSULFIL FORTE. (Wyeth-Ayerst) Sulfamethizole 0.5 Gm/Tab. Bot. 100s.
Use: Urinary anti-infective, analgesic.

•**THIOTEPA,** U.S.P. XXII. For Inj., U.S.P. XXII. Thiophosphoramide. N, Tris(1-Aziridinyl phosphine sulfide. (Lederle) Triethylenethiophosphoramide 15 mg/Vial.
Use: Antineoplastic agent.

THIOTEPA. (Lederle) The ethylenimine-type N, N; N"-Triethylene thiophosphoramide. Pow. for reconstitution: Thiotepa powder 15 mg, sodium Cl 80 mg, sodium bicarbonate 50 mg/Vial.
Use: Antineoplastic agent.

•**THIOTHIXENE,** U.S.P. XXII. Cap., U.S.P. XXII. N,N,-Dimethyl-9-(3-(4-methyl-1-piperazinyl)pro-

pylidene)thioxanthene-2-sulfonamide. As HCl salt.
Use: Psychotherapeutic agent.
See: Navane, Cap., Vial (Roerig).
Navane Concentrate Soln. (Roerig).

•**THIOTHIXENE HCl,** U.S.P. XXII. Inj., Oral Soln., U.S.P. XXII.
Use: Antipsychotic.
See: Navane Hydrochloride (Pfizer).

THIOURACIL. 2-Thiouracil.
Use: Antithyroid agent.

THIOUREA. (City Chem.) Pow., Bot., lb.
Use: Antithyroid agent.

THIOXANTHENE DERIVATIVE.
See: Taractan, Preps. (Roche).

THIOXOLONE. B.A.N. 6-Hydroxy-1,3-benzoxathiol-2-one.
Use: Keratolytic agent.

THIPHENAMIL. F.D.A. S-[2-(Diethylamino)-ethyl]-diphenylthioacetate.

•**THIPHENCILLIN POTASSIUM.** USAN. (1) Potassium 3,3-dimethyl-7-oxo-6-[2-(phenylthio)acetamido]-4-thia-1-azabicyclo[3.2.0] heptane-2-carboxylate; (2) Potassium 6-(phenylmercaptoacetamido)penicillanate.
Use: Antibacterial.

THIPYRI-12. (Sig) Vitamins B_1 1000 mg, B_6 1000 mg, cyanocobalamin (B_{12}) 10,000 mcg, sodium Cl 0.5%, sodium bisulfite 0.1%, benzyl alcohol (as preservative) 0.9%. Univial 10 ml.
Use: Vitamin supplement.

•**THIRAM.** USAN. Bis(dimethylthiocarbamoyl) disulfide.
Use: Antifungal.

THIXO-FLUR TOPICAL GEL. (Hoyt) Acidulated phosphate sodium fluoride in gel base 1.2%. Bot. 4 oz, 8 oz, 32 oz.
Use: Dental caries preventative.

•**THONZONIUM BROMIDE,** U.S.P. XXII. Hexadecyl {2-[(p-methoxybenzyl)-2-pyrimidinylamino]ethyl} dimethylammonium bromide.
Use: Detergent.
W/Colistin base, neomycin base, hydrocortisone acetate, polysorbate 80, acetic acid, sodium acetate.
See: Coly-Mycin-S, Otic, Liq. (Warner-Chilcott).
W/Isoproterenol.
See: Nebair, Aerosol (Warner-Chilcott).
W/Neomycin sulfate, gramicidin, thonzylamine HCl, phenylephrine HCl.
See: Biomydrin, Spray, Drops (Warner-Chilcott).

THONZYLAMINE. B.A.N. 2-[N-p-Anisyl-N-(pyrimidin-2-yl)amino]ethyldimethylamine.
Use: Antihistamine.

•**THONZYLAMINE HYDROCHLORIDE.** 2[[2-(Dimethylamino)ethyl](p-methoxybenzyl)amino]pyrimidine monohydrochloride.
Use: Antihistamine.

THOR SYRUP. (Towne) Dextromethorphan HBr 90 mg, pyrilamine maleate 22.5 mg, phenylephrine HCl 10 mg, ephedrine sulfate 15 mg, sodium citrate 325 mg, ammonium Cl 650 mg, guaifenesin 50 mg/fl oz. Bot. 4 oz.
Use: Antitussive, antihistamine, decongestant, expectorant.

THORADEX HCl. (Cenci) Chlorpromazine 10 mg, 25 mg, 50 mg or 100 mg/Tab. Bot. 100s, 1000s.
Use: Antipsychotic agent, antiemetic/antivertigo.

THORAZINE. (SmithKline) Chlorpromazine HCl.
Tab.: 10 mg, 25 mg, 50 mg, 100 mg or 200 mg. Bot. 100s, 1000s, Single unit pkg. 100s.
Amp.: 25 mg, ascorbic acid 2 mg, sodium bisulfite 1 mg, sodium sulfite 1 mg, sodium Cl 6 mg/1 ml. Amp. 1 ml, 2 ml, Box 10s, 100s, 500s; Vial 10 ml, Box 1s, 20s, 100s.
Spansule: 30 mg, 75 mg, 150 mg or 200 mg. Bot. 50s, 100s (S.U.P.), 500s. 300 mg Bot. 50s, 100s (S.U.P.).
Syr.: 10 mg/5 ml. Bot. 4 oz. **Supp.:** Chlorpromazine base, glycerin, glyceryl monopalmitate, glyceryl monostearate, hydrogenated coconut oil fatty acids, hydrogenated palm kernel oil fatty acids. 25 mg or 100 mg. Box 12s. **Conc.:** 30 mg/ml. Bot. 4 oz. in Ctn. 36s, 1 gal; 100 mg/ml. Bot. 8 oz.
Use: Antipsychotic agent, antiemetic/antivertigo.

THORETS. (Buffington) Benzocaine loz. Sugar, lactose and salt free. Dispens-A-Kits 500s.
Use: Local anesthetic.

THOR-PROM TABS. (Major) Chlorpromazine **10 mg, 25 mg, 50 mg or 100 mg/Tab.:** Bot. 100s, 1000s; **200 mg/Tab.:** Bot. 250s, 1000s.
Use: Antiemetic/antivertigo, antipsychotic agent.

•**THOZALINONE.** USAN. 2-Dimethylamino-5-phenyl-2-oxazolin-4-one.
Use: Antidepressant.
See: Stimsen (Lederle).

THREAMINE DM. (Various Mfr.) Phenylpropanolamine HCl 12.5 mg, chlorpheniramine maleate 2 mg, dextromethorphan HBr 10 mg/5 ml. Syr. Bot. pt, gal.
Use: Decongestant, antihistamine, antitussive.

THREE-AMINE TD. (Vitarine) Phenylpropanolamine HBr 50 mg, pheniramine maleate 25 mg, pyrilamine maleate 25 mg/TR Cap.
Use: Decongestant, antihistamine.

•**THREONINE,** U.S.P. XXII. $C_4H_9NO_3$ as L-threonine.
Use: Amino acid.

THREONINE. (Various Mfr.) Threonine 500 mg/Cap. or Tab. **Cap.:** Bot. 60s, 100s. **Tab.:** Bot. 100s, 250s.
Use: Nutritional supplement.

THROAT DISCS. (Marion) Capsicum, peppermint, anise, cubeb, glycyrrhiza, linseed. Box 60s.
Use: Minor throat irritations.

THROAT-EZE. (Faraday) Cetylpyridinium Cl 1:3000, cetyl dimethyl benzyl ammonium Cl 1:3000, benzocaine 10 mg/Wafer. Loz., foil wrapped.
Use: Local anesthetic.

•**THROMBIN,** U.S.P. XXII. Thrombin, topical, mammalian origin.
(Parke-Davis)—Thrombin, Topical (Bovine).
(Upjohn)—Vial (1000 units) 30 ml.
Use: Local hemostatic.

THROMBINAR. (Armour) Thrombin topical. Vial 1000, 5000, 10,000, 50,000 U.S. Standard Units.
Use: Hemostatic.

THROMBOPLASTIN.
Use: Diagnostic aid (prothrombin estimation).

THROMBOSTAT. (Parke-Davis) Prothrombin is activated by tissue thromboplastin in the presence of calcium Cl. **1000** U.S. (N.I.H.) units: Vial 10 ml. **5000** U.S. units: Vial 10 ml w/5 ml diluent. **10,000** U.S. units: Vial 20 ml w/10 ml diluent. **20,000** U.S. units: Vial 30 ml w/20 ml diluent.
Use: Local hemostatic.

THURFYL NICOTINATE. B.A.N. Tetrahydrofurfuryl nicotinate. Trafuril.
Use: Topical vasodilator.

THYCAL. (Mills) Thermoloid (thyroid) 2 gr, iodized calcium 2 gr, peptone 1 gr/Tab. Bot. 1000s.
Use: Thyroid hormone.

THYLOX. (C.S. Dent) Medicated bar soap w/absorbable sulfur. Bar 3.4 oz.
Use: Cleansing aid.

•**THYMOL,** N.F. XVII. Phenol, 5-methyl-2-(1-methylethyl)- p-Cymen-3-ol. (Various Mfr.) 0.25 lb, 1 lb.
Use: Antifungal, anti-infective local anesthetic, antitussive, nasal decongestant.
See: Vicks Regular and Wild Cherry Medicated Cough Drops (Vicks).
Vicks Vaporub, Oint. (Vicks).
W/Combinations.
See: Listerine Antiseptic, Soln. (Warner-Lambert).

THYMOL IODIDE.
Use: Antifungal; anti-infective.

THYMOXAMINE. B.A.N. 4-(2-Dimethylamino-ethoxy)-5-isopropyl-2-methylphenyl acetate. Moxisylyte (I.N.N.) Opilon [hydrochloride].
Use: Peripheral vasodilator.

THYODATIL. Name used for Nifuratel.

THYPINONE. (Abbott Diagnostics) Protirelin 500 mcg/1 ml. Adjunctive agent in the diagnostic assessment of thyroid function. Amp.
Use: Diagnostic aid.

THYRAR. (Rorer) Bovine thyroid preparation 0.5 gr, 1 gr or 2 gr/Tab. Bot. 100s.
Use: Thyroid hormone.

THYRO-BLOCK. (Wallace) Potassium iodide 130 mg/Tab. In 14s.
Use: Thyroid hormone.

THYROBROM. (Mills) Brominated thyroid 1 gr, 2 gr, 3 gr or 4 gr/Tab. or SC Tab. Bot. 1000s.
Use: Thyroid hormone.

•**THYROGLOBULIN,** U.S.P. XXII. Tab., U.S.P. XXII. Substance obtained by fractionation of thyroid glands from hog, *Sus scrofa* Linne' var. domesticus Gray (Fam. Suidae), containing not less than 0.7% iodine.
Use: Thyroid hormone.
See: Proloid, Tab. (Parke-Davis).
Thyrar, Tab. (Armour).

•**THYROID,** U.S.P. XXII. Tab., U.S.P. XXII.
Use: Thyroid hormone.
See: Arco Thyroid, Tab. (Arco).
Armour Thyroid, Tab. (Rorer).
Dathroid 0.05 and 3, Tab. (Scrip).
Delcoid, Tab. (Delco).
Marion Thyroid, Tab. (Marion).
S-P-T., Cap. (Fleming).
Thermoloid, Tab. (Mills).
Thyrocrine, Tab. (Lemmon).

THYROID BROMINATED.
See: Thyrobrom, Tab. (Mills).

THYROID COMBINATIONS.
See: Henydin, Preps. (Arcum).
Thycal, Tab. (Mills).

THYROID HORMONES.
See: Liothyronine Sodium
Thyroxin (Various Mfr.).

THYROID PREPARATIONS.
See: Proloid, Tab. (Parke-Davis).
Thyrar, Tab. (Rorer).
Thyrobrom, Tab. (Mills).
Thyroxin, Preps. (Various Mfr.).

THYROLAR. (Rorer) Liotrix. **0.25 gr/Tab.:** Bot. 100s; **0.5 gr, 1 gr, 2 gr or 3 gr/Tab.:** Bot. 100s, 1000s.
Use: Thyroid hormone.

•**THYROMEDAN HYDROCHLORIDE.** USAN. 2-(Die- thylamino)ethyl [3,5-diiodo-4-(3-iodo-4-methoxy-phenoxy) phenyl] acetate hydrochloride.
Use: Thyromimetic.

THYROPROPIC ACID. 4-(4-Hydroxy-3-iodophenoxy)-3,5-diiodohydrocinnamic acid. Triopron (Warner Chilcott).
Use: Anticholesteremic.

THYROTROPHIN. B.A.N. Thyrotrophic hormone. Thytropar; Thytrophin.

THYROTROPIC PRINCIPLE OF BOVINE ANTERIOR PITUITARY GLANDS.
See: Thytropar, Vial (Armour Labs.).

•**THYROXINE I-125.** USAN.
Use: Radioactive agent.

•**THYROXINE I-131.** USAN.
Use: Radioactive agent.

L-THYROXINE, SODIUM.
See: Levoid, Vial (Pharmex).
Synthroid, Tab., Inj. (Flint).

THYROZYME-II A. (Abbott Diagnostics) T-4 diagnostic kit. Quantitative measurement of unsaturated thyroxine binding globulin in serum. Test unit 100s, 500s.
Use: Diagnostic aid.

THYTROPAR. (Armour) Thyrotropin from bovine anterior pituitary glands. Thyrotropin, B.A.N. Thyroid myxedema due to pituitary insufficiency. Vial 10 IU.

Uso: Diagnostic aid.

TIACRILAST. USAN.
Use: Anti-allergic.

•**TIAMENIDINE HYDROCHLORIDE.** USAN.
Use: Antihypertensive.

•**TIAMULIN.** USAN.
Use: Antibacterial.

•**TIAMULIN FUMARATE.** USAN.
Use: Antibacterial.

•**TIAPAMIL HYDROCHLORIDE.** USAN.
Use: Antagonist (to calcium).

•**TIARAMIDE HYDROCHLORIDE.** USAN.
Use: Anti-asthmatic.

•**TIAZOFURIN.** USAN.
Use: Antineoplastic.

•**TIAZURIL.** USAN.
Use: Coccidiostat.

•**TIBENELAST SODIUM.** USAN.
Use: Anti-asthmatic; bronchodilator.

•**TIBOLONE.** USAN. (1) 17-Hydroxy-7α-methyl-19-nor-17α-pregn-5(10)-en-20-yn-3-one; (2) 17α-Ethynyl-17-hydroxy-7α-methyl-5 (10)-estren-3-one.
Use: Anabolic.

•**TIBRIC ACID.** USAN. 2-Chloro-5-(cis-3,5-dimethylpiperidinosulfonyl)benzoic acid.
Use: Treatment of hyperlipemia.

•**TIBROFAN.** USAN. 4,4′,5-Tribromo-2-thiophenecarboxanilide. Under study.
Use: Disinfectant.

•**TICABESONE PROPIONATE.** USAN.
Use: Glucocorticoid.

TICAR. (Beecham Labs) Ticarcillin disodium. 1 Gm, 3 Gm, 6 Gm/Vial in 10s. Piggyback Vials 3 Gm in 10s. Bulk Pharmacy Pkg. 20 Gm in 10s. Bulk Pharmacy Pkg. 30 Gm/Vial, 10s. ADD-Vantage 3 Gm Pkg. 10s.
Use: Antibacterial, penicillin.

TICARBODINE, USAN. α,α,α-Trifluoro-2,6-dimethylthio-1-piperidinecarboxy-m-toluidide. 2,6-Dimethylpiperidino-3′-(trifluoromethyl)thioformanilide.
Use: Anthelmintic.

TICARCILLIN CRESYL SODIUM. USAN.
Use: Antibacterial.

TICARCILLIN DISODIUM, STERILE, U.S.P. XXII. 6-[2-Carboxy-2-(3-thienyl)-acetamido]penicillanic acid.
Use: Antibiotic.
See: Ticar, inj. (Beecham Labs.).

TICARCILLIN DISODIUM AND CLAVULANATE POTASSIUM, STERILE, U.S.P. XXII.
Use: Antibiotic, inhibitor (β-*lactamase*).

TICLATONE. USAN. 6-Chloro-1,2-benzisothiazolin-3-one.
Use: Antibacterial, antifungal.

TICLOPIDINE HYDROCHLORIDE. USAN.
Use: Inhibitor (platelet).

TICONAZOLE CREAM, U.S.P. XXII.

TICRYNAFEN. USAN.
Use: Diuretic, uricosuric, antihypertensive.

TIDEX. (Allison) Dextroamphetamine sulfate 5 mg/Tab. Bot. 100s, 1000s.
Use: CNS stimulant.

TIDEXSOL TABLETS. (Winthrop Products) Acetaminophen.
Use: Analgesic.

TIEMONIUM IODIDE. B.A.N. 4-[3-Hydroxy-3-phenyl-3-(2-thienyl)propyl]-4-methylmorpholinium iodide.
Use: Antispasmodic; anticholinergic.

•**TIFURAC SODIUM.** USAN.
Use: Analgesic.

TIGAN. (Beecham Labs) Trimethobenzamide hydrochloride. **Cap.:** 100 mg. Bot. 100s; 250 mg. Bot. 100s. **Amp.:** (100 mg/ml) 2 ml. Box 10s. Vial 20 ml. **Supp.:** 200 mg. Box 10s, 50s. **Pediatric Supp.:** 100 mg Box 10s.
Use: Anticholinergic.

•**TIGEMONAM DICHOLINE.** USAN.
Use: Antimicrobial.

•**TIGESTOL.** USAN. (1) 19-Nor-17α-pregn-5(10)-en-20-yn-17-ol; (2) 17-α-Ethynyl-5(10)-estren-17-ol. Under study.
Use: Progestin.

TIGLOIDINE. B.A.N. Tiglylpseudotropeine. Tiglyssin [hydrobromide].
Use: Treatment of the Parkinsonian syndrome.

TIGO. (Burlington) Polymixin B sulfate 5000 units, zinc bacitracin 400 units, neomycin sulfate 5 mg/Gm. Oint. Tube 0.5 oz.
Use: Anti-infective, external.

TIHIST-DP. (Vita Elixir) d-methorphan HBr 10 mg, pyrilamine maleate 16 mg, sodium citrate 3.3 gr/5 ml.
Use: Antitussive, antihistamine.

TIHIST NASAL DROPS. (Vita Elixir) Pyrilamine maleate 0.1%, phenylephrine HCl 0.25%, sodium bisulfite 0.2%, methylparaben 0.02%, propylparaben 0.01%/30 ml.
Use: Antihistamine, decongestant.

TIJA TABLETS. (Vita Elixir) Oxytetracycline HCl 250 mg/Tab.
Use: Antibacterial, tetracycline.

TIJA SYRUP. (Vita Elixir) Oxytetracycline HCl 125 mg/5 ml.
Use: Antibacterial, tetracycline.

TIJECT-20. (Mayrand) Trimethobenzamide HCl 100 mg/ml. Vial 20 ml.
Use: Antiemetic/antivertigo.

•**TILETAMINE HCl,** USAN. 2-(Ethylamino)-2-(2-thienyl)cyclohexanone HCl.
Use: Anesthetic; anticonvulsant.

TILIDATE. B.A.N. Ethyl 2-dimethylamino-1-phenylcyclohex-3-ene-1-carboxylate.
Use: Analgesic.

•**TILIDINE HCl.** USAN. (±)-Ethyl trans-2-(dimethylamino)-1-phenyl-3-cyclohexene-1-carboxylate HCl.
Use: Analgesic.

•**TILOMISOLE.** USAN.
Use: Immunoregulator.

•**TILORONE HCl.** USAN. 2,7-Bis[2-(diethylamino)ethoxy]fluoren-9-one dihydrochloride.
Use: Antiviral.

TIMED REDUCING AIDS-CAFFEINE FREE. (Weeks & Leo) Phenylpropanolamine HCl 75 mg/TR Cap. Bot. 28s, 56s.
Use: Diet aid.

•**TIMEFURONE.** USAN.
Use: Anti-atherosclerotic.

TIMENTIN. (Beecham Labs) Ticarcillin disodium 3 Gm, clavulanic acid (as potassium salt) 0.1 Gm. Vial 3.1 Gm, Box 10s. Piggyback Vials 3.1 Gm, Box 10s.
Use: Antibacterial, penicillin.

•**TIMOBESONE ACETATE.** USAN.
Use: Adrenocortical steroid (topical).

TIMOLIDE. (Merck Sharp & Dohme) Timolol maleate 10 mg, hydrochlorothiazide 25 mg/Tab. Bot. 100s.
Use: Antihypertensive.

•**TIMOLOL.** USAN.
Use: Anti-adrenergic (beta-receptor).

•**TIMOLOL MALEATE,** U.S.P. XXII. Ophth. Soln., Tab., U.S.P. XXII. (S)-1-[Cl, 1-dimethyl-ethyl) amino]-3-[[4-(4 morpholinyl)-1,2,5-thiadiazol-3-yl]oxy]-2-propanol, (Z)-butenedioate (1:1) salt.
Use: Treatment of chronic open angle, aphakic and secondary glaucoma, antihypertensive, prevention of recurrent M.I.
See: Blocadren, Tab. (Merck Sharp & Dohme)
Timoptic, Ophth. (Merck Sharp & Dohme).
Timoptic In Ocudose, Ophth. (Merck Sharp & Dohme).

•**TIMOLOL MALEATE AND HYDROCHLOROTHIAZIDE TABLETS,** U.S.P. XXII.
Use: Antihypertensive.
See: Timolide,Tab. (Merck Sharp & Dohme).

TIMOPTIC. (Merck Sharp & Dohme) Timolol maleate 0.25% or 0.5% soln. Ocumeter Ophthalmic Dispenser 2.5 ml, 5 ml, 10 ml, 15 ml.
Use: Beta-adrenergic blocking agent.

TIMOPTIC IN OCUDOSE. (Merck Sharp & Dohme) Timolol maleate 0.25% or 0.5%. Preservative-free in sterile occudose ophthalmic UD dispenser.
Use: Beta-adrenergic blocking agent.

•**TINABINOL.** USAN.
Use: Antihypertensive.

TINACTIN. (Schering) **Soln. 1%:** Tolnaftate (10 mg/ml) w/butylated hydroxytoluene, in nonaqueous homogeneous PEG 400. Plastic squeeze bot. 10 ml. **Cream 1%:** Tolnaftate (10 mg/Gm) in homogeneous, nonaqueous vehicle of PEG-400, propylene glycol, carboxypolymethylene, monoamylamine, titanium dioxide, butylated hydroxytoluene. Tube 15 Gm, 30 Gm, UD 0.7 Gm. **Pow. 1%:** Tolnaftate w/corn starch, talc. Plastic container 45 Gm, 90 Gm. **Pow. Aerosol 1%:** Tolnaftate w/butylated hydroxytoluene, talc, polyethylene-polypropylene glycol monobutyl ether, denatured alcohol, inert propellant of isobutane. Spray can 100 Gm. **Liq. Aerosol 1%:** Tolnaftate w/butylated hydroxytoluene, polyethylene-polyproplyene glycol monobutyl ether, alcohol 36%, inert propellant of isobutane. Spray can 120 ml.
Use: Antifungal, external.

TINASTAT. (Vita Elixir) Sodium hyposulfite, benzethonium Cl/2 oz.
Use: Keratolytic.

TINAVAL POWDER. (Vale) Tolnaftate 1%. Bot. 45 Gm.
Use: Antifungal, external.

TINDAL. (Schering) Acetophenazine maleate 20 mg/Tab. Bot. 100s.
Use: Antipsychotic agent.

TINE TEST, OLD TUBERCULIN, Rosenthal. (Lederle).
See: Tuberculin Tine Test (Lederle).

TINE TEST, PURIFIED PROTEIN DERIVATIVE. (Lederle).
See: Tuberculin Tine Test (Lederle).

TIN FLUORIDE. Stannous Fluoride, U.S.P. XXII.

TING. (Pharmacraft) **Cream:** Benzoic acid, boric acid, zinc oxide, zinc stearate, alcohol 18.7%. Tube 0.9 oz, 1.8 oz. **Pow.:** Boric acid, benzoic acid, zinc stearate, zinc oxide. Can 2.5 oz. **Spray Pow.:** Total undecylenate 19% as undecylenic acid and zinc undecylenate. Can 2.5 oz.
Use: Antifungal, external.

•**TINIDAZOLE.** USAN. 1-[2-(Ethylsulfonyl)-ethyl]-2-methyl-5-nitroimidazole.
Use: Antiprotozoal.
See: Fasigyn (Pfizer).
Simplotan (Pfizer).

TINSET. (Janssen) Oxatomide.
Use: Antiallergenic, antiasthmatic.

TINVER LOTION. (Barnes-Hind) Sodium thiosulfate 25%, salicylic acid 1%, isopropyl alcohol 10%, propylene glycol, menthol, disodium edetate, colloidal alumina. Bot. 4 oz, 6 oz.
Use: Antifungal, external.

•**TIOCONAZOLE,** U.S.P. XXII.
Use: Antifungal.
See: Vagistat (Fujisawa SmithKline).

•**TIODAZOSIN.** USAN.
Use: Antihypertensive.

•**TIODONIUM CHLORIDE.** USAN.
Use: Antibacterial.

•**TIOPERIDONE HYDROCHLORIDE.** USAN.
Use: Antipsychotic.

•**TIOPINAC.** USAN.
Use: Anti-inflammatory, analgesic.

•**TIOSPIRONE HYDROCHLORIDE.** USAN.
Use: Antipsychotic.

•**TIOTIDINE.** USAN.
Use: Antagonist.

•**TIOXIDAZOLE.** USAN.
Use: Anthelmintic.

•**TIPENTOSIN HYDROCHLORIDE.** USAN.
Use: Antihypertensive.

TIPRAMINE TABS. (Major) Imipramine 10 mg, 25 mg or 50 mg/Tab. **10 mg:** Bot. 250s; **25 mg or 50 mg:** Bot. 250s, 1000s.
Use: Antidepressant.

TIPREDANE. USAN.
Use: Adrenocortical steroid (topical).

TIPRENOLOL. B.A.N. 3-Isopropylamino-1-[2-(methylthio)phenoxy]propan-2-ol.
Use: Beta-adrenergic receptor blocking agent.

TIPRENOLOL HCl. USAN. (±)-1-(Isopropylamino)-3-[o-(methylthio)-phenoxy]-2-propanol HCl.
Use: Anti-adrenergic (β-receptor).

TIPRINAST MEGLUMIDE. USAN. A Mead Johnson investigative drug.
Use: Anti-allergenic agent.

TIPROPIDIL HYDROCHLORIDE. USAN.
Use: Vasodilator.

TIQUINAMIDE HYDROCHLORIDE. USAN.
Use: Anticholinergic.

TIREND. (Norcliff Thayer) Caffeine 100 mg/Tab. Bot. 12s, 25s, 50s.
Use: Analeptic.

TIRILAZAD MESYLATE. USAN.
Use: Inhibitor, lipid peroxidation.

TI-SCREEN. (TI Pharmaceuticals) Ethylhexyl-p-methoxy-cinnamate 7.5%, oxybenzone 5%, SPF 15. PABA free. Lot. Bot. 120 ml.
Use: Sunscreen.

TISIT. (Pfeiffer) Pyrethrins 0.3%, piperonyl butoxide technical 3%, petroleum distillate 1.2%, benzyl alcohol 2.4%. Shampoo. Bot. 118 ml.
Use: Pediculicide.

TISSUE FIXATIVE AND WASH SOLUTION. (Wampole-Zeus) A modified Michel's tissue fixative and buffered wash solution.
Use: To facilitate the transport and processing of fresh tissue biopsies.

TISSUE RESPIRATORY FACTOR (TRF). (International Hormone) RSF, SRF, LYCD, PCO, Procytoxid marketed as 2000 units. Supplied as bulk liquid concentrate.
Use: Promotion of cellular oxidation.

TIS-U-SOL. (Travenol) Pentalyte irrigation containing sodium Cl 800 mg, potassium Cl 40 mg, magnesium sulfate 20 mg, sodium phosphate 8.75 mg, monobasic potassium phosphate 6.25 mg/100 ml. Bot. 250 ml, 1000 ml.
Use: Sterile irrigating solution.

TITAN. (Barnes-Hind) Benzalkonium Cl, EDTA, nonionic cleaner buffers. Bot. 1 oz, 2 oz.
Use: Hard contact lens care.

•**TITANIUM DIOXIDE,** U.S.P. XXII.
Use: Solar ray protectant.

TITICUM RIPENS.
W/Oxyquinoline sulfate, charcoal.
See: Triticoll, Tabs. (Western Research).

TITRACID. (Trimen) Calcium carbonate 420 mg/Tab. Bot. 100s.
Use: Antacid.

TITRALAC. (3M Products) Glycine 150 mg, calcium carbonate 0.42 Gm/Tab. Bot. 40s, 100s, 1000s.
Use: Antacid.

•**TIXANOX.** USAN.
Use: Anti-allergic.

•**TIXOCORTOL PIVALATE.** USAN.
Use: Anti-inflammatory (topical).

T-KOFF. (T.E. Williams) Phenylpropanolamine HCl 20 mg, phenylephrine HCl 20 mg, chlorpheniramine maleate 5 mg, codeine phosphate 10 mg/5 ml. Syr. Bot. 480 ml. Grape flavor.
Use: Antihistamine, decongestant, antitussive.

T-MATINIC. (Tennessee) Iron 100 mg, desiccated liver 200 mg, stomach powder 100 mg, vitamins B_{12} 10 mcg, C 50 mg, folic acid 1 mg/Cap. Bot. 100s, 1000s. Vial 30 ml.
Use: Vitamin/mineral supplement.

TOBRADEX. (Alcon) Tobramycin 0.3%, dexamethasone 0.1%. Susp. 5 ml.
Use: Corticosteroid, anti-infective, ophthalmic.

•**TOBRAMYCIN,** U.S.P. XXII. Ophth. Oint., Ophth. Soln., U.S.P. XXII. An antibiotic obtained from cultures of *Streptomyces tenebrarius.*
Use: Antibiotic.
See: Tobrex, Soln., Oint. (Alcon).

•**TOBRAMYCIN AND DEXAMETHASONE OPHTHALMIC SUSPENSION,** U.S.P. XXII.
Use: Antibiotic.

•**TOBRAMYCIN SULFATE INJECTION,** U.S.P. XXII.
Use: Antibiotic.
See: Nebcin, Amp., Hyporet (Lilly).

TOBREX OPHTHALMIC OINTMENT. (Alcon) Tobramycin 0.3% in sterile ointment base. Tube 3.5 Gm.
Use: Anti-infective, ophthalmic.

TOBREX SOLUTION. (Alcon) Tobramycin 0.3%. Ophthalmic soln. Bot. 5 ml w/dropper.
Use: Anti-infective, ophthalmic.

•**TOCAINIDE.** USAN.
Use: Antiarrhythmic, cardiac depressant.
See: Tonocard, Tab. (Merck Sharp & Dohme).

•**TOCAINIDE HYDROCHLORIDE,** U.S.P. XXII. Tab., U.S.P. XXII.
Use: Antiarrhythmic, cardiac depressant.

•**TOCAMPHYL.** USAN. 1-p, α-Dimethyl-benzyl camphorate 1:1 salt with 2,2′-iminodiethanol.
Use: Choleretic.
See: Gallogen, Tab. (Beecham-Massengill).

TOCLONOL EXPECTORANT. (Cenci) Carbetapentane citrate 7.25 mg, terpin hydrate 16.65 mg, menthol 0.83 mg, alcohol 7.2%, sodium citrate 66.15 mg, citric acid 6.65 mg, glycerin 45 min/5 ml. Bot. 3 oz, 6 oz, 16 oz.
Use: Expectorant.

TOCLONOL W/CODEINE ELIXIR. (Cenci) Same as Toclonol Expectorant plus codeine 10 mg/5 ml. Bot. pt, gal.
Use: Expectorant, antitussive.

TOCOPHEROL-DL-ALPHA. Vitamin E, U.S.P. XXII. 5,7,8-Trimethyltocol, alpha-Tocopherol, dl-alpha-tocopherol, Vit. E, wheat germ oil. dl-2,5,7,8-Tetramethyl-2-(4′,8′,12′-trimethyltridecyl)-6-chromanol.

Cap. and Tab.:
Denamone, Cap. (3 min., 10 min.) wheat germ oil (Vio-Bin).
Ecofrol, Cap. (O'Neal).
Eprolin, Gelseal (Lilly).
Epsilan M, Cap. (Warren-Teed).
Lib-E, Cap. (AVP).
Oint.:
Myopone (Drug Prods.).
Soln.:
Aquasol E, Soln. (USV Pharm.).

•**TOCOPHEROLS EXCIPIENT,** N.F. XVII.

•**TOCOPHERSOLAN.** USAN. (+)-α-Toco-pheryl polyethylene glycol 1000 succinate.
Use: Vitamin E supplement.

TOCOPHERYL ACETATE-d-ALPHA. Vitamin E, U.S.P. XXII.
See: Aquasol E, Prods. (USV Labs.).
E-Ferol, Prep. (Fellows).
Epsilan-M, Cap. (Warren-Teed).
Lib-E-400, Cap. (AVP).
Tocopher, Cap. (Quality Generics).
Tokols, Cap. (Ulmer).
Vit. E. (Various Mfr.).

TOCOPHERYL ACETATES, CONC. D-ALPHA. Vitamin E, U.S.P. XXII. d-alpha-Toco-pheryl acetate.

TOCOPHERYL ACID SUCCINATED D-ALPHA. Vitamin E, U.S.P. XXII.
See: E-Ferol Succinate, Tab., Cap. (Fellows).
Vitamin E (Various Mfr.).

TOCOSAMINE. (Trent) Sparteine sulfate 150 mg, sodium Cl 4.5 mg/ml. Amp. 1 ml. Box 12s, 100s.
Use: Oxytocic.

TODAY VAGINAL CONTRACEPTIVE SPONGE. (VLI) Nonoxynol-9, citric, sorbic, benzoic acid, sodium dihydrogen, citrate, sodium metabisulfite, polyurethane foam sponge. 3s, 6s, 12s.
Use: Contraceptive.

TODRAZOLINE. B.A.N. Ethyl 3-phthalazin-1-yl-carbazate. Binazine.
Use: Antihypertensive.

TOFENACIN. B.A.N. N-Methyl-2-(2-methyl-benzhydryloxy)ethylamine. Elamol hydrochloride.
Use: Treatment of the Parkinsonian syndrome.

•**TOFENACIN HCl.** USAN. N-Methyl-2-[(o-methyl-a-phenyl-benzyl)oxy]-ethylamine HCl.
Use: Anticholinergic.

TOFRANAZINE. (Geigy) Combination of imipramine and promazine. Pending release.

TOFRANIL. (Geigy) Imipramine HCl. **Tab.:** 10 mg. Bot. 100s, 1000s; 25 mg or 50 mg. Bot. 100s, 1000s, UD 100s, Gy-Pak 100s, 1 unit (12×100); 6 units (72×100). **Amp.:** 25 mg/2 ml w/ascorbic acid 2 mg, sodium bisulfite 1 mg, sodium sulfite 1 mg and Amp 2 ml.
Use: Antidepressant, anti-enuretic.

TOFRANIL-PM. (Geigy) Imipramine pamoate. **75 mg/Cap.** Bot. 30s, 100s, 1000s, UD 100s. **100 mg or 125 mg/Cap.:** Bot. 30s, 100s. **150 mg/Cap.:** Bot. 30s, 100s, UD 100s.
Use: Antidepressant.

TOLAMIDE TABS. (Major) Tolazamide. **100 mg/Tab.:** Bot. 100s, 250s; **250 mg/Tab.:** 200s, 500s; **500 mg/Tab.:** Bot. 100s, 500s.
Use: Antidiabetic.

•**TOLAMOLOL.** USAN. 4-[2-(2-Hydroxy-3-o-tolyloxypropylamino)ethoxy]benzamide.
Use: Beta-adrenergic receptor blocking agent, coronary vasodilator, antiarrhythmic.

•**TOLAZAMIDE,** U.S.P. XXII. Tab., U.S.P. XXII. (Upjohn) 1-(Hexahydro-1-azepinyl)-3-(p-tolylsulfonyl) urea. 1-Perhydroazepin-1-yl-3-toluene-p-sul- phonylurea. Tolanase. Benzenesulfonamide, N-[[(hexahydro-1H-azepin-1-yl)amino]carbonyl]-4-methyl-. 1-(Hexahydro-1H-azepin-1-yl)-3-(p-tolylsulfonyl) urea.
Use: Hypoglycemic agent.
See: Ronase, Tab. (Solvay).
Tolinase, Tab. (Upjohn).

•**TOLAZOLINE HYDROCHLORIDE,** U.S.P. XXII. Inj., Tab., U.S.P. XXII. Benzazoline HCl, 2-Benzyl-2- imidazoline HCl. Vasimid, Vasodil.
Use: Anti-adrenergic, vasodilator (peripheral).
See: Priscoline, Prep. (Ciba).
Tazol, Tab. (Durst).
Toloxan, Tab. (Kenyon).
Tolzol, Tab. (Robinson).

•**TOLBUTAMIDE,** U.S.P. XXII. Tab. U.S.P. XXII. N-Butyl-N′-toluene-p-sulfonylurea. Benzenesulfonamide, N-[(butylamino)carbonyl]-4-methyl-. 1-Butyl-3-(p-tolylsulfonyl)urea.
Use: Hypoglycemic.
See: Orinase, Preps. (Upjohn).

•**TOLBUTAMIDE SODIUM, STERILE,** U.S.P. XXII.
Use: Diagnostic aid (diabetes).
See: Orinase Diagnostic (Upjohn).

•**TOLCICLATE.** USAN.
Use: Antifungal.

TOLDIMFOS. B.A.N. 4-Dimethylamino-o-tolylphosphinic acid. Tonophosphan (sodium salt).
Use: Phosphorus source, Veterinary medicine.

TOLECTIN 200. (McNeil Pharm) Tolmetin sodium 200 mg/Tab. Bot. 100s.
Use: Nonsteroidal anti-inflammatory drug; analgesic.

TOLECTIN 600. (McNeil Pharm) Tolmetin sodium 600 mg/Tab. Bot. 100s.
Use: Nonsteroidal anti-inflammatory drug; analgesic.

TOLECTIN DS. (McNeil Pharm) Tolmetin sodium 400 mg/Cap. Bot. 100s, 500s, UD 100s.
Use: Nonsteroidal anti-inflammatory drug; analgesic.

•**TOLFAMIDE.** USAN.
Use: Enzyme inhibitor.

TOLFRINIC. (Ascher) Ferrous fumarate 200 mg, vitamins B_{12} 25 mcg, C 100 mg/Tab. Bot. 100s.
Use: Vitamin/mineral supplement.

•**TOLGABIDE.** USAN.
Use: Anti-epileptic (control of abnormal movements).

•**TOLIMIDONE.** USAN.
Use: Anti-ulcerative.

TOLINASE. (Upjohn) Tolazamide 100 mg, 250 mg or 500 mg/Tab. **100 mg or 500 mg.** Bot. 100s. **250 mg:** Bot. 100s, UD 100s.
Use: Antidiabetic.

•**TOLINDATE.** USAN.
Use: Antifungal.
See: Dalnate (USV Pharm.).

•**TOLIODIUM CHLORIDE.** USAN.
Use: Food additive.

•**TOLMETIN.** USAN.
Use: Anti-inflammatory.

•**TOLMETIN SODIUM,** U.S.P. XXII. Cap., Tab., U.S.P. XXII. Sodium 1-Methyl-5-p-toluoylpyrrole-2-acetic acid.
Use: Anti-inflammatory.
See: Tolectin, Tab. (McNeil).
Tolectin DS, Cap. (McNeil).

•**TOLNAFTATE,** U.S.P. XXII. Topical Aerosol Powder, Cream, Gel, Powder, Topical Soln., U.S.P. XXII. o-2-Naphthyl m,N-dimethyl-thiocarbanilate. Naphthiomate-T; Tinaderm. Carbamothioic acid, methyl(3-methylphenyl)-, 0-2-naphthalenyl ester.
Use: Topical antifungal agent.
See: Aftate, Prods. (Schering-Plough).
Tinactin, Soln., Cream, Pow., Pow. Aerosal (Schering).

•**TOLOFOCON A.** USAN.
Use: Contact lens material (hydrophobic).

TOLONIUM CHLORIDE. 3-Amino-7-dimethylamino-2-methyl-phenazathionium. Blutene Chloride.

TOLOXAN. (Kenyon) Tolazoline HCl 25 mg/Tab. Bot. 100s, 1000s.
Use: Antihypertensive.

TOLOXYCHLORINAL. 1,1′-[[(o-Tolyloxy)-methyl]ethylenedioxy]bis[2,2,2-trichloro-ethanol].1,1′-[3-o-Tolyloxypropylenedioxy]bis (2,2,2-trichloroethanol. Propoxychlorinol.
Use: Sedative.

TOLPENTAMIDE. B.A.N. 1-Cyclopentyl-3-toluene-p-sulfonylurea.
Use: Hypoglycemic agent.

TOLPERISONE. B.A.N. 2-Methyl-3-piperidino-1-p-tolylpropan-1-one. Mydocalm.
Use: Muscle relaxant.

TOLPIPRAZOLE. B.A.N. 5-Methyl-3-[2-(4-m-tolylpiperazin-1-yl)ethyl]pyrazole.
Use: Tranquilizer.

•**TOLPOVIDONE I-131.** USAN.α-(p-Iodobenzyl)-poly[1-(2-oxo-1-pyrrolidinyl)ethylene]-^{131}I.
Use: Differential diagnosis of source of hypoalbuminemia.
See: Raovin (Abbott).

TOLPRONINE. B.A.N. 1-(1,2,3,6-Tetrahydro-1-pyridyl)-3-o-tolyloxypropan-2-ol. Proponesin [hydrochloride]
Use: Analgesic.

TOLPROPAMINE. B.A.N. NN-Dimethyl-3-phenyl-3-p-tolypropylamine. Tylagel [hydrochloride]
Use: Antipruritic.

•**TOLPYRRAMIDE.** USAN. N-p-tolylsulfonyl-1-pyrrolidinecarboxamide. 1-Tetramethylene-3-p-tolysulfonylurea.
Use: Oral hypoglycemic.

•**TOLRESTAT.** USAN.
Use: Inhibitor (aldose reductase).

•**TOLTRAZURIL.** USAN.
Use: Coccidiostat (veterinary).

•**TOLU BALSAM,** U.S.P. XXII.
Use: Pharmaceutic necessity for Compound Benzoin Tincture, expectorant.
See: Vicks Regular and Wild Cherry Medicated Cough Drops (Vicks).

•**TOLU BALSAM SYRUP,** N.F. XVII. (Lilly) Bot. 16 fl oz.
Use: Vehicle.

•**TOLU BALSAM TINCTURE,** N.F. XVII.
Use: Flavor.

TOLUIDINE BLUE O CHLORIDE.
See: Blutene Chloride.

TOLU-SED (No Sugar). (Scherer) Codeine phosphate 10 mg, guaifenesin 100 mg/5 ml, alcohol 10%. Bot. 4 oz, pt.
Use: Antitussive, expectorant.

TOLU-SED DM (No Sugar). (Scherer) d-Methorphan HBr 10 mg, guaifenesin 100 mg/5 ml, alcohol 10%. Bot. 4 oz, pt.
Use: Antitussive, expectorant.

TOLYCAINE. B.A.N. Methyl 2-diethylaminoacetamido-m-toluate. Baycain [hydrochloride]
Use: Local anesthetic.

TOLZOL. (Robinson) Tolazoline HCl 25 mg/Tab. Bot. 100s, 1000s, Bulk pack 5000.
Use: Antihypertensive.

TOMOCAT. (Lafayette) CT barium sulfate 1.5% w/v. Case of 24 Bot.
Use: Radiopaque agent.

TOMOCAT 1000. (Lafayette) Barium sulfate suspension concentrate 5% w/v/Bot. for dilution to 1.5% w/v at time of use. Bot. 225 ml w/1000 ml dilution Bot. Case 24 Bot. and 2 Dilution Bot.
Use: Radiopaque agent.

•**TOMOXETINE HYDROCHLORIDE.** USAN.
Use: Antidepressant.

TONAMINE. (Kenyon) Liver, vitamin B_{12} equivalent 1 mcg, ferrous gluconate 44 mg, B_2 0.5 mg, folic acid 2 mg, d-panthenol 2.5 mg, dl-methionine 10 mg, niacinamide 100 mg, procaine HCl 2%/2 ml. Vial 30 ml.
Use: Vitamin/mineral supplement.

TONAVITE-M ELIXIR. (Goldline) Bot. 12 oz, pt, gal.
Use: Dietary supplement.

•**TONAZOCIN MESYLATE.** USAN.
Use: Analgesic.

TONBEC TABLETS. (A.V.P.) Vitamins B_1 15 mg, B_2 10 mg, B_6 5 mg, nicotinamide 50 mg, calcium pantothenate 10 mg, ascorbic acid 300 mg/Tab. Bot. 60s.
Use: Vitamin supplement.

TONECOL. (A.V.P.) Promethazine w/expectorant and vasoconstrictor. Bot. pt.
Use: Antihistamine, expectorant, vasoconstrictor.

TONECOL COUGH SYRUP. (A.V.P.) Dextromethorphan HBr 10 mg, phenylephrine HCl 5 mg, chlorpheniramine maleate 1 mg, sodium citrate 15 mg, guaifenesin 25 mg/5 ml, alcohol 7%. Bot. pt.
Use: Antitussive, decongestant, antihistamine, expectorant.

TONELAX TABLETS. (A.V.P.) Danthron 75 mg, calcium pantothenate 25 mg/Tab. Bot. 100s, 1000s.
Use: Laxative.

TONO-B PEDIATRIC. (Vale) Iron 5 mg, thiamine HCl 0.167 mg, riboflavin 0.133 mg/Tab. Bot. 1000s.
Use: Vitamin/mineral supplement.

TONOCARD. (Merck Sharp & Dohme) Tocainide HCl 400 mg or 600 mg/Tab. Bot. 100s, UD 100s.
Use: Antiarrhythmic.

TONOJUG 2000. (Lafayette) Barium sulfate powder 1200 Gm for suspension to make 2000 ml. Bot. 2000 Gm Case: 8 Bot.
Use: Radiopaque agent.

TONOPAQUE ORAL BARIUM. (Lafayette) Barium sulfate powder 180 Gm for suspension. Bot. 180 Gm Case 24s.
Use: Radiopaque agent.

TOOTHACHE RELIEF-3 IN 1. (C.S. Dent) Toothache gum, toothache drops, benzocaine lotion.
Use: Local anesthetic.

TOP BRASS ZP-11. (Revlon) Zinc pyrithione 0.5% in cream base.
Use: Antiseborrheic.

TOP-FORM. (Hoyt) Topical formfitting gel applicators. Disposable trays for topical fluoride office treatments, plus permanent trays for topical fluoride home self treatments. Box 100s.
Use: Topical fluoride applications in home or office.

TOPIC. (Syntex) Benzyl alcohol 5% in greaseless gel base containing camphor, menthol, isopropyl alcohol 30%. Tube 2 oz.
Use: Antipruritic.

TOPICAL FLUORIDE. (Pacemaker) Acidulated phosphate fluoride. Flavors: orange, bubblegum, lime, raspberry, grape cinnamon. Liq. Bot. 4 oz, pt.
Use: Dental caries preventative.

TOPICORT CREAM. (Hoechst) Desoximetasone 0.25% emollient cream consisting of isopropyl myristate, cetyl stearyl alcohol, white petrolatum, mineral oil, lanolin alcohol and purified water. Tube 15 Gm, 60 Gm, 120 Gm.
Use: Corticosteroid, topical.

TOPICORT GEL. (Hoechst) Desoximetasone 0.05% in gel base, alcohol 20%. Tube 15 Gm, 60 Gm.
Use: Corticosteroid, topical.

TOPICORT LP CREAM. (Hoechst) Desoximetasone 0.05%. Tube 15 Gm, 60 Gm.
Use: Corticosteroid, topical.

TOPICORT OINTMENT. (Hoechst) Desoximetasone 0.25% in ointment base. Tube 15 Gm, 60 Gm,
Use: Corticosteroid, topical.

TOPICYCLINE. (Norwich Eaton) Tetracycline HCl 2.2 mg/ml, 4-epitetracycline HCl, sodium bisulfite. Bot. 70 ml w/diluent.
Use: Anti-acne.

•**TOPIRAMATE.** USAN.
Use: Anticonvulsant.

TOPOCAINE.
See: Surfacaine (Lilly).

•**TOPOTECAN HYDROCHLORIDE.** USAN.
Use: Antineoplastic.

•**TOPTERONE.** USAN.
Use: Anti-androgen.

•**TOQUIZINE.** USAN.
Use: Anticholinergic.

TORADOL. (Syntex) Ketorolac tromethamine 15 mg or 30 mg/ml. Inj. 15 mg/ml in Cartrix syringes 1 ml, 2 ml, 30 mg/ml in Cartrix syringes 1 ml. Alcohol 10%.
Use: Nonsteroidal anti-inflammatory drug; analgesic.

TORECAN. (Boehringer Ingelheim) Thiethylperazine. **Tab.:** 10 mg w/tartrazine. Bot. 100s. **Amp.:** 10 mg/2 ml w/sodium metabisulfite 0.5 mg, ascorbic acid 2 mg, sorbitol 40 mg, q.s. carbon dioxide. **Supp.:** 10 mg w/cocoa butter. Box 12s.
Use: Antiemetic/antivertigo.

•**TOREMIFENE CITRATE.** USAN.
Use: Antineoplastic, anti-estrogen.

TORGANIC-DM. (Major) Dextromethorphan HBr 10 mg, iodinated glycerol 30 mg/5 ml. Liq. Bot. 473 ml. Alcohol free.
Use: Antitussive, expectorant.

TORNALATE INHALER. (Winthrop Pharm) Bitolterol mesylate metered inhaler. Bot. 16.4 Gm w/oral inhaler. Refill 16.4 Gm.
Use: Bronchodilator.

TORNALATE TABLETS. (Winthrop Products) Bitolterol mesylate.
Use: Bronchodilator.

TORULA YEAST, DRIED, Obtained by growing *Candida (torulopsis) utilis* yeast on wood pulp wastes (Nutritional Labs.) Concentrate 100 lb. drums.
Use: Nutritional supplement.

•**TOSIFEN.** USAN.
Use: Anti-anginal.

TOTACILLIN. (Beecham Labs) Ampicillin trihydrate equivalent to: **Cap.:** 250 mg or 500 mg. Bot. 500s. **Susp.:** 125 mg/5 ml. Bot. 100 ml, 150 ml, 200 ml; 250 mg/5 ml. Bot. 100 ml, 200 ml.
Use: Antibacterial, penicillin.

TOTACILLIN-N. (Beecham Labs) Ampicillin sodium 250 mg, 500 mg, 1 Gm or 2 Gm/Vial in

10s; Piggyback Vial 500 mg, 1 Gm or 2 Gm, in 25s; Bulk pharm. pkg. 10 Gm in 25s.
Use: Antibacterial, penicillin.

TOTAL. (Allergan) Polyvinyl alcohol, edetate disodium, benzalkonium Cl in a sterile, buffered, isotonic solution. Bot. 2 fl oz, 4 fl oz.
Use: Hard contact lens care.

TOTAL ECLIPSE COOLING ALCOHOL. (Dorsey) Padimate O, oxybenzone, glyceryl PABA, alcohol 77%. SPF 15. Lot. Bot. 120 ml.
Use: Sunscreen.

TOTAL ECLIPSE MOISTURIZING. (Dorsey) Padimate O, oxybenzone, octyl salicylate. Moisturizing base. SPF 15. Lot. Bot. 120 ml.
Use: Sunscreen.

TOTAQUINE, Alkaloids from Cinchona bark, 7% to 12% quinine anhydrous, 70% to 80% total alkaloids (cinchonidine, cinchonine, quinidine and quinine).
Use: Antimalarial.

TOTOMYCIN HYDROCHLORIDE. Tetracycline, U.S.P. XXII.

•**TOXIN, DIPHTHERIA FOR SCHICK TEST,** U.S.P. XXII.
Use: Diagnostic aid (dermal reactivity indicator).

TOXO. (Wampole-Zeus) *Toxoplasma* antibody test system. An IFA test system for the detection of antibodies to *Toxoplasma gondii.* Test 120s.
Use: Diagnostic aid.

•**TOXOID, DIPHTHERIA,** U.S.P. XXII.
Use: Immunizing agent (active).
See: Diphtheria Toxoid, Aluminum Hydroxide, Adsorbed.

•**TOXOID, TETANUS ADSORBED,** U.S.P. XXII.
Use: Immunizing agent (active).

TOXOID MIXTURE.
See: Tri-Solgen, Vial (Lilly).

T.P.L. TROCHES. (Kasdenol) Triamite. Loz. 5 Gm 15s.
Use: Mouth and throat preparation.

TPM-TEST. (Wampole) Indirect hemagglutination test for the qualitative and quantitative determination of antibodies to *Toxoplasma gondii* in serum. Kit 120s.
Use: Diagnostic aid.

TPN ELECTROLYTES. (Abbott Hospital Prods) Multiple electrolyte additive: Sodium Cl 321 mg, calcium Cl 331 mg, potassium Cl 1491 mg, magnesium Cl 508 mg, sodium acetate 2420 mg. 20 ml in Fliptop or Pintop Vial 50 ml or Univ. Add. Syringe 20 ml.
Use: Electrolyte replacement.

TPN ELECTROLYTES II. (Abbott) Na^+ 15 mEq/L, K^+ 18 mEq/L, Ca^{++} 4.5 mEq/L, Mg^{++} 5 mEq/L, Cl^- 35 mEq/L, acetate 7.5 mEq/L. 20 ml Fill in Fliptop and Pintop Vial 50 ml and Fill Syringe 20 ml.
Use: Fluid/electrolyte replacement.

TPN ELECTROLYTES III. Na^+ 25 mEq/L, K^+ 40.6 mEq/L, Ca^{++} 5 mEq/L, Mg^{++} 8 mEq/L, Cl^- 33.5 mEq/L, acetate 40.6 mEq/L, gluconate 5 mEq/L. 20 ml fill in Fliptop and Pintop Vial 50 ml and Fill Syringe 20 ml.
Use: Fluid/electrolyte replacement.

TP TROCHES. (EJ Moore) Triamite. Jar 500s, Box 15s.
Use: Mouth and throat preparation.

•**TRACAZOLATE.** USAN.
Use: Sedative.

TRACE. (Lorvic) Erythrosine concentrated soln. Squeeze Bot. 30 ml, 60 ml, Dispenser Packet 200s.
Use: Plaque dye soln.

TRACE-4. (IMS) Zinc 4 mg, copper 1 mg, manganese 0.5 mg, chromium 10 mcg. Vial 5 ml, 20 ml.
Use: Mineral supplement.

TRACE 28 LIQUID. (Lorvic) D & C Red No. 28 in aqueous soln. Bot. 30 ml, 60 ml.
Use: Diagnostic aid.

TRACE 28 TABLETS. (Lorvic) D & C Red No. 28. Tab. Box 30s, 180s, 700s.
Use: Diagnostic aid.

TRACELYTE. (Lyphomed) A combination of electrolytes and trace elements additive. Vial 20 ml.
Use: Fluid/electrolyte replacement.

TRACELYTE WITH DOUBLE ELECTROLYTES. (Lyphomed) A combination of electrolytes and trace elements additive. Vial 40 ml.
Use: Fluid/electrolyte replacement.

TRACELYTE-II. (Lyphomed) A combination of electrolytes and trace elements additive. Vial 20 ml.
Use: Fluid/electrolyte replacement.

TRACELYTE-II WITH DOUBLE ELECTROLYTES. (Lyphomed) Combination of electrolytes and trace elements additive. Vial 40 ml.
Use: Fluid/electrolyte replacement.

TRACEPLEX. (Enzyme Process) Iron 30 mg, iodine 0.1 mg, copper 0.5 mg, magnesium 40 mg, zinc 10 mg, vitamin B_{12} 5 mcg/4 Tab. Bot. 100s, 250s.
Use: Vitamin/mineral supplement.

TRACRIUM INJECTION. (Burroughs Wellcome) Atracurium besylate 10 mg/ml. Amp. 5 ml. Box 10s; 10 ml MDV. Box 10s.
Use: Muscle relaxant.

TRAC TABS 2X. (Hyrex) Atropine sulfate 0.06 mg, hyoscyamine 0.03 mg, methenamine 120 mg, methylene blue 6 mg, phenyl salicylate 30 mg, benzoic acid 7.5 mg/Tab. Bot. 100s, 1000s.
Use: Urinary anti-infective.

•**TRAGACANTH,** N.F. XVII.
Use: Pharmaceutical aid (suspending agent).

•**TRALONIDE.** USAN.
Use: Glucocorticoid.

•**TRAMADOL HYDROCHLORIDE.** USAN.
Use: Analgesic.

•**TRAMAZOLINE,** USAN. 2-[(5,6,7,8-Tetrahydro-1-naphthyl)amino]-2-imidazoline.
Use: Adrenergic.

TRANCIN. Fluphenazine.
Use: Antipsychotic agent.

TRANCOGESICO TABLETS. (Winthrop Products) Dipyrone, chlormezanone.
Use: Analgesic, muscle relaxant.

TRANCOPAL. (Winthrop Pharm) Chlormezanone 100 mg or 200 mg/Cap. **100 mg:** w/saccharin. Bot. 100s. **200 mg:** Bot. 100s, 1000s.
Use: Antianxiety agent.

TRANDATE INJECTION. (Allen & H) Labetalol HCl 5 mg/ml. Vial 20 ml, 40 ml. Box 1s. Prefilled Syringe 4 ml, 8 ml.
Use: Antihypertensive.

TRANDATE TABLETS. (Glaxo) Labetalol HCl 100 mg, 200 mg or 300 mg/Tab. Bot. 100s, 500s, 100s.
Use: Antihypertensive.

TRANDATE HCT. (Glaxo) Labetalol 100 mg, 200 mg or 300 mg, hydrochlorothiazide 25 mg/Tab. Bot. 100s.
Use: Antihypertensive, diuretic.

•**TRANEXAMIC ACID.** USAN.
Use: Hemostatic for hemophiliacs.
See: Cyclokapron, Tab., Inj. (KabiVitrum).

•**TRANILAST.** USAN.
Use: Anti-asthmatic.

TRANQUIL. (Kenyon) Mephenesin 400 mg, mephobarbital 10 mg, hyoscine HBr 0.25 mg/Tab. Bot. 1000s.
Use: Muscle relaxant, sedative/hypnotic, anticholinergic/antispasmodic.

TRANQUILIZERS.
See: A-poxide, Cap. (Abbott).
Atarax, Preps. (Roerig).
Centrax, Cap. (Parke-Davis).
Compazine, Preps. (SmithKline).
Equanil, Tab. (Wyeth-Ayerst).
Fenarol, Tab. (Winthrop Products).
Haldol, Tab., Inj., Concentrated Soln. (McNeil).
Harmonyl, Tab. (Abbott).
Librium, Cap., Inj. (Roche).
Loxitane, Prod. (Lederle).
Mellaril, Tab., Soln. (Sandoz).
Meprobamate (Various Mfr.).
Miltown, Preps. (Wallace).
Permitil, Preps. (Schering).
Proketazine Maleate, Preps. (Wyeth-Ayerst).
Prolixin, Preps. (Squibb).
Sparine HCl, Preps. (Wyeth-Ayerst).
Stelazine, Preps. (SmithKline).
Taractan, Preps. (Roche).
Thorazine HCl, Preps. (SmithKline).
Tindal, Tab. (Schering).
Trancopal, Cap. (Winthrop Pharm).
Tranxene, Cap. (Abbott).
Trilafon, Preps. (Schering).
Tybatran, Cap. (Robins).
Ultran, Preps. (Lilly).
Valium, Preps. (Roche).
Vesprin, Preps. (Squibb).
Vistaril, Preps. (Pfizer).

TRANQUILS CAPSULES. (Blue Cross) Pyrilamine maleate 25 mg/Cap. Bot. 30s.
Use: Sleep aid.

TRANQUILS TABLETS. (Blue Cross) Acetaminophen 300 mg, pyrilamine maleate 25 mg/Tab. Bot. 30s.
Use: Analgesic, sleep aid.

•**TRANSCAINIDE.** USAN.
Use: Antiarrhythmic, cardiac depressant.

TRANSCLOMIPHENE. (E)-2-[p-(2-Chloro-1, 2-diphenylvinyl) phenoxy] triethylamine.

TRANSDERM-NITRO. (Ciba) Nitroglycerin 2.5 mg, 5 mg, 10 mg or 15 mg. **2.5 mg:** 2.5 mg/24 hr. Pkg. 30s. **5 mg:** 5 mg/24 hr. Pkg. 30s. **10 mg:** 10 mg/24 hr. Pkg. 30s. **15 mg:** 15 mg/24 hr. Pkg. 30s.
Use: Antianginal.

TRANSDERMSCOP. (Ciba) Scopolamine 0.5 mg per 2-unit blister pkg. (programmed delivery over 3-day period).
Use: Antiemetic/antivertigo agent.

TRANSTHYRETIN EIA. (Abbott Diagnostics) Enzyme immunoassay for the quantitative determination of transthyretin in human serum or plasma. Test kit 100s.
Use: Diagnostic aid.

TRANS-VER-SAL. (Minnetonka Medical) Salicylic acid 15%/Transdermal patch. 6 mm, 12 mm. 40s.
Use: Keratolytic.

TRANXENE CAPSULES. (Abbott) Clorazepate dipotassium 3.75 mg, 7.5 mg or 15 mg/Cap. UD 100s.
Use: Antianxiety agent.

TRANXENE T-TAB TABLETS. (Abbott) Chlorazepate dipotassium 3.75 mg, 7.5 mg or 15 mg/Tab. Bot. 100s, 500s.
Use: Antianxiety agent.

TRANXENE-SD. (Abbott) Chlorazepate dipotassium 22.5 mg/Tab. Bot. 100s.
Use: Antianxiety agent.

TRANXENE-SD HALF STRENGTH TABLETS. (Abbott) Chlorazepate dipotassium 11.25 mg/Tab. Bot. 100s.
Use: Antianxiety agent.

TRANYLCYPROMINE. B.A.N. (±)trans-2-Phenylcyclopropylamine. Parnate (sulfate).
Use: Monoamine oxidase inhibitor; antidepressant.

TRANYLCYPROMINE SULFATE, U.S.P. XXI. Tab., U.S.P. XXI. Trans-dl-2-phenylcyclopropylamine sulfate (±)-trans-2-phenylcyclopropylamine sulfate (2:1).
Use: Antidepressant.
See: Parnate, Tab. (SmithKline).

TRAPENS. (Mills) Triticum 4 gr, oxyquinoline sulfate 1/20 gr, pow. charcoal 0.5 gr/Tab. Bot. 100s.

TRASICOR. (Ciba) Oxprenolol HCl, B.A.N.
Use: Beta-adrenergic blocking agent.

TRAUMACAL. (Mead Johnson Nutrition) Nutritionally complete formula for traumatized patients. Vanilla flavor. Can 8 oz.
Use: Enteral nutritional supplement.

TRAUM-AID HBC. (American McGaw) Advanced high branched chain amino acids diet. Assorted flavors. Packet 132 Gm.
Use: Enteral nutritional supplement.

T-RAU TABLET. (Tennessee Pharm.) Rauwolfia serpentina 50 mg or 100 mg/Tab. Bot. 100s, 1000s.
Use: Antihypertensive.

TRAVAMULSION 10% INTRAVENOUS FAT EMULSION. 1.1 kcal/ml, 270 mOsm/liter. Bot. 500 ml.
Use: Parenteral nutritional supplement.

TRAVAMULSION 20% INTRAVENOUS FAT EMULSION. (Travenol) 2 kcal/ml, 300 mOsm/liter. Bot. 500 ml.
Use: Parenteral nutritional supplement.

TRAVASE. (Flint) Proteolytic enzyme ointment, from bacillus subtilis; 82,000 casein units of proteolytic activity/Gm. Tube 14.2 Gm.
Use: Topical enzyme preparation.

TRAVASOL. (Travenol) Crystalline L-amino acids injection 5.5% or 8.5% (with or without electrolytes). IV Bot. 500 ml, 1000 ml, 2000 ml.
Use: Parenteral nutritional supplement.

TRAVASOL 3.5% M INJECTION WITH ELECTROLYTE #45. (Travenol) Crystalline L-amino acids 3.5% Soln. IV Bot. 500 ml, 1000 ml.
Use: Parenteral nutritional supplement.

TRAVASOL 10%. (Travenol) Crystalline L-amino acids injection 10%. Bot. 200 ml, 500 ml, 1000 ml, 2000 ml.
Use: Parenteral nutritional supplement.

TRAVASORB HEPATIC DIET. (Travenol) 378 kcal/Pkt. Carton 6s.
Use: Enteral nutritional supplement.

TRAVASORB HN PEPTIDE DIET. (Travenol) High nitrogen defined peptide 333 kcal/Pkt. Carton 6s.
Use: Enteral nutritional supplement.

TRAVSORB MCT LIQUID DIET. (Travenol) Digestible protein medium chain triglyceride diet. Packet 89 Gm.
Use: Enteral nutritional supplement.

TRAVASORB MCT POWDER DIET. (Travenol) Digestible protein medium chain triglyceride diet 400 kcal/Pkt. Carton 6s.
Use: Enteral nutritional supplement.

TRAVASORB RENAL DIET. (Travenol) 467 kcal/Pkt. Carton 6s. Packet 112 Gm.
Use: Enteral nutritional supplement.

TRAVASORB STANDARD DIET. (Travenol) Defined peptide diet, 333 kcal/pkt. Carton 6s.
Use: Enteral nutritional supplement.

TRAVASORB WHOLE PROTEIN LIQUID DIET. (Travenol) Lactose free complete nutrition 250 kcal/Can. Can 8 oz.
Use: Enteral nutritional supplement.

TRAVEL AIDS. (Faraday) Dimenhydrinate 50 mg/Tab. Bot. 30s.
Use: Antiemetic/antivertigo agent.

TRAVEL-EZE. (Approved) Pyrilamine maleate 25 mg, hyoscine hydrobromide 0.325 mg/Tab. Pkg. 20s.
Use: Antiemetic/antivertigo agent.

TRAVEL SICKNESS. (Walgreen) Dimenhydrinate 50 mg/Tab. Bot. 24s.
Use: Antiemetic/antivertigo agent.

TRAVELTABS. (Geneva) Dimenhydrinate 50 mg/Tab. Bot. 100s.
Use: Antiemetic/antivertigo agent.

TRAVERT. (Travenol) Invert sugar injection 10% in water or saline. Plastic Bot. 500 ml, 1000 ml. W/electrolyte No. 2 Bot. 500 ml, 1000 ml, W/electrolyte No. 4 Bot. 250 ml, 500 ml Soln. (10%).
Use: Fluid/electrolyte replacement.

•**TRAZODONE HYDROCHLORIDE.** USAN. 2-[3-[4-(m-Chlorophenyl)-1-piperazinyl]propyl]-1,2,4-triazolo[4,3-a]pyridin-3(2H)-one monohydrochloride.
Use: Antidepressant.
See: Desyrel, Tab. (Mead Johnson).

•**TREBENZOMINE HYDROCHLORIDE.** USAN.
Use: Antidepressant.

TRECATOR S.C. (Wyeth-Ayerst) Ethionamide. 2-Ethyl thioisonicotinamide. 250 mg/Tab. Bot. 100s.
Use: Antituberculous agent.

•**TRELOXINATE.** USAN.
Use: Antihyperlipoproteinemic.

TRENBOLONE. V.B.A.N. 17β-Hydroxyoestra-4,9,11-trien-3-one.
Use: Anabolic steroid, veterinary medicine.

•**TRENBOLONE ACETATE.** USAN.
Use: Anabolic steroid for veterinary use.

TRENDAR. (Whitehall) Ibuprofen 200 mg/Tab. Bot. 20s, 40s.
Use: Nonsteroidal anti-inflammatory drug; analgesic.

TRENTAL TABLETS. (Hoechst) Pentoxifylline 400 mg/CR Tab. Bot. 100s, UD 100s.
Use: Hemorheologic agent.

TREOSULFAN. B.A.N.L-Threitol 1,4-dimethanesul-phonate.

•**TREPIPAM MALEATE.** USAN.
Use: Sedative.

•**TRESTOLONE ACETATE.** USAN.
Use: Antineoplastic, androgen.

TRETAMINE. B.A.N. 2,4,6-Tri(aziridin-1-yl)-1,3,5-triazine. Triethanomelamine; Triethylene Melamine; TEM.
Use: Antineoplastic agent.

TRETHINIUM TOSYLATE. B.A.N. 2-Ethyl-1,2,3,4-tetrahydro-2-methylisoquinolinium toluene-p-sulfonate.
Use: Hypotensive.

TRETHOCANOIC ACID. 3-Hydroxy-3,7,11-trimethyldodecanoic acid.
Use: Anticholesteremic.

•**TRETINOIN,** U.S.P. XXII. Cream, Gel, Topical Soln., U.S.P. XXII. 3,7-Dimethyl-9-(2,6,6-trimet-

hylcyclohex-1-enyl)nona-2,4,6,8-all-transtetrae-noicacid. All trans-Retinoic acid. Vitamin A acid.
Use: Keratolytic.
See: Retin-A, Cream, Gel, Soln. (Ortho).

TREXAN TABLETS. (Du Pont) Naltrexone HCl 50 mg/Tab. Bot. 50s.
Use: Antidote, opioid antagonist.

TREXIN. (A.V.P.) Tetracycline HCl 250 mg/Cap. Bot. 100s.
Use: Antibacterial, tetracycline.

TRIAC. (Vitarine) Triprolidine HCl 2.5 mg, pseudoephedrine HCl 60 mg/Tab. Bot. 100s, 1000s.
Use: Antihistamine, decongestant.

TRIACET CREAM. (Lemmon) Triamcinolone acetonide 0.025%, 0.1% or 0.5%. **0.025%:** Tube 15 Gm, 80 Gm, 1 lb; **0.1%:** Tube 15 Gm, 80 Gm, 480 Gm; **0.5%:** Tube 15 Gm.
Use: Corticosteroid, topical.

•**TRIACETIN,** U.S.P. XXII. Glyceryl triacetate.
Use: Topical antifungal.
See: Enzactin, Preps. (Wyeth-Ayerst).
Fungacetin, Oint. (Blair).

TRIACETYLOLEANDOMYCIN. Troleandomycin.
Use: Antibiotic.

TRIACIN C. (Various Mfr.) Pseudoephedrine HCl 30 mg, triprolidine HCl 1.25 mg, codeine phosphate 10 mg/5 ml, alcohol 4.3%. Syr. Bot. pt, gal.
Use: Decongestant, antihistamine, antitussive.

TRIACT LIQUID. (Winthrop Products) Aluminum, magnesium hydroxide, simethicone.
Use: Antacid, antiflatulent.

TRIACT TABLETS. (Winthrop Products) Aluminum, magnesium hydroxide, simethicone.
Use: Antacid, antiflatulent.

•**TRIAFUNGIN.** USAN.
Use: Antifungal.

•**TRIAMCINOLONE,** U.S.P. XXII. Tab., U.S.P. XXII. 9-Alpha fluoro-16-alpha hydroxy-prednisolone. 9-Fluoro-11β, 16α,17,21-tetrahydroxy-pregna-1,4-diene-3, 20-dione.
Use: Adrenocortical steroid (anti-inflammatory).
See: Aristocort, Tab., Syr. (Lederle).
Aristoderm, Foam (Lederle).
Aristospan, Parenteral (Lederle).
Kenacort, Tab., Syr. (Squibb Mark).
SK-Triamcinolone, Tab. (SmithKline).

•**TRIAMCINOLONE ACETONIDE,** U.S.P. XXII. Topical Aerosol, Cream, Oint., Dental Paste, Lot., Sterile Susp., U.S.P. XXII. 9-α-fluoro-16-α-17-α-isopropylidenedioxy-Δ′ hydrocortisone. Pregna-1,4-diene-3,20-dione,8-fluoro-11,21-dihydroxy-16-17-[(1-methylethylidene)bis(oxy)]-,(11β,16α)-. 9-Fluoro-11β,16α,17,21-tetrahydroxypregna-1,4-diene-3,20-dione cyclic 16,17-acetal with acetone.
Use: Glucocorticoid, topical anti-inflammatory.
See: Aristocort, Cream, Oint. (Lederle).
Aristoderm Foam (Lederle).
Aristogel, Gel (Lederle).
Kenalog Preps. (Squibb Mark).
Triacet, Cream (Lemmon).
Tramacin, Cream (Johnson & Johnson).
Tri-Kort, Inj. (Keene).
W/Neomycin, gramicidin, Nystatin.
See: Mycolog, Preps. (Squibb).

•**TRIAMCINOLONE ACETONIDE SODIUM PHOSPHATE.** USAN.
Use: Glucocorticoid.

•**TRIAMCINOLONE DIACETATE,** U.S.P. XXII. Sterile Susp., Syrup, U.S.P. XXII. 9-Alpha-fluoro-16-alpha-hydroxyprednisolone diacetate. 9-Fluoro-11β, 16α, 17,21-tetrahydroxy-pregna-1,4-diene-3,20-dione-16,21-diacetate.
Use: Glucocorticoid.
See: Amcort, Inj. (Keene).
Aristocort Diacetate Forte (Lederle).
Aristocort Diacetate Intralesional, Inj. (Lederle).
Kenacort, Syr. (Squibb Mark).
Tracilon, Susp. (Savage).
Triam-Forte, Inj. (Hyrex).

•**TRIAMCINOLONE HEXACETONIDE,** U.S.P. XXII. Sterile Susp., U.S.P. XXII. 9-Fluoro-11β,16α,17,21-tetra hyroxypregna-1,-4-diene-3,20-dione cyclic 16, 17-acetal with acetone, 21-(3,3-dimethylbutyrate).
Use: Injectable glucocorticoid.
See: Aristospan, Preps. (Lederle).

TRIAM-FORTE. (Hyrex) Triamcinolone diacetate 40 mg/ml. Vial 5 ml.
Use: Corticosteroid.

TRIAMINIC. (Dorsey) Pyrilamine maleate 25 mg, pheniramine maleate 25 mg, phenylpropanolamine HCl 50 mg/TR Tab. Bot. 100s, 250s.
Use: Antihistamine, decongestant.
W/Dormethan, terpin hydrate.
See: Tussaminic, Tab. (Dorsey).

TRIAMINIC ALLERGY TABLETS. (Dorsey) Phenylpropanolamine HCl 25 mg, chlorpheniramine maleate 4 mg/Tab. Blister pk. 24s.
Use: Decongestant, antihistamine.

TRIAMINIC CHEWABLES. (Sandoz Consumer) Phenylpropanolamine HCl 6.25 mg, chlorpheniramine maleate 0.5 mg/Chew. tab. Blister pkg. 24s.
Use: Decongestant, antihistamine.

TRIAMINIC COLD SYRUP. (Dorsey) Phenylpropanolamine HCl 12.5 mg, chlorpheniramine maleate 2 mg/5 ml, sorbitol. Bot. 4 oz, 8 oz.
Use: Decongestant, antihistamine.

TRIAMINIC COLD TABLETS. (Dorsey) Phenylpropanolamine HCl 12.5 mg, chlorpheniramine maleate 2 mg/Tab. Blister pkg. 24s.
Use: Decongestant, antihistamine.

TRIAMINIC-DM COUGH FORMULA. (Dorsey) Phenylpropanolamine HCl 12.5 mg, dextromethorphan HBr 10 mg/5 ml, sorbitol. Bot. 4 oz, 8 oz.
Use: Decongestant, antitussive.

TRIAMINIC EXPECTORANT. (Dorsey) Phenylpropanolamine HCl 12.5 mg, guaifenesin 100 mg/5 ml, alcohol 5%, saccharin, sorbitol. Bot. 4 oz, 8 oz.

Use: Decongestant, expectorant.
TRIAMINIC EXPECTORANT W/CODEINE. (Dorsey) Phenylpropanolamine HCl 12.5 mg, codeine phosphate 10 mg, guaifenesin 100 mg/5 ml, alcohol 5%, saccharin, sorbitol. Bot, pt.
Use: Decongestant, antitussive, expectorant.
TRIAMINIC EXPECTORANT DH. (Dorsey) Guaifenesin 100 mg, phenylpropanolamine HCl 12.5 mg, pheniramine maleate 6.25 mg, pyrilamine maleate 6.25 mg, hydrocodone bitartrate 1.67 mg/5 ml, alcohol 5%, saccharin, sorbitol. Bot, pt.
Use: Expectorant, decongestant, antihistamine, antitussive.
TRIAMINIC NITE LIGHT LIQUID. (Sandoz) Pseudoephedrine 15 mg, chlorpheniramine maleate 1 mg, dextromethorphan HBr 7.5 mg. Bot. 120 ml, 240 ml.
Use: Decongestant, antihistamine, antitussive.
TRIAMINIC ORAL INFANT DROPS. (Dorsey) Phenylpropanolamine HCl 20 mg, pheniramine maleate 10 mg, pyrilamine maleate 10 mg/ml. Dropper bot. 15 ml.
Use: Decongestant, antihistamine.
TRIAMINIC-12 TABLETS. (Dorsey) Phenylpropanolamine HCl 75 mg, chlorpheniramine maleate 12 mg/SR Tab. Pkg. 10s, 20s.
Use: Decongestant, antihistamine.
TRIAMINIC TR TABLETS. (Dorsey) Phenylpropanolamine HCl 50 mg, pheniramine maleate 25 mg, pyrilamine maleate 25 mg/TR Tab. Bot. 100s, 250s.
Use: Decongestant, antihistamine.
TRIAMINICIN TABLETS. (Sandoz Consumer) Phenylpropanolamine HCl 25 mg, acetaminophen 650 mg, chlorpheniramine maleate 4 mg/Tab. Pkg. 12s, 24s, 48s, 100s. Industrial pkg. 200 × 1s.
Use: Decongestant, analgesic, antihistamine.
TRIAMINICOL MULTI SYMPTOM COLD SYRUP. (Dorsey) Phenylpropanolamine HCl 12.5 mg, chlorpheniramine maleate 2 mg, dextromethorphan HBr 10 mg/5 ml, saccharin, sorbitol. Bot. 4 oz, 8 oz.
Use: Decongestant, antihistamine, antitussive.
TRIAMINICOL MULTI-SYMPTOM COLD TABLET. (Sandoz Consumer) Phenylpropanolamine HCl 12.5 mg, chlorpheniramine maleate 2 mg, dextromethorphan HBr 10 mg/Tab. Blister pkg. 24s.
Use: Decongestant, antihistamine, antitussive.
TRIAMINILONE-16,17-ACETONIDE.
See: Triamcinolone acetonide.
TRIAMOLONE 40. (Forest) Triamcinolone diacetate 40 mg/ml. Vial 5 ml.
Use: Corticosteroid.
TRIAMONIDE 40. (Forest) Triamcinolone acetonide 40 mg/ml. Vial 5 ml.
Use: Corticosteroid.
•**TRIAMPYZINE SULFATE.** USAN. 2-(Di-methylamino)-3,5,6-trimethylpyrazine sulfate.
Use: Anticholinergic.
•**TRIAMTERENE,** U.S.P. XXII. Caps., U.S.P. XXII. 2,4,7-Triamino-6-phenyl-pteridine. 2,4,7-Pteridinetriamine,6-phenyl-Dytac.
Use: Diuretic.
See: Dyrenium, Cap. (SmithKline).
•**TRIAMTERENE AND HYDROCHLOROTHIAZIDE CAPSULES,** U.S.P. XXII.
Use: Diuretic.
See: Dyazide, Cap. (SmithKline).
TRIANIDE. (Seatrace) Triamcinolone acetonide 40 mg/ml. Vial 5 ml.
Use: Corticosteroid.
TRIAPRIN. (Dunhall) Acetaminophen 325 mg, butalbital 50 mg/Cap. Bot. 100s, 500s.
Use: Analgesic, sedative/hypnotic.
TRI-AQUA. (Pfeiffer) Caffeine 100 mg, extracts of buchu, uva ursi, zea, triticum/Tab. Bot. 50s, 100s.
Use: Diuretic.
TRIASYN B. (Lannett) Vitamins B_1 2 mg, B_2 3 mg, B_3 20 mg/Cap or Tab. **Cap.:** Bot. 100s, 500s. **Tab.:** Bot. 1000s.
Use: Vitamin supplement.
TRIATROPHENE. (Lannett) Magnesium trisilicate 7.5 gr, phenobarbital ⅛ gr, atropine sulfate 1/1000 gr/Tab. Bot. 1000s.
Use: Antacid, sedative/hypnotic, anticholinergic/antispasmodic.
TRIAVIL. (Merck Sharp & Dohme) Perphenazine 2 mg, amitriptyline HCl 10 mg/blue Tab.; perphenazine 4 mg, amitriptyline HCl 10 mg/salmon-colored Tab.; perphenazine 2 mg, amitriptyline HCl 25 mg/orange Tab.; perphenazine 4 mg, amitriptyline 25 mg/yellow Tab. Bot. 100s, 500s, UD 100s. Perphenazine 4 mg, amitryptyline 50 mg/orange Tab. Bot. 60s, 100s, UD 100s.
Use: Psychotherapeutic agent.
TRI-A-VITE F. (Major) Fluoride 0.5 mg, vitamins A 1500 IU, D 400 IU, C 35 mg/ml. Drops. Bot. 50 ml.
Use: Vitamin supplement, dental caries preventative.
TRIAZIQUONE. B.A.N. Tri(aziridin-1-yl)-1,4-benzoquinone. Trenimon.
Use: Antineoplastic agent.
•**TRIAZOLAM,** U.S.P. XXII. Tab., U.S.P. XXII.
Use: Sedative, hypnotic.
See: Halcion, Tab. (Upjohn).
TRI-BARBS. (Lannett) Phenobarbital 32 mg, butabarbital sodium 32 mg, secobarbital sodium 32 mg/Cap. Bot. 1000s.
Use: Sedative/hypnotic.
•**TRIBENOSIDE.** USAN. Ethyl 3,5,6-tri-O-benzyl-D-glucofuranoside. Glyvenol. Not available in U.S.
Use: Venoprotective agent.
TRI-BIOCIN. (Approved) Bacitracin 400 units, polymyxin B sulfate 5000 units, neomycin 5 mg/Gm. Tube 0.5 oz.
Use: Anti-infective, external.

TRI-BIOTIC OINTMENT. (Standex) Polymyxin B sulfate 5000 units, bacitracin 400 units, neomycin sulfate 5 mg/Gm. Tube 0.5 oz.
Use: Anti-infective, external.

TRIBROMOETHANOL. 2,2,2-Tribromoethanol.
Use: Anesthetic (inhalation).

TRIBROMOMETHANE. Bromoform.

•**TRIBROMSALAN.** USAN. 3,4′,5-Tribromosalicylanilide. Hilomid.
Use: Germicide, disinfectant.
See: Diaphene (or ASC-4) (Stecker).
Tuasol 100 (Merrell Dow).

•**TRICETAMIDE.** USAN. 3,4,5-Trimethoxybenzoylglycine diethylamide.
Use: Sedative.

TRI-CHLOR. (Gordon) Trichloracetic acid 80%. Bot. 15 ml.
Use: Cauterizing agent.

TRICHLORAN.
See: Trichloroethylene.

•**TRICHLORMETHIAZIDE,** U.S.P. XXII. Tab., U.S.P. XXII. 3-Dichloromethyl-6-chloro-7-sulfamyl-3,4-dihydro-1,2,4-benzothiadiazine-1,1-dioxide. 6-Chloro-3-(dichloromethyl)-3,4-dihydro-2H-1,2,4-benzothiadiazine-7-sulfonamide-1,1-Dioxide.
Use: Diuretic; antihypertensive.
See: Aquex, Tab. (Lannett).
Metahydrin, Tab. (Merrell Dow).
Naqua, Tab. (Schering).
Rochlomethiazide, Tab. (Robinson).
W/Reserpine.
See: Metatensin, Tab. (Merrell Dow).
Naquival, Tab. (Schering).

TRICHLORMETHINE (I.N.N.).
See: Trimustine, B.A.N.

TRICHLOROACETIC ACID, U.S.P. XXI. Acetic acid, trichloro.
Use: Topical, as a caustic.

TRICHLOROBUTYL ALCOHOL.
See: Chlorobutanol.

TRICHLOROCARBANILIDE. W/Salicylic acid, sulfur.

•**TRICHLOROMONOFLUOROMETHANE,** N.F. XVII.
Use: Aerosol propellant.

TRICHOLINE CITRATE.
See: Choline citrate.

TRICHOTINE. (Reed & Carnrick) **Pow.**: Sodium lauryl sulfate, sodium perborate, chloride, aromatics. Pkg. 5 oz, 20 oz. **Liq.**: Sodium lauryl sulfate, sodium borate, ethyl alcohol 8%, aromatics. Bot. 4 oz, 8 oz.
Use: Vaginal preparation.

•**TRICIRIBINE PHOSPHATE.** USAN.
Use: Antineoplastic.

•**TRICITRATES ORAL SOLUTION,** U.S.P. XXII.

TRICLOBISONIUM. Triburon, Oint. (Roche).

TRICLOBISONIUM CHLORIDE. Hexamethylenebis[dimethyl[1-methyl-3-(2,2,6-tri-methylcyclohexyl)propyl]-ammonium] Dichloride.
Use: Anti-infective, external.

•**TRICLOCARBAN.** USAN. 3,4,4′-Trichloro- carbanilide.
Use: Germicide, disinfectant.
See: Artra Beauty Ban (Schering-Plough).
W/Clofulcarban.
See: Safeguard Bar Soap (P & G).

•**TRICLOFENOL PIPERAZINE.** USAN. Piperazine (1:2) with (2,4,5-trichlorophenol).
Use: Anthelmintic (nematodes).

TRICLOFOS. B.A.N. 2,2,2-Trichloroethyl dihydrogen phosphate. Tricloryl (mono-sodium salt).
Use: Hypnotic.

•**TRICLONIDE.** USAN.
Use: Anti-inflammatory.

•**TRICLOSAN.** USAN. 5-Chloro-2-(2,4-dichlorophenoxy)phenol.
Use: Antibacterial.
See: Clearasil Soap (Vicks).

TRICODENE LIQUID. (Pfeiffer) Chlorpheniramine maleate 0.5 mg, dextromethorphan HBr 10 mg, ammonium Cl 90 mg, sodium citrate, sorbitol, mannitol/5 ml. Liq. Bot. 120 ml.
Use: Antihistamine, antitussive, expectorant.

TRICODENE SYRUP. (Pfeiffer) Pyrilamine maleate 4.17 mg, codeine phosphate 8.1 mg, terpin hydrate, menthol/5 ml. Syr. Bot. 120 ml.
Use: Antihistamine, antitussive, expectorant.

TRICODENE FORTE. (Pfeiffer) Phenylpropanolamine HCl 12.5 mg, chlorpheniramine maleate 2 mg, dextromethorphan HBr 10 mg/5 ml. Liq. Bot. 120 ml.
Use: Decongestant, antihistamine, antitussive.

TRICODENE NN. (Pfeiffer) Phenylpropanolamine HCl 5 mg, chlorpheniramine maleate 0.5 mg, dextromethorphan HBr 10 mg, ammonium Cl 90 mg, sodium citrate/5 ml. Syr. Bot. 120 ml.
Use: Decongestant, antihistamine, antitussive, expectorant.

TRICODENE PEDIATRIC. (Pfeiffer) Phenylpropanolamine HCl 12.5 mg, dextromethorphan HBr 10 mg/5 ml. Liq. 120 ml.
Use: Decongestant, antitussive.

TRICOMINE. (Major) Pseudoephedrine HCl 60 mg, carbinoxamine maleate 4 mg, dextromethorphan HBr 15 mg/5 ml, alcohol 5%. Bot. 120 ml.
Use: Decongestant, antihistamine, antitussive.

TRICONSIL. (Geneva Generics) Aluminum hydroxide 80 mg, magnesium trisilicate 80 mg, sodium bicarbonate 200 mg/Tab, sodium 50.6 mg. Bot. 100s.
Use: Antacid.

TRICYCLAMOL CHLORIDE. B.A.N. 1-(3-Cyclohexyl-3-hydroxy-3-phenylpropyl)-1-methylpyrroidinium Cl. Elorine Chloride; Lergine.
Use: Anticholinergic.

TRICYLATATE HCl. 1-Methyl-3-pyrrolidylmethyl benzilate HCl.

TRIDERM CREAM. (Del-Ray) Triamcinolone acetonide 0.1%. Tube 1 oz, 3 oz.
Use: Corticosteroid, topical.

TRIDESILON CREAM. (Miles Pharm) Desonide 0.05% in vehicle buffered to the pH range of normal skin, glycerin, methylparaben, sodium lauryl sulfate, aluminum sulfate, calcium acetate, cetyl stearyl alcohol, synthetic beeswax, white petrolatum, mineral oil. Tube 15 Gm, 60 Gm.
Use: Corticosteroid, topical.

TRIDESILON OTIC. (Miles Pharm) Desonide 0.05%, acetic acid 2% in vehicle. Bot. 10 ml.
Use: Otic preparation.

TRIDEX TAB., TIMED TRIDEX CAP., TIMED TRIDEX JR. CAP. (Fellows) Changed to Daro Tab., Daro Timed Cap., Daro Jr. Timed Cap.

•**TRIDIHEXETHYL CHLORIDE,** U.S.P. XXII. Inj., Tab., U.S.P. XXII. (3-Cyclohexyl-3-hydroxy-3-phenylpropyl)-tri-ethylammonium Cl.
Use: Anticholinergic.
W/Meprobamate.
See: Milpath, Tab. (Wallace).
Pathibamate, Tab. (Lederle).
W/Phenobarbital.
See: Pathilon w/Phenobarbital Tab., Cap. (Lederle).

TRIDIL 0.5 mg/ml (American Critical Care) Nitroglycerin 0.5 mg/ml, alcohol 10%, water for injection, buffered with sodium phosphate. Amp. 10 ml. Box 20s.
Use: Antianginal.

TRIDIL 5 mg/ml (American Critical Care) Nitroglycerin 5 mg/ml, alcohol 30%, propylene glycol 30%, water for injection. Amp. 5 ml, 10 ml. Vial 5 ml, 10 ml. Box 20s. Special administration set w/10 ml Amp.
Use: Antianginal.

TRIDIONE. (Abbott) Trimethadione (Troxidone) **300 mg/Cap.:** Bot. 100s. **150 mg/Dulcet Tab.:** Bot. 100s. **Soln.:** 1.2 Gm/fl oz. Bot, pt.
Use: Anticonvulsant.

TRIDRATE BOWEL EVACUANT KIT. (Mallinckrodt) Magnesium citrate soln. 300 ml, bisacodyl 5 mg/Tab. (3s), bisacodyl 10 mg/Supp. (1). Kit.
Use: Laxative.

•**TRIENTINE HYDROCHLORIDE.** USAN.
Use: Wilson's disease therapy adjunct.
See: Cuprid, Cap, (Merck Sharp & Dohme).

TRIENZYME. (Fellows) Amylolytic 30 mg, proteolytic 10 mg, celluloytic 3 mg/Tab. Bot. 1000s.
Use: Digestive aid.

TRI-ESTROGEN. (Rocky Mtn.) Potassium estrone sulfate 1 mg, estrone 2 mg, estradiol 0.2 mg/10 ml. Vial 10 ml.
Use: Estrogen.

TRIETHANOLAMINE,
See: Trolamine, N.F. XVII.

TRIETHANOLAMINE POLYPEPTIDE OLEATE CONDENSATE.
See: Cerumenex, Drops (Purdue Frederick).

TRIETHANOLAMINE SALICYLATE.
See: Aspercreme, Cream (Thompson).
Aspergel, Oint. (LaCrosse).
Myoflex, Cream (Warren-Teed).

TRIETHANOLAMINE TRINITRATE BIPHOSPHATE. Trolnitrate Phosphate.

•**TRIETHYL CITRATE,** N.F. XVII.

TRIETHYLENEMELAMINE. Tretamine TEM. 2,4,6-Tris(1-aziridinyl)-5-triazine.
Use: Antineoplastic agent.

TRIFED. (Geneva Generics) Pseudoephedrine HCl 60 mg, triprolidine HCl 2.5 mg/Tab. Bot. 100s, 1000s.
Use: Decongestant, antihistamine.

TRIFED-C. (Geneva Generics) Pseudoephedrine HCl 30 mg, triprolidine HCl 1.25 mg, codeine phosphate 10 mg/5 ml, alcohol 4.3%. Syr. Bot. pt, gal.
Use: Decongestant, antihistamine, antitussive.

•**TRIFENAGREL.** USAN.
Use: Antithrombotic.

•**TRIFLOCIN.** USAN. 4-(α,α,α-Trifluoro-m-toluidino) nicotinic acid.
Use: Diuretic.

•**TRIFLUBAZAM.** USAN.
Use: Tranquilizer.

•**TRIFLUMIDATE.** USAN. Ethyl m-benzoyl-N-[(trifluoromethyl)sulfonyl]carbanilate.
Use: Anti-inflammatory.

TRIFLUOMEPRAZINE. V.B.A.N. NN-Dimethyl-2-(2-trifluoromethylphenothiazin-10ylmethyl) propylamine. Nortran.
Use: Tranquilizer, veterinary medicine.

TRIFLUOPERAZINE. B.A.N. 10-[3-(4-Methyl-piperazin-1-yl)propyl]-2-trifluoromethylphenothiazine.
Use: Tranquilizer, antiemetic.

•**TRIFLUOPERAZINE HCl,** U.S.P. XXII. Inj., Syr., Tab., U.S.P. XXII. 10-[3-(1-Methyl-4-piperazinyl)- propyl]-2-trifluoromethyl phenothiazine HCl. 10-(3-(4-Methyl-1-piperazinyl)propyl)-2-(trifluoromethyl)phenothiazine dihydrochloride.
Use: Tranquilizer, sedative, antipsychotic.
See: Stelazine Inj., Liq., Tab. (SmithKline).

•**TRIFLUPERIDOL.** USAN.
Use: Antipsychotic.

•**TRIFLUPROMAZINE,** U.S.P. XXII. Oral Susp., XXII.
Use: Tranquilizer, antipsychotic agent.

•**TRIFLUPROMAZINE HCl,** U.S.P. XXII. Inj., Tab., U.S.P. XXII. 10-[3-Di-methylamino)propyl]-2-(trifluoromethyl)phenothiazine HCl. Fluopromazine, B.A.N.
Use: Tranquilizer, antipsychotic agent.
See: Vesprin Prods. (Princeton).

•**TRIFLURIDINE.** USAN.
Use: Antiviral used to treat herpes simplex eye infections.
See: Viroptic Ophthalmic Soln., (Burroughs Wellcome).

TRIGELAMINE. (EJ Moore) Pyrilamine maleate, pheniramine maleate, chloropheniramine maleate, benzalkonium Cl, menthol. Tube. 1.25 oz.
Use: Antihistamine, topical.

TRIGESIC. (Squibb Mark) Acetyl-p-aminophenol 125 mg, aspirin 230 mg, caffeine 30 mg/Tab. Bot. 100s.
Use: Salicylate analgesic combination.

TRIGLYCERIDE REAGENT STRIP. (Ames) Seralyzer reagent strip. A quantitative strip test for triglycerides in serum or plasma. Bot. 25s.
Use: Diagnostic aid.

TRI-GRAIN. (Pharmex) Isometheptene tartrate. **Inj.**: 100 mg/ml. Vial 10 ml. **Tab.**: Bot. 24s, 100s.
Use: Antispasmodic, vasoconstrictor.

TRIHEMIC-600. (Lederle) Vitamins C 600 mg, B_{12} 25 mcg, intrinsic factor concentrate 75 mg, folic acid 1 mg, E 30 IU, ferrous fumarate 115 mg, dioctyl sodium succinate 50 mg/Tab. Bot. 30s, 500s.
Use: Vitamin/mineral supplement.

TRIHEXANE. (Rugby) Trihexyphenidyl 2 mg/Tab. Bot. 100s, 1000s.
Use: Antiparkinson agent.

TRIHEXIDYL. (Schein) Trihexyphenidyl 2 mg/Tab. Bot. 100s, 1000s.
Use: Antiparkinson agent.

TRIHEXY-2. (Geneva Generics) Trihexyphenidyl 2 mg/Tab. Bot. 100s, 1000s.
Use: Antiparkinson agent.

TRIHEXY-5. (Geneva Generics) Trihexyphenidyl 5 mg/Tab. Bot. 100s, 1000s.
Use: Antiparkinson agent.

•**TRIHEXYPHENIDYL HYDROCHLORIDE,** U.S.P. XXII. Elix., Extended-release Cap., Tab. U.S.P. XXII. α-Cyclohexyl-α-phenyl-1-piperidinepropanol HCl. 1-Piperidine-propanol, α-cyclohexyl-α-phenyl-, HCl. Benzhexol, B.A.N.
Use: Anticholinergic, antiparkinsonian.
See: Artane, Elix., Tab. (Lederle).
Hexyphen-2, Tab. (Robinson).
Hexyphen-5, Tab. (Robinson).

TRI-HISTIN. (Recsei) **25 mg/Tab.:** Pyrilamine maleate 10 mg, chlorpheniramine maleate 1 mg. Bot 100s, 500s, 1000s. **50 mg/Tab.:** Pyrilamine maleate 20 mg, methapyrilene HCl 15 mg, chlorpheniramine maleate 2 mg. Bot. 1000s. **100 mg SA Cap.:** Pyrilamine maleate 40 mg, pheniramine maleate 25 mg. Bot. 100s, 500s, 1000s. **Expectorant:** Pyrilamine maleate 5 mg, chlorpheniramine maleate 0.5 mg, guaifenesin 20 mg, phenylpropanolamine 7.5 mg, phenylephrine HCl 2.5 mg, sodium citrate 100 mg/5 ml. Bot. pt. gal. **Liq.:** Pyrilamine maleate 5 mg, chlorpheniramine maleate 0.5 mg/5 ml. Bot. pt. gal.
Use: Antihistamine, expectorant, decongestant.

W/Benzyl alcohol, chlorobutanol, isopropyl alcohol.
See: Derma-Pax, Liq. (Recsei).

W/Codeine phosphate, guaifenesin, phenylpropanolamine, phenylephrine HCl, sodium citrate.
See: Trihista-Codeine, Liq. (Recsei).

W/Ephedrine HCl, aminophylline, mephobarbital.
See: Asmasan, Tab. (Recsei).

TRIHYDROXYESTRINE. Trihydroxyestrin.

TRIHYDROXYETHYLAMINE. Triethanolamine.

TRI-IMMUNOL. (Lederle) Diphtheria and tetanus toxoids and pertussis vaccine combined, aluminum phosphate-adsorbed purogenated. Vial 7.5 ml.
Use: Agent for immunization.

TRIIODOMETHANE.
See: Iodoform. (Various Mfr.).

L-TRIIODOTHYRONINE SOD.
See: Cytomel, Tab. (SmithKline).
Liothyronine Sodium

dl-TRIIODOTHYRONINE SODIUM.

TRI-K. (Century) Potassium acetate 0.5 Gm, potassium bicarbonate 0.5 Gm, potassium citrate 0.5 Gm/fl oz. Saccharin. Bot. pt, gal.
Use: Potassium supplement.

•**TRIKATES ORAL SOLUTION,** U.S.P. XXII.
Use: Potassium deficiency.

TRIKATES ORAL SOLUTION. (Lilly) Potassium 15 mEq from potassium acetate, potassium bicarbonate, potassium citrate/5 ml, saccharin. Bot. 16 fl oz, gal.
Use: Potassium supplement.

TRI-KORT. (Keene) Triamcinalone acetonide suspension 40 mg/ml. Vial 5 ml.
Use: Corticosteroid.

TRILAFON. (Schering) Perphenazine. **Tab.**: 2 mg, 4 mg, 8 mg or 16 mg. Bot. 100s, 500s. **Inj.**: 5 mg/ml w/disodium citrate 24.6 mg, sodium bisulfite 2 mg, water for injection/ml. Amp. 1 ml. **Concentrate:** 16 mg/5 ml. Bot. 4 oz w/dropper.
Use: Antipsychotic, antiemetic/antivertigo agent.

TRILAX. (Drug Industries) Docusate sodium 200 mg, yellow phenolphthalein 30 mg, dehydrocholic acid 20 mg/Cap. Bot. 100s, 500s.
Use: Laxative, choleretic.

TRI-LEVLEN 21 TABLETS. (Berlex) **Group 1:** Levonorgestrel 0.05 mg, ethinyl estradiol 0.03 mg/Tab. **Group 2:** Levonorgestrel 0.075 mg, ethinyl estradiol 0.04 mg/Tab. **Group 3:** Levonorgestrel 0.125 mg, ethinyl estradiol 0.03 mg/Tab. Slidecase 21s. Box 3s.
Use: Oral contraceptive.

TRI-LEVLEN 28 TABLETS. (Berlex). **Group 1:** Levonorgestrel 0.05 mg, ethinyl estradiol 0.03 mg/Tab. **Group 2:** Levonorgestrel 0.075 mg, ethinyl estradiol 0.04 mg/Tab. **Group 3:** Levonorgestrel 0.125 mg, ethinyl estradiol 0.03 mg/Tab. **Group 4:** Inert tablets. Slidecase 28s. Box 3s.
Use: Oral contraceptive.

TRILISATE LIQUID. (Purdue Frederick) Choline magnesium trisalicylate from choline salicylate 293 mg, magnesium salicylate 362 mg/tsp. to provide 500 mg salicylate/tsp. Bot. 8 oz.
Use: Salicylate analgesic combination.

TRILISATE TABLETS. (Purdue Frederick) Choline magnesium trisalicylate. **500 mg/Tab.:** of salicylate from choline salicylate 293 mg, magnesium salicylate 362 mg. Bot. 100s. **750 mg/**

Tab.: of salicylate from choline salicylate 400 mg and magnesium salicylate 544 mg. Bot. 100s. **1000 mg/Tab.:** of salicylate from choline salicylate 587 mg, magnesium salicylate 725 mg. Bot. 60s.
Use: Salicylate analgesic combination.

TRILOG. (Hauck) Triamcinolone acetonide 40 mg/ml. Vial 5 ml.
Use: Corticosteroid.

TRILONE. (Century) Triamcinalone diacetate susp. Amp. 10 ml.
Use: Corticosteroid.

TRILONE. (Hauck) Triamcinolone diacetate 40 mg/ml. Vial 5 ml.
Use: Corticosteroid.

•**TRILOSTANE.** USAN.
Use: Adrenocortical suppressant.
See: Modrastane, Cap. (Winthdrop-Breon).

TRIMAHIST ELIXIR. (Tennessee Pharm.) Phenylephrine HCl 5 mg, prophenpyridamine maleate 12.5 mg, l-menthol 1 mg, alcohol 5%/5 ml. Bot. pt, gal.
Use: Antihistamine.

TRIMAX GEL. (Winthrop Products) Aluminum, magnesium hydroxide, simethicone.
Use: Antacid, antiflatulent.

TRIMAX TABLET. (Winthrop Products) Aluminum, magnesium hydroxide, simethicone.
Use: Antacid, antiflatulent.

TRIMAZIDE. (Major) Trimethobenazamide. **Cap.:** 250 mg. Bot. 100s. **Supp.:** 100 mg or 200 mg. 10s.
Use: Antiemetic/antivertigo agent.

TRIMAZINOL. α-{[(4,6-Diaminos-triazin-2-yl)-aminol]-methyl} benzyl alcohol.
Use: Anti-inflammatory agent.

•**TRIMAZOSIN HYDROCHLORIDE.** USAN.
Use: Antihypertensive.

TRIMCAPS. (Mayrand) Phendimetrazine tartrate 105 mg/SR Cap. Bot. 30s, 100s.
Use: Anorexiant.

TRIMEDINE. (Trimen) Phenylephrine HCl 5 mg, chlorpheniramine maleate 1 mg, dextromethorphan HBr 15 mg/5 ml, sorbitol. Liq. Bot. pt, gal.
Use: Decongestant, antihistamine, antitussive.

TRIMEPERIDINE. B.A.N. 1,2,5-Trimethyl-4-phenyl-4-piperidyl propionate.
Use: Narcotic analgesic.

TRIMEPRAZINE. B.A.N. 10-(3-Dimethylamino-2-methylpropyl)phenothiazine. Alimemazine (I.N.N.) Vallergan.
Use: Tranquilizer; antihistamine.

TRIMEPRAZINE TARTRATE, U.S.P. XXII. Syr., Tab., U.S.P. XXII. (±)-10-(3-Dimethylamino-2-methylpro-pyl)-phenothiazine tartrate (2:1) 10H-Phenothiazine-10-propanamine N,N,β-trimethyl-2,3-dihydrox- ybutanedioate (2:1).
Use: Antipruritic.
See: Temaril, Prods. (Herbert).

TRIMETAMIDE. Trimethamide.

TRIMETAPHAN CAMSYLATE. B.A.N. 1,3-Dibenzyldecahydro-2-oxoimidazo[4,5-c]thieno[1,2-a]-thiolium(+)-camphor-10-sulfonate.
Use: Hypotensive.

TRIMETAZIDINE. B.A.N. 1-(2,3,4-Trimethoxybenzyl)piperazine.
Use: Vasodilator.

•**TRIMETHADIONE,** U.S.P. XXII. Cap., Oral Soln., Tab., U.S.P. XXII. 3,5,5-Trimethyl-2,4-oxazolidinedione.
Use: Anticonvulsant.
See: Tridione, Preps. (Abbott).

TRIMETHADIONE (I.N.N.). Troxidone, B.A.N.

TRIMETHAMIDE. N-[(2-Amino-6-methyl-3-pyridyl)methyl]3,4,5-trimethoxybenzamide.
Use: Antihypertensive.

TRIMETHAPHAN CAMPHOR SULFONATE. Trimethaphan Camsylate, U.S.P. XXII.

•**TRIMETHAPHAN CAMSYLATE,** U.S.P. XXII. Inj., U.S.P. XXII. d-3,4-(1′,3′-Dibenzyl-2′-ketoimidazolido)-1,2-trimethylenethiophanium d-camphorsulfonate. Trimethaphan camphorsulfonate. (+)-1,3-Dibenzyldecahydro-2-oxoimidazo[4,5-c]thieno-[1,2-α]-thiolium 2-oxo-10-bornanesulfonate.
Use: Antihypertensive.
See: Arfonad, Amp. (Roche).

TRIMETHIDINIUM METHOSULFATE. B.A.N. d-(N-methyl-N-(gamma-trimethyl-ammonium-propyl))-1-methyl-8,8-di-methyl-3-azabicyclo-(3,2,1) octane dimethosulfate. 1,3,8,8-Tetramethyl-3-(3-(trimethylammonio)propyl)-3-azoniabicyclo(3.2.1)octane. Tab.
Use: Antihypertensive.

•**TRIMETHOBENZAMIDE HCl,** U.S.P. XXII. Cap., Inj., U.S.P. XXII. N- {p-[2-(Dimethylamino) ethoxy]-benzyl} -3,4,5-trimethoxybenzamide HCl.
Use: Antiemetic.
See: Tegamide, Supp. (G & W).
Tigan, Preps. (Beecham Labs.).

TRIMETHOBENZAMIDE HYDROCHLORIDE AND BENZOCAINE SUPPOSITORIES.
Use: Antiemetic/antivertigo agent.

•**TRIMETHOPRIM,** U.S.P. XXII. Tab., U.S.P. XXII. 2,4-Diamino-5-(3,4,5-trimethoxybenzyl)pyrimidine. Syraprim.
Use: Antibacterial agent.
See: Proloprim, Tab. (Burroughs Wellcome).
Trimpex, Tab. (Roche).
W/Sulfamethoxazole.
See: Bactrim, Oral Susp., Pediatric Susp., Tab. (Roche).
Septra, Tab. (Burroughs Wellcome).
Septra DS, Tab. (Burroughs Wellcome).

•**TRIMETHOPRIM SULFATE.** USAN.
Use: Antibacterial.

TRIMETHYLENE. Cyclopropane, U.S.P. XXII.

•**TRIMETOZINE.** USAN.
Use: Sedative.

•**TRIMETREXATE.** USAN.
Use: Antineoplastic.

TRIMETTE. (Wesley) Phenobarbital 0.25 gr, atropine sulfate 2/300 gr, dextroamphetamine sul-

fate 15 mg, aloin 0.25 gr/Cap. or Tab. Bot. 1000s.
Use: Sedative/hypnotic, anticholinergic/antispasmodic, CNS stimulant.

TRIMEX. (Mills) Dextroamphetamine sulfate 15 mg, amobarbital 60 mg, thyroid 3 gr/Cap. Bot. 50s. **No. 2:** Dextroamphetamine sulfate 10 mg, amobarbital 60 mg, thyroid 2 gr/Cap. Bot. 50s.
Use: CNS stimulant, sedative/hypnotic, thyroid hormone.

TRIMINOL. (Rugby) Phenylpropanolamine HCl 12.5 mg, chlorpheniramine maleate 2 mg, dextromethorphan HBr 10 mg/5 ml. Syr. Bot. 120 ml.
Use: Decongestant, antihistamine, antitussive.

•**TRIMIPRAMINE.** USAN. 5-[3-(Dimethylamino)-2-methylpropyl]-10,11-dihydro-5H-dibenz[b,f]-azepine.
Use: Antidepressant.

•**TRIMIPRAMINE MALEATE.** USAN. 5-[3-(Dimethylamino)-2-methylpropyl]-10,11-dihydro-5H-dibenz [b,f]azepine maleate (1:1).
Use: Antidepressant.
See: Surmontil (Wyeth-Ayerst).

TRIMIXIN. (Hance) Bacitracin 200 units, polymyxin B sulfate 4000 units, neomycin sulfate 3 mg/Gm. Oint. Tube 0.5 oz.
Use: Anti-infective, external.

•**TRIMOPROSTIL.** USAN.
Use: Gastric antisecretory.

TRIMO-SAN. (Milex) Oxyquinoline sulfate, sodium lauryl sulfate 0.0084%, boric acid 1%, borax 0.7%. Tube 4 oz w/boilable nylon jel Jector; Refill tube 4 oz.
Use: Vaginal preparation.

TRIMOX. (Squibb Mark) Amoxicillin trihydrate. **Cap.:** 250 mg. Bot. 100s, 500s; 500 mg. Bot. 50s, 500s, UD 100s. **Oral Susp.:** 125 mg/5 ml. Bot. 80 ml, 100 ml, 150 ml, Unimatic Bot. 5 ml, Ctn. 4 × 25s; 250 mg/5 ml. Bot. 80 ml, 100 ml, 150 ml, Unimatic Bot. 5 ml, Ctn. 4 × 25s.
Use: Antibacterial, penicillin.

•**TRIMOXAMINE HYDROCHLORIDE.** USAN. α-Allyl-3,4,5-trimethoxy-N-methylphenethylamine HCl.
Use: Antihypertensive.

TRIMPEX. (Roche) Trimethoprim 100 mg/Tab. Bot. 100s, Tel-E-Dose 100s.
Use: Urinary anti-infective.

TRIM-QWIK. (O'Connor) Powder based meal food supplement. Can 10 oz.
Use: Meal replacement.

TRIMSTAT. (Laser) Phendimetrazine tartrate 35 mg/Tab. Bot. 100s, 1000s.
Use: Anorexiant.

TRIM SULF D/S. (Metro Med) Sulfamethoxazole 800 mg, trimethoprim 160 mg/Tab. Bot. 100s, 500s.
Use: Urinary anti-infective.

TRIM SULF S/S. (Metro Med) Sulfamethoxazole 400 mg, trimethoprim 80 mg/Tab. Bot. 100s, 500s.
Use: Urinary anti-infective.

TRIMTABS. (Mayrand) Phendimetrazine tartrate 35 mg/Tab. Bot. 100s, 500s.
Use: Anorexiant.

TRIMUSTINE. B.A.N. Tri-(2-chloroethyl)amine. Trichlomethine (I.N.N.) Trillekamin hydrochloride.
Use: Antineoplastic agent.

TRINALIN REPETABS. (Schering) Azatadine maleate 1 mg, pseudoephedrine sulfate 120 mg/Tab. Bot. 100s.
Use: Antihistamine, decongestant.

TRIND. (Mead Johnson Nutrition) Phenylpropanolamine HCl 12.5 mg, chlorpheniramine maleate 2 mg/5 ml, alcohol 5%, sorbitol. Bot. 5 oz.
Use: Decongestant, antihistamine.

TRIND DM. (Mead Johnson Nutrition) Phenylpropanolamine HCl 12.5 mg, dextromethorphan HBr 7.5 mg, chlorpheniramine maleate 2 mg/5 ml, alcohol 5%, sorbitol. Bot. 5 oz.
Use: decongestant, antitussive, antihistamine.

TRI-NEFRIN EXTRA STRENGTH. (Pfeiffer) Phenylpropanolamine HCl 25 mg, chlorpheniramine maleate 4 mg/Tab. Bot. 24s, 50s.
Use: Decongestant, antihistamine.

TRINIAD. (Kasar) Isoniazid 300 mg/Tab. Bot. 30s, 100s, 1000s.
Use: Antituberculous agent.

TRINIAD PLUS 30. (Kasar) Isoniazid 300 mg, pyridoxine HCl 30 mg/Tab. Bot. 30s, 100s, 1000s.
Use: Antituberculous agent.

TRINITRIN TABLETS.
See: Nitroglycerin Tablets, U.S.P. XXII.

TRINITROPHENOL. Picric acid. 2,4,6-Trinitrophenol.
See: Picric Acid (Various Mfr.).

TRI-NORINYL. (Syntex) Norethindrone 1 mg, ethinyl estradiol 0.035 mg/Tab. Norethindrone 0.5 mg, ethinyl estradiol 0.035 mg/Tab. 21 and 28 day. (7 inert tabs) Wallette.
Use: Oral contraceptive.

TRINOTIC. (Forest Pharm.) Secobarbital 65 mg, amobarbital 40 mg, phenobarbital 25 mg/Tab. Bot. 1000s.
Use: Sedative/hypnotic.

TRIO-BAR. (Jenkins) Butabarbital sodium 33⅓%, phenobarbital sodium 33⅓%. Total barbiturates 0.25 gr, ¾ gr or 1.5 gr/Tab. Bot. 1000s.
Use: Sedative/hypnotic.

TRIOBEAD-125. (Abbott Diagnostics) T3 diagnostic kit. T3 uptake radioassay for the measurement of thyroid fuction by indirectly determining the degree of saturation of serum thyroxine binding globulin (TBG). Test unit 50s, 100s, 500s.
Use: Diagnostic aid.

TRIOCIL.
See: Hexetidine.

TRIOFED SYRUP. (Various Mfr.) Pseudoephedrine HCl 30 mg, triprolidine HCl 1.25 mg/5 ml. Syr. Bot. 120 ml, pt, gal.

Use: Antihistamine, decongestant.

•**TRIOLEIN I-125.** USAN.
Use: Radioactive agent.

•**TRIOLEIN I-131.** USAN.
Use: Radioactive agent.

TRI-ORAPIN. (Standex) Estrone 2 mg, estradiol 0.2 mg, potassium estrone 1 mg/10 ml.
Use: Estrogen.

TRIOXANE.
See: Trioxymethylene (Various Mfr.).

•**TRIOXIFEN MESYLATE.** USAN.
Use: Anti-estrogen.

•**TRIOXSALEN,** U.S.P. XXII. Tab., U.S.P. XXII. 6-Hydroxy-β,2,7-trimethyl-5-benzofuranacrylic acid,δ-lactone; 4,5,-8-trimethylpsoralen. 2,5,9-Trimethyl-7H-furo-(3,2-g)(1)benzopyran-7-one. 7H-Furo[3,2-g][1]-benzopyran-7-one, 2,5,9-trimethyl-.
Use: Pigmenting and phototherapeutic agent.
See: Trisoralen, Tab. (Elder).

TRIOXYMETHYLENE. Name is incorrectly used to denote paraformaldehyde in some pharmaceuticals.
See: Paraformaldehyde (Various Mfr.).
W/Sodium oleate, triethanolamine, docusate sodium, stearic acid, aluminum silicate.
See: Cooper Creme (Whittaker).

•**TRIPAMIDE.** USAN.
Use: Antihypertensive, diuretic.

TRI-PAIN. (Ferndale) Acetaminophen 162 mg, aspirin 162 mg, salicylamide 162 mg, caffeine 16.2 mg/Tab. Bot. 100s.
Use: Salicylate analgesic combination.

TRIPARANOL. B.A.N. 2-(p-Chlorophenyl)-1-[p-[2-(diethylamino)ethoxy]phenyl]-1-p-tolylethanol.
Use: Blood lipid lowering agent.

TRIPELENNAMINE. B.A.N. 2-(N-Benzyl-N-2-pyridyl)ethyldimethylamine.
Use: Antihistamine.
See: Pyribenzamine citrate or hydrochloride. (Geigy).

•**TRIPELENNAMINE CITRATE,** U.S.P. XXII. Elix., U.S.P. XXII. 2-(Benzyl[2-dimethylamino-ethyl]-amino) pyridine dihydrogen citrate. 1,2-Ethanediamine, N,N-dimethyl-N′-(phenylmethyl)-N′-2-pyridinyl-,2-hydroxy-1,2,3-propanetricarboxylate (1:1).
Use: Antihistamine.

•**TRIPELENNAMINE HYDROCHLORIDE,** U.S.P. XXII. Tab. U.S.P. XXII.
Use: Antihistamine.
See: Pyribenzamine Hydrochloride, Preps. (Geigy).
Ro-Hist, Tab. (Robinson).

TRIPHASIL-21. (Wyeth-Ayerst) Three drug phases in 21 day cycle: **Phase I:** 6 brown tab. Levonorgestrel 0.05 mg, ethinyl estradiol 0.03 mg/Tab. **Phase II:** 5 white tab. Levonorgestrel 0.075 mg, ethinyl estradiol 0.04 mg/Tab. **Phase III:** 10 yellow tab. Levonorgestrel 0.125 mg, ethinyl estradiol 0.03 mg/Tab.
Use: Oral contraceptive.

TRIPHASIL-28. (Wyeth-Ayerst) Three drug phases and one inert phase in 28 day cycle: **Phase I:** 6 brown tab. Levonorgestrel 0.05 mg, ethinyl estradiol 0.03 mg/Tab. **Phase II:** 5 white tab. Levonorgestrel 0.075/mg, ethinyl estradiol 0.04 mg Tab. **Phase III:** 10 yellow tab. Levonorgestrel 0.125 mg, ethinylestradiol 0.03 mg/Tab. **Phase IV:** 7 inert green tablets.
Use: Oral contraceptive.

TRI-PHEN-CHLOR. (Rugby) Phenylpropanolamine HCl 20 mg, phenylephrine HCl 5 mg, chlorpheniramine maleate 2.5 mg, phenyltoloxamine citrate 7.5 mg/5 ml. Syr. Bot. pt, gal.
Use: Antihistamine, decongestant.

TRIPHENYL. (Rugby) Phenylpropanolamine HCl 12.5 mg, chlorpheniramine maleate 2 mg/5 ml, alcohol free. Syr. Bot. 120 ml, pt.
Use: Decongestant, antihistamine.

TRIPHENYL EXPECTORANT. (Rugby) Phenylpropanolamine HCl 12.5 mg, guaifenesin 100 mg/5 ml, alcohol 5%. Bot. 120 ml, pt, gal.
Use: Decongestant, expectorant.

TRIPHENYLMETHANE DYES.
See: Fuchsin.
Methylrosaniline Chloride.

TRIPHENYL T.D. (Rugby) Phenylpropanolamine HCl 50 mg, pyrilamine maleate 25 mg, pheniramine maleate 25 mg/Tab. Bot. 100s, 1000s.
Use: Decongestant, antihistamine.

TRIPHENYLTETRAZOLIUM CHLORIDE. TTC.
See: Uroscreen (Pfizer).

TRIPHEX CAPSULES. (Tennessee Pharm.) Dextroamphetamine sulfate 15 mg, amobarbital 100 mg/Cap. Bot. 100s.
Use: CNS stimulant, sedative/hypnotic.

TRIPIPERAZINE DICITITRATE, HYDROUS.
See: Piperazine Citrate, U.S.P. XXII.

TRIPLAN-D. (Eastwood) Antibiotic ointment. Tube 0.5 oz, Jar 4 oz.
Use: Anti-infective, external.

TRIPLE ANTIBIOTIC OINTMENT. (Walgreen) Bacitracin 400 units, polymyxin B sulfate 5000 units, neomycin sulfate 5 mg/Gm. Tube 0.5 oz, 1 oz.
Use: Anti-infective, external.

TRIPLE BROMIDES, EFFERVESCENT TABLETS.
W/Phenobarbital.
See: Palagren, Liq. (Westerfield).

TRIPLE DYE. (Kerr) Gentian violet, proflavine, hemisulfate, brilliant green in water. Dispensing Bot. 15 ml. Single Use Dispos-A-Swab 0.65 ml. Box 10s. Case 10×50 Box.
Use: Umbilical area antiseptic.

TRIPLE DYE. (Xttrium) Brilliant green 2.29 mg, proflavine hemisulfate 1.14 mg, gentian violet 2.29 mg/ml. Bot. 30 ml.
Use: Umbilical area antiseptic.

TRIPLE-GEN SUSPENSION. (Goldline) Hydrocortisone 1%, neomycin sulfate 0.35%, polymyxin B sulfate 10,000 units/ml, benzalkonium Cl, cetyl alcohol, glyceryl monostearate, po-

lyoxyl 40 stearate, propylene glycol, mineral oil. Bot. 7.5 ml.
Use: Ophthalmic corticosteroid, anti-infective.

TRIPLEN. (Interstate) Tripelennamine HCl 50 mg/Tab. Bot. 100s, 1000s.
Use: Antihistamine.

TRIPLE PASTE. (Torch) Burow's soln. 1 part, absorption base 2 parts, Lassar's zinc oxide paste 3 parts. Jar 2 oz, lb.
Use: Antieczematic, diaper rash product.

TRIPLE SULFA No. 2. (Standex; Kenyon) Sulfadiazine 167 mg, sulfamethazine 167 mg, sulfamerazine 167 mg/Tab. Bot. 100s. (Kenyon) Bot. 100s, 1000s.
Use: Antibacterial, sulfonamide.

TRIPLE SULFA SUSPENSION. (Standex) Sulfamethazine 2.5 gr, sulfadiazine 2.5 gr, sulfamerazine 2.5 gr, sodium citrate 0.75 gr/5 ml. Bot. pt.
Use: Antibacterial, sulfonamide.

TRIPLE SULFA TABLETS. (Century; Stanlabs) Sulfadiazine 2.5 gr, sulfamerazine 2.5 gr, sulfamethazine 2.5 gr/Tab. Bot. 100s, 1000s.
Use: Antibacterial, sulfonamide.

•**TRIPLE SULFA VAGINAL CREAM,** U.S.P. XXII.
Use: Antibacterial.

•**TRIPLE SULFA VAGINAL TABLETS,** U.S.P. XXII.
Use: Antibacterial.

TRIPLE SULFOID. (Vale) Sulfadiazine 167 mg, sulfamerazine 167 mg, sulfamethazine 167 mg/5 ml or Tab. **Liq.:** Bot. pt, 2 oz. 12s. **Tab.:** Bot. 100s, 1000s.
Use: Antibacterial, sulfonamide.

TRIPLE SULFONAMIDE. Dia-Mer-Thia Sulfonamides. Meth-Dia-Mer Sulfonamides.
Use: Antibacterial, sulfonamide.

TRIPLE VITA. (PBI) Vitamins A 1500 IU, D 400 IU, C 35 mg/ml, alcohol free. Drops. Bot. 50 ml.
Use: Vitamin supplement.

TRIPLE VITA-FLOR. (PBI) Fluoride 0.5 mg, vitamins A 1500 IU, D 400 IU, C 35 mg/ml, alcohol free. Drops. Bot. 50 ml.
Use: Dental caries preventative, vitamin supplement.

TRIPLE X. (Youngs Drug) Pyrethrins 0.3%, piperonyl butoxide 3%, petroleum distillate 1.2%, benzyl alcohol 2.4%. Bot. 2 oz, 4 oz.
Use: Pediculicide.

TRIPODRINE. (Danbury) Pseudoephedrine HCl 60 mg, triprolidine HCl 2.5 mg/Tab. Bot. 100s, UD 100s.
Use: Decongestant, antihistamine.

TRIPOLE-F. (Spanner) Testosterone 25 mg, estrone 6 mg, progesterone 25 mg/ml. Vial 10 ml.
Use: Androgen, estrogen, progestin combination.

TRIPOSED SYRUP. (Blue Cross) Triprolidine HCl 1.25 mg, pseudoephedrine HCl 30 mg/5 ml. Bot. 120 ml, 240 ml, pt, gal.
Use: Antihistamine, decongestant.

TRIPOSED TABLETS. (Blue Cross) Triprolidine HCl 2.5 mg, pseudoephedrine HCl 60 mg/Tab. Bot. 100s, 1000s.
Use: Antihistamine, decongestant.

TRIPOTASSIUM CITRATE.
See: Potassium Citrate, U.S.P. XXII.

TRIPROFED. (Robinson) Triprolidine HCl, pseudoephedrine. Syr. Bot. 100s, 1000s.
Use: Antihistamine, decongestant.

TRIPROFED EXPECTORANT WITH CODEINE. (Robinson) Triprolidine HCl, pseudoephedrine, codeine, expectorant. Bot. pt, gal.
Use: Antihistamine, decongestant, antitussive, expectorant.

TRIPROFED SYRUP. (Robinson) Triprolidine HCl, pseudoephedrine. Bot. pt, gal.
Use: Antihistamine, decongestant.

•**TRIPROLIDINE HCl,** U.S.P. XXII. Syrup, Tab., U.S.P. XXII. Trans 1-4-methylphenyl)-1-(2-pyridyl)-3-pyr- rolidino-prop-1-ene HCl. Trans-2-[3-(1-pyrrolidinyl)-1-(p-tolyl)-propenyl]pyri-dine hydrochloride. (E)-2-(3-(1-Pyrrolidinyl)-1-p-tolypropenyl)pyridine monohydrochloride monohydrate.
Use: Antihistiminic.
See: Actidil, Syr. (Burroughs Wellcome).
W/Codeine phosphate, pseudoephedrine HCl, guaifenesin.
See: Actifed-C, Syr. (Burroughs Wellcome).

TRIPROLIDINE AND PSEUDOEPHEDRINE HYDROCHLORIDE SYRUP. U.S.P. XXII.
Use: Antihistamine, decongestant.
See: Actifed, Syr. (Burroughs Wellcome).

TRIPROLIDINE AND PSEUDOEPHEDRINE HYDROCHLORIDE TABLETS, U.S.P. XXII.
Use: Antihistamine, decongestant.
See: Actifed, Tab., (Burroughs Wellcome).
Atridine, Tab. (Interstate).
Sudahist, Tab. (Upsher-Smith).
Suda-Prol, Tab., Cap. (Quality Generics).
Triphed, Tab. (Lemmon).
Triphedrine, Tab. (Redford).
Triprofed, Tab. (Robinson).

TRIPTIFED. (Weeks & Leo) Triprolidine HCl 2.5 mg, pseudoephedrine HCl 60 mg/Tab. Bot. 36s, 100s.
Use: Antihistamine, decongestant.

TRIPTONE CAPLETS. (Commerce) Dimenhydrinate 50 mg/Tab. Bot. 12s.
Use: Antiemetic/antivertigo agent.

•**TRIPTORELIN.** USAN.
Use: Antineoplastic.

TRISOL. (Buffington) Borax, sodium Cl, boric acid. Irrigator Bot. 1 oz, 4 oz.
Use: Artificial tear solution.

TRISORALEN. (Elder) Trioxsalen 5 mg/Tab. Tartrazine. Bot. 28s, 100s.
Use: Psoralen.

TRI-STATIN. (Rugby) Triamcinolone acetonide 0.1%, neomycin sulfate 0.25%, granicidin 0.25 mg, nystatin 100,000 units/Gm. Cream. 15 Gm, 30 Gm, 60 Gm, 120 Gm, 480 Gm.
Use: Topical corticosteroid, anti-infective.

TRISTOJECT. (Mayrand) Triamcinolone diacetate 40 mg/ml. Vial 5 ml.
Use: Corticosteroid.

•**TRISULFAPYRIMIDINES.** Oral Susp., Tab., U.S.P. XXII.
Use: Antibacterial.
See: Meth-Dia-Mer Sulfonamides (Various Mfr.).
Neotrizine, Preps. (Lilly).
Terfonyl, Liq., Tab. (Squibb Mark).

TRITANE. (Econo-Rx) Brompheniramine maleate 2 mg, guaifenesin 100 mg, phenylephrine HCl 5 mg, phenylpropanolamine HCl 5 mg, alcohol 3.5%/5 ml. Bot. gal.
Use: Antihistamine, expectorant, decongestant.

TRITANE DC. (Econo-Rx) Brompheniramine maleate 2 mg, guaifenesin 100 mg, phenylephrine HCl 5 mg, phenylpropanolamine HCl 5 mg, alcohol 3.5%, codeine phosphate 10 mg/5 ml. Bot. gal.
Use: Antihistamine, expectorant, decongestant, antitussive.

•**TRITIATED WATER.** USAN.
Use: Radioactive agent.
See: Tritiotope (Squibb).

TRITUSSIN COUGH SYRUP. (Towne) Pyrilamine maleate 40 mg, pheniramine maleate 20 mg, citric acid 100 mg, codeine phosphate 58 mg/fl oz. menthol and glycerin in flavored base. Bot. 4 oz.
Use: Antihistamine, expectorant, antitussive.

TRIURISUL. (Sheryl) Sulfacetamide 250 mg, sulfamethizole 250 mg, phenazopyridine HCl 50 mg/Tab. Bot. 100s.
Use: Urinary anti-infective, analgesic.

TRIVA DOUCHE POWDER. (Boyle) Alkyl aryl sulfonate 35%, sodium sulfate 52.5%, oxyquinoline sulfate 2%, lactose 9.67%, disodium ethylene hydrated silica, EDTA 0.33%. Packet 3 Gm, 24s.
Use: Vaginal preparation.

TRI-VERT. (T.E. Williams) Dimenhydrinate 25 mg, niacin 50 mg, pentylenetetrazol 25 mg/Cap. Bot. 100s.
Use: Antiemetic/antivertigo agent.

TRI-VI-FLOR 0.25 mg DROPS. (Mead Johnson Nutrition) Fluoride 0.25 mg, vitamins A 1500 IU, D 400 IU, C 35 mg/ml. Drop. Bot. 50 ml.
Use: Dental caries preventative, vitamin supplement.

TRI-VI-FLOR 0.25 mg WITH IRON DROPS. (Mead Johnson Nutrition) Fluoride 0.25 mg, vitamins A 1500 IU, D 400 IU, C 35 mg, iron 10 mg/ml. Drop. Bot. 50 ml.
Use: Dental caries preventative, vitamin/mineral supplement.

TRI-VI-FLOR 0.5 mg DROPS. (Mead Johnson Nutrition) Fluoride 0.5 mg, vitamins A 1500 IU, D 400 IU, C 35 mg/ml. Bot. 50 ml.
Use: Dental caries preventative, vitamin supplement.

TRI-VI-FLOR 1.0 mg CHEWABLE TABLETS. (Mead Johnson Nutrition) Fluoride 1 mg, vitamins A 2500 IU, D 400 IU, C 60 mg/Tab. Bot. 100s, 1000s.
Use: Dental caries preventative, vitamin supplement.

TRI-VI-SOL DROPS. (Mead Johnson Nutrition) Vitamin A 1500 IU, D 400 IU, C 35 mg/ml. Drop. Bot. 30 ml, 50 ml with calibrated "Safti-dropper."
Use: Vitamin supplement.

TRI-VI-SOL WITH IRON DROPS. (Mead Johnson Nutrition) Vitamins A 1500 IU, C 35 mg, D 400 IU, iron 10 mg/ml. Bot. 50 ml.
Use: Vitamin/mineral supplement.

TRI-VITAMIN WITH FLUORIDE. (Rugby) Fluoride 0.5 mg, vitamins A 1500 IU, D 400 IU, C 35 mg/ml. Drop. Bot. 50 ml.
Use: Dental caries preventative, vitamin supplement.

TRI-VITE. (Foy) Thiamine HCl 100 mg, pyridoxine HCl 100 mg, cyanocobalamine 1000 mcg/ml. Vial 10 ml.
Use: Vitamin supplement.

TROBICIN. (Upjohn) Spectinomycin HCl equivalent to spectinomycin activity: **2 Gm/Vial:** w/Ampule of diluent containing bacteriostatic water for injection 3.2 ml, benzyl alcohol 0.945% in ampule. **4 Gm/Vial:** w/Ampule of diluent containing bacteriostatic water for injection 6.2 ml, benzyl alcohol 0.945%.
Use: Anti-infective.

TROCAL. (Hauck) Dextromethorphan HBr 7.5 mg, guaifenesin 50 mg/Loz. Bot. 500s.
Use: Antitussive, expectorant.

•**TROCLOSENE POTASSIUM.** USAN. (1) 1,3-Dichloro-s-triazine-2,4,6 (1H,3H,5H)trione potassium salt; (2) Potassium dichloroisocyanurate.
Use: Topical anti-infective.

•**TROLAMINE,** N.F. XVII. 2,2″,2″-Nitrilotri- ethanol Ethanol, 2,2′,2″-nitrilotris-. Triethanolamine.
Use: Pharmaceutic aid (alkalinizing agent).
W/Ortho-iodobenzoic.
See: Progonasyl (Saron).

•**TROLEANDOMYCIN,** U.S.P. XXII Cap., Oral Susp., U.S.P. XXII. Triacetyloleandomycin.
Use: Antibiotic.
See: Tao (Roerig).

TROLNITRATE PHOSPHATE, B.A.N. Di[tri-(2-nitratoethyl)ammonium]hydrogen phosphate. Praenitrona.
Use: Vasodilator.
See: Nitretamin (Squibb).

TROMAL. Butacetin. 4′-tert-Butoxyacetanilide.
Use: Analgesic, antidepressant.

TROMETAMOL. B.A.N. 2-Amino-2-hydroxymethyl-propane-1,3-diol. Tromethamine, Talatrol, Trizma.
Use: Treatment of gastric hyperacidity.

•**TROMETHAMINE,** U.S.P. XXII. For Inj., U.S.P. XXII. 2-Amino-2(hydroxymethyl)-1,3-propanediol. Trometamol, B.A.N.
Use: Alkalinizer.

TRONOLANE CREAM. (Ross) Pramoxine HCl 1% in cream base. Tubes 1 oz, 2 oz.
Use: Anorectal preparation.

TRONOLANE SUPPOSITORIES. (Ross) Pramoxine 1% as pramoxine and pramoxine HCl in a lubricating suppository base. Pkg. 10s, 20s.
Use: Anorectal preparation.

•**TROPANSERIN HYDROCHLORIDE.** USAN.
Use: Seratonin receptor antagonist (specific in migraine).

TROPHAMINE INJECTION. (Kendall McGaw) Nitrogen 4.65 Gm, amino acids 30 Gm, protein 29 Gm/500 ml. Bot 500 ml IV infusion.
Use: Nutritional supplement.

TROPH-IRON. (SmithKline Prods) Vitamins B_{12} 25 mcg, B_1 10 mg, iron 20 mg/5 ml. Saccharin. Bot. 4 fl oz.
Use: Vitamin/mineral supplement.

TROPHITE. (SmithKline Prods) Vitamins B_{12} 25 mcg, B_1 10 mg/5 ml. Elix.: Bot. 4 oz.
Use: Vitamin supplement.

TROPICACYL. (Akorn) Tropicamide soln. 0.5% or 1%. **0.5%:** In 15 ml. **1%:** In 2 ml, 15 ml.
Use: Cycloplegic, mydriatic.

TROPICAL BLEND. (Schering-Plough) A series of products is marketed under the Tropical Blend name including: Hawaii Blend Oil SPF 2 (Bot. 8 oz); Hawaii Blend Lotion SPF 2 (Bot. 8 oz); Rio Blend Oil SPF 2 (Bot. 8 oz); Rio Blend Lotion SPF 2 (Bot. 8 oz); Jamaica Blend Oil SPF 2 (Bot. 8 oz); Jamaica Blend Lotion SPF 2 (Bot. 8 oz). All contain homosalate in various oil and lotion bases.
Use: Sunscreen.

•**TROPICAMIDE,** U.S.P. XXII. Ophth. Soln., U.S.P. XXII. N-Ethyl-2-phenyl-N-(4-pyridylmethyl)hydracrylamide. Benzeneacetamide, N-ethyl-α-(hydroxymethyl)-N-(4-pyridinylmethyl)-. Formerly Bis-Tropamide.
Use: Anticholinergic, ophthalmic.
See: Mydriacyl, Drop. (Alcon).

TROPIGLINE. B.A.N. Tiglytropeine.
Use: Treatment of the Parkinsonian syndrome.

TROPINE BENZOHYDRYL ESTER METHANESULFONATE. (also named benztropine methane-sulfonate).

•**TROSPECTOMYCIN SULFATE.** USAN.
Use: Antibacterial.

TROVIT. (Sig) Vitamins B_2 0.3 mg, B_6 1 mg, choline Cl 25 mg, panthenol 2 mg, dl-methionine 10 mg, inositol 20 mg, niacinamide 50 mg, B_{12} 10 mg/ml. Vial 30 ml.
Use: Vitamin supplement.

TROXERUTIN. B.A.N. 3′,4′,7-Tri-[0-(2-hydroxyethyl)]rutin.
Use: Treatment of venous disorders.

TROXIDONE. B.A.N. 3,5,5-Trimethyloxazolidine-2,4-dione.
Use: Anticonvulsant.
See: Trimethadione (I.N.N.) Tridione.

TROXONIUM TOSYLATE. B.A.N. Triethyl-2-(3:4:5-trimethoxybenzoyloxy)ethylammonium toxylate (Tosylic acid is the trivial name for p-toluenesulfonic acid).
Use: Hypotensive.

TROXYPYRROLIUM TOSYLATE. B.A.N. N-Ethyl-N-2-(3:4:5-trimethyoxybenzoyloxy)-ethylpyrrolidinium toxylate (Tosylic acid is the trivial name for p-toluenesulphonic acid).
Use: Hypotensive.

TRUPHYLLINE. (G & W) Aminophylline 250 mg/Supp. (equivalent to theophylline 198 mg). UD 10s, 25s.
Use: Bronchodilator.

TRYMEGEN. (Medco Supply) Chlorpheniramine maleate 4 mg/Tab. Bot. 1000s.
Use: Antihistamine.

TRYNISIN COLD SYRUP. (Halsey) Bot. 4 oz, 8 oz.
Use: Antihistamine.

•**TRYPSIN, CRYSTALLIZED,** U.S.P. XXII. For Inhalation Aerosol, U.S.P. XXII.
Use: Proteolytic enzyme.
W/Castor oil.
See: Granulex (Hickam).
W/Chymotrypsin.
See: Chymolase, Tab. (Warren-Teed).
Orenzyme, Tab. (Merrell Dow).

TRYPARSAMIDE. Monosodium N-(Carbamylmethyl)arsanilate.

TRYPTACIN. (Arther Inc.) L-tryptophan 500 mg or 1000 mg/Tab. Bot. 100s, 250s, UD 100s.
Use: Nutritional supplement.

TRYPTIZOL HYDROCHLORIDE. Amitriptyline HCl, U.S.P XXII.
Use: Antidepressant.

•**TRYPTOPHAN,** U.S.P. XXII. $C_{11}H_{12}N_2O_2$ as L-tryptophan.
Use: Amino acid.

TRYSUL. (Savage) Sulfathiazole 3.42%, sulfacetamide 2.86%, sulfabenzamide 3.7%, urea 0.64%. Tube 78 Gm.
Use: Anti-infective, vaginal.

T-SERP TABLET. (Tennessee Pharm.) Reserpine alkaloid 0.25 mg/Tab. Bot. 100s, 1000s.
Use: Antihypertensive.

T-STAT. (Westwood) Erythromycin 20 mg/ml, alcohol 71%. Bot. 60 ml.
Use: Anti-acne.

TTC. Triphenyltetrazolium Chloride.
See: Uroscreen, Tube (Pfizer).

•**TUAMINOHEPTANE,** U.S.P. XXII. Inhalant, U.S.P. XXII.
Use: Adrenergic.

•**TUBERCULIN.** U.S.P. XXII.
Use: Diagnostic aid (dermal reactivity indicator).
See: Aplisol (Parke-Davis), Aplitest (Parke-Davis).

TUBERCULIN, MONO-VACC TEST. (Lincoln) Mono-Vacc test is a sterile, disposable multiple puncture scarifier with liquid Old Tuberculin on the points. Box test 25s.
Use: Diagnostic aid.

TUBERCULIN PURIFIED PROTEIN DERIVATIVE. (Squibb/Connaught) A concentrated solution for multiple puncture testing. Vial 1 ml.
Use: Diagnostic aid.

TUBERCULIN PURIFIED PROTEIN DERIVATIVE.
See: Tubersol, Inj. (Squibb/Connaught).

TUBERCULIN TINE TEST. (Lederle) **Old Tuberculin (OT):** Each disposable test unit consists of a stainless steel disc, with four tines (or prongs) 2 millimeters long, attached to a plastic handle. The tines have been dip-dried with antigenic material. The entire unit is sterilized by ethylene oxide gas. The test has been standardized by comparative studies, utilizing 0.05 mg US Standard Old Tuberculin (5 International Units) or 0.0001 mg US Standard (5 International Units) by the Mantoux technique. The reliability appears to be comparable to the standard Mantoux. Test in a jar 25s. Package 100s. Bin Package 250s. **Purified Protein Derivative (PPD):** Equivalent to or more potent than 5 TU PPD Mantoux test. Test in a jar 25s. Package 100s.
Use: Diagnostic aid.

TUBERLATE. (Heun) Sodium p-aminosalicylate 12 gr, succinic acid 4 gr/Tab. Bot. 500s.
Use: Antituberculous agent.

TUBERSOL. (Squibb/Connaught) Tuberculin purified protein derivative (Mantoux) 1 TU, 5 TU or 250 TU. Vial 1 ml, 5 ml.
Use: Diagnostic aid.

TUBEX. (Wyeth-Ayerst) The following drugs are available in various Tubex sizes:
Ativan
Bicillin C-R
Bicillin C-R 900/300
Bicillin Long-Acting
Codeine Phosphate
Cyanocobalamin
Digoxin
Dimenhydrinate
Diphenhydramine HCl
Diphtheria and Tetanus Toxoids Adsorbed (Pediatric)
Epinephrine
Furosemide
Heparin Flush Kits
Heparin Lock Flush
Heparin Sodium Soln.
Hydromorphone HCl
Hydroxyzine HCl
Influenza Virus Vaccine, Trivalent
Mepergan
Meperidine HCl
Morphine Sulfate
Naloxone Inj.
Naloxone Inj., Neonatal
Oxytocin
Pentobarbital Sodium
Phenergan
Phenobarbital Sodium
Prochlorperazine Edisylate
Secobarbital Sodium
Sodium Cl, Bacteriostatic
Sparine HCl
Tetanus and Diphtheria Toxoids Adsorbed (Adult)
Tetanus Immune Globulin (Human)
Tetanus Toxoid Aluminum Phosphate Adsorbed.
Tetanus Toxoid, Fluid
Thiamine HCl
Wycillin

TUBOCURARINE CHLORIDE, U.S.P. XXII. Inj., U.S.P. XXII. Tubocuraranium, 7′,12′-dihydroxy-6,6′-dimethoxy-2,2′,2′-trimethyl-, Cl, hydrochloride, pentahydrate. d-Tubocurarine Cl. (Various Mfr.)
Metubine Iodide (Lilly) 3 mg/ml. Amp. 10 ml.
(Abbott) 3 mg/ml. Fliptop vial 10 ml;
15 mg in Abboject Syringe 5 ml.
Use: Skeletal muscle relaxant.

TUBOCURARINE CHLORIDE, DIMETHYL. Dimethyl ether of d-tubocurarine Cl.

(±)-TUBOCURARINE CHLORIDE HYDROCHLORIDE PENTAHYDRATE. Tubocurarine Chloride, U.S.P. XXII.

TUBOCURARINE IODIDE, DIMETHYL. Dimethyl ether of d-tubocurarine iodide.
Use: Skeletal muscle relaxant.
See: Metubine, Vial (Lilly).

•**TUBULOZOLE HYDROCHLORIDE.** USAN.
Use: Antineoplastic.

TUCKS. (Parke-Davis Prods) Pads saturated with solution of witch hazel 50%, glycerin 10%, methylparaben 0.1%, benzalkonium Cl 0.003%. Jar 40s, 100s.
Use: Anorectal preparation.

TUCKS CREAM. (Parke-Davis Prods) Witch hazel 50% in cream base. Tube 40 Gm w/rectal applicator.
Use: Anorectal preparation.

TUCKS TAKE-ALONGS. (Parke-Davis Prods) Non-woven wipes saturated with solution of witch hazel 50%, glycerine 10%, purified water, methylparaben 0.1%, benzalkonium Cl 0.003%. Box 12s.
Use: Anorectal preparation.

TUINAL. (Lilly) Equal parts Seconal Sodium and Amytal Sodium 100 mg or 200 mg/Pulvule. **100 mg:** Bot. 100s, 1000s, Blister Pkg. 10 × 10s. Dispenser roll 40 × 25s; **200 mg:** Bot. 100s, 1000s, UD 100s, 1000s.
Use: Sedative/hypnotic.

TUMS. (Norcliff Thayer) Calcium carbonate 500 mg/Tab. Available in peppermint and assorted flavors in various package sizes. Roll 12s singles, 3-roll wraps. Bot. 75s, 150s.
Use: Antacid.

TUMS EXTRA STRENGTH. (Norcliff Thayer) **Chew. Tab.:** Calcium carbonate 750 mg, sodium ≤ 2 mg. Pkg. 12s, 48s, 96s. **Liq.:** Cal-

cium carbonate 1000 mg/5 ml, sodium >5 mg/5 ml. Bot. 360 ml.
Use: Antacid.

TUMS LIQUID EXTRA STRENGTH W/SIMETHICONE. (Norcliff-Thayer) Calcium carbonate 1000 mg, simethicone 30 mg, sorbitol. Bot. 360 ml.
Use: Antacid, antiflatulent.

TUR-BI-KAL NASAL DROPS. (Emerson) Phenylephrine HCl in a saline solution. Dropper Bot. 1 oz, 12s.
Use: Decongestant.

TURBILIXIR. (Burlington) Chlorpheniramine maleate 2 mg, phenylephrine HCl 5 mg, phenylpropanolamine HCl 5 mg/5 ml. Bot. pt, gal.
Use: Antihistamine, decongestant.

TURBINAIRE.
See: Decadron Phosphate, Preps. (Merck Sharp & Dohme).

TURBISPAN LEISURECAPS. (Burlington) Chlorpheniramine maleate 12 mg, 1-phenylephrine HCl 15 mg, phenylpropanolamine HCl 15 mg/SR Cap. Bot. 30s.
Use: Antihistamine, decongestant.

TURGASEPT AEROSOL. (Wyeth-Ayerst) Ethyl alcohol 44.25%, essential oils 0.9%, n-alkyl (50% C-14, 40% C-12, 10% C-16) dimethyl benzylammonium Cl 0.33%, o-phenylphenol 0.25% w/propellant. Spray can 11.5 oz. in bouquet, fresh lemon, leather, citrus blossom scents.
Use: Disinfectant, deodorant.

TURPENTINE OIL W/COMBINATIONS.
See: Sloan's Liniment, Liq. (Warner-Lambert).

TUSAL. (Hauck) Sodium thiosalicylate 50 mg/ml. Vial 30 ml.
Use: Salicylate analgesic.

TUS-F. (Orbit) Dextromethorphan HBr 10 mg/5 ml. Bot. 4 oz, pt.
Use: Antitussive.

TUSILAN. Dextromethorphan HBr.
Use: Antitussive.

TUSQUELIN. (Circle) Dextromethorphan HBr 15 mg, chlorpheniramine maleate 2 mg, phenylpropanolamine 5 mg, phenylephrine HCl 5 mg, fluid-extract ipecac 0.17 min., potassium guaiacolsulfonate 44 mg/5 ml, alcohol 5%. Syr. Bot. pt.
Use: Antitussive, antihistamine, decongestant, expectorant.

TUSREN. (Wren) Guaifenesin 200 mg/Tab. Bot. 100s, 1000s.
Use: Expectorant.

TUSSABAR. (Tennessee) Acetaminophen 400 mg, salicylamide 500 mg, potassium guaiacolsulfonate 120 mg, pyrilamine maleate 30 mg, ammonium Cl 500 mg, sodium citrate 500 mg, phenylephrine HCl 30 mg/oz. Bot. pt, gal.
Use: Analgesic, expectorant, antihistamine, decongestant.

TUSSABID. (Ion) Guaifenesin 200 mg, dextromethorphan HBr 30 mg/Cap. Bot. 24s, 100s.
Use: Expectorant, antitussive.

TUSSACOL. (Jenkins) Dextromethorphan HBr 7.5 mg, pyrilamine maleate 8.0 mg, chlorpheniramine maleate 0.3 mg, phenylephrine HCl 5 mg, acetaminophen 100 mg, guaifenesin 50 mg/Tab. Bot. 1000s.
Use: Antitussive, antihistamine, decongestant, analgesic, expectorant.

TUSSAFED DROPS. (Everett) Carbinoxamine maleate 2 mg, pseudoephedrine HCl 25 mg, dextromethorphan HBr 4 mg/ml. Bot. 30 ml with calibrated dropper.
Use: Antihistamine, decongestant, antitussive.

TUSSAFED EXPECTORANT. (Calvital) Chlorpheniramine maleate 2 mg, pseudoephedrine HCl 30 mg, guaifenesin 100 mg/5 ml. Bot. pt, gal.
Use: Antihistamine, decongestant, expectorant.

TUSSAFED SYRUP. (Everett) Dextromethorphan HBr 15 mg, pseudoephedrine HCl 60 mg, carbinoxamine maleate 4 mg/5 ml. Bot. 4 oz, 16 oz.
Use: Antitussive, decongestant, antihistamine.

TUSSAHIST. (Defco) Codeine phosphate 10 mg, phenylpropanolamine HCl 12.5 mg, chlorpheniramine maleate 2 mg, pyrilamine maleate 7.5 mg, guaifenesin 100 mg/5 ml. Bot. 4 oz, pt, gal.
Use: Antitussive, decongestant, antihistamine, expectorant.

TUSS ALLERGINE MODIFIED T.D. (Rugby) Phenylpropanolamine HCl 75 mg, caramiphen edisylate 40 mg/TR Cap. Bot. 100s, 500s, 1000s.
Use: Decongestant, antitussive.

TUSSANIL. (Misemer) Chlorpheniramine maleate 4 mg, phenylephrine HCl 10 mg/5 ml, alcohol 5%. Bot. pt.
Use: Antihistamine, decongestant.

TUSSANIL DH. (Misemer) Phenylpropanolamine HCl 25 mg, guaifenesin 100 mg, hydrocodone bitartrate 1.66 mg, salicylamide 300 mg/Tab. Bot. 100s.
Use: Decongestant, expectorant, antitussive, analgesic.

TUSSANIL DH SYRUP. (Misemer) Phenylephrine HCl 10 mg, chlorpheniramine maleate 4 mg, hydrocodone bitartrate 2.5 mg/5 ml, alcohol 5%. Bot. pt.
Use: Decongestant, antihistamine, antitussive.

TUSSANIL EXPECTORANT SYRUP. (Misemer) Hydrocodone bitartrate 2.5 mg, phenylephrine HCl 10 mg, guaifenesin 100 mg/5 ml, alcohol 5%. Bot. pt.
Use: Antitussive, decongestant, expectorant.

TUSSANOL. (Tyler) Pyrilamine maleate $\frac{3}{4}$ gr, codeine phosphate 1 gr, ammonium Cl 7.5 gr, sodium citrate 5 gr, menthol $\frac{1}{10}$ gr/fl oz. Bot. 4 fl oz, pt, gal.
Use: Antihistamine, antitussive, expectorant.

TUSSANOL with EPHEDRINE. (Tyler) Ephedrine sulfate 2 gr, pyrilamine maleate $\frac{3}{4}$ gr, codeine phosphate 1 gr, ammonium Cl 7.5 gr, sodium citrate 5 gr, menthol $\frac{1}{10}$ gr/30 ml. Bot. 16 fl oz.

Use: Bronchodilator, antihistamine, antitussive, expectorant.

TUSSAR-2 SYRUP. (Rorer) Codeine phosphate 10 mg, carbetapentane citrate 7.5 mg, chlorpheniramine maleate 2 mg, guaifenesin 50 mg, sodium citrate 130 mg, citric acid 20 mg/5 ml, alcohol 5%, methylparaben 0.1%. Bot. pt.
Use: Antitussive, antihistamine, expectorant.

TUSSAR DM. (Rorer) Dextromethorphan HBr 15 mg, chlorpheniramine maleate 2 mg, phenylephrine HCl 5 mg/5 ml, methylparaben 0.1%. Bot. 4 oz, pt.
Use: Antitussive, antihistamine, decongestant.

TUSSAR SF. (Rorer) Codeine phosphate 10 mg, carbetapentane citrate 7.5 mg, chlorpheniramine maleate 2 mg, guaifenesin 50 mg, sodium citrate 130 mg, citric acid 20 mg/5 ml, methylparaben 0.1%, alcohol 12%. Sugar free. Bot. 4 oz, pt.
Use: Antitussive, antihistamine, expectorant.

TUSSCIDIN EXPECTORANT. (Cenci) Guaifenesin 100 mg/5 ml. Bot. 4 oz, pt, gal.
Use: Expectorant.

TUSSCIDIN EXPECTORANT-D. (Cenci) Dextromethorphan HBr 15 mg, guaifenesin 100 mg/5 ml. Bot. 4 oz, pt, gal.
Use: Antitussive, expectorant.

TUSSEX COUGH. (Various Mfr.) Phenylephrine HCl 5 mg, dextromethorphan HBr 10 mg, guaifenesin 100 mg/5 ml. Syr. Bot. 120 ml, gal.
Use: Decongestant, antitussive, expectorant.

TUSS-GENADE MODIFIED CAPS. (Goldline) Phenylpropanolamine HCl 75 mg, caramiphen edisylate 40 mg. Bot. 100s, 1000s.
Use: Decongestant, antitussive.

TUSSGEN EXPECTORANT. (Goldline) Bot. pt, gal.
Use: Expectorant.

TUSSGEN LIQUID. (Goldline) Pseudoephedrine HCl 60 mg, hydrocodone bitartrate 5 mg/5 ml. Bot. 100s, 1000s.
Use: Decongestant, antitussive.

TUSSIDRAM. (Dram) Dextromethorphan 10 mg, phenylpropanolamine 12.5 mg, guaifenesin 50 mg, chlorpheniramine maleate 2 mg/5 ml. Bot. pt.
Use: Antitussive, decongestant, expectorant, antihistamine.

TUSSIGON. (Daniels) Hydrocodone bitartrate 5 mg, homatropine methylbromide 1.5 mg/Tab. Bot. 100s, 500s.
Use: Antitussive, anticholinergic/antispasmodic.

TUSSIONEX. (Pennwalt) Hydrocodone (as polistivex) 10 mg, chlorpheniramine 8 mg. Liq. Bot. 473 ml, 900 ml.
Use: Antitussive, antihistamine.

TUSSI-ORGANIDIN LIQUID. (Wallace) Codeine phosphate 10 mg, organidin 30 mg/5 ml, saccharin, sorbitol. Bot. pt, gal.
Use: Antitussive, expectorant.

TUSSI-ORGANIDIN DM LIQUID. (Wallace) Dextromethorphan HBr 10 mg, organidin 30 mg/5 ml, saccharin, sorbitol. Bot. pt, gal.
Use: Antitussive, expectorant.

TUSSIREX. (Scot-Tussin) Phenylephrine HCl 4.2 mg, pheniramine maleate 13.3 mg, codeine phosphate 10 mg, sodium citrate 83.3 mg, sodium salicylate 83.3 mg, caffeine citrate 25 mg/5 ml. Syr. Bot. 120 ml, 240 ml, pt, gal.
Use: Decongestant, antihistamine, antitussive, expectorant, salicylate analgesic.

TUSSIREX SUGAR FREE LIQUID. (Scot-Tussin) Codeine phosphate 10 mg, pheniramine maleate 13.33 mg, phenylephrine HCl 4.17 mg, sodium citrate 83.33 mg, sodium salicylate 83.33 mg, caffeine citrate 25 mg/5 ml. Bot. 120 ml, pt, gal.
Use: Antitussive, antihistamine, decongestant, expectorant, salicylate analgesic.

TUSSI-R-GEN DM LIQUID. (Goldline) Dextromethorphan HBr 10 mg, iodinated glycerol 30 mg Bot. 120 ml pt.
Use: Antitussive, expectorant.

TUSSI-R-GEN LIQUID EXPECTORANT. (Goldline) Codeine phosphate 10 mg, iodinated glycerol 30 mg/5 ml. Bot. pt.
Use: Antitussive, expectorant.

TUSS-LA. (Hyrex) Pseudoephedrine HCl 120 mg, guaifenesin 500 mg/LA Tab. Bot. 100s.
Use: Decongestant, expectorant.

TUSSOGEST. (Major) Phenylpropanolamine HCl 75 mg, caramiphen edisylate 40 mg/TR Cap. Bot. 100s, 500s, 1000s.
Use: Decongestant, antitussive.

TUSS-ORNADE LIQUID. (SmithKline) Caramiphen edisylate 6.7 mg, phenylpropanolamine HCl 12.5 mg/5 ml, alcohol 5%. Bot. pt.
Use: Antitussive, decongestant.

TUSS-ORNADE SPANSULE. (SmithKline) Caramiphen edisylate 40 mg, phenylpropanolamine HCl 75 mg/Cap. Bot. 50s, 500s.
Use: Antitussive, decongestant.

TUSSTAT EXPECTORANT. (Century) Diphenhydramine HCl 80 mg, ammonium Cl 12 gr, sodium citrate 5 gr, menthol 1/10 gr, alcohol 5%/oz. Bot. 4 fl oz, pt, gal.
Use: Antihistamine, expectorant.

T-VITES. (Freeda) Vitamins B_1 25 mg, B_2 25 mg, B_3 150 mg, B_5 25 mg, B_6 25 mg, C 100 mg, biotin 30 mcg, PABA 30 mg, K, Mg, Mn, zinc 20 mg/Tab. Bot. 100s.
Use: Vitamin/mineral supplement.

TWEEN 20, 40, 60, 80. (ICI Americas) Polysorbates, N.F. XVII.
Use: Surface active agents.

12 HOUR COLD CAPSULES. (Nature's Bounty) Phenylpropanolamine HCl 75 mg, chlorpheniramine maleate 4 mg/Cap. Pkg. 10s.
Use: Decongestant, antihistamine.

TWENDEX PB. (Allison) Dextroamphetamine sulfate 20 mg, phenobarbital 1 gr/Tab. Bot. 30s, 100s.

Use: CNS stimulant, sedative/hypnotic.
TWICE-A-DAY. (Major) Oxymetazoline 0.05%. Soln. 15 ml, 30 ml.
Use: Decongestant.
TWILITE. (Pfeiffer) Diphenhydramine HCl 50 mg/ Tab. Pkg. 20s.
Use: Sleep aid.
TWIN-K LIQUID. (Boots) Potassium ions 20 mEq/15 ml. Bot. pt.
Use: Treatment of hypokalemia.
2-TONE DISCLOSING SOLUTION. (Lorvic) Dropper Bot. 2 oz.
Use: Disclosing solution.
2-24. (Walgreen) Belladonna alkaloids 0.2 mg, phenylpropanolamine HCl 50 mg, chlorpheniramine maleate 4 mg/Cap. Bot. 10s.
Use: Anticholinergic/antispasmodic, decongestant, antihistamine.
TWO-CAL HN HIGH NITROGEN LIQUID NUTRITION. (Ross) High nitrogen liquid nutrition (2 calories/ml). 1900 calories (1 quart) provide 100% US RDA for vitamins and minerals for adults and children over 4 yrs. Can 8 fl oz.
Use: Enteral nutritional supplement.
TWO-CAL IM. (Fellows) Calcium glycerophosphate 10 mg, calcium levulinate 15 mg/ml. Vial 100 ml.
Use: Calcium supplement.
TWO-DYNE CAPSULES. (Hyrex) Butalbital 50 mg, caffeine 40 mg, acetaminophen 325 mg/ Cap. Bot. 100s, 1000s.
Use: Sedative/hypnotic, analgesic.
TY-CAPLETS. (Major) Acetaminophen 500 mg/ Tab. Bot. 100s.
Use: Analgesic.
TY-CAPS. (Major) Acetaminophen 500 mg/Cap. Bot. 100s, 1000s, UD 100s.
Use: Analgesic.
TY-COLD TABLETS. (Major) Pseudoephedrine 30 mg, chlorpheniramine maleate 2 mg, dextromethorphan HBr 15 mg, acetaminophen 325 mg. Pkg. 24s.
Use: Decongestant, antihistamine, antitussive, analgesic.
TYFORMIN. B.A.N. 4-Guanidinobutyramide.
Use: Oral hypoglycemic agent.
TYLENOL CHILDREN'S CHEWABLE TABLETS. (McNeil Prods) Acetaminophen 80 mg/ Tab. Bot. 30s, 48s. Blisters 2s. Hospital pack 250 × 1.
Use: Analgesic.
TYLENOL CHILDREN'S ELIXIR. (McNeil Prods) Acetaminophen 160 mg/5 ml. Bot. 2 oz, 4 oz, pt. UD 100 × 5 ml, 100 × 10 ml.
Use: Analgesic.
TYLENOL EXTRA-STRENGTH. (McNeil Prods) Acetaminophen 500 mg/Tab. or Capl. **Tab.:** Bot. 30s, 60s, 100s, 200s. **Capl.:** Bot. 24s, 50s, 100s, 175s.
Use: Analgesic.
TYLENOL EXTRA-STRENGTH ADULT LIQUID. (McNeil Prods) Acetaminophen 1000 mg/30 ml, alcohol 8.5%. Bot. 8 oz. Hosp. Bot. 8 oz.
Use: Analgesic.
TYLENOL INFANTS' DROPS. (McNeil Prods) Acetaminophen 80 mg/0.8 ml. Bot. w/dropper 15 ml.
Use: Analgesic.
TYLENOL JUNIOR STRENGTH SWALLOWABLE TABLETS. (McNeil Prods) Acetaminophen 160 mg/Tab. Box. 30s. Hosp. 250 × 1.
Use: Analgesic.
TYLENOL MAXIMUM STRENGTH SINUS MEDICATION. (McNeil Prods) Acetaminophen 500 mg, pseudoephedrine HCl 30 mg/Tab. or Capl. Bot. 24s, 50s.
Use: Analgesic, decongestant.
TYLENOL REGULAR STRENGTH. (McNeil Prods) Acetaminophen 325 mg/Tab. or Capl. **Tab.:** Tin 12s. Vial 12s. Bot. 24s, 50s, 100s, 200s. **Capl.:** Bot. 24s, 50s.
Use: Analgesic.
TYLENOL WITH CODEINE. (McNeil Pharm) **No. 1:** Acetaminophen 300 mg, codeine phosphate 7.5 mg/Tab. Bot. 100s. **No. 2:** Acetaminophen 300 mg, codeine phosphate 15 mg/Tab. Bot. 100s, 500s, UD 20 × 25s. **No. 3:** Acetaminophen 300 mg, codeine phosphate 30 mg/Tab. Bot. 100s, 500s, 1000s, UD 500s. **No. 4:** Acetaminophen 300 mg, codeine phosphate 60 mg/ Tab. Bot. 100s, 500s, UD 500s.
Use: Narcotic analgesic combination.
TYLENOL WITH CODEINE ELIXIR. (McNeil Pharm) Acetaminophen 120 mg, codeine phosphate 12 mg/5 ml, alcohol 7%. Bot. 4 oz, pt, UD Cups 10 × 5 ml, 10 × 15 ml.
Use: Narcotic analgesic combination.
TYLOSIN. V.B.A.N. An antibiotic derived from an actinomycete resembling Streptomyces fradie. Tylan.
Use: Antibiotic, veterinary medicine.
TYLOSTERONE. (Lilly) Diethylstilbestrol 0.25 mg, methyltestosterone 5 mg/Tab. Bot. 100s.
Use: Estrogen, androgen combination.
TYLOX. (McNeil Pharm) Oxycodone HCl 5 mg, acetaminophen 500 mg/Cap. Bot. 100s, UD 4 × 25s.
Use: Narcotic analgesic combination.
TYMATRO THROAT TROCHES. (Bowman) Benzocaine 5 mg, cetylpyridinium Cl 1.5 mg/Loz. Bot. 1000s.
Use: Local anesthetic, antiseptic.
TYMAZOLINE. B.A.N. 2-(5-Isopropyl-2-methylphenoxymethyl)-2-imidazoline. Pernazene hydrochloride.
Use: Vasoconstrictor.
TYMPAGESIC. (Adria) Phenylephrine HCl 0.25%, antipyrine 5%, benzocaine 5%, in propylene glycol. Liq. Bot. w/dropper 13 ml.
Use: Otic preparation.
TY-PAP. (Major) **Elix.:** Acetaminophen 160 mg/5 ml. Bot. pt, gal. **Supp.:** Acetaminophen 120 mg or 650 mg. Pkg. 12s.

Use: Analgesic.

•**TYPHOID VACCINE,** U.S.P. XXII. (Wyeth-Ayerst)—Vial 5 ml, 10 ml, 20 ml.
Use: Active immunizing agent.

TYROBENZ. (Mallard) Benzocaine 10 mg/Loz. Bot. 500s.
Use: Local anesthetic.

TYRO-LOZ. (Kenyon) Tyrothricin 2 mg, benzocaine 5 mg/Loz. Bot. 100s, 1000s.
Use: Local anesthetic.

•**TYROPANOATE SODIUM,** U.S.P. XXII. Cap., U.S.P. XXII. Sodium 3-butyramido-α-ethyl-2,4,6-triiodohydrocinnamate.
Use: Diagnostic aid (radiopaque medium, cholecystographic).
See: Bilopaque (Winthrop Pharm).

TYROPAQUE CAPS. (Winthrop Products) Tyropanoate sodium.
Use: Radiopaque agent.

•**TYROSINE,** U.S.P. XXII. L-Tyrosine.
Use: Amino acid.

TYROSUM SKIN CLEANSER. (Summers) Isopropanol 50%, polysorbate 80 2%, acetone 10%. Bot. 4 oz, pt. Towlettes 24s, 50s.
Use: Anti-acne.

•**TYROTHRICIN,** U.S.P. XXII. Spray. Soln., Troches: An antibiotic from *Bacillus brevis.* Tyrodac; Tyroderm.
Use: Antibacterial.

TY-TABS. (Major) Acetaminophen with codeine #2, #3 or #4. Bot. 100s, 500s or 1000s.
Use: Narcotic analgesic combination.

CHILDREN'S TY-TABS. (Major) Acetaminophen 80 mg/Tab. Bot. 30s, 100s.
Use: Analgesic.

TY-TABS EXTRA STRENGTH. (Major) Acetaminophen 500 mg/Tab. Bot. 100s, 1000s.
Use: Analgesic.

TYZINE NASAL SOLUTION. (Key) Tetrahydrozoline HCl 0.1%. Bot. pt, oz.
Use: Nasal decongestant.

TYZINE NASAL SPRAY. (Key) Tetrahydrozoline HCl 0.1%. Bot. 0.5 oz.
Use: Nasal decongestant.

TYZINE PEDIATRIC NASAL DROPS. (Key) Tetrahydrozoline HCl 0.05%. Bot. 0.5 oz.
Use: Nasal decongestant.

U

UAA. (Econo Med) Methenamine 40.8 mg, phenyl salicylate 18.1 mg, methylene blue 5.4 mg, benzoic acid 4.5 mg, atropine sulfate 0.03 mg, hyoscyamine 0.03 mg/Tab. Bot. 100s, 1000s.
Use: Urinary anti-infective.

UBT. (NMS) For detection of blood in the urine.
Use: Diagnostic aid.

UCEPHAN. (Kendall-McGaw) Sodium benzoate 10%, sodium phenylacetate 10% (10 Gm/100 ml). Liq. Bot. 100 ml.
Use: For urea cycle enzymopathies.

UCG-BETA SLIDE MONOCLONAL II. (Wampole) Two-minute latex agglutination inhibition slide test for the qualitative detection of B-hCG/hCG (sensitivity 0.5 IU hCG/ml) in urine. Kit 50s, 100s, 300s.
Use: Diagnostic aid.

UCG-BETA STAT. (Wampole) One-hour passive hemagglutination inhibition tube test for the qualitative detection and quantitative determination of B-hCG/hCG (sensitivity 0.2 IU hCG/ml) in urine. Kit 50s, 300s.
Use: Diagnostic aid.

UCG-LYPHOTEST. (Wampole) One-hour passive hemagglutination inhibition tube test for the qualitative or quantitative determination of human chorionic gonadotropin (sensitivity 0.5-1 IU hCG/ml) in urine. Kit 10s, 50s, 300s.
Use: Diagnostic aid.

UCG-SLIDE TEST. (Wampole) Rapid latex agglutination inhibition slide test for the qualitative detection of human chorionic gonadotropin (Sensitivity: 2 IU hCG/ml) in urine. Kit 30s, 100s, 300s, 1000s.
Use: Diagnostic aid.

UCG-TEST. (Wampole) Two-hour hemagglutination inhibition tube test for the determination of human chorionic gonadotropin (sensitivity 0.5 IU hCG/ml undiluted specimen. 1.5 IU hCG/ml 1:3 diluted specimen) in urine and serum. Kit 10s, 25s, 100s, 300s.
Use: Diagnostic aid.

UCG-TITRATION SET. (Wampole) A two-hour hemagglutination inhibition tube test for the determination of human chorionic gonadotropin (Sensitivity 1 IU hCG/ml) in urine or serum. Kit 45s.
Use: Diagnostic aid.

ULACORT. (Fellows) Prednisolone 5 mg/Tab. Bot. 1000s.
Use: Corticosteroid.

ULACORT (AQUASPENSION INJECTIONS). (Fellows) Prednisolone acetate 25 mg or 50 mg/ml. Vial 10 ml.
Use: Corticosteroid.

ULCERIN P TABLETS. (Winthrop Products) Aluminum hydroxide.
Use: Antacid.

ULCERIN TABLETS. (Winthrop Products) Aluminum hydroxide.
Use: Antacid.

ULCER THERAPY.
See: Antacids.
Anticholinergic Agents.

•**ULDAZEPAM.** USAN.
Use: Sedative.

ULTRA B50. (Nature's Bounty) Vitamins B_1 50 mg, B_2 50 mg, B_3 50 mg, B_5 50 mg, B_6 50 mg, B_{12} 50 mcg, folic acid 0.1 mg, PABA 50 mg, inositol 50 mg, biotin 50 mcg, choline 50 mg, lecithin 50 mg/Tab. Bot. 60s, 180s.
Use: Vitamin supplement.

ULTRA B100. (Nature's Bounty) Vitamins B_1 100 mg, B_2 100 mg, B_3 100 mg, B_5 100 mg, B_6 100 mg, B_{12} 100 mcg, folic acid 0.1 mg, PABA 100 mg, inositol 100 mg, biotin 100 mcg, choline bitartrate 100 mg/TR Tab. Bot. 50s.
Use: Vitamin supplement.

ULTRABEX. (Approved) Vitamins B_1 20 mg, C 50 mg, B_2 2 mg, B_6 0.5 mg, niacinamide 35 mg, calcium pantothenate 0.5 mg, wheat germ oil 30 mg, B_{12} 20 mcg, liver desiccated 150 mg, iron 11.58 mg, calcium 29 mg, phosphorus 23 mg, dicalcium phosphate 100 mg, magnesium 1.11 mg, manganese 1.3 mg, potassium 2.24 mg, zinc 0.68 mg, choline 25 mg, inositol 25 mg, pepsin 32.5 mg, diastase 32.5 mg, hesperidin 25 mg, biotin 20 mcg, hydrolyzed yeast 81.25 mg, protein digest 47.04 mg, amino acids 34.21 mg/Cap. Bot. 50s, 100s, 1000s.
Use: Vitamin/mineral supplement.

ULTRA CAP. (Weeks & Leo) Acetaminophen 300 mg, guaifenesin 100 mg, chlorpheniramine maleate 4 mg, phenylephrine HCl 10 mg, dextromethorphan HBr 6 mg/Cap. Vial 18s.
Use: Analgesic, expectorant, antihistamine, decongestant, antitussive.

ULTRACEF. (Bristol Labs) **Cap.:** Cefadroxil monohydrate 500 mg. Bot. 50s, 100s, UD 100s. **Tab.:** 1 Gm. Bot. 24s, UD 100s. **Pow. for oral susp.:** 125 mg/ml or 250 mg/5 ml. Bot. 50 ml, 100 ml.
Use: Antibacterial, cephalosporin.

ULTRACORTINOL. (Ciba) Agent to suppress overactive adrenal glands. Pending release.

ULTRA-DERM BATH OIL. (Baker/Cummins) Bot. 8 oz.
Use: Emollient.

ULTRA-DERM MOISTURIZER. (Baker/Cummins) Bot. 8 oz.
Use: Emollient.

ULTRA-FREEDA. (Freeda) Vitamins A 3333 IU, D 133 IU, E 66.6 mg, B_1 16.7 mg, B_2 16.7 mg, B_3 33 mg, B_5 33 mg, B_6 16.7 mg, B_{12} 33 mcg, C 333 mg, iron 5 mg, folic acid 0.27 mg, calcium 66.7 mg, zinc 7.5 mg, choline 33 mg, inositol 33 mg, beta carotene 833 IU, bioflavonoids complex 33 mg, PABA 16.7 mg, biotin 100 mcg, Cr, I, K, Mg, Mn, Mo, Se/Tab. Bot. 90s, 180s, 270s.
Use: Vitamin/mineral supplement.

ULTRAGESIC. (Stewart-Jackson) Acetaminophen 500 mg, hydrocodone bitartrate 5 mg/Cap. Bot. 100s.
Use: Narcotic analgesic combination.

ULTRALENTE INSULIN.
See: Iletin (Lilly).

ULTRA MIDE 25. (Baker/Cummins) Bot. 8 oz.
Use: Emollient.

ULTRAPEN POTASSIUM SALT.
See: Propicillin, B.A.N.

ULTRAPRED. (Horizon) Prednisolone acetate 1%. Susp. Bot. 5 ml.
Use: Corticosteroid, ophthalmic.

ULTRASONE. (Gordon) Ultrasonic contact cream. Bot. qt, gal. Plastic Bot. 8 oz.
Use: Ultrasonic contact cream.

ULTRA TEARS. (Alcon) Hydroxypropyl methylcellulose 1%, benzalkonium Cl 0.01%/15 ml. Drop-tainer disp. 15 ml.
Use: Artificial tears.

ULTRAVATE. (Westwood Squibb) Halobetasol propionate.
Use: Corticosteroid, topical.

ULTRAZYME ENZYMATIC CLEANER. (Allergan) Subtilisin A, effervescing, buffering and tableting agents for dilution in hydrogen peroxide 3%. Tab. Pkg. 5s, 10s.
Use: Soft contact lens care.

ULTRUM. (Towne) Vitamins A 5000 IU, E 30 IU, C 90 mg, folic acid 400 mcg, B_1 2.25 mg, B_2 2.6 mg, niacinamide 20 mg, B_6 3 mg, B_{12} 9 mcg, biotin 45 mcg, D 400 IU, pantothenic acid 10 mg, calcium 162 mg, phosphorus 125 mg, iodine 150 mcg, iron 27 mg, magnesium 100 mg, copper 3 mg, manganese 7.5 mg, potassium 7.5 mg, zinc 22.5 mg/Tab. Bot. 100s.
Use: Vitamin/mineral supplement.

ULTRUM WITH SELENIUM. (Towne) Vitamins A 5000 IU, E 30 IU, C 90 mg, folic acid 2.25 mg, B_1 2.25 mg, B_2 2.6 mg, niacinamide 20 mg, B_6 3 mg, B_{12} 9 mcg, D 400 IU, biotin 45 mcg, pantothenic acid 10 mg, calcium 162 mg, phosphorus 125 mg, iodine 150 mcg, iron 27 mg, magnesium 100 mg, copper 3 mg, manganese 7.5 mg, potassium 7.7 mg, chloride 7 mg, molybdenum 15 mcg, selenium 15 mcg, zinc 22.5 mg/Tab. Bot. 130s.
Use: Vitamin/mineral supplement.

UNASYN. (Roerig) Ampicillin sodium 1 Gm, sulbactam sodium 0.5 Gm, ampicillin sodium 2 Gm, sulbactam sodium 1 Gm. Pow. for inj. Vial, piggyback vial.
Use: Antibacterial, penicillin.

10-UNDECENOIC ACID. Undecylenic Acid, U.S.P. XXII.
Use: Antifungal, external.

10-UNDECENOIC ACID, ZINC (2+) SALT. Zinc Undecylenate, U.S.P. XXII.
Use: Antifungal, external.

UNDECOYLIUM CHLORIDE-IODINE. 1-[[(2-Hydroxyethyl) carbamoyl]methyl]-pyridimium Cl alka-noates compound with I_2 (1:1). Virac, Preps. (Ruson).
Use: Anti-infective, external.

•**UNDECYLENIC ACID,** U.S.P. XXII. Compound Oint. U.S.P. XXII. 10-Undecenoic acid. (Lannett) Cap. 0.44 Gm, Bot. 100s, 500s, 1000s.
Use: Topical antifungal.
See: Desenex Liquid, Penetrating Foam (Pharmacraft).
W/Benzethonium Cl, benzalkonium Cl, tannic acid, isopropyl alcohol.
See: Tulvex, Liq. (Commerce).
W/Dichlorophene.
See: Fungicidal Talc (Gordon).

Onychomyootin, Liq. (Gordon).
W/Salicylic acid.
See: Sal-Dex, Liq. (Scrip).
W/Salicylic acid, benzoic acid, sulfur, dichlorophene.
See: Fungicidal, Oint. (Gordon).
W/Salicylic acid, dichlorophene, hexachlorophene.
See: Podiaspray, Aerosol Pow. (Dalin).
W/Sodium propionate, sodium caprylate, propionic acid, salicylic acid, copper undecylenate.
See: Verdefam, Soln. (Texas).
W/Zinc undecylenate.
See: Cruex Cream, Spray Pow. (Pharmacraft)
Desenex, Preps. (Pharmacraft).
Ting, Aerosol (Pharmacraft).
Undoguent, Cream (Torch).

UNDECYLENIC ACID SALTS. Calcium, copper, zinc.

UNDELENIC OINTMENT. (Gordon) Undecylenic acid 5%, zinc undecylenate 20%. Jar oz, lb.
Use: Antifungal, external.

UNDELENIC TINCTURE. (Gordon) Undecylenic acid 10%, chloroxylenol 0.5%. Brush Bot. oz. Bot. pt.
Use: Antifungal, external.

UNDEX CREAM. (Durel) Undecylenic acid 5%, zinc undecylenate 5% in duromantel cream.
Use: Antifungal, external.

UNDOGUENT. (Torch) Undecylenic acid 5%, zinc undecylenate 20% in a non-greasy, water-washable cream base. Jar 2 oz, lb.
Use: Antifungal, external.

UNDULANT FEVER DIAGNOSIS. Brucella Abortus Antigen. Brucellergen.

UNGUENTINE OINTMENT "ORIGINAL FORMULA." (Mentholatum) Phenol 1% in ointment base. Tube oz.
Use: Minor skin irritations.

UNGUENTINE PLUS FIRST AID CREAM. (Mentholatum) Parachlorometaxylenol 2%, lidocaine HCl 2%, phenol 0.5% in a moisturizing cream base. Tube ½ oz, 1 oz, 2 oz.
Use: Minor skin irritations.

UNGUENTINE SPRAY. (Mentholatum) Benzocaine, alcohol. Can 5 oz.
Use: Minor skin irritations.

UNGUENTUM BOSSI. (Doak) Ammoniated mercury 5%, hexamethylene tetramine sulfosalicylic acid 2%, tar distillate "Doak" 5%, Doak oil 40%, nonionic emulsifiers 5%, unguentum "Doak" 48%. Tube 2 oz. Jar 16 oz.
Use: Antipsoriatic.

UNIAD. (Kasar) Isoniazid 100 mg/Tab. Bot. 100s, 1000s.
Use: Antituberculous agent.

UNIAD-PLUS. (Kasar) Isoniazid 100 mg, pyridoxine HCl 5 mg or 10 mg/Tab. Bot. 1000s.
Use: Antituberculous agent.

UNIBASE. (Parke-Davis) Water-absorbing oint. base. Jar lb.
Use: Ointment base.

UNICAP. (Upjohn) Vitamins A 5000 IU, D 400 IU, E 16.5 mg, C 60 mg, folic acid 400 mcg, B_1 1.5 mg, B_2 1.7 mg, niacin 20 mg, B_6 2 mg, B_{12} 6 mcg, tartrazine/Tab. or Cap. **Tab.:** Bot. 90s, 120s. **Cap.:** Bot. 90s, 120s, 240s, 1000s.
Use: Vitamin supplement.

UNICAP JUNIOR CHEWABLE. (Upjohn) Vitamins A 5000 IU, D 400 IU, E 15 IU, C 60 mg, folic acid 400 mcg, B_1 1.5 mg, B_2 1.7 mg, niacin 20 mg, B_6 2 mg, B_{12} 6 mcg/Tab. Bot. 90s, 120s.
Use: Vitamin supplement.

UNICAP M. (Upjohn) Vitamins A 5000 IU, D 400 IU, E 33 mg, C 60 mg, folic acid 400 mcg, B_1 1.5 mg, B_2 1.7 mg, niacin 20 mg, B_6 2 mg, B_{12} 6 mcg, pantothenic acid 10 mg, iodine 150 mcg, iron 18 mg, copper 2 mg, zinc 15 mg, calcium 60 mg, phosphorus 45 mg, manganese 1 mg, potassium 5 mg, tartrazine/Tab. Bot. 30s, 90s, 180s, 500s.
Use: Vitamin/mineral supplement.

UNICAP PLUS IRON. (Upjohn) Vitamins A 5000 IU, D 400 IU, E 16.5 mg, C 60 mg, folic acid 400 mcg, B_1 1.5 mg, B_2 1.7 mg, niacin 20 mg, B_6 2 mg, B_{12} 6 mcg, pantothenic acid 10 mg, iron 18 mg/Tab. Bot. 90s.
Use: Vitamin/mineral supplement.

UNICAP SENIOR. (Upjohn) Vitamins A 5000 IU, D 200 IU, E 16.5 mg, C 60 mg, folic acid 400 mcg, B_1 1.2 mg, B_2 1.4 mg, niacin 16 mg, B_6 2.2 mg, B_{12} 3 mcg, pantothenic acid 10 mg, iodine 150 mcg, iron 10 mg, copper 2 mg, zinc 15 mg, calcium 100 mg, phosphorus 77 mg, magnesium 30 mg, manganese 1 mg, potassium 5 mg/Tab. Bot. 90s.
Use: Vitamin/mineral supplement.

UNICAP T. (Upjohn) Vitamins A 5000 IU, D 400 IU, E 33 mg, C 500 mg, folic acid 400 mcg, B_1 10 mg, B_2 10 mg, niacin 100 mg, B_6 6 mg, B_{12} 18 mcg, pantothenic acid 25 mg, iodine 150 mcg, iron 18 mg, copper 2 mg, zinc 15 mg, manganese 1 mg, potassium 5 mg, selenium 10 mcg/Tab. Bot. 60s, 500s.
Use: Vitamin/mineral supplement.

UNICOMPLEX-M. (Rugby) Iron 18 mg, vitamins A 5000 IU, D 400 IU, E 15 mg, B_1 1.5 mg, B_2 1.7 mg, B_3 20 mg, B_5 10 mg, B_6 2 mg, B_{12} 6 mcg, C 60 mg, folic acid 0.4 mg, Ca, Cu, I, K, Mn, Zn/Tab. Bot. 90s, 1000s.
Use: Vitamin/mineral supplement.

UNICOMPLEX-T WITH MINERALS. (Rugby) Iron 10 mg, vitamins A 5000 IU, D 400 IU, E 15 mg, B_1 10 mg, B_2 10 mg, B_3 100 mg, B_5 20 mg, B_6 2 mg, B_{12} 4 mcg, C 300 mg, folic acid 0.4 mg, Ca, Cu, I, K, Mg, Mn/Tab. Bot. 60s, 1000s.
Use: Vitamin/mineral supplement.

•**UNIFOCON A.** USAN.
Use: Contact lens material.

UNIPEN. (Wyeth-Ayerst) Sodium nafcillin. **Cap.:** 250 mg. Bot. 100s, Redipak 100s. **Tab.:** 500 mg. Bot. 50s. Cap. and Tab. buffered w/calcium carbonate. **Vial:** Vial 2 Gm, Piggyback Vial 2

Gm, Bulk vial 10 Gm. **Oral Soln.** 250 mg/5 ml w/alcohol 2%. Bot. to make 100 ml.
Use: Antibacterial, penicillin.

UNIPHYL TABLETS. (Purdue Frederick) Theophylline 200 mg or 400 mg/Controlled-release Tab. **200 mg:** Bot. 60s, 100s, UD 100s. **400 mg:** Bot. 60s, 100s, 500s, UD 100s.
Use: Bronchodilator.

UNIPRES. (Solvay) Hydralazine HCl 25 mg, hydrochlorothiazide 15 mg, reserpine 0.1 mg/Tab. Bot. 100s, 1000s.
Use: Antihypertensive.

UNISOL. (CooperVision) Buffered isotonic solution with sodium Cl, boric acid, sodium borate. Bot. 15 ml.
Use: Soft contact lens care.

UNISOL 4 STERILE SALINE. (CooperVision) Buffered isotonic solution with sodium Cl, boric acid, sodium borate. Bot. 120 ml.
Use: Soft contact lens care.

UNISOM. (Leeming) Doxylamine succcinate 25 mg/Tab. Blister 8s, 16s, 32s, 48s.
Use: Sleep aid.

UNISOM DUAL RELIEF. (Leeming) Acetaminophen 650 mg, diphenhydramine HCl 50 mg/Tab. Blister 8s, 16s, 32s.
Use: Analgesic, sleep aid.

UNITROL. (Republic Drug) Phenylpropanolamine HCl 75 mg/TR Cap. Pkg. 28s.
Use: Diet aid.

UNI-TUSSIN SYRUP. (United Research Laboratories) Dextromethorphan HBr 15 mg, guaifenesin 100 mg, alcohol 1.4%. Bot. 120 ml.
Use: Antitussive, expectorant.

UNNA'S BOOT.
See: Zinc Gelatin, U.S.P. XXII.

UNPROCO CAPSULES. (Solvay) Dextromethorphan HBr 30 mg, guaifenesin 200 mg/Cap. Bot. 100s.
Use: Antitussive, expectorant.

UNSATURATED ACIDS.
See: Fatty acids, unsaturated; fats, unsaturated.

UPLEX. (Arcum) Vitamins A 5000 IU, D 400 IU, B_1 3 mg, B_2 3 mg, B_6 1 mg, B_{12} 2.5 mcg, nicotinamide 20 mg, calcium pantothenate 5 mg, C 50 mg/Cap. Bot. 100s, 1000s.
Use: Vitamin supplement.

UPLEX NO. 2. (Arcum) Vitamins A palmitate 10,000 IU, D 400 IU, B_1 5 mg, B_2 5 mg, C 100 mg, B_6 2 mg, B_{12} 3 mcg, E 2.5 IU, niacinamide 25 mg, calcium pantothenate 5 mg/Cap. Bot. 100s, 1000s.
Use: Vitamin supplement.

URABETH TABS. (Major) Bethanechol 5 mg, 10 mg, 25 mg or 50 mg/Tab. **5 mg:** Bot. 100s. **10 mg:** Bot. 250s. **25 mg:** Bot. 250s, 1000s. **50 mg:** Bot. 100s, UD 100s.
Use: Urinary tract product.

URACID. (Wesley) dl-Methionine 0.2 Gm/Cap. Bot. 100s, 1000s.
Use: Diaper rash product.

•**URACIL MUSTARD,** U.S.P. XXII. Cap., U.S.P. XXII. 5-[Bis(2-Chloroethyl)amino]uracil. (Upjohn) 1 mg/Cap. Bot. 50s.
Use: Antineoplastic.

URADAL.
See: Carbromal (Various Mfr.)

URAMUSTINE. B.A.N. 5-Di-(2-chloroethyl) aminouracil.
Use: Antineoplastic agent.

URAPINE TABS. (Major) Bot. 1000s.
Use: Urinary analgesic.

URDEX. (Pharmex) Phenylpropanolamine 12.5 mg, atropine sulfate 0.2 mg, chlorpheniramine 5 mg/ml. Vial 10 ml.
Use: Decongestant, anticholinergic/antispasmodic, antihistamine.

•**UREA,** U.S.P. XXII. Sterile U.S.P. XXII. Carbamide.
Use: Topically for dry skin; diuretic.
See: Aquacare, Cream, Lot. (Herbert).
Aquacare-HP, Cream, Lot. (Herbert).
Artra Ashy Skin, Cream (Schering-Plough).
Calmurid, Cream (Pharmacia).
Carmol, Cream (Ingram).
Carmol Ten, Lot. (Ingram).
Elaqua 10% or 20%, Cream (Elder).
Gormel, Cream (Gordon).
Nutraplus, Cream, Lot. (Owen).
Rea-lo, Lot. (Whorton).
W/Benzocaine, benzyl alcohol, p-chloro-m-xylenol, propyleneglycol.
See: 20-Cain Burn Relief (Alto).
W/Hydrocortisone acetate.
See: Carmol-HC, Cream (Ingram).
W/Glycerin.
See: Kerid Ear Drops, Liq. (Blair).
W/Sulfur colloidal, red mercuric sulfide.
See: Teenac, Cream, Oint. (Elder).
W/Zinc oxide, sulfur, salicylic acid, benzalkonium Cl, isopropyl alcohol.
See: Akne Drying Lotion (Alto).

UREACIN-10 LOTION. (Pedinol) Urea 10%. Bot. 8 oz.
Use: Emolllent.

UREACIN-20 CREME. (Pedinol) Urea 20%. Jar 2.5 oz.
Use: Emollient.

UREACIN-40 CREME. (Pedinol) Urea 40%. Jar oz.
Use: Treatment of nail destruction and dissolution.

UREA PEROXIDE.

UREAPHIL. (Abbott Hospital Prods) Sterile urea 40 Gm, citric acid 1 mg/150 ml. Bot. 150 ml.
Use: Osmotic diuretic.

URECHOLINE. (Merck Sharp & Dohme) Bethanechol Cl. **Inj.:** 5 mg/ml Vial 1 ml, 6s. **Tab.:** 5 mg, 10 mg, 25 mg or 50 mg. Bot. 100s, UD 100s.
Use: Urinary tract product.

•**UREDEPA.** USAN. Ethyl[bis(1-aziridinyl)-phosphinyl]carbamate.

Use: Antineoplastic.
See: Avinar (Armour).
p-UREIDOBENZENEARSONIC ACID.
See: Carbarsone, U.S.P. XXII.
•**UREDOFOS.** USAN.
Use: Anthelmintic.
See: Sansalid (Beecham).
URELIEF. (Rocky Mtn.) Methenamine 2 gr, salol 0.5 gr, methylene blue 1/10 gr, benzoic acid 1/8 gr, hyoscyamine sulfate 1/2000 gr, atropine sulfate 1/1000 gr/Tab. Bot. 100s.
Use: Urinary anti-infective.
URESE. (Roerig)
See: Benzthianide.
URETHAN. Ethyl Carbamate, Ethyl Urethan, Urethane.
Use: Antineoplastic agent.
UREX TABLETS. (Riker) Methenamine hippurate 1 Gm/Tab. Bot. 100s, 500s.
Use: Urinary anti-infective.
URICOSURIC AGENTS.
See: Anturane, Tab., Cap. (Geigy).
Benemid, Tab. (Merck Sharp & Dohme).
ColBenemid, Tab. (Merck Sharp & Dohme).
U.R.I. (Sig) Atropine sulfate 0.2 mg, chlorpheniramine maleate 5 mg, phenylpropanolamine HCl 12.5 mg/ml. Vial 10 ml.
Use: Anticholinergic/antispasmodic, antihistamine, decongestant.
URIC ACID REAGENT STRIPS. (Ames) Seralyzer reagent strip. For uric acid in serum or plasma. Bot. 25s.
Use: Diagnostic aid.
URIDINE, 2-DEOXY-5-IODO-. Idoxuridine, U.S.P. XXII.
URIDIUM. (Ferndale; Pharmex) Phenylazodiamine pyridine HCl 75 mg, sulfacetamide 250 mg/Tab. Bot. 30s, 100s, 1000s. (Ferndale) 100s.
Use: Urinary anti-infective.
URIDON MODIFIED. (Rugby) Methenamine 40.8 mg, phenylsalicylate 18.1 mg, atropine sulfate 0.03 mg, hyoscyamine 0.03 mg, benzoic acid 4.5 mg, methylene blue 5.4 mg/Tab. Bot. 100s, 1000s.
Use: Urinary anti-infective.
URIFON-FORTE. (T.E. Williams) Sulfamethizole 450 mg, phenazopyridine HCl 50 mg/Cap. Bot. 100s, 1000s.
Use: Urinary anti-infective.
URIGEN. (Fellows) Calcium mandelate 0.2 Gm, methenamine 0.2 Gm, phenazopyridine HCl 50 mg, sodium phosphate 80 mg/Cap. Bot. 100s, 1000s.
Use: Urinary anti-infective.
URINARY ANTISEPTIC #2. (Vitarine) Atropine sulfate 0.03 mg, hyoscyamine 0.03 mg, methenamine 40.8 mg, methylene blue 5.4 mg, phenylsalicylate 18.1 mg, benzoic acid 4.5 mg/Tab. Bot. 100s, 1000s.
Use: Urinary anti-infective.
URINARY ANTISEPTIC #2 S.C.T. (Lemmon) Atropine sulfate 0.03 mg, hyoscyamine sulfate 0.03 mg, methenamine 40.8 mg, methylene blue 5.4 mg, phenyl salicylate 18.1 mg, bonzoic acid 4.5 mg/Tab. Bot. 100s, 1000s.
Use: Urinary anti-infective.
URINARY ANTISEPTIC #3 S.C.T.. (Lemmon) Atropine sulfate 0.06 mg, hyoscyamine sulfate 0.03 mg, methenamine 120 mg, methylene blue 6 mg, phenyl salicylate 30 mg, benzoic acid 7.5 mg/Tab. Bot. 100s, 1000s.
Use: Urinary anti-infective.
URINE.
See: Diagnostic agents.
URINE SUGAR TEST.
See: Clinistix (Ames).
URIN-TEK. (Ames) Tubes, plastic caps, adhesive labels, collection cups, and disposable tube holder. Package 100×5.
URISAN-P. (Sandia) Atropine sulfate 0.03 mg, hyoscyamine 0.03 mg, gelsemium 6.1 mg, methenamine 40.8 mg, salol 18.1 mg, benzoic acid 4.5 mg, methylene blue 5.4 mg, phenylazodiaminopyridine HCl 100 mg/Tab. Bot. 100s, 1000s.
Use: Urinary anti-infective.
URISED. (Webcon) Atropine sulfate 0.03 mg, hyoscyamine 0.03 mg, methenamine 40.8 mg, methylene blue 5.4 mg, benzoic acid 4.5 mg, phenyl salicylate 18.1 mg/Tab. Bot. 100s, 500s, 1000s.
Use: Urinary anti-infective.
URISEDAMINE. (Webcon) Methenamine mandelate 500 mg, l-hyoscyamine 0.15 mg/Tab. Bot. 100s.
Use: Urinary anti-infective.
URISEPT. (Robinson) Urinary antiseptic. Tab. Bot. 100s, 1000s.
Use: Urinary tract product.
URISPAS. (SmithKline) Flavoxate HCl 100 mg/Tab. Bot. 100s, UD 100s.
Use: Urinary antispasmodic.
URISTIX 4 REAGENT STRIPS. (Ames) Urinalysis reagent strip test for glucose, protein, nitrite, leukocytes. Bot. 100s.
Use: Diagnostic aid.
URISTIX REAGENT STRIPS. (Ames) Urinalysis reagent strip test for protein and glucose. Bot. 100s.
Use: Diagnostic aid.
URI-TET. (American Urologicals) Oxytetracycline HCl 250 mg/Cap. Bot. 100s, 1000s.
Use: Antibacterial, tetracycline.
URITIN. (Richlyn) Methenamine 40.8 mg, atropine sulfate 0.03 mg, hyoscyamine sulfate 0.03 mg, salol 18.1 mg, benzoic acid 4.5 mg, methylene blue 5.4 mg, gelsemium 6.1 mg/Tab. Bot. 1000s.
Use: Urinary anti-infective.
URITIN FORMULA. (Vangard) Atropine sulfate 0.03 mg, hyoscyamine 0.03 mg, methenamine 40.8 mg, methylene blue 5.4 mg, phenyl salicylate 18.1 mg, benzoic acid 4.5 mg/Tab. Bot. 1000s.

Use: Urinary anti-infective.

URITROL. (Kenyon) Atropine sulfate 0.03 mg, hyoscyamine 0.03 mg, gelsemium 6.1 mg, methenamine 40.8 mg, salol 18.1 mg, benzoic acid 4.5 mg, methylene blue 5.4 mg/Tab. Bot. 100s, 1000s. Double Strength Tab. Bot. 100s, 1000s.
Use: Urinary anti-infective.

URIZOLE. (Jenkins) Sulfisoxazole 7.7 gr/Tab. Bot. 1000s.
Use: Antibacterial, sulfonamide.

UROBAK. (Shionogi) Sulfamethoxazole 500 mg/Tab. Bot. 100s, 1000s.
Use: Antibacterial, sulfonamide.

UROBIOTIC. (Roerig) Oxytetracycline as the HCl equivalent to oxytetracycline 250 mg, sulfamethizole 250 mg, phenazopyridine HCl 50 mg/Cap. Bot. 50s, UD pack Box 100s.
Use: Urinary anti-infective.

UROCIT-K. (Mission) Potassium citrate 540 mg/Tab. Bot. 100s.
Use: Urinary tract product.

URODINE. (Interstate) Phenazopyridine HCl 100 mg/Tab. Bot. 1000s.
Use: Urinary analgesic.

URODINE. (Kenyon) Phenylazodiaminopyridine HCl 100 mg/Tab. Bot. 100s, 1000s.
Use: Urinary analgesic.

URODINE. (Robinson) Phenylazodiaminopyridine HCl 1.5 gr/Tab. Bot. 100s, 1000s.
Use: Urinary analgesic.

•**UROFOLLITROPIN.** USAN.
Use: Hormone (follicle-stimulating). Induction of ovulation in patients with polycystic ovary disease.
See: Metrodin, Inj. (Serono).

UROGESIC. (Edwards) Phenazopyridine HCl 100 mg, hyoscyamine HBr 0.12 mg, atropine sulfate 0.08 mg, scopolamine HBr 0.003 mg/Tab. Bot. 100s, 500s.
Use: Urinary analgesic.

UROGRAPHY AGENTS.
See: Diodrast.
Iodohippurate Sodium, Inj.
Iodopyracet.
Iodopyracet Compound.
Methiodal, Inj.
Renografin (Squibb).
Renovist (Squibb).
Renovue (Squibb).
Sodium Acetrizoate, Inj.
Sodium Iodomethamate, Inj.

•**UROKINASE.** USAN. Plasminogen activator isolated from human kidney tissue.
Use: Plasminogen activator.

URO-KP-NEUTRAL. (Star) Sodium (as dibasic sodium phosphate) 1361 mg, potassium 298.6 mg, phosphorus (as dibasic potassium phosphate) 1037 mg/6 Tab. Bot. 100s.
Use: Phosphorus supplement.

UROLENE BLUE. (Star) Methylene blue 65 mg/Tab. Bot. 100s, 1000s.
Use: Urinary anti-infective.

UROLOGIC SOL G. (Abbott Hospital Prods) Bot. 1000 ml.
Use: Irrigating solution.
See: Thiosulfi, Preps. (Wyeth-Ayerst).

URO-MAG. (Blaine) Magnesium oxide 140 mg/Cap. Bot. 100s, 1000s.
Use: Antacid.

URONAL.
See: Barbital (Various Mfr.).

URO-PHOSPHATE. (Poythress) Sodium biphosphate 500 mg, methenamine 300 mg/Film Coated Tab. Bot. 100s, 1000s.
Use: Urinary anti-infective.

UROPLUS DS. (Shionogi) Trimethoprim 160 mg, sulfamethoxazole 800 mg/Tab. Bot. 100s, 500s.
Use: Anti-infective.

UROPLUS SS. (Shionogi) Trimethoprim 80 mg, sulfamethoxazole 800 mg/Tab. Bot. 100s, 500s.
Use: Anti-infective.

UROQID-ACID. (Beach) Methenamine mandelate 350 mg, sodium acid phosphate 200 mg/Tab. Bot. 100s, 500s.
Use: Urinary anti-infective.

UROQID-ACID NO. 2. (Beach) Methenamine mandelate 500 mg, sodium acid phosphate 500 mg/Tab. Bot. 100s, 500s.
Use: Urinary anti-infective.

UROTROL. (Mills) Sulfacetamide 250 mg, sulfamethizole 250 mg, phenazopyridine HCl 50 mg/Tab. Bot. 100s.
Use: Urinary anti-infective.

UROTROPIN NEW. Methenamine Anhydromethylene Citrate (Various Mfr.).

URO-VES. (Mallard) Methenamine 40.8 mg, phenyl salicylate 18.1 mg, atropine sulfate 0.03 mg, hyoscyamine 0.03 mg, benzoic acid 4.5 mg, methylene blue 5.4 mg/Tab. Bot. 1000s.
Use: Urinary anti-infective.

UROVIST CYSTO. (Berlex) Diatrizoate meglumine 300 mg, edetate calcium disodium 0.05 mg/ml. Dilution bot. 500 ml w/300 ml soln.
Use: Radiopaque agent.

UROVIST CYSTO PEDIATRIC. (Berlex) Diatrizoate meglumine 300 mg, edetate calcium disodium 0.1 mg/ml. Dilution bot. 300 ml w/100 ml soln.
Use: Radiopaque agent.

UROVIST MEGLUMINE DIU/CT. (Berlex) Diatrizoate meglumine 300 mg, edetate calcium disodium 0.05 mg/ml. Bot. 300 ml, Ctn. 10s.
Use: Radiopaque agent.

UROVIST SODIUM 300. (Berlex) Diatrizoate sodium 500 mg, edetate calcium disodium 0.1 mg/ml. Vial 50 ml, Box 10s.
Use: Radiopaque agent.

URSINUS INLAY-TABS. (Sandoz Consumer) Pseudoephedrine HCl 30 mg, aspirin 325 mg/Tab. Bot. 24s, 100s.
Use: Decongestant, salicylate analgesic.

URSODIOL. Ursodeoxycholic acid.
Use: Gallstone solubilizing agent.
See: Actigall (Ciba).

URSULFADINE NO. 1. (Kenyon) Phenylazodiaminopyridine HCl 50 mg, sulfacetamide 250 mg/Tab. Bot. 100s, 1000s.
Use: Urinary anti-infective.

UTICORT CREAM. (Parke-Davis) Betamethasone benzoate 0.025%. Tube 15 Gm, 60 Gm.
Use: Corticosteroid.

UTICORT GEL. (Parke-Davis) Betamethasone benzoate 0.025% in solubilized gel base. Tube 15 Gm, 60 Gm.
Use: Corticosteroid.

UTICORT LOTION. (Parke-Davis) Betamethasone benzoate 0.025%. Bot. 15 ml, 60 ml.
Use: Corticosteroid.

UTIMOX. (Parke-Davis) Amoxicillin trihydrate. **Cap.:** 250 mg Bot. 100s, 500s, UD 100s; 500 mg Bot. 100s, UD 100s; **Oral susp.:** 125 mg or 250 mg/5 ml Bot. 80 ml, 100 ml, 150 ml, 200 ml.
Use: Antibacterial, penicillin.

U-TRAN. (Scruggs) Atropine sulfate 0.03 mg, hyoscyamine 0.03 mg, methenamine 40.8 mg, benzoic acid 4.5 mg, salol 18.1 mg, methylene blue 5.4 mg/Tab. Bot. 100s, 1000s.
Use: Urinary anti-infective.

U-TRI SPECIAL FORMULA OINTMENT. (U-Tri) Oint. Jar 4 oz, 7 oz.
Use: External analgesic.

UVALERAL.
See: Bromisovalum.

UVASAL POWDER. (Winthrop Products) Sodium bicarbonate, tartaric acid.
Use: Antacid.

UVA URSI. Leaves. (Sherwood Labs.) Fluidextract. Bot. pt, gal.

UVIBAN. Sodium Actinoquinol.
Use: Treatment of flash burns (ophthalmic).

UVINUL MS-40. (General Aniline & Film)
See: Sulisobenzone.

V

VACCINE, MUMPS. Mumps Virus Vaccine Live, U.S.P. XXII.
Agent for immunization.

VACCINE, PERTUSSIS. Pertussis Vaccine, U.S.P. XXII.
Use: Active immunizing agent.

VACCINE, PERTUSSIS, ADSORBED. Pertussis Vaccine Adsorbed, U.S.P. XXII.
Use: Active immunizing agent.
See: Pertussis Vaccine, Aluminum Hydroxide Adsorbed.

VACCINE, PERTUSSIS, ALUM PRECIPITATED.
Use: Agent for immunization.
See: Pertussis Vaccine, Alum Precipitated (Various Mfr.).

VACCINE, POLIOMYELITIS. Poliovirus Vaccine Inactivated, U.S.P. XXII.
Use: Active immunizing agent.

•**VACCINE, RABIES (DUCK EMBRYO),** Rabies Vaccine U.S.P. XXII.
Use: Active immunizing agent.

•**VACCINE, SMALLPOX.** Smallpox Vaccine, U.S.P. XXII.
Use: Active immunizing agent.

VACCINE, WHOOPING COUGH. Pertussis Vaccine, U.S.P. XXII.
Use: Active immunizing agent.

•**VACCINIA IMMUNE GLOBULIN,** U.S.P. XXII. (Hyland) Gamma globulin fraction of serum of healthy adults recently immunized w/vaccinia virus 16.5%. Vial 5 ml.
Use: Prevention or modification of smallpox or vaccinia infections; passive immunizing agent.

VACOCIN. Under study.
Use: Antibiotic.

VADEMIN-Z. (Hauck) Vitamin A 12,500 IU, D 50 IU, E 50 mg, B_1 10 mg, B_2 5 mg, B_3 25 mg, B_5 10 mg, B_6 2 mg, C 150 mg, zinc 20 mg, Mg, Mn/Cap. Bot. 60s, 500s.
Use: Vitamin/mineral supplement.

VAGILLA TRIPLE SULFA. (Lemmon) Sulfathiazole 3.42%, sulfacetamide 2.86%, sulfabenzamide 3.7%, urea 0.64% in cream base. Tube 78 Gm.
Use: Anti-infective, vaginal.

VAGINEX CREME. (Schmid) Benzocaine, resorcinol in cream base.
Use: Vaginal preparation.

VAGISAN CREME. (Sandia) Sulfanilamide 15%, 9-aminoacridine HCl 0.2%, allantoin 1.5% in a dispersible base. Tube 4 oz w/applicator.
Use: Anti-infective, vaginal.

VAGISEC. (Schmid) Polyoxyethylene nonyl phenol, sodium ethylene diamine tetraacetate, docusate sodium. Plastic Bot. 4 oz. Liq. Packette 12s.
Use: Vaginal preparation.

VAGISEC PLUS SUPPOSITORIES. (Schmid) Polyoxyethylene nonyl phenol 5.25 mg, sodium edetate 0.66 mg, docusate sodium 0.07 mg, 9-aminoacridine HCl 6 mg, in a polyethylene glycol base w/glycerin, citric acid. Box 28s.
Use: Vaginal preparation.

VAGISTAT. (Fujisawa SmithKline) Tioconazole 6.5%. Vaginal oint. Prefilled applicator 4.6 Gm.
Use: Antifungal, vaginal.

VAGISUL CREME. (Sheryl) Sulfanilamide 15%, aminoacridine 0.2%, allantoin 1.5%. Tube 4 oz.
Use: Anti-infective, vaginal.

VAGITROL. (Lemmon) Sulfanilamide 15% in cream base. Tube 113 Gm.
Use: Anti-infective, vaginal.

VALACET. (Vale) Hyoscyamus 10.8 mg, aspirin 259.2 mg, caffeine anhydrous 16.2 mg, gelsemium extract 0.6 mg/Tab. or Cap. Bot. 100s, 1000s, 5000s.
Use: Anticholinergic/antispasmodic, salicylate analgesic.

VALADOL. (Squibb Mark) Acetaminophen 5 gr/Tab. Bot. 100s, 500s.

Use: Analgesic.

VALERGEN. (Hyrex) Estradiol valerate 10 mg, 20 mg or 40 mg/ml. Vial 10 ml.
Use: Estrogen.

VALERIAN. (Lilly) Tincture, alcohol 68%. Bot. 4 fl oz, 16 fl oz.
W/Phenobarbital, passiflora, hyoscyamus.
See: Aluro, Tab. (Foy).

VALERTEST. (Hyrex) **No. 1:** Estradiol valerate 4 mg, testosterone enanthate 90 mg/ml. Vial 10 ml. **No. 2:** Double strength. Vial 10 ml. Amp. 2 ml, 10s.
Use: Estrogen, androgen combination.

VALETHAMATE BROMIDE. 2-Diethylaminoethyl 3-methyl-2-phenylvalerate methylbromide. Diethyl(2-hydroxyethyl)methyl-ammonium bromide 3-methyl-2-phenylvalerate. Murel.
Use: Anticholinergic.

VALIHIST TABLETS. (Otis Clapp) Phenylephrine 5 mg, acetaminophen 325 mg, chlorpheniramine maleate 2 mg, caffeine 45 mg/Tab. Bot. 500s.
Use: Decongestant, analgesic, antihistamine.

•**VALINE,** U.S.P. XXII. $C_5H_{11}NO_2$ as L-valine.
Use: Amino acid.

VALISONE. (Schering) Betamethasone valerate.
Cream: 1 mg/Gm Hydrophilic cream of water, mineral oil, petrolatum, polyethylene glycol 1000 monocetyl ether, cetostearyl alcohol, monobasic sodium phosphate, phosphoric acid, 4-chloro-m-cresol as preservative. Tube 15 Gm, 45 Gm, 110 Gm. Jar 430 Gm.
Oint.: 1 mg/Gm Base of liquid and white petrolatum and hydrogenated lanolin. Tube 15 Gm, 45 Gm.
Lot.: 1 mg/Gm w/isopropyl alcohol 47.5%, water slightly thickened w/carboxy vinyl polymer, pH adjusted w/sodium hydroxide. Bot. 20 ml, 60 ml.
Reduced Strength Cream 0.01%: Hydrophilic cream of water, mineral oil, petrolatum, polyethylene glycol 1000 monocetyl ether, cetostearyl alcohol, monobasic sodium phosphate, phosphoric acid, 4-chloro-m-cresol as preservative. Tube 15 Gm, 60 Gm.
Use: Corticosteroid.

VALIUM TABLETS. (Roche) Diazepam 2 mg, 5 mg or 10 mg/Tab. Bot. 100s, 500s, Tel-E-Dose 100s (10×10), (4×25) RPN (Reverse Numbered Packages), Prescription Pak 50s.
Use: Antianxiety agent.

VALIUM INJECTABLE. (Roche) Diazepam 5 mg/ml, propylene glycol 40%, ethyl alcohol 10%, sodium benzoate, benzoic acid 5%, benzyl alcohol 1.5%. Amp. 2 ml, 10s. Vial 10 ml, Box 10s. Tel-E-Ject (Disposable syringe) 2 ml, Box 10s.
Use: Antianxiety agent.

VALLERGINE.
See: Promethazine HCl, U.S.P. XXII.

VALNAC CREAM. (NMC Labs) Betamethasone valerate 0.1%. Cream Tube 15 Gm, 45 Gm.
Use: Corticosteroid.

VALNAC OINTMENT. (NMC Labs) Betamethasone valerate 0.1%. Oint. Tube 15 Gm, 45 Gm.
Use: Corticosteroid.

•**VALNOCTAMIDE.** USAN.
Use: Tranquilizer.

VALORIN. (Otis Clapp) Acetaminophen 325 mg/Tab. Sugar, caffeine, lactose and salt free. Safety pack 500s, Aidpack 100s.
Use: Analgesic.

VALORIN EXTRA. (Otis Clapp) Acetaminophen 500 mg/Tab. Sugar, caffeine, lactose and salt free. Safety pack 500s, Aidpack 100s.
Use: Analgesic.

VALORIN SUPER. (Otis Clapp) Acetaminophen 500 mg/Tab. w/caffeine. Sugar, salt, lactose free. Safety pack 500s.
Use: Analgesic.

VALPIN 50. (Du Pont) Anisotropine methylbromide 50 mg/Tab. Bot. 100s.
Use: Anticholinergic/antispasmodic.

VALPIPAMATE METHYLSULFATE.
See: Pentapiperide Methylsulfate.

•**VALPROATE SODIUM.** USAN.
Use: Anticonvulsant.

•**VALPROIC ACID,** U.S.P. XXII. Cap., Syr., U.S.P. XXII. 2-Propylpentanoic acid.
Use: Anticonvulsant.
See: Depakene, Cap., Liq. (Abbott).
Myproic Acid Syr. (PBI).

VALRELEASE. (Roche) Diazepam 15 mg/SR Cap. Bot. 100s, Prescription Pak 30s.
Use: Antianxiety agent.

VALUPHED. (H.L. Moore) Pseudoephedrine HCl 60 mg, triprolidine HCl 2.5 mg/Tab. Pkg. 24s.
Use: Decongestant, antihistamine.

VAMATE. (Major) Hydroxyzine pamoate 50 mg/Cap. Bot. 100s, 250s, 500s, UD 100s.
Use: Antianxiety agent.

VANADRYX TR. (Vangard) Dexbrompheniramine maleate 6 mg, psuedoephedrine sulfate 120 mg/Tab. Bot. 100s, 500s.
Use: Antihistamine, decongestant.

VANCENASE AQ NASAL. (Schering) Beclomethasone dipropionate monohydrate 0.042%. Bot. 25 Gm with metering atomizing pump and nasal adapter.
Use: Intranasal steroid.

VANCENASE NASAL INHALER. (Schering) Metered-dose aerosol unit containing beclomethasone dipropionate in propellants. Each actuation delivers 42 mcg. Canister 16.8 Gm w/nasal adapter.
Use: Intranasal steroid.

VANCERIL INHALER. (Schering) Metered-dose aerosol unit of beclomethasone dipropionate in propellants. Each actuation delivers 42 mcg of beclomethasone dipropionate. Canister 16.8 Gm w/oral adapter. Box 1s.
Use: Respiratory inhalant.

VANCOCIN CAPSULES. (Lilly) Vancomycin HCl 125 mg or 250 mg/Pulvule. Bot. 10s, 20s.

Use: Anti-infective.

VANCOCIN IV. (Lilly) Vancomycin HCl 500 mg/Vial. 1s; 1 Gm/Vial. 10s; ADD-Vantage 500 mg or 1 Gm/Vial. 1s.
Use: Anti-infective.

VANCOCIN ORAL. (Lilly) Vancomycin HCl for oral soln. Traypak 1 Gm, Container 10 Gm.
Use: Anti-infective.

VANCOLED INJECTION. (Lederle) Vancomycin HCl equivalent to vancomycin 500 mg/10 ml reconstituted soln. Vial 10 ml.
Use: Anti-infective.

VANCOMYCIN HCl, U.S.P. XXII. Cap., For Oral Soln., Sterile, U.S.P. XXII. An antibiotic from *Streptomyces orientalis.*
Use: (I.V.) Gram-positive (staph.) infection; antibacterial.
See: Vancocin, Prods. (Lilly).
Vancoled, Vial (Lederle).

VANILLA, N.F. XVII. Tinct. N.F. XVII.
Use: Pharmaceutic aid (flavor).

VANILLAL.
See: Ethyl Vanillin.

VANILLIN, N.F. XVII. 4-Hydroxy-3-methoxy-benzaldehyde.
Use: Pharmaceutic aid (flavor).

VANICREAM. (Pharmaceutical Specialties) Oil in water vanishing cream containing white petrolatum, cetearyl alcohol, ceteareth-20, sorbitol, propylene glycol, simethicone, glyceryl monostearate, polyethylene glycol monostearate, sorbic acid. Oint. lb.
Use: Ointment base.

VANIROME.
See: Ethyl Vanillin.

VANODONNAL TIMECAPS. (Drug Industries) Phenobarbital 50 mg, atropine sulfate 0.0582 mg, hyoscyamine sulfate 0.311 mg, hyoscine hydrobromide 0.0195 mg/SR Cap. Bot. 100s.
Use: Sedative/hypnotic, anticholinergic/antispasmodic.

VANOXIDE. (Dermik) Benzoyl peroxide 5%, propylene glycol, hydroxyethyl cellulose, FD & C color, cholesterol-sterol, cetyl alcohol, propylene glycol stearate, polysorbate 20, lanolin alcohol, propylparaben, decyl oleate, purcelline oil syn., antioxidants, vegetable oil, methylparaben, tetrasodium EDTA, buffers, cyclohexanediamine tetraacetic acid, calcium phosphate, silicone emulsion, silica. Bot. 25 Gm, 50 Gm.
Use: Anti-acne.

VANOXIDE-HC. (Dermik) Hydrocortisone alcohol 0.5%, benzoyl peroxide 5%/25 Gm in lotion w/ same ingredients as Vanoxide. Bot. 25 Gm.
Use: Anti-acne.

VANQUISH. (Glenbrook) Aspirin 227 mg, acetaminophen 194 mg, caffeine 33 mg, dried aluminum hydroxide gel 25 mg, magnesium hydroxide 50 mg/Tab. Capsule shaped tablets. Bot. 15s, 30s, 60s, 100s.
Use: Salicylate analgesic combination, antacid.

VANSEB DANDRUFF SHAMPOO. (Herbert) Sulfur 2%, salicylic acid 1%, surfactants, protein. **Cream:** Tube 3 oz. **Lot.:** Bot. 4 oz.
Use: Antidandruff, antiseborrheic.

VANSEB-T TAR DANDRUFF SHAMPOO. (Herbert) Sulfur 2%, salicylic acid 1%, coal tar solution 5%, surfactants, protein. **Cream:** Tube 3 oz. **Lot.:** Bot. 4 oz.
Use: Antidandruff, antiseborrheic.

VANSIL. (Pfizer Laboratories) Oxaminiquine 250 mg/Cap. Bot. 24s.
Use: Anthelmintic.

•**VAPIPROST HYDROCHLORIDE.** USAN.
Use: Platelet aggregation inhibitor.

VAPOCET TABLETS. (Major) Hydrocodone 5 mg, acetaminophen 500 mg/Tab. Bot. 100s.
Use: Narcotic analgesic combination.

VAPONEFRIN SOLUTION. (Fisons) A 2.25% solution of bioassayed racemic epinephrine as HCl, chlorobutanol 0.5%. Vial 7.5 ml, 15 ml, 30 ml.
Use: Bronchodilator.

VAPORIZER IN A BOTTLE. (O'Connor) Wick dispensed medicated vapors.
Use: Cough, cold, sinus, hayfever treatment.

VAPORUB. (Vicks).
See: Vicks Vaporub (Vicks).

VAPOSTEAM. (Vicks).
See: Vicks Vaposteam (Vicks).

•**VAPREOTIDE.** USAN.
Use: Antineoplastic.

VARICELLA-ZOSTER IgG IFA TEST SYSTEM. (Wampole-Zeus) Test for the qualitative or semi-qualitative detection of VZ IgG antibody in human serum. Test kit 100s.
Use: Diagnostic aid.

•**VARICELLA-ZOSTER IMMUNE GLOBULIN,** U.S.P. XXII. A sterile buffered solution of the globulin fraction of human plasma containing 99% immunoglobulin G with traces of immunoglobulins A and M. It is derived from adult human plasma selected for high titers of varicella-zoster antibiodies.
Use: Passive immunizing agent.

VARICELLA ZOSTER IMMUNE GLOBULIN, HUMAN. (Massachusetts Public Health Biologic Labs) Varicella-zoster virus antibody 125 units/] 2.5 ml. Vial, single dose.
Use: Immune serum.

VARI-FLAVORS. (Ross) Flavor packets to provide flavor variety for patients on liquid diets. Dextrose, artificial flavor, artificial color. Packet 1 Gm, Ctn. 24s.
Use: Liquid nutrition flavoring aid.

VARIPLEX-C. (Nature's Bounty) Vitamins B_1 15 mg, B_2 10 mg, B_3 100 mg, B_5 20 mg, B_6 5 mg, B_{12} 10 mcg, C 500 mg/Tab. Bot. 100s.
Use: Vitamin supplement.

VARITOL. (Kenyon) Atropine sulfate 0.03 mg, hyoscyamine 0.03 mg, gelsemium 6.1 mg, methenamine 40.8 mg, salol 18.1 mg, benzoic acid

4.5 mg, methylene blue 5.4 mg/Tab. Bot. 100s, 1000s.
Use: Urinary anti-infective.

VARITOL-D.S. (Kenyon) Atropine sulfate 0.06 mg, hyoscyamine 0.06 mg, gelsemium 12.2 mg, methenamine 81.6 mg, salol 36.2 mg, benzoic acid 9 mg, methylene blue 10.8 mg/Tab. Bot. 100s, 1000s.
Use: Urinary anti-infective.

VASCOR. (McNeil) Bepridil HCl.
Use: Antianginal.

VASCUNITOL. (Apco) Mannitol hexanitrate 0.5 gr/Tab. Bot. 100s.
Use: Vasodilator.

VASCUSED. (Apco) Mannitol hexanitrate 0.5 gr, phenobarbital 0.25 gr/Tab. Bot. 100s.
Use: Vasodilator.

VASELINE DERMATOLOGY FORMULA CREAM. (Chesebrough-Pond's) Petrolatum, mineral oil, dimethicone. Jar 3 oz, 5.25 oz.
Use: Emollient.

VASELINE DERMATOLOGY FORMULA LOTION. (Chesebrough-Pond's) Petrolatum, mineral oil, dimethicone. Bot. 5.5 oz, 11 oz, 16 oz.
Use: Emollient.

VASELINE FIRST AID CARBOLATED PETROLEUM JELLY. (Chesebrough-Pond's) Petrolatum, chloroxylenol. Plastic Jar 1.75 oz, 3.75 oz. Plastic Tube 1 oz, 2.5 oz.
Use: Medicated antibacterial.

VASELINE PURE PETROLEUM JELLY SKIN PROTECTANT. (Chesebrough-Pond's) White petrolatum. Tube 1 oz, 2.5 oz. Jar 1.75 oz, 3.75 oz, 7.75 oz, 13 oz.
Use: Protectant for minor skin irritations.

VASERETIC. (Merck Sharp & Dohme) Enalapril maleate 10 mg, hydrochlorothiazide 25 mg/Tab. Bot. 100s.
Use: Antihypertensive.

VASIMID.
See: Tolazoline HCl, U.S.P. XXII.

VASOCIDIN OPHTHALMIC OINTMENT. (CooperVision) Prednisolone acetate 5 mg, sulfacetamide sodium 100 mg/Gm. Tube 3.5 Gm.
Use: Corticosteroid, anti-infective.

VASOCIDIN OPHTHALMIC SOLUTION. (CooperVision) Prednisolone sodium phosphate 0.25% (equivalent to prednisolone phosphate 0.23%), sulfacetamide sodium 10%, thimerosal 0.01%. Plastic dropper-tip squeeze bot. 5 ml, 10 ml.
Use: Corticosteroid, anti-infective.

VASOCLEAR. (CooperVision) Naphazoline HCl 0.02% in Lipiden polymeric vehicle, benzalkonium Cl 0.01%. Bot. 15 ml.
Use: Vasoconstrictor/mydriatic.

VASOCLEAR A. (CooperVision) Naphazoline HCl 0.02%, zinc sulfate 0.25%, polyvinyl alcohol 0.25%. Bot. 15 ml.
Use: Vasoconstrictor/mydriatic.

VASOCON-A OPHTHALMIC SOLUTION. (CooperVision) Naphazoline HCl 0.05%, antazoline phosphate 0.5%. Plastic squeeze bot. w/dropper tip 15 ml.
Use: Vasoconstrictor/mydriatic.

VASOCON REGULAR. (CooperVision) Naphazoline HCl 0.1%. Bot. plastic squeeze w/dropper tip 15 ml.
Use: Vasoconstrictor/mydriatic.

VASOCONSTRICTOR.
See: Epinephrine Preps.

VASCORAY. (Mallinckrodt) Iothalamate meglumine 52%, iothalamate sodium 26% (40% iodine). Vial 25 ml, 50 ml. Bot. 100 ml, 200 ml.
Use: Radiopaque agent.

VASODILAN. (Mead Johnson) Isoxsuprine HCl 10 mg or 20 mg/Tab. **10 mg:** Bot. 100s, 1000s, UD 100s. **20 mg:** Bot. 100s, 500s, 1000s, UD 100s.
Use: Peripheral vasodilator.

VASODILATORS.
See: Amyl Nitrite.
Apresoline, Tab., Amp. (Ciba).
Arlidin, Tab. (USV).
Cardilate, Tab. (Burroughs Wellcome).
Cyclospasmol, Tab., Cap. (Wyeth).
Erythrityl Tetranitrate, Tab.
Glyceryl Trinitrate Preps.
Isordil, Tab. (Wyeth).
Kortrate, Cap. (Amid).
Mannitol Hexanitrate.
Metamine, Tab. (Pfizer).
Nisane, Elix. (Amid).
Nitroglycerin.
Pentritol, Cap., Tempule (Armour).
Peritrate, Tab. (Parke-Davis).
Sodium Nitrate.
Sorbitrate, Tab. (Stuart).
Vasodilan, Tab., Amp. (Mead Johnson).

VASODILATORS, CORONARY.
See: Glyceryl Trinitrate, Preps. (Various Mfr.).
Isordil, Tab. (Wyeth).
Khellin (Various Mfr.).
Papaverine, Inj., Tab. (Various Mfr.).
Pentaerythritol Tetranitrate, Tab.
Peritrate, Tab. (Parke-Davis).
Roniacol Elix., Tab. (Roche).
Sorbitrate, Tab. (Stuart).

VASOFLO. (Hauck) Papaverine HCl 150 mg/Cap. Bot 100s.
Use: Peripheral vasodilator.

VASOLATE. (Parmed) Pentaerythritol tetranitrate 30 mg/Cap. Bot. 100s, 1000s.
Use: Antianginal.

VASOLATE-80. (Parmed) Pentaerythritol tetranitrate 80 mg/Cap. Bot. 100s, 1000s.
Use: Antianginal.

VASOMIDE TABLETS. (Lannett) Niacin 50 mg, salicylamide 300 mg, ascorbic acid 15 mg, vitamins B_1 3 mg, dl-desoxyephedrine HCl 2.5 mg, B_{12} 3 mcg/Tab. Bot. 100s, 1000s.

VASOMINIC-T.D. (A.V.P.) Phenylpropanolamine HCl 40 mg, chlorpheniramine maleate 5 mg,

phenylephrine HCl 10 mg, phenyltoloxamine citrate 15 mg/TR Tab. Bot. 100s.
Use: Decongestant, antihistamine.

•**VASOPRESSIN INJECTION,** U.S.P. XXII. beta-Hypophamine. Posterior pituitary pressor hormone.
Use: Posterior pituitary hormone (antidiuretic).
See: Pitressin, Amp. (Parke-Davis).

VASOPRESSIN TANNATE INJECTION. beta-Hypophamine tannate.
See: Pitressin Tannate, Amp. (Parke-Davis).

VASOSULF. (CooperVision) Sulfacetamide sodium 15%, phenylephrine HCl 0.125%. Bot. 5 ml, 15 ml.
Use: Anti-infective, decongestant (ophthalmic).

VASOTEC. (Merck Sharp & Dohme) Enalapril maleate 2.5 mg, 5 mg, 10 mg or 20 mg/Tab. Bot. 100s, UD 100s.
Use: Antihypertensive.

VASOTEC I.V. (Merck Sharp & Dohme) Enalaprilat 1.25 mg/ml. Inj. Vial 2 ml.
Use: Antihypertensive.

VASOTHERM INJ. (Pharmex) Niacin as sodium salt 100 mg, benzyl alcohol 1.5%/ml. Vial 30 ml.
Use: Vasodilator.

VASOTUS LIQUID. (Sheryl) Codeine phosphate 1/6 gr, phenylephrine HCl, prophenpyridamine maleate. Liq. Bot. pt.
Use: Antitussive, decongestant, antihistamine.

VA-TRO-NOL. (Vicks).
See: Vicks Va-Tro-Nol (Vicks).

VAZEPAM. (Major) Diazepam 2 mg, 5 mg or 10 mg/Tab. Bot. 100s, 500s, 1000s.
Use: Antianxiety agent.

VAZOSAN. (Sandia) Papaverine HCl 150 mg/Tab. Bot. 100s, 1000s.
Use: Peripheral vasodilator.

V-CILLIN-K. (Lilly) Penicillin V potassium 125 mg, 250 mg or 500 mg/Tab. **125 mg:** Bot. 100s. **250 mg:** Bot. 100s, 500s. **500 mg:** Bot. 24s, 100s, 500s.
Use: Antibacterial, penicillin.

V-CILLIN-K FOR ORAL SOLUTION. (Lilly) Penicillin V potassium 125 mg or 250 mg/5 ml. **125 mg:** Bot. 100 ml, 150 ml, 200 ml, UD 5 ml. **250 mg:** Bot. 100 ml, 150 ml, 200 ml.
Use: Antibacterial, penicillin.

V-DEC-M. (Seatrace) Pseudoephedrine HCl 120 mg, guaifenesin 500 mg/SR Tab. Bot. 100s.
Use: Decongestant, expectorant.

VDRL ANTIGEN. (Laboratory Diagnostics) VDRL antigen with buffered saline. Blood test in diagnosis of syphillis. **Vial:** Sufficient for 500 tests. **Amp.:** 10 × 0.5 ml sufficient for 500 tests.
Use: Diagnostic aid.

VDRL SLIDE TEST. (Laboratory Diagnostics) VDRL antigen. Slide flocculation and spinal fluid test for syphilis. Vial 5 ml Complete kit, reactive control, nonreactive control, 5 ml.
Use: Diagnostic aid.

VE-400. (Western Research) Vitamin E 400 IU/Cap. Bot. 1008s.
Use: Vitamin E supplement.

•**VECURONIUM BROMIDE.** USAN.
Use: Blocking agent (neuromuscular).

VEETIDS. (Squibb) Penicillin-V potassium. **Soln.:** 125 mg or 250 mg/5 ml Bot. 100 ml, 200 ml. **Tab.:** 250 mg or 500 mg. Bot. 100s, 1000s, Unimatic 100s.
Use: Antibacterial, penicillin.

VEETIDS "500'. (Squibb) Penicillin V potassium 500 mg/Tab. Bot. 100s, 1000s, UD 100s.
Use: Antibacterial, penicillin.

•**VEGETABLE OIL, HYDROGENATED,** U.S.P. XXII.
Use: Pharmaceutic aid (tablet lubricant).

VEHICLE/N AND VEHICLE/N MILD. (Neutrogena) Topical vehicle system for compounding. Appliderm Applicator Bot. oz.
Use: Extemporaneous compounding.

VELACYCLINE. N-Pyrrolidinomethyl tetracycline.
Use: Antibacterial, tetracycline.

VELBAN. (Lilly) Extract from Vinca rosea Linn. Vinblastine sulfate, lyophilized. Vial 10 mg/10 ml. Box 1s.
Use: Antineoplastic agent.

VELLADA TABLETS. (Fellows) Phenobarbital 0.25 gr, hyoscyamus extract 1/8 gr, passiflora extract 0.25 gr, valerian extract 0.25 gr/Tab. Bot. 1000s.
Use: Sedative/hypnotic, anticholinergic/antispasmodic.

VELMATROL. (Kenyon) Sulfisoxazole 500 mg/Tab. Bot. 100s, 1000s.
Use: Antibacterial, sulfonamide.

VELMATROL-A. (Kenyon) Sulfisoxazole 500 mg, phenylazodiaminopyridine HCl 50 mg/Tab. Bot. 100s, 1000s.
Use: Urinary anti-infective.

VELOSEF. (Squibb) Cephradine. **Oral Susp.:** 125 mg or 250 mg/5 ml. Bot. 100 ml, 200 ml. **Cap.:** 250 mg or 500 mg Bot. 24s, 100s, UD Unimatic 100s. **Inj.:** (w/anhydrous sodium carbonate. Sodium equivalent to 136 mg/Gm of cephradine) 250 mg, 500 mg, 1 Gm or 2 Gm/vial. 2 Gm vial is sodium free for infusion. Bot. 200 ml.
Use: Antibacterial, cephalosporin.

VELOSULIN. (Nordisk) Purified pork insulin injection 100 IU/ml.
Use: Antidiabetic agent.

VELOSULIN HUMAN. (Nordisk) Human insulin injection 100 IU/ml.
Use: Antidiabetic agent.

VELSAR. (Adria) Vinblastine sulfate 10 mg. Pow. for inj. Vial.
Use: Antineoplastic agent.

VELTANE. (Lannett) Brompheniramine maleate 4 mg/Tab. Bot. 1000s.
Use: Antihistamine.

VELTAP. (Lannett) Brompheniramine maleate 4 mg, phenylephrine HCl 5 mg, phenylpropanolamine HCl 5 mg, alcohol 3%/5 ml. Bot. pt, gal.
Use: Antihistamine, decongestant.

VELVACHOL. (Owen) Hydrophilic ointment base petrolatum, mineral oil, cetyl alcohol, cholesterol, parabens, stearyl alcohol, purified water, sodium lauryl sulfate. Jar lb.
Use: Hydrophilic ointment base.

VELVEDERM CLEANSER. (Torch) Sulfonated detergent with a stable emulsion of vegetable oil. Lot. Bot. 8 oz.
Use: Cleanser.

VELVEDERM-HANDORA NORMALIZER. (Torch) Glycerin, fatty alcohols, fatty acid in hydrophilic base w/pH of 5.0 to 5.5. Cream. Jar 4 oz, 8 oz. Lot. Bot. 8 oz.
Use: Emollient.

VELVEDERM MOISTURIZER. (Torch) Mineral oil, emulsifiers, fatty alcohol, propylene glycol, hydroxymethylcellulose, water. Bot. 4 oz.
Use: Emollient.

VENESETIC.
See: Amobarbital Sodium, Preps. (Various Mfr.).

VENETHENE. No mfr. listed.

VENOGLOBULIN-I. (Alpha Therapeutic) Immune Globulin Intravenous (IGIV). Pow. for Inj. Vial 2.5 Gm, 5 Gm.
Use: Immune serum.

VENOMIL. (Hollister-Stier) Diagnostic 1 mcg/ml, Maintenance 100 mcg/ml. Individual patient kit.
Use: Allergenic extract.

VENSTAT. (Seatrace) Brompheniramine maleate 10 mg/ml. Vial 10 ml.
Use: Antihistamine.

VENTOLIN AEROSOL. (Allen & H) Albuterol 90 mcg/acutation. Aerosol canister 17 Gm containing 200 metered inhalations. Canister 17 Gm w/oral adapter.
Use: Bronchodilator.

VENTOLIN ROTACAPS. (Allen & Hanburys) Microfine albuterol 200 mg. Cap. for inhalation. Bot. UD 96s. For use with the Rotohaler inhalation device.
Use: Bronchodilator.

VENTOLIN INHALATION SOLUTION. (Allen & Hanburys) Albuterol sulfate 5 mg/ml. Bot. 20 ml w/calibrated dropper.
Use: Bronchodilator.

VENTOLIN SYRUP. (Allen & Hanburys) Albuterol sulfate 2 mg/5 ml. Bot. pt.
Use: Brondilator.

VENTOLIN TABLET(Allen & Hanburys) Albuterol sulfate 2 mg or 4 mg/Tab. Bot. 100s, 500s.
Use: Brondilator.

VEPESID. (Bristol-Myers/Bristol Oncology) Etoposide. **Vial:** 100 mg/Vial. **Cap.:** 50 mg/Cap. Bot.20s.
Use: Antineoplastic agent.

VERACOLATE. (Numark) Bile salts 1.07 gr, phenolphthalein 0.5 gr, capsicum oleoresin 0.05 min, cascara extract 1 gr/Tab. Bot. 100s.
Use: Laxative.

VERACTIL. Methotrimeprazine, B.A.N.

•**VERADOLINE HYDROCHLORIDE.** USAN.
Use: Analgesic.

•**VERAPAMIL.** USAN. 5-[3,4-Di-methoxyphenethyl)methylamino]-2-(3,4-dimethoxyphenyl)-2-isopropylvaleronitrile. Isoptin. Cordilox HCl.
Use: Coronary vasodilator.

•**VERAPAMIL HYDROCHLORIDE.** USAN.
Use: Antianginal, cardiac depressant (antiarrhythmic).
See: Calan, Tab., Inj. (Searle).
Calan SR, Capl. (Searle).

VERATRUM ALBA.
See: Protoveratrines A and B (Various Mfr.).

VERAZEPTOL. (Femco) Chlorothymol, eucalyptol, menthol, phenol, boric acid, zinc sulfate. Pow. Bot. 3 oz, 6 oz, 10 oz.
Use: Vaginal preparation.

VERAZIDE. B.A.N. 2′-Veratrylideneisonicotino-hydrazide.
Use: Treatment of tuberculosis.

VERAZINC. (Forest) Zinc sulfate 220 mg/Cap. Bot. 100s, 1000s.
Use: Zinc supplement.

VERCYTE. (Abbott) Pipobroman 25 mg/Tab. Bot. 100s.
Use: Antineoplastic agent.

VERGO OINT. (Daywell) Calcium pantothenate 8%, ascorbic acid 2%, starch. Tube 0.5 oz.
Use: Keratolytic.

•**VERILOPAM HYDROCHLORIDE.** USAN.
Use: Analgesic.

VERIN. (Hauck) Aspirin (Acetylsalicylic Acid; ASA) 650 mg/TR Tab. Bot. 100s.
Use: Salicylate analgesic.

•**VERLUKAST.** USAN.
Use: Antiasthmatic.

VERMICIDE. (Pharmex) Tube 2 oz.
Use: Pediculicide.

VERMOX. (Janssen) Mebendazole 100 mg/Tab. Box 12s.
Use: Anthelmintic.

VERNACEL. (Professional Pharmacal) Prophenpyridamine maleate 0.5%, phenylephrine HCl ⅛% in a methylcellulose solution. Plastic Bot. 15 ml, 30 ml.
Use: Antihistamine, decongestant, ophthalmic.

VERNAMYCINS. Under study.
Use: Antibiotic.

VERNOLEPIN. A sesquiterpene dilactone. Under study.
Use: Against Walker carcinosarcoma 256.

•**VEROFYLLINE.** USAN.
Use: Bronchodilator, antiasthmatic.

VERONAL SODIUM.
See: Barbital Sodium (Various Mfr.).

VERR-CANTH. (C & M Pharmacal) Cantharidin 0.7%, penederm 0.5%. Bot. 7.5 ml.
Use: Keratolytic.

VERREX. (C & M Pharmacal) Salicylic acid 30%, podophyllin 10%. Bot. 7.5 ml w/applicator tip.
Use: Keratolytic.

VERSACAPS. (Seatrace) Brompheniramine maleate 4 mg, pseudoephedrine HCl 60 mg, guaifenesin 300 mg/Cap. Bot. 100s, 1000s.

Use: Antihistamine, decongestant, expectorant.

VERSAL. (Suppository) Bismuth subgallate, balsam peru, zinc oxide, benzyl benzoate/Supp. Box 12s, 100s, 1000s.
Use: Anorectal preparation.

VERSA-QUAT. (Ulmer) Quaternary ammonium one-step cleaner-disinfectant-sanitizer-fungicide-virucide for general housekeeping. Bot. gal.
Use: Cleanser, disinfectant.

VERSED. (Roche) Midazolam HCl 1 mg or 5 mg/ml, sodium Cl 0.8%, disodium edetate 0.01%, benzyl alcohol 1%. **1 mg/ml:** Vial 2 ml, 5 ml, 10 ml. Box 10s. **5 mg/ml:** Vial 1 ml, 2 ml, 5 ml, 10 ml. Box 10s. Disposable Syringe 2 ml Box 10s.
Use: General anesthetic.

VERSENATE, CALCIUM DISODIUM.
See: Calcium Disodium Versenate, Amp. (Riker).

VERSENATE DISODIUM.
See: Disodium Versenate, Amp. (Riker).

VERSIDYNE. Methopholine. 1-(p-Chlorophenethyl)-2-methyl-6,7-dimethoxy-1,2,3,4-tetrahydroisoquinoline.
Use: Analgesic.

VERSTAT. (Saron) Pheniramine maleate 12.5 mg, nicotinic acid 50 mg/Cap.
Use: Antihistamine, vitamin B_3 supplement.

VERSTRAN. (Parke-Davis) Prazepam.
Use: Antianxiety agent.
See: Centrax, Tab. (Parke-Davis).

VERV ALERTNESS CAPSULES. (APC) Caffeine 200 mg/Cap. Vial 15s.
Use: Analeptic.

•**VESNARINONE.** USAN.
Use: Cardiotonic.

VERUKAN-20. (Syosset) Salicylic acid 16.7%, lactic acid in flexible collodione 16.7%. Bot. 15 ml.
Use: Keratolytic.

VETALAR. (Parke-Davis) Ketamine HCl 100 mg/ml. Bot. 10 ml.
Use: Anesthetic (veterinary).

V-GAN. (Hauck) Promethazine HCl 25 mg or 50 mg/ml. Vial 10 ml.
Use: Antiemetic, antihistamine.

VIACAPS. (Manne) Vitamins A (soluble) 45,000 IU, C 500 mg/Cap. Bot. 60s, 120s, 1000s.
Use: Vitamin supplement.

VIBESATE. Polvinate 9.3%, molrosinol 3.1% with propellant.

VIBRAMYCIN. (Pfizer Laboratories) Doxycycline. **Cap.:** 50 mg Bot. 50s, UD pak 100s, X-Pack (10 Cap.) 5s; 100 mg Bot. 50s, 500s; UD pak 100s, V-Pak (5 Cap) 5s, Nine-Pak 10s. **Pediatric Oral Susp.:** 25 mg/5 ml. Bot. 2 oz. **Syr.:** 50 mg/5 ml. Bot. oz, pt.
Use: Antibacterial, tetracycline.

VIBRA-TABS. (Pfizer Laboratories) Doxycycline hyclate 100 mg/Tab. Bot. 50s, 500s, UD Pack 100s.
Use: Antibacterial, tetracycline.

VICAM INJECTION. (Keene) Vitamins B_1 50 mg, B_2 5 mg, B_3 125 mg, B_5 6 mg, B_6 5 mg, B_{12} 1000 mcg, C 50 mg/ml. Inj. Vial 10 ml.
Use: Vitamin supplement.

VICAM IV. (Keene) Vitamins B_1 50 mg, B_2 5 mg, B_{12} 1000 mcg, B_6 5 mg, dexpanthenol 6 mg, niacinamide 125 mg, C 50 mg/ml, benzyl alcohol 1% as preservative in water for injection. Vial multiple dose.
Use: Parenteral nutritional supplement.

VICEF. (Drug Industries) Thiamine HCl 10 mg, pyridoxine HCl 10 mg, B_{12} 50 mcg, C 100 mg, E 100 IU, niacinamide 25 mg, folic acid 1.5 mg, ferrous fumarate 45 mg/2 Cap. Bot. 100s.
Use: Vitamin/mineral supplement.

VICKS CHILDRENS COUGH SYRUP. (Vicks) Dextromethorphan HBr 3.5 mg, guaifenesin 50 mg/5 ml, alcohol 5%. Bot. 3 oz.
Use: Antitussive, expectorant.

VICKS COUGH SILENCERS. (Vicks) Dextromethorphan HBr 2.5 mg, benzocaine 1 mg, Special Vicks Medication (menthol, peppermint oil, anethole) 0.35%/Loz. Box 14s.
Use: Antitussive, anesthetic.

VICKS DAYCARE CAPLETS. (Vicks) Acetaminophen 325 mg, pseudoephedrine HCl 30 mg, guaifenesin 100 mg, dextromethorphan HBr 10 mg/Cap. Bot. 20s.
Use: Analgesic, decongestant, expectorant, antitussive.

VICKS DAYCARE LIQUID. (Vicks) Acetaminophen 650 mg, dextromethorphan HBr 20 mg, pseudoephedrine HCl 60 mg, guaifenesin 200 mg/oz, alcohol 10%. Bot. 6 oz, 10 oz.
Use: Analgesic, antitussive, decongestant, expectorant.

VICKS FORMULA 44. (Vicks) Dextromethorphan HBr 30 mg, chlorpheniramine maleate 40 mg/10 ml, alcohol 10%. Bot. 4 oz, 8 oz.
Use: Antitussive, antihistamine.

VICKS FORMULA 44 COUGH CONTROL DISCS. (Vicks) Dextromethorphan (HBr equivalent) 5 mg/Disc. Pkg. 24s.
Use: Antitussive.

VICKS FORMULA 44D. (Vicks) Dextromethorphan HBr 30 mg, pseudoephedrine HCl 60 mg, guaifenesin 200 mg/15 ml, alcohol 10%. Bot. 4 oz, 8 oz.
Use: Antitussive, decongestant, expectorant.

VICKS FORMULA 44M. (Vicks) Dextromethorphan HBr 30 mg, pseudoephedrine HCl 60 mg, guaifenesin 200 mg, acetaminophen 500 mg/20 ml, alcohol 20%. Bot. 4 oz, 8 oz.
Use: Antitussive, decongestant, expectorant, analgesic.

VICKS ICE BLUE. (Vicks) Menthol. Loz. Pkg. 14s, 40s.
Use: Local anesthetic.

VICKS ICE BLUE THROAT DROPS. (Vicks) Menthol in a soothing sugar base. Drop. Box 14s. Bag 40s.
Use: Local anesthetic.

VICKS INHALER. (Vicks) l-Desoxyephedrine 50 mg, Special Vicks Medication (menthol, camphor, bornyl acetate) 150 mg. Inhaler 0.007 oz.
Use: Nasal decongestant.

VICKS NYQUIL. (Vicks) Acetaminophen 1000 mg, doxylamine succinate 7.5 mg, pseudoephedrine HCl 60 mg, dextromethorphan HBr 30 mg/30 ml, alcohol 25%. Regular and cherry flavors. Regular contains FD&C Yellow #5 tartrazine. Bot. 6 oz, 10 oz, 14 oz.
Use: Analgesic, antihistamine, decongestant, antitussive.

VICKS ORACIN. (Vicks) Benzocaine 6.25 mg, menthol (Regular 0.1%, cherry 0.08%) in a cooling sorbitol base/Loz. Regular or Cherry flavor. Regular flavor lozenge contains FD&C Yellow #5 tartrazine. Pkg. 18s.
Use: Local anesthetic.

VICKS SINEX. (Vicks) Phenylephrine HCl 0.5%, cetylpyridinium Cl 0.04%, thimerosal 0.001% preservative. Nasal Spray. Plastic Squeeze Bot. 0.5 oz, 1 oz.
Use: Nasal decongestant.

VICKS SINEX LONG-ACTING. (Vicks) Oxymetazoline HCl 0.05% in aqueous soln., thimerosal 0.001%. Nasal Spray. Plastic Squeeze Bot. 1 oz, 0.5 oz.
Use: Nasal decongestant.

VICKS THROAT DROPS. (Vicks) Menthol in soothing Vicks sugar base. Regular, cherry, lemon flavor. Bag 40s, Box 14s.
Use: Local anesthetic.

VICKS THROAT LOZENGES. (Vicks) Benzocaine 5 mg, cetylpyridinium Cl 1.66 mg, Special Vicks Medication (menthol, eucalyptus oil, camphor). Loz. 12s.
Use: Local anesthetic.

VICKS VAPORUB. (Vicks) Special Vicks Medication 14% (camphor 4.73%, menthol 2.67%, spirits of turpentine 4.5%, eucalyptus oil 1.2%). Jar 1.5 oz, 3 oz. 6 oz. Tube 2 oz.
Use: Decongestant vaporizing ointment.

VICKS VAPOSTEAM. (Vicks) Eucalyptus oil 1.5%, camphor 6.2%, menthol 3.2%, alcohol 74%. Bot. 4 oz, 6 oz.
Use: Steam medication, decongestant, antitussive.

VICKS VA-TRO-NOL. (Vicks) Ephedrine sulfate 0.5%, Special Vicks Aromatic Blend in an aqueous base (menthol, eucalyptol, camphor) 0.06%, thimerosal 0.001%. Drop. Bot. 0.5 oz, 1 oz.
Use: Nasal decongestant.

VICODIN. (Knoll) Hydrocodone bitartrate 5 mg, acetaminophen 500 mg/Tab. Bot. 100s, 500s. Hospital pack 100s.
Use: Narcotic analgesic combination.

VICODIN ES. (Knoll) Hydrocodone bitartrate 7.5 mg, acetaminophen 750 mg/Tab. Bot. 100s, UD 100s.
Use: Narcotic analgesic combination.

VICON-C. (Russ) Ascorbic acid 300 mg niacinamide 100 mg, zinc sulfate 80 mg, magnesium sulfate 70 mg, thiamine mononitrate 20 mg, d-calcium pantothenate 20 mg, B_2 10 mg, B_6 5 mg/Cap. Bot. 60s, 500s, UD 100s.
Use: Vitamin/mineral supplement.

VICON FORTE. (Russ) Vitamins A 8000 IU, E 50 IU, C 150 mg, niacinamide 25 mg, thiamine mononitrate 10 mg, d-calcium pantothenate 10 mg, B_2 5 mg, B_6 2 mg, B_{12} 10 mcg, folic acid 1 mg, zinc sulfate 80 mg, magnesium sulfate 70 mg, manganese Cl 4 mg/Cap. Bot. 60s, 500s, UD 100s.
Use: Vitamin/mineral supplement.

VICON PLUS. (Russ) Vitamins A 4000 IU, e 50 IU, C 150 mg, niacinamide 25 mg, thiamine mononitrate 10 mg, d-calcium pantothenate 10 mg, B_2 5 mg, zinc sulfate 80 mg, magnesium sulfate 70 mg, manganese Cl 4 mg, B_6 2 mg/Cap. Bot. 60s.
Use: Vitamin/mineral supplement.

VICRYL SUTURES. (Ethicon) Polyglactin 910.

VICTORS. (Vicks) Special Vicks Medication (menthol, eucalyptus oil) in a soothing Vicks sugar base. Regular or Cherry flavor drops. Stick-Pack 10s, Bag 40s.
Use: Local anesthetic.

VICTOR'S VAPOR COUGH. (Vicks) Menthol, eucalyptus oil. Loz. Pkg. 10s.
Use: Local anesthetic.

•**VIDARABINE PHOSPHATE.** USAN.
Use: Antiviral.

•**VIDARABINE, STERILE,** U.S.P. XXII., Conc. for Inj., Ophth. Oint., U.S.P. XXII. 9-β-D-Arabinofuranosyladenine.
Use: Antiviral.
See: Vira-A Ophthalmic, Oint. (Parke-Davis).
Vira-A, Inj. (Parke-Davis).

•**VIDARABINE SODIUM PHOSPHATE.** USAN.
Use: Antiviral.

VI-DAYLIN ADC DROPS. (Ross) Vitamins A 1500 IU, C 35 mg, D 400 IU/ml. Bot. 30 ml, 50 ml. Bot. 50 ml w/dropper.
Use: Vitamin supplement.

VI-DAYLIN ADC PLUS IRON DROPS. (Ross) Vitamins A 1500 IU, C 35 mg, D 400 IU, iron 10 mg/ml. Bot. 50 ml w/dropper.
Use: Vitamin/mineral supplement.

VI-DAYLIN CHEWABLE. (Ross) Vitamins A 2500 IU, D 400 IU, E 15 IU, C 60 mg, folic acid 0.3 mg, B_1 1.05 mg, B_2 1.2 mg, niacin 13.5 mg, B_6 1.05 mg, B_{12} 4.5 mcg/Tab. Bot. 100s.
Use: Vitamin supplement.

VI-DAYLIN CHEWABLE W/FLUORIDE. (Ross) Fluoride 1 mg, vitamins B_1 1.05 mg, B_2 1.2 mg, niacinamide 13.5 mg, B_6 1.05 mg, C 60 mg, A 2500 IU, B_{12} 4.5 mcg, E 15 IU, folic acid 0.3 mg, D 400 IU/Tab. Bot. 100s.
Use: Dental caries preventative, vitamin/mineral supplement.

VI-DAYLIN DROPS. (Ross) Vitamins A 1500 IU, D 400 IU, E 5 IU, C 35 mg, B_1 0.5 mg, B_2 0.6

mg, niacin 8 mg, B_6 0.4 mg, B_{12} 1.5 mcg/ml. Bot. 50 ml.
Use: Vitamin supplement.

VI-DAYLIN/F ADC DROPS. (Ross) Vitamins A 1500 IU, D 400 IU, C 35 mg, fluoride 0.25 mg/ml. Bot. 50 ml.
Use: Vitamin supplement, dental caries preventative.

VI-DAYLIN/F ADC PLUS IRON DROPS. (Ross) Vitamins A 1500 IU, C 35 mg, D 400 IU, iron 10 mg, fluoride 0.25 mg/ml. Bot. 50 ml.
Use: Vitamin/mineral supplement, dental caries preventative.

VI-DAYLIN/F DROPS. (Ross) Vitamins A 1500 IU, D 400 IU, E 5 IU, C 35 mg, B_1 0.5 mg, B_2 0.6 mg, niacin 8 mg, B_6 0.4 mg, fluoride 0.25 mg/ml. Bot. 50 ml.
Use: Vitamin supplement, dental caries preventative.

VI-DAYLIN/F PLUS IRON. (Ross) **Drops:** Fluoride 0.25 mg, vitamins A 1500 IU, D 400 IU, E 4.1 mg, B_1 0.5 mg, B_2 0.6 mg, B_3 8 mg, B_6 0.4 mg, C 35 mg, iron 10 mg/ml, alcohol $>$ 0.1%. Bot. 50 ml. **Chew. Tab.:** Fluoride 1 mg, vitamins A 2500 IU, D 400 IU, E 15 mg, B_1 1.05 mg, B_2 1.2 mg, B_3 13.5 mg, B_6 1.05 mg, B_{12} 4.5 mcg, C 60 mg, folic acid 0.3 mg, iron 12 mg. Bot. 100s.
Use: Dental caries preventative, vitamin/mineral supplement.

VI-DAYLIN LIQUID. (Ross) Vitamins A 2500 IU, B_1 1.05 mg, B_2 1.2 mg, B_6 1.05 mg, B_{12} 4.5 mcg, C 60 mg, D 400 IU, E 20.4 mg (as d-alpha tocopheryl acetate), niacin 13.5 mg/5 ml. Bot. 8 oz, pt.
Use: Vitamin supplement.

VI-DAYLIN PLUS IRON CHEWABLE. (Ross) Vitamins A 2500 IU, D 400 IU, E 15 IU, C 60 mg, folic acid 0.3 mg, B_1 1.05 mg, B_2 1.2 mg, niacin 13.5 mg, B_6 1.05 mg, B_{12} 4.5 mcg, iron 12 mg/Tab. Bot. 100s.
Use: Vitamin/mineral supplement.

VI-DAYLIN PLUS IRON DROPS. (Ross) Vitamins A 1500 IU, D 400 IU, E 5 IU, C 35 mg, B_1 0.5 mg, B_2 0.6 mg, niacin 8 mg, B_6 0.4 mg, iron 10 mg/ml. Bot. 50 ml w/dropper.
Use: Vitamin/mineral supplement.

VI-DAYLIN PLUS IRON LIQUID. (Ross) Vitamins A 2500 IU, D 400 IU, C 60 mg, E 15 IU, B_1 1.05 mg, B_2 1.2 mg, niacin 13.5 mg, B_6 1.05 mg, B_{12} 4.5 mcg, iron 10 mg/tsp. Bot. 8 oz, 16 oz.
Use: Vitamin/mineral supplement.

VIDECON. (Vita Elixir) Vitamin D 50,000 units/Cap.
Use: Vitamin D supplement.

VI-DERM SOAP. (Arthrins) Extract of Amaryllis 10%. Pkg. cake 1s. Bar 3.5 oz.
Use: Skin cleanser.

•**VIFILCON A.** USAN.
Use: Contact lens material.

•**VIFILCONB.** USAN.
Use: Contact lens material (hydrophilic).

VIFLUORINEED. (Hanlon) Vitamins A 5000 IU, D 400 IU, C 75 mg, B_1 2 mg, B_2 3 mg, niacinamide 20 mg, fluoride 1 mg/Chew. Tab. Bot. 100s.
Use: Vitamin/mineral supplement.

•**VIGABATRIN.** USAN.
Use: Anticonvulsant.

VIGEROLAN. (Lannett) Geriatric vitamin-mineral capsule with choline, inositol, methionine. Bot. 100s, 500s, 1000s.
Use: Vitamin/mineral supplement.

VIGORTOL. (Rugby) Vitamins B_1 2.5 mg, B_2 1.25 mg, B_3 25 mg, B_5 5 mg, B_6 0.5 mg, B_{12} 0.5 mcg, iron 10 mg, choline 50 mg, inositol 50 mg, zinc 1 mg, I, K, Mg, Mn/15 ml, alcohol 18%. Liq. Bot. pt, gal.
Use: Vitamin/mineral supplement.

VILEX. (Dunhall) Vitamin B_1 100 mg, riboflavin phosphate sodium 1 mg, B_6 10 mg, panthenol 5 mg, niacinamide 100 mg/ml. Amp. 30 ml.
Use: Vitamin supplement.

VILIVA. (Vita Elixir) Ferrous fumarate 3 gr.
Use: Iron supplement.

VILOXAZINE. B.A.N. 2-(2-Ethoxyphenoxymethyl)-tetrahydro-1,4-oxazine.
Use: Treatment of mental disease.
See: Vivalan hydrochloride.

•**VILOXAZINE HCL.** USAN.
Use: Antidepressant.

VIMINAL CAPSULES. (Cenci) Vitamins A 5000 IU, D 400 IU, B_1 3 mg, B_2 2.5 mg, niacinamide 20 mg, B_6 1.5 mg, calcium pantothenate 5 mg, B_{12} 2.5 mcg, C 50 mg, E 3 IU, calcium 215 mg, phosphorus 166 mg, iron 13.4 mg, magnesium 7.5 mg, manganese 1.5 mg, potassium 5 mg, zinc 1.4 mg/Cap. Bot. 30s, 100s, 500s.
Use: Vitamin/mineral supplement.

VIMINAL G CAPSULES. (Cenci) Vitamins A 12,500 IU, D 400 IU, B_1 5 mg, B_2 2.5 mg, niacinamide 40 mg, B_6 1 mg, calcium pantothenate 4 mg, B_{12} 2 mcg, C 75 mg, E 2 IU, choline bitartrate 31.4 mg, inositol 15 mg, calcium 75 mg, phosphorus 58 mg, iron 30 mg, magnesium 3 mg, manganese 0.5 mg, potassium 2 mg, zinc 0.5 mg/Cap. Bot. 30s, 100s, 500s.
Use: Vitamin/mineral supplement.

VIMINAL T. (Cenci) Vitamins A 25,000 IU, D 400 IU, B_1 10 mg, B_2 5 mg, niacinamide 100 mg, B_6 1 mg, B_{12} 5 mcg, C 150 mg, calcium 103.6 mg, phosphorus 80.2 mg, iron 10 mg, magnesium 5.5 mg, manganese 1 mg, potassium 5 mg, zinc 1.4 mg/Cap. Bot. 100s, 500s.
Use: Vitamin/mineral supplement.

VIMINATE. (Various Mfr.) Vitamins B_1 2.5 mg, B_2 1.25 mg, B_3 25 mg, B_5 5 mg, B_6 0.5 mg, B_{12} 0.5 mcg, iron 7.5 mg, zinc 1 mg, choline 50 mg, inositol 50 mg, I, K, Mg, Mn/15 ml, alcohol 18%. Liq. Bot. pt, gal.
Use: Vitamin/mineral supplement.

VIMIN-CO. (Jenkins) Vitamins A 5000 IU, D 400 IU, B_1 3 mg, B_2 2.5 mg, B_6 1 mg, B_{12} 2 mcg, C 50 mg, niacinamide 20 mg, calcium 46 mg,

phosphorus 35 mg, iron 13.4 mg, calcium pantothenate 2 mg, magnesium 1 mg, manganese 1.5 mg, potassium 5 mg, zinc 1.4 mg/Cap. Bot. 1000s.
Use: Vitamin/mineral supplement.

VI-MIN-FOR-ALL. (Barth's) Vitamins A 3 mg, D 10 mcg, C 120 mg, B_1 35 mg, B_{12} 15 mcg, biotin, niacin 2.33 mg, E 30 IU, B_6, pantothenic acid, calcium 375 mg, phosphorus 180 mg, iron 20 mg, iodine 0.1 mg, rutin 10 mg, hesperidin-lemon bioflavonoid complex 10 mg, choline, inositol 2.4 mg, copper 10 mcg, manganese 2 mg, zinc 110 mcg, silicone 210 mcg/Tab. Bot. 100s, 500s.
Use: Vitamin/mineral supplement.

VIMMS-38. (Approved) Vitamins A 12,500 IU, D 1200 IU, B_1 15 mg, B_2 10 mg, C 75 mg, niacinamide 30 mg, calcium pantothenate 2 mg, B_6 0.5 mg, E 5 IU, Brewer's yeast 10 mg, B_{12} 15 mcg, iron 11.58 mg, desiccated liver 15 mg, choline bitartrate 30 mg, inositol 30 mg, calcium 59 mg, phosphorus 45 mg, zinc 0.68 mg, dicalcium phosphate 200 mg, manganese 1.11 mg, magnesium 1 mg, potassium 0.68 mg, pepsin 16.5 mg, diastase 16.5 mg, yeast 40.63 mg, protein digest 23.52 mg, amino acids 34.22 mg/Cap. Bot. 50s, 100s, 1000s.
Use: Vitamin/mineral supplement.

VINACTANE SULFATE. (Ciba) Viomycin Sulfate.

•**VINAFOCON A.** USAN.
Use: Contact lens material.

VINBARBITAL. 5-Ethyl-5-(1-methyl-1-butenyl)barbituric acid.
Use: Sedative/hypnotic.

VINBARBITAL SODIUM. 5-Ethyl-5-(1-methylbut-1-enyl)-barbiturate sodium
Use: Sedative/hypnotic.

VINBARBITONE. B.A.N. 5-Ethyl-5-(1-methylbut-1- enyl)barbituric acid.
Use: Hypnotic; sedative.

VINBLASTINE SULFATE. (Lyphomed) Vinblastine sulfate 10 mg/vial. Pow. for inj.
Use: Antineoplastic agent.

•**VINBLASTINE SULFATE,** U.S.P. XXII. Inj., Sterile, U.S.P. XXII. Vincaleukoblastine. Alkaloid extracted from *Vinca rosea* Linn.
Use: Antineoplastic.
See: Velban, Amp., Vial (Lilly).

VINCALEUKOBLASTINE, 22-OXO-, SULFATE (1:1)(SALT). Vincristine Sulfate, U.S.P. XXII.

VINCASAR PFS. (Adria) Vincristine sulfate 1 mg/ml. Vial 1 ml.
Use: Antineoplastic agent.

•**VINCOFOS.** USAN.
Use: Anthelmintic.

•**VINCRISTINE SULFATE,** U.S.P. XXII. Inj., U.S.P. XXII. (Lilly) Vincaleukoblastine, 22-oxo-,sulfate (1:1)(salt) Leurocristine. An alkaloid extracted from *Vinca rosea Linn.*
Use: Antineoplastic.
See: Oncovin, Amp. (Lilly).
Vincasar PFS, Vial (Adria).

•**VINDESINE.** USAN.
Use: Antineoplastic.

•**VINDESINE SULFATE.** USAN.
Use: Antineoplastic.

•**VINEPIDINE SULFATE.** USAN.
Use: Antineoplastic.

•**VINGLYCINATE SULFATE.** USAN. 4-Deacetylvincaleukoblastine 4-(N,N-dimethylglycinate) (ester) sulfate (1:1.5)(salt).
Use: Antineoplastic.

•**VINLEUROSINE SULFATE.** USAN. Sulfate salt of an alkaloid extracted from *Vinca rosea* Linn. Also see Vinblastine.
Use: Antineoplastic.

•**VINPOCETINE.** USAN. Ethyl apovincamin-22-oate.
Use: Antineoplastic.

•**VINROSIDINE SULFATE.** USAN. Sulfate salt of an alkaloid extracted from *vinca rosea* Linn.
See: Vinblastine.
Use: Antineoplastic.

VINYLACETATE-POLYVINYLPYRROLIDONE.
See: Ivy-Rid Spray (Mallard).

VINYL ALCOHOL POLYMER, U.S.P. XXII.
See: Polyvinyl alcohol.

VINYLBITONE. B.A.N. 5-(1-Methylbutyl)-5-vinylbarbituric acid.
Use: Hypnotic; sedative.

VINYL ETHER, U.S.P. XXI.
Use: General anesthetic (inhalation.).
See: Vinethene, Liq.

VINYZENE. Bromchlorenone.
Use: Fungicide, bactericide.

•**VINZOLIDINE SULFATE.** USAN.
Use: Antineoplastic.

VIO-BEC. (Solvay) Vitamins B_1 25 mg, B_2 25 mg, niacinamide 100 mg, calcium pantothenate 40 mg, B_6 25 mg, C 500 mg/Cap. Bot. 100s.
Use: Vitamin supplement.

VIO-BEC FORTE. (Solvay) Vitamins B_1 25 mg, B_2 25 mg, B_6 25 mg, C 500 mg, calcium pantothenate 40 mg, niacinamide 100 mg, E 30 IU, B_{12} 5 mcg, folic acid 0.5 mg, zinc 25 mg, copper 3 mg/Tab. Bot. 100s.
Use: Vitamin/mineral supplement.

VIODO HC. (NMC Labs) Iodochlorhydroxyquin 3%, hydrocortisone 1% in cream base. Tube 20 Gm.
Use: Corticosteroid, antifungal (external).

VIOFORM. (Ciba) Clioquinol. **Cream:** 3%. Tube oz. **Oint.:** 3% in petrolatum base. Tube oz.
Use: Antifungal, external.

VIOFORM-HYDROCORTISONE. (Ciba) **Cream:** Clioquinol 3%, hydrocortisone 1% in water-washable base w/stearyl alcohol, cetyl alcohol, stearic acid, sodium lauryl sulfate, glycerin, petrolatum. Tube 20 Gm. **Oint.:** Clioquinol 3%, hydrocortisone 1% in petrolatum base. Tube 20 Gm. **Mild Cream:** Clioquinol 3%, hydrocortisone 0.5% w/ingredients included in Cream. Tube 0.5 oz, 1 oz.
Use: Antifungal, corticosteroid (external).

VIOGEN-C. (Goldino) Vitamins B_1 20 mg, B_2 10 mg, B_3 100 mg, B_5 20 mg, B_6 5 mg, C 300 mg, Mg, zinc 18 mg/Cap. Bot. 60s, 500s, UD 100s.
Use: Vitamin/mineral supplement.

VIOKASE. (Robins) **Tab.:** Lipase 8000 units, protease 30,000 units, amylase 30,000 units/Tab. Bot. 100s, 500s. **Pow.:** Lipase 16,800 units, protease 70,000 units, amylase 70,000 units/0.7 Gm (0.25 tsp.).
Use: Digestive enzymes.

VIOPAN-T. (Trimen) Vitamins A 8000 IU, D 400 IU, E 30 mg, B_1 10 mg, B_2 10 mg, B_3 100 mg, B_5 5 mg, B_6 2 mg, B_{12} 6 mcg, C 200 mg, iron 15 mg, folic acid 0.4 mg, calcium 100 mg, zinc 15 mg, choline 25 mg, L-lysine 25 mg, biotin 10 mcg, Cu, I, K, Mg, Mn, phosphorus 42 mg/Tab. Bot. 100s.
Use: Vitamin/mineral supplement.

VIOSTEROL W/HALIBUT LIVER OIL. Vitamins A 50,000 IU, D 10,000 IU/Gm. (Abbott)—Bot. 5 ml, 20 ml, 50 ml. Cap.: Vitamins A 5000 IU, D 1000 IU (Ives) Cap.: Vitamins A 5000 IU, D 1700 IU.
Use: Vitamin supplement.

•**VIPROSTOL.** USAN.
Use: Hypotensive, vasodilator.

VIPRYNIUM EMBONATE. B.A.N. 6-Dimethylamino-2-[2-(2:5-dimethyl-1-phenyl-3-pyrrolyl)vinyl]-1-methylquinolinium embonate. (Embonic acid is adopted as the trivial name for 4:4′ methylenebis-(3-hydroxymaphthalene-2-carboxylic acid). Vanquin. Pyrvinium Pamoate.
Use: Anthelmintic.

VIRA-A FOR INFUSION. (Parke-Davis) Vidarabine for infusion 200 mg/ml. Vial 5 ml.
Use: Antiviral.

VIRA-A OPHTHALMIC. (Parke-Davis) Vidarabine 3% in a sterile inert base. Tube 3.5 Gm.
Use: Antiviral.

VIRAC. (Ruson) Undecoylium Cl-iodine. Iodine complexed with a cationic detergent. Surgical soln. Bot. 2 oz, 8 oz, 1 gal.
Use: Antiseptic.

VIRACIL. (Approved) Phenylephrine HCl 5 mg, hesperidin 50 mg, thenylene HCl 12.5 mg, pyrilamine maleate 12.5 mg, vitamin C 50 mg, salicylamide 2.5 gr, caffeine 0.5 gr, sodium salicylate 1.25 gr/Cap. Bot. 16s, 36s.
Use: Decongestant, vitamin supplement, antihistamine, analgesic.

VIRAMISOL. (Seatrace) Adenosine phosphate 25 mg/ml. Vial 10 ml.
Use: Relief of varicose vein complications.

VIRANOL. (American Dermal) Salicylic acid 16.7%, lactic acid 16.7% in flexible collodion vehicle. Bot. 10 ml.
Use: Keratolytic.

VIRAZOLE. (ICN) Ribavirin 6 Gm/Vial.
Use: Antiviral.

•**VIRGINIAMYCIN.** USAN. An antibiotic produced by *Streptomyces virginie*}.
Use: Antibacterial.

VIRIDIUM. (Vita Elixir) Phenylazodiaminopyridine HCl 100 mg/Tab.
Use: Urinary tract product.

•**VIRIDOFULVIN.** USAN.
Use: Antifungal.

VIRILON. (Star) Methyltestosterone 10 mg/SR Cap. Bot. 100s, 1000s.
Use: Androgen.

VIROGEN HERPES SLIDE TEST. (Wampole) Latex agglutination slide test for the detection of herpes simplex virus antigens directly from lesions or cell culture. Test kit 100s.
Use: Diagnostic aid.

VIROGEN ROTATEST. (Wampole) Latex agglutination slide test for the qualitative detection of rotavirus in fecal specimens. Test kit 50s.
Use: Diagnostic aid.

VIROGEN RUBELLA SLIDE TEST. (Wampole) Latex agglutination slide test for the detection of rubella virus antibody in serum. Test kit 100s, 500s, 5000s.
Use: Diagnostic aid.

VIROGEN RUBELLA MICROLATEX TEST. (Wampole) Latex agglutination microlatex test for the detection of rubella virus antibody in serum. Test kit 500s, 5000s.
Use: Diagnostic aid.

VIROGEN RUBELLA SLIDE TEST WITH FAST TRAK SLIDES. (Wampole) Latex agglutination slide test for the detection of rubella virus antibody in serum.
Use: Diagnostic aid.

VIRO-MED TABLETS. (Whitehall) Acetaminophen 500 mg, chlorpheniramine maleate 2 mg, pseudoephedrine HCl 30 mg, dextromethorphan HBr 15 mg/Tab. Bot. 20s, 48s.
Use: Analgesic, antihistamine, decongestant, antitussive.

VIROPTIC OPHTHALMIC SOLUTION. (Burroughs Wellcome) Trifluridine 1%. Bot. 7.5 ml.
Use: Antiviral.

•**VIROXIME.** USAN.
Use: Antiviral.

VIROZYME INJECTION. (Marcen) Sodium nucleate 2.5%, phenol 0.5%, protein hydrolysate 2.5%, benzyl alcohol 0.2%. Vial 5 ml, 10 ml.
Use: Promote leukocytosis and phagocytosis.

VIRUGON. Under study. Anhydro bis-(beta-hydroxyethyl) biguanide derivative.
Use: Treatment of influenza, mumps, measles, chicken pox and shingles.

VISALENS SOAKING & CLEANING SOLUTION. (Leeming) Sterile soln. containing cleaning agents, benzalkonium Cl, buffered soln. Bot. 4 oz.
Use: Hard contact lens care.

VISALENS WETTING SOLUTION. (Leeming) Sterile soln. containing polyvinyl alcohol with hydroxypropyl methylcellulose, edetate disodium, sodium Cl, benzalkonium Cl 1:25,000. Bot. 2 oz.
Use: Hard contact lens care.

VISCARIN W/IODINE, BORIC ACID, PHENOL, CHLOROPHYLL.
See: Triophyll, Liq. (Schaffer).

VISCOAT SOLUTION. (Cilco) Sodium chondroitin sulfate 40 mg, sodium hyaluronate 30 mg, sodium dihydrogen phosphate hydrate 0.45 mg, disodium hydrogen phosphate 2.65 mg, sodium Cl 4.3 mg/ml. Glass syringe disposable 0.25 ml, 0.5 ml.
Use: Viscoelastic solution.

VISCUM ALBUM, EXTRACT. Visnico.
Use: Vasodilator.

VISINE. (Leeming) Tetrahydrozoline HCl 0.05%, sodium Cl, boric acid, sodium borate, benzalkonium Cl 0.01%, disodium ethylenediamine tetraacetate 0.1%. Dropper Bot. 0.5 oz, Plastic bot. 0.5 oz, ¾ oz, 1 oz.
Use: Vasoconstrictor/mydriatic (ophthalmic).

VISINE AC. (Leeming) Tetrahydrozoline HCl 0.05%, zinc sulfate 0.25%, benzalkonium Cl 0.01%, sodium Cl, boric acid, sodium citrate, ethylenediamine tetraacetate 0.1%. Bot. 0.5 oz, 1 oz.
Use: Vasoconstrictor/mydriatic (ophthalmic).

VISKEN. (Sandoz) Pindolol 5 mg or 10 mg/Tab. Bot. 100s.
Use: Antihypertensive.

VISNADINE. B.A.N. 10-Acetoxy-9,10-dihydro-8,8-dimethyl-9-α-methylbutyryloxy-2H,8H-benzo-[1,2-b:3,4-b′]dipyran-2-one. Cardine.
Use: Coronary vasodilator.

VIPROSTOL. USAN.

VISTACON. (Hauck) Hydroxyzine HCl 50 mg/ml. Vial 10 ml.
Use: Antianxiety agent.

VISTAJECT 25 & 50. (Mayrand) Hydroxyzine HCl 25 mg or 50 mg/ml. Vial 10 ml.
Use: Antianxiety agent.

VISTAQUEL 50. (Pasadena) Hydroxyzine HCl 50 mg/ml. Vial 10 ml.
Use: Antianxiety agent.

VISTARIL. (Pfizer Laboratories) Hydroxyzine pamoate equivalent to hydroxyzine HCl. **Cap.:** 25 mg, 50 mg or 100 mg. Bot. 100s, 500s, UD 100s. **Oral Susp.:** 25 mg/5 ml. Bot. 120 ml, pt.
Use: Antianxiety agent.

VISTARIL I.M. (Roerig) Hydroxyzine HCl. **25 mg/ml:** Vial 10 ml, Box 1s. **50 mg/ml:** Vial 10 ml, Box 1s.; Vial 1 ml, UD 25s. **100 mg/2 ml:** Vial 2 ml, UD 25s.
Use: Antianxiety agent.

VISTARIL ISOJECT I.M. (Roerig) Hydroxyzine HCl 50 mg/ml or 100 mg/2 ml Amp. 1 ml, 2 ml.
Use: Antianxiety agent.

VISTAZINE 50. (Keene) Hydroxyzine HCl 50 mg/ml. Vial 10 mg/ml.
Use: Antianxiety agent.

VITA-BEE C-800. (Rugby) Vitamins E 45 mg, B_1 15 mg, B_2 17 mg, B_3 100 mg, B_5 25 mg, B_6 25 mg, B_{12} 12 mcg, C 800 mg/Tab. Bot. 60s.
Use: Vitamin supplement.

VITA-BEE W/C. (Rugby) Vitamins B_1 15 mg, B_2 10 mg, B_3 50 mg, B_5 10 mg, B_6 5 mg, C 300 mg/TR Cap. Bot. 50s, 100s.
Use: Vitamin supplement.

VITABIX. (Spanner) Vitamins B_1 100 mg, B_2 2 mg, B_6 5 mg, B_{12} 30 mcg, niacinamide 100 mg, panthenol 10 mg/ml. Vial 10 ml. Multiple dose vial 30 ml.
Use: Vitamin supplement.

VITA-BOB CAPSULES. (Scot-Tussin) Vitamins A 5000 IU, D 400 IU, E 30 mg, B_1 1.5 mg, B_2 1.7 mg, B_3 20 mg, B_6 2 mg, B_{12} 6 mcg, C 60 mg, folic acid 0.4 mg/Cap. Bot. 100s.
Use: Vitamin supplement.

V-I TABS. (Kenyon) Vitamins A 5000 IU, D-2 500 mg, B_1 3 mg, B_2 2.5 mg, B_6 1 mg, B_{12} 1 mg, C 50 mg, niacinamide 20 mg, calcium pantothenate 1 mg, iron 15 mg/Tab. Bot. 100s, 1000s.
Use: Vitamin/mineral supplement.

VITA-C. (Freeda) Ascorbic acid 4 Gm/tsp. Crystals 100 Gm, 500 Gm, 1000 Gm.
Use: Vitamin C supplement.

VITACARN. (Kendall McGaw) L-Carnitine 1 Gm/10 ml. UD Box 50s, 100s.
Use: L-carnitine supplement.

VITA-CEBUS. (Cenci) Vitamins A 10,000 IU, D 1000 IU, C 100 mg, B_1 5 mg, B_2 5 mg, B_6 1 mg, B_{12} 1 mcg, niacin and niacinamide 30 mg, calcium pantothenate 5 mg, E 3 mg, yeast 1 gr, liver 1 gr, hesperidin complex 10 mg, calcium 200 mg, copper 0.75 mg, magnesium 5 mg, manganese 1 mg, potassium 5 mg, zinc 0.3 mg/2 Tab. Bot. 100s, 250s. Liq. 4 oz, 8 oz.
Use: Vitamin/mineral supplement.

VITACREST. (Nutrition) Vitamins A 25,000 IU, D 400 IU, E 10 IU, B_1 25 mg, B_2 12 mg, B_6 10 mg, B_{12} 10 mcg, biotin 10 mcg, folic acid 0.1 mg, calcium pantothenate 25 mg, niacinamide 50 mg, inositol 25 mg, l-glutamic acid 10 mg, l-lysine HCl 20 mg, p-aminobenzoic acid 25 mg, C 250 mg, wheat germ oil 10 mg, brewers yeast (dried) 10 mg, whole liver desiccated 10 mg, soybean lecithin 50 mg, iron 10 mg, calcium carbonate 625 mg, copper 0.2 mg, zinc 0.2 mg, magnesium 10 mg, manganese 0.2 mg, potassium 10 mg/Cap. Bot. 100s.
Use: Vitamin/mineral supplement.

VIT-A-DROPS. (Vision Pharm.) Vitamin A 5000 IU, polysorbate 80. Bot. 15 ml.
Use: Ocular lubricant.

VITADYE. (Elder) FD & C yellow No. 5, D. & C. red. No. 40, FD & C blue No. 1 dyes and dihydroxyacetone 5%. Bot. 0.5 oz, 2 oz.
Use: Cosmetic cover for hypopigmented skin.

VITA ELIXIR. (Vita Elixir) Alcohol 25%, vitamins A palmitate 5000 IU, D-2 500 IU, iron 10 mg/45 ml w/multivitamins and minerals.
Use: Vitamin/mineral supplement.

VITAFOL. (Everett) Iron 65 mg, vitamins A 6000 IU, D 400 IU, E 30 mg, B_1 1.1 mg, B_2 1.8 mg, B_3 15 mg, B_6 2.5 mg, B_{12} 5 mcg, C 60 mg, folic acid 1 mg, calcium/Tab. Bot. 100s, 1000s.

Use: Vitamin/mineral supplement.

VITAFORT. (Kessel) Vitamins A 4000 IU, D 400 IU, E 15 IU, C 70 mg, folic acid 1 mg, B_1 2 mg, B_2 2 mg, niacinamide 20 mg, B_6 2 mg, B_{12} 5 mcg, calcium pantothenate 10 mg/Cap. Bot. 60s.
Use: Vitamin supplement.

VITA-IRON FORMULA. (Barth's) Iron 120 mg, vitamins B_1 5 mg, B_2 10 mg, C 20 mg, niacin 2 mg, B_{12} 25 mcg, lysine, desiccated liver 200 mg, bromelain/Tab. Bot. 100s, 500s.
Use: Vitamin/mineral supplement.

VITAJEN. (Jenkins) Vitamins B_1 12 mg, B_2 4 mg, B_{12} 10 mcg, B_6 2 mg, calcium pantothenate 6 mg, nicotinic acid 40 mg/fl oz. Bot. 4 oz, gal.
Use: Vitamin supplement.

VITA-KAPS FILMTABS. (Abbott) Vitamins A 5000 IU, D 400 IU, B_1 3 mg, B_2 2.5 mg, nicotinamide 20 mg, B_6 1 mg, C 50 mg, B_{12} 3 mcg/Filmtab. Bot. 100s, 1000s.
Use: Vitamin supplement.

VITAKAPS-M. (Abbott) Vitamins A 5000 IU, D 400 IU, B_1 3 mg, B_2 2.5 mg, nicotinamide 20 mg, B_6 1 mg, B_{12} 3 mcg, C 50 mg, iron 10 mg, copper 1 mg, iodine 0.15 mg, manganese 1 mg, zinc 7.5 mg/Filmtab. Bot. 100s.
Use: Vitamin/mineral supplement.

VITAL B50. (Goldline) Vitamins B_1 50 mg, B_2 50 mg, B_3 50 mg, B_5 50 mg, B_6 50 mg, B_{12} 50 mcg, folic acid 0.1 mg, biotin 50 mcg, PABA 50 mg, choline bitartrate 50 mg, inositol 50 mg, bromelain 20 mg/TR Tab. Bot 60s.
Use: Vitamin supplement.

VITAL HIGH NITROGEN. (Ross) Amino acids, partially hydrolyzed whey, meat and soy, hydrolyzed cornstarch, sucrose, safflower oil, MCT mono and diglycerides, soy lecithin, vitamins A, B_1, B_2, B_3, B_5, B_6, B_{12}, C, D, E, K, folic acid, biotin, choline, Ca, P, Mg, Fe, Cu, Zn, Mn, I, Cl. Packet 80 Gm.
Use: Enteral nutritional supplement.

VITALAX. (Vitalax) Candy base, gumdrop flavored. Pkg. 20s.
Use: Laxative.

VITAMEL-M. (Eastwood) Liq. Bot. 16 oz.

VITAMEL WITH IRON. (Eastwood) Drops 50 ml. Chew. Tab. Bot. 100s.

VITAMIN A, U.S.P. XXII. Cap., U.S.P. XXII. Oleovitamin A.
Use: Anti-xerophthalmic vitamin, emollient.
Amp.
Aquasol A, Preps. (USV Pharm.).
Cap.
Acon (Du Pont).
Alphalin (Lilly).
Aquasol A (USV Labs.).
Vi-Dom-A (Miles Pharm).
Oint.
Aquasol A (USV Pharm.).
Retin-A (Johnson & Johnson).
Tab.
Dispatabs (Person & Covey).
Vial
Aquasol A (USV Labs.).

VITAMIN A, ALPHALIN. (Lilly) Vitamin A 50,000 IU/Gelseal. Bot. 100s.
Use: Vitamin A supplement.

VITAMIN A, WATER MISCIBLE, OR SOLUBLE. Water miscible vitamin A.
Use: Vitamin A supplement.

VITAMIN Bc.
See: Folic Acid (Various Mfr.).

VITAMIN B1. Thiamine HCl, U.S.P. XXII.
Use: Vitamin B_1 supplement.

VITAMIN B1 MONONITRATE. Thiamine mononitrate.
Use: Vitamin B_1 supplement.

VITAMIN B1 & B12. (Pharmex) Vitamins B_1 100 mg, B_{12} 1000 mcg/ml. Vial 10 ml.
Use:Vitamin supplement.

VITAMIN B1 W/PANCREATIN, OX BILE EXTRACT PEPSIN, GLUTAMIC ACID HCl.
See: Maso-Gestive, Tab. (Mason).

VITAMIN B1 W/THYROID.
See: T & T, Tab. (Mason).

•**VITAMIN B2.** Riboflavin, U.S.P. XXII.
Use: Vitamin B_2 supplement.

•**VITAMIN B3.** Niacinamide, U.S.P. XXII. Nicotinamide.
Use: Vitamin B_3 supplement.

•**VITAMIN B5.** Calcium Pantothenate U.S.P. XXII.
Use: Vitamin B_5 supplement.

•**VITAMIN B6.** Pyridoxine HCl, U.S.P. XXII.
Use: Vitamin B_6 supplement.
See: Hexa-Betalin, Tab. (Lilly).
Hexavibex, Vial (Parke-Davis).

VITAMIN B6 & B1. (Pharmex) Vitamins B_6 100 mg, B_1 100 mg/ml. Vial 10 ml.
Use: Vitamin supplement.

VITAMIN B-8.
See: Adenosine phosphate.

•**VITAMIN B12.** Cyanocobalamin, U.S.P. XXII. Cobalamine.
See:
Cap., Tab.
Redisol (Merck Sharp & Dohme).
Vial, Amp.
Bedoce (Lincoln).
Berubigen (Upjohn).
Betalin-12 (Lilly).
Cabadon-M (Solvay).
Cobadoce Forte (Solvay).
Crysto-Gel (Solvay).
Cyano-Gel, Liq. (Maurry).
Dodex (Organon).
Poyamin (Fellows).
Redisol (Merck Sharp & Dohme).
Rubramin (Squibb).
Ruvite 1000 (Savage).
Sigamine (Sig).
Sytobex-H (Parke-Davis).
Vi-Twel, Inj. (Berlex).
W/Ferrous-sulfate, ascorbic acid, folic acid.
See: Intrin, Cap. (Merit).

W/Folic acid, niacinamide, liver.
See: Hepfomin 500, Inj. (Keene Pharm.).
W/Thiamine.
See: Cobalin, Vial (Ulmer).
Cyamine, Vial (Keene).
W/Thiamine, vitamin B_6.
See: Orexin, Tab. (Stuart).

VITAMIN B12 a & b.
See: Hydroxocobalamin (Various Mfr.).

VITAMIN B15. Pangamic acid, betaglucono-dimethylaminoacetic acid.
Use: Alleged to increase oxygen supply in blood. Not approved by FDA as a vitamin or drug. Illegal to sell Vitamin B_{15}.

VITAMIN B COMPLEX. Concentrated extract of dried brewer's yeast and extract of corn processed w/*Clostridium acetobutylicum*}.
See: Becotin, Pulvules (Lilly).
Betalin Complex, Amp. (Lilly).
Savaplex, Vial (Savage).

VITAMIN B COMPLEX NO. 104. (Century) Vitamins B_1 100 mg, B_2 2 mg, B_6 2 mg, d-panthenol 10 mg, niacinamide 125 mg, benzyl alcohol 1%, gentisic acid ethanolamide 2.5%/Vial 30 ml.
Use: Vitamin supplement.

VITAMIN B COMPLEX, BETALIN COMPLEX, ELIXIR. (Lilly) Vitamins B_1 2.7 mg, B_2 1.35 mg, B_{12} 3 mcg, B_6 0.555 mg, pantothenic acid 2.7 mg, niacinamide 6.75 mg, liver fraction 500 mg/5 ml, alcohol 17%. Bot. 16 oz.
Use: Vitamin supplement.

VITAMIN B COMPLEX W/VITAMIN C. (Century) Vitamins B_1 25 mg, B_2 5 mg, B_6 5 mg, niacinamide 50 mg, panthenol 5 mg, calcium 50 mg, propethylene glycol 300 10%, gentisic acid ethanolamide 2.5%, benzyl alcohol 2%/Vial 30 ml.
Use: Vitamin supplement.

VITAMIN B COMPLEX, BETALIN COMPLEX CAPSULES. (Lilly) Vitamins B_1 1 mg, B_2 2 mg, B_6 0.4 mg, pantothenic acid 3.333 mg, niacinamide 10 mg, B_{12} 1 mcg/Pulvule. Bot. 100s.
Use: Vitamin supplement.

VITAMIN C.
See: Ascorbic Acid Preps.

VITAMIN C, CEVALIN. (Lilly) Ascorbic acid 250 mg or 500 mg/Tab. Bot. 100s.
Use: Vitamin C supplement.

VITAMIN C W/COMBINATIONS.
See: Allbee C-800, Prods. (Robins).
Allbee with C, Cap. (Robins).
Allbee-T, Tab. (Robins).
Anti-therm, Tab. (Scrip).
Bejectal w/Vitamin C (Abbott).
Colrex, Cap. (Solvay).
Nialexo-C, Tab. (Mallard).
Thex, Cap. (Ingram).
Thex Forte, Cap. (Ingram).
Vicon-C, Cap. (Glaxo).
Vicon Forte, Cap. (Glaxo).
Vicon Plus, Cap. (Glaxo).
Vi-Zac, Cap. (Glaxo).
Z-BEC, Tab. (Robins).

VITAMIN D. Cholecalciferol, U.S.P. XXII.
Use: Vitamin D supplement.

VITAMIN D, DELTALIN. (Lilly) Vitamin D-2 50,000 units (1.25 mg)/Gelseal. Bot. 100s.
Use: Vitamin D supplement.

VITAMIN D, SYNTHETIC.
See: Activated 7-Dehydro-cholesterol Calciferol.

VITAMIN D-1.
See: Dihydrotachysterol.

VITAMIN D-2. Activated ergasterol, Ergocalciferol.
See: Calciferol, Preps. (Various Mfr.).
Drisdol, Liq. (Winthrop Pharm).
Viosterol (Various Mfr.).

VITAMIN D-3.
See: Activated 7-dehydrocholesterol.
Calciferol Prep. for related activity.

VITAMIN D-3-CHOLESTEROL. Compound of crystalline vitamin D-3 and cholesterol.
Use: Vitamin supplement.

VITAMIN D-4.
See: Dihydrotachysterol, Preps. (Various Mfr.).

•**VITAMIN E,** U.S.P. XXII. Cap., U.S.P. XXII. It may consist of: d- or dl-alpha tocopherol, d-or dl-alpha tocopheryl acetate, d- or dl-alpha tocopheryl acid succinate, mixed tocopherols concentrate, or d-alpha tocopheryl acetate concentrate.
Use: Vitamin E supplement.
See: Aquasol E (USV).
Eprolin, Gelseal (Lilly).
E-Vites, Cap. (Quality Generics).
Pertropin Cap. (Lannett).
Solucap E. Cap. (Jamieson-McKames).
Tega-E-Cream (Ortega).
Tocopher, Prod. (Quality Generics).
Tocopherol, Preps. (Various Mfr.).
Wheat Germ Oil (Various Mfr.).

VITAMIN E, EPROLIN. (Lilly) Alpha-tocopherol 100 units/Gelseal. Bot. 100s.
Use: Vitamin E supplement.

VITAMIN E W/QUININE SULFATE, NIACIN.
See: Myodyne, Tab. (Paddock).

VITAMIN F.
See: Fats, Unsaturated.
Fatty Acids, Unsaturated.

VITAMIN G.
See: Riboflavin.

VITAMIN K.
See: Hykinone, Amp. (Abbott).
Menadiol, Sodium Diphosphate, Preps. (Various Mfr.).
Menadione, Preps. (Various Mfr.).
Menadione Sodium Bisulfite, Preps. (Various Mfr.).

VITAMIN K-1.
See: Phytonadione, U.S.P. XXII.

VITAMIN K-3.
See: Menadione, U.S.P. XXII.

VITAMIN K OXIDE. Not available, but usually K-1 is desired.

VITAMIN M.

See: Folic Acid, U.S.P. XXII.

VITAMIN P. Citrin.
See: Bio-Flavonoid Compounds (Various Mfr.).
Hesperidin Preps. (Various Mfr.).
Quercetin (Various Mfr.).
Rutin, Preps. (Various Mfr.).

VITAMIN T. Sesame seed factor, termite factor.
Use: Claimed to aid proper blood coagulation and promote formation of blood platelets. Not approved by FDA as an active vitamin.

VITAMIN U. Present in cabbage juice.

VITAMIN, MAINTENANCE FORMULA.
See: Stuart Formula, Tab., Liq. (Stuart).
Vi-Magna, Cap. (Lederle).

VITA-MINS. (Mills) Vitamins A 5000 IU, D 200 IU, C 30 mg, B_1 1 mg, B_2 2 mg, B_6 0.1 mg, B_{12} 1 mcg, d-calcium pantothenate 0.5 mg, niacinamide 20 mg, folic acid 0.1 mg, ferrous gluconate 25 mg, copper gluconate 5 mg, zinc gluconate 5 mg, manganese gluconate 5 mg/Tab. Bot. 100s.
Use: Vitamin/mineral supplement.

VITAMINS: STRESS FORMULA.
See: Cebefortis, Tab. (Upjohn).
Folbesyn, Tab., Vial (Lederle).
Probec-T, Tab. (Stuart).
Stresscaps, Cap. (Lederle).
Stresscaps With Iron (Lederle).
Stresscaps With Zinc (Lederle).
Stresstabs-600 (Lederle).
Thera-combex Kap. (Parke-Davis).

VITAMINS W/ANTIOBESITY AGENTS.
See: Fetamin, Tab. (Mission).
Obedrin, Cap. or Tab. (Massengill).

VITAMINS W/LIVER & LIPOTROPIC AGENTS.
See: Heptuna, Cap. (Roerig).
Lederplex, Preps. (Lederle).
Livitamin, Preps. (Beecham Labs).
Metheponex, Cap. (Rawl).
Methischol, Cap. (USV Pharm.).

VITA NATAL. (Scot-Tussin) Folic acid 1 mg/Tab. Bot. 100s.
Use: Folic acid supplement.

VITANEED. (Biosearch) P-beef, Ca and Na caseinates, CHO-maltodextrin. F-partially hydrogenated soy oil, mono and diglycerides, soy lecithin. Protein 35 Gm, CHO 125 Gm, fat 40 Gm, sodium 500 mg, potassium 1250 mg/L, 1 Cal/ml, 375 mOsm/kg H_20. Liq. Ready-to-use 250 ml.
Use: Enteral nutritional supplement.

VITAON. (Vita Elixir) Vitamin B_{12} 25 mcg, thiamine HCl 10 mg, ferric pyrophosphate 250 mg/5 ml.
Use: Vitamin supplement.

VITA PLUREX FORTE. (Standex) Vitamins B_1 1.5 mg, B_2 2 mg, B_6 0.1 mg, calcium pantothenate 1 mg, niacinamide 10 mg/Tab. Bot. 100s.
Use: Vitamin supplement.

VITA PLUREX W/C CAPSULES. (Standex) Vitamins B_1 15 mg, B_2 10 mg, B_6 5 mg, niacinamide 50 mg, calcium pantothenate 10 mg, C 300 mg/Cap. Bot. 100s.
Use: Vitamin supplement.

VITA-PLUS B12. (Scot-Tussin) Vitamin B_{12} 1000 mcg/ml. Inj.
Use: Vitamin B_{12} supplement.

VITA-PLUS E. (Scot-Tussin) Vitamin E 294 mg as d-alpha tocopheryl acetate/Cap.
Use: Vitamin E supplement.

VITA-PLUS G. (Scot-Tussin) Vitamins A 10,000 IU, D 400 IU, E 2 mg, B_1 5 mg, B_2 2.5 mg, B_3 40 mg, B_5 4 mg, B_6 1 mg, B_{12} 2 mcg, C 75 mg, iron 30 mg, calcium 75 mg, zinc 0.5 mg, choline 31.4 mg, inositol 15 mg, K, Mg, Mn, phosphorus 58 mg/Cap. Bot. 100s.
Use: Vitamin/mineral supplement.

VITA-PLUS H CAPSULES. (Scot-Tussin) Vitamins B_1 17.5 mg, B_2 8.5 mg, B_3 35 mg, B_5 5 mg, B_6 0.25 mg, B_{12} 5 mcg, iron 11.7 mg, C 60 mg, choline, inositol, dessicated liver/Cap. Bot. 100s.
Use: Vitamin/mineral supplement.

VITA-PLUS H LIQUID SUGAR FREE. (Scot-Tussin) Vitamins B_1 30 mg, l-lysine monohydrochloride 300 mg, B_{12} 75 mcg, B_6 15 mg, iron pyrophosphate soluble 100 mg/5 ml. Bot. 4 oz, 8 oz, pt, gal.
Use: Vitamin/mineral supplement.

VITA-RAY CREME. (Gordon) Vitamins E 3000 IU, A 200,000 IU/oz w/aloe 10%. Jar 0.5 oz, 2.5 oz.
Use: Emollient.

VITAREX. (Pasadena Research) Vitamins A 10,000 IU, D 200 IU, B_1 15 mg, B_2 10 mg, B_6 5 mg, B_{12} 5 mcg, C 250 mg, niacinamide 100 mg, calcium pantothenate 20 mg, E 15 mg, iron 15 mg, iodine 0.15 mg, calcium 50 mg, phosphorus 40 mg, copper 0.1 mg, manganese 0.1 mg, magnesium 5 mg, potassium 2 mg/Tab. Bot. 100s.
Use: Vitamin/mineral supplement.

VITA-SUP. (Kenyon) Vitamins A 12,500 IU, D 1000 IU, B_1 5 mg, B_2 2.5 mg, B_6 1 mg, B_{12} 2 mcg, C 75 mg, niacinamide 40 mg, calcium pantothenate 4 mg, E 3 IU, dicalcium phosphate 260 mg, choline bitartrate 31.4 mg, inositol 15 mg, liver protein fraction 25 mg, ferrous sulfate 102 mg, manganese sulfate 1.5 mg, potassium sulfate 4.5 mg, zinc sulfate 1.4 mg, magnesium sulfate 21.6 mg/Cap. Bot. 100s, 1000s.
Use: Vitamin/mineral supplement.

VITATONE DROPS. (Winthrop Products) Multivitamin.
Use: Dietary supplement.

VITATRUM. (Halsey).
Use: Dietary supplement.

VITAZIN. (Mesemer) Ascorbic acid 300 mg, niacinamide 100 mg, thiamine mononitrate 20 mg, d-calcium pantothenate 20 mg, riboflavin 10 mg, pyridoxine HCl 5 mg, magnesium sulfate 70 mg, zinc 25 mg/Cap. Bot. 100s.

Use: Vitamin/mineral supplement.

VITA-ZOO. (Towne) Vitamins A 2500 IU, D 400 IU, E 15 IU, C 60 mg, folic acid 0.3 mg, B_1 1.05 mg, B_2 1.2 mg, niacin 13.5 mg, B_6 1.05 mg, B_{12} 4.5 mcg/Tab. Bot. 100s.
Use: Vitamin supplement.

VITA-ZOO PLUS IRON. (Towne) Vitamins A 2500 IU, D 400 IU, E 15 IU, C 60 mg, folic acid 0.3 mg, B_1 1.05 mg, B_2 1.2 mg, niacin 13.5 mg, B_6 1.05 mg, B_{12} 4.5 mcg, iron 15 mg/Tab. Bot. 100s.
Use: Vitamin supplement.

VITEC. (Pharmaceutical Specialties) Dl-alpha tocopheryl acetate in a vanishing cream base. Cream. 120 Gm.
Use: Emollient.

VI-TESTROGEN. (Pharmex) Testosterone 10 mg, estrogenic substance (natural) 1 mg, vitamins B_1 50 mg, B_2 2 mg, B_6 5 mg, panthenol 10 mg, niacinamide 100 mg, inositol 25 mg, choline Cl 25 mg, d,l-methionine 25 mg/cc, sodium carboxymethylcellulose 0.05%, procaine HCl 1%, benzyl alcohol 2%. Vial 10 ml.
Use: Androgen, estrogen, vitamin supplement.

VITORMAINS. (Hauck) Tab. Bot. 100s.
Use: Vitamin supplement.

VITRAMONE. (Harvey) Natural estrogenic hormone 1 mg, vitamins B_1 10 mg, B_2 2 mg, B_6 5 mg, niacinamide 40 mg, inositol 50 mg, choline Cl 10 mg, methionine 10 mg/ml 10 ml.
Use: Estrogen, vitamin B supplement.

VITRON-C. (Fisons) Ferrous fumarate 200 mg, ascorbic acid 125 mg/Tab. Bot. 100s, 1000s.
Use: Vitamin/mineral supplement.

VITRON-C PLUS TABLETS. (Fisons) Ferrous fumarate 400 mg, vitamin C 250 mg/Tab. Bot. 30s, 100s, 500s.
Use: Vitamin/mineral supplement.

VIVACTIL. (Merck Sharp & Dohme) Protriptyline HCl 5 mg or 10 mg/Tab. **5 mg:** Bot. 100s. **10 mg:** Bot. 100s, UD 100s.
Use: Antidepressant.

VIVALAN. Viloxazine HCl (Orphan Drug).
Use: Narolepsy, cataplexy.
Sponsor: Stuart.

VIVARIN. (Beecham Products) Caffeine alkaloid 200 mg/Tab. Blister Pk. 16s, 40s, 80s.
Use: Analeptic.

VIVIKON. (Brown) Vitamins B_1 5 mg, B_2 2 mg, B_6 10 mg, d-panthenol 5 mg, niacinamide 10 mg, procaine HCl 2%/ml. 100 ml.
Use: Vitamin supplement.

VIVONEX FLAVOR PACKETS. (Norwich Eaton) Non-nutritive flavoring for Vivonex diets when consumed orally. Orange-pineapple, lemon-lime, strawberry and vanilla. Pkg. 60s.
Use: Flavoring.

VIVONEX, STANDARD. (Norwich Eaton) Free amino acid/complete enteral nutrition. Six packets provide kilocalories 1800, available nitrogen 5.88 Gm as amino acids 37 Gm, fat 2.61 Gm, carbohydrate 407 Gm, and full day's balanced nutrition. Calorie:nitrogen ratio is 300:1. Unflavored pow. Packet 80 Gm, Pkg. 6s.
Use: Enteral nutritional supplement.

VIVONEX T.E.N. (Norwich Eaton) Free amino acid, high nitrogen/high branched chain amino acid complete enteral nutrition. Ten packets provide kilocalories 3000, available nitrogen 17 Gm, amino acids 115 Gm, fat 8.33 Gm, carbohydrate 617 Gm and full day's balanced nutrition. Calorie:nitrogen ratio is 175:1. Unflavored pow. Packet 80 Gm, Pkg. 10s.
Use: Enteral nutritional supplement.

VIVOTIF BERNA. (Berna) Typhoid vaccine (oral). *S. typhi* Ty21a (viable) 2 to 6 X 10^9 colony forming units and *S. typhi* Ty21a[2] (non-viable) 5 to 50 X 10^9 colony forming units/Cap. Single foil blister with 4 doses.
Use: Agent for immunization.

VI-ZAC. (Glaxo) Vitamins A 5000 IU, C 500 mg, E 50 IU, zinc sulfate 80 mg/Cap. Bot. 60s.
Use: Vitamin/mineral supplement.

V-LAX. (Century) Psyllium mucilloid (hydrophilic) 50%, dextrose 50%. Pow. 0.25 lb, 1 lb.
Use: Laxative.

VLEMASQUE. (Dermik) Sulfurated lime topical solution 6% (Vleminck's Soln.), alcohol 7% in drying clay mask. Jar 4 oz.
Use: Anti-acne.

VM. (Last) Vitamins B_1 6 mg, B_2 4 mg, niacinamide 40 mg, iron 100 mg, calcium 188 mg phosphorus 188 mg, manganese 4 mg, alcohol 12%. Bot. 16 oz.
Use: Vitamin/mineral supplement.

V-M CAPSULES. (Vale) Vitamins A, D, B_1, B_2, B_6, C, niacinamide, Ca, Fe, calcium pantothenate, Mg, Mn, K, Zn, P/Tab. Bot. 100s, 1000s.
Use: Vitamin/mineral supplement.

V-M TAB. (Kenyon) Vitamins A palmitate 5000 IU, D-2 500 IU, B_1 2.5 mg, B_2 2.5 mg, B_6 0.5 mg, B_{12} 1 mcg, C 50 mg, niacinamide 15 mg, E 0.5 IU, d-calcium pantothenate 5 mg, iron 25 mg, copper 0.375 mg, manganese 0.5 mg, zinc 0.15 mg, potassium 2.5 mg, magnesium 2.5 mg, iodine 0.05 mg/Tab. Bot. 100s, 1000s.
Use: Vitamin/mineral supplement.

•**VOLAZOCINE.** USAN. 3-(Cyclopropylmethyl)-1,2,3,4,5,6-hexahydro-cis-6,11-dimethyl-2,6-methano-3-benzazocine. Under study.
Use: Analgesic.

VOLIDAN. (British Drug House) Megestrol acetate.

VOLITANE. (Trent) Parethoxycaine 0.2%, hexachlorophene 0.025%, dichlorophene 0.025%. Aerosol spray can 3 oz.
Use: Counterirritant, antiseptic.

VOLMAX TABLETS. (Glaxo) Albuterol sufate 4 mg or 8 mg/Tab. Box 100s.
Use: Bronchodilator.

VOLTAREN. (Geigy) Diclofenac sodium 25 mg, 50 mg, 75 mg/Tab. Bot. 60s, 100s, 1000s, UD 100s.

Use: Nonsteroidal anti-inflammatory drug; analgesic.
VONEDRINE HYDROCHLORIDE. Vonedrine (phenylpropylmethylamine) HCl.
Use: Decongestant.
VONTROL. (Smith Kline & French) Diphenidol 25 mg as HCl/Tab. Bot. 100s.
Use: Antiemetic/antivertigo agent.
VORTEL. Clorprenaline HCl.
Use: Bronchodilator.
VOSOL OTIC SOLUTION. (Wallace) Propylene glycol diacetate 3%, acetic acid 2%, benzethonium Cl 0.02%, sodium acetate 0.015%. Bot. 15 ml, 30 ml.
Use: Otic preparation.
VOSOL HC OTIC SOLUTION. (Wallace) Propylene glycol diacetate 3%, acetic acid 2%, benzethonium Cl 0.02%, hydrocortisone 1%. Bot. 10 ml.
Use: Otic preparation.
VOXSUPRINE TABS. (Major) Isoxsuprine HCl 10 mg or 20 mg/Tab. Bot. 100s, 250s, 1000s, UD 100s.
Use: Vasodilator.
V-TUSS EXPECTORANT. (Vangard) Hydrocodone bitartrate 5 mg, pseudoephedrine HCl 60 mg, guaifenesin 200 mg/5 ml, alcohol 12.5%.
Use: Antitussive, decongestant, expectorant.

W

WADE GESIC BALM. (Wade) Menthol 3%, methyl salicylate 12%, petrolatum base. Tube oz, Jar lb.
Use: External analgesic.
WADE'S DROPS. Compound Benzoin Tincture.
WAKESPAN. (Weeks & Leo) Caffeine 250 mg/TR Cap. Vial 15s.
Use: Analeptic.
WAL-FINATE ALLERGY TABS. (Walgreen) Chlorpheniramine maleate 4 mg/Tab. Bot. 50s.
Use: Antihistamine.
WAL-FINATE DECONGESTANT TABS. (Walgreen) Chlorpheniramine maleate 4 mg, pseudoephedrine sulfate 60 mg/Tab. Bot. 50s.
Use: Antihistamine, decongestant.
WAL-FORMULA COUGH SYRUP WITH d-METHORPHAN. (Walgreen) Dextromethorphan HBr 15 mg, doxylamine succinate 7.5 mg, sodium citrate 500 mg/10 ml. Bot. 6 oz, 8 oz.
Use: Antitussive, antihistamine, expectorant.
WAL-FORMULA D COUGH SYRUP. (Walgreen) Dextromethorphan HBr 20 mg, phenylpropanolamine HCl 25 mg, guaifenesin 100 mg/10 ml, alcohol 10%. Bot. 6 oz, 8 oz.
Use: Antitussive, decongestant, expectorant.
WAL-FORMULA M COUGH SYRUP. (Walgreen) Dextromethorphan HBr 30 mg, pseudoephedrine HCl 60 mg, guaifenesin 200 mg, acetaminophen 500 mg/20 ml Bot. 8 oz.
Use: Antitussive, decongestant, expectorant, analgesic.
WAL-FRIN NASAL MIST. (Walgreen) Phenylephrine HCl 0.5%, pheniramine maleate 0.2% Bot. 0.5 oz.
Use: Decongestant, antihistamine.
WALGREEN ARTIFICIAL TEARS. (Walgreen) Hydroxypropyl methylcellulose 0.5%. Bot. 0.5 oz.
Use: Artificial tear solution.
WALGREENS FINEST IRON TABLETS. (Walgreen) Iron 30 mg/Tab. Bot. 100s.
Use: Iron supplement.
WALGREEN SODA MINTS. (Walgreen) Sodium bicarbonate 300 mg/Tab. Bot. 100s, 200s.
Use: Antacid.
WALGREEN'S FINEST VIT B_6. (Walgreen) Pyridoxine HCl 50 mg/Tab. Bot. 100s.
Use: Vitamin B_6 supplement.
WAL-MINIC. (Walgreen) Phenylpropanolamine HCl 12.5 mg, guaifenesin 100 mg/5 ml, alcohol 5%. Bot. 6 oz, 8 oz.
Use: Decongestant, expectorant.
WAL-MINIC COLD RELIEF MEDICINE. (Walgreen) Phenylpropanolamine HCl 12.5 mg, chlorpheniramine maleate 2 mg/5 ml Bot. 6 oz, 8 oz.
Use: Decongestant, antihistamine.
WAL-MINIC DM. (Walgreen) Phenylpropanolamine HCl 12.5 mg, dextromethorphan HBr 10 mg/5 ml Bot. 6 oz, 8 oz.
Use: Decongestant, antitussive.
WAL-PHED PLUS. (Walgreen) Pseudoephedrine HCl 60 mg, chlorpheniramine maleate 4 mg/Tab. Bot. 50s.
Use: Decongestant, antihistamine.
WAL-PHED SYRUP. (Walgreen) Pseudoephedrine HCl 30 mg/5 ml. Bot. 4 oz.
Use: Decongestant.
WAL-PHED TABLETS. (Walgreen) Pseudoephedrine HCl 30 mg/Tab. Bot. 50s, 100s.
Use: Decongestant.
WAL-TAP ELIXIR. (Walgreen) Brompheniramine maleate 2 mg, phenylpropanolamine HCl 12.5 mg/5 ml. Bot. 4 oz.
Use: Antihistamine, decongestant.
WAL-TUSSIN. (Walgreen) Guaifenesin 100 mg/5 ml. Bot. 4 oz.
Use: Expectorant.
WAL-TUSSIN DM. (Walgreen) Guaifenesin 100 mg, dextromethorphan HBr 15 ml/5 ml. Bot. 4 oz, 8 oz.
Use: Expectorant, antitussive.
WARFARIN. B.A.N. (Various Mfr.) Comp. 42. 3-(alpha-Acetonylbenzyl)-4-hydroxycoumarin. 4-Hydroxy-3-(3-oxo-1-phenylbutyl)coumarin.
Use: Rodenticide, anticoagulant.
See: Coumadin.
Marevan (sodium derivative).
•**WARFARIN SODIUM,** U.S.P. XXII. For Inj., Tab., U.S.P. XXII. 2H-1-Benzopyran-2-one, 4-hydroxy-3-(3-oxo-1-phenylbutyl)-, sodium salt. 3-

(alpha-Acetonyl-benzyl)-4-hydroxycoumarin and its sodium salt athrombin.
Use: Anticoagulant.
See: Coumadin Sodium, Tab., Inj. (Du Pont).
Sofarin, Tab. (Lemmon).
Panwarfin, Tab. (Abbott).

WART-AID. (Republic) Calcium pantothenate, ascorbic acid, starch. 15 Gm.
Use: Keratolytic.

WART FIX. (Last) Castor oil 100%. Bot. 0.3 fl oz.
Use: Wart removal.

WART-OFF. (Leeming) Salicylic acid 17% in flexible collodion, alcohol 20.5%, ether 54.2%. Bot. 0.5 oz.
Use: Keratolytic.

WARTGON. (E.J. Moore) Castor oil. Tube 0.5 oz.
Use: Wart removal.

•**WATER,** U.S.P. XXII is found in the following grades of purity:
Bacteriostatic Water for Injection, U.S.P. XXII.
Purified Water, U.S.P. XXII.
Sterile Water For Inhalation, U.S.P. XXII.
Sterile Water For Injection, U.S.P. XXII.
Sterile Water For Irrigation, U.S.P. XXII.
Water, U.S.P. XXII.
Water For Injection, U.S.P. XXII.
Use: Pharmaceutic aid (solvent), irrigation therapy, vehicle, fluid.
See: Abbott Labs. for sizes of each available.
Upjohn for sizes available.

WATER BABIES SUNBLOCK LOTION BY COPPERTONE SPF-15. (Schering-Plough) Ethylhexyl-P-methoxycinnamate, oxybenzone in lotion base, SPF-15. Bot. 8 fl oz.
Use: Sunscreen.

WATERMELON SEED EXTRACT. Citrin (Table Rock).

WATERMELON SEED EXTRACT W/Phenobarbital, theobromine. Cithal (Table Rock).

WATER-MISCIBLE VITAMIN A.
See: Acon, Cap. (Du Pont).
Aquasol Vitamin A, Cap. (USV Labs.).
Testavol-S, Cap. (Fellows).
Vi-Dom-A, Cap. (Miles Pharm).

•**WAX, CARNAUBA,** N.F. XVII.
Use: Pharmaceutic aid (tablet polishing agent).

•**WAX, EMULSIFYING,** N.F. XVII.
Use: Emulsifying agent, stiffening agent.

•**WAX, MICROCRYSTALLINE,** N.F. XVII.
Use: Pharmaceutic aid (stiffening agent).

•**WAX, WHITE,** U.S.P.XVII.
Use: Pharmaceutic aid (stiffening agent).

•**WAX, YELLOW,** N.F. XVII.
Use: Stiffening agent.

WAXSOL. Docusate Sodium, U.S.P. XXII.

WAYDS. (Wayne) Docusate sodium 100 mg/Cap. Bot. 100s.
Use: Laxative.

WAYDS-PLUS CAPSULES. (Wayne) Docusate w/casanthranol. Bot. 50s.
Use: Laxative.

WAYNADE T-D CAPSULES. (Wayne) Antihistamine compound. Bot. 100s.
Use: Antihistamine.

WAYNE-E CAPSULES. (Wayne) Vitamin E **100 IU or 200 IU/Cap.:** Bot. 1000s. **400 IU/Cap.:** Bot. 100s.
Use: Vitamin E supplement.

WAYSED TABLETS. (Wayne) Bot. 100s, 1000s.

WEHDRYL. (Hauck) Diphenhydramine HCl 50 mg/ml. Inj. Vial 10 ml.
Use: Antihistamine.

WEHGEN. (Hauck) Estrogenic substance or estrogens (mainly estrone) 2 mg/ml, sodium carboxymethylcellulose, polysorbate 80, methyl and propyl parabens. Inj. Aqueous susp. Vial 10 ml.
Use: Estrogen.

WEHLESS. (Hauck) Phendimetrazine tartrate 35 mg/Cap. Bot. 100s.
Use: Anorexiant.

WEHLESS-105 TIMECELLES. (Hauck) Phendimetrazine tartrate 105 mg/SA Cap. Bot. 100s.
Use: Anorexiant.

WEHYDRYL. (Hauck) Diphenhydramine HCl 50 mg/ml. Vial 10 ml.
Use: Antihistamine.

WELDERS EYE LOTION. (Weber) Tetracaine, potassium Cl, boric acid, camphor, glycerin, disodium edetate, benzalkonium Cl as preservatives. Bot. oz.
Use: Burn preparation.

WELLBUTRIN. (Burroughs Wellcome) Bupropion 75 mg or 100 mg/Tab. Bot. 100s.
Use: Antidepressant.

WELLCOVORIN. (Burroughs Wellcome) Leucovorin 5 mg or 25 mg as calcium/Tab. **5 mg:** Bot. 100s. **25 mg:** Bot. 25s.
Use: Prophylaxis and treatment of the undesired hematopoietic effects of folic acid antagonists.

WELLDORM. Dichloralphenazone. B.A.N.

WELLFERON. Interferon alfa-n1. (Orphan Drug).
Use: Kaposi's sarcoma in AIDS patients.
Sponsor: Burroughs Wellcome.

WERNET'S ADHESIVE CREAM. (Block) Carboxymethylcellulose gum, ethylene oxide polymer, petrolatum in mineral oil base. Cream. Tube 1.5 oz.
Use: Denture adhesive.

WERNET'S POWDER. (Block) Karaya gum, ethylene oxide polymer. Bot. 0.63 oz, 1.75 oz, 3.55 oz.
Use: Denture adhesive.

WES-B/C. (Western Research) Vitamins B_1 15 mg, B_2 10 mg, B_6 5 mg, niacinamide 50 mg, calcium pantothenate 10 mg, C 300 mg/Cap. Bot. 1000s.
Use: Vitamin supplement.

WESCOHEX. (West) Bot. 5 oz, pt, gal.
Use: Antibacterial skin cleanser.

WESMATIC FORTE TABLETS. (Wesley) Phenobarbital ⅛ gr, ephedrine sulfate 0.25 gr, chlor-

pheniramine maleate 2 mg, guaifenesin 100 mg/Tab. Bot. 100s, 1000s.
Use: Sedative/hypnotic, decongestant, antihistamine, expectorant.

WESPRIN BUFFERED. (Wesley) Aspirin 325 mg, aluminum hydroxide, magnesium hydroxide. Tab. Bot. 1000s.
Use: Analgesic.

WESTCORT CREAM. (Westwood) Hydrocortisone valerate 0.2% in a hydrophilic base with white petrolatum. Tube 15 Gm, 45 Gm, 60 Gm, 120 Gm.
Use: Corticosteroid, topical.

WESTCORT OINTMENT. (Westwood) Hydrocortisone valerate 0.2% in hydrophilic base with white petrolatum, mineral oil. Tube 15 Gm, 45 Gm, 60 Gm.
Use: Corticosteroid, topical.

WESTHROID. (Western Research) Thyroid 0.5 gr, 1 gr, 2 gr, 3 gr or 4 gr/Tab.; 5 gr/SC Tab. Handicount 28s (36 bags of 28s).
Use: Thyroid hormone.

WESTRIM. (Western Research) Phenylpropanolamine HCl 37.5 mg/Tab. Bot. 100s.
Use: Diet aid, decongestant.

WESTRIM-LA 50. (Western Research) Phenylpropanolamine HCl 50 mg/TR Cap. Bot. 1000s.
Use: Diet aid, decongestant.

WESTRIM-LA 75. (Western Research) Phenylpropanolamine HCl 75 mg/TR Cap. Bot. 1000s.
Use: Diet aid, decongestant.

WESVITE. (Western Research) Vitamins B_1 10 mg, B_2 5 mg, B_6 2 mg, pantothenic acid 10 mg, niacinamide 30 mg, B_{12} 3 mcg, C 100 mg, E 5 IU, A 10,000 IU, D 400 IU, iron 15 mg, copper 1 mg, iodine 0.15 mg, manganese 1 mg, zinc 1.5 mg/Tab. Bot. 1000s.
Use: Vitamin/mineral supplement.

WET-N-SOAK. (Allergan) Polyvinyl alcohol, edetate disodium, benzalkonium Cl 0.004% soln. Bot. 4 oz, 6 oz.
Use: Hard and RGP contact lens care.

WET-N-SOAK PLUS. (Allergan). Polyvinyl alcohol, edetate disodium, benzalkonium Cl 0.003%. Soln. Bot. 30 ml, 120 ml.
Use: Contact lens care.

WHEAT GERM OIL. (Viobin) **Liq.:** Bot. 4 oz, 8 oz, pt, qt. **Cap.: 3 min.** Bot. 100s, 400s; **6 min.** Bot. 100s, 225s, 400s; **20 min.** Bot. 100s.
Use: Vitamin E supplement.

WHEAT GERM OIL. (Various Mfr.).
See: Natural Wheat Germ Oil, Cap., Oint. (Spirt).
Natural Viobin Wheat Germ Oil, Liq. (Spirt).
Tocopherol Preps. (Various Mfr.).
Use: Vitamin E supplement.

WHEAT GERM OIL CAPSULES. (Robinson) Soft gelatin, oblong, clear 3, 6, 14 min/Cap. 100s, 1000s.
Use: Vitamin E supplement.

WHEAT GERM OIL CONCENTRATE. (Thurston) Perles. 6 min. Bot. 100s.
Use: Heart disorders, heart muscle fatigue.

WHIRL-SOL. (Sween) Moisturizing bath additive. Bot. 2 oz, 8 oz, 16 oz, 21 oz, gal, 5 gal, 30 gal, 55 gal.
Use: Emollient.

WHITE IODINE. (Pharmex) Bot. 0.5 oz.

•**WHITE LOTION,** U.S.P. XXII. Lotio Alba.
Use: Astringent, topical protectant.
See: Lotioblanc, Lot. (Arnar-Stone).

•**WHITE OINTMENT,** U.S.P. XXII.
Use: Pharmaceutic aid (oleaginous ointment base).

WHITE PRECIPITATE.
See: Ammoniated Mercury, U.S.P. XXII.

WHITFIELD'S OINTMENT. (Various Mfr.) Benzoic acid 6%, salicylic acid 3%.
Use: Anti-infective, external.

WHITSPHILL. (Torch) Salicylic acid 6%, benzoic acid 12% in hydrophilic vehicle. Jar 2 oz, lb. Also available in half-strength.
Use: Anti-infective, external.

WHOOPING COUGH VACCINE.
See: Pertussis Vaccine, U.S.P. XXII.

WHORTON'S CALAMINE LOTION. (Whorton) Calamine, zinc oxide, glycerin (U.S.P. strength) in carboxymethylcellulose lotion vehicle. Bot. 4 oz, gal.
Use: Minor skin irritations.

WHORTON'S SKIN CARE CREAM. (Whorton) 5 oz, 16 oz.

WIBI LOTION. (Owen) Purified water, SD alcohol 40, glycerin, PEG-4, PEG-6-32 stearate, PEG-6-32, glycol stearate, carbomer 940, PEG-75, methylparaben, propylparaben, triethanolamine, menthol, fragrance. Bot. 8 oz, 16 oz.
Use: Emollient.

WIDOW SPIDER SPECIES ANTIVENIN (LATRODECTUS MACTANS). Antivenin, Lactrodectus mactans, U.S.P. XXII.
Use: Passive immunizing agent.

WIGRAINE. (Organon) Ergotamine tartrate 1 mg, caffeine 100 mg/Tab. or Supp. **Tab.:** Box 20s, 100s. **Supp.:** Box 12s.
Use: Agent for migraine.

WILD CHERRY.
Use: Flavored vehicle.

WILPOWR. (Foy) Phentermine HCl 30 mg/Cap. Bot. 100s, 500s, 1000s.
Use: Anorexiant.

WILPOR-CLEAR. (Foy) Phentermine HCl 30 mg/Cap. Bot. 1000s.
Use: Anorexiant.

WINADOL SYRUP. (Winthrop Products) Paracetemol.
Use: Analgesic.

WINADOL TABLETS. (Winthrop Products) Paracetamol.
Use: Analgesic.

WINASMA TABLETS. (Winthrop Products) Theophylline anhydrous, ephedrine sulfate, chlormezanone.
Use: Antiasthmatic.

WINASORB DROPS. (Winthrop Products) Paracetamol.
Use: Analgesic.
WINASORB SUSPENSION. (Winthrop Products) Paracetamol.
Use: Analgesic.
WINASORB SYRUP. (Winthrop Products) Paracetamol.
Use: Analgesic.
WINASORB TABLETS. (Winthrop Products) Paracetamol.
Use: Analgesic.
WINAVIT TABLETS. (Winthrop Products) Stanozolol, vitamins.
Use: Anabolic steroid, vitamins.
WINGEL. (Winthrop Consumer Products) Short polymer, hexitol stabilized aluminum-magnesium hydroxide equivalent to aluminum hydroxide 180 mg and magnesium hydroxide 160 mg/5 ml or Tab. **Liq.:** Saccharin, sorbitol. Bot. 6 oz, 12 oz. **Chew. Tab.:** Box 50s, 100s.
Use: Antacid.
WINORYLATE SACHET. (Winthrop Products) Benorylate.
Use: Analgesic.
WINOLATE SUSPENSION. (Winthrop Products) Benorylate.
Use: Analgesic.
WINSTEROID TABLETS. (Winthrop Products) Stanozolol.
Use: Anabolic steroid.
WINSTROL. (Winthrop Pharm) Stanozolol 2 mg/Tab. Bot. 100s.
Use: Anabolic steroid.
WINTERGREEN OINTMENT. (Wisconsin) Bot. 2 oz, lb.
Use: External analgesic.
WINTHROCIN SUSPENSION. (Winthrop Products) Erythromycin stearate.
Use: Anti-infective.
WINTHROCIN TABLETS. (Winthrop Products) Erythromycin stearate.
Use: Anti-infective.
WINTODON TABLETS. (Winthrop Products) Glycobiarsoln.
Use: Amebicide.
WINTOMYLON CAPS. (Winthrop Products) Nalidixic acid.
Use: Urinary anti-infective.
WINTOMYLON SUSPENSION. (Winthrop Products) Nalidixic acid.
Use: Urinary anti-infective.
WINTOMYLON TABLETS. (Winthrop Products) Nalidixic acid.
Use: Urinary anti-infective.
WINTON TABLETS. (Winthrop Products) Aluminum and magnesium hydroxide.
Use: Antacid.
WINTOSIN COUGH SYRUP. (Winthrop Products) Dextromethorphan HBr.
Use: Antitussive.
WINTRAMOX CAPSULES. (Winthrop Products) Amoxicillin trihydrate.
Use: Antibacterial, penicillin.
WINTRAMOX SUSPENSION. (Winthrop Products) Amoxicillin trihydrate.
Use: Antibacterial, penicillin.
WINTREX CAPSULES. (Winthrop Products) Tetracycline HCl.
Use: Antibacterial, tetracycline.
WINTROPLEX TABLETS. (Winthrop Products) Aspirin, chlormezanone.
Use: Salicylate analgesic, antianxiety agent.
WITCH HAZEL. (Various Mfr.) Hammamelis water (Witch Hazel). Bot. 120 ml, 240 ml, 280 ml, 480 ml, 960 ml, gal.
Use: Astringent.
WITHIN. (Miles) Vitamins A 5000 IU, E 30 IU, C 60 mg, folic acid 0.4 mg, B_1 1.5 mg, B_2 1.7 mg, niacin 20 mg, B_6 2 mg, B_{12} 6 mcg, pantothenic acid 10 mg, D 400 IU, iron 27 mg, calcium 450 mg, zinc 15 mg/Tab. Bot. 60s, 100s.
Use: Vitamin/mineral supplement.
WNS SUPPOSITORIES. (Winthrop Products) Sulfamylon HCl.
Use: Anorectal preparation.
WOLFINA. (Forest) Whole root rauwolfia 100 mg/Tab. Bot. 100s.
Use: Antihypertensive.
WONDERFUL DREAM SALVE. (Kondon) Phenylmercuric nitrate 1:5000, oils of tar, turpentine, olive and linseed oil, rosin, burgundy pitch, camphor.
WONDRA. (Procter & Gamble) Petrolatum, lanolin acid, glycerin, stearyl alcohol, cyclomethicone, EDTA, hydrogenated vegetable glycerides phosphate, cetyl alcohol, isopropyl palmitate, stearic acid, PEG-100 stearate, carbomer-934, dimethicone, titanium dioxide, imidazolidinyl urea, parabens. Lot. Bot. 180 ml, 300 ml, 450 ml.
Use: Emollient.
WOOD CHARCOAL TABLETS. (Cowley) 5 gr or 10 gr/Tab. Bot. 1000s.
WOOD CREOSOTE.
See: Creosote (Various Mfr.).
WORMAL TABLETS. (Salsbury) Phenothiazine 500 mg, piperazine 50 mg, dibutyltin dilaurate 125 mg/Tab. Bot. 100s, 1000s, 10,000s.
Use: Anthelmintic for poultry.
WOOL FAT. Lanolin, Anhydrous.
W/W-ANTI-SPAS. (Whiteworth) Antispasmodic compound Bot. 16 oz.
Use: Antispasmodic.
W/W-BROMINE. (Whiteworth) Brompheniramine. Elix. Bot. 16 oz, gal.
Use: Expectorant.
W/W-BROMINE DS. (Whiteworth) Brompheniramine DC. Bot. 16 oz.
Use: Expectorant.
W/W-FED LIQUID. (Whiteworth) Triprolidine, pseudoephedrine. Syr. Bot. 16 oz, gal.
Use: Antihistamine, decongestant.

W/W-FED TABLETS. (Whiteworth) Triprolidine, pseudoephedrine. Tab. Bot. 100s, 1000s.
Use: Antihistamine, decongestant.

W/W FED w/C. (Whiteworth) Triprolidine, pseudoephedrine, codeine. Bot. 16 oz, gal.
Use: Antihistamine, decongestant, antitussive.

W/W HISTINE DH. (Whiteworth) Phenylhistine DH. Elix. Bot. 16 oz.
Use: Antihistamine.

W/W-HISTINE ELIXIR. (Whiteworth) Phenylhistine. Elix. Bot. 16 oz.
Use: Antihistamine.

W/W-HISTINE EXPECTORANT. (Whiteworth) Phenylhistine expectorant. Bot. 16 oz.
Use: Antihistamine.

WYAMINE SULFATE INJECTION. (Wyeth-Ayerst) Mephentermine sulfate 15 mg or 30 mg, methylparaben 1.8 mg, propylparaben 0.2 mg/ml. Vial 10 ml. Amp. 2 ml.
Use: Vasopressor.

WYAMYCIN-S TABLETS. (Wyeth-Ayerst) Erythromycin **250 mg as stearate/Tab.:** Bot. 100s, 500s. **500 mg as stearate/Tab.:** Bot. 100s.
Use: Anti-infective.

WYANOIDS. (Wyeth-Ayerst) Ephedrine sulfate 3 mg, belladonna extract 15 mg, boric acid, zinc oxide, bismuth oxyiodide and subcarbonate, balsam peru, beeswax, cocoa butter/Supp. Box 12s.
Use: Anorectal preparation.

WYCILLIN. (Wyeth-Ayerst) Penicillin G procaine susp. 600,000 units/ml in a stabilized aqueous susp. w/lecithin, povidone, methylparaben, propylparaben. Tubex 1 ml, 2 ml, 4 ml.
Use: Antibacterial, penicillin.

WYCILLIN INJECTION AND PROBENECID TABLETS. (Wyeth-Ayerst) Combination pkg. containing two disposable syringes of procaine penicillin G 2,400,000 units/4 ml size and two probenecid tablets 0.5 Gm each.
Use: Antibacterial.

WYDASE LYOPHILIZED. (Wyeth-Ayerst) Hyaluronidase. Vial 150 units/ml or 1500 units/10 ml with lactose and thimerosal.
Use: Hyaluronidase.

WYDASE STABILIZED SOLUTION. (Wyeth-Ayerst) Hyaluronidase 150 units in sterile saline soln. with sodium Cl, EDTA, thimerosal. Vial 1 ml, 10 ml.
Use: Hyaluronidase.

WYOVIN HYDROCHLORIDE. Dicyclomine. B.A.N.

WYGESIC. (Wyeth-Ayerst) Propoxyphene HCl 65 mg, acetaminophen 650 mg/Tab. Bot. 100s, 500s, Redipak 100s.
Use: Narcotic analgesic combination.

WYMOX. (Wyeth-Ayerst) Amoxicillin as trihydrate. **Cap.:** 250 mg Bot. 100s, 500s; 500 mg Bot. 50s, 500s. **Oral Susp.:** 125 mg/5 ml Bot. to make 80 ml, 100 ml, 150 ml; 250 mg/5 ml Bot. to make 80 ml, 100 ml, 150 ml.
Use: Antibacterial, penicillin.

WYTENSIN. (Wyeth-Ayerst) Guanabenz acetate. **4 mg/Tab.:** Bot. 100s, 500s, Redipak 100s. **8 mg/Tab.:** Bot. 100s. **16 mg/Tab.:** Bot. 100s.
Use: Antihypertensive.

X

•**XAMOTEROL.** USAN.
Use: Cardiac stimulant.

XANAX. (Upjohn) Alprazolam 0.25 mg, 0.5 mg or 1 mg/Tab. Bot. 100s, 500s, UD 100s. Visipack 4 × 25s.
Use: Antianxiety agent.

•**XANOXATE SODIUM.** USAN.
Use: Bronchodilator.

•**XANTHAN GUM,** N.F. XVII.
Use: Suspending agent.

XANTHINE DERIVATIVES.
See: Caffeine.
Theobromine.
Theophylline.

•**XANTHINOL NIACINATE.** USAN. 7-{2-Hydroxy-3-[(2-hydroxyethyl))methylamino]-propyl} theophylline compound with nicotinic acid.
Use: Vasodilator (peripheral).
See: Complamex.
Complamin.

XANTHIOL HCl. 4-[3-(2-Chlorothioxanthene-9-yl)-propyl]-1-pipera zinepropanol dihydrochloride.
Use: Antinauseant.
See: Daxid (Roerig).

XANTHOCILLIN. B.A.N. Antibiotics obtained from the mycelium of *Penicillium notatum* (Xanthocillin X is 2:3-Diisocyano1:4-di(p-hydroxyphenyl)buta-1:3-diene).

XANTHOTOXIN. Methoxsalen.

X-DRIN. (Pharmex) **Cap.:** Bot. 72s. **Pellet:** Bot. 144s. **Tab.:** Bot. 21s, 90s.
Use: Dietary.

•**XENBUCIN.** USAN.
Use: Antihypercholesteremic.

•**XENON Xe 127,** U.S.P. XXII.
Use: Radioactive agent.

•**XENON Xe 133,** U.S.P. XXII.
Use: Radioactive agent.

XENTHIORATE HCl. 2-Diethylaminoethyl-2(4-biphenylyl)thiobutyrate HCl.

XENYSALATE. B.A.N. 2-Diethylaminoethyl 3-phenylsalicylate. Sebaclen is the hydrochloride.
Use: Treatment of seborrhea.

XERAC. (Person & Covey) Isopropyl alcohol 44%, microcrystalline sulfur 4%. Tube 1.5 oz.
Use: Anti-acne.

XERAC AC. (Person & Covey) Aluminum Cl hexahydrate 6.25% in anhydrous ethanol 96%. Bot 35 ml, 60 ml.
Use: Anti-acne.

XERAC BP5. (Person & Covey) Benzoyl peroxide 5% in hydrogel. Tube 1.5 oz, 3 oz.
Use: Anti-acne.

XERAC BP10. (Person & Covey) Benzoyl peroxide 10% in hydrogel. Tube 1.5 oz, 3 oz.
Use: Anti-acne.

XEROFORM OINTMENT 3%.
(City) Pow. 0.25 lb, 1 lb.
(Consolidated) Jar 1 lb, 5 lb.
(Robinson) Jar 1 lb, 5 lb.

XERO-LUBE. (Scherer) Monobasic potassium phosphate, dibasic potassium phosphate, magnesium Cl, potassium Cl, calcium Cl, sodium Cl, sodium fluoride, sorbitol soln., sodium carboxymethylcellulose, methylparaben. Bot. 6 oz.
Use: Mouth and throat product.

•**XILOBAM.** USAN.
Use: Relaxant (muscle).

•**XIPAMIDE.** USAN.
Use: Antihypertensive, diuretic.

•**XORPHANOL MESYLATE.** USAN.
Use: Analgesic.

X-PREP BOWEL EVACUANT KIT-1. (Purdue Frederick) Kit contains Senokot S tab., X-Prep liquid, Rectolax supp.
Use: Laxative.

X-PREP BOWEL EVACUANT KIT-2. (Purdue Frederick) Kit contains citralax granules, X-Prep liquid, Rectolax supp.
Use: Laxative.

X-PREP LIQUID. (Gray) Senna extract with alcohol 7%, sucrose 50 Gm. Bot. 2.5 oz.
Use: Laxative.

X-RAY CONTRAST MEDIA.
See: Iodine Products, Diagnostic.

X SEB SHAMPOO. (Baker/Cummins) Salicylic acid 4%, coal tar soln. 10% in a blend of surface-active agents. Bot. 4 oz.
Use: Antiseborrheic.

X SEB T. (Baker/Cummins) Coal tar soln. 10%, salicylic acid 4%. Bot. 4 oz.
Use: Antiseborrheic.

XTRACARE. (Sween) Bot. 2 oz, 4 oz, 8 oz, 21 oz, gal.
Use: Emollient.

XTRA-VITES. (Barth's) Vitamins A 10,000 IU, D 400 IU, C 150 mg, B_1 5 mg, B_2 1 mg, niacin 3.33 mg, pantothenic acid 183 mcg, B_6 250 mcg, B_{12} 215 mg, E 15 IU, rutin 20 mg, citrus bioflavonoid complex 15 mg, choline 6.67 mg, inositol 10 mg, folic acid 50 mcg, biotin, aminobenzoic acid/Tab. Bot. 30s, 90s, 180s, 360s.
Use: Vitamin supplement.

X-TROZINE CAPSULES. (Rexar) Phendimetrazine tartrate 35 mg/Cap. Bot. 1000s.
Use: Anorexiant.

X-TROZINE S.R. CAPSULES. (Rexar) Phendimetrazine tartrate 105 mg/SR Cap. Bot. 100s, 200s, 1000s.
Use: Anorexiant.

X-TROZINE TABLETS. (Rexar) Phendimetrazine tartrate 35 mg/Tab. Bot. 1000s.
Use: Anorexiant.

•**XYLAMIDINE TOSYLATE.** USAN. N-[2-(m-Methoxyphenoxy)propyl]-2-m-tolylacetamidine mono-p-toluenesulfonate hemihydrate.
Use: Antiserotonin.

XYLAZINE. V.B.A.N. N-(5,6-Dihydro-4H-1,3-thiazin-2-yl)-2,6-xylidine.
Use: Analgesic, veterinary medicine.

•**XYLAZINE HYDROCHLORIDE.** USAN.
Use: Analgesic, relaxant (muscle).

•**XYLITOL,** N.F. XVII.

XYLOCAINE HYDROCHLORIDE. (Astra) Lidocaine HCl. **Amp.:** (1%): 2 ml, 5 ml, 30 ml; w/epinephrine 1:200,000 30 ml. (1.5%): 20 ml; w/epinephrine 1:200,000 30 ml. (2%): 2 ml, 10 ml; w/epinephrine 1:200,000 20 ml. (4%): 5 ml. **Multi-dose Vial:** (0.5%): 50 ml; w/epinephrine 1:200,000 50 ml. (1%): 20 ml, 50 ml; w/epinephrine 1:100,000 20 ml, 50 ml. (2%): 20 ml, 50 ml; w/epinephrine 1:100,000 20 ml, 50 ml. **Single-dose Vial:** (1%): 30 ml. (1.5%) 20 ml; w/epinephrine 1:200,000 10 ml, 30 ml. (2%) w/epinephrine 1:200,000 20 ml.
Use: Local anesthetic.

XYLOCAINE HYDROCHLORIDE FOR CARDIAC ARRHYTHMIA. (Astra) **Intravenous:** Lidocaine 2%. Amp 5 ml, disp. syringe 5 ml. Continuous infusion 1 Gm/25 ml Vial; 2 Gm/50 ml Vial. Prefilled syringe 100 mg/5 ml, 12s. Continuous infusion prefilled syringe 1 Gm, 2 Gm. **Intramuscular:** Amp. 10%, 5 ml.
Use: Local anesthetic.

XYLOCAINE HYDROCHLORIDE 4% SOLUTION. (Astra) Topical use. Bot. 50 ml.
Use: Local anesthetic.

XYLOCAINE HYDROCHLORIDE FOR SPINAL ANESTHESIA. (Astra) Lidocaine HCl 1.5% or 5%, glucose 7.5%, sodium hydroxide to adjust pH. Specific gravity 1.028-1.034. Amp. 2 ml. Box 10s.
Use: Local anesthetic.

XYLOCAINE JELLY. (Astra) Lidocaine HCl 2% in sodium carboxymethylcellulose with parabens. Tube 30 ml.
Use: Local anesthetic.

XYLOCAINE OINTMENT. (Astra) Lidocaine base 5%. Tube 3.5 Gm, 35 Gm. Ointment base of polyethylene glycols and propylene glycol.
Use: Local anesthetic.

XYLOCAINE VISCOUS. (Astra) Lidocaine HCl 2%, sodium carboxymethylcellulose, parabens. Bot. 20 ml (25s), 100 ml, 450 ml.
Use: Local anesthetic.

•**XYLOFILCON A.** USAN.
Use: Contact lens material.

•**XYLOMETAZOLINE HCl,** U.S.P. XXII. Nasal Soln., U.S.P. XXII. 2-(4-tert-Butyl-2,6-dimethyl benzyl)-2- imidazoline HCl.
Use: Adrenergic (vasoconstrictor).
See: Isohalent L.A., Liq. (Elder).
Long Acting Neo-Synephrine, Prods. (Winthrop Consumer Products).
Otrivin Spray (Geigy).

Rhinall L.A., Liq. (First Texas).
Sine-Off, Spray (Menley & James).
Vicks Sinex Long Acting, Nasal Spray (Vicks).

XYLO-PFAN. (Adria) Xylose 25 Gm/Bot.
Use: Diagnostic aid.

XYLOPHAN D-XYLOSE TOLERANCE TEST. (Pfanstiehl) D-xylose 25 Gm/UD bot.
Use: Diagnostic aid.

•**XYLOSE,** U.S.P. XXII.
Use: Diagnostic aid (intestinal function determination).

Y

YAGER'S LINIMENT. (Yager) Oil of turpentine and camphor w/clove oil fragrance, emulsifier, emollient, ammonium oleate (less than 0.5% free ammonia) penetrant base.
Use: Rubefacient.

YATREN.
See: Chiniofon, Tab.

YDP LICE SPRAY. (Youngs Drug) Synthetic pyrethroid in aerosoln. Can 5 oz.
Use: Pediculicide for inanimate objects.

YEAST ADENYLIC ACID. An isomer of adenosine 5-monophosphate, has been found inactive.
See: Adenosine 5-Monophosphate, Preps. for active compounds.

YEAST, DRIED.
Use: Protein and vitamin B Complex source.

YEAST TABLETS, DRIED.
Use: Supplementary source of B complex vitamins.
See: Brewer's Yeast, Tab.

YEAST, TORULA.
See: Torula Yeast.

YEAST W/IRON.
See: Natural Super Iron Yeast Powder (Spirt) (Pharmex) Bot. 200s.

YELETS. (Freeda) Iron 60 mg, vitamins A 10,000 IU, D 400 IU, E 10 IU, B_1 10 mg, B_2 10 mg, B_3 25 mg, B_5 10 mg, B_6 10 mg, B_{12} 10 mcg, C 100 mg, folic acid 0.1 mg, PABA, lysine, glutamic acid, Ca, I, Mg, Mn/Tab. Bot. 100s, 250s, 500s.
Use: Vitamin/mineral supplement.

YELLOW ENZYME.
See: Riboflavin (Various Mfr.).

•**YELLOW FERRIC OXIDE,** N.F. XVII.
Use: Pharmaceutic aid (color).

YELLOW FEVER VACCINE, U.S.P. XXII.
Use: Active immunizing agent.
See: YF-VAX, Inj. (Squibb/Connaught).

•**YELLOW OINTMENT,** U.S.P. XXII.
Use: Pharmaceutic aid (ointment base).

YELLOW WAX, N.F. XVII.
Use: Pharmaceutic aid (stiffening agent).

YF-VAX. (Squibb/Connaught) Yellow fever vaccine. Vial 1 dose, 5 dose with diluent.
Use: Agent for immunization.

YOCON. (Palisades) Yohimbine HCl 5.4 mg/Tab. Bot. 100s, 1000s.
Use: Impotence.

YODORA DEODORANT CREAM. (Norcliff Thayer) Jar 2 oz.
Use: Deodorant.

YODOXIN. (Glenwood) Iodoquinol 210 mg or 650 mg/Tab. Bot. 100s, 1000s. Pow. Bot. 25 Gm.
Use: Amebicide.

YOHIMBINE HCl. Indolalkylamine alkaloid. Available as 5.4 mg tab. under the tradenames Aphrodyne (Star), Yocon (Palisades) and Yohimex (Kramer).
Yohimbine has no FDA sanctioned indications.
W/Methyltestosterone, nux vomica extract.
See: Climactic, Tab. (Burgin-Arden)
Rochor, Tab. (Rocky Mtn.)

YOHIMEX. (Kramer) Yohimbine HCl 5.4 mg/Tab. Bot. 100s.
Use: Impotence.

YOMESAN. (Farbenfabriken Bayer) Niclosamide. B.A.N. Under study.
Use: Anthelmintic.

•**YTTERBIUM Yb 169 PENTETATE INJECTION,** U.S.P. XXII.
Use: Radioactive agent.

YUTOPAR. (Astra) Ritodrine HCl. **Tab.:** 10 mg Bot. 60s, UD 100s. **Inj.:** 10 mg/ml, Amp. 5 ml; 15 mg/ml, vial 10 ml, syringe 10 ml.
Use: Uterine relaxant.

Z

•**ZACOPRIDE HYDROCHLORIDE.** USAN.
Use: Antiemetic, stimulant (peristaltic).

•**ZALTIDINE HYDROCHLORIDE.** USAN.
Use: Antagonist to histamine H_2 receptors.

ZANOSAR. (Upjohn) Streptozocin sterile pow. 100 mg/ml. Vial 1 Gm.
Use: Antineoplastic agent.

ZANTAC INJECTION. (Glaxo Pharmaceuticals) Ranitidine 25 mg as HCl/ml. Vial 2 ml, 10 ml, 40 ml, syringe 2 ml.
Use: Histamine H_2 antagonist.

ZANTAC SYRUP. (Glaxo) Ranitidine 15 mg as HCl/ml, alcohol 7.5%. Bot. pt.
Use: Histamine H_2 antagonist.

ZANTAC TABLETS. (Glaxo) Ranitidine 150 mg or 300 mg as HCl/Tab. **150 mg:** Bot. 60s, UD 100s. **300 mg:** Bot. 30s, UD 100s.
Use: Histamine H_2 antagonist.

ZANTINE. (Metro Med) Dipyridamole 25 mg, 50 mg or 75 mg/Tab. Bot. 1000s.
Use: Coronary vasodilator.

ZANTRYL. (Ion) Phentermine HCl 30 mg/SR Cap. Bot. 100s.
Use: Anorexiant.

ZARONTIN. (Parke-Davis) Ethosuximide. **Cap.:** 250 mg. Bot. 100s. **Syr.:** 250 mg/5 ml. Bot. pt.
Use: Anticonvulsant.

ZAROXOLYN. (Pennwalt) Metolazone 2.5 mg, 5 mg or 10 mg/Tab. Bot. 100s, 500s, 1000s, UD 100s.
Use: Diuretic.

•**ZATOSETRON MALEATE.** USAN.
Use: Antimigraine.

Z-BEC. (Robins) Vitamins E 45 mg, C 600 mg, B_1 15 mg, B_2 10.2 mg, B_3 100 mg, B_6 10 mg, B_{12} 6 mcg, pantothenic acid 25 mg, zinc 22.5 mg/Tab. Bot. 60s, 100s, 500s.
Use: Vitamin/mineral supplement.

ZBT BABY. (Glenwood) Talc, mineral oil, magnesium stearate, propylene glycol, BHT. Pow. 120 Gm.
Use: Diaper rash product.

ZEASORB-AF POWDER. (Stiefel) Tolnaftate 1%, talc. Can 2.5 oz.
Use: Antifungal, external.

ZEASORB POWDER. (Stiefel) Talc, microporous cellulose, supersorb carbohydrate acrylic copolymer. Sifter-top Can 2.5 oz, 8 oz.
Use: Moisture absorbent.

ZECAPS. (Everett) Vitamin E 200 mg, zinc 9.6 mg as gluconate/Cap. Bot. 60s.
Use: Vitamin/mineral supplement.

ZEFAZONE. (Upjohn) Cefmetazole sodium 1 Gm or 2 Gm/vial. Pow. for inj.
Use: Anti-infective.

ZEIN, N.F. XVII.

ZEMALO. (Barre) Sulfur, zinc oxide, camphor, titanium oxide. Bot. 4 oz, pt, gal.
Use: Minor skin irritations.

ZENATE. (Reid-Rowell) Vitamins A 5000 IU, D 400 IU, E 30 mg, C 80 mg, folic acid 1 mg, thiamine 3 mg, riboflavin 3 mg, niacin 20 mg, B_6 10 mg, B_{12} 12 mcg, calcium 300 mg, iodine 175 mcg, iron 65 mg, magnesium 100 mg, zinc 20 mg/Tab. Bot. 100s.
Use: Vitamin/mineral supplement.

•**ZENAZOCINE MESYLATE.** USAN.
Use: Analgesic.

ZENDIUM. (Oral-B) Sodium fluoride 0.22%. Tube 0.9 oz, 2.3 oz.
Use: Dental caries preventative.

•**ZENIPLATIN.** USAN.
Use: Antineoplastic.

ZENTRON. (Lilly) Iron (as ferrous sulfate) 20 mg, vitamins B_1 1 mg, B_2 1 mg, B_6 1 mg, B_{12} 5 mcg, pantothenic acid 1 mg, niacinamide 5 mg, C 100 mg/5 ml, alcohol 2%. Bot. 8 fl oz.
Use: Vitamin/mineral supplement.

ZENTRON CHEWABLE. (Lilly) Elemental iron (as ferrous fumarate) 20 mg, vitamins B_1 1 mg, B_2 1 mg, B_6 1 mg, B_{12} 5 mcg, pantothenic acid 1 mg, niacinamide 5 mg, C 100 mg/Chew. tab. Bot. 50s.
Use: Vitamin/mineral supplement.

ZEPHIRAN. (Winthrop Pharm) **Aqueous soln.:** Benzalkonium Cl 1:750. Bot. 240 ml, gal. **Disinfectant concentrate:** 17% in 120 ml, gal. **Tincture:** 1:750 in gal. **Tincture spray:** 1:750 in 30 Gm, 180 Gm, gal.
Use: Antiseptic, germicide.

ZEPHIRAN TOWELETTES. (Winthrop Pharm) Moist paper towels with soln. of zephiran Cl 1:750. Box 20s, 100s, 1000s.
Use: Antiseptic, germicide.

ZEPHREX TABLETS. (Bock) Pseudoephedrine HCl 60 mg, guaifenesin 400 mg/SR Tab. Bot. 100s.
Use: Decongestant, expectorant.

ZEPHREX-LA TABLETS. (Bock) Pseudoephedrine HCl 120 mg, guaifenesin 600 mg/Tab. Bot. 100s.
Use: Decongestant, expectorant.

ZEPINE. (Foy) Reserpine alkaloid 0.25 mg/Tab. Bot. 100s, 500s, 1000s.
Use: Antihypertensive.

•**ZERANOL.** USAN. (1) (3S, 7X)-3,4,5,6,7,8,9,10,11,12- Decahydro-7, 14, 16-trihydroxy-3-methyl-1H-2-benzoxacyclotetradecin-1-one; (2) (6X, 10S)-6-(6,-10-dihyroxyundecyl)-b-resorcylic acid lactone.
Use: Anabolic.

ZEROXIN-10. (Syosset) Benzoyl peroxide 10%. Gel 45 Gm, 120 Gm.
Use: Anti-acne.

ZESTORETIC. (ICI Pharma) Lisinopril 20 mg, hydrochlorothiazide 12.5 mg or lisinopril 20 mg, hydrochlorothiazide 25 mg/Tab. Bot. 100s.
Use: Antihypertensive combination.

ZESTRIL. (Stuart) Lisinopril 5 mg, 10 mg or 20 mg/Tab. Bot. 100s, UD 100s.
Use: Antihypertensive.

ZETAR EMULSION. (Dermik) Colloidal whole coal tar 30% (300 mg/ml) in polysorbates. Bot. 6 oz.
Use: Antiseborrheic.

ZETAR SHAMPOO. (Dermik) Colloidal whole coal tar 1% in a shampoo. Bot. 6 oz.
Use: Antiseborrheic.

ZETRAN. (Hauck) Diazepam 5 mg/ml. Inj. Vial 10 ml.
Use: Antianxiety agent.

Z-GEN. (Goldline) Vitamins E 45 mg, B_1 15 mg, B_2 10.2 mg, B_3 100 mg, B_5 25 mg, B_6 10 mg, B_{12} 6 mcg, C 600 mg, zinc 22.5 mg/Tab. Bot. 60s, 100s.
Use: Vitamin/mineral supplement.

•**ZIDOMETACIN.** USAN.
Use: Anti-inflammatory.

•**ZIDOVUDINE.** USAN. (Formerly azidothymidine, AZT).
Use: Antiviral for management of certain AIDS and other serious HIV infections.
See: Retrovir, Cap. (Burroughs Wellcome).

ZILACTIN MEDICATED GEL. (Zila) Tannic acid 7%, suspended in alcohol 80.8%. Tube 0.25 oz.
Use: Treatment of cold sores.

•**ZILANTEL.** USAN.
Use: Anthelmintic.

•**ZILEUTON.** USAN.
Use: Inhibitor (5-lipoxygenase).
ZIMCO. (Sterwin) Vanillin.
•**ZIMELDINE HYDROCHLORIDE.** USAN.
Use: Antidepressant.
ZINACEF. (Glaxo) Cefuroxime 750 mg, 1.5 Gm or 7.5 Gm as sodium for parenteral administration. **750 mg:** Tray 25s. Infusion Pack Tray 10s. **1.5 Gm:** Tray 25s. Infusion Pack Tray 10s. **7.5 Gm:** Pharmacy Bulk Pkg. Tray 6.s
Use: Anti-infective.
ZINCATE. (Paddock) Zinc sulfate 220 mg/Cap. Bot. 100s, 500s, 1000s.
Use: Emetic, astringent.
ZINC-220. (Alto) Zinc sulfate 220 mg/Cap. Bot. 100s, 1000s, UD 100s.
Use: Zinc supplement.
•**ZINC ACETATE,** U.S.P. XXII. Acetic acid, zinc salt, dihydrate.
Use: Pharmaceutic necessity for Zinc-Eugenol Cement.
ZINCA-PAK. (SoloPak) Zinc 1 mg or 5 mg/ml. Inj. **1 mg:** Vial 10 ml, 30 ml. **5 mg:** Vial 5 ml.
Use: Parenteral nutritional supplement.
ZINCATE. (Paddock) Zinc sulfate 220 mg (elemental zinc 50 mg)/Cap. Bot. 100s, 1000s.
Use: Zinc supplement.
ZINC BACITRACIN. Bacitracin Zinc, U.S.P. XXII.
Use: Antibiotic.
•**ZINC CHLORIDE,** U.S.P. XXII. Inj., U.S.P. XXII.
Use: Astringent, desensitizer for dentin, replacement therapy.
W/Formaldehyde.
See: Forma Zincol Concentrate (Ingram).
•**ZINC CHLORIDE Zn 65.** USAN.
Use: Radioactive agent.
•**ZINC-EUGENOL CEMENT,** U.S.P. XXI.
Use: Dental protectant.
ZINCFRIN. (Alcon) Zinc sulfate 0.25%, phenylephrine HCl 0.12% in buffered soln. Droptainer 15 ml.
Use: Astringent, decongestant, ophthalmic.
•**ZINC GELATIN,** U.S.P. XXI. Zinc gelatin boot. Unna's Boot.
Use: Topical protectant.
•**ZINC GELATIN IMPREGNATED GAUZE,** U.S.P. XXI.
Use: Topical protectant.
ZINC-GLENWOOD. (Glenwood) Zinc Sulfate 220 mg/Cap. Bot. 100s.
Use: Zinc supplement.
•**ZINC GLUCONATE,** U.S.P. XXII.
Use: Supplement (trace mineral).
ZINCHLORUNDESAL. Zincundesal.
ZINC INSULIN.
See: Insulin Zinc, Preps. (Various Mfr.).
ZINCON SHAMPOO. (Lederle) Pyrithione zinc 1%, sodium methyl cocoyltaurate, sodium Cl, magnesium aluminum silicate, sodium cocoyl isethionate, glutaral, water w/pH adjusted. Bot. 4 oz, 8 oz.
Use: Antiseborrheic.

•**ZINC OXIDE,** U.S.P. XXII. Flowers of zinc.
Use: Mild astringent and antiseptic in skin diseases.
See: Calamine Preps.
W/Combinations.
See: Akne, Drying Lot. (Alto).
Almophen, Oint. (Bowman).
Anecal, Cream (Lannett).
Anocaine, Supp. (Mallard).
Anoids Rectal Supp. (Scrip).
Anugesic, Oint., Supp. (Parke-Davis).
Anulan, Vial (Lannett).
Anusol, Oint., Supp. (Parke-Davis).
Anusol-HC, Supp. (Parke-Davis).
Aracain Rectal Oint., Supp. (Commerce).
Biscolan, Supp. (Lannett).
Bonate, Supp. (Suppositoria).
Calamatum, Preps. (Blair).
Cala-Zinc-Ol, Liq. (Emerson).
Caldesene, Oint. (Pharmacraft).
Caleate HC Cream, Oint. (Elder).
Caloxol, Oint. (Bowman).
CZO, Lot. (Elder).
Dereq Medicone HC, Supp. (Medicone).
Dermatrol, Oint. (Gordon).
Desitin, Oint. (Leeming).
Diaprex, Oint. (Moss, Belle).
Doctient, Supp. (Suppositoria).
Elder Diaper Rash Oint. (Elder).
Epinephricaine, Oint. (Upjohn).
Ergophene, Oint. (Upjohn).
Hemocaine, Oint. (Mallard).
Hemorrhoidal Oint. (Towne).
Hydro Surco, Lot. (Alma).
Ladd's Paste (Paddock).
Lanaburn, Oint. (Lannett).
Lasan, Oint. (Stiefel).
Medicated Powder (Johnson & Johnson).
Medicated Foot Powder (Upjohn).
Mexsana, Pow. (Plough).
Nullo Foot Cream (DePree).
Obtundia Calamine Cream (Otis Clapp).
Pazo, Oint., Supp. (Bristol-Myers).
Petrozin Compound Oint. (Bowman).
Pile-Gon, Oint. (E.J. Moore).
PZM Oint. (Wendt-Bristol).
Rectal Medicone HC, Supp. (Medicone).
RVPaque, Oint. (Elder).
Saratoga, Oint. (Blair).
Schamberg, Lot. (Paddock).
Sebasorb, Lot. (Summer).
Supertah, Oint. (Purdue Frederick).
Taloin, Tube (Warren-Teed).
Ting, Cream, Pow. (Pharmacraft).
Unguentine Oint. "Original Formula" (Norwich-Eaton).
Versal, Supp. (Suppositoria).
Wyanoids, Preps. (Wyeth-Ayerst).
Xylocaine Supp. (Astra).
Zinc Boric Lotion, Liq. (Emerson).
Zonox Colloidal, Liq. (Scrip).

•**ZINC OXIDE OINTMENT,** U.S.P. XXII. (Norwich Eaton) Tube 1 oz, 2.25 oz.
Use: Protective coating for minor skin irritations.
•**ZINC OXIDE PASTE,** U.S.P. XXII.
Use: Topical protectant, astringent.
•**ZINC OXIDE AND SALICYLIC ACID PASTE,** U.S.P. XXII.
Use: Topical protectant, astringent.
ZINC PHENOLSULFONATE.
Use: Astringent.
W/Belladonna leaf extract, kaolin, pectin, sodium carboxymethylcellulose.
See: Gelcomul, Liq. (Commerce).
W/Bismuth subgallate, kaolin, pectin, opium pow.
See: Diastay,Tab. (Elder).
W/Bismuth subsalicylate, salol, methyl salicylate.
See: Pepto-Bismol, Liq. (Norwich Eaton).
W/Kaolin, pectin.
See: Pectocel, Liq. (Lilly).
W/Opium pow., bismuth subgallate, pectin, kaolin.
See: Bismuth, Pectin & Paregoric (Lemmon).
ZINC PYRITHIONE. Bis-[1-hydroxy-2(1H)-pyridinethionato] zinc.
Use: Bactericide, fungicide, antiseborrheic.
See: Breck One, Shampoo (Breck).
Zincon, Shampoo (Lederle).
ZP-11, Liq. (Revlon).
•**ZINC STEARATE,** U.S.P. XXII. Octadecanoic acid, zinc salt.
Use: Dusting powder.
W/Combinations.
See: Ting, Cream, Pow. (Pharmacraft).
ZINC SULFANILATE. Zinc sulfanilate tetrahydrate. Nizin, Op-Isophrin-Z, Op-Isophrin-Z-M (Broemmel).
Use: Antibacterial.
•**ZINC SULFATE,** U.S.P. XXII. Inj., Ophth. Soln. U.S.P. XXII. Sulfuric acid, zinc salt (1:1), heptahydrate.
Use: Astringent (ophthalmic).
See: Op-Thal-Zin Ophth. (Alcon).
Scrip-Zinc, Cap. (Scrip).
Zinc-Glenwood, Cap. (Glenwood).
Zin-Cora, Cap. (Elder).
W/Boric acid, phenylephrine HCl.
See: Phenylzin Drops, Ophth. Soln. (Smith, Miller & Patch).
W/Calcium lactate.
See: Zinc-220, Cap. (Alto).
W/Menthol, methyl salicylate, alum, boric acid, oxyquinoline citrate.
See: Maso pH Powder (Mason).
W/Phenylephrine HCl, polyvinyl alcohol.
See: Prefrin-Z, Liquifilm (Allergan).
W/Piperocaine HCl, boric acid, potassium Cl.
See: M-Z Drops (Smith, Miller & Patch).
W/Sodium Cl.
See: Bromidrosis Crystals (Gordon).
W/Sulfur, hexachlorophene.
See: Acnederm, Lot. (Lannett).
W/Vitamins.
See: Neovicaps TR, Cap. (Scherer).
Vicon-C, Cap. (Glaxo).
Vicon Forte, Cap. (Glaxo).
Vicon Plus, Cap. (Glaxo).
Vi-Zac, Cap. (Glaxo).
Z-Bec, Tab. (Robins).
ZINC SULFIDE, LOTION.
See: White Lotion, U.S.P.
ZINC SULFOCARBOLATE.
W/Aluminum hydroxide, pectin, kaolin, bismuth subsalicylate, salol.
See: Wescola Antidiarrheal-Stomach Upset (Western Research).
ZINC TRACE METAL ADDITIVE. (IMS) Zinc 4 mg/ml. Inj. Vial. 10 ml.
Use: Parenteral nutritional supplement.
ZINCUNDESAL.
See: Zinchlorundesal.
ZINC-10-UNDECENOATE.
See: Zinc Undecylenate, U.S.P. XXII.
•**ZINC UNDECYLENATE,** U.S.P. XXII. 10-Undecenoic acid, zinc (2+) salt. Zinc 10-undecenoate. (Various Mfr.).
Use: Antifungal.
W/Benzocaine, hexachlorophene.
See: Fung-O-Spray (Scrip).
W/Benzocaine, undecylenic acid, menthol.
See: Decyl-Cream LBS (Scrip).
W/Caprylic acid, sodium propionate.
See: Deso-Cream (Quality Generics).
Deso-Talc, Foot Pow. (Quality Generics).
W/Undecylenic acid.
See: Cruex Cream, Spray Pow. (Pharmacraft).
Desenex, Prods. (Pharmacraft).
Ting, Aerosol (Pharmacraft).
Quinsana, Med. Oint. (Mennen).
•**ZINDOTRINE.** USAN.
Use: Bronchodilator.
•**ZINOCANAZOLE HYDROCHLORIDE.** USAN.
Use: Antifungal.
•**ZINOSTATIN.** USAN.
Use: Antineoplastic.
•**ZINTEROL HYDROCHLORIDE.** USAN.
Use: Bronchodilator.
•**ZINVIROXIME.** USAN.
Use: Antiviral.
ZIRADRYL LOTION. (Parke-Davis Prods) Benadryl HCl 2%, zinc oxide 2%, alcohol 2%. Bot. 6 oz.
Use: Antihistamine-containing preparation, external.
ZIRCONIUM CARBONATE OR OXIDE.
See: Dermaneed, Lot. (Hanlon).
W/Benzocaine, menthol, camphor.
See: Rhulicream, Oint. (Lederle).
W/Benzocaine, menthol, camphor, calamine, pyrilamine maleate.
See: Ivarest, Cream (Carbisulphoil).
W/Benzocaine, menthol, camphor, calamine, isopropyl alcohol.
See: Rhulispray, Aerosol (Lederle).
W/Benzocaine, pyrilamine maleate, povidone.
See: Poison Ivy Cream (McKesson).

W/Calamine, zinc oxide, pyrilamine maleate.
See: Zircostan, Creme (Standex).
W/Parethoxycaine, calamine.
See: Zotox, Spray, Oint. (Commerce).

ZIRCOSTAN CREME. (Standex) Zirconium oxide 4.5%, calamine 6%, zinc oxide 4%, pyrilamine maleate 0.5%.
Use: Minor skin irritations.

ZIXORYN. Flumecinol (Orphan Drug).
Use: Hyperbilirubinemia in infants unresponsive to phototherapy.
Sponsor: Farmacon.

ZNG. (Western Research) Zinc gluconate 35 mg/Tab. Handicount 28s (36 bags of 28 tab.).
Use: Zinc supplement.

ZNP BAR. (Stiefel) Zinc pyrithione 2%. Bar 4.2 oz.
Use: Antiseborrheic.

Zn-PLUS PROTEIN. (Miller) Zinc in a zinc-protein complex made with isolated soy protein 15 mg/Tab. Bot. 100s.
Use: Zinc supplement.

ZODEAC-100. (Econo Med) Iron 60 mg, vitamins A 8000 IU, D 400 IU, E 30 IU, B_1 1.7 mg, B_2 2 mg, B_3 20 mg, B_5 11 mg, B_6 4 mg, B_{12} 8 mcg, C 120 mg, folic acid 1 mg, biotin 300 mcg, Ca, Cu, I, K, Mg, Zn. Bot. 100s.
Use: Vitamin/mineral supplement.

ZOFENOPRIL CALCIUM. USAN.
Use: Enzyme inhibitor (angiotensin-converting).

ZOFENOPRILAT ARGININE. USAN.
Use: Antihypertensive.

ZOFRAN. (Glaxo) Ondansetron HCl.
Use: Antiemetic (cancer chemotherapy).

ZOLADEX. (ICI).
Use: LHRH agonist.

ZOLAMINE HCl. USAN. 2-[[2-(Dimethylamino)ethyl]-(p-methoxybenzyl)-amino]thiazole monohydrochloride.
Use: Antihistamine, local anesthetic.
W/Eucupin dihydrochloride.
See: Otodyne, Soln. (Schering).

ZOLAZEPAM HYDROCHLORIDE. USAN.
Use: Sedative.

ZOLERTINE HYDROCHLORIDE. USAN. 1-Phenyl-4-[2-(1H-tetrazol-5-yl)ethyl]piperazine HCl.
Use: Antiadrenergic, vasodilator.

ZOLICEF. (Bristol Labs) Cefazolin 500 mg. Pow. for inj. Vial 10 ml.
Use: Antibacterial, cephalosporin.

ZOLPIDEM TARTRATE. USAN.
Use: Hypnotic, sedative.

ZOLYSE. (Alcon Surgical) Lyophilized alpha-chymotrypsin 750 units with 9 ml balanced salt solution.
Use: Enzyme, ophthalmic.

ZOMEPIRAC SODIUM, U.S.P. XXI. Tab., U.S.P. XXI. Sodium 5-(4-chlorobenzoyl)-1, 4-dimethyl-1H-pyrrole-2-acetate dihydrate.
Use: Non-steroidal, anti-inflammatory, analgesic agent.

ZOMETAPINE. USAN.
Use: Antidepressant.

ZONE-A LOTION. (UAD Labs) Hydrocortisone acetate 1%, pramoxine HCl 1%. Bot. 2 oz.
Use: Corticosteroid, local anesthetic.

•**ZONISAMIDE.** USAN.
Use: Anticonvulsant.

ZONITE LIQUID DOUCHE CONCENTRATE. (Norcliff Thayer) Benzalkonium Cl 0.1%, propylene glycol, menthol, thymol, EDTA in buffered soln. Bot. 8 fl oz, 12 fl oz.
Use: Vaginal preparation.

ZONIUM CHLORIDE. (Lannett) Benzalkonium Cl 12.8%, 17% or 50%. Bot. pt, gal. 12.8%, 17%; also Bot. 4 oz. Also as 1:1,000, Bot. pt, gal.
Use: Antiseptic.

•**ZOPOLRESTAT.** USAN.
Use: Antidiabetic.

•**ZORBAMYCIN.** USAN.
Use: Antibacterial.

ZORPRIN. (Boots) Aspirin 800 mg/SR Tab. Bot. 100s.
Use: Salicylate analgesic.

•**ZORUBICIN HYDROCHLORIDE.** USAN.
Use: Antineoplastic.

ZOSTRIX (GenDerm) Capsaicin 0.025%. Cream 45 Gm.
Use: External analgesic.

ZOVIRAX CAPSULES. (Burroughs Wellcome) Acyclovir 200 mg/Cap. Bot. 100s, UD 100s.
Use: Antiviral.

ZOVIRAX OINTMENT 5%. (Burroughs Wellcome) Acyclovir 50 mg/Gm. Tube 15 Gm.
Use: Antiviral, external.

ZOVIRAX STERILE POWDER. (Burroughs Wellcome) Acyclovir sodium 500 mg/Vial. Vial 10 ml.
Use: Antiviral.

ZOXAZOLAMINE. B.A.N. 2-Amino-5-chlorobenzoxazole. Flexin.
Use: Skeletal muscle relaxant, uricosuric.

Z-PRO-C. (Person & Covey) Zinc sulfate 200 mg (elemental zinc 45 mg), ascorbic acid 100 mg/Tab. Bot. 100s.
Use: Vitamin/mineral supplement.

Z-TEC. (Seatrace) Iron equivalent 50 mg/ml from iron dextran complex. Vial 10 ml.
Use: Iron supplement.

•**ZUCLOMIPHENE.** USAN. Transclomiphene.
Use: None given.

ZURINOL. (Major) Allopurinol. **100 mg/Tab.:** Bot. 100s, 500s, 1000s, UD 100s. **300 mg/Tab.:** Bot. 100s, 500s, UD 100s.
Use: Agent for gout.

ZYDERM I. (Collagen Corp.) Highly purified bovine dermal collagen 35 mg/ml implant. Sterile syringe 0.1 ml, 0.5 ml, 1 ml, 2 ml.
Use: Collagen implant.

ZYDERM II. (Collagen Corp.) Highly purified bovine dermal collagen 65 mg/ml implant. Syringe 0.75 ml.
Use: Collagen implant.

ZYDONE. (DuPont) Hydrocodone bitartrate 5 mg, acetaminophen 500 mg/Cap. Bot. 100s.
Use: Narcotic analgesic combination.

ZYLOPRIM. (Burroughs Wellcome) Allopurinol. **100 mg/Tab.:** Bot. 100s, 1000s, UD 100s; **300 mg/Tab.:** Bot. 30s, 100s, 500s, UD 100s.
Use: Agent for gout.

ZYMACAP. (Upjohn) Vitamins A 5000 IU, D 400 IU, E 15 mg, C 90 mg, folic acid 400 mcg, B_1 2.25 mg, B_2 2.6 mg, niacin 30 mg, B_6 3 mg, B_{12} 9 mcg, pantothenic acid 15 mg/Cap. Bot. 90s, 240s.
Use: Vitamin supplement.

ZYMASE. (Organon) Lipase 12,000 units, protease 24,000 units, amylase 24,000 units. Cap. Bot. 100s.
Use: Digestive enzyme.

ZYMENOL. (Houser) Mineral oil 50%, yeast, cellulose gum, sorbitol, saccharin. Bot. 14 oz.
Use: Laxative.

ZYNOXUN OINTMENT. (Alton) Tube 5 oz. Jar lb.
Use: Protective ointment.

ZYPAN TABLETS. (Standard Process) Pancreatin 1.5 Gm, pepsin (1:3000) 1.5 Gm, betaine HCl 2.75 Gm, ammonium Cl 0.15 Gm/Tab. Bot. 100s.
Use: Digestive aid.

Reference Information

Common Abbreviations

Word	Abbreviation	Meaning
ana	$\overline{aa}$, aa	of each
ante cibum	a.c.	before meals or food
ad	ad	to, up to
aurio dextra	a.d.	right ear
ad libitum	ad lib.	at pleasure
aurio laeva	a.l.	left ear
ante meridiem	A.M.	morning
aqua	aq.	water
aqua destillata	aq. dest.	distilled water
aurio sinister	a.s.	left ear
aures utrae	a.u.	each ear
bis in die	b.i.d.	twice daily
bowel movement	b.m.	bowel movement
blood pressure	b.p.	blood pressure
cong	C.	a gallon
cum	$\overline{c}$	with
capsula	caps.	capsule
	cc.	cubic centimeter
compositus	comp.	compound
dies	d.	day
dilue	dil.	dilute
dispensa	disp.	dispense
divide	div.	divide
dentur tales doses	d.t.d.	give of such a dose
elixir	el.	elixir
	e.m.p.	as directed
et	et	and
	ex aq.	in water
fac, fiat, fiant	f., ft.	make, let be made
Food and Drug Administration	FDA	Food and Drug Administration
gramma	Gm., g.	gram
granum	gr.	grain
gutta	gtt.	a drop
hora	h.	hour
hora somni	h.s., hor. som.	at bedtime
	i.m., I.M	intramuscular
	i.v.	intravenous
liquor	liq.	a liquor, solution
	mcg.	microgram
	mg.	milligram
	ml.	milliliter
misce	M.	mix
more dictor	m. dict.	as directed
mixtura	mixt.	a mixture
National Formulary	N.F.	National Formulary
numerus	no.	number
nocturnal	noc.	in the night
non repetatur	non. rep.	do not repeat, no refills
octarius	O, Oct.	a pint
oculus dexter	o.d.	right eye
oculus laevus	o.l.	left eye
oculus sinister	o.s.	left eye
oculo uterque	o.u.	each eye
post cibos	p.c., post. cib.	after meals
post meridiem	P.M.	afternoon or evening
per os	p.o.	by mouth

Word	Abbreviation	Meaning
pro re nata	p.r.n.	as needed
pulvis	pulv.	a powder
quoque alternis die	q.a.d.	every other day
	q.d.	every day
quiaque hora	q.h.	every hour
quater in die	q.i.d.	four times a day
	q.o.d.	every other day
quantum sufficiat	q.s.	a sufficient quantity
	q.s. ad	a sufficient quantity to make
quam volueris	q.v.	as much as you wish
recipe	Rx	take, a recipe
repetatur	rep.	let it be repeated
sine	s̄, s	without
secundum artem	s.a.	according to art
sataratus	sat.	saturated
signa	Sig.	label, or let it be printed
solutio	sol.	solution
	solv.	dissolve
semis	s̄s̄., ss	one-half
si opus sit	s.o.s.	if there is need
statim	stat.	at once, immediately
suppositorium	supp.	suppository
syrupus	syr.	syrup
tabella	tab.	tablet
	tal.	such
	tal. dos.	such doses
ter in die	t.i.d.	three times a day
tincture	tr., tinct.	tincture
tritura	trit.	triturate
	tsp.	teaspoonful
unguentum	ung.	ointment
United States Adopted Names	USAN	official adopted names
United States Pharmacopeia	U.S.P.	United States Pharmacopeia
ut dictum	ut. dict.	as directed
while awake	w.a.	while awake

[NOTE: *The listing of commonly used abbreviations is included as an aid in interpreting medical orders.]

Common Systems of Weight and Measure*

METRIC SYSTEM

Metric Weight

1 microgram†	μg (mcg)	=	0.000,001	g
1 milligram	mg	=	0.001	g
1 centigram	cg	=	0.01	g
1 decigram	dg	=	0.1	g
1 gram	g	=	1.0	g
1 dekagram	Dg	=	10.0	g
1 hectogram	Hg	=	100.0	g
1 kilogram	Kg	=	1000.0	g

Metric Liquid Measure

1 microliter	μl	=	0.000,001	L
1 milliliter	ml	=	0.001	L
1 centiliter	cl	=	0.01	L
1 deciliter	dl	=	0.1	L
1 liter	L	=	1.0	L
1 dekaliter	Dl	=	10.0	L
1 hectoliter	Hl	=	100.0	L
1 kiloliter	Kl	=	1000.0	L

APOTHECARY SYSTEM

Apothecary Weight

1 grain‡	gr	=	1 gr		
1 scruple	℈	=	20 gr		
1 dram	ʒ	=	60 gr	=	3℈
1 ounce	℥	=	480 gr	=	8ʒ
1 pound	℔	=	5760 gr	=	12℥

Apothecary Liquid Measure

1 minim	♏	=	1 ♏		
1 fluidram	fʒ	=	60 ♏		
1 fluidounce	f℥	=	480 ♏	=	8 fʒ
1 pint	pt	=	7680 ♏	=	16 f℥
1 quart	qt	=	15630 ♏	=	32 f℥
1 gallon	gal	=	61440 ♏	=	8 pt℥

AVOIRDUPOIS SYSTEM

Avoirdupois Weight

1 ounce = 1 oz = 437.5 grains (gr)

1 pound = 1 lb = 16 ounces (oz) = 7000 grains (gr)

*The listing of common systems of weight and measure is included to aid the practitioner in calculating dosages.

†Note: The abbreviation μg or mcg is used for microgram in pharmacy rather than gamma (γ) as in biology.

‡Note: The grain in each of the above systems has the same value, and thus serves as a basis for the interconversion of the other units.

Approximate Practical Equivalents*

Weight Equivalents

1 grain	= 1 gr	= 64.8	milligrams
1 gram	= 1 Gm or g	= 15.432	grains
1 kilogram	= 1 Kg	= 2.20	pounds avoirdupois (lb)
1 ounce avoirdupois	= 1 oz	= 28.35	grams
1 ounce apothecary	= 1 ℥	= 31.1	grams
1 pound avoirdupois	= 1 lb	= 454.	grams

Measure Equivalents

1 milliliter	= 1 ml	= 16.23	minims (♏)
1 fluidram†	= 1 fʒ	= 3.4	ml
1 teaspoonful†	= 1 tsp	= 5.00	ml
1 tablespoonful	= 1 tbs or tbsp	= 15.	ml
1 fluidounce	= 1 f℥	= 29.57	ml
1 wineglassful	= 2 f℥	= 60.	ml
1 teacupful	= 4 f℥	= 120.	ml
1 tumblerful	= 8 f℥	= 240.	ml
1 pint	= 1 pt or O or Oct	= 473.	ml
1 liter	= 1 L	= 33.8	fluidounces (f℥)
1 gallon	= 1 gal or C or Cong	= 3785.	ml

*The listing of approximate practical equivalents is included to aid the practitioner in calculating and converting dosages among the various systems.

†Note: On prescription a fluidram is assumed to contain a teaspoonful which is 5 ml.

International System of Units

The *Système international d'unités* (International System of Units) or *SI* is a modernized version of the metric system. The primary goal of the conversion to SI units is to revise the present confused measurement system and to improve test-result communications.

The SI has 7 basic units from which other units are derived:

Base Units of SI		
Physical Quantity	Base Unit	SI Symbol
length	meter	m
mass	kilogram	kg
time	second	s
amount of substance	mole	mol
thermodynamic temperature	kelvin	K
electric current	ampere	A
luminous intensity	candela	cd

Combinations of these base units can express any property although, for simplicity, special names are given to some of these derived units.

Representative Derived Units		
Derived Unit	Name and Symbol	Derivation from Base Units
area	square meter	m^2
volume	cubic meter	m^3
force	newton (N)	$kg \cdot m \cdot s^{-2}$
pressure	pascal (Pa)	$kg \cdot m^{-1} \cdot s^{-2}$ (N/m^2)
work, energy	joule (J)	$kg \cdot m^2 \cdot s^{-2}$ ($N \cdot m$)
mass density	kilogram per cubic meter	kg/m^3
frequency	hertz (Hz)	s^{-1}
temperature	degree Celsius (°C)	°C = °K -273.15
concentration		
mass	kilogram/liter	kg/L
substance	mole/liter	mol/L
molality	mole/kilogram	mol/kg
density	kilogram/liter	kg/L

Prefixes to the base unit are used in this system to form decimal multiples and submultiples. The preferred multiples and submultiples listed below change the quantity by increments of 10^3 or 10^{-3}. The exceptions to these recommended factors are outlined by the rectangle.

Prefixes and Symbols for Decimal Multiples and Submultiples		
Factor	Prefix	Symbol
10^{18}	exa	E
10^{15}	peta	P
10^{12}	tera	T
10^9	giga	G
10^6	mega	M
10^3	kilo	k
10^2	hecto	h
10^1	deka	da
10^{-1}	deci	d
10^{-2}	centi	c
10^{-3}	milli	m
10^{-6}	micro	μ
10^{-9}	nano	n
10^{-12}	pico	p
10^{-15}	femto	f
10^{-18}	atto	a

To convert drug concentrations to or from SI units:

$$\text{Conversion factor (CF)} = \frac{1000}{\text{mol wt}}$$

Conversion *to* SI units: μg/ml x CF = μmol/L

Conversion *from* SI units: μmol/L ÷ CF = μg/ml

Normal Laboratory Values

In the following tables, normal reference values for commonly requested laboratory tests are listed in traditional units and in SI units. The tables are a guideline only. Values are method dependent and "normal values" may vary between laboratories.

BLOOD, PLASMA or SERUM		
	Reference Value	
Determination	Conventional Units	SI Units
Ammonia	10-80 μg/dl	5-50 μmol/L
Amylase	0-130 U/L	0-130 U/L
Antinuclear antibodies	negative at 1:8 dilution of serum	
Bilirubin: direct total	≤0.2 mg/dl 0.1-1 mg/dl	≤4 μmol/L 2-18 μmol/L
Calcitonin, male female medullary carcinoma	0-14 pg/ml 0-28 pg/ml >100 pg/ml	0-4.1 pmol/L 0-8.2 pmol/L >29.3 pmol/L
Calcium[1]	8.8-10.3 mg/dl	2.2-2.6 mmol/L
Carbon dioxide content	22-28 mEq/L	22-28 mmol/L
Chloride*	95-105 mEq/L	95-105 mmol/L
Coagulation screen: Bleeding time Prothrombin time Partial thromboplastin time (activated)	 3-9.5 min <2 sec from control 25-38 sec	 180-570 sec <2 sec from control 25-38 sec
Copper, total	70-140 μg/dl	11-22 μmol/L
Corticotropin (ACTH)	20-100 pg/ml	4-22 pmol/L
Cortisol: 8 am 8 pm 4 hr ACTH test Overnight suppression test	5-25 μg/dl <10 μg/dl 30-45 μg/dl <5 μg/dl	0.14-0.69 μmol/L <0.28 μmol/L 0.83-1.24 μmol/L <0.14 μmol/L
Creatine phosphokinase, total (CK, CPK)	≤130 U/L	≤130 U/L
Creatine phosphokinase isoenzymes	CK-MB = ≤5% total CK	≤0.05
Creatinine	0.6-1.2 mg/dl	50-110 μmol/L
Follicle stimulating hormone (FSH), female peak production male	 2-15 mIU/ml 20-50 mIU/ml 1-10 mIU/ml	 2-15 IU/L 20-50 IU/L 1-10 IU/L
Glucose, fasting	70-110 mg/dl	3.9-6.1 mmol/L
Hematologic tests: Hematocrit (Hct), female male	 33%-43% 39%-49%	 0.33-0.43 0.39-0.49
Hemoglobin (Hb), female male	12-15 g/dl 13.6-17.2 g/dl	120-150 g/L 136-172 g/L
Leukocyte count (WBC)	3200-9800/mm³	3.2-9.8 x 10^9/L
Erythrocyte count (RBC), female male	3.5-5 million/mm³ 4.3-5.9 million/mm³	3.5-5 x 10^{12}/L 4.3-5.9 x 10^{12}/L
Mean Corpuscular Volume (MCV)	76-100 μm³/cell	76-100 fl/cell
Mean Corpuscular Hemoglobin (MCH)	27-33 pg/RBC	27-33 pg/RBC
Mean Corpuscular Hemoglobin Concentration (MCHC)	33-37 g/dl	330-370 g/L

[1] Slightly higher in children.

(Table continued on following page)

BLOOD, PLASMA or SERUM (Cont.)		
	Reference Value	
Determination	**Conventional Units**	**SI Units**
Hematologic tests (cont.):		
Erythrocyte sedimentation rate		
(sedrate, ESR): female	≤ 30 mm/hr	≤ 30 mm/hr
male	≤ 20 mm/hr	≤ 20 mm/hr
Erythrocyte enzymes:		
Glucose-6-phosphate dehydrogenase (G6PD)	5-15 U/g Hb	5-15 U/g Hb
Pyruvate kinase	13-17 U/g Hb	13-17 U/g Hb
Ferritin (serum): Iron deficiency	0-12 ng/ml	0-4.8 nmol/L
Borderline	13-20 ng/ml	5.2-8 nmol/L
Iron excess	> 400 ng/L	> 160 nmol/L
Folic acid: normal	> 3.3 ng/ml	> 7.3 nmol/L
borderline	2.5-3.2 ng/ml	5.75-7.39 nmol/L
Platelet count	150,000-450,000/mm³	150-450 x 10^9/L
Vitamin B_{12}: normal	205-876 pg/ml	150-674 pmol/L
borderline	140-204 pg/ml	102.6-149 pmol/L
Iron		
female	60-160 μg/dl	11-29 μmol/L
male	80-180 μg/dl	14-32 μmol/L
Iron Binding Capacity	250-460 μg/dl	45-82 μmol/L
Lactic Acid	0.5-2.2 mmol/L	0.5-2.2 mmol/L
Lactic dehydrogenase	50-150 U/L	50-150 U/L
Lead	≤ 50 μg/dl	≤ 2.4 μmol/L
Lipids: Cholesterol		
< 29 yr	< 200 mg/dl	< 5.2 mmol/L
30-39 yr	< 225 mg/dl	< 5.85 mmol/L
40-49 yr	< 245 mg/dl	< 6.35 mmol/L
> 50 yr	< 265 mg/dl	< 6.85 mmol/L
Triglycerides	40-150 mg/dl	0.4-1.5 g/L
LDL	50-190 mg/dl	1.3-4.9 mmol/L
HDL		
female	30-90 mg/dl	0.8-2.35 mmol/L
male	30-70 mg/dl	0.8-1.8 mmol/L
Magnesium	1.8-3 mEq/L	0.8-1.2 mmol/L
Osmolality	280-296 mOsm/kg water	280-296 mmol/kg
Oxygen saturation (arterial)	96%-100%	0.96-1
PCO_2, Arterial	35-45 mm Hg	4.7-6 kPa
pH, Arterial	7.35-7.45	7.35-7.45
PO_2, Arterial: breathing room air[2]	75-100 mm Hg	10-13.3 kPa
on 100% O_2	> 500 mm Hg	
Phosphatase (acid), total:	≤ 3 King-Armstrong units/dl	≤ 5.5 U/L
	≤ 3 Bodansky units/dl	≤ 16.1 U/L
Phosphatase (alkaline)[3]	30-120 U/L	30-120 U/L
Phosphorus, inorganic[4]	3-4.5 mg/dl	1-1.5 mmol/L
Potassium	3.5-5 mEq/L	3.5-5 mmol/L

[1] Higher in males.
[2] Age dependent.
[3] Infants and adolescents up to 104 U/L.
[4] Infants in the first year up to 6 mg/dl.

BLOOD, PLASMA or SERUM (Cont.)		
	Reference Value	
Determination	**Conventional Units**	**SI Units**
Progesterone Follicular phase Luteal phase	 < 2 ng/ml 2-20 ng/ml	 < 6 nmol/L 6-64 nmol/L
Prolactin	2-15 ng/ml	0.08-6 nmol/L
Protein: Total Albumin Globulin	6-8 g/dl 4-6 g/dl 2.3-3.5 g/dl	60-80 g/L 40-60 g/L 23-35 g/L
Rheumatoid factor	< 60 IU/ml	
Sodium	135-147 mEq/L	135-147 mmol/L
Testosterone, female male	< 0.6 ng/ml 4-8 ng/ml	< 2 nmol/L 14-28 nmol/L
Thyroid Hormone Function Tests: Thyroid-stimulating hormone (TSH) Thyroxine-binding globulin capacity Total triiodothyronine (T_3) Total thyroxine by RIA (T_4) T_3 resin uptake	 0.5-5 μU/ml 15-25 μg T_4/dl 75-220 ng/dl 4-12 μg/dl 25%-35%	 0.5-5 arb unit 193-322 nmol/L 1.2-3.4 nmol/L 52-154 nmol/L 0.25-0.35
Transaminase, AST (Aspartate aminotransferase, SGOT)	7-27 U/L	117-450 nmol/sec/L
Transaminase, ALT (Alanine aminotransferase, SGPT)	1-21 U/L	17-350 nmol/sec/L
Urea nitrogen (BUN)	8-18 mg/dl	3-6.5 mmol/L
Uric acid	2-7 mg/dl	120-420 μmol/L
Vitamin A	0.15-0.6 μg/ml	0.5-2.1 μmol/L
Zinc	75-120 μg/dl	11.5-18.5 μmol/L

URINE					
		Reference Value			
Determination		**Conventional Units**		**SI Units**	
Catecholamines: Epinephrine Norepinephrine		< 20 μg/day < 100 μg/day		< 109 nmol/day < 590 nmol/day	
Creatinine		15-25 mg/kg/day		0.13-0.22 mmol/kg/day	
Potassium[1]		25-125 mEq/day		25-125 mmol/day	
Protein, quantitative		< 150 mg/day		< 0.15 g/day	
Sodium[1]		40-220 mEq/day		40-220 mmol/day	
Steroids:		(mg/day)		(μmol/day)	
	Age (yrs)	male	female	male	female
17-Ketosteroids	10	1-4	1-4	3-14	3-14
	20	6-21	4-16	21-73	14-56
	30	8-26	4-14	28-90	14-49
	50	5-18	3-9	17-62	10-31
	70	2-10	1-7	7-35	3-24
17-Hydroxycorticosteroids (as cortisol), female		2-8 mg/day		5-25 μmol/day	
male		3-10 mg/day		10-30 μmol/day	

[1] Varies with intake.

DRUG LEVELS†		
	Reference Value	
Drug Determination	Conventional Units	SI Units
Aminoglycosides (peak levels):		
Amikacin	8-16 µg/ml	nd
Gentamicin	4-8 µg/ml	nd
Kanamycin	8-16 µg/ml	nd
Netilmicin	0.5-10 µg/ml	nd
Streptomycin	25 µg/ml	nd
Tobramycin	4-8 µg/ml	nd
Antiarrhythmics:		
Amiodarone	0.5-2.5 µg/ml	nd
Bretylium	0.5-1.5 µg/ml	nd
Digitoxin	9-25 µg/L	11.8-32.8 nmol/L
Digoxin	0.5-2.2 ng/ml	0.6-2.8 nmol/L
Disopyramide	2-6 µg/ml	6-18 µmol/L
Flecainide	0.2-1 µg/ml	nd
Lidocaine	1-5 µg/ml	4.5-21.5 µmol/L
Mexiletine	0.5-2 µg/ml	nd
Phenytoin	10-20 µg/ml	40-80 µmol/L
Procainamide	4-8 µg/ml	17-34 µmol/L
Propranolol	50-200 ng/ml	190-770 nmol/L
Quinidine	1.5-3 µg/ml	4.6-9.2 µmol/L
Tocainide	4-10 µg/ml	nd
Verapamil	0.08-0.3 µg/ml	nd
Anticonvulsants:		
Carbamazepine	4-12 µg/ml	17-51 µmol/L
Phenobarbital	15-40 µg/ml	65-172 µmol/L
Phenytoin	5-20 µg/ml	40-80 µmol/L
Primidone	6-10 µg/ml	25-46 µmol/L
Valproic acid	50-100 µg/ml	350-7000 µmol/L
Chloramphenicol	10-20 µg/ml	31-62 µmol/L
Ethanol[1]	0 mg/dl	0 mmol/L
Lithium	0.5-1.5 mEq/L	0.5-1.5 mmol/L
Salicylate	100-200 mg/L	724-1448 µmol/L
Sulfonamide	5-15 mg/dl	nd
Theophylline	10-20 µg/ml	55-110 µmol/L

† The values given are generally accepted as desirable for achieving therapeutic effect without toxicity for most patients. However, exceptions are not uncommon.

[1] Toxic: 50-100 mg/dl (10.9-21.7 mmol/L).

nd – No data available.

Trademark Glossary

Many companies use trademarks to identify specific dosage forms or unique packaging materials. The following list is provided as a guide to the interpretation of these descriptions.

Abbo-Pac (Abbott)
Unit dose package

Accu-Pak (Ciba)
Unit dose blister pack

Act-O-Vial (Upjohn)
Vial system

ADD-Vantage (Abbott)
Sterile dissolution system for admixture

ADT (Upjohn)
Alternate day therapy

Arm-A-Med (Armour)
Single-dose plastic vial

Arm-A-Vial (Armour)
Single-dose plastic vial

Aspirol (Lilly)
Crushable ampule for inhalation

Back-Pack (MSD)
Unit-of-use package

bidCAP (Bristol Labs)
Double strength capsule

Bristoject (Bristol Labs)
Unit dose syringe

Caplet (Various)
Capsule shaped tablet

Carpuject (Winthrop Pharm.)
Cartridge needle unit

Chronosule (Schering)
Sustained action capsule

Chronotab (Schering)
Sustained action tablet

Clinipak (Wyeth-Ayerst)
Unit dose package

ControlPak (Sandoz)
Unit dose rolls, tamper resistant

Delcap (Ortho)
Unit dispensing cap

Detecto-Seal (Winthrop Pharm.)
Tamper resistant parenteral package

Dialpak (Ortho)
Compliance package

Dis-Co Pack (Robins)
Unit dose package

Disket (Lilly)
Dispersible tablet

Dispenserpak (Burroughs Wellcome)
Unit-of-use package

Dispertab (Abbott)
Particles in tablet

Dispette (Lederle)
Disposable pipette

Divide-Tab (Abbott)
Scored tablet

Dividose (Mead Johnson)
Tablet, bisected/trisected

D·Lay (Lemmon)
Timed release tablet

Dosette (Elkins-Sinn)
Single dose ampule or vial

Dosepak (Upjohn)
Unit of use package

Drop Dose (Burroughs Wellcome)
Ophthalmic dropper dispenser

Drop-Tainer (Alcon)
Ophthalmic dropper dispenser

Dulcet (Abbott)
Chewable tablet

Dura-Tab (Berlex)
Sustained release tablet

Enduret (Boehringer Ingelheim)
Prolonged action tablet

Enseal (Lilly)
Enteric coated tablet

EN-tabs (Pharmacia)
Enteric coated tablet

Extencap (Robins)
Controlled release capsule

Extentab (Robins)
Continuous release tablet

Filmlok (Squibb)
Veneer coated tablet

Filmseal (Parke-Davis)
Film coated tablet

Filmtab (Abbott)
Film coated tablet

Flo-Pack (Burroughs Wellcome)
Vial for preparation of IV drips

Gelseal (Lilly)
Soft gelatin capsule

Gradumet (Abbott)
Controlled release tablet

Gy-Pak (Geigy)
Unit-of-issue package

Gyrocap (Rhone-Poulenc Rorer)
Timed release capsule

Hyporet (Lilly)
Unit dose syringe

Identi-Dose (Lilly)
Unit dose package

Infatab (Parke-Davis)
Chewable pediatric tablet

Inject-all (Bristol Labs)
Prefilled disposable dilution syringe

Inlay-Tabs (Dorsey/Sandoz)
Inlaid tablets

Isoject (Pfizer)
Unit dose syringe

Kapseal (Parke-Davis)
Banded (sealed) capsule

Kronocap (Ferndale)
Sustained release capsule

Lederject (Lederle)
Disposable syringe

Liquitab (Mission)
Chewable tablet

Memorette (Syntex)
Compliance package

Mix-O-Vial (Upjohn)
Two compartment vial

Mono-Drop (Winthrop Pharm.)
Ophthalmic plastic dropper

Ocumeter (MSD)
Ophthalmic dropper dispenser

Ovoid (Winthrop Pharm.)
Sugar coated tablet

Perle (Forest)
Soft gelatin capsule

Pilpak (Wyeth-Ayerst)
Compliance pack

Plateau CAP (Marion Merrell Dow)
Controlled release capsule

Pulvule (Lilly)
Bullet-shaped capsule

Rediject (Organon)
Unit dose syringe

Redipak (Wyeth-Ayerst)
Unit dose or unit-of-issue package

Redi Vial (Lilly)
Dual compartment vial

Repetabs (Schering)
Extended-release tablet

Rescue Pak (Burroughs Wellcome)
Unit dose packaging

Respihaler (MSD)
Aerosol for inhalation

Robicap (Robins)
Capsule

Robitab (Robins)
Tablet

SandoPak (Sandoz)
Unit dose blister package

Sani-Pak (Hauck)
Sanitary dispensing box

Secule (Wyeth-Ayerst)
Single dose vial

Sequels (Lederle)
Sustained release capsule or tablet

SigPak (Sandoz)
Unit-of-use package

Snap Tabs (Sandoz)
Tablet with facilitated bisect

Softab (Stuart)
Chewable tablet

Solvet (Lilly)
Soluble tablet

Spansule (SmithKline Beecham)
Sustained release capsule

Stat-Pak (Adria)
Unit dose package

Steri-Dose (Parke-Davis)
Unit dose syringe

Steri-Vial (Parke-Davis)
Ampule

Supprette (Webcon)
Suppository

Supule (Lemmon)
Suppository

Tabloid (Burroughs Wellcome)
Branded tablet (with raised lettering)

Tamp-R-Tel (Wyeth-Ayerst)
Tubex, tamper resistant

Tel-E-Amp (Roche)
Single dose amp

Tel-E-Dose (Roche)
Unit dose strip package

Tel-E-Ject (Roche)
Unit dose syringe

Tel-E-Pack (Roche)
Packaging system

Tel-E-Vial (Roche)
Single dose vial

Tembid (Wyeth-Ayerst)
Sustained action capsule

Tempule (Armour)
Timed release capsule or tablet

Ten-Tab (3M Pharmaceuticals
Controlled release tablet

Thera-Ject (SmithKline Beecham)
Unit dose syringe

Tiltab (SmithKline Beecham)
Tablet shape

Timecap (Schwarz Pharma Kremers Urban)
Sustained release capsule

Timecelle (Hauck)
Timed release capsule

Timespan (Roche)
Timed release tablet

Titradose (Wyeth-Ayerst)
Scored tablet

Traypak (Lilly)
Multivial carton

Tubex (Wyeth-Ayerst)
Cartridge-needle unit

Turbinaire (MSD)
Aerosol for nasal inhalation

UDIP (Marion Merrell Dow)
Unit dose indentification pak

U-Ject (Upjohn)
Disposable syringe

Uni-Amp (Winthrop Pharm.)
Single dose ampule

Unimatic (Squibb)
Unit dose syringe

Uni-nest (Winthrop Pharm.)
Ampule

UNI-Rx (Marion Merrell Dow)
Unit dose packages and containers

Unisert (Upsher-Smith)
Suppository

Vaporole (Burroughs Wellcome)
Crushable ampule for inhalation

Visipak (Upjohn)
Reverse numbered pack

Wyseal (Wyeth-Ayerst)
Film coated tablet

Glossary

Abduction—the act of drawing away from a center.
Abstergent—a cleansing application or medicine.
Acaricide—an agent lethal to mites.
Achlorhydria—the absence of hydrochloric acid from gastric secretions.
Acidifier, systemic—a drug used to lower internal body pH in patients with systemic alkalosis.
Acidifier, urinary—a drug used to lower the pH of the urine.
Acidosis—an accumulation of acid in the body.
Acne—an inflammatory disease of the skin accompanied by the eruption of papules or pustules.
Addison's Disease—a condition caused by adrenal gland destruction.
Adduction—the act of drawing toward a center.
Adenitis—a gland or lymph node inflammation.
Adjuvant—an ingredient added to a prescription which complements or accentuates the action of the primary agent.
Adrenergic—a sypathomimetic drug that activates organs innervated by the sympathetic branch of the autonomic nervous system.
Adrenocorticotropic Hormone—an anterior pituitary hormone that stimulates and regulates secretion of the adrenocortical steroids.
Adrenocortical steroid, anti-inflammatory—an adrenal cortex hormone that participates in regulation of organic metabolism and inhibits the inflammatory response to stress; a glucocorticoid.
Adrenocortical steroid, salt regulating—an adrenal cortex hormone that maintains sodium-potassium electrolyte balance by stimulating and regulating sodium retention and potassium excretion by the kidneys.
Adsorbent—an agent that binds chemicals to its surface; it is useful in reducing the free availability of toxic chemicals.
Alkalizer, systemic—a drug that raises internal body pH in patients with systemic acidosis.
Allergen—a specific substance that causes an unwanted reaction in the body.
Amblyopia—pertaining to a dimness of vision.
Amebiasis—an infection with a pathogenic amoeba.
Amenorrhea—an abnormal discontinuation of the menses.
Amphiarthrosis—a joint in which the surfaces are connected by discs of fibrocartilage.
Anabolic—an agent that promotes conversion of simple substance into more complex compounds; a constructive process for the organism.
Analeptic—a potent central nervous system stimulant used to maintain vital functions during severe central nervous system depression.
Analgesic—a drug that selectively suppresses pain perception without inducing unconsciousness.
Ancyclostomiasis—the presence of hookworms in the intestine.
Androgen—a hormone that stimulates and maintains male secondary sex characteristics.
Anemia—a deficiency of red blood cells.
Anesthetic, general—a drug that eliminates pain perception by inducing unconsciousness.
Anesthetic, local—a drug that eliminates pain perception in a limited area by local action on sensory nerves; a topical anesthetic.
Angina pectoris—a sharp chest pain starting in the heart, often spreading down the left arm. A symptom of coronary disease.
Angiography—an X-ray of the blood vessels.
Anhydrotic—a drug that checks perspiration flow systemically; an antidiaphoretic.
Anodyne—a drug which acts on the sensory nervous system, either centrally or peripherally, to produce relief from pain.
Anorexiant—a drug that suppresses appetite, usually secondary to central stimulation of mood.
Anorexigenic—an agent promoting a dislike or aversion to food.
Antacid—a drug that neutralizes excess gastric acid locally.
Anthelmintic—a drug that kills or inhibits worm infestations such as pinworms and tapeworms (nematodes, cestodes, trematodes).
Antiadrenergic—a drug that prevents response to sympathetic nervous system stimulation and adrenergic drugs; a sympatholytic or sympathoplegic drug.
Antiamebic—a drug that kills or inhibits the pathogenic protozoan *Entamoeba histolytica,* the causative agent of amebic dysentery.
Antianemic—a drug that stimulates the production of erythrocytes in normal size, number and hemoglobin content; useful in treating anemias.
Antiasthmatic—an agent that relieves the symptoms of asthma.
Antibacterial—a drug that kills or inhibits pathogenic bacteria, the causative agents of many systemic gastrointestinal and superficial infections.
Antibiotic—an agent produced by or derived from living cells of molds, bacteria or other plants, which destroy or inhibit the growth of microbes.
Anticholesteremic—a drug that lowers blood cholesterol levels.
Anticholinergic—a drug that prevents response to parasympathetic nervous system stimulation and cholinergic drugs; a parasympatholytic or parasympathoplegic drug.

Anticoagulant—a drug that inhibits clotting of circulating blood or prevents clotting of collected blood.
Anticonvulsant—a drug that selectively prevents epileptic seizures; a central depressant used to arrest convulsions by inducing unconsciousness.
Antidepressant—a psychotherapeutic drug that induces mood elevation, useful in treating depressive neuroses and psychoses.
Antidiabetic—a drug used to prevent the development of diabetes.
Antidote—a drug that prevents or counteracts the effects of poisons or drug overdoses, by adsorption in the gastrointestinal tract (general antidotes) or by specific systemic action (specific antidotes).
Antieczematic—a topical drug that aids in the control of exudative inflammatory skin lesions.
Antiemetic—a drug that prevents vomiting, especially that of systemic origin.
Anti-fibrinolytic—an agent (drug) that inhibits liquifaction of fibrin.
Antifilarial—a drug that kills or inhibits pathogenic filarial worms of the superfamily *Filarioidea,* the causative agents of diseases such as loaiasis.
Antiflatulant—an agent inhibiting the excessive formation of gas in the stomach or intestines.
Antifungal—a drug that kills or inhibits pathogenic fungi, the causative agents of systemic, gastrointestinal, and superficial infections.
Antihemophilic—a blood derivative containing the clotting factors absent in the hereditary disease hemophilia.
Antihistaminic—a drug that prevents response to histamine, including histamine released by allergic reactions.
Antihypercholesterolemic—a drug that lowers blood cholesterol levels, especially elevated levels sometimes associated with cardiovascular disease.
Antihypertensive—a drug that lowers blood pressure, especially diastolic blood pressure in hypertensive patients.
Anti-infective, local—a drug that kills a variety of pathogenic microorganisms and is suitable for sterilizing the skin or wounds.
Anti-inflammatory—a drug which counteracts or suppresses inflammation, and produces suppression of the pain, heat, redness and swelling of inflammation.
Antileishmanial—a drug that kills or inhibits pathogenic protozoa of the genus *Leishmania,* the causative agents of diseases such as kala-azar.
Antileprotic—an agent which fights leprosy, a generally chronic skin disease.
Antilipemic—an agent reducing the amount of circulating lipids.
Antimalarial—a drug that kills or inhibits the causative agents of malaria.
Antimetabolite—a substance that competes with or replaces a certain metabolite.
Antimethemoglobinemic—a drug that reduces non-functional methemoglobin (Fe^{+++}) to normal hemoglobin (Fe^{++}). normal hemoglobin (Fe^{++}).
Antimycotic—an agent inhibiting the growth of fungi.
Antinauseant—a drug that suppresses nausea, especially that due to motion sickness.
Antineoplastic—a drug that is selectively toxic to rapidly multiplying cells and is useful in destroying malignant tumors.
Antioxidant—an agent used to reduce decay or transformation of a material from oxidation.
Antiperiodic—a drug that modifies or prevents the return of malarial fever; an antimalarial.
Antiperistaltic—a drug that inhibits intestinal motility, especially for the treatment of diarrhea.
Antipruritic—a drug that prevents or relieves itching.
Antipyretic—a drug employed to reduce fever temperature of the body; a febrifuge.
Antirheumatic—a drug that alleviates inflammatory symptoms of arthritis and related connective tissue diseases.
Antirickettsial—a drug that kills or inhibits pathogenic microorganisms of the genus Rickettsia, the causative agents of diseases such as typhus (e.g. Chloramphenicol USP).
Antischistosomal—a drug that kills or inhibits pathogenic flukes of the genus *Schistosoma,* the causative agents of schistosomiasis.
Antiseborrheic—a drug that aids in the control of seborrheic dermatitis ("dandruff").
Antiseptic—a substance that will inhibit the growth and development of microorganisms without necessarily destroying them.
Antisialagogue—a drug which diminishes the flow of saliva.
Antispasmodic—an agent used to quiet the spasms of voluntary and involuntary muscles; a calmative or antihysteric.
Anti-syphilitic—a remedy used in the treatment of syphilis.
Antitoxin—a biological drug containing antibodies against the toxic principles of a pathogenic microorganism, used for passive immunization against the associated disease.
Antitrichomonal—a drug that kills or inhibits the pathogenic protozoan *Trichomonas vaginalis,* the causative agent of trichomonal vaginitis.
Antitrypanosomal—a drug that kills or inhibits pathogenic protozoa of the genus *Trypanosoma,* the causative agents of diseases such as West African trypanosomiasis.
Antitussive—a drug that suppresses coughing.
Antivenin—a biological drug containing antibodies against the venom of a poisonous animal; an antidote for a venomous bite.

Anxiety—a feeling of apprehension, uncertainty and fear.
Aperient—a mild laxative.
Aphasia—the inability to use and/or understand written and spoken words, due to damage of cortical speech centers.
Aphonia—a whisper voice due to disease of the larynx or its innervation.
Apnea—the absence of breathing.
Areola—a pigmented ring on the skin.
Arsenical—having to do with arsenic.
Arteriosclerosis—a hardening of the arteries.
Arthritis—an inflammation of a joint.
Ascariasis—a condition caused by roundworms in the intestine.
Ascaricide—an agent that kills roundworms of the genus *Ascaris*.
Aspergillus—a fungi genus including many types of molds.
Astasia—the ability to stand up without help.
Asthma—a disease characterized by recurring breathing difficulty due to bronchial muscle constriction.
Astringent—a mild protein precipitant suitable for local application to toughen, shrink, blanch, wrinkle and harden tissue, diminish secretions and coagulate blood.
Ataractic—an agent having a quieting, tranquilizing effect.
Ataxia—incoordination, especially of gait.
Atheroma—a fatty granular degeneration of an artery wall.
Atrophy—a wasting away.
Avitaminosis—a disease caused by lack of one or more vitamins in the diet.
Axilla—armpit.
Bacteriostatic—an agent that inhibits the growth of bacteria.
Basedow's disease—a form of hyperthyroidism, also known as Grave's disease and Parry's disease.
Biliary Colic—a sharp pain in the upper right side of the abdomen due to a gallstone impaction.
Bilirubin—a bile pigment.
Billuria—the presence of bile in the urine.
Blood Calcium Regulator—a drug that maintains the blood level of ionic calcium, especially by regulating its metabolic disposition elsewhere.
Blood Volume Supporter—an intravenous solution whose solutes are retained in the vascular system to supplement the osmotic activity of plasma proteins.
Bradycardia—a slow heart rate.
Bright's Disease—a disease of the kidneys, including the presence of edema and excessive urine protein formation.
Bromidrosis—foul smelling perspiration.
Bronchitis—an inflammation of the bronchi.
Bronchodilator—a drug which can dilate the lumina of air passages of the lungs.
Bruit—an arterial sound audible with a stethoscope.
Buerger's Disease—a thromboangiitis obliterans inflammation of the walls and surrounding tissue of the veins and arteries.
Bursitis—an inflammation of the bursa.
Callus—a hard bonelike material developing around a fractured bone.
Calmative—a sedative.
Candidiasis—an infection by the yeastlike organism *Candida albicans*.
Carbonic Anhydrase Inhibitor—an enzyme inhibitor, the therapeutic effects of which are diuresis and reduced formation of intraocular fluid.
Carcinoma—a malignant growth.
Cardiac Depressant—a drug that depresses myocardial function so as to supress rhythmic irregularities characterized by fast rate; an antiarrhythmic.
Cardiac Stimulant—a drug that increases the contractile force of the myocardium, especially in weakened conditions such as congestive heart failure; a cardiotonic.
Cardiopathy—a disease of the heart.
Caries—decay of the teeth.
Carminative—an aromatic or pungent drug that mildly irritates the gastrointestinal tract and is useful in the treatment of flatulence and colic. Peppermint Water is a common carminative.
Caruncle—a small fleshy projection on the skin.
Cathartic—a drug that promotes defecation, usually by enhancing peristalsis or by softening and lubricating the feces.
Caudal—pertains to the distal end or tail.
Caustic—a topical drug that destroys tissue on contact and is suitable for removal of abnormal skin growths.
Central Depressant—a drug that reduces the functional state of the central nervous system and with increasing dosage induces sedation, hypnosis, and general anesthesia; respiration is depressed.
Central Stimulant—a drug that increases the functional state of the central nervous system and with increasing dosage induces restlessness, insomnia, disorientation, and convulsions; respiration is stimulated.
Cerebral—pertaining to the brain.
Cerumen—earwax.
Chloasma—skin discoloration.
Cholagogue—a drug that stimulates the emptying of the gallbladder and the flow of bile into the duodenum.
Cholecystitis—an inflammation of the gallbladder.
Cholecystokinetic—an agent that promotes emptying of the gallbladder.
Cholelithiasis—the presence of calculi (stones) in the gallbladder.
Choleretic—a drug that increases the production and secretion of dilute bile by the liver.

Chorea—a disorder, usually of childhood, characterized by uncontrolled spasmotic muscle movements; sometimes referred to as St. Vitus' dance.
Chymotrypsin—a proteinase in the gastrointestinal tract; its proposed use has been the treatment of edema and inflammation.
Claudication—limping.
Climacteric—a time period in women just preceding termination of the reproductive processes.
Clonus—a spasm in which rigidity and relaxation succeed each other.
Coagulant—a drug that replaces a deficient blood factor necessary for coagulation; clotting factor.
Coccidiostat—a drug used in the treatment of coccidal (protozoal) infections in animals, especially birds; used in veterinary medicine.
Colitis—an inflammation of the colon.
Colloid—a disperse system of particles larger than those of true solutions but smaller than those of suspensions (1 to 100 millimicrons in size).
Collyrium—an eyewash.
Colostomy—the surgical formation of a more or less permanent opening into the colon.
Corticoid—a term applied to hormones of the adrenal cortex or any substance, natural or synthetic, having similar activity.
Corticosteroid—a steroid produced by the adrenal cortex.
Coryza—a headcold.
Counterirritant—an agent (irritant) which causes irritation of the part to which it is applied, and draws blood away from a deep seated area.
Cranial—pertaining to the skull.
Crepitation—the grating of a joint.
Cryptitis—an inflammation of a follicle or glandular tubule, usually in the rectum.
Cryptococcus—a genus of fungi which does not produce spores, but reproduces by budding.
Cryptorchidism—the failure of one or both testes to descend.
Cutaneous—pertaining to the skin.
Cyanosis—a blue or purple skin discoloration due to oxygen deficiency.
Cycloplegia—the loss of accommodation.
Cyclopegic—a drug which paralyzes accommodation of the eye.
Cystitis—an inflammation of the bladder.
Cystourethography—the examination by x-ray of the bladder and urethra.
Cytostasis—a slowing of the movement of blood cells at an inflamed area, sometimes causing capillary blockage.
Debridement—the cutting away of dead or excess skin from a wound.
Decongestant—a drug which reduces congestion caused by an accumulation of blood.
Decubitus—the patient's position in bed; the act of lying down.
Demulcent—an agent used generally internally to sooth and protect mucous membranes.
Dermatitis—an inflammation of the skin.
Dermatomycosis—lesions or eruptions caused by fungi on the skin.
Detergent—an emulsifying agent useful for cleansing wounds and ulcers as well as the skin.
Dextrocardia—when the heart is located on the right side of the chest.
Diagnostic Aid—a drug used to determine the functional state of a body organ or the presence of a disease.
Diaphoretic—a drug used to increase perspiration; a hydroticorsudorfice.
Diarrhea—an abnormal frequency and fluidity of stools.
Digestive Enzyme—an enzyme that promotes digestion by supplementing the naturally occurring counterpart.
Digitalization—the administration of digitalis to obtain a desired tissue level of drug.
Diplopia—double vision.
Disinfectant—an agent that destroys pathogenic microorganisms on contact and is suitable for sterilizing inanimate objects.
Distal—farthest from a point of reference.
Diuretic—a drug that promotes renal excretion of electrolytes and water, thereby increasing urine volume.
Dysarthria—difficulty in speech articulation.
Dysmenorrhea—pertaining to painful menstruation.
Dysphagia—difficulty in swallowing.
Dyspnea—difficult breathing.
Ecbolic—a drug used to stimulate the gravid uterus to the expulsion of the fetus, or to cause uterine contraction; an oxytocic.
Eclampsia—a toxic disorder occurring late in pregnancy involving hypertension, weight gain, edema and renal dysfunction.
Ectasia—pertaining to distension or stretching.
Ectopic—out of place; not in normal position.
Eczema—an inflammatory disease of the skin with infiltrations, watery discharge, scales and crust.
Effervescent—bubbling; sparkling; giving off gas bubbles.
Embolus—a blood clot in the blood stream lodged in a vessel, thus obstructing circulation.
Emetic—a drug that induces vomiting, either locally by gastrointestinal irritation or systemically by stimulation of receptors in the central nervous system.
Emollient—a topical drug, especially an oil or fat, used to soften the skin and make it more pliable.
Endometrium—the uterine mucous membrane.
Enteralgia—an intestinal pain.
Enterobiasis—a pinworm infestation.
Enuresis—involuntary urination, as in bedwetting.
Epidermis—the outermost layer of the skin.

Episiotomy—a surgical incision of the vulva when deemed necessary during childbirth.
Epistaxis—a nosebleed.
Erythema—redness.
Erythrocyte—a red blood cell.
Escharotic—corrosive.
Estrogen—a hormone that stimulates and maintains female secondary sex characteristics and functions in the menstrual cycle to promote uterine gland proliferation.
Etiology—the cause of a disease.
Euphoria—an exaggerated feeling of well being.
Eutonic—having normal muscular tone.
Exfoliation—a scaling of the skin.
Exophthalmos—a protrusion of the eyeballs.
Expectorant—a drug that increases secretion of respiratory tract fluid, thereby lowering its viscosity and cough-inducing irritancy and promoting its ejection.
Extension—the movement of a joint to move 2 body parts away from each other.
Exteroceptors—receptors on the exterior of the body.
Fasciculations—the visible twitching movements of muscle bundles.
Fibroid—a tumor of fibrous tissue, resembling fibers.
Filariasis—the condition of having round worm parasites reproducing in the body tissues.
Fistula—an abnormal opening leading from a body cavity to the outside of the body or to another cavity.
Flexion—the movement of a joint in which 2 moveable parts are brought toward each other.
Fungistatic—inhibiting the growth of fungi.
Furunculosis—a condition marked by the presence of boils.
Gallop Rhythm—a heart condition where 3 separate beats are heard instead of 2.
Gastralgia—a stomach pain.
Gastritis—inflammation of the stomach lining.
Gastrocele—a hernial protrusion of the stomach.
Gastrodynia—pain in the stomach, a stomach ache.
Geriatrics—a branch of medicine which treats problems peculiar to old age.
Germicidal—an agent that is destructive to pathogenic microorganisms.
Gingivitis—an inflammation of the gums.
Glaucoma—a disease of the eye evidenced by an increase in intraocular pressure and resulting in hardness of the eye, atrophy of the retina and eventual blindness.
Glossitis—an inflammation of the tongue.
Glucocorticoid—a corticoid which increases gluconeogenesis, thereby raising the concentration of liver glycogen and blood sugar.
Glycosuria—an abnormal quantity of glucose in the urine.
Gout—a disorder which is characterized by a high uric acid level and sudden onset of recurrent arthritis.
Granulation—the formation of small round fleshy granules on a wound in the healing process.
Hematemesis—the vomiting of blood.
Hematinic—a drug that promotes hemoglobin formation by supplying a factor essential for its synthesis.
Hemiplegia—a condition in which one side of the body is paralyzed.
Hematopoietic—a drug that stimulates formation of blood cells, especially by supplying deficient vitamins.
Hemoptysis—expectoration of blood.
Histoplasmosis—a lung infection caused by the inhalation of fungus spores, often resulting in pneumonitis.
Hodgkin's Disease—a disease marked by chroniclymph node enlargement sometimes including spleen and liver enlargement.
Hydrocholeresis—putting out a thinner, more watery bile.
Hypercholesterolemia—the condition of having an abnormally large amount of cholesterol in the body cells.
Hemorrhage—copious bleeding.
Hemostatic—a locally acting drug that arrests hemorrhage by promoting clot formation or by serving as a mechanical matrix for a clot.
Hepatitis—an inflammation of the liver.
Hyperemia—an excess of blood in any part of the body.
Hyperesthesia—an increase in sensations.
Hyperglycemic—a drug that elevates blood glucose level, especially for the treatment of hypoglycemic states.
Hypertension—blood pressure above the normally accepted limits, high blood pressure.
Hypertriglyceridemia—an increased level of triglycerides in the blood.
Hypnotic—a central depressant which, with suitable dosage, induces sleep.
Hypodermoclysis—a subcutaneous injection with a solution.
Hypoesthesia—a diminished sensation of touch.
Hypoglycemic—a drug that promotes glucose metabolism and lowers blood glucose level, useful in the control of diabetes mellitus.
Hypokalemia—an abnormally small concentration of potassium ions in the blood.
Hyposensitize—to reduce the sensitivity to an agent, referring to allergies.
Hypotensive—a drug which diminishes tension or pressure, to lower blood pressure.
Ichthyosis—an inherited skin disease characterized by dryness and scales.
Idiopathic—denoting a disease of unknown cause.
Ileostomy—the establishment of an opening from the ileum to the outside of the body.
Immune Serum—a biological drug containing antibodies for a pathogenic microorganism, use-

ful for passive immunization against the associated disease.

Immunizing Agent, active—an antigenic preparation (toxoid or vaccine) used to induce formation of specific antibodies against a pathogenic microorganism, which provides delayed but permanent protection against the associated disease.

Immunizing Agent, passive—a biological preparation (antitoxin, antivenin or immune serum) containing specific antibodies against a pathogenic microorganism, which provides immediate but temporary protection against the associated disease.

Impetigo—an inflammatory skin infection with isolated pustules.

Insulin—one of the hormones that regulate carbohydrate metabolism, used as replacement therapy in diabetes mellitus.

Inversion—a turning inward.

Irrigating solution—a solution for washing body surfaces and/or various body cavities.

Isoniazid—a compound effective in tuberculosis treatment.

Kakidrosis—foul smelling perspiration.

Keratitis—an inflammation of the cornea.

Keratolytic—a topical drug that softens the superficial keratin-containing layer of the skin to promote exfoliation.

Lacrimal—pertaining to tears.

Laxative—a gentle purgative medicine; a mild cathartic.

Leishmaniasis—a number of types of infections transmitted by sand flies.

Leucocytopenia—a decrease in the number of white cells.

Leucocytosis—an increased white cell count.

Leukoderma—an absence of pigment from the skin.

Libido—sexual desire or creative energy.

Leucocyte—a white blood cell.

Lipoma—a fatty tumor.

Lipotropic—a drug, especially one supplementing a dietary factor, that prevents the abnormal accumulation of fat in the liver.

Lochia—a vaginal discharge of mucus, blood and tissue after childbirth.

Lues—a plague; specifically syphilis.

Macrocyte—a large red blood cell.

Malaise—a general feeling of illness.

Melasma—a darkening of the skin.

Melena—black feces or black vomit from altered blood in the higher GI tract.

Meninges—the membranes covering the brain and spinal cord.

Metastasis—the shifting of a disease or its symptoms from one part of the body to another.

Mastitis—an inflammation of the breast.

Miotics—agents which constrict the pupil of the eye; a myotic.

Moniliasis—an infection with any of the species of monilia types of fungi *(Candida)*.

Mucolytic—an agent that can destroy or dissolve mucous membrane secretions.

Myalgia—a pain in the muscles.

Myasthenia Gravis—a chronic progressive muscular weakness caused by myoneural conduction, usually spreading from the face and throat.

Myelocyte—an immature white blood cell in the bone marrow.

Myelogenous—originating in bone marrow.

Myoclonus—involuntary, sudden and rapid unpredictable jerks; faster than chorea.

Mydriatic—a drug that dilates the pupil of the eye, usually by anticholinergic or adrenergic mechanism.

Myoneural—pertaining to muscle and nerve.

Myopia—nearsightedness.

Narcotic—a drug that produces insensibility or stupor; a class of drug regulated by law.

Neonatal—pertaining to the first four weeks of life.

Neoplasm—an abnormal tissue growing more rapidly than usual showing a lack of structural organization.

Nephritis—an inflammation of the kidney.

Nephrosclerosis—a hardening of the kidney tissue.

Neuralgia—a pain extending along the course ofone or more of the nerves.

Neurasthenia—nervous prostration.

Neuroglia—the supporting elements of the nervous system.

Neuroleptic—a substance that acts on the nervous system.

Neurosis—a functional disorder of the nervous system.

Nocturia—urination at night.

Normocytic—pertaining to anemia due to some defect in the blood-forming tissues.

Nuchal—the nape of the neck.

Nystagmus—a rhythmic oscillation of the eyes.

Oleaginous—oily or greasy.

Omphalitis—an inflammation of the navel in a newborn.

Onychomycosis—a ringworm or fungus infection of the nails.

Ophthalmic—pertaining to the eye.

Oral—pertaining to the mouth.

Orthopnea—a discomfort in breathing in any but the upright sitting or standing positions.

Osmidrosis—foul smelling perspiration.

Ossification—a formation of, or conversion to, bone.

Osteomyelitis—an inflammation of the marrow of the bone.

Osteoporosis—a reduction in bone quantity; skeletal atrophy.

Otalgia—pain in the ear; an earache.

Otitis—inflammation of the ear.

Otomycosis—an ear infection caused by fungus.

Otorrhea—a discharge from the ear.

Oxytocic—a drug that selectively stimulates uterine motility and isuseful in obstetrics, especially in the control of postpartum hemorrhage.
Ozochrotia—foul smelling perspiration.
Palpitations—an awareness of one's heart action.
Paget's Disease—a disease characterized by lesions around the nipple and areola found in elderly women.
Pallor—the lack of the normal red color imparted to the skin by the blood of the superficial vessels.
Parasympatholytic—See Anticholinergic.
Parasympathomimetic—See Cholinergic.
Parenteral—pertaining to the administration of a drug by means other than through the alimentary canal; subcutaneous, intramuscular or intravenous administration of drug.
Parkinsonism—a group of neurological disorders marked by hypokinesia, tremor, and muscular rigidity.
Paroxysm—a sudden recurrence or intensification of symptoms.
Pathogenic—giving origin to disease.
Pediatric—pertaining to children's diseases.
Pediculicide—an insecticide suitable for erradicating louse infestations in humans (pediculosis).
Pediculosis—an infestation with lice.
Pellagra—characterized by GI disturbances, mental disorders, and skin redness and scaling due to niacin deficiency.
Pernicious—particularly dangerous or harmful.
Phlebitis—an inflammation of a vein.
Pleurisy—an inflammation of the membrane surrounding the lungs and the thoracic cavity.
Pneumonia—an infection of the lungs.
Poikilocytosis—a condition in which pointed or irregularly shaped red blood cells are found in the blood.
Polydipsia—excessive thirst.
Posology—the science of dosage.
Posterior Pituitary Hormone(s)—a multifunctional hormone with oxytocic-milk ejection, and antidiuretic-vasopressor fractions.
Progestin—a hormone that functions in the menstrual cycle and during pregnancy to promote uterine gland secretion and to reduce uterine motility.
Pronation—the act of turning the palm downward or backward.
Prophylactic—a remedy that tends to prevent disease.
Protectant—a topical drug that remains on the skin and serves as a physical barrier to the environment.
Proteolytic Enzyme—an enzyme used to liquefy fibrinous or purulent exudates.
Psoriasis—an inflammatory skin disease accompanied with itching.
Psychotherapeutic—a drug that selectively affects the central nervous system to alter emotional state. See Antidepressant; Tranquilizer.
Ptosis—a drooping or sagging of the muscle.
Pulmonary—pertaining to the lungs.
Purulent—containing or forming pus.
Pyelitis—a local inflammation of renal and pelvic cells due to bacterial infection.
Pylorospasm—a spasmodic muscle contraction of the pyloric portion of the stomach.
Pyoderma—any skin discharge characterized by pus formation.
Radiopaque Medium—a diagnostic drug, opaque to X rays, whose retention in a body organ or cavity makes X-ray visualization possible.
Raynaud's Phenomenon—spasms of the digital arteries with blanching and numbness of the fingers, usually with another disease.
Reflex Stimulant—a mild irritant suitable for application to the nasopharynx to induce reflex respiratory stimulation.
Rheumatoid—a condition resembling rheumatism.
Rhinitis—an inflammation of the mucous membrane of the nose.
Rubefacient—a topical drug that induces mild skin irritation with erythema, sometimes used to relieve the discomfort of deep-seated inflammation.
Rubeola—a synonym popularly used for both measles and rubella.
Saprophytic—getting nourishment from dead material.
Sarcoma—a malignant tumor derived from connective tissue.
Scabicide—an insecticide suitable for the erradication of itch mite infestations in humans (scabies).
Schistosomacide—an agent which destroys schistosomes; destructive to the trematodic parasites or flukes.
Schistosomiasis—an infection with *Schistosoma haematobium* involving the urinary tract and causing cystitis and hematuria.
Scintillation—a visual sensation manifested by an emission of sparks.
Sclerosing Agent—an irritant suitable for injection into varicose veins to induce their fibrosis and obliteration.
Scotomata—an area of varying size and shape within the visual field in which vision is absent or depressed.
Seborrhea—a condition arising from an excess secretion of sebum.
Sebum—the fatty secretions of sebaceous glands.
Sedative—a central depressant which, in suitable dosage, induces mild relaxation useful in treating tension.
Sinusitis—an inflammation of a sinus.
Skeletal Muscle Relaxant—a drug that inhibits contraction of voluntarymuscles, usually by interfering with their innervation.
Smooth Muscle Relaxant—a drug that inhibits

contraction of involuntary (e.g., visceral) muscles, usually by action upon their contractile elements.

Sociopath—a psychopathic person who, due to his unaccepted attitudes, is badly adjusted to society.

Spasmolytic—an agent that relieves spasms and involuntary contraction of a muscle; an antispasmodic.

Sputum—mucous spit from the mouth.

Stenosis—the narrowing of the lumen of a blood vessel.

Stomachic—a d rug which is used to stimulate the appetite and gastric secretion.

Stomatitis—an inflammation of the mouth.

Subcutaneous—under the skin.

Sudorific—causing perspiration.

Superacidity—an increase of the normal acidity of the gastric secretion; hyperacidity.

Supination—the act of turning the palm forward or upward.

Suppressant—a drug useful in the control, rather than the cure, of a disease.

Surfactant—a surface active agent that decreases the surface tension between two miscible liquids; used to prepare emulsions, act as a cleansing agent, etc.

Synarthrosis (fibrous joint)—a joint in which the bony elements are united by continuous fibrous tissue.

Syncope—fainting.

Synovia—clear fluid which lubricates the joints; joint oil.

Systole—the ventricular contraction phase of a heartbeat.

Tachycardia—a rapid contraction rate of the heart.

Taeniacide—an agent used to kill tapeworms.

Taeniafuge—agent to expel tapeworms.

Therapeutic—a treatment of disease.

Thoracic—pertaining to the chest.

Thyroid Hormone—a drug containing one or more of the iodinated amino acids that stimulate and regulate the metabolic rate and functional state of body tissues.

Thyroid Inhibitor—drug that reduces excessive thyroid hormone production, usually by blocking hormone synthesis.

Tics—a repetitive twitching of muscles, often in the face and upper trunk.

Tinea—a fungal infection of the skin.

Tonic—an agent used to stimulate the restoration of tone to muscle tissue.

Tonometry—the measurement of tension in some part of the body.

Topical—the local external application of a drug to a particular place.

Toxoid—a modified bacterial toxin, less toxic than the original form, used to induce active immunity to bacterial pathogens.

Tranquilizer—a psychotherapeutic drug that induces emotional repose without significant sedation, useful in treating certain neuroses and psychoses.

Tremors—involuntary rhythmic tremulous movements.

Trichomoniasis—an infestation with parasitic flagellate protozoa of the genus *Trichomonas.*

Trypanosomiasis—a disease caused by protozoan flagellates in the blood.

Uricosuric—drug that promotes renal uric acid excretion; used to treat gout.

Urolithiasis—a condition marked by the formation of stones in the urinary tract.

Urticaria—a rash of hives generally of systemic origin.

Vaccine—preparation of live attenuated or dead pathogenic microorganisms, used to induce active immunity.

Vasoconstrictor—an adrenergic drug used locally in the nose to constrict blood vessels and reduce tissue congestion.

Vasodilator—a drug that relaxes vascular smooth muscles, expecially for the purpose of improving peripheral or coronary blood flow.

Vasopressor—an adrenergic drug used systemically to constrict blood vessels and raise blood pressure.

Verruca—a wart.

Vertigo—illusion of movement.

Vesicant—an agent which, when applied to the skin causes blistering and the formation of vesicles; an epispastic.

Visceral—pertaining to the internal organs.

Vitamin—an organic chemical essential in small amounts for normal body metabolism, used therapeutically to supplement the naturally occurring counterpart in foods.

Container Requirements for U.S.P XXII Drugs

Legend:

WC	= well closed container	TP	= tamper-proof
T	= tight container	In	= inert atmosphere
LR	= light resistant container	U	= unit dose
+	= controlled temperature	S	= separate ingredient
P	= plastic specified	U	= packaging before mixing
G	= glass specified	A	= pressurized container
C	= collapsible tubes	OT	= Ophthalmic Tube
S/M	= Single Dose/Multi Dose	SC	= Radioactive Shielding
H	= Reduced Moisture	R	= Remote from fire
SP	= Special consideration		

a = Tablets	g = Ointment	m = Vaginal	t = Gel/Jelly
b = Capsules	h = Lotion	n = Lozenges	v = Otic
c = Solution	i = Suppository	o = Powder	w = Intraocular solution
d = Syrup	j = Suspension	p = Enema	x = Veterinary use
e = Elixir	k = Ophthalmic	r = Inhalation	y = Emulsion
f = Cream	l = Aerosol	s = Nasal	z = Tincture

Drug (Dosage Form)	WC	T	LR
Acetaminophen	X[i t]	X[a b c e]	
Acetaminophen Oral		X[e j]	
Acetaminophen & Aspirin (tab)		X	
Acetaminophen, Aspirin & Caffeine	X[a]	X[b]	
Acetaminophen & Caffeine		X[a b]	
Acetaminophen & Codeine Phosphate		X[a b e]	X[a b e]
Acetaminophen & Diphenhydramine Citrate (tab)		X	
Acetaminophen for Effervescent Oral Soln.		X	
Acetohydroxamic Acid (tab)		X[a o +]	
Acetazolamide (tab)	X		
Acetic Acid Otic Soln.		X	
Acetohexamide (tab)	X		
Acetophenazine Maleate		X[a o]	X[a o]
Acetylcysteine & Isoproterenol HCl Inhalation Soln.		G/P	
Acrisorcin (cream)		C	
Acyclovir		X[o]	
Albuterol	X[o]		X[o]
Albuterol Sulfate	X[o]		X[o]
Alcohol		R	
Alcohol, Dehydrated		R	
Alcohol, Rubbing		R	
Alclometasone Dipropionate		C[f g]	

Drug (Dosage Form)	WC	T	LR
Allopurinol (tab)	X		
Alprazolam	X[o]	X[a]	X[a]
Alum	X		
Ammonium Alum	X		
Potassium Alum	X		
Alumina & Magnesia	X[a]	X[j +]	
Alumina & Magnesium Carbonate		X[a]	X[j +]
Alumina and Magnesium Carbonate and Magnesium Oxide (tab)		X	
Alumina & Magnesium Trisilicate		X[j + a]	
Alumina, Magnesia, Calcium Carbonate, Simethicone (tab)	X		
Alumina, Magnesia & Simethicone Oral		X[j +]	
Aluminum Acetate Topical Soln.		X	
Aluminum Carbonate Gel, Basic	X[a b]	X[+]	
Aluminum Hydroxide Gel	X[a b]	X[j +]	
Aluminum Phosphate Gel	X[a]	X[j +]	
Aluminum Subacetate Topical Soln.		X	
Amantadine HCl		X[b d]	
Amdinonide		X[f g]	
Amiloride HCl (tab)	X		
Amiloride HCl & Hydrochlorothiazide (tab)	X		

*The listing of container requirements for Compendial drugs is included as an aid to the practitioner in storing and dispensing.

Drug (Dosage Form)	WC	T	LR
Aminobenzoic Acid		X[t c]	X[t c]
Aminobenzoate Potassium	X[b a]	X[c]	
Aminocaproic Acid		X[a d]	
Aminoglutethimide (tab)	X		X
Aminophylline	X[i +]	X[a]	
Aminophylline, Oral		X[c]	
Aminosalicylate Sodium (tab)		X[+]	X[+]
Aminosalicylic Acid (tab)		X[+]	X[+]
Amitriptyline HCl (tab)	X		
Aromatic Ammonia Spirit		X[+]	X[+]
Ammonium Chloride Delayed Release (tab)		X	
Amobarbital (tab)	X		
Amobarbital Sodium (cap)		X	
Amodiaquine		X	
Amodiaquine HCl (tab)		X	
Amoxapine		X[o]	
Amoxicillin		X[a b +]	
Amoxicillin for Oral Susp.		X[+]	
Amoxicillin Oral Susp.	M[+]		
Amoxicillin & Clavulanate Potassium		X[h + a]	
Amoxicillin & Clavulanate Potassium for Oral Susp.		X[+]	
Amphetamine Sulfate (tab)		X	
Amphotericin B	X[h]	C[f g]	
Ampicillin (all dosage forms)		X	
Ampicillin Boluses		X[x]	
Ampicillin Soluble Powder		X[x]	
Ampicillin & Probenecid (cap)		X	
Ampicillin & Probenecid for Oral Susp.		U	
Amprolium (all dosage forms)		X	
Amyl Nitrate (inhalant)		UG[+]	UG[+]
Anileridine HCl (tab)		X	
Anthralin		X[f g +]	X[f g +]
Antimony Sodium Tartrate		X	
Antipyrine & Benzocaine Otic Soln.			X
Antipyrine, Benzocaine & Phenylephrine HCl Otic Soln.		X	X
Apomorphine HCl (tab)		X	
Apraclonidine HCl		X[o]	X[o]
Apraclonidine Ophthalmic		X[c]	X[c]
Ascorbic Acid		X[a c]	X[a c]
Aspirin	X[i +]	X[a b]	
Aspirin, Buffered		X[a]	
Aspirin, Delayed Release		X[a b]	
Aspirin, Effervescent Tablets for Oral Soln.		X	
Aspirin, Extended Release (tab)		X	
Aspirin, Alumina & Magnesia (tab)		X	
Aspirin, Alumina & Magnesium Oxide (tab)		X	
Aspirin, Caffeine & Dihydrocodeine (cap)		X	
Aspirin & Codeine Phosphate (tab)	X		X
Aspirin, Codeine Phosphate, Alumina & Magnesia (tab)	X		X
Aspirin, Codeine Phosphate & Caffeine	X[a b]		
Atropine Sulfate	X[a]	C[k g]	
Attapulgite, Activated	X		
Attapulgite, Colloidal Activated	X		
Azatadine Maleate (tab)	X		
Azathioprine (tab)			X
Aztreonam		X[o]	
Bacampicillin HCl (tab)		X	
Bacampicillin HCl for Oral Susp.		X	
Bacitracin (ointment)	X[g +]	COT[k +]	
Bacitracin & Polymyxin B Sulfate, Topical		A[l +]	
Bacitracin Methylene Disalicylate, Soluble	X[x]	X[o x]	
Bacitracin Zinc Soluble Powder		X[x]	
Bacitracin Zinc	X[g +]		
Bacitracin Zinc & Polymyxin B Sulfate (ointment)	X	COT[k]	X
Baclofen	X[a]	X[o]	
Barium Sulfate	X[j]		
Beclomethasone Dipropionate	X		
Belladonna Extract (tab)		X	X
Belladonna (tincture)		X[+]	X[+]
Bendroflumethiazide (tab)		X	
Benoxinate HCl Ophthalmic Soln.		X	
Benzethonium Chloride		X[c z]	X[c z]
Benzocaine		X[f g +]	X[f g +]
Benzocaine Otic Soln.		X[+]	X[+]
Benzocaine, Topical		X[c l +]	X[c +]
Benzoic & Salicylic Acid (oint.)	X[+]		
Benzoin Tincture Compound		X[+]	X[+]
Benzonatate (cap)		X	X
Benzoyl Peroxide		X[h t]	
Benzthiazide (tab)		X	

Drug (Dosage Form)	WC	T	LR
Benztropine Mesylate (tab)	X		
Benzyl Benzoate (lot)		X	X
Benzylpenicilloyl Polylysine Concentrate			X
Beta Carotene (cap)		X	X
Betaine HCl	X		
Betamethasone	X[a,d]	C[f]	
Betamethasone Benzoate (gel)		XC	
Betamethasone Dipropionate	XC[g]	X[h,i]	C[f]
Betamethasone Valerate	C[f,g]	X[f,g]	X[h]
Betaxolol HCl		X[o]	
Betaxolol HCl Ophthalmic		X[c]	
Bethanechol Chloride (tab)	X		
Biotin		X[o]	
Biperiden HCl (tab)	X		
Bisacodyl	X[a,i,+]		
Bismuth Subgallate		X[o]	X[o]
Bismuth, Milk of	X[+]		
Bromodiphenhydramine HCl		X[b]	X[e]
Bromocriptine Mesylate		X[a,o,+]	X[a,o,+]
Brompheniramine Maleate	X[e]	X[a]	X[e]
Brompheniramine Maleate & Pseudoephedrine Sulfate Syrup	X		X
Bumetanide		X[a,o]	X[a,o]
Busulfan (tab)	X		
Butalbital, Acetaminophen & Caffeine (tab)		X	
Butabarbital & Aspirin (tab)		X	
Butamben	X		
Butoconazole Nitrate	X[o]	C[f,+]	X[o]
Calamine (lot)		X	
Calamine, Phenolated (lot)		X	
Calciferol (cap)		X	X
Calcium Acetate		X	
Calcium Carbonate	X[a,o]		
Calcium Carbonate Oral Susp.		X[t]	
Calcium Carbonate & Magnesia (tab)	X		
Calcium & Magnesium Carbonates (tab)	X		
Calcium Carbonate, Magnesia & Simethicone (tab)	X		
Calcium Citrate	X[o]		
Calcium Glubionate		X[d,+]	
Calcium Gluconate (tab)	X		
Calcium Hydroxide Topical Soln.		X	

Drug (Dosage Form)	WC	T	LR
Calcium Lactate (tab)	X		
Calcium Lactobionate	X[o]		
Calcium Pantothenate (tab)		X	
Calcium Phosphate, dibasic (tab)	X		
Camphor Spirit		X	
Candicidin	XT[g,+]	X[m,+]	
Captopril		X[o,a]	
Carbachol Soln.		X[k,w,+]	
Carbamazepine (tab)		GH	
Carbamide Peroxide		X[o,+]	X[o,+]
Carbamide Peroxide Topical Soln.		X[+]	X[+]
Carbenicillin Indanyl Sodium (tab)	X		
Carbidopa & Levodopa (tab)	X		X
Carbinoxamine Maleate (tab)		X	X
Carbol-Fuchsin Topical Soln.		X	X
Carbomer 910		X	
Carbomer 934		X	
Carbomer 934a		X	
Carbomer 940		X	
Carbomer 1341		X	
Carboxymethylcellulose Sodium Paste	X[+]		
Carboxymethylcellulose Sodium (tab)		X	
Carisoprodol	X[a]	X[o]	
Carisoprodol & Aspirin (tab)	X		
Carisoprodol, Aspirin & Codeine Phosphate (tab)	X		
Carphenazine Maleate Oral Soln.		X	X
Casanthranol		X[o,+]	X[o,+]
Cascara (tab)		X	
Cascara, Aromatic Fluidextract		X[+]	X[+]
Cascara Sagrada Extract		X[+]	X[+]
Cascara Sagrada Fluidextract		X[+]	X[+]
Castor Oil		X[b,y,+]	
Castor Oil Aromatic		X	
Cefaclor		X[b]	
Cefaclor for Oral Susp.		X	
Cefadroxil		X[a,b]	
Cefadroxil for Oral Susp.		X	
Cefixime		X[a,o]	
Cefixime for Oral Susp.		X[j]	
Cefoperazone Sodium		X[o]	
Cefotaxime Sodium		X[o]	
Cefoxitin Sodium		X[o]	
Cefpiramide		X[o]	
Ceftazidime		X[o]	

Drug (Dosage Form)	WC	T	LR
Cefuroxime Axetil	X[a]	X[o]	
Cefuroxime Sodium		X[o]	
Cellulose, Microcrystalline		X	
Cellulose, Microcrystalline & Carboxymethylcellulose Sodium		X	
Cellulose Sodium Phosphate	X		
Cephalexin		X[a b]	
Cephalexin for Oral Susp.		X	
Cephalexin HCl		X[o]	
Cephalothin Sodium		X[o]	
Cephradine		X[a b j]	
Cetylpyridinium Chloride	X[n]	X[c]	
Charcoal, Activated	X		
Chloral Hydrate		X[b]	X[d]
Chlorambucil (tab)	X		X
Chloramphenicol (all dosage forms)		X	
Chloramphenicol Ophthalmic		CTP[c g +]	
Chloramphenicol Palmitate Oral Susp.		X	X
Chloramphenicol & Hydrocortisone Acetate for Ophthalmic Susp.		X	
Chloramphenicol & Polymyxin B Sulfate Ophthalmic Oint.		COT	
Chloramphenicol, Polymyxin B Sulfate & Hydrocortisone Acetate Ophthalmic Oint.		COT	
Chloramphenicol & Polymyxin B Sulfate Ophthalmic Oint.		COT	
Chloramphenicol & Prednisolone Ophthalmic Oint.		COT	
Chlordiazepoxide (tab)		X	X
Chlordiazepoxide & Amitriptyline HCl (tab)		X	X
Chlordiazepoxide HCl (cap)		X	X
Chlordiazepoxide HCl & Clidinium Bromide (cap)		X	X
Chloroquine Phosphate (tab)	X		
Chlorothiazide (tab)	X		
Chlorothiazide Oral Susp.		X	
Chlorotrianisene	H[b +]	X[o]	
Chloroxylenol	X[o]		
Chlorpheniramine Maleate		X[a d]	X[d]
Chlorpheniramine Maleate Extended-Release		X	
Chlorpromazine HCl	X[a]	X[d]	X[a]
Chlorpromazine HCl Oral Concentrate		X	X
Chlorpromazine HCl (supp)	X[+]		X[+]
Chlorpropamide (tab)	X		
Chlorprothixene (tab)	X		X
Chlorprothixene Oral Susp.		X	X
Chlortetracycline HCl	C[g]	X[a b]	C[g]X[a b]
Chlortetracycline & Sulfamethazine Soluble Pow.		X[x]	X[x]
Chlortetracycline HCl Ophthalmic Oint.		COT	
Chlortetracycline HCl Soluble Pow.		X[x]	X[x]
Chlorthalidone (tab)	X		
Chlorzoxazone (tab)		X	
Cholestyramine Oral Susp.		X	
Chymotrypsin for Ophthalmic Soln.		UG[+]	
Ciclopirox Olamine Cream	C[+]		
Cimetidine		X[a o +]	X[a o +]
Ciprofloxacin HCl	X[a]	X[o]	X[o]
Cinoxacin (cap)	X		
Cinoxate Lotion		X	X
Cisplatin		X[o]	X[o]
Clavulanate Potassium		X	
Clemastine Fumarate (tab)	X		
Clindinium Bromide (cap)		X	X
Clindamycin HCl (cap)		X	
Clindamycin Palmitate HCl Oral Soln.		X	
Clindamycin Phosphate		X[o t]	
Clindamycin Phosphate, Topical		X[c j]	
Clioquinol (Iodochlorhydroxyquin)	X[o]	C[f g]	C[f g]
Clioquinol & Hydrocortisone		XC[f g]	X[f g]
Clocortolone Pivalate		C[f]	C[f]
Clofibrate (cap)	X		X
Clomiphene Citrate (tab)	X		X
Clonazepam		X[a +]	X[a +]
Clonidine HCl (tab)	X		
Clonidine HCl & Chlorthalidone (tab)	X		
Clorazepate Dipotassium		In[o]	In[o]
Clotrimazole	X[m]	X[c h +]	X[c +]
Clotrimazole (cream)		C[+]	
Clotrimazole & Betamethasone Dipropionate (cream)		XC	
Cloxacillin Benzathine		X[o x]	
Cloxacillin Sodium (cap)		X	
Coal Tar		X[c g]	
Cocaine HCl Tablets for Topical Soln.	X		

Drug (Dosage Form)	WC	T	LR
Cod Liver Oil		In	
Codeine Phosphate (tab)	X		X
Codeine Sulfate (tab)	X		
Colchicine (tab)	X		X
Colestipol HCl for Oral Susp.		XU	
Colistin Sulfate for Oral Susp.		X	X
Colistin & Neomycin Sulfates & Hydrocortisone Acetate Otic Susp.		X	
Collodion		X	
Collodion, Flexible		X[+]	
Copper Gluconate	X[o]		
Cortisone Acetate (tab)	X		
Cromolyn Sodium for Inhalation		X[+]	X[+]
Cromolyn Sodium Soln.		X[s]	X[s]
Cromolyn Sodium Ophthalmic		S/M[o]	S/M[o]
Croscarmellose Sodium		X	
Crotamiton (cream)		C	X
Cyanocobalamin Co-57	X[b]	X[c]	X[b c]
Cyanocobalamin Co-60	X[b]	U[c]	X[b c]
Cyclacillin (tab)		X	
Cyclacillin for Oral Susp.		X	
Cyclizine HCl (tab)		X	X
Cyclobenzaprine HCl (tab)	X		
Cyclopentolate HCl Ophthalmic Soln.		X[+]	
Cyclophosphamide		X[a o +]	
Cycloserine HCl (tab)		X	
Cyclosporine		X[o]	X[o]
Cyclosporine Oral Soln.		X	
Cyclothiazide	X[a o]		
Cyproheptadine HCl	X[a]	X[d]	
Danazol (cap)	X		
Dapsone (tab)	X		X
Dehydrocholic Acid (tab)	X		
Demecarium Bromide Ophthalmic Soln.		X	X
Demeclocycline HCl		X[a b]	X[a b]
Demeclocycline HCl & Nystatin		X[a b]	X[a b]
Demeclocycline Oral Susp.		X	X
Desipramine HCl		X[a b]	
Desoximetasone	C[f g t +]	C[f t +]	C[f]
Desoxycorticosterone Acetate Pellets		U	
Dexamethasone	X[a]	X[e k]C[t +]	
Dexamethasone Sodium Phosphate		C[f]X[r t]	C[k]
Dexchlorpheniramine Maleate		X[a d]	X[d]
Dextroamphetamine Sulfate	X[a]	X[e b]	X[e]

Drug (Dosage Form)	WC	T	LR
Dextromethorphan HBr (syr)		X	X
Diatrizoate Meglumine & Diatrizoate Sodium Soln.		X	X
Diatrizoate Sodium Soln.		X	X
Diazepam		X[a b]	X[a b]
Diazepam Extended Release (cap)		X	X
Diazoxide (cap)	X	X	
Diazoxide Oral Susp.		X	X
Dibucaine		XC[f g]	XC[f g]
Dichlorphenamide	X[a o]		
Dicloxacillin Sodium (cap)	X		
Dicloxacillin Sodium for Oral Susp.		X	
Dicumarol (tab)	X		
Dicyclomine HCl	X[a b]	X[d]	
Dienestrol (cream)		C	
Diethylcarbamazine Citrate (tab)		X	
Diethylpropion HCl (tab)	X		
Diethylstilbestrol (tab)	X		
Diethyltoluamide Topical Soln.		X	
Diflorasone Diacetate		C[f g +]	C[f g +]
Diflunisal (tab)	X		
Digitalis		X[a b]	
Digitoxin (tab)	X		
Digoxin		X[a e +]	
Dihydrocodeine Bitartrate		X[o]	
Dihydrostreptomycin Sulfate (Boluses)		X[x]	
Dihydrotachysterol	X[a b]		X[a b]
Dihydrotachysterol Oral Soln.		X	X
Dihydroxyaluminum Aminoacetate (tab)	X		
Dihydroxyaluminum Aminoacetate Magma	X[+]		
Dihydroxyaluminum Sodium Carbonate (tab)	X[+]		
Diltiazem HCl		X[a o]	X[a o]
Dimenhydrinate	X[a]	X[d]	
Dimethyl Sulfoxide		X[+]	X[+]
Dinoprost Tromethamine (tab)		X	
Dioxybenzone & Oxybenzone (cream)		X	
Diperodon (ointment)		X	
Diphemanil Methylsulfate (tab)		X	
Diphenhydramine & Pseudoephedrine (cap)		X	
Diphenhydramine HCl		X[b]	X[e]
Diphenhydramine Citrate		X	X
Diphenoxylate HCl & Atropine Sulfate (tab)	X		X

Drug (Dosage Form)	WC	T	LR
Diphenoxylate HCl & Atropine Sulfate Oral Soln.		X	X
Diphylline	X	X[a c]	
Dipivefrin HCl		X[k o]	X[k o]
Dipyridamole (tab)		X	X
Disopyramide Phosphate (cap)	X		
Disopyramide Phosphate Extended-Release (cap)	X		
Disulfiram (tab)		X	X
Docusate Calcium (cap)		X[+]	
Docusate Potassium (cap)		X[+]	
Docusate Sodium	X[a]	X[b + d c]	X[d]
Doxepin HCl (cap)	X		
Doxepin HCl Oral Soln.		X	X
Doxycycline for Oral Susp.		X	X
Doxycycline Calcium Oral Susp.		X	X
Doxycycline Hyclate		X[a b]	X[a b]
Doxycycline Hyclate Delayed-Release (cap)		X	X
Doxylamine Succinate	X[a]	X[d]	X[a d]
Dusting Powder, Absorbable	X		
Dyclonine HCl Topical Soln.		X	X
Dyclonine HCl (gel)		P/G	G
Dydrogesterone (tab)	X		
Dyphylline Elixir		X	
Dyphylline & Guaifenesin		X[a c]	
Echothiophate Iodide for Ophthalmic Soln.		G[+]	
Econazole Nitrate	X[o]		X[o]
Enalapril Maleate	X[a o]		
Enalaprilat	X[o]		
Ephedrine Sulfate	X[a]	X[b d s]	X[b d s]
Ephedrine Sulfate & Phenobarbital (cap)	X		
Epinephrine		X[k r s]	X[k r s]
Epinephrine Bitartrate		X[k]	X[k]
Epinephrine Bitartrate Inhalation Aerosol	X	X	
Epinephrine Inhalation Aerosol		X	X
Epinephryl Borate Ophthalmic Soln.		X	X
Ergocalciferol		X[a b]	X[a b]
Ergocalciferol Oral Soln.		X	X
Ergoloid Mesylates (tab)		X	X
Ergoloid Mesylates Oral Soln.		X[+]	X[+]
Ergonovine Maleate (tab)	X		
Ergotamine Tartrate (tab)	X		
Ergotamine Tartrate Inhalation Aerosol		X	X

Drug (Dosage Form)	WC	T	LR
Ergotamine Tartrate & Caffeine	X[a]	X[i +]	X[a]
Erythrityl Tetranitrate (tab)		X[+]	
Erythrityl Tetranitrate, Diluted		X[+]	
Erythromycin (tab)		X	
Erythromycin Delayed-Release		X[a b]	
Erythromycin (oint)		CX[+]	
Erythromycin Ophthalmic		COT[g]	
Erythromycin Pledgets		X	
Erythromycin Topical		X[c t]	
Erythromycin & Benzoyl Peroxide Topical		SX[t]	
Erythromycin Estolate		X[a b j]	
Erythromycin Estolate for Oral Soln.		X	
Erythromycin Estolate Oral Susp.		X[+]	
Erythromycin Estolate & Sulfisoxazole Acetyl Oral		X[j]	
Erythromycin Ethylsuccinate (tab)		X	
Erythromycin Ethylsuccinate Oral Susp.	X		
Erythromycin Ethylsuccinate for Oral Susp.		X	
Erythromycin Ethylsuccinate & Sulfisoxazole Acetyl for Oral Susp.	X		
Erythromycin Stearate (tab)		X	
Erythromycin Stearate for Oral Susp.		X	
Erythrosine Sodium		X[a c]	X[a c]
Estradiol (cream)		C[m]	
Estradiol (tab)		X	X
Estrogens, Conjugated (tab)	X		
Estrogens, Esterified (tab)	X		
Estropipate	X[a]	C[m f]	
Ethacrynic Acid (tab)	X		
Ethambutol HCl (tab)	X		
Ethchlorvynol (cap)		X	X
Ethinamate (cap)		X	
Ethinyl Estradiol (tab)	X		
Ethionamide (tab)	X		
Ethopropazine HCl (tab)	X	X	
Ethosuximide (cap)		X	
Ethotoin		X[a o]	
Ethylcellulose Aqueous Dispersion		X[+]	
Ethynodiol Diacetate & Ethinyl Estradiol (tab)	X		

Drug (Dosage Form)	WC	T	LR
Ethynodiol Diacetate & Mestranol (tab)	X		
Etidronate Disodium (tab)		X	
Eucatropine HCl Ophthalmic Soln.		X	
Eugenol	X	X	
Famotidine	X[a o]		X[a o]
Fenoprofen Calcium	X[a b]		
Fentanyl Citrate		X[o]	
Ferrous Fumarate (tab)		X	
Ferrous Gluconate		X[a b e]	X[a b e]
Ferrous Sulfate		X[a c d]	X[c]
Floxuridine		X[o]	X[o]
Flucytosine (cap)		X	X
Fluhydrocortisone Acetate (tab)	X		
Flumethasone Pivalate (cream)		C	
Flunisolide Nasal Soln.		X[+]	X[+]
Fluocinolone Acetonide		C[f g]	
Fluocinolone Acetate Topical Soln.		X	
Fluocinonide	C[f g t]		
Fluorescein Sodium & Benoxinate HCl Ophthalmic		X[c]	X[c]
Fluorescein Sodium & Proparacaine HCl Ophthalmic		G[+]	G[+]
Fluorometholone (cream)		C	
Fluorometholone Ophthalmic Susp.		X	
Fluorouracil		XT[c f +]	
Fluoxymesterone (tab)	X		X
Fluphenazine HCl		X[a e]	X[a e]
Fluphenazine HCl Oral Soln.		X	X
Flurandrenolide		X[f g h]	X[f g h]
Flurandrenolide (tab)	X[+]		
Flurazepam HCl (cap)		X	X
Flurbiprofen Sodium		X[o]	
Flurbiprofen Sodium Ophthalmic Soln.		X	
Folic Acid (tab)	X		
Formaldehyde Soln.		X[+]	
Furazolidone		X[j +]	X[j +]
Furosemide (tab)	X		X
Gauze (all)	X		
Gemfibrozil (cap)		X	
Gentamicin Sulfate		X[d]C[f g]	
Gentamicin Sulfate Ophthalmic		COT[g]	
Gentamicin & Prednisolone Acetate Ophthalmic	OT[g +]	X[j]	
Gentian Violet		X[c]C[f t]	
Glutaral Concentrate		X[+]	X[+]
Glutethimide	X[a b]		
Glycerin Oral Solution		X	
Glycerin Suppository	X[+]		

Drug (Dosage Form)	WC	T	LR
Glycerin Ophthalmic Soln.		TPG/P	X
Glycopyrrolate (tab)		X	
Gold Sodium Thiomalate		X[o]	X[o]
Green Soap Tincture		X	
Griseofulvin		X[a b]	
Griseofulvin Oral Susp.		X	
Griseofulvin, Ultramicrosize (tab)		X	
Guaifenesin		X[a b d]	
Guanabenz Acetate		X[a o]	X[a o]
Guanadrel Sulfate	X[o]	X[a]	X[a]
Guanethidine Monosulfate (tab)	X		
Halazepam	X[a o]		
Halazone Tablets for Soln.		X	X
Halcinonide	X[a f g]		
Haloperidol (tab)		X	X
Haloperidol Oral Soln.		X	X
Haloprogin		X[+ f]	X[f]
Haloprogin Topical Soln.		X[+]	X
Halothane		G[+]	X[+]
Heparin Sodium		X[o +]	
Hetacillin (tab)		X	
Hetacillin for Oral Susp.		X	
Hetacillin Potassium		X[b]	X[a x]
Hetacillin Potassium Oral Susp.		X	
Hexachlorophene Cleansing Emulsion		X	X
Hexachlorophene Liquid Soap		X	X
Hexylcaine HCl Topical Soln.		X	
Hexylresorcinol		X[o]	X[o]
Homatropine Hydrobromide Ophthalmic Soln.		X	
Homatropine Methylbromide (tab)		X	X
Hydralazine HCl (tab)		X	X
Hydrochlorothiazide (tab)	X		
Hydrocodone Bitartrate (tab)		X	X
Hydrocortisone (Cortisol)	X[a g]	X[f h p t]	
Hydrocortisone Acetate	X[f g]	X[h]	
Hydrocortisone Acetate Ophthalmic		X	
Hydrocortisone Butyrate	X[f o]		
Hydrocortisone Cypionate Oral Susp.		X	X
Hydrocortisone Valerate (cream)	X		
Hydrocortisone & Acetic Acid Otic Soln.		X	X
Hydroflumethiazide (tab)		X	
Hydrogen Peroxide Concentrate	SP[+]		

Drug (Dosage Form)	WC	T	LR
Hydrogen Peroxide Topical Soln.		X[+]	X[+]
Hydromorphone HCl (tab)		X	X
Hydroquinone (cream)	X		X
Hydroquinone Topical Soln.		X	X
Hydroxyamphetamine HBr Ophthalmic Soln.		X	X
Hydroxychloroquine Sulfate (tab)		X	X
Hydroxypropyl Cellulose Ocular System		U[+]	
Hydroxypropyl Methylcellulose Ophthalmic Soln.		X	
Hydroxyurea (cap)		X	
Hydroxyzine HCl		X[a d]	X[d]
Hydroxyzine Pamoate (cap)	X		
Hydroxyzine Pamoate Oral Susp.		X	X
Hyoscyamine (tab)	X		X
Hyoscyamine Sulfate (tab)		X	X
Hyoscyamine Sulfate Oral Soln.		X[+]	X[+]
Ibuprofen (tab)	X		
Ichthammol (ointment)		C[+]	
Idoxuridine Ophthalmic	C[g t]	X[c]	X[c]
Imipramine HCl (tab)		X	
Indapamide	X[o a]		
Indium In^{111} Oxyquinoline		U[c +]	
Indomethacin	X[b i +]		
Indomethacin Extended-Release (cap)	X		
Indomethacin Oral		X[j]	X[j]
Indomethacin Sodium	X[o]		X[o]
Insulin		X[+]	X
Insulin Human		X[+]	X
Iocetamic Acid (tab)		X	
Iodide, Sodium, I-123, I-125, I-131 (cap)	X		
Iodine (all Soln. & Tinct.)		X[+]	X[+]
Iodoquinol (tab)	X		
Iopamidol	X[o]		X[o]
Iopanoic Acid (tab)		X	X
Ipecac Syrup		X[+]	
Ipodate Calcium for Oral Susp.	X		
Iopodate Sodium (cap)		X	
Isocarboxazid (tab)	X		X
Isoetharine Inhalation Soln.		X	X
Isoetharine Mesylate Inhalation Aerosol			X
Isoflurophate Ophthalmic		C[g]	
Isoniazid	X[a]	X[d]	X[a d]
Isopropamide Iodide (tab)	X		
Isopropyl Alcohol (all)		X[+]	
Isoproterenol Inhalation Soln.		X	X
Isoproterenol HCl	X[a]	X[r l]	X[a r l]
Isoproterenol HCl & Phenylephrine Bitartrate Inhalation Aerosol		X	X
Isoproterenol Sulfate Inhalation		X[c l]	X[c l]
Isosorbide Concentrate		X	X
Isosorbide Dinitrate (tab)	X		
Isosorbide Dinitrate Chewable (tab)	X		
Isosorbide Dinitrate, Diluted		X	
Isosorbide Dinitrate, Extended-Release	X[a b]		
Isosorbide Dinitrate, Sublingual (tab)	X		
Isosorbide Oral Soln.	X		
Isotretinoin		I[m o]	X[o]
Isoxsuprine HCl (tab)		X	
Kanamycin Sulfate (cap)		X	
Ketoconazole (tab)	X		
Labetolol HCl		X[o a t]	X[o a t]
Lactic Acid		X	
Lactulose (syr/conc)		X[+]	
Lanolin		X[+]	
Lanolin, Anhydrous	X[+]		
Levobunolol HCl	X[o]		
Levobunolol HCl Ophthalmic Soln.		X	
Levocarnitine		X[o]	
Levocarnitine, Oral Soln.		X	
Levodopa		X[a b +]	X[a b +]
Levonorgestrel (tab)	X		X
Levonorgestrel & Ethinyl Estradiol (tab)	X		
Levopropoxyphene Napsylate (tab)		X	X
Levopropoxyphene Napsylate Oral Susp.		X[+]	X[+]
Levorphanol Tartrate (tab)	X		
Levothyroxine Sodium (tab)		X	X
Lidocaine		X[g l]	
Lidocaine Oral Topical Soln.		X	
Lidocaine HCl Oral Topical Soln.		X	
Lidocaine Topical Soln.		X	
Lidocaine HCl Jelly		X	
Lime		X	
Lincomycin HCl		X[b d]	
Lindane		X[f h]	
Lindane Shampoo		X	
Liothyronine Sodium (tab)		X	

Drug (Dosage Form)	WC	T	LR
Liotrix (tab)		X	
Lisinopril	X[a o]		
Lithium Carbonate	X[a b]		
Lithium Carbonate Extended-Release (tab)	X		
Lithium Citrate (syr)		X	
Loperamide HCl (cap)	X		
Lorazepam		X[a o]	X[a o]
Loxapine (cap)		X	
Loxapine Succinate		X[o]	
Lypressin Nasal Soln.		P	
Mafenide Acetate (cream)		X[+]	X[+]
Magaldrate	X[a]	X[j]	
Magaldrate & Simethicone (tab)	X		
Magaldrate & Simethicone Oral Susp.		X[+]	
Magnesia (tab)	X		
Magnesium Carbonate & Sodium Bicarbonate for Oral Susp.		X	
Magnesium Citrate Oral Soln.		SP[+]	
Magnesium Gluconate	X[a o]		
Magnesium Hydroxide Paste		X	
Magnesium Oxide	X[a b]		
Magnesium Salicylate (tab)		X	
Magnesium Trisilicate (tab)	X		
Malathion		X[o]G[h]	X[o]
Manganese Carbonate	X[o]		
Maprotiline HCl (tab)	X		
Mazindol (tab)		X[+]	
Mebendazole (tab)	X		
Mecamylamine HCl	X[a]	X[o]	
Mechlorethamine HCl		X	X
Meclizine HCl (tab)	X		
Meclocycline Sulfosalicylate Cream		X	X
Meclofenamate Sodium (cap)		X	X
Medroxyprogesterone Acetate (tab)	X		
Medrysone Ophthalmic Susp.		X	X
Mefenamic Acid		X[b o]	X[o]
Megestrol Acetate (tab)	X		
Melphalan (tab)	X		
Menadiol Sodium Diphosphate (tab)	X		X
Mepenzolate Bromide	X[a]	X[d o]	X[d]
Meperidine HCl	X[a]	X[d]	X[a d]
Mephenytoin (tab)	X		
Mephobarbital (tab)	X		
Meprobamate (tab)	X		

Drug (Dosage Form)	WC	T	LR
Meprobamate Oral Susp.		X	
Mercaptopurine (tab)	X		
Mercury, Ammoniated (oint.)	X	C[k]	X
Mesoridazine Besylate (tab)	X		X
Mesoridazine Besylate Oral Soln.		X[+]	X[+]
Metaproterenol Sulfate	X[a]	X[o r l d]	X[o r d l a]
Metaraminol Bitartrate	X[o]		
Methacycline HCl (cap)		X	X
Methacycline HCl Oral Susp.		X	X
Methadone HCl (tab)	X		
Methadone HCl Oral Concentrate		X[+]	X[+]
Methadone HCl Oral Soln.		X[+]	X[+]
Methamphetamine	X[a o]		X[a o]
Methamphetamine HCl (pow)		X	X
Methantheline Bromide (tab)	X		
Metharbital (tab)		X	
Methazolamide (tab)	X		
Methdilazine (tab)		X	X
Methdilazine HCl		X[a d]	X[a d]
Methenamine	X[a]	X[e]	
Methenamine & Monobasic Sodium Phosphate (tab)		X	
Methenamine Hippurate (tab)	X		
Methenamine Mandelate (tab)	X		
Methenamine Mandelate for Oral Soln.	X[c]	X[j]	
Methimazole (tab)	X		X
Methocarbamol (tab)		X	
Methotrexate (tab)	X		
Methoxsalen (cap)		X	X
Methoxsalen Topical Soln.		X	X
Methscopolamine Bromide (tab)		X	
Methsuximide (cap)		X	
Methyclothiazide (tab)	X		
Methylbenzethonium Chloride	X[e]	X[h]C[g]	
Methylcellulose	X[a]	X[k +]	
Methylcellulose Oral Soln.		X[+]	X[+]
Methyldopa (tab)	X		
Methyldopa Oral Susp.		X[+]	X[+]
Methyldopa & Chlorothiazide (tab)	X		
Methyldopa & Hydrochlorothiazide (tab)	X		

Drug (Dosage Form)	WC	T	LR
Methylergonovine Maleate (tab)		X	X
Methylphenidate HCl (tab)		X	
Methylphenidate HCl Extended-Release (tab)		X	
Methylprednisolone (tab)		X	
Methylprednisolone Acetate	X[p]	XC[f]	X[f]
Methyltestosterone	X[a b]		
Methyprylon		X[a b]	X[a b]
Methysergide Maleate (tab)		X	
Metoclopramide HCl		X[a o]	X[a o]
Metoclopramide Oral Soln.		X[+]	X[+]
Metolazone		X[a o]	X[a o]
Metoprolol Tartrate (tab)		X	X
Metoprolol Tartrate & Hydrochlorothiazide (tab)		X	X
Metronidazole	X[a]	CP[t +]	X[a]
Metyrapone (tab)		X[+]	X[+]
Metyrosine (cap)	X		
Mexiletine HCl		X[b o]	
Miconazole Nitrate		X[m i] C[f]	
Miconazole Nitrate, Topical	X[o]		
Mineral Oil		X[p y]	
Mineral Oil, Light, Topical		X	
Minocycline HCl		X[a b]	X[a b]
Minocycline HCl Oral Susp.		X	X
Minoxidil	X[o]	X[a]	
Mitotane (tab)		X	X
Mitoxantrone HCl		X[o]	
Monobenzene (cream)		X[+]	
Nadolol	X[o]	X[a]	
Nadolol & Bendroflumethiazide (tab)		X	
Nafcillin Sodium		X[a b]	X[a]
Nafcillin Sodium for Oral Soln.		X	
Nalidixic Acid (tab)		X	
Nalidixic Acid Oral Susp.		X	
Nandrolone Phenpropionate		X[o]	X[o]
Naphazoline HCl Soln.		X[k s]	X[k s]
Naproxen (tab)	X		
Naproxen Sodium (tab)	X		
Natamycin Ophthalmic Susp.		TP	
Neomycin Sulfate	X[f g +]	X[a c +]	X[c +]
Neomycin Sulfate Ophthalmic Oint.		COT[+]	
Neomycin Sulfate & Bacitracin		X[g +]	X[g +]
Neomycin Sulfate & Bacitracin Zinc	XC[g]		
Neomycin Sulfate & Dexamethasone Sodium Phosphate		X[f]	
Neomycin Sulfate & Dexamethasone Sodium Phosphate Ophthalmic	X[c +]	COT[g]	X[c +]
Neomycin Sulfate & Fluocinolone Acetonide		XC[f]	
Neomycin Sulfate & Fluorometholone	CX[g]		
Neomycin Sulfate & Flurandrenolide		CX[f g h]	X[f g h]
Neomycin Sulfate & Gramicidin	CX[g]		
Neomycin Sulfate & Hydrocortisone	CX[f g]		
Neomycin Sulfate & Hydrocortisone Otic Susp.	X	X	
Neomycin Sulfate & Hydrocortisone Acetate	CX[f g h]		
Neomycin Sulfate & Hydrocortisone Acetate Ophthalmic		X[j]COT[g]	
Neomycin Sulfate & Methylprednisolone Acetate		CX[f]	X[f]
Neomycin Sulfate & Prednisolone Acetate Ophthalmic		COTX[j]	X[h]
Neomycin Sulfate & Prednisolone Sodium Phosphate Ophthalmic Oint.		COT	
Neomycin Sulfate, Sulfacetamide Sodium & Prednisolone Acetate, Ophthalmic		COT[g]	
Neomycin Sulfate & Triamcinolone Acetonide		XCT[f]	
Neomycin Sulfate & Triamcinolone Acetonide Ophthalmic Oint.		COT	
Neomycin & Polymyxin B Sulfates Ophthalmic	COT[g +]		X[c +]
Neomycin & Polymyxin B Sulfate & Bacitracin Zinc	CX[g]	CX[g]	X[g +]
Neomycin & Polymyxin B Sulfate & Bacitracin Zinc & Hydrocortisone Acetate Ophthalmic Oint.		COT	
Neomycin & Polymyxin B Sulfate & Bacitracin Zinc & Hydrocortisone Acetate Oint.	CX[+]		

Drug (Dosage Form)	WC	T	LR
Neomycin & Polymyxin B Sulfates, Bacitracin & Lidocaine	X[g +]		
Neomycin & Polymyxin B Sulfates, Bacitracin Zinc & Hydrocortisone Acetate Ointment	X[g k +]		
Neomycin & Polymyxin B Sulfate & Hydrocortisone Otic Soln.		X	X
Neomycin & Polymyxin B Sulfates & Dexamethasone Ophthalmic	COT[g]X[j]	X[j]	
Neomycin & Polymyxin B Sulfate & Gramicidin	CX[f]		
Neomycin & Polymyxin B Sulfate & Gramicidin Ophthalmic Soln.		X	
Neomycin & Polymyxin B Sulfates, Gramicidin & Hydrocortisone Acetate Cream	X		
Neomycin & Polymyxin B Sulfates & Hydrocortisone Susp.		TP[k v]	X[k v]
Neomycin & Polymyxin B Sulfate & Hydrocortisone Soln.		TP[k v]	X[k v]
Neomycin & Polymyxin B Sulfates & Hydrocortisone Acetate Ophthalmic Susp.		X	
Neomycin & Polymyxin B Sulfates & Prednisolone Acetate Ophthalmic Susp.		X	
Neostigmine Bromide		X[a o]	
Neostigmine Methylsalicylate		X[o]	
Niacin (tab)	X		
Niacinamide (tab)		X	
Nifedipine (cap)		X[+]	X[+]
Nitrofurantoin		X[a b j]	X[a b j]
Nitrofurazone		X[f g]	X[f g]
Nitrofurazone Topical Soln.		X	X
Nitroglycerin		G[a +]	X[g]
Nitromersol Topical Soln.		X	X
Nizatidine		X[b o +]	X[b o +]
Nonoxynol 9		X	
Norethindrone (tab)	X		
Norethindrone & Ethinyl Estradiol (tab)	X		
Norethindrone & Mestranol (tab)	X		
Norethindrone Acetate (tab)	X		
Norethindrone Acetate & Ethinyl Estradiol (tab)	X		
Norfloxacin	X[a]	X[o]	X[o]
Norgestrel (tab)	X		
Norgestrel & Ethinyl Estradiol (tab)	X		
Nortriptyline HCl		X[a c]	X[c]
Novobiocin Calcium Oral Susp.		X	X
Nylidrin HCl (tab)		X	
Nystatin	X[g +]	X[a h + n]	X[a h + n]
Nystatin Cream		XC[+]	
Nystatin for Oral Susp.		X	
Nystatin Oral Susp.		X	X
Nystatin Vaginal		X[a i +]	X[a i +]
Nystatin & Clioquinol Ointment		XC[+]	
Nystatin & Iodoquinol (Iodochlorhydroxyquin)		X[g]	X[g +]
Nystatin, Neomycin Sulfate, Gramicidin & Triamcinolone Acetonide		X[f g]	
Nystatin & Triamcinolone Acetonide		X[f g]	
Ointment, White and/or Yellow	X		
Oleovitamin A & D (cap)		X	X
Ophthalmic Oint., Bland Lubricating	OT[g]		
Opium Powder	X		
Opium Tincture		X[+]	X[+]
Oxacillin Sodium (cap)		X[+]	
Oxacillin Sodium for Oral Soln.		X[+]	
Oxamniquine (cap)		X	
Oxandrolone (tab)		X	X
Oxazepam	X[a b]		
Oxprenolol HCl	X[o]	X[a]	X[a]
Oxprenolol Extended-Release (tab)		X	X
Oxtriphylline	X[e o]		
Oxtriphylline Delayed-Release (tab)		X	
Oxtriphylline Extended-Release (tab)		X	
Oxybutynin Chloride	X[o]	X[a d]	X[a d]
Oxycodone (tab)		X	X
Oxycodone & Acetaminophen		X[a b]	X[a b]
Oxycodone & Aspirin (tab)		X	X
Oxycodone HCl		X[o]	
Oxycodone HCl Oral Soln.		X	X
Oxymetazoline HCl Soln.		X[k s]	
Oxymetholone (tab)	X		
Oxymorphone HCl Suppositories	X[+]		

Drug (Dosage Form)	WC	T	LR
Oxyphenbutazone (tab)		X	
Oxyphencyclimine HCl (tab)		X	
Oxytetracycline (tab)		X	X
Oxytetracycline Calcium Oral Susp.		X	X
Oxytetracycline HCl (cap)		X	X
Oxytetracycline & Nystatin (cap)		X	X
Oxytetracycline & Nystatin for Oral Susp.		X[+]	X[+]
Oxytetracycline HCl & Hydrocortisone Ointment	X		X
Oxytetracycline HCl & Hydrocortisone Acetate Ophthalmic Susp.		X	X
Oxytetracycline & Phenazopyridine Hydrochlorides & Sulfamethizole (cap)		X	X
Oxytetracycline HCl & Polymyxin B Sulfate	X[g,o,m]		X[g]
Oxytetracycline HCl & Polymyxin B Ophthalmic Oint.		COT	
Pancreatin		X[a,b,+]	
Pancrelipase		X[a,b,+]	
Papain Tablets for Topical Soln.		X[+]	X[+]
Papaverine HCl (tab)		X	
Parachlorophenol Camphorated		X	X
Paramethadione (cap)		X	
Paramethadione Oral Soln.		X	X
Paramethasone Acetate (tab)	X		
Paregoric		X[+]	X[+]
Pargyline HCl (tab)	X		
Paromomycin Sulfate		X[b,d]	
Pectin	X		
Penicillamine		X[a,b]	
Penicillin G Benzathine (tab)		X	
Penicillin G Benzathine Oral Susp.		X	
Penicillin G Potassium (tab)		X	
Penicillin G Potassium Tablets for Oral Soln.		X	
Penicillin G Procaine, Neomycin & Polymyxin B Sulfates & Hydrocortisone Acetate Topical Susp.	X		
Penicillin V (tab)		X	
Penicillin V for Oral Susp.		X	
Penicillin V Benzathine		X[l,+]	

Drug (Dosage Form)	WC	T	LR
Penicillin V Benzathine, Oral Susp.		X[+]	
Penicillin V Potassium (tab)		X	
Penicillin V Potassium for Oral Soln.		X	
Pentaerythritol Tetranitrate (tab)		X	
Pentazocine HCl (tab)		X	X
Pentazocine HCl & Aspirin (tab)		X	X
Pentazocine & Naloxone HCl (tab)		X	X
Pentobarbital Elixir		X	
Pentobarbital Sodium (cap)		X	
Peppermint Spirit		X	
Perphenazine	X[d]	X[a]	X[a,d]
Perphenazine Oral Soln.	X		X
Perphenazine & Amitriptyline HCl (tab)	X		
Phenacemide (tab)	X		
Phenazopyridine HCl (tab)		X	
Phendimetrazine Tartrate	X[a]	X[b]	
Phenelzine Sulfate (tab)		X[+]	X[+]
Phenindione (tab)	X		
Phenmetrazine HCl (tab)		X	
Phenobarbital	X[a]	X[e]	X[e]
Phenol		X	X
Phenol, Liquefied		X	X
Phenolphthalein (tab)		X	
Phenoxybenzamine HCl (cap)	X		
Phenprocoumon (tab)	X		
Phensuximide (cap)		X	
Phentermine HCl		X[a,b]	
Phenylbutazone		X[a,b]	
Phenylephrine HCl Soln.		X[k,s]	X[k,s]
Phenylephrine HCl Nasal Jelly		X	
Phenylpropanolamine HCl Extended-Release		X[a,b]	X[a,b]
Phenytoin (tab)	X		
Phenytoin Oral Susp.		X[+]	
Phenytoin Sodium, Extended (cap)		X	
Phenytoin Sodium, Prompt (cap)		X	
Physostigmine Salicylate Ophthalmic Soln.		X	X
Physostigmine Sulfate Ophthalmic Ointment		COT	
Phytonadione (tab)	X		X
Pilocarpine HCl Ophthalmic Soln.		X	
Pilocarpine Nitrate Ophthalmic		X	X
Pimozide		X[a,o]	X[a,o]

Drug (Dosage Form)	WC	T	LR
Pindolol	X[a,o]		X[a,o]
Piperacetazine (tab)	X		X
Piperazine Citrate		X[a,d]	
Pipobroman (tab)	X		
Piroxicam		X[b,o]	X[b,o]
Podophyllum Resin		X[o]	X[o]
Podophyllum Resin Topical Soln.		X	X
PEG 3350 & Electrolytes for Oral Soln.		X	
Polyethylene Oxide		X	X
Polymyxin B Sulfate & Bacitracin Zinc Topical	X[o]	A[l,t]	
Polymyxin B Sulfate & Hydrocortisone Otic Soln.		X	X
Polythiazide (tab)		X	X
Potassium Bicarbonate Effervescent Tabs for Oral Soln.		X[+]	
Potassium Bicarbonate & Potassium Chloride for Effervescent Oral Soln.		X[+,a,o]	
Potassium & Sodium Bicarbonate & Citric Acid Effervescent for Oral Soln. (tab)		X	X
Potassium Carbonate	X[o]		
Potassium Chloride Oral Soln.		X	
Potassium Chloride for Oral Soln.		X	
Potassium Chloride Extended-Release		X[a,b,+]	
Potassium Chloride, Potassium Bicarbonate, & Potassium Citrate Effervescent Tablets for Oral Soln.		X[+]	
Potassium Citrate & Citric Acid Oral Soln.		X	
Potassium Gluconate		X[a,e]	X[e]
Potassium Gluconate & Potassium Chloride for Oral Soln.	X		
Potassium Gluconate & Potassium Chloride Oral		X	
Potassium Gluconate & Potassium Citrate Oral Soln.	X		
Potassium Gluconate, Potassium Citrate & Ammonium Chloride, Oral Soln.		X	
Potassium Iodide (tab)		X	
Potassium Iodide Oral Soln.		X	X
Povidone Iodide Topical Soln.		X[+]	

Drug (Dosage Form)	WC	T	LR
Povidone-Iodine Oint.		X	
Povidone-Iodine Cleansing Soln.		X	
Pralidoxime Chloride (tab)	X		
Pramoxine HCl		X[f,t]C[t]	
Prazepam		X[a,b]	X[a,b]
Praziquantel	X[o]	X[a]	X[o]
Prazosin HCl (cap)	X		X
Prednisolone	X[a]	X[c,d,f]	X[d]
Prednisolone Acetate Ophthalmic Susp.		X	
Prednisolone Sodium Phosphate Ophthalmic Soln.		X	X
Prednisone	X[a]	X[d]	
Prednisone Oral Soln.		X	
Primaquine Phosphate (tab)	X		X
Primidone (tab)	X		
Primidone Oral Susp.		X	X
Probenecid (tab)	X		
Probenecid & Colchicine (tab)	X		X
Probucol	X		X
Procainamide HCl		X[a,b]	
Procainamide HCl Extended Release (tab)		X	
Procarbazine HCl (cap)		X	X
Prochlorperazine Edisylate Oral Soln.		X	X
Prochlorperazine Edisylate Syr.		X	X
Prochlorperazine Maleate (tab)	X		X
Prochlorperazine Suppositories		X	
Procyclidine HCl (tab)		X[+]	
Promazine HCl		X[a,c,d]	X[a,c,d]
Promethazine HCl		X[a,d,i,+]	X[a,d,i,+]
Propantheline Bromide (tab)	X		
Proparacaine HCl Ophthalmic Soln.		X	X
Propiomazine HCl		X[o]	X[o]
Propoxyphene HCl (cap)		X	
Propoxyphene HCl & Acetaminophen (tab)		X	
Propoxyphene HCl, Aspirin & Caffeine (cap)		X[+]	
Propoxyphene Napsylate		X[a,o]	
Propoxyphene Napsylate Oral Susp.		X	X
Propoxyphene Napsylate & Acetaminophen (tab)		X[+]	
Propoxyphene Napsylate & Aspirin (tab)		X	
Propranolol HCl (tab)	X		

Drug (Dosage Form)	WC	T	LR
Propranolol HCl Extended-Release (cap)	X		
Propranolol HCl & Hydrochlorothiazide (tab)	X		
Propranolol HCl & Hydrochlorothiazide Extended-Release (cap)	X		
Propylene Glycol		X	
Propylhexedrine Inhalant		X[+]	
Propylthiouracil (tab)	X		
Protamine Sulfate		X[+]	X[+]
Protriptyline HCl (tab)		X	
Pseudoephedrine HCl		X[a d]	X[d]
Psyllium Hydrophilic Mucilloid for Oral Susp.		X	
Pyrantel Pamoate Oral Susp.		X	X
Pyrazinamide (tab)	X		
Pyridostigmine Bromide		X[a d]	X[d]
Pyridoxine HCl (tab)	X		
Pyrilamine Maleate (tab)	X		
Pyrimethamine (tab)		X	X
Pyroxylin			SP
Pyrvinium Pamoate		X[a j]	X[a j]
Quinacrine HCl (tab)		X	
Quinestrol (tab)	X		
Quinethazone (tab)		X	
Quinidine Gluconate Extended-Release	X[a o]		X[a o]
Quinidine Sulfate	X[a]	X[b]	X[a b]
Quinidine Sulfate Extended-Release (tab)	X		X
Quinine Sulfate	X[a]	X[b]	
Racepinephrine		X[o]	X[o]
Racepinephrine Soln.		X[r +]	X[r +]
Ranitidine HCl		X[a o]	X[a o]
Ranitidine Oral Soln.		X[+]	X[+]
Rauwolfia Serpentina (tab)		X	X
Oral Rehydration Salts		SX[a +]	
Reserpine		X[a e]	X[a e]
Reserpine & Chlorothiazide (tab)		X	X
Reserpine & Hydrochlorothiazide (tab)		X	X
Reserpine, Hydralazine & Hydrochlorothiazide (tab)		X	X
Resorcinol, Compound (oint)		X[+]	
Resorcinol & Sulfur (lot)	X		
Ribavirin		X[o]	
Ribavirin for Inhalation Soln.		H[+]	
Riboflavin (tab)		X	X
Rifampin (cap)		X[+]	X[+]

Drug (Dosage Form)	WC	T	LR
Rifampin & Isoniazid (cap)		X[+]	X[+]
Ritodrine HCl (tab)		X[+]	
Rose Water Oint.		X	X
Saccharin Sodium	X[a]	X[c]	
Safflower Oil		X	X
Salicylamide	X[o]		
Salicylic Acid Collodion		X[+]	
Salicylic Acid Gel		XC[+]	
Salicylic Acid Plaster	X[+]		
Salicylic Acid Topical Foam		X	
Scopolamine HBr Ophthalmic		X[c]C[g]	
Scopolamine HBr (tab)		X	X
Secobarbital Elixir		X	
Secobarbital Sodium (cap)		X	
Secobarbital Sodium & Amobarbital (cap)	X		
Selenious Acid		X	
Selenium Sulfide Lotion		X	
Senna Syrup		X[+]	
Sennosides (tab)	X		
Silver Nitrate Ophthalmic Soln.		X	X
Silver Nitrate, Toughened		X	X
Silver Sulfadiazine	X[o]	CT[f]	
Simethicone	X[a]	X[y]	
Simethicone Oral Susp.		X	X
Sodium Acetate Soln.		X	
Sodium Bicarbonate	X[a o]		
Sodium Chloride	X[a]	C[k]	
Sodium Chloride & Dextrose (tab)	X		
Sodium Citrate & Citric Acid Oral Soln.		X	
Sodium Fluoride (tab)		X	
Sodium Fluoride Oral Soln.		XP	
Sodium Fluoride & Phosphoric Acid		P[t]	
Sodium Fluoride & Phosphoric Acid Topical Soln.		P	
Sodium Gluconate	X[o]		
Sodium Lactate Soln.		X	
Sodium Phosphate	X[p]		
Sodium Phosphates Oral Soln.		X	
Sodium Polystyrene Sulfonate Susp.	X[+]		
Sodium Salicylate (tab)	X		
Sorbitol Soln.		X	
Spironolactone (tab)		X	X
Spironolactone & Hydrochlorothiazide		X[a]	X[o]
Squalane		X	
Stannous Fluoride Gel	X		

Drug (Dosage Form)	WC	T	LR
Stanozolol (tab)		X	X
Topical Starch	X		
Sulfacetamide Sodium Ophthalmic	COT[g]	X[c +]	X[c +]
Sulfacetamide Sodium & Prednisolone Acetate Ophthalmic		TP[j] CTP[g]	
Sulfadiazine (tab)	X		X
Sulfadoxine & Pyrimethamine (tab)	X		X
Sulfamerazine (tab)	X		
Sulfamethizole (tab)	X		
Sulfamethizole Oral Susp.		X	X
Sulfamethoxazole (tab)	X		X
Sulfamethoxazole Oral Susp.		X	X
Sulfamethoxazole & Trimethoprim	X		X
Sulfamethoxazole & Trimethoprim Oral Susp.		X	X
Sulfapyridine (tab)	X		X
Sulfasalazine (tab)	X		
Sulfathiazole, Sulfacetamide & Sulfabenzamide Vaginal	C[f]X[a]		X[a f]
Sulfinpyrazone	X[a b]		
Sulfisoxazole (tab)	X		X
Sulfisoxazole Acetyl Oral Susp.		X	X
Sulfisoxazole Diolamine Ophthalmic		C[g]X[c]	X[c]
Sulfoxone Sodium (tab)		X	X
Sulfur Ointment	X[+]		
Sulindac (tab)	X		
Suprofen	X[o]		
Suprofen Ophthalmic		X[c]	
Sutilains Ointment		CX[+]	
Talbutal (tab)		X	
Talc	X		
Tamoxifen Citrate (tab)	X		X
Tape, Adhesive	X[+]		
Terbutaline (tab)		X[+]	
Terfenadine		X[a o]	X[a o]
Terpin Hydrate Elixir		X	
Terpin Hydrate & Codeine Elixir		X	
Terpin Hydrate & Dextromethorphan HBr Elixir		X	
Testolactone (tab)		X	
Tetracaine Oint.		C	
Tetracaine Ophthalmic Oint.		C	
Tetracaine & Menthol Oint.		C	
Tetracaine HCl		C[f]	

Drug (Dosage Form)	WC	T	LR
Tetracaine HCl Topical Soln.		X	X
Tetracaine HCl Ophthalmic Soln.		X	X
Tetracycline Boluses		X[x]	
Tetracycline HCl Ophthalmic	COT[g]		
Tetracycline HCl Soluble Pow.		X[x]	
Tetracycline HCl & Novobiocin Sodium (tab)		X[x]	
Tetracycline Phosphate Complex & Novobiocin Sodium (cap)		X[x]	
Tetracycline Oral Susp.		X	X
Tetracycline HCl (tab/cap/ophthalmic susp/topical soln)		X	X
Tetracycline HCl & Nystatin (cap)		X	X
Tetracycline Phosphate Complex (cap)		X	X
Tetrahydrozoline HCl Soln.		X[k s]	
Theophylline	X[a b]		
Theophylline Extended Release (cap)	X		
Theophylline, Ephedrine HCl & Phenobarbital (tab)	X		
Theophylline & Guaifenesin		X[b c]	
Theophylline Sodium Glycinate	X[a]	X[e]	
Thiabendazole (tab)		X	
Thiabendazole Oral Susp.		X	
Thiamine HCl		X[a o]	X[a e]
Thiamine Mononitrate Elixir		X	X
Thiethylperazine Maleate		X[a i o +]	X[a i o]
Thimerosol, Topical		X[c l +]	X[c l +]
Thimerosal, Tincture		X[+]	X[+]
Thioguanine (tab)	X		
Thioridazine, Oral		X[c j +]	X[c j +]
Thioridazine HCl (tab)		X	X
Thiothixene (cap)	X		X
Thiothixene HCl Oral Soln.		X	X
Thyroglobulin (tab)		X	
Thyroid (tab)		X	
Ticarcillin Monosodium		X[o]	
Timolol Maleate Ophthalmic Soln.		X	
Timolol Maleate (tab)	X		X
Timolol Maleate & Hydrochlorothiazide (tab)	X		X

Drug (Dosage Form)	WC	T	LR
Tioconazole		X[a f o]	
Tobramycin Ophthalmic		X[c]COT[g]	
Tobramycin & Dexamethasone Ophthalmic		X[j]	
Tobramycin & Fluorometholone Acetate Ophthalmic		X[c]	
Tocainide HCl	X[a o]		
Tolazamide (tab)		X	
Tolazoline HCl (tab)	X		
Tolbutamide (tab)	X		
Tolmetin Sodium	X[a]	X[b]	
Tolnaftate		X[f o t]	
Tolnaftate, Topical		X[c l +]	
Tolu Balsam		X[+]	
Trazodone HCl		X[o]	X[o]
Trazodone (tab)		X[a]	X[a]
Tretinoin		C[f]X[c]	X[c f t]
Triamcinolone (tab)	X		
Triamcinolone Acetonide	X[g]	X[f h]	
Triamcinolone Acetonide Dental Paste		X	
Triamcinolone Acetonide Topical		X[i +]	
Triamcinolone Diacetate (syr)		X	X
Triamterene (cap)		X	X
Triamterene & Hydrochlorothiazide		X[a b]	X[a b]
Triazolam (tab)		X	X
Trichlormethiazide (tab)		X	
Tricitrates Oral Soln		X	
Tridihexethyl (tab)	X		
Trientine HCl		X[a o +]	In[o]
Trifluoperazine HCl	X[a]	X[d]	X[a d]
Triflupromazine Oral Susp.		X	X
Triflupromazine HCl (tab)	X		X
Trihexyphenidyl HCl		X[a c]	
Trihexyphenidyl HCl Extended-Release (cap)		X	
Trikates Oral (soln)		X	X
Trimeprazine Tartrate	X[a]	X[d]	X[a d]
Trimethadione		X[a b c +]	
Trimethobenzamide HCl (cap)	X		
Trimethoprim (tab)		X	X
Trioxsalen (tab)	X		X
Tripelennamine HCl (tab)	X		
Tripelennamine Citrate Elixir		X	X
Triprolidine HCl		X[a d]	X[a d]
Triprolidine & Pseudoephedrine Hydrochlorides		X[a d]	X[a d]
Trisulfapyrimidines (tab)	X		
Trisulfapyrimidines Oral Susp.		X[+]	
Troleandomycin (cap)		X	
Troleandomycin Oral Susp.		X[+]	
Tropicamide Ophthalmic Soln.		X[+]	
Tuaminoheptane Inhalant		X[+]	
Tyropanoate Sodium (cap)		X	X
Undecylenic Acid, Compound Ointment		X[+]	
Uracil Mustard (cap)		X	
Valproic Acid		X[bd+]	
Vancomycin HCl (cap)		X	
Vancomycin HCl for Oral Soln.		X	
Verapamil HCl (tab)		X	X
Vidarabine Ophthalmic Ointment		COT[+]	
Vinblastine Sulfate		X[+]	X[+]
Vincristine Sulfate		X[+]	X[+]
Vitamin A (cap)		X	X
Vitamin E (cap)		X	X
Vitamin E Preparation		In	X
Warfarin Sodium (tab)		X	
Water, purified		X	
White Lotion		X	
Xylometazoline HCl Nasal Soln.		X	X
Xylose		X[+]	
Zinc Gluconate	X[a o]		
Zinc Oxide (oint/paste)	X[+]		
Zinc Oxide & Salicylic Acid Paste	X		
Zinc Sulfate Ophthalmic Soln.		X	

Provided by Dr. Kenneth S. Alexander, Associate Professor of Pharmacy, College of Pharmacy, University of Toledo.
The listing of container requirements for Compendial drugs is included as an aid to the practitioner in storing and dispensing.

Container and Storage Requirements for Sterile U.S.P. XXII Drugs

*Legend:

I = Containers for sterile solids as described under injections
N = Intact Flexible Container Meeting The General Requirements
S = Single dose
M = Multiple dose
U = Unspecified
P = Plastic
A = Type I glass
B = Type II glass
C = Type III glass
Sy = Syringe
O = Original Package
T = Avoid Toxic Substances
X = Colorless
D = Type II or III Glass Depending on Final Soln. pH
IN = Inert atmosphere
M = Protect from moisture
LR = Light Resistant
L = Protect From Light
R = Refrigerator (2°–8°C)
F = Freezer (−4°C)
H = Protect from Heat
RT = Controlled Room Temperature
TP = Tamper-Proof
W = Transparent
SC = Radioactive Shielding
Tr = Treated To Prevent Adsorption

Drugs	Container	Glass Type	Storage Conditions
Acetazolamide Sodium, Sterile	I	C	
Acetic Acid Irrigation	S,P	A,B	
Acetylcysteine Solution	S,M	A,P	O_2 excluded
Acetylcholine for Ophthalmic Soln.	I		
Dehydrated Alcohol Inj.	S	A	
Alcohol and Dextrose Inj.	S	A,B	
Alphaprodine HCl Inj.	S,M	A	
Alprostadil Inj.	S	A	R
Amdinocillin, Sterile	I		
Amikacin Sulfate Inj.	S,M	A,C	
Aminoacetic Acid Irrigation	S	A,B	
Aminocaproic Acid Inj.	S,M	A	
Aminohippurate Sodium Inj.	S,M	A	
Aminophylline Inj.	S	A	CO_2 excluded
Amitriptyline HCl Inj.	S,M	A	
Ammonia N 13 Inj.	S,M		SC
Ammonium Chloride Inj.	S,M	A,B	
Ammonium Molybdate Inj.	S,M	A,B	
Amobarbital Sodium, Sterile	I	D	
Amoxicillin, Sterile	I		
Amphotericin B for Inj.	I		R,L
Ampicillin, Sterile	I		
Ampicillin Sodium, Sterile	I		R,L
Ampicillin Sodium and Sulbactam Sodium, Sterile	I		
Anileridine Inj.	S,M	A	L
Anticoagulant Citrate Dextrose Solution	S,M,P	A,B	
Anticoagulant Citrate Phosphate Dextrose Adenine Solution	S,P	A,B	X,W
Anticoagulant Sodium Citrate Soln.	S	A,B	
Anticoagulant Heparin Soln.	S,P	A,B	
Antihemophilic Factor			R

*The listing of container and storage requirements for sterile Compendial drugs is included as an aid to the practitioner in storing and dispensing.

Drugs	Container	Glass Type	Storage Conditions
Antihemophilic Factor, Cryoprecipitated			F (−18°C)
Antirabies Serum	U		R
Antivenin (Latrodectus mectans)	S		H
Antivenin (Crotalidae) Polyvalent	S		H
Antivenin (Micrurus fulvius)	S		H
Arginine HCl Inj.	S	B	
Ascorbic Acid Inj.	S	A,B	LR
Atropine Sulfate Inj.	S,M	A	
Aurothioglucose Susp., Sterile	S,M	A	L
Azathioprine Sodium for Inj.	I	C	RT
Azlocillin Sodium, Sterile	I		
Aztreonam for Inj.	I		
Aztreonam Inj.	I		F
Aztreonam, Sterile	I		
Bacitracin, Sterile	I	D	R
Bacitracin Zinc, Sterile	I		R (cool place)
BCG Vaccine	U	A	R
Benztropine Mesylate Inj.	S,M	A	
Benzylpenicilloyl Polylysine Inj.	S,M	A	R
Betamethasone Sodium Phosphate Inj.	S,M	A	
Betamethasone Sodium Phosphate and Betamethasone Acetate (Susp.), Sterile	M	A	
Bethanechol Chloride Inj.	S	A	
Biological Indicator for Dry Heat Sterilization, Paper Strip	O		L,H,M,T
Biological Indicator for Ethylene Oxide Sterilization, Paper Strip	O		L,H,M,T
Biological Indicator for Steam Sterilization, Paper Strip	O		L,H,M,T
Biperiden Lactate Inj.	S	A	L
Bleomycin Sulfate, Sterile	I	B	
Blood Grouping Serums (All)	U		R
Botulism Antitoxin	S		R
Brompheniramine Maleate Inj.	S,M	A	L
Bumetanide Inj.	S,M	A	L
Bupivacaine HCl Inj.	S,M	A	
Bupivacaine and Epinephrine Inj.	S,M	A	L
Bupivacaine in Dextrose Inj.	S	A	
Butorphanol Tartrate Inj.	S,M	A	L
Caffeine and Sodium Benzoate Inj.	S	A	
Calcium Chloride Inj.	S	A	
Calcium Gluceptate Inj.	S	A,B	
Calcium Gluconate Inj.	S	A	
Calcium Levulinate Inj.	S	A	
Capreomycin Sulfate, Sterile	I	B	R
Carbenicillin Disodium, Sterile	I	D	
Carboprost Tromethamine Inj.	S,M	A	R
Cefamandole Naftate for Inj.	I	D	
Cefamandole Sodium, Sterile	I		
Cefamandole Sodium for Inj.	I		
Cefazolin Sodium, Sterile	I	B	
Cefazolin Sodium Inj.	I		F
Cefanocid Sodium, Sterile	I		
Cefmenoxime for Inj.	I		
Cefmenoxime HCl, Sterile	I		
Cefmetazole Sodium, Sterile	I		
Cefoperazone Sodium, Sterile	I		
Cefoperazone Sodium Inj.	I		F

Drugs	Container	Glass Type	Storage Conditions
Cefotaxime Sodium, Sterile	I	B	
Cefotaxime Sodium Inj.	S,M		F
Cefotetan Disodium, Sterile	I		
Ceforanide for Inj.	I		
Cefoxitin Sodium, Sterile	I	B	
Cefoxitin Sodium Inj.	I		F
Cefpiramide for Inj.	I		
Ceftazidime Inj.	I		F
Ceftazidime for Inj.	I		L
Ceftazidime, Sterile	I		L
Ceftizoxime Sodium Inj.	I		F
Ceftizoxime Sodium, Sterile	I		
Ceftriaxone Sodium Inj.	I		
Ceftriaxone Sodium, Sterile	I		F
Cefuroxime Sodium Inj.	I		F
Cefuroxime Sodium, Sterile	I		
Cellulose Oxidized (all)	I		L,R
Cephalothin Sodium Inj.	I		F
Cephapirin Sodium, Sterile	I	D	
Cephradine for Inj.	I		
Cephradine, Sterile	I		
Chloramphenicol Inj.	S,M		
Chloramphenicol, Sterile	I		
Chloramphenicol Sodium Succinate, Sterile	I	B	
Chlordiazepoxide HCl, Sterile	I	B	L
Chloroprocaine HCl Inj.	S,M	A	
Chloroquine HCl Inj.	S	A	
Chlorothiazide Sodium for Inj.	I	C	
Chlorpheniramine Maleate Inj.	S,M	A	L
Chlorpromazine HCl Inj.	S,M	A	L
Chlorprothixene Inj.	S		L
Chlortetracycline HCl, Sterile	I		L
Cholera Vaccine	U		R
Sodium Chromate Cr 51 Inj.	S,M		
Chromic Chloride Inj.	S,M	A,B	
Cisplatin for Inj.	I		
Citric Acid, Magnesium Oxide Sodium Carbonate Irrigation	S	A,B	
Clavulanate Potassium, Sterile	I		
Clindamycin Phosphate, Sterile	I	D	
Clindamycin Phosphate Inj.	S,M	A,P	
Cloxacillin Benzathine, Sterile	U(tight)		
Cloxacillin Sodium, Sterile	U(tight)		
Cloxacillin Sodium Intramammary Infusion	Sy		TP
Coccidioidin			R
Codeine Phosphate Inj.	S,M	A	L
Colchicine Inj.	S	A	L
Colistimethate Sodium, Sterile	I	D	
Corticotropin Inj.	S,M	A	R
Corticotropin for Inj.	I	B	
Corticotropin Inj., Repository	S,M	A	
Corticotropin Zinc Hydroxide, (Susp.), Sterile	S,M	A	RT
Cortisone Acetate Susp., Sterile	S,M	A	
Cromolyn Sodium Inhalation	S(double-ended ampule)	A,B,P	
Cupric Chloride Inj.	S,M	A,B	
Cupric Sulfate Inj.	S,M	A,B	

Drugs	Container	Glass Type	Storage Conditions
Cyanocobalamin Inj.	S,M	A	LR
Cyclophosphamide for Inj.	I		RT
Cyclosporin Concentrate for Inj.	S,M		
Cyclizine Lactate Inj.	S	A	
Cyclophosphamide for Inj.	I	B	RT
Cysteine HCl Inj.	S,M	A	
Cytarabine, Sterile	I	B	
Dacarbazine for Inj.	S,M, or I	A	L
Dactinomycin for Inj.	I	B	LR
Daunorubicin HCl for Inj.	I	B	LR
Deslanoside Inj.	S	A	
Dexamethasone Acetate Suspension, Sterile	S,M	A	
Dextrose and Sodium Chloride Inj.	S	A,B	
Diatrizoate Meglumine Inj.	S,M	A,C	L
Diatrizoate Meglumine and Diatrizoate Sodium Inj.	S	A,C	L
Diatrizoate Sodium Inj.	S,M	A,C	L
Diazepam Inj.	S,M	A	L
Diazoxide Inj.	S	A	L
Dibucaine HCl Inj.	S,M	A	L
Dicloxacillin Sodium, Sterile	I	D	
Dicyclomine HCl Inj.	S,M	A	
Diethylstilbestrol Inj.	S,M	A	LR
Digitoxin Inj.	S	A	Avoid excessive heat
Digitoxin Inj.	S,M	A	L
Digoxin Inj.	S	A	LR,H
Dihydroergotamine Mesylate Inj.	S	A	Avoid heat
Dihydroergotamine Mesylate, Heparin Sodium and Lidocaine HCl Inj.	S,M	A	
Dihydrostreptomycin Sulfate, Sterile	I		
Dimenhydrinate Inj.	S,M	A,C	
Dimercaprol Inj.	S,M	A,C	
Dimethyl Sulfate Irrigation	S		RT,L
Dinoprost Tromethamine Inj.	S,M	A	
Diphenhydramine HCl Inj.	S,M	A	L
Diphtheria Antitoxin	U		R
Diphtheria Toxoid	U		R
Diphtheria Toxoid Adsorbed	U		R
Diphtheria and Tetanus Toxoids/Adsorbed	U		R
Diphtheria and Tetanus Toxoids and Pertussis Vaccine/Adsorbed	U		R
Dobutamine HCl for Inj.	I	B	RT
Dopamine HCl Inj.	S	A	
Dopamine HCl and Dextrose Inj.	S	A,B	
Doxapram HCl Inj.	S,M	A	
Doxorubicin HCl Inj.	S,M	A	LR,R (not to exceed 250 ml if multidose)
Doxorubicin HCl for Inj.	I	B	(Not to exceed 250 ml if multidose)
Doxorubicin HCl for Inj.	I		
Doxycycline Hyclate for Inj.	I	B	L
Doxycycline Hyclate, Sterile	I		L
Droperidol Inj.	S,M	A	L
Dyphylline Inj.	S,M	A	RT,L
Edetate Calcium Disodium Inj.	S	A	
Edetate Disodium Inj.	S	A	
Edrophonium Chloride Inj.	S,M	A	

Drugs	Container	Glass Type	Storage Conditions
Elements Inj., Trace	S,M	A,B	
Emetine HCl Inj.	S	A	LR
Ephedrine Sulfate Inj.	S,M	A	LR
Epinephrine Bitartrate for Ophthalmic Soln.	I		
Epinephrine Inj.	S,M	A	LR
Epinephrine Oil Susp., Sterile	S	A,C	LR
Ergonovine Maleate Inj.	S	A	LR,R
Ergotamine Tartrate Inj.	S	A	LR
Erythromycin Ethylsuccinate Inj.	S,M	A	
Erythromycin Ethylsuccinate, Sterile	I		
Erythromycin Gluceptate, Sterile	I	D	
Erythromycin Lactobionate, Sterile	I		
Erythromycin Lactobionate for Inj.	I	D	
Estradiol Cypionate Inj.	S,M	A	LR
Estradiol Suspension, Sterile	S,M	A	
Estradiol Valerate Inj.	S,M	A,C	LR
Estrone Inj.	S,M	A	
Estrone Suspension, Sterile	S,M	A	
Ethacrynate Sodium for Inj.	I	D	
Ethiodized Oil Inj.	S,M		LR
Ethylnorepinephrine HCl Inj.	S,M	A	LR
Evans Blue Inj.	S	A	
Fentanyl Citrate Inj.	S	A	L
Ferrous Citrate Fe 59 Inj.	S,M		
Floxuridine, Sterile	M	A	L (discard after 2 weeks when reconstituted)
Fludeoxyglucose F 18 Inj.	S,M		SC
Fluorescein Sodium Inj.	S	A	
Fluorouracil Inj.	S	A	RT,L
Fluphenazine Enanthate Inj.	S,M	A,C	L
Fluphenazine HCl Inj.	S,M	A	L
Folic Acid Inj.	S,M	A	
Fructose Inj.	S	A,B	
Fructose and Sodium Chloride Inj.	S	A,B	
Furosemide Inj.	S,M	A	LR
Gallamine Triethiodide Inj.	S,M	A	L
Gallium Citrate Ga 67 Inj.	S,M		
Gallium Citrate Ga 67 Inj., Sterile	I	D	
Gentamicin Sulfate Inj.	S,M	A	
Globulin Serum, Anti-Human	U		R
Glucagon for Inj. w/solvent	I/S,M w/solvent		
Glycine Irrigation	S	A,B	
Glycopyrrolate Inj.	S,M	A	
Gold Sodium Thiomalate Inj.	S,M	A	L
Gonadotropin, Chorionic for Inj.	I	D	
Haloperidol Inj.	S,M	A	L
Heparin Calcium Inj.	S,M	A	R
Heparin Lock Flush Soln.	S,M	A	
Heparin Sodium Inj.	S,M	A	
Hepatitis B Virus Vaccine Inactivated	U		R
Hetacillin Potassium, Sterile	I		
Histamine Phosphate Inj.	S,M	A	L
Hyaluronidase for Inj.	I	A,C	RT
Hyaluronidase Inj.	S,M	A	R
Hydralazine HCl Inj.	S,M	A	
Hydrocortisone (Cortisol) Suspension, Sterile	S,M	A	

Drugs	Container	Glass Type	Storage Conditions
Hydrocortisone (Cortisol) Acetate Suspension, Sterile	S,M	A	
Hydrocortisone (Cortisol) Sodium Phosphate Inj.	I	C	
Hydrocortisone (Cortisol) Sodium Succinate for Inj.	I	C	
Hydromorphone HCl Inj.	S,M	A	L
Hydroxyocobalamin Inj.	S,M	A	L
Hydroxyprogesterone Caproate Inj.	S,M	A,C	
Hydroxystilbamidine Isethionate, Sterile	I	D	LR
Hydroxyzine HCl Inj.	S,M		L
Hyoscyamine Sulfate Inj.	S,M	A	
Imipramine HCl Inj.	S	A	LR
Indigotindisulfonate Sodium Inj.	S	A	LR
Indium In-111 Pentetate Inj.	S		
Indocyanine Green, Sterile	I	B	
Indomethacin Sodium, Sterile	I		
Insulin Inj.	M		R
Isophane Insulin Suspension	M		R
Insulin Zinc Suspension	M		R
Insulin Zinc Suspension, Extended	M		R
Insulin Zinc Suspension, Prompt	M		R
Insulin Suspension, Protamine Zinc	M		R
Insulin Human Inj.	M		R
Insulin and Sodium Chloride Inj.	S	A,B	
Iodinated I 125 Albumin Inj.	S,M		R
Iodinated I 131 Albumin Inj.	U		
Iodinated I 131 Albumin Aggregated Inj.	S,M		R
Iodipamide Inj.	S	A	L
Iodipamide Meglumine Inj.	S	A,C	
Iodohippurate Sodium I 123 Inj.	S,M		SC
Iodohippurate Sodium I 131 Inj.	S,M		
Iopamidol Inj. (Intravascular/Intrathecal)	S	A	L
Iophendylate Inj.	S	A	
Iothalamate Meglumine Inj.	S	A	L
Iothalamate Meglumine and Sodium Iothalamate Inj.	S	A	L
Iothalamate Sodium Inj.	S	A	L
Iron Dextran Inj.	S,M	A,B	
Iron Sorbitex Inj.	S	A	
Isoniazid Inj.	S,M	A	L
Isoproterenol HCl Inj.	S	A	L
Isoxsuprine HCl Inj.	S,M	A	
Kanamycin Sulfate, Sterile	I		
Kanamycin Sulfate Inj.	S,M	A,C	
Ketamine HCl Inj.	S,M	A	L,H
Labetolol HCl Inj.	S,M(60 ml max)	A	R,RT,L
Leucovorin Calcium Inj.	S	A	LR
Levorphanol Tartrate Inj.	S,M	A	
Lidocaine HCl, Sterile	I		
Lidocaine HCl Inj.	S,M	A	
Lidocaine HCl and Dextrose Inj.	S	A,B	
Lidocaine and Epinephrine Inj.	S,M	A	LR
Lincomycin HCl, Sterile	I		
Lincomycin HCl Inj.	S,M	A	
Lorazepam Inj.	S,M	A	L
Magnesium Sulfate	S,M	A	
Manganese Chloride Inj.	S,M	A,B	

Drugs	Container	Glass Type	Storage Conditions
Manganese Sulfate Inj.	S,M	A,B	
Mannitol Inj.	S	A,B	
Mannitol and Sodium Chloride Inj.	U	D	
Measles Virus Vaccine Live	S,M		LR,R
Measles and Mumps Virus Vaccine, Live	S,M		LR,R
Measles, Mumps and Rubella Virus Vaccine, Live	S,M		LR,R
Measles and Rubella Virus Vaccine, Live	S,M		LR,R
Mechlorethamine HCl for Inj.	I	B	
Medroxyprogesterone Acetate Susp., Sterile	S,M	A	
Menadiol Sodium Diphosphate Inj.	S	A	LR
Menadione Inj.	S,M	A	
Meningococcal Polysaccharide Vaccine (Group A)	M		R
Meningococcal Polysaccharide Vaccine (Group C)	M		R
Meningococcal Polysaccharide Vaccine (Groups A and C combined)	M		R
Meperidine HCl Inj.	S,M	A	
Mephentermine Sulfate Inj.	S,M	A	
Mepivacaine HCl Inj.	S,M	A	
Mepivacaine HCl and Levonordefrin Inj.	S,M	A	
Meprobamate Inj.	S	A	
Meprylcaine HCl and Epinephrine Inj.	S	A	L
Mesoridazine Besylate Inj.	S	A	L
Metaraminol Bitartrate Inj.	S,M	A	L
Methadone HCl Inj.	S,M	A	LR
Methantheline Bromide, Sterile	I	D	
Methicillin Sodium, Sterile	I		RT
Methicillin Sodium for Inj.	I		L,RT
Methocarbamol Inj.	S	A	
Methohexital Sodium for Inj.	I	C	
Methotrexate Sodium for Inj.	I		L
Methotrexate Sodium Inj.	S,M	A	L
Methotrimeprazine Inj.	S,M	A	L
Methoxamine HCl Inj.	S,M	A	L
Methydopate HCl Inj.	S	A	
Methylene Blue Inj.	S	A	
Methylergonovine Maleate Inj.	S	A	LR
Methylprednisolone Acetate Susp., Sterile	S,M	A	
Methylprednisolone Sodium Succinate for Inj.	I	C	
Metoclopramide Inj.	S,M	A	LR(no antioxidant)
Metocurine Iodide Inj.	S,M	A	
Metoprolol Tartrate Inj.	S	A,B	L
Metronidazole Inj.	S,P	A,B	L
Mezlocillin Sodium, Sterile	I		
Miconazole Inj.	S	A	RT
Minocycline HCl, Sterile	I		L
Mitomycin for Inj.	I	D	L
Mitoxantrone for Inj. Conc.	S	A	
Morphine Sulfate Inj.	S,M	A	L
Morphine Sulfate Inj. (Preservative Free)	S	A	L
Morrhuate Sodium Inj.	S,M	A	

Drugs	Container	Glass Type	Storage Conditions
Moxalactam Disodium for Inj.	I		
Mumps Virus Vaccine Live	S,M		LR,R
Nafcillin Sodium, Sterile	I		
Nafcillin Sodium Inj.	I		F
Nafcillin Sodium for Inj.	I	D	
Nalorphine HCl Inj.	S,M	A	
Naloxone HCl Inj.	S,M	A	L
Nandrolone Decanoate Inj.	S,M	A	L
Nandrolone Phenpropionate Inj.	S,M	A	L
Neomycin Sulfate, Sterile	I		
Neostigmine Methylsulfate Inj.	S,M		L
Netilmicin Sulfate Inj.	S,M	A	
Niacin Inj.	S,M	A	
Niacinamide Inj.	S,M	A	
Nitroglycerin Inj.	S,M	A,B	
Norepinephrine Bitartrate Inj.	S	A	LR
Nylidrin HCl Inj.	S,M	A	
Orphenadrine Citrate Inj.	S,M	A	L
Oxacillin Sodium for Inj.	I	D	RT
Oxacillin Sodium Inj.	I		F
Oxacillin Sodium, Sterile	I		
Oxymorphone HCl Inj.	S,M	A	L
Oxytetracycline, Sterile	I		L
Oxytetracycline HCl for Inj.	I	B	L
Oxytetracycline Inj.	S,M		L
Oxytetracycline HCl, Sterile	I		L
Papaverine HCl Inj.	S,M	A	
Penicillin G Benzathine, Sterile	I		
Penicillin G Benzathine Susp., Sterile	S,M	A,B	R
Penicillin G Benzathine and Penicillin G Procaine Susp., Sterile	S,M	A,C	
Penicillin G Potassium for Inj.	I	D	
Penicillin G Potassium, Sterile	I	D	
Penicillin G Procaine, Sterile	I		
Penicillin G Procaine for Susp., Sterile	S,M	A,C	
Penicillin G Procaine Susp., Sterile	S,M	A,C	R
Penicillin G Procaine Intramammary Infusion	Sy(well closed)		
Penicillin G Procaine w/Aluminum Stearate Susp., Sterile	S,M	A,C	
Penicillin G Procaine and Dihydrostreptomycin Sulfate Susp., Sterile	S,M(tight)		
Penicillin G Procaine Dihydrostreptomycin Sulfate Intramammary Infusion	Sy(well closed)		
Penicillin G Procaine, Dihydrostreptomycin Sulfate & Prednisolone Susp., Sterile	S,M(tight)		
Penicillin G Procaine, Dihydrostreptomycin Sulfate, Chlorpheniramine Maleate, and Dexamethasone Susp., Sterile	S,M(tight)		R
Penicillin G Sodium for Inj.	I	D	
Penicillin G Sodium for Inj.	I		
Penicillin G Sodium, Sterile	I	D	
Pentazocine Lactate Inj.	S,M	A	
Pentobarbital Sodium Inj.	S,M	A	
Perphenazine Inj.	S,M	A	L
Pertussis Vaccine	U		R

Drugs	Container	Glass Type	Storage Conditions
Pertussis Vaccine Adsorbed	U		R
Phenobarbital Sodium, Sterile	I	D	
Phenobarbital Sodium Inj.	I	D	
Phentolamine Mesylate for Inj.	I	B	
Phenylephrine HCl Inj.	S,M	A	L
Phenytoin Sodium Inj.	S,M	A	RT
Phosphate P^{32}, Chromic Susp.	S,M		
Phosphate P^{32}, Sodium Soln.	S,M	Tr	
Physostigmine Salicylate Inj.	S	A	L
Phytonadione Inj.	S,M	A	L
Pilocarpine Ocular System	S		R
Piperacillin Sodium, Sterile	I		
Plicamycin for Inj.	I	D	L
Poliovirus Vaccine Inactivated	U		R
Polymyxin B Sulfate, Sterile	I	D	L
Posterior Pituitary Inj.	S,M	A	
Potassium Acetate Inj.	S,M	A,B	
Potassium Chloride Inj.	S,M	A,B	
Potassium Chloride in Dextrose Inj.	S	A,B	
Potassium Chloride in Dextrose and Sodium Chloride Inj.	S	A,B,P	
Potassium Chloride in Sodium Chloride Inj.	S	A,B,P	
Potassium Phosphates Inj.	S,M	A	
Pralidoxone Chloride, Sterile	I	B	
Prednisolone Acetate Susp., Sterile	S,M	A	
Prednisolone Sodium Phosphate Inj.	S,M	A	L
Prednisolone Sodium Succinate for Inj.	I	D	
Prednisolone Tebutate Susp., Sterile	S,M	A	
Prilocaine HCl Inj.	S,M	A	
Prilocaine & Epinephrine Inj.	S,M	A	L
Procainamide HCl Inj.	S,M	A	
Procaine HCl Inj.	S,M	A,B	
Procaine HCl, Sterile	I	D	
Procaine HCl and Epinephrine Inj.	S,M	A,B	LR
Procaine and Phenylephrine HCl Inj.	S,M	A	
Procaine HCl, Tetracycline HCl and Levonordefrin Inj.	S,M	A	
Prochlorperazine Edisylate Inj.	S,M	A	L
Progesterone Inj.	S,M	A,C	
Progesterone Susp., Sterile	S,M	A	
Progesterone Intrauterine Contraceptive Sys.	S		
Promazine HCl Inj.	S,M	A	L
Promethazine HCl Inj.	S,M	A	L
Propantheline Bromide, Sterile	S	D	
Propiomazine HCl Inj.	S	A	RT,L
Propoxycaine HCl, Procaine HCl and Levonordefrin Inj.	S,A		
Propoxycaine HCl, Procaine HCl and Norepinephrine Bitartrate Inj.	S,M	A	
Propranolol HCl Inj.	S	A	LR
Propyliodone Oil Susp., Sterile	S	D	LR
Protamine Sulfate for Inj.	I	D	
Protamine Sulfate Inj.	S	A	R
Protein Hydrolysate Inj.	S	A,B	H
Pyridostigmine Bromide Inj.	S	A	L
Pyridoxine HCl Inj.	S,M	A	L

Drugs	Container	Glass Type	Storage Conditions
Quinidine Gluconate Inj.	S,M	A	
Rabies Immune Globin	U		R
Rabies Vaccine	U		R
Ranitidine Inj.	S,M	I	LR,RT
Ranitidine in Sodium Chloride Inj.	N		LR,RT
Reserpine Inj.	S	A	LR
Riboflavin Inj.	S,M	A	LR
Rifampin for Inj.	I		
Ringer's Inj.	S	A,B	
Lactated Ringer's Inj.	S	A,B	
Ritodrine HCl Inj.	S	A	RT
Rolitetracycline for Inj.	I	B	L
Rolitetracycline, Sterile	I		L
Rubella Virus Vaccine Live	S,M		LR,R
Rubella and Mumps Virus Vaccine Live	S,M		LR,R
Scopolamine Hydrobromide Inj.	S,M	A	LR
Secobarbital Sodium, Sterile	I	D	
Secobarbital Sodium Inj.	S,M	A	L,R
Selenious Acid Inj.	S,M	A,B	
Selenomethionine Se75 Inj.	U		R
Sisomicin Sulfate Inj.	S,M	A	
Smallpox Vaccine	U		R
Sodium Acetate Inj.	S	A	
Sodium Bicarbonate Inj.	S	A	
Sodium Chloride Inhalation Soln.	S		
Sodium Chloride Inj.	S	A,B	
Sodium Chloride Inj., Bacteriostatic	S,M	A,B	
Sodium Lactate Inj.	S	A,B	
Sodium Nitrate Inj.	S	A	
Sodium Nitroprusside, Sterile	I	D	L
Sodium Pertechnetate Tc99m Inj.	S,M		R
Sodium Phosphates Inj.	S,M	A	
Sodium Sulfate Inj.	S	A	
Sodium Thiosulfate Inj.	S	A	
Spectinomycin HCl, Sterile	I		
Spectinomycin HCl for Suspension, Sterile	I		
Streptomycin Sulfate, Sterile	I	D	
Streptomycin Sulfate Inj.	S,M	A	
Succinylcholine Chloride, Sterile	I	D	
Succinylcholine Chloride Inj.	S,M	A,B	R
Invert Sugar Inj.	S,P	A,B	
Sulbactam Sodium, Sterile	I		
Sulfadiazine Sodium Inj.	S	A	LR
Sulfamethoxazole & Trimethoprim Concentrate for Inj.	S,M	A	L
Sulfisoxazole Diolamine Inj.	S,M	A	L
Sulfobromophthalein Sodium Inj.	S	A	
Technetium Tc99m Albumin Inj.	S,M		R
Technetium Tc99m Albumin Aggregated Inj.	S,M		R
Technetium Tc99m Albumin Colloid Inj.	S,M		R
Technetium Tc99 Disofenin Inj.	S,M		In
Technetium Tc99m Etiodonate Inj.	S,M		
Technetium Tc99m Ferpentate Inj.	S,M		R,L
Technetium Tc99m Gluceptate Inj.	S,M		R
Technetium Tc99m Lidofenin Inj.	S,M		R
Technetium Tc99m Medronate Inj.	S,M		
Technetium Tc99m Oxidronate Inj.	S,M		

Drugs	Container	Glass Type	Storage Conditions
Technetium Tc99m Penetate Inj.	S,M		R
Technetium Tc99m Pyrophosphate Inj.	S,M		R
Technetium Tc99m (Pyro- and trimeta-) Phosphates Inj.	U		D
Technetium Tc99m Succimer Inj.	S		RT,L
Technetium Tc99m Sulfur Colloid Inj.	S,M		
Terbutaline Sulfate Inj.	S	A	L,RT
Testolactone Susp., Sterile	S,M	A	
Testosterone Pellets	S		
Testosterone Susp., Sterile	S,M	A	
Testosterone Cypionate Inj.	S,M	A	L
Testosterone Enanthate Inj.	S,M	A	
Testosterone Propionate Inj.	S,M	A	
Tetanus Antitoxin	U		R
Tetanus Immune Globulin	U		R
Tetanus Toxoid	U		R
Tetanus Toxoid Adsorbed	U		R
Tetanus and Diphtheria Toxoids Adsorbed (for adult use)	U		R
Tetracaine HCl, Sterile	I	A	
Tetracaine HCl Inj.	S,M	A	R,L
Tetracaine HCl in Dextrose Inj.	S,M(up to 100 ml)	A	R,L,RT(tray for 12 months)
Tetracycline HCl, Sterile	I		L
Tetracycline HCl for Inj.	I	B	L
Tetracycline Phosphate Complex for Inj.	I		L
Tetracycline Phosphate Complex for Inj.	I	B	L
Tetracycline Phosphate Complex, Sterile	I		L
Thallous Chloride Tl 201 Inj.	S,M		
Theophylline in Dextrose Inj.	S	A,B,P	
Thiamine HCl Inj.	S,M	A	L
Thiamylal Sodium for Inj.	I	C	
Thiethylperazine Maleate Inj.	S	A	L
Thiopental Sodium for Inj.	I	C	
Thiotepa for Inj.	I	D	R,L
Thiothixene HCl Inj.	S	A	L
Thiothixene HCl for Inj.	I		LR
Ticarcillin Disodium, Sterile	I	D	
Ticarcillin Disodium & Clavulanate Potassium, Sterile	I		
Ticarcillin Disodium & Clavulanate Potassium, Inj.	I		F
Tobramycin Sulfate, Sterile	I		
Tobramycin Sulfate Inj.	S,M	A	
Tolazoline HCl Inj.	S,M	A	
Tolbutamide Sodium, Sterile	I	D	
Triamcinolone Diacetate Susp., Sterile	S,M	A	
Triamcinolone Hexacetonide Susp., Sterile	S,M	A	
Tridihexethyl Chloride Inj.	S	A	
Trifluoperazine HCl Inj.	M	A	L
Trifluopromazine HCl Inj.	S,M	A	L
Trimethaphan Camsylate Inj.	S,M	A	R
Trimethobenzamide HCl Inj.	S,M	A	
Tromethamine for Inj.	I	C	
Tubocurarine Chloride Inj.	S,M		
Typhoid Vaccine	U		R

Drugs	Container	Glass Type	Storage Conditions
Urea, Sterile	I	D	
Vaccinia Immune Globulin	U		R
Vancomycin HCl, Sterile	I	B	
Vancomycin HCl for Inj.	I		
Varicella-Zoster Immune Globulin	U		R
Vasopressin Inj.	S,M	A	
Verapamil (HCl) Inj.	S	A	LR
Vidarabine Concentrate for Inj.	S,M	A	
Vinblastine Sulfate, Sterile	I	D	R
Vincristine Sulfate Inj.	U	U	L,R
Vincristine Sulfate for Inj.	U		L,R
Warfarin Sodium for Inj.	I	D	LR
Water for Inhalation, Sterile	S		
Water for Inj., Bacteriostatic	S,M	A,B	
Water for Inj., Sterile	S	A,B	
Water for Irrigation, Sterile	S	A,B	
Xenon Xe 127	S (leakproof stoppers)		RT,SC
Xenon Xe 133	S (leakproof stoppers)		RT,SC
Xenon Xe 133 Inj.	S (totally filled)		RT,SC
Yellow Fever Vaccine	U (nitrogen filled ampuls®)		R
Ytterbium Yb 169 Pentetate Inj.	S		RT
Zinc Chloride Inj.	S,M	A,B	
Zinc Sulfate Inj.	S,M		

Provided by Dr. Kenneth S. Alexander, Associate Professor of Pharmacy, College of Pharmacy, University of Toledo.

*The listing of container and storage requirements for sterile Compendial drugs is included as an aid to the practitioner in storing and dispensing.

Oral Dosage Forms That Should Not Be Crushed

Drug Product	Manufacturer	Dosage Form	Reason/Comments
Accutane	Roche	Capsule	Mucous membrane irritant
Actifed 12 Hour	Burroughs Wellcome	Capsule	Slow release (i)
Acutrim	Ciba	Tablet	Slow release
Aerolate SR, JR, III	Fleming & Co.	Capsule	Slow release* (i)
Afrinol Repetabs	Schering	Tablet	Slow release
Allerest 12-Hour	Fisons	Caplet	Slow release
Android Buccal	ICN/Brown	Tablet	Buccal tablet
Artane Sequels	Lederle	Capsule	Slow release* (i)
Arthritis Bayer Timed-Release	Glenbrook	Capsule	Slow release
ASA Enseals	Lilly	Tablet	Enteric-coated
Asbron G Inlay	Sandoz	Tablet	Multiple compressed tablet (i)
Atrohist L.A.	Adams	Tablet	Slow release
Atrohist Sprinkle	Adams	Capsule	Slow release
Azulfidine Entabs	Pharmacia Labs	Tablet	Enteric-coated
Betapen-VK	Bristol	Tablet	Taste (c)
Biphetamine	Fisons	Capsule	Slow release
Bisacodyl	Various	Tablet	Enteric-coated (a)
Bisco-Lax	Schein	Tablet	Enteric-coated (a)
Bontril-SR	Carnrick	Capsule	Slow release
Breonesin	Breon	Capsule	Liquid filled (b)
Brexin L.A.	Savage	Capsule	Slow release
Bromfed	Muro	Capsule	Slow release (l)
Bromfed PD	Muro	Capsule	Slow release (l)
Calan SR	Searle	Tablet	Slow release (h)
Cama Arthritis Pain Reliever	Dorsey	Tablet	Multiple compressed tablet
Cardizem	Marion Merrell Dow	Tablet	Slow release
Cardizem SR	Marion Merrell Dow	Capsule	Slow release*
Carter's Little Pills	Carter-Wallace	Tablet	Enteric-coated
Cefal Filmtab	Abbott	Tablet	Enteric-coated
Charcoal Plus	Kramer	Tablet	Enteric-coated
Chloral Hydrate	Various	Capsule	Liquid in capsule (i)
Chlorpheniramine Maleate T-D	Lederle	Capsule	Slow release
Chlor-Trimeton Repetab	Schering	Tablet	Slow release (i)
Choledyl SA	Parke-Davis	Tablet	Slow release (i)
Cipro	Miles	Tablet	Taste (c)
Codimal-LA	Central	Capsule	Slow release
Coffee Break	Columbia	Tablet	Slow release
Colace	Mead Johnson	Capsule	Taste (c)
Comhist-LA	Norwich	Capsule	Slow release*
Compazine Spansule	SKF	Capsule	Slow release
Congess SR, JR	Fleming & Co.	Capsule	Slow release
Constant-T	Geigy	Tablet	Slow release*
Contac	SmithKline Beecham	Capsule	Slow release*
Cotazym-S	Organon	Capsule	Enteric-coated*
Creon	Reid-Rowell	Capsule	Enteric-coated*
Dallergy	Laser	Capsule	Slow release (i)
Dallergy - D	Laser	Capsule	Slow release
Dallergy - JR	Laser	Capsule	Slow release
Deconamine-SR	Berlex	Capsule	Slow release (i)

The listing of oral dosage forms that should not be crushed is included as an aid to the practitioner in dispensing drugs and consulting with patients.

Drug Product	Manufacturer	Dosage Form	Reason/Comments
Deconsal L.A.	Adams	Tablet	Slow release
Demazine Repetabs	Schering	Tablet	Slow release (i)
Depakene	Abbott	Capsule	Slow release-mucous membrane irritant (i)
Depakote	Abbott	Capsule	Enteric coated
Desoxyn Gradumets	Abbott	Tablet	Slow release
Desyred	Mead Johnson	Tablet	Taste (c)
Dexedrine Spansule	SmithKline Beecham	Capsule	Slow release
Diamox Sequels	Lederle	Capsule	Slow release
Diet-Aid	Columbia	Capsule	Slow release
Diet-Aid with Vitamin C	Columbia	Capsule	Slow release
Dilatrate-SR	Reed & Carnrick	Capsule	Slow release
Dimetane Extentab	Robins	Tablet	Slow release (i)
Disobrom	Geneva	Tablet	Slow release
Disophrol Chronotab	Schering	Tablet	Slow release
Dital	UAD	Capsule	Slow release
Donnatal Extentab	Robins	Tablet	Slow release (i)
Donnazyme	Robins	Tablet	Enteric-coated
Drisdol	Winthrop	Capsule	Liquid filled (b)
Drixoral	Schering	Tablet	Slow release (i)
Dulcolax	Boehringer Ingelheim	Tablet	Enteric-coated (a)
Easprin	Parke Davis	Tablet	Enteric-coated
Ecotrin	SmithKline Beecham	Tablet	Enteric-coated
E.E.S. 400 Filmtab	Abbott	Tablet	Enteric-coated (i)
Elixophyllin SR	Berlex	Capsule	Slow release* (i)
E-Mycin	Boots	Tablet	Enteric-coated
Endafed	UAD	Capsule	Slow release
Enkaid	Bristol	Capsule	Taste (c)
Entex LA	Norwich	Tablet	Slow release (i)
Entolase-HP	Robins	Capsule	Enteric-coated
Entozyme	Robins	Tablet	Enteric-coated
Equanil	Wyeth	Tablet	Taste (c)
Ergostat	Parke-Davis	Tablet	Sublingual form (g)
Eryc	Parke-Davis	Capsule	Enteric-coated*
Ery-tab	Abbott	Tablet	Enteric-coated
Erythrocin Stearate Filmtab	Abbott	Tablet	Enteric-coated
Erythromycin Base Filmtab	Abbott	Tablet	Enteric-coated
Eskalith CR	SmithKline Beecham	Tablet	Slow release
Fedahist Timecaps	Schwarz Pharma	Capsule	Slow release (i)
Feldene	Pfizer	Capsule	Mucous membrane irritant
Feocyte	Dunhall	Tablet	Slow release
Feosol	SmithKline Beecham	Tablet	Enteric-coated (i)
Feosol Spansule	SmithKline Beecham	Capsule	Slow release* (i)
Feratab	Upsher-Smith	Tablet	Enteric-coated (i)
Fergon	Winthrop	Capsule	Slow release* (i)
Fero-Grad 500 mg	Abbott	Tablet	Slow release
Fero-Gradumet	Abbott	Tablet	Slow release
Ferro-Sequels	Lederle	Capsule	Slow release*
Festal II	Hoechst	Tablet	Enteric-coated
Feverall Sprinkle Caps	Upsher-Smith	Capsule	Taste* (j)
Fumatinic	Laser	Capsule	Slow release
Gastrocrom	Fisons	Capsule	Dissolve in water (k)
Geocillin	Roerig	Tablet	Taste
Gris-Peg	Herbert	Tablet	Crushing may precipitate (l)
Guaifed	Muro	Capsule	Slow release
Guaifed-PD	Muro	Capsule	Slow release
Hydergine LC	Sandoz	Capsule	Liquid in capsule (i)
Hydergine Sublingual	Sandoz	Tablet	Sublingual route (i)
Hytakerol	Winthrop	Capsule	Liquid-filled (b) (i)
Iberet	Abbott	Tablet	Slow release (i)

Drug Product	Manufacturer	Dosage Form	Reason/Comments
Iberet-500	Abbott	Tablet	Slow release (i)
Ilotycin	Dista	Tablet	Enteric-coated
Inderal-LA	Ayerst	Capsule	Slow release
Inderide-LA	Ayerst	Capsule	Slow release
Indocin SR	MSD	Capsule	Slow release* (i)
Ionamin	Fisons	Capsule	Slow release
Isoclor Timesule	Fisons	Capsule	Slow release (i)
Isoptin SR	Knoll	Tablet	Slow release
Isordil Chewable 10 mg	Wyeth	Tablet	Crushing prevents absorption in mouth
Isordil Sublingual	Wyeth	Tablet	Sublingual form (g)
Isordil Tembid	Wyeth	Tablet	Slow release
Isuprel Glossets	Breon	Tablet	Sublingual form (g)
Kaon-CL 6.7 mEq	Adria	Tablet	Slow release (i)
Kaon-CL 10	Adria	Tablet	Slow release (i)
K-Lease	Adria	Capsule	Slow release* (i)
Klor-Con	Upsher-Smith	Tablet	Slow release (i)
Klor-Con/EF	Upsher-Smith	Tablet	Effervescent tablet (d) (i)
Klorvess	Sandoz	Tablet	Effervescent tablet (d) (i)
Klotrix	Mead Johnson	Tablet	Slow release (i)
K-Lyte	Mead Johnson	Tablet	Effervescent tablet (d)
K-Lyte CL	Mead Johnson	Tablet	Effervescent tablet (d)
K + 10	Alra	Tablet	Slow release (i)
K + Care	Alra	Tablet	Effervescent tablet (d) (i)
K-Tab	Abbott	Tablet	Slow release (i)
Levsinex Timecaps	Schwarz Pharma	Capsule	Slow release
Lithobid	Ciba-Geigy	Tablet	Slow release (i)
Mag-Tab Sr	Adria	Tablet	Slow release
Measurin	Winthrop	Tablet	Slow release
Meprospan	Wallace	Capsule	Slow release*
Mestinon Timespan	Roche	Tablet	Slow release (i)
MI-Cebrin	Dista	Tablet	Enteric-coated
MI-Cebrin T	Dista	Tablet	Enteric-coated
Micro-K	Robins	Capsule	Slow release* (i)
Motrin	Upjohn	Tablet	Taste (c)
MS Contin	Purdue Frederick	Tablet	Slow release (i)
MSC Triaminic	Dorsey	Tablet	Enteric-coated
Naldecon	Bristol	Tablet	Slow release (i)
Nico 400	Marion	Capsule	Slow release
Nicobid	Rhone-Poulenc Rorer	Capsule	Slow release
Nitro-Bid	Marion Merrell Dow	Capsule	Slow release*
Nitrocine Timecaps	Schwarz Pharma	Capsule	Slow release
Nitroglyn	Kenwood	Capsule	Slow release*
Nitrong	Rhone-Poulenc Rorer	Tablet	Sublingual route (g)
Nitrostat	Parke-Davis	Tablet	Sublingual route (g)
Noctec	Squibb	Capsule	Liquid in cap. (i)
Nolamine	Carnrick	Tablet	Slow release
Nolex LA	Carnrick	Tablet	Slow release
Norflex	Riker	Tablet	Slow release
Norpace CR	Searle	Capsule	Slow release
Novafed	Dow	Capsule	Slow release
Novafed A	Dow	Capsule	Slow release
Novahistine LP	Lakeside	Tablet	Slow release (i)
Optilets 500 Filmtab	Abbott	Tablet	Enteric-coated
Optilets M 500 Filmtab	Abbott	Tablet	Enteric-coated
Oragrafin	Squibb	Capsule	Liquid in cap.
Ornade Spansule	SmithKline Beecham	Capsule	Slow release
Pabalate	Robins	Tablet	Enteric-coated
Pabalate SF	Robins	Tablet	Enteric-coated
Pancrease	McNeil	Capsule	Enteric-coated*

Drug Product	Manufacturer	Dosage Form	Reason/Comments
Pancrease MT	McNeil	Capsule	Enteric-coated*
Panmycin	Upjohn	Capsule	Taste
Papaverine Sustained Action	Various	Capsule	Slow release
Pathilon Sequels	Lederle	Capsule	Slow release*
Pavabid Plateau	Marion Merrell Dow	Capsule	Slow release*
PBZ-SR	Geigy	Tablet	Slow release (i)
Perdiem	Rhone-Poulenc Rorer	Granules	Wax-coated
Peritrate SA	Parke-Davis	Tablet	Slow release (h)
Permitil Chronotab	Schering	Tablet	Slow release (i)
Phazyme	Carnrick	Tablet	Slow release
Phazyme 95	Carnrick	Tablet	Slow release
Phazyme PB	Carnrick	Tablet	Slow release
Phenergan	Wyeth	Tablet	Taste (c) (i)
Phyllocontin	Purdue Frederick	Tablet	Slow release
Polaramine Repetabs	Schering	Tablet	Slow release (i)
Prelu-2	Boehringer Ingelheim	Capsule	Slow release
Preludin	Boehringer Ingelheim	Tablet	Slow release
Prilosec	MSD	Capsule	Slow release
Pro-Banthine	Searle	Tablet	Taste
Procainamide HCl S.R.	Various	Tablet	Slow release
Procan SR	Parke-Davis	Tablet	Slow release
Procardia	Pfizer	Capsule	Delays absorption (e) (b)
Procardia XL	Pfizer	Tablet	Slow release, AUC unaffected
Pronestyl-SR	Squibb	Tablet	Slow release
Proventil Repetabs	Schering	Tablet	Slow release (i)
Quadra-Hist	Harvey	Tablet	Slow release
Quibron-T/SR	Mead Johnson	Tablet	Slow release (i)
Quinaglute Dura-Tabs	Berlex	Tablet	Slow release
Quinalan S.R.	Lannett	Tablet	Slow release
Quinidex Extentabs	Robins	Tablet	Slow release
Respaire S.R.	Laser	Capsule	Slow release
Respbid	Boehringer Ingelheim	Tablet	Slow release
Rhinex D-Lay	Lemmon	Tablet	Slow release
Ritalin-SR	Ciba	Tablet	Slow release
Robimycin Robitab	Robins	Tablet	Enteric-coated
Rondec-TR	Ross	Tablet	Slow release (i)
Roxanol-SR	Roxane	Tablet	Slow release (i)
Ru-Tuss	Boots	Tablet	Slow release
Ru-Tuss DE	Boots	Tablet	Slow release
Singlet	Dow	Tablet	Slow release
Slo-Bid Gyrocaps	Rhone-Poulenc Rorer	Capsule	Slow release*
Slo-Niacin	Upsher Smith	Tablet	Slow release
Slo-Phyllin GG	Rhone-Poulenc Rorer	Capsule	Slow release (i)
Slo-Phyllin Gyrocaps	Rhone-Poulenc Rorer	Capsule	Slow release* (i)
Slow-FE	Ciba	Tablet	Slow release (i)
Slow-K	Ciba	Tablet	Slow release (i)
Slow-Mag	Searle	Tablet	Slow release
Sorbitrate S.A.	Stuart	Tablet	Slow release
Sparine	Wyeth	Tablet	Taste (c)
S-P-T	Fleming	Capsule	Liquid gelatin susp.
Sudafed 12 hour	Burroughs Wellcome	Capsule	Slow release (i)
Sustaire	Pfizer	Tablet	Slow release (i)
Tavist-D	Sandoz	Tablet	Muliple compressed tablet
Tedral SA	Parke-Davis	Tablet	Slow release
Teldrin	SmithKline Prods.	Capsule	Slow release*
Tepanil Ten-Tab	Riker	Tablet	Slow release
Tessalon Perles	DuPont	Capsule	Slow release
Theo-24	Searle	Tablet	Slow release (i)
Theobid	Russ	Capsule	Slow release* (i)

Drug Product	Manufacturer	Dosage Form	Reason/Comments
Theobid Jr.	Russ	Capsule	Slow release* (i)
Theoclear-LA	Central	Capsule	Slow release (i)
Theo-Dur	Key	Tablet	Slow release (i)
Theo-Dur Sprinkle	Key	Capsule	Slow release* (i)
Theolair-SR	Riker	Tablet	Slow release (i)
Theo-Sav	Savage	Tablet	Slow release (h)
Theovent	Schering	Capsule	Slow release (i)
Theox	Carnrick	Tablet	Slow release
Therapy Bayer	Glenbrook	Caplet	Enteric-coated
Thorazine Spansule	SmithKline Beecham	Capsule	Slow release
T-Phyl	Purdue Frederick	Tablet	Slow release
Trental	Hoechst	Tablet	Slow release
Triaminic	Sandoz	Tablet	Enteric-coated (i)
Triaminic-12	Sandoz	Tablet	Slow release (i)
Triaminic TR	Sandoz	Tablet	Multiple compressed tablet (i)
Trilafon Repetabs	Schering	Tablet	Slow release (i)
Triptone Caplets	Commerce	Tablet	Slow release
Tuss-LA	Hyrex	Tablet	Slow release
Tuss-Ornade Spansule	SmithKline Beecham	Capsule	Slow release
ULR-LA	Geneva Marsam	Tablet	Slow release
Uniphyl	Purdue Frederick	Tablet	Slow release
Valrelease	Roche	Capsule	Slow release
Verelan	Lederle	Capsule	Slow release*
Wellbutrin	Burroughs Wellcome	Tablet	Anesthetize mucous membrane
Wyamycin-S	Wyeth	Tablet	Slow release
Wygesic	Wyeth	Tablet	Taste
ZORprin	Boots	Tablet	Slow release
Zymase	Organon	Capsule	Enteric-coated

The listing is included to alert the health care practitioner about oral dosage forms that should not be crushed, and to serve as an aid in consulting with patients. Reprinted from Mitchell, John F: Hospital Pharmacy 24: 91, 1989 and revised by John F. Mitchell, Pharm. D. and Kathleen S. Pawlicki, M.S.

* Capsule may be opened and the contents taken without crushing or chewing; soft food such as applesauce or pudding may facilitate administration; contents may generally be administered via nasogastric tube using an appropriate fluid provided entire contents are washed down the tube.

(a) Antacids and/or milk may prematurely dissolve the coating of the tablet.

(b) Capsule may be opened and the liquid contents removed for administration.

(c) The taste of the product in a liquid form would likely be unacceptable to the patient; administration via nasogastric tube should be acceptable.

(d) Effervescent tablets must be dissolved in the amount of diluent recommended by the manufacturer.

(e) If the liquid capsule is crushed or the contents expressed, the active ingredient will be, in part, absorbed sublingually.

(f) Acid contents of the stomach may prematurely activate the ingredients.

(g) Tablets are made to disintegrate under the tongue.

(h) Tablet is scored.

(i) Liquid dosage forms of the product are available; however, dose, frequency of administration and manufacturers may differ from that of the solid dosage form.

(j) Capsule contents intended to be placed in a teaspoonful of water or soft food.

(k) Contents may be dissolved in water for administration.

(l) Crushing may result in precipitation of larger particles.

Pharmaceutical Company Labeler Code Index

LISTED IN NUMERICAL ORDER

00002
Eli Lilly and Co.

00003
Apothecon

00004
Roche Laboratories

00005
Lederle Laboratories

00006
Merck Sharp and Dohme

00007
SmithKline Beecham Pharm.

00008
Wyeth-Ayerst Laboratories

00009
The Upjohn Company

00011
Hynson, Westcott & Dunning

00013
Adria Laboratories

00014
Searle & Company

00015
Mead Johnson Oncology Products

00016
Pharmacia Inc.

00017
Wampole Laboratories

00019
Mallinckrodt Medical, Inc.

00021
Reed & Carnrick

00023
Allergan Pharmaceuticals

00023
Herbert Laboratories

00024
Winthrop Pharmaceuticals

00024
Winthrop Consumer

00025
Searle Laboratories

00025
Searle Consumer Products

00026
Miles Inc.

00028
Geigy Pharmaceuticals

00029
SmithKline Beecham Pharm.

00031
A. H. Robins Company, Inc.

00031
A.H. Robins Cons. Prod. Div.

00032
Reid-Rowell

00033
Syntex Laboratories

00034
Purdue Frederick Co.

00037
Wallace Laboratories

00038
Stuart Pharmaceuticals

00039
Hoechst-Roussel Pharm., Inc.

00041
Oral-B Laboratories, Inc.

00043
Sandoz Pharmaceutical Corp.

00044
Knoll Pharmaceuticals

00045
McNeil Pharmaceutical

00045
McNeil Consumer Products Co.

00046
Warner Chilcott Laboratories

00048
Boots-Flint

00049
J. B. Roerig Division

00052
Organon, Inc.

00053
Armour Pharmaceutical Company

00054
Roxane Laboratories, Inc.

00056
DuPont Pharmaceutical

00058
Iolab Pharmaceuticals

00060
Dupont Phamaceuticals,Caribe

00062
Ortho Pharmaceutical Corp.

00062
Ortho Diagnostic Systems

00062
Ortho Dermatologic

00065
Alcon Laboratories, Inc.

00066
Dermik Laboratories, Inc.

00067
Rhone-Poulenc Rorer Pharm Inc.

00068
Marion Merrell Dow Inc.

00068
Marion Merrell Dow Inc.

00069
Pfizer Laboratories

00071
Parke-Davis

00071
Parke-Davis Consumer Products

00072
Westwood Pharmaceuticals

00074
Abbott Laboratories

00074
Abbott Hospital Products

00074
Ross Laboratories

00074
Abbott Diagnostics

00075
Rhone-Poulenc Rorer Pharm Inc.

00076
Star Pharmaceuticals, Inc.

00077
Sola/Barnes-Hind

00078
Sandoz Pharmaceuticals

The "Pharmaceutical Company Labeler Code Index" is presented to aid the practitioner in the identification of drug products. In this section the codes are listed in numerical order. Additionally, the pharmaceutical labeler codes are also listed with the alphabetical listing of Pharmaceutical Manufacturers and/or Drug Distributors.

00081
Burroughs Wellcome Co.

00083
Ciba Pharmaceutical

00083
Ciba Consumer Pharmaceuticals

00085
Schering-Plough Corporation

00085
Key Pharmaceuticals

00085
Schering-Plough Corporation

00086
Carnrick Laboratories, Inc.

00087
Mead Johnson Nutritionals

00087
Bristol-Myers U.S. Pharm.

00087
Mead Johnson Laboratories

00088
Marion Merrell Dow Inc.

00089
3M Pharmaceutical

00089
3M Personal Care Products

00091
Schwarz Pharma Kremers Urban

00093
Lemmon Company

00094
DuPont Critical Care

00095
Poythress Laboratories. Inc.

00096
Person and Covey, Inc.

00098
Kirkman Sales Company

00102
Regal Laboratories

00115
Richlyn Laboratories, Inc.

00116
Xttrium Laboratories. Inc.

00118
Hollister-Stier

00121
Pharmaceutical Associates, Inc

00122
Rexall Group

00126
Colgate-Hoyt

00127
Ulmer Pharmacal

00128
SmithKline Beecham Con Brands

00131
Central Pharmaceuticals, Inc.

00132
C. B. Fleet Co., Inc.

00137
Johnson & Johnson

00140
Roche Products Inc.

00143
West-Ward, Inc.

00145
Stiefel Laboratories, Inc.

00147
Camall Company, Inc.

00149
Norwich Eaton Pharm.

00150
Murray Drug Corporation

00152
Gray Pharmaceutical Co.

00154
Blair Laboratories

00161
Cutter Medical

00161
Cutter Biological

00163
ICN Pharmaceuticals, Inc.

00164
Carter Products

00165
Blaine Company, Inc.

00168
E. Fougera and Co.

00172
Zenith Laboratories, Inc.

00173
Glaxo, Inc.

00173
Allen & Hanburys

00178
Mission Pharmacal Company

00182
Goldline Laboratories, Inc.

00185
Vitarine Pharmaceuticals, Inc.

00186
Astra Pharmaceutical Prod. Inc

00187
ICN Pharmaceuticals, Inc.

00191
Ortega Pharm. Co., Inc.

00192
Miles Inc.

00193
Ames Company

00195
Rhone-Poulenc Pharmaceuticals

00196
Rachelle Laboratories, Inc.

00212
Sandoz Nutrition

00217
Dunhall Pharmaceuticals, Inc.

00222
Boyle and Company Pharm.

00223
Consolidated Midland Corp.

00224
Konsyl Pharmaceuticals

00224
Lafayette Pharmaceuticals

00225
B. F. Ascher and Company

00228
Purepac Pharmaceutical Co.

00234
Schmid Products Co.

00235
Fisons Consumer Health

00244
Medicone Company

00245
Upsher-Smith Labs., Inc.

00248
Brown Pharmaceutical Company

00249
Geriatric Pharmaceutical Corp.

00252
JMI-Canton Pharmaceuticals Inc

00256
Fleming & Co.

00258
Inwood Laboratories

00259
Mayrand, Inc.

00261
Drug Industries Co.

00263
Rystan Company, Inc.

00264
McGaw, Inc.

00268
Center Laboratories

00273
Lorvic Corporation

00274
Scherer Laboratories,Inc.

00275
Arco Pharmaceuticals, Inc.

00276
Misemer Pharmaceuticals, Inc.

00277
Laser, Inc.

00281
Savage Laboratories

00283
Beutlich, Inc.

00288
Fluoritab Corp.

00295
Denison Laboratories, Inc.

00298
Vortech Pharmaceuticals

00299
Owen/Galderma Laboratories Inc

00299
Allercreme

00300
Tap Pharmaceuticals

00302
Gentco, Inc.

00304
J.J. Balan, Inc.

00310
ICI Pharma

00314
Hyrex Pharmaceuticals

00316
Del-Ray Laboratory, Inc.

00317
Whorton Pharmaceuticals, Inc.

00327
Guardian Laboratories

00332
Biocraft Laboratories, Inc.

00338
Baxter Healthcare Corporation

00338
Clintec Nutrition

00346
Ciba Vision Care

00348
Medtech Laboratories, Inc.

00349
Parmed Pharmaceuticals Inc.

00362
Novocol Chemical Mfr. Co.

00364
Schein Pharmaceutical, Inc.

00372
Scot-Tussin Pharmacal Co., Inc

00374
Lyne laboratories

00377
Pal-Pak, Inc.

00378
Mylan Pharmaceuticals

00386
Gebauer Chemical Company

00394
Mericon Industries, Inc.

00395
Humco Laboratory,Inc.

00396
Milex Products, Inc.

00398
C & M Pharmacal, Inc.

00402
Steris Laboratories Inc.

00418
Pasadena Research Labs

00421
The Fielding Company

00433
Research Industries Corp.

00436
Century Pharmaceuticals, Inc.

00444
Scrip, Inc.

00451
Muro Pharmaceutical, Inc.

00454
Lexis Pharmaceuticals Inc.

00456
Forest Pharmaceutical, Inc.

00462
Pharmaderm

00463
C. O. Truxton Inc.

00466
Macsil, Inc.

00469
Lyphomed

00472
National Pharmaceutical Mfr.

00477
Obetrol Pharmaceuticals

00482
Kenwood Laboratories

00485
Edwards Pharmaceuticals Inc.

00486
Beach Pharmaceuticals

00487
Nephron Corporation

00496
Ferndale Laboratories, Inc.

00502
Genentech, Inc.

00514
Dow B. Hickam, Inc.

00516
Glenwood Inc.

00517
American Regent

00521
Chesebrough-Pond's, Inc.

00524
Boots Pharmaceuticals, Inc.

00527
The Lannett Co., Inc.

00534
Health & Medical Techniques

00536
Rugby Labs., Inc.

00537
Spencer-Mead, Inc.

00539
American Urologicals, Inc.

00548
I.M.S. Ltd.

00551
The Seatrace Company

00554
Pharmakon Laboratories, Inc.

00555
Barr Laboratories, Inc.

00556
H.R. Cenci Labs., Inc.

00563
Bock Pharmacal Company

00573
Whitehall Laboratories

00574
Paddock Laboratories

00575
Baker Cummins Pharm., Inc.

00585
Fisons Corp.

00586
Heather Drug Company Inc.

00588
Keene Pharmaceuticals Inc.

00590
DuPont Pharmaceuticals

00591
Danbury Pharmacal

00597
Boehringer Ingelheim, Inc.

00598
Approved Pharmaceuticals Corp

00601
KabiVitrum, Inc.

00615
Vangard Labs, Inc.

00619
Walker Pharmacal Company

00641
Elkins-Sinn, Inc.

00642
Everett Laboratories, Inc.

00659
Circle Pharmaceuticals, Inc.

00663
Pfizer Laboratories

00665
International Laboratories

00677
United Research Laboratories

00684
Primedics Laboratories

00686
Raway Pharmacal, Inc.

00689
Daniels Pharmaceuticals, Inc.

00713
G & W Labs.

00725
Bolar Pharmaceutical Company

00729
Fidelity Halsom

00731
Alto Pharmaceuticals, Inc.

00737
Life Labs

00741
Walker, Corp and Co., Inc.

00744
Daywell Laboratories Corp.

00766
SmithKline Beecham Con Brands

00777
Dista Products Co.

00781
Geneva Marsam

00785
UAD Laboratories, Inc.

00803
Eclipse

00813
Pharmics Icorporated

00814
Interstate Drug Exchange

00822
Boots Laboratories

00832
Pharmaceutical Basics, Inc.

00832
Pharmaceutical Basics Inc.

00837
Columbia Laboratories, Inc.

00839
H. L. Moore Drug Exchange,Inc.

00879
Halsey Drug Company

00884
Pedinol Pharmacal, Inc.

00904
Major Pharmaceutical Inc.

00905
Schiapparelli Searle

00917
Wesley Pharmacal Co., Inc.

00918
Whittaker General Medical

00927
Pfeiffer Company

00938
Davis and Geck

00944
Hyland Therapeutics

00961
Cook-Waite Laboratories, Inc.

00978
Smith Kline Diagnostics

00995
Pfipharmecs

00998
Webcon Products

01020
Cumberland Packing Corp.

05128
Zila Pharmaceuticals, Inc.

05551
Amgen Inc.

05745
Nastech Pharmaceutical Co.,Inc

08026
Smith+Nephew United

08535
Kyoto Diagnostics, Inc.

08880
Sherwood Medical

10003
A.V.P. Pharmaceuticals, Inc.

10019
Anaquest

10038
Ambix Laboratories Inc.

10106
J. T. Baker, Inc.

10119
Bausch and Lomb, Inc.

10119
Bausch and Lomb Pharm.

10157
Blistex, Inc.

10158
Block Drug Company, Inc.

10160
Bluco Inc./Med. Discnt. Outlet

10223
Cetylite Industries, Inc.

10244
Otis Clapp & Son, Inc.

10244
Buffington

10310
Commerce Drug Company

10356
Beiersdorf, Inc.

10432
Freeda Vitamins, Inc.

10481
Gordon Laboratories

10486
C. S. Dent & Co. Division

10651
Lavoptik Co., Inc.

10706
Kenneth A. Manne Co.

10712
Marlyn Company Inc.

10719
Maurry Biological Co., Inc.

10742
Mentholatum Co., Inc.

10797
Oakhurst Company

10812
Neutrogena Dermatologies

10888
Advanced Nutrit. Tech. Inc.

10952
Recsei Laboratories

10956
Reese Chemical Co.

10960
Republic Drug Company

10961
Requa

10974
Pegasus Medical, Inc.

11012
Schaffer Laboratories

11086
Summers Laboratories, Inc.

11089
McGregor Pharmaceuticals, Inc.

11290
Thompson Medical Co.

11299
Torch Laboratories, Inc.

11311
Trimen Laboratories, Inc.

11370
Warner Lambert Consumer Prod.

11414
Willen Drug Co.

11444
W. F. Young, Inc.

11509
Combe Incorporated

11584
International Ethical Labs

11588
DEP Corporation

11704
Survival Technology, Inc.

11720
Super-X Drug Corporation

11808
ION Laboratories, Inc.

11845
Mason Distributors, Inc.

11940
Medco Lab, Inc.

11980
Allergan Americana

12071
Richie Pharmacal Co., Inc.

12120
Wisconsin Pharmacal Co.

12136
Bird Corporation

12463
Abana Pharmaceuticals

12622
Olin Corporation

12758
Mason Pharmaceuticals, Inc.

12843
Glenbrook Labs.

12934
Nion Corporation

14362
Mass. Public Health Bio. Lab.

16500
Miles Inc.

17022
Veratex Corp.

17156
Medi-Physics, Inc.

17204
Miller Pharmacal Group Inc.

17236
Dixon-Shane Inc.

17271
Deseret Medical, Inc.

17314
Alza Corporation

17478
Akorn, Inc.

18393
Lehn & Fink

19458
Eckerd Drug Company

19810
Bristol-Myers Products

19810
Bristol-Myers Oncology Div.

21406
Columbia Laboratories, Inc.

22200
Mennen Company

22840
Greer Laboratories, Inc.

23317
NMC Laboratories

23900
Vicks Health Care Products Div

24208
Pharmafair, Inc.

25077
The Hudson Corporation

25332
Legere Pharmaceuticals, Inc.

25358
Donell DerMedex

25866
Vicks Pharmacy Products Div.

28851
Kendall Company

30103
Randob Laboratories, Ltd.

31280
Becton Dickinson & Company

31795
Fibertone Co.

32954
MiLance Laboratories, Inc.

35470
Gen-King

37000
The Procter and Gamble Co.

38083
Campbell Laboratories

38130
Econo Med Pharmaceuticals, Inc

38137
Spectrum Chemical Mfg. Corp.

38245
Copley Pharmaceutical, Inc.

38697
Berkeley Biologicals

39506
Somerset Pharmaceuticals

39769
SoloPak Laboratories

39769
Smith & Nephew SoloPak

39822
Pharma-Tek, Inc.

41100
Plough, Inc.

41383
LactAid Inc.

41470
Loma Linda Foods, Inc.

42021
Sclavo, Inc.

42987
W. E. Hauck, Inc.

44081
Med-Corp

44087
Serono Laboratories, Inc.

44437
Bolan Pharmaceutical, Inc.

45334
Pharmaceutical Specialties Inc

45565
Med-Derm Pharmaceuticals, Inc.

45809
Shionogi USA

46287
Carolina Medical Products Co.

46500
Rydelle Laboratories

47679
Baxter Healthcare Corporation

47854
Syosset Laboratories Co., Inc.

48017
Hermal Pharmaceutical Labs Inc

48028
Redi-Products Labs, Inc.

48532
Delmont Laboratories, Inc.

48558
Arther, Inc.

48663
Unitek Corporation

48723
Apothecus, Inc.

49072
McGuff Company, Inc.

49158
Thames Pharmacal Co., Inc.

49281
Connaught Laboratories, Inc.

49447
Chattem Consumer Products

49502
Dey Laboratories, Inc.

49669
Alpha Therapeutic Corp.

49692
SmithKline Beecham Con Brands

49727
Vita-Rx Corporation

49731
Sherman Laboratories, Inc.

49884
Par Pharmaceuticals

49938
Jacobus Pharmaceutical Co.

50111
Sidmak Laboratories, Inc.

50185
McHenry Laboratories Inc.

50242
Genentech, Inc.

50272
General Generics, Inc.

50330
Mastar Pharmaceutical Co.

50349
American Therapeutics, Inc.

50361
Merieux Institute, Inc.

50419
Berlex Laboratories, Inc.

50445
Nordisk-USA

50458
Janssen Pharmaceutica, Inc.

50474
Whitby Pharmaceuticals, Inc.

50486
Blairex Labs., Inc.

50520
Optimox Corporation

50694
Seres Laboratories

50732
LuChem Pharaceuticals, Inc.

50893
Westport Pharmaceuticals, Inc.

50914
Iso Tex Diagnostics, Inc.

50924
Boehringer Mannheim Diags.

50930
Parnell Pharmaceuticals, Inc.

50962
Xactdose, Inc.

51079
UDL Laboratories, Inc.

51081
Nutripharm Laboratories, Inc.

51189
T.E. Williams Pharmaceuticals

51201
American Dermal Corp.

51244
I.C.P. Pharmaceuticals

51285
Duramed Pharmaceuticals, Inc.

51301
Great Southern Laboratories

51309
Quad Phamaceuticals, Inc.

51318
Stellar Pharmacal Corp.

51353
The Sanitube Company

51432
Harber Pharmaceutical Co.

51479
Dura Pharmaceuticals

51552
Gallipot Inc.

51626
US Products, Inc.

51641
Alra Laboratories, Inc.

51655
Pharmaceutical Corporation

51662
Healthfirst Corporation

51672
Taro Pharmaceuticals U.S.A,Inc

51687
T/I Pharmaceuticals

51801
Nomax, Inc.

51803
Anbex, Inc.

52041
Dayton Laboratories,Inc.

52152
Amide Pharmaceuticals, Inc.

52189
Invamed Incorporated

52238
Optopics Laboratories, Corp.

52268
Braintree Laboratories Inc.

52273
Quantum Pharmics, Ltd.

52311
Biosearch Medical Products Inc

52446
Qualitest Products Inc.

52489
Chemi-Tech Laboratories

52544
Watson Laboratories

52555
Martec Pharmaceutical, Inc.

52584
General Inj. & Vac., Inc.

52604
Jones Medical Industries

52747
US Pharmaceutical Corp.

52761
GenDerm Corporation

52836
Milance Laboratories, Inc.

52891
Medical Market Specialties

53014
Adams Laboratories

53118
Millgood Laboratories, Inc.

53124
Praxis Biologics, Inc.

53159
Palisades Pharmaceuticals Inc.

53191
Bio-Tech

53258
VHA Supply Company

53335
Tyson & Associates, Inc.

53385
Standard Drug Company

53443
Americal Pharmaceutical Inc.

53489
Mutual Pharmaceutical Co.,Inc.

53506
Redi-Med, Inc.

53885
Lifescan

53905
Cetus

54022
Vitaline Corporation

54027
Spectra Pharmaceutical Service

54274
Best Generics

54323
Flander Incorporated

54391
R & D Laboratories, Inc.

54429
Chase Laboratories

54482
Sigma-Tau Pharmaceuticals

54569
Allscripts

54627
ValMed, Inc.

54686
Ethitek Pharmaceuticals

54765
GynoPharma Laboratories

54807
R.I.D. Inc., Distributor

54891
Vision Pharmaceuticals Inc.

54977
Scripts America Corp.

55077
Inter-Hermes Pharma, Inc.

55084
Doctor's Pharmacy, Inc.

55326
Curatek (Limited Partnership)

55390
Loch Pharmaceuticals

55425
Dal-Med Pharmaceuticals, Inc.

55437
Nelson Pharmaceutical,Inc.

55499
Numark Laboratories, Inc.

55505
Kramer Laboratories, Inc.

55515
Oclassen

55516
Dyna Pharm, Inc.

55559
Calgon Vestal Laboratories

55566
Ferring Laboratories, Inc.

55953
Novopharm, Inc.

57267
Summit Medical Products, Inc.

57284
Galen Pharma Inc.

57317
Fujisawa SmithKline Corp.

57506
American Drug Industries, Inc.

57665
Enzon, Inc.

58177
Ethex Corporation

58178
US Bioscience

58337
Berna Products Corporation

58468
Genzyme Corporation

60077
Young Dental

60104
Pioneer Pharmaceuticals Inc.

72363
Brimss Incorparated

74300
Leeming/Pacquin

74312
Nature's Bounty, Inc.

74684
Goody's Manufacturing Corp.

76611
Navaco Laboratories

76660
Richardson-Vicks, Inc.

79511
Triton Consumer Products Inc.

87900
Menley and James Laboratories

89169
Canaan Laboratories

89709

Amcon Laboratories

99207
Medicis Dermatologicals, Inc.

12463
Abana Pharmaceuticals
230 Oxmoor Circle, Ste. 1111
Birmingham, AL 35209
205-942-1808

00074
Abbott Laboratories
One Abbott Road
Abbott Park, IL 60064
708-937-6100

Acme United Corporation
75 Kings Highway Cutoff
Fairfield, CT 06430
203-332-7330

53014
Adams Laboratories
14801 Sovereign Road
Ft. Worth, TX 76155-2645
817-545-7791

Adolphs
Ragu Foods Inc.
75 Merritt Blvd.
Trumbull, CT 06611
203-381-3500

00013
Adria Laboratories
P.O. Box 16529
Columbus, OH 43216-6529
614-764-8100

Advanced Care Products Div.
Route 202
Raritan, NJ 08869
201-524-0171

10888
Advanced Nutrit. Tech. Inc.
P.O. Box 3225
Elizabeth, NJ 07207
201-354-2740

17478
Akorn, Inc.
100 Akorn Drive
Abita Springs, LA 70420
504-893-9300

00065
Alcon Laboratories, Inc.
6201 South Freeway
Ft. Worth, TX 76134
817-293-0450

Alk America
132 Research Dr.
Milford, CT 06460
203-877-4782

00173
Allen & Hanburys
5 Moore Drive
Research Triangle Pk., NC 27709
919-248-2500

00299
Allercreme
P.O. Box 6600
Ft. Worth, TX 76115
817-293-0450

11980
Allergan Americana
Homigueros, PR 00660
714-752-4500

00023
Allergan Pharmaceuticals
2525 DuPont Drive
Irvine, CA 92714-1599
714-752-4500

49669
Alpha Therapeutic Corp.
5555 Valley Blvd.
Los Angeles, CA 90032
213-225-2221

51641
Alra Laboratories, Inc.
3850 Clearview Court
Gurnee, IL 60031
708-244-9440

00731
Alto Pharmaceuticals, Inc.
P.O. Box 1910
Landolakes, FL 34639-1910
813-949-7464

Alva Laboratories
6625 Avondale Ave.
Chicago, IL 60631
312-792-0200

17314
Alza Corporation
950 Page Mill Road
Palo Alto, CA 94304
415-494-5000

10038
Ambix Laboratories Inc.
210 Orchard Street
East Rutherford, NJ 07073
201-939-2200

89709
Amcon Laboratories
40 N. Rock Hill Rd.
St. Louis, MO 63119
314-961-5758

53443
Americal Pharm. Inc.
1340 N. Jefferson St.
Anaheim, CA 92807
504-893-9300

51201
American Dermal Corp.
P.O. Box 900
Plumsteadville, PA 18949-0900
215-766-2110

57506
American Drug Industries
8510-20 S. Perry Ave.
Chicago, IL 60621
312-667-7070

00517
American Regent
1 Luitpold Drive
Shirley, NY 11967
516-924-4000

50349
American Therapeutics, Inc.
83 Carlough Rd.
Bohemia, NY 11716
516-563-1830

00539
American Urologicals, Inc.
7881 Hollywood Blvd., Suite 4
Pembroke Pines, FL 33024
305-651-6575

00193
Ames Company
P.O. Box 70
Elkhart, IN 46515
219-264-8111

05551
Amgen Inc.
1900 Oak Terrace Lane
Thousand Oaks, CA 91320-1789
805-499-5725

*A Pharmaceutical Labeler Code appears before the address for each company. This code has been added as an aid in the identification of drug products.

52152
Amide Pharmaceuticals, Inc.
101 East Main Street
Little Falls, NJ 07424
201-890-1440

10019
Anaquest
2005 W. Beltline Hwy.
Madison, WI 53173
608-273-0019

51803
Anbex, Inc.
15 W. 75th Street
New York, NY 10023
212-556-3223

Apothecary Products, Inc.
11531 Rupp Drive
Burnsville, MN 55337
612-890-1940

00003
Apothecon
P.O. Box 4000
Princeton, NJ 08543-4000
609-987-6800

48723
Apothecus, Inc.
132 South Street
Oyster Bay, NY 11771
516-624-8200

00598
Approved Pharm. Corp.
1643 E. Genesee St.
P.O. Box 6669
Syracuse, NY 13217-6669
315-478-2121

00275
Arco Pharmaceuticals, Inc.
90 Orville Drive
Bohemia, NY 11716
516-567-9500

00053
Armour Pharm. Co.
P.O. Box 511
Kankakee, IL 60901
215-628-6085

48558
Arther, Inc.
P.O. Box 1455
W. Caldwell, NJ 07007
201-263-2050

00225
B. F. Ascher and Company
15501 West 109th St.
Lenexa, KS 66219
913-888-1880

00186
Astra Pharmaceutical Prod.
50 Otis
Westborough, MA 01581
508-366-1100

10003
A.V.P. Pharmaceuticals, Inc.
9829 Main Street, P.O. Box N
Clarence, NY 14031
716-688-9676

10106
J. T. Baker, Inc.
222 Red School Lane
Phillipsburg, NJ 08865
201-859-2151

00575
Baker Cummins Pharm., Inc.
8800 Northwest 36th Street
Miami, FL 33178-2404
305-590-2282

00304
J.J. Balan, Inc.
5725 Foster Ave.
Brooklyn, NY 11234
718-251-8663

00555
Barr Laboratories, Inc.
2 Quaker Road
Pomona, NY 10970
914-362-1100

10119
Bausch and Lomb Pharm.
1400 North Goodman Street
Rochester, NY 14692
716-338-6000

00338
Baxter Healthcare Corp.
1425 Lakecook Rd. LC 1-3
Deerfield, IL 60015
708-940-5000

00486
Beach Pharmaceuticals
P.O. Box 128
Conestee, SC 29636
813-837-5044

31280
Becton Dickinson & Co.
One Becton Drive
Franklin Lakes, NJ 07417-1881
201-848-6900

10356
Beiersdorf, Inc.
P.O. Box 5529
S. Norwalk, CT 06856
203-853-8008

38697
Berkeley Biologicals
1831 Second St.
Berkeley, CA 94710
415-843-6846

50419
Berlex Laboratories, Inc.
300 Fairfield Rd.
Wayne, NJ 07470
201-694-4100

58337
Berna Products Corporation
4216 Ponce De Leon Blvd.
Coral Gables, FL 33146
305-443-2900

54274
Best Generics
19589 N.E. 10th Avenue
North Miami Beach, FL
33179-3501
305-653-2378

00283
Beutlich, Inc.
7149 North Austin Avenue
Niles, IL 60648
708-647-8110

00332
Biocraft Laboratories, Inc.
18-01 River Road
Fair Lawn, NJ 07410
201-703-0400

00719
Bioline Labs
1900 W. Commercial Blvd.
Ft. Lauderdale, FL 33309
305-772-2332

Biomerica, Inc.
1533 Monrovia Avenue
Newport Beach, CA 92663
714-645-2111

52311
Biosearch Medical Products
P.O. Box 1700
Somerville, NJ 00876
201-722-5000

53191
Bio-Tech
Fayetteville, AR 72701

12136
Bird Corporation
3101 E. Alejo Road
Palm Springs, CA 92262
714-327-1571

00165
Blaine Company, Inc.
2700 Dixie Highway
Fort Mitchell, KY 41017
606-341-9437

00154
Blair Laboratories
100 Connecticut Ave.
Norwalk, CT 06856
203-853-0123

50486
Blairex Labs., Inc.
4810 Tecumseh Ln.
P.O. Box 15190
Evansville, IN 47716-0190
812-476-8077

10157
Blistex, Inc.
1800 Swift Drive
Oak Brook, IL 60521
708-571-2870

10158
Block Drug Company, Inc.
257 Cornelison Ave.
Jersey City, NJ 07302
201-434-3000

10160
Bluco Inc./Med. Discnt. Outlet
14849 W. McNichols
Detroit, MI 48235
313-273-0322

00563
Bock Pharmacal Company
P.O. Box 8519
St. Louis, MO 63126-0519
314-343-0994

00597
Boehringer Ingelheim, Inc.
90 East Ridge
Ridgefield, CT 06877
203-798-9988

50924
Boehringer Mannheim Diags.
9115 Hague Rd.
Indianapolis, IN 46250-0100
317-845-2000

Boehringer Mannheim Pharmaceuticals
15204 Omega Drive
Rockville, MD 20850-3241
301-990-2700

44437
Bolan Pharmaceutical, Inc.
415 W. Pipeline
Hurst, TX 76053
817-589-7061

00725
Bolar Pharmaceutical Co.
33 Ralph Avenue
Copiague, NY 11726-0030
516-842-8383

00048
Boots Company
300 Tri-State Internat. Center
Lincolnshire, IL 60069-4415
708-405-7400

00222
Boyle and Company Pharm.
1030 S. Arroyo Parkway
Pasadena, CA 91105
818-441-0284

52268
Braintree Laboratories Inc.
60 Columbian, P.O. Box 361
Braintree, MA 02184
617-843-2202

72363
Brimms Incorporated
425 Fillmore Ave.
Tonawanda, NY 14150
716-694-7100

19810
Bristol-Myers Oncology Div.
P.O. Box 4755
Evansville, IN 47721-0001
812-429-5000

19810
Bristol-Myers Products
1350 Liberty Ave.
Hillside, NJ 07205
201-851-2400

00003
Bristol-Myers Squibb Co.
P.O. Box 4000
Princeton, NJ 08543-4000
609-921-4000

00087
Bristol-Myers U.S. Pharm.
2404 West Pennsylvania St.
Evansville, IN 47721-0001
812-429-5000

00248
Brown Pharmaceutical Co.
3300 Hyland Ave.
Costa Mesa, CA 92626
213-389-1394

10244
Buffington
115 Shawmut Rd.
Canton, MA 02021-9160
617-821-5400

00081
Burroughs Wellcome Co.
3030 Cornwallis Road
Research Triangle Pk, NC 27709
919-248-3000

00398
C & M Pharmacal, Inc.
1721 Maple Lane
Hazel Park, MI 48030-2696
313-548-7846

55559
Calgon Vestal Laboratories
P.O. Box 147
St. Louis, MO 63166-0147
314-535-1810

00147
Camall Company, Inc.
P.O. Box 307
Romeo, MI 48065-0307
313-752-9683

38083
Campbell Laboratories
P.O. Box 812 FDR Station
New York, NY 10150
212-688-7684

J.R. Carlson Labs, Inc.
15 College Drive
Arlington Heights, IL 60004
708-255-1600

00086
Carnrick Laboratories, Inc.
65 Horse Hill Road
Cedar Knolls, NJ 07927
201-267-2670

46287
Carolina Medical Products
P.O. Box 147
Farmville, NC 27828
919-753-7111

00164
Carter Products
One-Half Acre Road
Cranbury, NJ 08512
609-655-6000

00556
H.R. Cenci Labs., Inc.
1420 Tuolumne St.
P.O. Box 12524
Fresno, CA 93778-2524
209-268-4401

00268
Center Laboratories
35 Channel Drive
Port Washington, NY 11050
516-767-1800

00131
Central Pharmaceuticals
120 East Third Street
P.O. Box 328
Seymour, IN 47274-9985
812-522-3915

00436
Century Pharmaceuticals
10377 Hague Road
Indianapolis, IN 46256
317-849-4210

53905
Cetus
1400 53rd Street
Emeryville, CA 94608
415-420-3300

10223
Cetylite Industries, Inc.
9051 River Road
P.O. Box CN6
Pennsauken, NJ 08110
609-665-6111

54429
Chase Laboratories
280 Chestnut Street
Newark, NJ 07105-1598
201-589-8181

49447
Chattem Consumer Products
1715 W. 38th Street
Chattanooga, TN 37409
615-821-4571

00521
Chesebrough-Pond's, Inc.
33 Benedict Place
Greenwich, CT 06830
203-661-2000

00083
Ciba Consumer Pharm.
Raritan Plaza III
Edison, NJ 08837
201-225-6000

00083
Ciba Pharmaceutical
556 Morris Avenue
Summit, NJ 07901
201-277-5000

00346
Ciba Vision Care
2910 Amwiler Court
Atlanta, GA 30360
404-448-1200

00659
Circle Pharmaceuticals, Inc.
10377 Hague Road
Indianapolis, IN 46256
317-842-5463

City Chemical Corporation
132 W. 22nd Street
New York, NY 10011
212-929-2723

10244
Otis Clapp & Son, Inc.
115 Shawmut Road
Canton, MA 02021-9160
617-868-1950

00338
Clintec Nutrition
Three Parkway North, Ste. 500
Deerfield, IL 60015
708-940-5000

00126
Colgate-Hoyt
1 Colgate Way
Canton, MA 02021
617-769-6850

Colgate-Palmolive Co.
300 Park Avenue
New York, NY 10022
212-310-2000

Collagen Corporation
2500 Faber Place
Palo Alto, CA 94303
415-856-0200

21406
Columbia Laboratories, Inc.
4000 Hollywood Blvd.
3rd Fl South
Hollywood, FL 33021
305-944-3666

11509
Combe Incorporated
1101 Westchester Ave.
White Plains, NY 10604
914-694-5454

10310
Commerce Drug Company
565 Broad Hollow Road
Farmingdale, NY 11735
516-293-7070

49281
Connaught Laboratories
Route 611, P.O. Box 187
Swiftwater, PA 18370-0187
717-839-7187

00223
Consolidated Midland Corp.
195 E. Main St.
Brewster, NY 10509
914-279-6108

00003
ConvaTec Research/ Development
P.O. Box 5254
Princeton, NJ 08543-5254
201-359-9200

00961
Cook-Waite Laboratories
90 Park Avenue
New York, NY 10016
212-907-2712

CooperBiomedical, Inc.
One Technology Court
Malvern, PA 19355
215-251-2000

CooperVision
3495 Winton Place
Rochester, NY 14623-2807
408-434-7000

38245
Copley Pharmaceutical, Inc.
25 John Road
Canton, MA 02021
617-268-1208

01020
Cumberland Packing Corp.
#2 Cumberland St.
Brooklyn, NY 11205
914-835-4826

55326
Curatek (Limited Partnership)
1965 Pratt Boulevard
Elk Grove Village, IL 60004
708-806-7680

00161
Cutter Biological
400 Morgan Lane
West Haven, CT 06516-4175
203-937-2000

00161
Cutter Medical
2200 Powell St.
Emeryville, CA 94662
415-420-4000

55425
Dal-Med Pharmaceuticals
P.O. Box 1545
Dania, FL 33004
305-989-5005

00591
Danbury Pharmacal
12 Stoneleigh Avenue
Carmel, NY 10512
914-225-1700

00689
Daniels Pharmaceuticals
2517 25th Avenue North
St. Petersburg, FL 33713
813-323-5151

00938
Davis and Geck
One Cyanamid Plaza
Wayne, NJ 07470
201-831-2000

52041
Dayton Laboratories, Inc.
3307 N.W. 74th Ave.
Miami, FL 33122
305-594-0988

00744
Daywell Laboratories Corp.
78 Unquowa Place
Fairfield, CT 06430
203-255-3154

48532
Delmont Laboratories, Inc.
P.O. Box 269
Swarthmore, PA 19081
215-543-3365

00316
Del-Ray Laboratory, Inc.
27-20th Avenue N.W.
Birmingham, AL 35215
205-853-8247

00295
Denison Laboratories, Inc.
60 Dunnell Lane
Pawtucket, RI 02860
401-723-5500

10486
C. S. Dent & Co. Division
317 E. Eighth St.
Cincinnati, OH 45202
513-241-1677

11588
DEP Corporation
2101 East Via Arado
Rancho Dominguez, CA 90220
213-604-0777

00066
Dermik Laboratories, Inc.
920A Harvest Drive, Ste. 200
Blue Bell, PA 19422
215-540-8300

17271
Deseret Medical, Inc.
9450 South State
Sandy, UT 84070
801-255-6851

49502
Dey Laboratories, Inc.
2751 Napa Valley Corp. Dr.
Napa, CA 94558
707-224-3200

00777
Dista Products Co.
Bldg. 11/3 Lilly Corp. Center
Indianapolis, IN 46285
317-276-4000

17236
Dixon-Shane Inc.
256 Geiger Road
Philadelphia, PA 19115
215-673-7770

55084
Doctor's Pharmacy, Inc.
2275 Cassens Drive
Fenton, MO 63026
314-349-1600

25358
Donell DerMedex
342 Madison Ave., Ste. 1422
New York, NY 10173

00261
Drug Industries Co.
3237 Hilton Road
Ferndale, MI 48220
313-547-3784

00217
Dunhall Pharm.
P.O. Box 100
Gravette, AR 72736
501-787-5232

00094
DuPont Critical Care
Barley Mill Plaza
P.O. Box 80027
Wilmington, DE 19880-0027
302-892-1688

00590
DuPont Pharmaceuticals
Barley Mill Pl P26-2172
P.O. Box 80026
Wilmington, DE 19880-0026
302-892-7050

51479
Dura Pharmaceuticals
11175 Flintkote Ave.
San Diego, CA 92121-1203
619-457-2553

51285
Duramed Pharm.
5040 Lester Road
Cincinnati, OH 45213
513-731-9900

55516
Dyna Pharm, Inc.
P.O. Box 2141
Del Mar, CA 92014-2141
619-792-9523

Eagle Vision, Inc.
6485 Poplar Ave.
Memphis, TN 38119
901-767-3937

Eaton Medical Corporation
2288 Dunn Ave.
Memphis, TN 38114
901-744-8024

19458
Eckerd Drug Company
8333 Bryan Dairy Rd.
P.O. Box 4689
Clearwater, FL 34618
813-397-7461

38130
Econo Med Pharm.
4305 Sartin Rd.
Burlington, NC 27217-7522
919-226-1091

00485
Edwards Pharmaceuticals
111 Mulberry St.
Ripley, MS 38663
601-837-8182

00641
Elkins-Sinn, Inc.
555 East Lancaster Pike
St. Davids, PA 19087
215-971-5539

57665
Enzon, Inc.
40 Cragwood Road
South Plainfield, NJ 07080
201-668-1800

58177
Ethex Corporation
10888 Metro Court
St. Louis, MO 63043-2413
314-567-3307

54686
Ethitek Pharmaceuticals
7855 Gross Point Road
Skokie, IL 60077
708-675-6611

00642
Everett Laboratories, Inc.
76 Franklin Street
East Orange, NJ 07017-3004
201-674-8455

00496
Ferndale Laboratories, Inc.
780 W. Eight Mile Road
Ferndale, MI 48220-1218
313-548-0900

55566
Ferring Laboratories, Inc.
75 Montebello Road
Suffern, NY 10901
914-368-2244

31795
Fibertone Co.
6324 Ferris Sq.
San Diego, CA 92121
619-452-3100

00729
Fidelity Halsom
1330 Farr Drive at Stanley
Dayton, OH 45404
513-224-7636

00421
The Fielding Company
94 Weldon Parkway
Maryland Heights, MO 63043
314-567-5462

Fiske
14 Yale Drive
New York, NY 10956

00235
Fisons Consumer Health
P.O. Box 1212
Rochester, NY 14603-1212
716-475-9000

00585
Fisons Corp.
P.O. Box 1766
Rochester, NY 14623
716-475-9000

54323
Flander Incorporated
P.O. Box 39143
Charleston, SC 29047
803-571-6768

00132
C. B. Fleet Co., Inc.
4615 Murray Place
Lynchburg, VA 24506
804-528-4000

00256
Fleming & Co.
1600 Fenpark Drive
Fenton, MO 63026
314-343-8200

00288
Fluoritab Corp.
P.O. Box 507
Temperance, MI 48182-0507
313-847-3985

00456
Forest Pharmaceutical, Inc.
2510 Metro Blvd.
Maryland Heights, MO 63043-9979
314-569-3610

00168
E. Fougera and Co.
60 Baylis Road
Melville, NY 11747
516-454-6996

10432
Freeda Vitamins, Inc.
36 East 41st St.
New York, NY 10017-6203
212-685-4980

57317
Fujisawa SmithKline Corp.
3 Parkway North Center
Deerfield, IL 60015-2548
708-317-0600

00713
G & W Labs.
111 Coolidge St.
South Plainfield, NJ 07080
201-753-2000

57284
Galen Pharma Inc.
2905 MacArthur Blvd.
Northbrook, IL 60062
708-498-0045

51552
Gallipot Inc.
2401 Pilot Knob Rd.
St. Paul, MN 55120
612-681-9517

Gambro Hospal, Inc.
1185 Oak St.
Lakewood, CO 80215

00386
Gebauer Chemical Company
9410 St. Catherine Ave.
Cleveland, OH 44104
216-271-5252

00028
Geigy Pharmaceuticals
556 Morris Avenue
Summit, NJ 07901
201-277-5000

52761
GenDerm Corporation
425 Huehl Road
Northbrook, IL 60062
708-564-5435

00502
Genentech, Inc.
460 Point San Bruno Blvd.
South San Francisco, CA
94080
415-266-1000

50272
General Generics, Inc.
P.O. Box 510
Oxford, MS 38655
601-234-0130

52584
General Inj. & Vac., Inc.
U.S. Highway 52/P.O. Box 9
Bastian, VA 24314-0009
703-688-4121

00302
Genetco, Inc.
1 Baiting Place Rd.
Farmingdale, NY
11735-5002
516-293-2214

00781
Geneva Marsam
2599 W. Midway Blvd.
P.O. Box 469
Broomfield, CO 80038-0469
303-466-2400

35470
Gen-King
80-25 Cornish Ave.
Elmhurst, NY 11373
718-478-8800

58468
Genzyme Corporation
One Kendall Square
Cambridge, MA 02139
617-252-7500

00249
Geriatric Pharm. Corp.
P.O. Box 99
Butler, WI 53007
414-272-2552

00173
Glaxo, Inc.
Five Moore Dr.
Research Triangle Pk, NC
27709
919-248-2100

12843
Glenbrook Labs.
90 Park Avenue 17th Floor
New York, NY 10016
212-907-2000

00516
Glenwood Inc.
83 N. Summit St.
Tenafly, NJ 07670
201-569-0050

00182
Goldline Laboratories, Inc.
1900 W. Commercial Blvd.
Ft. Lauderdale, FL 33324
305-491-4002

74684
Goody's Manufacturing Corp.
436 Salt Street
Winston-Salem, NC 27108
919-723-1831

10481
Gordon Laboratories
State and Parkview Roads
Upper Darby, PA
19082-1694
215-789-3055

Graham-Field, Inc.
400 Rabro Drive East
Hauppauge, NY 11788
516-582-5900

00152
Gray Pharmaceutical Co.
100 Connecticut Ave.
Norwalk, CT 06856
203-853-0123

51301
Great Southern Laboratories
10863 Rockley Road
Houston, TX 77099
713-530-3077

22840
Greer Laboratories, Inc.
P.O. Box 800
Lenoir, NC 28645-0800
704-754-5327

00327
Guardian Laboratories
P.O. Box 2500
Smithtown, NY 11787-2500
516-273-0900

Gulf Bio-Systems, Inc.
1415 Michigan Street
Adrian, MI 49221-3445
214-386-0442

54765
GynoPharma Laboratories
50 Division Street
Somerville, NJ 08876
201-725-3100

00879
Halsey Drug Company
1827 Pacific Street
Brooklyn, NY 11233
718-467-7500

51432
Harber Pharmaceutical Co.
350 Meadowlands Pkwy.
Secaucus, NJ 07094
201-348-3700

43797
W.E. Hauck, Inc.
P.O. Box 1065
Alpharetta, GA 30239-1065
404-475-4758

HDC Corporation
2109 O'Toole Ave.
San Jose, CA 95131
408-954-1909

00534
Health & Medical Techniques
P.O. Box A
Rahway, NJ 07065-1175
201-382-9300

51662
Healthfirst Corporation
P.O. Box 279
Edmonds, WA 98020
206-771-5733

00586
Heather Drug Company Inc.
1 Fellowship Road
Cherry Hill, NJ 08003
609-424-3663

Helena Laboratories
P.O. Box 572
Beaumont, TX 77704-0752
409-842-3714

00023
Herbert Laboratories
18600 Von Karman Avenue
Irvine, CA 92713-9534
714-955-6200

48017
Hermal Pharmaceutical Labs
163 Delaware Avenue
Delmar, NY 12460
518-475-0175

00514
Dow B. Hickam, Inc.
P.O. Box 2006
Sugarland, TX 77478
713-491-1900

Hirsch Industries, Inc.
4912 West Broad St., Ste. 201
Richmond, VA 23230
804-355-4500

00039
Hoechst-Roussel Pharm.
Route 202-206, P.O. Box 2500
Somerville, NJ 08876-1258
201-231-2000

Holles Laboratories
30 Forest Notch
Cohasset, MA 02025-1198
617-383-0741

00118
Hollister-Stier
P.O. Box 3145
Spokane, WA 99220-3153
509-489-5656

25077
The Hudson Corporation
Bohemia, NY 11716

00395
Humco Laboratory, Inc.
P.O. Box 2550
Texarkana, TX 75503
903-793-3174

00944
Hyland Therapeutics
550 North Brand Blvd.
Glendale, CA 91203
818-956-3200

00011
Hynson, Westcott & Dunning
250 Schilling Circle
Cockeysville, MD 21030
301-771-0100

00314
Hyrex Pharmaceuticals
P.O. Box 18385
Memphis, TN 38181-0385
901-794-9050

00310
ICI Pharma
Concord Pike and Murphy Road
Wilmington, DE 19897
302-886-2231

00187
ICN Pharmaceuticals, Inc.
3300 Hyland Avenue
Costa Mesa, CA 92626
714-545-0100

51244
I.C.P. Pharmaceuticals
P.O. Box 294
Cudahy, WI 53110
414-521-4647

Immuno U.S., Inc.
1200 Parkdale Rd.
Rochester, MI 48063
313-652-7872

00548
I.M.S. Ltd.
1886 Santa Anita Ave.
South El Monte, CA 91733
818-442-6757

55077
Inter-Hermes Pharma, Inc.
4 Reuten Drive
Closter, NJ 07624
201-784-1436

11584
International Ethical Labs
Reparto Metropolitano
Rio Piedras, PR 00921
809-765-3510

00665
International Laboratories
901 Sawyer Road
Marietta, GA 30062
404-578-2007

Interpro
P.O. Box 1823
Haverhill, MA 01831
508-373-2438

00814
Interstate Drug Exchange
1500 New Horizons Blvd.
Amityville, NY 11701-1130
516-957-8300

52189
Invamed Incorporated
12 Dwight Place
Fairfield, NJ 07006
201-575-3303

00258
Inwood Laboratories
300 Prospect Street
Inwood, NY 11696
516-371-1155

00058
Iolab Pharmaceuticals
500 Iolab Drive
Claremont, CA 91711
714-624-2020

11808
ION Laboratories, Inc.
7171 Pebble Drive
Fort Worth, TX 76118
817-589-7257

50914
Iso Tex Diagnostics, Inc.
Box 909
Friendswood, TX 77546
713-482-1231

49938
Jacobus Pharmaceutical Co.
37 Cleveland Lane
Princeton, NJ 08540
609-921-7447

50458
Janssen Pharmaceutica, Inc.
40 Kingsbridge Road
Piscataway, NJ 08854
201-524-9100

00252
JMI-Canton Pharm.
119 Schroyer Ave., S.W.
Canton, OH 44702
216-456-2873

Johnson & Johnson Medical, Inc.
P.O. Box 130
Arlington, TX 76140-0130
817-465-3141

52604
Jones Medical Industries
P.O. Box 46903
St. Louis, MO 63146-6903
314-432-7557

KabiVitrum
See Clintec

00588
Keene Pharmaceuticals Inc.
P.O. Box 7
Keene, TX 76059-0007
817-645-8083

28851
Kendall Company
One Federal Steet
Boston, MA 02110-2003
617-574-7000

00482
Kenwood Laboratories
383 Rt. 46 West
Fairfield, NJ 07006-2402
201-882-1505

00085
Key Pharmaceuticals
Galloping Hill Road
Kenilworth, NJ 07033
201-298-4000

Kingswood Laboratories
1119 Third Ave. S.W.
P.O. Box 567
Carmel, IN 46032
317-846-7452

00098
Kirkman Sales Company
P.O. Box 1009
Wilsonville, OR 97070
503-694-1600

00044
Knoll Pharmaceuticals
30 N. Jefferson Rd.
Whippany, NJ 07981
201-887-8300

00224
Konsyl Pharmaceuticals
4200 South Hulen Street
Fort Worth, TX 76109
817-763-8011

55505
Kramer Laboratories, Inc.
8778 S.W. 8th Street
Miami, FL 33174-9990
305-223-1287

08535
Kyoto Diagnostics, Inc.
P.O. Box 800457
Houston, TX 77280-0457
219-925-6719

41383
LactAid Inc.
P.O. Box 111
Pleasantville, NJ 08232
609-653-6100

00224
Lafayette Pharmaceuticals
P.O. Box 4499
Lafayette, IN 47903
317-447-3129

00527
The Lannett Co., Inc.
9000 State Rd.
Philadelphia, PA 19136
215-333-9000

00277
Laser, Inc.
P.O. Box 905
2000 N. Main St.
Crown Point, IN 46307
219-663-1165

10651
Lavoptik Co., Inc.
661 Western Ave. N.
St. Paul, MN 55103
612-489-1351

00005
Lederle Laboratories
North Middletown Road
Pearl River, NY 10965-1299
914-732-5000

74300
Leeming/Pacquin
235 East 42nd St.
New York, NY 10017
212-573-3131

25332
Legere Pharmaceuticals, Inc.
7326 E. Evans Rd.
Scottsdale, AZ 85260
602-991-4033

19200
Lehn & Fink
225 Summit Avenue
Montvale, NJ 07645
201-573-5700

P. Leiner Nutritional Products
1845 W. 205th St.
Torrance, CA 90501
213-328-9610

Lemar Laboratories, Inc.
10 Perimeter Way
N.W. Bldg. B-200
Atlanta, GA 30339
404-952-3922

00093
Lemmon Company
P.O. Box 30
Sellersville, PA 18960
215-723-5544

00454
Lexis Pharmaceuticals Inc.
100 Congress Ave., Suite 400
Austin, TX 78701
512-474-7724

00737
Life Labs
9380 San Fernando Rd.
Sun Valley, CA 91532
213-875-0330

Life's Finest
P.O. Box 5610
Clearwater, FL 33518-5610
813-536-7650

53885
Lifescan
2443 Wyandotte Street
Mountainview, CA
94043-2313

00002
Eli Lilly and Co.
Bldg. 11/3 Lilly Corp. Center
Indianapolis, IN 46285
317-276-2000

55390
Loch Pharmaceuticals
270 Northfield Rd.
P.O. Box 46568
Bedford, OH 44146
516-742-7040

41470
Loma Linda Foods, Inc.
11503 Pierce St.
Riverside, CA 92505
714-687-7800

00273
Lorvic Corporation
8810 Frost Ave.
St. Louis, MO 63134-1095
314-524-7444

50732
LuChem Pharmaceuticals
8910 Linwood Ave.
P.O. Box 6038
Shreveport, LA 71106
318-688-4800

00374
Lyne Laboratories
260 Tosca Drive
Stoughton, MA 02072

00469
Lyphomed
Parkway N. Center 3
Deerfield, IL 60015-2548
708-317-8800

00466
Macsil, Inc.
1326 Frankford Ave.
Philadelphia, PA
19125-0976
215-739-7300

00904
Major Pharmaceutical Inc.
3720 Lapeer Road
Auburn Hills, MI 48321
313-370-0680

00019
Mallinckrodt Medical, Inc.
675 McDonnell Blvd.
Box 5840
St. Louis, MO 63134
314-895-2000

10706
Kenneth A. Manne Co.
1522 Cleveland Ave., N.W.
Canton, OH 44711
216-455-5717

00068
Marion Merrell Dow Inc.
P.O. Box 8480
Kansas City, MO 64114
816-966-4000

Marlin Industries
P.O. Box 560
Grover City, CA 93483-0560
213-393-3644

10712
Marlyn Company Inc.
6324 Ferris Square
San Diego, CA 92121
619-453-5600

52555
Martec Pharmaceutical, Inc.
1800 N. Topping
Kansas City, MO 64120
816-241-4144

11845
Mason Distributors, Inc.
5105 N.W. 159th Street
Hialeah, FL 33014-6370
305-624-5557

12758
Mason Pharmaceuticals, Inc.
4425 Jamboree
Newport Beach, CA 92660
714-851-6860

14362
Mass. Public Health Bio. Lab.
305 South St.
Jamaica Plains, MA 02130
617-522-3700

50330
Mastar Pharmaceutical Co.
P.O. Box 3144
Bethlehem, PA 18017
215-258-8770

10719
Maurry Biological Co., Inc.
6109 South Western Ave.
Los Angeles, CA 90047
213-759-1127

00259
Mayrand, Inc.
P.O. Box 8869
Greensboro, NC 27419
919-292-5347

00264
McGaw, Inc.
ASC2 P.O. Box 19791
Irvine, CA 92713-9791
714-660-2000

11089
McGregor Pharmaceuticals
8420 Ulmenton Road #305
Largo, FL 34641
813-530-4361

49072
McGuff Company, Inc.
3617 W. MacArthur Blvd.
#507
Santa Ana, CA 92704
714-545-2491

50185
McHenry Laboratories Inc.
118 N. Wells-Lee Bldg.
Edna, TX 77957
512-782-5438

00045
McNeil Consumer Products
Camp Hill Road
Fort Washington, PA
19034-2292
215-233-7000

00045
McNeil Pharmaceutical
Welsh and McKean Rds.
Spring House, PA
19477-0776
215-628-5000

00087
Mead Johnson Laboratories
2404 Pennsylvania Street
Evansville, IN 47721
812-426-6000

00087
Mead Johnson Nutritionals
2404 Pennsylvania St.
Evansville, IN 47721
812-426-6000

00015
Mead Johnson Oncology Products
2400 West Lloyd Expressway
Evansville, IN 47721-0001
812-429-5000

MedChem
444 Washington St.
Woburn, MA 01801
617-938-9328

11940
Medco Lab, Inc.
P.O. Box 864
Sioux City, IA 51102-0864
712-255-8770

44081
Med-Corp
5001 Spring Valley Road
Dallas, TX 75244-3910
214-385-7214

45565
Med-Derm Pharmaceuticals
P.O. Box 5193
Kingsport, TN 37663
615-477-3991

Medi Aid Corporation
8250 S. Akron Street
Suite 205
Englewood, CO 80155
303-790-1655

Medical Frontiers
7560 McEwen Road
Centerville, OH 45459
513-434-3363

52891
Medical Market Specialties
P.O. Box 150
Boonton, NJ 07005
201-263-4243

Medical Technology Corporation
71 Veronica Avenue
Somerset, NJ 08875-0218
201-246-3366

99207
Medicis Dermatologicals
100 East 42nd St.
New York, NY 10017
212-599-2000

00244
Medicone Company
225 Varick St.
New York, NY 10014
212-924-5166

17156
Medi-Physics, Inc.
140 East Ridgewood
P.O. Box 289
Paramus, NJ 07653-0289
201-599-8931

00348
Medtech Laboratories, Inc.
P.O. Box 1108
3510 N. Lake Creek
Jackson, WY 83001
307-733-1680

87900
Menley and James Laboratories
100 Tournament Drive
Horsham, PA 19044
215-441-6509

22200
Mennen Company
Hanover Ave., Box 1000
Morristown, NJ 07960
201-631-9000

10742
Mentholatum Co., Inc.
1360 Niagara St.
Buffalo, NJ 14213
716-882-7660

00006
Merck Sharp and Dohme
WP 38M-2
West Point, PA 19486
215-661-5000

00394
Mericon Industries, Inc.
8819 N. Pioneer Road
Peoria, IL 61615
309-676-0744

50361
Merieux Institute, Inc.
7855 N.W. 12th St.
Suite #114
Miami, FL 33126-1818
305-593-9577

32954
MiLance Laboratories, Inc.
P.O. Box 39
Maplewood, NJ 07040
201-580-1591

16500
Miles Labs.
1127 Myrtle St., P.O. Box 340
Elkhart, IN 46515-0340
219-264-8111

00026
Miles Pharm.
400 Morgan Lane
West Haven, CT 06516
203-937-2000

00396
Milex Products, Inc.
5915 Northwest Highway
Chicago, IL 60631-1032
312-631-6484

17204
Miller Pharmacal Group Inc.
245 W. Roosevelt Rd.
West Chicago, IL
60186-0279

53118
Millgood Laboratories, Inc.
P.O. Box 170159
Atlanta, GA 30317
404-377-6538

00276
Misemer Pharmaceuticals
4553 S. Campbell
Springfield, MO 65810-5918
417-881-0660

00178
Mission Pharmacal Co.
P.O. Box 1676
San Antonio, TX 78296-1676
512-650-3273

Monoclonal Antibodies, Inc.
2319 Charleston Rd.
Mountain View, CA 94043
408-739-2700

00839
H. L. Moore Drug Exchange
389 John Downey Dr.
New Britain, CT 06050
203-826-3600

Morton Salt
110 North Wacker Dr.
Chicago, IL 60606
312-621-5200

Murdock Pharmaceuticals
1400 Mountain Springs Park
Springvale, UT 84663
801-489-3633

00451
Muro Pharmaceutical, Inc.
890 East St.
Tewksbury, MA 01876-9987
508-851-5981

00150
Murray Drug Corporation
415 S. 4th Street
Murray, KY 42071
502-753-6654

53489
Mutual Pharmaceutical Co.
1100 Orthodox Street
Philadelphia, PA 19124
215-288-6500

00378
Mylan Pharmaceuticals
P.O. Box 4310
Morgantown, WV 26505
304-599-2595

National Patent Medical
P.O. Box 419
Dayville, CT 06241

00472
National Pharmaceutical Mfr.
7205 Windsor Blvd.
Baltimore, MD 21207
301-298-1000

74312
Nature's Bounty, Inc.
105 Orville Drive
Bohemia, NY 11716
516-567-9500

76611
Navaco Laboratories
512 Ash Avenue
McAllen, TX 78501
512-682-0188

55437
Nelson Pharmaceutical, Inc.
3101 Louisiana Avenue N.
Minneapolis, MN 55424
612-542-3232

00487
Nephron Corporation
P.O. Box 1974
Tacoma, WA 98401-1974
206-475-3452

NeuroGenesis/MATRIX Tech. Inc.
1020 Bay Area Boulevard
Houston, TX 77058
713-488-7687

10812
Neutrogena Dermatologies
5760 W. 96th Street
Los Angeles, CA 90045
213-642-1150

Newport Pharmaceuticals
897 West 16th
Newport Beach, CA 92663
714-642-7511

12934
Nion Corporation
11581 Federal Drive
El Monte, CA 91731
213-686-2105

Nix-O-Tine Pharmaceuticals Ltd.
2320 W. Peoria Ave.
Suite B-146
Phoenix, AZ 85029-4753
602-870-9977

23317
NMC Laboratories
70-36 83rd Street
Glendale, NY 11385
718-326-1500

51801
Nomax, Inc.
40 North Rock Hill Rd.
St. Louis, MO 63119
314-961-2500

50445
Nordisk-USA
3202 Tower Oaks Blvd.
Suite 100
Rockville, MD 20852-4219
301-897-9220

00149
Norwich Eaton Pharm.
P.O. Box 191
Norwich, NY 13815
607-335-2111

00362
Novocol Chemical Mfr. Co.
485-09 S. Broadway
Hicksville, NY 10801
516-496-7200

55953
Novopharm, Inc.
165 E. Commerce
Suite 100/200
Schaumberg, IL 60173-5326
708-882-4200

55499
Numark Laboratories, Inc.
P.O. Box 6321
Edison, NJ 08818

51081
Nutripharm Laboratories
8 Bartles Corner Road
Suite 101
Flemington, NJ 08822
908-806-8954

10797
Oakhurst Company
3000 Hemstead Turnpike
Levittown, NY 11756
516-731-5380

00477
Obetrol Pharmaceuticals
396 Rockaway Ave.
P.O. Box 397
Valley Stream, NY 11582
516-561-7662

55515
Oclassen
San Rafael, CA 94901
415-258-4500

Ocular Pharmaceuticals, Inc.
712 Ginesi Drive
Morganville, NJ 07751
201-972-8585

OHM Laboratories, Inc.
P.O. Box 279
Franklin Park, NJ 08823
908-297-3030

12622
Olin Corporation
120 Long Ridge Road
Stamford, CT 06904-1355
203-356-2000

Optikem International
2172 S. Jason Street
Denver, CO 80223
303-936-1137

50520
Optimox Corporation
2720 Monterey, Suite 406
Torrance, CA 90503
213-618-9370

52238
Optopics Laboratories Corp.
Main Street, P.O. Box 210
Fairton, NJ 08320-0210
609-451-9350

00041
Oral-B Laboratories, Inc.
170 S. Whisman Road
Mountain View, CA 94041
415-961-8130

00052
Organon, Inc.
375 Mt. Pleasant Ave.
West Orange, NJ 07052
201-325-4500

Organon Teknika Corp.
100 Akzo Avenue
Durham, NC 27704
919-620-2000

00191
Ortega Pharm. Co., Inc.
586 S. Edgewood Ave.
Jacksonville, FL 33205
904-387-0536

00062
Ortho Diagnostic Systems
Route 202
Raritan, NJ 08869
201-218-6000

00062
Ortho Pharmaceutical Corp.
Route 202, P.O. Box 300
Raritan, NJ 08869
201-524-0400

00299
Owen/Galderma Labs. Inc.
P.O. Box 6600
Fort Worth, TX 76115
817-293-0450

00574
Paddock Laboratories
3101 Louisiana Ave. North
Minneapolis, MN 55427
612-546-4676

53159
Palisades Pharmaceuticals
219 County Road
Tenafly, NJ 07670
201-569-8502

00377
Pal-Pak, Inc.
1201 Liberty St.
P.O. Box 299
Allentown, PA 18105
215-433-7579

49884
Par Pharmaceuticals
One Ram Ridge Rd.
Spring Valley, NY 10977
914-425-7100

00071
Parke-Davis
201 Tabor Road
Morris Plains, NJ 07950
201-540-2000

00071
Parke-Davis Consumer Products
201 Tabor Road
Morris Plains, NJ 07950
201-540-2000

00349
Parmed Pharmaceuticals
4220 Hyde Park Blvd.
Niagara Falls, NY 14305
716-284-5666

50930
Parnell Pharmaceuticals, Inc.
373-G Vintage Park Drive
Foster City, CA 94404
415-574-1500

The Parthenon Co., Inc.
3311 West 2400 South
Salt Lake City, UT 84119
801-972-5184

00418
Pasadena Research Labs
940 Calle Amancer, Suite L
San Clemente, CA 92672
714-492-4030

00884
Pedinol Pharmacal, Inc.
30 Banfi Plaza North
Farmingdale, NY 11735
516-293-9500

10974
Pegasus Medical Service
16 Technology Dr., Suite 122
Irvine, CA 92718-2325

00096
Person and Covey, Inc.
616 Allen Avenue
Glendale, CA 91201
818-240-1030

00927
Pfeiffer Company
P.O. Box 100
Wilkes-Barre, PA 18773
717-826-9000

00995
Pfipharmecs
235 East 42nd St.
New York, NY 10017
212-573-7775

00069
Pfizer Laboratories
235 E. 42nd St.
New York, NY 10017-5755
212-573-2323

00121
Pharmaceutical Associates
P.O. Box 128
Conestee, SC 29636
803-277-7282

00832
Pharmaceutical Basics Inc.
6451 West Main Street
Morton Grove, IL 60053
708-967-5600

00832
Pharmaceutical Basics, Inc.
(Solid Dosage Forms)
8755 W. Higgins Rd.
Suite 810
Chicago, IL 60631
312-380-0080

51655
Pharmaceutical Corporation
12348 Hancock
Carmel, IN 46032
317-573-8000

45334
Pharmaceutical Specialties
P.O. Box 729
Rochester, MN 55903-0729
507-288-8500

00016
Pharmacia Inc.
800 Centennial Ave.
Piscataway, NJ 08855-1327
201-457-8000

00462
Pharmaderm
60 Baylis Road
Melville, NY 11747
516-454-7677

24208
Pharmafair, Inc.
205C Kelsey Lane
Tampa, FL 33619
813-972-7705

00554
Pharmakon Laboratories
6050 Jet Port Industrial Blvd.
Tampa, FL 33634
813-886-3216

39822
Pharma-Tek, Inc.
P.O. Box AB
Huntington, NY 11743
516-757-5522

00813
Pharmics Incorporated
1878 South Redwood Rd.
Salt Lake City, UT 84104
801-972-4138

60104
Pioneer Pharmaceuticals Inc.
209 40th Street
Irvington, NJ 07111
201-372-6200

41100
Plough, Inc.
P.O. Box 377
3030 Jackson Ave.
Memphis, TN 38151
901-320-2011

Polymer Technology Corporation
100 Research Drive
Wilmington, MA 01887

00095
Poythress Laboratories, Inc.
16 N. 22nd St.
Richmond, VA 23261
804-644-8591

53124
Praxis Biologics, Inc.
30 Corporate Woods
Suite 300
Rochester, NY 14623-1493
716-272-7000

Precision-Cosmet
500 Iolab Drive
Claremont, CA 91711
612-933-1215

00684
Primedics Laboratories
1852 West 169th Street
Gardenia, CA 90247
213-770-3005

00003
Princeton Pharmaceutical Products
P.O. Box 4000
New Brunswick, NJ
08543-4000
609-243-6000

37000
The Procter and Gamble Co.
P.O. Box 599
Cincinnati, OH 45201-0599
513-530-2153

Professional Supplies, Inc.
1153 Main St.
Stevens Point, WI 54481
715-345-0404

00034
Purdue Frederick Co.
100 Connecticut Ave.
Norwalk, CT 06856
203-853-0123

00228
Purepac Pharmaceutical Co.
200 Elmora Ave.
Elizabeth, NJ 07207
201-527-9100

51309
Quad Pharmaceuticals, Inc.
6340 LaPas Trail
Indianapolis, IN 46268
317-299-6611

52446
Qualitest Products Inc.
1025 Jordan Road
Huntsville, AL 35811
205-859-4011

52273
Quantum Pharmics, Ltd.
26 Edison Street
Amityville, NY 11701
516-842-4200

54391
R & D Laboratories, Inc.
4204 Glencoe Avenue
Marina Del Rey, CA
90292-5612
213-305-8053

00196
Rachelle Laboratories, Inc.
P.O. Box 187
Culver, IN 46511
219-842-3305

30103
Randob Laboratories, Ltd.
508 Franklin Ave.
Mt. Vernon, NY 10550
914-699-3131

00686
Raway Pharmacal, Inc.
Lower Granit Road
Accord, NY 12404
914-626 8133

10952
Recsei Laboratories
330 S. Kellogg Bldg. M
Goleta, CA 93117-3875
805-964-2912

53506
Redi-Med, Inc.
801-N N. Blacklawn Rd.
P.O. Box 1407
Conyers, GA 30207
404-929-0961

48028
Redi-Products Labs, Inc.
Prichard Industrial Park
P.O. Box 126
Prichard, WV 25555
304-486-5656

00021
Reed & Carnrick
One New England Ave.
Piscataway, NJ 08855
201-981-0070

10956
Reese Chemical Co.
10617 Frank Ave.
Cleveland, OH 44106
216-231-6441

00102
Regal Laboratories
1925 Enterprise Parkway
Twinsburg, OH 44087
216-425-9811

00032
Reid-Rowell
901 Sawyer Road
Marietta, GA 30062-2224
404-578-9000

10960
Republic Drug Company
P.O. Box 186
Buffalo, NY 14216
716-874-5060

10961
Requa
1 Seneca Place, Box 4008
Greenwich, CT 06830
203-869-2445

00433
Research Industries Corp.
1847 West 2300 South
Salt Lake City, UT 84119
801-972-5500

00122
Rexall Group
4031 N.E. 12th Terrace
Ft. Lauderdale, FL 33334
305-561-2187

00195
Rhone-Poulenc Pharm.
174 Clover Lane
Princeton, NJ 08540
609-395-8300

00067
Rhone-Poulenc Rorer Pharm.
500 Virginia Drive
Fort Washington, PA 19034
215-628-6000

76660
Richardson-Vicks, Inc.
1 Far Mill Crossing
P.O. Box 854
Shelton, CT 06484-0925
203-925-6000

12071
Richie Pharmacal Co., Inc.
197 State Avenue
P.O. Box 460
Glasgow, KY 42141
502-651-6150

00115
Richlyn Laboratories, Inc.
Castor and Kensington Aves.
Philadelphia, PA 19124
215-289-2220

54807
R.I.D. Inc., Distributor
525 Mednik Avenue
Los Angeles, CA 90022
213-268-0635

54092
Roberts Pharm. Corp.
Meridian Center III
6 Industrial Way West
Eatontown, NJ 07724
908-389-1182

00031
A. H. Robins Company, Inc.
P.O. Box 8299
Philadelphia, PA
19101-1245
215-688-4400

00031
A.H. Robins Cons. Prod. Div.
1211 Sherwood Ave.
Richmond, VA 23261-6609
804-257-2735

00004
Roche Dermatologics Prod.
340 Kingsland St.
Nutley, NJ 07110-1199
201-812-2000

00004
Roche Laboratories
340 Kingsland St.
Nutley, NJ 07110-1199
201-235-7536

00140
Roche Products Inc.
State Road #670 Km 2.7
Manati, Puerto Rico 00701
809-854-3020

00049
J. B. Roerig Division
235 E. 42nd St.
New York, NY 10017
212-573-2323

00074
Ross Laboratories
625 Cleveland Ave.
Columbus, OH 43215
614-227-3333

00054
Roxane Laboratories, Inc.
P.O. Box 16532
Columbus, OH 43216-6532
614-276-4000

00536
Rugby Labs., Inc.
898 Orlando Ave.
West Hempstead, NY 11552
516-536-8565

50474
Russ Pharmaceuticals
See Whitby

46500
Rydelle Laboratories
1525 Howe Street
Racine, WI 53403-5011
414-631-2000

00263
Rystan Company, Inc.
P.O. Box 214
Little Falls, NJ 07424-0214
201-256-3737

00043
Sandoz Pharmaceutical Corp.
59 Route 10
East Hanover, NJ 07936
201-503-7500

00212
Sandoz Nutrition
5320 W. 23rd Street
Minneapolis, MN 55440
612-925-2100

51353
The Sanitube Company
19 Concord St.
S. Norwalk, CT 06854
203-853-7856

00281
Savage Laboratories
60 Baylis Road
Melville, NY 11747-2006
516-454-9071

00364
Schein Pharmaceutical, Inc.
26 Harbor Park Dr.
Port Washington, NY 11050
516-625-9000

00274
Scherer Laboratories, Inc.
14335 Gillis Road
Dallas, TX 75244-3718
214-233-2800

00085
Schering-Plough Corporation
Galloping Hill Road
K-6-2 H9A
Kenilworth, NJ 07033
201-298-4000

00905
Schiapparelli Searle
P.O. Box 5110
Chicago, IL 60680-5110
708-982-7000

Schiff Bio Foods
121 Moonachie Avenue
Moonachie, NJ 07074
201-933-2282

00234
Schmid Products Co.
Route 46 West
Little Falls, NJ 07424
201-256-5500

Scholl, Inc.
3030 Jackson, P.O. Box 377
Memphis, TN 38151
901-320-2011

00091
Schwarz Pharma Kremers Urban
5600 W. County Line
Mequon, WI 53092
414-354-4300

42021
Sclavo, Inc.
5 Mansard Court
Wayne, NJ 07470
201-696-8300

00372
Scot-Tussin Pharmacal Co.
50 Clemence St., Box 8217
Cranston, RI 02920-0217
401-942-8555

00444
Scrip, Inc.
101 South St.
Peoria, IL 61602-1986
309-674-3488

54977
Scripts America Corp.
5317 N.W. 35 Terrace
Fort Lauderdale, FL 33309
305-486-7880

00014
Searle & Company
Box 5110
Chicago, IL 60680
708-470-9710

00551
The Seatrace Company
P.O. Box 363
Gadsden, AL 35902-0363
205-442-5023

50694
Seres Laboratories
3331 Industrial Drive
Box 470
Santa Rosa, CA 95401
707-526-4526

44087
Serono Laboratories, Inc.
100 Longwater Circle
Norwell, MA 02061
617-982-9000

S.G. Labs, Inc.
500 North Broadway
Jericho, NY 11753
516-822-2900

49731
Sherman Laboratories, Inc.
P.O. Box 368
Abita Springs, LA 70420
504-893-0007

08881
Sherwood Medical
1831 Olive Street
St. Louis, MO 63103
314-621-7788

45809
Shionogi USA
3848 Carson St., #206
Torrance, CA 90503
213-540-1161

50111
Sidmak Laboratories, Inc.
17 West St., P.O. Box 371
East Hanover, NJ 07936
201-386-5566

54482
Sigma-Tau Pharmaceuticals
200 Orchard Ridge Drive
Gaithersburg, MD 20878
301-948-1041

39769
Smith & Nephew SoloPak
1845 Tonne Road
Elk Grove Village, IL
60007-5125
708-806-0080

08026
Smith & Nephew United
11775 Starkey Rd.
P.O. Box 1970
Largo, FL 34649-1970
813-392-1261

00766
SmithKline Beecham Consumer Brands
100 Beecham Drive
Pittsburgh, PA 15205
412-928-1000

00029
SmithKline Beecham Pharm.
P.O. Box 7929
Philadelphia, PA 19103
215-751-4000

00978
SmithKline Diagnostics
225 Baypointe Parkway
San Jose, CA 95134-1622
408-435-2660

Soft Rinse Corp.
2411 Third Street South
Wisconsin Rapids, WI 54494

00077
Sola/Barnes-Hind
810 Kifer Road
Sunnyvale, CA 94086-5200
619-277-9873

Solgar Company, Inc.
P.O. Box 330
Lynbrook, NY 11563
516-599-2442

39506
Somerset Pharmaceuticals
400 Morris Avenue, Suite 7S
Denville, NJ 07834
201-586-2310

54027
Spectra Pharmaceutical Service
155 Webster Street
Hanover, MA 02339
617-871-3991

38137
Spectrum Chemical Mfg. Corp.
14422 S. San Pedro St.
Gardena, CA 90248-9985

00537
Spencer-Mead Medical Supply Co.
865 Merrick Ave.
Westbury, NY 11590
718-338-6664

Sphinx Pharmaceutical Corp.
P.O. Box 52330
Durham, NC 27717
919-489-9090

00003
Squibb Diagnostic Division
P.O. Box 4500
Princeton, NJ 08543-4500
609-987-1813

00003
Squibb-Marsam
P.O. Box 1022
Cherry Hill, NJ 08034
609-424-5600

00003
Squibb-Novo, Inc.
211 Carnegie Center
Princeton, NJ 08540
609-921-8989

53385
Standard Drug Company
P.O. Box 710
Riverton, IL 62561
217-629-9884

00076
Star Pharmaceuticals, Inc.
1990 N.W. 44th Street
Pompano Beach, FL
33064-1278
305-971-9704

51318
Stellar Pharmacal Corp.
1990 N.W. 44th Street
Pompano Beach, FL 33064
305-972-6060

00402
Steris Laboratories Inc.
620 North 51st Avenue
Phoenix, AZ 85043
602-278-1400

00145
Stiefel Laboratories, Inc.
2801 Ponce de Leon Blvd.
Coral Gables, FL 33134
305-443-3807

Storz Ophthalmics
3365 Tree Court Industrial
St. Louis, MO 63122-6694
314-225-5051

00038
Stuart Pharmaceuticals
Concord Pike and New Murphy Rd.
Wilmington, DE 19897
302-886-2231

11086
Summers Laboratories, Inc.
Morris Rd. and Wissahickon Creek
Fort Washington, PA 19034
215-646-1477

57267
Summit Medical Products
1075 Central Park Ave.
Scarsdale, NY 10583
914-472-2737

11720
Super-X Drug Corporation
175 Tri-County Parkway
Cincinnati, OH 45246
513-782-3001

11704
Survival Technology, Inc.
8101 Glenbrook Rd.
Bethesda, MD 20814
301-656-5600

00033
Syntex Laboratories
3401 Hillview Ave.
Palo Alto, CA 94304
415-855-5050

47854
Syosset Laboratories Co.
150 Eileen Way
Syosset, NY 11791
516-921-6306

Syva Company
929 Queensbridge
St. Louis, MO 63021
314-391-5374

Tambrands Incorporated
1 Marcus Ave.
Lake Success, NY 11042
516-358-8300

Tanning Research Labs. Inc.
1190 U.S. 1 North
Ormond Beach, FL 32174
904-677-9559

00300
Tap Pharmaceuticals
2355 Waukegan Road
Deerfield, IL 60015
708-317-5700

51672
Taro Pharmaceuticals U.S.A.
Six Skyline Drive
Hawthorne, NY 10532
914-345-9001

49158
Thames Pharmacal Co., Inc.
2100 Fifth Avenue
Ronkonkoma, NY 11779-6906
516-737-1155

11290
Thompson Medical Co.
222 Lakeview Ave.
West Palm Beach, FL 33401
407-820-9900

00089
3M Personal Care Products
3M Center, Bldg. 223-4N-10
St. Paul, MN 55144-1000
612-733-1110

00089
3M Pharmaceutical
225-IN-07 3M Center
St. Paul, MN 55144-1000
612-736-4930

51687
T/I Pharmaceuticals
15231 Barranca Parkway
Irvine, CA 92718
714-727-7466

11299
Torch Laboratories, Inc.
P.O. Box 248
Reistertown, MD 21136
301-363-6350

11311
Trimen Laboratories, Inc.
80-26th Street
Pittsburgh, PA 15222
412-261-0339

79511
Triton Consumer Products
5105 Tollview Dr., Suite 190
Rolling Meadows, IL 60008
708-577-5900

00463
C. O. Truxton Inc.
P.O. Box 1594
Camden, NJ 08101
609-365-4118

Tsumura Medical
104 Peavey Road
Chaska, MN 55318
612-448-4181

53335
Tyson & Associates, Inc.
12832 Chadron Ave.
Hawthorne, CA 90250-5525
213-675-1080

00785
UAD Laboratories, Inc.
P.O. Box 10587
8839 Highway 18 W
Jackson, MS 39289-0587
601-372-7773

51079
UDL Laboratories, Inc.
P.O. Box 10319
Rockford, IL 61131-3019
815-282-1201

00127
Ulmer Pharmacal
2440 Fernbrook Lane
Plymouth, MN 55447-9987
612-559-3333

00677
United Research Laboratories
3600 Meadow Lane
Bensalem, PA 19020-8546
215-638-2626

48663
Unitek Corporation
2724 South Peck Rd.
Monrovia, CA 91016
213-445-7960

00009
The Upjohn Company
7000 Portage Rd.
Kalamazoo, MI 49001
616-323-4000

00245
Upsher-Smith Labs., Inc.
14905-23rd Ave. N.
Minneapolis, MN 55447
612-473-4412

58178
US Bioscience
One Tower Bridge
100 Front St.
West Conshohocken, PA
19428
215-832-4502

US Packaging Corp. Medical Div.
506 Clay Street
LaPorte, IN 46350
219-362-9782

52747
US Pharmaceutical Corp.
2500 Park Central Blvd.
Decatur, GA 30035
404-987-4745

51626
US Products, Inc.
16636 N.W. 54th St.
Miami Lakes, FL 33014
305-620-9540

54627
ValMed, Inc.
410 Great Road
Littleton, MA 01460
508-486-8300

00615
Vangard Labs, Inc.
31-E Bypass
Glasgow, KY 42141
502-651-6188

17022
Veratex Corp.
1304 E. Maple Road
P.O. Box 4031
Troy, MI 48084
313-588-2970

53258
VHA Supply Company
320 Deker Dr.
P.O. Box 160909
Irving, TX 75016
214-650-4444

23900
Vicks Health Care Products Div.
One Far Mill Crossing
Shelton, CT 06484
203-925-7701

25866
Vicks Pharmacy Products Div.
One Far Mill Crossing
Shelton, CT 06484
203-929-2500

54891
Vision Pharmaceuticals Inc.
P.O. Box 400
Mitchell, SD 57301-0400
605-996-3356

54022
Vitaline Corporation
722 Jefferson Avenue
Ashland, OR 97520
503-482-9231

00185
Vitarine Pharmaceuticals
227-15 North Conduit Ave.
Springfield Gardens, NY
11413-3199
718-276-8600

49727
Vita-Rx Corporation
P.O. Box 8229
Columbus, GA 31908
404-568-1881

Vivan Pharmacol Inc.
1000 Bennett Blvd.
Lakewood, NJ 08701
201-364-9700

00298
Vortech Pharmaceuticals
6851 Chase Rd., Box 189
Dearborn, MI 48121
313-584-4088

00741
Walker, Corp. and Co., Inc.
P.O. Box 1320
Syracuse, NY 13201
315-463-4511

00619
Walker Pharmacal Company
4200 Laclede Ave.
St. Louis, MO 63108
314-533-9600

00037
Wallace Laboratories
P.O. Box 1
Cranbury, NJ 08512
609-655-6000

00017
Wampole Laboratories
Half Acre Rd., P.O. Box 1001
Cranbury, NJ 08515-0181
609-655-6000

00047
Warner Chilcott Laboratories
201 Tabor Road
Morris Plains, NJ 07013
201-540-2000

11370
Warner Lambert Consumer
170 Tabor Road
Morris Plains, NJ 07950
201-540-2000

52544
Watson Laboratories
132-A Business Center Drive
Corona, CA 91720
714-736-8444

00998
Webcon Products
6201 South Freeway T4-4
Ft. Worth, TX 76134-2099
817-293-0450

00917
Wesley Pharmacal Co., Inc.
114 Railroad Dr.
Ivyland, PA 18974
215-953-1680

50893
Westport Pharmaceuticals
1 Turkey Hill Rd. South
Westport, CT 06880
203-226-0622

00143
West-Ward, Inc.
465 Industrial Way
Eatontown, NJ 07724
201-542-1191

00003
Westwood-Squibb Pharmaceutical
100 Forest Avenue
Buffalo, NY 14213
716-887-3400

50474
Whitby Pharmaceuticals
P.O. Box 27426
Richmond, VA 23261-7426

00573
Whitehall Laboratories
685 Third Avenue
New York, NY 10017-4076
212-878-5500

00918
Whittaker General Medical
8741 Landmark Rd.
Richmond, VA 23261
804-264-7500

00317
Whorton Pharmaceuticals
4202 Gary Avenue
Fairfield, AL 35064
205-786-2584

11414
Willen Drug Co.
18 North High Street
Baltimore, MD 21202-4785
301-752-1865

51189
T.E. Williams Pharm.
P.O. Box 312
Divide, CO 80814-0312
719-687-3092

00024
Winthrop Consumer
90 Park Avenue
New York, NY 10016
212-907-2000

00024
Winthrop Pharmaceuticals
90 Park Avenue
New York, NY 10016
212-907-2000

12120
Wisconsin Pharmacal Co.
2977 Hwy. 60
Jackson, WI 53037
414-677-4121

00008
Wyeth-Ayerst Laboratories
P.O. Box 8299
Philadelphia, PA 19101
215-688-4400

50962
Xactdose, Inc.
722 Progressive Lane
South Beloit, IL 61080
815-624-8523

00116
Xttrium Laboratories, Inc.
415 West Pershing Road
Chicago, IL 60609
312-268-5800

60077
Young Dental
13705 Shoreline Court East
St. Louis, MO 63045
314-344-0010

11444
W.F. Young, Inc.
111 Lyman Street
Springfield, MA 01101
413-737-0201

00172
Zenith Laboratories, Inc.
140 Legrand Avenue
Northvale, NJ 07647
201-767-1700

05128
Zila Pharmaceuticals, Inc.
5227 North 7th St.
Phoenix, AZ 85014-2800
602-266-6700

Notes

Notes

ISBN 0-932686-29-X

90000

9 780932 686299